HANDBUCH DER ALLGEMEINEN PATHOLOGIE

HERAUSGEGEBEN VON

F. BÜCHNER   E. LETTERER   F. ROULET

FÜNFTER BAND

HILFSMECHANISMEN DES STOFFWECHSELS

ERSTER TEIL

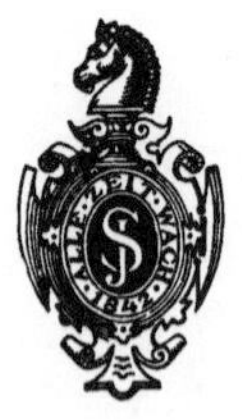

SPRINGER-VERLAG

BERLIN · GÖTTINGEN · HEIDELBERG

1961

HILFSMECHANISMEN DES STOFFWECHSELS

I

BEARBEITET VON

H. BENNHOLD · W. BOLT · F. BÜCHNER · M. H. F. FRIEDMAN
W. GIESE · F. GROSSE-BROCKHOFF · H. HEINLEIN
E. JECKELN · H. W. KNIPPING · U. C. LUFT · H. OTT
W. SCHOEDEL · J. E. THOMAS

REDIGIERT VON

E. LETTERER

MIT 326 ZUM TEIL FARBIGEN ABBILDUNGEN

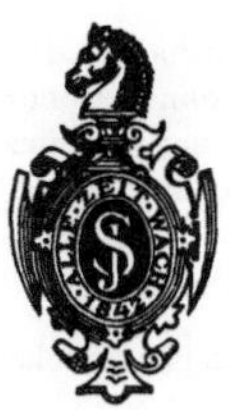

SPRINGER-VERLAG

BERLIN · GÖTTINGEN · HEIDELBERG

1961

ISBN-13: 978-3-642-94825-1   e-ISBN-13: 978-3-642-94824-4
DOI: 10.1007/ 978-3-642-94824-4

Druck der Universitätsdruckerei H. Stürtz AG, Würzburg

Inhaltsverzeichnis.

Die Pathologie der Verdauung und Resorption. Von Professor Dr. E. JECKELN-Lübeck.

Inhaltsverzeichnis. XV

The normal physiology of the digestive system.

By

J. EARL THOMAS*-Loma Linda (Cal.) USA

and

M. H. F. FRIEDMAN**-Philadelphia (Pa.) USA.

With 6 figures.

1. Mastication.

The physiological process of digestion begins with mastication which serves to reduce the size of the food particles, moisten and lubricate dry food, distribute the salivary enzymes through the food mass and provide stimuli for reflexes that are important in subsequent stages of digestion.

Mechanics of mastication. In the human the lower jaw can be moved antero-posteriorly, laterally or vertically. Any one or all of these movements may be utilized in chewing, depending upon the type of food and the purpose to be accomplished. The up and down motion merely approximates or separates the upper and lower teeth and is used for crushing food particles, whereas the lateral movements are used in grinding. The antero-posterior motion may also be used in grinding but is chiefly important for aligning the upper and lower incisor teeth for biting.

The force of the bite is apparently limited by the ability of the peridental membrane to withstand pressure without undue pain and not necessarily by the power of the muscles of mastication. Maximum total force between the molars in excess of 270 pounds (122 + kg.) has been recorded in the human[1]. In the dog a maximum force of 165 kg. has been observed[2], but for obvious reasons there is no assurance that this represents the maximum of which the dog is capable.

The masticatory reflex. Mastication may be initiated and controlled voluntarily but for the most part it is a self-regulating reflex. The dual nature of the nervous mechanism is indicated by the fact that chewing movements may be elicited by electrical stimulation of appropriate areas in the cerebral cortex[3] as well as by sensory stimulation of the mouth in decerebrate animals[4]. According to MAGNUS (1945), who has recently reviewed the subject, a bulbar center produces rhythmic movements of the jaw in response to stimulation of receptors in the mouth; this center is subordinate to a thalamocortical center which is responsible for the finer regulation of the movements.

---

* Professor of Physiology, The College of Medical Evangelists, Loma Linda, California.
** Professor of Physiology, The Jefferson Medical College, Philadelphia, Pennsylvania.

[1] BLACK 1895.   [2] TRISKA 1924.   [3] FERRIER 1886, MAGOUN et al. 1933, RIOCH 1934.
[4] SHERRINGTON 1917, BAZETT and PENFIELD 1922.

2. Deglutition.

Magendie (1838) described the act of swallowing as occurring in three stages which we shall designate as the oral, pharyngeal, and esophageal stages respectively, indicating the anatomical area through which the food is being propelled at each stage. The mechanics of swallowing are influenced by the consistency of the material swallowed, and are somewhat different for liquids than for solids. This description will be based on swallowing a solid or semi-solid bolus; incidental mention will be made of the difference in mechanism when liquids are swallowed.

The first or oral stage.

In the first or oral stage the bolus is manipulated into position on the upper surface of the tongue by the action of the muscles of the cheeks and tongue. The tongue is then made firm by contraction of its musculature and pressed against the teeth and hard palate to prevent escape of the bolus anteriorly or laterally. Pressure in the mouth is increased through contraction of the mylohyoid muscle and the bolus is projected into (or through) the pharynx very much as one might project a slippery object like a pumpkin seed by squeezing it between the thumb and forefinger. The mechanism is equally effective with liquids since only one avenue of escape is provided, namely that into the pharynx.

The second or pharyngeal stage.

This stage is complicated by the fact that provision must be made for closing the airway, both above and below the oral pharynx during the passage of the bolus in order to prevent the entrance of food into the nose or into the trachea. It is obvious also that respiration must be interrupted momentarily during this stage. Closure of the communication between the oral pharynx and nasopharynx is accomplished by approximation of the soft palate to the post-pharyngeal wall, a movement that is aided by contraction of the tensor palatini and levator palatini muscles as well as by the pressure of the bolus against the oral surface of the palate. Protection of the laryngeal opening is a more complicated process and there is no general aggreement as to the manner in which it is accomplished. The following description is based on several observations[1].

The mechanisms involved will be more easily understood if we bear in mind the facts that except during the act of swallowing, the lumen of the laryngeal pharynx into which the bolus must enter is a mere slit between its anterior and posterior walls so that no true lumen exists and that the posterior wall is relatively immobile because it is in contact with the prevertebral muscles and fascia. The only way an opening can be made for the oncoming bolus is by moving the anterior wall forward along with the structures placed anterior to it, namely the larynx and hyoid bone. A forward movement of the larynx thus becomes a necessity during the passage of the bolus; the base of the tongue and the epiglottis at the same time move backward and the larynx comes to lie beneath these structures which, together, form an effective covering for its upper surface. Probably the intrinsic muscles of the larynx aid by closing the glottic opening through approximation of both the true and the false vocal cords. Apparently the function of the epiglottis is to serve as a sort of water shed to divert the swallowed material to one side or the other, or, if a large amount of liquid is swallowed, to both sides or even over its end in a full stream, but in any case well away from the larynx.

---

[1] Küpferle 1913, Dessecker 1923, Mosher 1927, Barclay 1930, Hegner 1936, Dahm and Schorre 1937, Pancoast, Pendergrass and Schaeffer 1940, and others.

The upper esophageal sphincter (the cricopharyngens muscle) is caused to relax, possibly by a reflex from the laryngeal mucosa[1], permitting the esophagus to open and receive the bolus (Fig. 1). During the pharyngeal stage the bolus is propelled with great speed and often gains enough momentum to carry it deep into the esophagus. Forces other than those already mentioned may be involved. Some writers speak of a peristaltic action of the pharyngeal muscles but the movement is much too rapid to be peristalsis as ordinarily conceived. Doubtless the pharyngeal muscles assist by forming the pharynx into an appropriately shaped passage-way but their action is not essential[2] and the major factors must be sought elsewhere. Probably the bolus is carried through the pharynx chiefly by the momentum imparted to it by forces developed during the oral stage. This view is supported by the fact that denervation of the mylohyoid mucle causes serious impairment of swallowing in the dog whereas denervation of the pharyngeal muscles has little effect[3]. An additional factor may be negative pressure produced in the laryngeal pharynx by the forward movements of the larynx and hyoid bone[4]. Liquids may be projected all the way to the cardia, particularly in the human in the upright position; in this situation the transit is aided by gravity[5].

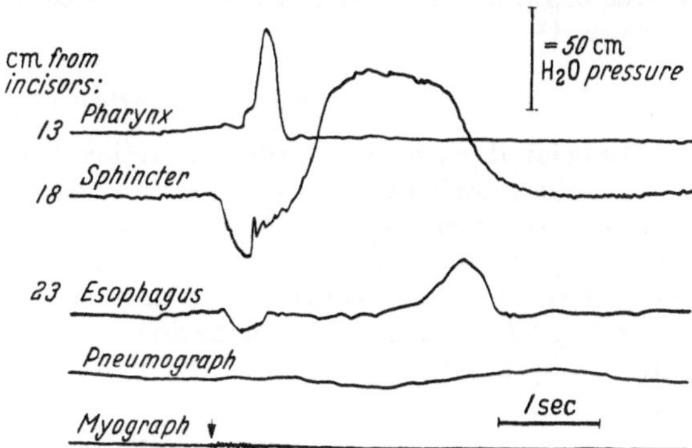

Fig. 1. Simultaneously recorded pressures at different levels in the pharynx and esophagus during the 2nd stage of swallowing. Increase in pressure signifies contraction and decrease, relaxation at the indicated level. Relaxation of the pharyngo-esophageal sphincter is clearly shown. Deglutition pressures at the pharyngo-esophageal junction. Recorded at high speed (5 cm./sec.). From CODE et al. 1958. Courtesy of C. C. Thomas Company, Springfield, Illinois.

The oral and pharyngeal stages of swallowing are not separated by any appreciable time interval and constitute, in fact, a single coordinated act. For this reason they are often described together as a single "buccopharyngeal" stage[6].

The third or esophageal stage.

If a single act of swallowing is allowed to go on to completion a peristaltic contraction appears at the upper end of the esophagus immediately following the pharyngeal stage and progresses downward to the cardia. However, if two or more swallowing efforts are made in rapid succession the third stage follows only the last of the series[7]. If a peristaltic wave is already in progress it is inhibited by a new swallowing effort. This significant fact serves to bring the swallowing mechanism into accord with the "Law of the Intestine" as formulated by BAYLISS and STARLING (1899). In the case of the esophagus the "descending inhibition" serves to accomodate the esophagus to the oncoming bolus.

The progress of a bolus through the esophagus depends, in large measure, upon the consistency of the material swallowed. As mentioned previously, liquids may be projected all the way to the cardia. Depending on the state of the cardia, some of the liquid may pass directly into the stomach or it may remain in the lower

---

[1] DESSECKER 1923, CODE et al. 1958.   [2] MELTZER 1908.
[3] KRONECKER and MELTZER 1883.   [4] BARCLAY 1930, FYKE jr. and CODE 1955.
[5] CANNON and MOSER 1898.   [6] KÜPFERLE 1913.
[7] KRONECKER and MELTZER 1883, MELTZER 1899.

portion of the esophagus until it is carried through the carida by the advancing peristaltic wave[1]. Solids are propelled, at least in a major part of their transit, by peristalsis. Peristalsis progresses more rapidly in the upper, striped muscle part of the esophagus than in the lower, smooth muscle portion[2]. Altogether, from six to nine seconds are required for a peristaltic wave to travel the length of the esophagus. If, for any reason, the primary peristaltic wave initiated by the swallowing reflex fails to empty the esophagus additional ("secondary") waves begin at the level of the remaining contents and continue until the lumen is cleared[2].

Receptive relaxation of the stomach.

Associated with the swallowing reflex there is a temporary decrease in the tone of the gastric muscle resulting in a decrease in intragastric pressue; this has been described as the "receptive relaxation" of the stomach[3]. This relaxation commonly involves the first portion of the diodenum also[4] where, in the dog at least, it persists for a considerable time after the last swallow. In the stomach, the effect of the receptive relaxation is to prevent an increase in intragastric pressure by adapting the size of the organ to the volume of its contents.

The swallowing reflex.

Swallowing, like chewing, may be initiated voluntarily but is normally a reflex act. Like chewing it may be produced by stimulation of appropriate cortical areas[5] or by stimulation of local receptors, even in the decerebrate preparation[6]. In the human the receptors are distributed in a ring-like fashion around the entrance to the oral pharynx and are found in the mucous membrane covering the anterior and posterior pillars of the fauces, the tonsils, soft palate, base of the tongue and post-pharyngeal wall. According to POMMERENKE (1928) the most sensitive areas are in the vicinity of the anterior and posterior pillars and the tonsils.

The coordination of the numerous somatic and visceral muscles involved in the act of swallowing is controlled by a group of neurones in the floor of the fourth ventricle known as the swallowing center. According to MARKWALD (1889) this center is situated above and lateral to the alae cinereae and is closely associated with, though distinct from, the respiratory center.

Because of the close anatomical association of the swallowing center with the respiratory center, dysphagia is a clinical sign of grave prognostic significance in progressive lesions of the brain such as occur in bulbar polyomyelitis. Cortical regulation of swallowing is indicated by the fact that psychogenic dysphagia is a frequent symptom of neurosis[7].

The peripheral nerve fibers involved in the act of swallowing are chiefly in the hypoglossal, glossopharyngeal, and vagus nerves. The vagus supplies the esophagus, hence one of the more serious consequences of cutting these nerves above the origin of the main esophageal branches is interference with swallowing. The striped muscle of the esophagus is permanently paralyzed after a high vagotomy, for example, in the neck, but the smooth muscle of the lower third shows some degree of recovery and peristalsis in this portion may return and swallowing again becomes possible[8]. Peristalsis occurring under these circumstances has

---

[1] MELTZER 1897.   [2] CANNON and MOSER 1898, MELTZER 1899.
[3] CANNON and LIEB 1910.   [4] THOMAS and CRIDER 1935.
[5] MILLER 1920, RIOCH and BRENNER 1938.   [6] FERRIER 1886, BAZETT and PENFIELD 1922.
[7] WINKELSTEIN 1944.   [8] CANNON 1907.

been referred to as tertiary esophageal peristalsis*. In those animals, for example the dog and rabbit, in which the entire esophagus is made up of striped muscle high vagotomy results in permanent inability to swallow. The innervation of the esophagus has been described in detail by GREVING (1919).

3. Gastric motility.

The principal functions of the stomach are to store food and prepare it for intestinal digestion. These may be designated the "reservoir function" and the "digestive function" of the stomach respectively. There is also a "propulsive function" since the food must eventually be passed on into the intestine. We propose in this section to consider only the contribution of the gastric musculature to the performance of these functions.

The periodic activity of the empty stomach.

The smooth muscle of the stomach is seldom completely inactive but its activity increases during gastric digestion and, periodically, when the stomach is empty. The activity of the empty stomach was first observed by SCHIROKICH (1901) whose observations were extended by TSCHESCHKOV (1902) and later by BOLDYREFF (1904) and by CANNON and WASHBURN (1912). CANNON (1911a, p. 204) recognized the relation between the motor activity of the empty stomach and the sensation of hunger. Later, the "hunger contractions" were studied and described in detail by CARLSON (1916) and his co-workers and numerous pupils. Hunger contractions occur during "hunger periods" wich are periods of increased gastric motor activity, lasting from 15 to 30 minutes, intervening between rest periods of 1 to $2^1/_2$ hours duration. The hunger contractions are in the nature of peristaltic waves superimposed on contractions of the gastric smooth muscle as a whole. In contrast to digestive peristalsis, which is evident chiefly in the distal portion of the body and in the pyloric portion of the stomach, the hunger waves travel the entire length of the stomach. During hunger periods individual contractions occur about every half-minute. They usually give rise to unpleasant sensations which vary all the way from a vague feeling of emptyness to easily recognized pain of a cramp-like nature.

The motor activity of the upper small intestine is also increased during hunger periods and typical hunger contractions appear in the duodenum[1]. Probably hunger contractions, particularly those of the duodenum, are an important factor contributing to the pain of peptic ulcer. This pain is described by patients as a feeling of intense hunger and, as is well known, is relieved by taking food.

Digestive peristalsis.

Wheen food is taken hunger contractions, if present, cease abruptly. At the same time there is a decrease in the tonus of the gastric muscle, including the cardiac and pyloric sphincters (see "receptive relaxation of the stomach", above). After a variable time, which in the dog may range from a few minutes to a half-hour after the last food is taken, the tonus of the gastric muscle returns and digestive peristalsis begins.

The outstanding characteristic of this type of gastric peristalsis is the constancy of its rhythm. When the stomach contains food, peristaltic waves occur

---

* The term "tertiary peristalsis" is used by some radiologists in a different sense to designate incoordinated or writhing movements of the lower third that may be seen in the aged or in certain disease states (TEMPLETON 1944).

[1] IVY, VLOEDMAN and KEANE 1925, THOMAS and CRIDER 1935.

regularly at a frequency of about three per minute. Each wave begins as a slight circular constriction of the stomach in some part of the corpus ventriculi; the exact point of origin varies with conditions, one of which is the amount of food in the stomach[1]. The constriction appears in the x-ray silhouette as a slight indentation on the greater and lesser curvatures. It travels toward the pylorus, becoming deeper meanwhile, until it finally ends with a contraction of the pyloric sphincter[2].

Not all gastric waves reach the pylorus in this manner. Some appear to terminate at the preantral sphincter or at some point on the pyloric antrum, most frequently in the region of the pyloric canal. When this happens the portion of the stomach beyond the point of termination of the wave appears to contract concentrically, expelling its contents either into the duodenum or back into the more proximal portion of the stomach. This behavior is probably best explained by the assumption that some of the waves are deep enough to obliterate the lumen of the stomach at some point; when such obliteration occurs the consequent sudden rise in pressure distal to the constriction stimulates the remainder of the muscle to execute a simultaneous contraction. The points at which this is most likely to occur are at the preantral sphincter and the beginning of the pyloric canal, a fact which accounts for the frequency with which concentric contractions beyond these points have been described. It is probably significant that the antral muscle shows a greater tendency to contract in response to the stimulus of stretching, than does the other gastric muscle[3].

During digestion the body and fundus of the stomach, which serve the reservoir function primarily, behave quite differently from the antral portion which serves mainly the functions of digestion and propulsion. The muscle of the body and fundus is relatively thin and participates to only a slight extent in visible peristalsis. It is this portion of the stomach that undergoes the greatest changes in size and shape, accommodating itself through changes in tonus to the volume of its contents.

The tonic contraction of the muscle of the body and fundus of the stomach exerts a more or less constant pressure on the gastric contents. Probably the pressure is increased periodically through the rhythmic changes in tone described by Cole (1911). According to this author in addition to peristaltic contractions, the whole stomach contracts and relaxes rhythmically approximately every 20 seconds. Cole applied the terms "systole" and "diastole" to these contractions and relaxations. During each systole the peristaltic waves are abserved to increase in force as indicated by deeper indentations on the greater and lesser curvatures, as seen in the x-ray silhouette; a decrease in the vigor of peristalsis is associated with the phase of "diastole".

Either hyper- or hypomotility of the stomach may be seen clinically but specific diseases involving these conditions as a principal feature are not well defined in the literature. Such changes are frequently psychogenic and result from acute or chronic emotional disturbances. Acute emotional upsets such as occur in sudden anger, fear or pain are usually associated with relaxation of the gastric muscle[4]. This is attributed to increased activity of the thoraco-lumbar sympathetic nerve fibers which reach the stomach via the splanchnics and have a predominantly inhibitory effect. Hypermotility is said to occur more frequently in prolonged or chronic emotional states involving resentment or prolonged anger[5]. Hyperperistalsis is also seen in pyloric obstruction; in this situation it

---

[1] Cannon 1911 b.   [2] Wheelon and Thomas 1921.   [3] Gellhorn and Budde 1923.
[4] Cannon 1936.   [5] Wolf and Wolff 1943.

is due in part to absence of inhibitory reflexes from the duodenum[1] and probably also in part to continued stimulation by retained gastric contents.

4. The mechanics of gastric evacuation.

KELLING'S (1900) remark that: "because of the hydrostatic relations in the abdomen, gravity can have no effect" on the movement of the gastrointestinal contents* and CANNON'S (1911a) deduction that: "muscular contraction is necessary to create a difference in pressure" in order that "the food may move onward through the alimentary canal" suggest the fundamental considerations on which any discussion of the mechanics of gastric emptying must be based. The problem is to define the nature and source of the pressure differences that serve to move the gastric contents into the duodenum.

A careful study of intraluminal pressures in the antrum of the stomach and first portion of the duodenum has been made by QUIGLEY and his associates[2]. These authors distinguish between basal pressures and phasic pressures; the basal pressures are observed in the intervals between peristaltic waves or in the absence of peristalsis; the phasic pressures are developed as a consequence of the rhythmic activity of the gastric muscle and are associated in time with the peristaltic waves. Basal pressures are in part due to the tension developed by the tonic contraction of the gastrointestinal muscle and in part to the pressure external to the organs, i.e., the intra-abdominal pressure. They are usually low, being (in the dog) slightly above or below the atmospheric pressure. The most important fact is that they are slightly higher, by 1 to 2 cm. H_2O, in the gastric antrum than in the duodenum. This difference indicates the existence of some sort of barrier between the stomach and duodenum even when the pyloric sphincter is apparently relaxed; this may possibly be a fold of mucous membrane as postulated by COLE (1928).

Phasic increases in pressure above the basal level occur as a result of the passage of peristaltic waves. The phasic pressure wave is initiated by an increase in the antral pressure followed by a rise in the duodenal pressure; subsequently both pressures fall to the basal level. "Typically", according to QUIGLEY (1944), "the antral phasic wave begins slightly in advance of the bulbar wave; they reach a maximum simultaneously and the bulbar pressure returns to the basal level before the antral". Contraction of the pyloric sphincter begins during the progress of the antral peristaltic wave, increasing the resistance to the outflow of chyme and in this way favoring an increase in the antral pressure which may rise to between 5 cm. and 30 cm. H_2O. The sphincter remains contracted during the period of increased bulbar pressure and therefore helps to prevent regurgitation of the duodenal contents. These cyclic changes are illustrated in Figure 2.

The passage of gastric chyme into the duodenum begins before the phasic increase in antral pressure is apparent, that is, with only basal pressure difference to serve as a driving force. This could only result from either a decrease in resistance at the pyloric orifice or from an increase in the pressure gradient too small to be detected by the methods employed. QUIGLEY and associates define the

---

* This statement is applicable to the normal situation in which the gastrointestinal contents have approximately the same specific gravity as the body fluids and tissues. If the contents have a higher specific gravity, as do most radio-opaque mixtures used in roentgen diagnosis, they will be affected by gravity; the results observed under these artificial conditions should not be confused with the normal mechanism.

[1] THOMAS, CRIDER and MOGAN 1934.
[2] BRODY, WERLE, MESCHAN and QUIGLEY 1940, QUIGLEY 1944, QUIGLEY and BRODY 1950.

period during which evacuation occurs without an evident increase in the pressure gradient as "evacuation period A". This is followed at once (without interruption of the flow) by "evacuation period B" which coincides in time with the rising phase of antral pressure and the beginning of the contraction of the pyloric sphincter. It continues only so long as the rising pressure in the antrum is sufficient to overcome the increasing resistance at the pylorus caused by the contracting sphincter and the rise in bulbar pressure. Although it is apparent that a hyperactive sphincter might slow evacuation by shortening evacuation period B, other evidence to be presented indicates that the pyloric sphincter is not an important regulator of gastric emptying.

Regulation of gastric emptying.

The early studies of Hirsch (1893) and v. Mering (1893) indicated that emptying of the stomach is regulated through stimuli resulting from the presence of various substances in the duodenum. They found that presence in the duodenum of physiological salt solution, HCl (Hirsch), water, milk, or sugar-peptone solution (Mering) caused a delay in gastric emptying. They raised the question of whether the effect was due to closure of the pylorus or to diminished gastric peristalsis, but left it unanswered. Subsequent investigators in Europe[1] generally favored the view that inhibition of gastric peristalsis was the sole, or at least a secondary, cause of the delayed emptying. In the United States, largely due to the influence of Cannon (1911a), the opposite view prevailed. According to Cannon's "acid control" theory, acid in the stomach causes the pylorus to open whereas acid in the duodenum causes closure of the pylorus and thus prevents further exit of gastric contents until a neutral reaction again appears in the duodenum.

More recent studies have shown that the presence in the duodenum of substances known to retard gastric emptying do so by inhibiting gastric motility[2]. They cause relaxation of the pyloric sphincter[3] and not contraction as postulated by Cannon. It is true that acid in the duodenum may cause a brief, temporary contraction of the pyloric sphincter under certain conditions but the threshold for the "pyloric reflex" is higher than for inhibition of the stomach[4], hence the "pyloric reflex" is not a factor in regulation of gastric emptying.

The concept that the pyloric sphincter is the main, if not the sole, regulator of gastric emptying, even though proved to be in error, has been difficult to

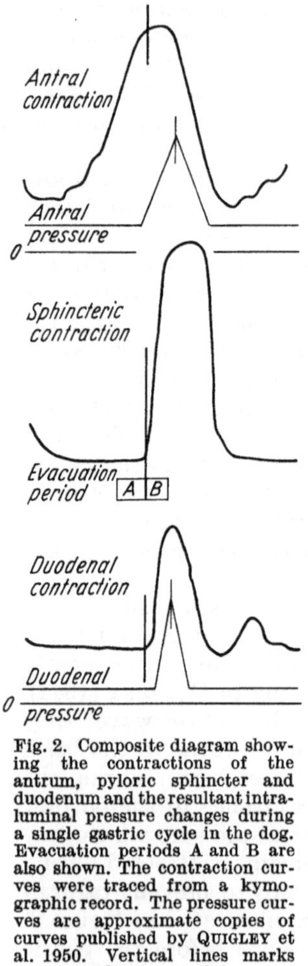

Fig. 2. Composite diagram showing the contractions of the antrum, pyloric sphincter and duodenum and the resultant intraluminal pressure changes during a single gastric cycle in the dog. Evacuation periods A and B are also shown. The contraction curves were traced from a kymographic record. The pressure curves are approximate copies of curves published by Quigley et al. 1950. Vertical lines marks simultaneous points.

[1] Moritz 1901, Kelling 1900, 1903, Katsch 1926.
[2] Thomas and Mogan 1931, Quigley, Zettelman and Ivy 1934.
[3] Thomas, Crider and Mogan 1934, Quigley and Meschan 1937, Quigley et al. 1942.
[4] Thomas, Crider and Mogan 1934.

eradicate, especially from the clinical literature. Gastric retention due to various conditions now known to be associated with gastric inhibition and relaxation of the sphincter[1] is still frequently described as pylorospasm. Probably the most important of these is the situation following section of the vagus nerves. For some weeks or months following vagotomy the tonus of the whole gastric muscle, including the pyloric sphincter, is decreased[2,3] and propulsive peristalsis is diminished or absent. The sphincter may appear to be contracted on x-ray examination but only because it has relaxed less, perhaps, than be remainder of the gastric muscle. Pylorospasm doubtless occurs in other circumstances but it is not common and should never be diagnosed as a cause of gastric retention in the absence of vigorous antral peristalsis.

Acid and other substances that act in the intestine to inhibit gastric motility do so through a dual mechanism involving a reflex over the vagi (the enterogastric reflex of THOMAS and MOGAN 1931) and a hormone (enterogastrone) which is liberated from the duodenal mucosa especially by fat[4] or carbohydrate[5]. Whether acid, peptone, and hypertonic solutions which are believed to act reflexly also excite the humoral mechanism is not known for certain, nor do we know the extent to which fat and carbohydrate may excite the reflex mechanism.

The assumption that a reflex mechanism is involved is based on the observation that certain substances are without effect after the vagi are cut and the response to acid greatly decreased; for example in the dog, 10 ml. N/10 HCl in the duodenum was without effect in vagotomized dogs (dogs weighing 20 to 25 Kilo were used) and 20 ml. causes only a brief and uncertain inhibition. Recently SHAPIRO and WOODWARD (1955) have reported that vagotomy is without effect on the inhibitory action of acid in human subjects. Since they regularly used 100 ml. N/10 acid their experiments are not comparable to those reported in dogs even if the amount of acid is calculated on a per Kilo basis. Obviously, in order to detect a change in a reflex which is merely depressed and not abolished by vagotomy it is necessary to test it with a submaximal stimulus.

Coordination of stomach and duodenum.

The first portion of the duodenum is a relatively quiescent structure in the human. However, in the dog it exhibits vigorous rhythmic contractions except during a certain phase of the gastric cycle, specifically, when a peristaltic wave is approaching the pylorus. At this time the activity of the first part of the duodenum is, apparently, inhibited and the duodenum relaxes, as though in preparation for receiving a part of the gastric contents[6]. A somewhat similar phenomenon has been observed in rabbits and has been called "the receptive relaxation of the duodenum"[7]. The activity in the duodenum is resumed immediately after the gastric peristaltic wave reaches the pylorus, giving rise to the impression that the wave passes over the pylorus and continues in the duodenum as a wave of intestinal peristalsis[8].

Whether the increased duodenal activity that follows each gastric cycle in the dog is, in fact, a continuation of the gastric peristaltic wave is still undetermined. Of much greater interest is the question of whether a similar phenomenon occurs in the human duodenum. Unfortunately, the investigations that would be necessary to establish the facts have not been done. Nevertheless certain observations by IVY and VLOEDMAN (1925) indicate that a mechanism for gastroduodenal coordination similar to that found in the dog exists also in man. In

---

[1] QUIGLEY et al. 1943.　　[2] CODE et al. 1952.　　[3] QUIGLEY and LOUCKES 1951.
[4] LIM 1933.　　[5] QUIGLEY and PHELPS 1934.　　[6] WHEELON and THOMAS 1922.
[7] JOSEPH and MELTZER 1910.　　[8] MESCHAN and QUIGLEY 1938.

a study of hunger activity in the human intestine they noted that in the first four or five inches of the duodenum contractions occur simultaneously with, or immediately following, contractions of the stomach. Certain of their records obtained with balloons in the stomach and duodenum of human subjects are similar to records obtained from dogs by Wheelon and Thomas (1922) and later by Thomas and Crider (1935) using similar methods. Brody and Quigley (1947) studied the gastroduodenal pressure cycle in humans and found it to be similar to that in dogs; since the pressure cycle is dependant on a motility cycle it is probable that the motility cycle is likewise similar in the two species.

Vomiting.

Vomiting is a reflex which serves to relieve the uppor gastrointestinal tract of its contents; this may occur either because the contents are irritating or because the organs themselves are not in a normal state. In either case there is excessive stimulation (irritation) of some part of the tract. The most irritable area is the first portion of the duodenum[1] but adequate stimulation of other parts of the intestine or of the stomach can induce the reflex.

The sensory impulses initiated in the gut are transmitted over visceral afferent nerves which accompany the vagi and splanchnics, and eventually reach the vomiting center in the medulla. They are also conveyed to receptive areas in the brain where they give rise to a conscious sensation interpreted as nausea. From the vomiting center, motor impulses are transmitted over visceral and somatic efferent nerves to the smooth muscle of the viscera and the voluntary muscles of the thorax, abdomen, neck and mouth. These impulses are coordinated in such a way as to bring about muscular movements resulting in evacuation of the contents of the upper intestine and stomach through the mouth.

The first muscular movement to occur is a strong sustained contraction of the jejunum, followed by similar contractions of the duodenum. Next the pyloric sphincter contracts and then the pyloric portion of the stomach. These changes all take place during the period of nausea and result in emptying the contents of the jejunum, duodenum and pyloric portion of the stomach into the fundus and body of the stomach, which are relaxed and dilated. At this point the voluntary muscles come into play, and at the same time the cardiac sphincter, esophagus and esophago-pharyngeal sphincter relax. Following an inspiratory movement, the glottis is closed and the abdominal muscles contract, compressing the stomach between the contracted diaphragm and the abdominal organs. The pressure on the gastric contents causes their evacuation through the relaxed esophagus.

Vomiting may be induced by abnormal stimulation of sensory receptors outside the gastrointestinal tract, for example, in the uterus, kidneys, heart, semicircular canals, eyes, nose, and mouth. It may also occur as a result of direct stimulation of the vomiting center. Certain of the emetic drugs act in this way but most important clinically is the "central" vomiting caused by traumatic stimulation of the center due to head injuries, increased intracranial pressure, brain tumors or meningeal irritation. This type of vomiting is characterized by the great force with which the contents are ejected ("projectile vomiting") and a minimum of nausea and contraction of the voluntary muscles.

5. Movements of small intestine.
Rhythmic contractions.

The dominant characteristic of the muscle of the small intestine is its rhythmicity which it manifests under appropriate conditions by alternating contractions

---

[1] Luckhardt, Phillips and Carlson 1919.

and relaxations at a remarkably regular frequency. The rhythmic contractions may occur at regularly spaced intervals along a section of the intestine, dividing it into short segments (the "segmenting contractions" of CANNON 1902) or they may occut singly or in pairs or in a variety of other arrangements. The area involved in each contraction may be less than one cm. or several cms. long. The rhythmic nature of this activity reminded LUDWIG (1861) of a pendulum, hence the name "pendulum movements"* often applied to these contractions.

The frequency of the rhythmic contractions varies with the species of animal and with the region of the intestine in which they occur. In the rabbit the contractions recur at a frequency of about 20 per minute in the duodenum and about 10 per minute in the lower ileum[1]; the frequency in other parts of the intestine is intermediate between these extremes, becoming less the greater the distance from the pylorus. In the dog's duodenum the frequency is about 18 per minute and in the human probably somewhat less. The frequency is surprisingly constant in any one area and is not affected by stimulation of the extrinsic nerves or by neurotropic drugs. In excised material the frequency varies with the temperature.

According to DOUGLAS (1949) the frequency of rhythmic contractions in the dog's jejunum may drop from 18 to 12 per minute if the jejunum is cut off from the duodenum. This observation suggests that the rhythm of the pendular contractions is not determined locally but by some sort of conducted impulse which is initiated at a higher level at a frequency corresponding to the frequency of the rhythmic contractions, and which is conducted along the intestine in an aboral direction as a wave of excitation. The electrical studies of AMBACHE (1947), BOZLER (1949a and b) and of MILTON, SMITH and ARMSTRONG (1955) lend strong support to this view. These authors have described the electrical activity of the intestine as consisting of (1) slow waves which are not necessarily associated with muscular contraction and (2) rapid spike-like waves which appear only when the muscle contracts. The slow waves occur at a frequency corresponding to the frequency of the rhythmic contractions, whether or not these are evident and, they are regularly conducted along the intestine in an aboral direction at a velocity corresponding to the velocity of a peristaltic wave. AMBACHE (1947) has suggested that they arise in a "pacemaker" which he does not further identify. When ryhthmic activity is present a slow wave precedes each rhythmic contraction and a series of rapid spike-like waves is then superimposed on the slow wave. The frequency of the slow waves, like that of the rhythmic contractions, is not affected by neurotropic drugs. These observations strongly suggest the existence of a pacemaker[2] or pacemakers for the intestine which send down the intestine regularly spaced impulses that serve to increase the excitability of the muscle but are, of themselves, subthreshold for contraction. Actual contractions may result from summation of local stimuli with these conducted impulses (see Fig. 4).

Rhythmic contractions may be induced in a quiescent portion of the intestine by mechanical or chemical stimulation of the mucosa, or stimulation of the muscle by stretching; hence the intestinal contents are adequate stimuli. Probably the

---

* LUDWIG used the pendulum as a symbol of rhythm only but some authors have attempted to apply the simile in the sense of the to and fro motion of a pendulum. Swaying movements of the intestinal coils are to be seen at times as well as a to and fro motion of opaque masses within the intestine as seen with a fluoroscope. However, to identify only these as "pendulum movements" is confusing since the term as originally used and commonly applied is synonymous merely with "rhythmic movements" without regard to the effect of the activity on the intestinal coils or their contents.

AlVAREZ 1948.   [2] MILTON and SMITH 1956.

function of the rhythmic contractions is to agitate the intestinal contents and bring the digesting mass into intimate contact with the absorbing surface of the mucosa.

Intestinal peristalsis.

The term peristalsis has been used to describe a variety of contractile phenomena which have one thing in common, namely, they progress along the intestine in an aboral direction. Any strong contraction in the intestine tends to spread, both orally and aborally; however, the oral spread is inhibited and the aboral spread is facilitated by some means, possibly the conducted impulses described in the preceding section. Rhythmic contractions may, while retaining their rhythmic character, recur at successively· more aboral levels and appear to travel along the intestine as a wave of "peristalsis". In other situations the rhythmic contractions remain localized while the "tonus" of the muscle is increased in a particular area; if the tonic contraction spreads in the aboral direction and fades out orally it becomes a "peristaltic wave" which progresses without interrupting the rhythmic contractions. The tonic contraction may be powerful enough to obscure the relaxation phase of the rhythmic cycle and appear to progress along the intestine as a smooth, progressive contraction. Nevertheless, a rhythm persists as Bozler (1949b) has shown form a study of the electrical variations accompanying peristalsis. Peristaltic waves of this character which sweep rapidly over the entire small intestine were described by van Braam Houckgeest (1872) under the name "Rollbewegungen" are described in the more recent literature as rush waves or "Peristaltic Rush" after the terminology proposed by Meltzer and Auer (1907).

Wheter the conditions that give rise to rhythmic contractions on the one hand and to peristaltic movements on the other, differ qualitatively or only quantitatively is not known. It is known that both mechanical and chemical stimuli are effective in promoting peristalsis and that mild stimulation favors rhythmic activity. Doubtless not only the nature and strength of the stimuli but also the irritability of the intestinal neuromuscular mechanism play a significant part in determining the nature and location of the activity. The latter may be influenced by local and central reflexes and by circulating hormones and metabolites as well as by the previous history of the muscle, for example, by refractoriness or fatigue following a period of activity.

The gradients of the intestine.

The physiological functions of the small intestine that can be measured such as rate of rhythmic contractions, respiratory metabolism[1], etc., are of greater magnitude in the duodenum than elsewhere and decrease progressively toward the lower end of the gut. Thus a gradient may be said to exist with respect to these functions; the gradient of rhythmicity is illustrated in Figure 3. The intestinal gradients have been described by Alvarez and his co-workers in numerous publications (see Alvarez 1948). A similar gradient in the physical features of the intestine is obvious even on casual inspection; thus the duodenum is pinker (better blood supply) and larger than the jejunum or ileum. Alvarez (1948) has stressed the importance of the gradients in establishing the normal aboral direction of peristalsis and he considers that many disturbances of function may be traced to local temporary reversals of the gradients associated with alterations in irritability due to disease.

---

[1] Wilson and Wiseman 1954.

However the gradients do not of themselves satisfactorily account for the direction of conduction of the peristaltic waves. Indeed, if the gradient of irritability has any influence on conduction it should favor conduction in the direction of increasing irritability; this is opposite to the direction in which conduction actually occurs. Elsewhere, as in the heart, where both a gradient of irritability and unidirectional conductions are manifest, the direction of conduction is not determined by the gradient but by the site of origin of the stimulus; if the pacemaker shifts position, for example to the atrioventricular node in the heart, backward conduction readily occurs.

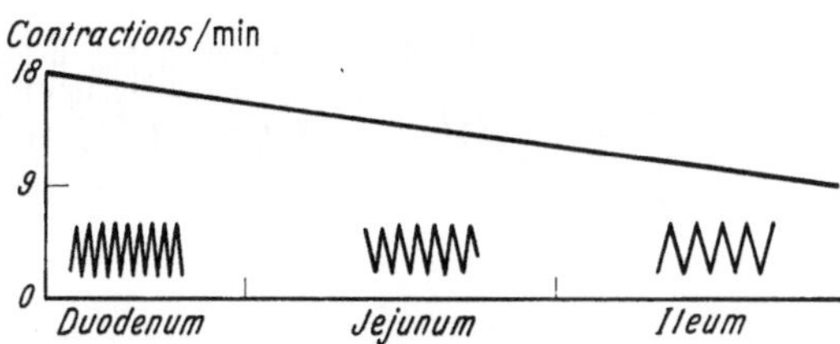

Fig. 3. Diagram illustrating the relative frequency of rhythmic contractions in the duodenum, jejunum and ileum respectively. The slope of the curve is represented as being uniform; acutally, the slope may vary at different levels. Gradient of rhythmicity in small intestine. From THOMAS 1955.

The existence of gradients of structure and function in the intestine is now universally recognized but their functional significance remains obscure. Quite possibly they represent nothing more than an evolutionaly adaptation to the greater functional demands made on the more proximal segments of the intestine.

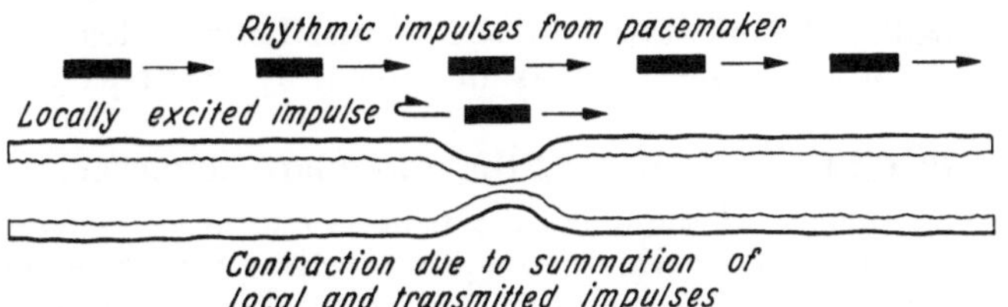

Fig. 4. Diagram illustrating the concept of a pacemaker mechanism for intestinal rhythmic contractions and peristalsis. The black rectangles represent waves of excitation transmitted from the hypothetical pacemaker. An excitatory process arising locally could not be conducted upstream because it would encounter a refractory phase following a wave of excitation from the pacemaker. From THOMAS 1955.

On the other hand, if the existence of a pacemaker or pacemakers is established by further study, the gradients would insure that the conducted impulses were always initiated at the highest possible level, as in the heart, and thus determine the forward or aboral direction of peristalsis (Fig. 4).

The myenteric reflex.

BAYLISS and STARLING (1899, 1901) observed that the response of the small intestine of the dog to local stimuli consists of a contraction of the smooth muscle above and relaxation below the stimulated area. "This", they said, "is the law of the intestine". The response occurs after complete extrinsic denervation of the gut but does not appear in its characteristic form if the myenteric plexus is paralyzed by cocaine or nicotine. For these reasons BAYLISS and STARLING attributed the reaction to a reflex involving the myenteric plexus. CANNON (1912) later reported similar observations and proposed that the reflex involved be designated the "myenteric reflex".

The observations and conclusions cited in the preceding paragraph have been the subject of a more or less continuous controversy since they were first reported, with a majority of observers contending either that the myenteric reflex does not exist, that it occurs only under exceptional circumstances[1], or that only the contraction phase can be elicited consistently[2]. Much of the evidence cited is unconvincing having been obtained under conditions in which the delicate reflex mechanism of the intestine could not be expected to function normally.

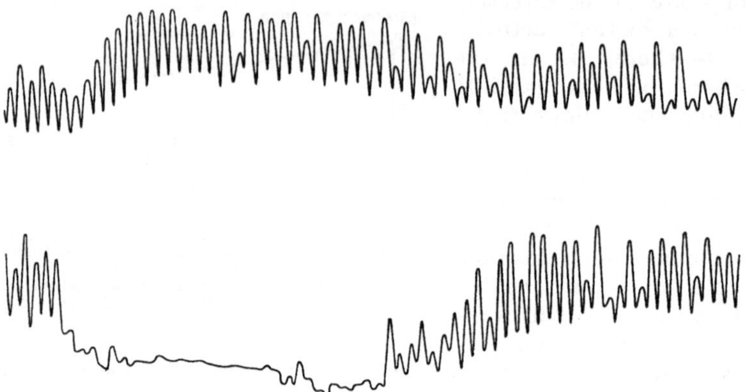

Fig. 5. Kymographic record of a myenteric reflex in a dog. Two balloons in the upper jejunum, about 5 cm. apart, were connected to water manometers recording on a kymograph. One cc. of soap solution injected between the balloons caused contraction above (upper record) and relaxation below (lower record) the stimulated point. From Thomas 1955.

The reflex is readily demonstrated in the unanesthetized dog with duodenal fistula[3] where it occurs essentially as described by Bayliss and Starling (Fig. 5).

The intestinal villi and the muscularis mucosae.

The absorbing surface of the small intestine is enormously increased by the superabundance of the mucosa which, except when the gut is distended, is thrown into circular folds called plicae circulares. A still greater increase in surface is provided by the intestinal villi; these are tit-like projections of the mucous membrane about 1 mm. in length which cover the circular folds as well as the intervening spaces and, macroscopically, resemble the pile on a piece of velvet. Our intest in these structures at this point has to do with the activities of the muscularis mucosae which lies everywhere directly beneath the mucous membrane, following its folds, and axtending into each villus as a fine filament of smooth muscle fibers.

The activities of the muscularis mucosae, including those of the villi, have been studied by a number of investigators[4] beginning with Gruby and Delafond (1843). It has generally been observed that in the fasting animal the villi are inactive and lie flat on the mucosal surface when first exposed for study. Covering them with liquids of various sorts, such as solutions of sugar, salt, amino acids, weak alkalis or even with distilled water causes them to become active. In the fed animal activity of the villi can be observed without special stimulation.

The activity is of two kinds, a lashing movement and a more or less rhythmical shortening and lengthening. It is generally believed that these movements accelerate the flow of blood and lymph and that they increase absorption. Although King, Arnold and Church (1922) were unable to find evidence for any of these functions, more recent studies, especially those of v. Kokas and v. Ludany (1933a), leave little doubt that efficient absorption of food stuffs from the intestine is dependent to some extont on the activity of the villi.

[1] Alvarez 1948.   [2] Bozler 1949a.   [3] Thomas 1951, 1955.
[4] Exner 1902, Müller 1904, Magnus 1904, Hambleton 1914, King and Arnold 1922, Verzár 1931, Kokas and Ludány 1932, 1933a, 1933b, 1934, 1938.

The movements of the villi are partly under nervous control[1], being augmented by stimulation of the splanchnic (but not the vagus) nerves and by sympathomimetic drugs and depressed by atropine and nicotine. Their activity is also increased by villikinine[2], one of the intestinal hormones.

No regular or consistent activity of the main sheet of muscle comprising the muscularis mucosae has been described but it is believed to be active during digestion and to be in part responsible for the various mucosal patterns seen in roentgenograms of the small intestine. One function of this muscle is, apparently, to withdraw the mucosa from contact with sharp objects by forming pits or grooves with a firm base[3] which is difficult to penetrate.

Abnormal motility patterns in the small intestine are seen in some nervous and endocrine disturbances and in vitamin deficiencies[4]; their significance, when they occur, is not always clear. Paralysis of the intestine sometimes follows abdominal surgery or other trauma. This has been shown by CANNON and MURPHY (1906) to be due to reflexes over the splanchnic nerves and, to some extent, the intrinsic plexuses in the intestinal wall.

6. Movements of the large intestine.

The movements of the large intestine are not basically different from those of the small intestine but due to the relative infrequency of muscular activity in the colon, detailed knowledge of its movements is largely lacking. Species differences are also considerable so that observations made on experimental animals are not necessarily applicable to the human. Studies on human subjects are difficult because the periods of activity of the colon, always brief and infrequent, are apt to be prevented by the anxiety of the subject incident to the study; consequently, fluoroscopic observations are often disappointing. Various types of local rhythmic contractions, slow contractions involving whole segments of the colon, antiperistalsis and peristalsis have been observed in experimental animals.

BARCROFT and STEGGERDA (1932) studied the exteriorized colon of dogs, and saw what they described as "kneading movements" in the proximal colon. These appear to correspond roughly to the segmenting contractions of the small intestine but involve larger areas of the gut and occur at a slower rate, about 2 cantractions per minute. These movements usually appeared first in the cecum, and then spread to the region of the ileocoecal valve; they were accompanied by an increase in tone of the affected area which diminished its volume capacity and forced the contents into more distal segments. When a distally placed segment became distended antiperistalsis appeared and drove the contents back into the cecum which, by this time, had relaxed. A similar to-and-fro motion of the contents of the proximal colon was observed in cats by CANNON (1902), using the x-ray method. He attributed the forward motion to mass contractions of the cecum and ascending colon or to forward peristalsis; the return flow was caused by antiperistalsis.

Probably mechanisms exist in the human colon with functions similar to those seen in laboratory animals but the observations are so unsatisfactory that nothing can be stated with confidence. TODD (1930) made x-ray studies of the colon in about 100 medical students. Although he noted peristalsis and mass contractions of the cecum he was unable to account for the observed forward progress of the contents. OPPENHEIMER (1940) has described a slow progression

[1] KING and ARNOLD 1922.   [2] KOKAS and LUDÁNY 1938.
[3] EXNER 1902, KING and ARNOLD 1922.   [4] FELDMAN 1948.

of the haustral contractions which he thinks moves the contents forward somewhat in the manner of the conveyors in a dredge. Antiperistalsis was rarely seen[1] except in the spastic colon, in spite of the fact that it is probably the most frequent type of activity seen in laboratory animals[2].

Mass movements.

The function of the movements decribed in the preceding paragraphs is, evidently, to agitate the colonic contents and to promote absorption, chiefly of water, by a continuous exchange of the material that is in contact with the mucosa. When the contents of the proximal colon have reached a certain consistency due to the loss of water, they are transferred to the more distal parts of the colon by means of a mass movement or mass peristalsis; as described by Hurst (1907) this is a true peristaltic wave, sometimes progressing over the entire length of the colon in a few seconds time. According to Code et al. (1954) these movements are propulsive but are not true peristaltic waves, since they involve simultaneous contraction of large segments of the colon; however, since they accomplish a forward movement of the colonic contents, it is evident that they comprise in a functional sense, all the essential features of peristalsis. Mass movements occur only at infrequent intervals, once or twice in 24 hours; the most favorable time is after a meal. The movement itself is not normally associated with any conscious sensation but it is frequently followed by a desire to defecate. The association of mass movements of the colon with the act of eating was studies by Hertz and Newton (1913) who ascribed it to a reflex effect of filling the stomach; they named this the "gastro-colic reflex"*.

Abnormal motor activity in the colon is one of the most common conditions for which the physician may be consulted. It may express itself as constipation or diarrhea. The causes may be local only or they may involve more fundamental disease states. Psychic factors are important and it can be safely asserted that no other part of the gastrointestinal tract is so frequently involved in emotional disturbances as is the large intestine. This statement is supported, not only by lay observation and clinical experience but also by experimental observations on suitable human subjects in which it has been seen that experimentally induced emotional reactions are nearly always accompanied by changes in tone motility or vascularity of the large intestine[3].

Defecation.

The occurrence of mass movements in the colon may give rise to a desire to defecate. The sensation is due to passage into the rectum of feces previously accumulated in the pelvic colon. The act of defecation is, in the adult, preceded by a voluntary effort consisting of assumption of an appropriate posture, voluntary relaxation of the external anal sphincter and, usually, compression of the abdominal contents by means of straining efforts. These movements in turn probably give rise to stimuli which augment the visceral reflexes which originate primarily in the distended rectum. As a result of these reflexes peristaltic waves appear

---

* A similar response of the ileum to feeding, which had been seen by several observers, was named by Hertz the "gastro ileac reflex". Douglas and Mann (1939, 1940) found that the entire small intestine manifests increased motility under these circumstances but the stimulus is transmitted along the intestine and not exclusively by way of the central nervous system.

[1] Todd 1930.   [2] Elliott and Barclay-Smith 1904, and many others.
[3] Friedman and Snape 1946, Wolff et al. 1949, Miner 1954.

in the entire colon[1], and the internal anal sphincter relaxes. The peristalsis in the descending colon carries its contents into the pelvic colon which in turn transfers them to the rectum eventually to be evacuated by way of the anus. Hence the entire distal colon from the splenic flexure to the anus may be emptied at one time.

A prominent mechanical feature of the final act of evacuation is contraction of the longitudinal muscle of the distal colon which is most pronounced in the rectum itself. The shortening of the distal colon tends to elevate the pelvic colon and obliterate the angle which it normally makes with the upper end of the rectum; this straightening of the passage doubtless facilitates evacuation. Shortening of the rectum itself, assuming that it has a firm grip on its contents at the upper end, is an important factor in expelling the feces through the anal orifice.

The act of defecation provides another instance of a reflex that is under some degree of voluntary control. The voluntary regulation consists of the ability to inhibit the reflex under normal circumstances and to initiate it voluntarily provided the necessary visceral stimulus (recent distention of the rectum) is present. Reflex centers for defecation have been located in the hypothalamus[2], in the lower lumbar and upper sacral segments of the spinal cord and in the ganglionic plexus of the gut[3].

7. Nervous regulation of gastro-intestinal motility.

The gastrointestinal tract is capable of carrying on its major functions in the absence of the extrinsic innervation. This automaticity may be attributed partly to the local nervous mechanism comprising the myenteric and submucous plexuses and partly to the properties of the smooth muscle. The exact division of labor between these mechanisms has never been determined but it has been suggested that the essentially rhythmic functions such as gastric peristalsis, segmenting contractions of the small intestine and antiperistalsis in the colon are myogenic[4] and that the more highly coordinated functions such as forward peristalsis in the small and large intestine are dependent on the functional integrity of the myenteric plexus[5].

Both the neurogenic and myogenic functions are subject to regulatory reflexes through the central nervous system by way of the extrinsic nerves. These nerves belong to either the cranio-sacral or the thoraco-lumbar division of the autonomic system. The cranio-sacral nerves are the vagi and pelvic visceral nerves; their fibers are preganglionic and terminate in the gut by making synaptic connection with certain neurones of the intrinsic plexuses. The preganglionic thoraco-lumbar fibers run chiefly in the splanchnic nerves and end in either the celiac, superior mesenteric or inferior mesenteric ganglia. Smaller rami from the lumbar sympathetic chain, principally to the aortic plexus and inferior mesenteric ganglia, are also involved. From the ganglia the path is continued through post-ganglionic fibers, generally associated with the blood vessels; these fibers end directly on the muscle or gland cells[6]. The vagi and splanchnics supply mainly the esophagus, stomach and small intestine. The exact limits are, however, uncertain particularly in the case of the vagi which seem to supply the proximal colon in some animals but not in others. Branches of the superior mesenteric plexus are distributed to both the small intestine and the proximal colon; the

---

[1] HERTZ 1909.　　　[2] HESS 1945.　　　[3] MÜLLER 1911; cited by KUNTZ 1953.
[4] THOMAS and KUNTZ 1926a and b.　　　[5] BAYLISS and STARLING 1899, 1901.
[6] KUNTZ 1953, p. 212.

distal colon and rectum receive their thoraco-lumbar autonomic fibers from the inferior mesenteric plexus and their cranio-sacral fibers from the pelvic visceral nerves.

Functionally, the nerves are often classified as parasympathetic (cranio-sacral nerves) or sympathetic (thoraco-lumbar nerves), but it is more in keeping with modern thought to consider them as cholinergic or adrenergic, depending on whether they liberate acetylcholine or an adrenin-like substance at their final termination on the muscles. In this sense most parasympathetics are cholinergic and the sympathetics are adrenergic, but there is considerable mixing since cholinergic fibers have been demonstrated in considerable abundance in the sympathetics.

Attempts to classify the extrinsic nerves as excitatory or inhibitory to the intestinal muscle have given rise to confusion. Such a simple approach fails to take account of the true relation of the visceral nerves to the peripheral neuro-muscular mechanism. The latter comprises a local relfex mechanism with its effectors, and is possessed of a high degree of autonomy in its response to local stimuli. The extrinsic nerves influence this mechanism in such a way as to increase or decrease its excitability, much as the descending tracts of the spinal cord facilitate or inhibit spinal reflexes[1]. Considered in this light, it is not surprising that both "motor" and "inhibitory" effects have been described as resulting from stimulation of either the sympathetic or parasympathetic nerves. It is true that, generally, the cholinergic nerves tend to increase and the adrenergic nerves to decrease the reactivity of the local mechanism; to the extent that this occurs the parasympathetics are chiefly "excitatory" and the sympathetics (but less consistently) "inhibitory" to the muscle. It is much more firmly established that the results of stimulation of the extrinsic nerves are unpredictable and largely dependent on the state of the reacting mechanism; when the muscle is active or in high tonus inhibitory effects tend to predominate and vice versa.

Summary of gastrointestinal reflexes affecting motility.

The following reflexes have been described in the preceding sections: receptive relaxation of the stomach, the enterogastric reflex, receptive relaxation of the duodenum, the myenteric reflex, and the pyloric reflex.

Another reflex, which may be elicited by stimuli within the normal range, is the inhibition of stomach and small intestine that occurs during the act of defecation[2] or in response to stimuli in the anorectal region which normally tend to induce defecation. This is an adrenergic, sympathetic reflex since it is abolished by division of the splanchnic nerves.

Reflex responses to noxious stimuli remain to be described. Painful stimuli applied to almost any part of the body may cause inhibition of motility in the whole gastrointestinal tract. The peritoneal surfaces seem to be particularly sensitive to stimuli causing this type of inhibition and this fact accounts for the remarkable absence of intestinal motility when the abdomen is opened for surgical or experimental purposes[3]. The path for this reflex involves the sympathetic nerves since section of the splanchnic nerves eliminates the response unless the stimuli are applied directly to the viscera[3]. In the conscious animal strong emotions cause a similar result.

Strong stimulation of the intestine inhibits motility in the remainder of the tract; if the stimulus is intraluminal pressure the reflex is called the "intestino-

---

[1] Carlson et al. 1922.   [2] For literature see Youmans 1949.
[3] Cannon and Murphy 1906.

intestinal inhibitory reflex"[1]. It is necessary to distinguish this reflex from the inhibitory effect of more moderate stimuli which affects only those segments immediately aboral to the stimulated area and is a part of the myenteric reflex. The intestino-intestinal reflex is a response to mechanical stimuli which are either abnormal in intensity or, according to YOUMANS, in the upper range of normal, whereas, the myenteric reflex may be elicited with either mechanical or chemical stimuli which are definitely submaximal for the normal range. The nervous mechanisms of the two reflexes are also different; the myenteric reflex is unaffected by extrinsic denervation whereas the intestino-intestinal reflex is either abolished by cutting the extrinsic nerves or its threshold is raised to such an extent as to amount practically to abolition of the reflex.

The varied responses of the gastrointestinal muscle to reflex stimulation tend to be confusing; however, if we take account of the intensity and distribution of the stimulus evoking each type of reflex, a certain degree of consistency can be distinguished. Localized, moderate stimuli tend to be confined to the local nerve plexus and to cause contraction above and relaxation below the stimulated area. This is the first law of the intestine. The classical example is the myenteric reflex. Similar normal stimuli when applied over a wider area, in addition to causing local myenteric reflexes, affect the extrinsic innervation. They modify the activity of whole segments of the gut at a distance from the stimulated area, chiefly through an effect on the parasympathetic efferents. Segments above the stimulated area are inhibited; insofar as the activity of distal segments is affected, it tends to be increased. Examples are the enterogastric and the gastro-colic reflexes. These phenomenona are so consistent that they may be said to comprise a second law of the intestine.

If the stimuli are of abnormal intensity the reactions do not conform to the normal pattern. Strong chemical stimuli applied to the mucosa may cause hyperperistalsis, antiperistalsis or vomiting. The local mechanism is adequate for hyperperistalsis and antiperistalsis but vomiting is a central nervous system reflex. Normal stimuli may elicit responses of this nature in an abnormally irritable intestine. Overdistention causes generalized inhibition of the whole gut as do noxious stimuli acting elsewhere; the efferent path is in the sympathetic nerves.

The relation of autonomic reflexes to visceral disease processes cannot be developed fully in this brief discussion. It may be pointed out, however, that emotional expression involves, among other things a discharge of impulses over the autonomic nerves. Such impulses may, at times, produce reactions in the viscera which are not appropriate to the local, functional requirements and thus give rise to various types of malfunction. Gastric stasis, anorexia, vomiting, diarrhoea or constipation when due to emotional states are manifestations of such inappropriate responses to stimulation of autonomic mechanisms. Hyperemia, hypermotility and hypersecretion of the stomach has been observed in association with emotional states involving chronic anxiety and resentment[2]. There seems no reason to doubt that a disturbance of this character, if sufficiently intense or prolonged can give rise to organic disease.

8. Salivary secretion.

Characteristics of secretion.

The salivary glands are compound organs composed of different types of secretory epithelia, each producing its characteristic secretion. The secretory cells are arranged as alveoli and discharge their secretions into the lumen of the

---

[1] YOUMANS 1949.   [2] WOLF and WOLFF 1942, 1947.

alveolus. The contents of the alveoli are collected by a series of branching ducts into large ducts and ultimately pass to the buccal cavity by way of the large gland ducts. In addition, the epithelial cells of the small collecting ducts may contribute their secretions. The alveoli may consist of many mucous cells (notably the small buccal glands) or only serous cells (notably the parotid gland), but in the submaxillary and sublingual glands the alveoli are mixed, some consisting of purely mucous cells, others of purely serous cells, and still other of mucous cells interspersed with serous cells. In the last case, the serous cells assume a position next to the basement membrane, peripheral to the mucous cells, and because of their shape are known as demilune cells. The demilune cells discharge their secretion into the alveolus or lumen by means of canaliculi which pass between the mucous cells. The proportion of serous and mucous cells varies in each type of gland as with the species.

In the dog and cat, the secretion of saliva is intermittant, occurring in response to some appropriate stimulus[1]. In ruminating animals, the secretion from the parotid gland is continuous and spontaneous even though the secretion from the submaxillary gland in these animals is intermittent. The secretion from the unstimulated parotid gland, often at hourly rates in excess of 60 cc. in the goat and 2000 cc. in the ox[2], serves as a constant source of alkali for neutralizing the abomasum content. In man salivary secretion also appears to be continuous although the question of its spontaneity is still unsettled. In healthy young people, the modal value for secretion rate in the absence of discernable stimuli was found to be 0.24 cc. per minute[3]. The pre-breakfast unstimulated morning mixed saliva may be produced at rates ranging from 1 to 111 cc. per hour while chewing can produce in some individuals a salivary flow of almost 200 cc. per hour[4, 5]. Pregnancy per se, unassociated with nausea, does not result in increased salivary activity.

The saliva secreted by man normally is slightly acid (p_H 6.64). Both hourly and seasonal fluctuations in p_H values are encountered[5]. In humans, the mixed salivary secretions have a diastatic power which is more or less in proportion to the nitrogen content. This is true also in pregnant women exhibiting ptyalism.

The most important function of saliva is that of moistening and lubricating the food. Salivary digestion of starch plays a minor role: although reduced in elderly people there is no impairment in starch digestion since the pancreatic and intestinal digestion are adequate[6]. Under certain conditions the salivary glands may have an excretory role, shown by the elevated urea and NPN contents of saliva in kidney impairment and the "sweet taste" in patients with diabetes. Recent evidence also points to the salivary glands playing a role in iodine metabolism[7].

Nervous regulation.

The salivary glands are exclusively under nervous control. Secretory activity is initiated reflexly, the most important reflex being the bucco-salivary reflex due to the action of food on the taste buds of the mouth. The activity of the salivary center is integrated with the activities of the centers of mastication and deglutition. Stimulation of the rostral parts of the center provokes the submaxillary glands while the caudal part provokes the parotid gland[8].

[1] Babkin 1928.   [2] Mangold 1929.   [3] Spealman 1943.   [4] Becks et al. 1939, 1943.
[5] Eisenbrandt 1943.   [6] Meyer and Necheles 1940,
[7] Fawcett and Kirkwood 1954.   [8] Walker and Green 1938, Wang 1943.

An esophago-salivary reflex is responsible for a profuse secretion of saliva when the esophagus is distended, as by a bolus of food. The accumulated saliva is swallowed, and, as described earlier, the act of swallowing results in a peristaltic wave along the esophagus which may carry the bolus into the stomach. The profuse salivation seen in patients with carcinoma of the esophagus probably is due to this reflex also. Irritation of the gastric mucosa may result in reflex salivary secretion and the profuse salivation experienced during nausea may in part be due to this reflex. Conditioned reflex salivary secretion occurring on presentation of appropriate conditioned stimuli to the olfactory, visual and auditory sense organs play an extremely important role in the digestive processes. No secretory inhibitory fibers to the salivary glands have been demonstrated satisfactorily. The drying of the mouth and cessation of salivary secretion which occur in such emotional states as fright, probably are the result of decreased blood flow to the glands rather than nervous inhibition of secretory activity. Since phonation is impaired when the mouth is dry, it may be said that the salivary glands also play a part in speech mechanics.

Histologic studies[1] support the view that each type of secretory cell receives fibers from only one division of the autonomic nervous system. In the submaxillary gland, for example, the mucous cells receive parasympathetic fibers while the serous cells receive sympathetic. The effects of direct nerve stimulation are complicated, however, by the fact that the parasympathetic and sympathetic nerves carry vasodilator and vasoconstrictor fibers respectively to the salivary glands[2], so that the secretory effect of autonomic nerve stimulation may be influenced by the altered blood supply to the various glandular elements. In addition, it is probable that not all secretory cells of an alveolus participate in the secretory processes at any one time and therefore the composition of the secretion will vary as new secretory units become activated.

Paralytic secretion.

The salivary glands offer a good example of the phenomenon of *paralytic secretion* first described by CLAUDE BERNARD in 1864. Following section of the chorda tympani the submaxillary gland secretes continuously for about 5 or 6 weeks. The secretion comes from the demilune and not the mucous cells. A paralytic secretion may also be obtained in cats which have been subjected to pretreatment for 10 to 13 days with atropine rather than severance of the chorda tympani[3]. Whether the paralytic secretions produced by atropine and by denervation are identical awaits further study.

A "paralytic secretion" has also been described as occurring in the small intestine after sympathetic denervation. The salivary paralytic secretion differs from this in that it is not simply a release from tonic constritor vasomotor action. Neither is it an example of the phenomenon of "sensitization by denervation" so well described by CANNON (1949) and his collaborators. The cholinesterase content of the denervated gland is apparently not decreased[4] but there may be an increase in the excitability of the secretory cells[5]. This phenomenon merits further study, not only for its own sake but as a means of furthering our knowledge of the influence of denervation on gastrointestinal processes in general.

---

[1] RAWLINSON 1933, 1935.
[2] LANGLEY 1885, CHAUCHARD and CHAUCHARD 1929, ANREP 1922, HOLZLÖHNER and HOFFMANN 1931.
[3] EMMELIN and MUREN 1951a, 1951b.   [4] MACINTOSH 1937.
[5] FLEMING and MACINTOSH 1935.

9. Electric stimulation.

Electric stimulation of the autonomic nerves to the salivary glands causes characteristic changes in the electrical potentials[1] that may be observed by placing electrodes in various positions on or within the gland and connecting them to a suitable recording device. With one electrode on the hilus and another on the outer surface of the submaxillary gland stimulation of either the sympathetic or parasympathetic nerves causes the hilus of the gland to become electropositive to the outer surface after a comparatively long latent period. The latent period is 0.2 to 0.3 second with the parasympathetic and somewhat longer when the sympathetic is stimulated. Following parasympathetic stimulation the hilus positivity rapidly declines and may change to a negative potential; there is another sharp rise in hilus positivity when the current is turned off. The potential caused by sympathetic stimulation is more consistently hilus-positive.

Since this gland is composed of several different types of cells, each of which may have its own electrical characteristics, it is doubtful what significance should be ascribed to the external secretory potential. More precise information may be obtained from the use of a microelectrode with the tip placed in the interior of a single cell. With this Lundberg (1957) has obtained three types of response representing, presumably, three types of cells: alveolar cells, demilune cells, and duct cells. In all cases the interior of the cell was electronegative to the external medium. In the case of the alveolar cells, stimulation of either the parasympathetic or sympathetic caused a sustained increase in internal negativity or "hyperpolarization" of the cell membrane. This followed a time course roughly parallel to that already described for the external secretory potential. When the microelectrode was in what was believed to be a demilune cell the parasympathetic caused hyperpolarization but the sympathetic caused a decrease in the internal negativity of the cell (apparent depolarization). With the electrode in what was thought to be a cell of the striated ducts both sympathetic and parasympathetic nerves caused apparent depolarization.

In the sublingual gland microelectrodes picked up currents corresponding to those obtained from alveolar cells of the submaxillary but the external secretory potential was of a polarity opposite to that of the submaxillary gland, that is, the hilus became electro-negative. This difference was believed to be due to differences in the cellular composition of the two glands and not to any difference in the electrical response of corresponding individual cells.

These electrical phenomena are remarkable in several respects. They are evidently not analagous to the familiar action potentials of nerve and muscle. They appear not to be concerned with the excitatory process, which must be quite different in gland cells than in muscle cells for example, but with the functional work of the cell. Lundberg has presented good evidence that the hyperpolarization associated with secretory activity is caused by an active transport of chloride ions through the outer cell membrane which is triggered by the release of neurohormone at the autonomic nerve endings. The apparent depolarization, when it occurs, is not a self propagating disturbance of the cell membrane of the sort we are accustomed to associate with depolarization but is probably due to the sustained activity of an ion transport mechanism opposite to that causing hyperpolarization.

As a corollary to these observations, Lundberg (1958) has suggested that secretion of water and salt by the alveolar cells is accomplished through the activity of an active chloride ion transport mechanism in the outer cell membrane

---

[1] Lundberg 1958.

which pumps chloride ions into the cell from the surrounding interstitial fluid. Electrical forces cause sodium to accompany chloride and osmotic forces take in water. As a result of the increased hydrostatic pressure within the cell the salt and water escape through the inner membrane (where there may also be an ion pump) into the lumen of the alveolus. He has suggested further that the rodded epithelial cells of the ducts actively absorb sodium from the secretion. Sodium absorption at this point would account for the apparent depolarization of these cells (decreased internal negativity) and also for the fact that saliva may be hypotonic with respect to the blood.

10. Esophageal secretion.

Two types of secretory glands are found in the esophagus: esophageal glands occurring throughout the whole esophagus and cardiac glands extending from the cardia of the stomach into the lower part of the esophagus. The secretory nerve for these glands is the vagus[1]. On stimulation of the vagus with a strong faradic current an alkaline (p_H 7.5 to 8.3) viscous material is secreted but as stimulation is continued the secretion, particularly from the glands in the lower esophagus, gradually becomes less viscid. The serous secretion is also alkaline and neither the mucous or serous secretions exhibit enzymatic activities. Reflex esophageal secretion from stimulating the mouth with food, particularly tasty food, can be elicited. The main function of the esophageal secretion is lubrication of the food while in transit from the mouth to the stomach.

11. Gastric secretion.
Formation and secretion of acid.

The hydrochloric acid would appear to be elaborated at the membrane surface of the intracellular canaliculus of the parietal cell. The acidity of the parietal secretion, often referred to as the "primary acidity", is usually accepted as being of constant unvarying concentration, only slightly hypertonic to blood[2]. It is postulated that the all-or-none law applies to the secretory activity of the parietal cell and that variations in the observed rates of secretion of juice are due to differences in the number of cells participating in secretion.

The probable source of the hydrogen and chloride ions which are secreted are the water and chlorides of the plasma and lymph but the mechanism of acid formation is still a matter of uncertainty. The chief differences between the major theories concern the manner in which hydrogen ion, chloride ion, and water are transferred from parietal cell into the gastric tubule[3]. Most recent workers subscribe to the view that the immediate step leading to the production of hydrogen ion is an oxidation-reduction reaction[4,5,6]. The electrical potential differences existing across the mucosa are believed by some investigators[4,5] to regulate the oxidation-reduction reaction and hence acid secretion. Attempts to relate hydrogen ion formation to oxygen consumption[5,7] in isolated stomachs have not provided a critical test of the oxidation-reduction hypothesis. More recently it has been demonstrated that in addition to active transport of the hydrogen ion

---

[1] Vineberg and Komarov 1933.

[2] Babkin 1950 and Heinz and Öbrink 1954 and James 1957, present extensive reviews of the literature.

[3] Hollander 1943.

[4] Rehm 1950, Rehm, Hokin, de Graffenried, Bajandas and Coy jr. 1951, Crane, Davies and Longmuir 1948.

[5] Davies and Ogston 1950.   [6] Conway 1953.   [7] Davenport 1957.

there is also active transport of the chloride ion. It is this active transport of chloride which is the source of the distinctive electrical potential[1, 2]. As yet we have still much to learn about the forces determining water movement in gastric secretion. One hypothesis suggests that water is pumped into the canaliculus and that the water in turn pulls chloride and hydrogen with it[3], but another hypothesis suggests the opposite; namely that water movement through the parietal cell is passive and secondary to solute secretion[4].

The process of acid production involves an unusually large share of all the metabolic resources of the parietal cell. Thus it is not surprising that many metabolic poisons are able to block acid secretion. To date drugs and other agents which interfere with the special metabolism of the cell must usually be given in concentrations which affect basal cell metabolism as well and hence are toxic.

The secretory activity of the parietal cell may be maintained at high levels and without fatigue if an adequate supply of water and chloride is assured[5]. In the dog under adequate stimulation the secretory rate may reach 0.08 ml. of 0.16 N HCl per minute per square centimeter of mucosa[6]. On the basis of the dry weight of the whole mucosa, the human stomach has been calculated to secrete at rates as high as 100 ml per milligram per hour[7]. This makes the parietal cell one of the most active cells in the body and activity can be maintained only at a high rate of blood flow. The production of 1 ml. of gastric juice has been calculated to involve an anverage flow of 50 ml. of blood[8]. In a patient with gastric hypersecretion, this would mean that the daily supply of blood to the stomach would be in excess of twenty-five times his total blood volume.

The vascular system of the gastric mucosa is peculiarly constructed to supply these prodigious volumes of blood. A vast mucosal capillary network with many freely inter-anastomatic connections, absence of end arteries, and numerous arterio-venous shunts of large caliber are ideal for supplying tremendous volumes of blood during secretory activity[9]. Attempts to reduce gastric secretion permanently by devascularization of the stomach to an extent just short of development of necrosis have been ineffective[10], no doubt due to establishment of an adequate collateral circulation within a few weeks.

Because of its extreme diffusibility, urea may be found in the gastrointestinal tract in the same concentration as in the blood plasma[11]. By the action of urease the urea of the stomach is the source of most of the ammonium ion of the gastric juice. The possibility that the hydrogen ions of the hydrochloric acid are derived from ammoium ions[12] has been dismissed by a mass of contrary evidence. More recently it has been suggested that protection of the gastric cells from acid-pepsin action by intramucosal neutralization with ammonia may be a major function of gastric urease. A similar view holds that development of "tissue acidoses" through failure in this homeostatic mechanism may be a contributory factor in gastritis. These views all fail, however, when it is pointed out that normal frogs, rats, cats, and pigs may secrete acid without evidence of any gastric urease and, furthermore, that gastric urease according to recent investigations is actually bacterial origin.

[1] Rehm 1950, Rehm, Hokin, de Graffenried, Bajandas and Coy jr. 1951, Crane, Davies and Longmuir 1948.
[2] Hogben 1952, 1955.   [3] Hollander 1943, 1949.   [4] Teorell 1939, Öbrink 1956.
[5] Friedman 1939.   [6] Friedman 1955.   [7] Davies 1948.   [8] Crane and Davies 1951.
[9] Barlow 1953.
[10] Babkin, Armour and Webster 1943, Layne and Bergh 1943, Somerville 1945, Wood 1949.
[11] Hessel 1933, v. Korff and Glick 1951, Linderstrom-Lang and Ohlsen 1936.
[12] Mathews 1920.

Secretion of mucus, pepsin and lipase.

Two types of mucus have been identified in gastric juices; one of which is believed to be secreted by the surface epithelial cells and the other by the neck chief cells[1]. While both appear to be secreted spontaneously and continuously, their rates of secretion may be greatly increased by local mechanical and chemical irritants and by reflexes. In the corpus and fundus, the secretion from the neck chief cells and surface epithelium is more profuse on parasympathetic stimulation while in the pyloric area, the mucus secretion is more profuse on sympathetic stimulation[2]. Undoubtedly, during strong motor activities of the gastric musculature there is also expression into the lumen of mucus from the mucosal folds[3].

The formation and extrusion of pepsinogen granules by the chief cells appear to be continuous processes. The energy requirements for these processes have not been determined. When the zymogen secretion rate exceeds the restitution as it does on prolonged vagus stimulation, the chief cells show reduction in numbers of granules and show vacuolization[4]. Under such conditions the juice consists of acid with only low peptic activity. Whether the chemically identical enzyme is secreted by all species of vertebrates is unknown since the result of immunologic studies are inconclusive. It is of interest to note that only in the mammalian species has the pepsin been identified as emanating from a distinct specialized cellular unit, the chief cell. In all other vertebrates the gland body consists of only a single kind of cell[5] so that the pepsin must be secreted also by either this cell or else by cells of the surface epithelium.

The near identity of the structure of gastric juice pepsin and one of the gastric mucins has recently been proposed as suggestive evidence for a common secretory apparatus. This gastric mucin has been identified tentatively as coming from the neck cells which, in the organogenesis of the stomach, serve as the source of the peptic chief cells. (In this connection it is interesting to note that measurements of roentgen ray absorptions show the mucous- and enzyme-secreting cells to have similar masses, and much greater than mass of the parietal cell[6].) On the other hand, the parietal cells do not have any visible precursors but arise *de novo*. It is interesting to note that even in the achlorhydric juice of pernicious anemia patients there is usually found appreciable amounts of pepsin and mucus.

Pepsin secretion may be augmented above the basal rate by appropriate stimuli, the most important of which are reflexes from higher centers (i.e., condition reflexes) and from the gastrointestinal tract. Evidently the chief cells are capable of liberating pepsinogen into the blood stream directly: the finding that blood peptic activity parallels gastric pepsin secretion[7] supports this view. A substance with optimum proteolytic activity at p_H 2.0—3.4 is found in alkaline or slightly acid urine and probably represents excreted pepsinogen[8] and hence has been designated uropepsin. The determination of uropepsin as a reflection of gastric gland activities offers interesting possibilities as a function test[9].

A lipolytic enzyme with optimun activity on substrates of lower triglycerides at p_H 5.5 and higher triglycerides at p_H 7.5 is known to be present in gastric juice but its role in digestion is uncertain. Gastric lipase has been demonstrated histochemically to be present in the gastric mucous membrane so that it does not represent regurgitated pancreatic lipase which it resembles closely. Apparently

[1] Babkin 1950.   [2] Baxter 1939.   [3] Oushakov 1896, Hollander and Stein 1943.
[4] Bowie and Vineberg 1935.   [5] Biedermann 1911.
[6] Engström and Glick 1950.   [7] Spiro, Ryan and Jones 1955.
[8] Bucher 1947, Brucke 1861, Grutzner 1891.
[9] Mirsky, Kaplan and Broh-Kahn 1950.

there is no basis for the belief that gastric lipase plays an important role in fat digestion in the infant.

Rennin, the enzyme acting to clot milk, is also found in gastric juice, particularly in infants. Since acid and pepsin also clot milk a specific role for rennin in digestion is not certain.

Phases of gastric secretion.

The course of gastric secretion in response to a meal may be described as occurring in three overlapping phases which are designated according to the nature or the site of action of the secretory stimulus. These are the initial reflex phase, the gastric phase, and the intestinal phase. The sequence, magnitude, and duration of the phases are shown in Figure 6 which is a composite of data obtained from animal experiments and from humans subjected to various surgical procedures.

The term initial reflex phase denotes the initial response of the gastric glands to food; it involves unconditioned and conditioned reflexes and is abolished by bilateral vagotomy. The unconditioned or inborn reflex secretion is elicited by stimulation

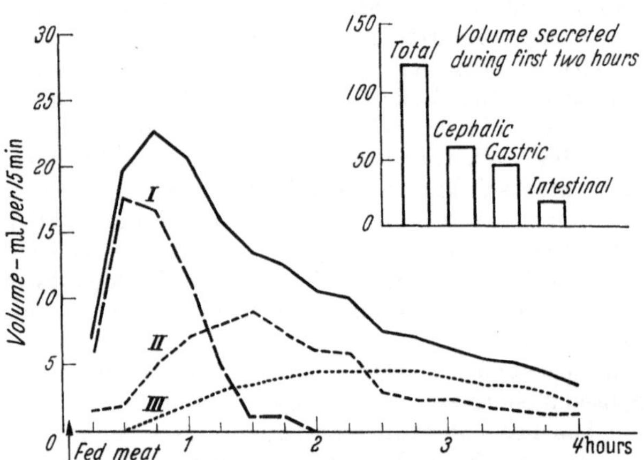

Fig. 6. Reconstructed curves to show the approximate distribution between the several phases of the gastric secretion in a dog after a meal of 300 gm. of meat. *I* Cephalic or initial reflex phase. *II* Gastric or pyloric phase. *III* Intestinal phase.

of gustatory receptors and perhaps also by swallowing movements. Conditioned or acquired reflex secretion of what has been appropriately called "appetite juice"[1] is provoked by the odor, sight, or thought of food or the sound of food being prepared. This phase of secretion has been called also the psychic, cephalic or nervous phase[2] but its nature is best decribed by "initial reflex phase"[3].

The initial reflex gastric secretion usually starts within three minutes after eating commences. In a dog with an esophageal fistula the feeding of ground raw meat for a period of only five minutes elicites a secretion which continues for one and one-half hours or longer[4] (Fig. 6). A state of central excitation is apparently set up which lasts for at least this length of time. The nature of central excitation of the vagal nuclei is not known but suggested explanations based on alteration in concentration of (or permeability to) choline esterase of central nervous tissue[5] and the participation of neural reverberating circuits have been offered.

It is believed that the more complex nervous development of man explains why the greater proportion of the gastric secretory response in man is neurogenic. In addition, because man chews his food, stimulation of the tast and olfactory receptors is prolonged and hence reflex secretion of gastric juice occurs over a greater length of time. Indeed it may be that in man a major faction of chewing is the reflex initiation of secretion of an acid gastric juice of high peptic activity.

[1] PAVLOV 1910.   [2] PAVLOV 1910, 1927, IVY 1925,   [3] BABKIN 1950.
[4] THOMAS and FRIEDMAN 1950.   [5] FRIEDMAN 1954, FRIEDMAN, APPERT and BEAMER 1955.

Absence of an initial reflex phase of gastric secretion has been reported in ruminants such as the sheep and goat[1]. Acid secretion also is said not to be provoked in these species by insulin hypoglycemia[2]. Gastric acid secretion is continuous and possibly the only nervous control in these species is one of inhibition via sympathetic vaso regulatory fibers.

The gastric phase of gastric secretion results from mechanical distension[3] and secretogogues present in or derived from food[4]. The site of action of both the mechanical and chemical stimuli is the pyloric antrum and for this reason this phase of secretion is often referred to as the pyloric phase. The gastric phase commences soon after food is eaten and therefore there is temporal overlapping with the preceding initial reflex phase. Furthermore, evacuation of the stomach, as described earlier, begins after gastric digestion has been in progress for only a short time, so that the gastric phase overlaps also succeeding intestinal phase (see below, and Figure 6). Since the gastric phase is produced by contact of the food with the pyloric antrum, it may be expected to be of greater magnitude and duration the longer the meal remains in the stomach, as when the meal is of large size or of a consistency which delays evacuation[5].

It is highly probable that two distinct hormones of gastric origin participate in the gastric phase of gastric secretion. These hormones are dealt with separately below but may here be identified as gastrin[6] which excites the parietal cell, and gastrozymin[7], which excites the chief cell. (The reader will readily note later the similarity between the activities of gastrin and gastrozymin on the stomach and secretin and pancreozymin on the pancreas.) For this reason the secretion of the gastric phase, resulting from pyloric antrum stimulation, always shows a greater peptic activity than does that due to administration of gastrin.

The intestinal phase of gastric secretion is associated with the presence of food in the intestine. This would appear to be due in part to direct excitation of the gastric glands by the absorbed food digestion products and in part by central vagus stimulation[8]. While certain amino acids do indeed have a gastric secretogogue action when given intravenously[9], the required blood threshold levels are for greater than intra-intestinal threshold levels for the same effect[10]. These findings, together with the observation that distension of the intestine may provoke gastric secretion in a manner similar to distension of the antrum[11], suggests the intervention of an intestinal "gastrin". In support of this concept is the demonstration that gastrin-like activity is exhibited by certain intestinal mucosa extrects. Since the secretion during the intestinal phase shows peptic activity it is possible that a gastrozymin-like hormone participates in this phase.

Variations in gastric secretory activity.

The parietal cell becomes distinguishable in the human fetal stomach by the end of the fourth month so that the stomach is potentially able to secrete acid at birth. Studies on premature as well as normal fullterm unfed newborn infants have revealed that acid of relatively high concentration is present even before the first meal is taken[12]. The gastric glands at birth respond well to histamine[13] and gastrin[14] and a cephalic or initial reflex phase becomes soon established.

[1] Popov 1932, Espe and Cannon 1937.　　[2] Hill 1952.　　[3] Savitch and Zeliony 1913.
[4] Babkin 1927, Cowgill and Smith 1933.　　[5] Friedman and Pincus 1945.
[6] Keeton, Koch and Luckhardt 1920, Komarov 1942, Friedman and King 1947.
[7] Harper and Raper 1943.　　[8] Babkin 1934.
[9] Okada et al. 1930, LaBarre and Destrée 1935.　　[10] Ivy and Javois 1924/25.
[11] Beamer, Friedman, Thomas and Rehfuss 1944.
[12] Pollitzer 1921, Hess 1913, Griswold and Shohl 1941, Taylor 1917.
[13] Cutter 1938, Ritter 1941.　　[14] Sutherland 1921.

The acidity of the gastric contents appears to be highest shortly after birth. The acidity of both histamine and food-stimulated secretions falls progressively during the first week and rises again only after the 10th day[1]. Whether this is due to exhaustion of a stored secretory stimulant (e.g. gastrin) acquired from the mother[2], or to the dehydration which is so general in this period of life, is purely speculative.

It has been generally accepted that gastric hypersecretion characterizes the patient with duodenal ulcer. Tests made by a single aspiration of the stomach, or by a series of intermittant aspirations, show that more gastric juice may be recovered from the duodenal ulcer patient than from the non-ulcer subject[3]. This, however, often reflects retention of gastric contents in the ulcer patient (due to gastric atony, pyloric stenosis, etc.). A more accurate picture is revealed when the gastric contents are aspirated continuously over a period of time, obviating the effect of alterations in gastric evacuation through the pylorus[4].

While the interdigestive gastric secretion may be found in the ulcer patient to be in excess of that in the non-ulcer subject, it is usual to find the gastric secretion in response to food to be unaltered. One explanation may be that the continuous interdigestive secretion in the healthy person is minimal but in the ulcer patient, due to processes as yet ill understood, it is submaximal. Upon the gastric glands being maximally stimulated, as by a meal of adequate composition and amount, the secretion in both the ulcer and non-ulcer subjects is maximal, and hence the total output of acid is the same in both. This explanation is supported by the findings of several groups of investigators that no statistically significant differences in either volume or acid output of continuously aspirated gastric secretion existed between duodenal ulcer and normal subjects for a period of about 8 to 10 hours following a meal[5].

The foregoing, of course, does not exclude hypersecretion in duodenal ulcer patients with gastric hyperplasia. While such conditions have not been demonstrated to be common[6], they must, however, be considered and may well explain the different nocturnal secretory curves found by numerous investigators in ulcer patients[7]. Experimental gastric hyperplasia has been produced in guinea pigs by constant stimulation of the gastric glands with histamine[8] but similar experiments on cats and dogs have given negative results[9].

A discussion of the variations in secretory activity of the gastric glands would not be complete without some reference to species differences. Data obtained in animal experiments should be applied to man only with caution. In man there is a continuous "basal" or "interdigestive" secretion of acid. We do not, however, know whether this secretion is truly spontaneous or the result of indiscernible stimuli[10] (e.g., conditioned reflexes, minor infections, etc.). In some species, such as the marmot[11] and rat[12], acid secretion is continuous. This apparently spontaneous process appears to be an innate property of the parietal cell and may be augmented by appropriate stimuli. In other species, notably the cat[13] and dog[14], acid secretion is intermittent and occurs only in response to a specific stimulus.

---

[1] Miller 1941.   [2] Friedman 1942.

[3] Ihre 1938, Bloomfield, Chen and French 1940, Sandweiss et al. 1946b, Atkinson and Henley 1955.

[4] Sandweiss et al. 1946a, 1946b, Friedman et al. 1956, Olson and Bridgwater 1954, Brown et al. 1952. Kirsner et al. 1948.

[5] Sandweiss et al. 1946a, Friedman at el. 1956, Olson and Bridgwater 1954, Brown et al. 1952.

[6] Cox, A. J. 1945.

[7] Henning and Norpoth 1933, Winkelstein 1935, Val dez 1942, Levin et al. 1952.

[8] Cox, A. J., jr., and V. R. Barnes, 1945.   [9] Friedman and Hoffard 1952.

[10] Babkin 1932.   [11] Friedman and Armour 1936.   [12] Friedman 1943.

[13] Friedman 1950.   [14] Pavlov 1910.

The gastrin mechanism. The gastric phase is due principally to the hormone gastrin which is elaborated by the mucosa of the antrum and acts to stimulate the parietal cells selectively. EDKINS (1906) postulated the existence of a "gastric secretin" (now called gastrin) analogous to the pancreatic secretin discovered several years earlier by BAYLISS and STARLING (1902) but for many years the identity of this hormonal agent was in doubt. The presence of the powerful gastric stimulant, histamine, in extracts of stomach tissue led many investigators[1] to the view that "gastrin" was probably only histamine. This view was shown to be erroneous when in recent years several investigators[2] showed independently that a histaminefree gastrin could indeed be prepared from the mucous membrane of the pyloric antrum.

While there are numerous experiments which indicate that the gastric phase is nearly wholly hormonal in origin, evidence has been presented to suggest that the elaboration or release of the hormone, gastrin, from the pyloric antrum in response to stimuli acting locally involves reflexes over a local nervous network in the antrum. Neither mechanical stimulation of the antrum nor irrigation of the antrum with chemical secretagogues evokes the secretion of acid if the antral mucosa has been painted with coceine or atropine[3]. Acid secretion on antral stimulation is still obtained however if only the fundic glands are painted with procaine[4]. The gastrinforming cells apparenly are activated through stimulation of special receptors in the antral epithelium: gastrin is not released into the circulation when the receptor cells cannot be excited as when the mucosa is anesthetized. This is consistent with the view that excitation of the pyloric glands involves an adeno-enteric reflex[5].

The secretory response to vagal stimulation is decreased if the pyloric antrum has been removed[6]. Fibers from the vagus innervate the parietal cell and acid secretion results from vagus nerve stimulation. In addition, the nerve plexus innervating the gastrin-forming cells of the antrum is also in synaptic connection with vagal fibers. Gastrin release conceivably occurs not only when the antrum is stimulated but also when vagus is stimulated. In other words, the effects of vagus stimulation on acid secretion are two-fold: first, direct action on the parietal cell and second, indirect action through the intervention of gastrin. The total effect of vagus nerve stimulation would therefore be reduced if the pyloric region were removed or if its main blood supply were obstructed. If however, the vagus stimulation were intense, as it can be in insulin-induced hypoglycemia, the direct response of the parietal cells may be maximal and therefore mask the effects of antrumectomy.

The mode of action of gastrin on the parietal cell is not known but similarities in action to histamine suggest some relationship. The possibility must be entertained that gastrin acts through the intervention of locally liberated histamine.

Effects of nerve stimulation.

Although in the lower vertebrates (e.g., elasmobranch fishes[7] and tailed amphibia[8]) the gastric musculature is well innervated, the gastric glands do not respond to stimulation of either the vagus or sympathetic nerves[9]. The gastric

---

[1] KEETON, KOCH and LUCKHARDT 1920, SACKS, IVY, BURGESS and VANDOLAH 1932.
[2] KOMAROV, 1938, 1942, UVNÄS 1945, HARPER 1946, FRIEDMAN and KING 1947.
[3] ZELJONY and SAVITCH 1911/12, GREGORY and IVY 1941, WOODWARD, LYON, LANDOR and DRAGSTEDT 1954.
[4] GREGORY and IVY 1941.   [5] LIM and MOZER 1950.
[6] UVNÄS 1942, WOODWARD, LYON, LANDOR and DRAGSTEDT 1954.
[7] BABKIN, FRIEDMAN and MacKAY-SAWYER 1935/36.   [8] FRIEDMAN 1942.
[9] BABKIN, CHAISSON and FRIEDMAN 1935/36.

secretory response to nerve stimulation is also weak in certain reptiles but becomes well established in most birds[1] and mammals. The result of electrical stimulation of the vagus nerve, directly in the dog and indirectly (as in shock therapy[2]) in man, show it to be the secretory nerve to the gastric glands. A weak current yields a secretion of mucus only while a strong current yields a flow of acid and pepsin as well[3]. Pavlov (1910) assumed the presence of inhibitory fibers to the gastric gland but this view has not received support from recent investigations. Histophysiological studies reveal that during stimulation of the vagus nerve with a current of appropriate strength there is a discharge of pepsinogen granules from the chief cells corresponding in extent to the peptic activity of the secreted juice[4]. The surface epithelial cells discharge similarly their mucous precursor substance following administration of acetylcholine[5].

Besides secretory fibers to the gastric glands, there are in the vagus nerve also dilator fibers to the gastric arterioles so that their synchronous action results in increased blood flow during active secretion. In addition, metabolic products of glandular activity probably also serve as local vasodilator stimuli.

The mucous-secreting cells of the pyloric antrum are said to be under control of the sympathetic nervous system[6]. Current evidence does not support the view that in the cat, dog, or man there are any sympathetic secretory fibers to the acid- and pepsin-secreting cells but critical experiments to elucidate this are rather scanty. Sympathetic vasoconstrictor fibers supply the gastric arterioles and their excitation may bring about reduction in gastric secretion as a consequence of reduction in blood flow. The inhibitory effects of adrenaline are similarly explained. The presence in either the vagus or sympathetic of inhibitory secretory fibers, in the sense of acting in an "antisecretory" capacity on the parietal or chief cells, has never been demonstrated.

Direct electrical excitation of certain circumscribed areas in the brain of the dog and cat has provoked gastric secretion[7] but this alone does not identify a particular "gastric secretion" center. The influence of central excitation on acid and pepsin secretion has been further studied in animals and man indirectly by the use of insulin. Hypoglycemia induced by insulin results in excitation of the whole central nervous system, including the hypothalamus which is generally regarded as the integrating center of the autonomic nervous system. In the cat[8], dog[5] and man[4] insulin hypoglycemia, through its action on the autonomic centers, is a potent vagus stimulus, resulting in the secretion of an enzyme-rich acid gastric juice. This effect is abolished by vagotomy[9], and constitutes the basis of a clinical test for the integrity of continuity of the vagus nerves supplying the gastric glands[10].

Since insulin hypoglycemia excites the whole nervous system, a secretory effect on the gastric glands will be obvious only where parasympathetic stimulation predominates as in the dog and man. In ruminant herbinova such as the sheep and goat, however, no gastric secretion is obtained following insulin because of the predominance of central sympathetic stimulation[11].

Effects of histamine.

Histamine provokes the secretion of an acid juice which, after an initial "washing out" of the crypts, is practically free of pepsin and mucus. Indeed, not only

---

[1] Friedman 1939.   [2] Fetter 1944.   [3] Vineberg 1931.
[4] Bowie and Vineberg 1935.   [5] Morton and Stavraky 1948.   [6] Baxter 1934a, 1934b.
[7] Beattie, Brow and Long 1930, Beattie 1932, Davey and Kaoda 1950.
[8] Friedman 1950.   [9] La Barre and Cespédès 1931, Babkin 1939.
[10] Hollander 1946.   [11] Hill 1952.

does histamine appear to stimulate the parietal cell selectively, but under certain conditions may actually depress the secretion of pepsin[1] and mucus[2].

The role of histamine in normal gastric secretion is obscure. BABKIN[3] proposed the hypothesis that histamine participates in all phases of gastric secretion, including those which are predominantly nervous in origin. He believed that acetylcholine liberated from the cholinergic fibers on vagus stimulation affected the parietal cell by first causing the liberation of histamine locally. On the other hand, the effect of vagus stimulation on mucus and pepsin secretion was due to the action of acetylcholine directly on the cells. Under certain conditions only the vagal fibers supplying the parietal cells appear to be excited selectively since in such experiments vagus stimulation yields a gastric secretion identical in composition to that due to histamine[4].

That a relationship between histamine and vagal activity exists, is the conclusion from experiments showing a correlation between secretory response to nervous stimuli and the presence of histamine, particularly in the gastric juice[5]. The greater increase in histamine content of the juice than of the blood noted after vagus stimulation[6] or feeding has been explained by the great permeability of the parietal cells to histamine[7], so that the formed histamine enters into the stomach lumen before it is taken up by the gastric veins. Some histamine, however, does enter into the circulation and is excreted by the kidneys accounting for the increase in the urinary histamine found to occur following gastric stimulation. Additional support for the view of the inter-dependence of vagus and histamine effects comes from studies in comparative physiology. Many species of lower vertebrates, such as the elasmobranchs and salamanders, are refractory to histamine and it is in these species that autonomic nerve stimulation does not provoke acid secretion[8]. Whether the foregoing point to histamine as the *immediate* or *final* mediator of nervous stimuli on the parietal cell is however in doubt. The secretion of acid from a stomach perfused with blood was at a low rate when histamine was introduced directly into the perfusion system[9] and apparently depended on some interaction between the histamine and the blood[10].

Neither histaminase, a diamine oxidase which inactivates histamine, nor the synthetic antihistaminics have a depressant effect on gastric secretion excited by histamine or food. Failure of the antihistaminic compounds to inhibit secretion when given parenterally may be due to non-penetration to the receptor elements of the parietal cell[11]. The results of clinical trials have shown that antihistaminics actually augment rather than inhibit gastric secretion[12]. Probably this is due on one hand to the fact that most antihistaminics are themselves potent histamine release agents and on the other hand to the increased blood flow to the glands brought about by the anti-edemic effect of these agents.

Regulatory mechanism of acid secretion.

The levels of acidity in the digestive tract are regulated by (1) dilution or partial neutralization of the acid secreted by the parietal cells and (2) inhibition of the activity of the acid secretory mechanism. These processes normally occur in an integrated manner to maintain gastroenteric homeostasis and prevent damage to the integrity of the intestinal mucosa by unduly high acidities. Per-

---

[1] ALLEY 1935.   [2] GROSSBERG et al. 1950.   [3] BABKIN, B. P. 1950.
[4] SCHACTER 1949, BALLEM, NOBLE and WEBSTER 1948.
[5] EMMELIN and KAHLSON 1944, CODE et al. 1947.   [6] MacINTOSH 1938.
[7] KAHLSON 1948.   [8] BABKIN, CHAISSON and FRIEDMAN 1935/36, FRIEDMAN 1942.
[9] FRIEDMAN and APPERT 1956.   [10] BORN and VANE 1953.   [11] LINDE 1950.
[12] ASHFORD 1949, LINDE 1950.

haps it is when these fail that the patient is forced to have recourse to the use of antacids and anti-secretory drugs.

The concentration of acid of the gastric juice which is withdrawn from the lumen of the stomach is almost alsways less than the primary acidity and usually is referred to as the "secondary acidity". Of the intragastric mechanisms operating to reduce the acidity below that of the primary acidity, the "two component" system and the "back-diffusion" system are the most important. In the former it is believed that the acid of the parietal secretion is diluted and neutralized partially by mucus and other non-parietal secretions, such as those of the neck chief cells[1]. Alternative, or parhaps supplemental, is the process involving diffusion of the secreted hydrogen ion back through the mucosa into the blood plasma in exchange for sodium ion diffusion from the blood into the gastric lumen[2].

Further reduction of the acidity of the gastric contents is brought about by dilution and neutralization with fluids of extragastric origin. Regurgitation of intestinal, pancreatic, and biliary secretions into the stomach occurs frequently. The free acidity is also appreciably reduced by the acid-binding capacity of the mucus of swallowed salivary and esophageal secretions.

In addition to mechanisms which reduce the *acidity*, there are mechanisms which effectively reduce the *rate* of the parietal cell secretion. These latter appear to be adjusted to the level of acidity in the pyloric antrum[3] and intestine[4], and come into play when local acid concentrations reach values that may be interpreted as possibly deleterious. The *antral* acidity is said to regulate acid secretion due to the pyloric phases[5] and not that which is purely nervous in origin[6] (i.e., the initial reflex phase). The inhibitory effect of the acid in contact with the antrum may be due to direct interference with formation or release of gastrin[7]. The *intestinal* acidity appears most effective in regulating gastric secretion of nervous origin. Gastric secretion elicited by food or insulin hypoglycemia is found to be markedly inhibited when the intestinal p_H is as low as 2.5[8] but histamine-stimulated secretion is not affected[9]. The threshold level of intestinal p_H necessary for the onset of secretory inhibition has not been determined but it should be noted that to inhibit gastric tonus and motility an intestinal p_H of 3.0 or lower is required[10].

Normally the acidity of the duodenal contents of either dog or man is rarely as low as p_H 3.0[11] even though the acidity of the antral contents is as low as p_H 1.2[12]. In great part this is due to the secretin mechanism. As soon as the duodenal p_H drops below 4.0 there is elicited a secretion of alkaline pancreatic juice which prevents effectively a further drop in intestinal p_H[13]. Apparently the intestinal mechanism for controlling gastric secretion is for emergency use, to be set in operation to reduce acid secretion when there is failure to reduce adequately the acid concentration. It would be interesting to determine whether dysfunction of the regulatory mechanisms discussed above may account for the gastric hypersecretion exhibited by patients with active duodenal ulcer.

---

[1] Pavlov 1910, Babkin 1931, 1931 b, Hollander 1952.
[2] Teorell 1935, 1939, Öbrink 1948, Friedman 1951, 1952.
[3] Sokolov 1904, Pavlov 1910, Farrell 1928, Goldberg 1932.
[4] Day and Webster 1935, Griffiths 1936, Pincus, Thomas and Rehfuss 1942, Shay et al. 1942.
[5] Dragstedt, Oberhelman, Zubiran and Woodward 1953.
[6] Wilhelmj, McCarthy and Hill 1937.   [7] Woodward et al. 1954.
[8] Pincus, Thomas and Rehfuss 1942.   [9] Pincus, Friedman, Thomas and Rehfuss 1944.
[10] Thomas and Crider 1940.   [11] Thomas and Crider 1936.
[12] Thomas and Crider 1937.   [13] Thomas and Crider 1940.

In addition to acid, certain foodstuffs, especially neutral fats, acting in the intestine also depress gastric secretion. EWALD and BOAS in 1886 reported that inclusion of fat in a meal inhibited gastric secretion and this was amply verified by several workers in PAVLOV'S laboratory (see BABKIN 1928). It soon became evident that the site of action of the fat is the small intestine and not the stomach. The inhibition of acid secretion following administration of neutral fat in the intestine is in duration proportional to the quantity of fat used, and is usually followed by a subsequent phase of rebound secretion.

The inhibitory action of the fat is due to the formation and/or liberation of enterogastrone[1] from the intestinal mucosa and possibly also to inhibitory enterogastric reflexes. The neutral fat in the intestine soon undergoes digestion (particularly pertinant is the fact that soap in the intestine is a potent stimulus to pancreatic secretion and gall bladder evacuation) and, because of the lowered intragastric pressure at this time[2], is regurgitated into the stomach. The products of fat digestion acting in the pyloric antrum[3] probably ecite the formation of gastrin giving rise to the secondary augmented or rebound phase of gastric secretion[4].

Concentrated solutions of sugars when ingested or introduced directly into the small intestine also depress gastric secretion[5] but in most experiments the effects of the high osmotic activity of the solution have been overlooked. Small bowel irritation by hypertonic salt solutions or by condiments may depress gastric secretion, usually after an initial excitatory phase.

One important difference between the effects of lipids, concentrated sugar solutions, and acids applied to the intestine and the effects of intravenous administration of "enterogastrone" concentrates must be noted. Whereas such concentrates inhibit gastric secretion provoked by a variety of stimuli, including histamine[6], acids, carbohydrates and fats in the intestine depress gastric secretion due to food, shamfeeding, and insulin hypoglycemia but not that due to histamine[7].

Influence of endocrines and vitamins.

The role of the endocrine glands on gastrointestinal functions, based on data obtained from the use of various gland preparations, needs restudy. Investigators have not always appreciated that a "potent" gland extract may be heavily contaminated with other fractions of high pharmacologic activity. For example, the gastric secretory depressant action attributed to urinary chorionic gonadotropin[8] was eventually found to be due mainly to urogastrone[9]* present as a contaminant. Furthermore the results obtained from administration of a particular "hormone" are not always those which one would expect from the effects of ablation of the test gland or its excitation in situ. Thus, while gastric secretion is heightened during normal lactation[10], the administration of an anterior pituitary extract with marked lactogenic activity has been found to be without effect on the gastrointestinal cytology[11] or gastric secretion[12].

Hypophysectomy in the experimental animals is followed by a number of atrophic changes in structure of the digestive glands. In the pigeon[13], cat[14] and

---

* A gastric secretory depressant resembling enterogastrone, found in urine.

[1] FENG, HOU and LIM 1929, LIM 1933. WALAWSKI 1928, KOSAKA et al. 1932, LIM, LING and LIU 1934.   [2] THOMAS and MOGAN 1931.   [3] SOKOLOV 1904.
[4] KOMAROV and KOMAROV 1940, THOMAS and FRIEDMAN 1950.
[5] MILLER, BERGEIM, REHFUSS and HAWK 1920, FRIEDMAN 1939.
[6] GRAY, BRADLEY and IVY 1937
[7] DAY and KOMAROV 1939, SHAY, GERSHON-COHEN and FELS 1939.
[8] FRIEDMAN et al. 1939, GRAY et al. 1939.   [9] SANDWEISS 1945, FRIEDMAN 1951.
[10] KLEIN 1933.   [11] FRIEDMAN and PODOLSKY 1942.
[12] McCARTHY et al. 1955.   [13] SCHOOLEY, RIDDLE and BATES 1941.
[14] AHLSTROM, HAEGER, JACOBSOHN and KAHLSON 1950.

rat[1] there is marked dimunition in the size of the gastrointestinal tract, particularly in the height of the intestinal villi[1, 2]. The chief cells of the stomach[3] and the acinar cells of the pancreas are definitely affected. As may be expected, these atrophic changes are reflected by depressed secretion and absorption, functions dependant on the integrity of a normal mucosa. The intestinal secretin content[4] and alkaline phosphatase activity[5], as well as the intestinal absorption of sugars[6] and electrolytes[7] are reduced following hypophysectomy. A decreased secretion of gastric juices[8], is also noted. Since adrenalectomy may result in similar atrophic changes and dysfunction[9] it is probable that the effects of hypophysectomy may be secondary to removal of adrenocorticotrophic stimuli of pituitary origin[10].

The influence of other endocrine glands on gastric secretion has not been explored thoroughly. Gonadectomy is without significant effect on the gastric cytology or secretion[11] and neither is the state of uncomplicated pregnancy[12]. During lactation, however, there is a period of gastric hypersecretion[13]. Thyroid-parathyroidectomy in the dog increases gastric secretion[14] while administration of parathormone was found by Babkin et al. (1940) to decrease both the volume and acidity. The parathormone effects appear dependent on the raised blood calcium level and may be duplicated by administration of calcium gluconate[14].

A complete achlorhydria may be developed experimentally in animals maintained on a diet deficient in the vitamin B complex[15]. Feeding yeast or vitamin B_1 (thiamin) restores normal gastric secretory function in the deficient animal but does not result in hypersecretion when administered in excess to normal animals. Deficiencies in other members of the B complex also affect gastric secretion adversely but this may be part of generalized metabolic disturbances.

Administration of vitamin D (as activated ergosteral) results in depression of gastric secretion provided that hypercalcemia develops[16]. Hypercalcemia affects secretion of nervous origin in particular, perhaps due to failure in transganglionic transmission of the nerve impulse by high calcium levels.

Attempts to control the gastric hypersecretion of ulcer patients by inducing either a vitamin B complex deficiency or a hypercalcemia with parathomone, calcium lactate or vitamin D have met with failure.

Effects of roentgen rays, hyperthermia and stress.

Exposure of the stomach to ionizing radiations beyond a certain dosage results in suppression of gastric secretion[17]. The histological changes in the gastric mucosa range from degeneration of the parietal cells only, to atrophy, metaplasia, infiltration, and complete replacement of the mucous membrane by fibrous connective tissue. Achlorhydria may be complete but usually is only temporary: in patients the effects are unpredictable. X-rays have been used for treatment of ulcer[18] since the early reports of Wilms in 1916 and Bruegel in 1917. The beneficial effects are said to be due to the ensuing achlorhydria rather than direct promotion

[1] Schooley, Riddle and Bates 1940.   [2] Friedman 1953.   [3] Baker and Abrams 1954.
[4] Dorchester and Haist 1953.   [5] Verzár 1936.   [6] Soulianoc 1954.
[7] Verzár 1931.   [8] Cutting at el. 1937, Crafts and Walker 1947.
[9] Tuerkischer and Wertheime 1945, Verzár 1931, 1936.
[10] Baker and Bridgman 1954.   [11] Abrams and Baker 1954.
[12] McCarthy, Evans and Dragstedt 1955.
[13] Klein 1933, McCarthy, Evans and Dragstedt 1955.   [14] Schiffrin 1942.
[15] Webster and Armour 1934.   [16] Babkin 1950, p 540.
[17] Regaud, Nogier and Lacassagne 1912, Miescher 1923, Portis and Ahrens 1924, Ivy, McCarthy and Orndorff 1924, Case and Boldyreff 1928, Snell and Bollman 1934, Palmer and Templeton 1939.
[18] Jenkins and MacGeorge 1940, Ricketts et al. 1948.

of proliferation and healing. Treatment is not without danger unless protection of the intestine, liver and pancreas is assured. There is now mounting interest in the possibilities of γ and β radiations from radioactive isotopes such as A^{41}, Kr^{87}, P^{32}, and I^{131}, introduced into the stomach in a thin-walled rubber balloon[1].

Depression of gastric secretion results from induction of fever by injection of bacterial pyrogens[2] and, less effectively, use of diathermy apparatus[3]. Bacterial pyrogens may inhibit secretion when raising the temperature by only 1^0 as effectively as when raising it 4^0 C. In some instances a depressant gastric secretory effect in the dog[4] and rat[5] have obtained when the bacterial pyrogen was administered in doses too small to affect body temperature. It is apparent that the explanation for the effects of hyperthermia on the gastric glands will not be available without further investigation. However, attention should be called to the fact that many agents inhibit gastric secretion when administered parenterally probably through the associated hyperpyrexia. Included in this category of non-specific secretory depressants are milk proteins and certain tissue extracts advocated for use in peptic ulcer therapy.

The factor of stress has long been recognized as playing an important role in the regulation of gastric secretion. Direct observations of the human gastric mucosa through a gastric fistula, made over a century ago by BEAUMONT (1834) and more recently be a number of other investigators[6], have shown that anxiety, fear resentment, and other emotional states have a marked influence. In experimental animals, chronic emotional states and chronic stress have been shown to affect gastric secretion[7] and to produce erosions of the gastrointestinal mucosa[8]. The particular gastric responses of the human subject to emotions such as fear or anger depend on personality factors: thus in the high anxiety individual it may be inhibited[9]. These observations do not offer direct evidence that hypersecretion induced by stress is responsible for the erosive lesions. It must be borne in mind that damage may be due to any one or more of the numerous tissue changes, including local redistribution of blood flow, which are associated with stress and the accompanying hormonal imbalances.

Influence of age and sex on gastric secretion.

The principal differences in gastric secretion between men and women and in different age groups is in the volume and acidity of the gastric juice secreted in response to various stimuli. The differences due to either age or sex are evident only in the averages since there is a wide individual variation and a great deal of overlap, both between the sexes and in different age groups. On the average, men secrete more acid than women and the incidence of achlorhydria is higher in women than in men by a factor of about 3 per cent[10]. Achlorhydria is extremely rare in males under 20 years of age. Vanzant and his associates (1932) did not find a single case of achlordhydria in a group of 111 young men ranging in age from 20 to 25 years which they studied at the Mayo Clinic. HOWEVER, BENNETT and RYLE (1921) found four cases in one hundred apparently healthy male students. VANZANT and his associates (1932) found about 3 per cent of achlorhydria in young women. In both sexes the incidence of achlorhydria increases rapidly with age,

[1] McKENDRY 1950, SIMON 1949 STEINFELD 1952, LUSHBAUGH and HOUCK 1955.
[2] MEYER, COHEN and CARLSON 1918, VANZANT and SNELL 1932, BLICKENSTAFF and GROSSMAN 1950.
[3] BANDES, HOLLANDER and BIERMAN 1948.   [4] NECHELES 1943.
[5] McGINTY, WILSON and RODNEY 1949.
[6] WOLF and WOLFF 1943.   [7] MAHL 1949.   [8] SELYE 1951.
[9] EICHHORN and TRACKTIR 1955.   [10] VANZANT and associates 1932.

attaining at age 65, about 25 per cent in males and about 28 per cent in females[1]. Even higher percentages have been reported[2, 3]. Curiously enough, in the series of over 3000 cases studied by Vanzant et al. (1932) the incidence of achlorhydria declined after age 65; the authors suggest that this decline may be due to a possible higher death rate among achlorhydrics.

Bloomfield and Keefer (1928) found that the average acidity of the gastric juice collected after an alcohol test meal declined from 75 clinical units (mEq/1) at age 20 to about 25 clinical units in the group past 60 years of age. Their averages, especially in the older age group, were influenced by their inclusion of achlorhydrics. When these are excluded, as they were in the Vanzant series, the decline in acidity with age is not so marked and indeed is not evident in females. In males, these authors found a decline of only about 10 clinical units in average acidity between ages 20 and 70. Polland and Bloomfield (1931) found that the volume as well as the acidity of the gastric secretion induced by histamine declined with age, apparently in a linear fashion. These authors did not include achlorhydrics but they did not separate their subjects as to sex. These authors reported their values in per cent of normal and their curves show a decline in acidity of about 25 per cent between ages 20 and 70; in the same period of time there was a decline in the average volume of secretion obtained in the histamine test of something over 35 per cent. It is evident that differences in the population and the methods used preclude the drawing of any precise conclusions but it is certain that the incidence of achlorhydria increases with age in both men and women and that young men secrete more hydrochloric acid than young women but suffer a greater decline in their gastric secretory function with advancing age.

Gastric secretion in disease.

Changes in gastric secretion observed in duodenal ulcer patients have already been mentioned. Although the average gastric and duodenal acidity in duodenal ulcer patients is higher than in normal controls, gastric ulcer patients have, on the average a lower than normal acidity[4]. It has been suggested that the hypo-acidity in gastric ulcer may be secondary to an associated chronic gastritis. Hypoacidity is also the usual finding in gastric carcinoma. Indeed, canacer in any part of the body is often associated with gastric anacidity or hypoacidity[5], probably due to the accompanying general cachexia.

Gastric secretion is depressed in many kinds of extragastric disease, for example, acute fevers, malnutrition from any cause, gall bladder disease, Addisons disease, sprue, acne rosaceae and chronic arthritis[6]. In acute fevers the depression of secretion is probably mainly due to the pyrexia since an increase in body temperature from any cause has been shown to depress gastric secretion; however, the influence of bacterial toxins cannot be ruled out. In the other diseases mentioned the hyposecretion is probably to be attributed to cachexia to which the parietal cells, with their high metabolic rate, seem to be particularly susceptible.

Anacidity or hypoacidity is usually associated with severe anemia of any type. In pernicious anemia anacidity is always present and is probably associated with the etiology since absence of "intrinsic" factor, probably due to atrophic changes in the gastric mucosa, is responsible for failure to absorb vitamin B_{12}. While the parietal cells probably do not produce "intrinsic factor", they suffer atrophy along with the rest of the mucosa. Adequate treatment of the anemia does not cure the achlorhydria.

---

[1] Bloomfield and Keefer 1928.   [2] Polland and Bloomfield 1931.
[3] Vanzant and associates 1932.   [4] Atkinson and Henley 1955.   [5] Carlson 1923.
[6] Taylor 1955.

12. Secretion of pancreatic juice.
Properties and function of pancreatic juice.

The pancreas secretes an alkaline fluid of low viscosity in which the character-istic inorganic constituents are sodium and potassium bicarbonate and sodium and potassium chloride. The sodium and potassium concentrations correspond to those of the blood plasma[1] but the bicarbonate-chloride ratio varies with the rate of secretion[2, 3]. The bicarbonate content ranges from a maximum of about 150 milliequivalents per liter to a minimum approximating the bicarbonate of blood plasma[3]. The chloride varies reciprocally with the bicarbonate in such a way that the sum of the two expressed in milliequivalents approximates a con-stant[1, 2, 3]. The bicarbonate increases (and the chloride decreases) with increasing rates of secretion. A linear negative correlation has recently been shown to exist between the logarithim of the bicarbonate (mEq./l.) and the reciprocal of the rate of secretion[4].

Inorganic constituents of the juice other than chloride and bicarbonate are similar to those of the blood plasma except that calcium and phosphate are relatively low[5]. The calcium content, which is 3 to 4 mg. per cent, probably corres-ponds to the diffusible calcium of the blood[6].

The p_H of dogs' pancreatic juice, when collected without exposure to air ranges from 8.0 to 8.3[7]. Values outside this range have been reported, particularly in human pancreatic juice, but the p_H of the juice as secreted by the normal human subject, without contamination or exposure to air, has probably never been measured.

In addition to water and inorganic salts the pancreatic juice contains a variable amount of protein which consists of a mixture of digestive enzymes. Three of these are well known: trypsin, lipase and amylase; but by suitable methods of analysis it is possible to show the presence of some eight or ten separate proteins in the juice[8, 9] each of which probably represents a different enzyme. Some of these can be identified; for example, what was formerly called trypsin has been shown by KUNITZ and NORTHROP (1935, 1936) to comprise at least two enzymes which they called trypsin and chymo-trypsin respectively; both digest native protein but they differ in their specificity, solubility, crystalline form, etc. Recent work by WALDRON (1952) suggests the possibility of two amylases, a suggestion strongly supported by the electrophoretic analysis recently reported by GROSS-BERG and co-workers (1952). A carboxy-peptidase has been identified and crystallized[10]. Even with these additions the list falls short of the number of separate components believed to be present in the juice and we may look forward to the discovery of additional pancreatic enzymes.

The proteolytic enzymes do not occur in the juice in active form but as pro-enzymes or zymogens[11] which are designated respectively, trypsinogen, chymo-trypsinogen and procarboxy-peptidase. Trypsinogen is changed to active trypsin when mixed with the secretion of the intestinal mucosa which contains an activating agent called enterokinase[12]. The active trypsin in turn converts chymo-trypsinogen and procarboxypeptidase into the active form. Trypsin is also able to activate trypsinogen but the process is less efficient than activation by enterokinase since a considerable amount of inactive protein is always produ-

---

[1] GAMBLE and McIVER 1928a.   [2] BALL 1930.
[3] HART and THOMAS 1945, CONLY et al. 1955.   [4] CONLY, CRIDER and THOMAS 1955.
[5] GAMBLE aud McIVER 1928a.   [6] KOMAROV, LANGSTROTH and McRAE 1939.
[7] HART and THOMAS 1945.   [8] MUNRO and THOMAS 1945.
[9] GROSSBERG, KOMAROV and SHAY 1952.   [10] ANSON 1935.   [11] HEIDENHAIN 1875.
[12] SCHEPOWALNIKOW 1899.

ced[1]. Any active trypsin that may be formed in the pancreas is inactivated, probably by trypsin inhibitor, a protein substance found in pancreatic tissue by Kunitz and Northrop (1936). The inhibitor is present also in pancreatic juice[2]. Trypsin inhibitor combines with trypsin to produce an inactive protein; in the intestine this reaction is prevented by some constituent of the intestinal secretion which has not been identified but is apparently not enterokinase[2].

The amylases depend for their activity on the presence of neutral salts, the most active of which are the chlorides. All the pancreatic enzymes are most active in neutral or slightly alkaline media but their activity is not destroyed by a moderate degree of acidity. It is interesting in this connection that the intestinal contents are usually acid in reaction[3] (p_H 2.5 to 6.0), hence the pancreatic enzymes do not ordinarily have an optimal medium for their activity.

Under certain conditions pancreatic enzymes may escape into the tissues surrounding the acini or into the blood[4]. Apparently there is always some diffusion of enzymes from the acinous cells into the blood[5] and this diffusion may be increased during active secretion even under normal circumstances. However the quantities are unimportant unless there is obstruction to the normal flow of juice from ducts into the intestine[6] or an increase in the permeability of the ducts or the acini to the enzymes in the juice or in the acinous cells[7]. Even under these conditions there is no digestion of the tissues unless the inactive proenzmes become activated.

The mechanism of activation of extracellular pancreatic enzymes is obscure; probably tissue kinases, which may be released from injured cells, play a part[8] in activating the proteolytic enzames. It is commonly believed that reflux of bile[9] into the pancreatic ducts may cause sufficient tissue damage to activate the proteolytic enzymes whereas the bile itself serves to activate the lipase. In acute pancreatitis from whatever cause there is always the danger of extensive tissue destruction and fat necrosis brought about by activated pancreatic enzymes.

The function of the pancreatic secretion can be inferred from the disturbances that appear when it is absent from the intestine[10]. These comprise deficiency in absorption of the various foodstuffs, affecting chiefly fat, and the appearence of undigested fat, meat fibers and starch in the stools. The absorption deficit is sufficient to bring about a serious impairment of nutrition. If the pancreatic juice is diverted to the outside of the body while the pancreas remains functional, as in total pancreatic fistula, other serious consequences follow such as dehydration, loss of base from the blood and finally death in 5 to 8 days (in dogs)[11].

Regulation of pancreatic secretion.

Secretion of pancreatic juice is intermittent in some animals, for example the dog and cat, and continuous in others such as the rabbit[12]. In man the secretion is probably continuous but in all species the rate of secretion is increased during digestion. The increase is due to specific stimuli associated with the digestive process. Except for a brief and relatively unimportant episode of

[1] Kunitz 1939.   [2] Kalser and Grossman 1955.
[3] Mann and Bollman 1930, Thomas and Crider 1936.   [4] Cherry and Crandall jr. 1932.
[5] Zucker, Newburger and Berg 1932.
[6] Lagerlöf 1945, Burke, Plummer and Bradford 1950.
[7] Popper, Necheles and Russell 1948, Popper 1948, Comfort 1937.
[8] Troll and Doubilet 1951.   [9] Bernard 1856, Opie 1910, Archibald 1919.
[10] Bernard 1856, v. Mering and Minkowski 1889, Handelsman, Golden and Pratt 1934, Hoerner 1935.
[11] Pavlov 1902, Elman and McCaughan 1927, Camble and McIver 1928b.
[12] Heidenhain 1883.

secretion during the act of eating[1], induced by the sight, smell and taste of food, the effective stimuli act only from the small intestine. By analogy with the three well known phases of gastric secretion we may say that there is a cephalic phase and an intestinal phase but no gastric phase of pancreatic secretion[2].

The substances that act as stimuli in the intestine comprise various constituents of the gastric chyme. They include water[3], acid[3], products of protein digestion[4], products of starch digestion[5], fat[3] and products of fat digestion. When used singly each of these stimuli produces a characteristic type of pancreatic juice. For example HCl in the intestine produces an abundant watery secretion low in enzymes. The carbohydrates will not usually induce secretion in a resting gland but in the presence of other stimuli they increase, moderately, the enzyme output[6]. Products of protein digestion, fats, and fatty acids are powerful stimuli for enzyme secretion but only moderately stimulate secretion of fluid.

Stimuli may act on the pancreas either through the nervous system or by means of hormones. Nervous stimulation occurs during the act of eating and possibly as a result of the presence in the intestine of certain types of stimuli but the latter possibility lacks positive proof. The efferent fibers involved are in the vagi[7] and, to a smaller extent, in the splanchnic nerves; they are all cholinergic[8]. The principal effect of the secretory nerves is to increase the enzyme output of the pancreas but the secretion of water and salts is also moderately increased. Cutting the splanchnic nerves has little effect on pancreatic function but cutting the vagi (in dogs) permanently reduces the enzyme output by from 50 to 80 per cent, depending on the method of stimulation employed in the study[9].

The hormones concerned in secretion of pancreatic juice are secretin[10] and pancreozymin[11]. Secretin is present in the mucous membrane of the upper small intestine where it is released into the blood by the action of acid and to a lesser degree by other substances in the intestine. It is carried by the blood to the pancreas where it causes an abundant secretion of dilute pancreatic juice with a high bicarbonate and low enzyme content. Excess secretin is destroyed by an enzyme[12], secretinase, present in the blood and tissues. Secretin may be extracted from the excised intestine by means of HCl. Extracts of this nature, purified to the extent that they are free from toxic substances, are available commercially and are used in tests of pancreatic function[13].

Although highly purified secretin is mainly a stimulus for secretion of water and salts, crude preparations increase the output of enzymes as well. HARPER and RAPER (1943) have shown that the latter effect is due to the presence of a specific substance which they call pancreozymin. Presumably, pancreozymin is a hormone, which, like secretin, is released from the intestinal mucosa by specific stimuli and serves to increase the enzyme content of the pancreatic juice. Effective stimuli include water, HCl, peptone, amino acids, fats and soaps[14].

Acid in the intestine is the most effective stimulus for secretion of fluid by the pancreas[15]; furthermore, no other stimulus, with the possible exception of soap, when used singly in the fasting animal is capable of inducing secretion at a rate comparable to that formed during digestion. For these reasons it is commonly

---

[1] WALTHER 1897, 1899, KREWER 1899.   [2] IVY 1926.   [3] For literature see BABKIN 1928.
[4] THOMAS and CRIDER 1941.   [5] HARPER and VASS 1941, THOMAS and CRIDER 1947.
[6] BABKIN and SAVICH 1921, HARPER and VASS 1941, THOMAS and CRIDER 1947.
[7] HEIDENHAIN 1875, 1883, PAVLOV 1893.
[8] BABKIN, HEBB and SERGEYEVA 1939, BABKIN 1946.
[9] CRIDER and THOMAS 1944, PINCUS, THOMAS and LACHMAN 1948a.
[10] BAYLISS and STARLING 1902.   [11] HARPER and RAPER 1943.
[12] GREENGARD, STEIN and IVY 1941a and b.   [13] AGREN, LAGERLÖF and BERGLUND 1936.
[14] WANG and GROSSMAN 1950.   [15] BABKIN 1928, p. 500.

believed that the digestive secretion is largely due to the acidity of the intestinal contents, and as a corollary, that pancreatic secretion is regulated to a great extent by the secretin mechanism. If this is true the rate of secretion during digestion should fluctuate with the acidity of the intestinal contents. However, Pincus et al. (1948b) were unable to detect any significant correlation between the p_H of the duodenal contents of dogs and the volume of pancreatic juice secreted during digestion of various types of food. Other stimuli that are active during digestion, particularly the vagus impulses are known to greatly augment the effect of secretin[1]. These stimuli may be the determining factor in the quantitative response to circulating secretin, completely overshadowing the affect of the actual concentration of secretin in the blood.

The mechanism of pancreatic secretion.

Secretion of enzymes by the pancreas involves two distinct processes: (1) synthesis within the cell of the enzymes or their precursors and (2) discharge of enzymes from the secretory cells into the ducts. Synthesis is a continuous process believed not to be subject to nervous or humoral regulation and to be controlled only by the laws that govern chemical equilibria in general[2]. The synthesized material appears within the acinous cells as zymogen granules which accumulate in the resting gland until they come to occupy most of the available space within the cells[3].

Under the influence of appropriate stimuli the zymogen granules diminish in number and in size; at the same time enzymes appear in the secretion. The exact mechanism is not known but at some point the granules dissolve in the intracellular fluid and are discharged through the cell wall into the ducts. Stimuli such as HCl and secretin which produce a watery secretion with a low enzyme content have little effect on the granules while stimuli which call forth secretion rich in enzymes deplete the granules and may, if they act over a long period of time leave the cells almost free of zymogen granules[4].

It has long been assumed that the inorganic constituents of the juice are secreted by the same cells that produce the enzymes, namely the acinous cells. However, the fact that fluid secretion and enzyme secretion are separately regulated raises a theoretical objection to this view. All current theories of stimulation require that cells shall respond to a stimulus with a characteristic type of functional activity regardless of the nature of the stimulus. It would be difficult to imagine an excititory mechanism that would cause the cell to give one type of response to one stimulus and a totally different response to another type of stimulus. In the other digestive glands about which we have more information each component of the secretion that is independently regulated is formed by a different type of cell.

We must also take account of the clinical observation that in certain types of pancreatic disease enzyme secretion may be depressed or absent while secretion of fluid and bicarbonate remains normal[5]. On the other hand, in glands injured by alloxan, fluid secretion may be subnormal while enzymes are secreted normally. This latter observation, reported by Grossman and Ivy[6], contains a hint as to a possible solution of the problem. Histological examination of the glands which

---

[1] Gayet and Guillaumie 1930, Thomas 1950, p. 109.

[2] Langstroth, McRae and Komarov 1939.

[3] Heidenhain 1875, 1883. For more recent observations and the extensive modern literature see Hirsch 1939, 1948, 1957 and Sluiter 1944.

[4] Babkin, Rubaschkin and Savich 1909.   [5] Lagerlöf 1939, Friedman and Snape 1950.

[6] Grossman and Ivy 1946.

failed to respond normally to secretin showed no injury to the acinous cells but the cells of the intralobular ducts appeared abnormal; in particular they exhibited vacuolization. The intralobular duct cells are continuous with the centroacinous cells that line the alveoli and are identical with these cells in their cytological structure. It is possible that cells of this type secrete water and bicarbonate while the acinous cells secrete only enzymes [1].

13. Secretions of the small intestine.

Methods of study of intestinal secretion.

The secretion of the intestine may be collected in anesthetized, operated animals by simply opening the abdomen and inserting a suitable collecting tube into a portion of the intestine. This method is unsatisfactory because operative trauma and anesthetic drugs, especially the latter [2], greatly depress the secretory activity of the intestinal glands. These difficulties may be partially overcome by decerebrating or decapitating the animal under anesthesia and then allowing time for the anesthetic to be eliminated, as was done by WRIGHT and his co-workers (1940). The situation is further improved if the animal is immered in physiological saline; this eliminates the irritant effects on the intestine of drying and exposure. The same results can be achieved by cutting the spinal cord and allowing the animal to recover from the necessary anesthesia as was done by SAVITCH in 1904. The best results are obtained by use of an unanesthetized animal with a surgically isolated loop of intestine. The animal is prepared by cutting through the intestine at two points and re-establishing its continuity by end to end anastomosis. If one end of the isolated segment is closed and the other end brought out through the abdominal wall to form a fistula, the loop of intestine involved is described as a Thiry loop (1864). The preparation was modified in 1888 by VELLA by bringing both ends of the intestine out through the skin of the abdominal wall; such a preparation is known as a Thiry-Vella loop. These loops retain so much of their innervation as reaches them through the mesentery but are separated from their connections through the myeneteric and sub-mucous plexuses with the intestine above and below. Intestinal loops without a nerve supply have been prepared [3] by isolating a segment of intestine as in the preparation of a Thiry loop and implanting it under the skin of a mammary gland of a lactating female animal. At first the mesenteric pedicle is left intact but after the local blood vessels have invaded the intestine the mesenteric pedicle is cut. Since the intestine so prepared is entirely deprived of nervous influences, it may be used to decide whether or not hormonal influences affect secretion.

In man, and in animals with a simple intestinal fistula, it is possible to collect intestinal secretion by means of a multilumen intestinal tube [4]. Two of the lumens of the tube are used to inflate balloons; a third lumen having an opening between the balloons can be used to collect the secretion which accumulates in this area. The method has the obvious disadvantage of placing foreign bodies in the intestine which are known to profoundly influence secretion. However, it is useful for studying the composition of secretions obtained under these circumstances. In all studies of intestinal secretion it is important to remember that mechanical stimulation, and especially distension of the intestine, is a profound stimulus to secretion; consequently, when the quantity of secretion is to be determined,

---

[1] THOMAS 1952.   [2] WRIGHT, JENNINGS, FLOREY and LIUM 1940.
[3] IVY, FARRELL and LUETH 1927, NASSET, PIERCE and MURLIN 1935, FLOREY and HARDING 1935, SONNENSCHEIN, GROSSMAN and IVY 1947.
[4] MILLER and ABBOTT 1934, ABBOTT and MILLER 1936.

or when quantitative differences in secretion obtained under different circumstances are sought, it is essential that mechanical stimulation of the mucosa be avoided. For example, a Thiry fistula into which a catheter has been inserted for collecting the secretion will produce a greater than normal amount of succus entericus[1].

14. Morphology.

The mucous membrane of the small intestine is everywhere covered with villi which are minute projections on the mucosa about 1 mm. in height and somewhat less in diameter. The villi are invested by a layer of columnar cells, of the type characteristic of the small intestine, set upon a basement membrane beneath which is a fine layer of a smooth muscle fibers; the muscle is continuous with the muscularis mucosae. Between the villi are the openings of the intestinal glands, or crypts of Lieberkühn. These are simple tubular glands which do not penetrate the muscularis mucosae. The epithelium covering the villi and that lining the crypts is of the same columnar type, The free end of each columnar cell, next to the lumen of the intestine, is provided with a specialized cuticular border resembling the brush border of certain renal tubular cells[2]. Its appearance suggests that it contains fine pores or is contituted of substances of varied chemical nature arranged in the form of columns. This border may play some essential role in absorption.

Interspersed among the columnar cells are goblet cells and certain other specialized types. The goblet cells secrete mucus. Also among the columnar cells are certain cells which stain with silver, known as argentaffine or enterochromaffine[3] cells and other cells with large acidophile granules known as Paneth cells. It is now known that the argentaffine cells produce serotonin[4] or at least synthesize its precursor.

In the bottoms of the crypts many of the epithelial cells may be seen to be undergoing mitosis and at the tips of the villi one can see that cells are being shed into the lumen of the intestine[5]. It seems reasonable then, to believe that there is going on in the intestinal mucous membrane a process of continuous replacement of the epithelial lining, new cells being produced in the bottoms of the crypts and the older cells continuously shed at the tips of the villi. The importance of this process will be more evident when we come to consider the mechanism of secretion of the intestinal enzymes.

In the first part of the duodenum, in addition to the regular intestinal glands, are special mucous glands known as Brunner's glands. These are similar in structure to the pyloric glands of the stomach. They are made up of long tubules frequently branched and often tortuous which penetrate the muscularis mucosae. Their ducts empty into the crypts of Lieberkühn. Brunner's glands are very numerous in the duodenum between the pylorus and the entrance of the bile and pancreatic ducts. Below this level they are seen less frequently and none are found beyond the duodenojejunal junction.

15. Duodenal secretion. Brunner's glands.

The secretion of the duodenum consists of mucus and an alkaline fluid containing sodium bicarbonate. The composition of this secretion was studied by Florey and Harding (1933, 1934) who found the principal organic constituent to be mucus, although traces of lipase were present in the secretions from dogs

---

[1] Thiry 1864.   [2] Vérzar and McDougall 1936.   [3] Macklin and Macklin 1932.
[4] Erspamer and Asero 1952, Olson and Gray 1958.   [5] Leblond and Stevens 1948.

and a pepsin-like enzyme in the secretions from dogs and goats. The presence of a proteolytic enzyme resembling pepsin emphasizes the relation between these glands and the pyloric glands of the stomach which also secrete mucus and pepsin. Previous investigators have reported the finding of numerous other enzymes in the secretion, but FLOREY and HARDING attributed their presence to contamination of the juice with desquamated epithelial cells. The mucus is doubtless secreted by BRUNNER's glands but the source of the alkaline fluid is not clear; it is probably secreted by the glands of LIEBERKÜHN, although in the rabbit, in which duodenal secretion is abundant, the BRUNNER's glands contain serous as well mucous cells. The outstanding characteristic of the alkaline fluid is its high bicarbonate content which may be as much as 0.1 normal. The p_H of the secretion is in the neighborhood of 8.2 when it is collected without exposure to air.

Control of BRUNNER's gland secretion. The secretion of BRUNNER's glands increases on stimulation of the vagus nerves and administration of parasympathomimetic drugs such as pilocarpine and physostigmine; it is not augmented by stimulation of the sympathetic nerves[1]. The amount of secretion is increased after meals, even in transplanted denervated pouches of the duodenum[2]. This proves that there is a humoral mechanism for regulating the secretion in addition to whatever nervous mechanism there may be. The nature of the hormone has been the subject of some discussion and is still undetermined; FLOREY and HARDING (1935a) were convinced that it is pancreatic secretin. They were led to this conclusion by the fact that practically all the stimuli which increase pancreatic secretion, including contact of hydrochloric acid with the duodenal mucous membrane, also increase the secretion of BRUNNER's glands. They also found that what they considered to be a highly purified secretin preparation stimulated duodenal secretion when given intravenously. SONNENSCHEIN and his associates (1947) were unable to confirm the results with secretin. Using what they believed was a crystalline picrolonate of secretin they observed little effect on BRUNNER's glands, although crude secretin caused an abundant secretion. GROSSMAN (1950) has suggested that there is a special hormone for these glands which he proposes to call *"duocrinin"*; however, writing in 1958, he still considers the subject to be *subjudice*.

Functions of the duodenal secretion. FLOREY and HARDING (1933) emphasized the protective function of the secretion of BRUNNER's glands and considered it an important factor in preventing duodenal ulceration. In addition it may assist in emulsification and suspension of fat and other food particles. Since, like other intestinal secretions, it contains enterokinase it helps to activate the trypsinogen of pancreatic juice. Duodenal secretion is said to contain "intrinsic factor" and therefore, probably assists in absorption of vitamin B_{12}. The various hormones known to be produced by the duodenal mucosa are probably not secreted into the lumen of the intestine except incidentally and in small quantities and are not functional in this situation.

16. Intestinal secretion or succus entericus.

In general the secretion of the small intestine is a thin, colorless, or slightly straw-colored fluid somewhat opalescent and containing flecks of mucus. On centrifuging and examination of the sediment it can be seen that the cloudly appearance of the juice is partially due to cellular debris, including some intact cells of the type characteristic of the intestinal mucous membrane[3]. In chemical

---

[1] FLOREY and HARDING 1934.   [2] FLOREY and HARDING 1935b.
[3] FLOREY, WRIGHT and JENNINGS 1941.

composition, the juice consists of water, inorganic salts, and organic material. The inorganic salts are those commonly present in body fluids, except that the bicarbonate concentration is higher than it is in blood or interstitial fluid. The alkalinity on titration is said to vary between 0.02 and 0.67 per cent sodium bicarbonate equivalent. Various estimates of the p_H of the intestinal secretion have been given ranging from 6.3 to 9. The higher values undoubtedly are the result of loss of carbon dioxide from the juice. It is generally considered to be an alkaline fluid and may probably have a true p_H as high as 8.3.

The quantity of fluid secreted by the small intestine is never very great, a few cc. per hour being the usual amount that it is possible to obtain experimentally, even under conditions of stimulation. It is difficult to determine with accuracy the amount actually secreted because of the tremendous absorptive capacity of the intestine. Many times more than the amount that it is possible to collect may be secreted and reabsorbed during an observation period. That the mucosa is capable of passing into the lumen of the intestine enormous amounts of fluid is evidenced from the great water loss that occurs through the intestine in pathologic states such as cholera, diarrhea, or intestinal obstruction. The organic matter of the juice consists of mucus, enzymes and cellular debris. The mucus is contributed by the goblet cells which are present everywhere in the mucous membrane and, in the upper end of the intestine, by the BRUNNER's glands of the duodenum.

Intestinal enzymes.

The source of the enzyme is unknown but is assumed that they are produced by the columnar cells, although the argentaffine cells or the Paneth cells may be responsible for some of them. A really formidable array of enzymes have been reported as occurring in intestinal secretion. A pepsin like protese (from the duodenum only), an amylase, a lipase, at least two peptidases, sucrase (invertase), maltase, lactase, enterokinase, alkaline phosphatase, nucleo-phophatases, and nucleosidases have been described.

Peptidases. One of the major functions of intestinal digestion is the final reduction of the products of peptic and tryptic digestion to amino acids; this is accomplished by intestinal peptidases. The presence of peptidases has been reported by all investigators who have studied the problem[1]. The ones usually described[2] are amino peptidase, which act on the peptide linkages of terminal amino acids possessing a free amino group; tri-peptidases and di-peptidases which split tri- and di-peptides respectively into their constituents amino acids.

Lipase. Most investigators[3] have reported finding a weak lipase action in intestinal secretion.

Di-saccharides. The various di-saccharidases, sucrase, lactase and maltase are present in succus entericus under all normal circumstances.

Enterokinase. Enterokinase the enzyme which converts trypsinogen to trypsin (see under Pancreatic secretion) is present in the intestinal secretion under normal circumstances[4]. However SAVICH (1904) stated that if pancreatic juice was excluded from the intestine, or in an intestinal loop in which the pancreatic juice did not circulate, enterokinase gradually disappeared from the secretion. WALDSCHMIDT-LEITZ and HARTENECK (1925) and WALDSCHMIDT-LEITZ and LINDER-STRÖM-LANG (1927) likewise concluded that pancreatic juice was necessary for liberation of enterokinase from the epithelial cells. FLOREY. WRIGHT and JEN-

---

[1] SALASKIN 1902, KUTSCHER and SEEMAN 1902, WALDSCHMIDT-LEITZ and WALDSCHMIDT-GRASER 1927.

[2] FLOREY, WRIGHT and JENNINGS 1941.   [3] BOLDYREFF 1904, 1912.

[4] SCHEPOWALNIKOW 1899.

NINGS (1941) and BABKIN[1] considered that the evidence in niether case was
sufficient. The point is of considerable interest and merits firther investigation.

The studies of WRIGHT, JENNINGS, FLOREY and LIUM in 1940, raised a
question as to a source of the enzymes ordinarily found in intestinal secretion.
They reported that when they took precautions to prevent injury to the mucous
membrane while collecting the secretion and then immediately centrifuged the
collected secretion so as to remove cellular debris, only amylase and enterokinase
were consistently present in the supernatant fluid. They consider that these
enzymes and possible maltase, are secreted by the intestinal glands in the usual
sense. The others, they believe, are intracellular enzymes which exist in the cells
of the mucous membrane and appear in the juice only as a result of the shedding
of these cells and their distintegration in the intestine. They point to the opinions
of many physiologists that most of the digestion of peptides and di-saccharides
takes place in the epithelial cells while these substances are being absorbed. This
is not, however, a necessary conclusion from the observed facts. The rapid rate
of mitosis in the depths of the glands of LIEBERKÜHN and the continuous shedding
of epithelial cells from the tips of the villi[2] may represent a special kind of holocrine
secretory process by which endocellular enzymes are secreted into the intestinal
juice, the secretory product being the entire epithelial cell with its contained
enzymes. Under normal circumstances the presence of active trypsin in the
intestinal contents would seem to insure the rapid disintegration of these cells
and liberation of their contained enzymes into the intestinal secretion. In this
connection it may be significant that enterokinase is secreted directly and so
insures that activation of trypsinogen does not depend on the disintegration of
shed epithelial cells.

17. Regulation of intestinal secretion.

Nervous regulation. It was demonstrated in PAVLOV'S laboratory[3], that
stimulation of the vagus nerve in animals in which the spinal cord has been
severed in the neck caused, after a latent period of from 1 to $1^1/_2$ hours, a moderate
secretion of intestinal juice from the duodenum and also from the rest of the small
intestine. Wright and his co-workers[4] were unable to obtain clear evidence that
the vagal stimulation caused secretion from the jejunum or ileum. Stimulation
of the sympathetic caused no secretion but cutting the nerves resulted in a marked
increase in secretion, but in different parts of the intestine depending upon which
nerves were severed; for example, cutting the splanchnics only caused an increase
in secretion from the duodenum; cutting all the pre-ganglionic sympathetic
fibers was followed by secretion from the entire small intestine[5]. If only the pre-
ganglionic fibers were cut, the secretion stopped after a few days but was again
resumed if the sympathetic ganglia were removed, thus severing the post-ganglionic fibers. Paralytic secretion is increased by physostigmine and inhibited
by atropine; it is therefore considered to be dependent upon some cholinergic
mechanism in the intestine[6]. Parasympathomimetic drugs, in general, increase
the secretion and sympathomimetic drugs tend to inhibit it[6]. From these observations we can conclude that secretion from the intestinal epithelium is augmented
by a cholinergic mechanism involving the vagi and the enteric plexuses and that
this mechanism is antagonized by the sympathetic. Whether this antagonism

---

[1] B. P. BABKIN — personal communication to the author (J. E. T.).
[2] LEBLOND and STEVENS 1948.   [3] SAVITCH and SOCHESTVENSKY 1917.
[4] WRIGHT, JENNINGS, FLOREY and LIUM 1940.
[5] WRIGHT, JENNINGS, FLOREY and LIUM 1940.
[6] WRIGHT, JENNINGS, FLOREY and LIUM 1940.

is a direct one or in indirect, depending on the influence of the sympathetic vasomotor nerves on the blood supply to the intestinal glands, remain uncertain. One interpretation of the paralytic secretion is that section of the sympathetic nerves results in dilatation of the blood vessels of the intestine and in this way greatly increases the blood flow. Such an increase in blood flow would provide a greater amount of fluid for secretion and presumably, might produce the augmentation of secretion seen on section of the sympathetic nerves[1]. BABKIN (1950) has pointed out that cutting the sympathetic nerves to the small intestine increases its motility, which undoubtedly has a massaging effect on the mucous membrane; in view of the fact that one of the most effective stimuli for intestinal secretion is mechanical stimulation of the mucosa, this factor alone may be sufficient to account for the increased secretion.

The fact that the paralytic juice contains the usual enzymes and mucin and that it is inhibited by atropine suggests that it is a true secretion and not a transudate such as might be expected to result from vascular congestion[2]. However, in an equilbrium situation such as probably exists between secretion and absorption in the small intestine, the displacement of a single major factor, such as the blood flow through the capillaries, which would favor one element in the equilibrium, in this case secretion, might well cause a shift in favor of secretion such as is seen after denervation of the intestine.

The most effective stimulus for secretion of succus entericus is local, mechanical or chemical stimulation of the intestinal mucous membrane. Such stimuli are always present in the digesting intestine due to the presence of chyme and the food particles which it contains[3]. Feeding is not very effective in increasing the rate of intestinal secretion from an isolated intestinal loop, provided the nerve supply is intact, but if the sympathetic nerves have been severed a noticeable increase in secretion takes place when animal is fed[4]. This indicates that some factor, either nervous or humoral, operates to increase the secretion during digestion.

The early investigators were of the opinion that pancreatic secretin was an effective stimulus for intestinal secretion[5]. This point of view was a result of experiments in which injections of secretin containing preparations resulted in undoubted increases in secretion of intestinal juice. However, as more highly purified preparation of secretin became available the influence on intestinal secretion became less so that it is now very doubtful whether secretin as such acts upon the intestinal glands[6]. However, intestinal extracts, from which secretin has been totally eliminated remain potent stimuli for intestinal secretion. This subject has been investigated most fully by NASSET and his co-workers (1938) who have prepared an extract of the intestinal mucous membrane which is free from secretin, from vasodilator material and from other toxic substances but has a powerful effect upon the secretion of the small intestine when given intravenously. Subcutaneous injection is less effective but in large doses produces some secretion[7]. They believe that this material is a hormone which normally augments the intestinal secretion and for which they propose the name "entero-crinin". The fact that a hormonal mechanism is involved has been amply demonstrated both by NASSET and his co-workers (1935) and by FLOREY et al. (1935) by means of denervated loops of intestine; such loops secrete when acid and certain other substances are placed in the intact portions of the intestine, and also after meals.

---

[1] STARLING 1906.   [2] FLOREY, WRIGHT and JENNINGS 1941.   [3] THIRY 1864.
[4] WRIGHT, FLOREY, JENNINGS and LIUM 1940.
[5] DELENZENNE and FROUIN 1904, ÅGREN 1934, FLOREY and HARDING 1935.
[6] NASSET, E. S. Personal communication to the author (J. E. T.) THOMAS 1950.
[7] SCHIFFRIN and NASSET 1939.

18. The function of succus entericus.

Enzymatic digestion of food, in all its phases, is a hydrolytic process; an abundance of water to serve as one of the reacting substances is therefore essential. The succus entericus provides this water in the area in which the major part of digestion of food occurs. Water is also necessary to serve as a solvent and as a medium of suspension and transport for the solids which are either dissolved or suspended in the chyme. The enzymes, either in the secretion or in the cells, complete the digestion of protein and carbohydrate by reducing the peptides, resulting from peptic and tryptic digestion, to amino acids and the di-saccharides, resulting from amylolytic digestion of starch, to glucose. Other disaccharides that may be present in the food are likewise digested, liberating their constituent monosaccharides. In fat digestion the succus entericus serves as a source of water and as a medium for suspension and emulsification of the fat particles; it also provides a certain amount of lipase.

19. Secretion of the colon.

The mucosa of the mammalian caecum and colon is in many respects similar to that of the small intestine; crypts are present but there are no villi. As in the small intestine, the cells at the bottoms of the crypts exhibit numerous mitoses, suggesting the continuous replacement of shed epithelial cells. Goblet cells are more numerous than in the small intestine and the epithelial cells between the goblet cells differ among themselves but in the majority the protoplasm is clear and free from secretory granules. The secretion is scanty[1] as is to be expected from the fact that a major function of the large intestine is absorption of water. The decrease in volume of intestinal contents that occurs in this area indicates that secretion does not keep pace with absorption. Actually, it is usually not possible to collect any secretion from a colonic fistula unless the mucous membrane is stimulated mechanically by insertion of a catheter or other instrument. Even with this stimulation only a few tenths of a cc. per hour can be collected. When anything can be collected it consists of a watery fluid with clumps of white mucus; often it is viscous and opalescent. The reaction is alkaline due to sodium bicarbonate which may be present in concentrations as high as 80—90 mEq./l., according to DE BEER et al. (1935). The specific gravity was stated by these authors to be 1.0613; the fluid part of the secretion contained 98.6 per cent water. Of the solids 0.63 per cent was organic and the remainder inorganic material.

The secretion of the caecum apparently contains enzymes corresponding to those found in the small intestine, with the exception of enterokinase which is not present. The secretion of enzymes becomes progressively less and ultimately disappears toward the distal colon. The large intestine has an extraordinary capacity to secrete mucus and under certain circumstances may secrete a surprisingly large amount of this material[2]. As elsewhere in the intestine, mucus is secreted in response to strong local stimulation or irritation, hence, mucus, is likely to be secreted in unusual amounts in the presence of bacterial infection or other causes of local irritation, such as irritant cathartics. The secretion is an active process involving utilization of oxygen; it is inhibited by perfusion of the intestine with cyanide.

Nervous control of colonic secretion. FLOREY (1930) and WRIGHT et al. (1938) found that stimulation of the nervus erigens caused the colon to secrete a clear mucoid fluid; in contrast to the practical absence of spontaneous secretion,

---

[1] WRIGHT, FLOREY and JENNINGS 1938.   [2] WRIGHT, FLOREY and JENNINGS 1938.

stimulation produced as much as 55 cc. in one 8 hour period from the distal half of
the colon; the average rate was about 5 cc. per hour. Reflex secretion was observed
on stimulation of the cut end of one nervus erigens, the other being intact; the
reflex center was in the lumbar spinal cord. Larson and Bargen (1933) observed
secretion of mucus in an isolated segment of the colon at the time of defecation.
It should be recalled that the nervus erigens supplies only the distal portion of the
colon with parasympathetic fibers; the parasympathetic supply for the proximal
colon comes from the vagi. Acetylcholine and pilocarpine increase colonic secretion
whereas atropine inhibits it. Histamine has been reported to cause a slight
increase in secretion. The secretion is reduced by anesthetics. Cutting the sympathetics does not produce paralytic secretion in the large intestine, but stimulation
of the sympathetics diminishes the secretory response to stimulation of the nervus
erigens[1].

The relationship of the secretory function of the colon to the autonomic nerves
has a bearing upon the occurrence of certain diseases of the colon in which there
is excessive secretion of mucus; for example, mucous colitis. This is a disease in
which excessive amounts of mucus appear in the stools constituting, in some cases,
tubular casts of the colon. This has often been considered a psychosomatic
disease and has a close relationship to abnormal emotional states.

20. Absorption.

Absorption of the products of digestion is limited of to the small intestine. The
intestinal villi, which carry out important functions in the absorptive process,
are confined to the small intestine and are most numerous in the duodenum.
The presence of 18 to 40 villi per square millimeter increases the absorptive
surface to over 700 square centimeters in the rat intestine, which is about 100 cm.
long and 0.25 cm. in circumference. In man, the mucosal surface is about
10 square meters, while the serosal area is only 0.6 suqare meters. In addition the
intestinal villi show remarkable functional regenerative powers and so too do
the intestinal lacteals. In the dog, for example, almost normal fat absorption is
present one week after resection of the mesenteric lymph nodes.

The physiochemical factors of absorption are poorly understood, but it is
obvious that filtration, osmosis and diffusion play only limited roles. The
phenomenon of the selective absorption of some substances with the rejection
of others of identical solubility and molecular weight has still not been explained
satisfactorily. Structural configuration of the molecule appears to be a most determining factor. In addition participation of specific enzymatic processes is involved.

Mechanical factors which influence absorption include the movements of the
villi, the segmenting and peristaltic movements of the intestine, and the respiratory movements which alter intraluminal pressures in the intestine. Villikinin
which controls movements of the villi, and enterocin, which excites movements
of the intestinal musculature, are said to be two local hormones which influence
absorption but unequivocal proof of their existence is wanting[2].

The intestinal villi perform movements designed to pump into, and pass
along, the central lacteals and capillaries such materials as have been absorbed
through the intestinal epithelium. Their movements are of a coordinated nature
and are affected by injury to Meisner's plexus but not by bowel denervation.
Even during activity only a fraction of the villi capillary vessels are seen to be
open at one time. Opening of the maximum number of capillaries and dilatation

---

[1] Wright, Florey and Jennings 1938.
[2] Grossman 1950.

of the main artery and vein occur when the intestinal mucosa is irritated. To what degree dysfunction of movements of the villi may account for the mal-absorption observed in certain clinical conditions such as coeliac disease and sprue is not known. Nervous regulation of absorptive processes has been suggested by several investigators, but this probably is an indirect effect of the autonomic nervous system on intestinal movements. Parasympathetic drugs, such as atropine, which are used in ulcer therapy, are known to interfere with intestinal absorption[1], probably by arresting movements of the villi and intestine.

The "absorptive state" of the organism is one factor determining selective absorption. A particular substance may be absorbed more readily if the substance being absorbed from an adjacent loop of intestine is the same, but delayed if the two are of different composition. Competition between the two absorbing substances, either as substrates for a common enzyme system or for a common carrier system, has been suggested as the basis for the delay. Within rather broad limits, the rate of absorption from the intestine is not determined for most foods by their previous absorption. In general food materials may be absorbed readily even against a concentration gradient (viz., dextrose) and a state of "absorptive saturation" is encountered only in the absorption of inorganic ions, especially iron.

Lipid absorption. The phenomena of fat absorption present problems of special interest. It would appear that lipids are absorbed by an intracellular process, with the material passing directly through the substance of the columnar striated epethelial cells. In contrast, absorption of aqueous-soluble material is an intercellular process. Modified lymphatics specially adapted to the task of lipid absorption occur in the lacteals of the villi. During fat digestion the epithelial cells of the villi fill with fat droplets which either stream to the base of the cell or form larger aggregates which leave the cells more slowly. How these fat droplets reach the lacteals is not well understood but the view that leucocytes participate in fat transport from epithelium to lactal has been shown to be untenable[2]. Movements of the villi[3] and rhythmic contractions of the valved lacteal lymphatics themselves[4] undoubtedly promote transfer of fat towards the thoracic duct.

The lacteals appear to be the preferred route but fat absorption may not be restricted to them. In the lower vertebrates substantial fat absorption must occur through the portal system and subepithelial lymphatics since intestinal villi are poorly developed or absent. In the dog[5] and cat[6] with experimentally ligated thoracic and right lymphatic ducts, fat absorption from the intestine may continue practically undiminished but the possibility that the lymph ducts establish new openings into the blood stream must not be overlooked (DRINKER and GOFFEY 1941).

Lipolysis, as noted below, is not essential for fat absorption but it may determine the route of transit and the ultimate destination of the absorbed fat. While neutral fat is taken up by the lacteals and transferred to the systemic circulation by way of the thoracic duct lymph, about 20 per cent of the dietary fat is absorbed as fatty acids by way of the portal system and passed directly to the liver[7]. Lipid digestion and absorption is known to be impaired in the absence of bile. The role of bile is primarily that of lowering surface tension and this function may be assumed by other surface-active agents such as synthetic detergents. Steroid

---

[1] LAJOS 1938, INGELFINGER et al. 1943.   [2] LEACH 1938.   [3] DRINKER and GOFFEY 1941.
[4] FLOREY 1926/27.   [5] HALL 1913.   [6] HAMBURGER 1900.   [7] LING 1937.

hormones are absorbed in the absence of bile[1] and so also is liquid petrolatum if emulsified sufficiently fine[2, 3].

In the classic concept, dietary fat is hydrolyzed to glycerol and fatty acids. The glycerol is absorbed as such, while the fatty acids form with bile absorbable water-soluble choleic acid complexes. Within the epithelial cell phospholipid is synthesized by dissociation of the complex and recombination of the freed fatty acid with glycero-phosphate. Before being taken up by the lacteals the phospholipid is reconverted to neutral fat by dephosphorylation.

The above description is not wholly in agreement with experimental findings. Frazer (1946) has proposed a partition hypothesis in which dietary fat may be also absorbed as neutral fat providing it is finely enough emulsified. Fatty acids may also pass directly into the portal circulation without prior conversion to neutral fat. Since normally the upper intestine is acid rather than alkaline, the emulsifying agents which can reduce and keep fat particles at absorbable size are limited. Frazer (1946) and his co-workers have concluded that no single physiological substance but only a combination of substances have this property. They found this property in a combination of bile, fatty acids and monoglycerides. Thus as soon as lipolysis has progressed far enough to produce fatty acids and glycerine the conditions are created for the absorption of neutral fat.

Following a fat meal the presence in the systemic circulation of lipid droplets or chylomicrons gives the serum a milky appearance, the so-called post-prandial lipemia. This alimentary lipemia may be abolished by small doses of heparin[4], certain other anticoagulants[5], and a tissue anti-lipemic factor[6]. In older age groups the chylomicrons are larger in size and reflect perhaps a difference in the degree of intestinal lipolysis[7].

The role of fat absorption in the etiology of disease has long been of paramount interest. In atherosclerosis the deposition of fat substances in the arterial intima may be related to an abnormality in the size of the absorbed particles, making the disease a matter of intestinal dysfunction rather than antecedent pathology of the arterial wall[8]. This becomes a matter for reflection since cholesterol, the substance usually implicated in atherosclerosis, is transported entirely by the thoracic duct lymph and is not modified by the liver before entering the systemic circulation[9].

Impaired fat absorption is found in the vitamin-deficiency states only when the condition of the patient is nutritinally poor[10]. While clinical improvement may be shown by patients with sprue when under liver therapy[11], the impaired absorption of fat persists until the patient's nutritional state is corrected. From experiments on animals maintained on diets deficient in various members of the B complex of vitamins, it would appear that the defective fat absorption seen clinically may be secondary to alterations in the structure of the intestinal epithelium. As already noted, the impaired gastric secretion in vitamin B deficiency states has been similarly explained. In any event, the indiscriminate administration of vitamins to promote fat absorption is justified only in the face of a frank vitamin deficiency.

Although lipid absorption in man is fundamentally an intestinal process, the stomach plays an ill-understood role. Intestinal absorption of lipids is low in patients with total gastrectomy[12], or atrophic gastritis, and also in patients with

[1] Selye 1943, Hoffman, Masson and Desbarats 1948.   [2] Frazer and Stewart 1942.
[3] Stryker 1941.   [4] Hahn 1943.   [5] Waldron and Friedman 1948.   [6] Spitzer 1952.
[7] Marder, Becker, Maizel and Necheles 1952.   [8] Moreton 1950.
[9] Biggs, Friedman and Byers 1951.   [10] Irwin et al. 1936.
[11] Barker and Rhoads 1937.   [12] Jones et al. 1948, Rekers et al. 1943.

delayed gastric evacuation due to pyloric stenosis[1] or vagotomy[2]. A shortened intestinal transit time sometimes found in these patients can explain the malabsorption only in part.

The defective fat absorption and steatorrhea in coeliac disease, chronic pancreatitis, and fibrocystic disease of the pancreas are dealt with in another section. The role of bile need be mentioned again but only briefly. Although absorption of fats, cholesterol, and fat-soluble vitamins in the emulsified state occurs in experimental exclusion of bile from the intestine, it must be borne in mind that bile is the only surface-active agent available normally and its absence accounts for the marked disturbances in the absorption of fat and fat-soluble vitamins (especially vitamin K) seen clinically in biliary tract obstructions.

Carbohydrate and protein absorption. Digestion of carbohydrate and protein is completed in the upper part of the small intestine and the digestion products are absorbed from this region as soon as formed. Through operation of the law of mass action, the ready removal of the end products of enzymatic degradation ensures completion of digestion. Translocation of the digestion products is proportional to the area of mucosal surface and hence absorption is normally geratest in the duodenum and jejunum. The ileum, however, affords absorbing facilities for sugars and amino-acids should the duodenum and/or jejunum be unavailable, as in gastroenterostomies and enterectomies. In one patient with only one meter of intestine remaining, absorption (as determined by utilization of test meals) was 87 per cent complete for carbohydrate and 80 per cent for protein 27 years after operation[3]. (As would be expected from the preceding, fat absorption was impaired most.)

Monosaccharides are readily absorbed but other carbohydrates in food must undergo either preliminary hydrolysis (e. g., sucrose) or bacterial digestion (e. g., cellulose). The absence of specific cellulose splitting bacteria from the human intestine accounts for the "bulk laxative" effects of raw vegetables and medical preparations conteining methyl cellulose.

Carbohydrate absorption from the intestine occurs at a steady rate, which, within limits, is independent of concentration in the intestine[4]. Normally, however, the carbohydrate concentration in the intestine is not excessive due to the delay in gastric evacuation produced by concentrated solutions of sugar in the small intestine[5]. The phenomenon of absorptive selectivity is exhibited for sugars to a marked degree: each sugar is absorbed at a rate determined only by its molecular configuration so that the dextro and laevulo forms of a particular sugar have different rates of absorption[6]. The order of intestinal acceptance for different sugars varies with the species.

Polypeptides and even native proteins probably are absorbed from the intestine to only a limited extent[7] but the greatest part of the protein is absorbed as amino acid. The intracellular peptidases of the epithelium may act as a chemical barrier to the uptake of proteins in their native state but is possible that certain proteins may be reconstituted from their constituent amino acids after transit through the intestinal mucosa. No good evidence has supported the belief that native proteins may be absorbed more readily when the epithelium of the intestine is eroded. The chief route of amino acid transport is the portal system so that all dietary proteins are subjected to liver metabolic activities. This may be expected to affect the therapeutic value of parentrally useful protein preparations when they are given by mouth.

---

[1] HEJDA 1930.   [2] Fox and GRIMSON 1950.   [3] NOCKER 1950.   [4] CORI and CORI 1928.
[5] THOMAS 1957.   [6] CORI 1925, 1931, HEWITT 1924.
[7] SALTER and LERMAN 1935, NEWEY and SMITH 1957.

Absorption of inorganic salts. The phenomenon of selective absorption is well exhibited by inorganic ions. Ammonium, sodium and potassium are the most readily absorbed cations and magnesium and barium the least[1]. Of the anions, the halogens and acetate are aborbed readily while sulfate, phosphate, citrate and oxalate radicles are absorbed in small amounts only[2]. Unabsorbable salts (such as magnesium sulfate) may exert sufficient osmotic activity to prevent the reabsorption of the digestive secretions from the stomach, pancreas, and liver. The retained fluid, by distension of the intestine, may thus act as a stimulus to initiate rush peristalsis or catharsis. The osmotic activity of the unabsorable salt may be great enough to even withdraw fluid from the tissues and lead to dehydration. Other inorganic salts may be unabsorbable because they form large colloidal complexes. The colloidal phosphates and hydroxides of aluminum are prominent examples of therapeutic use.

The concentration at which salts are absorbed at optimum rates is not well known. For sodium chloride this is said to be between 0.6 and 0.8 per cent. When ingested in concentrations other than this, the optimum concentration is said to be attained by adjustments in the rate of water absorption and possibly by active secretion of water. More recent work with radio-active sodium, however, casts grave doubts on the validity of many older experiments and one may expect great advances in this field of absorption to be made in the near future.

The so-called "co-absorptive functions" of the digestive secretions have an important influence on the uptake of iron and calcium salts. Unless ingested in readily ionizable form, these minerals remain largely undissociated and unabsorbed. The absence of acid gastric juice, which is needed to provide the intestinal p_H levels for dissociation of these salts, may account for the development of nutritional anemias and osteoporosis in patients with achlorhydria or massive gastric resections. In pancreatic disease, however, the poor absorption of calcium may be secondary to the excretion of the calcium as soaps due to impariment in fat digestion and absorption.

Details about the process of iron absorption are still largely conjectural. It is well established that the ferrous form of iron is absorbed more readily than the ferric[3, 4] and that dietary iron, which is usually ferric, must first be prepared in the gastrointestinal tract by acid and reducing agents (e.g., ascorbic acid). Apparently iron absorption is regulated by the amount of iron stored in the gastrointestinal tissue. The gastrointestinal depot iron is in equilibrium with the plasma iron and when the latter is low, as in chronic anemia and hemorrhage, the intestinal absorption of iron may be increased 5 to 15 fold, especially if it is already in the ferrous form[5].

It is believed that some of the ferrous iron taken up by the intestinal epithelium combines with apoferritin to form ferritin[6], the intestinal depot iron, from which it is released into the circulation as needed. Some of the absorbed iron, however, passes directly into the portal system and is transferred to the liver mainly as a complex with serum globulin. Presumably the proportion of iron converted to ferritin is determined by the degree to which iron goes directly into the circulation and the amount of apoferritin available. Since all iron is absorbed by the capillary vessels and none by the lymphatics[7], the action of the liver on the absorbed iron will determine the gradient in concentrations between liver and intestine. The altered iron absorption in febrile states may reflect the role of the liver in iron utilization.

[1] Budolfsen 1956.   [2] Vischer et al. 1944.   [3] Moore et al. 1939.
[4] Hahn et al. 1945.   [5] Moore et al. 1944.   [6] Granick 1946.   [7] Labarre, J. 1942.

The concept of "physiological saturation" of iron storage depots, based on studies with radioactive iron, may explain failure to increase blood iron levels by dietary regimen above. Unless utilization processes call on and deplete gastro-intestinal iron depots, intestinal absorption will not necessarily be increased. Intestinal tissue saturation with iron may take only one or two hours but depletion is a matter of days[1]. During liver therapy of pernicious anemia patients, the serum iron falls because of increased hematopoiesis, but iron absorption from the intestine does not increase until much later[2]. Lest, however, the problem of iron absorption is made to appear as simply a matter of control by the intestinal mucosa, it should be noted that in untreated pernicious anemia iron absorption may be at high rates even though iron is not being utilized[3], and also that normal iron absorption may occur following extensive enterectomy.

Hemoglobin is readily digested in the gastrointestinal tract and its degradation products absorbed. In gastro-intestinal hemorrhage, therefore, an elevated serum iron level may accompany the azotemia even though the hemoglobin level is reduced[4].

Absorption from the stomach and colon. The stomach is not primarily an organ for the absorption of digestion products but under experimental conditions appears to have this property to a limited degree. Dextrose and sucrose are not absorbed from the stomach of the cat, rat, dog and man if the gastric mucosa is not hyperaemic and not distended[5]. From chemical studies it is concluded that the absorption of neutral fats from the stomach is likewise negligible[6] but this is not supported by the histological appearance of the gastric mucosa showing fat droplets[7]. The studies on fat absorption are all fairly old and one may expect that the use of isotope-tagged lipids will yield a wealth of important new information.

Intestinal contents reaching the colon are essentially a liquid mass of feces from which all absorbably nutrient has already been removed. The principle function of the colon is the reabsorption of water and electrolytes: the importance of this function is made striking by the dehydration of the patient with diarrhea.

Literature.

ABBOTT, W. O., and T. G. MILLER: Intubation studies of the human small intestine. J. Amer. med. Ass. **106**, 16 (1936). — ABRAMS, G. D., and B. L. BAKER: The cytology and secretory activity of gastric zymogenic cells after ablation of the ductless glands. Gastro-enterology **27**, 462 (1954). — AGREN, G: Über die pharmakodynamischen Wirkungen und chemischen Eigenschaften des Secretins. Skand. Arch. Physiol. **70**, 10 (1934). — AGREN, G., H. LAGERLÖF and H. BERGLUND: Secretin test of pancreatic function in diagnosis of pancreatic disease. Acta med. scand. **90**, 244—271 (1936). — AHLSTRÖM, C. G., K. HAEGER, D. JACOB-SOHN and G. KAHLSON: Atrophy of the gastrointestinal tract after hypophysectomy or adrenalectomy. Acta physiol. scand. **25**, Suppl. 89, 4 (1951). — ALLEY, A.: The inhibitory effect of histamine on gastric secretion. Amer. J. dig. Dis. **1**, 787 (1935). — ALVAREZ, W. C.: An introduction to gastroenterology, 4. edit. New York: Paul B. Hoeber 1948. — AMBACHE, N.: Electrical activity of isolated mammalian intestine. J. Physiol. (Lond.) **106**, 139 (1947). — ANREP, G. V.: Observations on augmented salivary secretion. J. Physiol. (Lond.) **56**, 263 (1922). — ANSON, M. L.: Crystalline carboxypolypeptidase. Science **81**, 467—468 (1935). — ARCHIBALD, E.: The experimental production of pancreatitis in animals as the result of the resistance of the common duct sphincter. Surg. Gynec. Obstet. **28**, 529—545 (1919). — ASHFORD, C. A., H. HELLER and G. A. SMART: Action of histamine on hydrochloric acid and pepsin secretion in man. Brit. J. Pharmacol. **4**, 153 (1949). ~ Effect of antihistamine substance on gastric secretions in man. Brit. J. Pharmacol. **4**, 157 (1949). — ATKINSON, M., and K. S. HENLEY: Levels of intragastric and intraduodenal acidity. Clin. Sci. **14**, 14 (1955).

---

[1] HAHN et al. 1943.   [2] HEMMELER 1943.   [3] DUBACH, CALLENDER and MOORE 1948.
[4] BLACK and POWELL 1942.
[5] LONDON and POLOWZOWA 1906, 1908, MADDOCK, TRIMBLE and CAREY jr. 1933.
[6] VOLHARD 1900.   [7] SCHILLING 1901.

Babkin, B. P.: Die Sekretorische Tätigkeit der Verdauungsdrüsen. In Handbuch der normalen und pathologischen Physiologie, Bd. 3, S. 689—818. Berlin: Springer 1927. ~ Die äußere Sekretion der Verdauungsdrüsen. Berlin: Springer 1928. ~ Address on factors regulating composition of gastric juice. Canad. med. Ass. J. 25, 134—139 (1931). ~ The factors regulating the composition of the gastric juice. Canad. med. Ass. J. 25, 134 (1931b). ~ Does the stomach secrete gastric juice continuously? Libman Anniversary volumes. Vol. 1, p. 113. New York: International Press 1932. ~ Chemical phase of gastric secretion and its regulation. Amer. J. dig. Dis. 1, 715 (1934). ~ Testing of the secretory activity of the gastric glands in man by means of histamine and insulin. Amer. J. dig. Dis. 5, 753 (1939). ~ Antagonistic and synergistic phenomena in the autonomic nervous system. Trans. roy. Soc. Can., Ser. III, Sec. V 40, 1—25 (1946). ~ Secretory mechanism of the digestive glands, 2. edit. New York: Paul Hoeber 1950. — Babkin, B. P., J. C. Armour and D. R. Webster: Restoration of functional capacity of stomach when deprived of its main arterial blood supply. (Louis Gross memorial lecture.) Canad. med. Ass. J. 48, 1—10 (1943). — Babkin, B. P., A. F. Chaisson and M. H. F. Friedman: Factors determining the course of the gastric secretion in elasmobranchs. J. biol. Board Canada 1, 251 (1935). — Babkin, B. P., M. H. F. Friedman and M. E. MacKay-Sawyer: Vagal and sympathetic innervation of the stomach of the skate. J. biol. Board Canada 1, 239 (1935/36). — Babkin, B. P., C. O. Hebb and M. A. Sergeyeva: Parasympathetic-like effect of splanchnic nerve stimulation on pancreatic secretion. Quart. J. exp. Physiol. 29, 217—237 (1939). — Babkin, B. P., O. Komarov and S. A. Komarov: Effect of activated ergosterol and of parathyroid hormone on gastric secretions in the dog. Endocrinology 26, 703 (1940). — Babkin, B. P., W. J. Rubaschkin u. W. W. Ssawitsch: Über die morphologischen Veränderungen der Pankreaszellen unter Einwirkung verschiedenartiger Reize. Arch. mikr. Anat. 74, 68—104 (1909). — Babkin, B. P., et W. W. Ssawitsch: L'influence des solutions acids du sucre sur la production des ferments pancréatiques. J. Russ. Physiol. 3, 143 (1921). Cited by Babkin, 1928. — Baker, B. S., and G. D. Abrams: Effect of hypophysectomy on the cytology of the fundic gland of the stomach and on the secretion of pepsin. Amer. J. Physiol. 177, 409—412 (1954). — Baker, B. S., and R. M. Bridgman: The histology of the gastrointestinal mucosa after adrenolectomy or administration of adrenocorticoid hormones. Amer. J. Anat. 94, 363 (1954). — Ball, E. G.: The composition of pancreatic juice and blood serum as influenced by injection of acid and base. J. biol. Chem. 86, 433—448 (1930). — Ballem, C. M., R. L. Noble and D. R. Webster: A new parasympathetic stimulantethyl 3:3 dimethylallyl barbituric acid. Canad. med. Ass. J. 58, 477 (1948). — Bandes, J., F. Hollander and W. Bierman: Effect of physically induced pyrexia on gastric acidity. Gastroenterology 10, 697—707 (1948). — Barclay, A. E.: The normal mechanism of swallowing. Brit. J. Radiol. 3, 534—546 (1930). — Barcroft, J., and F. R. Steggerda: Observations on the proximal portion of the exteriorized colon. J. Physiol. (Lond.) 76, 460—471 (1932). — Barker, W. H., and C. P. Rhoads: The effect of liver extract on the absorption of fat in sprue. Amer. J. med. Sci. 194, 804 (1937). — Barlow, T. E.: Vascular patterns in the alimentory canal. In: Visceral circulation, edit. by G. W. W. Wolstenholme. Boston: Little & Brown 1953, 278 p. — Baxter, S. G.: Sympathetic secretory innervation of gastric mucosa. Amer. J. dig. Dis. 1, 36 (1934a). ~ Role of the sympathetic nervous system in gastric secretion. Amer. J. dig. Dis. 1, 40 (1934b). Bayliss, W. M., and E. H. Starling: The movements and innervation of the small intestine. J. Physiol. (Lond.) 24, 99—143 (1899). ~ The movements and innervation of the small intestine. J. Physiol. (Lond.) 26, 125—138 (1901). ~ The mechanism of pancreatic secretion. J. Physiol. (Lond.) 28, 325—353 (1902). — Bazett, H. C., and W. G. Penfield: A study of the Sherrington decerebrate animal in the chronic as well as the acute condition. Brain 45, 185—265 (1922). — Beamer, W. D., M. H. F. Friedman, J. E. Thomas and M. E. Rehfuss: Factors responsible for the intestinal phase of gastric secretion. Amer. J. Physiol. 141, 613—618 (1944). — Beattie, J.: The relation of the tuber cinereum to gastric and cardiac functions. Canad. med. Ass. J. 26, 278 (1932). — Beattie, J., G. R. Brow and C. N. H. Long: Physiological and anatomical evidence for the existence of nerve tracts connecting the hypothalamus with spinal sympathetic centers. Proc. roy. Soc. B 106, 253 to 274 (1930). — Beaumont, W.: Experiments and observations on the gastric juice and the physiology of digestion. Plattsburgh, 1933, reprinted Boston 1929, p. 106. — Becks, H.: Human saliva. VII. A study of rate of flow of resting saliva. J. dent. Res. 18, 431—440 (1939). — Becks, H., W. W. Wainwright and D. Young: Further studies of the calcium and phosphorus content of resting and activated saliva of caries-free and caries active individuals. J. dent. Res. 22, 139—146 (1943). — Bennett, T. I., and J. A. Ryle: Studies in gastric secretion. V. A study of normal gastric function based on one hundred healthy men by means of the fractional method of gastric analysis. Guy's Hosp. Rep. 71, 286 (1921). Cit. by Vanzant et al. 1932. — Bernard, C.: Du rôle des actions réflexes paralysantes dans les phénomènes des sécrétions. J. Anat. (Paris) 1, 507 (1864). ~ Leçons de physiologie experimentale appliquées à la médicine, vol. II, p. 278. Paris: Martinet 1856. — Biedermann, W.:

Wintersteins Handbuch der vergleichenden Physiologie. Bd. 2: Die Aufnahme, Verarbeitung und Assimilation der Nahrung. Jena: Gustav Fischer 1911. — BIGGS, M. W., M. FRIEDMAN and S. O. BYERS: Intestinal lymphatic transport of absorbed cholesterol. Proc. Soc. exp. Biol. (N.Y.) 78, 641—643 (1951). — BLACK, D. A. K., and J. F. POWELL: Absorption of hemoglobin iron. Biochem. J. 36, 110 (1942). — BLACK, G. V.: An investigation of the physical characters of the human teeth, etc. II. The force exerted in the closure of the jaws. Dent. Cosmos 37, 496 (1895). — BLICKENSTAFF, D., and M. I. GROSSMAN: A quantitive study of the reduction of gastric acid secretion associated with pyrexia. Amer. J. Physiol. 160, 567—571 (1950). — BLOOMFIELD, A. L., C. K. CHEN and L. R. FRENCH: Basal gastric secretion as a clinical test of gastric function with special reference to peptic ulcer. J. clin. Invest. 19, 803 (1940). — BLOOMFIELD, A. L., and C. S. KEEFER: Gastric acidity. Relation to various factors such as age and physical fitness. J. clin. Invest. 5, 285 (1928). — BOLDYREFF, W. N.: Die periodische Tätigkeit des Verdauungsapparates außer der Verdauungszeit. Zbl. Physiol. 18, 489—493. ~ Über den Übergang des Darmsaftes und der Galle in den Magen. Die Bedingungen und wahrscheinliche Bedeutung dieser Erscheinung. Zbl. Physiol. 18, 457—460 (1904). ~ Diss. St. Petersburg 1904. Zit. bei BABKIN 1927. ~ Die Lipase des Darmsaftes und ihre Charakteristik. Hoppe-Seylers Z. physiol. Chem. 50, 394 (1912). Zit. bei BABKIN 1927. — BORN, G. V. R., and J. R. VANE: Gastric secretion induced by histamine. J. Physiol. (Lond.) 121, 445—451 (1953). — BOWIE, D. J., and A. M. VINEBERG: The selective action of histamine and the effect of prolonged vagal stimulation on the cells of gastric glands in the dog. Quart. J. exp. Physiol. 25, 247 (1935). — BOZLER, E.: Myenteric reflex. Amer. J. Physiol. 157, 329—336 (1949a). ~ Reflex peristalsis of the intestine. Amer. J. Physiol. 157, 338—342 (1949b). — BRODY, D. A., and J. P. QUIGLEY: Intralumen pressure of stomach and duodenum in health and disease. Gastroenterology 9, 570 (1947). — BRODY, D. A., J. M. WERLE, I. MESCHAN and J. P. QUIGLEY: Intralumen pressures of the digestive tract, especially the pyloric region. Amer. J. Physiol. 130, 791—801 (1940). — BROWN, G. M., E. C. R. PURCHASE and T. J. BRESNAHAN: Nocturnal gastric contents in duodenal ulcer and non-ulcer dyspepsia. Gastroenterology 21, 333 (1952). — BRUCKE, E.: Beiträge zur Lehre von der Verdauung. S.-B. Akad. Wiss. 43 (2), 601 (1861). Zit. bei W. SAHLI, Pflügers Arch. ges. Physiol. 36, 209 (1885). — BRUEGEL, C.: Die Beeinflussung des Magenchemismus durch Röntgenstrahlen. Münch. med. Wschr. 64, 379 (1917).— BUCHER, G. R.: Uropepsin: A review of the literature and report of some experiental findings. Gastroenterology 8, No 5 (1947). — BUDOLFSEN, S. E.: The influence of different ions on the intestinal absorption of sodium and chloride. Acta physiol. scand. 38, 31 (1956). — BURKE, J. O., K. PLUMMER and S. BRADFORD: Serum amylase response to morphine, mecholyl and secretin as a test of pancreatic function. Gastroenterology 15, 699—707 (1950).

CANNON, W. B.: The movements of the intestine studied by means of the röntgen ray. Amer. J. Physiol. 6, 251—277 (1902). ~ Oesophageal peristalsis after bilateral vagotomy. Amer. J. Physiol. 19, 436—444 (1907). ~ The mechanical factors of digestion. New York: Longmans 1911a. ~ The nature of gastric peristalsis. Amer. J. Physiol. 29, 250—266 (1911b). ~ Peristalsis, segmentation and the myenteric reflex. AmerJ. Physiol. 30, 114—128 (1912). ~ Digestion and health. New York: Norton 1936. — CANNON, W. B., and C. W. LIEB: The receptive relaxation of the stomach. Amer. J. Physiol. 27 (proc.), xiii 1910). — CANNON, W. B., and A. MOSER: The movements of food in the esophagus. Amer. J. Physiol. 1, 435—444 (1898). — CANNON, W. B., and F. T. MURPHY: The movements of the stomach and intestines in some surgical conditions. Ann. Surg. 43, 512—526 (1906). — CANNON, W. B., and A. ROSENBLUEHT: The supersensitivity of denervated structures. A law of denervation. New York: Macmillan 1949. — CANNON, W. B., and A. L. WASHBURN: An explanation of hunger. Amer. J. Physiol. 29, 441—454 (1912). — CARLSON, A. J.: The control of hunger in health and disease. Chicago, Ill.: University Chicago Press 1916. ~ The secretion of gastric juice in health and disease. Physiol. Rev. 3, 1 (1923). — CARLSON, A. J., T. E. BOYD and J. F. PEARCY: Studies on visceral sensory nervous system; innervation of cardia and lower end of esophagus in mammals. Amer. J. Physiol. 61, 14—41 (1922). — CASE, J. T., and W. N. BOLDYREFF: Influence of roentgen rays in gastric secretion. Amer. J. Roentgenol. 19, 61—70 (1928). — CHAUCHARD, A., et B. CHAUCHARD: Etude comparative de l'excitabilité des fibres sécrétoires et des fibres vasodilatatrices de la corde du tympan. C. R. Soc. Biol. (Paris) 100, 825 (1929). — CHERRY, I. S., and L. A. CRANDALL jr.: The specificity of pancreatic lipase; its appearance in the blood after pancreatic injury. Amer. J. Physiol. 100, 266—273 (1932). — CODE, C. F.: The inhibition of gastric secretion. Pharmacol. Rev. 3, 59—106 (1951). — CODE, C. F., B. CREAMER, J. F. SCHLEGEL and others: An atlas of esophageal motility. Springfield, Ill.: Ch. C. Thomas 1958. — CODE, C. F., G. A. HALLENBECK and R. A. GEGORY: Histamine content of canine gastric juice. Amer. J. Physiol. 151, 593—605 (1947). — CODE, C. F., N. C. HIGHTOWER jr. and C. G. MORLOCK: Motility of the alimentary canal in man. Review of recent studies. Amer. J. Med. 13, 328 (1952). — CODE, C. F., G. R. WILKINSON jr. and W. G. SAUER: Normal and some abnormal colonic motor patterns in man. Ann. N.Y. Acad. Sci. 58, 317 (1954). — Cole, L. G.: The complex motor phenomena of various types of unobstructed gastric peristalsis. Arch. Roentg. Ray 16, 242—247, 259—261 (1911). ~ The living stomach and its motor phenomenon. Acta radiol. (Stockh.) 9, 533—545 (1928). — Comfort, M. W.: Serum lipase: its diagnostic value. Amer. J. dig. Dis. 3, 817—821 (1937). — Conly, S. S., J. O. Crider and J. E. Thomas: Relation of bicarbonate concentration of pancreatic juice to rate of secretion. Amer. J. Physiol. 182, 97 (1955). — Conway, E. J.: The biochemistry of gastric acid secretion. Springfield, Ill.: Ch. C. Thomas 1953. 185 pp. — Cori, C. F.: Fate of sugar in the animal body. Rate of absorption of hexoses and pentoses from the intestinal tract. J. biol. Chem. 66, 691 (1925). ~ Mammalian carbohydrate metabolism. Physiol. Rev. 11, 143 (1931). — Cori, C. F., and G. T. Cori: Relation between absorption and utilization of galactose. Proc. Soc. exp. Biol. (N.Y.) 25, 402 (1928). — Cowgill, G. R., and E. R. Smith: Protein as a stimulant for secretion of pepsin. Proc. Soc. exp. Biol. (N.Y.) 30, 1228 (1933). — Cox, A. J.: Variations in size of the human stomach. Calif. west. Med. 63, 267 (1945). — Cox jr., A. J., and V. R. Barnes: Experimental hyperplasia of the stomach mucosa. Proc. Soc. exper. Biol. (N.Y.) 60, 118 (1945). — Crafts, R. C., and B. S. Walker: The effects of hypophysectomy on gastric acidity of adult female rats. Endocrinology 40, 395 (1947). — Crane, E. E., and R. E. Davies: Chemical and electrical energy relations of stomach. Biochem. J. 49,169—175 (1951).— Crane, E. E., R. E. Davies and N. M. Longmuir: Relations between hydrochloric acid secretion and electrical phenomena in frog gastric mucosa. Biochem. J. 43, 321—336 (1948). — Crider, J. O., and J. E. Thomas: Secretion of pancreatic juice after cutting the extrinsic nerves. Amer. J. Physiol. 141, 730—737 (1944). — Crider, R., and S. Walker: Physiological studies on the stomach of a woman with a gastric fistula. Arch. Surg. (Chicago) 57, 1—1 (1948). — Cutter, R. D.: The normal gastric secretion of infants and small children following stimulation with histamine. J. Pediat. 12, 1—15 (1938). — Cutting, W. C., E. C. Dodds, R. L. Moble and P. C. Williams: Pituitary control of alimentary blood flow and secretion; gastric secretion and blood flow in hypophysectomized animals. Proc. roy. Soc. Lond. 123, 49 (1937).

Dahm, M., u. E. Schorre: Das Röntgenbewegungsbild bei Schlucklähmungen. Fortschr. Röntgenstr. 56, 598—615 (1937). — Davenport, H. W.: Metabolic aspects of gastric acid secretion. In: Metabolic aspects of transport accross cell membranes, edit. Q. R. Murphy, p. 295. Madison, Wisconsin: University of Wisconsin Press 1957. — Davey, L., B. Kaoda and J. Fultem: Effect on gastric secretion of frontal lobe stimulation. Res. Publ. Ass. nerv. ment. Diss. 29, 617 (1950). — Davies, R. E.: Hydrochloric acid production by isolated gastric mucosa. Biochem. J. 42, 621—627 (1948). — Davies, R. E., and A. G. Ogsten: On the mechanism of secretion of ione by the gastric mucosa and by other tissues. Biochem. J. 46, 324 (1950). — Day, J. J., and S. A. Komarov: Glucose and gastric secretion. Amer. J. dig. Dis. 6, 169 (1939). — Day, J. J., and D. R. Webster: The autoregulation of the gastric secretion. Amer. J. dig. Dis. 2, 527 (1935/36). — De Beer, E. J., C. G. Johnston and D. W. Wilson: Composition of intestinal secretions. J. biol. Chem. 108, 113 (1935). — Delenzenne, C., et A. Frouin: La secretion physiologique du suc intestinal. Action l'acide chlorhydrique sur le secretion duodenale. C. R. Soc. Biol. (Paris) 56, 319 (1904). Cit. by Babkin 1950. — Dessecker, C.: Beitrag zur pathologischen Physiologie des Schluckaktes und zur Füllung des Bronchialbaumes mit Röntgenbrei. Mitt. Grenzgeb. Med. Chir. 37, 41—50 (1923). — Dorchester, J. E. C., and R. E. Haist: The secretin content of the intestine in normal and hypophysectomized rats. J. Physiol. 118 (2), 188 (1952). — Doscherholmen, A.: On the action of the anti histamine agent lergitin on the gastric secretion of hydrochloric acid. Acta med. scand. 135, 195 (1949). — Douglas, D. M.: The decrease in frequency of contraction of the jejunum after transplantation to the ileum. J. Physiol. (Lond.) 110, 66—75 (1949). — Douglas, D. M., and F. C. Mann: The activity of the lower part of the ileum in the dog in relation to the ingestion of food. Amer. J. dig. Dis. 6, 434—439 (1939). ~ The gastro-ileac reflex: Further experimental observations. Amer. J. dig. Dis. 7, 53—57 (1940). — Dragstedt, L. R., H. A. Oberhelman, J. M. Zubiran and E. R. Woodward: Antrum motility as a stimulus for gastric secretion. Gastroenterology 24, 71 (1953). — Drinker, C. K., and J. M. Goffey: Lymphatics, lymph and lymphoid tissue, Vol. 1, p. 529—531. Cambridge: Harvard University Press 1941. — Dubach, R., S. T. E. Callender and C. V. Moore: Iron transport and metabolism. Blood 3, 526—540 (1948).

Edkins, J. S.: The chemical mechanism of gastric secretion. J. Physiol. (Lond.) 34, 183 (1906). — Eichhorn, R., and J. Tracktir: The relationship between anxiety, hypnotically induced emotions and gastric secretion. Gastroenterology 29, 422—431 (1955). — Eisenbrandt, L. L.: Variation in p_H of saliva of 5 individuals. J. dent. Res. 22, 147, 293 (1943). — Elliott, T. R., and E. Barclay-Smith: Antiperistalsis and other muscular activities of the colon. J. Physiol. 31, 272—304 (1904). — Elman, R., and J. M. McCaughan: Collection of entire external secretion of pancreas under sterile conditions and fatal effect of total loss of pancreatic juice. J. exp. Med. 45, 561—570 (1927). — EMMELIN, N., and G. S. KAHLSON: Histamine as a physiological excitant of acid gastric secretion. Acta physiol. scand. 8, 289—304 (1944). — EMMELIN, N., and A. MUREN: Paralytic secretion in cats after treatment with atropine. Acta physiol. scand. 22, 2—3 (1951). ~ Sensitization of the submaxillary gland to chemical stimuli. Acta physiol. scand. 24, 2—3 (1951). — ENGSTRÖM, A., and D. GLICK: The mass of gastric mucosa cells measured by x-ray absorption. Science 111, 379—380 (1950). —ERSPAMER, V., and B. ASERO: Identification of enteramine, the specific hormone of the enterochromaffin system as 5-hydroxytryptamine. Nature (Lond.) 169, 800 (1952). — ESPE, D. L., and C. Y. CANNON: Gastric secretion in ruminants. Amer. J. Physiol. 119, 720 (1937). — EWALD, C. A., u. J. BOAS: Beiträge zur Physiologie und Pathologie der Verdauung. Virchows Arch. path. Anat. 104, 271—305 (1886). — EXNER, A.: Wie schützt sich der Verdauungstrakt vor Verletzungen durch spitze Fremdkörper? Pflügers Arch. ges. Physiol. 89, 253—280 (1902).

FARRELL, J. I.: Contributions to the physiology of gastric secretion. XIII. The response of the glands to substances applied to gastric mucosa. Amer. J. Physiol. 85, 672, 684 (1928). — FAWCETT, D. M., and S. KIRKWOOD: Tyrosine Iodinase. J. biol. Chem. 209, 249—256 (1954).— FELDMAN, M.: Clinical roentgenology of the digestive tract, 3. edit. Baltimore: Williams & Wilkins Company 1948. — FENG, T. P., H. C. HAU and R. K. S. LIM: On the mechanism of the inhibition of gastric secretion by fat. Chin. J. Physiol. 3, 371 (1929). — FERRIER: The functions of the brain, 2. edit., p. 260. New York: G. P. Putnam's Sons 1886. — FETTER, D.: Studies of gastric secretion during electro shock therapy. Amer. J. dig. Dis. 11, 405—406 (1944). — FLEMING, A. J., and F. C. MacINTOSH: The effect of sympathetic stimulation and of autonomic drugs on the paralytic submaxillary gland of the cat. Quart. J. exp. Physiol. 25, 2278 (1935). — FLOREY, H.: Observations on the contractility of lacteals. J. Physiol. (Lond.) 62, 267 (1926/27). ~ Secretion of mucus by the colon. Brit. J. exp. Path. 11, 348 (1930). — FLOREY, H. W., and H. E. HARDING: Observations on the functions of mucus and the early stages of bacterial invasion of the intestinal mucosa. J. Path. Bact. 37, 283 (1933). — FLOREY, H. W., and H. E. HARDING: The functions of Brunner's glands and the pyloric end of the stomach. J. Path. Bact. 37, 431 (1933). ~ Further observations on the secretion of Brunner's glands. J. Path. Bact. 39, 255 (1934). ~ The nature of the hormone controlling Brunner's glands. Quart. J. exp. Physiol. 25, 329 (1935a). ~ Humoral control of secretion of Brunner's glands. Proc. roy. Soc. B 117, 68 (1935b). — FLOREY, H. W., R. D. WRIGHT and M. A. JENNINGS: Secretions of the intestine. Physiol. Rev. 21, 36 (1941). — FOX, H. J., and K. S. GRIMSON: Defective fat absorption following vagotomy. J. Lab. clin. Med. 35, 362—365 (1950). — FRAZER, A. C.: Absorption of triglyceride fat from the intestine. Physiol. Rev. 26, 103 (1946). — FRAZER, A. C., and H. STEWART: Emulsification and absorption of fats and paraffins in the intestine. Nature (Lond.) 149, 167 (1942). — FRIEDMAN, M. H. F.: Gastric secretion in birds. J. cell. comp. Physiol. 13, 219 (1939). ~ Gastric reabsorption of hydrogen ion as mechanism reducing the acidity of parietal secretion. Fed. Proc. 10, 45 (1951). ~ Urinary gastric secretory depressant (urogastrone). In: Vitamins and hormones, Chapt. 9. New York: Academic Press 1951. ~ Gastric secretion in necturus. J. cell. comp. Physiol. 20, 379 (1942). ~ Gastric secretion in the newborn. Amer. J. dig. Dis. 9, 275 (1942). ~ Histamine ineffective in the rat as a gastric secretory stimulant. Proc. Soc. exp. Biol. (N.Y.) 54, 42 (1943). ~ Gastric secretion in the cat. Amer. J. Physiol. 163, 712 (1950). ~ Gastric reabsorption of hydrogen ion as mechanism reducing the acidity of parietal secretion. Fed. Proc. 10, 45 (1951). ~ Mécanismes régularisant l'acidité et la sécrétion gastriques. Acta gastro-ent. belg. 12, 820—824 (1952). ~ Action of anticholinesterase agents on gastric secretion. Fed. Proc. 13, III (1954). — FRIEDMAN, M. H. F., and H. APPERT: Acid secretion by the perfused stomach. Fed. Proc. 15, 67 (1956). — FRIEDMAN, M. H. F., H. APPERT and W. D. BEAMER: Central action of anticholinesterase agents on gastric secretion, heart rate, and blood pressure. Fed. Proc. 14, 50—51 (1955). — FRIEDMAN, M. H. F., and J. C. ARMOUR: Gastric secretion in the ground hog (marmota monax) during hibernation. J. cell. comp. Physiol. 8, 201 (1936). — FRIEDMAN, M. H. F., and E. N. KING: Presence of a specific gastric hormone (gastrin) in the dog's pyloric mucosa. Fed. Proc. 6, 107 (1947). — FRIEDMAN, M. H. F., and I. J. PINCUS: Influence of consistency of food on gastric secretion. Exp. Med. Surg. 3, 100 (1945). — FRIEDMAN, M. H. F., and H. M. PODOLSKY: Prolactin and healing of experimental peptic ulcer. Endocrinology 31, 689 (1942). — FRIEDMAN, M. H. F., R. O. RECKNAGEL, D. J. SANDWEISS and T. L. PATTERSON: Inhibitory effects of urine extracts on gastric secretion. Proc. Soc. exp. Biol. (N.Y.) 41, 509 (1939). — FRIEDMAN, M. H. F., and W. J. SNAPE: Dissociation of secretion of pancreatic enzymes and bicarbonate in patients with chronic pancreatitis. Gastroenterology 15, 296—303 (1950). ~ Color changes in the mucosa of the colon in children as affected by food and psychic stimuli. Fed. Proc. 5, 30 (1946). — FYKE jr., F. E., and C. F. CODE: Resting and deglutition pressures in the pharyngoesophageal region. Gastroenterology 9, 24 (1955).

GAMBLE, J. L., and M. A. McIVER: Acid-base composition of pancreatic juice and bile. J. exp. Med. 48, 849—857 (1928a). ~ Body fluid changes due to continued loss of the external secretion of the pancreas. J. exp. Med. 48, 859—869 (1928b). — Gayet, P., et M. Guillaumie: Sur les modifications de l'excrétion pancréatique consécutives, à l'hyperglycémie des centres encéphaliques. C. R. Soc. Biol. (Paris) 105, 373 (1930). — Gellhorn, E., u. W. Budde: Beiträge zur Physiologie der Magenmuskulatur. Pflügers Arch. ges. Physiol. 200, 604—619 (1923). —Goldberg, S. L.: Intrinsic regulation of gastric acidity. Arch. intern. Med. A 9, 816—825 (1932). — Gordon, O. L., and Y. M. Chernya: (Physiology of the gastric secretion in man): Studies on patients with gastric fistula and artificial esophagus. Klin. Med. (Moskau) 18, 63 (1940). — Granick, S.: Ferritin, increase of protein apoferritin in gastrointestinal mucosa as direct response to iron feeding. Function of ferritin in regulation of iron absorption. J. biol. Chem. 164, 737—746 (1946). — Gray, J. S., W. B. Bradley and A. C. Ivy: On the preparation and biological assay of enterogasterone. Amer. J. Physiol. 118, 463 (1937). — Gray, J. S., E. Wieczorowski and A. C. Ivy: Inhibition of gastric secretion by extracts of normal male urine. Science 89, 489 (1939). — Greengard, H., I. F. Stein jr. and A. C. Ivy: Modification of the pancreatic response to secretin by urine and urine concentrates. Amer. J. Physiol. 134, 245—250 (1941 a, b). ~ Secretinase in blood serum. Amer. J. Physiol. 133, 121—127 (1941a). — Gregory, R. A., and A. C. Ivy: The humoral stimulus of gastric secretion. Quart. J. exp. Physiol. 31, 111 (1941). — Greving, R.: Die Innervation der Speiseröhre. Z. angew. Anat. 15, 327—357 (1919/20). — Griffiths, W. J.: The duodenum and the automatic control of gastric acidity. J. Physiol. (Lond.) 87, 34 (1936). — Griswold, C., and A. T. Shohl: Gastric digestion in new-born infants. Amer. J. Dis. Child. 30, 544—549 (1925). — Grossberg, A. L., S. A. Komarov and H. Shay: Distribution of proteins and enzymatic activities in electrophoretic components of canine pancreatic juice. Amer. J. Physiol. 168, 269—282 (1952). ~ Mucoproteins of gastric juice and mucus and mechanism of their secretion. Amer. J. Physiol. 162, 136 (1950). ~ Proteins of canine gastric juice. Amer. J. Physiol. 165, 1—9 (1951). — Grossman, M. I.: Gastrointestinal Hormones. Physiol. Rev. 30, 33—90 (1950). — Grossman, M. I., and A. C. Ivy: Effect of alloxan upon external secretion of the pancreas. Proc. Soc. exp. Biol. (N.Y.) 63, 62—63 (1946). — Gruby and Delafond: C. R. Acad. Sci. (Paris) 16, 1125 (1843). — Grutzner, P.: Über Fermente im Harn. Dtsch. med. Wschr. 17, 10 (1891).

Hahn, P. F.: Abolishment of alimentary lipemia following injection of heparin. Science 98, 19—20 (1943). — Hahn, P. F., W. F. Bale, J. F. Ross, W. M. Balfour and G. H. Whipple: Radioactive iron absorption by gastrointestinal tract; influence of anemia, anoxia, and antecedent feeding distribution in growing dogs. J. exp. Med. 78, 169—188 (1943). — Hahn, P. F., E. Jones, R. C. Lowe, G. R. Meneely and W. Peacock: Relative absorption and utilization of ferrous and ferric iron in anemia as determined with radioactive isotope. Amer. J. Physiol. 143, 191—197 (1945). — Hall, K.: On fat absorption after ligation of the lacteals. Z. Biol. 62, 448 (1913). — Hambleton, B. F.: Note on movements of the intestinal villi. Amer. J. Physiol. 34, 446—447 (1914). — Hamburger, H. J.: Über das Verhalten des Blasenepithels gegenüber Harnstoff. Arch. Anat. u. Physiol. 1—2, 9—21 (1900). — Handelsman, M. B., L. A. Golden and J. H. Pratt: Effect of variations in diet on absorption of food in absence of pancreatic digestion. J. Nutr. 8, 479—495 (1934). — Harper, A. A.: The effect of extracts of gastric and intestinal mucosa on the secretion of HCl by the cat's stomach. J. Physiol. (Lond.) 105, 31 p. (1946). — Harper, A. A., and H. W. Raper: Pancreozymin, stimulant of secretion of pancreatic enzymes in extracts of small intestine. J. Physiol. (Lond.) 102, 115—125 (1943). — Harper, A. A., and C. C. N. Vass: The control of the external secretion of the pancreas in cats. J. Physiol. (Lond.) 99, 415—435 (1941). — Hart, W. M., and J. E. Thomas: Bicarbonate and chloride of pancreatic juice secreted in response to various stimuli. Gastroenterology 4, 409—420 (1945). — Hegner, K.: Untersuchungen über die Schluckstraße. Arch. Ohr.-, Nas.- u. Kehlk.-Heilk. 140, 387—396 (1936). — Heidenhain, R.: Beiträge zur Kenntnis des Pankreas. Pflügers Arch. ges. Physiol. 10, 557—632 (1875). ~ Hermanns Handbuch der Physiologie, vol. V, part 1. Leipzig 1883. — Heinz, E., and K. J. Öbrink: Acid formation and acidity control in the stomach. Physiol. Rev. 34, 643—673 (1954). — Hejda, B.: Alimentary hyperlipemia; study of lipemic curve. Amer. J. med. Sci. 180, 84—90 (1930). — Hemmeler, G.: L'anémie hypochrome après resection d'estomac. Schweiz. med. Wschr. 72, 1105 (1942). — Henning, N., u. L. Norpoth: Untersuchungen über die sekretorische Funktion des Magens während des nächtlichen Schlafes. Arch. Verdau.-Kr. 53, 64 (1933). — Hertz, A. F.: The passage of food along the alimentary canal. Guy's Hosp. Rep. 61 (46 of S. III), 389—427 (1907). ~ Constipation and allied intestinal disorders. London: Oxford University Press 1909. — Hertz, A. F., and A. Newton: The movements of the colon in man. J. Physiol. (Lond.) 47, 57—65 (1913). — Hess, Alfred F.: The gastric secretion of infants at birth. Amer. J. dig. Dis. 6, 264—276 (1913). — Hess, W. R.: Von den höheren Zentren des vegetativen Funktionssystems. Bull. schweiz. Akad. med. Wiss. 1, 138—164 (1945). — Hessel, G.: Untersuchungen über die Ausscheidung harnfähiger Stoffe in den Magendarmkanal bei nephrektomierten Hunden etc. Z. ges. exp. Med. 91, 267 (1933). — Hewitt, J. A.: The metabolism of carbohydrates. Pt. III. The absorption of glucose, fructose and galactose from the small intestine. Biochem. J. 18,

161 (1924). — HILL, J. K.: The effect of insulin on the secretion of gastric juice in the goat. Quart. J. exp. Biol. 37, 143—190 (1952). — HIRSCH, A.: Weitere Beiträge zur motorischen Funktion des Magens nach Versuchen an Hunden mit Darmfisteln. Zbl. klin. Med. 14, 377—383 (1893). — HIRSCH, G. C.: Form- und Stoffwechsel der Golgi-Körper. Protoplasma-Monogr. 18. Berlin: 1939. ~ Dynamik der Sekretions-Systeme. Verh. der Dtsch. Zool. in Kiel. Leipzig: Geist & Portig 1948. — HIRSCH, G. C., L. C. U. JUNQUEIRA, H. A. ROTHSCHILD u. S. R. DOHI: Die Pankreassaft-Sekretion bei der Ratte. Die kontinuierliche, irreguläre Hungersekretion und ihre Ursachen. Pflügers Arch. ges. Physiol. 264, 78 (1957). — HOERNER, M. T.: Effect of exclusion of pancreatic secretions by avulsion of pancreatic ducts on reaction of the duodenal content. Amer. J. dig. Dis. 2, 295—297 (see also p. 298, 300, 302) (1935). — HOFFMAN, M. M., G. MASSON and M. L. DESBARATS: Role of bile in absorption of steroid hormones from the gastrointestinal tract. Endocrinology 42, 279 (1948). — HOGBEN, C. A.: Gastric anion exchange: its relation to the immediate mechanism of hydrochloric acid secretion. Proc. nat. Acad. Sci. (Wash.) 38, 13—18 (1952). — HOGBEN, C. A. M.: Active transport of chloride by isolated frog gastric epithelium: origin of the gastric mucosal potential. Amer. J. Physiol. 180, 641—649 (1955). — HOLLANDER, F.: The chemistry and mechanics of hydrochloric acid formation in the stomach. Gastroenterology 1, 401—430 (1943). ~ The insulin test for the presence of intact nerve fibers after vagal operations for peptic ulcer. Gastroenterology 7, 607 (1946). ~ The composition and mechanism of formation of gastric acid secretion. Science 110, 57—63 (1949). ~ Gastric secretion of electrolytes. Fed. Proc. 11, 706 (1952). — HOLLANDER, F., and J. STEIN: Mucus, acid and water secretion in the stomach following the injection of pilocarpine. Amer. J. Physiol. 190, 136 (1943). — HOLZLÖHNER, E., u. F. HOFFMANN: Die Drüsentätigkeit bei Nervenreizung. II. Die Beziehungen zwischen Blutstrom und Sekretstrom der Glandula submaxillaris bei Chordareizung. Z. Biol. 91, 522 (1931). — HOUCKGEEST, B. v.: Pflügers Arch. ges. Physiol. 6, 266 (1872). Zit. bei MELTZER u. AUER 1907.

IHRE, B.: Human gastric secretion. Acta med. scand., Suppl. 95 (1938). — INGELFINGER, F. J., R. E. MOSS and J. D. HELM jr.: Effect of atropine upon absorption of vitamin A. J. clin. Invest. 22, 699 (1943). — IRWIN, M. H., H. STEENBOCK and A. R. KEMMERER: Influence of vitamins A, B or D, anemia or fasting upon rate of fat absorption in the rat. J. Nutr. 12, 357 (1936). — IVY, A. C.: Contributions to physiology of stomach; causes of gastric secretion; their practical significance and mechanisms concerned. J. Amer. med. Ass. 85, 877 (1925). ~ Recent advances in physiology of gastric and pancreatic secretion. Northw. Med. (Seattle) 25, 589—592 (1926). — IVY, A. C., J. I. FARRELL and H. C. LUETH: Contributions to the physiology of the pancreas. III. A hormone for external pancreatic secretion. Amer. J. Physiol. 82, 27 (1927). — IVY, A. C., and A. J. JAVOIS: Contributions to the physiology of gastric secretion, etc. Amer. J. Physiol. 71, 583, 591, 604 (1924/25). — IVY, A. C., J. B. MCCARTHY and B. H. ORNDORFF: Effect of exposure of abdominal and thoracic areas to roentgen rays on gastric secretion. J. Amer. med. Ass. 83, 1977—1984 (1924). — IVY, A. C., D. A. VLOEDMAN and J. KEANE: Small intestine in hunger. Amer. J. Physiol. 72, 99—108 (1925).

JAMES, A. H.: The physiology of gastric digestion. London: Edward Arnold 1957. — JENKINS, R., and M. MACGEORGE: Control by radium for gastric acidity. Arch. intern. Med. 70, 714—721 (1940). — JONES, C. M., P. J. CULVER, G. D. DRUMMEY and A. E. RYAN: Modification of fat absorption in the digestive tract by the use of emulsifying agent. Ann. intern. Med. 29, 1 (1948). — JOSEPH, D. R., and S. J. MELTZER: Inhibition of the duodenum coincident with the movements of the pyloric part of the stomach. Amer. J. Physiol. 27 (proc.), XXXI (1910/11).

KAHLSON, G.: The nervous and humoral control of gastric secretion. Brit. med. J. 1948 II, 1091. — KALSER, M. H., and M. I. GROSSMAN: Secretion of trypsin inhibitor in pancreatic juice. Gastroenterology 29, 35 (1955). — KATSCH, G.: Handbuch der inneren Medizin von BERGMANN and STAEHELIN, Bd. 3/1, S. 245. Berlin: Springer 1926. — KELLING, G.: Untersuchungen über die Spannungszustände der Bauchwand, der Magen- und der Darmwand. Z. Biol., N.S. 26, 161—258 (1903). ~ Zur Chirurgie der chronischen, nicht malignen Magenleiden. Arch. Verdau.-Kr. 6, 438—470 (1900). — KEETON, R. W., F. C. KOCH and A. B. LUCKHARDT: Gastrin studies. III. The response of the stomach mucosa of various animals to gastrin bodies. Amer. J. Physiol. 51, 454 (1920). — KING, C. E., and L. ARNOLD: The activities of the intestinal mucosal motor mechanism. Amer. J. Physiol. 59, 97—121 (1922). — KING, C. E., L. ARNOLD and J. G. CHURCH: The physiological role of the intestinal mucosal movements. Amer. J. Physiol. 61, 80—92 (1922). — KIRSNER, J. B., E. LEVIN and W. L. PALMER: Observations on excessive nocturnal gastric secretion in patients with duodenal ulcer. Gastroenterology 11, 598—617 (1948). — KLEIN, EUGENE: Increased acid secretion in a transplanted pouch during lactation. Arch. Surg. (Chicago) 26, 235 (1933). — KOKAS, E. v., u. G. v. LUDÁNY: Die Beobachtung der Zottenbewegung am überlebenden Darm. Pflügers Arch. ges. Physiol. 231, 20—23 (1932). ~ Die hormonale Regelung der Darmzottenbewegung. Pflügers

Arch. ges. Physiol. **232**, 293—298 (1933b). ~ Die hormonale Regelung der Darmzottenbewegung; das *Villikinin*. Pflügers Arch. ges. Physiol. **234**, 182—186 (1934). ~ Die Wirkung der Gewürzmittel auf die Bewegung der Darmzotten und die Glykoseresorption. Naunyn-Schmiedeberg's Arch. exp. Path. Pharmak. **169**, 140—145 (1933a). ~ Relation between villikinine and absorption of glucose from intestine. Quart. J. exp. Physiol. **28**, 15—22 (1938). — Komarov, O., and S. A. Komarov: Effect of olive oil and of cod liver oil on gastric secretion in the dog. Canad. med. Assoc. J. **43**, 129 (1940). — Komarov, S. A.: Gastrin. Proc. Soc. exp. Biol. (N.Y.) **38**, 514 (1938). ~ Studies on gastrin. I. Methods of isolation. Rev. canad. Biol. **1**, 191 (1942). ~ Studies on gastrin. II. Physiological properties. Rev. canad. Biol. **1**, 377 (1942). — Komarov, S. A., G. O. Langstroth and D. R. McRae: The secretion of crystalloids and protein material by the pancreas in response to secretin administration. Canad. J. Res. **17**, 113—123 (1939). — Korff, R. W. v., and D. Glick: Role of urease in gastric mucosa; plasma urea as source of ammonium ion in gastric juice of histamine-stimulated dog. Amer. J. Physiol. **165**, 688 (1951). — Kosaka, T., R. K. S. Lim, S. M. Ling and A. C. Liu: On the mechanism of the inhibition of gastric secretion by fat. A gastric inhibitory agent obtained from the intestinal mucosa. Chin. J. Physiol. **6**, 107 (1932). — Krewer, A. R.: Diss. St. Petersburg 1899. Zit. bei Babkin 1928, S. 526. — Kronecker, H., u. S. J. Meltzer: Der Schluckmechanismus, seine Erregung und seine Hemmung. Arch. Physiol. (DuBois-Raymond) Suppl.-Bd. 1883, S. 328—362. — Küpferle, L.: Zur Physiologie des Schluckmechanismus nach Röntgen-kinematographischen Aufnahmen. Pflügers Arch. ges. Physiol. **152**, 579—588 (1913). — Kunitz, M.: Effect of the formation of an inert protein on the kinetics of the autocatalytic formation of trypsin from trypsinogen. J. gen. Physiol. **22**, 293—310 (1939). — Kunitz, M., and J. H. Northrop: Crystalline chymo-trypsin and chymo-trypsinogen; isolation, crystallization and general properties of new proteolytic encyme and its precursor. J. gen. Physiol. **18**, 433—458 (1935). ~ Isolation from beef pancreas of crystalline trypsinogen, trypsin, trypsin inhibitor, and trypsin-inhibitor compound. J. gen. Physiol. **19**, 991—1007 (1936). — Kuntz, A.: The autonomic nervous system, 4. edit. Philadelphia 1953. — Kutscher, F., and J. Seeman: Hoppe-Seylers Z. physiol. Chem. **35**, 432 (1902). Zit. bei Florey et al. 1942.

Labarre, J.: Absorption et action hématinique du phosphogluconate ferreux. Rev. canad. Biol. **1**, 104 (1942). — Labarre, J., et C. de Cespédes: Rôle du système nerveux central dans l'hypersécrétion gastrique consécutive a l'administration d'insuline. C. R. Soc. Biol. (Paris) **106**, 1249 (1931). — Labarre, J., et P. Destrée: Les functions contractiles et sécrétoires de l'estomac au cours de l'hyperaminoacidémie experimentale. Arch. int. Physiol. **41**, 490 (1935). — Lagerlöf, H.: Normal esterases and pancreatic lipase in the blood· study with new chemical and clinical methods (second secretin test). Acta med. scand. **120**, 407—436 (1945). ~ The secretin test of pancreatic function. Quart. J. Med. **8**, 115—126 (1939). — Lajos, S.: Glucoseresorption aus dem Darm unter der Wirkung von Opium und Atropin. Biochem. Z. **295**, 132 (1938). — Langley, J. N.: On the physiology of the salivary secretion. III. The paralytic secretion of saliva. J. Physiol. (Lond.) **6**, 71 (1885). — Langstroth, G. O., D. R. McRae and S. A. Komarov: The synthesis and secretion of protein material by the pancreas. Canad. J. Res. **17**, 137—149 (1939). — Larsson, L. M., and J. A. Bargen: Action of cathartics on isolated dog's colon. Arch. Surg. (Chicago) **27**, 1120 (1933). — Layne, J. A., and G. S. Bergh: The effect of ligation of the arteries of the stomach upon gastric secretion and upon the endoscopic appearance of the gastric mucosa in dog. Surgery **13**, 136 (1943). — Leach, E. H.: The role of leucocytes in fat absorption. J. Physiol. (Lond.) **93**, 1 (1938). — Leblond, C. P., and C. E. Stevens: The constant renewal of the intestinal epithelium in the albino rat. Anat. Rec. **100**, 357 (1948). — Levin, E., J. B. Kirsner and W. L. Palmer: Differences in gastric secretion in normal individuals and in patients with peptic ulcer. Rev. Gastroent. **19**, 226 (1952). — Lim, R. K. S.: Observations on the mechanism of inhibition of gastric function by fat. Quart. J. exp. Physiol. **23**, 263—268 (1933). — Lim, R. K. S., S. M. Ling and A. C. Liu: Depressor substance in extracts of the intestinal mucosa. Purification of enterogastrone. Chin. J. Physiol. **8**, 219 (1934). Lim, R. K. S., and P. Mozer: Mechanism of excitation of internal secretion of pylorus and adenteric reflex. Amer. J. Physiol. **163**, 730 (1950). — Linde, S.: Studies on the stimulation mechanism of gastric secretion. Acta physiol. scand. **21**, Suppl., 74 (1950). — Linderstrom-Lang, K., and A. S. Ohlsen: Distribution of urease in dog's stomach (studies on enzymatic histochemistry). Entymologia **1**, 92 (1936). — Ling, S. M.: On the question of the portal absorption of fat. Chin. J. Physiol. **12**, 493 (1937). — London, E. S., u. W. W. Polowzowa: Zum Chemismus der Verdauung im tierischen Körper, etc. Z. physiol. chem. Strassb. **54**, 429 (1907/08). — Luckhardt, A. B., H. T. Phillips and A. J. Carlson: Contributions to the physiology of the stomach: LI. The control of the pylorus. Amer. J. Physiol. **50**, 57—66 (1919). — Ludwig, C.: Lehrbuch der Physiologie des Menschen, vol. II, S. 615. Leipzig u. Heidelberg: Wintersche 1861. — Lundberg, A.: Secretory potentials in the sublingual glands of the cat. Acta physiol. scand. **40**, 21 (1957). ~ Electrophysiology of salivary glands. Physiol. Rev. **38**, 21 (1958). — Lushbaugh, C. C., and C. Houck:

Pathology of monkeys exposed to massive doses of total gamma radiation. Fed. Proc. 14, 420 (1955).
MacIntosh, F. C.: Choline-esterase content of normal and denervated submaxillary gland of the cat. Proc. Soc. exp. Biol. (N.Y.) 37, 248 (1937). ~ Histamine as a normal stimulant of gastric secretion. Quant. J. exp. Physiol. 28, 87 (1938). — Macklin, C. C., and M. T. Macklin: The intestinal epithelium: in special cytology, E. V. Cowdry, editor, 2. edit., vol 1, p. 233—325. New York: Paul B. Hoeber 1932. — Maddock, S. J., H. C. Trimble and B. W. Carey jr.: Is d-glucose absorbed from stomach of dog? J. biol. Chem. 103, 285 (1933). — Magendie, F.: Précis élémentaire de physiologie. Paris 1836. Trans. by Revere, 5. edit. New York: Harper Bros 1838. — Magnus, R.: Versuche am überlebenden Dünndarm von Säugetieren. Pflügers Arch. ges. Physiol. 102, 123, 349 (1904). — Magnus, W. O. C.: Über die Zentren für Lecken und Kauen. Mschr. Psychiat. Neurol. 110, 193—235 (1945). — Magoun, H. W., S. W. Ranson and C. Fisher: Cortifugal pathways for mastication, lapping and other motor functions in the cat. Arch. Neurol. Psychiat. (Chicago) 30, 292—308 (1933).— Mahl, G. F.: Effect of chronic fear on the gastric secretion of HCl in dogs. Psychosom. Med. 11, 30 (1949).—Mangold, E.: Handbuch der Ernährung und des Stoffwechsels der landwirtschaftlichen Nutztiere, Bd. 2. Berlin: Springer 1929. — Mann, F. C., and J. L. Bollman: Reaction of content of gastrointestinal tract. J. Amer. med. Ass. 95, 1722—1724 (1930). — Marder, L., G. H. Becker, B. Maizel and H. Necheles: Fat absorption and chylomicronemia. Gastroenterology 20, 43—59 (1952). — Markwald, M.: Über die Ausbreitung der Erregung und Hemmung vom Schluckzentrum auf das Atemzentrum. Z. Biol. 7, 1—54 (1889). — Mathews, A. P.: Physiological chemistry, 3. edit., p. 375. New York: Wood 1920. — McCarthy, J. D., S. O. Evans and L. R. Dragstedt: Gastric secretion in dogs during pregnancy and lactation. Gastroenterology 27, 275—280 (1954). — McGinty, D. A., M. L. Wilson and G. Rodney: The ulcer-inhibiting action of pyrogens. Proc. Soc. exp. Biol. (N.Y.) 70, 334 (1949). — McKendry, J. B. R.: Intracavitary visceral radiation: Effect on gastric acid secretion. Proc. Soc. exp. Biol. (N.Y.) 75, 25 (1950). — Meltzer (1908): Zit. bei Schreiber, Arch. Verdau.-Kr. 21, 1—15 (1915). — Meltzer, S. J.: A further experimental contribution to the knowledge of the mechanism of deglutition. J. exp. Med. 2, 453—464 (1897). ~ On the causes of the orderly progress of the peristaltic movements in the esophagus. Amer. J. Physiol. 2, 266—272 (1899). — Meltzer, S. J., and J. Auer: Peristaltic rush. Amer. J. Physiol. 20, 259—281 (1907). — Mering, J. v.: Über die Funktion des Magens. Verh. Kongr. inn. Med. 12, 471—487 (1893). — Mering, J. v., u. O. Minkowski: Diabetes mellitus nach Pankreasexstirpation. Naunyn-Schmiedeberg's Arch. exp. Path. Pharmak. 26, 371—387 (1889). — Meschan, I., and J. P. Quigley: Spontaneous motility of the pyloric sphincter ans adjacent regions of the gut in the unanesthetized dog. Amer. J. Physiol. 121, 350—357 (1938). — Meyer, J., S. J. Cohen and A. J. Carlson: Contribution to the physiology of the stomach. XLVI. Gastric secretion during fever. Arch. intern. Med. 21, 354—365 (1918). — Meyer, J., and H. Necheles: Studies in old age. IV. The clinical significance of salivary, gastric and pancreatic secretion in the aged. J. Amer. med. Ass. 115, 2050—2053 (1940). — Meyer, J., E. Spier and F. Newelt: Basal secretion of digestive enzymes in old age. Arch. intern. Med. 65, 171—177 (1940). — Miescher, G.: Über den Einfluß der Röntgenstrahlen auf die Sekretion des Magens. Strahlentherapie 15, 252—272 (1923). — Miller, F. R.: The cortical paths for mastication and deglutition. J. Physiol. (Lond.) 53, 473—478 (1920). — Miller, R. A.: Observations on the gastric acidity during the first month of life. Arch. Dis. Childh. 16, 22—30 (1941). — Miller, R. J., O. Bergeim, M. E. Rehfus and P. B. Hawk: Gastric response to foods, etc. Amer. J. Physiol. 51, 322; 52, 1, 28, 248; 53, 65 (1920). — Miller, T. G., and W. O. Abbott: Intestinal intubation: a practical technique. Amer. J. med. Sci. 187, 595 (1934). — Milton, G. W., and A. W. M. Smith: The pacemaking area of the duodenum. J. Physiol. (Lond.) 132, 100 (1956). — Milton, G. W., A. W. M. Smith and H. I. O. Armstrong: The origin of the rhythmic electropotential changes in the duodenum. Quart. J. exp. Physiol. 40, 79 (1955). — Miner, R. W. (Editor of symposium): The colon: Its normal and abnormal physiology and therapeutics. Ann. N.Y. Acad. Sci. 58, 293 (1954). — Mirsky, I. A., S. Kaplan and Broh-Kahn: Pepsinogen excretion (uropepsin) as index of influence of various life situations on gastric secretion. Res. Publ. Ass. nerv. ment. Dis. 29, 628—646 (1950). — Moore, C. V., W. R. Arrowsmith, J. Welch and V. Minnick: Studies in iron transportation and metabolism; observations on absorption of iron from gastrointestinal tract. J. clin. Invest. 18, 553—580 (1939). — Moore, C. V., R. Dubach, V. Minnick and H. K. Roberts: Absorption of ferrous and ferric radioactive iron by human subjects and by dogs. J. clin. Invest. 23, 756—766 (1944). — Moreton, J. R.: Chylomicronemia, fat tolerance, and atherosclerosis. J. Lab. clin. Med. 35, 373—384 (1950). — Moritz, S.: Studien über die motorische Tätigkeit des Magens. Z. Biol., N. S. 42, 565—611 (1901). — Morton, G. M., and G. W. Stavraky: A histo-physiological study of the effect of intraarterial injection of acetylcholine upon the gastric mucosa of the dog. Gastroenterology 12, 808—820 (1948). —

Mosher, H. P.: X-ray study of movements of the tongue, epiglottis and hyoid bone in swallowing followed by a discussion of difficulty in swallowing caused by retropharyngeal divirticulum, postcricoid webs and exostoses of cervical vertebrae. Laryngoscope (St. Louis) 37, 235—262 (1927). — Müller, A.: Beiträge zur Kenntnis von den Schutzeinrichtungen des Darmtraktes gegen spitze Fremdkörper. Pflügers Arch. ges. Physiol. 102, 206—216 (1904). — Müller, L. R.: Die Darminnervation. Dtsch. Arch. klin. Med. 105, 1—43 (1911). — Munro, M. P., and J. E. Thomas: The number and relative concentration of protein constituents of canine pancreatic juice as determined by electrophoresis. Amer. J. Physiol. 145, 140—146 (1945).

Nasset, E. S.: Enterocrinin, a hormone which excites the glands of the small intestine. Amer. J. Physiol. 121, 481 (1938). — Nasset, E. S., H. B. Pierce and J. R. Murlin: Proof of a humoral control of intestinal secretion. Amer. J. Physiol. 111, 145 (1935). — Necheles, H.: Depression of the stomach by non-specific substances. Proc. Inst. Med. Chicago 14, 345—346 (1943). — Nocker, J.: Stoffwechseluntersuchungen bei ausgedehnter Dünndarmresektion. Dtsch. Z. Verdau.- u. Stoffwechselkr. 10, 77—79 (1950).

Öbrink, K. J.: Studies on the kinetics of the parietal secretion of the stomach. Acta physiol. scand. 15, 106 (1948). ~ Water permeability of the isolated stomach of the mouse. Acta physiol. scand. 36, 229—244 (1956). — Okada, S., K. Kuramochi, T. Tsukahara and T. Ooinoue: Pancreatic function: secretory mechanism of digestive juices. Arch. intern. Med. 45, 783 (1930). — Olson, W. H., and A. B. Bridgwater: Nocturnal and insulin gastric secretion. J. Amer. med. Ass. 154, 977—981 (1954). — Olson, T. E., and S. J. Gray: Serotonin and gastroenterology. Amer. J. Gastroent. 29, 280 (1958). — Oppenheimer, A.: Ileocecal region. Radiology 34, 545—559 (1940). — Oushakov, V. G.: The effect of the vagus on the secretion of gastric juice. Doctorate dissertation, 1896. Cit. by Babkin 1950.

Palmer, W. L., and F. Templeton: The effect of radiation therapy on gastric secretion. J. Amer. med. Ass. 112, 1424—1434 (1939). — Pancoast, H. K., E. P. Pendergrass and J. P. Schaeffer: The head and neck in roentgen diagnosis, p. 797—798. Springfield, Ill.: Ch. C. Thomas 1940. — Pavlov, I. P.: Beiträge zur Physiologie der Absonderung: Innervation der Bauchspeicheldrüse. Arch. Physiol. Suppl.-Bd.. 176—200 (1893). ~ The work of the digestive glands. Translation by Thompson. London: C. Griffin & Company 1902. ~ The work of the digestive glands. Translated by W. H. Thompson, 2. edit. London: C. Griffin & Company 1910. ~ Conditioned reflexes. Translated by G. V. Anrep. Oxford: University Press 1927. — Pincus, I. J., M. H. F. Friedman, J. E. Thomas and M. E. Rehfuss: A quantitative study of the inhibitory effect of acid in the intestine on gastric secretion. Amer. J. dig. Dis. 11, 205—208 (1944). — Pincus, I. J., J. E. Thomas, D. Hausman and P. O. Lachman: Relationship between the pH of the duodenal content and pancreatic secretion. Proc. Soc. exp. Biol. (N.Y.) 67, 497—501 (1948b). — Pincus, I. J., J. E. Thomas and P. O. Lachman: The effect of vagotomy on secretion of pancreatic juice after ingestion of various foodstuffs. Fed. Proc. 7, 94 (1948a). — Pincus, I. J., J. E. Thomas and M. E. Rehfuss: A study of gastric secretion as influenced by changes in duodenal acidity. Proc. Soc. exp. Biol. (N.Y.) 51, 367 (1942). — Polland, W. S., and A. L. Bloomfield: Normal standards of gastric function. J. clin. Invest. 9, 651 (1931).—Pollitzer, R.: Gastric secretion in the newborn. Pediatrica 29, 253—259 (1921). — Pommerenke, W. T.: A study of sensory areas eliciting the swallowing reflex. Amer. J. Physiol. 84, 36—41 (1928). — Popov, N. A.: Physiology of the Sheep. Moscow 1932. Zit. bei W. Lenkeit, Ergebn. Physiol. 35, 573 (1933). — Popper, H. L.: Acute pancreatitis; evaluation of classification, symptomatology, diagnosis and therapy. Amer. J. dig. Dis. 15, 1—4 (1948).—Popper, H. L., H. Necheles and K. C. Russell: Transition of pancreatic edema into pancreatic necrosis. Surg. Gynec. Obstet. 87, 79—82 (1948). — Portis, S. A., and R. Ahrens: The effect of shorter wave-length roentgen rays on the gastric secretion dogs. Amer. J. Roentgenol. 11, 272—280 (1924).

Quigley, J. P.: Digestive tract: Intralumen pressures with special reference to gastrointestinal propulsion and gastric evacuation. Medical physics, vol. 1, p. 310—318. Chicago: Yearbook Publ. 1944. — Quigley, J. P., H. J. Bavor, M. R. Read and B. L. Brofman: Evidence that body irritations or emotions retard gastric evacuation, not by producing pylorospasm but by depressing gastric motility. J. clin. Invest. 22, 839 (1943). — Quigley, J. P., and D. A. Brody: Digestive tract. Intralumen pressures: Gastrointestinal propulsion, gastric evacuation, pressure-wall tension relationships. Medical Physics, vol. II, p. 280—292. Chicago: Yearbook Publ. 1950. — Quigley, J. P., and M. S. Louckes: The effects of complete vagotomy on the pyloric sphincter and the gastric evacuation mechanisms. Gastroenterology 19, 533 (1951). — Quigley, J. P., and I. Meschan: Action of fats introduced into the duodenum on the pyloric sphincter and adjacent portions of the gut. Amer. J. Physiol. 119, 386 (1937). — Quigley, J. P., and K. R. Phelps: The mechanism of gastric motor inhibition from ingested carbohydrates. Amer. J. Physiol. 109, 133—138 (1934). —

QUIGLEY, J. P., M. R. READ, K. H. RADZON, I. MESCHAN and J. M. WERLE: The effect of hydrochloric acid on the pyloric sphincter, the adjacent portions of the digestive tract and on the process of gastric evacuation. Amer. J. Physiol. 137, 153—159 (1942). — QUIGLEY, J. P., H. J. ZETTELMAN and A. C. IVY: Analysis of the factors involved in gastric motor inhibition by fats. Amer. J. Physiol. 108, 643 (1934).

RAWLINSON, H. E.: Cytological changes after autonomic and adrenalin stimulation of the cat's submaxillary gland. Anat. Rec. 57, 289 (1933). ~ The changes in the alveolar and demilune cells of the simple and the stimulated paralytic submaxillary gland of the cat. J. Anat. (Lond.) 70, 143 (1935). — REGAUD, C., I. NOGIER et A. LACASSAGNE: Sur les effects redoutables des irradiations étendus de l'abdomen et sur les lésions du tube digestif determinées par les rayons des rœntgen. Arch. Elect. méd. 21, 321 (1912). Zit. bei RICKETS et al., Gastroenterology 11, 818 (1948). — REHM, W. S.: A theory of the formation of HCl by the stomach. Gastroenterology 14, 401 (1950). — REHM, W. S., L. E. HOKIN, T. P. DE GRAFFENRIED, F. J. BAJANDAS and F. E. COY jr.: Relationship between potential difference of the resting and secreting stomach. Amer. J. Physiol. 164, 187—201 (1951). — REKERS, P. E., J. C. ABELS and C. P. RHOADS: Metabolic studies in patients with gastrointestinal cancer: fat metabolism, method of study. J. clin. Invest. 22, 243 (1943). — RICKETTS, W. E., W. L. PALMER, J. B. KIRSNER and A. HAMANN: Radiation therapy in peptic ulcer. Gastroenterology 11, 789—806 (1948). — RIOCH, J. McK.: The neural mechanism of mastication. Amer. J. Physiol. 108, 168—176 (1934). — RIOCH, D. McK., and C. BRENNER: Experiments on the corpus striatum and rhinencephalon. J. comp. Neurol. 68, 491—507 (1938). — RITTER, J. A.: Fractional gastric analysis in the newborn. Penn. med. J. 44, 1321 (1941).

SACKS, J., A. C. IVY, J. P. BURGESS and J. E. VANDOLAH: Histamine as the hormone for gastric secretion. Amer. J. Physiol. 101, 331 (1932). — SALASKIN, S. S.: Über das Vorkommen des Peptons bzw. albumosenspaltenden Ferments (Erepsin von Conheim) im reinen Darmsaft vom Hunde. Hoppe-Seylers Z. physiol. Chem. 35, 419 (1902). Zit. bei FLOREY et al. 1941. — SALTER, W. T., and J. LERMAN: Metabolic effects of human thyroglobulin and its proteolytic cleavage products. J. clin. Invest. 14, 691 (1935). — SANDWEISS, D. J.: Enterogastrone, anthelone and urogastrone. Gastroenterology 5, 404 (1945). — SANDWEISS, D. J., M. H. F. FRIEDMAN, M. H. SUGARMAN and H. M. PODOLSKY: Nocturnal gastric secretion. II. Studies on normal subjects and patients with duodenal ulcer. Gastroenterology 7, 38 (1946b). — SANDWEISS, D. J., M. H. SUGARMAN, H. M. PODOLSKY and M. H. F. FRIEDMAN: Nocturnal gastric secretion in duodenal ulcer. J. Amer. med. Ass. 130, 258 (1946a). — SAVITCH, V. V.: The secretion of intestinal juice. Thesis, St. Petersburg 1904. Cit. by BABKIN 1950. ~ Russki vratch. Nr 38, 1912. Cit. by BABKIN 1928. — SAVITCH, V. V., et N. A. SOCHESTVENKY: L'influence du nerf vague sur la sécrétion de l'intestin. C. R. Soc. Biol. (Paris) 80, 508 (1917). — SAVITCH, V., u. G. ZELIONY: Zur Physiologie des Pylorus. Pflügers Arch. ges. Physiol. 150, 128 (1913). — SCHACTER, M.: Anesthesia and gastric secretion. Amer. J. Physiol. 156, 248—255 (1949). — SCHAPIRO, H., and E. R. WOODWARD: Inhibition of gastric motility by acid in duodenum. J. appl. Physiol. 8, 121 (1955). — SCHEPOWALNIKOW, N. P.: Die Physiologie des Darmsaftes [russisch]. Diss. St. Petersburg 1899. Reviewed by WALTHER: Jber. Fortschr. Thier-Chemie 29, 378 (1899). — SCHIFFRIN, M. J.: Relationship between the parathyroid and the gastric glands in the dog. Amer. J. Physiol. 135, 660—669 (1942). — SCHIFFRIN, M. J., and E. S. NASSET: Response of jejunum and ieleum to food and enterocrinin. Amer. J. Physiol. 128, 70 (1939). — SCHIROKICH, P. O.: Zur Frage von dem Übertritt der Speise aus dem Magen in den Darm. Prot. XI. Kongr. Russ. Naturforscher u. Ärzte, 1901, Nr 10, S. 488. Zit. bei BABKIN 1928, S. 833. — SCHOOLEY, J. P., O. RIDDLE and R. W. BATES: Replacement therapy in hypophysectomized juvenile pigeons. Amer. J. Anat. 69, 123 (1941). — SELYE, H.: Role of bile in absorption of steroids. Endocrinology 32, 279 (1943). ~ The general adaptation syndrome. In: Peptic Ulcer, DAVID SANDWEISS, Editor. p. 125. Philadelphia: W. B. Saunders Company 1951. — SHAY, H., J. GERSHON-COHEN and S. S. FELS: A self regulatory duodenal mechanism for gastric acid control and an explanation for the pathologic gastric physiology in uncomplicated duodenal ulcer. Amer. J. dig. Dis. 9, 124—128 (1942). ~ The role of the upper small intestine in the control of gastric secretion, etc. Ann. intern. Med. 13, 294 (1939). — SHEEHAN, C.: The hypothalamus and gastrointestinal regulation. Res. Publ. Ass. nerv. ment. Dis. 20, 589 (1940). — SHERRINGTON, C. S.: Reflexes elicitable in the cat from the pinna, vibrissae and jaws. J. Physiol. (Lond.) 51, 404—431 (1917). — SIMON, N.: Suppression of gastric acidity with beta particles of P^{32}. Science 109, 503—564 (1949). — SLUITER, J. W.: Das Restitutionsproblem in der Pankreaszelle. I. Die Bedeutung des Golgi-Apparates. Z. Zellforsch., Abt. A 33, 187—224 (1944). — SNELL, A. M., and J. L. BOLLMAN: Gastric secretion following irradiation of the exposed stomach and the upper abdominal viscera by roentgen rays. Amer. J. dig. Dis. 1, 164—168 (1934). — SOKOLOV, A. P.: Analysis of the secretory work of the stomach in the dog. Thesis St. Petersburg 1904. — SOMERVILLE, T. H.: Physiological gastrectomy: the operation of ligature of the arteries of the stomach to relieve gastric hyperacidity and to prevent recurrent ulceration after gastro-enterostomy. Brit. J. Surg. **33**, 146 (1945). — Sonnenschein, R. R., M. I. Grossman and A. C. Ivy: The humoral regulation of Brunner's glands. Acta med. scand. **28**, Suppl. 196, 296 (1947). — Soulairac, A.: La régulation neuro-endocrinienne de l'absorption intestinale des glucides. Ann. Endocr. (Paris) **8**, 377—393 (1947). — Spealman, C. R.: Volume flow of resting salivary secretion. Amer. J. Physiol. **139**, 225—229 (1943). — Spiro, H. M., A. E. Ryan and C. M. Jones: The utility of the blood pepsin assay in clinical medicine. New Engl. J. Med. **253**, 261—266 (1955). — Spitzer, J. J.: Properties of heparin-produced lipemia clearing factor. Amer. J. Physiol. **171**, 492 (1952). — Starling, E. H.: Recent advances in the physiology of digestion. London: A. Constable Co. 1906. Cit. by Babkin 1950. — Steinfeld, W.: Suppression of gastric acidity by radio Krypton. Proc. Soc. exp. Biol. (N.Y.) **81**, 636—638 (1952). — Stryker, W. A.: Absorption of liquid petrolatum (mineral oil) from the intestine. Arch. Path. (Chicago) **31**, 670 (1941). — Sutherland, G. F.: The response of the stomach glands to gastrin before and shortly after birth. (Physiology of stomach 57.) Amer. J. Physiol. **55**, 390—403 (1921).

Taylor, N. B.: Physiological basis of medical practice by Best and Taylor, 6. edit., p. 519. Baltimore: Williams & Wilkins 1955.—Taylor, Rood: Hunger and appetite secretion of gastric juice in infant's stomach. Amer. J. Dis. Child. **14**, 258—266 (1917). — Templeton, H. E.: X-ray examination of the stomach. p. 114, 116, 458 and 459. Chicago, Ill.: Chicago University Press 1944. — Teorell, T.: Duodenal regurgitation "versus" electrolyte diffusion in the gastric juice. Acta med. scand. **85**, 518 (1935). ~ On the permeability of the stomach mucosa for acids and some other substances. J. gen. Physiol. **23**, 263 (1939). ~ Transport processes and electrical phenomena in ionic membranes: In Progress in biophysics, edit. by Butler and Randall. New York: Academic Press 1953. — Thiry, L.: Eine neue Methode, den Dünndarm zu isolieren. S.-B. Akad. Wiss. Wien, math.-nat. Kl. 1, **50**, 77 (1864). Zit. bei Babkin 1927. — Thomas, J. E.: The external secretion of the pancreas. Springfield, Ill.: Ch. C. Thomas 1950. ~ Myenteric reflex in dog's duodenum. Fed. Proc. **10**, 136 (1951). ~ Physiology of the external secretion of the pancreas. Trans. N.Y. Acad. Sci., Ser. II 14, 310—313 (1952). ~ The gradient theory versus the reflex theory of intestinal peristalsis. Amer. J. Gastroent. **23**, 13 (1955). ~ Mechanics and regulation of gastric emptying. Physiol. Rev. **37**, 453 (1957). — Thomas, J. E., and J. O. Crider: Carbohydrates as stimuli for secretion of pancreatic enzymes. Fed. Proc. **6**, 214 (1947). ~ The effect of fat on the p_H of the contents of the duodenum. Amer. J. Physiol. **114**, 603—608 (1936). ~ A quantitative study of acid in the intestine as a stimulus for the pancreas. Amer. J. Physiol. **131**, 349 (1940). ~ Rhythmic changes in duodenal motility associated with gastric peristalsis. Amer. J. Physiol. **111**, 124—129 (1935). ~ The pancreatic secretagogue action of products of protein digestion. Amer. J. Physiol. **134**, 656—663 (1941). — Thomas, J. E., J. O. Crider and C. J. Mogan: A study of reflexes involving the pyloric sphincter and antrum their role in gastric evacuation. Amer. J. Physiol. **108**, 683—700 (1934). — Thomas, J. E., and M. H. F. Friedman: Physiology of the upper gastrointestinal tract as it relates to peptic ulcer. In peptic ulcer in general practice, edit. by D. J. Sandweiss and committee of American Gastroenterological Association, Chap. 3, p. 33—60. Philadelphia: W. B. Saunders Company 1950. — Thomas, J. E., and A. Kuntz: Gastrointestinal motility in relation to enteric nervous system. Amer. J. Physiol. **76**, 606—626 (1926a). ~ Study of vagoenteric mechanism by means of nicotine. Amer. J. Physiol. **76**, 598—605 (1926b). — Thomas, J. E., and C. J. Mogan: The enterogastric reflex. Proc. Soc. exp. Biol. (N.Y.) **28**, 968—969 (1931). — Todd, T. W.: Behavior patterns of the alimentary tract. Baltimore: Williams & Wilkins Company 1930. — Trach, B., C. F. Code and O. H. Wangensteen: Histamine in human gastric mucosa. Amer. J. Physiol. **141**, 78—82 (1944). — Triska, W.: Experimentelle Studien über die Beiß-kraft. Pflügers Arch. ges. Physiol. **204**, 660—667 (1924). — Troll, W., and H. Doubilet: The determination of proteolytic enzymes and proenzymes in human pancreatic juice. Gastroenterology 19, 326—330 (1951). — Tscheschkov, A. M.: Neunzehnmonatige Lebens-fristung eines Hundes nach gleichzeitiger Durchschneidung beider Nn. vagi. am Halse. Diss. St. Petersburg 1902. Zit. bei Babkin 1928, S. 833. — Tuerkischer, E., and E. Werthei-mer: Adrenalectomy and gastric secretion. J. Endocr. 4, 143 (1945).

Uvnäs, B.: Further attempts to isolate a gastric secretory excitant from the pyloric mucosa of pigs. Acta physiol. scand. **9**, 296 (1945). ~ The part played by the pyloric region in the cephalic phase of gastric secretion. Acta physiol. scand. 4, Suppl. 13, 1—86 (1942).

Val Dez, F. C.: Night secretion of free hydrochloric acid in stomach. Illinois med. J. 81, 149 (1942). — Vanzant, F. R., W. C. Alvarez, G. B. Eustenman, H. L. Dunn and J. Berkson: The normal range of gastric acidity from youth to old age. Arch. intern. Med. **49**, 345 (1932). — Vanzant, F. R., and A. M. Snell: The effect of injection of nonspecific protein on the pain of ulcer and on gastric secretion: A clinical and experimental study. J. clin. Invest. 11, 647—659 (1932). — Vella, L.: Unters. Naturl. Mensch. Tiere. 13, 40 (1888a), 13, 432 (1888b). Zit. bei Florey et al. 1941. — Verzár, F.: Probleme und Ergebnisse auf dem Gebiete der Darmresorption. Ergebn. Physiol. **32**, 391—471 (1931). — VERZÁR, F., and J. M. McDOUGALL: Absorption from the intestine. London and New York: Longmans Green & Co. 1936. — VINEBERG, A. M.: The activation of different elements of the gastric secretion by variation of vagal stimulation. Amer. J. Physiol. **96**, 363 (1931). — VINEBERG, A. M., and S. A. KOMAROV: Influence of the vagus nerve on esophageal secretion. Amer. J. Physiol. **104**, 73 (1933). — VISSCHER, M. B., E. S. FETCHER, C. W. CARR, H. P. GREGOR, M. S. BUSHEY, and D. E. BARKER: Amer. J. Physiol. **142**, 550 (1944). — VOLHARD, F.: Über Resorption und Fettspaltung im Magen. Münch. med. Wschr. **47**, 141, 194 (1900).

WALAWSKI, J.: Les biodialysates intestinaux, agenti inhibiteurs de la sécrétion gastrique. C. R. Soc. Biol. (Paris) **99**, 1169 (1928). — WALDRON, J. M.: Amylase activity of canine pancreatic juice. Amer. J. Physiol. **168**, 283—286 (1952). — WALDRON, J. M., and M. H. F. FRIEDMAN: The dual effect of anticoagulants on lipemia. Rev. canad. Biol. **7**, 201 (1948). — WALDSCHMIDT-LEITZ, E., u. A. HARTENECK: Zur Kenntnis der spontanen Aktivierung des Trypsins. Hoppe-Seylers Z. physiol. Chem. **149**, 221 (1925). — WALDSCHMIDT-LEITZ, E., u. K. LINDERSTRØM-LANG: Spezifität tierischer Proteasen; über Störungen der Reaktion zwischen Trypsin und Enterokinase. Hoppe-Seylers Z. physiol. Chem. **166**, 247 (1927). Zit. bei FLOREY et al. 1941. — WALDSCHMIDT-LEITZ, E., u. J. WALDSCHMIDT-GRASER: Über die enzymatischen Wirkungen von Pankreas und Darmsekret. Hoppe-Seylers Z. physiol. Chem. **166**, 247 (1927). — WALKER, A. E., and H. D. GREEN: Electrical excitability of the motor face area: A comparative study in primates. J. Neurophysiol. **1**, 152—165 (1938). — WALTHER, A. A.: Arch. des sciences biol. (St. Petersburg) **7**, 1 (1899). Cit. by BABKIN 1927, p. 754. ~ Diss. St. Petersburg 1897. Zit. bei BABKIN 1928, S. 526. — WANG, S. C.: Localization of the salivatory center in the medulla of the cat. J. Neurophysiol. **6**, 195—202 (1943). — WANG, C. C., and M. I. GROSSMAN: Physiological determination of release of secretin and pancreozymin from intestine of dogs with transplanted pancreas. Amer. J. Physiol. **164**, 527—545 (1950). — WEBSTER, D. R., and J. C. ARMOUR: Vitamin B complex and gastric secretion. Proc. Soc. exp. Biol. (N.Y.) **31**, 463—464 (1934). — WHEELON, H., and J. E. THOMAS: Rhythmicity of the pyloric sphincter. Amer. J. Physiol. **54**, 460—473 (1921). ~ Motility of the duodenum and relation of duodenal motility to that of the pars pylorica. Amer. J. Physiol. **59**, 72—96 (1922). — WILHELMJ, C. M., H. H. McCARTHY and F. C. HILL: Acid inhibition and the cephalic (psychic) phase of gastric secretion. Amer. J. Physiol. **120**, 619 (1937). — WILMS, H.: Röntgenbestrahlung bei Pylorospasmus. Münch. med. Wschr. **63**, 1073 (1916). — WILSON, T. H., and G. WISEMAN: Metabolic activity of the rat and gloden hamster. J. Physiol. (Lond.) **123**, 126—130 (1954). — WINKELSTEIN, A.: One hundred and sixty-nine studies in gastric secretion during night. Amer. J. dig. Dis. **1**, 778 (1935). ~ Some general observations on cardiospasm. Med. Clin. N. Amer. 589—592 (1944). — WOLF, S., and H. G. WOLFF: Evidence on the genesis of peptic ulcer in man. J. Amer. med. Ass. **120**, 670—675 (1942). ~ Human gastric function. An experimental study of a man and his stomach. New York: Oxford University Press 1943. ~ Human gastric function. New York: Oxford University Press 1947. — WOLFF, H. G., W. J. GRACE and S. WOLF: Life situations, emotions and the large bowel. Trans. Ass. Amer. Phycus. **62**, 192 (1949). — WOOD, W. Q.: Treatment of peptic ulceration by vascular ligation. Arch. Surg. (Chicago) **58**, 455 (1949). — WOODWARD, E. R., E. S. LYON, J. LANDOR and L. R. DRAGSTEDT: Physiology of the gastric antrum: experimental studies on isolated antrum pouches in dogs. Gastroenterology **27**, 766—785 (1954). — WRIGHT, R. D., H. W. FLOREY and M. A. JENNINGS: The secretion of the colon of the cat. Quart. J. exp. Physiol. **28**, 207 (1938). — WRIGHT, R. D., M. A. JENNINGS, H. W. FLOREY and R. LIUM: The influence of nerves and drugs on secretion by the small intestine and an investigation of the enzymes in intestinal juice. Quart. J. exp. Physiol. **30**, 73 (1940).

YOUMANS, W. B.: Nervous and neurohumoral regulation of intestinal motility. New York: Interscience Publ. 1949.

ZELIONY, G., and V. SAVITCH: Proc. Soc. Russian Physicians. St. Petersburg 1911/12. [Russian.] Cit. by BABKIN 1944. — ZUCKER, T. H., P. G. NEWBURGER and B. N. BERG: The amylase of serum in relation to functional states of the pancreas. Amer. J. Physiol. **102**, 209—221 (1932).

Die Pathologie der Verdauung und Resorption.

Von

E. JECKELN.

Mit 19 Abbildungen.

Einleitung.

Wer es heute unternimmt, eine Darstellung der Pathologie der Verdauung und Resorption zu geben, erfährt sehr bald, daß es kaum möglich ist, ein auch nur einigermaßen geschlossenes Bild zu erzielen. Dies gilt besonders für den Pathologen, der gemäß Schulung und Denken die gestaltlichen Veränderungen zu erfassen sucht, mit welchen die krankhaften Störungen einhergehen. Bei manchen Abschnitten des Verdauungskanales ist die Ausbeute reichlich; lebensfrische Fixierungen von Operationsmaterial im Verein mit für experimentelle Untersuchungen günstigen Vorbedingungen haben, etwa beim Magen, eine Fülle von Ergebnissen gezeitigt, die auch für eine allgemeinpathologische Betrachtung eine breite Grundlage abgeben. Aber gerade bei dem Hauptresorptionsorgan, dem Dünndarm, liegen die Dinge recht ungünstig, und wenn in einem der bekanntesten Lehrbücher der Verdauungskrankheiten aus dem Jahre 1949 der Satz steht: „Der Dünndarm hat sich der modernen anatomischen Diagnostik bisher mit bemerkenswertem Erfolg widersetzt"[1], so gilt dies auch heute noch, wenigstens was die Erforschung von gestaltlichen Veränderungen in ihrer Beziehung zu gestörten Funktionen betrifft. Es ist hier nicht der Ort, den Gründen für die Schwierigkeiten nachzugehen, die eine Kenntnis der feineren Morphologie der Dünndarmstörungen bisher vereitelt haben; sie dürften überwiegend technischer Natur sein.

Wie sehr die Notwendigkeit empfunden wird, eine Korrelation zwischen Funktion und gestaltlichen Veränderungen herzustellen, wird durch die Erfindung neuer Methoden zur Feststellung geweblicher Veränderungen deutlich. Es seien hier cytodiagnostische Untersuchungen mittels einer Zelltupfsonde von HENNING u. WITTE (1957) und Dünndarmbiopsien mittels der Sonde von SHINER (1959) angeführt.

Ich bin mir also bewußt, daß die einzelnen Abschnitte dieses Beitrags von wechselnder Vollständigkeit sind, zumal ich es vermieden habe, Arbeiten rein klinischen, physiologisch-chemischen oder experimentellen Charakters stärker in den Vordergrund zu stellen, als es der Blick auf die gestaltlichen Manifestationen der Vorgänge gestattet.

A. Die krankhaften Störungen der Verdauung (und besonders dieser) und Resorption infolge von Veränderungen in der Bildung, der Abgabe und dem Transport der Verdauungssäfte.

1. Die Störungen der Kautätigkeit und die Dyschylien der Kopfspeicheldrüsen.

Die Vorgänge der Verdauung und Resorption beginnen mit der Aufnahme, Zerkleinerung und Speicheldurchsetzung der Nahrung in der Mundhöhle. Mangelhafte Kautätigkeit, wie sie vor allem bei Schäden des Gebisses erfolgt, führt

---

[1] HENNING und BAUMANN 1949.

zu einer Beeinträchtigung der bereits in der Mundhöhle beginnenden Verdauung der Kohlenhydrate und der Eiweißverdauung im Magen, wie seit langem bekannt und von klinischer Seite immer wieder beobachtet worden ist[1]. Schlecht zerkaute Speisen reizen die Magenschleimhaut und sollen zu Entzündungen führen. WÜNSCHE (1939) stellte fest, daß es bei Gesunden nach Kauen zu einem deutlichen Anstieg der Säure kommt; bei chronischer Gastritis blieb diese Kausekretion meist aus. Die Motilität des Magens war bei Beobachtung vor dem Röntgenschirm während des Kauaktes gesteigert. — Im einzelnen dürfte es schwer sein festzustellen, in welcher Weise und in welchem Ausmaße mangelnde Zerkauung der Speisen Störungen der Verdauung und Resorption nach sich ziehen.

Krankhafte Veränderungen der Sekretion der Kopfspeicheldrüsen sind schon lange bekannt, wenngleich sich unsere Kenntnisse bisher auf relativ grobe Abweichungen, überwiegend solche quantitativer Natur, bezogen. FABIAN (1938) stellte fest, daß bei Kranken mit organischen Magenachylien, mit isolierter Lungentuberkulose, Basedowerkrankung und Diabetes mellitus mit und ohne Insulinbehandlung, also bei Erkrankungen, die mit einer Minderung der Magenfunktion einhergehen, eine Herabsetzung der Speichelmenge eintritt; am stärksten war sie bei Kranken mit perniziöser Anämie. Die Erklärung dieses Verhaltens geht über Hypothesen nicht hinaus. Nicht alle Partialfunktionen des Speichels sind in derselben einfachen Weise wie die Absonderung der Speichelmenge mit dem Funktionszustande der Magendrüsen verknüpft. So konnte FABIAN (1938) auch in Fällen Histamin-refraktärer Magenachylie durch Histamin die Speichelsekretion noch erheblich verstärken. Genauere Kenntnisse über Funktionsstörungen der Kopfspeicheldrüsen und vor allem auch solche der gestaltlichen Äquivalente der gestörten Funktion sind erst neueren Datums.

Der Leitgedanke der zugrunde liegenden Forschungen, um die sich besonders SEIFERT und GEILER (1956) verdient gemacht haben, geht bemerkenswerterweise von Beobachtungen an der Bauchspeicheldrüse aus. Seit man erkannt hatte, daß der unter dem Bilde der cystischen Pankreasfibrose zunächst beschriebenen Störung eine Sekretionsanomalie nicht nur der Bauchspeicheldrüse, sondern auch der Kopfspeicheldrüsen sowie der Schleimdrüsen der Luftwege und des Darmes zugrunde liegt, die in dem neueren Schrifttum deshalb mit der übergeordneten Bezeichnung „Mucoviscidose"[2] belegt wurde, nachdem ferner SEIFERT (1954) in größerem Umfang bei ernährungsgestörten Säuglingen analoge Veränderungen der Bauchspeicheldrüse auch ohne das Vollbild der cystischen Pankreasfibrose festgestellt hatte, war es nur ein logischer Schritt, die Kopfspeicheldrüsen von Säuglingen und Kindern systematisch auf das Vorkommen von Veränderungen zu untersuchen, die als Ausdruck einer Dyschylie zu gelten haben. Diesen Schritt haben SEIFERT und GEILER (1956) getan und sind zu folgenden Feststellungen gekommen: Unter Dyschylien sind alle Strukturänderungen des Drüsengewebes zu verstehen, die als morphologisches Äquivalentbild einer Störung der Sekretproduktion, der Sekretabgabe und des Sekretabtransportes zu betrachten sind. Entsprechend der Gliederung des Drüsenaufbaus ist zwischen einer *acinären* und einer *canaliculären* Dyschylie unterschieden worden. Bei der acinären Dyschylie der mukösen Endstücke sind eine Aufquellung des Cytoplasmas und eine Anhäufung von Schleimkügelchen verschiedener Größen der Beginn der Veränderung, die zum Platzen des Zelleibes und zur Verschleimung ganzer Endstücke führen kann. Sie wird als die Folge gesteigerter Sekretion gedeutet, die schließlich zur Zellerschöpfung führt. Bei Übertreten des Schleimes in das Zwischengewebe kann es zu serös-zelliger Reaktion und zur Bildung von

---

[1] TROPP 1940, HENNING und BAUMANN 1949.   [2] FARBER 1944 u. a.

Schleimhautgranulomen kommen. Diese Veränderungen wurden bei Infektionskrankheiten, bei Ernährungsstörungen, Leukämien und Krankheiten des zentralen Nervensystems beobachtet. Durch Eindickung und Viscositätszunahme des Sekretes kann es zur Verstopfung der Drüsenlichtung und zur Entwicklung dyschylischer Acinuscysten mit Einlagerung zwiebelschalenartig geschichteter Mikrolithenkugeln kommen, wie das am eindrucksvollsten bei der Mucoviscidose der Fall ist. Die Schleimzellen selbst verfallen der Druckatrophie. Bei chronischen Mangelerkrankungen kommt aber auch im Rahmen allgemeiner Dystrophie eine einfache Atrophie der Drüsenendstücke mit verminderter Sekretbildung und -abgabe vor.

Auch bei den dyschylisch bedingten Veränderungen der serösen Endstücke folgt einer zunächst feststellbaren Hypersekretion (dichte Anfüllung der lumenwärts gelegenen Teile des Cytoplasmas mit Proencymgranula) ein Erschöpfungszustand mit Abnahme der Granula, der zum Bilde der hydropisch-vacuolären Umwandlung führt. Entweder erfolgt eine Restitution oder die Veränderung geht in Zellnekrose über. Infolge Rückganges der Speichelsekretion kann eine aufsteigende Infektion eine erneute Belastung und Schädigung des Drüsengewebes bringen. Dieser Vorgang erklärt das häufige Auftreten von Speicheldrüsenentzündungen nach Operationen. Auch die bei den mukösen Drüsen infolge Mangelernährung auftretende Atrophie ist bei den serösen Drüsen zu beobachten, und zwar häufiger als bei den mukösen. Bei der canaliculären Dyschylie der Speicheldrüsen finden sich die gesteigert beanspruchten Gangepithelien in hydropisch-vacuolärer Umwandlung, in besonders schweren Fällen in Nekrose. Auch hier kann Austritt von Speichelmassen in das umgebende Gewebe mit Bildung von Granulomen oder eines Speichelödems erfolgen. Darüber hinaus kann es zur Bildung von Becherzellen kommen.

Im Zustande der Hypersekretion besteht zunächst nur eine starke Gangfüllung; hier gehen bei dyschylischen Zuständen Entmischungs- und Eindickungsvorgänge mit Viscositätsänderungen vor sich. Die Färbbarkeit des Sekretes ändert sich infolge physikalisch-chemischer Zustandsänderungen („dyschylische Metachromasie" von Seifert und Geiler). Auch hier können infolge der veränderten Viscosität Mikrolithen gebildet werden und dyschylische Gangcysten entstehen. Mit der Ausreifung des Drüsengewebes scheint die Häufigkeit der dyschylischen Speicheldrüsenveränderungen zuzunehmen, so daß schwächste Grade bei Frühgeburten gefunden wurden. — Aus den vorliegenden Grundkrankheiten folgern die Autoren, daß es sich bei „der Dyschylie" nicht um eine ätiologische Einheit handele, sondern um den örtlichen Ausdruck allgemeiner Schädigungen, die — mit Ausnahme der aufsteigenden Entzündung — auf dem Blutwege ausgelöst werden.

Wieweit diese Vorgänge auch für die allgemeine Pathologie der Verdauung beim Erwachsenen Bedeutung haben, müssen weitere Untersuchungen zeigen.

2. Die Dyschylien des Magens.

a) Veränderungen in der Menge und Zusammensetzung des Magensaftes.

Diese werden als Hypersekretion oder Hyposekretion bezeichnet, wenn die Menge des abgesonderten Magensaftes gegenüber der Norm vermehrt oder vermindert ist. Dabei spielt der Gehalt an Salzsäure die Hauptrolle, so daß die Hyperacidität oder die Hypacidität im Vordergrunde steht. Für das Verständnis der auf Veränderungen der Magensaftzusammensetzung beruhenden Erkrankungen ist weiterhin die Berücksichtigung der Magenfermente von Bedeutung. Es ist zu unterscheiden zwischen den Fermenten des Magens als Organ und denen des Magensaftes. Neben den bekannten Fermenten der Magenschleimhaut Pepsin, Kathepsin, Chymase, Mucinasen u. a. ist für die menschliche Krankheitslehre der Castlesche intrinsic-factor bedeutungsvoll geworden, bei dem es sich vielleicht um ein eiweißspaltendes Ferment handelt, was aber noch nicht ganz geklärt ist[1]. Auf seine Rolle bei der Entstehung der perniziösen Anämie wird noch zurückzukommen sein. — Ein vollständiges Versiegen der Magensaftsekretion wird als Achylie bezeichnet, wobei ein Fehlen der Sekretion auch nach Histamininjektion als Histamin-refraktäre Achylie bezeichnet wird. — Die Ursachen für eine fehlerhafte Magensaftsekretion können mannigfaltig sein; nur ein Teil von ihnen ist dem morphologischen Nachweis zugängig. Ein Teil von ihnen ist nur mit biochemischen Untersuchungsmethoden faßbar, doch soll nicht vergessen werden, daß bei Störungen der Magenverdauung außer Änderungen der chemischen Verhältnisse auch mechanische Vorgänge, also die endogen und exogen bedingten Magenbewegungen eine Rolle spielen[1]. Das komplizierte Zusammenspiel sekretorischer und neuraler Vorgänge und die Einwirkung sekretionsfördernder und sekretionshemmender Stoffe in den verschiedenen Phasen der Magensekretion können hier nur gestreift werden. Ihre Ursachen wie auch ihre Folgen haben sich der morphologischen Forschung nur zum Teil erschlossen.

Bei Verzögerung der Magenentleerung kreisen die chemischen Saftstromerreger länger im Blut; es erfolgt eine Vermehrung der abgesonderten Saftmenge. Gastritis und Erosionen können folgen[2]. Starke Magensaftsekretion führt auch zur Herabsetzung des Chloridgehaltes des Blutes. Salzsäuremangel setzt die Desinfektionswirkung des Magensaftes herab und begünstigt die Entstehung einer Avitaminose B. Die antiseptische Wirkung des Magensaftes darf aber nicht überschätzt werden, denn gerade Gärungs- und Fäulniserreger werden nur in verhältnismäßig geringem Maße abgetötet[1].

b) Die chronische Gastritis als Ursache von Dyschylien.

Sekretorische Fehlleistungen, die krankhafte Störungen der Verdauung und Resorption nach sich ziehen können, sind zweifellos bei chronischen Entzündungen der Magenschleimhaut vorhanden und wenigstens zum Teil mit kennzeichnenden Schleimhautveränderungen verbunden. Aber auch hier pflegen vor dem Eintritt eindeutiger organischer Veränderungen zunächst Hypersekretion und Hyperacidität und erst späterhin Hyposekretion und Hypacidität vorzuherrschen, bis dann schließlich die Magensaftsekretion versiegen und Achylie eintreten kann. Zunächst, nämlich bei Hypersekretion und bei Hyperacidität und im Beginn der Hyposekretion und Hypacidität, wurde bei Versuchen an Hunden von THOMSEN[3] histologisch vor allem an den Drüsenepithelien nichts gefunden, und erst bei Vorliegen einer Atrophie ließ cystischer Umbau der Schleimhaut mit zunehmendem Schwund der sekretbildenden Epithelien den Rückschluß auf eine morphologisch verursachte Sekretionsstörung zu. Beim Menschen ist der entsprechende Rückschluß bei der chronischen Umbaugastritis möglich. Hier ist der charakteristische Vorgang eine in der Zone der Pylorusdrüsen beginnende, auf die Korpusdrüsenschleimhaut fortschreitende Schleimhautumwandlung in heterotope Formationen mit indifferenten, dunkelkernigen Epithelien, oder es entstehen Dünndarmdrüsen mit Becherzellen, im Korpusdrüsenbereich auch Pylorusdrüsen. Damit einhergeht eine Abnahme der Secretinbildung, und es kommt zu einer Einschränkung der Magensaft- und Salzsäureproduktion; bei hochgradigem Umbau der Pylorusdrüsenschleimhaut kann auch schon auf diesem

---

[1] KRZYWANEK und FLASCHENTRÄGER 1954.   [2] ZUKSCHWERDT 1931.
[3] Zit. nach BÜCHNER 1950.

Wege eine Achylie die Folge sein. Durch Histamin kann bei erhaltenen Korpusdrüsen noch eine Magensaftsekretion ausgelöst werden; wenn auch diese zerstört sind, tritt eine Histamin-refraktäre Achylie ein[1].

Andererseits können entzündliche Prozesse der Magenschleimhaut zu einer Resorptionsbeschleunigung führen, wie es Henning (1949) mit einer besonderen Methode für das Jodion festgestellt hat. In Fällen akuter gastritischer Schübe ließ sich eine Ausscheidung von in den Magen eingebrachtem Jodnatrium oder Jodkalium durch den Speichel messen, die im entsprechenden Zeitraum bei Gesunden nicht eintrat. Eine solche positive „Resorptionsprobe" bewies entzündliche Veränderungen im Korpusabschnitt. Die diffus atrophische Magenschleimhaut verhielt sich in diesen Versuchen wie die normale.

Henning (1955) wies auch darauf hin, daß die Störungen der Pepsinproduktion viel weniger studiert worden sind als die der Säuresekretion. Gleichzeitig mit Hyperacidität und Hypersekretion ist oft „Hyperpepsinie" zu beobachten. Bei progredienter Schleimhautschädigung soll die Pepsinproduktion viel länger unangetastet bleiben als die Salzsäurebereitung. Man soll Pepsinogen fast regelmäßig im achylischen Mageninhalt finden; es fehlt nur bei extremem Drüsenschwund.

c) Das akute und chronische Geschwür als Ursache von Dyschylien.
Geschwürentstehung und sekretorische Fehlleistung.

Sekretionsstörungen beim akuten und chronischen Geschwür des Magens und des Zwölffingerdarmes sind altbekannt. Bei einer großen Zahl von Ulcuskranken finden sich Hypersekretion und Hyperacidität, wenngleich normale Magensaftwerte und verminderte Sekretion mit verminderter Säurebildung vorkommen. Durch die fraktionierte Ausheberung haben unsere Kenntnisse über die Sekretion des Ulcusmagens eine wesentliche Vertiefung erfahren. Nach Henning (1955) unterscheidet man etwas schematisch das pylorusnahe und das pylorusferne Geschwür. Ersteres zeigt häufig hyperaciden und hypersekretorischen Typus; beim Ulcus duodeni pflegen die Säurewerte hoch zu sein. — Eine bedeutungsvolle Sekretionsstörung ist die nächtliche Dauersekretion, wie sie für das Zwölffingerdarmgeschwür als besonders charakteristisch angesehen wird. „Der supersekretorische Ulcusmagen hält mit Zähigkeit an seinem Sekretionstyp fest. Man kann die gleichen Aciditätskurven vor Beginn und nach Abschluß einer erfolgreichen Kur, ja nach narbiger Heilung des Geschwürs erheben. Direkte Beziehungen zwischen Höhe und Form der Aciditätskurve zu den Beschwerden lassen sich nicht nachweisen. Bei alten Geschwüren der kleinen Kurvatur, insbesondere bei kardianahen Defekten, sieht man Säuremangel[2]."

Im allgemeinen wird man erwarten dürfen, daß die im Geschwürmagen eintretenden sekretorischen Fehlleistungen nicht unmittelbar dem Geschwür ihre Entstehung verdanken. Wenn man von gastritischen Veränderungen als Ursache solcher Fehlleistungen absieht, ergibt sich als eine der wichtigsten, mit der Ulcusgenese im Zusammenhang stehenden Fragen die nach Abweichungen der menschlichen Magensaftsekretion von der bei Säugern festgestellten[3]. Bekanntlich erfolgt beim Menschen die Absonderung des Salzsäure-Pepsingemisches in einer durch nervöse Impulse (Vagus) erregten ersten Phase; die Erregung geschieht durch den Kauakt, durch Geschmacksempfindungen und den Schluckakt bei der Nahrungsaufnahme. Die zweite Phase ist durch die chemische Erregung der Körperdrüsenschleimhaut vom Blute her durch das in der Pylorusdrüsenschleimhaut gebildete Secretin bestimmt. Beim Tier ist ebenfalls — von besonderen

---

1 Büchner 1950.   3 Henning 1955.   2 Babkin 1928.

Bedingungen abgesehen — die Magensaftsekretion dem Verdauungsakt zugeordnet. Beim Menschen muß dieser Vorgang als die Regel angesehen werden; die Wirksamkeit der Magensalzsäure wird durch die Bindung an Bestandteile der Nahrung, besonders Abbaustoffe des Eiweißes, die Wirkung der Schleimdecke des Magens und des oberen Duodenums und die salzsäureverdünnende Wirkung von Speichel, Galle und Pankreassaft auf das notwendige Maß beschränkt[1]. Für den gesunden Menschen ist die ohne klinische Kontrolle getroffene Feststellung einer interdigestiven Leersekretion nach Büchner (1951) als fragwürdig anzusehen. Indessen ist nach den Arbeiten von Büchner und seinen Schülern nicht zu bezweifeln, daß rezidivierende Leersekretionen beim Menschen vorkommen. Sie bilden das wichtigste pathogenetische Moment in der Frage der peptischen Geschwürentstehung.

Die Theorien der Geschwürentstehung dürfen als bekannt gelten und sollen hier nur kurz gestreift werden; auch können die zahllosen experimentellen Untersuchungen auf diesem Gebiet hier nicht im einzelnen berücksichtigt werden. — Virchow hat 1853 die Gefäßtheorie der Geschwürentstehung begründet. Nach ihr entstehen nach Gefäßverschluß Infarkte, die geschwürig zerfallen. Die Rolle des Magensaftes sollte nur eine sekundäre sein, indem der Magensaft ein einmal entstandenes Geschwür unterhalten und vertiefen könne. Eine vorherige Gewebsschädigung infolge Durchblutungsstörung sei aber die Voraussetzung. Dieser Theorie stehen die Tatsachen entgegen, daß Gefäßverschlüsse als Ursache einer Geschwürbildung kaum jemals nachgewiesen worden sind, und daß ferner bei chronischen Stauungen der Magenschleimhaut, die zu Durchblutungsschäden führen könnten, im allgemeinen chronische Geschwüre vermißt werden[2]. Das letzte Wort über die Rolle von Durchblutungsschäden der Magenschleimhaut bei der Geschwürsentstehung dürfte aber noch ausstehen. — v. Bergmann hat 1913 die Theorie entwickelt, daß neurogen bedingte Spasmen der Magenwandgefäße oder der Magenwandmuskulatur die initialen Durchblutungsstörungen herbeiführen können. Für diese neurogene Gefäßtheorie werden die Ulcera bei Hirnerkrankungen angeführt.

Einen starken Impuls erfuhr die Ulcusforschung durch die Arbeiten von Puhl[3] und Konjetzny[4], die auf Grund sehr ausgedehnter geweblicher Untersuchungen das morphologische Bild der Gastritis und Duodenitis ausführlich beschrieben und zur Grundlage der Entzündungstheorie der Geschwürentstehung gemacht haben. Während Konjetzny zunächst für die Entstehung der Erosionen in den gastritisch veränderten Schleimhäuten dem Magensaft eine mitwirkende Bedeutung zuerkannte, hat er später eine Mitwirkung des Magensaftes bei der Entstehung der Erosionen nachdrücklich abgelehnt. Der entscheidende histologische Befund, auf den sich weitere Folgerungen aufbauen, ist die Nekrose im Grunde der Erosion. Solche Nekrosen sind zweifelsfrei wiederholt nachgewiesen worden[2] und nach ihrem Charakter von Büchner und Hamperl (1932 [zit. bei Büchner 1951]) als „Quellungsnekrosen" bezeichnet worden, die nur auf die Einwirkung des Magensaftes zurückgeführt werden könen. Sie finden sich nur da, wo Magensaft zur Einwirkung kommen kann, fehlen also bei akuter Cholecystitis, Appendicitis und Salpingitis[1]. Die Nekrosen werden offenbar bald abgestoßen, und so kommt es, daß bei der erosiven Gastro-Duodenitis häufig das Bild der nekrosefreien Erosion gefunden wird. Es ist durch das Regenerationsepithel in der Umgebung der Epitheldefekte gekennzeichnet. „Die akute erosive Gastritis und Duodenitis ist hiernach eine akute, durch den Magensaft hervorgerufene peptische Gastro-Duodenitis, die in der Regel bald über das Stadium der nekrosefreien Erosion ausheilt[1]." Die alte Günsburgsche Ätz- oder Säuretheorie der Geschwürentstehung ist also durch die neuesten Untersuchungen wieder in den Mittelpunkt der Ulcusforschung gerückt, freilich unter Heranziehung sehr zahlreicher und subtiler humanhistologiser und experimentellhistologischer Studien.

---

[1] Büchner 1951. [2] Büchner 1951 (Lit.). [3] Puhl 1932, 1933.
[4] Konjetzny 1923, 1926, 1930, 1947.

Die Frage, die zunächst der Klärung bedurfte, war die, ob der hyperaktive Magensaft die *gesunde* Schleimhaut andauen kann. Auf frühere Untersuchungen will ich hier nicht eingehen, da sie zum Teil mit unzureichenden Versuchsanordnungen erfolgten. Hingegen scheinen neuere Untersuchungen von Remé (1951) den schlüssigen Beweis erbracht zu haben, daß schon die bloße Einwirkung von Magensaft das Bild der peptischen Erosionen und Geschwüre am normalen Darm und Magen hervorrufen kann.

Remé hat sich dabei unter anderem der Methode der Erzeugung einer kontinuierlichen Leersekretion eines hyperaciden Magensaftes mit allmählich absinkendem Pepsingehalt durch intramuskuläre Injektion von Histamin in Bienenwachs bedient. Die erzielten Veränderungen wurden nicht als Gefäßwirkungen des Histamins erklärt, sondern als Folge dauernder Hypersekretion, zumal hämorrhagische Infarzierungen und Ödeme fehlten, wie sie als erstes morphologisches Substrat des Histaminkollapses bei intravenöser Anwendung hoher Histamindosen beobachtet wurden. Der histologische Befund der erzielten Zottenspitzennekrosen und der ausgebildeten Ulcera entsprach in allen Teilen dem, der uns aus der Pathologie des Ulcus pepticum beim Menschen bekannt ist.

Von besonderer Bedeutung ist in diesem Zusammenhang auch die Beobachtung von Puhl und Brodersen (1931), die bei einem Hund durch 2mal 0,5 mg Histamin subcutan eine reichliche Leersekretion und dann das Bild einer ausgesprochenen akuten ulcerösen Gastritis erzeugten, wenn sie vorher eine Oesophagostomie anlegten und dadurch die Verdünnung des Leersekretes durch verschluckten Speichel verhinderten. — Freilich ist zu sagen, daß die Deutung der durch Histamin hervorgerufenen Geschwüre als reine Folgen der Hypersekretion durch verschiedene Autoren angegriffen wurde[1] und gefolgert wurde, daß die kombinierte Wirkung eines auf Durchblutungsstörungen beruhenden Gewebsschadens und des Magensaftes für die Pathogenese des Geschwüres zu fordern sei[2]. Büchner (1951) ist aber, besonders nach dem Ausfall der Reméschen Versuche, davon überzeugt, daß „große Mengen eines salzsäurereichen Leersekretes bei normaler Schleimhaut alle Übergänge von der akuten erosiven Gastro-Duodenitis bis zum perforierten und chronischen Geschwür des Magens und Duodenums verursachen können". Es ist interessant, daß Remé bei Setzung intramuskulärer, in Bienenwachs eingeschlossener Histamindepots bei stündlicher Ausheberung beim Hund über 2000 cm³ Magensaft im Laufe eines Tages gewinnen konnte.

Koch (1959) glaubt, eine Beziehung zwischen der „so überaus häufigen Mucoviscidosis der Erwachsenen" und der Ulcuskrankheit gefunden zu haben. Eine besondere Häufigkeit der Mucoviscidosis bei Erwachsenen kann bisher nicht angenommen werden und bedürfte noch weiterer Beweise. Es ist zudem nicht erwiesen, daß die von Koch in den Mittelpunkt der Ulcusgenese gestellte „minderwertige Schleimhaut" als „das lang gesuchte genetische und morphologische Substrat" etwas mit Mucoviscidosis zu tun hat. Über die Mucoviscidosis der Erwachsenen und ihre Häufigkeit siehe unter „Dyschylien des Pankreas".

Die Frage der Hyperchylie als Ursache des chronischen Magen-Zwölffingerdarmgeschwüres wird, worauf wiederum Büchner (1951) mit besonderem Nachdruck hingewiesen hat, durch einige Beispiele aus der menschlichen Pathologie beleuchtet. Hier sind zunächst die chirurgischen Erfahrungen bei Pylorusausschaltung nach v. Eiselsberg zu nennen, nach welcher bis zu 44% Mißerfolge durch das Auftreten postoperativer peptischer Jejunalgeschwüre angegeben wurden. In diesen Fällen wird die Magensaftsekretion des Fundusteiles vom Antrum pylori aus noch zu einer Zeit unterhalten, in welcher die aufgenommenen Speisen und Eiweißabbauprodukte, die imstande wären, die Verdauungsenzyme zu binden, den Magen längst wieder verlassen haben[3]. Aus Versuchen

---

[1] Literatur s. bei Büchner 1951.
[2] Konjetzny und Puhl 1926, Staemmler und Merkel 1943.
[3] Enderlen, Freudenberg und v. Redwitz 1923.

von ZUKSCHWERDT und BECKER (1933) geht hervor, daß nicht das Zurückbleiben des Pförtners, sondern der Rückstrom von Duodenalinhalt in den Pyloruskanal die Ursache des postoperativen Jejunalgeschwüres, und zwar durch Verbindung von Leersekretion und Verhaltung des in das Jejunum einströmenden Magensaftes ist.

Schließlich sind in diesem Zusammenhang Beobachtungen von Bedeutung, in denen Fehlbildungen des Darmrohres durch das Auftreten von Magenschleimhautinseln, mit einer Geschwürbildung vergesellschaftet, beobachtet wurden. BÜCHNER (1951, 1958) wies auf das Geschwür des unteren Dünndarmes neben dem mit Korpusschleimhaut ausgekleideten Meckelschen Divertikel hin, ferner auf die Beobachtung PUHLs (1933) über ein chronisches peptisches Geschwür des unteren Dünndarmes unterhalb einer Insel von Korpusschleimhaut. Besonders eindrucksvoll ist auch eine Beobachtung von ROSSET (1938) bei einem Säugling mit einem 3fachen Magen und Blindverschluß eines Nebenmagens. Sehr bald nach der Geburt hatte sich in dem verschlossenen Magenteil ein peptisches Geschwür entwickelt, an dessen Folgen das Kind starb.

Es kann nicht Aufgabe dieser Darstellung sein, die Gedankengänge näher zu erörtern, welche von der Theorie der peptischen Geschwürentstehung zur Betrachtung weiterer pathogenetischer Momente, also etwa psychisch-nervöser Faktoren führen. Auch auf das Problem der geographischen Unterschiede im Auftreten von Magen- und Zwölffingerdarmgeschwüren[1] kann hier nicht eingegangen werden. Es bleibt festzustellen, daß das chronische peptische Geschwür ein einleuchtendes Beispiel ist für die Beziehungen zwischen sekretorischen Fehlleistungen und manifesten, in Gewebsänderungen sich äußernden Störungen.

In diesem Zusammenhang ist ein Syndrom zu erwähnen, das von ZOLLINGER u. ELLISON (1955) beschrieben wurde. Es besteht aus der Trias: Nicht-insulinproduzierender Inselzelltumor des Pankreas, Hypersekretion und Hyperacidität des Magens und peptische Ulcerationen des Jejunum. Von späteren Beschreibern[2] wurden auch Magen- und Duodenalgeschwüre mitgeteilt. Auch Adenome anderer endocriner Drüsen (Hypophyse, Nebennieren) wurden dabei gefunden. Die Beziehungen zu den Sekretionsstörungen des Magens sind noch ungeklärt.

d) Die Dyschylie beim Resektionsmagen.

Die Störungen der Sekretion nach Magenresektion sind mit solchen der Motorik und Entleerung vergesellschaftet. Sie sind naturgemäß vor allem von klinischer Seite untersucht und beschrieben worden. Zunächst haben gastroskopische und histologische Untersuchungen ergeben, daß im Restmagen nahezu regelmäßig eine chronische Gastritis besteht, und daß auch in den oberen Dünndarmschlingen chronisch-entzündliche Veränderungen vorhanden sind. MEYER-BURGDORFF (1934) hob hervor, daß diese Veränderungen unabhängig von dem Grundleiden, also gleichgültig, ob ein Carcinom oder Ulcus vorgelegen hat, oder ob eine schwere Gastritis im Ulcusmagen bestand, sich regelmäßig sowohl im Restmagen wie auch in der Anastomose und im Duodenum und Jejunum finden. Sie können demnach nicht primärer Natur sein, sondern müssen sich erst sekundär ausgebildet haben und mit den veränderten Verdauungsvorgängen in Zusammenhang stehen. Mit der schließlichen morphologischen Umstellung der Schleimhaut ist untrennbar ihre funktionelle verknüpft, vor allem ihre sekretorische Leistung. Durch Ausfall des Pylorus und des Antrumteiles, also des sog. Säureweckers,

---

[1] STRAUB und SCHORNAGEL 1959.
[2] FISHER und FLANDREAU 1957, v. PLANTA 1957, PRIEST und ALEXANDER 1957, DONALDSON jr., VOM EIGEN und DWIGHT 1957, OBERHELMAN jr., NELSEN und DRAGSTEDT 1958, ELLISON, ABRAMS und SMITH 1959.

hat Meyer-Burgdorff bei 70 Magenresezierten nach mindestens 4jähriger Beobachtungszeit in 80% Anacidität gefunden, in den restlichen 20% bestanden normale Säurewerte. Da auch die Tätigkeit der großen Verdauungsdrüsen von der Aufbereitung des Mageninhalts abhängt, liegt in der ersten Zeit nach der Resektion auch die Gallensekretion darnieder. Ein schwacher Reiz zur Gallensekretion wird immerhin vom oberen Jejunum ausgelöst, so daß nach Monaten eine gewisse Anpassung an die veränderten Verhältnisse erfolgt. Auch die Pankreassekretion leidet nicht auf die Dauer, so daß sich die äußere Sekretion des Restmagens, der Leber und des Pankreas überraschend gut ausgleicht. Allerdings ist die Nahrungsausnutzung trotzdem eingeschränkt, da Verweildauer und Resorption des Verdauten nach Magenresektion gestört sind. Ist es also zweifellos nicht nur eine fehlerhafte Zusammensetzung der Verdauungssäfte, welche nach Magenresektion Störungen hervorruft, so bildet sie doch eine Quelle dieser Störungen. Interessant in diesem Zusammenhang ist die nach totaler Magenresektion von Bürger gemeinsam mit Konjetzny[1] bei einer 40jährigen Frau untersuchte Nahrungsausnutzung.

Der Calorienverlust betrug im ganzen zwischen 7 und 12%, hielt sich also in mäßigen Grenzen. Die Kohlenhydratresorption war normal, die Fettverluste schwankten zwischen 11,9 und 19,3%, die Stickstoffverluste im Stuhl zwischen 7,6 und 33,3%.

Die nicht ohne weiteres selbstverständliche schlechte Fettausnutzung wurde von Bürger durch den Fortfall des chemischen Salzsäurereflexes erklärt (herabgesetzte Pankreassaft- und Gallenabsonderung). — Die Erscheinungen der veränderten Magenentleerung (Sturzentleerung) mit ihren Folgen für die Darmverdauung seien nur gestreift; sie haben mit der veränderten Magensaftsekretion insofern etwas zu tun, als der Ausfall der chemischen Phase der Sekretion durch Verlust der Pförtnergegend Anteil an der Zusammensetzung der in den Dünndarm gelangenden, schwer resorbierbar gewordenen Nahrungsbestandteile hat.

Kurz erwähnt sei ein nach Magenresektion beschriebener Zustand, der im angloamerikanischen Schrifttum als „dumping-syndrome" bezeichnet wird und in Völlegefühl, Herzklopfen, Schmerzen in der linken Mittelbauchgegend, Schwindel und Schweißausbrüchen nach Mahlzeiten besteht. Er wird, wenigstens zum Teil, auf eine von hypoglykämischen Zuständen gefolgte Hyperglykämie zurückgeführt, die durch vermehrte Zuckerresorption im oberen Dünndarm hervorgerufen wird[2].

Die nach Magenresektionen auftretenden Anämien werden unter Magenachylie abgehandelt. Meist liegen hypochrome Anämien vor, doch sind auch der perniziösen Anämie entsprechende Blutbefunde erhoben worden. Es dürften dann weitgehend Schleimhautveränderungen verantwortlich zu machen sein, die zur Zerstörung der Bildungsstätte des Castleschen intrinsic-factors führen bzw. die Entfernung von solchen Abschnitten[2]. Weshalb die Anämie nicht selten erst spät und auch nur in einem Bruchteil der Fälle auftritt, hängt wahrscheinlich damit zusammen, daß die Stapelform des antianämischen Prinzips bei einem erstaunlich geringen Bedarf lange Zeit ausreicht[3].

e) Die Magenachylie.

Als Ursache des Magensaftmangels ist, falls es sich nicht nur um vorübergehende Zustände handelt, eine diffuse organische Schädigung der Magenschleimhaut oder gänzliches Fehlen der spezifisch sezernierenden Drüsen zu

---

[1] Bürger 1951.   [2] Henning 1955, Lindenschmidt 1955.   [3] Meyer-Burgdorff 1934.

erwarten. Es ist nicht bekannt, ob eine primäre Atrophie der Magenschleimhaut vorkommt. Sicher ist, daß Magensaftmangel eine der wichtigsten Erscheinungen der chronischen Magenschleimhautentzündungen ist. Nach HENNING (1951) kann bei allen gastroskopisch faßbaren Formen der chronischen Gastritis, auch bei der hypertrophischen, Achylie angetroffen werden; bei der atrophischen Gastritis ist sie stets vorhanden. Auch die Achylien bei alten Ulcera und Carcinomen beruhen auf Gastritis. Hinsichtlich der Diagnose der Gastritis bedürfen unsere Feststellungen einer Revision. Seit Einführung der Magenbiopsie und histologischer Untersuchung des gewonnenen Materials zeigt sich mehr und mehr, daß die bisherigen, überwiegend auf gastroskopischen Befunden beruhenden Gastritisdiagnosen in sehr vielen Fällen nicht zutreffen[1].

Eine besondere Rolle spielt die Magenachylie bei der *perniziösen Anämie*. Sie beruht zweifellos auf einer Atrophie der Fundusschleimhaut mit Ersatz der spezifisch-sezernierenden Drüsen durch Schleimdrüsen[2], einer Veränderung, die regelmäßig zu erheben ist. Die Achylie pflegt dem Ausbruch der Bluterkrankung jahrelang vorauszugehen, was dafür spricht, daß der Umbau der Magenschleimhaut nicht die Folge der perniziösen Anämie ist[3]. Er wird heute als ihre Ursache angesehen. Die sekretorische Fehlleistung beruht auf der Zerstörung der Bildungsstätte des intrinsic-factors CASTLEs in den Korpusdrüsen. Der mit der Nahrung zugeführte extrinsic-factor, das Vitamin B_{12}, der durch den intrinsic-factor resorptionsfähig gemacht wird, kann also bei der perniziösen Anämie nicht resorbiert werden.

In diesem Zusammenhang sei eine Beobachtung FEYRTERS (1952) erwähnt. Eine 45jährige Frau bekam nach einer im 34. Lebensjahr durchgemachten „ausgiebigen" Dünndarmresektion eine perniziöse Anämie. Sie reagierte gut auf Leber und starb Jahre später an einer Hirnhauttuberkulose. Histologisch zeigte die Fundusdrüsenschleimhaut nur geringe Atrophie und interstitielle Entzündung. Die Fundusdrüsen waren aus Hauptzellen und reichlichen Belegzellen aufgebaut. Epikritisch wurde die perniziöse Anämie darauf zurückgeführt, daß bei intakter Magensekretion die Resorption des sog. Antiperniciosa-Prinzips infolge der Dünndarmresektion gestört war („enterogene Perniciosa").

Eine Achylie ist auch in manchen Fällen voll ausgebildeter Addisonscher Krankheit beobachtet worden[4], wobei in den histologisch untersuchten Fällen die Fundusschleimhaut Atrophie, interstitielle Entzündung und Ersatz der Fundusdrüsen durch mukoide Drüsen mit fast völligem bzw. völligem Schwund der Belegzellen aufwies. Diese Veränderungen sind aber nicht die Regel. Im Beginn mancher Fälle von Addisonscher Krankheit kann nach FEYRTER und KLIMA (1952) das Verhalten gegensätzlich sein, d. h. es bestehen Normacidität und auch Hyperacidität.

Wenngleich nicht durch völlige Achylie verursacht, soll im Zusammenhang mit den durch fehlerhafte Magensekretion bedingten Anämien noch eine weitere Form erwähnt werden, die zweifellos auch beim Resektionsmagen eine Rolle spielt. Gemeint sind die auf mangelnde Eisenresorption zurückzuführenden Vorgänge. Im einzelnen wird auf die grundlegende Darstellung von M. B. SCHMIDT (1940) verwiesen. Nach den dort zitierten Untersuchungen LINTZELs wird die Resorption des Nahrungseisens oder des Eisens in Präparaten, solange dieses nicht in schleimhautschädigenden Dosen verabfolgt wird, dadurch bestimmt, in welchem Grade es durch die Berührung mit der Salzsäure des Magens ionisiert wird. Der Körper läßt Eisen nur oder fast nur in ionisierter Form aus dem Darmrohr übertreten, und zwar in Form von Ferroionen. „Der Salzsäure kommt also eine wichtige Rolle bei der Versorgung des Körpers mit Eisen zu, und damit

---

[1] HENNING 1956, KABISCH und GRUNER 1958, KÜHN 1960.
[2] FEYRTER und KLIMA 1952.   [3] BÜCHNER 1955.   [4] FEYRTER und KLIMA 1952.

wird es verständlich, daß trotz ausreichender Zufuhr mit der Nahrung bei Störung der Magensaftsekretion doch die Aufnahme ungenügend bleibt und eine Verarmung der Gewebe eintritt und in unvollkommener Blutbildung zum Ausdruck kommt[1]." So ergibt sich als eine Möglichkeit für das Zustandekommen hypochromer Anämie das Fehlen genügender Salzsäureproduktion im Magen. Die hypochromen Formen der „agastrischen Anämie", wie sie beim Resektionsmagen vorkommen, müssen hierher gerechnet werden.

Die Histamin-refraktäre Achylie kann für nutritive *Allergien* dadurch Bedeutung haben, daß in der Nahrung enthaltene Allergene nicht durch die Salzsäure des Magens zerstört werden. In neueren Versuchen hat Hansen (1955) ihre außerordentlich schnelle Resorption nachgewiesen; bereits 1—2 min nach duodenaler Applikation eines Test-Proteins ließ sich im Prausnitz-Küster-Versuch eine Änderung der Wärmestrahlung am Erfolgsort registrieren.

3. Die Dyschylien des Pankreas.

a) Die Dyschylien durch fehlerhafte Sekretbildung. Die cystische Pankreasfibrose.

Störungen in der äußeren Sekretion der Bauchspeicheldrüse sind schon lange bekannt, doch haben erst die Forschungen der letzten Jahre tiefere Einblicke in die Häufigkeit und Bedeutung solcher Störungen erbracht und unsere Kenntnisse pathogenetischer Einzelheiten erheblich erweitert. Dies gilt vor allem für die Störungen der Pankreassaftabgabe bei Säuglingen und jungen Kindern sowie für das Gebiet der sog. Fermententgleisungen. Im Gegensatz zu anderen Gebieten der Stoffwechselpathologie hat hier die pathologische Histologie besonders förderlich wirken können.

Obwohl bereits 1925 Burghard bei der Mitteilung einer Beobachtung von fibrocystischen Pankreasveränderungen bei einem $3^1/_2$ Monate alten Säugling mit „Dekomposition" die Forderung erhoben hatte, bei allen ernährungsgestörten Säuglingen und Kleinkindern, die zur Sektion kommen, das Pankreas histologisch zu durchforschen, ist diese Untersuchung in der Folgezeit offensichtlich etwas vernachlässigt worden. Auf Grund von Durchmusterungen der Bauchspeicheldrüsen ernährungsgestörter Kleinkinder und Säuglinge kam Mahrburg (1934) zu der Feststellung von Veränderungen, die wir heute als dyschylisch bezeichnen, und hob auch ihre Bedeutung für die Magen- und Darmstörungen hervor. Auch er beklagte sich, wohl mit Recht, über eine zu geringe Beachtung des Pankreas am Sektionstisch. Zum Teil wird man diese darauf zurückführen müssen, daß bei nicht bald nach dem Tode vorgenommener Sektion und bei routinemäßiger Untersuchung autolytische Vorgänge die Auswertung der histologischen Bilder zu beeinträchtigen pflegen. Durch frühzeitige Entnahme nach dem Tode oder bei Anfixierung unmittelbar nach dem Tode durch Formalin ist dieser Fehler zu vermeiden[2]. Nach den Untersuchungen von Ilgner und Würkert (1952) (histochemische Darstellung der Thymonucleinsäure in den Kernen des Pankreasparenchyms) bei chronischen Ernährungsstörungen war eine Abnahme der Fermentproduktion zu erwarten, wie die Verminderung der Thymonucleinsäure folgern ließ. Systematisch ist Seifert (1954) durch die Auswertung eines großen kindlichen Sektionsgutes diesen Veränderungen nachgegangen und hat bei akut ernährungsgestörten Säuglingen folgende wesentliche Merkmale festgestellt: eiweißreiches, herdförmig interstitielles Exsudat in der Nachbarschaft der Gefäße, Sekretansammlungen in den Gängen sowie im Bereich intraacinärer Cystenbildungen; nur geringe interstitielle Fibrose. Im Gegensatz zu den akuten Ernährungsstörungen bestand an den Bauchspeicheldrüsen von

---

[1] M. B. Schmidt 1940.   [2] Seifert 1954.

Säuglingen mit einer chronischen rezidivierenden Ernährungsstörung sehr häufig eine unterschiedlich starke interstitielle Fibrose sowohl inter- als auch intralobulär, meist in Verbindung mit einem herdförmigen eiweißreichen Exsudat in Nachbarschaft der Gefäße bei völligem Fehlen entzündlicher Zellinfiltrate. Eine Pankreassklerose oder gar -cirrhose mit Umbau der Läppchenstruktur war aber in keinem Falle erreicht. Auch fanden sich nirgends Zeichen einer Sialangitis oder Perisialangitis, dagegen in etwa einem Drittel der Fälle geringe cystische Erweiterungen des Gangsystems und teilweise intraacinäre Cystenbildungen mit Ansammlungen

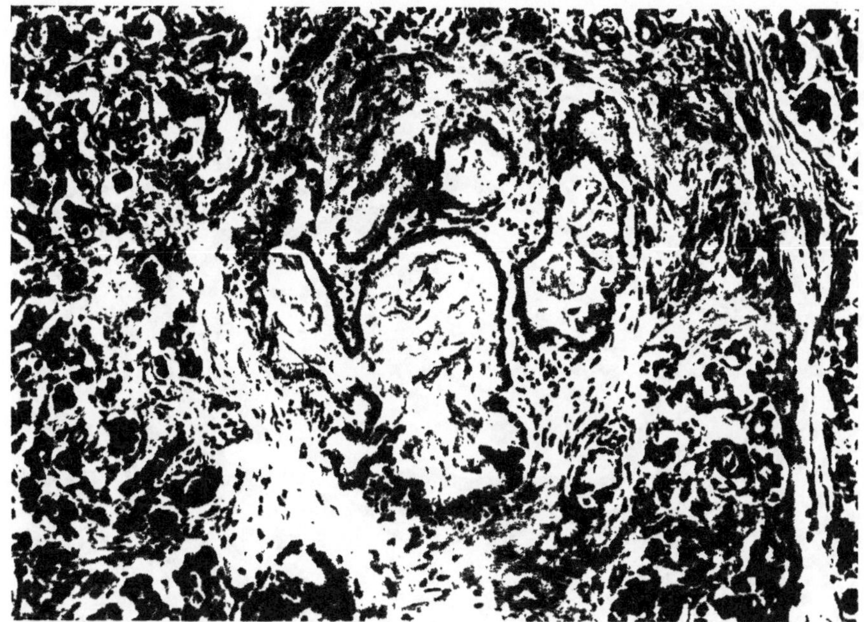

Abb. 1. Pankreas eines 6 Monate alten, ernährungsgestörten Säuglings. Gangektasien mit eingedicktem Sekret. HE-Färbung.

acidophilen Sekretes. In ähnlicher Weise wie bei den Dyschylien der Kopfspeicheldrüsen ist auch bei den Dyschylien des Pankreas eine Trennung in acinäre und canaliculäre Dyschylien von SEIFERT (1956) durchgeführt worden. — Die Veränderungen gingen mit einem unterschiedlich starken Verlust der Kerne des exkretorischen Parenchyms an Thymonucleinsäure einher. Sie wurden als Zeichen einer Sekretionsstörung („Dyschylie") mit seröser, in den chronischen Fällen zu Organsklerosen führender Begleitpankreatitis gedeutet und auf bakteriell-toxische Einwirkungen zurückgeführt.

Aus der Gruppe der sog. chronischen Ernährungsstörungen hob SEIFERT (1954) solche heraus, bei denen es sich um eine *cystische Pankreasfibrose* handelte. Diese Erkrankung ist schon seit längerer Zeit bekannt, wenngleich erst in den letzten Jahren in ihren verschiedenen Erscheinungsformen und hinsichtlich ihrer pathogenetischen Dignität eingehender untersucht. Seit der Mitteilung LANDSTEINERs (1905) über schwere cystische Pankreasveränderungen mit Sekreteindickungen beim Meconiumileus ist eine große Zahl von weiteren Beobachtungen cystischer Pankreasfibrose mitgeteilt worden. Von älteren Beobachtungen über Cystenpankreas bei Neugeborenen sind in dem Handbuchbeitrag von GRUBER (1929) die von KAUFMANN (1901) und BENCKER (1901) aufgeführt, doch ist es sehr wahrscheinlich, daß die Veränderung viel häufiger vorkommt, als bisher angenommen wurde. Da sie nicht immer mit bloßem Auge erkennbar ist, muß vermutet werden, daß sie bisweilen übersehen wird. Seifert (1954) gab eine Zusammenstellung über die Häufigkeit der cystischen Pankreasfibrose, nach der sie in 1,5—8% aller Säuglingsobduktionen in verschiedenen Ländern entdeckt wurde. Einer Mitteilung von Schulze-Jena (1955) ist zu entnehmen, daß die Pankreasfibrose in den USA in 3—4% aller Sektionen gefunden wird. Fanconi, Knauer und Uehlinger (1936) wiesen als erste auf die Kombination von cystischer Pankreasfibrose mit Bronchiektasen hin. Die erste zusammen-

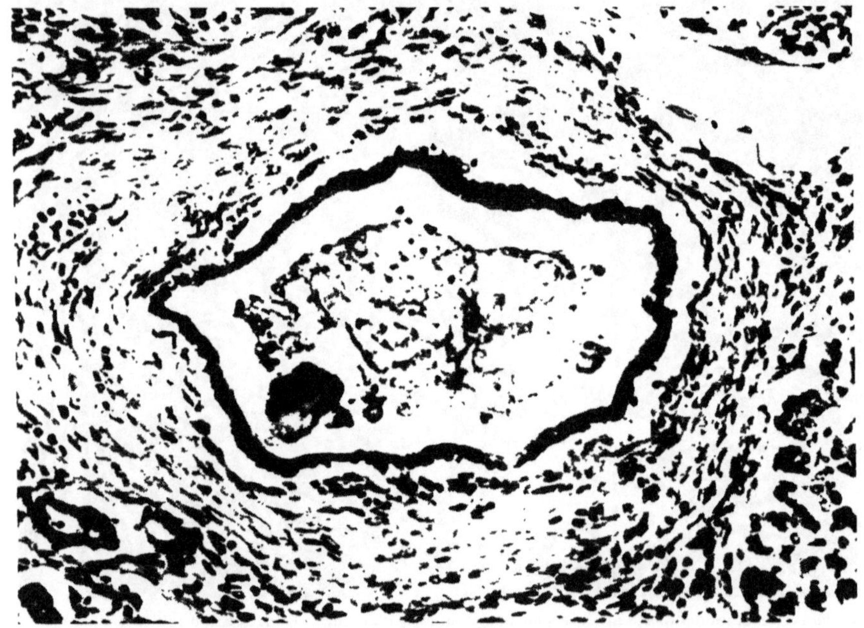

Abb. 2. Pankreas eines 6 Monate alten, ernährungsgestörten Säuglings. Mit eingedicktem Sekret gefüllter erweiterter Gang. Beginnende Mikrolithenbildung. HE-Färbung.

fassende Arbeit über cystische Pankreasfibrose stammt von Andersen (1938); sie enthält die heute noch gültige Einteilung der Erkrankungsformen in 3 Gruppen:

1. Meconiumileus (bei Neugeborenen, Tod in der 1.—2. Lebenswoche).

2. Pneumonisch-dyspeptische Form (Säuglingsalter, Tod bis zum 6. Lebensmonat an Bronchopneumonie).

3. Cöliakieähnliche Form (späteres Säuglings- und Kindesalter bis zur Pubertät).

Nachdem festgestellt war, daß nicht nur am Pankreas, sondern gleichzeitig am Darm, an den Speicheldrüsen und an den Bronchien Veränderungen vorlagen[1], gab Glanzmann (1946) der Erkrankung den Namen *Dysporia* [2] *entero-broncho-pancreatica*.

Seit etwa 1945 ist eine große Zahl von Arbeiten erschienen, die sich mit dem Problem der genannten Krankheit befassen; nur die für die Frage der Dyschylie wichtigen können hier Berücksichtigung finden. Es erscheint zunächst notwendig, auf die Frage der Cystenbildungen im Pankreas einzugehen. Hiermit hat sich

---

[1] Farber 1944.

[2] $\delta v\sigma\pi o\varrho i\alpha$ = ,,des schwierigen Weges'' (Glanzmann) = ,,schwierige Passage''.

vor allem in Deutschland SEIFERT[1] eingehender befaßt. Aus der Vielfalt der im Pankreas beobachteten cystischen Bildungen verdienen in diesem Zusammenhang die Retentionscysten nähere Betrachtung. Bei der cystischen Pankreasfibrose spielen die häufigsten Ursachen der Cystenentstehung wie Steinbildung, Tumoren, Sialangitis, Gewächse der Nachbarschaft, Restzustände schwerer sklerosierender Pankreasaffektion und dergleichen keine Rolle. SEIFERT (1954) wies mit Recht darauf hin, daß nach experimentellen Untersuchungen eine rein mechanische Erklärung für die Cystenbildungen nicht ausreicht, da die Unterbindung des Ausführungsganges im Anfang zu einem interstitiellen Ödem sowie Anstieg der Serumamylase und im Endstadium zu einer völligen Atrophie des Parenchyms und Sklerose des Interstitiums, dagegen nur vorübergehend zur cystischen Gangerweiterung führe. Dagegen haben die Nachprüfungen der Befunde von BAGGENSTOSS[2] im wesentlichen zu einer Bestätigung geführt: Eine Sekretretention und Cystenbildung ist auch ohne mechanische Gangverlegung dann zu beobachten, wenn es zu Irritation des Gefäßnervensystems durch bakterielle, toxische oder andere Noxen kommt. Dies soll darauf beruhen, daß entweder infolge Wasserverarmung bei häufigem Erbrechen eine Störung der

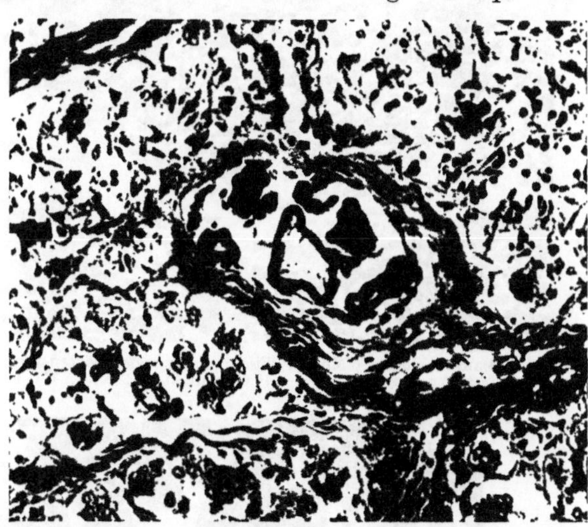

Abb. 3. Pankreas eines 6 Monate alten, ernährungsgestörten Säuglings. Gang mit geschichteten Sekretmassen. Azanfärbung.

Secretinproduktion der Darmschleimhaut oder eine abnorme neurale Reizung eintritt. In diesem Zusammenhang sind Versuche FARBERs[3] zu erwähnen, dem es gelang, durch wochenlange Pilocarpingaben bei Katzen der cystischen Pankreasfibrose analoge Bilder zu erzeugen. Jedenfalls dürfte sicher sein, daß die Cystenbildungen bei der cystischen Pankreasfibrose von den Retentionscysten zu unterscheiden sind und eine Gruppe für sich bilden, bei der eine primäre Störung der Sekretionsbildung vorliegt („dyschylische Pankreascysten" nach SEIFERT). Da sie gelegentlich auch zur mechanischen Verlegung des Sekretabflusses führen können, sind Beziehungen zu den sog. Retentionscysten gegeben, und der Gedanke SEIFERTs, daß auch bei den letzteren Anomalien der Sekretbildung durch mannigfache Schädigungen des Pankreasparenchyms eine Rolle spielen können, erscheint nicht abwegig.

Bei der *cystischen Pankreasfibrose* beginnt die Cystenbildung mit einer Ausweitung der Drüsenendstücke mit Umgestaltung des Drüsenepithels und Einbeziehung der centroacinären Zellen in das erweiterte Gangsystem. Kennzeichnend ist eine Veränderung der Struktur des Sekretes, die auf eine Veränderung seiner Zusammensetzung und Konsistenz hindeutet. Es zeigen sich eigentümlich zwiebelschalenartig geschichtete Sekretmassen sowie mikrolithenartige Gebilde, die auch färberisch (z. B. bei Azanfärbung) gewisse Rückschlüsse

---

[1] SEIFERT 1954, 1956.
[2] BAGGENSTOSS 1948, zit. nach SEIFERT 1954.
[3] FARBER 1944, zit. nach SEIFERT 1954.

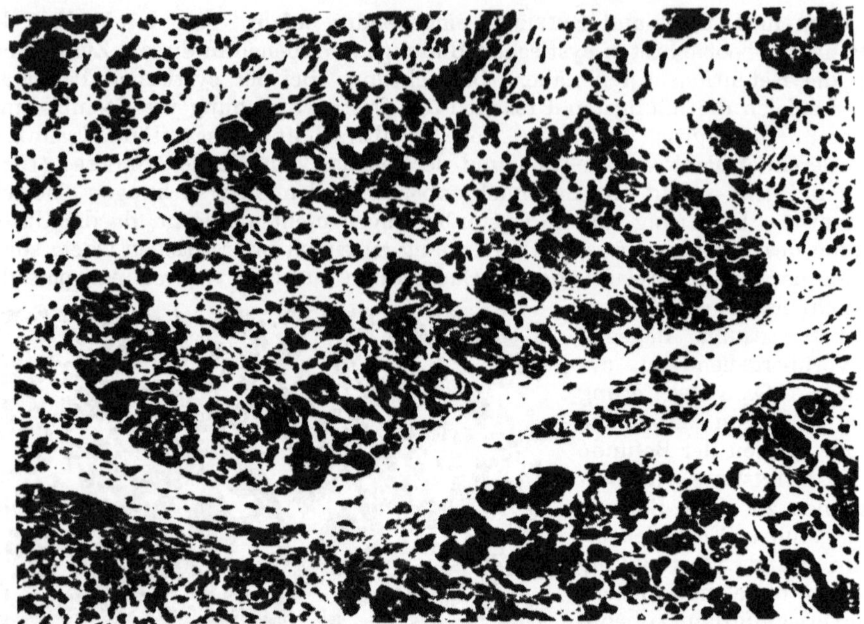

Abb. 4. Pankreas eines 6 Monate alten, ernährungsgestörten Säuglings. Ausfüllung der erweiterten Acini mit eingedicktem Sekret. HE-Färbung.

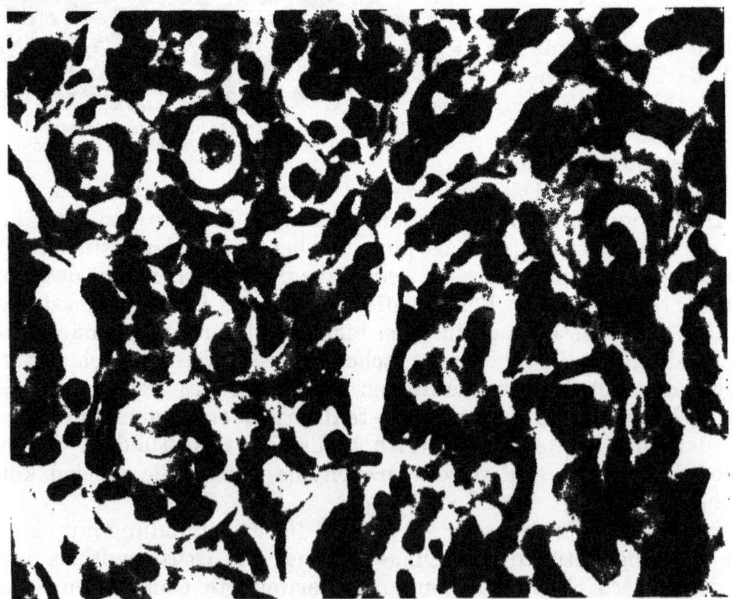

Abb. 5. Pankreas eines 6 Monate alten, ernährungsgestörten Säuglings. Ausfüllung der erweiterten Acinuslichtungen mit eingedicktem Sekret bei stärkerer Vergrößerung. HE-Färbung.

auf den physikalischen Zustand des veränderten Sekretes gestatten[1]. Hier ist die Beobachtung von Glanzmann und Berger (1954) anzuführen, die beim Meconiumileus einen pathologischen Eiweißstoff im Meconium fanden, der mit

---

[1] Seifert 1954.

fettartigen Stoffen in Gegenwart von Wasser eine feste Gallerte bildet. Dieser Befund wurde von FREUDENBERG (1955) bestätigt.

Auf Grund der Theorie FARBERs (1944) einer angeborenen generalisierten Sekretionsstörung wurde die Bezeichnung „Mucoviscidosis" eingeführt. SAEGESSER und Mitarbeiter (1955), die diesen Ausdruck übernahmen, machten neben den im Pankreas gelegenen Störungen vor allem die Produktion eines vermehrten und dicken Schleimes durch die Darmdrüsen für die Entstehung des Meconiumileus verantwortlich und subsumierten unter das Krankheitsbild der Mucoviscidose die Sekretionsanomalien zahlreicher Schleimdrüsen. Die Konzeption einer Sekretionsanomalie der Schleimdrüsen ist in den letzten Jahren erweitert worden. Wie zahlreiche Untersucher mitteilen, liegt eine Erkrankung vor, bei deren Vollbild alle exokrinen Drüsen fehlerhaft arbeiten. Der histologische Nachweis ist zwar bisher nur für die schleimproduzierenden Drüsen erbracht, doch werden auch der Schweiß, der Mundspeichel und die Tränenflüssigkeit in ihrer Zusammensetzung stark verändert angegeben (abnorm hoher Elektrolytgehalt)[1]. Die Erkrankung scheint rezessiv vererbt zu werden[2]; ihre Häufigkeit schwankt

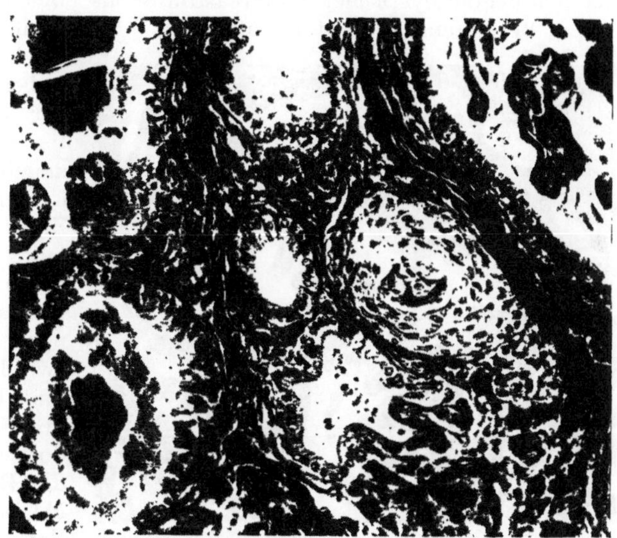

Abb. 6. Cystische Pankreasfibrose. 5 Monate alter Säugling. Pankreas mit Epithelmetaplasie und mikrolithenartigen Sekretkugeln. HE-Färbung. (Beobachtung von SEIFERT, Leipzig.)

innerhalb weiter Grenzen. Auf etwa 1000 Geburten kommt durchschnittlich ein krankes Kind. Nach DI SANT'AGNESE (1957) erscheint bei Homocygoten das Vollbild, während bei Heterocygoten sich die Krankheit nur zum Teil oder gar nicht offenbart. So erklärt es sich vielleicht auch, daß es Fälle von sicherer Mucoviscidose gibt, in denen die Störung der Pankreasexkretion nicht nachweisbar ist[3]. Im allgemeinen wird man aber eine solche Störung nur selten vermissen. — In Japan ist die Erkrankung unbekannt, auch bei der Negerbevölkerung und in jüdischen Familien in der USA. sind nur wenige Fälle beobachtet worden[4].

Besonderes Interesse verdient das Verhalten der Leber bei Mucoviscidose. Noch vor wenigen Jahren war hierüber wenig bekannt. Es wurden Erweiterungen und Ausfüllungen der Gallengänge mit eingedickter Galle beschrieben und Ausgang in Cirrhose angegeben[5]. In den letzten vier Jahren wurde in zahlreichen Veröffentlichungen eine Beteiligung der Leber geschildert[6]. Neben erhöhtem

---

[1] DI SANT'AGNESE und Mitarbeiter 1956—1959, RENDLE-SHORT 1956.
[2] PRINZ 1950, WERTHEMANN, GROGG und FREY 1952.
[3] DUBOIS-MANNE, VAN GEFFEL und ZYLBERSZAG 1956.
[4] BACHMANN 1957.   [5] SCHULZE-JENA 1955.
[6] GLOOR und WERTHEMANN 1955, CLAIREAUX 1956, BACHMANN 1957, NORRIS 1957, OEHLERT 1957, HOWANIETZ 1958, STRAUB und ZIEGLER 1958, BECKMANN 1959, DI SANT'AGNESE und ANDERSEN 1959.

Fettgehalt der Leber sind Schleimeindickungen in den Gallenwegen mit oder ohne cholangitische Veränderungen, pericholangioläre Fibrosen und Cirrhose, auch mit portaler Hypertension geschildert worden. Nach Beckmann (1959) fand di Sant'Agnese, einer der besten Kenner der Mucoviscidosis, bei 116 Patienten Leberveränderungen sowohl autoptisch wie auch bioptisch, die sich als herdförmige biliär-cirrhotische Veränderungen mit Konkrementen oder als multilobuläre biliäre Cirrhose darboten. Im allgemeinen wird auch hier die generalisierte Sekretionsstörung als primum movens angesehen. Oehlert (1957) führt die Lebercirrhose auf den allgemeinen, resorptionsbedingten Eiweißmangel zurück, der sich bei der cystischen Pankreasfibrose als Folge eines Mangels an proteolytischen Verdauungsfermenten entwickelt. Gloor u. Werthemann (1955) betrachten die herdförmige biliäre Lebercirrhose nicht als eine Folge der Mucoviscidose, sondern halten sie für eine Mißbildung mit angeborener Hyperplasie und Cystenbildung. Auch Straub u. Ziegler (1958) nahmen eine primäre Fehlbildung des hepatischen Drüsengewebes an.

Es ist jedenfalls sicher, daß noch nicht alle Zusammenhänge zwischen Pankreaserkrankung und Beteiligung anderer Organe im Formenkreis der Mucoviscidosis geklärt sind. So sei erwähnt, daß Reemtsma, di Sant'Agnese, Malm u. Barker (1958) bei ihren Patienten eine deutliche Abnahme der Neutralfettresorption im Dünndarm feststellten, in gerin-

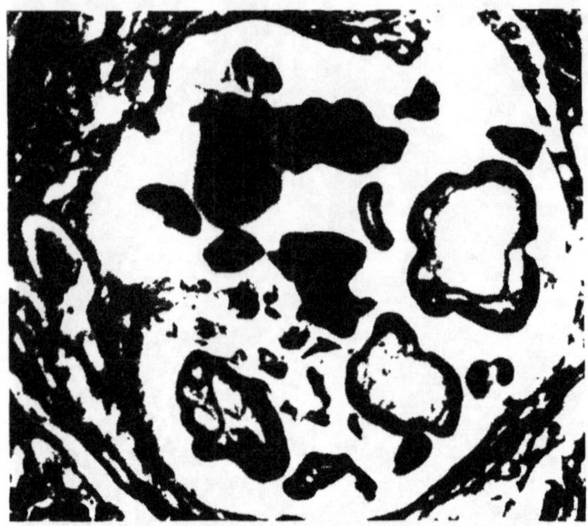

Abb. 7. Cystische Pankreasfibrose. 5 Monate alter Säugling. Metachromasie des Sekretes. Azanfärbung. (Beobachtung von Seifert, Leipzig.)

gerem Grade auch eine solche von Fettsäuren. Hieraus ergibt sich die Vermutung, daß bei der cystischen Pankreaserkrankung nicht nur eine Störung der äußeren Pankreassekretion vorliegt, sondern noch eine weitere Störung der fermentativen Tätigkeit, die im Dünndarm zu lokalisieren ist.

Die zunehmende Bedeutung des Krankheitsbildes der Mucoviscidosis wird besonders durch Veröffentlichungen deutlich, die sich mit dem Auftreten dieser Erkrankung bei Erwachsenen in jüngster Zeit befaßt haben. An früheren diesbezüglichen Beobachtungen sind mir lediglich die von Frischauf (1952) und Seifert (1954) bekannt. Frischauf berichtete von einem 16jährigen Mädchen, bei dem auf Grund der Anamnese und „des charakteristischen Fermentbefundes" die Diagnose einer cystischen Pankreasfibrose gestellt wurde. Es bestand eine tiefgreifende Störung der Nahrungsausnutzung mit dauernden Fettstühlen. Die Beobachtung von Seifert betraf eine 49jährige Frau, die an einer schweren akuten Gastroenteritis bei ulceröser Cholecystitis gestorben war. Die histologischen Veränderungen der Bauchspeicheldrüse entsprachen weitgehend denen der kindlichen cystischen Pankreasfibrose. Über die Entstehung der Veränderungen (seit Kindheit bestehend oder erst später entstandene Sekretionsstörung?) ließ sich leider nichts aussagen. — Die neueren Feststellungen einer Mucoviscidose bei Erwachsenen beruhen überwiegend auf dem Schweißtest (erhöhter Gehalt des Schweißes an Na-Ionen), der nach di Sant'Agnese u. Andersen (1959) in 99% aller Fälle positiv ausfällt.

Die genannten Autoren behandelten von 1939 bis 1958 550 Patienten mit Mucoviscidosis; von diesen waren 106 über 10 Jahre alt, der älteste 24 Jahre. Die Kranken von BAUMGARTNER und DE VOOGD (1959) waren 17 und 25 Jahre alt. Die Patientin von HENDRIX und GOOD (1956), bei der mit 11 Jahren die Diagnose einer cystischen Pankreasfibrose gestellt worden war, erreichte ein Alter von 17 Jahren. Die charakteristischen Sektionsbefunde waren in diesem Falle: Bronchiektasen, starke Erweiterung der Bronchialdrüsen und Ausfüllung mit viscösem Schleim, chronische Pneumonie, Cor pulmonale, völliger Schwund des exkretorischen Pankreasparenchyms bei Erweiterung der Ausführungsgänge. Biliäre Lebercirrhose.

Eine besondere Stellung nehmen die Arbeiten von KOCH (1959), BOHN u. KOCH (1959) sowie KOCH u. LAPP (1959) ein. Diese Autoren vertreten den Standpunkt, daß die Mucoviscidose auch eine „überaus häufige, dominant erbliche

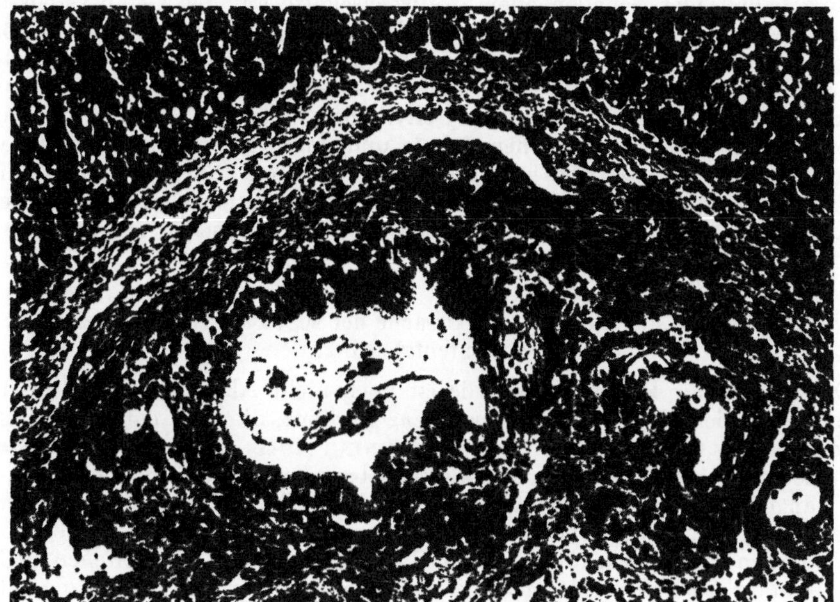

Abb. 8. 3 Wochen alter Säugling. Mucoviscidose. Leber. Erweiterung der Gallengänge und Ausfüllung mit dicker, zäher Galle. HE-Färbung.

Krankheit" im Erwachsenenalter darstellt. Das Leiden soll bei Erwachsenen diskretere Erscheinungen aufweisen als im Kindesalter, die Störungen treten nur partiell in Erscheinung (besonders herabgesetzte Carboxypeptidase des Pankreasspeichels); sekundäre Spätschäden können im Vordergrunde stehen (Osteoporose, Tetanie, Erkrankung der Atmungsorgane).

Pathologisch-anatomisch wird von 3 Fällen berichtet, bei denen mikroskopisch eine cystische Pankreasfibrose diagnostiziert wurde. Mit Recht weist jedoch SEIFERT in einem Referat der Arbeit von KOCH u. LAPP darauf hin, daß die geschilderten Pankreasveränderungen sowie die beigefügten Abbildungen der im Erwachsenenalter relativ häufigen chronisch-rezidivierenden Pankreatitis entsprechen. — Die von den genannten Autoren vermutete Häufigkeit der Erwachsenen-Mucoviscidosis ist somit bis jetzt nicht durch anatomische Befunde gestützt.

Es ist nicht unwahrscheinlich, daß die äußere Sekretion des Pankreas nicht unwesentlich von der Ernährung abhängt. Eiweißmangelernährung kann sich störend auf die Fermentproduktion auswirken, und experimentell ließen sich Veränderungen des Pankreasgewebes durch Eiweißmangelernährung hervorrufen[1]. Bei dem malignen Typ der Fehlernährung, welche in tropischen Gegenden

---

[1] POPPER 1952.

vorkommt und als *Kwashiorkor* bezeichnet wird, ist Pankreasatrophie anzutreffen. Davis[1] betrachtete diese Atrophie als das Ergebnis von Anforderungen an das Pankreas während der Kindheit, wenn unmittelbar nach der Entwöhnung eine hochcalorische Nahrung gegeben wird, die hauptsächlich aus Kohlenhydraten besteht, während Eiweiß fehlt oder von biologisch geringer Qualität ist. In Westindien und Ungarn sind ähnliche Beobachtungen an Kindern gemacht worden, die eiweißarm ernährt wurden[2]. Neuere Untersuchungen hierzu finden sich bei Trowell (1957).

Im übrigen sind als Ursache der Dyschylien des Pankreas vielfältige Faktoren angeführt worden, unter denen akute und chronische Intoxikationen durch Einwirkung bakterieller Schäden oder Stoffwechselgifte auf das Gefäßsystem und Drüsengewebe nach Seifert (1956) die Hauptrolle spielen. Hierher gehören auch die dyschylischen Veränderungen, wie sie bei der sog. (serösen) Begleitpankreatitis gefunden wurden. Seifert wies ferner auf die Bedeutung des Sauerstoffmangels für die kausale Genese dyschylischer Veränderungen hin, die durch Untersuchungen der Büchnerschen Schule und durch Popper und Doerr aufgedeckt wurde. Glanzmanns (1946) Hypothese einer Rhesusinkompatibilität als Ursache der fehlerhaften Sekretbildung dürfte heute als widerlegt gelten[3].

Auf die Beteiligung des Inselapparates bei der cystischen Pankreasfibrose gehe ich hier nicht ein.

b) Dyschylien des Pankreas als Ursache der sog. Pankreasinsuffizienz. Fermententgleisung.

Der Begriff der Pankreasdyschylie ist noch nicht Allgemeingut; die Klinik ist an die Bezeichnung *Pankreasinsuffizienz* gewöhnt, die vom pathogenetischen Standpunkt aus nicht allzuviel besagt. Henning (1949) definierte die Pankreasinsuffizienz als einen Zustand verminderter Absonderung von Bauchspeichel, die eine mangelhafte Spaltung der Nahrung zur Folge hat. Ihre Ursache ist stets organischer Natur. Unter den mechanischen Ursachen werden Gallen- oder Pankreassteine, Pankreaskopf- oder Gallengangscarcinom, in seltenen Fällen auch ein in die Ausführungsgänge eingedrungener Spulwurm besonders angeführt. Der gleiche Effekt wird in einem Versiegen der Quelle des Saftflusses durch Parenchymschäden (Pankreatitis, Pankreascirrhose, Pankreasatrophie) gesehen. Es wird bemerkt, daß leichtere Funktionsstörungen den Ernährungszustand und das Wohlbefinden nicht zu beeinträchtigen brauchen. Klinisch am besten faßbar ist die Störung der Fettverdauung. Bei der pankreatogenen Steatorrhoe wird die fehlende Fettspaltung durch das Auftreten von Neutralfetten im Stuhl deutlich im Gegensatz zu Steatorrhoe bei Gallenmangel (Fettsäurenadeln). Auf die nachweisbare Verminderung der *Fettspaltung* bei Pankreaserkrankung gegenüber schwerster Störung der *Fettresorption* bei normaler Spaltung der Nahrungsfette bei Sprue hat Bürger (1951) besonders hingewiesen. Fehlende Absonderung von Pankreassaft infolge Gangverlegung führt weiterhin zur mangelhaften Verdauung der mit der Nahrung aufgenommenen Eiweißstoffe, so daß Eiweißfäulnis im Darm erfolgt. — So erheblich die Zahl pathologisch-anatomischer Beobachtungen von Erkrankungen der Bauchspeicheldrüse ist, die zu einer ungenügenden Bildung von Bauchspeichel oder zu einer Erschwerung seines Abflusses in den Darm führen, so wenig verwertbare Angaben findet man im Schrifttum auf Grund von Einzelbeobachtungen, die in jeder Hinsicht, also stoffwechselmäßig und pathologisch-anatomisch, so durchuntersucht sind, daß die anatomischen Äquivalente der gestörten Funktion mit dieser in befriedigende

---

[1] Zit. nach Popper 1952.   [2] Popper 1952.   [3] Werthemann, Grogg und Frey 1952.

Beziehung gebracht werden können. Dieser Mißstand dürfte 2 Wurzeln haben: einmal die Unmöglichkeit, während des Lebens reinen Pankreassaft zu gewinnen (wenn nicht eine Fistel besteht) und zum anderen die rasch einsetzende Autolyse der Bauchspeicheldrüse, die bei nicht sehr frühzeitiger Sektion die Befunde trübt und die Klärung mancher Frage vereitelt.

Indes hat ANDERSEN (1942) die Fermente bei der kindlichen Pankreasinsuffizienz (Cöliakie-Syndrom) im Duodenalsaft untersucht und ist zu der Feststellung gekommen, daß Trypsin und Lipase verringert zu sein pflegen; die Prüfung der Amylase stieß auf Schwierigkeiten, weil sie schon normalerweise gering zu sein pflegt und nicht von der Mundspeichel-Amylase zu trennen ist.

POPPER (1952) hat darauf hingewiesen, daß der Verschluß kleinerer Pankreaswege zu einer chronisch-rezidivierenden Pankreatitis führt und eine viel größere Bedeutung, als gemeinhin angenommen wird, dadurch gewinnt, daß die interstitielle fibroblastische Entzündung zu einem Circulus vitiosus führt: durch Drosselung der kleinen Gänge, ihre cystische Erweiterung und Atrophie des exkretorischen Parenchyms wird die interstitielle Entzündung weiter gefördert. Er nennt als Folgen der chronischen rezidivierenden Pankreatitis

1. Dyskinesie der Gallenwege und Cholecystitis durch Übergreifen der Entzündung auf den Ductus choledochus,

2. Ernährungsschäden durch schlechte Ausnutzung der Speisen,

3. Diabetes mellitus (in 20%) durch Übergreifen der verödenden Prozesse auf die Langerhansschen Inseln.

Als Besonderheit sei eine Beobachtung ZINKGRÄFs (1951) erwähnt, in der exkretorische und inkretorische Pankreasinsuffizienz infolge stenosierender Pankreatitis auf dem Boden einer Pankreasmißbildung eintrat und zum Tode führte.

Während klinische Autoren[1] geneigt sind, hämatogen-infektiösen oder toxischen Einflüssen für die Entstehung pankreatitischer Prozesse eine gewisse Bedeutung zuzuerkennen, bezeichnet noch GRUBER (1929) die Ausbeute des Schrifttums über Beobachtungen zu diesem Kapitel als äußerst dürftig, und erst die anatomischen Forschungen der letzten Jahre haben hier unsere Auffassung geändert. Als Beispiel sei angeführt, daß BALL, BAGGENSTOSS und BARGEN (1950) bei chronischer ulceröser Colitis in 53% ihrer Fälle interstitielle Pankreatitis feststellten.

Auch für das Verständnis der akuten Pankreasnekrose sind neuere Untersuchungen bedeutungsvoll geworden. Ausgehend von dem zunächst klinischen Begriff einer „*Fermententgleisung*" im Pankreas[2], die mit einer Veränderung der Blutfermentwerte einhergeht[3] und unter dem Bilde einer serösen Entzündung als sog. Begleit- und Infektpankreatitis verläuft, hat sich insbesondere DOERR (1953, 1954) um die Erforschung der zugrunde liegenden gestaltlichen Umwandlungen verdient gemacht. Er hat die Möglichkeit der Stoffabgabe aus der Blutbahn durch die endothelähnlichen Uferzellen der initialen Speichelröhrchen in den Gangbaum bei Zuständen von Begleitpankreatitis des Menschen und bei experimenteller Gangunterbindung und akuter sekretorischer Reizung beim Hunde untersucht und über bestimmte histologische Äquivalentbilder der sog. Fermententgleisung bei der experimentellen Pankreatitis durch Äthionin berichtet. In Fällen fieberhafter Allgemeininfektion wurde sehr häufig eine seröse Begleitpankreatitis gefunden, wobei die histologischen Befunde nicht nur an eine Permeation in die Ganglichtung, sondern auch aus dieser heraus in das Interstitium denken ließen. Als Modell diente die Gangunterbindung beim Hunde und

---

[1] HENNING und BAUMANN 1946.   [2] KATSCH und GÜLZOW 1953.
[3] BRINCK und GÜLZOW 1937.

Reizung des Pankreas durch Sekretin[1] mit dem Erfolge des sog. Speichelödems
als eines Spezialfalles der serösen Entzündung. Mittels des Reduktionsindicators
Triphenyltetrazoliumchlorid (TTC)[2] und gestützt auf die erwähnten Befunde hat
Doerr (1954) den Weg der Fermententgleisung aufgezeigt. Einmal kann sie
durch eine Abschmelzung der basalen Abschnitte der Acinusepithelien erfolgen,
häufiger aber geschieht ein Übertritt von Bauchspeichel in die Blut- und Lymphbahn im Bereich der Wände der kleinen Ausführungsgänge (Isthmen). Von diesen
Störungen aus ergeben sich fließende Übergänge zur serösen Pankreatitis und
zur Pankreasnekrose (Modellfall einer parenteralen Verdauung)[3]. Von den zahlreichen neuen, meist experimentellen Untersuchungen über die Entstehung der
chronischen rezidivierenden Pankreatitis sind besonders die Arbeiten anzuführen
von Becker (1955), Becker u. Schaefer (1957, Stein und Powers jr. (1958),
Bartholomew (1959), Becker (1959), Grossman (1959).

c) Die Pankreasnekrose.

In der *akuten Pankreasnekrose* sehen wir die großartigste Form der Selbst-
verdauung des sekretliefernden Organs, deren Gefahr in der unmittelbaren
tödlichen Vergiftung des Organismus durch das frei werdende Trypsin oder in
Komplikationen innerhalb des Bauchraumes (Peritonitis) liegt. Es handelt sich,
wie allgemein bekannt, um eine Aktivierung des unter normalen Bedingungen
in inaktivem Zustand zur Sekretion kommenden Trypsins innerhalb des Pankreas
und um eine schlagartig sich entwickelnde Nekrose, vor allem im Schwanzteil
des Organs. Entscheidend ist dabei der Übertritt des Fermentes in das benachbarte
Gewebe, wodurch dieses der Eiweißverdauung anheimfällt und sekundär blutig
durchsetzt werden kann. Durch Verflüssigung und Abstoßung der abgestorbenen
Massen können diese in die Bauchhöhle gelangen. Mit dem Freiwerden von
Pankreassaft in dem Organ selbst werden Lipasen frei und führen zu Fettgewebs-
nekrosen bis weit in die Umgebung hinein. — Als Ursachen dieses Geschehens
werden seit langem Gallerückfluß, vor allem bei gemeinsamer Mündung des
Gallen- und Pankreasganges, Gefäßerkrankungen (sehr fraglich[4]), Trauma u. a.
angeschuldigt. Gelegentlich kommen auch seltenere Mechanismen zur Wirkung.
So hat Walthard (1935) die Invasion von 2 Ascariden in die Pankreasgänge
bei einem 56jährigen adipösen Manne als auslösende Ursache des Geschehens
mitgeteilt. Auch Gruber (1929) erwähnte derartige Vorkommnisse; es ist aber
bemerkenswert, daß nach ihm ein Einwandern von Würmern ziemlich häufig
ohne gröbere Schädigungen des Parenchyms erfolgen kann. In neuerer Zeit
mehren sich die Mitteilungen über das Auftreten von Pankreasnekrose auf andere
Weise bzw. Beobachtungen, die Zweifel aufkommen lassen müssen, ob dem sog.
Gallereflux[5] wirklich die entscheidende Bedeutung beizumessen ist, die ihm bisher
zuerkannt wurde. So bezweifelt W. W. Meyer (1950) auf Grund einer eindrucksvollen Beobachtung, daß das Eindringen von Galle in die Pankreasgänge als
pathogenetischer Faktor für die Entstehung einer Pankreasnekrose genügt. Er
wies darauf hin, daß bei der Kontrastmitteleinführung in die Gallenwege nicht
selten (nach Mirizzi und Hulton in 10%, nach Leven in 23%) eine Füllung des
Endteiles des Ductus pancreaticus erfolgt. Nach den Untersuchungen von
Wainright (1951) sind als Ursache für die Entstehung einer akuten hämorrhagischen Pankreatitis nur in einem kleinen Prozentsatz anatomische Besonderheiten

---

[1] Popper, zit. nach Doerr 1954.   [2] Doerr 1953.   [3] Doerr 1954, Seifert 1956.
[4] Gruber 1929.
[5] *Anmerkung:* Die von W. W. Meyer (1950) vorgeschlagene Bezeichnung „Influx" trifft den
Vorgang besser; von einem „*Zurück*strömen" oder einer „*Rück*stauung" kann ja keine
Rede sein.

im Bereich der Papilla Vateri und das Vorhandensein von Gallensteinen festzustellen. Unter 81 Fällen wurden 50mal intrapankreatische Veränderungen aufgedeckt (Dilatation der Acini und kleinen Gänge, Metaplasie des Gangepithels). Folge dieser Veränderung seien Rupturen der Acini mit Austritt von Pankreassaft. HICKEN und McALLISTER (1952) beobachteten bei Untersuchung von 100 Patienten mit nachgewiesener Gallenerkrankung und Reflux zum Pankreas nur in 3 Fällen eine akute oder subakute Pankreatitis und kamen zu dem Schluß, daß der Galleninflux in die Pankreasgänge ein normaler, physiologischer Vorgang sei und nur selten „entzündliche" Veränderungen im Pankreas hervorrufe. So wendet sich der Blick der neueren Forschung mehr den Vorgängen zu, die durch experimentell herbeigeführte hypoxydotische Zellschädigungen die akute Pankreasnekrose aus dem Speichelödem bedingen[1]. Es ist zu erwarten, daß auch die Humanpathologie vor neuen Ergebnissen steht.

Treten bei dem akuten Anfall von Pankreasnekrose die Störungen der äußeren Sekretion gegenüber dem dramatischen Geschehen der Organerkrankung oft in den Hintergrund, so sind auch bei Ausheilung des Prozesses die Folgen für die Produktion und Lieferung des Bauchspeichels offenbar nicht beträchtlich[2]. Es scheint, daß die Sekretionsleistungen des verbliebenen Drüsenanteils sich den Erfordernissen des Körpers anzupassen vermögen. Interessant ist in diesem Zusammenhang, daß nach SEBENING[3] bei 21 Patienten in dem ersten halben Jahr nach einer Operation wegen Pankreasnekrose auch eine innersekretorische Pankreasstörung nachzuweisen war, aber in keinem Fall eine Dauerschädigung des Inselapparates zurückblieb. Diese Feststellung läßt vielleicht den Gedanken an eine Parallele einer kompensatorischen oder Ausgleichsleistung des exkretorischen Parenchyms zu.

d) Folgen exkretorischer Pankreasinsuffizienz.

Es wurde schon erwähnt, daß bei der chronischen Entzündung des Pankreas eine Dyskinesie der Gallenwege eintreten kann, die in der Pathogenese der Gallenwegsentzündung Bedeutung erlangen kann. Die Frage, ob ein Einströmen von Pankreassaft eine Rolle bei der Entstehung der *Cholecystitis* spielt, wird verschiedentlich bejaht. BÜCHNER (1950) bringt Abbildungen von schwerer ulceröser Cholecystitis bei Kaninchen aus einer Dissertation von SCHILLING (1944). Die Gallenblasenentzündung war durch Injektion einer geringen Menge von Pankreassaft in die Gallenblase hervorgerufen worden. Diese Untersuchungen bestätigen frühere Wahrnehmungen[4], vor allem aber die Mitteilungen MEHNENs (1938) über das gehäufte Auftreten von entzündlichen Gallensteinen bei gemeinsamer Mündung der Gänge. Der Einstrom von Pankreassaft in die Gallenblase soll zu einer Verminderung der Gallensäuren und dadurch zur Ausfällung von Cholesterin führen. Unter 29 Fällen sog. Stippchengallenblase sah Verfasser 25 mit Rückflußmöglichkeit. — Pankreassaft, durch eine Transplantation des Ductus pancreaticus in die Gallenblase von Hunden gebracht, zeigte keine Wirkung auf die Gallenblase, solange beide Sekrete durch den Gallengang abfließen konnten. Wurde jedoch der Ductus cysticus abgebunden, so traten schwere Störungen bis Nekrosen auf[5]. Auch UNGER (1957) konnte experimentell keine Schädigung der Gallenblasenwand durch den Bauchspeichel feststellen.

Die Beziehungen zwischen exkretorischer Pankreasinsuffizienz und *Leberstoffwechsel* sind noch nicht restlos geklärt. Aus Tierversuchen[6] ist zu schließen

---

[1] POPPER 1952, DOERR 1954, BECKER 1957.   [2] GRUBER 1929.
[3] SEBENING, zit. nach GRUBER 1929.   [4] POPPER 1933.
[5] REID, zit. nach KRZYWANEK und FLASCHENTRÄGER 1954.   [6] Literatur bei MÄDER 1948.

daß im Pankreas ein den Transport und die Verwertung von Fetten regulierender
hormonähnlicher Stoff vorkommt, der von Dragstedt *Lipocaic* genannt wurde,
und der aus mehreren Faktoren zusammengesetzt sein muß. Bei cystischer
Pankreasfibrose ist Leberverfettung nicht selten (s. unter „Dyschylien des
Pankreas"). Eine Beobachtung Mäders (1948) ist geeignet, ein Schlaglicht
auf diese Beziehungen zu werfen. Es handelte sich um eine sehr seltene,
chronisch verlaufende Krankheit, die unter Zeichen exkretorischer Pankreasinsuffizienz (histologische Pankreasatrophie mit Vermehrung der Langerhansschen Inseln und Reichtum an A-Zellen) zu hochgradiger Kachexie führte.
Diesem Geschehen lief eine ständig zunehmende Leberverfettung parallel.
Als Ursache des Leidens nahm Verfasserin Pankreas- und Magensekretionsstö-
rungen an, die auf noch unbekannte Weise zu einem Absinken des Blutfett-
spiegels und Fettansammlung in der Leber führten. Die neben der Störung
der äußeren Sekretion bestehenden Inselveränderungen legten den Gedanken
nahe, daß auch Störungen der inneren Sekretion bei der Fettspeicherung im
Spiele waren (daher die vielleicht nicht ganz glückliche Bezeichnung „Inselfettleber"). Sanes und Mitarbeiter (1950) sind in der Bewertung von Pankreasveränderungen für die Entstehung einer Fettleber vorsichtiger, da übergeordnete
Faktoren die Leberveränderungen bewirkt haben können (Diabetes, Alkoholismus,
Unterernährung, Infektion). Nach dieser Auffassung darf nur dann ein „pan-
kreato-hepatisches Syndrom" angenommen werden, wenn die Leberveränderungen mit kongenitalen cystischen Pankreasveränderungen gekoppelt sind,
wobei dann das Versagen der Bauchspeicheldrüse als primärer pathogenetischer
Faktor für die Lebererkrankung anzusehen wäre. Bei cystischer Pankreasfibrose
ist zentrale Leberverfettung auf das Fehlen von Lipocaic zurückgeführt worden[1].
Auch in Fällen interstitieller Pankreatitis bei chronischer ulceröser Colitis fanden
Ball, Baggenstoss und Bargen (1950) regelmäßig Leberverfettung. Die Beziehungen scheinen allerdings hier wegen der Grundkrankheit nicht ganz klar.
Seifert (1951) sowie Stinson jr., Baggenstoss und Morlock (1952) untersuchten
den Zusammenhang zwischen Lebercirrhose und Pankreasveränderungen. Nach
diesen Untersuchungen scheint die portale Stauung auf die Ausbildung fibrotischer Zustände des Pankreas Einfluß zu haben; auch Erweiterungen der Drüsenendstücke und Gangerweiterungen mit Sekreteindickung sind von den amerikanischen Autoren erwähnt. — Über hieraus sich ergebende Störungen in der Zusammensetzung der Verdauungssäfte können keine Aussagen gemacht werden.

4. Die Dyschylien durch fehlerhafte Gallebildung und -absonderung.

Das zweite Sekret, das auf den Dünndarminhalt ergossen wird, ist das Sekret
der Leber, die Galle. So umfangreich das Schrifttum der speziellen Pathologie
der Leber und der Gallenwege ist, so wenig vollständig sind unsere Kenntnisse
über die den einzelnen krankhaften Abläufen zugeordneten Störungen in der
Bereitung und Lieferung der Galle. In der großen Zahl der Leberfunktions-
prüfungen, die physiologische Chemie und Klinik erarbeitet haben, nehmen die
der exkretorischen Leberleistung nur einen bescheidenen Raum ein (Ausscheidung
von Farbstoffen oder Röntgenkontrastmitteln, Bilirubinausscheidung nach intravenöser Bilirubinbelastung). Im Vergleich zu der quantitativen und qualitativen
Vielfalt der vorkommenden Störungen sind aber alle diese Prüfungen noch recht
grob und geben höchstens Aufschluß über eine vorhandene mehr oder weniger
schwere Störung, ohne die Grundlagen für eine wissenschaftliche Systematik
liefern zu können. Die Darstellung einer allgemeinen Pathologie der Sekretions-

---

[1] Michaud 1952.

störungen der Leber muß also notgedrungen recht lückenhaft ausfallen, wozu noch kommt, daß Störungen im Bereich der Gallenblase, ja sogar der völlige Funktionsausfall des Organs, keinen nachhaltigen Einfluß auf die Lieferung des Verdauungssekretes der Leber zu haben brauchen (vgl. die Angaben von GROGG und STAUB in Teil II dieses Bandes unter: Die Physiologie der Gallenblase und der Gallenwege). Die Störungen der Gallebereitung und -sekretion sind in dem Beitrag von KÜHN. (Die Pathologie der Ausscheidung der Leber) geschildert, auf den verwiesen wird.

Eine Verminderung der Gallensekretion erfolgt bei allen Zuständen mit Parenchymschädigung einhergehender diffuser Leberentzündung. Der Übertritt aller Gallenbestandteile ins Blut kann als Maßstab für die verminderte Lieferung von Galle in den Darm gelten. Die schwersten Störungen dieser Art sind also bei der diffusen toxischen Leberdystrophie zu erwarten, doch ist grundsätzlich eine gleichartige, dem Grade nach allerdings wechselnde Störung bei jedem mit Parenchymschädigung der Leber einhergehenden Prozeß zu erwarten, also bei allen Formen von Hepatitis.

Eine Vermehrung der Gallemenge ist nach HENNING (1955) unter regelhaften Bedingungen noch nicht mit Sicherheit festgestellt worden; lediglich eine Vermehrung des Gallenfarbstoffes (Pleiochromie) infolge erhöhten Blutfarbstoffangebotes an die Leber bei Blutzerfall verschiedenster Ursache ist bekannt.

Am bedeutungsvollsten für die Verdauung und Resorption ist zweifellos die Behinderung des Galleabflusses in den Zwölffingerdarm durch Drosselung oder Verlegung der Galleabflußwege. Die Ursachen dieser Störung sind bekannt (Steineinklemmung, Gewächsbildungen, besonders der Krebs des Pankreaskopfes) und bedürfen keiner weiteren Ausführungen. Entscheidend ist das Fehlen der Gallensäuren im Darm, welche für die Emulgierung der Fette notwendig sind und der Aktivierung der Pankreaslipase und Steigerung ihrer Wirksamkeit dienen. Ein großer Teil der Nahrungsfette kann dann nicht resorbiert werden und wird ungenützt mit dem Stuhl ausgeschieden (Fettstühle). Im Stuhl sieht man Massen von Fettsäurenadeln, da die Fettsäuren — die auch ohne die Wirkung der Galle durch Fettspaltung entstanden sein können — durch die „hydrotrope" Wirkung der Gallensäuren nicht wasserlöslich gemacht und nicht resorbiert werden können. Nach VERZÁR (1935) spielen die Gallensäuren auch bei der *Resorption* der Fette eine große Rolle. Sie sind normalerweise nur selten nachzuweisen[1]. — Auch das fettlösliche Vitamin K kann nicht resorbiert werden und gelangt nicht in die Leber; es kommt zu einer K-Hypo- bzw. -Avitaminose, der Aufbau von Prothrombin aus K-Vitamin unter Mitwirkung der Leberzellen ist gestört, und die Hypoprothrombinämie geht schließlich in den Zustand der hämorrhagischen Diathese über[1].

Eine Störung der Eiweiß- und Kohlenhydratspaltung bei Fehlen von Galle im Darm ist nicht bekannt.

Auf die Rolle einer fehlerhaften Zusammensetzung der Blasengalle für die Steinbildung in der Gallenblase soll in diesem Zusammenhang nicht eingegangen werden. Hingegen sei auf die Beteiligung der Leber bei der Mucoviscidose hingewiesen (s. Pankreasdyschylien).

Ob eine mangelhafte Alkalisierung des in den Dünndarm gelangenden Mageninhalts bei fehlerhafter Galleneinströmung in den Darm von Bedeutung ist, muß als nicht entschieden gelten. HUG (1939) hat diese Frage für die Erklärung peptischer Jejunalerosionen angeschnitten.

---

[1] HENNING und BAUMANN 1949.

5. Die Dyschylien durch fehlerhafte Darmsekretion.

Auch der Dünndarm gehört zu den großen Verdauungsdrüsen, wenngleich seine Bedeutung als Resorptionsorgan ungleich größer ist. Unsere Kenntnisse über die Darmsekretion des Menschen sind gering, was, wie Henning (1955) hervorhebt, darauf beruht, daß uns das reine menschliche Darmsekret fast unbekannt ist. Durch besondere Kunstgriffe (Ausschaltung einer Darmschlinge mit Fistelbildung) gelingt es, am Versuchstier reines Darmsekret zu gewinnen. Als Produktionsquellen kommen die Lieberkühnschen Drüsen, im Duodenum die Brunnerschen Drüsen in Frage[1]. Eine Reihe für die Verdauung wichtiger Fermente des Darmsaftes oder der Darmwand ist bekannt (Proteasen, Esterasen, Carbohydrasen, Nukleasen); die Ergebnisse wurden fast ausschließlich an Tieren (Hund, Schwein) gewonnen. Ferner werden in der Darmschleimhaut Hormone oder hormonartige Substanzen gebildet, welche auf andere Verdauungsdrüsen sowie die Sekretion und Motilität des Magens und auf die Zottentätigkeit wirken[2].

Über eine Verminderung oder Vermehrung des Darmsekretes haben wir keine genauen Kenntnisse, zumal Sekretion und Resorption immer nebeneinander hergehen. Verminderung der Sekretion ist bei schweren, chronischen, mit Drüsenatrophie einhergehenden Schleimhautentzündungen zu erwarten, wenn auch nicht bewiesen; Vermehrung der Sekretion bei akuten Entzündungen. Hier ist die Unterscheidung von der Absonderung entzündlichen Exsudates in den Darmentleerungen schwierig[1]. Vermehrte Sekretion ist stets bei erhöhter Peristaltik vorhanden.

Bei den sog. Darmdyspepsien (Gärungs- und Fäulnisdyspepsie) können dyschylische Komponenten eine Rolle spielen, z. B. Störungen in der Abscheidung diastatischer Fermente bei der Gärungsdyspepsie, Achylie des Magens bei der Fäulnisdyspepsie, doch ist anderen Einflüssen wie der mangelhaften mechanischen Aufbereitung der Digesta, der veränderten Darmflora, Darmentzündung, beschleunigter Peristaltik und Resorptionsstörungen eine erhebliche Bedeutung zuzuschreiben, deren Rolle freilich im einzelnen nicht immer zu klären ist. Ist schon die Kenntnis der pathologischen Physiologie dieser Störungen unvollständig, so ist die pathologische Anatomie an ihrer Klärung bisher so gut wie unbeteiligt geblieben

Bei der sog. Mucoviscidose der Neugeborenen in Form des Meconiumileus können die Darmdrüsen an der allgemeinen Sekretionsstörung durch Produktion vermehrten und eingedickten Schleimes beteiligt sein[3].

B. Die krankhaften Störungen der Verdauung und Resorption (und besonders dieser) bei ungestörter Lieferung der Verdauungssäfte.

1. Störungen infolge veränderter Motilität und bei Lichtungsänderungen des Darmrohres.

Diese Störungen, die Henning (1955) nicht zu den eigentlichen Störungen der Darmresorption rechnet, weil man unter Störung der Darmresorption im engeren Sinne nur die fehlerhafte Leistung des Resorptionsapparates selbst rechnen dürfe, beruhen auf einem zu kurzen Kontakt des resorptionsfähigen Materials mit dem Resorptionsorgan; sie haben sich weitgehend der anatomischen Forschung entzogen. Die Resorption wird also in allen Fällen gesteigerten Dünndarmtransportes leiden müssen; die möglichen Ursachen sollen hier nicht besprochen werden.

---

[1] Henning 1955.   [2] Krzywanek und Flaschenträger 1954.
[3] Saegesser und Mitarbeiter 1955.

Von besonderer Bedeutung für die Resorption sind die Bewegungsvorgänge in der Schleimhaut selbst, also die durch die Zotten und die Muscularis mucosae hervorgerufenen. Nach VERZÁR (1933) ist die sog. Zottenpumpe in qualitativer und sind die Muscularis mucosae-Bewegungen hauptsächlich in quantitativer Hinsicht für die Resorption von Bedeutung. Die pumpenden Zottenbewegungen werden durch lokale Blutungen gelähmt; sie hängen überhaupt weitgehend von einer vollkommenen Blutversorgung ab und werden vom CO_2-Gehalt des Blutes beeinflußt. Überventiliert man ein Tier, so daß es nach dem Aufhören der Ventilation sich in Apnoe befindet, so hört die Zottenbewegung auf und erscheint erst nach dem Eintritt der Spontanatmung wieder[1]. Auch Herabsetzung der Temperatur um 1—2° wirkt bereits lähmend auf die Zottentätigkeit. Bei Splanchnicusreizung wird die Schleimhaut anämisch, und die Zottenbewegung sistiert. Auch allgemeine Asphyxie wirkt lähmend, lokale hingegen steigert die Zottenbewegung. Das lokale chemische Milieu scheint der natürliche Reiz der Zottenbewegung zu sein; dafür spricht, daß sie beim hungernden Tier überhaupt nicht vorhanden oder nur sehr geringfügig ist, während des Resorptionsvorgangs aber stets sehr lebhaft wird. Besonders interessant ist die von KOKAS (1948) getroffene Feststellung, daß an einem transplantierten Darmstück nur dann Zottenbewegung wahrnehmbar war, wenn das Versuchstier sich im Stadium der Verdauung und Resorption befand. Die Zottentätigkeit wird durch ein in der Darmschleimhaut als unwirksames Proferment vorhandenes Hormon, das *Villikinin*, gesteuert.

Aus diesen Feststellungen wird für die menschliche Pathologie zu folgern sein, daß Umstände, welche die Bewegungsfähigkeit des Zottenapparates einschränken, also vor allem lokale Exsudatbildungen und zellige Infiltrate, ihre Resorptionsleistungen herabsetzen müssen. Meßbare Ergebnisse hierüber liegen allerdings nicht vor.

Selbst die Änderung der Resorption bei Ileus ist im einzelnen nicht erforscht, sowohl was die Phase erhöhter Motilität als auch die der Darmruhe betrifft. Freilich ist hier einer systematischen Auswertung durch die Vielfalt der Möglichkeiten in anatomischem Sitz, Komplikationen durch Darmwandentzündung, Darmwandhypertrophie, örtliche Kreislaufstörungen, Zersetzungsvorgänge im Darmrohr usw. eine Grenze gesetzt.

In 2 Fällen von Stenosenileus des Dünndarmes, in denen klinisch Fettstühle und ein sprueähnliches Bild beobachtet worden war, konnte ich bei Untersuchung der Operationspräparate nichts erkennen, was diese Erscheinungen erklärt hätte.

Ganz allgemein stellt man sich die Pathogenese der gestörten Resorption bei Ileuszuständen so vor, daß mit zunehmender Dehnung der Darmwand eine Kompression der feinen Blut- und Lymphgefäße erfolgt[2]. — Auf die Resorption von Darmgiften gehe ich hier nicht ein.

Eine Abnahme der alkalischen Phosphatase in den Darmepithelien nach Adrenalektomie war in Versuchen mit einer Verminderung der selektiven Glucoseresorption verbunden[3].

2. Störungen durch Kreislaufänderungen und entzündliche Vorgänge des Darmes.

Auf die Beeinträchtigung der Zottentätigkeit durch Kreislaufstörungen wurde oben hingewiesen. Auf die Bedeutung von Zirkulationsstörungen für die Resorption, und zwar sowohl von allgemeinen Kreislaufstörungen wie von

---

[1] KOKAS 1948.   [2] HENNING und BAUMANN 1949, BÜRGER 1951.
[3] VERZÁR und SAILER 1952, VERZÁR, SAILER und RICHTERICH 1952.

örtlichen Störungen in der Zottendurchblutung hat in neuerer Zeit DE Langen (1953, 1956) hingewiesen und gezeigt, daß auch leichtere, kurzfristige Intoxikationen, Infektionen und Diätfehler infolge fehlerhafter Zottenzirkulation zu deutlichen Resorptionsstörungen mit Fettdiarrhoen führen können. Näheres hierüber im Absatz „Sprue-Komplex". Nach Bürger (1951) ist bei Ödemkrankheit die Resorption der gesamten Nahrung erheblich verschlechtert. Fette und besonders Eiweißstoffe werden mangelhaft resorbiert; mit zunehmender Ausschwemmung der Ödeme nähern sich die Werte wieder der Norm. Für die schlechte Ausnutzung wird außer der Herabsetzung der zirkulierenden Blutmenge und der ödematösen Durchtränkung der Darmzotten auch eine mangelhafte fermentative Aufschließung der Digesta angeschuldigt [1].

Bei Enteritis ist nach den übereinstimmenden Befunden älterer und neuerer Autoren das Stuhlbild ein Beweis für mangelhafte Aufschließung und Resorption der Nahrungsbestandteile, gleichgültig, ob es sich um durchfällige oder geformte Stühle handelt. Durch Vermehrung oder Verminderung von Tonus und Peristaltik im ganzen Darm oder in einzelnen Abschnitten können mannigfaltige Bilder entstehen, die nicht einer bestimmten Enteritisform zugeordnet werden können. Auch der alte Dyspepsie-Begriff (Gärungs- und Fäulnisdyspepsie) mit der Annahme rein funktioneller Störungen dürfte heute weitgehend zugunsten einer Anschauung verlassen sein, die alle diese Störungen auf enteritische bzw. enterokolitische Vorgänge bezieht [1]. Welchen Umständen im einzelnen bei der akuten und chronischen Enteritis eintretende Resorptionsstörungen ihre Entstehung verdanken, ist nicht geklärt. Ausgedehnte flächenhafte Veränderungen bilden eine andere Voraussetzung als umschriebene Prozesse. Bei Geschwürsbildungen können Resorptionsstörungen ganz ausbleiben [2]. So erscheint es wenig aussichtsreich, eine Beziehung zwischen Art und Schwere der Störung einerseits und anatomischer Ausprägung enteritischer Zustände andererseits zu finden. Bestimmte, experimentell geprüfte Resorptionsstörungen (gestörte Resorption einzelner Stoffe, wie z. B. von Kalksalzen und isotonischen Lösungen [3]) besagen nichts Näheres über diese Beziehungen. Ob die Vorstellung einer auf der Schleimhaut sich bildenden „Schutzschicht" aus Schleim als resorptionverlangsamendes Moment [4] richtig ist, muß dahingestellt bleiben.

3. Störungen durch Ausschaltung wesentlicher Darmteile.

Einige Arbeiten haben sich mit dem Verhältnis von Darmlänge und Resorption befaßt [5, 6]. Gelegentlich scheint der Ausfall fast des gesamten Dünndarmes, wenigstens für einige Zeit, ohne schwerere Störungen vertragen zu werden.

Underhill (1955) erwähnte eine solche Beobachtung von Shonyo und Jackson: Bei einer 41jährigen Frau war wegen eines Adenocarcinoms des Jejunums mit Übergreifen auf die angrenzenden Darmschlingen fast der gesamte Dünndarm reseziert worden, so daß zwischen dem Pylorus und der Ileocöcalklappe nur ein 39 cm langes Darmstück verblieb. Bei einer Stoffwechseluntersuchung ein Jahr später war zwar ein Albumindefizit im Blut vorhanden, aber die Resorption und Ausnutzung von Wasser, Nahrung, Mineralien und Vitaminen war nicht ernstlich gestört.

Eine noch eindrucksvollere Beobachtung ist folgende: Bei einem damals 69jährigen Manne wurde im Februar 1948 wegen Darmbrandes eine subtotale Dünndarmresektion ausgeführt; es wurden 270 cm Dünndarm entfernt, so daß nur ein je 25 cm langes Stück des Jejunums und des Ileums verblieb. Nachdem in der ersten Zeit nach der Operation noch Fettstühle bestanden, ist nunmehr, nach 12 Jahren, keine nennenswerte Störung der Nahrungsausnutzung feststellbar [6].

---

[1] Henning und Baumann 1949.   [2] Bürger 1951.

[3] Catel 1938, Hetényi 1938, Bejul 1952.

[4] Nonnenbruch 1932.   [5] Mangold 1951.

[6] Sie wurde mir durch die Freundlichkeit der Herren Prof. Dr. Hansen und Dr. Lübbers zugänglich.

Im allgemeinen pflegen sich aber in solchen Fällen unstillbare Durchfälle einzustellen. Die Fettresorption wird schwer gestört, die Fette werden zwar gut verdaut, aber zu 45% mit dem Stuhl ausgeschieden, davon 80% in Form von Fettsäuren. Infolge des Verlustes von Calcium und Vitamin D mit den Fetten entwickelt sich leicht Tetanie. Die Kohlenhydratausnutzung pflegt ungestört zu bleiben, aber von dem Nahrungseiweiß verlassen 45% den Körper mit dem Stuhl. Auch die Bildung der Vitamine B_{12} und K durch bakterielle Tätigkeit im Colon bleibt aus. Bei manchen Patienten entsteht eine hyperchrome megaloblastische Anämie wie bei Sprue[1].

Die Folgen einer sehr ausgedehnten Dünndarmresektion können also denen der Umgehung des Dünndarmes entsprechen. Letztere tritt ein, wenn durch krankhafte Vorgänge eine abnorme Verbindung zwischen Magen bzw. Jejunum und Colon geschaffen wird, meist also wohl bei einem durchbrechenden Carcinom. Die gastro- bzw. jejunokolische Fistel, welche so entstehen kann, führt zu schweren Störungen der Resorption, besonders der Fette, und es bildet sich für gewöhnlich der Symptomenkomplex der Sprue heraus.

Über „enterogene Perniciosa" nach Dünndarmausfall siehe unter „Magenachylie".

4. Der Sprue-Komplex in seiner Beziehung zur Verdauung und Resorption.

Wohl bei keiner Erkrankung stehen Störungen der Darmresorption so im Vordergrund wie bei dem Komplex von Erscheinungen, der mit „Sprue" bezeichnet wird. Im anglo-amerikanischen Schrifttum hat sich die Bezeichnung „the malabsorption syndrome" eingebürgert. Die Forschung der letzten 30 Jahre hat sich mit diesem Krankheitsbild viel beschäftigt und, wenn auch keine restlose Klärung der Vorgänge bis ins einzelne, so doch viele wichtige Ergebnisse gezeitigt, die für die Kenntnis der Resorptionsleistungen unter normalen und gestörten Bedingungen sowie über die Folgen gestörter Darmresorption bedeutungsvoll geworden sind. Als grundlegend ist die Monographie von HESS-THAYSEN (1932) zu bezeichnen, der hervorgehoben hat, daß die nichttropische oder einheimische Sprue kein seltenes Vorkommen ist, und daß einheimische und tropische Sprue dieselbe Krankheit sind. Er betont auch, daß die Gee-Hertersche Cöliakie des Kindes in die gleiche Gruppe gehört, eine Auffassung, die jetzt wohl von den meisten Autoren geteilt wird[2].

Im Hinblick auf die zugrunde liegenden Störungen der Resorption ist an dieser Stelle nur von der sog. „idiopathischen" Sprue die Rede, d. h. von jenen Vorkommnissen, deren Hauptkennzeichen Fettstühle, Anämie und Auszehrung sind, und die nicht auf mangelhafter Verdauung infolge der Pankreassaftlieferung, auf Ausfall des Darmrohres oder auf Störungen des Lymphabflusses in der Darmwand oder im Gekröse beruhen, also auch nicht auf Darmwandamyloid oder Tuberkulose der Gekröselymphknoten (sog. symptomatische Sprue). Bei der „idiopathischen" Sprue ist, wie schon die Namengebung vermuten läßt, geradezu das Fehlen anatomischer Befunde kennzeichnend, welche die Resorptionsstörungen erklären könnten. Zwar werden bis in die neueste Zeit immer wieder Arbeiten veröffentlicht, welche sich bemühen, krankhafte Veränderungen des Darmes aufzudecken. So haben SVARTZ und Mitarbeiter (1947) sowie OEHLER (1953) neuerdings entzündliche Veränderungen der Darmwand beschrieben, OHELER mit Geschwüren und Wandsklerosierung, und dabei auf Veränderungen

---

[1] UNDERHILL 1955.
[2] HANSEN und v. STAA 1936, BÜRGER 1951, VERZÁR 1937, RIETSCHEL 1937, ROSENTHAL 1937, ADLERSBERG 1957, SAKULA und SHINER 1957.

der Zotten mit Bildung hyaliner Massen an den Zottenspitzen hingewiesen, wie sie schon früher beobachtet worden waren. Wenngleich diese Veränderungen in der Deutung zurückhaltend beurteilt werden, wird doch in Erwägung gezogen, daß die Resorptionsstörung hier ihre Ursache habe. Unspezifisch-entzündliche und geschwürige Schleimhautveränderungen des Dünndarmes sind bei Sprue schon früher häufig veröffentlicht worden, z. B. von Rosenthal (1937), während Luksch und Sachs (1937) besonderes Gewicht auf den weitgehenden Schwund des lymphatischen Gewebes speziell im Dünndarm legten. Diese Befunde gehören zu der Gruppe von Veränderungen, wie sie gleichfalls von manchen Autoren geschildert worden sind, nämlich den atrophischen[1]. Bei diesen bestand freilich oft die Schwierigkeit der Abgrenzung intravitaler Vorgänge von postmortalen, durch Fäulnis und Gasdehnung entstandenen[2]. Poursines und Dubarry (1950) glaubten aber, atrophische Veränderungen — neben entzündlichen — sicher verifizieren zu können, da sie sich bei einer 3 Std nach dem Tode vorgenommenen Leichenöffnung feststellen ließen. Wenngleich ein strenger Beweis für die intravitale Entstehung hierdurch noch nicht erbracht ist, so ist es doch durchaus wahrscheinlich, daß Atrophie der Darmschleimhaut vorkommt; sie ist ja auch schon an der Zunge intravital vorhanden. Zu ähnlichen Feststellungen kam Fahr (1937). — Andererseits ist festzustellen, daß eine Reihe von Autoren in Sprue-Fällen keinerlei charakteristische Veränderungen des Darmrohres fanden[3], was schon deutlich macht, daß in den Fällen, wo Geschwüre und dergleichen festzustellen waren, diese für die Entstehung der Resorptionsstörungen nicht maßgebend gewesen sein können. Man ist sich heute auch wohl darüber klar, daß es sich um sekundäre Vorkommnisse handelt, welche in erster Linie durch die veränderte Bakterienflora erklärt werden müssen, ebenso wie die von zahlreichen Autoren beschriebenen entzündlichen Infiltrate der Mucosa und Submucosa. Einen Fortschritt auf dem Gebiete der Morphologie brachte die Einführung der Shinerschen Jejunalsonde, mit der es gelang, Darmschleimhaut bioptisch zu gewinnen und histologisch zu untersuchen[4]. In einer Anzahl solcher Proben sowohl bei idiopathischer Steatorrhoe wie bei Cöliakie fand sich eine starke Atrophie der Schleimhautzotten. Diese Veränderungen werden, wenn auch mit Zurückhaltung, für primär bedeutungsvoll gehalten. Zu ähnlichen Ergebnissen kamen Salvesen u. Skogrand (1957) auf Grund histologischer Untersuchungen autoptisch gewonnenen Materials. — Daß bei Spruefällen mit langdauernder Behandlung mit Corticosteroiden geschwürige Veränderungen des Darmes beobachtet wurden[5], läßt sich für die Pathogenese der Erkrankung wohl kaum auswerten.

Es lag nahe, nach Zeichen der Chylusstauung als Ursache der Resorptionsstörungen zu suchen. Solche beschrieb Mohr (1939) und suchte durch sie Fettstühle wie Resorptionsstörungen zu erklären, nachdem ich kurze Zeit zuvor ähnliche Befunde wie Mohr bei einem klinisch als Sprue angesprochenen Fall erhoben hatte. Von meiner Beobachtung aus dem Jahre 1937 kann ich heute sagen, daß sie der Lipodystrophia intestinalis von Whipple zugerechnet werden muß, und so bleibt nur die Beobachtung Mohrs, in welcher sich bei Sprue Chylusstauung fand. Ich glaube aber, daß bei der „idiopathischen" Sprue Chylusstauung überhaupt keine Rolle spielt, sondern daß alle Fälle mit Chylusstauung eine Whipplesche Erkrankung darstellen. Die Schilderung, die Mohr von den

---

[1] Fahr 1936. [2] Boels und Tverdy 1950.
[3] Hess-Thaysen 1932, Froboese und Thoma 1933, Jeckeln 1937.
[4] Adlersberg 1957, Sakula und Shiner 1957, Himes und Adlersberg 1958, Shiner 1959.
[5] Himes, Gabriel und Adlersberg 1957.

Gekröselymphknoten seiner Beobachtung gab, ist zwar nicht sehr charakteristisch, bestärkt mich aber doch in der von mir geäußerten Annahme.

Zur Differentialdiagnose der „idiopathischen" Sprue ist zu sagen, daß auch noch andere Autoren unter dieser Diagnose oder als Sprue-ähnliche Zustände Veränderungen beschrieben haben, die nach unseren heutigen Kenntnissen dem Krankheitsbild der Lipodystrophia intestinalis zugehören und gerade im Hinblick auf die Störungen der Resorption gesondert betrachtet werden müssen. Die Bezeichnung Lipodystrophia intestinalis oder Whipplesche Krankheit ist im deutschsprachigen Schrifttum bis vor wenigen Jahren nicht bekannt gewesen. BOELS und TVERDY (1950) haben im belgischen Schrifttum darauf hingewiesen, daß meine schon erwähnte Mitteilung eine Whipplesche Erkrankung darstelle, und STAEMMLER (1953), der den gleichen Hinweis, auch bezüglich der Fälle von KLOOS (1939) u. a. auf seinem Freiburger Vortrag machte, konnte ich nur zustimmen[1]. Es bleibt also festzustellen, daß trotz großer klinischer Ähnlichkeiten Sprue und Whipplesche Krankheit zu trennen sind, und daß es für die „idiopathische" Sprue charakteristische, die Resorptionsstörungen erklärende morphologische Befunde am Darm nicht gibt. Die beschriebenen Zottenatrophien bedürfen hinsichtlich ihrer pathogenetischen Bedeutung wohl noch weiterer Klärung.

Hingegen haben klinische und physiologisch-chemische Untersuchungen zur Feststellung einer Reihe von Tatsachen geführt, die wichtig sind. Nach der Monographie von HESS-THAYSEN (1932) hat die Monographie von HANSEN und v. STAA (1936) einen wichtigen Fortschritt gebracht. Das Verdienst der letzteren liegt besonders in der Erkenntnis, daß bei der Sprue „eine Grundstörung — die Fettdiarrhoe — als eigentliche Krankheit und ferner die unter mannigfaltigen Bildern sich äußernde polysymptomatische Avitaminose als ‚zweite Krankheit' " zu unterscheiden sind. Hierauf muß etwas näher eingegangen werden, zumal diese Auffassung auch durch neuere Arbeiten nicht überholt oder in wesentlichen Punkten weitergetrieben ist. HANSEN und v. STAA kamen zu dem Schluß, daß die *primäre Störung* der enteralen Fettresorption ihrem Wesen nach unbekannt ist. — Hier ist zunächst zu fragen, ob die primäre Resorptionsstörung sich nur auf Fette oder auch auf andere Stoffe erstreckt. Alle Autoren sind sich darüber einig, daß eine Resorptionsstörung für Fette im Vordergrund der Erscheinungen steht. BÜRGER (1951) fand in langfristigen Untersuchungen, in denen sowohl die Zu- wie die Ausfuhr chemisch analysiert wurde, Fettverluste bis zu 89%. Primäre Störungen der Eiweißresorption sind nicht erwiesen. Von vielen Untersuchern, namentlich der Cöliakie, sind abnorm hohe N-Mengen im Stuhl gefunden worden, woraus auf eine mangelhafte Eiweißresorption geschlossen wurde; jedoch kamen HANSEN und v. STAA auf Grund kritischer Prüfungen der vorliegenden Mitteilungen zu dem Schluß, daß für die Annahme einer Störung des Eiweißstoffwechsels oder der Eiweißverdauung und -resorption nichts spräche, daß vielmehr derartige Annahmen offenbar auf unrichtiger Interpretation von Einzelbefunden beruhten. Auch BÜRGER (1951) lehnte eine Störung der Eiweißresorption ab; die hohen Stickstoffmengen des Stuhles entstehen nach ihm durch pathologisch gesteigerte Exkretion, weil die N-Verluste mehr von der Menge des Stuhles als von der Größe der Eiweißzufuhr abhängig sind. Was die Frage einer Störung des Kohlenhydratstoffwechsels betrifft, so hat bereits HESS-THAYSEN auf den flachen Verlauf der Blutzuckerkurve nach Glucosebelastung hingewiesen. Seine Feststellung ist von zahlreichen Beobachtern bestätigt worden. Die niedrige Blutzuckerkurve ist aber kein konstantes Symptom der Sprue und verhält sich

---

[1] JECKELN 1952, 1955.

unabhängig vom Grad der Steatorrhoe, so daß es abwegig erscheint, den Sitz der Störung für beide Symptome an einen Ort zu verlegen[1]. Die Kohlenhydratausnutzung liegt bei Sprue zwischen 94 und 98,2%, ist also normal[2]. Bei Sprue treten oft recht erhebliche Calciumverluste mit den Faeces auf, die offenbar aber nicht auf mangelnder Resorptionsfähigkeit der Darmschleimhaut für Calcium, sondern eher auf Bindung an freie Fettsäuren, andere freie Säuren und an unbekannte Komplexe beruhen. Auch ein erniedrigter Phosphorspiegel des Blutes beruht nicht auf einer primären Resorptionsstörung[1, 3]. Hingegen wurde neuerdings eine Verzögerung der Kochsalzresorption mittels Einbringung von radioaktivem Natrium in den Dünndarm wahrscheinlich gemacht[4].

Die *Sekundärschäden* bei der Sprue beruhen auf einer mangelhaften Resorption der mit der Nahrung zugeführten *Vitamine*. Für die fettlöslichen Vitamine ist dies leicht verständlich (vor allem Vitamin D); die Vitamine A, K und E werden wohl im allgemeinen in Mengen zugeführt, welche den Bedarf des Körpers bei weitem befriedigen, so daß klinische Ausfallserscheinungen bei Sprue selten sind. In dem bunten Bilde der sekundären Störungen finden sich aber auch Erscheinungen, die auf Mangel an nichtfettlöslichen Vitaminen beruhen, z. B. Hemeralopie (A-Mangel) oder hämorrhagische Diathese (C- oder K-Mangel)[5]. Unter dem Bilde der „zweiten Krankheit" bedarf die Anämie besonderer Erwähnung. Zum Teil handelt es sich um eine hypochrome Anämie; sie könnte mit Magensaft-Anacidität und einer Eisenresorptionsstörung in Zusammenhang gebracht werden, wie sie nach mangelnder Ionisierung des Nahrungseisens bei fehlender Säureproduktion des Magens eintritt[6]. Es handelt sich dabei also nicht um eine primäre Resorptionsstörung der Darmschleimhaut. Bei einem Teil der Sprue-Kranken besteht eine hyperchrome Anämie vom Typ der Perniciosa. Ihre Entstehung ist noch nicht restlos geklärt. Hansen und v. Staa denken an eine Hinderung der Synthese von B_{12} unter den veränderten biologischen Verhältnissen im Dünndarm oder an eine Zerstörung des synthetisierten Stoffes oder an eine Überführung in eine unresorbierbare Form. Eine eingehende Darstellung unserer jetzigen Kenntnisse über die gestörten Resorptionsverhältnisse findet sich in der von Adlersberg (1957) herausgegebenen Monographie des Mount-Sinai-Hospitals. Hier wird auch die interessante Tatsache erörtert, daß die Verdauungsstörung in vielen Fällen komplexer Natur ist und sowohl auf Störungen der Resorption wie auf gestörter Pankreassekretion beruht.

Steht also in dem skizzierten komplexen Bild der Sprue eine Störung der Fettresorption im Mittelpunkt, so daß diese als das eigentliche primäre Krankheitsgeschehen anzusprechen ist, so erhebt sich die Frage nach der Ursache dieser so markanten und bei unseren geringen Kenntnissen der enteralen Resorptionsstörungen besonders wichtigen und interessanten Erscheinung. Die morphologische Betrachtung läßt, wie schon aufgezeigt, hinsichtlich Ätiologie und Pathogenese im Stich. Auch die Annahme zunächst rein funktioneller Störungen, wie ich sie früher geäußert habe, ist nur hypothetisch. Die Theorie einer unspezifischen Infektion dürfte jetzt wohl allgemein verlassen sein, und auch ein primärer Vitaminmangel ist unwahrscheinlich.

Bei der Frage nach einer primären Störung der inneren Sekretion haben die Untersuchungen Verzárs und seiner Schule[7] eine gewisse Bedeutung erlangt, wenngleich sie nicht die Lösung des Problems brachten, wie es zunächst schien.

---

[1] Hansen und v. Staa 1936.   [2] Bürger 1951.   [3] Dumont-Ruyters 1950.
[4] Newsholme und French 1954.   [5] Hotz 1940.   [6] M. B. Schmidt 1940.
[7] Verzár 1933, 1935, 1937, Verzár und Jeker 1936, Verzár und Laszt 1936, Jeker 1936, Laszt und Verzár 1936.

Ausgehend von der Feststellung, daß die Prozesse, die in der Darmschleimhaut auf die Resorption von Glucose und Fett wirken, Phosphorylierungen sind, die im Tierversuch durch Monojodessigsäure gehemmt werden können, nahmen sie an, daß diese Phosphorylierungsprozesse inkretorisch durch die Nebennierenrinde reguliert werden. Das Resorptionsbild der Schleimhaut nach Nebennierenexstirpation entsprach dem bei Monojodessigsäure-Vergiftung. VERZÁR (1935) wies ferner auf Störungen der Fettresorption bei *Morbus Addison* hin, ohne allerdings beweisende Unterlagen hierfür zu liefern. BÜRGER (1951) hat Beziehungen zwischen Nebennierenrinde und Fettresorption bei Addisonscher Krankheit nicht bestätigen können. Sprue und Pellagra betrachtet VERZÁR als B_2-Avitaminosen und erwähnt in diesem Zusammenhang das Vorkommen von ausgesprochenen Veränderungen an den Nebennieren bei Mangel an Vitamin B. Er denkt daran, daß das Nebenniereninkret möglicherweise aus dem Vitamin aufgebaut wird. Auch die experimentell gewonnenen Tatsachen, daß bei B-Mangel die Resorption verschlechtert ist und daß Vitamin B in Form eines Hefepräparates den normalen Zustand wiederherstelle, wird in diesem Zusammenhang angeführt. Die Verzársche Hypothese des übergeordneten Funktionsausfalls der Nebennierenrinde bei Sprue hat keine allgemeine Zustimmung erfahren [1]. Weitere Einwände gegen eine primäre Störung der Nebennierenrindenfunktion sind:

1. Bei Sprue sind keine Veränderungen der Nebennieren anatomisch nachgewiesen worden, welche die Annahme einer Insuffizienz stützten [2]. Auch vermag VERZÁR in keiner Weise zu erklären, warum es bei Sprue-Kranken zu einer primären Nebennierenstörung mit Hypofunktion kommen soll [3].

2. Die Tatsache, daß an Cöliakie leidende Kinder völlig geheilt werden können, spricht gegen die Annahme eines primären Ausfalls der Nebennierenrinde [4].

Eine Störung von Phosphorylierungsvorgängen in der Darmwand bei Sprue ist nicht abzulehnen, wenngleich der Beweis dafür beim Menschen naturgemäß schwer zu erbringen ist. Soviel scheint sicher zu sein, daß im Mittelpunkt des pathogenetischen Geschehens bei der Sprue eine Störung der Resorption in der Wand des Dünndarmes, wahrscheinlich sogar in der Epithelzelle, vorliegt. Wie die primäre Störung in der Darmwand bzw. in der Epithelzelle zustande kommt, ist nach wie vor unklar. In älteren Arbeiten werden nur ziemlich allgemeine Vorstellungen darüber entwickelt, sie mögen trotzdem erwähnt werden. JECKELN (1937) hielt Störungen des Darmchemismus für entscheidend, die auf infektiöstoxische Vorgänge, Überwuchern von Gärungserregern, Mangelernährung und Änderungen der Darmmotilität zurückzuführen seien. Hierzu ist noch zu sagen, daß nach VERZÁR (1935) schon allein durch Änderungen der Motilitätsverhältnisse pathologische Resorption erfolgen kann (Abkürzung der Zeit für den Ablauf der enzymatischen Spaltungsprozesse einerseits und für den zeitlichen Ablauf der Diffusionsvorgänge andererseits). Auf die bei der Resorption tätigen Kräfte wie mechanische Kräfte (Peristaltik, Zottenbewegung, Darminnendruck, Durchblutungsgrad der Darmwand), ferner die aus der Lösung kommenden Kräfte und die durch die Oberfläche bedingten sowie die zelleigenen [4], in deren innigem Zusammenspiel mannigfaltige Störungen eintreten können, kann hier nur hingewiesen werden; wir wissen über Einzelheiten hierbei auftretender Störungen kaum etwas Sicheres. Für die Sprue nimmt FRAZER (1954) neben einer

---

[1] HANSEN 1936, 1937, RIETSCHEL 1937, HOTZ 1940, KOKAS 1948, MAGYAR und FÖLDI 1948, BÜRGER 1951.   [2] HANSEN und v. STAA 1936, RIETSCHEL 1937.
[3] RIETSCHEL 1937.   [4] STRACK 1954.

excessiven Schleimsekretion und verminderter Darmmotilität Veränderungen der Pumpbewegungen in den Zotten an. Ich verweise hierzu auf die oben erwähnten Beziehungen zwischen Zottenbewegung und Resorptionsprozessen[1] und führe die Ergebnisse von DE LANGEN (1953, 1956) hier an, die für die Pathogenese der Sprue bedeutungsvoll sind. Nach DE LANGEN beginnen die Störungen mit verminderter Blut- und Lymphzirkulation in der Darmschleimhaut, wobei sich durch verminderte Gasresorption Meteorismus entwickelt. Pathologisch-anatomisch braucht man hierbei keine Veränderungen zu finden. Die Steatorrhoen sind eine Folge der gestörten Zirkulation bzw. niedrigen Blutdruckes. Der Resorptionsvorgang selbst ist als ein diphasischer Prozeß zu betrachten, der dem der Nierensekretion ähnlich ist. Bei beiden ist der primäre Blutdruck von Bedeutung. Das Zusammenspiel von Blut- und Lymphstrom sowie Zottenbewegungen wird durch den CO_2-Gehalt des Gewebes, aber auch durch Histamin, Acetylcholin und Gallensäuren beeinflußt. Die Bedeutung von schädlichen Einflüssen, die von der Darmlichtung her einwirken, wird durch die Beobachtung sprueartiger Bilder bei Divertikulose des Jejunum unterstrichen[2]. Die Steatorrhoe, bei der sich später eine megaloblastische Anämie entwickelt, wird dadurch erklärt, daß der Effekt einer großen Zahl von Divertikeln mit ihrem stagnierenden Inhalt dem einer ausgeschalteten Dünndarmschlinge gleichkommt. In den Divertikeln entwickelt sich ein abnormes Bakterienwachstum, und ihr infizierter Inhalt kann in das Darmlumen gelangen, wodurch Funktionsstörungen mit fehlerhafter Resorption, besonders von Fetten, eintreten. Bei der tropischen Sprue, die in Südost-Asien in den letzten Jahren in großen Ausbrüchen bei Besatzungstruppen beobachtet wurde[3] und den Charakter einer akuten Massenerkrankung hatte, treten Störungen des Darmchemismus besonders in den Vordergrund. FRAZER (1950) schreibt dem Genuß ranzig gewordener Fette eine besondere Bedeutung zu.

Es dürfte feststehen, daß bestimmte Erreger in der Pathogenese der Sprue keine Rolle spielen. Darminfektionen, die unter Umständen lange Zeit vor Beginn der klinisch nachweisbaren Resorptionsstörung abgelaufen sind, können aber durchaus von Bedeutung sein, sei es, daß sie eine dauernde Änderung des Darmchemismus herbeiführen, sei es über eine veränderte Motilität. Auch RIETSCHEL (1937) ist der Ansicht, daß bei der Entstehung der Durchfälle (bei Cöliakie) die bakterielle, endogene Dünndarminfektion eine große Rolle spielt; die zweite wichtige Komponente sei das Chronischbleiben der Infektion mit Herabsetzung der bactericiden Kräfte des Darmes, wobei eine einseitige Schonkost mit einer vitaminarmen Diät, die diese bakteriellen Prozesse unterhält, besonders ungünstig wirke. Als drittes Moment, das für den ganzen Ablauf der Sprue von Wichtigkeit ist, wird die Acidose angesehen. Sie beruht auf einer bakteriellen Zersetzung der Nahrung mit alkalischem Saftstrom, der den Körper entmineralisiert, auf ungenügender intermediärer Verbrennung organischer Säuren und auf sauren Nahrungsmitteln.

Eine bedeutungsvolle Feststellung der letzten Jahre ist die gute Wirkung glutenfreier Nahrung auf den Verlauf der idiopathischen Sprue, vor allem der Coeliakie. Das Protein der Weizenklebersubstanz Gluten enthält eine glutaminsäurereiche Eiweißfraktion, das Gliadin. Nach HOTTINGER (1959) reagieren die Patienten auf Belastung mit Gliadin mit allergischen Symptomen, Steatorrhoe und Schock. Es ist heute als wahrscheinlich anzusehen, daß bei der Coeliakie

---

[1] KOKAS 1948.   [2] BADENOCH und Mitarbeiter 1955, DICK 1955, DE GEUS 1956, SCUDAMORE, HAGEDORN, WOLLAEGER und OWEN jr. 1958.
[3] AYREY 1947, STEFANINI 1949, FRAZER 1950.

(soweit sie nicht als Erscheinungsform der Mucoviscidosis auftritt) Antigen-Antikörper-Reaktionen mitspielen.

Die Beobachtung von SCUDAMORE, McCONAHEY u. PRIESTLEY (1958), daß bei einer 4 Jahre lang kranken 51jährigen Frau erst nach Entfernung eines Inselzellen-Adenoms des Pankreas die Sprueerscheinungen aufhörten, steht vereinzelt da. Die pathogenetischen Beziehungen sind ungeklärt.

Die Auffassung der Sprue als einer primären Avitaminose[1] dürfte heute verlassen sein.

In welcher Weise die primäre Störung der resorptiven Leistung des Darmes im einzelnen vor sich geht, ist ungeklärt. Für eine Störung in der Epithelzelle selbst spricht die Tatsache ungestörter Fettspaltung im Darm (im Gegensatz zur symptomatischen Sprue) und ferner das Fehlen einer nachgewiesenen Störung des Lymphabflusses. RIETSCHEL (1937) dachte in Verfolg der angeführten Gedankengänge daran, daß im Darm unter der bakteriellen Einwirkung auf die Nahrung pathologische Substanzen entstehen könnten, die das Darmepithel so schwer schädigen, daß eine entsprechende Resorptionsstörung resultiert. Von physiologisch-chemischer Seite[2] wurde der *mangelhaften Phosphorylierung* in der Epithelzelle die entscheidende Bedeutung zugeschrieben. Vielleicht dürfen in diesem Zusammenhang einige neuere Feststellungen der Physiologie der Fettresorption kurz angeführt werden: Nach VERZÁR (1935) wird das Neutralfett im Darm gespalten, und die Fettsäuren binden einen resorbierbaren Gallensäurenkomplex. In der Epithelzelle findet zuerst eine Spaltung dieses Komplexes statt, und die Fettsäure wird nun nach vorheriger oder nach nachträglicher Phosphorylierung des Glycerins zu einem Bestandteil eines Phosphatids umgewandelt. Damit wird einerseits das Diffusionsgefälle für die Fettsäuren in die Epithelzellen hinein ständig vergrößert, da sie ja durch die Synthese fortgeschafft werden, andererseits verwandelt diese Synthese das Fett bereits in körpereigenes Fett, und die toxischen Fettsäuren werden entgiftet.

Durch neuere Untersuchungen FRAZERs (1952) wird die Verzársche Erweiterung der alten Pflügerschen Hypothese allerdings in Frage gestellt. Nach FRAZER müssen wir heute 3 Phasen der Fettresorption unterscheiden, die abschließend erwähnt seien:

1. Die *intraluminäre* Phase. JOCHIMS und DOERKS (1955) unterteilen diese in eine Anlieferungsphase, in welcher die Beförderung der Nahrung zum Resorptionsorgan hin geschieht, und die intraluminäre Phase im engeren Sinne. Die kurzgliedrigen Fettsäuren können ziemlich vollständig hydrolysiert werden, die langgliedrigen normalerweise weder schnell noch vollständig. Die niedrigen Glyceride und Fettsäuren bilden mit Hilfe der gallensauren Salze ein feinverseiftes Material, das in die feinen Kanälchen an der Außenseite der Darmepithelien eintritt. Damit wird die 2., die *celluläre* Phase, eingeleitet, in welcher das fettige Material in die Zelle übertritt, wo eine Resynthese von Triglyceriden erfolgen kann. Die Bildung von Phospholipid ist nicht eine obligatorische Zwischenstufe, obwohl sie den Durchtritt durch die Zelle erleichtern kann. Die 3. Phase, die *Verteilungsphase*, verläuft so, daß elektrisch negativ geladene Teilchen die Darmzellen verlassen und ihren Weg in die Chylusgefäße nehmen und überwiegend nicht in das Portalblut. Kurzgliedrige Fettsäuren werden aber im Chylus nicht gefunden, sondern können zur Synthese anderer Substanzen gebraucht werden oder mit dem Portalblut in den Körper gelangen.

5. Die Whipplesche Krankheit und die aus ihren Erscheinungen sich ergebenden Fragen der gestörten Resorption.

Aus den im Rahmen eines allgemeinen Sprue-Komplexes auftretenden Erkrankungen ist die *Whipplesche Krankheit (Lipodystrophia intestinalis)* herauszuheben. Zwar steht auch hier die *Fettresorptionsstörung* durchaus im Mittelpunkt

---

[1] STEPP 1936, CASTLE zit. nach HANSEN und v. STAA 1936, VERZÁR 1935.
[2] VERZÁR und Mitarbeiter 1933—1952.

der Geschehnisse, auch ähnelt ihr klinisches Bild dem der „idiopathischen" Sprue so stark, daß sie nicht selten zu dieser gerechnet wurde, ehe ihre Besonderheiten in Europa bekannt wurden[1], doch ist sie durch ein gut umrissenes, anatomisches Bild gekennzeichnet.

Whipple beschrieb im Jahre 1907 erstmalig ein Krankheitsbild, das pathologisch-anatomisch durch hochgradige Speicherung von Fett, Fettsäuren und Lipoproteiden in Dünndarm und Gekröselymphknoten charakterisiert ist. Wegen ihrer grundsätzlichen Bedeutung sei seine Beobachtung kurz wiedergegeben.

Ein 36jähriger Arzt, der $5^1/_2$ Jahre an rheumatischen Gelenkschmerzen gelitten hatte, erkrankte 6 Monate vor seinem Tode plötzlich an unbeeinflußbaren Fettstühlen verbunden mit Gewichtsverlust und zunehmender Schwäche. Die klinische Untersuchung ergab eine tastbare Resistenz im rechten Oberbauch, eine hypochrome Anämie und Eosinophilie. Der Tod erfolgte durch Kachexie. Bei der Obduktion fand sich eine abgelaufene Entzündung der Aortenklappe und der serösen Häute. In der verdickten, von zahlreichen stecknadelkopfgroßen, gelbweißen Knötchen durchsetzten Darmschleimhaut waren Fette, Fettsäuen und Lipoproteide gespeichert, die teils in Schaumzellen, teils in erweiterten Lymphbahnen lagen. In den vergrößerten, auf dem Durchschnitt gelblich gesprenkelten und zum Teil kleincystisch umgewandelten mesenterialen und retroperitonealen Lymphknoten fanden sich mit Fett gefüllte Hohlräume, die von Schaumzellen und Riesenzellen umlagert waren. Das hochgradig reduzierte lymphatische Gewebe war zum Teil durch Bindegewebe ersetzt. Eine Verlegung des Ductus thoracicus bestand nicht.

Die Erkrankung wurde von Whipple als eine Störung der Fettresorption mit Ablagerung abnormer Fettsubstanzen aufgefaßt. Er wies in einem nach Levaditi gefärbten Milzschnitt Spirochäten-ähnliche Mikroorganismen nach, die er ursächlich für diese Störung verantwortlich machte. — Dieser ersten Veröffentlichung folgten im anglo-amerikanischen Schrifttum entsprechende oder ähnliche Beschreibungen. Jabusch (1952), die auf meine Veranlassung eine gleichartige Beobachtung — inzwischen habe ich zwei weitere Fälle gesehen — untersuchte und beschrieb, stellte etwa 36 Fälle des amerikanischen und 10 des deutschen Schrifttums fest; doch werden immer neue Beobachtungen mitgeteilt. Wie Staemmler (1953) und Jabusch hervorheben, sind auch im deutschsprachigen Schrifttum, wo der Name „Whipplesche Erkrankung" erst in den letzten Jahren in Gebrauch gekommen ist, Beobachtungen zu finden, die den Beschreibungen von Whipple und seinen Nachfolgern entsprechen[2].

Das klinische Bild ist, wie Staemmler zweifellos richtig meint, im allgemeinen so wenig bekannt, daß die Diagnose nur selten richtig gestellt wurde; meist wurde Sprue, Pankreastumor, chronische Pankreatitis oder Morbus Addison diagnostiziert. Die Erkrankung beginnt mit Leibschmerzen, die später in Diarrhoen übergehen. Diese gewinnen den Charakter ausgesprochener Fettdiarrhoen, gelegentlich mit Blutbeimengungen. Im Laufe der Krankheit stellen sich allgemeine Abmagerung, Körperschwäche und Ermüdbarkeit, mehr oder weniger deutliche, meist hypochrome Anämie, dazu Hypotonie und Pigmentierung der Haut ein; nicht selten werden Knotenbildungen im Leib getastet. Ascites kommt in etwa einem Fünftel der Fälle vor. Auffällig ist die Anamnese, die in vielen Fällen rheumatische Beschwerden meldet, gelegentlich begleitet von Endokarditis oder Pankarditis. Jabusch hat bei einer kritischen Wertung des Schrifttums in 62,5% der Fälle ein rheumatisches Leiden verzeichnet gefunden. Bemerkenswert ist ferner das Geschlechterverhältnis. Nach Jabusch sind in 84% Männer im 3.—5. Lebensjahrzehnt befallen. — Die pathologische Anatomie der Erkrankung ist in jüngster Zeit treffend von Staemmler auf der 36. Tagung der Deutschen Gesellschaft für Pathologie geschildert worden:

---

[1] Fahr 1933, Hansen und v. Staa 1936, Jeckeln 1937, Kloos 1939.
[2] Fleischmann 1930, Fahr 1928, 1936, Gärtner 1938, Korsch 1938, Jeckeln 1939, Kloos 1939, Schallock 1939, Frei 1947.

„Im anatomischen Bild treten regelmäßig 2 Veränderungen hervor:

1. Eine Erkrankung des Dünndarmes. Sie besteht gewöhnlich in einer diffusen Verdickung seiner Wand, im besonderen seiner Schleimhaut, die mit einer Unzahl gelblicher Knötchen (den verdickten Zotten) bedeckt ist und dadurch körnig erscheint, gelegentlich aber auch eine dunkelbraune, braungrüne oder fast schwarze Pigmentierung aufweist. Dazu kommen Erweiterungen der Chylusgefäße, die besonders in der Serosa hervortreten und lakunenartigen Charakter annehmen können.

2. Eine Erkrankung des Mesenteriums, das im ganzen verdickt und verhärtet sein kann, aber vor allem stark vergrößerte, nicht miteinander verbackene Lymphknoten umschließt, die sich derb anfühlen, auf dem Durchschnitt fleckig-gelb gesprenkelt, manchmal geradezu käseartig durchsetzt oder cystisch umgewandelt sind.

Mikroskopisch sehen wir 2 Prozesse, die gemeinsam oder mehr einzeln vorkommen können: a) starke Erweiterung der Chylusgefäße von der Zottenspitze bis in die abführenden Gefäße des Gekröses und die Sinus der Lymphknoten hinein, wobei die Hauptveränderung meist in den Lymphknoten sitzt, deren lymphatisches Gewebe weitgehend reduziert ist, während durch die hochgradig erweiterten, mit Fettsubstanzen gefüllten Sinus das Bild eines grobporigen Schwammes (Schweizer Käse) erzeugt wird; b) Fettspeicherungen in den Uferzellen der Chylusgefäße, die sich dabei in Schaumzellen oder Riesenzellen umwandeln, und in Stromazellen der Dünndarmschleimhaut, die zu ganzen Schaumzellenlagern, besonders an der Basis der Schleimhaut werden können. Als weitere Folge dieser Fettspeicherungen kommt es zur Bildung lipophager Granulome, besonders in den Lymphknoten. Oft besteht eine bindegewebig-schwielige Umwandlung in diesen. Bald steht nun die Erweiterung der Chylusgefäße, bald die zellige Fettspeicherung im Vordergrund, meist sind aber beide Prozesse, wenn auch in verschiedener Gradausprägung, nebeneinander zu sehen. Untersuchung der Fettsubstanzen hat immer ergeben, daß es sich um Lipoidgemische handelt, in denen die Neutralfette überwiegen und reichlich Kristallbildungen von Fettsäuren, spärlich Cholesterine nachweisbar sind. Daß sich in den Speicherzellen auch Glycoproteide finden, hat BLACK-SCHAFFER gezeigt.‘‘

Abb. 9. Dünndarm bei Whipplescher Krankheit. 54jähriger Mann.

Hierzu ist ergänzend zu sagen, daß die Angaben über die Natur der in den Schaumzellen gespeicherten Stoffe unterschiedlich sind. Während die meisten Autoren sowohl sudanophile wie sudanophobe Schaumzellen beschrieben, fanden andere nur sudanophile[1]. JABUSCH sah bei Betrachtung im Polarisationsmikroskop an der Basis der Schleimhaut einzelne anisotrope nadelförmige Kristalle, die übrigen Fettsubstanzen waren nicht doppeltbrechend. Einzelne der im Stroma der Schleimhaut gelegenen Schaumzellen und wenige spindelförmige Histiocyten der

---

[1] ROSEN und ROSEN 1947, REVENO 1950, KORSCH 1938, PLUMMER und Mitarbeiter 1950, STAEMMLER 1953.

Schleimhaut enthielten feintropfiges Fett, das sich mit Sudan III rot, mit Nilblau-
Sulfat dunkelblau färbte und keine Doppeltbrechung zeigte. Im größten Teil
der Schaumzellen waren mit den erwähnten Färbemethoden keine Fettstoffe

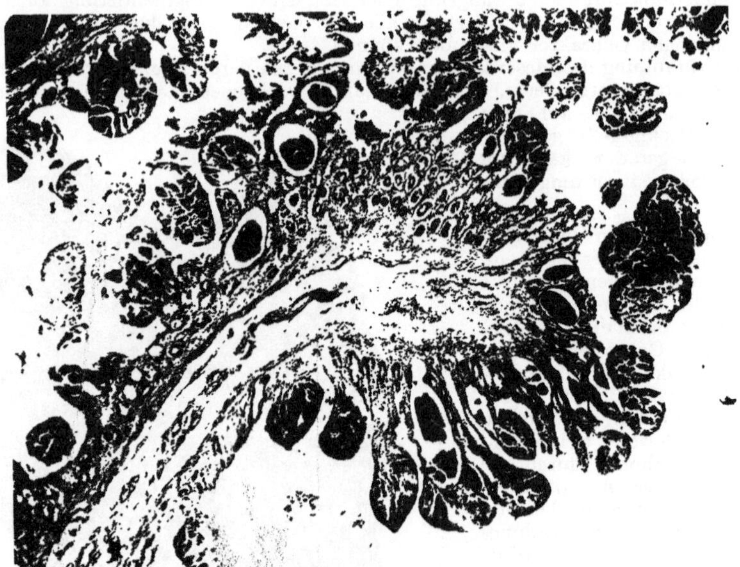

Abb. 10. Dünndarm bei Whipplescher Krankheit. (Beobachtung von STAEMMLER, Aachen.)

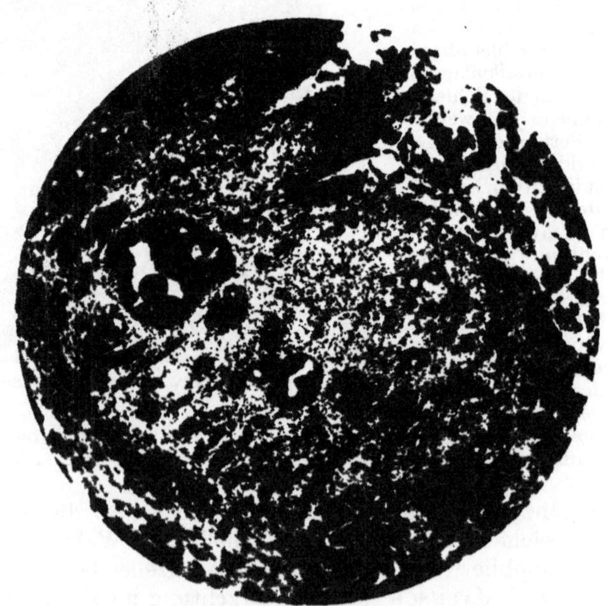

Abb. 11. Dünndarmschleimhaut bei Whipplescher Krankheit. 55jähriger Mann. Sudanfärbung.

nachweisbar. Ihr Cytoplasma färbte sich mit Mucicarmin blaßrötlich, mit Azan
schwach blau. Bei Anwendung der Feyrterschen Einschlußfärbung mit Thionin-
Weinsteinsäuregemisch fand sich in ihnen eine Rhodiochromie, in den tieferen

Schleimhautpartien von feingranulärem, in den oberen, autolytisch veränderten von diffusem Charakter. Nach Vorbehandlung der Gefrierschnitte mit absolutem Alkohol blieb eine Anfärbung aus. Auch bei Färbung mit Mucicarmin und mit Bestschem Carmin wurden die Schaumzellen nicht gefärbt. Es handelte sich also um Lipoproteide und nicht um Glucoproteide. — Diese Befunde waren im Bereich des gesamten Dünndarmes zu erheben. Die Schleimhäute von Magen und Dickdarm waren frei von Veränderungen. In den Gekröselymphknoten

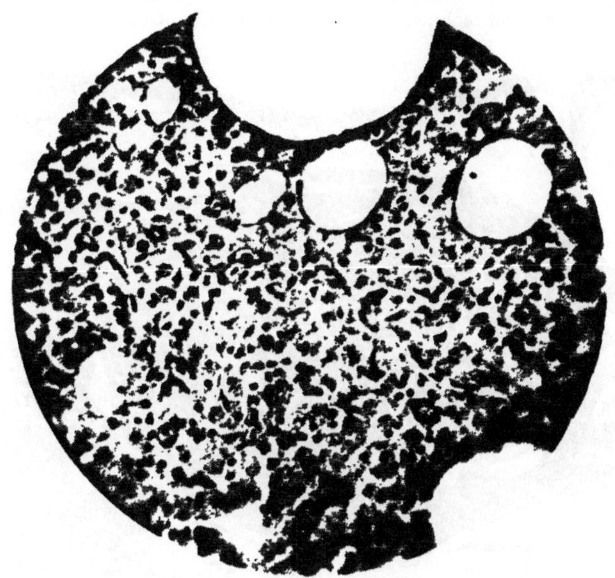

Abb. 12. Dünndarmschleimhaut bei Whipplescher Krankheit. 55jähriger Mann. HE-Färbung.

stellte JABUSCH gleichartiges färberisches Verhalten fest. Ich habe in der erwähnten früheren, zunächst als Sprue bezeichneten Beobachtung in den Schaumzellen der Dünndarmschleimhaut keine Fettstoffe nachweisen können. M. B. SCHMIDT hat damals bei Besichtigung meiner Präparate die Meinung geäußert, daß es sich bei den Schaumzellen um veränderte Reticulumzellen handele, und dachte daran, daß die vorliegende besondere Reaktion des R-Systems der Zotten auf die acidöse Beschaffenheit des Darminhalts gerichtet sein könnte. Auch heute noch scheint mir diese Auffassung nicht widerlegt zu sein.

Außer diesen Veränderungen der Darmschleimhaut scheinen noch weitere, wenigstens gelegentlich, vorzukommen.

Bei einer 68jährigen Frau, die unter der Diagnose eines fraglichen Pankreascarcinoms und einer Mitralstenose ad exitum kam, fanden sich autoptisch eine mäßige Stenose des Mitralostiums und totale Herzbeutelobliteration mit Myokardveränderungen, die, wie auch schon die Herzmuskelveränderungen im Fall von JABUSCH, an rheumatische Granulome erinnerten, jedoch feine Lipoidspeicherungen der gewucherten Histiocyten erkennen ließen. Im übrigen bestand das klassische Bild der Whippleschen Erkrankung mit Beteiligung mesenterialer, paraaortaler, pankreatischer und portaler Lymphknoten. An dem mikroskopischen Befund des Jejunums ist bemerkenswert, daß neben einer starken Schleimhautatrophie überall Zeichen chronischer Entzündung mit überwiegend lymphoplasmacellulärer Infiltration zu erkennen waren; dabei fanden sich auch Abschnitte mit sehr erheblicher Leukocytenbeteiligung und stärkerem Ödem. Die Submucosa zeigte die gleichen älteren und frischeren Zellinfiltrate mit starker Mastzellenbeteiligung. Durchweg bestand eine beträchtliche fibröse Sklerosierung dieser Wandschichten. Auch die Subserosa beteiligte sich hieran.

Das mikroskopische Bild der Whipple-Veränderungen ist also sehr charakteristisch und gestattet eine Diagnose aus probeexcidierten Lymphknoten. Jabusch zählte elf durch *Lymphknotenbiopsie* geklärte Fälle.

Eine eigene Beobachtung darf wohl ihrer Besonderheit wegen hier erwähnt werden: Ein 63jähriger Mann mit unauffälliger Vorgeschichte erkrankte mit den Zeichen peripherer Durchblutungsstörungen in den Zehen des rechten Fußes. Bei einer deshalb durchgeführten Grenzstrangresektion wurde ein dem Grenzstrang anliegender Lymphknoten mitentfernt. Dieser zeigte bei der feingeweblichen Untersuchung ganz charakteristische Whipple-Veränderungen. Wenige Tage danach erkrankte der Patient mit plötzlichem Erbrechen und Blähung des Leibes; die Stuhluntersuchung ergab positive Fettsäure- und Neutralfettbefunde. Auch nach der schnell wieder eingetretenen Genesung wurden gleichartige

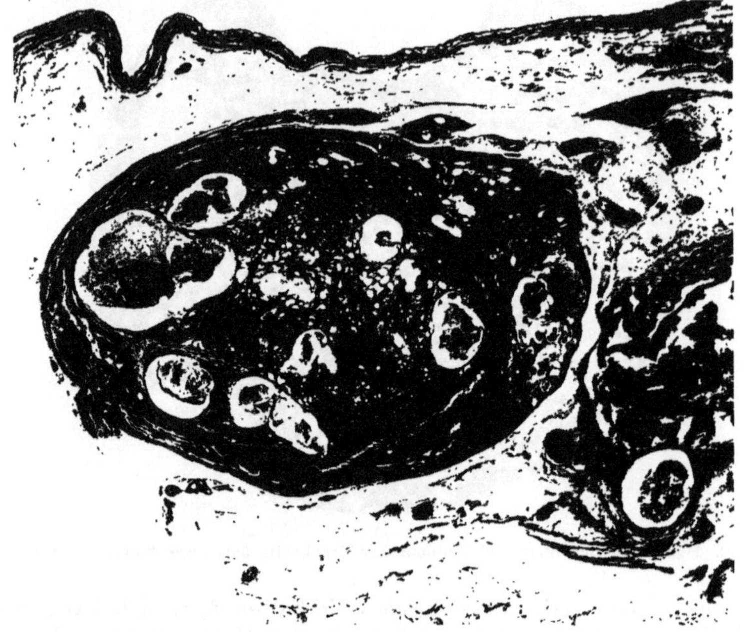

Abb. 13. Gekröselymphknoten bei Whipplescher Krankheit. (Beobachtung von Staemmler, Aachen.)

Stuhlbefunde zweimal erhoben. In der Folgezeit blieb der Mann erscheinungsfrei und zeigt auch jetzt, nach Ablauf von fast 5 Jahren, keine Zeichen einer Resorptionsstörung.

Offenbar können also entweder bereits vor Auftreten klinischer Erscheinungen von seiten des Darmes anatomische Veränderungen vorhanden sein, die auf eine Resorptionsstörung hinweisen, oder es gibt abortive Fälle.

Nach den vorliegenden histologischen Befunden liegt es nahe, die *Ursache* der Resorptionsstörung bei der Lipodystrophia intestinalis in einer *Behinderung des Chylusabflusses* aus dem Darm zu suchen. Das ist auch vielfach geschehen, indem man die sehr auffälligen und oft monströsen Lymphbahnerweiterungen zum Ausgangspunkt der Betrachtung machte. Eine entscheidende Rolle mußte hier eine Verlegung der abführenden Chylusgefäße spielen können. In zahlreichen Fällen von Whipplescher Erkrankung ist der Ductus thoracicus nicht untersucht worden. Kloos (1939) beschrieb bei einem Falle von Oesophaguscarcinom eine subtotale Obstruktion des Ductus thoracicus mit knolliger Auftreibung des Gekröses und Bildung polyblastischer Schaumzellen, fand aber keine Veränderungen, die dem Bilde der Whippleschen Krankheit entsprechen. In diesem Zusammenhang sei auf die Erfahrungen Walthers (1948) hingewiesen: Unter-

sucher, die ihr Augenmerk auf den Ductus thoracicus richteten, fanden gar nicht
so selten eine metastatische krebsige Erkrankung desselben. Aber auch ein völliger
Verschluß pflegte keine klinischen Symptome auszulösen, wohl wegen der vorhandenen Lymphkollateralen (Trunci mammarii int.). Von irgendwelchen anatomischen Befunden im Sinne der Whippleschen Krankheit erwähnt WALTHER
nichts. Dem stehen Beobachtungen über stenosierende Veränderungen des
Ductus thoracicus gegenüber, bei denen es zu den Erscheinungen der Whippleschen
Krankheit gekommen war. So berichtete SCHALLOCK (1939) über eine völlige
Verödung mesenterialer Lymphgefäße und eine Einengung des Ductus thoracicus

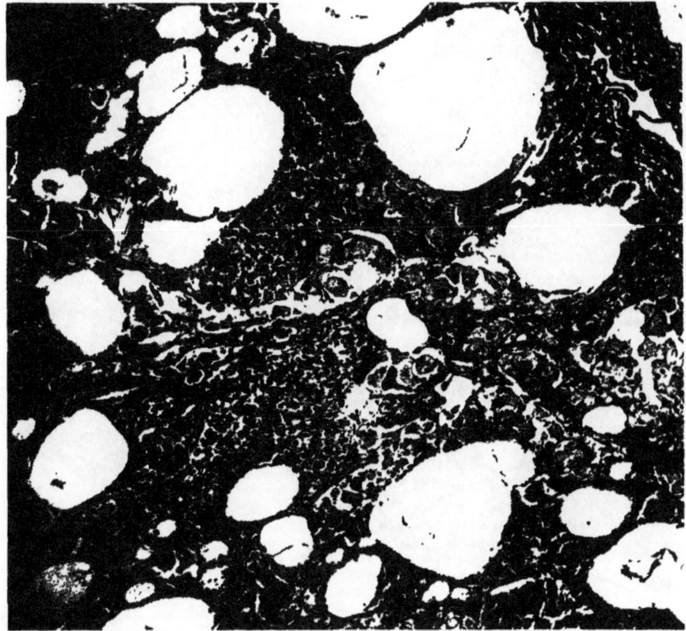

Abb. 14. Gekröselymphknoten bei Whipplescher Krankheit. 68jährige Frau. HE-Färbung.

bei einem 45jährigen Manne durch ein entzündlich gedeutetes Füllgewebe, die
als rheumatisch angesprochen wurden. SCHALLOCK gab den am Darm und den
Lymphknoten bestehenden Veränderungen, die ohne Zweifel denen der Whippleschen Krankheit entsprechen, folgende Deutung: „Durch einen teilweisen Ver-
ödungsvorgang des Ductus thoracicus im Bauchteil und eine weitgehende Obliteration der mesenterialen Lymphbahnen ist eine Chylusstauung im Darm und
den Gekröselymphknoten eingetreten. Durch diese Stauung wurden die betreffenden Abschnitte erweitert. Die starke Fettanhäufung läßt erkennen, daß
von der fetthaltigen Flüssigkeit die feiner dispersen Teile abgeleitet werden
konnten, und daß in den erweiterten Partien eine Art Filtration für die gröberen
Bestandteile mit nachfolgender Entmischung eintrat. Einzelne der ausgefallenen
Fettstoffe wirkten als Fremdkörper und führten zur Bildung von Ölsäure- oder
Cholesteringranulomen. Durch Überladung der abführenden Lymphknoten mit
diesen fetthaltigen Substanzen trat eine zunehmende Sperrung der Fettaufnahmen
durch den Darm ein. Die im Speisebrei enthaltenen Fette wurden daher in gleicher
Weise wie bei mangelnder Fermenteinwirkung, z. B. durch Pankreasinsuffizienz
oder bei Sprue, durch den Darm in Form der sprueähnlichen Durchfälle ausgeschieden.“

Diese Feststellungen Schallocks wurden durch neuere Beobachtungen Staemmlers (1953) gestützt.

Bei einem 43jährigen Manne, der zu Lebzeiten keine ausgesprochenen Fettstühle gehabt hatte, ergab sich autoptisch ein Befund, der eine Whipplesche Krankheit zu diagnostizieren zwang. Die wichtigste Veränderung war ein weitgehender Verödungsprozeß der abführenden Chyluswege, der in den mesenterialen Lymphknoten begann und sich von hier aus auf die Mesenterialwurzel erstreckte. Er ging mit hochgradiger Erweiterung der peripheren Chylusgefäße im Darm und Gekröse einher. — Die 2. Beobachtung Staemmlers betraf einen 47jährigen Mann, der nach einer Darmblutung starb. Auch hier bestand bei der Sektion der typische Befund einer Whippleschen Krankheit. Auffallend war wiederum die Veränderung in den

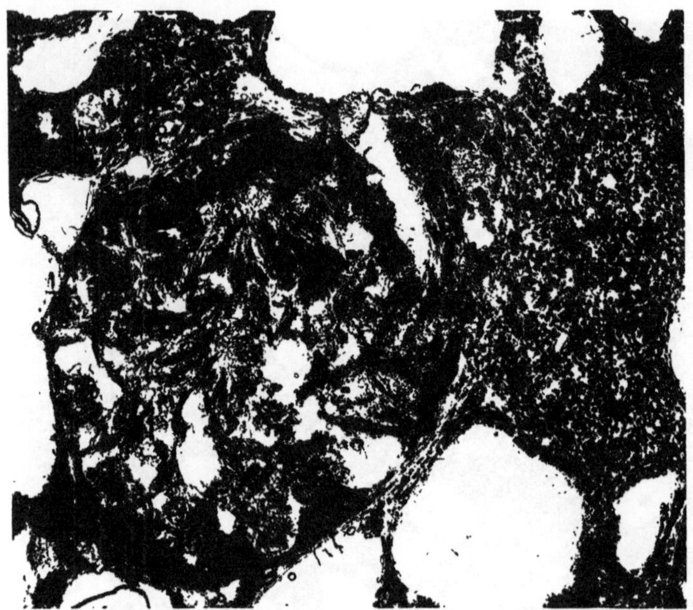

Abb. 15. Gekröselymphknoten bei Whipplescher Krankheit. 68jährige Frau. Gefrierschnitt,
Färbung: Thionin-Weinsteinsäure.

abführenden Chylusgefäßen der Gekrösewurzel. Ihre Wand war hochgradig teils strangförmig, teils knotig verdickt, die Lichtung eingeengt, aber nicht verschlossen. Die Wandverdickung hatte granulierenden Charakter und griff auch auf die nächste Umgebung über. Der Prozeß wurde als Perilymphangitis chronica granulomatosa mit Stenosierung der Lichtung bezeichnet.

Staemmler dachte — wenigstens in seinem zweiten Fall — ebenfalls an rheumatische Genese, während für seinen ersten Fall auch die Möglichkeit syphilitischer Entstehung angeführt wird. Die Veränderungen des Darmes und der Gekröselymphknoten sind nach ihm als Folgen des behinderten Chylusabflusses deutbar, während er der Vorstellung einer primären Störung des Fettstoffwechsels geringere Wahrscheinlichkeit einräumte.

Zum Beweis dieses Gedankens demonstrierte Staemmler Präparate eines 39jährigen Mannes, bei dem eine von einem primären Magencarcinom ausgehende Lymphgefäßcarcinose rein durch Stauung der Chylusflüssigkeit ähnliche Prozesse in den Lymphknoten, in den Chylusgefäßen und in der Darmwand zur Folge gehabt hatte.

Der Gedanke des gestörten Chylusabflusses ist also neuerdings wieder in den Mittelpunkt der pathogenetischen Betrachtungen bei der Whippleschen Erkrankung gerückt. Ob hiermit das primum movens in der Kette der Erscheinungen gefaßt ist, muß aber doch wohl noch als offen gelten. So ist es sicher nicht ungerechtfertigt, wenn Rössle (1939) und Korsch (1938) bei ihrer Beobachtung, die sicher eine Whipplesche Krankheit betraf, daran denken, daß eine chemische Veränderung des in den Lymphstrom gelangenden Fettes in den Lymphknoten als Fremdkörper wirkend zu Granulationen und Riesenzellenbildung geführt hat. Bestimmend für diesen Gedanken ist die Feststellung gewesen, daß sich die granulomatösen Veränderungen genau entsprechend dem Verlauf der Lymphbahnen fanden. CRANE u. AGUILA (1957) beschrieben bei Whipplescher Krankheit eine stenosierende chronische Entzündung der abführenden Lymphbahnen mit daraus hervorgehender Lymphstauung. — Auch ich habe in meinem früheren Fall an eine Behinderung des Chylusabflusses gedacht, der zum Teil schon in der

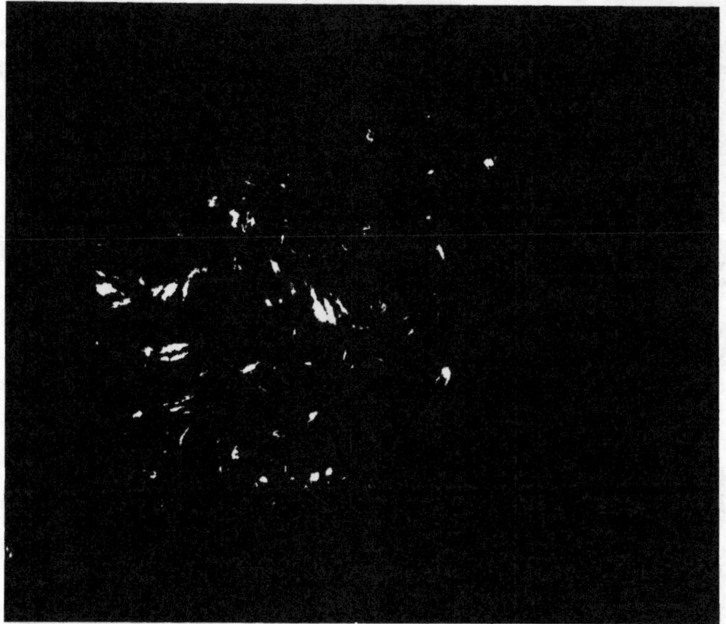

Abb. 16. Das gleiche Präparat wie bei Abb. 15 bei Polarisation.

Schleimhaut selbst eingetreten sein mußte. Die starken granulierenden Schleimhautveränderungen schienen mir eine solche mechanische Erklärung zuzulassen, wenngleich ich schon damals auch noch an andere, zur Zeit nicht übersehbare Momente dachte. Zum anatomischen Bilde der Whippleschen Krankheit gehört zweifellos eine chronische Entzündung der Darmschleimhaut. Diese kann sehr hohe Grade erreichen und auch zu weitgehender Sklerosierung der Darmwand führen. Aber es ist klar, daß damit nicht entschieden ist, ob die granulierenden Veränderungen das Primäre in der Kette der krankhaften Ereignisse bilden, oder ob sie, was durch die eigentümlichen, mit Speicherungsvorgängen einhergehenden Zellwucherungen nahegelegt wird, Reaktionen auf die Einwirkung fehlerhaft zusammengesetzter Stoffwechselprodukte sind. Das gilt nicht nur für die Darmwandveränderungen, sondern ebenso für die Erscheinungen an den abführenden Lymphwegen und den Lymphknoten. Schließlich ist es auch denkbar, daß unspezifische entzündliche Gewebswucherungen den Anfang des Geschehens bilden, die durch Behinderung des Chylusabflusses zu weiteren Veränderungen führen, wobei die Stellen der Abflußbehinderung bald in der Darmwand, bald in näherer oder weiterer Entfernung von ihr im Lymphgefäßsystem einsetzen können. Aber das sind nur Überlegungen, und wir haben keine gesicherten Kenntnisse über die

Einzelheiten der krankhaften Abläufe bei dieser für die Kenntnis der Resorptionsstörungen so wichtigen und geradezu als Modellfall imponierenden Erkrankung. Eines allerdings ist auffällig und kann vielleicht einen Schlüssel für weitere

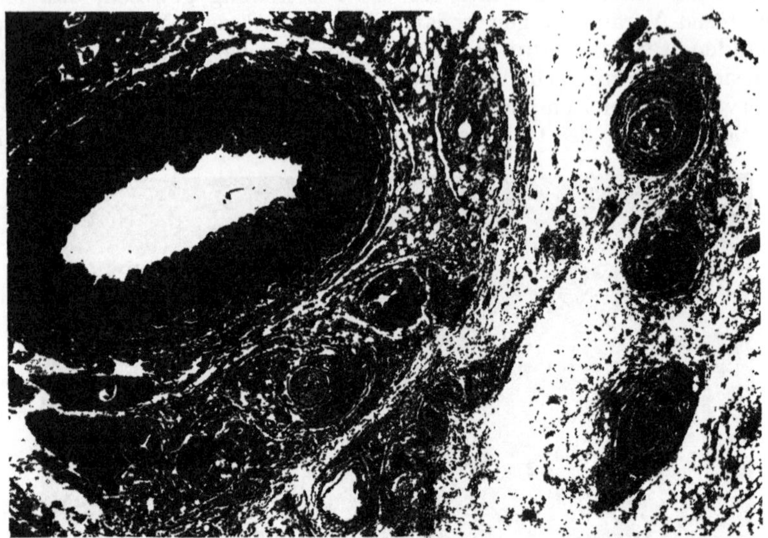

Abb. 17. Whipplesche Krankheit. Lymphangitis obliterans des Gekröses. (Beobachtung von Staemmler, Aachen.)

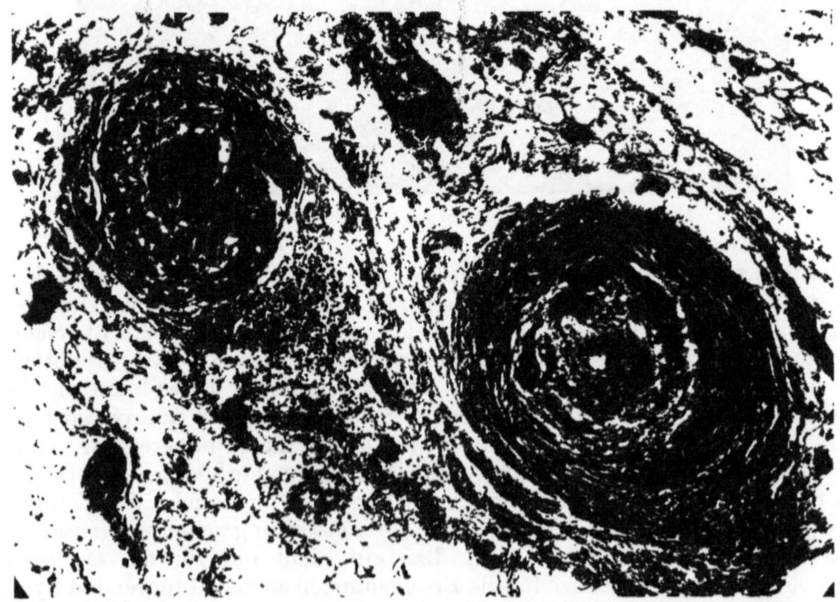

Abb. 18. Whipplesche Krankheit. Lymphangitis obliterans des Gekröses. (Beobachtung von Staemmler, Aachen.)

Untersuchungen bilden, nämlich die Tatsache, daß die Whipplesche Krankheit, wie schon erwähnt, in der Überzahl der Fälle bei Rheumatikern gefunden wird. Es erscheint in diesem Zusammenhang nicht uninteressant, daß schon Schallock (1939) die von ihm gefundenen Lymphgefäßveränderungen als Endzustände rheumatischer Lymphangitis deutete — damals war ja die merkwürdige Beziehung zum Rheumatismus kaum bekannt — und daß auch STAEMMLER neuerdings wieder an Rheumatismus denkt. In ähnlicher Weise kam JABUSCH zu der Erwägung „einer rheumatisch-allergischen Schädigung des Darmmesenchyms mit Fehlleistung des Darmepithels als Ursache der Whippleschen Erkrankung." Auch AMMANN (1957) wies auf die Beziehungen der Whippleschen Krankheit zum Rheumatismuskomplex (Kollagenkrankheit) hin. — Ob die Hypothese einer rheumatisch bedingten Schädigung als Ursache dieser höchst merkwürdigen und problemreichen Stoffwechselstörung, die auch RIEDERER (1956) vertrat, sich aufrecht erhalten läßt, müssen weitere Untersuchungen ergeben. Es ist vor allem

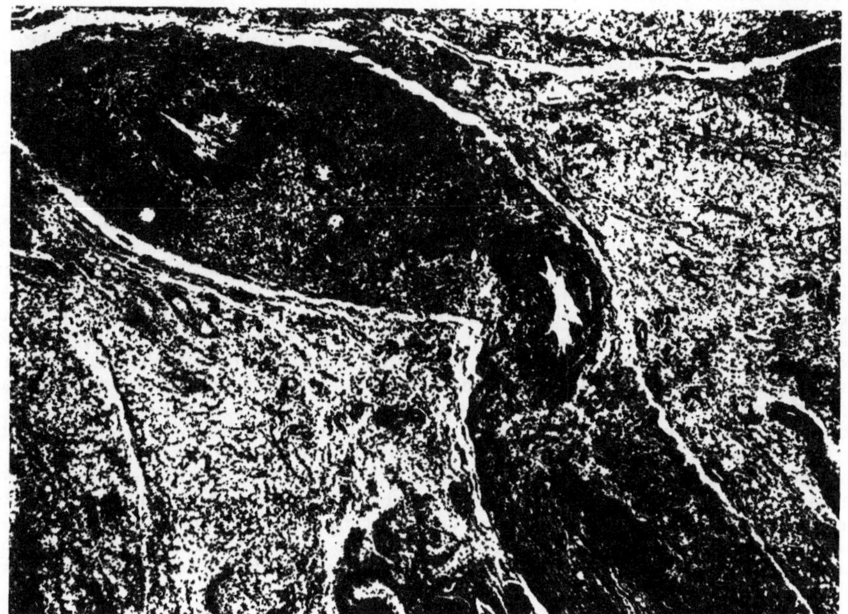

Abb. 19. Whipplesche Krankheit. Stenosierende Perilymphangitis. (Beobachtung von STAEMMLER, Aachen.)

zu prüfen, welche Bedeutung die Speicherung von Glyko- und Mucoproteiden hat, die auch in vom Darm entfernt liegenden Körpergegenden festgestellt wurde. UPTON (1952) und FARNAN (1958) erwogen die Herkunft dieser Stoffe aus Umsetzungen der bindegewebigen Grundsubstanz. — Die Forschungen der letzten Jahre haben eine generalisierte Reticuloendotheliose mit Speicherung von PAS-positiven Substanzen in den Vordergrund gestellt[1]. Unter diesen Umständen gewinnt die Lymphknotenbiopsie diagnostische Bedeutung[2]. Die als SPC (sickle-form-particle-containing) Zellen bezeichneten Makrophagen mit PAS-positiven Einschlüssen konnten sogar im Sediment der Peritonealflüssigkeit nachgewiesen werden[3]. — Trotz der Aufdeckung zahlreicher neuer geweblicher Besonderheiten wird man hinsichtlich der Ätiologie der Whippleschen Krankheit DRUBE (1959) zustimmen müssen, der in seinem Handbuchbeitrag schreibt: „Die Ätiologie der Whippleschen Erkrankung muß demnach genau so wie vor 50 Jahren als ungeklärt angesehen werden." Die Whipplesche Krankheit ist aber sicher eines der interessantesten Kapitel auf dem Gebiete der Störungen der Darmresorption.

[1] DICK 1957, FOROUHAR 1957, RUTISHAUSER und FOROUHAR 1957, RUTISHAUSER und DE WECK 1957, RUTISHAUSER und BORER 1959.
[2] PUITE und TESLUK 1955, SIERACKI und FINE 1959.   [3] SIERACKI 1958.

6. Weitere anatomische Befunde gestörter Darmresorption.

Eine der Whippleschen Erkrankung offenbar sehr nahestehende Krankheit beschrieben Faber, Meulengracht und Vimtrup (1952).

Ein 39jähriger Mann litt $1^1/_4$ Jahre vor seinem Tode an einer unaufhaltsamen Sprue-ähnlichen Krankheit: Durchfälle mit den Zeichen verminderter Fett- und Glucoseresorption und schließlich extreme Abmagerung. Bei der Sektion waren die Gekröselymphknoten vergrößert und zeigten mikroskopisch in den Sinus wie im lymphoiden Gewebe große Mengen ziemlich dunkler geschwollener Zellen mit Erythrocytenresten. Ihr Cytoplasma enthielt feine Vacuolen, aber keine fettigen oder schleimigen Substanzen. Ähnliche Zellanhäufungen fanden sich auch in Lymphbahnen sowie in Lymphknoten des Thorax und des Halses. Die Zellen wurden als freie speichernde Reticulumzellen oder endotheliale Elemente angesprochen. Weitere krankhafte Befunde waren eine entzündliche Zellinfiltration der Duodenalschleimhaut, Pankreasatrophie und dichte kleinzellige Infiltrate der Leber. Die Verff. dachten am ehesten an eine Verwandtschaft mit der Whippleschen Krankheit. Rheumatische Veränderungen fanden sich nirgends.

In diesem Zusammenhang ist auch eine Beobachtung Rössles (1938) anzuführen:

Hier lag eine sklerosierende Xanthomatose der gesamten Gekröseplatte des Dünndarmes mit Verlegung der Chylusgefäße bei einem 10 Monate alten Mädchen vor, das 4 Wochen vor der Klinikaufnahme mit Erbrechen, später Durchfällen ohne Blut und Schleim erkrankt war. Die Herde granulierender Xanthomatose, welche die Sektion aufdeckte, entsprachen den geweblichen Erscheinungen der Schüller-Christianschen Krankheit, doch fehlten weitere Lokalisationen der Veränderung. Auffällig war, daß nur bei mikroskopischer Untersuchung ein kleiner Gekröselymphknoten festzustellen war. — An diese Beobachtung knüpfte Rössle den Gedanken, daß eine schon im Darmgebiet sich auswirkende Störung des Lipoidstoffwechsels vorgelegen habe, welche die Chylusgefäße und Gekröselymphknoten geschädigt und zur Insuffizienz gebracht habe und so die pathologischen Fettstoffe zwang, sich um die undurchgängigen Lymphknoten abzulagern, wodurch dann ein Fremdkörperreiz und granulierende Entzündung entstanden. Als auffällige Besonderheit dieser Beobachtung ist zu erwähnen, daß auch in den erweiterten Lymphgefäßen des Gekröses Aufschwemmungen großer Schaumzellen lagen, während ihre Endothelien meist frei von Einlagerungen waren. Die Dünndarmwand hatte eine teils sklerotische, teils ödematöse Submucosa, und im Ödem fanden sich auffallend große Fibrocyten, öfter in Abrundung, möglicherweise mit beginnender Speicherung, in anderen Stücken starke Vergrößerung der Dünndarmzotten, im wesentlichen bedingt durch Erweiterung der Chylusgefäße bis unter das Epithel. Auch hier noch bestand der Inhalt zum Teil aus Schaumzellen, während solche nicht im Zwischengewebe und in der Submucosa vorhanden waren.

Rössle faßte diese Veränderungen als sekundär durch Chylusstauung bedingt auf, wies aber auf das auffällige Vorhandensein zahlreicher freier Xanthomzellen in den Wurzeln der Chylusgefäße selbst hin. — Im ganzen wird man wohl sagen müssen, daß der Ursprung des Prozesses nicht als geklärt gelten kann.

Weitere Befunde am Dünndarm, die auf eine gestörte Resorption schließen lassen, erstrecken sich auf einige wenige Beobachtungen der Speicherung fettiger Substanzen. Ihre Bedeutung ist durchweg hypothetisch. W. Fischer (1926) erwähnte bei der Darstellung der Chylusstauungen nach einer fettreichen Mahlzeit auch eine Anfüllung von *Zellen* mit Fettstoffen in der Darmschleimhaut. Offenbar handelte es sich um bindegewebige Speicherzellen. Feyrter (1929) beschrieb „Lipoidzellknötchen" der Duodenalschleimhaut, hervorgerufen durch gewucherte Speicherzellen. Froboese (1938) sah in 2 Fällen eine Veränderung, die in einer weißlichgelben, succulenten, lippenförmigen Schwellung aller Kerkringschen Querfalten des gesamten Dünndarmes bestand und durch Cholesterin-Speicherzellen in der Faltensubmucosa bei Freibleiben aller übrigen Darmschichten hervorgerufen war. In anderen Organen wurden keine Speicherzellansammlungen gefunden. Eine allgemeine Fettstoffwechselstörung wie auch chronische Chylusstauung als Ursachen dieser Veränderung waren unwahrscheinlich, und Froboese nahm in Anlehnung an Siegmund (1928) eine „Entgleisung im örtlichen Stoffwechsel und Fermentgeschehen bei der Veresterung der aufgenommenen Fette" an. Möglicherweise lag auch bei einer Beobachtung von FREI (1947) eine ähnliche Störung vor. Schließlich gehören hierher auch die von KÖBERLE (1940) in 15 Fällen beobachteten Ablagerungen von Lipoid-Cholesteringemisch im Stroma der Schleimhaut und Unterschleimhaut des Bulbus duodeni in pseudoxanthomartigen Speicherzellen. KÖBERLE nahm an, daß die Fette aus der Galle stammten und unter Begünstigung durch Chylusstauung infolge An- oder Hypacidität des Magensaftes bzw. vollständiger Ausschaltung des Duodenums von der Berührung mit Magensaft zur Ablagerung gelangten. Nach ihm ist eine Änderung der Wasserstoffionen-Konzentration die wichtigste Voraussetzung für das Zustandekommen der Ablagerungen.

Anhangsweise sei erwähnt, daß es nach BOELS und TVERDY (1950) STRYKER gelang, bei Kaninchen histologische Veränderungen zu erzeugen, die denen der Whippleschen Krankheit stark ähnelten, indem er der Nahrung Paraffinum liquidum zusetzte. Eine Nachprüfung dieser Versuche ist mir nicht bekannt.

7. Resorptionsstörungen und Vitamine.
Durch inkretorische Einflüsse bedingte Resorptionsstörungen.

Hier wäre der Ort, zunächst den *Sprue*-Komplex abzuhandeln. Es erschien mir aber zweckmäßig, die mit nicht-pankreatogenen Störungen der Fettresorption verbundenen Erkrankungen (Darmausschaltung, Sprue-Komplex, Whipplesche Erkrankung) geschlossen darzustellen, so daß der vorliegende Abschnitt nur ein Nachtrag zu den Abschnitten über diese mit avitaminotischen Erscheinungen einhergehenden Abläufe sein kann. Die Ausbeute an weiteren morphologischen Befunden ist gering und beschränkt sich im wesentlichen auf die *Pellagra*. Wenngleich heute klar ist, daß es sich bei ihr um eine im Mittelpunkt des Geschehens stehende B_2-Avitaminose handelt, so sind doch die auftretenden Störungen recht komplexer Natur; Fehlernährung, Stoffwechselstörungen durch Fermentinsuffizienz, innersekretorische Störungen sowie Änderungen der bakteriellen Darmbesiedlung haben Bedeutung. Viele Fragen sind aber noch ungelöst[1]. So bilden auch die anatomisch festgestellten Darmveränderungen nur einen Ausschnitt aus dem Geschehen, und ihre Rolle ist nicht restlos geklärt. Sie entwickeln sich erst im Laufe der Erkrankung und können kaum als ihre alleinige Ursache gelten. Der Dickdarm ist vorzugsweise betroffen; die hier sich abspielende, oft geschwürige chronische Schleimhautentzündung geht in Atrophie über. Als charakteristisch wird das Bild der Colitis cystica angesehen[2]. Am Dickdarm können alle Zeichen sekretorischer Tätigkeit fehlen, welchen Umstand EGER (1937) für die Entstehung der ulcerösen Colitis anschuldigte. Die entzündlichen, geschwürigen und atrophischen Veränderungen des Verdauungstraktes sind aber nicht auf den Dickdarm beschränkt, sondern können den gesamten Verdauungsschlauch von der Zunge an befallen[3]. — „Gastrogene" Pellagra (bei Achylia gastrica) ist beschrieben[4]. Im Laufe der Zeit können sich Erscheinungen einstellen, welche für Störungen der Darmsekretion sprechen. Nicht immer ist es möglich, in dem sich entwickelnden Circulus vitiosus die auf primärem Vitaminmangel beruhenden Erscheinungen von denen der sekundären, durch Resorptionsstörungen entstandenen Avitaminose zu trennen. Allerdings ist auf die geringe Beteiligung des Dünndarmes an den chronisch entzündlichen Vorgängen bei der Pellagra hinzuweisen; vielleicht ist dies ein Grund, weshalb sekundäre Resorptionsstörungen bei dieser Erkrankung nicht so im Vordergrund stehen wie bei der Sprue. Bei letzterer wurden auf pellagröse Störungen hindeutende Veränderungen, vielleicht auch Kombinationen

---

[1] MAINZER 1950.   [2] CEELEN 1931.   [3] HERZENBERG 1935.
[4] SEITZ 1943, MAASSEN 1943.

beider Erkrankungsformen beschrieben[1,2]. Auf die Bedeutung innersekretorischer Störungen bei der Pellagra sei in diesem Zusammenhang nur kurz hingewiesen; Sklerose der Nebennieren[3,4,5], aber auch Veränderungen anderer Drüsen (Hoden, Pankreas[4]), (Schilddrüse[5]), sind beschrieben. Für die Kenntnis gestörter resorptiver Leistungen des Verdauungskanales ist im ganzen unser Wissen über die Vorgänge bei Pellagra nicht bedeutend.

Da das fettlösliche *Vitamin A* nur in Anwesenheit von Fetten in der Nahrung resorbiert werden kann, sind Zeichen des Vitamin A-Mangels bei Störungen der Fettresorption zu erwarten. Als Früh- und Hauptsymptom ist die Nachtblindheit (Hemeralopie) anzusehen; diese kann allerdings auch andere Ursachen haben, da das Vitamin im Körper, besonders in der Leber, gespeichert wird.

Eine ungenügende Resorption von *Vitamin B₁* („Antineuritin", „Antineurin") soll bei mit Magen- und Darmstörungen verbundenen Krankheiten vorkommen und zu entsprechenden Ausfallserscheinungen wie Parästhesien und allgemeiner Muskelschwäche führen[6].

Über die Rolle des *Vitamin B₁₂* = intrinsic factor Castles siehe unter „Magendyschylien".

Eine ungenügende Resorption von *C-Vitamin* ist bei anacider Gastritis bekannt, da die Ascorbinsäure im alkalischen Milieu schnell abgebaut wird. Auch eine pathologische Colibesiedlung der obersten Dünndarmschlingen zerstört das Vitamin[7]. Bei chronischen Magen-Darmerkrankungen auftretende Hautpigmentierungen sind durch mangelhafte Resorption von C-Vitamin erklärt worden[8]. Von anderer Seite wurden diese Pigmentierungen auf Nebennierenstörungen infolge intestinaler Intoxikation bezogen[9].

Über Störungen der *Vitamin K*-Resorption s. unter „Dyschylien durch fehlerhafte Gallebildung und -absonderung".

Durch Resorptionsstörungen bedingte Ausfälle anderer Vitamine scheinen nicht genügend erforscht.

Über den Einfluß fehlerhafter Leistungen der Drüsen mit innerer Sekretion wurde schon oben (s. Abschnitt Sprue) einiges erwähnt; es handelte sich hier vor allem um die von Verzár (s. oben) inaugurierte Insuffizienz der *Nebennierenrinde* als Ursache von Resorptionsstörungen des Dünndarmes (Glucose- und Fettresorption). Auf die vor allem von klinischer Seite hiergegen gemachten Einwände wurde bereits hingewiesen. — Auch für den Morbus Addison machte Verzár (1925) den gleichen Einfluß der Nebennierenrinde geltend, denn auch bei dieser Krankheit werden gelegentlich Fettstühle beobachtet, und Addison-ähnliche Erscheinungen kommen bei Sprue vor. Pellagra wie Sprue wurden von Verzár als B₂-Avitaminose betrachtet; Pigmentation, Adynamie seien bei Pellagra Ausfallserscheinungen der Inkretion der Nebennierenrinde. — Wenn auch Veränderungen der Nebennierenrinde bei Pellagra beschrieben sind (s. oben) und die Nebennierenrinde in der Pathogenese der Erkrankung eine Rolle spielen kann (Verzár dachte an einen Aufbau des Inkretes aus dem Vitamin B₂, die Nebennierenrinde ist eine bevorzugte Ablagerungsstätte des Nicotinsäureamids[10]), so ist doch durchaus fraglich, ob der Nebenniere im Erkrankungsgeschehen die zentrale Rolle zukommt, die ihr Verzár zuschrieb.

Auch bei der Whippleschen Krankheit ist eine Erschöpfung der Nebennierenrindenfunktion angenommen worden, ohne daß diese Annahme durch anatomische Befunde gestützt werden konnte. Die gestörte Rindenfunktion soll hier zu

[1] Hansen und v. Staa 1936.   [2] Eger 1937.   [3] Froboese 1934.
[4] Herzenberg 1935.   [5] Froboese und Thoma 1933.   [6] M. B. Schmidt 1936.
[7] Mahlo und Müller 1936, Henning 1955.   [8] Hoff, zit. nach M. B. Schmidt 1936.
[9] Diehl 1933.   [10] Henning 1955.

einer Störung des humoralen Gleichgewichtes führen und den Stoffwechsel der Phospholipide beeinträchtigen. Durch Fettausflockung, z. B. in den Chylusgefäßen, soll es zu Lymphknoten- und Lymphbahnblockade kommen können. Diese Folgen wären dann die Ursache für die schlechte Fettresorption[1]. In dem von mir beschriebenen Whipple-Fall[2] untersuchte M. B. Schmidt die Nebennieren sehr eingehend und stellte nur geringfügige gewebliche Veränderungen in Form minimaler Atrophie und eine relative Fettarmut der Rinde fest. Für eine selbständige Erkrankung des Organs konnte er diese Veränderungen nicht halten.

Als Prototyp der endokrin bedingten Diarrhoen bezeichnete Henning (1949) die Durchfälle bei Morbus Basedow und Morbus Addison. Bei diesem soll infolge der fehlenden oder verringerten Adrenalinproduktion der hormonale Reiz für den Sympathicus fortfallen, bei jenem soll der erhöhte Vagotonus verantwortlich sein. Wieweit in schweren Fällen von Basedow, wo auch Fettdiarrhoen auftreten können, die Hyperperistaltik des Darmes allein oder noch andere Einflüsse wie Pankreasstörungen und thyreotoxisch bedingte Resorptionsstörungen[3] eine Rolle spielen, ist ungeklärt. Morphologische Äquivalente solcher Störungen sind nicht bekannt. Nach Rattenversuchen von Althausen und Stockholm (1938) wurde durch Einverleibung von Schilddrüsenhormon die Resorption von Traubenzucker, Galaktose, Xylose und Oleinsäure wesentlich gesteigert, Herausnahme der Schilddrüse hatte verringerte Traubenzuckerresorption zur Folge. Die Resorptionssteigerungen sollen vorzugsweise durch Beschleunigung der Magenentleerung und Steigerung der Phosphorylierungsvorgänge bedingt sein.

Schließlich sei noch die Beobachtung einer Epithelkörperchenhyperplasie bei Whipplescher Krankheit erwähnt[4]. Sie dürfte aber mit Veränderungen des Calcium- und Phosphorspiegels im Serum zusammenhängen, also sekundärer Natur sein.

Neue Fragestellungen auf dem Gebiete der gestörten Darmresorption ergeben sich aus den Untersuchungen Feyrters (1956, 1957, 1958) über das sog. GelbeZellen-Organ der Magen-Darmschleimhaut und seiner carzinoiden Geschwülste. Inwieweit Krankheiten der gestörten Darmresorption mit örtlichen Störungen des Gelbe-Zellen-Organes und des mit ihm eng verknüpften vegetativen Nervensystems zusammenhängen, bedarf noch eingehender Untersuchungen.

Literatur.

Adlersberg, D.: The malabsorption syndrome (Symposium). New York u. London 1957. Althausen, T. L., and M. Stockholm: Der Einfluß der Schilddrüse auf die Absorption im Verdauungstraktus. Amer. J. Physiol. 123, 577 (1938). — Ammann, R. W.: Zur Differentialdiagnose, Pathogenese und Ätiologie des Morbus Whipple. Helv. med. Acta 24, 118—143 (1957). — Andersen, D. H.: Cystic fibrosis of the pancreas and its relation to celiac disease. Amer. J. Dis. Childr. 56, 344—399 (1938). ~ Pancreatic enzymes in the duodenal juice in the celiac syndrome. Amer. J. Dis. Childr. 63, 643—658 (1942). — Ayrey, F.: Outbreaks of sprue during the Burma campaign. Trans. Roy. Soc. Trop. Med. (Lond.) 41, 377—406 (1947).
Babkin, B. P.: Die äußere Sekretion der Verdauungsdrüsen. Berlin 1928. — Bachmann, K. D.: Die sog. cystische Pankreasfibrose („Mucoviscidosis"). Ergebn. inn. Med. Kinderheilk., N.F. 8, 316—366 (1957). — Badenoch, J., P. D. Bedford and J. R. Evans: Massive diverticulosis of the small intestine with steatorrhoea and megaloblastic anaemia. Quart. J. Med., N. S. 24, 321—330 (1955). — Ball, W. P., A. H. Baggenstoss and J. A. Bargen: Pancreatic lesions associated with chronic ulcerative colitis. Arch. of Path. 50, 347—358 (1950). — Bartholomew, L. G.: Newer concepts in pancreatic disease. Gastroenterology 36, 122—127 (1959). — Baumgartner, U., u. K. K. de Voogd: Zwei Fälle von Mucoviscidosis im Erwachsenenalter. Schweiz. med. Wschr. 89, 130—134 (1959). — Becker, V.: Oedemstudien am Pankreas. Verh. dtsch. Ges. Path. 1955, 210—216. ~ Sekretionsstudien am Pankreas.

---

[1] Plummer und Mitarbeiter 1950.   [2] Jeckeln 1939.
[3] Henning und Baumann 1949.   [4] Odessky und Burdison 1950.

Stuttgart 1957. ~ Die chronische rückfällige und schleichende Pankreatitis. Med. Klin. **54**, 812—815, 822 (1959). ~ Über Papillitis stenosans Vateriana. Med Klin. **54**, 1417—1420 (1959). Becker, V., u. J. Schaefer: Die Bedeutung des Speichelödems für die Pankreasatrophie nach experimenteller Gangunterbindung. Virchows Arch. path. Anat. **330**, 243—266 (1957). — Beckmann, R.: Die Leber bei kongenitaler zystischer Pankreasfibrose. Acta hepato-splen. (Stuttg.) **6**, 65—76 (1959). — Bejul, E. A.: Untersuchungen des Resorptionsvermögens des Dünndarms bei chronischer Enteritis. Ref. Ber. allg. u. spez. Path. **18**, 229 (1953). — Black-Schaffer, B.: The tinctorial demonstration of a glycoprotein in Whipple's disease. Proc. Soc. Exper. Biol. a. Med. **72**, 225—227 (1949). — Boels, W., et G. Tverdy: Anatomopathologie de l'intestin grêle dans les diarrhées graisseuses idiopathiques. Acta gastro-enterol. belg. **13**, Suppl. 1, 481—505 (1950). — Bohn, H., u. E. Koch: Die Erwachsenen-Mucoviscidosis als überaus häufige, dominant erbliche Krankheit. Medizinische **1959**, 1139—1149. — Brinck, J., u. M. Gülzow: Fermententgleisung. Z. klin. Med. **131**, 747—758 (1937). — Büchner, F.: Allgemeine Pathologie. München u. Berlin 1950. ~ Über den heutigen Stand der Lehre von der Pathogenese des peptischen Geschwürs. Langenbecks Arch. u. Dtsch. Z. Chir. (Kongr.ber.) **297**, 302—318 (1951). ~ Spezielle Pathologie. München u. Berlin 1955. Die Pathogenese der Gastro-Duodenal-Geschwüre. Schweiz. Z. Path. **21**, 388—404 (1958). — Bürger, M.: Verdauungs- und Stoffwechselkrankheiten. Stuttgart 1951. — Burghard, E.: Pankreaserkrankungen im Säuglingsalter. Klin. Wschr. **1925**, 2305.

Catel, W.: Untersuchungen über Peristaltik und Resorption am entzündeten Darm. Klin. Wschr. **1936**, 1348—1350. — Ceelen, W.: Über Darmveränderungen bei „Pellagra". Beitr. path. Anat. **87**, 488—502 (1931). — Claireaux, A. E.: Fibrocystic disease of the pancreas in the newborn. Arch. Dis. Childh. **31**, 22—27 (1956). — Crane, J., and M. J. Aguilar: Obliterative lymphangitis of the mesentery in Whipple's disease. Gastroenterology **32**, 513 to 527 (1957).

Dick, A. P.: Association of jejunal diverticulosis and steatorrhoea. Brit. Med. J. **1955 I**, 145—148. — Dick, P.: Trois cas de maladie de Whipple. Gastroenterologia (Basel) **88**, 172—213 (1957). — Diehl, F.: Addisonismus bei chronischer Gastroenteritis. Dtsch. Arch. klin. Med. **175**, 177—187 (1933). — Doerr, W.: Indikatoruntersuchungen am Pankreas bei verschiedenen Funktionszuständen. Verh. dtsch. Ges. Path. (36. Tagg 1952) **1953**, 316—321. ~ Fermententgleisung im Pankreas, pathologisch-anatomisch gesehen. Ärztl. Wschr. **1953**, 681—690. ~ Pathologisch-anatomische Untersuchungen zum Problem der Fermententgleisung im Pankreas. Verh. dtsch. Ges. Path. (37. Tagg 1953) **1954**, 292—298. — Donaldson jr., R. M., P. R. vom Eigen and R. W. Dwight: Gastric hypersecretion, peptic ulceration and islet-cell tumor of the pancreas (the Zollinger-Ellison syndrom). Report of a case and review of the literature. New Engl. J. Med. **257**, 965—970 (1957). — Drube, H. Chr.: Die Whipplesche Krankheit (Lipodystrophia intestinalis). Ergebn. inn. Med. Kinderheilk. **12**, 605—633 (1959). — Dubois-Manne, R., R. van Geffel et S. Zylberszag: L'activité fermentaire du liquide duodénal dans la maladie coeliaque et dans la maladie fibro-kystique du pancréas. Rev. belge Path. **25**, 329—356 (1956). — Dumont-Ruyters, L.: Les diarrhées graisseuses idiopathiques. Étiopathogénie et sémiologie des d. g. i. Acta gastroenterol. belg. Suppl. 1, 45—82 (1950).

Eger, W.: Anatomische Befunde bei einem Fall von sporadischer Pellagra. Virchows Arch. **299**, 643—653 (1937). — Ellison, E. H., J. S. Abrams and D. J. Smith: A postmortem analysis of 812 gastroduodenal ulcers found in 20000 consecutive autopsies, with emphasis on associated endocrine disease. Amer. J. Surg. **97**, 17—30 (1959). — Enderlen, E., E. Freudenberg u. E. v. Redwitz: Experimentelle Untersuchungen über die Änderung der Verdauung nach Magen-Darmoperationen. Z. exper. Med. **32**, 41—97 (1923).

Faber, M., E. Meulengracht u. Bj. Vimtrup: A rapidly progressing sprue-like syndrome with hitherto undescribed pathological changes. Acta med. scand. (Stockh.) **142**, Suppl. 266, 381—392 (1952). — Fabian, G.: Physiologie und Pathologie der Speichelsekretion des Menschen in ihrer Beziehung zur Magenfunktion. Halle a. S. 1938. — Fahr, Th.: Zur Frage des Zusammenhanges zwischen Stoffwechselstörungen und morphologischen Veränderungen im reticulo-endothelialen System. Klin. Wschr. **1928**, 1787—1791. ~ Diskussionsbemerkung. Verh. dtsch. path. Ges. (29. Tagg 1936) **1937**, 288 ~ Diskussionsbemerkung. Verh. dtsch. path. Ges. (29. Tagg 1936) **1937**, 338. — Fanconi, G., C. Knauer u. E. Uehlinger: Das Cöliakiesyndrom bei angeborener cystischer Pankreasfibromatose und Bronchiektasien. Wien. med. Wschr. **1936**, 753—756. — Farber, S.: Pancreatic function and disease in early life. Arch. of Path. **37**, 238—250 (1944). — Farnan, P.: The systemic lesions of Whipple's disease. J. clin. Path. **11**, 382—390 (1958). — Feyrter, F.: Herdförmige Lipoidablagerung in der Schleimhaut des Magens (Lipoidinseln der Magenschleimhaut — Lubarsch). Lipoidzellenknötchen in der Schleimhaut des Darmes. Virchows Arch. **273**, 736—741 (1929).— Zur Pathologie und Klinik des Darmkarzinoides. Dtsch. med. Wschr. **1956**, 1073—1078. ~ Über die peripheren endokrinen (parakrinen) Drüsen. Medizinische **1957**, 663—669. ~ Zur Pathologie der sogenannten chronischen Dünndarmerkrankungen. Therapiewoche 8, 477—485

(1958). — FEYRTER, F., u. R. KLIMA: Über die Magenveränderungen bei der Addisonschen Krankheit. Dtsch. med. Wschr. 1952, 1173—1175. ~ Über die Histopathologie der Magenveränderungen bei der Anaemia perniciosa. Münch. med. Wschr. 1952, 145—150. — FISCHER, W.: Die Kreislaufstörungen des Magen-Darmkanals. In Handbuch der speziellen pathologischen Anatomie und Histologie, Bd. IV/1, S. 319. 1926. — FISHER, E. R., and R. H. FLANDREAU: Multiple endocrine tumors and peptic ulcer. Gastroenterology 32, 1075—1094 (1957). — FLEISCHMANN, R.: Über tumorbildende Fettgewebsgranulome im Gekröse des Dünndarms. Arch. klin. Chir. 158, 693—701 (1930). — FOROUHAR, B.: La réticulo-endotheliose de la maladie de Whipple. Ann. anat. path. 2, 402—431 (1957). — FRAZER, A. C.: Idiopathic steatorrhoe. Acta gastro-enterol. belg. 13, 876—884 (1950). ~ Lipid metabolism. Biochem. Soc. Symposia 1952, No 9. — Active transport and secretion. Symposia Soc. Exper. Biol. 1954, No 8. — FREI, R.: Über die histopathologischen Veränderungen am Dünndarm bei Störungen der Fettresorption (sog. Xanthomatose des Dünndarms). Schweiz. Z. Path. u. Bakter. 10, 685—702 (1947). — FREUDENBERG, E.: Die cystische Fibrose des Pankreas. Mschr. Kinderheilk. 103, 161—164 (1955). — FRISCHAUF, H.: Cystische Pankreasfibrose bei einer 16jährigen. Wien. klin. Wschr. 1952, 504—505. — FROBOESE, C.: Innere Sekretion und Pellagra. Verh. dtsch. path. Ges. (27. Tagg) 1934, 194—201. ~ Diffuses Xanthelasma der Darmschleimhaut (Cholesterinzellhyperplasie). Verh. dtsch. path. Ges. (31. Tagg 1938) 1939, 127—133. — FROBOESE, C., u. E. THOMA: Sprueähnliche oder pellagroide Erkrankung. Virchows Arch. 124, 478—489 (1933).

GÄRTNER, K.: Über einen Fall von hochgradiger Fettspeicherung in den Mesenteriallymphknoten. Frankf. Z. Path. 52, 529—537 (1938). — GEUS, A. DE: Jejunal diverticulosis. Arch. chir. neerl. 8, 181—191 (1956). — GLANZMANN, E.: Dysporia entero-broncho-pancreatica congenita familiaris. Cystische Pankreasfibrose. Ann. paediatr. (Basel 166, 289—313 (1946). — GLANZMANN, E., u. H. BERGER: Über Meconiumileus (Dysporia entero-bronchopancreatica congenita). Klinische, pathologisch-anatomische Beobachtungen und chemische Untersuchungen des Darminhaltes bei einem am 6. Lebenstage wegen Meconiumileus verstorbenen Neugeborenen. Ann. paediatr. (Basel) 175, 33—48 (1950). — GLOOR, F., u. A. WERTHEMANN: Über Leberveränderungen bei kongenitaler zystischer Pankreasfibrose. Schweiz. Z. Path. 18, 1244—1251 (1955). — GROSSMAN, M. I.: Experimental pancreatitis. Recent contributions. Symposium. J. Amer. med. Ass. 169, 1567—1570 (1959). — GRUBER, G. B.: Pathologie der Bauchspeicheldrüse. In Handbuch der speziellen pathologischen Anatomie und Histologie, Bd. V/2. Berlin 1929.

HAMPERL, H.: Zur Histologie der akuten Gastritis und der Erosionen der Magenschleimhaut. Beitr. path. Anat. 90, 85—141 (1932). — HANSEN, K.: Die einheimische Sprue. Zbl. inn. Med. 57, 425—431 (1936). ~ Einheimische —„europäische" — Sprue, ihre Symptomatologie und Pathogenese. Dtsch. med. Wschr. 1937, 849. ~ The rate of absorption of food allergenes proved by the method of PRAUSNITZ and KÜSTNER. Internat. Arch. Allergy 6, 356—360 (1955). — HANSEN, K., u. H. v. STAA: Die einheimische Sprue. Leipzig 1936. — HENDRIX, R. C., and D. M. GOOD: Fibrocystic disease of the pancreas after childhood: case report with necropsy at 17 years. Ann. intern. Med. 44, 166—173 (1956). — HENNING, N.: Die Verdauung und Resorption. Lehrbuch der speziellen pathologischen Physiologie, herausgeg. von L. HEILMEYER. Stuttgart 1955. ~ Die Schleimhautdiagnostik des Magens im Lichte bioptischer und zytologischer Untersuchungen. Münch. med. Wschr. 1956, 395 bis 398. — HENNING, N., u. W. BAUMANN: Lehrbuch der Verdauungskrankheiten. Stuttgart 1949. — HENNING, N., u. S. WITTE: Atlas der gastroenterologischen Cytodiagnostik. Stuttgart 1957. — HERZENBERG, H.: Pellagra. Beitr. path. Anat. 96, 97—110 (1935). — HESS THAYSEN, TH. E.: Non tropical sprue. London u. Kopenhagen 1932. — HETÉNYI, G.: Über Störungen der Kalkresorption und Auftreten von Tetanie im Laufe des chronischen Dünndarmkatarrhs. Klin. Wschr. 1938, 506—507. — HICKEN, N. F., and A. J. McALLISTER: Is the reflux of bile into pancreatic ducts a normal or abnormal physiologic process ? Amer. J. Surg. 83, 781—786 (1952). — HIMES, H. W., J. B. GABRIEL and D. ADLERSBERG: Previously undescribed clinical and postmortem observations in non-tropical sprue: possible role of prolonged corticosteroid therapy. Gastroenterology 32, 60—71 (1957). — HIMES, H. W., and D. ADLERSBERG: Pathologic changes in the small bowel in idiopathic sprue: biopsy and autopsy findings. Gastroenterology 35, 142—154 (1958). — HOTTINGER, A.: Enterale Allergie, Immunität und Zoeliakie. Dtsch. med. Wschr. 84, 1717—1724 (1959). — HOTZ, W.: Die einheimische Sprue. Stuttgart 1940. — HOWANIETZ, L.: Ein Fall von Mucoviscidose. Zbl. allg. Path. path. Anat. 97, 507 (1958). — HUG, O.: Peptische Erosionen im Jejunum. Virchows Arch. 304, 190—202 (1939).

ILGNER, G., u. R. WÜRKERT: Histochemische Thymonucleinsäureuntersuchungen bei ernährungsgestörten Säuglingen. Frankf. Z. Path. 63, 375—386 (1952).

JABUSCH, G.: Über die Whipplesche Erkrankung und ihre Beziehung zur Sprue. Inaug.-Diss. Hamburg 1953. — JECKELN, E.: Zur Pathologie der einheimischen Sprue. Virchows Arch. 303, 393—405 (1939). ~ Diskussionsbemerkung. Verh. dtsch. Ges. Path. (36. Tagg

1952) **1953**, 306. ~ Über neuere Ergebnisse der Dünndarmpathologie. Dtsch. med. J. **1955**, 137—142. ~ Fortschritte und Probleme in der Dünndarmpathologie. Verh. dtsch. Ges. inn. Med. **63** (Kongr.), 404—426 (1957). — JEKER, L.: Mikroskopische Untersuchungen über die Fettresorption im normalen Darm und bei Hemmung der Fettresorption durch Monojodessigsäure und Phlorrhizin. Pflügers Arch. **237**, 1—13 (1936). — JOCHIMS, J., u. G. DOERKS: Zur Methodik der Chylomikrographie und zur Physiologie der Fettresorption beim Säugling. Z. Kinderheilk. **77**, 278—292 (1955).

KABISCH, G., u. H. J. GRUNER: Die blinde Saugbiopsie der Magenschleimhaut in der klinischen Diagnostik. Ärztl. Wschr. **13**, 647—653 (1958). — KATSCH, G., u. M. GÜLZOW: Die Krankheiten der Bauchspeicheldrüse. In Handbuch der inneren Medizin, 4. Aufl., Bd. III/2, S. 295. Berlin-Göttingen-Heidelberg 1953. — KLOOS, K.: Über eine eigenartige Fettresorptionsstörung und ihre Beziehung zur Sprue. Virchows Arch. **304**, 625—658 (1939).— KOCH, E.: Die erbliche Erwachsenen-Mucoviscidosis und ihre Beziehungen zur Ulkuskrankheit. Dtsch. med. Wschr. **84**, 1773—1784 (1959). — KOCH, E., u. H. LAPP: Klinische und pathologisch-anatomische Befunde bei drei Erwachsenen mit Mucoviscidosis. Medizinische **1959**, 1149—1154, 1157—1158. — KÖBERLE, F.: Über diffuse Lipoidose des Duodenums. Beitr. path. Anat. **104**, 454—469 (1940). — KOKAS, E.: Die Bewegung der Darmzotten und ihre hormonale Regelung. Z. Vitamin-, Hormon- u. Fermentforsch. **2**, 98—112 (1948/49). — KONJETZNY, G. E.: Chronische Gastritis und Duodenitis als Ursache des Magenduodenalgeschwürs. Beitr. path. Anat. **71**, 595 (1923). ~ Die Entzündungen des Magens. In Handbuch der pathologischen Anatomie und Histologie, Bd. IV/2. Berlin 1926. ~ Die Deckepithelveränderungen der Magenschleimhaut bei akuter Gastritis. Virchows Arch. **275**, 816—827 (1930). ~ Die Geschwürsbildung im Magen, Duodenum und Jejunum. Stuttgart 1947. — KONJETZNY, G. E., u. H. PUHL: Das sog. Ulcus pepticum des Magens der Absatzkälber. Virchows Arch. **262**, 615—633 (1926). — KORSCH, H. J.: Fettstoffwechselstörung mit Granulombildung im Mesenterium. Zbl. Path. **71**, 337—344 (1938). — KRZYWANEK, F. W., u. B. FLASCHENTRÄGER: Die Biochemie der Verdauung. In Physiologische Chemie, herausgeg. von B. FLASCHENTRÄGER u. E. LEHNARTZ. Bd. 2, Teil 1: Der Stoffwechsel, S. 6—199. Berlin-Göttingen-Heidelberg 1954. — KÜHN, H. A.: Histologische Magenuntersuchung mit der Saugbiopsie. Fortschr. Med. **78**, 35—36 (1960).

LANDSTEINER, K.: Darmverschluß durch eingedicktes Mekonium. Pankreatitis. Zbl. Path. **16**, 903 (1905). — LANGEN, C. D. DE: Steatorrhoea and the intestinal circulation. Acta med. scand. (Stockh.) **146**, 7—19 (1953). ~ Die Vasomotilität bei Sprue und anderen Resorptionsstörungen. Gastroenterologia (Basel) **85**, 1—10 (1956). — LASZT, L., u. F. VERZÁR: Über chronische Jodessigsäurevergiftung und ihre Beziehung zur Gee-Herterschen Krankheit. Pflügers Arch. **237**, 483—493 (1936). — LINDENSCHMIDT, O.: Erkennung und Behandlung von Folgezuständen nach Magenoperationen. Medizinische **1955**, 1397—1400. — LUKSCH, F., u. H. W. SACHS: Sektionsbefund bei einem fraglichen Fall von einheimischer Sprue. Virchows Arch. **299**, 786—792 (1937).

MAASSEN, R.: Sekundäre Pellagra nach Gastroenterostomie (B_2-Komplex-Avitaminose). Dtsch. med. Wschr. **1938**, 1398—1399. — MÄDER, E.: Fettspeicherung der Leber bei exkretorischer Pankreasinsuffizienz. (Die Inselfettleber.) Frankf. Z. Path. **59**, 551—566 (1948). — MAGYAR, I., u. M. FÖLDI: Nebennierenrinde und Phosphorylierung. Z. Vitamin-, Hormonu. Fermentforsch. **2**, 134—140 (1948/49). — MAHLO u. MÜLLER: Über einen Zusammenhang zwischen gestörter Vitamin C-Resorption und pathologischer Pigmentierung bei Gastroenteritis und Achylia gastrica. Münch. med. Wschr. **1936**, 1276—1277. — MAHRBURG, ST.: Histologische Untersuchungen der Bauchspeicheldrüse bei Ernährungsstörungen bei Säuglingen. Virchows Arch. **293**, 682—696 (1934). — MAINZER, FR.: Fortschritte auf dem Gebiet der Pellagraforschung. Klin. Wschr. **1950**, 729—738. — MANGOLD, E.: Darmlänge, Durchgangszeit und Durchgangsgeschwindigkeit. Sitzgsber. dtsch. Akad. Wiss. Berlin, Kl. med. Wiss. **1951**, Nr 3. — MEHNEN, H.: Die Bedeutung der Mündungsverhältnisse von Gallen- und Pankreasgang für die Entstehung der Gallensteine. Arch. klin. Chir. **192**, 559—571 (1938). — MEYER, W. W.: Eindringen von Galle in die Pankreasgänge. Virchows Arch. **318**, 432—444 (1950). — MEYER-BURGDORFF, H.: Die pathologische Physiologie des Verdauungskanals nach Magenresektion. Chirurg **6**, 601—611 (1934). — MICHAUD, P.: Fibrose pancréatique et maladie coeliaque. Praxis (Bern) **1952**, 624—626. — MOHR, W.: Bericht über Vitamin C-Stoffwechseluntersuchungen und pathologisch-anatomische Dünndarmbefunde bei Sprue. Dtsch. Z. Verdgs. usw. Krkh. **2**, 142—151 (1939).

NEWSHOLME, G. A., and J. M. FRENCH: Absorption of $Na^{24}Cl$ from the small intestine in the sprue syndrome. Clin. Sci. **13**, 607—614 (1954). — NONNENBRUCH, W.: Über die Resorption aus dem entzündeten Darm. Dtsch. med. Wschr. **1932**, 1589—1590. — NORRIS, T. ST. M.: Intrahepatic portal hypertension due to mucoviscidosis. Proc. roy. Soc. Med. **50**, 507—516 (1957).

OBERHELMAN jr., H. A., TH. S. NELSEN and L. R. DRAGSTEDT: Peptic ulcer associated with tumors of the pancreas. A. M. A. Arch. Surg. **77**, 402—415 (1958). — ODESSKY,

L., and W. R. Burdison: Intestinal lipodystrophy (Whipples disease) occurring with parathyroid hyperplasia and nephrosis. Report of a case with autopsy. Arch. of Path. **49**, 307—320 (1950). — Oehler, V.: Sprue. Pathologisch-anatomische Untersuchungen bei 7 Beobachtungen von einheimischer und symptomatischer Sprue. Gastroenterologia (Basel) **79**, 257—282 (1953). — Oehlert, W.: Die Lebercirrhose bei der cystischen Pankreasfibrose des Säuglings. Beitr. path. Anat. **117**, 253—265 (1957).

Planta, F. v.: Nicht-insulinproduzierende Inselzellgeschwulst des Pancreas und Ulcus pepticum (Zollinger-Ellison-Syndrom). Schweiz. med. Wschr. **87**, 1272—1274 (1957). — Plummer, K., S. Russi, W. H. Harris jr. and Ch. M. Caravati: Lipophagic intestinal granulomatosis (Whipples disease). Clinical and pathologic study of thirty-four cases, with special reference to clinical diagnosis and pathogenesis. Arch. Int. Med. **85**, 280—310 (1950). — Popper, H.: The pathological aspects of pancreatic disease. Rev. Gastroenterol. **19**, 183—193 (1952). ~ Pankreassaft in den Gallenwegen. Seine pathogenetische Bedeutung für die Entstehung der akuten Pankreaserkrankungen. Arch. klin. Chir. **175**, 660—695 (1933). — Poursines, Y., et J.-J. Dubarry: A propos d'une autopsie de sprue réalisée dans des conditions exceptionnellement favorables. Acta gastro-enterol. belg. **13**, 924—927 (1950). — Priest, W. M., and M. K. Alexander: Islet-cell tumour of the pancreas with peptic ulceration, diarrhoea and hypokalaemia. Lancet **1957** II, 1145—1147. — Prinz, F.: Über cystische Pankreasfibrose. Verh. dtsch. Ges. Path. (34. Tagg 1950) **1951**, 338—341. ~ Über die gestaltlichen Veränderungen der Bauchspeicheldrüse bei der sogen. cystischen Pankreasfibrose. Beitr. path. Anat. **111**, 313—320 (1951). — Puhl, H.: Über die ursächliche Bedeutung des Magensaftes und des Hungerzustandes bei der Gastritis nach Scheinfütterung. Arch. klin. Chir. **169**, 597—625 (1952). ~ Primäres Jejunalgeschwür mit heterotoper Fundusschleimhaut. Zugleich ein Beitrag zur Frage der klinischen Bedeutung akzessorischer Pankreasanlagen. Dtsch. Z. Chir. **239**, 624—640 (1933). — Puhl, H., u. H. Brodersen: Zur Ätiologie der ulcerösen Gastritis und Duodenitis. Experimentelle Untersuchungen zur Frage der Einwirkung arteigenen Magensaftes auf die Magenduodenalschleimhaut. Arch. klin. Chir. **168**, 30—65 (1931). — Puite, R. H., and H. Tesluk: Whipple's disease. Amer. J. Med. **19**, 383—400 (1955).

Reemtsma, K., P. A. di Sant'Agnese, J. R. Malm and H. G. Barker: Cystic fibrosis of the pancreas: intestinal absorption of fat and fatty acid labeled with I^{131}. Pediatrics **22**, 525—532 (1958). — Remé, H.: Neuere chirurgische Experimente zum Problem des peptischen Geschwürs. Langenbecks Arch. u. Dtsch. Z. Chir. (Kongr.ber.) **267**, 357—362 (1951). ~ Experimentelle und histologische Untersuchungen zum Problem des peptischen Geschwürs an Hund und Katze. Beitr. path. Anat. **112**, 74—96 (1952). — Rendle-Short, J.: Fibrocystic disease of the pancreas presenting with acute salt depletion. Arch. Dis. Childh. **31**, 28—30 (1956). — Reveno, W. S.: Intestinal lipodystrophy (Whiplles disease). Report of a case. New England J. Med. **243**, 216—220 (1950). — Riederer, J.: Über Whipples intestinale Lipodystrophie, ihre Sonderstellung im Spruegeschehen, ihre Beziehung zum Rheumatismus und den Speicherkrankheiten. Dtsch. Z. Verdau.- u. Stoffwechselkr. **16**, 210—222 (1956). — Rietschel, H.: Die Cöliakie oder der intestinale Infantilismus (Gee-Herter-Heubnersche Erkrankung). Ber. physik.-med. Ges. Würzburg, N. F. **61**, 104—106 (1937). — Rössle, R.: Beitrag zur Frage der Speicherungskrankheiten. Verh. dtsch. path. Ges. (31. Tagg 1938) **1939**, 133—146. — Rosen, M. S., and S. H. Rosen: Intestinal lipodystrophy of Whipple. Report of a case and analysis of the literature. Amer. J. Path. **23**, 443—457 (1947). — Rosenthal, H.: Die Darmbefunde bei der einheimischen Sprue. Virchows Arch. **298**, 706—727 (1937). — Rosset, W.: Dreifachbildung des Magens mit peptischem Geschwür in einem Nebenmagen. Beitr. path. Anat. **100**, 382—386 (1938). — Rutishauser, E., et F. Borer: Cellules histiocytaires P.A.S.-positives dans la maladie de Whipple. J. suisse Méd. **89**, 397—410 (1959). — Rutishauser, E., u. B. Forouhar: Axilläre und inguinale Lymphdrüsen bei Morbus Whipple und Pneumatosis intestinalis. Schweiz. Z. Path. **20**, 98—102 (1957). — Rutishauser, E., et A. de Weck: Réticulo-endothéliose cutanée dans la maladie de Whipple. Dermatologica (Basel) **115**, No 3 (1957).

Saegesser, F., E. Juillard, G. Candardjis et P. Décosterd: L'iléus méconial, manifestation néonatale de la mucoviscidose. Arch. des Mal. Appar. digest. **44**, 63—74 (1955). — Sakula, J., and M. Shiner: Coeliac disease with atrophy of the small-intestine mucosa. Lancet **1957** II, 876—877. — Salvesen, H. A., and A. Skogrand: The pathology of steatorrhoea idiopathica. Report of a case with autopsy findings after intraperitoneal formalin fixation immediatly after death. Acta med. scand. **159**, 389—393 (1957). — Sanes, S., D. K. Miller, F. W. Breson and O. B. Geist: Fathy change and cirrhosis of the liver in patients with pancreatic lithiasis. Arch. Int. Med. **85**, 980—997 (1950). — Sant'Agnese, P. A. di: Fibrocytic disease of the pancreas, a generalized disease of exocrine glands. J. Amer. mes. Ass. **160**, 846—853 (1956). ~ Exocrine gland dysfunction in cystic fibrosis of the pancreas. Acta paediat. (Stockh.) **46**, 51—58 (1957). — Sant'Agnese, P. A. di, and D. H. Andersen: Cystic fibrosis of the pancreas in young adults. Ann. intern. Med. **50**, 1321—1330

(1959). — Schallock, G.: Über einen Fall von sprueartiger Erkrankung bei Lipoidgranulomen in den mesenterialen Lymphknoten infolge stenosierender (rheumatischer) Endangitis des Ductus thoracicus. Dtsch. Z. Verdgs. usw. Krkh. 2, 29—38 (1939). — Schmidt, M. B.: Über die Pathologie und die pathologische Anatomie der Avitaminosen. Ber. physik.-med. Ges. Würzburg, N. F. 60, 79—104 (1936). ~ Störungen des Eisenstoffwechsels und ihre Folgen. Erg. Path. 35, 105—208 (1940). — Schulze-Jena, B.: Neue Erkenntnisse über die Pankreasfibrose (Mucoviscidosis). Mschr. Kinderheilk. 103, 165—167 (1955). — Scudamore, H. H., A. B. Hagedorn, E. E. Wollaeger and C. A. Owen jr.: Diverticulosis of the small intestine and macrocytic anemia with report of two cases and studies on absorption of radioactive vitamin B_{12}. Gastroenterology 34, 66—84 (1958). — Scudamore, H. H., W. M. McConahey and J. T. Priestley: Nontropical sprue and functioning islet-cell adenoma of the pancreas. Report of a case. Ann. intern. Med. 49, 909—917 (1958). — Seifert, G.: Über Pankreasveränderungen bei Lebercirrhose und chronischer Blutstauung. Dtsch. Z. Verdgs-usw. Krkh. 11, 230—240 (1951). ~ Zur Pathologie des kindlichen Pankreas bei akuten und chronischen Ernährungsstörungen. Zugleich ein Beitrag zur cystischen Pankreasfibrose und zur Pathogenese der Pankreascysten. Beitr. path. Anat. 114, 1—47 (1954). ~ Die Pathologie des kindlichen Pankreas. Leipzig 1956. ~ Lipomatöse cystische Pankreasfibrose und lipomatöse Pankreasatrophie des Kindesalters. Beitr. path. Anat. 121, 64—80 (1959). — Seifert, G., u. G. Geiler: Zur Pathologie der kindlichen Kopfspeicheldrüsen. Zugleich ein weiterer Beitrag zur Dyschylie. Beitr. path. Anat. 116, 1—38 (1956). — Seitz, W.: Über gastroenterogene Pellagra. Dtsch. med. Wschr. 1943, 365—367. — Shiner, M.: Small intestinal biopsy: diagnostic and research value (Symposium). Proc. roy. Soc. Med. 52, 10—14 (1959). — Siegmund, H.: Lipoidzellhyperplasie der Milz bei chronischem Nierenleiden. Zbl. Path. 70, 328—332 (1928). — Sieracki, J. C.: Whipple's disease. Observation on systemic involvement. I. Cytologic observations. A. M. A. Arch. Path. 66, 464—467 (1958). — Sieracki, J. C., and G. Fine: Whipple's disease. Observations on systemic involvement. II. Gross and histologic observations. A. M. A. Arch. Path. 67, 81—83 (1959). — Staemmler, M.: Lipodystrophia intestinalis (Whipplesche Krankheit). Verh. dtsch. Ges. Path. (36. Tagg 1952) 1953, 294—311. ~ Lehrbuch der speziellen pathologischen Anatomie von Kaufmann, 11. u. 12. Aufl., Bd. I/1, S. 363—365. Berlin 1955. — Staemmler, M., u. H. Merkel: Die Ursachen der Ulcusentstehung im Magen und Duodenum. Klin. Wschr. 1943, 133—135. — Stefanini, M.: The diagnosis and pathogenesis of tropical sprue. Acta med. scand. (Stockh.) 133, 113—126 (1949). — Stein, A. A., and S. R. Powers jr.: Terminal pancreatitis. Arch. Path. (Chicago) 65, 445—448 (1958). — Stepp, W.: Vitaminmangel als Ursache und Folge von Magen-Darmerkrankungen. Münch. med. Wschr. 1936, 1119. — Stinson jr., J. C., A. H. Baggenstoss and C. G. Morlock: Pancreatic lesions associated with cirrhosis of the liver. Amer. J. Clin. Path. 22, 117—126 (1952). — Strack, E.: Die Biochemie der Resorption (Aufsaugung). In Physiologische Chemie, herausgeg. von B. Flaschenträger u. E. Lehnartz, Bd. 2, Teil 1, S. 200—254. 1954. — Straub, M., and H. E. Schornagel: General aetiology of gastro-duodenal ulcer. Schweiz. Z. Path. 21, 242—259 (1959). — Straub, W., et A. Ziegler: L'hépatomégalie dans la maladie fibrokystique. Praxis (Bern) 1958, 796—799. — Svartz, N., E. Nyman and T. Ernberg: Two cases of sprue with advanced lesions in the small intestine. Acta psychiatr. (Kobenh.) Suppl. 46, 307—311 (1947).

Tropp: Über den Zusammenhang zwischen Bezahnung und Nahrungsausnutzung. Dtsch. zahnärztl. Wschr. 1940, 222. — Trowell, H. C.: The world distribution of Kwashiorkor. Symposium. Acta Un. int. Cancer (Louvain) 13, 562—572 (1957).

Underhill, B. M. L.: Intestinal length in man. Brit. Med. J. 1955, 4950, 1243—1246. — Unger, K.: Tierexperimentelle Studien zur Frage der Pankreassaftschäden an den Gallenwegen. Langenbecks Arch. klin. Chir. 286, 218—248 (1957). — Upton, A. C.: Histochemical investigation of the mesenchymal lesions in Whipple's disease. Amer. J. Clin. Path. 22, 755—764 (1952).

Vandenbroucke, J., J. de Laet et E. Herpels: Les diarrhées graisseuses idiopathiques. Quelques aspects de la physiopathologie de l'intestin grêle, en particulier les processus de digestion et d'absorption. Acta gastro-enterol. belg. Suppl. 1, 5—44 (1950). — Verzár, F.: Über die Kräfte der Resorption aus dem Darm. Klin. Wschr. 1933, 489—494. ~ Die Pathologie der Darmresorption. Schweiz. med. Wschr. 1935, 1093. ~ Die Aktivität der Darmschleimhaut bei der Resorption. Schweiz. med. Wschr. 1935, 569—575. ~ Resorptionsstörungen durch Erkrankung der Nebennierenrinde. Schweiz. med. Wschr. 1937, 823. — Verzár, F., u. L. Jeker: Histologische Untersuchungen über die Fettresorption nach Exstirpation der Nebennieren. Pflügers Arch. 237, 14—18 (1936). — Verzár, F., u. L. Laszt: Der Zusammenhang zwischen Vitamin B_2 und dem Hormon der Nebennierenrinde. Pflügers Arch. 237, 476—482 (1936). — Verzár, F., u. E. Sailer: Glukose-Resorption und alkalische Phosphatase des Dünndarmes nach Adrenalektomie bei mit NaCl behandelten Tieren. Helvet. physiol. Acta 10, 247—258 (1952). — Verzár, F., E. Sailer u. R. Richterich: Einfluß der Nebennierenrinde auf die alkalische Phosphatase der Dünndarmschleimhaut. Helvet. physiol. Acta 10, 231—246 (1952).

WAINRIGHT, CH. W.: Intrapancreatic obstruction. New England J. Med. 244, 161—170 (1951). — WALTHARD, B.: Pancreatitis acuta haemorrhagica necroticans. Schweiz. med. Wschr. 1935, 1014. — WALTHER, H. E.: Krebsmetastasen, S. 84. Basel 1948. — WERTHE-MANN, A., E. GROGG u. W. FREY: Zur Pathogenese der cystischen Pankreasfibrose. Pathologisch-anatomischer Beitrag. Virchows Arch. 321, 411—457 (1952). — WÜNSCHE, H. W.: Die Beziehungen des Kauaktes zur Sekretion des gesunden und kranken Magens. Dtsch. Z. Verdgs- usw. Krkh. 2, 100—109 (1939).

ZINKGRÄF, E.: Über einen Fall von exkretorischer und inkretorischer Pankreasinsuffizienz infolge stenosierender Pankreatis auf dem Boden einer seltenen Pankreasmißbildung. Frankf. Z. Path. 62, 13—21 (1951). — ZOLLINGER, R. M., and E. H. ELLISON: Primary peptic ulcerations of the jejunum associated with islet cell tumors of the pancreas. Ann. Surg. 142, 709—728 (1955). — ZUKSCHWERDT, L.: Über Veränderungen der Magensaftsekretion als Folge verzögerter Entleerung. Z. exper. Med. 79, 578—606 (1931). — ZUKSCHWERDT, L., u. E. BECKER: Die Bedeutung des Pylorus für die Entwicklung des postoperativen peptischen Geschwüres. Dtsch. Z. Chir. 241, 39—54 (1933).

Die parenterale Verdauung.

Von

H. Heinlein-Köln.

Mit 4 Abbildungen.

I. Der Begriff der parenteralen Verdauung.

Der Begriff der parenteralen Verdauung wurde von Elias Metschnikoff (1892) geprägt und entwickelt. Er ging dabei von Untersuchungen an Einzellern aus, bei denen er feststellte, daß die von ihnen aufgenommenen Nahrungsteilchen von durchscheinenden Vacuolen umgeben wurden. In diesen Vacuolen wurden die Nahrungsteilchen mit Hilfe verdauender Fermente aufgeschlossen. Das gleiche geschah auch mit kleinsten Lebewesen (Bakterien), die ebenfalls in den Vacuolen verdaut wurden.

Weitere Untersuchungen an *Planarien*, die Blut gesaugt hatten, zeigten, daß dieses Blut intracellulär in den Darmepithelien, die große amöboide Zellen darstellten, durch Fermente verdaut wurde. Ein analoger Vorgang ließ sich auch bei den *Actinien* nachweisen.

Bei höherstehenden Wirbellosen wie den *Medusen* oder anderen Cölenteraten fand sich eine Analogie zwischen der eigentlichen Nahrungsverdauung, die in den Epithelzellen des Entoderms vor sich ging, und der Resorption von Fremdkörpern, die extrabuccal in den Körper eingedrungen waren. Letztere wurden von amöboiden Zellen, die die Funktion von Phagocyten besaßen, erfaßt und verdaut.

Bei den genannten Tierarten fand sich also kein so geschlossenes Verdauungssystem, bei dem die Verdauung extracellulär durch die von den Verdauungsorganen abgesonderten Sekrete vor sich geht, wie dies bei den Wirbeltieren der Fall ist.

Metschnikoff fragte sich nun, ob nicht auch dem Wirbeltier als Rest seiner Phylogenese neben seinem Verdauungssystem noch ein Zellsystem zur Verfügung stehe, das imstande sei, verdaubare Stoffe, die nicht enteral, sondern *parenteral* in den Organismus gelangten, zu verdauen. Er äußerte sich dazu folgendermaßen: „Ich stellte besonders den Gedanken in den Vordergrund, daß die intracelluläre Verdauung der einzelligen Organismen und vieler wirbelloser Tiere durch Heredität auf die Vertebraten übergegangen ist und sich in dieser Tierklasse noch deutlich bei den vom Mesoderm abstammenden amöboiden Zellen erhalten hat".

Bei der Injektion von Serum, Eiereiweiß, Milch und Fett in Säugetiere konnte er beobachten, daß dadurch eine beträchtliche aseptische Entzündung hervorgerufen wurde, „so daß man annehmen könnte, daß der Organismus die durch die Injektion zugeführten Mengen mittels einer entzündlichen Reaktion verdaut."

Auch nach der Injektion von roten Blutkörperchen, von Spermatozoen und Bakterien konnte er sehen, daß sie von Phagocyten (Mikrophagen und Makrophagen) aufgenommen und zerstört, d. h. verdaut wurden. Die Mikrophagen und die Makrophagen spielen nach Metschnikoff aber auch die Hauptrolle bei den Infektionskrankheiten, und zwar die Mikrophagen (Leukocyten) bei den akuten, die Makrophagen bei den chronischen Infektionskrankheiten, wobei der Schlußakt der Phagocytenreaktion auf der Verdauung der Bakterien beruht.

METSCHNIKOFF kam so zu dem Schluß, daß parenterale Verdauung und Entzündung gleich zu setzen seien, und daß dementsprechend entzündliche Reaktionen bis zu den Einzellern verfolgt werden könnten.

Eine solche Gleichsetzung von parenteraler Verdauung und Entzündung wurde von RÖSSLE (1923), der die Gedankengänge von METSCHNIKOFF aufnahm und weiter verfolgte, abgelehnt. Er postulierte mit Recht, daß für das Zustandekommen einer Entzündung das Vorhandensein eines — wenn auch primitiven — Mesenchyms unerläßlich sei. In seinen Arbeiten über die Entzündung, besonders ausführlich jedoch in seinem großen Referat auf der Tagung der Deutschen Pathologischen Gesellschaft in Göttingen 1923, ging er auf die Beziehungen zwischen parenteraler Verdauung und Entzündung ein. Er wies darauf hin, daß erst bei den Cölenteraten eine mesodermale Schicht vorhanden ist, und führte einen Versuch METSCHNIKOFFS an Schwämmen an, bei denen ein eingeführter Glassplitter von Ansammlungen mesodermaler Wanderzellen umgeben wurde; dasselbe geschah auch beim Eindringen von Pilzen. Hier sei die Entzündungsreaktion in einer Grundfunktion der tierischen Organisation, nämlich der Verdauung, verankert.

RÖSSLE prägte den Begriff der physiologischen Entzündung, die eine Reizantwort auf die Anwesenheit endogen entstandener Fremdkörper darstelle. Er rechnete hierzu den Abbau körpereigener Substanzen, z. B. ganzer Gewebe oder Glieder, wie bei der Metamorphose der Würmer oder Insekten. Hierbei handele es sich auch um eine Form der parenteralen Verdauung. In seinen eigenen experimentellen Untersuchungen gewann er jedoch den Eindruck, daß ein solcher Abbau nicht unbedingt durch Zellen geleistet werden müsse, sondern daß er — auch unabhängig von Zellen — durch chemische Stoffe vor sich gehen könne, wie er es bei der Überpflanzung von Hautlappen beim Axolotl beobachtete. Ähnliche Ansichten waren bereits über die Morphallaxien geäußert worden, die nach METSCHNIKOFF, dem sich einige Autoren anschlossen, durch Phagocytose, nach der Meinung anderer Untersucher[1] durch primäre Histolyse zustande kommen sollen.

Die engen Beziehungen zwischen parenteraler Verdauung und Entzündung veranlaßten RÖSSLE (1923) zur Definition der Entzündung als einer „krankhaft gesteigerten Funktion gewisser mesodermaler Abkömmlinge, die geeignet erscheint, das Bindegewebe der Organe von Fremdstoffen zu reinigen". Dementsprechend betrachtete er die geschlossenen Lymphknoten und die lymphadenoiden Organe als „Entzündungsorgane und organisierte Entzündung", die nicht nur der Verdauung von Nahrungsmaterial, sondern auch der Verarbeitung der zu Fremdstoffen gewordenen Abfallprodukte des normalen Gewebes, besonders der verbrauchten Zellen, dienen.

Hinsichtlich des Verhältnisses der parenteralen zur enteralen Verdauung führte RÖSSLE aus, daß man bisher die Verdauung als alleinige Leistung der Verdauungsdrüsen betrachtet habe, diese Auffassung jedoch vielleicht dahin abändern müsse, daß man zwischen einer enteroepithelialen Verdauung durch Sekrete und einer zweiten Verdauung durch die mesodermalen Organe unterscheiden müsse.

Er spannte den Bogen seiner Gedanken noch weiter zur Immunologie, indem er die Frage aufwarf, ob nicht die Entstehung der Immunstoffe ihr Analogon in der zur Histolyse dienenden parenteralen Verdauung habe. Die Immunkörper wären von diesem Standpunkt aus als Ergebnis einer parenteralen Verdauung zu bezeichnen. Eine Vergleichsmöglichkeit zwischen der „physiologischen" und der „pathologischen" Entzündung sieht RÖSSLE darin, daß entweder körpereigene, aber körperfremd gewordene oder fremde, in den Organismus gelangte Stoffe

---

[1] DUESBERG 1907, LOSS 1889.

durch die parenterale Verdauung entfernt werden sollen. Als körperfremde Stoffe betrachtete er z. B. auch Transplantate, Thromben oder Infarkte.

In neueren Untersuchungen an Schnecken[1] wurde nachgewiesen, daß den mesenchymalen Zellen und ihren Abkömmlingen gewebsreinigende Funktionen zukommen, die bei intrakardialer Injektion des Fremdstoffes (Tusche) von den Gefäßwandendothelien übernommen werden. Wenn Froschblutkörperchen in den Schneckenfuß injiziert wurden, so wurde dadurch eine entzündliche Reaktion ausgelöst, die dem entzündlichen Geschehen bei Wirbeltieren weitgehend ähnelte. Wurde diese Injektion von Froschblutkörperchen mehrmalig vorgenommen, so war die Abbaufunktion qualitativ gleich, jedoch quantitativ gesteigert. Ein solcher Wandel des Entzündungsbildes wurde teils als Folge einer spezifischen Umstimmung, teils als Folge einer unspezifischen Aktivierung der Abwehrkräfte aufgefaßt. Es wurde der Schluß gezogen, daß mit dem Auftreten eines Gefäßsystems in der Tierreihe nicht nur die Möglichkeit, sondern auch die Tatsache einer aus histiogener und hämatogener Komponente bestehenden Entzündung gegeben sei.

Wenn wir uns nun fragen, was unter *parenteraler* Verdauung zu verstehen ist, so handelt es sich dabei, wie aus dem früher Erörterten wohl schon hervorgegangen sein dürfte, einmal um den Abbau von körpereigenen Stoffen, die dem Körper aber fremd geworden sind, und zum anderen um körperfremde Stoffe, die nicht auf dem Weg über den Verdauungskanal in den Organismus gelangt sind. Bei der gewöhnlichen Verdauung geht die Spaltung der Nahrungsstoffe im Verdauungskanal durch verschiedene Fermente, die dort hervorgebracht werden, vor sich. Bei der parenteralen Verdauung handelt es sich um einen ähnlichen Prozeß, insofern als es auch hier einen extracellulären Abbau mit Hilfe von Fermenten gibt, die im Blut oder den Gewebssäften vorhanden sind. Die wichtigere Form der parenteralen Verdauung verhält sich jedoch insofern anders, als dabei eine intracelluläre Substanzverarbeitung vorliegt, bei der die Stoffe zunächst in die Zellen aufgenommen werden müssen, in denen dann ihre weitere Zerlegung durch die zelleigenen Fermente erfolgt. Welche Stoffe für die parenterale Verdauung in Frage kommen, an welchen Orten und durch welche Zellen die parenterale Verdauung vor sich geht, darüber wird im folgenden zu berichten sein.

II. Die Stoffe und ihr Schicksal.

A. Exogene Stoffe.

1. Belebte Stoffe.

An erster Stelle der von außen in den Organismus gelangenden Stoffe sind die belebten, vor allem die Krankheitserreger zu nennen. Wir wissen, daß zwar ein Teil dieser Krankheitserreger den Körper wieder verläßt, daß aber ein anderer Teil im Verlaufe der Auseinandersetzung zwischen Wirt und Gast vernichtet wird. Dabei spielt die Phagocytose eine wichtige Rolle.

Wiederum ist es Metschnikoff, dessen Untersuchungen wir wichtige Kenntnisse über diesen Vorgang und seine Bedeutung verdanken. Er konnte zeigen, daß die Phagocytose eine bedeutende Rolle im Kampf des Organismus gegen Krankheitserreger spielt. Seiner Meinung nach ist sie die Ursache der natürlichen Immunität mancher Tiere gegen bestimmte Bakterien. Wenn er Frösche, Hühner oder Hunde mit Milzbrandbacillen infizierte, so wurden diese von den Phagocyten aufgenommen und unschädlich gemacht. Mäuse und Meerschweinchen dagegen,

---

[1] Heinzel 1949/50.

die der Milzbrandinfektion erlagen, wiesen keine Phagocytose auf. METSCH-
NIKOFF deutet die Phagocytose als einen Abwehrvorgang. Er schreibt den
Phagocyten ein Wahlvermögen zu, das erklärt, warum nicht alle Bakterien der
Phagocytose unterliegen. Er unterscheidet 2 Arten von Phagocyten, die
Mikro- und Makrophagen. Die Mikrophagen sind identisch mit den neutrophilen
Leukocyten, während die Makrophagen aus den von SIEGMUND (1927) als „aktives
Mesenchym" bezeichneten Keimlagern stammen. Sowohl die natürliche als auch
die erworbene Immunität gegen Bakterien soll nach METSCHNIKOFF auf der
Phagocytose beruhen und Spezialfälle der parenteralen Verdauung darstellen.
Diese Anschauung kann jedoch heute als aufgegeben gelten, da gezeigt worden
ist[1], daß die Phagocyten nicht in allen Fällen imstande sind, die Bakterien an-
zugreifen; es wirken dabei noch besondere Serumstoffe, die Opsonine[2] und die
Bakteriotropine[3] mit, die die Bakterien für die Phagocytose geeignet machen.
Damit wurde bewiesen, daß bei der Immunisierung nicht eine Veränderung der
Leukocyten, wie METSCHNIKOFF glaubte, sondern eine solche des Serums eintritt.

Wenn wir nun eine etwas andere Vorstellung von der Phagocytose besitzen
als METSCHNIKOFF, so ändert das nichts an der Tatsache, daß wir auch heute die
Phagocytose und die intracelluläre Verdauung der Krankheitserreger als wesentlich für die Überwindung von Infektionskrankheiten, vor allem der bakteriell
bedingten, ansehen[4]. Nach Untersuchungen an Hunden mit experimenteller
Pneumokokkenpneumonie gibt es 2 Mechanismen, mit deren Hilfe der Orga-
nimus eine Bakteriämie abwehrt: 1. humorale Vorgänge im Blut und 2. die
Phagocytose durch Mikro- und Makrophagen[5]. Neuere Untersuchungen haben
bewiesen, daß sich unter den Mikrophagen vor allem die neutrophilen Leukocyten
an der Phagocytose beteiligen, und zwar 1,6mal stärker als die eosinophilen[6],
während die Lymphocyten im allgemeinen nicht phagocytieren und, wenn sie
es tun, dann weniger virulente Keime, wie etwa nichthämolysierende Strepto-
kokken[7].

Welche Vorstellung können wir uns nun heute vom Vorgang der Phagocytose
machen? Wenn auch, wie bereits oben erwähnt, dabei gewisse natürliche Antikörper, die Opsonine und Bakteriotropine, eine Rolle spielen, so ist es doch nicht
so, als ob die Phagocytose nicht auch ohne diese Stoffe möglich wäre. Wir kennen
die sich dabei abspielenden Vorgänge von den Untersuchungen über die Oberflächenphagocytose[8]. Während in einem flüssigen Milieu oder auf einer Glas-
unterlage Leukocyten die mit Kapseln versehenen Pneumokokken oder Strepto-
kokken oder Friedländer Bacillen nicht zu phagocytieren vermochten, gelang dies
auf rauhen Unterlagen wie Filtrierpapier oder auch Fibringerinnseln oder selbst
dann, wenn die Leukocyten nur dicht aneinander gedrängt waren.

Diese Oberflächenphagocytose wurde zwar von anderer Seite für möglich gehalten, jedoch für eine Erscheinung, die zwar in vitro, aber nicht in vivo
vorkomme[9]. Dieser Einwand konnte jedoch entkräftet werden[10]. Nach einer
dritten Meinung soll die Oberflächenphagocytose zwar eine Rolle spielen, jedoch
bei bekapselten Bakterien unterstützt durch die Tropinwirkung[11].

Wir dürfen somit die Oberflächenphagocytose als ein bewiesenes Phänomen
betrachten, ohne daß damit etwas gegen die Bedeutung der natürlichen Antikörper ausgesagt ist.

Die Annahme METSCHNIKOFFs, daß nur die Leukocyten Bakterien phagocytieren, während die Phagocytose von Gewebezellen die Aufgabe der Makro-

---

[1] DENYS 1898.   [2] WRIGHT 1910.   [3] NEUFELD 1929.
[4] ROBERTSON, COGGESHALL und TERRELL 1933.   [5] GREGG und ROBERTSON 1953.
[6] KÄRKI, SEPPÄLÄ und HALONEN 1951.   [7] SEITZER und SANDKÜHLER 1951.
[8] WOOD und SMITH 1947.   [9] HAEMERLI 1949.   [10] WOOD u. Mitarb. 1951.
[11] ROTH 1950.

phagen sei, kann heute nicht mehr als richtig angesehen werden, da die Makrophagen im allgemeinen ebensogut wie die Mikrophagen Bakterien phagocytieren.

Die zu phagocytierenden Bakterien werden von den Freßzellen aufgenommen. Wie das geschieht, ist keineswegs völlig klar. Es scheint, daß es dabei verschiedene Möglichkeiten gibt. So wird von mancher Seite angenommen, daß sie einfach ins Protoplasma einsinken, ohne daß man eine Tätigkeit der Zellen feststellen kann[1]. Ob dies tatsächlich der Fall ist und eine größere Rolle spielt, scheint

Abb. 1. Phagocytose von Gonokokken durch Leukocyten

jedoch zunächst noch fraglich. Auch wenn es so aussieht, als ob die Phagocyten ganz unbeteiligt wären, darf man doch nicht vergessen, daß zwischen den zu phagocytierenden Teilchen und den Phagocyten mancherlei physikalische Kräfte vorhanden sind, vor allem in Form der Oberflächenspannung, die wiederum bedingt ist durch verschiedene elektrische Ladung, durch verschiedene Viscosität. So kommt es wohl in den meisten Fällen zu einer Adsorption und schließlich zu einer Aufnahme des Teilchens. Dabei mag die amöboide Bewegung, d. h. die Fähigkeit des Umfließens eine mehr oder weniger große Rolle spielen. Jedenfalls darf man die Eigentätigkeit der phagocytierenden Zellen dabei nicht für gering erachten.

Wenn oben gesagt wurde, daß Bakterien sowohl von Mikro- wie von Makrophagen aufgenommen werden, so läßt sich doch nicht abstreiten, daß beiden ein gewisses Auswahlvermögen zukommt. Wie sollte man es sonst erklären, daß ganze Zellen oder besonders große Teilchen, wie wir sie als Dispersionskolloide von Kohle (Ruß) oder Quarzbestandteilen oder auch in der Form von makromolekularen organischen Kolloiden, etwa als Fett, gelegentlich im Organismus finden, fast nur von den Makrophagen phagocytiert werden? Hier scheint die Teilchengröße eine ausschlaggebende Rolle zu spielen.

---

[1] Heilbrunn 1943, McCutcheon 1948.

Es ist ganz sicher, daß die Bedingungen des Milieus die Phagocytose beeinflussen. Hierher gehört z. B. die Wasserstoffionenkonzentration, von der wir
wissen, daß ein p_H von etwa 7,0 das Phagocytoseoptimum darstellt[1].

Es wurde oben bereits auf die Wirkung natürlicher Antikörper, der Opsonine
und Bakteriotropine, für die Phagocytose hingewiesen. Ob es sich dabei tatsächlich

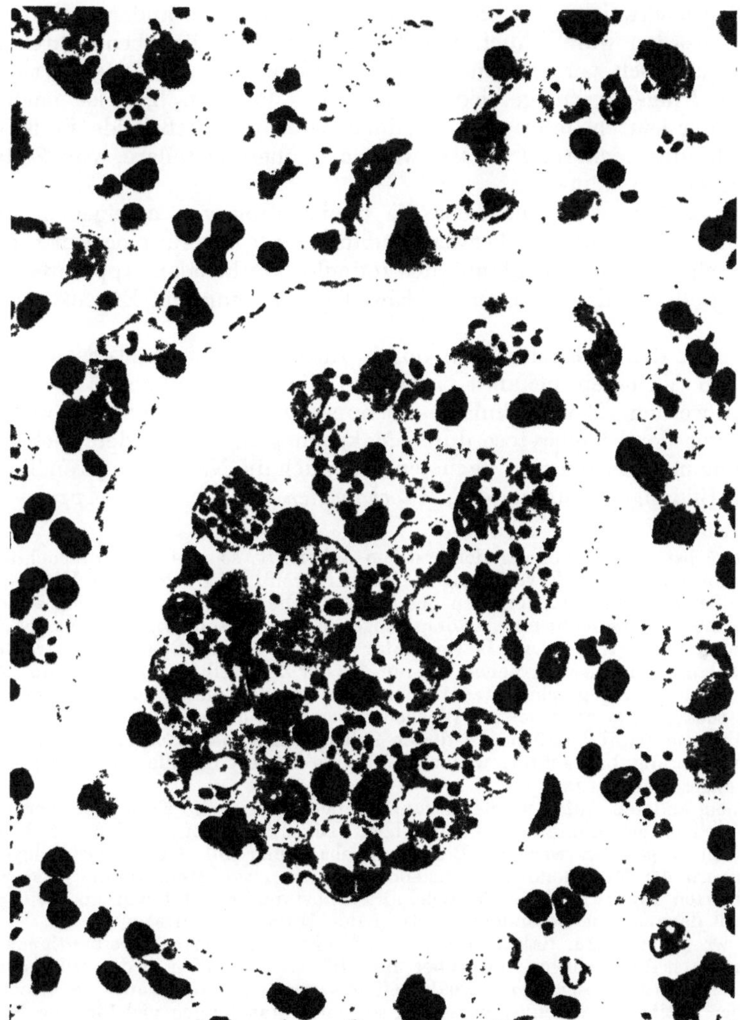

Abb. 2. Milz bei Histoplasmosis. Reticulumzellen in einer Milzvene, die Histoplasmen gespeichert haben.
(Aus G. HADFIELD: „Recent advances in pathology". London: Churchill 1953.)

um eine wirkliche Antikörpertätigkeit handelt, scheint sehr fraglich. Man könnte
sich sehr gut vorstellen, daß es sich dabei um eine völlig unspezifische Eiweißwirkung handelt, nämlich um denselben Effekt, der als Vehikelfunktion von
Eiweißkörpern beschrieben wurde[2]. Wenn kolloidal gelöste Farbstoffe mit Hilfe
des Eiweißvehikels in die Zelle einzudringen vermögen, in die sie sonst nicht
gelangen können, so kann dies wohl als „embatischer Effekt" bezeichnet werden.

[1] FENN 1922.　　[2] BENNHOLD 1932.

Ob dabei die Eiweißteilchen selbst in die Zelle hineingelangen oder nicht, scheint zunächst nicht völlig geklärt.

Bennhold (1932, 1938, 1951), dem wir Entscheidendes zur Frage der Vehikelfunktion zu verdanken haben, schien zunächst anzunehmen, daß ein Eindringen des Eiweißvehikels in die Zellen nicht in Frage komme. Nach Untersuchungen seines Schülers Seybold (1954) ergibt sich jedoch, daß eine Aufnahme von Eiweiß in die Zellen nachweisbar ist, so wie dies auch schon von anderen Untersuchern festgestellt worden war[1]. Auch Periston konnte in Zellen beobachtet werden. Während man noch vor einigen Jahren annahm, daß wohl das Periston N in Zellen einzudringen vermöge, jedoch nicht das Periston 3,5[2] ist nach Untersuchungen der letzten Jahre die Annahme berechtigt, daß beide Peristonarten, d. h. sowohl das niedermolekulare wie das höhermolekulare, von Zellen aufgenommen werden können[3].

Sollten sich die Versuche über die Speicherung von arteigenem und artfremdem Eiweiß als zutreffend erweisen, dann würde dies für eine außerordentlich starke Beteiligung wohl nicht nur des reticuloendothelialen Apparates, sondern eines sehr großen Zellsystems an der Eiweißspeicherung und Eiweißverarbeitung sprechen.

Schon von der Stoffaufnahme durch Einzeller ist seit Metschnikoff die Bildung von Vacuolen bekannt, in denen die aufgenommenen Teilchen eingeschlossen werden. Etwas Ähnliches ist nun auch von der Phagocytose bekannt, besonders von der Phagocytose durch Makrophagen. Wir finden auch hier eine Abscheidung in präformierten Vacuolen oder auch die Neubildung von Tröpfchen. Für diese Bildungen wurden die *Mitochondrien* und der *Golgi-Apparat* verantwortlich gemacht.

Was zunächst die Beteiligung der ersteren anbetrifft, so gibt es Untersuchungen, die nach Injektion von großen Eiweißmengen (Hühnereiweiß) bei Ratten, eine Wechselwirkung dieses Eiweißes mit den Mitochondrien beschreiben. Die Stäbchen sollen sich auflösen und die Speicherungstropfen nicht nur aus dem exogenen Eiweiß, sondern auch aus der Substanz der Mitochondrien bestehen. Als Beweis dafür wird die in den Speicherungstropfen nachgewiesene Ribonucleinsäure angesehen, die nur aus der Zelle selbst stammen kann. An durch temporäre Abklemmung geschädigten Rattennieren wurden die zugrunde gegangenen Teile des Hauptstückepithels nach etwa 3 Wochen durch neue atypische Epithelien ersetzt, die keinen Stäbchenapparat besaßen. In diesen Zellen wurde nach Eiweißeinspritzung keine tropfige Speicherung beobachtet, was ebenfalls als Beweis für die Bedeutung der Mitochondrien angesehen wurde[4].

Von einem anderen Autor wurde in ganz ähnlicher Weise die Eiweißspeicherung in den Hauptstückzellen der Mäuseniere beschrieben. Die Eiweißstoffe sollen im Innern der Mitochondrien gespeichert werden. Bei der Beobachtung mit dem Phasenmikroskop sah man im Innern der Mitochondrien glänzende Tröpfchen auftreten, die als Koacervate aus dem resorbierten Eiweiß und der Mitochondriensubstanz gedeutet wurden. Die Speicherfunktion soll danach eine besondere Leistung der Mitochondrien sein[5].

Fügen wir noch hinzu, daß Kaninchen radioaktiv markierte Eiweißantigene injiziert wurden und nach Aufarbeitung von Leber und Milz hauptsächlich in der Mikrosomen- und Mitochondrienfraktion dieser Organe wiedergefunden wurden[6], woraus auf eine mitochondriale Synthese der Antikörper geschlossen wurde, so scheint tatsächlich viel für eine Beteiligung der Mitochondrien zu sprechen.

Jedoch soll andererseits nicht übersehen werden, daß andere Untersucher keine Beteiligung der Mitochondrien an der Speicherung feststellen konnten. Bei Speicherungsversuchen mit Eiweiß und Mucin wurde trotz stärkster Speicherung keine Veränderung an den Mitochondrien entdeckt. Auch bei Umwandlung der Speicherzellen in Schaumzellen ließ sich keine Veränderung der Mitochondrien nachweisen[7].

Wenn so die Rolle der Mitochondrien bei der Speicherung und Segregation eine noch sehr fragliche ist, so liegen die Verhältnisse beim Golgi-Apparat etwas anders. Einmal ist schon oft auf die topographischen Beziehungen zwischen Golgi- und Segregationsapparat

---

[1] Heinlein und Zimmer 1955, Jancsó 1955. [2] Weese und Scholtan 1951.
[3] Jancsó 1955, Heinlein und Hübner 1958, [4] Oliver 1948.
[5] Zollinger 1948. [6] Haurowitz und Crampton 1952. [7] Jancsó 1955.

und auf die Abhängigkeit der ontogenetischen Entwicklung der Segregationsfähigkeit bei den Leukocyten von der Entwicklung des Golgi-Apparates hingewiesen worden[1], zum anderen konnte sogar kinematographisch beobachtet werden, wie bei der Pinocytose die aufgenommenen Substanzen nach der Mitte der Zellen, wo der Golgi-Apparat liegt, bewegt wurden[2]. Ähnliches ist auch bei der Phagocytose beobachtet worden.

Schließlich haben neuere Untersuchungen festgestellt, daß bei Speicherungsversuchen mit Trypanblau und Polyvinylpyrroiydon in den kanalisierten Epithelzellen der Froschniere, ein Zusammenhang zwischen der Ablagerung dieser Substanzen und dem Golgi-Apparat besteht. Der Golgi-Apparat war sichtlich verändert: die spezifische Golgi-Substanz umgab in Form von Brocken oder Fäden oder als dicke zusammenhängende Schicht die großen Vacuolen[3].

Daß die Phagocytose und die parenterale Verdauung eine große Rolle bei der Abwehr bzw. Überwindung von Infektionen spielen, wurde im vorhergehenden schon erwähnt. Die Bedeutung der Leukocyten ergibt sich ohne weiteres daraus, daß man sie am ersten dort auftreten sieht, wo als Abwehrreaktion sich eine Entzündung abspielt. Damit sind wieder die engen Beziehungen zwischen parenteraler Verdauung und Entzündung, wie sie Rössle (1923) dargestellt hat, erwiesen.

Den Lymphocyten kommt keine Rolle bei der Phagocytose zu. Zwar wurde ihre Umwandlung in makrophagen- und fibroblastenähnlichen Zellen behauptet[4], doch darf diese Hypothese als widerlegt gelten[5]. Es wäre aber durchaus möglich, daß sie zwar keine Krankheitserreger phagocytieren, aber vielleicht Abbauprodukte derselben aufnehmen und weiterverarbeiten. Dies dürfte noch vielmehr für die lymphocytären Plasmazellen gelten, die nach Moeschlin (1940, 1946) nicht von den Lymphocyten, sondern von eigenen Stammzellen in den Lymphknoten, den lymphatischen Reticulumzellen, abzuleiten sind. Auch diese können wohl solche Stoffe aufnehmen und verarbeiten, wie dies auch für die reticulären Plasmazellen von mancher Seite angenommen wird[6].

Schon Metschnikoff hatte neben den Mikrophagen den Makrophagen eine bedeutende Rolle bei der Phagocytose zugesprochen. Den Ursprung dieser Zellen sah er in Blut, Milz und Lymphknoten. Er schrieb, wie bereits erwähnt, den Mikro- und Makrophagen die Fähigkeit des Auswählens der zu resorbierenden Stoffe zu. Während die Mikrophagen ihre Wirkung besonders bei akuten Infektionskrankheiten ausüben sollten, sollen die Makrophagen imstande sein, vornehmlich die Erreger chronischer Infektionskrankheiten aufzunehmen (z. B. Leprabacillen, Tuberkulosebacillen, Actinomycespilze). Außerdem sollten sie tierische Zellen wie Blutkörperchen oder Spermatozoen phagocytieren. Beide Arten von Phagocyten sollten sich auch durch besondere Fermente, die Mikro- und Makrocytase, unterscheiden.

Die Makrophagentheorie von Metschnikoff wurde in der Folgezeit von Ribbert, Ranvier (1881—1891) und vor allem von Aschoff (1924) u. a. weitgehend ausgebaut. Besonders von letzterem — zusammen mit seinen Mitarbeitern — wurde der Begriff eines ganzen Makrophagensystems geschaffen, das unter dem Namen „Reticulo-endotheliales System" bekannt wurde. Maßgeblich für die Eingliederung von Organen in dieses System war ihre Fähigkeit zur Speicherung.

Da diese Gliederung mehr funktioneller als morphologischer Art war, unterlag das RES mancherlei Kritik. Aschoff unterschied ein Reticuloendothel im weiteren und eines im engeren Sinne. Unter letzterem verstand er:

1. die Reticulumzellen der Milzpulpa, der Rindenknötchen und der Markstränge der Lymphknoten sowie des übrigen lymphatischen Gewebes;

---

[1] Ehrich 1934. [2] Lewis 1931. [3] Jancsó 1955. [4] Maximow 1927, Bloom 1933.
[5] Seemann 1930, Pfuhl 1937. [6] Heinlein 1943, Büngeler 1951.

2. die Reticuloendothelien der Lymphsinus der Lymphknoten, der Blutsinus
der Milz, der Capillaren der Leberläppchen (Kupffersche Sternzellen), der Capillaren des Knochenmarks, der Nebennierenrinde und der Hypophyse.

Zum Reticuloendothel im weiteren Sinne rechnete ASCHOFF:

3. die Histiocyten, wie von ihm die beweglichen Bindegewebszellen (die
Clasmatocyten RANVIERS) im Gegensatz zu den fixen Bindegewebszellen (den
Fibroplasten bzw. Fibrocyten) genannt wurden;

4. die Splenocyten der Milzpulpa und die Monocyten des strömenden Blutes,
die aus der Gruppe 3, den Histiocyten, und der Gruppe 2, den Reticuloendothelien,
hervorgehen.

Bei stark gesteigerten Speicherungen treten schließlich auch noch die Endothelien der Blut- und Lymphgefäße sowie die Fibrocyten in Aktion. Diese beiden
letzten Gruppen speichern jedoch gewöhnlich nicht oder nur schwer. Aus diesem
Grunde glaubte ASCHOFF sie nicht zum RES rechnen zu dürfen, zumal sie sich
auch sonst verschieden verhalten sollten. Nicht dazu gerechnet wurden ferner
die Reticulumzellen des Thymus, die Gliazellen des Gehirns sowie die Wandzellen
der großen Körperhöhlen (Pleura, Peritoneum, Meningen), obwohl gerade diese
gut speichern.

Eine Revision dieser Einteilung hat neuerdings FRESEN (1946, 1954) vorgenommen, wobei er zu dem Ergebnis kam, daß die Capillarendothelien des
Knochenmarks, der Nebennieren und der Hypophyse im Gegensatz zu den Untersuchungen KIYONOS (1914) nicht speichern, während die pericapillären Histiocyten dies tun. Es verhalten sich danach die Capillarendothelien der genannten
Organe wie die Capillarendothelien an anderen Stellen. Die Endothelien der
Sinusoide der Lymphknoten und der Milz, die stark speichern, zeigen nach seinen
Angaben denselben reticulären Zusammenhang wie die Zellen des eigentlichen
Reticulums, so daß sie weder funktionell noch morphologisch als eigentliche
Endothelien, sondern als uferbildende Reticulumzellen (reticuläre Uferzellen) zu
betrachten sind. Die pericapillären Histiocyten könnten sich bei starker Reizung
als Uferzellen in die Endothelwand einlegen, so daß dadurch eine Speicherung
gewöhnlicher Endothelzellen vorgetäuscht werden könnte. Das RES im engeren
Sinne soll nach FRESEN aus einem einheitlichen reticulär-syncytialen fibrillären
Zellverband unter Ausschluß echter Endothelien bestehen.

Bei dieser Einteilung herrscht, wie man sieht, eine gewisse Willkür. SIEGMUND
(1927) u. a. lehnen diese deshalb auch ab, da es sich bei dem Speicherzellensystem
nicht um eine starre, sondern um eine fließende Struktur handele. Nach SIEG
MUND hängt die Ausdehnung des Speicherzellensystems von der funktionellen
Beanspruchung ab. So können Speicherzellen sowohl aus den ganz indifferenten,
pluripotenten, mesenchymalen Keimlagern, als auch aus den bereits weiterentwickelten, aber noch differenzierungsfähigen ruhenden Elementen des lockeren
Bindegewebes gebildet werden. Diese gesamte differenzierungsfähige Grundsubstanz bezeichnet SIEGMUND (1927) als „aktives Mesenchym". Die ruhenden
Mesenchymzellen können nach ihm in Abhängigkeit von der Funktion in Histiocyten, ja in Blutstammzellen mit sekundärer Umwandlung in Lymphocyten und
Leukocyten verwandelt werden. Sicher scheint dabei jedoch nur die Umwandlung
in Histiocyten zu sein, die in geringerer Menge als Bluthistiocyten oder Monocyten
im strömenden Blut erscheinen. Bei hochgetriebener Speicherung werden sie
jedoch in solchen Mengen ins Blut eingeschwemmt, daß man sogar von Monocytenschauern gesprochen hat. Diese Monocyten stellen zweifellos den Teil
der Makrophagen dar, der schon normalerweise im Blut vorhanden ist. Ihre
Abkunft war lange umstritten. Nach Auffassung von WEIDENREICH (1910),
MAXIMOW (1927) u. a. sollen sie von den Lymphocyten abstammen. Die Unter

suchungen von Aschoff (1913, 1924), Seemann (1930), Büngeler (1926), Schilling (1937), Masugi (1926) u. a. sprechen jedoch dafür, daß sie sich von den Reticulumzellen ableiten. Nach diesen Vorstellungen werden die Blutmonocyten im Knochenmark gebildet, sind also Abkömmlinge des Knochenmarkreticulums. Unter krankhaften Umständen wird ihre Zahl jedoch durch Bildung von Monocyten im Reticulum der Lymphknoten und des Gewebes (Histiocyten) vermehrt. Diese Monocyten besitzen nach den Untersuchungen von Pfuhl (1937) die Fähigkeit, sich in Fibroblasten umzuwandeln. Ihrer Abstammung entsprechend beteiligen sie sich an der Phagocytose, wobei sie gerade durch die chronisch verlaufenden Infektionskrankheiten auf den Plan gerufen werden. So wurde auf ihre Beteiligung bei der Bildung epitheloider Zellen im tuberkulösen Granulationsgewebe hingewiesen[1]. Es ist möglich, daß es dabei besonders die schwer verdaulichen Lipoide und Wachse der Tuberkelbacillen sind, die ihre Tätigkeit hervorrufen.

Was hier für die Blutmonocyten gesagt wurde, gilt in gleicher Weise auch für die anderen Zellen des RES. Handelt es sich dabei doch um ein Organ- bzw. Zellsystem, das die Aufgabe hat, unter anderem dadurch für den Schutz des Organismus zu sorgen, daß es ihn von Fremdstoffen befreit. Dies wird aber in erster Linie dadurch erreicht, daß solche Stoffe aufgenommen und verdaut oder eliminiert werden.

Wir kennen die Tätigkeit dieser Zellen besonders gut bei bakteriellen Allgemeininfektionen. Die Milzvergrößerung bei solchen Prozessen ist bekannt. Sie wird nicht nur durch die größere Blutmenge, sondern auch durch die Zellvermehrung verursacht. An der Zellvermehrung sind aus dem Blut eingeschwemmte Leukocyten, aber auch die vermehrten Endothelien und Reticulumzellen der Milz selbst beteiligt. Die Bakterien werden von den Endothelien resorbiert, wobei sich Resorptionsvacuolen in den Zellen bilden. Diese runden sich ab und werden aus dem Verband gelöst. Neben den Sinusendothelien sind auch die Reticulumzellen beteiligt, die vergrößert und vermehrt sind und zusammenhängende Stränge und Nester bilden. Welche Ausmaße die Reticulumzellwucherungen bei infektiösen Erkrankungen erreichen können, wissen wir von der Letterer-Siweschen Krankheit, die man ja als infektiöse Retikulose bezeichnet. Dabei finden sich die Reticulumzellwucherungen nicht nur in der Milz, sondern auch in der Leber, in den Lymphknoten und im Knochenmark.

Wir kennen solche Veränderungen bei chronischen Sepsisfällen, bei denen in der Milz so ausgedehnte Reticulumzellwucherungen auftreten, daß die Sinus klein und zusammengedrückt erscheinen. Gegenüber der starken Beteiligung von Endothelien und Reticulumzellen sind die Lymphfollikel verhältnismäßig unverändert. Gelegentlich kommen bei derartigen Vorgängen in den Capillaren der Leber Fibrinabscheidung vor, die von Dietrich (1943) als Zeichen des Mißerfolges der cellulären Reaktion gedeutet werden, da die größeren fleckweisen Ausfällungen mit Nekrosen von Stern- und Leberzellen verbunden seien.

Auch das Reticuloendothel der Leber nimmt an einer solchen Resorption und parenteralen Verdauung von Bakterien teil. In erster Linie sind es die Kupfferschen Sternzellen, die sich vergrößern und in ihrem Cytoplasma kleine und große Resorptionsvacuolen erkennen lassen, in denen manchmal noch Reste der aufgenommenen und verdauten Bakterien festzustellen sind. Es handelt sich also hier grundsätzlich um denselben Vorgang, der von Metschnikoff beim Verdauungsvorgang der Einzeller beschrieben wurde. Die Kupfferschen Sternzellen lösen sich dann aus dem Verband und werden unter Abrundung in die Sinusoide abgestoßen. Bekannt ist weiter das vermehrte Auftreten von

---

[1] Sabin und Mitarbeiter 1924.

Leukocyten in den Lebersinusoiden, das zu leukämieähnlichen Bildern führen kann. Es ist ja bekannt, daß Sternberg (1926) glaubte, die akuten Leukämien als Leukocytosen bei sepsisartigen Erkrankungen bezeichnen zu müssen.

Weiterhin müssen auch die Zellansammlungen in den Glissonschen Dreiecken mit der parenteralen Verdauung in Zusammenhang gebracht werden, wobei es sich allerdings weniger um die Verdauung der Bakterien als ihrer Stoffwechselprodukte handelt.

Auch die Lymphknoten zeigen eine erhöhte resorptive Leistung, die sich in ähnlichen Veränderungen kundtut, wie sie bei der Milz beschrieben wurden. Auch hier vergrößern sich in erster Linie die Sinusendothelien, die schließlich aus dem Verband gelöst werden. Ebenso kommt es zu einer Vergrößerung und Vermehrung der Reticulumzellen. In den Lymphfollikeln treten im Zentrum größere Zellen auf, die Speicherungserscheinungen aufweisen, wie man an Kerntrümmern feststellen kann. Diese Reaktionszentren scheinen besonders an der Resorption von Stoffen und ihrer Verarbeitung beteiligt zu sein.

Die Reaktion des Knochenmarks bei bakteriellen Allgemeininfektionen äußert sich ebenfalls in einer Vergrößerung und Schwellung der Reticulumzellen. Es werden jedoch nicht nur diese Zellen auf den Plan gerufen, sondern auch die Leukocyten und ihre Vorstufen, die Myelocyten und Myeloblasten, sowie die Megacaryocyten, die in verstärktem Maße Thrombocyten abstoßen. Das alles gehört zu dem Begriff des Reizmarks, das jedoch bei Überbeanspruchung in das Erschöpfungsmark übergehen kann.

Daß auch die Lungen an der Resorption und parenteralen Verdauung der Bakterien beteiligt sind, wird gewiß nicht überraschen, da bei bakteriellen Allgemeininfektionen die Bakterien in der Regel zunächst in die Lungencapillaren gelangen und auch die mit Bakterien beladenen Makrophagen zum Teil in der Lunge zerstört werden. Die Lunge wurde als „ein großartiges Verdauungsorgan, nicht nur den Fetten, sondern auch den Zellen gegenüber' bezeichnet[1]. Trotzdem sind die histologischen Veränderungen hier verhältnismäßig gering und bestehen hauptsächlich in der Bildung perivasculärer Zellmäntel.

Es sind aber nicht nur Bakterien, die in den Lungen festgehalten und parenteral verdaut werden, sondern auch andere Stoffe und Gewebe wie Thromben bei Lungenembolie, losgerissene Chorionzotten in der Schwangerschaft, Fettgewebszellen nach schweren Traumen, Geschwulstzellen u. a. Über das Schicksal dieser Stoffe wird später noch zu berichten sein.

Naturgemäß sind die Nieren als Ausscheidungsorgane an der Resorption und parenteralen Verdauung von Krankheitskeimen beteiligt, die sich in der Schwellung, Vergrößerung und Ablösung der Glomerulumendothelien ausdrücken. Eine hyaline Umwandlung und Aufquellung der Schlingen würde nach Dietrich (1943) einen Mißerfolg der Resorption anzeigen, woraus sich die Bilder einer gestörten Funktion, z. B. einer Nierenentzündung, ergeben würden. Eine solche Deutung würde allerdings den früher erwähnten Ansichten von Metschnikoff (1902) und Rössle (1923) widersprechen, die ja parenterale Verdauung und Entzündung mehr oder weniger gleichsetzen und daher der Ansicht sind, daß dementsprechend die Entzündung nicht eine gestörte, sondern eine erhöhte Funktion sein müsse.

Mit der Einbeziehung der Lungen und Nieren sind jedoch die Grenzen des Reticuloendothels im engeren wie im weiteren Sinne überschritten, und wir nähern uns hier der Ansicht von Siegmund, der ja, wie bereits erwähnt, eine viel weitere Auffassung von dem Speicherzellensystem hat, das sich der jeweiligen funktionellen Beanspruchung anpassen soll. Dies ist anscheinend, soweit es die Phagocyten betrifft, besonders bei veränderter Reaktionslage der Fall, wie wir

---

[1] Aschoff 1931.

sie im Experiment nach Sensibilisierung bzw. beim Menschen bei chronischen Infektionskrankheiten sehen. So konnte BIELING zeigen, daß bei Mäusen, die mit geringen Mengen pathogener Keime vorbehandelt waren, neuerdings eingespritzte Keime sehr viel rascher aus der Blutbahn verschwanden, als dies beim nichtvorbehandelten Tier der Fall war. Hier muß also ihre Resorption, Ausscheidung und vermutlich auch ihre Zerstörung verstärkt sein.

Bei seinen Untersuchungen an Menschen, die an Allgemeininfektionen gestorben waren, stellte SIEGMUND (1924/25) in zahlreichen Organen eine Endothelschwellung der Gefäße und Aufnahme von Bakterien in diese Zellen sowie eine Endothelablösung fest. Beim Untergang der Endothelien kommt es zum Auftreten von Fibrinknötchen. Auch experimentell konnte SIEGMUND (1925) durch Injektion steigender Mengen von Bakterien in den Venen der Leber, Milz und Lungen, aber auch der Haut und anderen Gefäßgebieten homogene Abscheidungen (hyaline Fibrinknötchen) feststellen. Er erzielte diese Veränderungen durch Injektion von lebenden und abgetöteten Colibakterien und Staphylokokken. Diese Bildungen sollen durch Zerfall von Endothelzellen mit nachfolgender Fibrinabscheidung entstehen und können durch Einwachsen von Endothelzellen organisiert werden. Außer diesen homogenen Abscheidungen kamen auch zellige Reaktionen in Form von Endothelpolstern vor, die umschriebene flache Knötchen bildeten oder über lange Strecken ausgedehnt waren.

Solche Endothelknötchen wurden auch am Endokard gefunden, und zwar sowohl am Wandblatt als auch an den Klappen. Hier ließen sich die im Tierexperiment hervorgerufenen Endokardveränderungen auch bei Menschen mit chronischen Infektionen nachweisen.

Alle hier geschilderten Veränderungen wurden als Reaktion des Mesenchyms auf den durch Bakterien hervorgerufenen Reiz in Form einer erweiterten Resorption und parenteralen Verdauung der Bakterien gedeutet.

Allerdings sind diese Feststellungen und ihre Deutung, die von SIEGMUND (1924/25) und DIETRICH (1927) gegeben wurde, nicht unwidersprochen geblieben. So konnte EWALD (1930) niemals sichere Zeichen einer primären Beteiligung des gewöhnlichen Gefäßendothels an der Bakterienphagocytose entdecken, und er betrachtete die Intimagranulome SIEGMUNDs als Fibrinthromben.

Es ist selbstverständlich, daß der intracellulären Verdauung die Aufnahme der Stoffe und eventuelle Speicherung vorausgehen muß, und so sehen wir, daß zahlreiche Arbeiten sich mit dem Problem der Speicherung in den Zellen befassen. Wenn auf der einen Seite der Kreis der speichernden Zellen sehr weit gezogen wurde — es sei nur erwähnt, daß von MÖLLENDORF (1927), DOMINICI (1920/21), HERINGA (1924) u. a. behaupteten, alle Bindegewebszellen, vor allem die Fibrocyten, besäßen die gleiche Speicherungsfähigkeit —, so muß auf der anderen Seite auch gesagt werden, daß der Begriff des RES von REINHARDT und RICKER (1933) und HOMUTH (1930) völlig abgelehnt wurde. Nach ihrer Ansicht kommt es für die Speicherung nur auf die schnellere oder langsamere Durchströmung und eventuell noch auf die Größe der Zellen an, während es gleichgültig ist, ob es sich bei den Zellen um Epithel- oder Bindegewebszellen handelt, die beide in gleicher Weise speichern können. Nach TANNENBERG (1930) sind dagegen die Kreislaufverhältnisse für die Speicherung zwar wesentlich, aber nicht ausschlaggebend. Er konnte in Gewebskulturen zeigen, daß nur die Blutmakrophagen, aber nicht die Fibroplasten Bakterien speichern.

Aus alledem kann man wohl als sicher schließen, daß organisierte Stoffe, wie sie Bakterien, Protozoen und Pilze darstellen, von Mikro- und Makrophagen aufgenommen und wenigstens zum Teil parenteral verdaut werden. Das Makrophagensystem ist das weitaus größere, und die Ausdehnung seiner Inanspruchnahme wird zum Teil von der Art der Keime und ihrer Menge abhängen, zum Teil aber auch davon, ob es sich um ein einmaliges oder wiederholtes Eindringen handelt.

Was geschieht nun mit den durch Phagocytose aufgenommenen Stoffen, oder mit anderen Worten, welche Mittel haben die Zellen zur Verfügung, um diese aufgenommenen lebenden Keime zu verdauen? Zweifellos besitzen die Mikrophagen wie die Makrophagen zahlreiche Fermente, die sie für die parenterale Verdauung einsetzen können. Es gibt in beiden Zellarten sowohl eiweiß- wie fett- wie kohlenhydratspaltende Fermente neben zahlreichen anderen.

Die von Rattenleukocyten aufgenommenen Friedländer-Bacillen sterben innerhalb von 30 min ab[1], und wir dürfen annehmen, daß sie ebenso schnell verdaut werden. Wenn wir etwa das Beispiel pyogener Kokken oder von Typhusbacillen heranziehen, so soll ihre Verdauung in etwa 1 Std vor sich gehen[2].

Freilich ist die Phagocytose nicht notwendigerweise schon ein sicheres Zeichen für die Abtötung und parenterale Verdauung von Keimen. Nicht selten ist es sogar so, daß die Keime sich in den Phagocyten vermehren und diese zum Absterben bringen[3]. Oder die Bakterien werden, wie dies bei den Tuberkelbacillen der Fall ist, zwar von Mikrophagen aufgenommen, aber keineswegs von diesen abgetötet, sondern zusammen mit den Mikrophagen von Makrophagen phagocytiert, worauf erst ihre mehr oder weniger vollständige Vernichtung gelingt.

Da die von den Phagocyten aufgenommenen und verdauten Bakterien zunächst ihre an die Ribo- oder Desoxyribonucleinsäure gebundene Färbbarkeit verlieren, ist es wahrscheinlich, daß die Phagocyten auch diese Säuren abbauen, da der Färbungsverlust durch Depolymerisierung bedingt ist[4].

Daß die Leukocyten aber nicht nur durch Phagocytose an der Vernichtung von Keimen sich beteiligen, sondern auch durch Fermente, die entweder von ihnen sezerniert werden, die sog. Leukine[5], oder die bei ihrem Zerfall frei werden, die Endolysine[6], wird seit längerem angenommen.

Weiter sollen im Serum bactericide bzw. bakteriolytische Stoffe vorkommen. So sind die β-Lysine beschrieben worden, die besonders wirksam gegen Subtilis-Milzbrand-Mycoides-Fränkel- und andere Bacillen sein sollen[7]. Es kommt zunächst zu einer Adsorption der Keime, worauf die Bakteriolyse erfolgt, bei der die Gramfärbbarkeit verschwindet. Das Lysin wird wieder frei und kann noch auf andere Bacillen einwirken.

Ein weiteres Lysin ist das X-Lysin von Wulff (1934) und Hjorth (1937), das im Blut fieberkranker Menschen vorkommt und eine thermostabile Substanz darstellt, die vornehmlich gramnegative Keime (Meningokokken, Paratyphus-Bacillen) angreift. Das X-Lysin ist nicht durch Bakterien adsorbierbar. Hjorth (1939) nimmt an, daß beim X-Lysin, beim β-Lysin und den bactericiden Leukocytenstoffen die gleiche Wirkungsweise vorliegt.

Bei allen diesen Stoffen handelt es sich um solche, die an der extracellulären Verdauung beteiligt sind. Jedoch ist gerade diese Lehre noch so verworren, daß eine weitere Klärung abgewartet werden muß.

2. Unbelebte Stoffe.

Wenn auch die belebten Stoffe die Hauptrolle bei der parenteralen Verdauung spielen, so ist doch nicht zu übersehen, daß auch die unbelebten von großer Bedeutung sind. An erster Stelle wäre hier das Eiweiß zu nennen. Die Gründe, weshalb man Eiweiß, oder besser gesagt, eiweißhaltige Flüssigkeit dem Organismus

---

[1] Smith und Wood 1947. [2] McCutcheon 1948. [3] Rogers und Tompsett 1952.
[4] Pollister und Leuchtenberger 1949. [5] Schneider und Huerler 1913.
[6] Petterson 1905. [7] Petterson 1934, 1936.

zuführt, sind verschiedener Art. Der wichtigste Zweck ist die Vermehrung der zirkulierenden Blutmenge, wenn sie zu stark abgesunken ist, wie wir dies vor allem im Kollaps sehen. Es ist dabei ziemlich gleichgültig, ob der Kollaps durch größere Blutungen nach außen oder innen, als Folge von Verbrennung oder Erfrierung, nach Hitzschlag oder als toxischer Kollaps bei Infektionskrankheiten aufgetreten ist. Immer kommt es dabei zu einem bedrohlichen Absinken der zirkulierenden Blutmenge. und es gilt nun, das Gefäßsystem schnellstens mit einem Stoff aufzufüllen, der vermöge seines hohen Molekulargewichts die Blutbahn nicht so rasch wieder verläßt, wie dies bei der Verwendung kristalliner Lösungen der Fall ist.

Ein anderer Grund ist nicht selten der, die Eiweißverluste auszugleichen, die bei lang dauernden Nephrosen entstehen. Schließlich darf die parenterale Eiweißzufuhr bei der sog. unspezifischen Therapie nicht vergessen werden. Sie stellt freilich nur einen Teil derselben dar und wird auch als Proteinkörpertherapie bezeichnet.

Betrachten wir zunächst die erstgenannten Gründe für die parenterale Eiweißzufuhr, nämlich die Verminderung der zirkulierenden Blutmenge im Kollaps und den Ausgleich von Eiweißverlusten. Die Gefäßbahn ist hier der gegebene Zuführungsweg. Die Form, in der eiweißhaltige Flüssigkeiten verabreicht werden, ist verschieden. In erster Linie kommt die Blutübertragung in Betracht, sei es als direkte Bluttransfusion vom Spender zum Empfänger oder als indirekte Form der Blutplasma- oder Serumkonserve, des Trockenplasmas oder des Serums. Jedenfalls handelt es sich immer um menschliches Blut oder Blutbestandteile.

Was geschieht nun damit im Organismus? Mit Hilfe der von MORAWITZ (1906) in die Untersuchungstechnik eingeführten „Plasmapheresis", worunter man die wiederholte Entnahme von Eigenblut und Ersatz durch fremdes Blut oder Blutersatzmittel versteht, konnte SCHÖRCHER (1939) zeigen, daß fast das gesamte Blut der Versuchstiere durch arteigenes Vollblut bzw. Heparin- oder Citratblut ersetzt werden konnte. Auch konserviertes Blut ließ sich mit gutem Erfolg verwenden, wobei sich jedoch erwies, daß der Erfolg von der Dauer der Konservierung abhing. Bei 10 Tage altem Heparin- oder Citratblut war ein Austausch nicht mehr möglich. Die Blutkörperchen blieben bei frischer Blutübertragung völlig erhalten, wie aus den Untersuchungen von WILLENEGGER (1937) hervorging, der noch nach 125 Tagen Spenderblutkörperchen im Blut des Empfängers nachwies.

Wir dürfen annehmen, daß die Eiweißstoffe des Serums oder Plasmas völlig für den Organismus ausgenützt werden. Dafür scheinen schon die Versuche von CARRELL und LINDBERGH (1935) zu sprechen, die isolierte Organe mit Serum durchströmten und sie dadurch am Leben erhielten. Alle Funktionen, einschließlich des Wachstums, blieben dabei erhalten. Weiter zeigten andere Autoren[1], daß eiweißfrei ernährte Hunde allein durch das transfundierte Plasma oder Serum anderer Hunde im Stickstoffgleichgewicht gehalten werden konnten. Daraus ergibt sich der zwingende Schluß, daß arteigenes Serum von den Zellen und Geweben des Organismus vollständig für den Stoffwechsel ausgenützt wird.

Aus neuesten experimentellen Untersuchungen mit dem Blutersatzmittel „Adaequan", das aus formyliertem Rinderserum besteht, und dessen Wert als Blutersatzmittel stark umstritten ist, geht hervor, daß das Adaequan in Zellen sichtbar gemacht werden kann[2]. Das Adaequan wurde in einer Menge von 3% des Körpergewichts den Versuchstieren (Mäusen, Meerschweinchen, Hunden) intravenös injiziert. Nach der Fixierung in der Susafixationsflüssigkeit wurden die Schnitte mit Kaliumpermanganat oxydiert, darauf mit Kaliummetabisulfit behandelt und schließlich mit Toluidinblau gefärbt. Nach 90 min färbte sich das Cytoplasma der Histiocyten im subcutanen Bindegewebe dunkel, und nach 3 Std begannen

---

[1] WHIPPLE und Mitarbeiter 1920.   [2] HEINLEIN und ZIMMER 1955.

blaue Granula sichtbar zu werden. Nach 24 Std hatte die Speicherung noch zugenommen. In der Leber war die Speicherung schon früher eingetreten, denn hier sah man bereits nach 60 min die Sternzellen dicht mit feinkörnigen Ablagerungen gefüllt, während gleichzeitig in den Leberepithelien Eiweißtropfen sichtbar wurden. Nach 3 Std hatte die Adaequanspeicherung ihren Höhepunkt erreicht. Die Leberepithelien waren jetzt mit großen Eiweißtropfen beladen, die sich zum Teil färberisch verschieden verhielten, so daß man den Eindruck hatte, daß sich an ihnen Umbauprozesse, vielleicht in Form eines fermentativen Abbaues, abspielten. Dafür könnte auch sprechen, daß die Eiweißtropfen in den Epithelien nach 24 Std fast ganz verschwunden waren, während die Sternzellen noch reichlich Granula enthielten.

Abb. 3. Adaequanspeicherung in Histiocyten der Cutis

Bereits 1907 wurde aus experimentellen Untersuchungen der Schluß gezogen, daß parenteral zugeführtes Eiweiß direkt verbrannt wird, oder daß zum mindesten eine äquivalente Menge von Körpereiweiß zerfällt[1].

Man könnte deshalb annehmen, daß parenteral zugeführtes Eiweiß gespeichert und intracellulär, vielleicht aber auch extracellulär abgebaut wird, so, wie dies auch von anderer Seite angenommen wurde[2]. Diese Annahme würde auch gut zu den Untersuchungen von Schoenheimer (1941) passen, aus denen auf einen rastlosen Umbau des Körpereiweißes geschlossen wurde. Dieser dauernde Umbau des Zelleiweißes wird als eine Art von Regeneration aufgefaßt.

Wenn wir also mit einer gewissen Wahrscheinlichkeit annehmen dürfen, daß parenteral zugeführtes Eiweiß auch parenteral verdaut werden kann — sei es intra- oder extracellulär —, so besteht doch auch noch eine andere Möglichkeit; es kann nämlich auch das intravenös injizierte Bluteiweiß aufgenommen werden, ohne zunächst weiter aufgespalten zu werden, ja vielleicht sogar in dieser Form in die Gewebsproteine eingebaut werden. Dafür sprechen Untersuchungen von Yuile, Lamson, Miller und Whipple (1951) über das Schicksal intravenös injizierter radioaktiver Plasmaeiweiße beim Hund. Dabei wurde festgestellt, daß nur wenig von C^{14} im ausgeatmeten CO_2 und im Harn erscheint, und daß die in den Organen gefundenen C^{14}-Konzentrationen auch den bei anderen Versuchsanordnungen festgestellten Stoffwechselgrößen entsprechen. Die Verfasser nehmen an, daß das intravenös injizierte Eiweiß vor dem Einbau in die Organe höchstens bis zur Stufe der Polypeptide abgebaut wird.

---

[1] Friedemann und Isaac 1907.   [2] Siegmund 1922, v. Gaza 1925.

Auch die Versuche von ABDOU und TARVER (1951) mit C^{14}-markiertem Eiweiß an Ratten hatten ein ähnliches Ergebnis; auch hier zeigte es sich, daß die Ausatmung von $C^{14}O_2$ nach peroraler Verabreichung stärker als nach intravenöser oder intraperitonealer Zufuhr war.

Auch der Mensch kann das parenteral zugeführte Eiweiß als Nahrungseiweiß ausnutzen, wie zahlreiche Untersuchungen gezeigt haben[1]. Ein Teil des infundierten Eiweißes wird im Stoffwechsel abgebaut, wie aus der Steigerung der N-Ausscheidung im Harn hervorgeht, während ein anderer Teil zur Bildung von Organeiweiß verwendet wird.

Seit langem hegte man die Ansicht, daß parenteral zugeführtes Protein von Speicherzellen aufgenommen wird. PFEIFFER und STANDENATH (1923) suchten das Schicksal des auf diesem Weg gegebenen Eiweißes zu erklären, indem sie Mäusen Rinderalbumin und Rinderglobulin, das sie vorher mit speicherungsfähigen Farbstoffen gefärbt hatten, intraperitoneal einspritzten. Die Färbung mit Eosin und Rose bengale erwies sich jedoch als zu schwach, so daß die damit behandelten Eiweißkörper in den Speicherzellen nicht mit Sicherheit nachgewiesen werden konnten. SCHULEMANN (1917) benutzte dann ein anderes Verfahren, bei dem er die parenteral zugeführten Eiweißstoffe mit einem basischen Farbstoff vital überfärbte. Es stellte sich dabei heraus, daß Eiweißstoffe in gleicher Weise wie andere negativ geladene Kolloide, z. B. Farbstoffe, gespeichert werden. Die Grundbedingung für die Speicherung scheint die negative Aufladung zu sein. Die Eiweißstoffe werden in der leicht alkalischen Flüssigkeit des Blutes negativ aufgeladen und wandern zur Anode. Solche natürliche Anoden sollen im Organismus die Speicherzellen sein.

Wie sollen wir uns nun den Vorgang der Aufnahme der Eiweißkörper in die Speicherzellen vorstellen? Vielleicht gelten hier ähnliche Regeln, wie sie für die Aufnahme anderer elektronegativ geladener Kolloide geschildert werden. So zeigte JANCSÓ (1934) bei Durchströmungsversuchen an der überlebenden Rattenleber mit verschiedenen kolloidalen Lösungen, daß die Speicherung in zwei Phasen verläuft. In der ersten Phase kommt es zur Anreicherung und Adsorption des Kolloides an der Oberfläche der Speicherzellen. In der zweiten Phase erfolgt dann die vacuoläre Speicherung der an der Oberfläche haftenden Substanzen im Inneren der Zellen. Auf Grund neuer Untersuchungen kamen N. JANCSÓ und A. JANCSÓ-GABOR (1952, 1955) zu folgenden Vorstellungen über die Proteinspeicherung in Zellen des Reticuloendothels: Durch vorausgegangene Versuche mit Germanin waren sie zu der Überzeugung gekommen, daß bei der Speicherung von Germanin weniger das RES von Milz, Leber und Knochen als der Histiocytenapparat des gesamten Bindegewebes beteiligt ist. Nach intravenöser Verabfolgung von Germanin war alsbald im ganzen Histiocytenapparat des subcutanen Bindegewebes eine ausgeprägte Germaninspeicherung festzustellen, in den Kupfferschen Sternzellen dagegen erst nach 2—4 Tagen. Das Germanin wird dabei nicht frei, sondern in einer an Proteinträger gebundenen Form nachgewiesen.

Mit Hilfe eines neuen mikrotechnischen Verfahrens konnten die Verfasser nun auch die Speicherung von artfremdem und arteigenem Eiweiß in den reticuloendothelialen Zellen nachweisen.

Das Verfahren beruht darauf, daß Zupfpräparate von Bindegewebe bzw. Quetschpräparate von Lebern mit 2%igem Goldchlorid übergossen und nach Auswaschen mit Methylalkohol fixiert werden. Dann werden sie mit May-Grünwaldscher Lösung gefärbt und mit absolutem Äthylalkohol differenziert, mit Xylol ausgewaschen und in Copaivabalsam eingebettet. Die Eiweißgranula werden in den reticuloendothelialen Zellen dunkelviolett gefärbt.

Nach diesen Untersuchungen ist der wichtigste Speicherungsort für die parenteral eingeführten nativen Proteine das Histiocytensystem des Binde-

---

[1] ECKARDT und DAVIDSON 1950.

gewebes. In diesen Zellen können sich überraschend schnell gewaltige Proteinmassen ablagern, die dann aber auch wieder abgebaut oder eliminiert werden.

Auch arteigenes Eiweiß wird in Histiocyten und Kupfferschen Zellen gespeichert. Diese Versuche deuten darauf hin, daß diese Zellen schon regelhaft Blutplasmaproteine in sich aufnehmen.

Nach der Vorstellung von Albert Fischer (1947) sind die Zellen nicht imstande, die Proteine enzymatisch anzugreifen, solange das Blut schnell an den Zellen vorbeifließt. Die Proteine müssen auf der Zelloberfläche niedergeschlagen werden, und zwar mit den mechanischen Mitteln des Blutgerinnungsvorganges. Es gibt Hinweise dafür, daß Proteine an der Zelloberfläche denaturiert werden. Der nächste Schritt ist dann der enzymatische Abbau. Nun hat sich jedoch aus den Untersuchungen von Anitschkow (1924), Pfeiffer (1921), Standenath (1928), Schittenhelm u. a. ergeben, daß für die mehr oder weniger diffusiblen semikolloidalen oder kolloidalen Lösungen neben der geschilderten granulären Speicherung auch noch eine andere Form der Abwanderung aus der Blutbahn in Frage kommt. Ein Großteil dieser Substanzen geht durch die Gefäße hindurch und imbibiert in diffuser Form das Bindegewebe. Auch in der Wand größerer Gefäße werden diese Stoffe in der Zwischensubstanz an die Oberfläche der elastischen Fasern adsorbiert und in den Gefäßwandzellen gespeichert.

Auch moderne Versuche mit markiertem Plasmaeiweiß zeigen, daß ein Teil des injizierten Eiweißes die Blutbahn rasch wieder verläßt und in die Lymphräume übertritt. Es stellt sich schließlich ein Gleichgewicht zwischen vasculärem und extravasculärem Eiweiß her. Dann erfolgt ein langsamer Abfall der Konzentration des markierten Eiweißes, der mit dem Abbau desselben und Ersatz durch unmarkierte Eiweißmoleküle erklärt wird[1].

Wir dürfen somit annehmen, daß mindestens ein Teil des parenteral zugeführten Eiweißes abgebaut wird, sei es nun extracellulär oder intracellulär. v. Gaza (1926) vertrat die Ansicht, daß nach der Speicherung von Eiweiß in den Zellen unter der Einwirkung von Fermenten aus den großen Eiweißmolekülen kleinere Moleküle (Peptide, Aminosäuren) entstehen. Aus den angeführten Untersuchungen von Whipple (1951) und seiner Schule wissen wir, daß Eiweiß gespeichert werden kann, und daß der größte Eiweißspeicher die Leber ist. Diese Theorie ist nicht neu, sie wurde schon seit langem in Deutschland vertreten[2]. Der Unterschied — wenn man überhaupt von einem solchen sprechen kann — liegt darin, daß eine früher nicht exakt beweisbare Annahme heute als gesichert gelten kann, und daß man sich das gespeicherte Eiweiß nicht als einen dem Stoffwechsel entzogenen Stoff vorstellen darf, sondern als Zelleiweiß, das sich an den Umsetzungen beteiligt. Ein solches Speicher- oder Reserveeiweiß findet sich in größter Menge im wachsenden Organismus, im erwachsenen dagegen vor allem im Zustand der Regeneration. Offenbar wird ein parenteraler Abbau und Umbau des aufgenommenen Eiweißes vorgenommen. Dafür sprechen vielleicht auch die Bildung von Eiweißkörpern, die an das Blut abgegeben werden, und die Zunahme des Bluteiweißes, die man nach parenteraler Eiweißzufuhr findet[3], vor allem die Zunahme des Fibrinogens und der Globuline. Dies würde der Ansicht vieler Forscher entsprechen, daß diese Bluteiweißkörper im Speicherzellensystem gebildet werden. Für eine sekretorische Tätigkeit spricht nach Siegmund auch die Ausstoßung stark färbbarer Tropfen bei eiweißverdauenden Zellen.

Mit der parenteralen Verdauung hängt auch die *Frage der Antikörperbildung* eng zusammen. Letztere hat zur Voraussetzung, daß Antigene in die Zellen

---

[1] Miller, Bale, Yuile, Masters, Tishkoff und Whipple 1949.
[2] Gross 1922.   [3] Berger 1922, Starlinger 1927, Heinlein 1934.

gelangen. Da die Antigene verhältnismäßig hochmolekulare Körper sind, so müssen wahrscheinlich auch die Zellen, von denen sie aufgenommen werden, groß sein. Daher wurde von einer Reihe von Autoren angenommen, daß es die Zellen des RES seien, von denen die Antigene aufgebaut und abgebaut werden, ein Vorgang, an den sich die Antikörperbildung anschließt. Man versuchte dies auch zu beweisen, etwa durch die Blockade des RES, worauf man eine Verminderung der Antikörperbildung fand. Da diese Antikörperbildung eng mit der Bildung der Globuline verknüpft ist, so dürfte die Annahme zutreffend sein, daß beide an der gleichen Stelle gebildet werden. Da die Antikörperbildung an anderer Stelle ausführlich abgehandelt wird, soll hier nur so weit davon die Rede sein, als sie sich mit der parenteralen Verdauung berührt.

Hier sind die Arbeiten von EHRICH u. Mitarb. (1946, 1949, 1955) zu nennen, nach denen Makrophagen zwar Antigene und Bakterien aufnehmen, jedoch keine Antikörper bilden. Bei der Untersuchung der Lymphknoten fanden sie in der abfließenden Lymphe mehr Antikörper als in der zufließenden und schlossen daraus, daß die Antikörper von den Lymphocyten der Lymphknoten gebildet werden. Nach ihrer Ansicht werden die antigenen Stoffe zunächst von polymorphkernigen Leukocyten und Zellen des RES aufgenommen und dort aufgeschlossen, also parenteral verdaut. Danach wird das so veränderte Antigen wieder frei und anschließend von Lymphocyten aufgenommen, in denen es nun die Antikörperbildung bewirkt. EHRICH (1955) scheint allerdings, nach neuester Interpretierung, unter Lymphocyten nicht die gewöhnlichen Lymphocyten, sondern die Plasmazellen zu verstehen.

Nach einer anderen Theorie[1] kommt die Antikörperbildung in der Weise zustande, daß jede Zelle einen Fermentapparat besitzt, mit dem sie an den Substraten, die in die Zellen hineingelangen, biochemische Änderungen hervorzurufen vermag, so daß das Substrat in den Stoffwechsel der Zelle einbezogen werden kann. Substraten gegenüber, die zunächst nicht fermentativ angegriffen werden können, werden adaptive Fermente gebildet, wozu es einer gewissen Zeitdauer bedarf. Eine solche Fermentadaptation wird dann auf die Tochterzelle vererbt. Wenn eine Fermentadaptation in der primitiven Reticulumzelle stattfindet, so reicht die Dauer der spezifischen Sensibilisierung weiter als die Lebensdauer individueller lymphoider oder plasmacellulärer Abkömmlinge, da diese die spezifische Fermentadaptation von der Reticulumzelle ererbt haben.

Obwohl die Meinungen über den Ort der Antikörperbildung weit auseinandergehen, scheint es doch recht wahrscheinlich, daß die Antigene von Zellen aufgenommen und verarbeitet, d. h. parenteral verdaut werden müssen, bevor die Antikörperbildung einsetzen kann.

Dafür scheinen auch neuere Untersuchungen mit markiertem Stickstoff zu sprechen[2]. Kaninchen wurden durch Injektion von Pneumokokken des Typ III immunisiert.

Nachdem die Antikörperbildung ihren Höhepunkt erreicht hatte, wurden sie mit N^{15}-Glykokoll gefüttert und dann mittels der spezifischen Polysaccharide das Antikörpereiweiß aus dem Serum entfernt. Während das Gesamtkörpereiweiß allmählich abnahm, fand gleichzeitig eine Aufspaltung und Resynthese wie bei den anderen Serumeiweißkörpern statt. Durch einen Prozeß, der ein Öffnen und Schließen der Peptidbindungen verlangt, wurde das verfütterte N^{15}-Glykokoll zunächst schnell in das Antikörpereiweiß eingefügt, langsamer nach Aufhören der Verfütterung. In Abänderung dieses Versuches wurden Kaninchen aktiv gegen Pneumokokkentyp III und außerdem, durch Transfusion homologen Immunserums, passiv gegen Pneumokokkentyp I immunisiert. Wenn zunächst der eine, dann der andere Antikörper mit spezifischen Polysacchariden entfernt wurde, dann enthielt der Typ III-Antikörper isotopen Stickstoff, der Typ I-Antikörper aber nicht.

BURNET 1949.
HEIDELBERGER, TREFFERS, RATNER, RITTENBERG und SCHOENHEIMER 1942.

Es wird angenommen, daß der strukturelle Unterschied zwischen Typ I- und Typ III-Antikörper, zumindest über große Teile ihrer molekularen Oberfläche, nur gering ist, da es noch nicht möglich war, irgendeinen Unterschied zwischen diesen beiden Eiweißkörpern — außer ihrer Spezifität — aufzufinden. Würde nun der Typ III-Antikörper des aktiv immunisierten Tieres durch teilweisen Ersatz von Aminosäuren abgebaut und wieder aufgebaut, so müßte der gleiche Vorgang auch den Typ I-Antikörper beeinflussen. Da aber der Umbau des Typ I-Antikörpers nicht stattfindet, so darf man der Annahme Raum geben, daß die Eiweißkörper vor der Resynthese aus ihren Bausteinen einem völligen Abbau unterliegen.

Die parenterale Verdauung spielt eine große Rolle bei der Zufuhr körperfremden Gewebes, sei es nun durch Transplantation ganzer Gewebsteile oder zerkleinerten Gewebes in Form von Gewebsbrei. Seitdem von BERTHOLD (1848) zum erstenmal Hoden beim Huhn und von KNAUER (1898) Ovarien beim Kaninchen transplantiert wurden, ist die Zahl der Transplantationen beim Tier und beim Menschen Legion geworden. Auf die Frage der Transplantation kann hier nicht näher eingegangen werden. Von der heteroplastischen Transplantation gilt es als Regel, daß die übertragenen Gewebe oder Organe schon nach kurzer Zeit dem parenteralen Abbau unterliegen. Aber auch das homoioplastisch transplantierte Gewebe scheint das gleiche Schicksal zu haben. Selbst übertragene Haut scheint nach kürzerer Zeit resorbiert und dann ersetzt zu werden. LEHMANN und TAMMANN (1926) berichteten über bessere Erfolge durch „Umstimmung" ihrer Versuchstiere. Diese „Umstimmung" wurde bei Mäusen erreicht durch Speicherung von Trypanblau. Danach gelang bei 32% die homoioplastische Transplantation.

Im allgemeinen kann man sagen, daß, abgesehen von so anspruchslosem Gewebe wie Sehnen, Fascien, Cornea, Knorpel oder Blutgefäßen, eine homoioplastische Übertragung von Geweben oder Organen, die dann auch dauernd ihre Funktion behalten, nicht gelingt.

Die Homoiotransplantate unterliegen mit der Zeit völligem Zerfall[1], werden fermentativ und cellulär abgebaut, also parenteral verdaut, und schließlich durch Bindegewebe ersetzt. Das gilt vor allem für die innersekretorischen Organe. Die behaupteten günstigen Ergebnisse der Hoden- und Ovarien-Transplantation[2] konnten durch Nachuntersuchungen nicht bestätigt werden[3]. Nach kürzerer oder längerer Zeit waren die transplantierten Organe resorbiert. Das gleiche gilt auch für andere Hormondrüsen. So wird von Probeexcisionen berichtet, die 3—5 Monate nach heteroplastischer Hypophysentransplantation vorgenommen wurden. Es wurde noch Bindegewebe gefunden, das kein Hypophysengewebe enthielt[4].

Man nimmt an, daß es sich dort, wo Homoiotransplantate zerfallen, d. h. parenteral verdaut werden, um Reaktionen aktiv erworbener Immunkörper handelt. Dafür sprechen z. B. folgende experimentelle Untersuchungen: Wenn beim Kaninchen zweimal ein Hauttransplantat vom gleichen Spendertier auf das gleiche Empfängertier übertragen wurde, so ging bei einer zweiten Übertragung das Transplantat schneller zugrunde als bei der ersten. Das entspricht einer Antigen-Antikörper-Reaktion, die mit dem Arthus-Phänomen verglichen wird[5].

Es gibt wohl kaum ein Organ, das man nicht zu transplantieren versucht hat. Auch die Niere wurde wiederholt als Homoiotransplantat bei Hunden und Katzen übertragen. Der Erfolg war jedoch zeitlich begrenzt. Schon nach 5 Tagen trat der Zerfall und die parenterale Verdauung des Organs ein.

Bei Hunden wurden schwere toxische Symptome beobachtet, wobei gleichzeitig um die Gefäße und die Glomerula Rundzelleninfiltrate auftraten[6].

---

[1] DEMPSTER 1951.   [2] STEINACH 1920, VORONOFF 1925.   [3] v. GAZA 1926.
[4] EHRHARDT und KITTEL 1937.   [5] GIBSON und MEDAWAR 1943, MEDAWAR 1944.
[6] DEMPSTER 1950.

Um so auffallender ist es nun, daß über die erfolgreiche Homoiotransplantation einer Niere beim Menschen berichtet wurde, bei der das transplantierte Organ über 2 Monate funktionierte[1]. Auf einer Art von Transplantation beruht auch die Gewebstherapie von FILATOV (1949) und vor allem die in letzter Zeit vielbesprochene Cellulartherapie von NIEHANS (1949).

Letzterer ging von der Vorstellung aus, daß Erkrankungen an Organen, die entweder selbst aktiv endokrin wirken oder in ihrer Funktion endokrin gesteuert werden, durch eine endokrinologisch gewählte Zelltherapie günstig beeinflußt werden können. Er stellte sich vor, daß dabei nicht eine Ersatztherapie wie etwa durch Injektion von Hormonpräparaten, sondern eine Wiederherstellung abgeschwächter Funktionen vorliege. Er nahm an, daß auch nach Gefriertrocknung die Zellen ihre Lebensfähigkeit behalten und funktionstüchtig bleiben würden. Über das weitere Schicksal dieser Zellen stellte er folgende Hypothesen auf: Die Zellen behalten ihre biologische Spezifität und wandern zu dem homologen Organ, wenn dieses ihrer bedarf, oder bleiben am Ort der Injektion leben, und das Blut bringt die Produkte ihrer spezifischen Tätigkeit zum bedürftigen Organ, oder die Zellen werden abgebaut und der Organismus verwendet ihre Abbaustoffe.

Durch neuere Untersuchungen[2] wurde nun festgestellt, daß injizierter Gewebsbrei schon nach kurzer Zeit abstirbt.

Bei der Injektion von zerkleinerter Hühnerleber in den Musculus quadriceps von Meerschweinchen konnte nach 48 Std beobachtet werden, daß die Struktur der Leberstückchen zwar noch einigermaßen erhalten, jedoch bereits ein Kernzerfall eingetreten war. Zwischen Leber und Muskulatur waren reichlich Rundzellen aufgetreten. Zum Teil waren es neutrophile Leukocyten, vorwiegend aber Zellen, deren Kern rund oder leicht gebuchtet war und bei denen es sich zweifellos um Makrophagen handelte. In den folgenden Tagen und Wochen zerfiel das Lebergewebe immer mehr und wurde durch ein Granulationsgewebe aufgesaugt.

Es handelt sich also hier um eine parenterale Verdauung der eingespritzten Gewebsteile.

Daraus wurde der Schluß gezogen, daß es sich bei der Cellulartherapie von NIEHANS nicht um eine Wirkung lebender Zellen, sondern irgendwelcher Abbauprodukte handelt. Das ging auch daraus hervor, daß PISCHINGER (1953) in eigenen Therapieversuchen dieselben Erfolge durch Injektion von Trockenleber erzielte. Bei der Deutung des Effektes legte er besonderen Wert auf die unspezifische Wirkung, ein sehr naheliegender Schluß, da wir die unspezifische Wirkung solcher Injektionen schon seit langem aus der besonders von WEICHARDT (1918, 1936), SCHITTENHELM (1919, 1921, 1922) u. a. inaugurierten, unspezifischen Therapie kennen.

Auch bei dieser unspezifischen Therapie handelt es sich — obwohl eine restlos befriedigende Erklärung noch aussteht — zum Teil wenigstens um die Folgen einer parenteralen Verdauung. Der ursprünglich von R. SCHMIDT (1916) als „Proteinkörpertherapie" bezeichneten Methode gab WEICHARDT (1919) den Namen „Protoplasmaaktivierung". Er verstand darunter „eine Reaktionsänderung im Sinne der Leistungssteigerung durch Eiweißspaltprodukte, welche primär aus dem eingespritzten Eiweiß oder sekundär vom Körpereiweiß herstammen". Daß auch Körpereiweiß dabei parenteral verdaut werden konnte, schloß man aus zahlreichen Untersuchungen; diese ergaben übereinstimmend bei Tieren, die sich im N-Gleichgewicht befanden, nach parenteraler Eiweißzufuhr eine N-Ausscheidung im Harn, die die eingeführte N-Menge bei weitem übertraf[3].

Andere Autoren fanden nach Proteininjektion ein Ansteigen des Aminosäurespiegels im Blut. So beobachteten DONATH und HEILIG (1924) eine Vermehrung um 61%. Außerdem wurde bei der Zufuhr artfremden Eiweißes ein Auftreten körpereigener Spaltprodukte in der Leber nachgewiesen, die man für Zerfallsprodukte des Körpereiweißes hielt[4].

---

[1] LAWLER, WEST, NULTY, CLANCY und MURPHY 1950.   [2] PISCHINGER 1953.
[3] KREHL und MATTHES 1895.   [4] PICK und HASHIMOTO 1916.

Durch die bei der parenteralen Verdauung entstehenden Spaltprodukte sollen Leistungssteigerungen sowohl des Gesamtorganismus als auch bestimmter Organe ausgelöst werden.

Nach F. Hoff (1944) liegt das Wesentlichste der unspezifischen Therapie in der Beeinflussung des vegetativen Systems („Vegetative Gesamtumschaltung"). Die grundlegenden Leistungen des Organismus werden im interstitiellen Bindegewebe vollzogen. Hier befindet sich als funktionelle Einheit das nervöse und capillare Endnetz, dessen Funktion vom Stammhirn in engster Wechselwirkung mit endokrinen Wirkstoffen (vor allem des Hypophysen-Nebennierensystems) gesteuert wird.

Die Vorgänge, die man bei parenteraler Eiweißzufuhr beobachten kann, sind ähnlich denjenigen, die bei der Phagocytose beschrieben wurden. Man sieht auch hier wieder, daß die Zellen sich vergrößern und in ihrem Innern häufig Vacuolen auftreten, die offenbar der morphologische Ausdruck für die Aufnahme und Verarbeitung, in diesem Falle von Eiweißstoffen, sind. In ganz ähnlicher Weise, wie dies früher bei Allgemeininfektionen beschrieben wurde, sieht man auch hier die Ablösung von Endothelzellen in der Leber und von Reticuloendothelien in der Milz, wobei gleichzeitig mit dieser Zellabstoßung eine Zellvergrößerung Hand in Hand geht. Büngeler (1926) hat diesen Vorgang als Endothelaktivierung bezeichnet. Auch in der Adventia von Gefäßen kann man solche Zellknötchen nachweisen.

Nicht unerwähnt darf bleiben, daß auch die parenterale Blutzufuhr hierher zu rechnen ist, und zwar sowohl die Zufuhr von Eigenblut als auch die von fremdem Blut. Soweit es sich dabei auch um Ersatz des Blutes handelt, wird darüber in einem anderen Kapitel berichtet. Hier interessiert die Blutzufuhr nur als eine Form der unspezifischen Therapie mit intramuskulären Blutinjektionen. Auch dabei kommt es zu einer parenteralen Verdauung, teils intra- und teils extracellulär, wobei die Erythrocytentrümmer von Speicherzellen aufgenommen werden.

Neben dem Eiweiß spielt für die parenterale Verdauung die Zufuhr anderer Stoffe eine verhältnismäßig geringe Rolle. Schon 1889 wurde von Coats eine Speicherung von Fettstoffen in reticulären Zellen bei diabetischer Lipämie beschrieben.

In der neueren englischen und amerikanischen Literatur ist von parenteralen Ernährungsversuchen mit verschiedenartigen Fettemulsionen viel die Rede. Die Versuche waren erfolgreich, da die Tiere die Infusion gut vertrugen, keine Fettembolien dabei gesehen wurden und die Ernährung gut war. Es wurden keine Lipoidgranulome in den Lungen festgestellt. Bei einem Hund fand sich jedoch eine Speicherung von Lipoidmaterial im Reticuloendothel[1]. Diese Untersuchungen erinnern an frühere Untersuchungen von Seemann (1930), der kolloidales Cholesterin intravenös bzw. intraarteriell injizierte. Das Cholesterin wurde dabei in den Lungengefäßen abgefiltert, wo es zu Cholesterinanhäufungen mit Entwicklung intravasculärer Riesenzellengranulome und allgemeiner Hyperplasie des Lungenparenchyms kam. In späteren Stadien wurden auch Anhäufungen des Cholesterins in Leber und Nieren festgestellt.

Ob überhaupt und inwieweit die parenterale Verdauung bei der Verarbeitung solcher Fettemulsionen eine Rolle spielt, läßt sich noch nicht überblicken.

Über die parenterale Verdauung von Kohlenhydraten ist verhältnismäßig wenig bekannt. Der einzige hier zu erwähnende Stoff ist das Dextran, das neuerdings als Blutersatzmittel von Bedeutung ist. Es ist, genau wie Stärke und Glykogen, nur aus Glucosemolekülen aufgebaut. Durch Bindung zwischen den Kohlenstoffatomen 1 und 6 sind die Glucosemoleküle zu langen Ketten aneinandergefügt, die aus Haupt- und Seitenketten bestehen. Das Dextran hat keine einheitliche Molekülgröße, sondern besteht aus verschieden großen Molekülen, deren Molekulargewicht zwischen 36000 und 141000 schwankt. Die ursprüngliche Annahme, daß das Dextran nicht gespeichert wird, hat sich nicht als völlig richtig

---

Lerner, Chaikoff und Entenman 1949.

erwiesen. Es hat sich herausgestellt, daß der größte Teil des Dextrans in den ersten Tagen nach der Infusion wieder ausgeschieden wird, ein kleiner Teil jedoch längere Zeit im Organismus zurückbleibt. Weiter hat eine Zuführung größerer Mengen auch zu morphologisch erkennbarer Speicherung geführt[1].

Bereits nach 30 min sind mit der Perjodsäure-Leukofuchsin-Methode (PAS) staubförmige Ablagerungen in den Histiocyten des subcutanen Bindegewebes nachzuweisen. Diese Speicherung hat nach 3 Tagen ihr Maximum erreicht. In der Leber finden sich 60 min nach der Injektion feine Granula in den Kupfferschen Sternzellen, während in den Leberepithelien größere Vacuolen mit tropfig kondensiertem Inhalt nachzuweisen sind. Nach 24 Std hat die Dextranspeicherung noch weiter zugenommen und erreicht nach 3 Tagen ihr Maximum. Auch nach 12 und 28 Tagen sind noch einzelne Zellen, die etwas Dextran enthalten, in der Leber vorhanden. Ganz ähnlich wie in der Leber verhält sich die Dextranspeicherung in der Milz.

Das Dextran wird in erster Linie durch die Nieren ausgeschieden; das sieht man daran, daß schon nach 30 min nach der Injektion PAS-positive Zylinder in den Sammelröhren und dichte granuläre Niederschläge auf der Oberfläche der Tubulusepithelien auftreten. Nach 24 Std sind die Tubulusepithelien der sezernierenden Nephrone dicht mit Dextrangranula gefüllt. Dagegen sind nach 3 Tagen nur noch ganz wenige Dextrangranula in den Epithelien vorhanden, und nach 12 Tagen ist kein Dextran mehr in den Nieren nachzuweisen[1]. Bei normaler Dosierung scheint dies jedoch nicht der Fall zu sein. Im allgemeinen wird man annehmen dürfen, daß das Dextran, soweit es nicht ausgeschieden wird, völlig abgebaut und zu Kohlensäure und Wasser verbrannt wird.

In den Untersuchungen von Cargill und Bruner (1951) mit radioaktivem Dextran wurde die Ausscheidung von $C^{14}O_2$ in der Exspirationsluft festgestellt. Es scheint, daß das Dextran parenteral bis zu den Endprodukten verdaut wird. Ob und wieweit dabei die Peroxydasen der Leukocyten eine Rolle spielen, wie dies Schmitz annimmt, scheint noch nicht völlig geklärt.

Neueste Untersuchungen[2] befassen sich mit dem Abbau von Polysacchariden in Lymphknoten.

Ratten wurde Glykogen, Dextran, Inulin und Glucose in verschiedenen Konzentrationen unter die Haut der Unterschenkel injiziert. Danach wurden die regionären Lymphknoten, Leber und Milz entnommen, in vergälltem absolutem Alkohol fixiert und in verschiedener Weise gefärbt. Die histologischen Befunde sind bei den verwendeten Polysacchariden im Prinzip die gleichen: Bereits vor Ablauf 1 Std nach Injektion setzen starke proliferative Vorgänge mit erheblicher Vermehrung besonders der aus dem Verband gelösten Reticulumzellen und Histiocyten ein, wobei eine große Zahl von Zellen

[1] Heinlein und Zimmer 1955.
[2] Lindner 1953.

Abb. 4. Dextran in der Subcutis

auffällt, die sich mit den verschiedenen spezifischen Färbungen als typische Gewebsmast-zellen identifizieren lassen. Die zugeführten Polysaccharide werden, wie eingehende papier-chromatographische Paralleluntersuchungen gezeigt haben, fermentativ gespalten; so ist nach kurzer Zeit innerhalb der Lymphknoten ein Stoffgemisch enthalten, das aus den zugeführten Polysacchariden und einer unterschiedlich großen Zahl von Auf-, Um- und Abbauprodukten besteht, die in dieser Form im Lymphknotenabflußgebiet weitergeleitet werden. Mit diesen verschiedenen Stoffgemischteilen sind offensichtlich die histiocytären Elemente beladen; neben der Aufnahme der Stoffe kann auch ihre Verarbeitung und ihre Abgabe von Stoffwechselprodukten histochemisch dargestellt werden. Die papierchromato-graphischen Paralleluntersuchungen haben den Beweis erbracht, daß der Lymphknoten imstande ist, auf Anforderung nicht nur Glucose von Glykogen und Dextran bzw. Fructose von Inulin sehr rasch in großer Menge abzuspalten — also Kohlenhydratabbauprozesse zu leisten —, sondern auch Glucose in Fructose umzubauen und schließlich aus den ab-gespaltenen Monosacchariden Di-, Tri- und Tetrasaccharide sowie höhermolekulare Kohlen-hydrate aufzubauen. Auch die Zwischenprodukte des Abbaus sind faßbar, z. B. die Maltose oder die nur kurze Zeit als Intermediärprodukte vorhandenen Phosphorsäureester. Die Fermentsysteme, welche der Lymphknoten offensichtlich bei derartigen Anforderungen aktivieren kann, sind durch den papierchromatographischen Nachweis von Abbau-, Um- und Aufbauprodukten indirekt erfaßt worden. Es gelang, Amylasen und Oligasen darzustellen.

Zusammenfassend kann gesagt werden, daß der Lymphknoten nicht nur im-stande ist, zugeführte Kohlenhydrate unabhängig von ihrem Polymerisations-grad abzubauen, sondern auch mannigfaltige Um- und Aufbauprozesse zu leisten, wobei die in auffällig großer Zahl neugebildeten Gewebsmastzellen eine besonders hohe Wirksamkeit entfalten, vielleicht in ähnlicher Weise wie die Plasmazellen bei bestimmten Eiweißstoffwechselvorgängen.

Was hier für den Lymphknoten nachgewiesen wurde, dürfte vice versa wohl auch für die anderen Teile des RES Geltung haben; wir dürfen annehmen, daß sie bei der parenteralen Verdauung von Kohlenhydraten eine größere Rolle spielen, als wir bisher anzunehmen geneigt waren.

Eine große Rolle haben sowohl bei Speicherungsversuchen als auch in der unspezifischen Therapie Stoffe gespielt, die größtenteils anorganischer Natur sind und infolgedessen nicht parenteral verdaut werden können, so daß sie streng-genommen nicht hierher gehören. Die Folgen einer solchen Behandlung sind ganz ähnlich wie bei der Zufuhr verdaubarer Stoffe; es kommt zwar nicht zu einer Verdauung der Stoffe selbst, dafür aber zu einer solchen der Speicherzellen, die derartige Stoffe gespeichert haben, so daß dieses Kapitel wenigstens kurz betrachtet werden soll. Es handelt sich auch hierbei um kolloidale Substanzen. Bei Speicherungsversuchen wurden vorzugsweise Farbstoffe wie Trypanrot oder Trypanblau, ferner Metallpräparate wie kolloidales Silber (Kollargol oder Elektro-kollargol), kolloidales Gold, Kupfer oder kolloidales Silicium benutzt. All diese Stoffe haben, wie Heinlein (1935) zeigen konnte, eine ganz ähnliche Wirkung auf die Blutproteine wie zugeführtes Eiweiß, nur noch in stärkerem Maße. Es kommt zu einer beträchtlichen Vermehrung des Fibrinogens und der Globuline bei gleichzeitiger Abnahme der Albumine. Er erklärte dies mit der starken Zell-mauserung, bei der die abgelösten Zellen parenteral verdaut werden. Die mor-phologischen Veränderungen entsprechen im wesentlichen den früher geschilderten Vorgängen am Speicherzellensystem, so daß darauf nicht mehr eingegangen zu werden braucht.

B. Endogene Stoffe.

Die im Organismus entstehenden Stoffe, die der parenteralen Verdauung unterliegen, sind von nicht geringerer Bedeutung als die von außen in den Körper gelangenden. Hier kommen alle Zellen in Frage, die mit dem Blut- oder Lymph-strom verschleppt werden, wie Geschwulstzellen, choriale Zellen, Chorionzotten, Fettgewebe, vor allem aber Thromben. Ferner müssen hier Vorgänge betrachtet werden, die eine Verdauung und Aufsaugung toten Materials nötig machen, also alle Prozesse, die wir als Folgezustände von Nekrosen beobachten können.

In der Schwangerschaft, vor allem bei der Erkrankung Schwangerer an puerperaler Eklampsie, kommt es zu einer Verschleppung von abgerissenen Chorionzotten. Sie werden in den Lungencapillaren festgehalten, gehen dort zugrunde und werden teils extra-, teils intracellulär verdaut. Ganz ähnlich ist dies auch bei der Verschleppung von Knochenmarksriesenzellen, wie sie bei allen möglichen Reizzuständen des Organismus vorkommt, oder auch bei der Einschwemmung von Knochenmarksgewebe mit Fettzellen. Knochenmarksgewebe oder gar Lebergewebe wird allerdings nur nach Zerstörung von Knochen bzw. Leber abgerissen und in die Blutbahn eingeschwemmt. Besonders verhängnisvoll ist die Verschleppung von Fettgewebe, das die Capillaren der Lunge verstopft und, wenn dies in größerem Ausmaß geschieht, durch Erhöhung des Widerstandes im Lungenkreislauf den Tod herbeiführt. Bei einem nichttödlichen Ausgang der Fettembolie wird dagegen das Fett extracellulär aufgespalten, oder es wird von Endothelzellen, auch unter Riesenzellenbildung, aufgenommen und verdaut.

Bei Geschwulstzellen muß man zwischen der Verschleppung einzelner Zellen und derjenigen ganzer Zellverbände unterscheiden. Es ist keineswegs sicher, daß schon aus verschleppten Einzelzellen Tochtergeschwülste entstehen. Vielmehr spricht die Wahrscheinlichkeit dafür, daß zunächst dem Organismus noch genügend Abwehrkräfte zur Verfügung stehen, um mit diesen Zellen fertig zu werden. Wir wissen aus zahlreichen Untersuchungen, daß Geschwulstzellen in die Lunge verschleppt werden[1]. Wir wissen aber auch seit den Untersuchungen von M. B. SCHMIDT (1903), daß diese Zellen in den Lungengefäßen zerstört werden. Er beschrieb den Untergang ganzer Geschwulstpfröpfe, die mit Fibrin umhüllt wurden und resorbiert wurden. Er mißt dieser Fibrinumhüllung für den Untergang der Geschwulstzellen große Bedeutung bei. Von anderer Seite wurden auch zugrunde gehende Einzelzellen in den Lungencapillaren nachgewiesen[2].

Auch in der Leber wurde eine Zerstörung von Geschwulstzellen beobachtet[3]. Dabei schienen die Kupfferschen Sternzellen an ihrem Abbau beteiligt zu sein. Sie waren dann aufgetrieben und enthielten Vacuolen.

Wir dürfen somit annehmen, daß verschiedene Organe die Fähigkeit besitzen, Geschwulstzellen teils extracellulär, teils intracellulär zu verdauen.

Weiter sehen wir die parenterale Verdauung bei Thrombosen und ihren Folgen. Wenn sich ein Thrombus in einem Gefäß gebildet hat, dann zeigt er einige Zeit später sekundäre Veränderungen. Diese Veränderungen können darin bestehen, daß der Thrombus anscheinend eitrig erweicht. Diese „puriforme" Erweichung des Thrombus ist aber keine eitrige Einschmelzung, sondern eine Form der parenteralen Verdauung, die durch die Fermente der Leukocyten hervorgerufen wird. Die Abbauprodukte werden dann mit dem Blutstrom fortgespült, so daß die Gefäßlichtung bald wieder durchlässig wird.

Häufiger sieht man jedoch, besonders bei großen Thromben, daß von der Gefäßwand her ein Gewebe in den Thrombus einsprießt und dessen Bestandteile in sich aufnimmt, d. h. parenteral verdaut. Jedoch handelt es sich dabei nicht um eine vollständige parenterale Verdauung, da der Thrombus als solcher zwar verschwindet, jedoch ersetzt wird durch ein Organisationsgewebe. Diese Organisation hat mit der parenteralen Verdauung nichts mehr zu tun, denn dabei handelt es sich, wie gesagt, um einen Austausch und Ersatz des ursprünglich vorhandenen Thrombus durch ein anderes Gewebe.

---

[1] SCHMIDT 1903.　　[2] STERN 1923, KOST 1936.　　[3] SCHAIRER 1939.

Nicht immer geschieht die parenterale Verdauung eines arteriellen Thrombus oder Embolus so rechtzeitig, daß das Leben in dem von der Arterie ernährten Gebiet aufrechterhalten werden kann. Sehr viel häufiger sehen wir, daß in dem betreffenden Gebiet ein Infarkt entsteht. Der Infarkt interessiert hier nur so weit, als er Beziehungen zur parenteralen Verdauung hat.

Das weitere Schicksal eines Infarktes ist wesentlich von seiner Größe abhängig. Bei Herz-, Nieren- und Milzinfarkten sieht man zunächst eine hyperämische Randzone auftreten, ein Zeichen, daß die benachbarten Arterien eingeschaltet werden, um das in seiner Ernährung gestörte Gebiet mitzuernähren. Das gelingt jedoch nicht, sondern es kommt in der Randzone zur Blutverlangsamung mit Austritt von Plasma und Leukocyten. Von dieser Randzone aus wird der Infarkt mehr oder weniger stark von Leukocyten durchwandert, die das tote Material parenteral verdauen. Dadurch kann es, besonders beim Herzmuskelinfarkt, zu einer so beträchtlichen Gewebsverflüssigung kommen, daß die Gefahr einer Herzruptur auftreten kann. Aber nicht nur Leukocyten durchdringen den Infarkt, sondern wir sehen von der Randzone aus auch ein zell- und gefäßreiches Gewebe eindringen, wobei die als Makrophagen tätigen Fibroplasten sich ebenfalls an der Beseitigung des toten Gewebes, also an der parenteralen Verdauung beteiligen.

Größere Infarkte können freilich nicht in dieser Weise durch parenterale Verdauung beseitigt und in Schwielengewebe umgewandelt werden. Sie schrumpfen vielmehr durch Wasserabgabe immer mehr zusammen, und in ihrer Umgebung bildet sich eine acelluläre Sklerose aus.

Was hier am Beispiel des Infarktes geschildert wurde, sehen wir in ähnlicher Weise auch bei anderen Nekrosen. Das Nekroseproblem soll dabei auch nur so weit erörtert werden, als es Beziehung zur parenteralen Verdauung hat. Grundsätzlich kann kein Zweifel darüber bestehen, daß das nekrotische Gewebe weitgehend verdaut wird und diese Verdauung extra- und intracellulär vor sich geht; dabei steht einmal mehr die eine, ein andermal die andere Form im Vordergrund.

Koagulationsnekrosen werden durch Proteinasen nur schwer verflüssigt; trotzdem kann aber auch ein solcher Herd in Erweichung und Verflüssigung übergehen. Anscheinend bedarf es dazu der Mitwirkung von Zellen, vor allem von Leukocyten. Dies sieht man z. B. bei der Verflüssigung tuberkulöser verkäster Bezirke. Auch bei anderen Koagulationsnekrosen, z. B. den Herzmuskelnekrosen bei Diphtherie, spielt die Verflüssigung des nekrotischen Gewebes eine Rolle, wie schon der Name der toxischen Myolyse besagt. Wahrscheinlich wirken dabei auch Leukocyten und mesenchymale Zellen mit.

Bei manchen Geweben steht dagegen die Verflüssigung von vorneherein so stark im Vordergrund, daß es gar nicht zur Gerinnung kommt. Dies gilt besonders für Nekrosen im Gehirn. Ob dieser Vorgang mit dem besonderen Flüssigkeitsreichtum oder dem besonders großen Gehalt an Fermenten zusammenhängt, ist ungeklärt.

Bei allen Nekrosen gehen nun, neben der mehr oder weniger deutlichen extracellulären Verdauung, wie sie bei der Colliquationsnekrose so besonders ausgeprägt ist, auch intracelluläre Verdauungsvorgänge einher. Wir sehen dies wieder besonders gut bei den Erweichungsherden im Gehirn, wo die Zerfallsprodukte von Zellen aufgenommen und abgebaut oder beseitigt werden, ferner aber auch beim Absterben einzelner Ganglienzellen, bei denen die einwandernden Mesenchym- und Gliazellen das Zerstörungswerk vollenden.

III. Die Verdauungsorte und die verdauenden Zellen.

In den vorhergehenden Kapiteln mußten wir schon die Frage nach den Organen, in denen die parenterale Verdauung vor sich geht, und nach den Zellen, die diese Arbeit übernehmen, kurz streifen. Es läßt sich infolgedessen diese Frage hier leichter beantworten. An der parenteralen Verdauung waren vor allem die Mikrophagen und die Makrophagen beteiligt, soweit die parenterale Verdauung nicht extracellulär vor sich ging. Es ergibt sich daraus, daß einerseits das Blut mit seinen Leukocyten und seinen verdauenden Fermenten daran beteiligt ist, andererseits die Organe, die wir zum RES rechnen, also vor allem die Milz, die Leber, das Knochenmark, die lymphatischen Organe. Welches dieser Organe am meisten bei der parenteralen Verdauung beteiligt ist, wird sich in erster Linie nach dem zu verdauenden Material und nach der Dauer des Verdauungsprozesses richten. Eingeleitet wird die Verdauung wohl immer von den Leukocyten, die bei längerer Dauer der parenteralen Verdauung von den Makrophagen abgelöst werden. Wenn es sich um besonders schwer zu verdauende Stoffe handelt, sehen wir als verdauende Zellen auch Riesenzellen in Erscheinung treten.

Die verdauende Tätigkeit von Riesenzellen kennen wir schon von den Osteoclasten des Knochenmarks und von den Riesenzellen des Chorionepithels. Von den ersteren wissen wir, daß sie imstande sind, Knochensubstanz abzubauen, und zwar sowohl bei normalen wie pathologischen Prozessen[1]. Bei experimentellen Untersuchungen an Ratten konnte beobachtet werden, daß sich die ersten Riesenzellen des Trophoblasten 5—6 Tage nach der Einnistung des Eies bildeten, und daß sie das Epithel der Uterindrüsen phagocytieren[2]. Auch an Mäuseeiern, die in die vordere Augenkammer transplantiert wurden, konnte die Riesenzellbildung am Trophoblasten und die Phagocytose von Erythrocyten durch diese Riesenzellen gesehen werden[3].

Am besten kann die verdauende Wirkung von Riesenzellen an den Fremdkörperriesenzellen beobachtet werden, die sich immer dort bilden, wo schwer resorbierbare körpereigene oder körperfremde Substanzen vorhanden sind, die ihrer Größe wegen nicht von den einkernigen Wanderzellen des Bindegewebes aufgenommen werden können[4].

Als solche körperfremde Substanzen, die eine Riesenzellenbildung auslösen, kommen alle möglichen Medikamente in öliger Lösung, chirurgisches Nahtmaterial, Talkumkristalle usw. in Frage; von körpereigenen Stoffen können vor allem verhornte Massen (z. B. in zerfallenden Atheromen), zerfallende fettige Substanzen, Cholesterin, Schleim-, Blut- und Fibringerinnsel und ähnliche Stoffe Anlaß zur Riesenzellenbildung geben.

Riesenzellenbildung kann durch Phagocytose und die damit verknüpfte parenterale Verdauung von Zellen geradezu bedingt sein; das lehren uns die oft ungewöhnlich großen Makrophagen in chronisch entzündeten Bezirken, deren Größe über 30 μ betragen kann, und die eine große Anzahl mehr oder weniger gut erhaltener Leukocytenkerne enthalten können. Auch bei den Typhuszellen ist es ganz ähnlich. Auch hier handelt es sich um riesig vergrößerte Makrophagen, Reticulumzellen der Lymphknoten, die oft eine große Anzahl von Lymphocyten phagocytiert haben.

Dagegen läßt sich wenig Sicheres darüber aussagen, ob etwa die Riesenzellenbildung bei den Masern etwas mit der Vermehrung des Masernvirus zu tun hat, ob es sich dabei um eine der Virusvermehrung gleichgeschaltete Reaktion handelt, oder ob darin eine Abwehrreaktion des Organismus zu sehen ist. Nach allem, was wir über die Riesenzellen und ihre Funktionen wissen, möchte man eher das letztere annehmen.

Auch bei anderen Riesenzellenbildungen wie den Sternbergschen Riesenzellen ist über ihre Bedeutung wenig bekannt. Da wir die Ursache der Lymphogranulomatose nicht kennen und man sich sogar darüber streitet, ob es sich dabei um eine Krankheit handelt, die zu den Geschwülsten oder besonderen Formen

---

[1] MAXIMOW 1927.   [2] ALDEN 1948.
[3] FAWCETT, WISLOCKI und WALDO 1947.   [4] MARCHAND 1924.

von Entzündungen zu rechnen ist, so vermögen wir auch nichts darüber zu sagen, ob die Riesenzellenbildung etwas mit einer Abwehrreaktion in Form einer parenteralen Verdauung eines fraglichen Erregers zu tun hat.

Ganz ähnlich ergeht es uns auch mit den Riesenzellen in Geschwülsten. Wir sehen nicht selten in ihnen Einschlüsse von Eiweißsubstanzen oder von Zelltrümmern. Wir vermögen jedoch nicht zu sagen, ob es sich dabei um Zeichen einer parenteralen Verdauung handelt.

In manchen Riesenzellen kommen Einschlüsse vor, von denen die sternförmigen (Astern), die sog. Schaumann-Körper und die als Centrosphären angesprochenen Gebilde erwähnt seien. Die sternförmigen Einschlüsse in Riesenzellen wurden zuerst 1890 beschrieben[1]. Sie fanden sich in der Randzone einer Dermoidcyste. Sie färben sich mit Elasticafarbstoffen[2], kommen häufig bei epitheloidzelliger Tuberkulose und bei Boeckschem Sarkoid vor, aber auch in Fremdkörpergranulomen und chronischen Entzündungen[3]. Nach den Untersuchungen von LINZBACH (1950) handelt es sich bei den Astern um strahlenartig angeordnete Traubsche Niederschlagsmembranen aus Elastin, die wahrscheinlich erst nach vorausgegangenem Abbau elastischer Fasern entstehen, die aus der Wand zugrunde gegangener Gefäße stammen und von Riesenzellen eingeschlossen wurden. Wir hätten es demnach auch hier mit einer Form der parenteralen Verdauung zu tun oder mindestens mit einem Versuch dazu.

Auch bei den Schaumann-Körpern handelt es sich um ovale und bohnengroße verkalkte Gebilde, die aus mehreren konzentrisch geschichteten Kalkschalen bestehen und sowohl intracellulär als auch in der Nachbarschaft der Riesenzellen vorkommen können.

LINZBACH wies nach, daß es sich bei den kleinen Schaumann-Körpern teils um verkalkte Capillarwandreste, teils um verkalkte Capillarthromben handelt, die von den Riesenzellen eingeschlossen wurden. Bei den größeren Schaumann-Körpern hat man es mit verkalkten Arteriolen- oder Venenthromben zu tun, an die sich sekundär Riesenzellen anlagern. Auch hier handelt es sich also mindestens um den Versuch einer parenteralen Verdauung.

IV. Die Resorption und die Resorptionswege.

Wir haben im Vorhergehenden gesehen, daß die parenterale Verdauung des Menschen ihr phylogenetisches Analogon in der parenteralen oder, besser gesagt, in der intraplasmatischen Verdauung der Protozoen hat. Diese intraplasmatische Verdauung der Protozoen erfolgt in einem besonderen Raum des Protoplasmas, in der Nahrungsvacuole, mit Hilfe von verdauenden Fermenten. Nach der Verdauung geht die Resorption, d. h. der Übertritt der gebildeten Verdauungsprodukte in das Plasma des Protozoons vor sich, während die nichtresorbierten Nahrungsteile im Verdauungsraum bleiben, um später nach außen entleert zu werden. Die resorbierten Nahrungsstoffe können auch als Reservematerial aufgespeichert werden.

Wir müssen uns dementsprechend fragen, in welcher Weise die bei der parenteralen Verdauung des Menschen entstehenden Verdauungsprodukte resorbiert werden. Da die parenterale Resorption in einem besonderen Kapitel behandelt wird, können wir uns hier damit begnügen, auf die Haupttatsachen hinzuweisen.

Jede Form der Verdauung, ob intraplasmatisch oder extraplasmatisch, dient dem Zweck, die Stoffe so vorzubereiten, daß sie in das lebende Plasma des Tieres oder des Menschen aufgenommen werden können. Diese Aufnahme wurde als *Permeation*[4] bezeichnet. Dieser weitgefaßte Begriff umschließt alle Formen und Arten des Übertrittes sowohl von Gasen wie Wasser und Salzlösungen, von mittelgroßen Energieträgern wie z. B. Aminosäuren, Fettsäuren, Glucose u. a. als auch von Großmolekülen. Diese Permeation ist ein sehr komplizierter physikalisch-chemischer Vorgang, der durch treibende Kräfte bestimmt wird.

---

[1] GOLDMANN 1890. [2] VOGEL 1911. [3] DE MONTMOLIN 1943. [4] HIRSCH 1955.

Diese Kräfte bestehen aus verschiedenen Faktoren, die in der Hauptsache folgendermaßen zusammengesetzt sind:

1. die molekularen Faktoren, d. h. die dem permeierenden Molekül innewohnenden Eigenschaften, also seine Größe, seine elektrische Ladung, die Eigenschaften der einzelnen Bausteine des Moleküls;

2. die Faktoren außerhalb der Zelle. Darunter ist vor allem der physikalisch-chemische Zustand des Zellmediums, z. B. der Gewebsflüssigkeit, zu verstehen, aber auch die nervöse und hormonale Beeinflussung der Permeation;

3. die Faktoren innerhalb der Zelle. Hierbei handelt es sich um solche, die durch den Zustand der Zellmembran und des Cytoplasmas bestimmt werden. Die Konstruktion ein und derselben Zellmembran muß man sich wechselnd, je nach den Umständen, vorstellen. Sowohl die Porengröße als auch die elektrische Ladung und die Anordnung ist variabel. Es herrscht hier kein stabiles, sondern ein dynamisches Gleichgewicht, das von außen wie von innen beeinflußbar ist.

Ähnlich wie bei der Zellmembran ist dies beim Cytoplasma. Auch hier haben wir mit einer dauernden Verschiebung des Gleichgewichts zu rechnen, wenn z. B. eingedrungene Teilchen an andere Moleküle gebunden werden und so neue komplexe Teilchen bilden. Dadurch, daß diese eingedrungenen Moleküle als Einzelteilchen verschwinden, wird aber auch der osmotische Druck innerhalb der Zelle verändert.

Aus dem Gesagten ergibt sich, wie kompliziert der Vorgang der Permeation ist. Das Verständnis wird erleichtert, wenn man die Permeation unterteilt in die passive Permeation oder Diffusion und in die aktive Permeation oder Resorption.

Um eine Diffusion handelt es sich beim Gas- und Flüssigkeitsaustausch. Daß mit dem Wasser auch molekular gelöste Stoffe wie NaCl, Glucose, Harnstoff u. a. diffundieren, wird nicht verwundern.

Bei der Resorption handelt es sich demgegenüber um einen Prozeß, der durch das aktive Mitwirken des Zellprotoplasmas zustande kommt. Das kann geschehen durch eine Änderung der physikalisch-chemischen Struktur der Zellmembran, z. B. ihres elektrischen Potentials, durch Veränderung ihrer Porenweite oder ihrer Oberflächenkräfte. Weiter kann das Plasma das permeierte Teilchen durch physikalische Adsorption an Micellen oder an Mitochondrien oder auch durch chemischen Einbau in Mikro- oder Makromoleküle der Grundsubstanz binden.

Ein großer Unterschied zwischen Diffusion und Resorption zeigt sich auch darin, daß letztere durch Stoffe verhindert werden kann, die auf die Diffusion keinen Einfluß ausüben wie z. B. Arsen, Jodacetat, Blausäure, Quecksilber u. a.

Die Resorption ist hormonal beeinflußbar, wie wir seit einiger Zeit wissen. Besonders kennen wir den Einfluß des Hypothalamus und der endokrinen Drüsen, der Hypophyse und der Schilddrüse, auf die Resorption der Glucose, die über die Phosphorylierung vor sich geht.

Auch die Aufnahme von Kolloiden ist ein resorptiver Prozeß. Allerdings reichen dabei die normalen Poren der Zellmembran, die eine Weite von 3—10 Å besitzen, nicht aus. Denn solche Makromoleküle haben einen Durchmesser zwischen 10 und 1000 Å. Man hat nicht nur eine Resorption von Dextrose, Lävulose und Stärke durch Protozoen, sondern auch eine Durchlässigkeit der Zellen im Nephron von Salamandra für Teilchen mit einem Durchmesser von 1000 Å nachgewiesen.

Von ganz besonderer Bedeutung ist natürlich auch bei der Resorption die Phagocytose, bei der die aufgenommenen Teilchen so groß sind, daß sie mikroskopisch gesehen werden können, also größer als $0{,}1\,\mu$. Dabei entsteht in der Zellmembran ein großes Tor, durch das das Partikelchen eingeschleust wird, wonach sich die Membran wieder schließt.

Eine sehr wichtige Form der Phagocytose ist die *Pinocytose,* worunter die Aufnahme von Wasser und Makromolekülen durch Makrophagen oder maligne Zellen in der Gewebskultur zu verstehen ist. Von der unsichtbaren Membran der Zelle wird eine kleine Wassermenge umgeben. Die Konstruktion dieser Membran ändert sich sehr schnell, wenn Pseudopodien ausgestreckt und zurückgezogen werden. Der von der Membran umhüllte Wassertropfen wird in wenigen Minuten zum Zellzentrum bewegt, die ihn umgebende Membran aufgelöst und das Wasser samt den darin enthaltenen Molekülen dem Plasma einverleibt. Das Wasser verschwindet dann, und die Moleküle werden zum Granulum verdichtet und verdaut. Diese Form der Resorption ist bedeutungsvoll für die Funktion der Makrophagen.

Schließlich wäre noch die Bedeutung gewisser Hilfsmechanismen der Resorption zu erwähnen, von denen nur die Hydrotropie und die Phosphorylierung genannt seien. Unter der Hydrotropie versteht man die Eigenschaft gewisser Substanzen, wasserunlösliche Stoffe wasserlöslich zu machen. Als die physiologisch wichtigsten wären hier die Gallensalze zu erwähnen, die Fett und fettähnliche Stoffe wasserlöslich und damit resorptionsbereit machen. Auch die Phosphorylierung durch Einwirkung des Fermentes Phosphatase ist für die Fettresorption wichtig.

Es scheint die Annahme berechtigt, daß bei der Resorption parenteraler Verdauungsprodukte keine anderen Gesetze herrschen als bei der Resorption normaler Verdauungsstoffe. Immerhin müssen wir in Betracht ziehen, daß die parenterale Verdauung mancher endogen entstandenen Stoffe größere Anforderungen an den Organismus stellt als etwa die enterale. Wir werden dies bei der Aufsaugung hämatogener Ergüsse sehen, die an anderer Stelle besprochen wird.

Was nun die Resorptionswege anbelangt, auf denen die resorbierten Stoffe transportiert werden, um schließlich in den Bau- und Betriebsstoffwechsel des Körpers eingeschaltet zu werden, so handelt es sich hier um die Lymph- und Blutbahnen, zwischen die als „Milieu intérieur" die Gewebsflüssigkeit geschaltet ist. In den Untersuchungen von Loeschcke u. Mitarb. (1934) mit kolloidalen Farbstoffen wurden die Resorptionsverhältnisse klarzustellen versucht und dabei ein System von Lymphscheiden nachgewiesen, dessen Ausbildung dem vorhandenen Capillarnetz proportional war.

Omentum maius, Appendices epiploicae und die Fettlager an anderen Körperstellen werden als Resorptionsorgane angesprochen. Die perivasculären Salträume sind nach Loeschcke ein über den ganzen Körper verbreitetes System, in dem sich die Flüssigkeitsbewegung in der Richtung von der Blutbahn zum Gewebe einerseits und in der Richtung vom Gewebe zur Lymphbahn andererseits vollzieht.

Im Gegensatz zu Loeschcke lehnt Pfuhl (1939, 1940) das Vorkommen perivasculärer Lymphscheiden ab. Er hält die zwischen den Zellen und Fasern vorhandenen und von Flüssigkeit durchströmten Spalten für nicht zum Lymphgefäßsystem gehörig, sondern es soll sich dabei um perivasculäre Ödeme handeln.

Wie diese Streitfrage in Zukunft auch entschieden werden mag, an der Bedeutung der Gewebsflüssigkeit wird dadurch nichts geändert.

Aus lang zurückliegenden Untersuchungen[1] ergab sich, daß auch die Abbaustoffe von Eiweiß wie Pepton, Glutaminsäure, Asparaginsäure, Alanin, Glykokoll mit verschiedener Geschwindigkeit resorbiert werden. Dabei handelt es sich um Resorptionsversuche aus der Bauchhöhle; jedoch kann dieses Beispiel wohl verallgemeinert werden. Es besagt soviel, daß endotheliale Scheidewände verhältnismäßig gut durchlässig sind und die Grenze anscheinend erst bei den hochmolekularen Eiweißkörpern erreicht wird. Dafür scheinen auch andere Untersuchungen[2] zu sprechen, die ebenfalls an der Bauchhöhle vorgenommen wurden, und aus denen hervorging, daß kristalloide Stoffe nicht nur aus der Bauchhöhle ins Blut aufgenommen werden, sondern daß auch der umgekehrte Weg möglich ist.

---

[1] Kjöllerfeldt 1917.   [2] Putnam 1923.

Aus diesen und anderen Untersuchungen[1] ist zu entnehmen, daß kristalloide Stoffe vornehmlich auf dem Blutwege, kolloidale Stoffe dagegen auf dem Lymphwege abtransportiert werden. Dementsprechend dürfen wir annehmen, daß auch die parenteral verdauten Eiweißstoffe und die Kohlenhydrate in ähnlicher Weise wie die enteral verdauten über den Blutweg, die verdauten Fettstoffe dagegen auf dem Lymphweg weiterbefördert werden.

V. Die Bedeutung der parenteralen Verdauung für den Organismus.

A. Humorale Veränderungen. (Veränderungen am Bluteiweiß.)

Die ursprünglichste und am leichtesten faßbare Bedeutung der parenteralen Verdauung liegt wohl darin, daß sie eine Art Selbstreinigung darstellt. Daß eine solche Tätigkeit nicht ohne Rückwirkung auf den Organismus bleiben kann, ist leicht verständlich.

So sehen wir bei vielen, wenn auch nicht allen Prozessen, bei denen eine parenterale Verdauung vor sich geht, eine Veränderung der Bluteiweißkörper in Form einer Vermehrung der Globuline und des Fibrinogens. Man findet eine derartige Vermehrung, die relativ, aber auch absolut sein kann, bei Infektionskrankheiten, Entzündungen, malignen Tumoren und anderen Krankheiten.

Die Albumine sind häufig entsprechend vermindert, brauchen dies jedoch nicht zu sein, so daß eine Vermehrung der Gesamtproteine die Folge sein kann.

So gut wir durch die modernen Untersuchungsmethoden, vor allem durch die Ultrazentrifugierung und die Elektrophorese, über die Zusammensetzung des Bluteiweißes unterrichtet sind, so wenig wissen wir im Grunde genommen auch heute noch darüber, in welchem Teil des Organismus es gebildet wird. Aus den Untersuchungen von CASPERSSON (1950) geht zwar hervor, welch großen Anteil die Desoxyribonucleinsäure des Kerns und die Ribonucleinsäure des Cytoplasmas an der Eiweißproduktion hat, aber wir können nur sagen, daß es sich dabei um die allgemeine Eiweißbildung handelt, also um die der Zelle, während wir keine Rückschlüsse daraus ziehen können, in welchen Organen die Produktion der Bluteiweißkörper stattfindet.

Über den Ort der Albuminbildung, die in der Leber stattfinden soll, herrscht noch eine gewisse Einigkeit; vom Fibrinogen glaubt man, daß es sowohl im Knochenmark als auch in der Leber produziert werden kann, dagegen ist man über den Ort der Globulinbildung recht verschiedener Meinung. Während man früher die Fibrinogenbildung[2] und auch die Globulinbildung[3] in das Reticuloendothel verlegte, nehmen heute zahlreiche Untersucher an, daß wenigstens das Globulin, oder besser gesagt die Globuline, in einem besonderen Zellsystem, nämlich den Plasmazellen gebildet werden[4]. Man zog diese Schlüsse aus Untersuchungen an Myelomen, bei denen man eine Globulinvermehrung im Blut fand. Da nun die Myelome aus Plasmazellen — wenn auch aus abnorm gebauten — zusammengesetzt sind, so folgerte man, daß auch das normale Globulin von Plasmazellen gebildet wird. Allerdings gehen auch hier die Meinungen auseinander, da die einen nur die reticulären Plasmazellen als Globulinbildner ansehen, während nach der Meinung anderer alle Plasmazellen dafür in Frage kommen. Gegen die Auffassung von der Rolle der Plasmazellen als alleinige Bildner der grobdispersen Eiweißkörper, vor allem der Globuline, scheint in

---

[1] KATSURA 1924.   [2] LESZLER und PAULICZKI 1933, HEINLEIN 1934.
[3] BERGER 1922, HEINLEIN 1935, STARLINGER 1927.
[4] APITZ 1939, 1940, FLEISCHHACKER und KLIMA 1936, HENNING 1938, ROHR 1940, BJØRNEBOE und GORMSEN 1941.

erster Linie auch die geringe Zahl der Plasmazellen zu sprechen. Der normale Plasmazellengehalt des Sternalmarks beträgt 1—2% der weißen Zellen[1].

Bereits 1934[2] wurde gezeigt, daß nach parenteraler Zufuhr von Pferdeserum, Shigavaccine, aber auch von kolloidalem Kupfer-Wismut, Siliquid, das Gesamteiweiß deutlich zunahm, im wesentlichen das Fibrinogen und die Globuline. Bei der mikroskopischen Untersuchung von Knochenmark und anderen Organen konnte keine Plasmazellenvermehrung nachgewiesen werden. Es wurde daraus der Schluß gezogen, daß die Behauptung, nur die Plasmazellen seien die Eiweißbildner, wenig Wahrscheinlichkeit hat. Etwas anderes wäre es dagegen, wenn man die Pasmazellen als einen Teil des Reticuloendothels ansähe, wie dies von mancher Seite geschieht[3].

Die Rolle der Plasmazellen im Eiweißstoffwechsel wird von anderer Seite dahin begrenzt, daß man glaubt, die Plasmazellen würden nicht Eiweiß sezernieren, sondern es resorbieren[4].

1950 hat Letterer bei Mäusen nachgewiesen, daß bereits nach einer Caseininjektion ein Anstieg des Globulins bei gleichzeitigem Abfall des Albumins erfolgt. Nach mehreren Injektionen wurden diese Veränderungen des Bluteiweißes, die auch elektrophoretisch festgestellt werden konnten, noch deutlicher. Über das gleichzeitige morphologische Bild sagte er aus, daß die Milz stets vergrößert war, und daß in der Leber und Niere mesenchymale Zellproliferationen vorhanden waren. Obwohl er sich nicht über die Beziehungen dieser Zellproliferationen zur Vermehrung der Globuline ausspricht, ist anzunehmen, daß er einen solchen Zusammenhang für möglich hält, da er an einer Stelle sagt, daß es bei Ausbleiben dieser Zellproliferationen fast nie zur Amyloidose komme, für die er eine Hyperproteinämie als Bedingung ansieht.

B. Morphische Veränderungen.

Über die bei der parenteralen Verdauung gefundenen morphologischen Veränderungen wurde bereits an früherer Stelle das Wesentliche gesagt, so daß hier nur noch einiges nachzuholen ist. Es wurde bereits dort von den Veränderungen in den verschiedenen Organen gesprochen, wie sie besonders von Siegmund, Dietrich, Pfeiffer u. Standenath (1925) u. a. aufgezeigt wurden. Es wurde festgestellt, daß die parenteral verdauenden Zellen sich in den Organen vermehren, und daß sie sogar Zellknötchen bilden können, wie dies in der Leber und in der Adventitia der Gefäße der Fall ist. Man kennt solche Zellknötchen besonders bei bakteriellen Infektionen[5], so daß die Parallele zwischen diesen Infektionen und der parenteralen Verdauung sehr nahe liegt und man annehmen darf, daß ein Teil der Abwehr eben auf der parenteralen Verdauung der Keime beruht, so wie dies schon früher erwähnt wurde. Weiterhin sieht man eine Vergrößerung solcher Zellen, in denen häufig Vacuolen auftreten, die offenbar eine ähnliche Bedeutung haben wie die Verdauungsvacuolen der Protozoen. Schließlich wäre noch die Ablösung der vergrößerten Reticulumzellen zu erwähnen, die besonders in der Milz so gut zu sehen ist. Man kann hier ihre Abrundung und Ablösung in den Sinus beobachten, so daß sie schließlich in vermehrter Menge im Blut kreisen.

Zusammenfassend kann man also sagen, daß es bei der parenteralen Verdauung zu einer Vermehrung der verdauenden Zellen kommt, die nicht an Ort und Stelle zu verbleiben brauchen, sondern an die Orte transportiert werden können, wo verdauungsfähige Stoffe vorhanden sind.

---

[1] Wuhrmann und Wunderly 1952.   [2] Heinlein 1943.
[3] Rohr 1949, Nägeli 1936, Bing 1940, Bing und Plum 1937.
[4] Büngeler und Rotter 1950, Dubois-Ferrière 1943, 1948, Heinlein 1943.
[5] Siegmund 1923, 1924, 1925.

VI. Die Bedeutung der parenteralen Verdauung für krankhafte Zustände.

1. Die Amyloidose.

Die parenterale Verdauung kann nicht nur, wie bereits früher geschildert wurde, krankhafte Zustände beseitigen, sondern auch hervorrufen oder wenigstens eine Teilursache für ihre Entstehung bilden. Es kann sich hier nur darum handeln, die vorhandenen Zusammenhänge zu streifen.

An erster Stelle wäre die Amyloidose zu nennen, die seit langem als eine Störung des Eiweißstoffwechsels bekannt ist. Schon seit den Untersuchungen von KUCZYNSKI (1923) weiß man, daß weiße Mäuse bei Fütterung eiweißreicher Nahrung an Amyloidose erkranken können. Ein wesentlich höherer Prozentsatz der Tiere erkrankte jedoch an Amyloidose, wenn den Tieren Eiweißlösungen eingespritzt wurden. KUCZYNSKI schloß aus diesen Untersuchungen, daß die Ursache der Amyloidentstehung in einem Übertritt von blutfremden, abbaubedürftigen Eiweißstoffen in den Kreislauf zu sehen sei. Die zweite Bedingung dafür soll das Vorhandensein von abbauenden Fermenten sein. An den Stellen, an denen die im Blut kreisenden Eiweißstoffe mit diesen Fermenten zusammentreffen, soll es zu einem Niederschlag, zur Amyloidbildung kommen.

Diese Fermenttheorie wurde jedoch bald verdrängt durch die überzeugendere Theorie, daß die Amyloidose das Produkt einer Antigen-Antikörperreaktion sei[1]. Als Antigen wurde zerfallendes Leukocyteneiweiß angesprochen[2]. Am Ort der Antikörperbildung komme es zur Antigen-Antikörperreaktion in der Form einer Präcipitation. Diese Präcipitation erfolge in den RES-reichen Organen wie Milz, Leber usw., die die Antikörper bilden, und zwar an der Stelle der Antikörperproduktion.

Durch die Untersuchungen von LETTERER (1934) wurde festgestellt, daß nicht allein das Leukocyteneiweiß, sondern überhaupt zerfallendes Körpereiweiß die Amyloidbildung hervorruft. Das gemeinsame Moment soll in dem starken parenteralen Reiz liegen, der zum Zerfall führe. Es würde sich also auch dabei um eine Form der parenteralen Verdauung handeln.

Für eine solche Erklärung der Amyloidentstehung könnten auch die Untersuchungen an Serumpferden, die an Amyloidose erkrankt waren, sprechen[3].

Es ist erklärlich, daß man die Amyloidentstehung auch in Beziehung zum RES brachte[4]. Eine Berechtigung ist dem auch nicht abzusprechen, vor allem, wenn man den Hauptsitz der Makrophagenbildung und der parenteralen Verdauung im reticuloendothelialen System sieht. Jedoch ist es fraglich, ob man diese Beziehung auf das RES im engeren Sinne begrenzen darf, und man wird LETTERER wohl recht geben müssen, wenn er ausführt: „Man kann höchstens sagen, daß auch die Amyloidose eine Krankheit des aktiven Mesenchyms, aber nicht des reticulo-endothelialen Systems im engeren Sinne ist."

Es ist hier nicht der Ort, um auf die verschiedenen Theorien der Amyloidbildung näher einzugehen. Kurz zusammengefaßt kann man sagen, daß die beiden Theorien, die heute die meisten Anhänger haben, entweder eine Hyperproteinämie annehmen[5] oder aber eine Paraproteinose mit Paraproteinämie[6].

LETTERER (1950, 1957) hält die Paraproteinämie für nicht ausschlaggebend für die Entstehung des Amyloids. Er vertritt die Anschauung, daß es sich dabei um eine Hyperproteinämie handle, die als Hyperglobulinämie sicher nachgewiesen sei. Von hier aus ergeben sich wieder Beziehungen zu den früher angeführten Tierversuchen mit experimentell erzeugtem Amyloid und zur parenteralen Verdauung.

---

[1] LOESCHCKE 1927, LETTERER 1926, 1934, 1949, 1950, LETTERER und SCHNEIDER 1953.
[2] LOESCHCKE 1927. [3] ARNDT 1931, WEIDLICH 1942.
[4] DOMAGK 1924, ARNDT 1931, PAGEL 1928, JAFFÉ 1926.
[5] LETTERER 1950, 1953.
[6] APITZ 1940, 1942, RANDERATH 1947, 1948, TERBRÜGGEN 1944, WUHRMANN 1946, WUHRMANN und WUNDERLY 1952.

Schließlich darf nicht unerwähnt bleiben, daß das Amyloid auch wieder verschwinden kann, und, wie manche glauben, sogar restlos, wenn die Ursache der Amyloidentstehung beseitigt wird.

Sicher ist jedenfalls, daß das Amyloid wieder abgebaut werden kann. Besonders eindrucksvoll sind hier noch immer die Untersuchungen von WALDENSTRÖM (1928), der durch wiederholte Leberpunktionen beim Menschen, die an chronisch eiternden Fisteln litten, die Bildung von Amyloid in der Leber verfolgte. Wenn es ihm nun gelang, die Eitersekretion herabzusetzen und die Fisteln zur Ausheilung zu bringen, so verschwand auch das Amyloid wieder. Nach seiner Meinung hält die Amyloidablagerung Schritt mit dem Eiterfluß, der reichlich sein und längere Zeit vor sich gehen muß, so daß der Patient dadurch stark heruntergebracht wird. Wenn es nicht gelingt, den Eiterfluß völlig zum Aufhören zu bringen, so verschwindet auch das Amyloid nicht vollständig. Die Auflösung des Amyloids sollte nach KUCZINSKI (1923) durch Plasmazellen vor sich gehen, die er „Amyloidoklasten" nannte. WALDENSTRÖM ist jedoch der Meinung, daß man sehr schwer spezielle Zellen unterscheiden könne und hält Täuschungen bei der ungleichmäßigen Auflösung des Amyloids für möglich.

Man kann über die Resorption des Amyloids nur sagen, daß sie theoretisch möglich ist bei Verschwinden der Grundursache der Amyloidentstehung. Es läßt sich jedoch nicht mit Bestimmtheit sagen, ob diese parenterale Verdauung des Amyloids intracellulär oder extracellulär vor sich geht.

2. Die Thrombose.

Wenn früher die Beseitigung von Thromben durch die parenterale Verdauung erwähnt wurde, so muß hier noch einiges über die Beziehung der Thrombenbildung zur parenteralen Verdauung nachgeholt werden. Zum Zustandekommen einer Thrombose gehören mehrere Faktoren: Stromverlangsamung, die Wandveränderung und die Änderung der Blutbeschaffenheit. Hier soll nur auf die letzten beiden Veränderungen eingegangen werden, da diese allein Beziehungen zur parenteralen Verdauung besitzen. Eine Reihe von Untersuchern[1] stimmt darin überein, daß durch parenterale Eiweißzufuhr im Experiment Thrombosen hervorgerufen werden können. Weiter ist aus zahlreichen Untersuchungen bekannt, daß die Bluteiweißkörper nach parenteraler Zufuhr von Eiweiß oder auch andersartigen Kolloiden ansteigen, wobei dieser Anstieg auf eine Vermehrung der grobdispersen Anteile, nämlich des Fibrinogens und der Globuline, zurückzuführen ist[2]. Vor allem die Fibrinogenvermehrung ist aber von wesentlicher Bedeutung für die Thromboseneigung. Man findet eine solche Fibrinogenvermehrung auch beim Menschen bei Infektionskrankheiten, akut entzündlichen Zuständen wie Pneumonie, Pleuritiden u. a. Hier handelt es sich aber um Veränderungen, bei denen die parenterale Verdauung von Infektionserregern, Gewebszerfallsprodukten oder Exsudaten eine besondere Rolle spielt.

Noch sehr viel eingehender ist die Gefäßwandveränderung als Ursache für die Thrombose untersucht worden. Schon RITTER (1926) hatte darauf hingewiesen, daß die Beziehungen zwischen Blut und Gefäßwand von wesentlicher Bedeutung für die Thrombose seien. Er hatte solche Thrombosen nach der intravenösen Injektion von Metallkolloiden, Farbstoffen, Fetten und Bakterienaufschwemmungen gesehen. Da er eine deutliche Speicherung dieser Stoffe im Venenendothel fand, kam er zu dem Schluß, daß die Ursache der Thrombose in der Störung der physikalisch-chemischen Grenzverhältnisse zwischen Endothel und Blut, und zwar hauptsächlich in einer primären Stoffwechselstörung des Endothels, zu suchen sei. Wenn bis dahin noch nicht von einer parenteralen Verdauung die Rede war, so wurde dies deutlich bei SIEGMUND (1923—1925), der in seinen bereits früher erwähnten Untersuchungen über Allgemeininfektionen,

---

[1] DIETRICH 1929, 1941, SIEGMUND 1923, 1924—1925, KUSAMA 1913.
[2] BERGER 1922, STARLINGER 1927, HEINLEIN 1934, 1935.

beim Menschen zellige Herde in der Gefäßintima und Fibrinknötchen fand. Diese Veränderungen brachte er mit der gelungenen Keimvernichtung, d. h. der parenteralen Verdauung, in Zusammenhang. Über die von ihm experimentell hervorgerufenen gleichartigen Veränderungen durch Injektionen von Colibakterien und Staphylokokken wurde ebenfalls schon früher gesprochen. Seiner Ansicht nach stehen diese Gewebsreaktionen zu der Bildung von Fibrinthromben nach Aschoff und Kusama in enger Beziehung.

Dietrich (1929—1941) suchte in ausgedehnten Untersuchungen den Beweis zu erbringen, daß ein Endotheluntergang für das Zustandekommen der Thrombose nicht unbedingt erforderlich sei. Er injizierte Kaninchen Coli- und Staphylokokkenvaccine in steigenden Dosen intravenös und unterband kurz vor der Einbringung der letzten Dosis ein Gefäßstück oder drosselte es vorsichtig. Gelegentlich verwendete er für die Vorbehandlung Caseosan und nur für die letzte Injektion Vaccine. An den auf diese Weise völlig ausgeschalteten Venen fand er in den ersten Stunden eine Verklumpung der Keime mit Anlagerung an der Intima, eine Vergrößerung der Endothelzellen und ein Auftreten kleiner Zellanhäufungen in der Gefäßwand feststellbar. Die Bakterienklümpchen lagen zum Teil innig an der Wand und waren an einigen Stellen mit einer homogenen Schicht bedeckt. Dietrich will diese Abscheidung mit homogenen Fibrinschichten gleichgesetzt wissen, die an mit Crotonöl geätzten Gefäßwandstellen auftreten. Er ist der Meinung, daß seine Untersuchungen zwar kein einwandfreier Beweis, aber doch ein wertvoller Hinweis in der Richtung seien, daß die Reaktion zwischen Gefäßwand und Blut unter geeigneter Abstimmung imstande ist, die Grundlage einer Thrombose zu bilden. Eine solche Reaktion würde ausgelöst durch Anpassung des Gefäßendothels an Resorptionsleistungen sowohl gegen feinste belebte Körperchen (Bakterien) als auch gegen kolloidal gelöste Eiweißstoffe. Sie führten zum Haften von körperlichen Teilchen und zur Abscheidung homogener Massen, die den Stromverhältnissen entsprechend zu Wirbeln geformt würden. Durch Einschluß von Leukocyten, Blutplättchen und roten Blutkörperchen könne vor einem Stromhindernis ein gemischter Thrombus entstehen. Die Reaktionsbereitschaft des Venenendothels gehe bei entsprechend langer Vorbehandlung den schon bekannten Reaktionen der kleinen Venen der Leber und anderer Gefäßgebiete parallel; ebenso stimme sie mit der Reaktion des Endokards überein, die bei geeigneten Bedingungen zu Endokarditis führen könne. Der Begriff einer Thrombosebereitschaft erhalte durch diese Beobachtung eine festere Grundlage. Sie beruhe nicht einseitig auf einer Strombehinderung, Wandveränderung oder bestimmter Blutbeschaffenheit, sondern auf einer Änderung der Beziehungen zwischen Gefäßwand und Blut, bei gleichzeitig begünstigender Stromverlangsamung.

Obwohl weder Siegmund noch Dietrich den Ausdruck „parenterale Verdauung" gebrauchen, besteht doch kein Zweifel darüber, daß das von ihnen beschriebene Geschehen durch eine parenterale Verdauung der corpusculären oder gelösten organischen Stoffe ausgelöst gedacht wird. Dietrich (1941) hat in einer neueren Arbeit die Theorie von der Bedeutung der Wandveränderung für die Thrombose noch einmal überprüft. Er verengte bei Kaninchen durch einen Fascienstreifen die V. jugularis und injizierte in die Ohrvene der gleichen Seite eine Aufschwemmung oder ein Filtrat von Coli oder Streptococcus viridans und machte 24 bzw. 48 Std später eine gleiche Injektion auf der anderen Seite. Nach der ersten Injektion fand sich keine Pfropfenbildung, nach der zweiten war an der Stenosestelle die Gefäßwand aufgelockert. Im Gefäß waren fädige Fibrinpfröpfe mit Einlagerung von Leukocyten vorhanden, jedoch keine Plättchenthromben. In einem Falle wurde ein größerer Embolus der Lunge beobachtet, der indessen auch keine Plättchenlamellen, sondern als Gerüst nur Fibrin aufwies. Obwohl Dietrich mit einiger Resignation sagt, daß „von der experimentellen Thrombose zur menschlichen Spontanthrombose noch ein weiter Schritt sei", wird die Bedeutung der Gefäßwandveränderungen für die Blutpfropfbildung nicht ernstlich angezweifelt. Es ist wahrscheinlich, daß es sich dabei nicht um grobmechanische Gefäßwandveränderungen handelt, sondern daß vielleicht noch viel häufiger gerade die feinsten, nur mikroskopisch sichtbaren Veränderungen eine Rolle spielen, die mit der Tätigkeit der Gefäßwandzellen bei der parenteralen Verdauung von Bakterien oder körperlicher Zerfallsprodukte zusammenhängen.

3. Die Speicherungskrankheiten.

In gewissem Zusammenhang mit der parenteralen Verdauung dürften Stoffwechselstörungen stehen, die man als Speicherungskrankheiten bezeichnet. Früher wurde bereits gesagt, daß der Organismus die Fähigkeit besitzt, Eiweiß in gewissem Ausmaß zu speichern. Noch viel mehr ist dies bei anderen organischen Stoffen wie Fetten, Kohlenhydraten, Vitaminen und auch bei anorganischen Stoffen der Fall.

Es wurde bereits früher erwähnt, daß bei den Plasmocytomen Paraproteinosen vorkommen, über deren Genese man verschiedener Meinung ist. Während von mancher Seite die Meinung vertreten wird, daß die Plasmocytome echte Geschwülste sind, deren Zellen Eiweißkörper sezernieren, sind andere Autoren der Auffassung, daß die Eiweißstörung das Primäre und die Resorption in den Plasmocytomzellen und die Zellanhäufung das Sekundäre ist. Bei der letzteren Ansicht würde es sich also um eine Eiweißstoffwechselstörung handeln, die man in ihrer Auswirkung vielleicht mit einem gewissen Recht als Eiweißspeicherungskrankheit bezeichnen könnte.

Bei den Plasmocytomen kommen nun, wie wir schon gesehen haben, lokale oder diffuse Eiweißablagerungen in der Form von Paramyloid vor. Die Paramyloidablagerung im Bereich der Plasmocytome selber zeigt einen Abbau, d. h. eine parenterale Verdauung vom Rande der Ablagerung her. Dieser Abbau geschieht durch Makrophagen mit hellem Protoplasma, nicht selten auch durch mehrkernige Riesenzellen. Nach der Meinung Büngelers und seiner Mitarbeiter (1955) sind auch die Plasmocytomzellen an diesem Abbau beteiligt.

Bei den eigentlichen Speicherungskrankheiten wäre die Thesauropathie von der Pathothesaurose zu unterscheiden. Bei der erstgenannten Erkrankung handelt es sich um die Speicherung eines bestimmten Stoffes, durch den Erkrankungen von Zellen, Geweben und Organen hervorgerufen werden, während im zweiten Fall eine krankhafte Stoffwechselstörung von Zellen und Geweben im Vordergrund steht, die dann Speicherungssymptome verschiedener Art nach sich zieht[1].

Hier interessiert nur die letztere Form. Leider wissen wir sehr wenig über die Ätiologie dieser Stoffwechselstörungen, ob es sich nun um Störungen des Lipoidstoffwechsels oder des Kohlenhydratstoffwechsels handelt. Was bis heute darüber gesagt wurde, ist Hypothese geblieben. So hat man bei der Glykogenspeicherungskrankheit ein abnorm gebautes Glykogen, eine Störung der inneren Sekretion oder einen gestörten Abbau durch mangelhafte Fermenteinwirkung auf das Substrat angenommen. Es scheint bewiesen, daß bei den Glykogenosen Fermente fehlen, und zwar entweder die Glucosidasen oder die Glucose-6-Phosphatase. Beim Fehlen der Glucosidasen kommt es zur Ablagerung abnorm strukturierten Glykogens, dessen Abbau hochgradig gestört ist[2].

Ähnliches gilt auch für die Lipoidosen. Die Meinung, daß eine primäre Vermehrung der Lipoide vorliege, ist immer mehr zugunsten der Ansicht zurückgetreten, daß es sich dabei um eine Störung des Zellstoffwechsels handelt. Welcher Art diese Störung ist, darüber besitzen wir freilich auch nur ungenügende Vorstellungen. In erster Linie könnte man wieder an eine fermentative Störung denken, an eine Unfähigkeit der Zellen, mit den in normalen oder auch in abnormen Mengen angebotenen Stoffen fertig zu werden. Eine solche Theorie würde demnach besagen, daß eine mangelhafte parenterale Verdauung vorliegt.

4. Die Entzündung.

Es wurde schon früher erwähnt, daß die parenterale Verdauung in enger Beziehung zur Entzündung steht, denn nach der Auffassung von Metschnikoff (1902) und Rössle (1923) war die Entzündung ja nichts anderes als eine Form der parenteralen Verdauung. Besonders auffallend ist dies bei der infektiösen Entzündung, wo der parenteralen Verdauung eine wesentliche Rolle bei der

---

[1] Letterer 1948.   [2] Zellweger 1956.

Unschädlichmachung der eingedrungenen Erreger zukommt. Wenn auch belebte Organismen die Hauptursache für Entzündungen beim Menschen darstellen, so sind sie doch nicht die einzige, und wir dürfen annehmen, daß auch bei Entzündungen, die durch chemische, physikalische oder mechanische Ursachen hervorgerufen werden, die parenterale Verdauung mitwirkt. Tatsächlich weiß man ja niemals genau, ob die scheinbare Erstursache der Entzündung, z. B. Einwirkung von Strahlen oder ätzenden Stoffen, auch unmittelbar die Entzündung hervorgerufen hat. Wir kennen aus den Untersuchungen von MENKIN (1950) die verschiedenen Stoffe, die bei der Entzündung eine Rolle spielen, wie das Leukotaxin, das Nekrosin, den „leucocytosis promoting factor", das Pyrexin und das Exudin. Hierbei handelt es sich um Stoffe, die Polypeptide zu sein scheinen. Diese Substanzen wurden aus Exsudaten, aus entzündeten Geweben und anscheinend auch aus Seren gewonnen. Wenn somit auch die Möglichkeit besteht, daß es sich um mehr oder weniger vorgebildete Substanzen handelt, so spricht doch manches dafür, daß sie erst im Laufe des Entzündungsprozesses gebildet bzw. frei werden. Man könnte sich gut vorstellen, daß sie beim Untergang bzw. der parenteralen Verdauung der unmittelbar durch das schädigende Agens betroffenen Zellen frei werden, wie dies HEINLEIN (1935, 1948) auch für andere Stoffe angenommen hat.

Noch sehr viel deutlicher wird die Beziehung der parenteralen Verdauung zur Entzündung in deren chronischer Phase, die LETTERER (1953) als „Zellverdauung" bezeichnet hat. Daß gerade diese Phase mit ihrer enormen Zellneubildung, die allmählich in die Reparation überleitet, die Phase der intracellulären Verdauung ist, wurde bereits früher angedeutet. Wenn wir nun noch die Beziehung der Entzündung zur nervösen und humoralen Steuerung betrachten, wie sie uns aus den Arbeiten von HOFF (1930), SELYE (1949, 1951, 1953), TONUTTI (1951, 1953) u. a. ersichtlich ist, so ergibt sich, daß auch die parenterale Verdauung, obwohl im wesentlichen ein örtlich begrenzter Prozeß, doch nicht nur von dieser lokalen Seite her betrachtet werden darf, sondern in den Rahmen einer höheren Ordnung eingefügt werden muß.

Wenn schon der parenteralen Verdauung bei der banalen, der normergischen Entzündung, eine solche Bedeutung zukommt, wieviel mehr muß dies dann bei der hyperergischen Entzündung der Fall sein. Hier liegt es geradezu im Wesen der Entzündung begründet, daß parenteral in den Organismus gelangte Stoffe auch parenteral verdaut werden und nun die Umstimmung des Organismus hervorrufen, so daß dieser, wenn er mit dem betreffenden Stoff nochmals in entsprechende Berührung kommt, überempfindlich reagiert. Daß diese allergische Reaktion sich in erster Linie in Form einer hyperergischen Entzündung manifestiert, beweisen uns menschliche allergische Krankheiten wie Bronchialasthma, Heuschnupfen, Urticaria, Ekzeme u. a. Die Stoffe, gegen die der Organismus überempfindlich geworden ist, können recht verschiedenartig sein, wenn es sich auch meist um Eiweißsubstanzen wie Gräserpollen, Schimmelsporen, Hautschuppen, Federn oder Tierhaare u. dgl. handelt. Neben solchen unbelebten spielen aber auch belebte Stoffe eine Rolle, wobei es auch hier die wiederholte Berührung mit bestimmten Substanzen ist, die die hyperergischen Entzündungserscheinungen hervorruft. Wir können uns den Prozeß wohl kaum anders vorstellen, als daß aus der parenteralen Verdauung dieser Allergene Antikörper entstehen, die zellständig sind, so daß nun jeder neue Kontakt mit dem Allergen zu einer Reizung der antikörpertragenden Zellen führt. Hierdurch werden dann die Antigen-Antikörperreaktionen ausgelöst, die bei entsprechender Reizbeantwortung des Organismus zur Krankheit führen. Eine wesentliche Rolle spielt dabei allerdings die Konstitution des Individuums.

Solche hyperergische Entzündungen kennen wir auch als Folge parenteraler Eiweißinjektionen, wie sie zu therapeutischen Zwecken oder im Tierexperiment vorgenommen werden. Die bekannteste Form einer solchen hyperergischen Entzündung ist beim Menschen die Serumkrankheit, wenn es sich dabei auch um ein verhältnismäßig seltenes Ereignis handelt.

Bei Seruminjektionen zur passiven Immunisierung treten gelegentlich schon nach der ersten Seruminjektion mehr oder weniger schwere Reaktionen auf, die sich bereits am 1. Tag einstellen können, die man in der Regel jedoch erst zwischen dem 6. und 10. Tag beobachtet. Es entstehen Urticaria, Ödeme der Haut, seltener der Schleimhäute, und oftmals Fieber. Der Blutdruck ist erniedrigt, der Puls beschleunigt. Die Lymphknoten sind geschwollen. Häufig stellen sich Schmerzen in der Muskulatur und den Gelenken ein; in seltenen Fällen kommt es zum Kollaps. Wie diese Erscheinungen entstehen, ist nicht ganz klar. Bei den sofort auftretenden Veränderungen hat man eine Überempfindlichkeit vermutet, wobei freilich meist eine Erklärung für diese Überempfindlichkeit fehlt. Bei der innerhalb von 6—11 Tagen einsetzenden Serumkrankheit hat bekanntlich bereits Pirquet (1910) angenommen, daß es sich um eine Antigen-Antikörperreaktion handelt, eine Ansicht, die auch heute noch gilt.

Oft tritt die Serumkrankheit des Menschen jedoch nach wiederholter Injektion artfremden Eiweißes auf. Auch dabei kann es, aber nur sehr selten, zum Serumschock kommen. Viel häufiger sind dagegen die bereits oben beschriebenen Erscheinungen der Serumkrankheit. Dabei handelt es sich zweifellos um Antigen-Antikörperreaktionen, die wiederum in Zusammenhang mit der parenteralen Verdauung des artfremden Eiweißes stehen, wobei eine Freisetzung kreislaufwirksamer bzw. entzündungserregender Stoffe erfolgt[1].

In ähnlicher Weise wie die beim Menschen auftretenden allergischen Krankheiten nach einmaliger oder häufiger wiederholter parenteraler Verdauung artfremden Eiweißes stellen sich auch bei manchen Tierarten, die dafür empfindlich sind, nach wiederholter experimenteller Eiweißzufuhr Veränderungen ein, die mit denjenigen des Menschen eine mehr oder weniger große Ähnlichkeit haben. Man spricht auch hier von allergisch-hyperergischer oder besser von anaphylaktischer Entzündung, um damit das Künstliche dieser Zustände hervorzuheben. Das bekannteste Beispiel der von Richet 1902 entdeckten Anaphylaxie ist das Arthussche Phänomen, das nach wiederholter Injektion von artfremdem Eiweiß in die Haut von Kaninchen oder Meerschweinchen entsteht. Man darf wohl annehmen, daß es sich hierbei um ein besonders auffallendes Beispiel einer lokalen Stoffverarbeitung, einer parenteralen Verdauung handelt; Rössle (1914, 1933, 1936) sieht den Zweck dieses Phänomens darin, daß durch die Schwere der Entzündung das Abströmen von Eiweiß in die Blutbahn und damit das Auftreten schwerer Allgemeinerscheinungen verhindert werden soll. Das ist zweifellos eine gute teleologische Erklärung, die obendrein auch mit der kausalen übereinstimmt; macht doch nach Menkin (1950) die Blockade der Lymph- und Blutgefäße durch Thromben und Fibrinbarrieren einen Abstrom unmöglich, und das Antigen wird somit an Ort und Stelle fixiert.

Wenn hier bisher davon die Rede war, daß solche anaphylaktischen Reaktionen durch Zufuhr artfremden Eiweißes hervorgerufen werden, so treten sie doch nicht allein im Verlauf von Fremdeiweißzufuhr auf. Letterer (1953) hat darauf hingewiesen, daß „nicht die Artfremdheit an sich, sondern der biologische Vorgang der verdauenden cellulären Arbeitsleistung das Maßgebende ist für die Hervorrufung einer anaphylaktischen Entzündung".

Er hatte in früheren Versuchen, ebenso wie sein Schüler Geissendörfer (1932), zeigen können, daß nach wiederholter Injektion von arteigenem Bluteiweiß das erstinjizierte Blut symptomlos versickert, während die zweite Injektion eine deutliche mit Ödem und

---

[1] Heinlein 1936, 1937, 1939, Menkin 1950.

Zellaustritten verbundene anaphylaktische Entzündung bewirkt. Auch HEINLEIN und MUSCHALLIK (1937) kamen mit der Injektion von Eigenserum bei Kaninchen zu ähnlichen Ergebnissen und stellten außer der lokalen Reaktion Veränderungen des Bluteiweißes fest, die in schwächerer Form den nach der Injektion von artfremdem Eiweiß entstandenen glichen.

Diese Beobachtungen sind ein Beweis dafür, daß die parenterale Verdauung auch hierbei von Bedeutung ist.

Auch die sog. spezifischen Entzündungen, von denen RÖSSLE geäußert hat, daß sie ihm auf allergische Genese verdächtig seien, haben sehr enge Beziehungen zur parenteralen Verdauung. Gerade die großzellige Granulombildung, die RÖSSLE mit den Epitheloid- und Riesenzellformen so verdächtig erschien, ist ein Beweis für eine intensive, wenn auch vielleicht besonders schwierige intracelluläre Verdauung. Am besten sehen wir das vielleicht am Beispiel der Tuberkulose. Es ist bekannt, daß tuberkulöses Granulationsgewebe nicht nur durch lebende, sondern auch durch abgetötete Tuberkelbacillen und daraus entstandene chemisch definierbare Substanzen hervorgerufen werden kann. Man braucht hier nur das A 3-Phosphatid von ANDERSON zu nennen. Mit dem Magnesiumsalz einer Phosphatidsäure, die dem A 3-Phosphatid von ANDERSON zugrunde liegt, konnte ROULET (1934, 1936) Granulome erzeugen, die histologisch Tuberkeln glichen. Nach den Untersuchungen amerikanischer Autoren gibt jede der drei Hauptkomponenten der Fettfraktion der Tuberkelbacillen, nämlich ein Phosphatid, ein acetonlösliches Fett und ein Wachs, eine charakteristische Gewebsreaktion.

Wenn man Kaninchen eine Suspension des Phosphatids in Wasser in die Bauchhöhle injizierte, so erfolgte innerhalb weniger Stunden eine Phagocytose des Lipoids durch Monocyten. Während der nächsten 3—4 Tage erschien das Fett in Form großer Vacuolen in den Zellen, zerteilte sich jedoch allmählich in immer feinere Vacuolen, so daß das Cytoplasma am 5.—7. Tag schaumig erschien. Bei Beginn der 3. Woche wurden Epitheloidzellen beobachtet, und danach bildeten sich rasch typische Langhanssche Riesenzellen. Anscheinend ist es die in allen Komponenten der Fettfraktion vorhandene Fettsäure, die Phthionsäure, die diese Epitheloid- und Riesenzellenreaktion bewirkt.

Man gewinnt jedoch aus den Untersuchungen von CATEL und SCHMIDT (1950) den Eindruck, daß nicht allein die Phthionsäure eine solche Reaktion hervorrufen kann, sondern daß auch Eiweißfraktionen aus den Tuberkelbacillen dazu imstande sind. Denn CATEL und SCHMIDT konnten mit gereinigtem Tuberkulin (GT Höchst), einem reinen Eiweißkörper, Epitheloidzellentuberkel hervorrufen. Auch BETTE (1953) sah nach Injektion der wasserlöslichen Fraktion von Tuberkelbacillen die stärkste Reaktion in Lymphknoten, und zwar in Form einer Aktivierung der Reticulumzellen mit Produktion zahlreicher histiocytärer Elemente, Epitheloidzellen und vergrößerter Endothelzellen. Bei den Kontrollen waren allerdings solche Zellen auch nach Anwendung von Lipoidfraktionen nachzuweisen.

Ähnliche Verhältnisse dürften auch für die cellulären Verdauungsvorgänge bei anderen sog. spezifischen Entzündungen, wie z. B. der Lues, der Lepra, der Lymphogranulomatose, vorliegen.

Es scheint sich dabei nicht um Vorgänge zu handeln, die für diese Erkrankungen spezifisch sind, sondern darum, daß die Erreger dieser Krankheiten bzw. ihre Stoffwechselprodukte so hohe Anforderungen an den cellulären Verdauungsapparat stellen. Vielleicht spielt dabei nicht nur die chemische Natur der Stoffe, sondern auch ihre Molekülgröße eine Rolle. Man könnte dies jedenfalls aus Untersuchungen von SCHALLOCK (1953) schließen, wonach die großen Globulinmoleküle die Bildung von epitheloidzellenähnlichen Histiocyten, sehr großen Histiocyten und Riesenzellen anregen.

Schlußbetrachtung.

Aus dieser Übersicht über die parenterale Verdauung, die viele Beziehungen nur andeuten konnte, da sich sonst zu große Überschneidungen mit anderen Kapiteln ergeben hätten, dürfte hervorgehen, daß die parenterale Verdauung eine recht bedeutungsvolle Rolle im Krankheitsgeschehen spielt. Es handelt sich dabei nicht um ein Schlagwort, das Metschnikoff erfand, und das dann wieder in Vergessenheit geriet, sondern um einen Begriff, der einen biologischen Vorgang eindeutig umschreibt. Über den Umfang des Begriffes „Parenterale Verdauung" wird man freilich verschiedener Meinung sein können, ebenso wie darüber, wieviel davon noch hypothetisch ist. Aus diesem Grunde wäre es sehr wünschenswert, wenn mit modernen Methoden, wobei besonders an die Markierung der Stoffe mit radioaktiven Isotopen zu denken wäre, manche Versuche nachgeprüft und erweitert würden. Dadurch könnte vieles aus dem Bereich der Hypothese auf den Boden der gesicherten Tatsache gestellt werden und die „Parenterale Verdauung" in Biologie und Pathologie noch mehr an Bedeutung gewinnen.

Literatur.

Abdou, J. A., and H. Tarver: Plasma protein; loss from circulation and catabolism to carbon dioxide. J. of Biol. Chem. 190, 769, 781 (1951). — Albright, F., A. F. Forbes, F. C. Bartter, E. C. Reifenstein jr., D. Bryant, L. D. Cox and E. F. Dempsey: Symposia on Nutrition 2, 155 (1950). — Alden, G. H.: Implantation of the rat egg. Amer. J. Anat. 83, 143 (1948). — Anitsckow, N.: Zur Frage der Verteilung intravenös eingeführter Kolloidsubstanzen im Organismus. Klin. Wschr. 1924 II, 1729. — Apitz, K.: Die Leukämien als Neubildungen. Virchows Arch. 299, 1. ~ Über die Bildung Russelscher Körperchen in den Plasmazellen multipler Myelome. Virchows Arch. 300, 113. ~ Die Paraproteinosen. Über die Störung des Eiweißstoffwechsels bei Plasmacytomen. Virchows Arch. 306, 631 (1940). ~ Allgemeine Pathologie der menschlichen Leukämien. Erg. Path. 35, 1 (1940). ~ Die neuen Anschauungen vom Plasmocytom des Knochenmarks, dem sog multiplen Myelom. Klin. Wschr. 1940 II, 1025. ~ Die Störungen des Eiweißstoffwechsels bei Plasmocytomträgern. Klin. Wschr. 1940, 1058. ~ Über Profibrin; die Agglutination von Blutplättchen durch Profibrin. Z. exper. Med. 105, 89 (1939). — Arndt, H. J.: Reticuloendothel und Amyloid. Verh. dtsch. path. Ges. (26. Tagg) 1931, 243. — Aschoff, L.: Das reticuloendotheliale System. Erg. inn. Med. 26, 1 (1924). ~ Vorträge über Pathologie. Jena: Gustav Fischer 1925. ~ Morphologie des reticuloendothelialen Systems. In Schittenhelms Handbuch der Krankheiten des Blutes und der blutbildenden Organe, Bd. II, S. 473. Berlin: Springer 1925. ~ Referat über die Monocytenentstehung auf der 1. Internat. Haemat. Tagg, Münster 1937. Disk.bem. Verh. dtsch. path. Ges. (26. Tagg) 1931, 149. — Aschoff, L., u. K. Kiyono: Zur Frage der großen Mononukleären. Fol. haemat. (Lpz.) 15, 383 (1913). ~ Ein Beitrag zur Lehre von den Makrophagen. Verh. dtsch path. Ges. 16, 107 (1913).

Bauer, J.: Modellversuche zur Koagulationsnekrose. Frankf. Z. Path. 57, 122 (1943). — Bennhold, H.: Über die Vehikelfunktion der Serumeiweißkörper. Erg. inn. Med. 42, 273 (1932). — Berger, W.: Das Verhalten des Serumproteins nach Seruminjektionen. Schweiz. med. Wschr. 1922, 225. ~ Über die Hyperproteinämie nach Eiweißinjektionen. Ein experimenteller Beitrag zur Pathologie des Serumproteins und zur Proteinkörpertherapie. Z. exper. Med. 28, 1 (1922). — Berthold: Über die Transplantation der Hoden. Göttinger Nachr. 1849, Nr 1. — Bette, H.: Über die Tuberkulose der Lymphknoten. Histologische Untersuchungen über die Wirkung der Tuberkulosebazillen am Retikulum der Lymphknoten. Inaug.-Diss. Münster 1953. — Bieling, R.: Immunitätsvorgänge bei akuter und chronischer Sepsis und die Entstehung rheumatischer Erkrankungen. Ann. Tomarkin Foundation 2 (1932). — Bieling, R., u. S. Isaac: Experimentelle Untersuchungen über die intravitale Haemolyse. II. Der Verlauf der intravitalen Haemolyse nach Milzexstirpation. Z. exper. Med. 26 (1922). ~ Experimentelle Untersuchungen über intravitale Haemolyse. III. Der Mechanismus der Ausscheidung artfremder und vergifteter arteigener Blutkörperchen. Z. exper. Med. 28 (1922). ~ Experimentelle Untersuchungen über intravitale Haemolyse. IV. Die Bedeutung des Reticuloendothels. Z. exper. Med. 28 (1922). — Bing, J.: Further investigations on hyperglobulinemia. (Occurence and degree of hyperglobulinemia in various diseases. Ratio between hyperglobulinemia, hyperproteinemia and hypoalbuminemia. Formolgelreaktion.) Acta med. scand. (Stockh). 103, 547 (1940. ~ Further investigations on hyperglobulinemia. (Is serumglobulin formed from plasma cells and reticulo endothelial cells ?) Acta med. scand. (Stockh.)

103, 565 (1940). — Bing, J., u. P. Plum: Serum proteins in leucopenia. (Contribution on question about place of formation of serum proteins.) Acta med. scand. (Stockh.) **92**, 415 (1937). — Bjørneboe, M., u. H. Gormsen: Untersuchungen über das Vorkommen von Plasmazellen bei experimenteller Hyperglobulinaemie bei Kaninchen. Klin. Wschr 1941 I, 314. — Bloom, W.: Ergebnisse der Züchtungsversuche von Blut und blutbildenden Organen. In Handbuch der allgemeinen Haematologie, Bd. 1, S. 1179. Berlin u. Wien: Urban & Schwarzenberg 1933. — Büngeler, W.: Experimentelle Untersuchungen über die Monocyten des Blutes und ihre Genese aus dem Reticulo-Endothel. Beitr. path. Anat. **76**, 181 (1926). ~ Experimentelle Untersuchungen über die Monocyten des Blutes und ihre Genese aus dem Reticulo-Endothel. Verh. dtsch. path. Ges. **21**, 308 (1926). ~ Die Wirkung der parenteralen Eiweißzufuhr auf das qualitative Blutbild des Kaninchens. Frankf. Z. Path. **34**, 350 (1926). ~ Der Organstoffwechsel bei Gewebsaktivierung und Anaphylaxie. Verh. dtsch. path. Ges. (25. Tagg) **1930**, 125. ~ Die Blutmonocyten im entzündlichen Exsudat und Granulationsgewebe. Verh. dtsch. path. Ges. (26. Tagg) **1931**, 148. ~ Geschwülste und regulierte abhängige Wachstumsstörungen (Hyperplasien), im Rahmen der Zellular- und Relationspathologie. Z. Krebsforsch. **58**, 72 (1951). ~ Die Definition des Geschwulstbegriffes und die Abgrenzung der Hyperplasien gegenüber den Geschwülsten. Verh. dtsch. Ges. Path. (35. Tagg) **1951**, 11. — Büngeler, W., u. W. Rotter: Blut und blutbildende Organe. In Lehrbuch der speziellen pathologischen Anatomie, herausgeg. von M. Staemmler. Berlin: W. de Gruyter & Co. 1955. — Burnet, F. M.: Production of Antibodies. Melbourne 1949.

Cain, H.: Hemmung des Eintrittes der Koagulationsnekrose an Implantaten durch Oxalat und durch Fermentgifte. Frankf. Z. Path. **58**, 171 (1944). — Cargill, W. H., and H. D. Bruner: Metabolism of C¹⁴-labeled dextran in the mouse. J. of Pharmacol. **103**, 339 (1951). — Carrel, A. U., and C. A. Lindbergh: Culture of whole organs. Science (Lancaster, Pa.) **81**, 621 (1935). — Caspersson, T. O.: Cell growth and cell function. New York 1950. — Catel, W., u. W. Schmidt: Klinische experimentelle Untersuchungen über das Wesen der lokalen Tuberkulinempfindlichkeit. Dtsch. med. Wschr. **1950**, 1140. — Coats: Zit nach Boyd, Pathology of internal diseases, 4. Philadelphia 1947. — Cohn, E.: Chemical, physiological and immunological properities and clinical use of blood derivates. Experientia (Basel) **3**, 125 (1947). — Coons, A. H., u. M. H. Kaplan: Localization of antigen in tissue cells. Improvements in method for delection of antigen by means of fluorecent antibody. J. of Exper. Med. **91**, 1 (1950). — Craddock jr., Ch. G., W. N. Valentine and J. S. Lawrence: The lymphocyte. Studies on its relationship to immunologic processes in the cat. J. Labor. a. Clin. Med. **34**, 158 (1949). — Cunningham, R. S., F. R. Sabin and C. A. Doan: The development of leucocytes, lymphocytes and monocytes from a specific stem cell in adult tissues. Contrib. Embryolog. **1925**, No 82.

Danielsen, W.: Über die Schutzvorrichtungen in der Bauchhöhle mit besonderer Berücksichtigung der Resorption. Beitr. klin. Chir. **54**, 458 (1907). — Dempster, W. J.: Observation on behavior of transplanted kidney in dogs. Ann. Roy. Coll. Surg. **7**, 275 (1950). ~ Problems involved in homotransplantation of tissues, with particular reference to skin. Brit. Med. J. **1951**, 1041. — Denys, J.: Compte-rendu des travaux exècutes sur le streptococcoque pyogène. Zbl. Bakt. (Jena) **24**, 685—691 (1898). — Denys, I., et I. Leclez: Sur le mechanisme de l'immunité chez le lapin vacciné contre le streptocoque pyogène. Cellule **11**, 175 (1895). — Dietrich, A.: Allgemeine Pathologie und Pathologische Anatomie. Leipzig: S. Hirzel 1943. ~ Die Entwicklung der Lehre von der Thrombose und Embolie seit Virchow. Virchows Arch. **235**, 212 (1921). ~ Thrombopathie mit parietaler Hirnthrombose und paradoxer Embolie. Virchows Arch. **254**, 830 (1925). ~ Endothelreaktion und Thrombose. Münch. med. Wschr. **1929**, 272. ~ Wesen und Bedingungen der Thrombose und Embolie. Klin. Wschr. **1931**, 54. ~ Thrombose, ihre Grundlage und ihre Bedeutung. Berlin: Springer 1932. ~ Gefäßwand und Thrombose. Dtsch. Ges. Kreislaufforsch. **7** (1934). ~ Allergische Reaktionen an Gefäßen. Verh. dtsch. Ges. Path. (30. Tagg) **1937**, 142. ~ Thrombose als reaktiver Vorgang. Münch. med. Wschr. **1939**, 1599. — Reaktive Thrombose im Tierversuch. Virchows Arch. **307**, 821 (1941). — Domagk, G.: Untersuchungen über die Bedeutung des Retikulo-Endothelialen Systems für die Vernichtung von Infektionserregern und für die Entstehung des Amyloids. Virchows Arch. **253**, 594 (1924). — Dominici, H.: Etudes sur le tissu conjonctif et les organes hématopoétiques des mammifères. Arch. d'Anat. microsc. **17**, 9 (1920/21). — Denys: Compte rendu des traveaux exécutés sur le streptocoque pyogène. Zbl. Bakter. Orig. **24**, 685 (1898). — Donath, J., u. R. Heilig: Über das Verhalten des Aminostickstoffes im künstlichen und natürlichen Fieber. Klin. Wschr. **1924**, 834. — Downey, H. u. F. Weidenreich: Über die Bildung der Lymphocyten in Lymphdrüsen und Milz. IX. Fortsetzung über die Studien über das Blut und die blutbildenden und blutzerstörenden Organe. Arch. mikroskop. Anat. **80**, 306 (1912). — Dubois-Ferrière, H.: La fonction des plasmocytes. Schweiz. med. Wschr. **1943**, 1346. ~ La genèse et la fonction des plasmocytes. Sang **19**, 574 (1948). — Duesberg: Contribution à l'étude des phénomènes histologiques de la métamorphose chez les amphibiens anoures. Archives de Biol. **22** (1906/07).

Eckardt, R. D., and C. S. Davidson: Sympiosa on nutrition. 2, 275 (1950). — Ehrhardt, C., u. C. Kittel: Zur Behandlung hypophysärer Störungen durch Hypophysenimplantation. Z. klin. Med. 132, H. 2 (1937). — Ehrich, W. E.: Die Leukocyten und ihre Entstehung. Erg. Path. 29, 1 (1934). ~ Die cellulären Bildungsstätten der Antikörper. Verh. dtsch. Naturforsch. 1955. — Ehrich, W. E., D. L. Drabkin and C. Forman: Nucleic acid and production of antibody by plasma cells. J. of Exper. Med. 90, 157 (1949). — Ehrich, W. E., T. N. Harris and E. Mertens: The absence of antibody in the macrophages during maximum antibody formation. J. of Exper. Med. 83, 373 (1946). — Ewald, W.: Zur Morphologie der Immunitätsreaktion mit besonderer Berücksichtigung des Gefäßendothels. Beitr. path. Anat. 83, 681 (1930).

Fagraeus, A.: The plasma cellular reaction and its relation to formation of antibodies in vitro. J. of Immun. 58, 1 (1948). — Fawcett, D. W., G. B. Wislocki and Ch. M. Waldo: The development of mouse ova in the anterior chamber of the eye and in the abdominal cavity. Amer. J. Anat. 81, 413 (1947). — Fenn, W. O.: Effect of the hydrogen ion concentration on the phagocytosis and adhesiveness of leucocytes. J. Gen. Physiol. 5, 169—179 (1923). — Filatov, V. P.: La thérapie tissulaire. Traitement par les stimulateurs biogènes. Med. franç. 9, 293 (1949). — Fischer, A.: Die Beteiligung der Blutproteine am Stoffwechsel der Gewebe. Biol. Rev. Cambridge Philos. Soc. 22, 178 (1947). — Fleischhacker, R., u. R. Klima: Beitrag zur Kenntnis des multiplen Myeloms der plasmacellulären Leukämie und des plasmazellulären Granuloms. Mit besonderer Berücksichtigung der bioptischen Knochenmarksuntersuchung. Fol. haemat. (Lpz.) 56, 5 (1936). — Fresen, O.: Zur Histomorphologie des Reticulo-Endothelialen Systems. Klin. Wschr. 1946, 24—25, 100. ~ Die Pathomorphologie des Retothelialen Systems. Verh. dtsch. Ges. Path. (37. Tagg) 1954, 26. — Friedemann, U., u. S. Isaac: Weitere Untersuchungen über parenteralen Eiweißstoffwechsel, Immunität und Überempfindlichkeit. Z. exper. Path. 4 (1907).

Gaza, W. v.: Wundheilung, Transplantation, Regeneration und Parabiose bei höheren Säugern und beim Menschen. In Handbuch der normalen und pathologischen Physiologie, Bd. 14/1. Berlin: Springer 1926. — Geissendörfer, H.: Über die Erzeugung geweblicher Überempfindlichkeit nach wiederholter Einspritzung arteigenen Blutes bei Meerschweinchen. Virchows Arch. 285, 385 (1932). — Gibson, T., and P. B. Medawar: Fate of skin homografts in men. J. of Anat. 77, 299 (1943). — Goldmann, E. E.: Eine ölhaltige Dermoidcyste mit Riesenzellen. Beitr. path. Anat. 7, 553 (1890). — Gregg, L. A., and O. H. Robertson: On the nature of bacteriemia in experimental pneumococcal pneumonie in the dog. II. Disappearance of pneumococci from the circulation in relation to the bactericidal action of the blood in vitro. J. of Exper. Med. 97, 297 (1953). — Gross, W.: Über Eiweißspeicherung in der Leber. Verh. dtsch. path. Ges. 21, 26 (1922). — Grote, L. R., u. B. Fischer-Wasels: Über totale Alymphocytose. Münch. med. Wschr. 1929, 2040.

Haemerli, M.: Spielt die „Surface phagocytosis" in der Sulfonamidtherapie die ihr von Wood zugedachte Rolle? Schweiz. Z. Path. u. Bakter. 12, 289 (1949). — Harris, T. N., E. Grimm, E. Mertens and W. E. Ehrich: The role of the lymphocyte in antibody formation. J. of Exper. Med. 81, 73 (1945). — Haurowitz, F., u. F. Breinl: Quantitative Untersuchungen der Verteilung eines arsenhaltigen Antigens im Organismus. Z. physiol. Chem. 205, 259 (1932). — Haurowitz, F., and C. F. Crampton: Fate in rabbits of intravenously injected I^{131}-iodoovalbumin. J. of Immun. 68, 73—85 (1952). — Haurowitz, F., u. F. Kraus: Die Verteilung chemisch markierter Antigene im Organismus normaler und sensibilisierter Tier. Z. physiol. Chem. 239, 76 (1936). — Heidelberger, N., H. P. Treffers, R. Schoenheimer, S. Ratner and D. Rittenberg: Behavior of antibody protein toward dietary nitrogen inactive and passive immunity. J. of Biol. Chem. 144, 555 (1942). — Heilbrunn, L. V.: An Outline of general physiology. Philadelphia: W. B. Saunders Company 1943, 1948. — Heinlein, H.: Chronische Histaminvergiftung und Entzündung. Virchows Arch. 296, 448 (1935). ~ Entzündung und körpereigene Wirkstoffe. 1. Mitt. Histamin und Acetylcholin. Beitr. path. Anat. 108, 58 (1943). ~ 2. Mitt. Adenylsäure und Leukotaxin. Frankf. Z. Path. 57, 316 (1943). ~ Reticuloendothel und Fibrinogenbildung. Verh. dtsch. path. Ges. 27, 177 (1934). ~ Das Verhalten der Bluteiweißkörper bei parenteraler Zufuhr von Eiweiß- und Nichteiweißkolloiden. Arch. exper. Path. u. Pharmakol. 179, 127 (1935). ~ Organveränderungen bei parenteraler Zufuhr von Eiweiß- und Nichteiweißkolloiden. Virchows Arch. 299, 667 (1937). ~ Morphologische Veränderungen durch parenterale Eiweißzufuhr. Erg. Hyg. 20, 274 (1937). ~ Die Bluteiweißbildung. Z. exper. Med. 112, 535 (1943). ~ Organveränderungen durch körpereigene kreislaufwirksame Substanzen. Verh. dtsch. Ges. Path. (29. Tagg) 1936, 93. — Heinlein, H., u. G. Hübner: Nachweis des Peristons in Blut, Harn und Gewebe. Beitr. path. Anat. 119, 301 (1958). — Heinlein, H., u. J. Korth: Tierexperimentelle Untersuchungen mit verschiedenen Blutersatzmitteln. Zbl. Path. 93, 82 (1955). — Heinlein, H., J. Korth, W. Flacke u. A. Zimmer: Die Pathogenese der Organschädigung bei experimenteller Diphtherie. Z. exper. Med. 123, 511 (1954). — Heinlein, H., J. Korth u. A. Zimmer: Über die Möglichkeit der Entgiftung des Organismus durch Periston N.

Ärztl. Wschr. 1957, 174. — HEINLEIN, H., u. H. W. MUSCHALLIK: Blut- und Organveränderungen durch parenterale Zufuhr von Eigenserum. Klin. Wschr. 1937 I, 873. — HEINLEIN, H., u. A. ZIMMER: Tierexperimentelle Untersuchungen über Speichererscheinungen nach Verabreichung verschiedener Blutersatzmittel. Zbl. Path. 93, 82 (1955). — HEINZEL, W.: Entzündung und allergisch-hyperergische Reaktion bei Mollusken (untersucht an der Hainschnecke). Virchows Arch. 317, 138 (1949/50). — HENNING, R.: Spezielle Pathologie des Sternalmarks in vivo. Med. Welt. 1938 I, 90. — HERINGA, G.: Untersuchungen über den Bau und die Bedeutung des Bindegewebes. Z. mikrosk.-anat. Forsch. 1, 607 (1924). — HIRSCH, G. C.: Die Lebensäußerungen der Tiere. In Handbuch der Biologie. Konstanz: Akademische Verlagsgesellschaft Athenaion 1955. — HJORTH, P.: Investigations of thermostabile baktericidal substance in human serum, demonstrated partikulary in serum of fever patients. Acta path. scand. (Københ.) 14, 412—426 (1937). ~ Preliminary report on baktericidal substances in normal human blood and thermostabil baktericidal substances exspecially in serum of fever patients. Ugeskr. Laeg. (dän.) 99, 192—201 (1937). ~ Studien über das X-Lysin, ein unter gewissen pathogenen Verhältnissen auftretendes thermostabiles Bakteriolysin. Z. Immun.forsch. 95, 360—379 (1939). — HOFF, F.: Unspezifische Therapie und natürliche Abwehrvorgänge. Berlin: Springer 1930. ~ Lehrbuch der speziellen pathologischen Physiologie. Jena: Gustav Fischer 1944. — HOMUTH, O.: Zur Kenntnis der Serumwirkung auf die innervierte Blutstrombahn nach Versuchen an lebenden Kaninchen. Z. exper. Med. 73, 251—281 (1930).

JAFFÉ, R. H.: Amyloidbildung bei Mäusen. Arch. of Path. 2, 149 (1926). — JANCSÓ, N.: Kolloidchemische Analyse des Speicherungsmechanismus reticulo-endothelialer Zellen mit Durchströmungsversuchen. Ber. Physiol. 81, 572 (1934). ~ Speicherung (Stoffanreicherung im Reticuloendothel und in der Niere). Budapest: Akadémiai Kladó 1955. ~ Storage of proteins and vinylpolymers in histiocytes and in the renal epithelium. Acta med. hung. 7, 173—210 (1955). — JANCSÓ, N., u. A. JANCSÓ-GABOR: Zelluläre Verteilung und Speicherungsmechanismus des „Bayer 205" (Germanin) in den Geweben. Acta physiol. hung. 3, 537 (1952). ~ Sichtbarmachung von Immunreaktionen in den Geweben. Acta physiol. hung. 3, 555 (1952). ~ Speicherung arteigener und artfremder Proteine in den Zellen des Reticuloendothels. Experientia (Basel) 8, 456 (1952). ~ Die Speicherung von Blutproteinen in den Histiocyten nach vorhergehender Histamineinwirkung. Experientia (Basel) 10, 256—258 (1954). — JANCSÓ-GABOR, A., u. N. JANCSÓ: Eiweißspeicherung in den Histiocyten beim Arthus-Phänomen. Schweiz. Z. allg. Path. 17, 585—591 (1954).

KÄRKI, N., T. SEPPÄLÄ u. P. L. HALONEN: Phagocytic activities of eosinophil leucocytes. Ann. med. exper. biol. et fenn. 197, 29 (1951). — KALLEE, E.. F. LOOHSS u. G. SEYBOLD: Albuminnachweis in Extracten von Lebermitochondrien. Verh. dtsch. Ges. inn. Med., (60. Kongr.) 1954. — KANZOW, U.: Über das Vorkommen von Russelschen Körperchen und Eiweißkristallen bei chronischen Entzündungen. Frankf. Z. Path. 62, 232 (1951). — KAPLAN, M. H., A. H. COONS and H. W. DEANE: Localization of antigens in tissue cells; cellular distribution of pneumococcal polysaccharides types II and III in mouse. J. of Exper. Med. 91, 15 (1950). — KATSURA, S.: Die Resorption der Farbstofflösungen aus der Bauch- und Pleurahöhle, mit besonderer Berücksichtigung des Ductus lymphaticus dexter. Tohoku J. Exper. Med. 5, 294 (1924). — KIYONO, K.: Die vitale Karminspeicherung. Jena 1914. ~ Zur Frage der histiocytären Blutzellen. Fol. haemat. (Lpz.) 18, 149 (1914). — KJÖLLERFELDT, M.: Untersuchungen über die Resorption des Eiweißes und einiger seiner Abbauprodukte in der Bauchhöhle des Kaninchens. Biochem. Z. 82, 188 (1917). — KLINGE, F.: Über die hyperergische (anaphylaktische) Entzündung. Klin. Wschr. 1927 II, 2265. ~ Die Merkmale der hyperergischen Entzündung. Klin. Wschr. 1927 I, 143. ~ Die Konstitution. 3. Ärztl. Fortbild.kurs, Bad-Salzuflen. Leipzig: Georg Thieme 1935. ~ Experimentelle Erzeugung von Arthritis deformans. Verh. dtsch. path. Ges. (26. Tagg) 1931, 216. — KNAUER, E.: Zur Ovarientransplantation. (Geburt am normalen Ende der Schwangerschaft nach Ovarientransplantation beim Kaninchen). Zbl. Gynäk. 8, 201 (1898).— KOST, G. F. W.: Das Schicksal eingeschwemmter Krebszellen in der Lunge. Z. Krebsforsch. 43, 291 (1936). — KREHL, L., u. M. MATTHES: Über die Wirkung von Albuminosen verschiedener Herkunft sowie einiger diesen nahestehenden Substanzen. Arch. exper. Path. 36, 437 (1895). — KRUSE, H., and P. D. McMASTER: Distribution and storage of blue antigenic azoproteins in tissues of mice. J. of Exper. Med. 90, 425 (1949). — KUCZYNSKI, M. H.: ERWIN GOLDMANNs Untersuchungen über zelluläre Vorgänge im Gefolge des Verdauungsprozesses. Virchows Arch. 239, 185 (1922). ~ Neue Beiträge zur Lehre vom Amyloid. Klin. Wschr. 1923 I, 727. ~ Weitere Beiträge zur Lehre vom Amyloid. Über die Rückbildung des Amyloides. Klin. Wschr. 1923 II, 2193. — KUSAMA, ST. H.: Über Aufbau und Entstehung der toxischen Thrombose und deren Bedeutung. Beitr. path. Anat. 55, 459 (1913).

LAWLER, R. H., J. W. WEST, P. H. McNULTY, E. J. CLANCY and R. P. MURPHY: Homotransplantation of kidney in human, preliminary report. J. Amer. Med. Assoc. 144, 844

(1950). — Lehmann, W., u. H. Tammann: Transplantation und Vitalspeicherung. Bruns' Beitr. 135, 259 (1926). — Lerner, S. R., J. U. Chaikoff and C. Entenman: A fat emulsion for intravenous feeding. Proc. Soc. Exper. Biol. a. Med. 70, 388 (1949). — Letterer, E.: Studien über Art und Entstehung des Amyloids. Beitr. path. Anat. 75 (1926). ~ Versuche über Umstimmung der Gewebsreaktion nach wiederholter Injektion von arteigenem Eiweiß. Verh. dtsch. path. Ges. 1931, 199 .~ Neuere Untersuchungen über die Entstehung des Amyloids. Virchows Arch. 293, 34 (1934). ~ Ein Beitrag zur experimentellen Amyloidforschung. Verh. dtsch. path. Ges. 1925. ~ Speicherungskrankheiten. Dtsch. med. Wschr. 73, 147 bis 152 (1948). ~ Probleme der Speicherung und der Speicherkrankheiten. Ärztl. Forsch. 2, 137—141 (1948). ~ Untersuchungen über den Einfluß verschiedenartiger Ernährung auf die experimentelle Amyloidose. Zugleich ein Beitrag zur Frage der Antikörperbildung in Abhängigkeit von der Ernährung. Virchows Arch. 317 (1949). ~ Die Amyloidose im Lichte neuer Forschungsmethoden. Dtsch. med. Wschr. 1950, 15. ~ Über normergische und hyperergische Entzündung. Dtsch. med. Wschr. 78, 759 (1953). — Letterer, E., u. G. Schneider: Die Bedeutung des Bluteiweißbildes bei der Amyloidkrankheit. Plasma 1, 263 (1953). — Leupold, E.: Organabbau und seine organspezifische Wirkung. Z. exper. Med. 95, 235 (1935). ~ Organschädigung durch organeigene Abbaustoffe. Verh. dtsch. path. Ges. (27. Tagg) 1934, 250. — Leszler, A., u. L. Pauliczki: Untersuchungen über die Rolle des reticuloendothelialen Systems in der Fibrinogenbildung. Z. exper. Med. 91, 86 (1933). — Lewis, W. H.: Pinocytosis. Bull. Johns Hopkins Hosp. 49, 17 (1931). — Lindner, H.: Experimentelle Untersuchungen zum Abbau von Polysacchariden in Lymphknoten. Verh. dtsch. path. Ges. (37. Tagg) 1953, 197. — Linzbach, A. I.: Über die Entstehung der Riesenzellen und ihrer Einschlüsse in epitheloidzelligen Granulomen. Verh. dtsch. Ges. Path. (38. Tagg) 1954, 187. — Loeschcke, H.: Vorstellungen über das Wesen von Hyalin und Amyloid auf Grund von serologischen Versuchen. Beitr. path. Anat. 77, 231 (1927). ~ Experimentelle Untersuchungen über Saftstrom- und Resorptionswege. Virchows Arch. 292, 281—309 (1934). — Loeschke, H., u. E. Loeschcke: Pericyten, Grundhäutchen und Lymphscheiden der Kapillaren. Z. mikrosk.-anat. Forsch. 35, 533—550 (1934). — Longcope, W. T.: The production of experimental nephritis by repeated proteid intoxication. J. of Exper. Med. 18, 678 (1913). — Loss, A.: Über Degenerationserscheinungen im Tierreich. Preisschrift der fürstl. Jablonowschen Ges. Leipzig 1889.

Marchand, F.: Die örtlichen reaktiven Vorgänge. In Krehl-Marchands Handbuch der allgemeinen Pathologie, Bd. 4, 1. Abt. Leipzig 1924. — Masugi, A.: Über die Beziehungen zwischen Monocyten und Histiocyten. Beitr. path. Anat. 76, 396 (1926). — Maximow, A.: Bindegewebe und blutbildende Gewebe. In Handbuch der mikroskopischen Anatomie des Menschen, Bd. 2, Teil 1. Berlin 1927. ~ Das Mesenchym als Quelle der verschiedenen Arten der Bindesubstanzen des Blutes, der blutbildenden Gewebe und des Endothels. In Handbuch der mikroskopischen Anatomie des Menschen, Bd. 2. Berlin: Springer 1927. — McCutcheon, M.: Inflamation. Pathology (Anderson). St. Louis: C. V. Mosby Comp. 1948. — McNeil, C.: Cellular changes in rabbits during antibody formation; responds to Eberthella typhosa. Amer. J. Path. 24, 1271 (1948). ~ Cellular changes in rabbits during antibody formation; multiple antigen injections. J. of Immun. 65, 359 (1950). — Medawar, P. B.: Behavior and fate of skin autografts and skin homografts in rabbits. (Report to War Wounds Commitee of Medical Research Council.) J. of Anat. 78, 176 (1944). — Menkin, V.: Newer concepts of inflammation. Springfield: Ch. C. Thomas 1950. — Metschnikoff, E.: L'inflammation. Paris 1892. ~ Immunität bei Infektionskrankheiten. Jena: Gustav Fischer 1902. — Milbradt, W.: Zum Verhalten der Leber und des nicht koagulablen Stickstoffs bei erhöhtem Eiweißzerfall. Z. exper. Med. 95 (1936). — Miller, L. L., W. F. Bale, C. L. Yuile, R. E. Masters, G. H. Tishkoff and G. H. Whipple: Use of radioaktive lysine in studies of protein metabolism. Syntesis and utilization of plasma proteins. J. of Exper. Med. 90, 297 (1949). — Möllendorff, W. v.: Handbuch der mikroskopischen Anatomie des Menschen. Berlin: Springer 1927. — Moeschlin, S. V.: Die Herkunft der Blutplasmazellen bei der Hepatitis epidemica an Hand von Milzpunktaten. Gastroenterologia (Basel) 71, 97 (1946). ~ Untersuchungen über Genese und Funktion der Blutplasmazellen an Hand von Lymphdrüsen- und Sternalpunktaten bei Rubeolen. Helvet. med. Acta 7, 227 (1940). — Montmolin, B. de: Über sternförmige Einschlüsse, welche Elastinreaktion geben. Ihr häufiges Vorkommen bei der Boeckschen Krankheit. Zbl. Path. 81, 277 (1943). — Morawitz, P.: Beobachtungen über den Wiederersatz der Bluteiweißkörper. Beitr. chem. Physiol. u. Path. 7, 153 (1906).

Nägeli, O.: Probleme des Reticulo-Endothelialen Systems (RES) in klinischer Betrachtung. Dtsch. med. Wschr. 1936 I, 797. — Neufeld, F.: Bakteriotropine und Opsonine. In Kolle-Wassermanns Handbuch der pathologischen Mikroorganismen, 3. Aufl., Bd. 2, S. 929. 1929. — Niehans, P.: Biologische Behandlung kranker Organe durch Einspritzung lebender Zellen. Bern 1949.

Oliver, J.: Structure of metabolic process in nephron. J. Mt. Sinai Hosp. 15, 175—222 (1948).

PAGEL, W.: Retikuloendothel-Amyloid-Tbc. Zbl. Tbk.forsch. **29**, 257 (1928). — PENTIMALLI, F.: Über chronische Proteinvergiftung und die durch sie bewirkte Veränderung der Organe. Experimentelle Untersuchungen. Virchows Arch. **275**, 193 (1929). ~ Versuche zur experimentellen Erzeugung der Leukämien. Verh. dtsch path. Ges. (37. Tagg) **1953**, 221. — PETERS, G.: Paraproteinosen und Zentralnervensystem. Dtsch. Z. Nervenheilk. **161**, 359 (1949). — PETTERSON, A.: Über die bakteriziden Leukozytenstoffe und ihre Beziehung zur Immunität. Zbl. Bakter. **39**, 423 (1905). ~ Die auf den Pneumokokkus wirkenden bakteriolytischen Substanzen im Tierkörper. Z. Immun.forsch. **83**, 335—344 (1934). ~ Les anticorps protecteurs contre quelques microbes sensibles à la bakteriolysine β. Schweiz. med. Wschr. **66**, 1255—1256 (1936). ~ Die thermostabilen Bakteriolysine und ihre Beziehungen zu den Mikroben. Z. Immun.-forsch. **88**, 210 (1936). — PFEIFFER, H.: Beobachtungen über Eiweißzerfallstoxikose. Wien. klin. Wschr. **1921** I, 69. — PFEIFFER, H., u. F. STANDENATH: Über biologische Wirkungen und Folgen der Speicherung des Reticuloendothels. Z. ges. exp. Med. **37**, 184—248 (1923). — PFUHL, W.: Referat über die Monocytenfrage auf der 1. Internat. Haematol. Tagg, Münster 1937. ~ Die vitale Darstellung der kleinen Lymphgefäße durch Trypanblau und die wissenschaftliche Auswertung der Methode. Anat. Anz. **89**, 177—186 (1939). ~ Die Lymphgefäße im entzündeten Bindegewebe (Trypanblauversuch). Z. mikrosk.-anat. Forsch. **48**, 387 bis 404 (1940). — PFUHL, W., u. W. WIEGAND: Die Lymphgefäße des großen Netzes beim Meerschweinchen und ihr Verhalten bei intraperitonealer Trypanblauinjektion. Z. mikrosk.-anat. Forsch. **47**, (1939). — PICK, E. P., u. H. HASHIMOTO: Über den intravitalen Eiweißabbau in der Leber sensibilisierter Tiere und dessen Beeinflussung durch die Milz. Arch. exper. Path. **76**, 89 (1914). — PIRQUET, CL. V.: Allergie. Berlin: August Hirschwald 1910. — PISCHINGER, A.: Schicksal und Wirkung körperfremden Gewebes im Organismus. Medizinische **1953**, 767. — POLLISTER, A. W., and C. LEUCHTENBERGER: The nature of the specifity of methyl green for chromatin. Proc. Nat. Acad. Sci. U.S.A. **35**, 111 (1949). — POMMERENKE, W. T., H. B. SLAVIN, D. H. KARIHER and G. H. WHIPPLE: Bloodplasma protein regeneration controled by diet; systematic standardization of food proteins for potency in protein regeneration. Fasting and iron feeding. J. of Exper. Med. **61**, 261 (1935). — PUTNAM, T. J.: The living peritoneum as a dialyzing membrane. Amer. J. Physiol. **63**, 548 (1923).

RANDERATH, E.: Zur pathologischen Anatomie der sog. Amyloidnephrosen. Zugleich ein Beitrag zur Frage der allgemeinen Amyloidose als Paraproteinose. Virchows Arch. **314**, 388 (1947). ~ Die Morphologie der Paraproteinosen. Verh. dtsch. path. Ges. (32. Tagg) **1948**. — RANVIER, L.: Les éléments et les tissus du système conjonctif. J. de Micrograph **1888—1891**. — RAU, L.: Über Vorkommen, Bedeutung und Entstehung der Riesenzellen. Erg. Path. **26**, 229 (1932). — REINHARDT, E., u. G. RICKER: Kritik der Lehre von der cellularen und der humoralen Reizung der Hautstrombahn. Virchows Arch. **288**, 393—454 (1933). — RIBBERT, H.: Die Bedeutung der Entzündung. Bonn: Cohen 1922. — RICHET, Ch.: L'anaphylaxie. Paris 1911. — RITTER, A.: Über die Bedeutung des Endothels für die Entstehung der Venenthrombose. Jena: Gustav Fischer 1926. ~ Endothel und Thrombenbildung. Dtsch. med. Wschr. **1928** II. — ROBERTSON, O. H., L. T. COGGESHALL and E. E. TERRELL: Experimental pneumococcus lobar pneumonia in dog; pathology. J. Clin. Invest. **12**, 433 (1933). — RÖSSLE, R.: Referat über Entzündung. Verh. dtsch. path. Ges. (19. Tagg) **1923**. ~ Über die Merkmale der Entzündung im allergischen Organismus. Verh. dtsch. path. Ges. **17**, 281 (1914). ~ Allergie und Pathologie. Klin. Wschr. **1933**, 574. ~ Die morphologischen Äquivalente der Allergie. Acta rheum. **8** (1936). — ROGERS, D. E., and R. TOMPSETT: Survival of staphylococci within human leukocytes. J. of Exper. Med. **95**, 209 (1952). — ROHR, K.: Das menschliche Knochenmark, 2. Aufl. Stuttgart: Georg Thieme 1949. — ROTH, W.: Immun- und Oberflächenphagocytose bei bekapselten pathogenen Bakterien. Schweiz. Z. Path. u. Bakter. **13**, 1 (1950). — ROULET, F. C.: Studien zur Histogenese des tuberkulösen Granuloms. Virchows Arch. **294**, 262 (1934). ~ Weitere Untersuchungen zur Histogenese des tuberkulösen Granuloms. Verh. dtsch. path. Ges. (29. Tagg) **193**, 194. ~ Die infektiösen „spezifischen" Granulome. In Handbuch der allgemeinen Pathologie, Bd. VII/1. Berlin: Springer 1956.

SABIN, F. R.: Cellular reactions to dye-protein with concept of mechanism of antibody formation. J. of Exper. Med. **70**, 67 (1939). — SABIN, F. R., C. A. DOAN and R. S. CUNNINGHAM: The separation of the phagocytic cells of the peritoneal exsudate into two distinct types. Proc. Soc. Exper. Biol. a. Med. **21** (1924). — The discrimination of two types of phagocytic cells in the connective tissues by the supervital technique. Contrib. Embryol. **1925**, 82. — SCHAIRER, E.: Über den Untergang der Tumorzellen in der menschlichen und tierischen Leber. Verh. dtsch. path. Ges. **31**, 463 (1939). — SCHALLOCK, G.: Die experimentellen Retikulosen. Verh. dtsch. path. Ges. (37. Tagg) **1953**, 86. — SCHILLING, V.: Monocytenreferat auf der 1. Internat. Haematologentagg Münster, 1937. — SCHITTENHELM, A.: Zur Proteinkörpertherapie. Münch. med. Wschr. **1919**, 1403. ~ Zur Frage der Proteinkörpertherapie. Münch. med. Wschr. **1921**, 1476. ~ Theorie und Praxis der Proteinkörperwirkung. Med.

Klin. 1922, 549. — Schmidt, M. B.: Die Verbreitungswege der Carcinome. Jena 1903. ~ Referat über Amyloid. Verh. dtsch. path. Ges. (7. Tagg) 1904, 2. — Schmidt, R.: Über Proteinkörpertherapie und über parenterale Zufuhr von Milch. Med. Klin. 1916, 171. ~ Proteinkörpertherapie. In Neue Deutsche Klinik von G. Klemperer, Bd. 12, S. 411. Berlin: Urban & Schwarzenberg 1943. — Schneider, R., u. K. Huerler: Weiterer Beitrag zur Frage der Bildung und Wirkung der Leukine. Arch. f. Hyg. 81, 372 (1913). — Schoenheimer, R.: The dynamic state of body constituents. Cambridge, Mass. 1941. — Schörcher, F.: Bluttransfusion, Bluttransfusionsapparate und Blutersatzflüssigkeiten. Münch. med. Wschr. 1939 II, 1268. — Schulemann, W.: Die vitale Färbung mit sauren Farbstoffen in ihrer Bedeutung für die Anatomie, Physiologie, Pathologie und Pharmakologie. Biochem. Z. 80 (1917). ~ Vitalfärbung, Tabulae, Biolog. 4, 511 (1927). ~ Die Problematik des reticuloendothelialen Systems und seiner Funktionen. Verh. Dtsch. Pharmak. Ges. Leipzig 1930. — Seemann, G.: Über die Beziehungen zwischen Lymphocyten, Monocyten und Histiocyten, insbesondere bei Entzündungen. Beitr. path. Anat. 85, 303 (1930). ~ Über die Herkunft der sog. Polyblasten (Histiocyten und Makrophagen). Verh. dtsch. path. Ges. (25. Tagg) 1930, 77. ~ Über das Schicksal des ins Blut eingeführten Cholesterins, insbesondere über die Filtrations- und die Abwehrvorgänge im Lungengewebe. Beitr. path. Anat. 83, 705—718 (1930). — Seitzer, K., u. St. Sandkühler: Über die Phagocytosefähigkeit der Lymphocyten. Arch. klin. Med. 198, 612 (1951). — Selye, H.: Das allgemeine Adaptationssyndrom als Grundlage für eine einheitliche Theorie der Medizin. Dtsch. med. Wschr. 1951, 963. — The physiology and pathology of exposure to stress. Acta Inc. Med. Publ. Montreal 1950. ~ Textbook of endocrinology, 2. Aufl. Montreal 1949. ~ Der heutige Stand der Stress-Konzeption. Münch. med. Wschr. 1953, 15. — Seybold, G.: Die Bedeutung der Mitochondrien und der Plasmaproteine für die Vitalspeicherung. Habil.-Schr. Tübingen 1954. — Siegmund, H.: Speicherung durch Reticulo-Endothelien, zelluläre Reaktion und Immunität. Klin. Wschr. 1922 II, 2566. ~ Reizkörpertherapie und aktives mesenchymatisches Gewebe. Münch. med. Wschr. 1923 I, 5. ~ Untersuchungen über Immunität und Entzündung. Verh. dtsch. path. Ges. (19. Tagg) 1923, 314. ~ Gefäßveränderung bei chronischer Streptococcensepsis. (Sepsis lenta.) Zbl. Path. 35, 276 (1924/25). ~ Über einige Reaktionen der Gefäßwände und des Endokards bei experimentellen und menschlichen Allgemeininfektionen. Verh. dtsch. path. Ges. (20. Tagg) 1925, 260. ~ Reticulo-Endothel und aktives Mesenchym. Beitr. klin. Med. 1927 I. ~ Plasmocytom des Magens mit sog. Amyloidtumor. Zbl. Path. 89, 451 (1952). — Smetana, H.: Permeability of renal glomeruli of several mammalian species to labelled proteins. Amer. J. Path. 23, 255 (1947). ~ Relation of the reticulo-endothel system into the formation of amyloid. Proc Soc. Exper. Biol. a. Med. 24, 187 (1946). — Smith, M. R., and W. B. Wood: Studies on the mechanism of recovery in pneumonia due to Friedlaender's bacillus. III. The role of "surface phagocytosis" in the destruction of the microorganismus in the lung. J. of Exper. Med. 86, 257 (1947). — Standenath, F.: Das Bindegewebe. Seine Entwicklung, sein Bau und seine Bedeutung für Physiologie und Pathologie. Erg. Path. 22, 2 (1928). — Starlinger, W.: Über die klinische Bedeutung des physico-chemischen Zustandes der zirkulierenden Eiweißkörper des Blutes und Gewebes. Klin. Wschr. 1927, 235. ~ Physiologisch-chemischer Zustand der zirkulierenden Eiweißkörper. Zbl. inn. Med. 1927, H. 77. — Steinach, E.: Verjüngung durch experimentelle Neubelebung der alternden Pubertätsdrüse. Roux' Arch. 46, 601 (1920). — Stern, A.: Das Schicksal eingeschwemmter Geschwulstzellen in der Lunge. Virchows Arch. 241 (1923). — Sternberg, C.: Blut. Lymphknoten. In Henke-Lubarsch' Handbuch der speziellen pathologischen Anatomie und Histologie, Bd. I, Teil 1. Berlin: Springer 1926.

Tannenberg, J.: Die Speicherung kolloidaler Körper nach mikroskopischen Beobachtungen am lebenden Tier und in der Gewebekultur. Verh. dtsch. path. Ges. (25. Tagg) 1930, 128. — Tannenberg, J., u. B. Fischer-Wasels: Die lokalen Kreislaufstörungen. In Handbuch der normalen und pathologischen Physiologie, Bd. 7/2. 1927. — Terbrüggen, A.: Zwei Grundformen der allgemeinen Amyloidose mit besonderer Berücksichtigung der Amyloidniere und Nephrose. Virchows Arch. 312 (1944). — Tompkins, E. H., and M. A. Grillo: Factors, favoring phagocytosis by reticulo-endothelial cells early in inflammation. Amer. J. Path. 29, 217 (1953). — Tonutti, E.: Über die strukturelle Funktionsanpassung der Nebennierenrinde. Endokrinologie 28, 1 (1951). ~ Experimentelle Untersuchungen zur Pathophysiologie der Nebennierenrinde. Verh. dtsch. Ges. Path. (36. Tagg) 1953, 123.

Vogel, K.: Über eigenartige Fremdkörperriesenzellen bei Bronchiolitis obliterans. Virchows Arch. 206, 157 (1911). — Voronoff, S.: Organverpflanzungen und ihre praktische Verwendung beim Haustier. Leipzig 1925.

Waldenström, H.: On the formation and disapearence of amyloid in man. Acta chir. scand. (Stockh.) 63, 479 (1928). — Weese, H., u. W. Scholtan: Pharmakologie des Periston N. Dtsch. med.Wschr. 76, 1492—1493 (1951). — Weichardt, W.: Über die Proteinkörpertherapie. Münch. med. Wschr. 1918, 581. ~ Über unspezifische Leistungssteigerungen. (Protoplasmaaktivierung.) Münch. med. Wschr. 1919, 289; 1920, 21. ~ Über die theoretische Grundlage der Proteinkörpertherapie. Wien. klin. Wschr. 1924, Nr 29 u. 30. ~ Die Grundlagen der unspezifischen Therapie. Berlin: Springer 1936. — WEIDENREICH, F.: Zur Kenntnis der Zellen mit basophilen Granulationen in Blut und Bindegewebe. Fol. haemat. (Lpz.) 5, 135 (1908). ~ Die Morphologie der Blutzellen und ihre Beziehungen zueinander. Anat. Rec. 4, 317 (1910). — WEIDLICH, N.: Beitrag zur Amyloidose der Rotlaufserumtiere. Z. Inf.krkh. Haustiere 58 (1942). — WHIPPLE, G. H., C. W. HOOPER and F. S. ROBSCHEIT: Blood regeneration following simple anemia. Amer. J. Physiol. 53, 151—282 (1920). — WHIPPLE, G. H., and F. S. ROBSCHEIT-ROBBINS: Anemia plus hypoproteinemia in dogs: various proteins in diet show various patterns in blood protein production; beef muscle, egg, lactalbumin, fibrin, viscera, and supplements. J. of Exper. Med. 94, 223—242 (1951). — WILLENEGGER, H.: Über den Gruppenstoff A des Schweins und der mit Schweinemagen hergestellten Pepton-Pepsin-Präparate und Impfstoffe. Diss. Bern 1937. — WOLLENSAK, J., u. G. SEYBOLD: Untersuchungen über die Bildungsstätten von Myelom-Proteinen bzw. γ-Globulinen. Z. Naturforsch. 11b, 588—592 (1956). ~ Serum-Protein-Nachweis durch fluoreszierende Antikörper in Leber und Niere. Z. Naturforsch. 12b, 147—150 (1957). — WOOD, W. B., and M. R. SMITH: Intracellular surface phagocytosis. Science 106, 86 (1947). — WOOD, W. B., M. R. SMITH, W. D. PARRY and J. W. BERRY: Studies on the cellular immunology of acute bacteriemia. I. Intravascular leucocytic reaktion and surface phagocytosis. J. of Exper. Med. 94, 521 (1951). — WRIGHT, A. E.: Studien über Immunisierung. Jena: Gustav Fischer 1910. — WUHRMANN, F.: Elektrophoreseuntersuchungen beim nephrotischen Syndrom und bei der Lebercirrhose und ihre klinische Bedeutung. Schweiz. med. Wschr. 1946, 251. — WUHRMANN, F., u. CH. WUNDERLY: Elekrophorese-Untersuchungen beim Plasmocytom und ihre klinische Bedeutung. Schweiz. med. Wschr. 1945, 234. ~ Die Bluteiweißkörper des Menschen. Basel: Benno Schwabe & Co. 1952. — WULFF, F.: On thermostabile baktericidal substance, demonstrated in human serum, partikulary in fever. J. of Immun. 27, 451—468 (1934). ~ On baktericidal substances against paratyphoid bacilli, demonstrated in human serum, exspecially in serum of fever patients. Acta path scand. (Københ.) 14, 530—537 (1937).

YUILE, C. L., B. G. LAMSON, L. MILLER and G. H. WHIPPLE: Conversion of plasma protein to tissue protein without evidence of protein break down; results of giving plasma protein labeled with carbon^{-14} parenterally to dogs. J. of Exper. Med. 93, 559 (1951).

ZELLWEGER, H.: Glykogenspeicherkrankheiten. Dtsch. med. Wschr. 1956, 1907. — ZOLLINGER, H. U.: Trübe Schwellung und Mitochondrien (Phasenmikroskopische Untersuchungen). Schweiz. Z. Path. u. Bakter. 11, 617—634 (1948). ~ Experimenteller Beitrag zur Frage der Mikrochondrienfunktion. Experientia (Basel) 4, 312—314 (1948).

Der Stofftransport.

Von

H. Bennhold und **H. Ott** (Tübingen).

Mit 6 Abbildungen.

Einleitung.

Transport dient in der Welt der Technik einerseits dazu, Stoffe dahin zu befördern, wo sie zum Aufbau höherer Einheiten dienen sollen *(,,Antransport")*; andererseits gibt es in der Technik auch Transport, der mehr den Zweck hat, Platz zu schaffen für den Raumbedarf weiterer Fabrikation; dazu gehört der *,,Abtransport"* von Fertigfabrikaten, ferner von überschüssigem Rohmaterial und von Abfällen, die während der Fabrikation entstehen. Das Wort Transport enthält also den Begriff der Zweckmäßigkeit: Antransport des Notwendigen, Abtransport des Fertigfabrikates sowie des Überflüssigen und des Schädlichen.

Analoges finden wir in der Welt des Lebendigen, im belebten Organismus. Transportvorgänge spielen sich hier sowohl im Bereich des Makroskopischen als auch im Bereich des Mikroskopischen ab. Die Endstationen der Antransporte besitzen meistens die Dimensionen von Zellen oder von ebenfalls nur mikroskopisch sichtbaren Gewebselementen. Mit zunehmender Empfindlichkeit der chemischen und physikalischen Nachweismethoden ist die Zahl der erfaßbaren Transportgüter immer größer geworden (Sauerstoff, Kohlensäure, Traubenzucker, Cholesterin, Fettsäuren, Eisen, Magnesium, Kobalt, Jod u. a. m., vgl. S. 183). Damit ist dann auch die Möglichkeit gegeben, den Zustand dieser Stoffe während der Passage in der Blutbahn näher zu studieren. Ferner lassen sich auf Grund des mikroskopischen Nachweises bestimmter Substanzen in Speicherorten (Reticuloendothel, Epithel der Nierentubuli) Transportvorgänge besonders gut verfolgen, z. B. von Bilirubin, Eisen, Vitalfarbstoffen oder von Substanzen, die mit Isotopen markiert wurden (Thyroxin). In anderen Fällen kann auf Transportvorgänge nur geschlossen werden aus dem Entstehungsort bestimmter Substanzen einerseits und ihren funktionellen oder morphologischen Effekten in entfernt liegenden Organen andererseits; dies trifft besonders zu für Fermente und Hormone (z. B. ACTH, Adiuretin, Thyroxin, Sexualhormone, Nebennierenrindenhormone).

Die Transportvorgänge im lebenden Organismus sind in kompliziertester Weise miteinander verflochten. Die Fertigfabrikate eines Organs — besser einer Zelle — werden sehr oft auf dem Strömungswege sogleich weiterbefördert als Antransportgut zu anderen Zellen, wo sie dann wiederum als Rohmaterial, als Nahrungsstoff, als Funktionsregler oder als notwendiger Zusatzstoff für physiologisch-chemische Prozesse eingesetzt werden. Schließlich müssen auch die reichlich entstehenden endgültigen Abfallstoffe den Ausscheidungsorganen wie Niere, Darm, Galle, Schweißdrüsen oder Lunge auf gut abgesicherten Wegen zugeführt werden.

Das geordnete Zusammenspiel der vielen, gleichzeitig im Organismus sich abspielenden Stofftransporte ermöglicht erst die Aufrechterhaltung der Lebensvorgänge. Insbesondere sind alle Stoffwechselprozesse auf das exakte Funktionieren der Transportbeziehungen angewiesen. Jede einzelne Zelle kann nur leben, wenn Antransport des Notwendigen sowie Abtransport der fertigen Produkte und der als Störfaktoren schädlichen Schlacken gewährleistet ist.

Die meisten Transportvorgänge im menschlichen Körper verlaufen automatisch, sind also dem Willen des Individuums nicht unterworfen; im Intestinaltrakt gilt dies allerdings nur für die Strecke zwischen Speiseröhre und Enddarm. Gesteuert werden diese Transportvorgänge vom vegetativen Nervensystem oft in Form von Reflexvorgängen, von hormonalen Einflüssen oder auch von unmittelbar wirkenden physikalischen oder chemischen Einwirkungen. Überall, wo makroskopisch oder mikroskopisch *Muskulatur* vorhanden ist, *die keiner willkürlichen Innervation unterliegt*, wird Veranlassung sein, nach Transportmechanismen zu fahnden, z. B. bei der Muskulatur von Herz, Blutgefäßen, Darm, von Ausführungsgängen der Drüsen und verschiedener Sekretions- und Exkretionsorgane. Natürlich gibt es auch hier Ausnahmen, z. B. die unwillkürliche Muskulatur der Sinnesorgane (Iris, M. stapedius), ferner die Arrectores pilorum, welche allerdings durch Druck auf die anliegenden Talgdrüsen nebenbei auch einen Sekrettransport mit auslösen können.

Die Energie beziehen die Transportmechanismen nicht nur von muskulären Elementen, sondern auch vom *Sekretionsdruck* der Drüsen, von den Bewegungen der *Flimmerhaare* mancher Schleimhäute oder von intracellulären Bewegungsphänomenen direkt, z. B. der Bewegung der Chromosomen durch Zugspindeln, oder von Geißelbewegungen.

Im Rahmen dieses Abschnittes der Allgemeinen Pathologie kann es nur Aufgabe sein, Transportwege von makroskopischem Ausmaß aufzuzeigen. Nur in einzelnen Fällen wird es möglich sein, sie bis in die mikroskopische Dimension etwa in der Größenordnung der Bindegewebsfaser oder der Zelle hinein zu verfolgen, z. B. wenn es sich um Endausläufer von makroskopischen Stoffverlagerungen bis an die Organellen der Zelle (z. B. an die Mitochondrien) handelt. Rein intracelluläre Bewegungsvorgänge, Protoplasmaströme, Granulabewegungen oder die Vorgänge bei der Mitose an den Kernspindeln sowie bei Muskelkontraktionen können hier nicht mit behandelt werden.

Die großräumigen Stofftransportvorgänge kommen zunächst durch Muskelbewegung zustande. Muskelbewegung befördert die Luft im Atmungssystem, die Nahrung und den Darminhalt im Verdauungssystem, Sekrete und Exkrete in den Ausführungsgängen der Drüsen und in den ableitenden Harnwegen. Auch die Bewegung der den Körper durchströmenden Flüssigkeiten im Zirkulationssystem ist eine Folge von Muskeltätigkeit. Jede bewegte Flüssigkeit im Körper fördert den Stoffaustausch und bildet einen Faktor im Transportgeschehen. Blut und Lymphe stellen dabei das eigentliche „Transportmilieu" des Körpers dar.

Stofftransporte ohne ausgesprochenes Transportmilieu.

Die *Transportvorgänge im Darm*, wo auf organeigenen Wegen der Speisebrei durch die glatte Muskulatur peristaltisch von Darmabschnitt zu Darmabschnitt, von Sekretquelle zu Sekretquelle weitergereicht wird, lassen sich ohne weiteres als direkte mechanische Fortbewegung verstehen. Die automatische Regulierung dieser Motorik geschieht durch Sympathicus und Vagus. Dabei geht der Stofftransport im Grobmakroskopischen hauptsächlich durch die *Peristaltik* vor sich. Die muskulär erfolgenden *Kontraktionen der Dünndarmzotten*, welche bei vielen Tieren nachgewiesen sind und beim Menschen wohl mit Recht vermutet werden, dienen weniger der Vorwärtsbewegung des Speisebreies als der mechanischen Bearbeitung seiner Randschichten im Sinne einer Durchmischung und Resorptionserleichterung; durch lokalen Rühreffekt soll einem zu langsamen Konzentrations-ausgleich an den resorbierenden Grenzflächen vorgebeugt werden.

Bei der *Sekretion von Drüsen* stellt zunächst der Sekretionsdruck als vis a tergo den hauptsächlichen Bewegungsimpuls dar. Gerade bei Drüsen sind Mischformen dieses Mechanismus mit der peristaltischen Bewegung häufig, insofern als außer dem Sekretionsdruck zusätzlich noch peristaltikartige Vorgänge an den Ausführungs-gängen (oder auch Kontraktionen von Myoepithelien) mitwirken: z. B. beim *Abtransport des Harns* aus Nierenbecken und Harnleiter, beim *Transport der Galle*, des *Pankreassaftes*, der *Darmdrüsensekrete*, der Absonderungen der *Speicheldrüsen*, der *Schweißdrüsen* und der *Geschlechtsdrüsen*. Bei den Speicheldrüsen scheinen die Myoepithelien als primitivste contractile, muskelartig wirkende Elemente zum Zweck der mechanischen Sekretentleerung eine wesentliche Rolle zu spielen.

Flimmerhaare und *Geißeln* bilden durch ihre Bewegung einen weiteren Transportmechanismus. Es handelt sich dabei um haar- und fadenförmige meta-plastische Differenzierungen der epithelialen Zellelemente. Von Flimmerhaaren spricht man, wenn sie relativ kurz (etwa 15μ) und in größerer Zahl von einer im Gewebe fixierten Zelle angelegt sind, und von Geißeln, wenn sie lang sind (50 bis 60μ) und der Fortbewegung der Zelle selbst dienen. Die beweglichen Flimmer-haare (Kinocilien) wurzeln dicht unter der Zelloberfläche in den dem Ektoplasma angehörenden Basalkörperchen (Blepharosomen), welche möglicherweise als moto-rische Zentren der in ihren Bewegungen erstaunlich aufeinander abgestimmten Cilien anzusehen sind. Transport durch Flimmerepithelien findet vor allem in sämtlichen *Luftwegen*, ferner in *Tube und Uterus* (Mitwirkung beim Transport des Eies nach der Ovulation) statt. Am ausgedehntesten ist der gesamte Respirations-tractus mit Flimmerepithel ausgestattet, welches das von den Schleimzellen abgesonderte Sekret und damit die eingeatmeten und niedergeschlagenen Fremd-körper (Staub) sowie abgeschilferte Epithelien nach außen befördert.

Der angestrebte Sekrettransport wird dadurch erreicht, daß die Cilien in der Richtung des Sekretstroms etwa 4—5mal schnellere Bewegungen ausführen als bei der Rückkehr in die Ausgangslage, weshalb nur dieser letztere Bewegungsvorgang mikroskopisch gut sichtbar ist.

Vor Betrachtung der Transportvorgänge mit einem besonderen Transport-milieu sei der in den *Luftwegen der Lunge* sich abspielenden Bewegungsprozesse gedacht. Das normale Transportgut ist hier der gasförmige Inhalt des gesamten Bronchialbaums bis in die feinsten Verzweigungen hinein. Durch Zufuhr von Frischluft wird eine ständige Anreicherung mit Sauerstoff und durch Abgabe von verbrauchter Luft eine Beseitigung der anfallenden Kohlensäure erzielt. Die Luftbewegungen in dem verzweigten Röhrensystem der Lungen werden ja grobmakroskopisch dadurch erzeugt, daß bei den Atemexkursionen im In-spirium das Zwerchfell nach unten tritt und gleichzeitig die beiden Thoraxhälften auseinanderweichen. Dem dadurch sehr stark sich vermehrenden Innenvolumen folgt die sauerstoffhaltige Außenluft, indem sie durch den Mund und die Nase in die Luftröhre einströmt. Die gegenläufigen Bewegungen von Thorax und Zwerchfell pressen dann im Exspirium die an Sauerstoff verarmte und an Kohlen-säure angereicherte Luft wieder heraus.

Beim Exspirium spielt die Elastizität der Rippenknorpel eine nicht unwesentliche Rolle: Im Inspirium werden sie durch den Zug der Atemmuskeln gedehnt und torquiert; im Ex-spirium setzen sie die so gespeicherte Energie in Bewegung um und unterstützen das Zu-sammenfallen des Brustkorbes. Die Elastizität ist hier im Rahmen des Atmungsprozesses als phasenmäßig arbeitender Energiespeicher im Exspirium ähnlich eingesetzt, wie es in der Aorta im Rahmen des Blutkreislaufes geschieht, wo in der Diastole durch die Windkessel-wirkung ein gleichmäßiger Druckablauf garantiert wird.

Ein Teil der Atemmuskulatur kann zwar willkürlich bewegt werden; dennoch verläuft die Atmung normalerweise unbewußt (natürlicher Schlaf, Ohnmacht,

Äthernarkose) und wird vom Atemzentrum am Boden der Rautengrube gesteuert. Der Gastransport bis zu den Alveolen als der Austauschrampe zur Blutbahn geschieht durch Sog und Ausstoß innerhalb eines feinverzweigten lufthaltigen Röhrensystems. Dabei wirkt die weitgehende Aufteilung des Wegesystems selbst transportbegünstigend; einerseits wird die Austauschfläche dadurch sehr vergrößert (etwa 100 m²) und wirkungsvoller, andererseits lassen die feinsten Luftwege einen Siebeffekt zustande kommen; so können Partikel über 1 μ Größe nicht bis in die Alveolen eindringen, ein für die Pathogenese der Pneumokoniosen wesentliches Faktum.

Schon an dieser Stelle begegnen wir Kollisionsmöglichkeiten bei 2 Stofftransporten. Die gleichen Bewegungsabläufe von Thorax und Zwerchfell dienen sowohl der Abgabe der Kohlensäure als auch der Aufnahme des Sauerstoffs. Die Koppelung dieser beiden lebenswichtigen Transporte stellt beim Gesunden einen sich sinnvoll ergänzenden, gewissermaßen doppelläufigen Transport dar.

Bei bestimmten pathologischen Zuständen kann es jedoch dadurch zu schweren Kollisionen kommen. Wenn z. B. eine arterielle Hypoxämie vorliegt, versucht der Organismus diesen Zustand durch eine vermehrte Ventilation zu verbessern. Durch die Hyperventilation kann zwar die erniedrigte Sauerstoffspannung normalisiert werden; gleichzeitig führt aber die Hyperventilation zu einer vermehrten Kohlensäureabgabe, obwohl hierfür keinerlei Bedürfnis vorliegt. Ja, die vermehrte Kohlensäureabgabe kann eine beträchtliche Alkalose des Blutes und damit eine Bedrohung der Integrität des Organismus verursachen. Auch bei Ventilationsstörungen (z. B. schweres Lungenemphysem) mit einer alveolären Hypoventilation (Störung des O_2- und CO_2-Transportes) besteht bei dem Versuch einer Sauerstofftherapie eine Kollisionsmöglichkeit. Die Sauerstoffatmung verbessert den gestörten O_2-Transport, die Dyspnoe und die mehr oder weniger vorhandene Cyanose verschwinden. Dieser therapeutische Teilerfolg führt aber gleichzeitig zu einer vermehrten Kohlensäure-Retention mit Verstärkung der respiratorischen Acidose durch eine verminderte Gesamtventilation. Die Ursache hierfür ist die Beseitigung der atemstimulierenden Wirkung der arteriellen Hypoxämie[1].

Stofftransporte mit besonderem Transportmilieu.

Die erweiterten Kenntnisse der Zusammensetzung des Blutplasmas, der Lymphe und der extracellulären Flüssigkeiten haben das Verständnis dafür wachgerufen, daß den zirkulierenden Körpersäften eine größere Bedeutung zukommt als nur die, ein sehr gut durchmischendes und dispergierendes Lösungsmittel zu sein.

Unter **Transportmilieu** *ist ein Milieu zu verstehen, in welchem — über die Summe der zu transportierenden Stoffe hinausgehend — auch Substanzen oder biologische Einheiten enthalten sind, welche dem Transportvorgang als solchem dienen (Erythrocyten, Serumeiweiß, z. T. auch Thrombocyten und Leukocyten).*

Vor HARVEY (1628) gab es keine gedankliche Abtrennung der Transportaufgaben von den nur spekulativ erfaßten Lebensvorgängen. Das sich Finden und sich räumlich in richtiger und harmonischer Weise zueinander Gliedern wurde als dem Lebendigen immanent angesehen und nicht als Problem empfunden.

GALEN (geb. 129 n. Chr.), dessen Lehre sich bis HARVEY gehalten hatte, stellte sich Blutentstehung und Blutbewegung folgendermaßen vor: Der Speisebrei (Chylos) sollte durch das Pfortadersystem vom Darm zur Leber gelangen; von dort zieht die Milz die verunreinigenden Substanzen an sich und verarbeitet sie zu schwarzer Galle. Der Rest des Chylos wird in der Leber unter Beihilfe des vegetativen Pneuma (Pneuma physikon) in Blut umgewandelt. Von der Leber gelangt dieses zum ersten Male gereinigte Blut dann teils direkt in den Körper, teils in das rechte Herz. Dort wird es durch die eingepflanzte Wärme („calor innatus") zum zweiten Male gereinigt und gibt seine Rückstände (als Ruß) durch die Lungenschlagader an die Lungen ab, wo sie bei der Ausatmung den Körper verlassen. Das so gereinigte Blut ernährt einesteils die Lungen; der andere Teil des Blutes geht durch die — entgegen allem Augenschein supponierten! — „Poren" der Kammerscheidewand in den linken Ventrikel. Dort wird das Blut mit einem Pneuma zootikon vermischt, welches mit der Einatmung in die Lunge aufgenommen wird. Schließlich wird es durch die Hauptschlagader in den ganzen Körper getrieben, wo

[1] RÜBSAM 1942, ROSSIER 1956.

dann in den blind endigenden feinen Adern aus dem hin und her wogenden Blute die geformten Gebilde, insbesondere Muskeln, entstehen, indem sie sich gewissermaßen aus dem flüssigen Blute absetzen, etwa wie am Strande des Meeres die auf und ab wogenden Wellen Schwemmgut ablagern. Diese ständig aus dem hin und her wogenden Blut sich neu bildenden Organmassen müßten aber nun rein mengenmäßig den Gesamtkörper sprengen.

Die 3 Arten des Pneuma sind Gestaltsformen der Seele: das dem Willen unterworfene Pneuma psychikon mit dem Sitz im Gehirn, das Pneuma zootikon mit dem Sitz im Herzen und das dem Willen nicht unterworfene Pneuma physikon mit dem Sitz in der Leber. Diese 3 Arten von Pneuma waren auf Grund von teleologischen Spekulationen mit allen *den* Fähigkeiten ausgestattet, welche für die zu erklärenden Sachverhalte notwendig oder wünschenswert waren. Ihre Eigenschaft als Gestaltsformen des Seelischen schützte sie wohl auch vor exakten, fast möchte man sagen, vor nichtadäquaten wissenschaftlichen — vielleicht sogar messenden — Erwägungen. Wenn nach Galen die Milz das in der Leber entstehende Blut reinigt, so ist es für ihn aber nur ein Spezialfall einer allgemeinen Konzeption. Er unterscheidet nämlich 4 Hauptkräfte im Organismus, welche für Stoffverlagerungen zuständig sind: eine anziehende, eine festhaltende, eine umwandelnde und eine ausstoßende Kraft. Auf das Wechselspiel dieser Kräfte werden alle Funktionen der einzelnen Organe zurückgeführt, wogegen — wenn man diese Kräfte als Prämisse anerkennt — kaum eine Einwendung möglich ist. Wie durch einen geheimnisvollen Sog kommen, meist auf direktem Wege, die Stoffe dorthin, wo sie gebraucht oder wo sie ausgeschieden werden. Ein echtes Transportproblem gab es damit eigentlich überhaupt nicht. Nur im kranken Körper kann es durch Störung der oben erwähnten Hauptkräfte zu einem „*error loci*" kommen.

Quantitativ messende Betrachtungen, welche auch vor den drei alt geheiligten Pneumata und vor den 4 Hauptkräften der Organe, wie Galen sie postuliert hatte, nicht haltmachten, führten Harvey dann zur Hypothese des Blutkreislaufs. Damit konnte er auf Grund rein mechanischer Vorstellungen die Bewegungen des Blutes im Organismus erklären und mit klinischen Beobachtungen in Einklang bringen. Die Hämodynamik und die Problematik der *Transportvorgänge waren damit der messenden Forschung erschlossen.* Eine fruchtbare und folgenreiche Idee in der Medizin war geboren. Schon vor Harvey hatten der Spanier Miguel Serveto († 1553) und ebenso der Italiener Realdo Colombo († 1559) die Passage des Blutes vom rechten Herzen über die Lunge zum linken Herzen angenommen und wahrscheinlich gemacht. Aber die Entdeckung der gesamten zirkulatorischen Vorgänge als des beherrschenden Prinzips aller Blutbewegungen bleibt das alleinige Verdienst William Harveys.

Als besonders formiertes und mit ausgesprochenem Transportmilieu (dem Blut) ausgestattetes Wegesystem imponiert in erster Linie die *Blutbahn.* Claude Bernard bezeichnet das Blut als wesentlichen Bestandteil des „milieu intérieur". Viel weniger ausgiebig nehmen am Stofftransport die langsam strömenden und schließlich die von nur geringen Impulsen bewegten Flüssigkeiten teil.

Es fällt in diesem Zusammenhang auf, daß bei den Körperflüssigkeiten des menschlichen Organismus mit zunehmender Strömungsgeschwindigkeit der Reichtum sowohl an Zellen als auch an Eiweiß stark zunimmt. Am ausgesprochensten gilt dies für das Blut, dessen reife rote Blutkörperchen sich ja normalerweise ausschließlich innerhalb der Blutgefäße befinden. Aber auch für den Eiweißgehalt trifft dies weitgehend zu. Dieser Parallelismus von Strömungsgeschwindigkeit einerseits und von Reichtum an Zellelementen und Eiweiß andererseits kann wohl als gewisser Hinweis dafür angeführt werden, daß Formelemente und kolloide Eiweißkörper irgendwie in den Transportmechanismus eingebaut sind. Ihr Zusammenarbeiten mit dem bewegten Suspensionsmittel scheint eine wesentliche funktionelle Komponente des Transportmilieus zu sein (vgl. Tabelle 1).

Es wäre nicht richtig, dem Liquor cerebrospinalis jede Transportfunktion abzusprechen, sind doch Strömungsrichtung, Geschwindigkeit und Materialabgabe in den verschiedenen Teilen der vom Liquor erfüllten Räume wohlbekannte Größen[1]. Natürlich kommen diesen Flüssigkeiten auch andere Aufgaben zu. Beim Kammerwasser findet sich komplette Stagnation; dann ist die Transportfunktion wohl nur gering.

---

[1] Meyer 1953, Lüthy 1953.

Tabelle 1. *Eiweißgehalt bewegter und stagnierender Körperflüssigkeiten.*

	g%
Plasma	6,5 —8,0
Lymphe (Hund)[1]	1,4 —4,6 (3,3)
Transsudat (bei Herzdekompensation)	1,2 —2,7
Ödemflüssigkeit (bei Herzdekompensation)	0,1 —1,3
(bei akuter Nephritis, Nephrose) . .	0,1 —1,1
Liquor cerebrospinalis	0,01 —0,025
Kammerwasser des Auges	0,006—0,018

Ehe auf die Rolle der Bewegungsvorgänge der Körperflüssigkeiten beim Transport eingegangen werden kann, soll die Strömungslehre, soweit sie dabei in Frage kommt, skizziert werden. Dieses kann nur in bezug auf das *Blut* als Transportmilieu geschehen. Für die sehr viel langsamer fließende Lymphe sind die physikalischen Strömungsfaktoren nur von geringer funktioneller Bedeutung. Obgleich RUSZNYÁK und seine Schüler 1957[1] einen nerval gesteuerten Tonus und eventuell auch reflektorische Spasmen der Lymphgefäße annehmen, so sind doch die Regulationsmechanismen der Lymphströmung erst sehr wenig erforscht. Das Lymphgefäßsystem als Transportweg soll deshalb erst in einem späteren Abschnitt zusammen mit der extracapillären Flüssigkeit besprochen werden (S. 232).

Strömungslehre.

Für die Austauschprozesse in den Capillaren ist die Art der dort herrschenden Strömungsverhältnisse von größter Bedeutung. Das Strömen von Blut und Lymphe, von Urin, Galle und Drüsenexkreten erfolgt in Röhren. Die extracelluläre Flüssigkeit der Gewebsspalten breitet sich unter dem Druck der bewegten Organe in Richtung des geringsten Widerstandes aus und gelangt, sofern sie nicht gemäß dem Starlingschen Prinzip durch den angestiegenen kolloidosmotischen Druck des Blutes in das venolennahe Capillarende eingesaugt wird, in das Interstitium und von dort eventuell in die Lymphgefäße.

Je nach Art der Flüssigkeit, der Form und der Art des Gefäßes und der wirkenden hydrostatischen Kraft ist die Art der Strömung verschieden. In einem Röhrensystem sind physikalisch 2 Strömungen möglich: die gleichmäßige, zur Röhrenachse parallel laufende, von der Rohrwandung zur Rohrmitte schneller werdende, *schlichte* oder *laminare*, und die völlig ungeordnete, *turbulente* Strömung. Laminare Strömung gibt es nur bis zu einer bestimmten Geschwindigkeit; wird diese überschritten, dann tritt — genau so wie durch eine Störung verursacht — Turbulenz auf. Im Gefäßsystem herrscht nur unmittelbar hinter den Herzklappen und in den Capillaren turbulente, sonst allenthalben laminare Strömung vor.

Für echte, *homogene Flüssigkeiten* beschreibt das Poiseuillesche Gesetz die Strömungsvorgänge und gibt das Flüssigkeitsvolumen (V), welches je Sekunde durch eine Röhre fließt, in Abhängigkeit von Länge (l), Röhrendurchmesser (r), Viscosität (η) und dem Druck (p) an: $V = \dfrac{\pi\, r^4\, p}{8\,\eta\, l}$. Es gilt aber nur für parabolische Geschwindigkeitsprofile während des Strömens und nicht für die Anfangsstrecke der Strömung. Während mit Strömungsbeginn sich die Flüssigkeitsteilchen gleich rasch bewegen, tritt bald am Rande des Gefäßes eine Verzögerung durch die Reibung an der Wand ein, die sich nach innen fortpflanzt. So entsteht der in der Mitte des Gefäßes am schnellsten fließende *Axialstrom*. Nach einer gewissen durchlaufenen Strecke hat sich das flächenhafte Strömungsprofil in ein parabolisches verwandelt.

Für die Strömung des Blutes gelten besondere Bedingungen, die sich daraus ergeben, daß das *Blut* keine homogene, sondern eine *heterogene* Flüssigkeit ist, und daß sich das Röhrensystem sehr stark verändert. Die Viscosität des Blutes ist keine Materialkonstante, sondern eine veränderliche Größe, die besser als „*scheinbare Viscosität*" bezeichnet wird[2]. Sie ist im Verhältnis zu anderen kolloidhaltigen Flüssigkeiten gering. Das ist dem einzigartigen Umstand zu verdanken,

[1] FÖLDI 1957, 1960.   [2] BARR 1931.

daß das Hämoglobin in den elastischen, leicht verformbaren corpusculären Elementen, den Erythrocyten, enthalten ist. Wäre der Blutfarbstoff frei, dann müßte die innere Reibung beträchtlich ansteigen[1]. Dem Poiseuilleschen Gesetz gehorcht das Blut bei laminarer Strömung in den Gefäßen mit großem Druckgefälle, nicht aber, wenn die Anzahl der roten Blutkörperchen stark ansteigt, oder in den Capillaren. Schon in kleinen Arterien und Arteriolen treten Abweichungen auf[2]. Dort verringert sich die Viscosität mit wachsender Strömungsgeschwindigkeit und abnehmendem Druckgefälle[3]. Andererseits nimmt bei Abnahme der Strömung das effektive Durchflußvolumen stärker ab, als dies das Gesetz zulassen würde.

Die innere Reibung verhält sich ja umgekehrt proportional der 4. Potenz des Röhrenradius, so daß kleinste Änderungen des Röhrendurchmessers große Änderungen des Gesamtstromwiderstandes mit sich bringen. Zusätzlich bewirkt die Änderung des Viscositätskoeffizienten eine Beeinflussung des Widerstandes. Man erklärt sie sich durch das Verhalten der Erythrocyten, die sich bei rascher Strömung säulenförmig aneinanderreihen, im Axialstrom rasch vorschießen und sich nur am Plasma reiben, bei langsamer werdender Strömung aber mehr und mehr hin- und herpendeln und sich dadurch bedeutend mehr aneinander stoßen. Es ist also nicht nur der enorm starke Effekt der Gefäßweite, sondern zusätzlich die momentane Beschaffenheit des Blutes (in der Anordnung der suspendierten Erythrocyten), welche auf die Strömung wirken. Der Angriff der Regulation erfolgt durch Veränderung des Gefäßlumens; die Viscosität ändert sich dann sekundär.

Auch für den venösen Rückfluß sind Abweichungen vom idealen Verhalten vorhanden, wenn die Druckunterschiede gering sind. Man kann deshalb sagen, daß die verschiedenen Gefäßgebiete durchaus unterschiedlich zu beurteilen sind, und daß dabei der Satz, daß „jedes Organ seinen individuellen Kreislauf besitzt"[4]) zu Recht besteht. In den kleinen Capillaren vom Durchmesser eines Erythrocyten herrscht wegen der corpuskulären Elemente völlig irreguläre Strömung. Die Blutsäule kann langsam oder rasch fließen, stillstehen, hin und her pendeln, ganz wie es der Öffnungszustand der Haargefäße bedingt, und einerlei, ob besondere Verschlußmechanismen vorhanden sind oder nicht.

Die Laminarströmung in den großen Gefäßen hat einen Effekt zur Folge, der für den Stofftransport von Bedeutung ist. Da bei gleichmäßiger Strömung keine Durchmischung erfolgt, fließen die Flüssigkeitssäulen, die sich aus kleineren Gefäßen in ein größeres sammeln, lange Zeit unvermengt nebeneinander. Teilt sich dieses größere Gefäß später wieder auf, dann können sich diese Ströme wie die Stränge eines Taues entflechten und in getrennte Capillargebiete abfließen. *Trotz der Sammlung in einem weiten Rohr ist eine vollständige Mischung ausgeblieben.* Nach den Versuchen von Bucher[5] muß man sogar annehmen, daß die Turbulenz im rechten Herzen und der A. pulmonalis zu gering ist, um zu verhindern, daß aus der V. cava cranialis kommende Partikel anders in den Lungen abgelagert werden als aus der caudalen Hohlvene kommende[6]. Es wird immer wieder diskutiert, ob diesem Umstand die Prädilektionslokalisation der Tuberkulose in den Lungenspitzen zuzuschreiben ist[7]. Auch das Blut in der V. portae ist nicht ideal gemischt, so daß bestimmte Leberareale aus bestimmten Quellgebieten versorgt werden können[8].

Die 3 Komponenten des Transportgeschehens im Bereich der Blutbahn.

Bleiben wir zunächst bei dem Prototyp eines strömenden Transportmilieus bei dem Blute.

Im Bereich des Blutes kann man den Transportvorgang in 3 Komponenten zerlegen:

---

[1] Suter 1942.   [2] Bayliss 1952.   [3] A. Müller 1942.   [4] Wertheimer 1938.
[5] Bucher 1951, 1952.   [6] Smith 1954.   [7] Esser 1955.   [8] Mumenthaler 1953.

I. Die **lokomotorische Komponente**. d. h. den *Bewegungsimpuls*; ihn steuert das Herz als zentrales Pumpwerk bei, dessen geregeltes Funktionieren durch eine Fülle von Regulationsmechanismen gesichert ist.

II. Die **vasomotorische Komponente**. Sie gewährleistet die äußerst *differenzierte Verteilung des Minutenvolumens* in der Peripherie entsprechend den jeweiligen regionalen Versorgungsbedürfnissen der Organe und ihrer Teile. Diese wird erzielt — ebenfalls unter Einschaltung zahlreicher nervaler, inkretorischer und chemischer Regulationsmechanismen — durch Kaliberänderungen der Arteriolen, Venolen und Capillaren.

III. Die **Vehikel**, welche eine sehr wesentliche Rolle als *lokale Abgaberegler* im Capillargebiet spielen. Dazu gehören in erster Linie die *Erythrocyten*, die *Thrombocyten* und die *Bluteiweißkörper*. Erst in zweiter Linie sind auch die weißen Blutkörperchen dazuzurechnen als Transporteure von Fermenten und Globulinen; sie haben dabei noch die Besonderheit, daß sie selbständige Zellelemente sind mit der Fähigkeit der Phagocytose, der amöboiden Bewegung und mit weitgehend eigenem Stoffwechsel. (**Zirkulierendes Transportmilieu** vgl. S. 180ff.)

Für den lokalen Abstrom aus den Capillaren spielen natürlich auch noch Eigenschaften eine Rolle, die den im Blut als Transportgut zirkulierenden Substanzen selbst sowie den Capillarmembranen und den Zellgrenzflächen eigen sind; bei den zirkulierenden Substanzen kommen Teilchengröße, Diffusionsfähigkeit und Löslichkeit in erster Linie in Frage, bei den Capillarmembranen und Zellgrenzflächen der gesamte Komplex der Adsorptions- und Permeabilitätsvorgänge einschließlich der fermentativ gesteuerten aktiven Transportprozesse in den Membranen.

Schließlich müssen hier auch *intracelluläre Prozesse* in Betracht gezogen werden, welche das Diffusionsgefälle in die Zelle hinein erhöhen oder erniedrigen können; in erster Linie handelt es sich dabei um fermentative Abbau- oder Aufbauvorgänge, eventuell mit Einschaltung von Trägersubstanzen (s. S. 237); in zweiter Linie um Adsorptionsvorgänge an intracelluläre Organellen, wobei die Mitochondrien offenbar im Vordergrund stehen[1]. — Die wichtigen physikalischen Eigenschaften des Transportgutes und der Empfangsstationen sowie die chemischen Prozesse, die einen Transport fördern oder behindern können, werden nicht dem großräumigen extracellulären Transportgeschehen zugerechnet und deshalb erst am Ende dieses Beitrages behandelt. Daß es bei den vielen verschiedenartigen *Transportvorgängen auch zu Kollisionen* kommen kann und daß daraus eventuell sogar therapeutische Folgerungen gezogen werden müssen, wird uns mehrfach beschäftigen (CO_2-Abgabe und O_2-Aufnahme [S. 169], Kollisionen der Regulationsmechanismen z. B. zwischen Aufrechterhaltung einerseits der Körpertemperatur und andererseits des Blutdrucks [S. 176], schließlich Verdrängungserscheinungen bezüglich der Bindung an ein Vehikel, z.B. bei CO-Vergiftung oder bei Kernikterus der Frühgeborenen [S. 200]).

Die beiden ersten oben aufgeführten Stufen der Transportapparatur bergen, wie im Folgenden gezeigt werden wird, so vielfach gestaffelte und miteinander verflochtene, ,,zweckmäßige'' Sicherungen und Regulationen in sich, daß sie zunächst in einer kurzen Übersicht dargestellt werden sollen. Nur so kann ein richtiger Maßstab für das Zusammenwirken der drei wichtigen Transportkomponenten und eine klare Vorstellung von der zu erwartenden Ausgestaltung und Bedeutung der bisher oft zu wenig beachteten dritten Komponente (Vehikelapparat) gewonnen werden.

Es ist selbstverständlich, daß eine solche Aufgliederung der einzelnen Regulationen sowohl bei der lokomotorischen als auch bei der vasomotorischen Komponente etwas Gewaltsames

---

[1] SEYBOLD 1958.

hat. Die Regulationen sind oft eng miteinander verflochten und vermascht. Regulatoren des Gefäßsystems können z. B. direkt oder auch indirekt das Herz mit beeinflussen (Adrenalin, Arterenol). Trotzdem schien eine gedrängte analytische Aufzählung nötig, einerseits um nicht durch eine zu ausführliche Darstellung den Rahmen dieses Beitrages zu durchbrechen, andererseits um doch zu zeigen, mit welcher Fülle schon jetzt bekannter Regulationen die beiden ersten Transportkomponenten ausgestattet sind. Man kann daraus ersehen, welche Ponderanz ihnen der Organismus zumißt, und daß es paradox wäre, bei der dritten Transportkomponente (Regelung der lokalen Stoffabgabe aus dem strömenden Blute) nicht auch mit vielfältigen und verschiedenartigen Sicherungsmaßnahmen zu rechnen.

Lokomotorik

als Komponente I des Transportapparates.

Durch die Pumparbeit des *Herzens* wird dem Gesamtorganismus das notwendige Blutvolumen angeboten.

Das rechte und das linke Herz stellen grob gesehen zwei gekoppelte, im gleichen Rhythmus arbeitende Pumpen dar. Der Mechanismus der Herzklappen sorgt für einen gerichteten Blutstrom analog den Verhältnissen bei einer technischen Pumpe. Die Volumenänderung des Innenraumes geschieht beim Herzen nicht durch Bewegung eines Stempels in einem starren Rohr, sondern mehr oder weniger durch konzentrische Kontraktion eines Hohlmuskels. Sehr schnell hat also schon hier die Analogie zur Pumpe ihre Grenze erreicht. Das Besondere des Herzens ist seine *Anpassungsfähigkeit an die jeweils zu bewältigenden Aufgaben.* In der Ruhe fördert jede Herzkammer etwa 70 cm³ Blut je Systole; dem Blutstrom wird dabei in der Aorta eine Geschwindigkeit von 40 cm je Sekunde gegeben.

Dabei scheint nach neueren Untersuchungen das Herz seinen Mechanismus als Pumpe je nach den Arbeitsbedingungen in verschiedener Weise ändern zu können. Das große, mit geringerer Frequenz schlagende Herz arbeitet systolisch durch Kontraktion der starken Ringmuskeln in der Gegend der Herzbasis. Die Füllung erfolgt alsdann durch die vis a tergo und durch die Vorhofskontraktionen (sofern nicht eine absolute Arrhythmie besteht) unter Mitwirkung formelastischer Kräfte der Ventrikelwand[1]. Bei abnehmender Füllung durch Orthostase oder durch Anzapfung des arteriellen Windkessels wird das Herz kleiner und schlägt frequenter. Die kurzen diastolischen Phasen genügen nicht mehr, um ausreichende Blutmengen in den Vorhöfen bereitzustellen. Deshalb tritt jetzt sehr viel mehr der von Böhme (1936) wiederentdeckte Ventilebenenmechanismus in Tätigkeit. Die spiralig longitudinalen Muskelzüge des Herzens geben dem Kontraktionsvorgang das Gepräge, wodurch die Ebenen der Atrioventrikularklappen sich systolisch in der Richtung auf die Herzspitze hin bewegen und dadurch ähnlich einem Spritzenstempel systolisch Blut aus den Venen in die Vorhöfe einsaugen und im gleichen Arbeitsgang das Blut aus dem Ventrikel in die Aorta und A. pulmonalis herausdrücken. Dieser Wechsel des Pumpmechanismus je nach der Menge des dem Herzen zuströmenden Blutes stellt einen durchaus eindrucksvollen Anpassungsvorgang des Herzens an anormale Arbeitsbedingungen dar.

Der systolische Druck in der Aorta des Gesunden beträgt 150 mm Hg, in der A. pulmonalis etwa $^1/_5$ dieses Betrages. Die elastischen Formelemente der Arterienwandungen lassen in dem Gefäßsystem Energiespeicher entstehen, so daß ein Blutdruckrest auch in der Diastole übrigbleibt; dadurch wird auch in dieser Phase der Herzaktion die Blutsäule weiter in das Gefäßrohr mit seinen unendlichen Verzweigungen hineingedrückt.

Von ganz besonderer Wichtigkeit ist der aus der Aortenelastizität stammende diastolische Druckverlauf für die Blutversorgung der Coronargefäße; sie haben ja ihre Abgangsstelle direkt peripher von den Ansatzlinien der Aortenklappen, also in der Zone des höchsten diastolischen Druckes; hinzukommt, daß der Herzmuskel gerade *das* Organ ist, welches wegen der starken systolischen Spannung der Muskulatur die Hauptblutmenge in der Diastole aufnimmt[2].

---

[1] Gauer 1956.
[2] Gregg 1950, dagegen Hochrein und Keller 1951 sowie Wiggers 1954.

Die *Regulationsmechanismen am Herzen* lassen sich folgendermaßen zusammenfassen:

Schon ein erhöhter diastolischer Füllungsdruck im Ventrikel und damit eine erhöhte Anfangsspannung erzeugen eine vergrößerte diastolische Faserlänge und führen zu verstärkter Ventrikelkontraktion mit erhöhtem Schlagvolumen (*Starlingsches Gesetz*, 1915). Spätere Untersuchungen haben gezeigt, daß auch unabhängig vom Druck im rechten Vorhof auf hormonalem Wege oder durch direkte Einflüsse des vegetativen Nervensystems[1] adaptative Steuerungen des Schlagvolumens vom Organismus erzielt werden können. Eine Drucksteigerung im rechten Vorhof und in der V. cava (d. h. Stauung venösen Blutes vor dem rechten Herzen, welches das anflutende Venenblut nicht vollständig abschöpfen kann) bewirkt Frequenzsteigerung der Herzaktion und dadurch Erhöhung des Minutenvolumens *(Bainbridge-Reflex)*.

Aus diesen beiden Regulationen, welche der Bewältigung einer größeren Menge zuströmenden Blutes aus dem großen Kreislauf dienen, hatte man geschlossen, daß dem Herzen sein Arbeitspensum vom Füllungszustand der Venen zudiktiert wird. Es zeigte sich aber später, daß auch Sympathicusreizung sowie Adrenalin eine Frequenzsteigerung und stärkere Verkürzung der contractilen Elemente bewirken *ohne* primäre Änderung von Füllungsvolumen und Füllungsdruck (vgl. unten). Ferner kann auf Grund von neueren röntgenkinematographischen Untersuchungen der Herztätigkeit und auf Grund des Studiums der Venenpulse im Cavagebiet angenommen werden, daß die *Herztätigkeit* (Schlagvolumen) *in der Hauptsache nicht durch die passive Füllung des Venensystems bestimmt wird, sondern daß dafür in erster Linie die Erfordernisse des arteriellen Kreislaufs und der zentrale Blutvorrat*, aus dem das Herz aktiv schöpft, *maßgebend sind*.

Bei längere Zeit hindurch bestehender vermehrter Anfangsspannung in der Systole entwickelt sich als Anpassung eine (konzentrische) *Hypertrophie* des Herzmuskels; ferner entsteht bei längere Zeit hindurch auftretender erhöhter Volumenbelastung des Ventrikels mit Anstieg des enddiastolischen Druckes und der enddiastolischen Wandspannung eine *Dilatation* der Herzkammern, welche eine Vergrößerung der Restblutmenge und damit eine sofort verfügbare Blutvolumen-Reserve im Ventrikel selbst bereitstehen läßt. [*Regulative Dilatation* nach REINDELL und DELIUS (1948)].

Je größere Herzleistungen der Organismus verlangt, um so größere Blutmengen führen die *Coronargefäße* dem Herzmuskel zu. — *Ausschüttung von Adrenalin und Arterenol* in normalen Dosen durch Aktivierung des NN-Markes bewirkt Frequenzsteigerung, Verstärkung der Herzkontraktion, Minderung des Restblutes und Steigerung des Minutenvolumens.

Aus dem Gebiete der funktionellen Pathologie ist zu erwähnen, daß Reizung von bestimmten Receptorfeldern im linken Ventrikel durch lokale Myokardschädigung (z. B. bei Infarkt, bei Vergiftung mit Veratrin u. a.) Schonung der geschädigten Ventrikelmuskulatur bewirkt. Das geschieht durch Bradykardie, Minderung des Energieumsatzes, Senkung des Blutdrucks, der zirkulierenden Blutmenge, Einschränkung der Willkürmotorik sowie zentralnervöser und psychischer Funktionen *(Bezold-Jarisch-Reflex)*.

Vasomotorik
als Komponente II des Transportapparates (Regulationsmechanismen der peripheren Blutverteilung).

Zur Sicherung der Versorgung der Gesamtperipherie müssen einige *extrakardiale hämodynamische Vorbedingungen* garantiert werden. Dies geschieht:

[1] KLEPZIG 1955, FRIEDBERG 1956.

a) Durch Bereitstellung der jeweils notwendigen zirkulierenden Blutmenge, d.h. des erforderlichen Volumens an „Transportmilieu".

Folgende Regulationen treten dabei in Wirksamkeit:

1. *Adiuretin* steht nicht nur im Dienste der Osmoregulation; über den Vagus werden auch elektrophysiologisch nachweisbare Impulse[1] aus Volumenreceptoren des linken Herzvorhofs[2] vermittelt. Je nach dem Dehnungsgrad des linken Vorhofs (während der Vorhofdiastole) kann auf diesem Wege die Freisetzung von Adiuretin und damit die *tubuläre Wasserrückresorption* gesteuert werden. In neuerer Zeit ist besonders die überragende Rolle des *Aldosterons*[3] für die *Volumenregulation* erkannt worden. Receptoren sind im Bereich der art. carotis communis und des rechten Herzvorhofs gelegen. Erfolgsorgan ist hier ebenfalls die Niere, in der bei Aldosteronzunahme die *Rückresorption von Natrium* ansteigt.

2. Die *Wasserabgabe und -aufnahme durch das Interstitium* hängt außerdem vom Elektrolytgehalt im Blut und Gewebe ab; auch hier können Hormone der Nebennierenrinde steuernd eingreifen.

3. Die *Bewirtschaftung der Blutdepots* in Lunge, Leber, subpapillärem Plexus der Haut[4] geschieht durch Sympathicus bzw. Vagus (eventuell auch via Acetylcholin). Dabei ist es unwichtig, ob man unter „Depots" nur wirklich *vollständig* stagnierende Blutbestände versteht oder auch Blut, welches nur besonders langsam fließt und daher ebenfalls geeignet ist, jederzeit durch vasomotorisch bedingte Erhöhung der regionalen Strömungsgeschwindigkeit als hämodynamische Reserve eingesetzt zu werden. — Als unmittelbar greifbare Blutreserven werden die 50—100 cm³ Restblut in den Ventrikeln angesehen; als weitere „Sofortdepots" sind neuerdings die intrathorakalen Blutvorräte besonders herausgestellt[5]; sie betragen etwa $^1/_3$—$^1/_4$ des Gesamtblutvolumens und sprechen auf Reaktionen der Receptorfelder im linken Vorhof besonders schnell und wirksam an. Vorübergehende kurzfristige Korrekturen des Blutvolumens im Sinne einer Verminderung geschehen durch Abschieben von komplettem Blut in Depots verschiedener Wertigkeit oder durch Verlagern von Blutplasma in das Interstitium. Nachhaltigere Regulationsvorgänge werden über die Diuresefunktionen der Tubuli bewerkstelligt. Das Ziel ist, durch Abstimmung von Blutvolumen und Gefäßtonus einen adäquaten intrathorakalen Blutvorrat aufrechtzuerhalten.

b) Durch Aufrechterhaltung des notwendigen zentralen Blutdrucks [Betriebsdruck nach R. Wagner (1954)], der das richtige Druckgefälle überall in die Peripherie gewährleistet:

1. Die erste Umformung der vom Herzen ausgeworfenen Pulswelle geschieht in der *Aorta* durch die Windkesselwirkung der elastischen Wandungen. Bei einem bestimmten Druck betragen die Weitbarkeitsanteile der Aorta 52% des gesamten arteriellen Systems[6]; direkt hinter den Semilunarklappen findet sich eine Partie der Aorta mit besonders hochgradiger Weitbarkeit und entsprechend starkem Glättungseffekt der Pulswelle gegenüber[7]. Diese gerade dort an der Abgangsstelle der Coronararterien lokalisierte, besonders starke Windkesselwirkung muß die hauptsächlich in der Diastole erfolgende Blutversorgung des Herzmuskels begünstigen. — Das sich peripherwärts an die Aorta anschließende arterielle Schlauchsystem hat nur einen viel geringeren Glättungseffekt. Ein Rest der Pulswelle dient in der Peripherie auch noch der Bewegung der interstitiellen Gewebsflüssigkeit. Es scheint eine Korrelation der Herztätigkeit mit der Kapazität des arteriellen Windkessels zu bestehen; Receptorfelder in der Bauchaorta werden als Ausgangspunkt für einen regulierenden Reflexmechanismus vermutet[8].

---

[1] Henry und Pearce 1956.   [2] Gauer und Henry 1956.   [3] Simpson 1954.
[4] Wollheim 1927.   [5] Sjöstrand 1952, Gauer 1956.
[6] Wetterer 1953.   [7] Remington 1952.   [8] Wagner 1954.

2. *Das Vasomotorenzentrum* (Boden des IV. Ventrikels) funktioniert als Zentralstelle der Blutdruckregulation; es empfängt :

a) Impulse von höheren cerebralen Zentren im Sinne einer Änderung des Schwellenwertes oder der Einstellung des Reglerniveaus des Vasomotorenzentrums[1].

b) Impulse von den pressosensiblen, auf Gefäßwandspannung ansprechenden Feldern im Sinus caroticus und Aortenbogen über den N. depressor vagi[2].

3. *Hormonale Einwirkungen* erfolgen vom NN-Mark und von der Hypophyse auf die Arteriolen. .

Im pathologischen Bereich ist hier der Schwiegksche „*Lungenentlastungsreflex*" (1935) zu erwähnen. Plötzliche Drucksteigerung im Gebiete der Lungenstrombahn (z. B. Lungenembolie) führt zu einer über den Vagus ausgelösten Blutdrucksenkung im Großen Kreislauf mit Verlagerung von Blut des Kleinen Kreislaufs in die Peripherie des Großen Kreislaufs.

Mit der bis hierher *durch Transportkomponente I und II* gebildeten Transportapparatur ist für die individuelle Versorgung der Myriaden von biologischen Einheiten (Zellen und Gewebsbestandteilen) nur eine ganz *schematische „Universalberieselung" mit dem monoton gelieferten, in der Zusammensetzung kaum modifizierbaren Inhalt des linken Ventrikels gewährleistet.* Nur ein Versorgungsgrad etwa wie bei einem Gradierwerk mit gut funktionierendem Pumpwerk und gleichmäßiger Verteilung der Sole auf die Reisigbündel ist erreicht. Eine solche Apparatur ist sehr geeignet, wenn es sich darum handelt, eine Sole zu konzentrieren und zu reinigen. Dabei kommt es ja nur darauf an, *irgendwo* auf den Reisigbündeln diese Teilchen zur Ablagerung zu bringen. Im Organismus liegen die Dinge aber viel komplizierter; dort besteht *an verschiedenen Orten ein sowohl qualitativ als auch quantitativ ganz verschiedener Bedarf,* der zudem noch vom augenblicklichen Funktionsgrad jeder Zelle abhängig ist. Im bisher geschilderten Transportsystem fehlt jede derartige echte Zuteilung entsprechend dem lokalen Bedarf, sowohl was grobe Zuteilung an einzelne Organe als auch was detaillierte individuelle Zuteilung an einzelne Zellen oder Zellbestandteile entsprechend ihrem momentanen Bedarfsstand anbelangt. Hier greifen nun weitere Transportmechanismen ein.

Eine *spezielle Blutzuteilung zu Orten besonderen Bedarfs mit Hilfe von genau dosierter Kalibereinstellung der kleinen und kleinsten* Blutgefäße bewirkt eine Etatisierung der einzelnen Gefäßprovinzen auf den für die Funktion notwendigen Anteil des vom Herzen gelieferten Minutenvolumens. Sie wird erreicht

1. durch *hormonale Einflüsse* (Nebennierenmark),

2. durch direkte *nervale Einflüsse* auf die vegetative Innervation der Arteriolen; so wird z. B. bei motorischer Innervation eines Muskels gleichzeitig nerval die Blutzufuhr durch Erweiterung der ihn versorgenden Arteriolen gesteigert.

3. durch *Änderungen der Reizschwelle* in der vasomotorischen Reaktion der Capillaren je nach dem Funktionszustand der Organe; so erweitert z. B. Arterenol die Blutbahn im *arbeitenden* Muskel und verengt sie im *ruhenden* Muskel; dadurch erfolgt Verschiebung des Blutes in Richtung auf das arbeitende Organ;

4. durch *Stoffwechselprodukte,* welche in den Capillaren der arbeitenden Organe entstehen und von sich aus vasomotorisch wirken (CO_2, Milchsäure, Muskeladenylsäure, Adenosintriphosphorsäure, Acetylcholin-Cholinesterase, Histamin).

Durch die Komponente I und II (vgl. S. 174 und 175) wird eine *Anpassung* der Blutzufuhr und der lokalen Dimensionierung der capillären Austauschfläche *an den momentanen Funktionszustand der Organe* erreicht. Allerdings ist dabei einschränkend zu berücksichtigen, daß sehr

---

[1] WAGNER 1954.   [2] HERING 1927, HEYMANS 1933.

komplizierende *Interferenzen* bei diesem vasomotorischen Geschehen auftreten können; z. B. können durch die sich mächtig durchsetzenden Ansprüche seitens der Wärmeregulation oder seitens der Chemoreceptoren im Glomus caroticum und in den Paraganglien der Aorta, welche auf CO_2-Zunahme oder O_2-Abnahme des vorbeiströmenden Blutes ansprechen, wichtige andere Anforderungen an das Vasomotorensystem ausgeschaltet werden. Der Organismus sucht zwar durch „kollaterale Vasokonstriktion"[1] — wobei von vornherein Coronargebiet und Hirngefäße ausgespart bleiben — einen aus solchen Interferenzen entstehenden Zusammenbruch zu vermeiden. Dennoch können solche Anspruchskollisionen unzweifelhaft zu Gefährdungen oder mindestens zu Verlangsamungen bei der Erfüllung bestimmter spezieller Transportaufträge führen[2].

Aber auch selbst mit einem geregelten, den lokalen Bedürfnissen angepaßten Blutangebot ist *noch kein kompletter Transportvorgang*, sondern *nur eine Vorbedingung dafür geschaffen*. Die Transportsicherung entspricht bisher etwa gut einregulierten Wasserstraßen, welche durch dichtbesiedelte Gebiete fließen. Ohne Zusammenfassung des Transportgutes in Lastkähnen wäre dabei nur eine verschwenderische Schwemmwirkung zu erwarten, etwa, wie wenn eine Ladung Getreide in einen Fluß geschüttet würde und stromabwärts ein Bedarfsort sich befände; das Getreide würde zur Hauptsache vorbeischwimmen und sich irgendwo anders verfangen, wo es verlorengeht.

Die Bindung im lebenden Organismus *an spezifische Trägersubstanzen* könnte bewirken, daß die transportierten Stoffe auf ihrem kreisförmig geschlossenen Transportwege verbleiben und schließlich, auch wenn sie vielfältige „große Umwege" machen sollten, doch nur an ihrem Bestimmungsort, dem Ort besonderer Affinität zur Ladung, aus der Blutbahn abgegeben werden.

Virchow ließ die im Zentrum aller Lebensvorgänge stehende Zelle einfach das „entnehmen, wessen sie bedurfte". Heute wissen wir, daß der Bedarf durch ein ökonomisches Transportsystem in besonderer Weise angeboten wird, und daß ferner die Aufnahme durch im einzelnen erklärbare physikalische und chemische Mechanismen der Zellstruktur und des Zellstoffwechsels zustande kommt. Diese alte „Potenz" der Zelle ist analysierbar, und der galenisch (s. S. 169) anmutende vitalistische Begriff einer „auswählenden Kraft" mußte zunehmender Kenntnis physikalischer und chemischer Zusammenhänge Platz machen.

Im Capillargebiet bestehen zwar durch maximal verlangsamte Blutströmung von etwa 0,05 cm/sec relativ günstige Vorbedingungen für Austauschvorgänge. Dennoch erscheint es kaum möglich, den Grenzmembranen der Capillaren und Zellen *alle die* qualitativen und quantitativen Auslesefunktionen aufzubürden, welche sowohl Kolloiden als auch echt gelösten sowie lipoidlöslichen Stoffen gegenüber zu gelten hätten. *Erst durch Einfügung eines Vehikelapparates erscheint eine Ökonomie im Transport und eine wesentliche Entlastung der Zellmembranen in ihren vielfältigen „Auslesefunktionen" möglich.*

Dazu kommt noch folgendes: Die vasomotorisch gesteuerte Blutzuteilung (Komponente II) in Richtung auf Orte besonderen Bedarfs hat ihren hauptsächlichen Geltungsbereich im Großen Kreislauf. Dort können die Umleitungen eines Teils des Blutes zu bestimmten Organen die Gefahr des „error loci" deutlich mindern (Abb. 1).

Die *Gefäßverbindungen* vom Herzen zu den Organen und die der Organe untereinander sind nun aber keineswegs gleich. Sie sind:

1. Direkt und total.

Dann erfolgt der Zustrom von Blut aus den vorgeschalteten Organen unmittelbar und praktisch quantitativ in das Empfangsorgan, und nur dort wirken die Vasomotoren. Es liegt in toto eine nebenweglose Direktverbindung

---

[1] Hess 1938.   [2] Rein 1949.

vor. (Beispiele: Darmblut—V. portae—Leber; Leber—rechter Ventrikel—Lunge; Lunge—linker Ventrikel).

2. *Direkt und partiell.*

Im großen Kreislauf strömt das im linken Herzen gemischte Lungenblut unmittelbar, aber aufgeteilt den verschiedenen Organen der Körperperipherie zu; bzw. das aus einem Organ abströmende venöse Blut stellt nur einen Teil der gegen Lungen und Herz zurückflutenden Blutmenge dar. (Beispiel: linker Ventrikel—Gehirn [oder Muskulatur . . .]).

3. *Partiell und indirekt.*

Verschiedene Organe der Kreislaufperipherie stehen zueinander nur in einer indirekten Verbindung. Die Leber empfängt ihren Anteil des Schlagvolumens des linken Ventrikels nur zum geringsten Teile direkt. Der Hauptteil ($^3/_4$ der überhaupt zuflutenden Menge) kommt erst indirekt *nach Passage der Milz* oder der *Mesenterialcapillaren* an. Das Organ liegt in einer Art Nebenschluß zum großen Kreislauf. (Beispiel: linker Ventrikel—Leber).

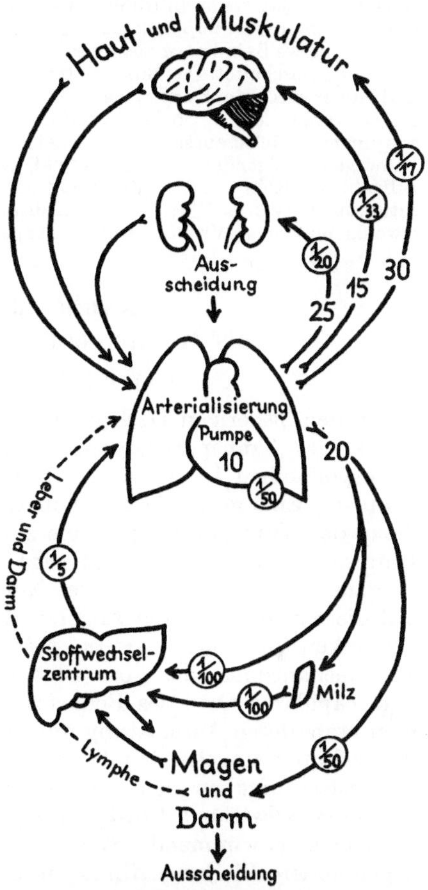

Im kleinen Kreislauf als Typus der Direktverbindung können Kaliberschwankungen der Blutgefäße nur en bloc wirken und nichts daran ändern, daß alles aus dem rechten Ventrikel herausströmende Blut quantitativ die Lunge passiert; nur die Gesamtmenge des durchfließenden Blutes je Minute kann geändert werden. Abzweigungen in andere Organe sind unmöglich; höchstens in die Blutspeicherräume der Lunge können Teile des zirkulierenden Blutes abgeschoben werden. Das gleiche gilt für den Pfortaderkreislauf und für die Blutzufuhr zur Leber. Im Großen Kreislauf kann der Organismus die Relation der Blutzuteilungen zu den einzelnen Organen sehr stark variieren.

Am schwierigsten liegen die Verhältnisse bei *Organen, die im Nebenschluß liegen*; erstens kann das vorgeschaltete Capillargebiet den Blutstrom entsprechend seinen eigenen Bedürfnissen dosieren, womit sich dann das nachfolgende Nebenschlußorgan abfinden muß; zweitens muß die Passage des vorgeschalteten Capillargebietes eine ausgesprochene Transportgefährdung bedeuten; es besteht die Gefahr, daß das Transportgut, dessen das im Nebenschluß befindliche Zweitorgan dringend bedarf, bereits im ersten Capillargebiet ausgesondert, gewissermaßen „abfiltriert" wird. Mit rein vasomotorischen Einwirkungen kann dieser Gefahr nicht begegnet werden. Gerade bei einem so vielfältig wichtigen Organ wie der Leber, die auch den im großen Kreislauf zirkulierenden Stoffwechselprodukten gegenüber wichtige chemische

Abb. 1. Schematische Darstellung des Blutkreislaufs und seiner größten Verzweigungsgebiete mit dem prozentualen Anteil der vom Herzen in Körperruhe geförderten Blutmenge. In den Kreisen Gehalt an Leberblut in Bruchteilen der hier strömenden Blutmenge.

Funktionen hat, ist diese ungünstige Antransportsituation besonders bemerkenswert. Das Beispiel des Bilirubins möge dies erläutern:

Beim Blutabbau entsteht im lebenden Organismus ständig Bilirubin. Es zirkuliert in einer Konzentration von 0,5—1 mg% im Plasma. Sein Bestimmungsort ist die Leber. Die hauptsächlichen Orte des Blutzerfalls gehören dem Großen Kreislauf an. Die Chancen, daß ein irgendwo im Knochenmark oder traumatisch aus einem Bluterguß entstandenes Bilirubinteilchen wirklich die Leber erreicht, sind gering (Abb. 1), wobei man besonders in Betracht ziehen muß, daß freies Bilirubin an sich eine große Affinität zu fast jeglichem Gewebe besitzt, mit dem man es in *wäßriger* Lösung in Berührung bringt. Nur durch Bindung des Bilirubins an Plasmaeiweiß sind normalerweise alle „transportgefährdenden" Affinitäten anderer Capillargebiete ausgeschaltet. Das Bilirubinteilchen zirkuliert in sicherer Bindung an das Albumin wieder und immer wieder im Körper, bis es einmal in die Leber gelangt, wo die Bindung an Plasmaeiweiß gelöst werden kann. So bewirkt die Bindung des Bilirubinteilchens an Plasmaeiweiß, daß aus einem zunächst aussichtslos erscheinenden Transportrisiko doch ein — allerdings auf vielen Umwegen erfolgender — im Endeffekt „gezielter" Transport wird. Die Ablagerungsorte des Bilirubins (RES und Tubulusepithel) entsprechen — außer bei hochpathologischen Situationen (vgl. S. 199f.) — den Hauptablagerungsorten des körperfremden, aber ebenfalls eiweißgebundenen Vitalfarbstoffes Trypanblau. Einzelheiten über den Bilirubintransport vgl. S. 198.

Zirkulierendes Transportmilieu
als Komponente III der Transportapparatur.
(Vehikel als lokale Abgabe-Regler.)

In den bisherigen Darlegungen wurde ein Überblick gegeben über die Problematik der Transportvorgänge, insbesondere soweit sie ein ausgesprochenes Transportmilieu in Form der Blut- oder Lymphströmung dafür in Anspruch nehmen. Eine große Anzahl von Regulationsmechanismen dient, wie wir sahen, dazu, den Transportvorgang bis zum fein regulierten *Angebot* des zirkulierenden Blutes zu sichern. Für die *Abgabe* von Stoffen aus der Blutbahn, welche gerade an ganz bestimmten Orten (des Notstandes) extravasculär gebraucht werden, ist mit diesem so geregelten Angebot des im Capillargebiet vorbeifließenden Inhalts des linken Ventrikels *nur eine primitive Vorbedingung* geschaffen. Es fehlt noch ein Mechanismus, der vom Blut her den Abstrom aus den Capillaren an die extracapillären Orte des Bedarfs mehr oder weniger selektiv freigibt. Die Zellmembran, deren Ausstattung mit Fermenten für aktive Transporte in den letzten Jahrzehnten eingehend untersucht wurde[1], kann der außerordentlichen Vielfalt an Ausleseaufgaben allein wohl kaum gerecht werden. Eine *Vorauslese im Flüssigkeitsstrom selbst durch Vehikel als lokale Abgaberegler ist notwendig.* Durch Bindung an solche schwimmende Speicher können die zu transportierenden Substanzen gegen andere Bindungsaffinitäten im durchströmten Gewebe abgesichert werden.

Erythrocyten als Vehikel.

Am deutlichsten ist dieses Vehikelprinzip als Bestandteil des Transportvorganges am größten Vehikel, dem *Erythrocyten,* und am besonders lebenswichtigen Transportgut, dem Sauerstoff, darstellbar.

Zunächst möge ein *phylogenetischer Rückblick* dies erläutern. Einzeller brauchen keinen Transportapparat für die Versorgung mit Sauerstoff; sie beziehen ihn rein nach den Gesetzen der Gaskinetik aus dem umgebenden Medium durch Diffusion. Mit der Ausbildung differenzierter Organe werden die Versorgungswege für einfache Diffusionsvorgänge zu weit. Ein strömendes Transportmilieu mit „schwimmenden Speichern" für Sauerstoff wird deswegen eingeschaltet. Bei niederen Tieren, z. B. bei den Regenwürmern, wird diese Funktion des Sauerstoffvehikels von eisenhaltigen Chromoproteiden (Erythrocruorinen) erfüllt; es handelt sich dabei um sauerstoffbindende Kolloide mit einem hohen Molekulargewicht von mehreren Millionen. Andere Würmer haben für den gleichen Zweck grüne, eisenhaltige, hochmolekulare

---

[1] Wilbrandt 1951.

Eiweißkörper (Chlorocruorine). Bei manchen Krebsen finden sich kupferhaltige Hämocyanine mit einem Molekulargewicht von 8 Millionen. Alle diese Chromoproteide verrichten ihre Vehikelfunktion als Sole ohne Einbau in mikroskopisch sichtbare corpusculäre Elemente. Sobald in der Phylogenese das letztere eintritt, geht das Molekulargewicht des Chromoproteids auf die Größenordnung des Hämoglobins mit 68000 herunter. Es hat den Anschein, als ob unter allen Umständen das Eindringen des Sauerstoffvehikels in die Zelle bzw. das Verlassen der Blutbahn verhindert werden soll, das eine Mal durch Bildung von Riesenmolekülen, das andere Mal durch Anheften von sehr viel kleineren Chromoproteidmolekülen an große Formelemente des Blutes, an die Erythrocyten.

Der Vorgang des Sauerstofftranportes soll offenbar in seinem letzten Stadium stets der eines Diffusionsprozesses bleiben; er wird dadurch noch besonders rationell gestaltet, daß durch CO_2-Anhäufung gerade in den sauerstoffbedürftigen Capillarbezirken eine Ansäuerung des Milieus stattfindet, welche die Sauerstoffbindungsfähigkeit des Hämoglobins stark herabsetzt, den Sauerstoff somit als besonders disponibel bereit hält. Die Erythrocyten funktionieren gewissermaßen als schwimmende Speicher. Die transportierende Grenzfläche der Erythrocyten eines Menschen ist für diesen weitverzweigten Transportvorgang mit etwa 3800 m², d. h. dem etwa 2000fachen der Körperoberfläche, sehr groß dimensioniert.

Ob auch noch andere im Erythrocyten enthaltene Substanzen als echtes Transportgut zu betrachten sind, ist zweifelhaft; am ehesten kämen noch die Fermente in Frage (Kohlensäureanhydrase, Cocarboxylase, Glyoxalase, Coenzym 1, Phosphatase, Cholinesterase, unter denen die Kohlensäureanhydrase hier wohl in erster Linie zu nennen wäre).

Die *Anreicherung mancher Kationen* im Erythrocyten ist oftmals recht hoch, wie aus dem Vergleich der jeweiligen Konzentration im Vollblut und im Plasma zu ersehen ist:

	Gehalt im Vollblut	Gehalt im Plasma
Kalium	175,2[1] mg%	16,34[2] mg%
Mangan	0,029 mg%	0,0029[3] mg%
Zink	0,880 mg%	0,300[4, 5] mg%

Es wäre aber durchaus verfrüht, auf Grund dieser Konzentrationsdifferenzen allein auf eine Vehikelfunktion der Erythrocyten diesen Kationen gegenüber schließen zu wollen. Von den *Medikamenten* haftet das Atebrin an den Erythrocyten; im isolierten Serum zeigt es auch deutliche Bindung an Albumin. Es ergeben sich somit Gleichgewichtszustände zwischen der Bindung an Erythrocyten und Bindung an Albumin, also Adsorptionskonkurrenz zwischen zwei Vehikeln im Transportmilieu, somit ein mehrgliedriges *Bindungsgleichgewicht*, dessen biologischer Bedeutung wir später noch mehrfach begegnen werden.

Thrombocyten.

Eine Rolle als mikroskopisch erfaßbare Vehikel scheinen ferner die *Blutplättchen* zu spielen. Das Transportgut der Thrombocyten ist besonders mannigfaltig: einerseits finden wir darin Faktoren der Blutgerinnung[6] wie Thromboplastin, ac.-Globulin, Plättchen-Antifibrinolysin und Accelerator der Fibrinbildung, andererseits vasoconstrictorische Substanzen wie Serotonin[7] und Noradrenalin[8]; schließlich noch eine Reihe von Enzymen[9] wie Katalase, Amylase, Tyrosinase, Hyaluronidase, alkalische und saure Phosphatase, β-Glucuronidase, Dopaoxydase, Acetylcholinesterase, Tryptase, Histaminase, Esterase; die 12 zuletzt aufgeführten Enzyme sind wohl als allgemeine Bestandteile der Zellausstattung und nicht als Transportgut aufzufassen. Serotonin und Noradrenalin werden durch aktive

---

[1] HALD 1947.　　[2] ELLIOTT und HOLLEY 1951.　　[3] KEHOE et al. 1940.
[4] VALLEE und GIBSON 1948.　　[5] HOCH und VALLEE 1949.　　[6] PERLICK 1960.
[7] HUMPHREY und JACQUES 1954, UDENFRIEND et al. 1955, SANO et al. 1958.
[8] WEIL-MALHERBE und BONE 1958.　　[9] WALLER et al. 1959.

Transportvorgänge in den Plättchen in hoher Konzentration gespeichert.[1] Reserpin hemmt diesen Speicherungsprozeß[2]. Für den lokalen Wundverschluß spielen einerseits die vasoconstrictorischen Substanzen und andererseits die Gerinnungsfaktoren der Plättchen, wie aus der Physiologie und Pathologie bekannt ist, eine hervorragende Rolle; in den Plättchen sind somit wichtige und sich ergänzende Reparaturfaktoren vereinigt, die durchaus geeignet sind, am Ort einer Verletzung baldigen Wundverschluß zu erzielen. Hinzu kommt noch, daß das Plättchen am Orte des Bedarfs bzw. des Notstandes „haltmacht"; die Lokomotorik (Komponente I der Transportvorgänge) reißt ab, das Plättchen haftet an der veränderten Gefäßwand, wird adhärent und agglutiniert; dabei geht es zugrunde; die Inhaltsstoffe werden frei und können am Ort des Bedarfes ihre regelhafte Wirkung entfalten. In den Thrombocyten ist das Serotonin gegenüber dem Plasma auf das Tausendfache angereichert[1]. Die Bindung scheint mit dem ATP-Gehalt der Plättchen in Zusammenhang zu stehen und hat einen intakten Energiestoffwechsel zur Voraussetzung[2]; enzymatische Prozesse spielen hier wohl eine entscheidende Rolle. Vergegenwärtige man sich im Gedankenexperiment einmal, welche Mengen von Serotonin und von Blutgerinnungsfaktoren in die Blutbahn eingeschwemmt werden müßten, um ohne das Plättchen-Vehikel *auch* an den Ort der Verletzung die lokal notwendige Menge dieser wichtigen Reparaturfaktoren — durch allgemeine Hebung des Blutspiegels — heranzubringen; welche gefährlichen Folgen müßte eine solche *generelle* Hebung des Blutspiegels an Serotonin und Gerinnungsfaktoren für den Gesamtorganismus haben! Auch an diesem Beispiel wird klar, wie sehr Vehikel zum Gesamtmechanismus der Transportapparatur im lebenden Organismus gehören.

Bei den *Leukocyten*, mit ihrem eigenen Stoffwechsel als komplette celluläre Elemente, ist das Problem, inwieweit sie als Vehikel anzusehen sind, viel komplexer. Die gezielte Zufuhr von Fermenten zu lokalen Entzündungen könnte an sich ebenfalls als Vehikelmechanismus interpretiert werden. Auf Einzelheiten in dieser Frage einzugehen, würde den Rahmen dieses Beitrags überschreiten.

Serumeiweißkörper.

Als weitere und betreffs des zu befördernden Transportgutes besonders ausgedehnte und *mannigfaltige* Vehikel sind die *Serumeiweißkörper* anzusehen. Als kolloide Trägersubstanzen mit einem Molekulargewicht von 69000 bis 1 Million verändern sie bei den von ihnen gebundenen Substanzen in fundamentaler Weise die Diffusions- und Abgabebedingungen. Sie sind in der Lage, zahlreiche körpereigene oder körperfremde Substanzen an sich zu binden, wie Bennhold mit Hilfe von Diffusions- und Kataphoreseversuchen (im Agar- bzw. Gelatinegel und im Michaelis-Apparat 1925—1932) zuerst zeigen konnte. Die Zahl der Substanzen, deren Bindung an Serumeiweißkörper beschrieben wurde, ist inzwischen sehr stark angewachsen (vgl. Tabelle 2, S. 183). Das Bluteiweißbild verschiedener Tiere zeigt große Unterschiede; das Serum mancher Schildkröten (Genus Pseudemys) z. B. hat keine dem menschlichen Albumin entsprechende Zacke[3]. — Die Serumeiweißkörper eines Menschen besitzen eine Grenzfläche in einer Größenordnung von etwa 700000 m². Durch ihre Bindungsfähigkeit bilden die Serumproteine ein regulierendes Moment im Stofftransport, beeinflussen die Verteilung im Körper, verhindern Überschwemmung und Verluste und regeln, gewissermaßen als „schwimmende Speicher", die lokale Abgabe der zu transportierenden Substanzen.

---

[1] Humphrey 1954, Weil-Malherbe und Bone 1958.
[2] Sano et al. 1958, Zucker 1961, Hughes 1959.   [3] Cohen 1958.

Tabelle 2. *Zusammenstellung von Stoffen, welche Bindungen mit Serumeiweiß eingehen.*

Erläuterungen. Die Zitate in der Tabelle sind in der Reihenfolge ihres Publikationsjahres angeordnet. Die Substanzen selbst folgen einander innerhalb der Gruppen alphabetisch. Das Symbol bedeutet, welches Protein auf seine Bindungsfähigkeit hin untersucht wurde. + = Bindung festgestellt, Ø = keine Bindung festgestellt, ? = Bindung fraglich. Die Reihenfolge der Serumproteine zeigt die Stärke der Bindungen an. P = Protein, Pl = Plasma, S = Serum ohne Berücksichtigung der Komponenten, A = Serumalbumin, A* = gereinigtes (kristallisiertes) Serumalbumin, G = Serumglobulin, α-, β-, γ-G = elektrophoretisch fraktioniertes α-, β- oder γ-Globulin. G-eu = Euglobulin, G-pseudo = Pseudoglobulin, Glyko = Glykoproteid, α_1-Lipo = α_1-Lipoproteid, β-Lipo = β-Lipoproteid. AL = durch Albumin wurde die Löslichkeit des untersuchten Stoffes erhöht. Die kursiven Symbole geben die Herkunft des Proteins an:

M = Mensch, *Pf* = Pferd, *R* = Rind, *H* = Hund, *K* = Kaninchen, *S* = Schwein, *Ra* = Ratte, *Ma* = Maus, *Me* = Meerschweinchen. † Siehe auch unter „Plasmaglobuline als Vehikel".

Wasser.

Bindung an verschiedene lösliche Proteine[1], an Aminogruppen[2].

Anorganische Stoffe.

Anionen.

Bromide A* *M* +[3]. Chloride A *Pf* +[4], S *Pf* +[5], S *H* Ø[6], A* *M* und *R* +[7], A +[8], A *M* +[9]. Fluoride A* *M* +[10]. Jod S *R* Ø[11], β-G und A *M* +[12], Inter-α-G und A *M* +[13]. Nitrate A* *M* +[14]. Perchlorate A* *M* +[15]. Phosphate S *Pf* +[16], A* *M* +[17], P +[18], Pl *M* +, *H* +[18a]. Rhodanid A* *M* +[19], A* *M* +[20], A +[21]. Sulfate S *M* Ø[22], S *M* ?[23], S *H* Ø[24], A* *M* und *R* +[25].

Kationen.

Barium α_1- und β-Lipo *M* +[26]. Blei, Bleisubacetat sr. Glyko *M* +[27]. Calcium S *M* +[28], S *Pf* +[29], A und G *M* +[30], G-eu *M* +[31], G (Thrombin) *Pf* +[32]. Casein +[33], A (verschiedene) +[34], α_1- und β-Lipo *M* +[35]. Eisen † S *R* + *S* +[36], β_1-G *M* +[37]. Gallium S *M* Ø[38]. Gold-Kolloid S *M* +[39], α_2-G, A, β- und γ-G *M* +[40], α- und β-G *M* +[41]. Kalium S *M* Ø[42]. Kobalt A, α- und β-G *Ma* +[43]. Kupfer † A *R*, *Pf*[43a] S *M* +[44], β-G *M* +[45], G *M* +[46], A* und G *R* +[47], Coeruloplasmin und A *M* +[48], Coeruloplasmin und A *Ma* +[49], Coerulo., A und α-, β-γ-G *H* + K + *Me* +[50]. Mangan S *Ma* und *M* Ø[51], Transmanganin *M*[51a]. Magnesium S *M* +[52], A *M* +[53], A, α-G *M* +[54]. Natrium S *M* Ø[55]. Quecksilber S *Pf* +[56], A* *M* +[57], S *M* +[58]. Selen A und G-pseudo +[59]. Silber A *M* +[60]. Silber-Kolloid S *M* +[61]. Thorium G *M*[62]. Zink A *Pf* +[63], S *M* +[64], A und α-, β-, γ-G *H* +[65].

[1] Starling 1896, Schade 1923, Cohn und Edsall 1943, Bull 1944, Schmidt 1944. [2] Mellon 1949. [3] Scatchard 1949a, 1957. [4] Pauli und Schön 1924. [5] Hayasida 1933. [6] Goudsmith 1939. [7] Scatchard 1949b, 1957. [8] Luck 1949. [9] Scatchard 1950. [10] Scatchard 1949a. [11] De Haan 1921a. [12] Bassett 1941, Taurog 1948, Maurer 1952. [13] Gordon 1952, Horst 1953a, Maurer 1953, Deiss 1952, 1953. [14] Scatchard 1949a. [15] Scatchard 1949, 1957. [16] Pearson 1936. [17] Ballou 1945. [18] Velick 1949. [18a] Walser 1960. [19] Scatchard 1949b, 1947. [20] Scatchard 1950, 1957. [21] Scatchard 1950. [22] Hayman 1932. [23] Bjering 1939. [24] Goudsmith 1939. [25] Boyer 1946. [26] Cohn 1953. [27] Cohn 1953. [28] Rona 1911, Greenberg 1930, Hopkins 1952, Müller 1953. [29] Pearson 1936. [30] Bendien 1933, McLean 1935, Gutmann 1937, Greenberg 1944. [31] Drinker 1939. [32] Widenbauer 1943, Martin 1950. [33] Chanutin 1942, Ludewig 1942. [34] Martin 1950, [35] Cohn 1953. [36] Laurell 1947. [37] Schade 1946, E. Cohn 1948, Cartwright 1949, Surgenor 1949, Wallenius 1952, Horst 1953b, Wuhrmann 1953. [38] Munn 1951, Horst 1954a. [39] v. Jancsó 1929. [40] Ott 1954. [41] Simon 1954. [42] Rona 1924, [43] Horst 1954a. [43a] Eisler 1936. [44] Macheboeuf 1944. [45] E. Cohn 1948, Surgenor 1949. [46] Keiderling 1950. [47] Klotz 1950a. [48] Holmberg 1947, Brendstrup 1953. [49] Gubler 1953, Horst 1954a. [50] Wolff 1955. [51] Horst 1954a. [51a] Cotzias 1960. [52] Augsberger 1925, Bernhard 1926. [53] Copeland 1952. [54] Prasad 1959. [55] Neuhausen 1922. [56] Taylor 1930. [57] Hughes 1947, Lonti 1948, Saroff 1949. [58] Kelley 1950. [59] McConnel 1950. [60] Neergaard 1923/24. [61] v. Jancsó 1929. [62] Bennhold 1938. [63] Pauli 1924. [64] Cohn 1953, Weitzel 1956. [65] Wolff 1955, 1956.

Organische Stoffe.
Körpereigene Stoffe.

Acetat A★ $M+$[66]. Acetalphosphatide α_1- und β-Lipo $M+$[67]. Acetylcholin „A" $H+$[68], α-G $M+$[69]. Acetyltryptophan A★ $M+$, $R+$[70]. Adenin, Adenosin, Adenylsäure A★ $R+$[71]. Neutrale Aminosäuren A, γ-G $M+$[72]. Bilirubin † S $M+$[73], A $M+$[74], S $M+$[75], A $R+$[76], α_1-G $M+$[77], A, α- und β-G $M+$[78]. Biliverdin† G-pseudo $M+$[79]. Cholesterin † und Ester G $M+$[80], S $M+$[81], A und G $R+$, $Pf+$[82], α_1-, β_1-G $M+$[83], α_1- und β_1-Lipo $M+$, $Ra+$[84]. Coproporphyrin A $M+$[85], Ferriprotoporphyrin IX A $M+$[86]. Fettsäuren A, α_1- und β-Lipo $M+$[87]. Gallensaure Salze S $M+$[88], S $Pf+$[89], A $M+$[90], S Pf Ø[91], S M und $Pf+$[92], A★ $M+$[93]. Hämatin A $M+$[94], β-G, A $M+$[94a]. Hämatoporph. A $M+$[95], A★ $M+$[96]. Harnsäure A M und *Gans* ?[97] und Urate S M und *Kücken*+[98], S[99], A $M+$[100]. Heparin α_2 und β-G $M+$[101]. Histamin A $M+$[102]. Lipoide † G $M+$, $R+$[103], α_1- und β_1-G $M+$[104]. Melanogen A $M+$[105]. Polysaccharide G $M+$[106], α-G $M+$[107]. Porphyrine A $M+$[108]. Phosphatide A $M+$[109]. Phosphorlipoproteide † α_1- und β_1-G $M+$[110]. Reststickstoffsubstanzen Blut $H+$[111], S $M+$[112], S M Ø[113], S $H+$[114], A★ R und $M+$[115]. Uroporphyrin S M Ø[116]. Zucker (Monosacchar.) S M Ø[117].

Hormone: Dijodtyrosin † S M Ø[118]. Corticosteroide† A $M+$[119]. Oestradiol S $R+$, $K+$, $M+$[120], S $M+$[121], S $M+$[122], β_1-Lipo $M+$[123], AL[124]. Progesteron † AL[124]. Testosteron † AL[124]. Thyroxin † (s. Jod) Inter-α-G und A $M+$[125]. 17-Ketosteroide † A (frakt.) $M+$[126], A $M+$[127]. Trijodthyronin † Inter-α-G und A $M+$[128].

Vitamine: Citrin A $M+$[129], Eriodictin A $M+$[129], (3. Stoff des Citrin) A $M+$[129]. Hesperidin A $M+$[129]. Laktoflavinphosphorsäure G-eu $M+$[130]. Nicotinamid G $M+$[131]. Thiochrome G-eu $M+$[131]. Vitamin A (Karotinoide) β_1-Lipo $M+$[132]. Vitamin C A $M+$[133]. Vitamin K A $M+$[133]. Vitamin B$_{12}$ † α_1-Seromucoid +[133a].

Körperfremde Stoffe.

a) Medikamente und Teststoffe: Aminopyrin S $Pf+$[134]. Atebrin A $M+$[135]. Atropin S $R+$ $K+$[136]. Aureomycin A $M+$[137]. Barbiturate A $M+$[138], A★ $M+$, $R+$[139]. Carcinogene Kohlenwasserstoffe Lipo $R+$[140]. Caronamid A $H+$[141]. Chloroform S+[142]. Chloromycetin A★ $R+$[143]. Cholin S Ø[144]. Cinchona Alkal. A★ $M+$[145]. Cinnamate A★ $R+$[146], A $R+$[147]. Cocain S $R+$, $Pf+$, $K+$[148]. Coffein S Pf[149], S Ø, A M Ø[150]. Digilanid A+[151]. Digitoxin und andere Glykoside S $M+$[152], S R und andere +[153], A $Ra+$[154], A *Frosch*+, $M+$[155], A★ $M+$[156], S (Frosch) + und $K+$[157]. Epinephrin S Ø[158], S $M+$[159]. Foliandrin A+[160].

[66] Ballou 1945, Cann 1958. [67] Leupold 1954. [68] Heim 1939. [69] Goldstein 1949. [70] Boyer 1947. [71] Klotz 1948a. [72] Hunter 1955. [73] Forrai 1927. [74] Bennhold 1929/30, Bendien 1933, Pedersen 1937. [75] Malloy 1937, Coolidge 1940, With 1945, Gray 1948. [76] Barac 1949. [77] Martin 1948/49. [78] Westphal 1949, Löffler 1949, Bennhold 1952. [79] Coolidge 1940. [80] Gardner 1927, Theorell 1930, Bennhold 1931, Bendien 1933. [81] Bruger 1935. [82] Mellander 1935. [83] E. Cohn 1948. [84] Gofman 1950, Kunkel 1952, Schettler 1955. [85] Gildemeister 1937. [86] Rosenfeld 1950. [87] Gordon 1955. [88] Brentano 1927. [89] Lecomte de Nouy 1928. [90] Bennhold 1938. [91] Laporta 1940. [92] Tayeau 1947. [93] E. Cohn 1948. [94] Fairly-Bromfield 1934, Keilin 1944. [94a] Aber 1960. [95] Gildemeister 1937. [96] Rosenfeld 1948, E. Cohn 1948. [97] Bennhold 1938. [98] Levine 1947, Wolfson 1947—1949. [99] Adlersberg 1942. [100] Morris 1958. [101] Hoch 1952, Blasius 1952. [102] Klamerth 1955. [103] Macheboeuf 1937. [104] Edsall 1947, E. Cohn 1948, Gofman 1950. [105] Bennhold 1938. [106] Meyer 1945, Stary 1953, Köiw 1952. [107] E. Cohn 1948, Schmid 1953, Knedel 1955. [108] Bennhold 1938. [109] Maurer 1953b. [110] Kunkel 1952, Schettler 1955. [111] Rosenthal 1926a. [112] Loiseleur 1937. [113] Bennhold 1938. [114] Malinow 1947. [115] Boyer 1945/46. [116] Gildemeister 1937. [117] De Haan 1921b, Bennhold 1938. [118] Horst 1954b. [119] Daughaday 1956. [120] Szego 1946. [121] Rakoff 1943. [122] Boettiger 1946. [123] Roberts 1946. [124] Bischoff 1948. [125] Horst 1954. [126] Gardner 1954. [127] Westphal 1956. [128] Deiss 1953, Horst 1954b. [129] Schubert 1947. [130] Schubert 1947. [131] Schubert 1947. [132] E. Cohn 1948. [133] Schubert 1947. [133a] Miller 1959. [134] Samson 1926. [135] Bennhold 1944. [136] Storm van Leeuwen 1921, Beutner 1925. [137] Sirota 1950. [138] Bennhold 1938, Ott 1952. [139] Goldbaum 1948, Klotz 1950b. [140] Avigan 1959. [141] Earle 1947, Beyer 1949. [142] Moore 1904/05. [143] Smith 1948. [144] Beutner 1924. [145] Hiatt 1946, Taggart 1949. [146] Duggan 1948. [147] Teresi 1948. [148] Beutner 1925, Pak 1926. [149] Pak 1926. [150] Breitinger 1956. [151] Farah 1945. [152] Oppenheimer 1913, Hoekstra 1931. [153] Lendle 1935, Haarmann 1940. [154] Fawaz 1944. [155] Fawaz 1944, Farah 1945. [156] Rothlin 1949. [157] Salter 1946. [158] Beutner 1925. [159] Barac 1949. [160] Farah 1945.

Germanin A (frakt.) Pf+, K +[161], S +[162], S M +[163],Pl + [164], G +[165], S +[166], Pl +[167], A M +[168]. Heparin A frakt. M +, Pf +[169],[170], α_2- und β-G M +[171] und Hippurate (p-amino) S M +[172], A R +[173]. Isonicotinsäurehydrazid S M Ø[174]. Jodkontrastmittel S Pf Ø[175], A M +[176], S M[177], A M +[178]. Mandelate A⋆ R +[179]. Morphin S Pf+, und R+ und K +[180]. Mustardgassulfon S M und K[181], P[182]. Must. gas. sulfoxin P[183]. Naphtochinone A⋆ M +[184], Pl (bes. A) +[185]. Neosalvarsan (Neosphenamin) A M +[186]. Oleate Blut H +[187], A⋆ R +[188], A⋆ M[189], A α_1- und β-Lipo M +[190]. p-Aminobenzoate S M +[191]. p-Aminosalicylsäure M Ø[192]. p-Aminosalicylate A M +[193]. Penicillin S M +[194], A M +[195], A⋆ R +[196]. Pilocarpin S Pf, K, R[197]. Procain S? [198]. Prontosil A M +[199]. Phenylbutazon A M +[200]. Prostigmin α-G +[202]. Physostigmin[203]. Salicylate S M und R[204], A M[205], S M[206], S M[207], A[208]. Salvarsan (vgl. Neosalvarsan) (Arsphen.) A[209]. Aureomycin A M[209a]. Streptomycin S M Ø[210], S M +[211], A +, G? [212], Pl M[213]. Strophantin S M Ø[214], S M Ø[215], A M Ø[216], S versch. Ø[217], Pl M Ø[218]. Sulfonamide A M +[219], A⋆ M +[220], A⋆ (versch.) +[221], A M +[222], S M + [222a]

b) *Farbstoffe.* Azofarbstoffe: Amaranth A R +[223]. Azorubin A M und R +[224]. Azosulfothiazol A R +[225]. Azoviolett A M +[226]. Benzoblau A M +[227]. Biebrich Scharlach Gelatine +[228]. Brillantkongorot A M +[229]. Brillantvitalrot S M +[230]. Carcinogene Azofarben A R +[231]. Buttergelb A G M +[232]. Diaminblau S +[233]. Diaminrot S +[234], A und G M +[235]. Evansblau A G M +[236]. Geigyblau A und G M +[237]. Kongorot S M +[238], A, α und β-G M +[239], Ovalbumin +[240]. Lachsrot A M +[241]. Methylorange A R und M +[242]. Niagarahimmelblau A M +[243]. Niagarahimmelblau 6 A M +[244]. o-Aminoazotoluol A und G M +[245]. Orange I und II A R +[246]. Orange I P +[247]. p-(2-hydroxy-5-methylphenylazo)-benzoesäure A M +[248]. Phenyl-(p-(p-dimethylaminobenzenazo)-benzoylamino)-azetat A M +[249]. Tropaeolin O A M +[250], Gelatine +[251]. Trypanblau A, β-G M +[252]. Trypanrot A, β-G M +[253]. Nitrofarbstoffe: Naphtolgelb A M +[254]. Picrinsäure A R +[255]. Phthaleinfarbstoffe: Bromphenolblau A M +[256]. Bromthymolblau S +[257]. Chromquecksilber P +[258].

[161] MAYER 1922. [162] KOCIAN 1936. [163] BOURSNELL 1939, DEWEY 1946, SPINKS 1948. [164] DEWEY 1948. [165] BOURSNELL 1948. [166] WILSON 1949. [167] TOWN 1950. [168] OTT 1954. [169] KLOPSTOCK 1932, BRINKHOUS 1938, QUICK 1938, CHARGAFF 1940, 1941. [170] COHEN 1940, FERGUSON 1940, WÖHLISCH 1940, ZIFF 1940, JACQUES 1943. [171] BLASIUS 1952, HOCH 1952. [172] SMITH 1945. [173] TERESI 1948. [174] EISFELD 1954. [175] ELSOM 1936. [176] SMITH 1938. [177] RIGGS 1947, 1949. [178] BENNHOLD 1950a, OTT 1956. [179] LUCK 1948. [180] STORM VON LEEUWEN 1921, BEUTNER 1925, PAK 1926. [181] FRANCIS 1947. [182] BANKS 1946. [183] BOURSNELL 1948. [184] BUEDING 1948, HEYMANN 1948, E. COHN 1948. [185] FIESER 1948. [186] BENNHOLD 1938. [187] ROSENTHAL 1926a. [188] DAVIS 1946. [189] GORDON 1953. [190] GORDON 1955. [191] LUNDQUIST 1945. [192] EISFELD 1954. [193] WAY 1948. [194] BIGGER 1944, EAGLE 1947/48, TEPPERMANN 1947. [195] TOMPSETT 1947, HORST 1954, OEFF 1954, 1955. [196] KLOTZ 1949. [197] STORM VON LEEUWEN 1921, 1924, PAK 1926, BEUTNER 1925. [198] BEUTNER 1925. [199] BENNHOLD 1938. [200] MOHRING 1958. [201] MILLER 1959. [202] GOLDSTEIN 1949. [203] KOELLE 1946. [204] STORM V. LEEUWEN 1924. [205] BENNHOLD 1938. [206] GALIMARD 1945. [207] SMITH 1946. [208] LUCK 1949. [209] OLIVER 1923. [209a] SIROTA 1950. [210] TOMPSETT 1947. [211] HENRY 1947. [212] KLOTZ 1949. [213] BOXER 1949. [214] OPPENHEIMER 1913. [215] LENDLE 1935. [216] HAARMANN 1940. [217] FARAH 1945, FAWAZ 1944. [218] ROTHLIN 1949. [219] BENNHOLD 1938, SCHÖNHOLZER 1940. [220] VAN DYKE 1945. [221] ANDERSEN 1945, DAVIS 1942, 1943, DEROUAX 1943, 1944, EARLE 1944, GILLIGAN 1943, HEINEMANN 1943, LUNDQUIST 1945, PAGET 1946. [222] REINHOLD 1944, GRASER 1949, SCHULZE 1955. [222a] NEWBOULD 1960. [223] KLOTZ 1946a und b, 1947. [224] BENNHOLD 1938, OTT 1952, KALLEE 1952, 1953. [225] KLOTZ 1946a und b, 1947. [226] BENNHOLD 1938. [227] WUNDERLY 1950a. [228] RAWLINS 1930. [229] BENNHOLD 1938, HOEKSTRA 1931. [230] DOW 1945, 1950. [231] BURKHARD 1955. [232] BENNHOLD 1947, WUNDERLY 1953a. [233] DOLADILHE 1939. [234] DOLADILHE 1939. [235] SCHUBERT 1950a. [236] DOW 1945, 1950, RAWSON 1943, GREGERSEN 1943, ALLEN 1950, WUNDERLY 1950a und b. [237] WUNDERLY 1950a, OTT 1951. [238] BENNHOLD 1923. [239] WUNDERLY 1950a und b, BENNHOLD 1950a. [240] HAUROWITZ 1952. [241] BENNHOLD 1938. [242] BENNHOLD 1938, KLOTZ 1946a und b, STRICKS 1949, LUCK 1949, KLOTZ 1950b, TERESI 1950, COLVIN 1952. [243] GREGERSEN 1937, RAWSON 1943. [244] GREGERSEN 1937, RAWSON 1943. [245] BENNHOLD 1947. [246] KLOTZ 1946a. [247] CAROLL 1950. [248] KARUSH 1950. [249] KARUSH 1954. [250] BENNHOLD 1938. [251] RAWLINS 1930. [252] DE HAAN 1922, SIENGALEWICZ 1924, SCHULTEN 1925, ALLEN 1950, BENNHOLD 1944, 1953, WUNDERLY 1950a. [253] BENNHOLD 1938, 1944, DE HAAN 1922, WUNDERLY 1950a. [254] BENNHOLD 1925, 1944. [255] TERESI 1948. [256] HEWITT 1927, BENNHOLD 1950a. [257] HEWITT 1927. [258] HIRSCHFELDER 1930.

Eosin S, A M + [259]. Erythrosin S + [260]. Fluorescein S + [261]. Phenolrot S M und R + [262]. Phenolphthalein S + [263]. Phenolsulphthalein S + [264]. Phloxinrot S + [265]. Rhodamin A M + [266]. Rose Bengale A M + [267]. Tetrabromphenolphthalein S M + [268], A M + [269], Leber-P +, A R, M + [270]. Tetrachlorphenolphthalein S + [271]. Thymolblau S + [271]. Triphenylmethanfarbstoffe: Bas. Fuchsin S + [272]. Brillantgrün S + [273]. Gentianaviolett S + [274]. Kristallviolett S + [275]. Malachitgrün S + [276]. Patentblau A M + [277]. Venediggrün S + [278]. Venedigviolett S + [278]. Viktoriablau S M + [279]. Verschiedene Farbstoffe: Acridinorange S + [280]. Anilinacridin S + [281]. Anilinonaphthalen S + [282]. Blau BZL α_1- und β-Lipo M + [283]. Chrysoidin A R + [284]. Indigocarmin A M + [285]. Lithiumcarmin α_1-G, A M +, K + [286]. Methylenblau S M + [287], A M + [288]. Neutralrot P + [289]. Ölrot α_1- und β-Lipo M + [290]. Sudanrot Lipo M + [291]. Sudanschwarz B α_1- und β-Lipo + [292].

c) Stoffe ohne wesentliche biologische Bedeutung, welche zur Erforschung der Bindung dienten: Äther S + [293]. Äthylen Blut M + [294]. Aliphat. Alkohole S + [295], S R + [296], A★ M + [297]. Amino-Acridin A M + [298], A M [299]. Ammoniumbasen (quarternär) A M + [300]. Aromat. Carboxylsäuren A★ R + [301]. Auxin (Indolacetat) A M + [302]. Benzoate A★ R [303]. Benzpyren Lipo M und andere A [304]. Bismutyltartrate S R + [305], G-eu [306]. Caprylate A★ R + [307]. Cyclopropan Blut M + [308]. Decylsulf. A R + [309]. Desoxyribonuclease A M Eier + [310]. Diamidin S [311]. Dodecylsulf. A★ Pf + [312], A★ M +, R + [313], A R [314], A + [315]. Fettsäuren mittl. Kettenlänge A + [316], A★ M, R + [317], A★ M, R + [318]. Guanidin A★ M, R [319]. Malonat (Di-Na-hexyl) A★ R [320]. Octylsulfat A R + [321]. m-Hydroxylbenzoate A★ R + [322]. o-Hydroxylphenylacetat A★ R + [322]. p-Hydroxylphenylacetat A★ R + [322]. p-dimethylaminoazobenzol Pl [323]. Phenole (substit.) S K [324], A, G M + [325], A★ R + [326], A★ M, R + [327], S Pf, R [328], A★ R + [329]. Phenylacetat A R + [330], A★ R + [331]. Phenylbutyrat A★ R + [332], A R + [333]. Pikrate A R + [334], A★ R + [335], A★ R + [336]. p-toluolsulfonat A★ M + [337]. Salicylurat S M [338]. Staub (Quarz-, Mineral-) β-G M + [339]. Sulfone A★ M + [340], A [341]. Trichloracetat A★ M, R + [342], A★ M + [343].

[259] BENNHOLD 1930, 1944, HEWITT 1927. [260] HEWITT 1927. [261] BUSCK 1906, DE HAAN 1921, 1922, HEWITT 1927, BENNHOLD 1938. [262] DE HAAN 1922, GROLLMANN 1925, ROSENTHAL 1925, HEWITT 1927, RICHARDS 1930, MARSHALL 1923, 1931, SHANNON 1935, GOLDRING 1936, PITTS 1938, SMITH 1938, ROBINSON 1941, BENNHOLD 1950a. [263] HEWITT 1927. [264] BRAUER 1948. [265] HEWITT 1927. [266] BENNHOLD 1938. [267] ROSENTHAL 1924, 1925, 1926, HEWITT 1927, BENNHOLD 1938. [268] HEWITT 1927, BRAUER 1949. [269] PEZOLD 1953. [270] BRAUER 1948, 1949, 1955. [271] HIRSCHFELDER 1930. [272] DOLADILHE 1939. [273] HIRSCHFELDER 1930. [274] DOLADILHE 1939. [275] HIRSCHFELDER 1930. [276] HIRSCHFELDER 1930, DOLADILHE 1939. [277] BENNHOLD 1938. [278] DOLADILHE 1939. [279] DOLADILHE 1939, WUNDERLY 1950. [280] DOLADILHE 1939. [281] WEBER 1954. [282] JOYCE 1954, WEBER 1954. [283] SWAHN 1952 OTT 1954. [284] KLOTZ 1947. [285] DE HAAN 1922 BLATTNER 1924, RICHARDS 1930, BENNHOLD 1950. [286] OTT 1953. [287] BECHHOLD 1907. [288] BENNHOLD 1950b. [289] DOLADILHE 1939. [290] DURRUM 1952. [291] WUNDERLY 1953b. [292] SWAHN 1952. [293] MOORE 1905. [294] ORCUTT 1937. [295] MOORE 1905. [296] BEUTNER 1929. [297] E. COHN 1948. [298] TAGGART 1948. [299] BENNHOLD 1938. [300] CHINARD 1948. [301] TERESI 1948. [302] THIMANN 1949. [303] LUCK 1948. [304] CHALMERS 1953. [305] SEI 1924. [306] BECHHOLD 1907. [307] DUGGAN 1948. [308] ORCUTT 1937. [309] KARUSH 1949. [310] CARTER 1946, STENHAGEN 1939. [311] FULLER 1942. [312] PUTNAM 1943. [313] DUGGAN 1948. [314] KARUSH 1949/50. [315] LUCK 1949. [316] DAVIS 1946, 1947. [317] BOYER 1946. [318] BOYER 1945, 1947. [319] BOYER 1946. [320] DUGGAN 1948. [321] KARUSH 1949. [322] MILLER 1949. [323] LUCK 1948. [324] BECHHOLD 1907. [325] BENNHOLD 1938. [326] TERESI 1948. [327] DUGGAN 1948. [328] BECHHOLD 1907. [329] BEUTNER 1925. [330] TERESI 1948. [331] LUCK 1948. [332] DUGGAN 1948. [333] TERESI 1948. [334] TERESI 1950. [335] TERESI 1948. [336] DUGGAN 1948. [337] SCATCHARD 1949a. [338] STORM V. LEEUWEN 1924. [339] SCHUMACHER 1956. [340] JACKSON 1948. [341] LUCK 1949. [342] DUGGAN 1948. [343] SCATCHARD 1949a.

Die Bindung an Plasmaeiweiß ist ein reversibler Prozeß, der sich rückläufig da abspielt, wo eine starke Affinität seitens fixer Zell- oder Gewebselemente zur Wirkung kommt. Die gebundenen Stoffe werden vom Bluteiweiß dort abgelöst, wo sich Eiweißstrukturen befinden, die selbst ein noch stärkeres Bindungsvermögen besitzen. Das ist in den fixen Speichern und besonders in den Ausscheidungsorganen der Fall; falls es sich um körpereigene Stoffe handelt, gilt dies auch für die Orte ihres normalen Umsatzes. Für den ganzen Vorgang der Ausscheidung genügt das Abhängen von einer Bindung an Plasmaeiweiß aber nicht überall. Die Zellen verfügen zusätzlich über energiefordernde Stoffwechselmechanismen, welche den intracellulären Weitertransport und schließlich die Eliminierung aus der Zelle bewerkstelligen können. Außerdem können offenbar auch fermentative Prozesse bei der Freisetzung oder Minderung der Bindungsfestigkeit gebundener Substanzen eine Rolle spielen (z. B. Kuppelung von Bilirubin, Thyroxin und Steroiden an Glucuronsäure).

In den letzten Jahren sind die Methoden des Bindungsnachweises von Substanzen an Serumeiweiß sehr verbessert worden; es sei z. B. an die verfeinerten Dialysemethoden, an die Einführung der Chromatographie, der Kationenaustauscher und an die Verwendung von Isotopenmarkierungen zum Spurennachweis gebundener Substanzen gedacht. Ferner hat die immer differenziertere Auftrennung der Serumeiweißkörper durch Elektrophorese[1] große Fortschritte gemacht; es sei an die Elektrophorese im flüssigen Milieu, an die Zonenelektrophorese auf Papier[2], in Pappe, in Stärke, in Agar, in Acetylcellulose und an die zweidimensionale Elektrophorese nach GRASSMANN 1953 gedacht. Schließlich bedeutete die Kombination von Elektrophorese mit immunbiologischen Reaktionen im Agarmilieu, wie sie in Form der Immunelektrophorese von GRABAR u. Mitarb. 1953 entwickelt wurden, einen weiteren großen methodischen Fortschritt; desgleichen die Elektrophorese im Stärkemilieu nach SMITHIES.

Etwa 23 Fraktionen können jetzt herausgetrennt werden. Deshalb bedürfen die in zurückliegenden Arbeiten gewonnenen Bindungsnachweise, insbesondere soweit sie sich auf Fällungsmethoden oder auf freie Elektrophorese im *Theorell*-Apparat gründen, einer Nachprüfung mit den neueren Methoden, ehe weitgehende Schlüsse daraus gezogen werden dürfen (vgl. S. 192).

Selbstverständlich ist mit dem Nachweis der Bindung eines Stoffes an Serumeiweiß noch keineswegs bewiesen, daß den Serumeiweißkörpern hierbei wirklich eine biologisch sich auswirkende Vehikelfunktion im Organismus zukommt. Das Bindungsvermögen ist zunächst *nur eine Voraussetzung* für die Möglichkeit solcher funktioneller Zusammenhänge.

Von manchen Seiten wurde Anstoß genommen an der teleologischen Formulierung „*Vehikel*", der wir in diesem Abschnitt immer wieder begegnen. Dagegen muß jedoch betont werden, daß wir bei der Darstellung funktioneller Vorgänge solche Formulierungen und Gleichnisse, die uns aus der unbelebten Natur geläufig sind, niemals ganz entbehren können. Sowohl aus Gründen einer klaren, zielgerichteten Darstellung als auch um neue Gedankengänge zur weiteren experimentellen Prüfung solcher biologischer Vorstellungen anzuregen, sind teleologische Formulierungen nicht nur erlaubt, sondern sogar geboten. Wer wird heutzutage noch Anstoß nehmen an den lebendigen Begriffen wie „Blutdruckzügler", Homöostase", an dem klinischen Begriff der „Kompensation" und „Dekompensation"? Auch das allgemein gefaßte Wort „Regulation" fällt in diese Kategorie; schon „Gleichgewicht" müßte den strikten Negierern aller teleologischen Formulierungen bei der Beschreibung biologischer Vorgänge suspekt sein. Ferner könnte man gegen das Wort „Vehikel" speziell einwenden, daß es streng genommen eine eigene Motorik und vorgeschriebene Fahrtrichtung mit festgelegter Endstation voraussetzen würde. Man könnte diesem Einwand ausweichen, indem man diese normale Rolle der Erythrocyten und der Serumeiweißkörper statt mit „Vehikel" mit der Bezeichnung „lokale Abgaberegler" charakterisieren würde. Trotzdem werden wir die Bezeichnung Vehikel im allgemeinen bevorzugen. Auch jedes physiologische Bild oder Gleichnis hat seine Begrenzung. Beim biologischen Vehikel liegt sie in der Form der Lokomotorik, welche in einer Schwemmwirkung statt in einer Eigenbewegung besteht. Demgegenüber wird ein bedeutsamer Inhaltsbestandteil der Lokomotorik, die Ortsverschiebung eines Stoffes und die lokale Anhäufung von Transportgut, durch das Wort „Vehikel" plastisch zur

---

[1] TISELIUS 1930.   [2] TURBA 1950, CREMER 1950, DURRUM 1950, GRASSMANN 1951.

Darstellung gebracht. Dies sind Faktoren, die für unsere Fragestellung von höchster biologischer Wichtigkeit sind. — Ebenso ist auch der später wiederholt gebrauchte Ausdruck „*gezielter Transport*" natürlich so zu verstehen, daß damit nur das *Endergebnis* eines komplizierten Transportvorganges mit Ablagerung in bestimmte Zellen (z. B. bei der Vitalfärbung) charakterisiert werden soll, also

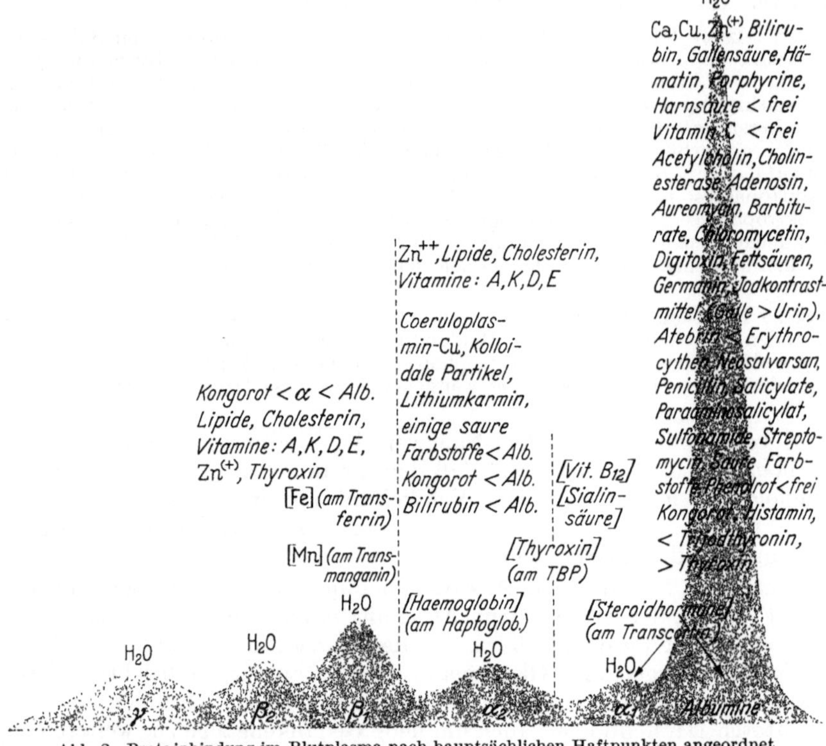

Abb. 2. Proteinbindung im Blutplasma nach hauptsächlichen Haftpunkten angeordnet.

Die eingezeichneten Bindungen sind schematisch aufzufassen; viele Stoffe weisen in ihrer Bindung Gleichgewichtszustände, z. B. zu ungebundenen oder zu an bestimmte Globulinfraktionen gebundenen Anteilen auf. Am deutlichsten ist dies bei der Bindung des Wassers an alle Serumproteinfraktionen festzustellen. Bei anderen Substanzen besteht nur ein Bindungsgleichgewicht zwischen freien und an Albumin gebundenen Anteilen in Abhängigkeit von der im Serum vorhandenen oder zum Serum zugesetzten Substanzmenge. Bei wieder anderen Stoffen besteht ein Bindungsgleichgewicht zwischen Albuminen und α-Globulinen oder auch zu α- sowie β-Globulinen. In solchen Fällen wurde im obigen Schema meistens nur das hauptsächliche Trägerprotein eingezeichnet. Nur bei einzelnen besonders prägnanten Beispielen (Vitamin C[1], Harnsäure[2], Atebrin[3], Kongorot[4], Bilirubin[4]) wurde das Gefälle zu freien Anteilen oder zu Anteilen, welche an andere Blutproteine gebunden sind, angegeben. So z. B. Harnsäure: Albumin < frei; Vitamin C: Albumin < frei; Atebrin: Albumin < Erythrocyten; Kongorot: Albumin > α-Globulin > β-Globulin (vgl. Abb. 4); Phenolrot: Albumin < frei; Bilirubin: Albumin > α- > β-Globulin (im Vollserum); Zink: fest am α_1 und α_2, lockerer am Albumin und am β-Globulin (+) (Hund).

Die mit eckigen Klammern eingefaßten Substanzen sind solche, von denen bekannt ist, daß sie nur an einer eng begrenzten Teilfraktion haften, welche im elektrischen Feld im Raum der α_1-, α_2-, β_1- oder β_2-Globuline wandert: z. B. das Vitamin B_{12}-bindende Globulin, welches im Rahmen der α_1-Glucoproteide wandert und dabei nur etwa 0,003 % der α_1-Globuline ausmacht (vgl. S. 218).

selbstverständlich kein „Direktschuß" nach Zielen über Kimme und Korn! Die kreisförmig geschlossene Strombahn mit dem automatisch immer wieder erfolgenden Stoffangebot (allerdings mit den großen Zufallsfaktoren der Strömung einhergehend) ersetzt hier das direkte Ansteuern eines bestimmten Organes und Organteiles, wie es Galen noch annehmen konnte.

---

[1] Schubert 1947.   [2] Bennhold 1938, Morris 1958.   [3] Hecht 1937.
[4] Bennhold 1950.

Als Vehikel kommen *Albumine, α-* und *β-Globuline* in Frage; *γ-Globuline* nur im Sinne eines Wassertransportes. Die Antikörpereigenschaften der *γ*-Globuline sind nach der heute vorherrschenden Meinung von charakteristischen und spezifischen Faltungseigentümlichkeiten, also Struktureigentümlichkeiten abhängig und nicht von einem besonderen substantiellen Faktor, welcher gebunden und transportiert wird. Auch das *Fibrinogen*, der Blutfaserstoff, geht, soweit wir wissen, keine Bindungen mit anderen Substanzen ein; regelhafte Transporteffekte sind also nicht zu erwarten. — Im Spektrum der Serumeiweiße, sinnfällig veranschaulicht durch das Elektrophoresebild, werden in den Albuminen offenbar chemisch gleichartige Proteine zusammengefaßt. $α_1$-, $α_2$- und *β*-Globuline sind aber Gemische einer ganzen Anzahl von Proteinen oder Proteiden, die als Gemeinsames nur die gleiche elektrophoretische Wanderungsgeschwindigkeit besitzen (Abb. 2). Wir müssen annehmen, daß die Albumine alle, die α- und β-Globuline nur zum Teil als Vehikel für bestimmte Substanzen dienen können. Dafür sind die Albuminvehikel relativ unspezifisch, während den Globulinvehikeln eine gewisse Spezifität in der Wechselwirkung mit einem bestimmten Transportgut zukommt. Man spricht von den eisen-, B_{12}- oder thyroxinbindenden Globulinen usw.

Der *Raum*, in dem sich die Serumproteine im Körper bewegen, ist keineswegs nur auf das Blutgefäßsystem beschränkt. Die Verfolgung radiomarkierter Eiweiße zeigt eindeutig, daß neben dem intravasalen eine fast gleich große Menge extravasalen Albumins vorhanden ist, zirkuliert und Räume erfüllt, die bedeutend ausgedehnter sind als das blutgefüllte Gefäßsystem. Zieht man noch eine gewisse Zelldurchdringung in Betracht, dann ergibt sich ein Kontakt zwischen Körperzellen und Eiweißvehikeln, der wesentlich größer ist als der mit dem Blute allein. Der Stoffaustausch wird dadurch gefördert. Noch unerforscht ist, welche Zeit das Serumeiweiß innerhalb und welche Zeit es außerhalb der Blutgefäße fließt, wo die Hauptaustrittstätten sich befinden, wie groß sein Anteil an der austretenden Flüssigkeit ist und ob nach dem Verlassen der arteriolennahen Capillare ein Rückfluß in den venösen Schenkel möglich ist. Die Lymphgefäße spielen dabei auch eine wichtige Rolle. Die aufschlußreichen Untersuchungen über die tubuläre Proteinrückresorption[1] in den Nieren und zahlreiche Nachweise von Blutproteinen in Nieren und Leberzellen[2] sind vorerst nur ein erster Hinweis auf noch nicht voll deutbare Mechanismen der Proteinbewegung.

Da die Eiweißbilder des Liquors, der Lymphe, des Kammerwassers, des Ödems und der auf einen Entzündungsreiz exsudierten Gewebsflüssigkeit nicht grob voneinander abweichen, müssen sich die Proteine der extravasculären Flüssigkeiten wenigstens in der Größenordnung der elektrophoretischen Fraktionen zueinander so verhalten wie einzelne Testeiweißstoffe und müssen genau so wie das untersuchte Albumin große Räume erfüllen. Allerdings ist es durchaus möglich, daß bestimmte Proteine am Verlassen des Gefäßsystems gehindert werden können. Die Anzahl der Stomata, durch welche die Eiweißkörper das Gefäßsystem verlassen, Verbrauch, Resorption, Abstrom, Druckverhältnisse und eventuelle celluläre Neubildung sind verantwortlich für einen wechselnden Gesamteiweißgehalt.

Durch Bindung eines Stoffes an ein Plasma-Protein entsteht das beladene Vehikel, welches sein Transportgut mit sich schleppt, bis es selbst abgebaut wird oder bis es an einen Ort gelangt, wo eine stärker wirkende Kraft die Last — oder einen Teil davon — ablöst. Die Abhängeorte zeichnen sich aus durch eine Affinität zum Transportgut, die etwa in der gleichen Größenordnung liegt oder stärker ist als die Affinität der Vehikel. Nun könnte man denken, daß es unendlich viele Abhängeorte mit unendlich vielen verschiedenen Affinitäten gäbe. Die Unordnung ist aber bei weitem nicht so groß, wie man vielleicht annimmt. Es hat sich nämlich gezeigt, daß die wirksamsten Abhängeorte die *Stellen des*

---

[1] SQUIRE 1953, SCHEURLEN 1961.   [2] PETERS 1950, BENNHOLD 1953, KALLEE 1954.

Stoffbedarfs, die *Ausscheidungsorgane* und die *Speicher* sind. Das Vehikel läßt also sein Transportgut so lange intra- und extravasculär zirkulieren, bis es zu einer Stelle kommt, wo es im Stoffwechsel gebraucht oder ausgeschieden oder gespeichert wird (Abb. 3). So nehmen die albumingebundenen Gallenfarbstoffe, sowie Bromsulfalein und die Gallenkontrastmittel ihren Weg zur Leber, ohne in die anderen Körperzellen einzudringen. Erst bei starker Belastung der Bindung an die zirkulierenden Serumeiweißkörper kann Transportgut auch an Orte des fixen Gewebes dort abgegeben werden, wo nur relativ schwache Affinitäten wirksam sind. Dann kommt es z. B. im Falle des Bilirubins zum Ikterus (vgl. S. 198—201). Entsprechend dem Gleichgewichtscharakter der adsorptiven Bindung haften die zuletzt gebundenen gleichartigen Teilchen am Eiweißvehikel lockerer als die ersten, welche in einem Stadium gebunden wurden, wo noch viele Bindungsplätze frei waren. Außerdem ist zu bedenken, daß viele Bindungen an Eiweiß stark abhängig vom p_H sind; lokale p_H-Änderungen können also Bindungsverhältnisse grundlegend ändern.

Verbrauch und Ausscheidung beseitigen den Stoff, im *Speicher* wird er dem Kreislauf entzogen und zurückgestellt.

Ein Stoff kann auch abseits vom Kreislauf in einem besonderen System zirkulieren, ohne in Zellen abgelagert oder anderweitig immobilisiert zu sein. Dabei kann trotzdem ein Gleichgewicht zum Transportsystem bestehen. Ein Beispiel dafür ist das Kupfer. Bis zu 2 mg werden täglich im Dünndarm resorbiert und sofort wieder durch die Galle ausgeschieden, um anschließend wieder resorbiert zu werden. Aus diesem *enterohepatischen Zirkel*, dem z. B. Urobilinogen, Urobilin, Gallensäuren, Cholesterin, Sulfonamide usw. auch manche Cortine unterliegen, besteht über die Leberzelle ein Zugang zum Blut. Ein im Blut oder in den Organen auftretender Mangel an diesen Stoffen könnte aus dem enterohepatischen Zirkel genau so gedeckt werden wie aus einem ruhenden Depot. Obwohl es sich um fundamental unterschiedliche Vorgänge handelt, sind sie im Endeffekt gleich; die Abgabe aus dem enterohepatischen Zirkel ist abhängig von zwei ganz verschiedenen Zellsystemen: von der Funktion der Leberzellen und von der der resorbierenden Darmzellen; wieweit eine solche denkbare „Speicherfunktion" des enterohepatischen Zirkels realisiert wird, wissen wir nicht.

In der Sicht von Bindungsgleichgewichten sind Speicher Orte besonderer Affinität, ausgestattet mit gelösten oder strukturellen Proteinen, welche ein Bindungsvermögen mit hoher Assoziationskonstante besitzen. Zweifellos ist das Speicherungsgeschehen nicht ausschließlich durch Gleichgewichtseinstellung erklärbar; für die Stoffaufnahme in Zellen sind fermentative Prozesse verschiedentlich nachgewiesen worden[1]. Die speichernde Zelle ist auch kein unveränderliches Gebilde, sondern kann durch das in ihr aufgehäufte Depot Rückwirkungen erleiden (Speicherschädigung) oder angeregt werden, z. B. zur Apoferritinsynthese bei einem hohen Eisenangebot. Vom Transportgeschehen aus bietet sich zwanglos eine vereinfachende Betrachtungsweise an.

Ein in den Kreislauf gelangter und *ohne* weitere Bindung zirkulierender Stoff wird sich ohne jede Gegenwirkung seitens des Transportmilieus überall dort anreichern, wo eine *Assoziationsmöglichkeit an fixes Gewebe* besteht. Ein Bindungsgleichgewicht stellt sich ein, wird aber immer wieder gestört, weil der Stoff an anderen Stellen verbraucht und abgebaut oder ausgeschieden wird. Der im Speicher gebundene Anteil, der im Gleichgewicht mit dem freien, im Kreislauf zirkulierenden Anteil steht, verringert sich. Das bewirkt, daß gebundener Stoff abdissoziieren muß, frei wird, den Speicher verläßt und zurückfließt. Durch die Speicher ist also einer zu starken Anreicherung in den durchströmten Körperräumen und Zellen vorgebeugt worden. Nicht an Bluteiweiß oder an Gewebe gebundene Stoffe breiten sich in ihrem ganzen Diffusionsraum aus.

---

[1] Wilbrandt 1951.

Anders verhält es sich, wenn der zirkulierende Stoff auch *Bindungen* mit *Bluteiweißkörpern* eingeht. *Den Vehikeln fällt* dann *die gleiche Rolle zu wie fixen Speichern*, nur daß sie den ins Blut gelangten Stoff *sofort* abfangen. Es stellt sich zuerst eine Vehikelbindung ein, welche zunächst einmal niedrige Affinitäten des fixen Gewebes ausschaltet und sich sekundär mit den Speichern in ein Gleichgewicht setzt. Der Stoff bleibt am transportierenden Serumprotein haften, bis er an Orten erhöhter Affinität abgegeben wird. Einer Überschwemmung ist vorgebeugt; die Speicher füllen sich, indem sich das Verteilungsgleichgewicht einstellt; im Blute kommt es dann durch Verbrauch und Ausscheidung zu einer Konzentrationsabnahme. Wenn sich die *Vehikel*, welche gewissermaßen als *zirkulierende Speicher* funktionieren, leeren, dann verschiebt sich das Verteilungsgleichgewicht, und aus fixen Speichern fließt die Substanz langsam zurück an die Vehikel, zu Verbrauchs- und Ausscheidungsorten. Beispiele dafür sind der Transport von Bilirubin über die Albuminbindung oder von Germanin, das über das Albuminvehikel seinen Weg zur Niere nimmt, oder die Fähigkeit des Kollidons, als kolloides „Fremdvehikel" den gespeicherten Farbstoff Diaminreinblau FF aus dem Gewebe in das Blut zurückzuholen und zur Ausscheidung zu bringen[1] (s. S. 227 f.).

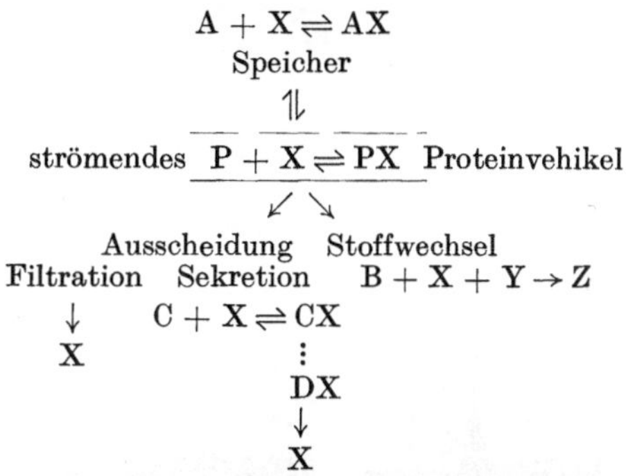

Daraus wird klar, daß die *Speicher* nicht nur Aufbewahrungsorte für einen späteren Verbrauch, sondern auch für spätere Ausscheidung sind. Sie sind

$$A + X \rightleftharpoons AX$$
Speicher
$$\Updownarrow$$
strömendes $\underline{P + X \rightleftharpoons PX}$ Proteinvehikel

Ausscheidung Stoffwechsel
Filtration Sekretion $\quad B + X + Y \to Z$
$\downarrow \qquad C + X \rightleftharpoons CX$
$X \qquad\qquad \vdots$
$$DX$$
$$\downarrow$$
$$X$$

Abb. 3. Schema eines Transportgleichgewichts durch reversible Bindung eines Stoffes (X) an Proteinvehikel (P), an Speichereiweißkörper (A) im Stoffwechsel (B) und bei der Ausscheidung (C). (Ohne Berücksichtigung reversibler Bindungen an Capillar- und Zellwände.)

wichtige Schutzeinrichtungen, Abstellgleise, die notwendig sind, weil die Niere und die Leber die Ausscheidung innerhalb einer Blutpassage nicht bewältigen. Es ist auch nötig, daß sie ubiquitär im Gefäßsystem eingelagert sind. So erfüllen sie ihren Zweck rasch. Daraus ergibt sich, daß ein Speicher nur richtig funktionieren kann, wenn sich die skizzierten Verteilungsgleichgewichte einstellen können. Dann, wenn die stark adsorbierende Außenbegrenzung der Speicherzellen dem Vehikel seine Last abnimmt oder diese nur so weit in die Zelle eingeschleust wird, daß immer noch ein unmittelbarer Kontakt mit den Vehikeln bestehenbleibt, wird der Weg eines Stoffes auf wenige Stationen beschränkt und eine ökonomische Verteilung gefördert. Ein klares Beispiel für die Bewegung zwischen Resorptionsort, Stoffwechsel sowie fixen und mobilen Speichern ist der Weg des Eisens (s. S. 202 f.). Die moderne Behandlung der Hämochromatose durch Aderlaß und Eisenentzug hat sich diese Erkenntnisse erfolgreich zunutze gemacht.

Plasmaalbumine als Vehikel.

Da die Beladung des Transportmittels mit dem Transportgut, d. h. die Bindung an die Vehikel im Mittelpunkt der Betrachtungen über das Transportgeschehen steht, kommt der Kenntnis der Wechselwirkung verschiedenster Stoffe mit den Plasmaeiweißkörpern besondere Bedeutung zu. Die Art der labilen Anheftung der transportierten Substanz an das Vehikel ist genau wie bei den Erythrocyten auch bei den Plasmaeiweißkörpern von größter Wichtigkeit für die Erklärung der damit zusammenhängenden Transportvorgänge.

---

[1] Schubert 1950.

In systematischen Untersuchungen hat sich Bennhold seit 1925 mit der Bindung von Stoffen (Farbstoffen, Bilirubin, Cholesterin) am Serumeiweiß beschäftigt. Er benützte dabei zunächst die Diffusion von Farbstoffen und Serumeiweißkörpern in Gelatinegallerte (embatischer Effekt des Serums) sowie seit 1930 als erster die Wanderungsunterschiede der freien und an Eiweiß gebundenen Farbstoffanteile im elektrischen Feld (Kataphorese in den

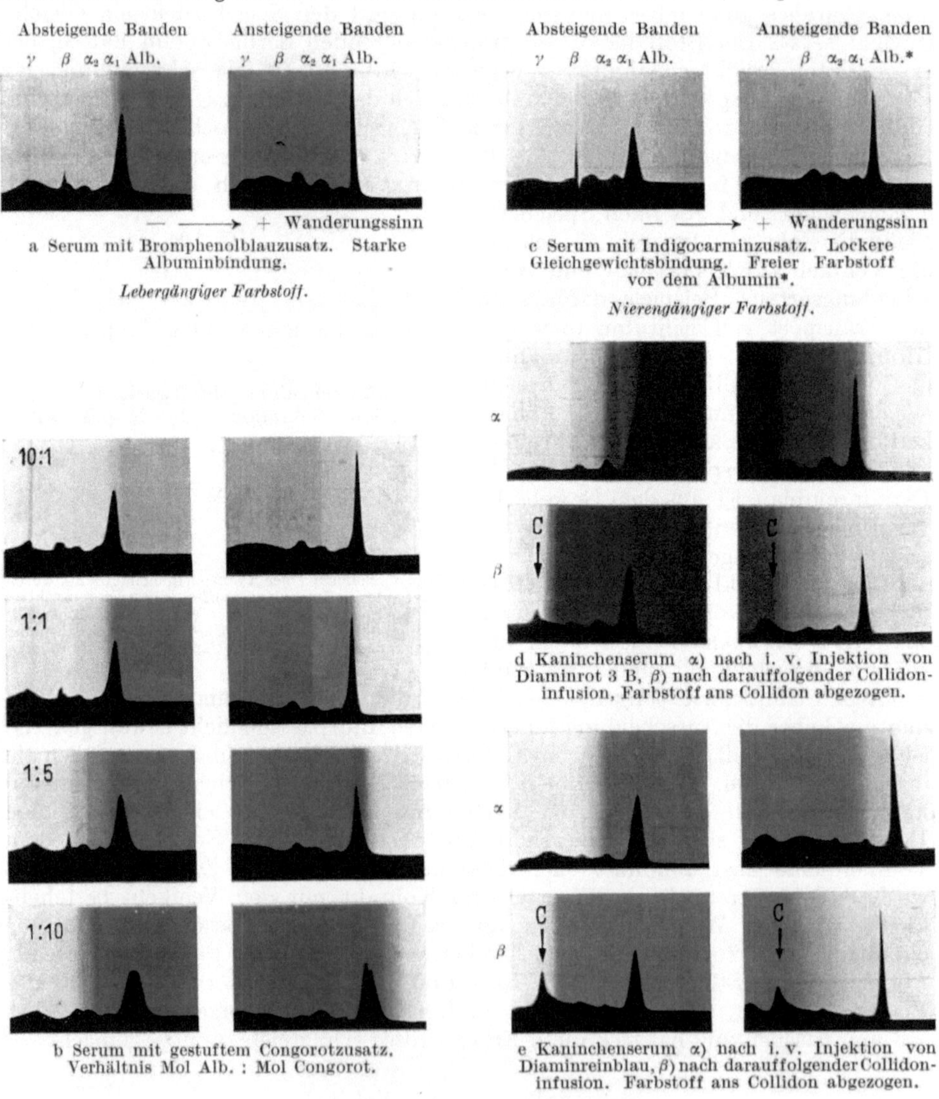

a Serum mit Bromphenolblauzusatz. Starke Albuminbindung.

Lebergängiger Farbstoff.

c Serum mit Indigocarminzusatz. Lockere Gleichgewichtsbindung. Freier Farbstoff vor dem Albumin*.

Nierengängiger Farbstoff.

d Kaninchenserum α) nach i. v. Injektion von Diaminrot 3 B, β) nach darauffolgender Collidon-infusion, Farbstoff ans Collidon abgezogen.

b Serum mit gestuftem Congorotzusatz. Verhältnis Mol Alb. : Mol Congorot.

e Kaninchenserum α) nach i. v. Injektion von Diaminreinblau, β) nach darauffolgender Collidon-infusion. Farbstoff ans Collidon abgezogen.

Abb. 4 a—e. Untersuchungen der Eiweißbindung mit Hilfe der Tiselius-Elektrophorese (Bennhold 1950).

Apparaten von Michaelis und von Theorell, später Elektrophorese nach Tiselius) und entwickelte daraus die Vorstellung einer Vehikelfunktion der Serumeiweißkörper (Abb. 4).

Es hatte sich bald herausgestellt, daß nicht alle Blutproteine gleichartig mit anderen, kleineren Molekülen reagieren. So binden z. B. einzelne Globuline in einer besonderen Weise Lipide, Schwermetalle oder Jod. Aus 2 Gründen steht aber das Albumin im Vordergrund der Betrachtungen. Es ist der Eiweißkörper, der in der höchsten Konzentration, d. h. mit der *größten bindenden Grenzfläche,* im Blute vorkommt und der außerdem in ganz ausgezeichneter Weise über *Bindungseigenschaften* verfügt. Die meisten quantitativen Bindungsstudien in vitro sind deshalb auch mit Albumin ausgeführt worden. Das Ergebnis dieser Untersuchungen ist natürlich nicht ohne weiteres auf das Blutmilieu zu übertragen. Jede Bindung steht in Abhängigkeit von Temperatur, p_H, Konzentration und Ionenstärke, und selbst die kleinste Verunreinigung kann im Experiment störende Einflüsse ausüben. Die zur Aufrechterhaltung des p_H notwendige Pufferkonzentration ist z. B. ihrerseits in wechselndem Ausmaß von Wirkung[1]. Es existieren daher überhaupt nur wenige absolute Daten, die mit isoionischem Albumin ermittelt wurden, welches außer H^+ und OH^- keine anderen Ionen enthält[2].

Im folgenden soll daher zuerst die Bindung an Albumin, in ihrer Vielfältigkeit abgehandelt werden. Über die physikalisch-chemischen Ergebnisse hinaus, die zum Verständnis der Bindung unerläßlich sind, soll dann am Beispiel des in erster Linie albumingebundenen Bilirubins, die Bedeutung dieser Bindung im Organismus dargelegt werden. Der Gallenfarbstoff ist deshalb ein besonders wichtiges erstes Beispiel, weil beim Kernikterus der Neugeborenen eine schwere Störung des Bilirubintransportes von großer pathogenetischer Bedeutung ist.

Albuminbindung.

Die Bindung an das Plasmaalbumin ist überwiegend eine reversible. Das will zuerst nicht mehr besagen, als daß die gebundenen Stoffe ohne tiefgreifende Veränderungen des Albuminmoleküls vorübergehend an seiner Oberfläche konzentriert werden können. Es ist heute nicht mehr gerechtfertigt, die Kräfte, welche die Adsorption bewirken, in physikalische und chemische zu unterteilen. Da der Vorgang nach dem Massenwirkungsgesetz einfach zu beschreiben ist, ist eine chemische Terminologie vorzuziehen. Sie wird allen Verhältnissen gerecht und ist klar[3]. KLOTZ[4] verallgemeinerte die nach dem Massenwirkungsgesetz erhaltenen Gleichungen für die Bindung von Ca-Ionen an Casein[5] und schuf neben einer einfachen rechnerischen Behandlung eine brauchbare allgemeine Modellvorstellung für eine Wechselwirkung zwischen Proteinen und anderen Stoffen. Er lehnte sich dabei an wesentlich ältere Theorien an[6].

Sein Modell ist ein Protein von der molaren Konzentration P, das identische Bindungsstellen besitzt. Diese Bindungsstellen sollen sich gegenseitig nicht beeinflussen, auch nicht, wenn ein Teil von ihnen bereits mit dem zu bindenden Stoff reagiert hat. Ist X die Konzentration des ungebundenen Stoffes, P_f die aller freien Bindungsstellen und nP die Gesamtzahl aller Bindungsstellen ($= P_f X + P_f$), dann ist $P_f = nP - P_f X$. Die einfache Gleichung des Massenwirkungsgesetzes

$$P_f + X = P_f X$$

mit der Assoziationskonstante $k = \dfrac{P_f X}{(P_f)(X)}$

läßt sich dann ausdrücken als

$$n P(X) k - (P_f X)(X) k = (P_f X)$$

$$n P(X) k = (P_f X)(1 + (X) k).$$

Benutzt man das Verhältnis r, Mol gebundener Farbstoffe je Mol Protein, dann wird

$$r = \frac{(P_f X)}{P} = \frac{n(X)}{\dfrac{1}{k} + (X)}.$$

In dieser Form ist die aus dem Massenwirkungsgesetz abgeleitete Gleichung identisch mit der Langmuirschen Adsorptionsisotherme, in der das Verhältnis von adsorbierter Substanz

---

[1] ALBERTY 1949, KLOTZ 1950b.   [2] SCATCHARD 1949a, b.   [3] LANGMUIR 1916.
[4] KLOTZ 1946c.   [5] CHANUTIN 1942.   [6] H. H. WEBER 1927, 1930.

zum Adsorptionsmittel gleich $\dfrac{b\,X}{\dfrac{1}{a}+X}$ ist. a und b sind Konstanten, X wieder die Kon-
zentration des ungebundenen Materials. Diese dem Massenwirkungsgesetz entsprechende Gleichung ist der empirischen Freundlichschen Adsorptionsisotherme k. $c^{1/n}$ vorzuziehen, die mit zunehmendem c eine unendliche Adsorption angibt, was eine physikalische Sinnlosigkeit wäre, da doch die adsorbierende Oberfläche endlich abgesättigt werden muß. Nach Langmuir wird das Ende der Adsorption mit b erreicht, was dem n, der maximalen Zahl der Bindungsstellen, entspricht.

Die Gleichung ist von verschiedenen Autoren etwas umgeformt worden, um vorteilhaft durch Extrapolation die Werte für k und n bestimmen zu lassen. Klotz[1] hat das reziproke $\dfrac{1}{r}=\dfrac{1}{k\,n}\cdot\dfrac{1}{X}+\dfrac{1}{n}$ verwandt und $\dfrac{1}{r}$ gegen $\dfrac{1}{X}$ aufgetragen. Er demonstrierte am Beispiel von Methylorange, daß sich eine gerade Linie mit der Neigung $\dfrac{1}{k\,n}$ ergibt, die die Ordinate im Abstand $\dfrac{1}{X}$ schneidet. Da der Wert für $\dfrac{1}{n}$ aber stets in der Nähe von Null liegt, müssen kleine experimentelle Ungenauigkeiten große Fehler in der Extrapolation zur Folge haben. Aus diesem Grunde benutzte Scatchard[2] $\dfrac{r}{X}=k\,n-k\,r$ und erzielte eine größere Sicherheit der Werte für n und k.

Da in weitaus den meisten Fällen das Protein mit mehr als einem Molekül unter Bindung reagiert, muß mit der Zahl der bereits besetzten Bindungsplätze die Wahrscheinlichkeit der Kombination abnehmen. Für gleichartige Bindungsplätze müssen die einzelnen Gleichgewichtskonstanten jeder Reaktion

$$k_1=\frac{(P\,X)}{(P)\,(X)},\quad k_2=\frac{(P\,X_2)}{(P\,X)\,(X)},\quad k_3=\frac{(P\,X_3)}{(P\,X_2)\,(X)}\ldots k_n\frac{(P\,X_n)}{(P\,X_{n-1}\,(X)}$$

voneinander abhängig sein. Klotz zeigte, daß sich diese Abhängigkeit einfach zum Ausdruck bringen läßt. Die i-te Assoziationskonstante $k_i=\dfrac{n-(i-1)\cdot k}{1}$. Ist k und n ermittelt, dann ergeben sich, gleichartige Bindungsplätze und keine Sekundäreffekte vorausgesetzt, ohne weiteres die einzelnen Gleichgewichtskonstanten k_1 bis k_n und damit auch die Bindungsenergie als Änderung der freien Energie $F_1\ldots_n=-RT\ln k_1\ldots_n$. Nach Feststellung der Temperaturabhängigkeit lassen sich aus den gewonnenen Daten thermodynamische Größen wie die Entropie und Enthalpie der Bindung ermitteln[3].

In den meisten Fällen konnten jedoch die experimentellen Daten nicht mit der einfachen Theorie in Übereinstimmung gebracht werden, die für die Erklärung der Bindung von Ca-Ionen an Casein[4] oder von Methylorange an Albumin[1] ausreichte. In erster Linie mußten Korrekturen für die elektrostatische Wechselwirkung benutzt und aus der Debye-Hückelschen Theorie berechnet werden, wobei allerdings zumeist eine Reihe von Annahmen über zwischenmolekulare Abstände, Molekülradien und die „effektive" Dielektrizitätskonstante der Reaktionspartner gemacht werden mußten[5]. Scatchard[2] erweiterte seine Gleichung (s. oben) zu $\dfrac{r\cdot e^{-2\omega Z}}{X}=k\,n-k\,r$ und ließ die experimentelle Bestimmung von w dem Korrekturglied für die elektrostatische Wechselwirkung zu, wenn sich die Unmöglichkeit der Berechnung ergab. Er wies aber auch darauf hin, daß eine Abweichung von der Linearität des klassischen Modells seine Ursache im Vorliegen von zwei oder mehreren Assoziationskonstanten haben kann, die beide zusammen den Bindungsvorgang beschreiben. Es war uns von unseren alten Untersuchungen her bekannt, daß viele Farbstoffe so an das Serumalbumin gebunden sind. daß eine Assoziationskonstante allein den Bindungsvorgang unmöglich beschreiben konnte. So zeigten Bromphenolblau, Azorubin, Bromsulfalein nur bis zu einem bestimmten Punkt eine starke „quantitative" Bindung an das Serumalbumin. Jenseits davon trat mit zunehmender Bindung sehr rasch auch ein beträchtlicher Anteil freien Farbstoffes in Erscheinung.

Es besteht kein Grund zur Annahme, daß jeden Bindungsvorgang nur eine Assoziationskonstante beschreiben darf. Karush und Sonnenberg stellten 1949 an der Albuminbindung von Na-Dodecyl, -Decyl- und -Octylsulfat fest, daß sich die Gleichgewichtskonstanten in einer Gaußschen Verteilerfunktion anordneten. K_0 ist eine mittlere Bindungskonstante und gibt Aufschluß über das Gebiet, in welchem die Konstanten variieren. Auch Nitrophenolate,

---

[1] Klotz 1946b.   [2] Scatchard 1949a.
[3] Klotz 1946b, Klotz und Curme 1948b, Teresi 1948, Scatchard 1949a, Karush 1949, 1950.
[4] Karush 1950.   [5] Klotz 1946b, Scatchard 1949a, Karush 1950.

2,4 Dichlorophenolate und Pikrat wiesen eine Bindung mit einer Gauß-Funktion der Assoziationskonstanten auf[1]. Diese Betrachtungsweise wurde von PAULING 1945 aus der Beschreibung der Heterogenität der Bindung des Haptens am Antikörper in Kongruenz mit dem Antigen übernommen. War dort die Heterogenität verknüpft mit Strukturunterschieden am Antikörpermolekül, so vermuteten KARUSH und SONNENBERG 1949 Differenzen in den Bindungsstellen am gleichen Albuminmolekül. Die *Heterogenitätstheorie* der Bindungsstellen an Proteinen, insbesondere am Serumalbumin, bewährte sich bei der Bindung des Farbstoffes p-(2-hydroxy-5-methylphenylazo)-benzoesäure, welcher zwei einfachen Bindungskonstanten folgte[2].

$$\frac{r}{X} = \frac{n_1 k_1}{1 + k_1 X} + \frac{n_2 k_2}{1 + k_2 X} \quad \text{und} \quad n = n_1 + n_2.$$

Mit 2 Konstanten beschrieb auch SCATCHARD[3] die Bindung von Cl- und Rhodanidionen an isoionisches Albumin. Von den 100 positiv geladenen N-Gruppen am Albumin besitzt eine kleine Gruppe ($n = 11$ und $k = 44$) eine höhere Assoziationskonstante und eine größere ($n = 30$ und $k = 1,1$) eine niedere Assoziationskonstante für Cl. — Für die Rhodanidbindung liegen 10 Plätze mit $k = 1000$ und 30 Plätze mit $k = 25$ vor.

Während der letzten Jahre ist die Zahl der untersuchten Stoffe, die mit dem Serumalbumin Bindungen eingehen, rasch angewachsen. Dabei war mehr das Interesse der Chemiker vorherrschend, Aufschluß über die Art der Wechselwirkung mit dem offenbar für solche Kombinationen geschaffenen Protein zu erhalten, als das Bedürfnis, die biologische Bedeutung dieses Faktums weiter zu erhellen. Das Studium der Proteinbindung schien Hinweise auf Eigenschaften der Proteinmoleküle zu geben, die bisher unbekannt waren. Die Antworten auf die Fragen: wieviel, wie stark, wo und warum bindet das Protein, sollten zur Beschreibung des Eiweißes beitragen.

Die Bindungsplätze des Albumins.

Die Salzbindung zwischen Proteinen und Ionen ist eine seit vielen Jahren bekannte Eigenschaft amphotärer Elektrolyte[4]. Wenn das zu bindende Ion durch Coulombsche Kräfte genügend nahe herangezogen wird, entfalten sich zusätzliche, weniger weitreichende, für jedes Molekül geradezu spezifische Bindungskräfte. Van der Waalssche Kräfte, Induktions- und Dispersionskräfte sowie Wasserstoffbrückenbindungen üben in den Dimensionen der Annäherung von 2—5 Å wechselnde Einflüsse aus (Tabelle 3). Bei großen Ionen spielt die elektrostatische Anziehung oder Abstoßung nicht unmittelbar zur Bindung benutzter Molekülteile eine Rolle[5]. Eine Verlängerung der Seitenketten verstärkt im allgemeinen die Haftfestigkeit; auch Verzweigungen sind von Bedeutung[6]. Diese vielfältige Kraftentfaltung und die geringen Kenntnisse über die feinere Textur der Proteinmoleküle sind die Gründe, weshalb Betrachtungen über das „Warum" der Bindung vorläufig nur sehr vorsichtig angestellt werden dürfen. Als sicher kann angesehen werden, daß die *Bindungsfähigkeit des Albumins in ihrer Mannigfaltigkeit die aller bisher untersuchten Eiweißstoffe übersteigt*[7]. Es sind in erster Linie die positiv geladenen Aminosäurereste des Lysins, Arginins und Histidins[8], welche wegen ihrer relativ hohen p_K-Werte bis weit in den alkalischen Bereich Ladungen tragen und elektrostatische Bindungen mit fast allen Anionen eingehen können. LUCK erklärte die besondere Kombinationsfähigkeit des Serumalbumins, das sich sogar mit einigen ungeladenen Substanzen[9] schwach verbinden kann, mit dem niederen Dipolmoment, d. h. der gleichmäßigen Ladungsverteilung am Protein. Unpolare Seitenketten des Eiweißes wie Leucin, Valin und Phenylalanin können Einfluß auf die Stabilisierung einer Bindung ausüben[10].

---

[1] TERESI 1948.   [2] KARUSH 1950.   [3] SCATCHARD 1950.
[4] WEBER 1927, 1930, 1931, SCHMIDT 1944.   [5] STEINHARD 1941, BOYER 1947.
[6] FIESER 1948.   [7] KLOTZ 1950b, LUCK 1951.   [8] BOYER 1947, KLOTZ 1950b.
[9] KARUSH 1950, LUCK 1949.   [10] DAVIS 1946, 1947.

Tabelle 3. *Reichweite der Kräfte und Phasen der Bindung nach* Otto (1955).

Anziehung zwischen	Wirkung	E = Kraft r = Feldradius	Reichweite in Ångström (Å) (1 Å = 10^{-8} cm)	Aufeinanderfolgende Phase
Anion und Kation	Elektrovalenz	$E = \dfrac{1}{r^2}$	~ 100	
Ion und permanentem Dipol	Ionenhydratation, Überdeckung von Dipolen im gleichen Molekül	$E = \dfrac{1}{r^3}$	$\underset{<}{\sim} 10$	1
aktiviertem Wasserstoff und Donator	H-Brücke	$E = \dfrac{1}{r^4}$	$\underset{<}{\sim} 5$	
koordinationsfähigem Metallatom und Donator	Komplexbildung	$E = \dfrac{1}{r^4}$	$\underset{<}{\sim} 5$	2
zwei permanenten Dipolen	Dipolattraktion	$E = \dfrac{1}{r^4}$	$\underset{<}{\sim} 5$	
permanentem Dipol und induziertem Dipol	van der Waalssche Kräfte	$E = \dfrac{1}{r^{4-5}}$	< 3	
zwei temporären Dipolen		$E = \dfrac{1}{r^{6-7}}$	< 2	3

Es nimmt auch die Adsorption von Fettsäuren mit ihrer Kettenlänge zu, weil hydrophobe Reste an den unpolaren Seitenketten durch van der Waalssche Kräfte zusätzlich gebunden werden können.

Aus der Entropiezunahme bei der Bindung hat Klotz[1] geschlossen, daß gebundene Wassermoleküle abgegeben werden, wodurch die Bindungsenergie eine Zunahme erfahren muß. Er hält diesen Umstand für wichtiger als van der Waalssche Kräfte. Da es unmöglich ist, aus der Anzahl ladungstragender Gruppen, die bei sehr vielen Proteinen sehr ähnlich ist, allein einen Schluß auf die Kombinationsfähigkeit des Proteins zu ziehen, hat der gleiche Autor eine interessante Hypothese entwickelt, nach welcher das Ausmaß der Bindung um so größer ist, je mehr NH_3^+-Gruppen und je weniger (OH—COO)-Gruppen vorhanden sind. Er nimmt an, daß die NH_3-Gruppen dann von H-Brücken-bindungen seitens der OH-Gruppen blockiert werden, wenn diese nicht an COO-Gruppen gebunden sind. Letztere haben eine größere Bindungsenergie, so daß die NH_3^+-Gruppen frei-gehalten werden (Abb. 5). Beim Albumin über-wiegen weitaus die NH_3^+-Gruppen über die Differenz von (OH—COO^-)-Gruppen, so daß ein hoher „Bindungsindex" resultiert. Alle anderen bisher untersuchten Proteine haben

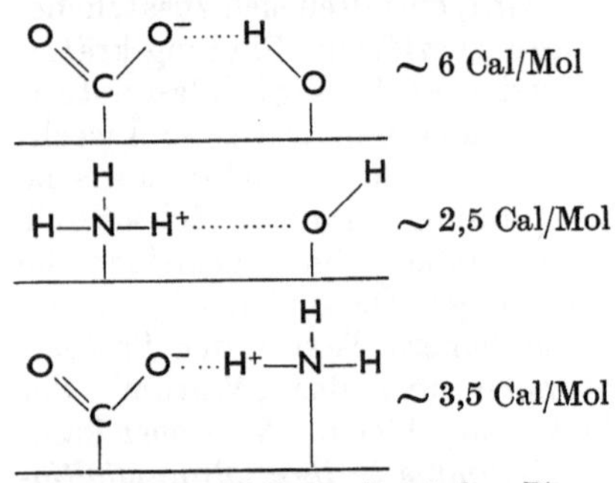

Abb. 5. Beeinträchtigung der starken Bindungsplätze an der Proteinoberfläche durch H-Brücken. Nach Klotz 1950

wesentlich kleinere Indices. Wegen der Behinderung der COO^--Gruppen ist auch die Wechselwirkung mit Kationen so gering. Karush[2] erklärt die besondere Befähigung zur Bindung mit so vielen verschiedenen Stoffen durch eine „konfigurationelle" Anpassungs-fähigkeit des Albumins, die wahrscheinlich durch lange, umfaltbare Seitenketten und durch ein Aufgehen von Interhelix-Bindungen zustande kommt. Im Vergleich mit der starren, nur auf das homologe Hapten abgestellten Oberfläche des Antikörpermoleküls vermutet er im Albumin strukturelle Faktoren, die eine Reihe von „konfigurationellen Alternativen" bedingen. Diese stehen miteinander im Gleichgewicht und besitzen ungefähr den gleichen Energiegehalt. Der zu bindende Stoff stabilisiert seiner Konstitution entsprechend das Protein, indem er mit mehreren ihm entgegenstehenden Gruppen reagiert. Dadurch wird der ganze Komplex widerstandsfähiger gegen Denaturierung durch Hitze oder Harnstoff.

---

[1] Klotz 1950.   [2] Karush 1950.

Kleinere Ionen müssen sogar in den Helix-Verband selbst aufgenommen werden können, also geradezu in das Molekül hineinschlüpfen. Diesen Überlegungen zufolge muß das gelöste Protein eine große konfigurationelle Entropie besitzen, was mit der ausgezeichneten, alle anderen Proteine übertreffenden Löslichkeit des Albumins übereinstimmt. Ist eine Wechselwirkung mit einem gebundenen Stoff durch 2 Assoziationskonstanten beschrieben, dann werden 2 Gruppen verschiedener Konfiguration an Albumin stabilisiert. Diese Eigenschaften kann man vielleicht als „Plastizität" des Albuminmoleküls ansprechen. Genaue Verdrängungsstudien haben diese Vorstellung bekräftigt. Durch Zusatz verschiedener farbloser, optisch isomerer Molekülteile eines Farbstoffs zu dem Albumin-Farbstoffgemisch ließ sich eine 3 Punkt-Fixierung wahrscheinlich machen. Die isomeren Farbteile gaben nur zu geringen Verdrängungen der gebundenen Farbe Anlaß[1]. Fast ohne Abhängigkeit von ihren Isomeren wurden die Teile gleichfalls am Eiweiß fixiert, während der gleichbleibende Rest der Farbe offenbar auch an der gleichen Stelle verankert blieb.

Die Bindungsstudien beweisen, daß durch die Wechselwirkung mit dem gebundenen Stoff das Protein sogar gewisse strukturelle Veränderungen erfahren kann. Auch die Eröffnung neuer Bindungsplätze ist möglich. Vorläufig ist noch nicht bekannt, bis zu welchem Grade der Belastung die Strukturausweitung reversibel ist. Für viele Farbstoffe muß man es bis zum Grade der Absättigung annehmen. Aggressiver verhielten sich Caprylat, Dodecylsulfat oder andere Alkylsulfate[2], welche eine Streckung des geknäulten Moleküls bewirkten[3].

So verständlich die Anionenbindung an kationische Bindungsplätze des Albumins ist, so überraschend ist die noch vorherrschende Unsicherheit in der Interpretation der Bindung von Kationen. Bei einem p_H von 7,8, bei dem die freien Carboxylgruppen der Asparagin- und Glutaminsäure vollständig ionisiert sind und wo ungefähr 130—135 saure Gruppen vorliegen, werden keine Komplexe mit aliphatischen Monoaminen von C_4 bis C_{12} gebildet[4]. Während keine Na-Bindung festgestellt werden konnte[5], fand sich für die gut untersuchte Cu^{++}-Bindung bei einem p_H von 4,5, daß COO^--Gruppen wesentlich beteiligt sein müssen[6].

Ein teilmethyliertes Albumin zeigt mit einer geringeren spezifischen Lichtabsorption auch eine geringere Bindung an. Aus der Verschiebung der Absorptionsmaxima der Cu-Albuminkomplexe bei p_H 7,0 schlossen die Autoren auf das Vorliegen von Chelatringen tetrakoordinierten Kupfers mit mindestens 2 Bindungen vom Albumin-Typ. Eine ganze Reihe von Cu-Aminosäurekomplexen absorbierte Licht genau so wie das Kupferalbumin.

Trotz dieser experimentellen Erhellung haftet den Betrachtungen über die Feinstruktur der Proteinoberfläche, an welche die Bindung erfolgt, noch viel Spekulatives an. Die aufgedeckten Unterschiede zwischen den einzelnen Eiweißstoffen sind aber schon heute sehr bemerkenswert. Die im wäßrigen Milieu so ganz verschieden bindenden Serumeiweißkörper zeigen überraschenderweise in essigsaurer, methanolischer Lösung an Fließpapier fixiert so gleichmäßige Bindung gegenüber dem sauren Farbstoff Amidoschwarz 10B, daß der gebundene Farbstoff nicht nur dem Protein-N jeder Serumfraktion proportional, sondern *sogar die relative Farbstoffbindung für alle elektrophoretischen Fraktionen nahezu gleich ist*. Die Technik der Papierelektrophorese benützt diese durch Denaturierung uniformierte Anfärbbarkeit zur Bestimmung der relativen Prozentwerte der Serumeiweißkörper[7]. Mit diesem etwas groben Hinweis soll gezeigt werden, wie außerordentlich milieuabhängig die Bindungsfähigkeit der Proteine ist. Die Frage, ob sich Albumine verschiedener Provenienz durch ihre Bindungsfähigkeit voneinander unterscheiden, wurde von KLOTZ bejaht. Auch wir fanden Unterschiede in der Bindung von Human-, Pferde- und Rinderalbumin für Azorubin[8] und MARTIN[9] für die Bindung von Ca^{++} gegenüber verschieden hergestellten Albuminen.

Kristallisationshilfen für Serumalbumin (z.B. Dekanol oder $HgCl_2$) besetzen in kristallisierten Präparaten Bindungsstellen. Eine solche Blockade kann unter Umständen auch in vivo eine Rolle spielen. Während eigene Untersuchungen bei einigen wenigen pathologischen Seren keine Unterschiede in der Azorubin-Bindefähigkeit des Serumalbumins erkennen ließen[10], konnten andere Autoren beim experimentellen Schock[11] bei Carcinomen[12] oder bei schweren Leberkrankheiten[13]

[1] KARUSH 1954.   [2] PUTNAM 1945, 1948.   [3] BOYER 1947.
[4] LUCK 1949.   [5] SCATCHARD 1950.   [6] KLOTZ 1950a.
[7] GRASSMANN 1950.   [8] OTT 1952, OPPERMANN 1957.   [9] MARTIN 1950.
[10] OTT 1952.   [11] WESTPHAL 1953.   [12] HUGGINS 1949.   [13] SCHULZE 1955.

ein Nachlassen dieser Testbindung des Albumins messen. Wann eine Blockade der Albumin-Bindungsplätze ins Gewicht fällt, ist schwer abzuschätzen. Die Kapazität der Moleküle ist jedenfalls sehr groß. Am ehesten wäre unter den Bedingungen starker Albuminverminderung eine Überlastung denkbar. Dann ist für viele Stoffe aber immer noch eine zusätzliche Gleichgewichtsbindung an bestimmte Globuline möglich. Das kann die Erklärung dafür abgeben, weshalb wir noch kaum ein umschriebenes klinisches Symptom eines fehlenden Serumeiweiß-Vehikels kennen. Die Albuminverminderung wirkt allerdings durch herabgesetzte Wasserbindung bei der Ödemgenese der Nephrosen mit; laboratoriumsmäßig ist der beschleunigte Kongoschwund aus der Blutbahn des Nephrotikers (Bennhold 1923 und 1925) zum größten Teil — bei den Analbuminämie-Patienten ausschließlich! — auf die Hypalbuminämie zurückzuführen.

Analbuminämie.

In diesem Zusammenhang muß auf die erstmalige Beobachtung einer familiären Analbuminämie[1] bei Bruder (28 Jahre alt) und Schwester (38 Jahre alt) hingewiesen werden, die einen nahezu symptomlosen Verlauf nahm. Dem Defekt im Eiweißbild entsprach zwar ein hochgradig pathologisch beschleunigter Schwund der albumingebundenen Farbstoffe Kongorot und in geringerem Maße auch Evansblue[2] in vivo; ferner fehlte in vitro die Azorubin- oder Germaninbindung[2]. Auswirkungen auf Funktion und Morphologie der Organe im Sinne einer krankhaften Leistungsminderung waren aber nicht vorhanden, wenn man von einer besonders prämenstruell in Erscheinung tretenden mäßigen Ödemneigung bei der Schwester absah. Obwohl der kolloidosmotische Druck des Serums auch beim Bruder stark herabgesetzt war, hatte der junge Mann keine Ödeme.

Bei dieser recessiv erblichen und offenbar schon embryonal einsetzenden Anomalie bestand offenbar noch die Möglichkeit, rechtzeitig Kompensationsfaktoren auszubilden, so daß der Wassertransport[3] und andere Funktionen der Albumine bis zur Homöostase geregelt werden konnten. Wie vielfältige biologische Mechanismen dafür herangezogen werden, wird im Abschnitt „Defektpathoproteinämien" (s. S. 241) dargelegt werden.

Bindung und Transport des Bilirubins.

Die Transportaufgaben, welche dem Organismus hinsichtlich des Bilirubins gestellt werden, sind aus verschiedenen Gründen interessant. Bilirubin fällt als Abbaustufe des Hämoglobins an. Man rechnet, daß täglich 1% des zirkulierenden Blutfarbstoffes abgebaut wird, wobei aus 1 g Hämoglobin 35 mg Bilirubin[4] entstehen, die auf gesicherten Wegen ausgeschieden werden müssen, da dieses die indirekte Diazoreaktion gebende Bilirubin in hoher Konzentration als Zellgift wirkt.

In den geringen Regel-Konzentrationen von 0,5—1,0 mg-% scheint es bei der Steuerung der Erythropoese eine „hormonähnliche" Rolle zu spielen[5]. Durch eine relativ feste Bindung am zirkulierenden Albumin wird das Bilirubin normalerweise gegen andere Bindungsplätze im Gewebe abgesichert. Bei dem pH 7,4 können maximal 2 Mole Bilirubin von einem Mol Albumin gebunden werden, d.h. auf 1 g Albumin kommen 15 mg Bilirubin[6]. Das Massenwirkungsgesetz ist auf diese Beziehung anwendbar. Das erste Mol haftet jeweils fester als das zweite.

---

[1] Bennhold 1954, 1958, 1959.   [2] Ott 1957.
[3] Scheurlen 1960, Bennhold 1960.
[4] Crosby 1955.   [5] Fellinger 1932, Patek 1934.   [6] Martin 1949.

Das gebundene Bilirubin gelangt nach mehr oder weniger vielfältigen Umwegen mit dem Blutstrom zur Leber, wo es abgehängt werden kann. Dort kommt es unter der Einwirkung mehrerer Fermente (insbesondere der in der Mikrosomenfraktion der Leber gebildeten Glucuronyltransferase) zu einer Koppelung des Bilirubins an die Glucuronsäure. Dieses Glucuronsäure-Bilirubin-Konjugat gibt die *direkte* Diazoreaktion und zeigt vor allem die funktionell wichtige Änderung, daß es nun *wasser*löslich geworden ist im Gegensatz zu dem nur *lipoid*löslichen unkonjugierten (indirekt reagierenden) Bilirubin[1]. Das konjugierte Bilirubin ist dadurch befähigt, im wäßrigen Milieu (mit der Galle und mit dem Urin) ausgeschieden zu werden, also auf Wegen, welche dem indirekt reagierenden Bilirubin praktisch verschlossen sind.

Das unkonjugierte (nicht veresterte) Bilirubin wird in der Literatur häufig als „freies" Bilirubin bezeichnet (weil es keine Bindung mit Glucuronsäure eingegangen ist); diese Bezeichnung hat aber gerade bei der Diskussion von Transportproblemen den großen Nachteil, daß dieses Bilirubin ja gerade eine ausgesprochene Bindung an Albumine aufweist. Dem Vorschlag von LATHE[2] auf Grund einer Umfrage bei namhaften Biochemikern ist deshalb zuzustimmen, daß der unveresterte Farbstoff als „*Bilirubin*", die Bilirubinglucuronide als „*konjugiertes Bilirubin*" zu bezeichnen sind.

Beide Arten von Bilirubin haften während des Transportes in der Blutbahn am Albumin, wie wir[3] nachweisen konnten, und wie es von PEDERSEN[4], GRAY[5] und KLATSKIN[6] späterhin mit verschiedenen Methoden bestätigt wurde. Die Bindung des wasserlöslichen Bilirubinglucuronids an Albumin ist anderer Art als diejenige des unveresterten Bilirubins. Die veresterten oder unveresterten Propionsäuregruppen des Bilirubins könnten Einfluß auf die Bindung haben. Das konjugierte Bilirubin haftet sehr viel lockerer am Albumin.

Bei normaler, niedriger Beladung mit Bilirubin ist die Bindung an das Albumin so fest, daß eine Abgabe an das Gewebe nicht zustande kommt. Steigt der Bilirubingehalt des Plasmas aber auf den hohen Wert von z.B. 20 mg-% an, dann ist bei Prüfung in vitro immer noch alles Bilirubin gebunden, es haftet jedoch *lockerer* am Albumin und geht sowohl intravasal an die α-Globuline über, als auch extravasal in erster Linie an die Elastinbestandteile der Haut und der Skleren[7].

Bei ganz hohen Bilirubinkonzentrationen von etwa 40 mg-% scheint sogar ein Teil des Bilirubins ungebunden zu sein (ältere eigene Untersuchungen). Es färbt in vivo das Gewebe dann fast ubiquitär. So bestimmt die konzentrationsabhängige Bindungsfestigkeit an das Albumin (und an die α- und schließlich auch β-Globuline) die Lokalisation der Abgabe des Farbstoffes im Gewebe. Mit Absinken des Bilirubinspiegels im Plasma geht der gleiche Prozeß rückläufig vor sich. Ausscheidung des Serumbilirubins bedeutet, daß sich das Bindungsgleichgewicht verschiebt in Richtung Elastin $\rightarrow$ Albumin $\rightarrow$ Ausscheidung; der Ikterus geht wieder zurück. Ob sich konjugiertes und unverestertes Bilirubin in ihren Affinitäten zu den erstrangigen und zweitrangigen Haftplätzen an Bluteiweiß und am fixen Gewebe verschieden verhalten, ist eine noch offene Frage.

Vor eine besonders geartete Transportaufgabe ist der *Organismus* des *Feten*, des *Frühgeborenen* und auch des *Neugeborenen* gestellt. Der Hämoglobinumsatz von der 3. Entwicklungswoche an führt zur Entstehung erheblicher Mengen von indirekt reagierendem, also unverestertem, nicht konjugiertem Bilirubin. In den 36 Wochen bis zur Geburt werden etwa 1000 mg Bilirubin gebildet[8]. Im Fruchtwasser findet sich keins, im Meconium des Neugeborenen lassen sich etwa 40 mg, in dem des Frühgeborenen nur wenige Milligramm nachweisen[9]. Nun würde

---

[1] SCHMID, R. 1956, TALAFANT 1956.   [2] LATHE 1956.   [3] BENNHOLD 1929.
[4] PEDERSEN 1937.   [5] GRAY 1948.   [6] KLATSKIN 1956.   [7] ROSENTHAL 1930.
[8] BETKE 1959.   [9] NAPP 1949.

dieser toxische Stoff, wenn er dank seiner Lipoidlöslichkeit in die Zelle gelangte, den fetalen Organismus gefährden. Das Bilirubin gelangt aber in Bindung an das Albumin zur Placenta und wird dort an das mütterliche Blut abgegeben; der Bilirubingehalt im Nabelarterienblut ist höher als der in der Nabelvene[1].

Bei dem Durchtreten des Pigmentes durch die Placentarschranke spielt vielleicht seine Lipoidlöslichkeit eine wichtige Rolle. Der höhere Bilirubin- und der wesentlich niedrigere Albumingehalt des fetalen Plasmas könnte ebenfalls die Abgabe des fetalen Bilirubins an das mütterliche bilirubinarme und albuminreichere Blut erleichtern[2]. Es handelt sich aber um einen aktiven Transport durch die Placentarschranke hindurch, denn auch bei ausgesprochenem Ikterus der Mutter wird das Plasma des Fetus in seiner Bilirubinabfuhr an das mütterliche Blut nicht behindert[3], allerdings läßt sich Glucuronyltransferase in der Placenta von Mensch und von Meerschweinchen nicht nachweisen[4]. Die Abgabe an den mütterlichen Organismus muß also in grundsätzlich anderer Weise bewerkstelligt werden, als die Ausscheidung beim Erwachsenen. In der Mutter wird das vom Fetus stammende Bilirubin dann konjugiert und durch die mütterliche Galle ausgeschieden. Erst das reife Neugeborene verfügt über den kompletten Mechanismus der Bilirubinausscheidung (aber auch bei normalem Geburtstermin tritt noch bei 50—75% der Neugeborenen Ikterus auf, weil die Synthese-Apparatur für die Fermente der Glucuronsäure-Bilirubin-Konjugierung doch nicht termingerecht fertig geworden ist[5]). Bei der Frühgeburt hört der fetale Abgabemechanismus an die Mutter mit der Unterbindung der Nabelschnur plötzlich auf, ohne daß die eigene normale Bilirubinausscheidung bereits funktioniert. Die Herstellung der 3 Fermente, welche die Konjugierung ermöglichen, insbesondere der Glucuronyltransferase, muß erst noch in Gang kommen. Bis diese Angleichung erreicht ist, häuft sich unkonjugiertes Bilirubin im Organismus des Frühgeborenen an. Bei Erythroblastose-Kindern kommt der vermehrte Erythrocytenzerfall mit zusätzlich vermehrtem Bilirubinanfall noch hinzu; aber auch ohne jede Erythroblastose kommen Fälle von schwerem Kernikterus vor[6]. Dazu kommt der niedrige Albuminspiegel bei Frühgeburten[7], der das Mißverhältnis von anfallendem Bilirubin zu den am Albuminvehikel verfügbaren Bindungsplätzen vergrößert. Ein Gefälle zur Zelle hin ist dadurch angebahnt und die Zellen des zentralen Nervensystems, insbesondere des Corpus striatum, Thalamus, Hippocampus[8] und des Myokards[9] sind der Giftwirkung des Bilirubins ausgesetzt, zumal das Gehirn der Frühgeborenen je nach dem Entwicklungsstadium besonders empfindlich zu sein scheint und außerdem die Bluthirn-Schranke besonders leicht passierbar sein soll[10]. Die Giftwirkung besteht hauptsächlich in einer Schädigung der Atmungskette und der damit gekoppelten Phosphorylierung, Vorgänge welche sich an Hirnschnitten und Hirnhomogenaten reproduzieren ließen[11]. Der von Orth[12] und von Schmorl[13] zuerst pathologisch-anatomisch beschriebene und von Kleinschmidt[14] klinisch bearbeitete, gefürchtete „Kernikterus" hat damit seine pathogenetische Grundlage[15] erhalten.

Die Albumine als Bilirubinvehikel sind beim Kernikterus so belastet, daß mehrere *Medikamente*, welche ebenfalls von den Albuminen gebunden werden, das schwach haftende Bilirubin zum Teil *verdrängen* und dadurch die Giftwirkung auf die Zellen verstärken. Auch Häm-Pigmente können ähnliche kompetitive Effekte auslösen[16]. Unter den Medikamenten ist vor allem Sulfi-

---

[1] Cserna 1923, Findlay 1947.   [2] Dancis 1959.   [3] Grodsky 1957.
[4] Dutton 1958, Smith Cl. A. 1959.   [5] Smith 1959.   [6] Aidin 1950.
[7] Plückthun 1959.   [8] Claireaux 1950.   [9] Diemer 1959.
[10] Patzer 1953, Zetterström 1959.   [11] Bowen 1957.   [12] Orth 1875.
[13] Schmorl 1904.   [14] Kleinschmidt 1951.
[15] Lathe 1957, Billing 1957, R. Schmid, 1956.   [16] Odell 1959.

soxazol („Gantrisin") anzuführen, welches früher oft bei der Behandlung von Frühgeburten prophylaktisch gegeben wurde, und bei dem sich nach einigen Jahren zeigte, daß es die Rate der Kernikterusfälle bis auf das 6fache erhöhte[1]! Ähnliche Verdrängungswirkungen fanden sich nach ebenfalls oft verabfolgten Medikamenten wie Sulfamethoxypyrimidin, Salicylsäure und bei Coffein-Natriumbenzoat[2]. Dieser kompetitive Effekt gegenüber der Bilirubinbindung zeigte sich auch darin, daß nach Gaben dieser Medikamente auch schon bei ungewöhnlich niedrigen Bilirubinwerten Kernikterus entstand[3].

Der kanadische Genetiker GUNN entdeckte einen Rattenstamm mit kongenitaler nicht hämolytischer Gelbsucht und mit angeborenem Mangel an Glucuronyltransferase[4]. Gab man diesen Ratten das Sulfonamid Gantrisin, dann fiel der Bilirubinspiegel ab und die Häufigkeit des Kernikterus stieg an[5]. Im Gegensatz hierzu wurde durch Albumingaben die Kernikterushäufigkeit bei diesen Ratten vermindert.

Aus diesen Beobachtungen und Überlegungen wurde von pädiatrischer Seite her schon die Folgerung gezogen, bei hochgradigem Ikterus Frühgeborener unter Umständen Serum therapeutisch zu verabreichen[6].

Die Plasmaglobuline als Vehikel.

Wenn auch das Albumin wegen seines universalen Bindungsvermögens die Hauptmenge der Plasmaeiweißvehikel stellt, erfährt die Bedeutung der Globuline im Transportgeschehen dadurch keine Minderung. In den Vordergrund ist das Vermögen bestimmter Globuline gerückt, ausschließlich mit einem ganz bestimmten Transportgut zu reagieren und so zu *spezifischen Vehikeln* zu werden. Aus der noch immer unübersehbaren Fülle verschiedener Globuline ließen sich, und zwar durch die Wechselwirkung mit dem Transportgut gekennzeichnet, das Transferrin als eisenbindendes, das Coeruloplasmin als kupferhaltiges, das Transcortin als cortisol- und desoxycorticosteronbindendes und das „Interalphaglobulin" als thyroxinbindendes Globulin elektrophoretisch lokalisieren und zum Teil isolieren. Das Vitamin B_{12}-bindende α-Globulin und zuletzt das Transmanganin, ein β-Globulin, sind in Spuren vorkommende Plasmaproteine, welchen offenbar nur als Transportmittel für ihr niedermolekulares Transportgut Bedeutung zukommt. Darüber hinaus sind die Plasmalipide, insbesondere die Neutralfette, stets an definierte Globuline gebunden und ihrerseits Vehikel für eine Anzahl hydrophober Plasmabestandteile (z. B. fettlösliche Vitamine).

Außer der spezifischen Kombinationsfähigkeit bestimmter Globuline besitzen andere α- und β-Globuline allgemeine Affinitäten zu einer bislang noch kaum überschaubaren Gruppe von Stoffen, welche auch mit dem Albumin Bindungen eingehen. Bei der Prüfung auf Bindung im Blutserum hatten sich viele saure Farbstoffe bei niedriger Farbkonzentration an das Serumalbumin gehängt; eine Bindung an Globuline konnte zunächst nicht festgestellt werden. Erst mit Erhöhung der Farbstoffkonzentration trat eine Mitbindung durch α- oder β-Globuline ein (z. B. bei Kongorot, Trypanblau, Evansblue, Diaminrot, Diaminreinblau, Geigyblau, Bilirubin)[7] (Abb. 4a—c). Nach Absättigung der Albuminbindung scheinen „Ersatzvehikel" zur Verfügung zu stehen, und bei Albuminmangel werden Vehikelfunktionen von Globulinen übernommen. Sonst albumingebundene Fettsäuren gehen dann Bindungen mit α_1- und β-Lipoproteiden ein, und sonst albumingebundene Farbstoffe haften an Globulinen. Wahrscheinlich geht der Lipidtransport bei A-β-Lipoproteidämie[8] viel stärker über albumingebundene Fettsäuren, zumal bei dem beobachteten Kind auch der α_1-Lipoproteidspiegel

---

[1] SILVERMANN 1956.   [2] ODELL 1958, 1959.   [3] BOWMANN 1957, HARRIS 1958, OPPE 1960.
[4] MALLOY 1940.   [5] JOHNSON 1957, BLANC 1959.   [6] DANCIS 1959, BLANC 1959.
[7] BENNHOLD 1938, 1947, 1950a, SCHUBERT 1950.   [8] SALT 1960.

sehr niedrig war. So konnten auch Albumine einen Teil der Funktionen der Globulinvehikel für Lipide übernehmen (s. S. 220 f.).

Der Umstand der hohen Albuminkonzentration des Serums hat das Studium der Globulinbindung erschwert und verzögert. Wenn auch die Menge Globulins, die vergleichbar dem Albumin unspezifisch bindende Eigenschaften hat, bedeutend unter der Menge zirkulierenden Albumins liegt, so hat doch das Studium analbuminämischer Seren[1] gezeigt, daß die Bindungsstärke etwa in der Größenordnung der Albuminbindung liegen dürfte. Erst wenn dem albuminfreien Serum die volle Menge Humanalbumin zugesetzt wurde, verschob sich der anfänglich globulingebundene Farbstoff Kongorot an das Albumin[1]. Daß die Bindefähigkeit der Globuline noch erhöht wird, wenn man sie entfettet, konnten wir am Beispiel der Kongorotbindung nachweisen[2].

Beobachtungen an ausschließlich globulingebundenen Farbstoffen sind selten. Eingehender untersucht ist der rote Farbstoff Lithiumcarmin[3], der bei niedrigen Farbzusätzen zum Serum (besonders deutlich bei Kaninchen-, Ratten- und Hundeseren) elektrophoretisch mit einem α_2-Globulin wandert und bei hohen Zusätzen vom Albumin mit gebunden wird.

Werden *kolloide Teilchen* im Serum emulgiert, dann wandern sie in Bindung mit den α_2-Globulinen[2]. So heterogene Stoffe wie Tusche-Partikeln, Goldsol, Berliner-Blau-Sol, durch Ultrabeschallung fein emulgierte Sudanfarbstoffe oder dem Serum zugesetzte Leberzellmikrosomen, welche in einem Kollidon- oder Dextranmilieu von p_H 8,5 ein durchaus unterschiedliches Verhalten zeigten, fanden sich an ein α_2-Humanserumglobulin fixiert. Das α_2-Globulin hatte hier ein stärkeres Bindungsvermögen als Albumin, und dieses war hohen Konzentrationen gegenüber wiederum wirksamer als γ-Globulin.

Ob der hier mehr unspezifischen Bindung an Globuline neben der Albuminbindung eine besondere Bedeutung zukommt, die über den Mechanismus eines „Ersatzvehikels" hinausgeht, ist vorläufig schwer abzuschätzen. Als spezifische Eiweißvehikel für Eisen, Kupfer, Jodhormone, Lipide, Cortine und das Vitamin B_{12} nehmen die bindenden Globuline einen festen Platz im Transportgeschehen ein.

Im folgenden soll die Bedeutung der Vehikelmechanismen der Globuline für den Stofftransport unter normalen und krankhaften Bedingungen an einigen besonders markanten Beispielen dargestellt werden. Dabei wird der Transport von Kupfer nach dem Eisentransport behandelt, wenn auch gerade das Transportkupfer albumingebunden ist und die Transportstörungen durch die Überlastung der Albumine mit Kupfer entstehen. Der Cu-Gehalt des im Plasma zirkulierenden Fermentes, Coeruloplasmin, soll für die Einteilung bestimmend sein. Die vielfältigen Beziehungen zwischen Vehikel, Speicher und Bedarfsort sind für das Eisen durch die Forschungen der letzten Jahre immer klarer geworden. Deshalb ist auch das Kapitel über Bindung und Transport von Eisen umfangreicher und behandelt ausführlicher die klinischen Folgen von Eisentransportstörungen.

Transportvorgänge im Eisenstoffwechsel.

An keinem lebenswichtigen Stoff läßt sich die Kompliziertheit der Transportvorgänge im Organismus so deutlich und paradigmatisch darstellen wie am Eisen; insbesondere läßt sich hier die Rolle der fixen Speicher (Apoferritin und Hämosiderin) und der mobilen Speicher (Transferrin-Vehikel) gut demonstrieren. In den letzten Jahrzehnten sind, seitdem Heilmeyer und Plötner 1937 die ersten zuverlässigen Eisenbestimmungsmethoden im Plasma ausgearbeitet hatten, sehr viele Daten gewonnen worden, welche die Transportbeziehungen dieses für den Organismus so kostbaren Metalls besonders klar erkennen lassen. — Im Bd. IV/2 dieses Handbuches sind alle wesentlichen Einzelheiten über Funktion und Stoffwechsel des Eisens mitgeteilt. Hier sollen nur kurz *die* Tatsachen zusammengefaßt werden, deren Kenntnis zur Darstellung der sich hierbei abspielenden *Transportvorgänge* notwendig ist.

Beim Eisen kennen wir die *Resorptionsorte* im Dünndarm und Duodenum. Von dort gelangt es via Pfortadersystem in die Leber; das Lymphgefäßsystem spielt dabei entgegen

---

[1] Ott 1957.   [2] Bennhold 1952b.   [3] Ott 1953.

früheren Vorstellungen[1] keine nennenswerte Rolle[2]. Als *Speicherorte* sind bekannt: Leber, Milz, Lymphdrüsen, Mucosa des Dünndarms und RES. — Wir wissen ferner, daß das Eisen in zwei verschiedenen Speicherformen abgelagert wird: erstens als Ferritin[3], welches im Zellplasma und nicht im Kern lokalisiert ist, zweitens als Hämosiderin[4]. Im Ouchterlony-Test verhalten sich die Eiweißkomponenten beider Eisenverbindungen immunbiologisch gleich[5]. Im *Ferritin* ist das Eisen an das hochmolekulare Zellprotein Apoferritin gebunden und ist in dieser eiweißreichen Bindung besonders gut disponibel.

Apoferritin, welches im elektrischen Feld mit der Geschwindigkeit der α_2-Globuline wandert, besitzt ein Molekulargewicht von 460000 und schließt das Eisen als Ferrihydroxyd und als Ferriphosphat micellär ein. Apoferritin wird intracellulär gebildet, sobald Eisen in die speichernde Zelle (z. B. der Mucosa) eindringt. Ferritin enthält 17—24% Eisen. *Hämosiderin* ist eine eisenreichere, wasserärmere und in den meisten Fällen auch stabilere Verbindung und enthält 29—36% Eisen[6]; es wird deshalb besonders reichlich gebildet bei relativem Apoferritin-Mangel, eventuell auch bei hochgradigem Eiweißmangel in der Nahrung[7]. Eisen, welches überstürzt und in großen Mengen zugeführt wird, kann zunächst als vorläufiges Hämosiderindepot abgelagert werden; von dort wird es dann erst allmählich in Ferritindepots umgelagert[8] oder direkt zum Aufbau von Hämoglobin, Myoglobin oder Zellfermenten abgegeben. Eisen, welches längere Zeit als Hämosiderin gespeichert war, kann fast völlig seine Mobilisierbarkeit verlieren.

Der *Eisenspiegel* im Plasma wird in erster Linie vom Resorptionsort in der Darmmucosa („Mucosal acceptor"[9]) aus gesteuert. Nervale und endokrine Mechanismen spielen dabei zweifellos eine wichtige Rolle[10]. Je nach dem Eisenbedarf des Organismus, der Füllung der Speicher, der Höhe des Plasmaeisenspiegels und der latenten Bindungskapazität[11] wird Eisen von der Mucosa resorbiert. Niedriger Eisenspiegel und hohe Werte der latenten Bindungskapazität führen oft zu starker Eisenresorption aus dem Darm und zu Eisenmobilisierung aus den Speichern, unabhängig vom Eisenangebot in der zugeführten Nahrung. Der normale Eisenspiegel beträgt 90—120 μg-% bei der Frau und 120—140 μg-% beim Mann.

Wie mühelos die Eisendepots bei Bedarf mobilisiert und die Resorption von Nahrungseisen entsprechend gesteigert werden können, zeigten LINTZEL und RADEFF 1930 in Rattenversuchen. Zwangen sie Ratten dadurch, daß sie sie einer Luftverdünnung von etwa 8000 m Höhenlage aussetzten, zur forcierten Hämoglobinbildung, dann konnten sie das Depoteisen in Milz und Leber von 10,6 mg/kg Körpergewicht auf 2,6 senken. Der Eiseneinbau in das neu zu produzierende Hämoglobin betrug 9,2 mg/kg Körpergewicht und stammte offenbar aus der gesteigerten Resorption im Darm. Voraussetzung des Hämoglobinaufbaus in den Erythroblasten und Reticulocyten des Knochenmarks ist, daß die aus Mobilisierung und Resorptionssteigerung dem zirkulierenden Blute zugeführten Eisenmengen auch wirklich im Knochenmark nutzbar abgeladen werden. Die lückenlose Regelung des Eisentransportes zwischen Resorptionsort, fixem Speicher und Verbrauchsort ist Voraussetzung für die Anpassung der Erythrocyten-Produktion bei plötzlichen hohen Anforderungen an den Sauerstofftransport. Interessanterweise steigt, wenn man Ratten in Luftdruckverhältnisse großer Höhenlage bringt, auch sogleich der Transferrinspiegel an[12]. — Dasselbe gilt für den Antransport des Eisens zu anderen Orten dringenden Bedarfs (Herstellung von Myoglobin oder von Fermenten mit Zellhämin-Charakter). In Versuchen am Hund hat man festgestellt, daß *normalerweise* 57% des Gesamteisens zum Aufbau des Hämoglobins dienen, 7% zum Aufbau des Myoglobins (in der Muskelzelle); 16% des Gesamteisens finden sich in den Zellhäminen, während die restlichen 20% als Speichereisen im Ferritin und Hämosiderin abgelagert sind[12]. Die Eisenversorgung befindet sich demnach in folgender allgemeiner Ausgangssituation: Der *Eisenzustrom* ins Blut setzt sich zusammen aus einem Anteil, der im Darm *resorbiert wurde* und aus einem weiteren, der aus dem Erythrocyten- bzw. *Hämoglobinabbau* (vorwiegend in der Milz), ferner aus dem Myoglobin- und Zellhäminabbau stammt; der *Antransport* zu den *Bedarfsstätten* ist ein fast ubiquitäres Bedürfnis seitens des Knochenmarks, der Muskelzelle und aller Zellen, welche der Zellhämine bedürfen; im Nebenschluß liegen die *Speicher* zur schnellen Abdeckung aller dringenden Eisenanforderungen.

Zwischen alle diese heterogenen Instanzen ist die Blutbahn eingeschaltet, welche geregelte Transportbeziehungen — ohne Error loci! — herstellen soll. Dies erscheint dadurch besonders kompliziert, daß das dreiwertige Eisen von sich aus hochdiffusibel ist und ohne ein Trägerprotein in seiner Abgabe aus dem Blut räumlich nicht zu steuern wäre. Insbesondere bestände

[1] McCallum 1891, Gilman, Moore 1939.
[2] Endicott 1949, Peters, Peterson 1952, Everett 1954.
[3] Granick 1942, 1946, Hahn 1943.   [4] Asher 1933.   [5] Wöhler 1959.
[6] Asher 1933, Behrens 1952, Thedering 1949.   [7] Keiderling 1959.
[8] Wöhler 1955.   [9] Granick 1946.   [10] Schäfer 1949, Thedering 1949.
[11] Laurell 1947.   [12] Hahn 1943.

dann die Gefahr großer Eisenverluste durch die Niere, welche jedoch normalerweise pro Tag nur etwa 48—64 μg Fe in den Harn durchtreten läßt[1].

Als Trägerprotein wurde von Schade und Caroline 1946 sowie von Laurell und Ingelmann 1947 das eisenbindende *Transferrin* (auch „Siderophilin"[2] oder „eisenbindendes β-Globulin" genannt) isoliert; es hat ein Molekulargewicht von etwa 90000 und wandert elektrophoretisch mit der Geschwindigkeit der β_1-Globuline. — Beim Gesunden findet man 0,2—0,32 g-% Transferrin im Plasma[3]. Jedes Transferrinmolekül bindet 2 Ferriionen und 2 Bicarbonationen[2]. Bei Menschen verschiedener Rassen und Volksgruppen fand Smithies 1958 mit seiner zweidimensionalen Elektrophorese im Stärkemilieu verschiedene Transferrintypen, welche er als β_1-Globulin B, C und D bezeichnete. Neuerdings sind sogar 10 Transferrin-Kombinationen festgestellt worden[4]. Die Transferrintypen sind zweifellos genetisch bedingt[5]. Normalerweise genügt der Transferringehalt von 100 cm³ Plasma, um 250—300 μg Eisen in vitro zu binden. Die unbenützte Bindungskapazität stellt offensichtlich eine Transportmittelreserve dar, gestattet aber vielleicht auch eine differenzierte Verteilung des Eisens an Abgabeplätze verschiedener Eisenaffinität (vgl. S. 208). Im Transferrinkomplex hat das Eisen eine deutlich geringere biologische Halbwertzeit (90 min) als die Eiweißkomponente (12 Tage)[6]. Diese beiden Feststellungen sind eindrucksvolle Belege für die biologisch ständig beanspruchte und mit Auswechselvorgängen einhergehende Eisenbindung am Transferrin. Die ungenützte Bindungskapazität des Transferrins scheint uns für den Eisentransport unter normalen Verhältnissen und bei bestimmten Krankheitsbildern von besonderer Wichtigkeit zu sein. Der Vorgang der Bindung des Eisens sowohl an das Transferrin im kompletten Serum als auch an isoliertes Transferrin ist in vitro ohne Zusatz irgendwelcher Fermente jederzeit reproduzierbar. Der Bindungsprozeß geht nach Untersuchungen mit immunbiologischen Methoden sehr schnell vor sich[7] und ist in vitro bei einem p_H von 7,2 sehr fest; die Bindungsfähigkeit ist jedoch stark milieuabhängig; bei einem p_H unter 7,2 wird ein Teil des Eisens frei, bei p_H 5,0 wird fast alles Eisen aus dem Transferrin herausgelöst und ist frei und ionisiert.

Auch durch Änderung des Redoxpotentials, durch Zusatz von Vitamin C[3] sowie durch Komplexbildner, wahrscheinlich auch durch Enzyme könnte im Organismus die Eisenbindung an das Transferrin lösbar sein. Neuerdings ist auch die Mitwirkung der Adenosintriphosphorsäure bei der Abhängung des Eisens vom Transferrin behauptet worden[8]. Wir finden also bei der Eisenbindung an Transferrin zunächst nicht die analogen einfachen Gleichgewichtszustände wie bei den sauren Farbstoffen.

In neuen Versuchen wurde festgestellt, daß auch in vitro ohne obige Milieuänderungen die Eisenbindung an Transferrin lösbar ist. Brachte man menschliches mit Fe⁵⁹ markiertes Serum mit nichtmarkiertem Kaninchenserum im Überschuß zusammen, dann gingen erhebliche Mengen Fe⁵⁹ in vitro (ohne Anwesenheit cellulärer Elemente) von menschlichem Transferrin auf das Kaninchentransferrin über, wie sich durch immunologische Fällung des Humantransferrins und durch Messung der noch verbliebenen Fe⁵⁹-Konzentration im Präcipitat nachweisen ließ[9].

Solange die Bindungskapazität des Trägerproteins nicht überschritten ist, zirkuliert das Eisen bei p_H 7,2 in fester Bindung an das Transferrin. Sobald jedoch die oben angeführten milieuändernden Faktoren in vivo extra- oder intracellulär gegeben sind, könnte ein Verhalten analog den Bindungsverhältnissen der sauren Farbstoffe einschließlich des Bilirubins (vgl. S. 188, 199) resultieren. Dies

---

[1] Cartwright 1954. [2] Schade 1949, Surgenor 1949.
[3] Turnbull 1961. [4] Horsfall 1958. [5] Gitlin 1956.
[6] Schade 1949. [7] Mazur 1960. [8] Lohss 1961, Kallee 1961.

bedeutet, daß in vivo bei entsprechender Milieuänderung, mit der gerade an den Zellmembranen durchaus zu rechnen ist, am Ort der Abhängung ebenfalls die Bindungslabilität mit dem Umfang der besetzten Bindungsplätze zunimmt. Der Befund, daß die beiden Bindungsplätze des Transferrins das Eisen mit unterschiedlichen Dissoziationskonstanten binden[1], könnte neue Gesichtspunkte über das Zustandekommen einer abgestuften Bindung beibringen. In der Nähe der Transferrin-Sättigung wird die Milieuänderung sich durch Freigabe von Fe am stärksten auswirken und daher auch am auffälligsten sein, selbst gegenüber an sich geringgradigen Bindungsaffinitäten irgendwo im fixen Gewebe. Demgegenüber wird bei geringer Inanspruchnahme der Transferrinkapazität ein spärlicheres Freiwerden von Eisen zu erwarten sein, so daß dieses nur an Orte höchster Affinität (Knochenmark) abgegeben (vgl. später Eisenmangelanämie) wird. Mit solchen Bindungsunterschieden ist es auch wohl zu erklären, daß intravenös appliziertes Ferrieisen hauptsächlich in der Leber deponiert wird; erfolgt die Injektion jedoch nach Bindung an zusätzliches Trägerglobulin, dann findet sich auch beim Gesunden hauptsächliche Eisenablagerung im Knochenmark[2].

Ganz anders ist es, wenn Eisen, an körperfremde große Moleküle geheftet, dem Organismus einverleibt wird. Nach Injektion von *Eisendextran (Myofer)* z. B. können diese Komplexe lange Zeit im Blute zirkulieren und bei Eisenanalysen des Blutes völlig anormale hohe Werte (900—3000 μg-%) ergeben, ohne daß toxische Symptome durch freies Eisen auftreten. Es zeigt sich sogar, daß bei so hohen Eisenwerten im Blute dennoch eine hohe latente Eisenbindungsfähigkeit erhalten geblieben war: Nach peroraler Gabe von Eisen stieg das „Serumeisen" noch um durchschnittlich weitere 166 γ-% Eisen an[3]. Der großmolekulare Dextrankomplex ist dann — als nicht richtig eingepaßtes „Fremdvehikel" — nur in der Lage, den Abstrom des Eisens durch die Niere zu verhindern; diese Eisenbindung ist aber nicht so abgestimmt, daß Eisen an den Orten des physiologischen Bedarfs (Knochenmark usw.) ohne weiteres direkt freigemacht werden kann, wie es beim Transferrin der Fall ist; zu dem Fremdvehikel Dextran fehlt gewissermaßen der physiologische „Abgabeschlüssel". Das Eisen des Myofers kann dem Organismus nicht direkt nutzbar gemacht werden, ehe das Molekül — wahrscheinlich im RES — abgebaut und das so frei gewordene Eisen in der Blutbahn an das Transferrin geheftet wird.

Das Transferrin kann man andererseits als Eisenvehikel teilweise ausschalten durch intravenöse Gaben von Äthylendiamintetraessigsäure (ADTE). Diese besitzt starke Affinität zum Eisen und bildet mit ihm eine harnfähige Komplexverbindung in Form von Metall-Chelaten unter Herauslösung des Eisens aus der Transferrinbindung; dadurch steigt die Eisenausscheidung durch die Niere auf das 10fache an[4]. Das Transferrin wird dann mindestens teilweise seiner eisenbewahrenden Vehikelfunktion und seiner spezifischen Abgabefunktion beraubt.

Am Beispiel des Myofers und des Kollidons als Fremdvehikel einerseits sowie der Chelatbildung andererseits sieht man, welche Wichtigkeit die intakten Vehikel für die Ausscheidungsvorgänge durch die Niere und für Clearance-Werte haben können.

Wie lassen sich nun pathologische Prozesse des Eisenstoffwechsels und entsprechende klinische Krankheitsbilder mit diesen Vorstellungen von der wichtigen Transportfunktion des Transferrins vereinbaren ? Zwei Krankheitsbilder kommen dabei in erster Linie in Frage:

1. die mit hohem Eisenspiegel im Blut einhergehende *Hämochromatose*;

2. die mit Hyposiderinämie einhergehende *Eisenmangelanämie*. Als weitere Krankheitsbilder werden schließlich noch das seltene Krankheitsbild der *sideroachrestischen Anämie* und der *perniziösen Anämie* auf Besonderheiten im Eisenstoffwechsel untersucht werden.

Bei der *Hämochromatose* ist nach übereinstimmender Ansicht der meisten Forscher die Regulation der intestinalen Eisenresorption durchbrochen. Wahr-

---

[1] WOODWORTH 1959, SCHADE 1960.   [2] HUFF 1951, LINTZEL 1953.
[3] SCHNEIDER 1959.   [4] FIGUEROA 1954, GREENWALT 1955.

scheinlich spielen genetische Faktoren eine wesentliche Rolle[1]. Auf dem Boden einer familiären Hypersiderinämie kann durch lange Zeit gegebene Eisenmedikation eine Hämochromatose manifest werden[2]. Heilmeyer[3] spricht von einer „Durchlöcherung der Einfuhrsperre". Dadurch muß es zu einer ungeregelten, stoßweisen, von der jeweiligen Nahrungsaufnahme abhängigen Eisenresorption durch den Darm kommen. Es findet sich ein deutlich erhöhter Eisenspiegel im Blute[4]. Erstaunlicherweise paßt sich in den schweren Krankheitsfällen der Transferrinspiegel diesem hohen Eisenangebote *nicht* an, sondern ist sogar abnorm niedrig, so daß in vielen Fällen von Hämochromatose ein hochgradiges Mißverhältnis zwischen Eisen- und Transferringehalt des Blutes besteht[5] und in fortgeschrittenen Fällen auch das periphere Blut des großen Kreislaufes eine nahezu vollständige Auffüllung der Bindungskapazität des Transferrins zeigt. Das besagt mit größter Wahrscheinlichkeit, daß schon bei den normalen täglichen Bluteisenspiegelschwankungen von 30—40 μg-%[6] — welche aber bei der fehlenden intestinalen Resorptionssteuerung im Falle der Hämochromatose sicherlich noch größer sind — mindestens zeitweise kleine, schnell vom Gewebe abgefangene Mengen *freien* Eisens zirkulieren.

Ganz besonders ungünstig müssen unter diesen Verhältnissen die Transportbedingungen im *Pfortadergebiet* sein, wo nach einer ungesteuerten Fe-Resorption aus eisenhaltiger Nahrung die Überschwemmung des Pfortaderblutes mit Eisen noch nicht durch Mischung mit dem Gesamtblutvolumen ausgeglichen ist. Die Leber wird also betreffs Zustroms von ungebundenem oder ungenügend gebundenem Eisen ganz besonders exponiert sein. Wie stark die Leber das frisch resorbierte Eisen abfängt, kann man aus der mehrfach bestätigten Tatsache ablesen, daß *peroral* eingenommenes Eisen bei Hämochromatose-Patienten (im Gegensatz zu Gesunden) kaum einen Anstieg des peripheren Bluteisens herbeiführt[7], während man bei der unregulierten „durchlöcherten Einfuhrsperre" an sich eher das Gegenteil erwarten sollte; die Leber fängt offenbar den größten Teil des intestinal resorbierten Eisens ab. Auch nach *intravenösen* Eisengaben sinkt der Bluteisengipfel wesentlich schneller ab als beim Normalen[8]: offenbar ebenfalls als Folge zeitweise frei zirkulierenden Eisens und einer eventuell auch weniger festen Eisenbindung in der Nähe des Transferrinsättigungsgrades.

Ebenso ist die abnorm hohe Siderourie bei der Hämochromatose (auf das 4—40fache der Norm) auf die Transportinsuffizienz des Transferrins zu beziehen[9]. Es findet sich ferner stets eine stark positive Eisenbilanz[10].

In welcher Beziehung stehen nun die *klinischen Erscheinungen der Hämochromatose* zu den geschilderten Transportstörungen? Wir finden: *Lebercirrhose, Pankreascirrhose* (oft mit *Diabetes mellitus*), *Nebennierenschädigungen* mit *Hypotonie, Herzschädigungen, Hodenatrophie* mit Potenzschwäche und schließlich auch psychische Störungen. Diesen klinischen Symptomen entsprechen genau die pathologischen Eisenablagerungsorte: allem voran die *Leber* mit 20—40 g pathologisch gespeicherten Eisens (bei einem Eisenbestand des normalen Gesamtorganismus von 4 g!), dann aber auch *Pankreas, Herzmuskel, Nebenniere, Hypophyse, Plexus chorioideus, Hirnhäute* und *Ependym*; ferner die retroperitonealen *Lymphdrüsen, Niere, Schweißdrüsen, Malpighi-Schicht der Haut*; auffallend gering Milz und Knochenmark. Dieses plötzliche Auftreten von Eisenablagerungen in

---

[1] Frisch 1922, Wegener 1928, Laferre 1934, Sheldon 1935, Lawrence 1949, Harvier 1950, Althausen 1951, Löhr 1952-1956, Hedinger 1953, Kappeler 1956.
[2] Fisher 1960.   [3] Heilmeyer 1954.   [4] Büchmann 1948.
[5] Rath 1948, Braunsteiner 1952, Davis 1952, Gillov 1952, Remy 1954.
[6] Valquist 1941, Skouge 1939, Heidel 1955, Bothwell 1955, Keiderling 1959.
[7] Hemmeler 1951, Lange 1958.   [8] Gitlow 1952, Remy 1954, Lange 1958.
[9] Morczek 1952.   [10] Marble 1939.

ganz verschiedenen Organen, deren Gewebe sich histologisch, chemisch und färberisch so ganz verschieden verhält, ist etwas sehr Merkwürdiges, gewissermaßen ein Error loci en bloc! Im Sinne LETTERERS[1] kann man von einer Thesauropathie und zwar von einer „multilokulären Thesauropathie" sprechen.

Es ist kaum vorstellbar, daß plötzlich ein so multilokulärer Eisenhunger von der Gewebsseite her auftritt. Eine gemeinsame Ursache muß diesem Phänomen zugrunde liegen, und diese muß zunächst im Transportapparat, und zwar in der nachgewiesenen Diskrepanz von Hypersiderinämie und Hypotransferrinämie, gesucht werden. Der verminderte, im Pfortadergebiet wahrscheinlich zum Teil aufgehobene Transferrinschutz für das zirkulierende Eisen führt zur Abgabe von Eisen an Orte, zu denen bei normaler Belastung der Eisenbindungskapazität des Transferrins niemals ein Ablagerungsgefälle hätte zustande kommen können. Eine *Insuffizienz des Transportmilieus für Eisen* führt so zu einem folgenschweren Error loci.

So verständlich die Eisenablagerungen auf Grund obiger Überlegungen sind, so unerklärt ist zunächst noch das Ausbleiben einer kompensatorischen Transferrinvermehrung anläßlich der Hypersiderinämie. Die wahrscheinlichste Deutung besteht in der Annahme, daß die erheblichen Schwankungen des Eisenspiegels in dem Pfortadergebiet als *erstes die Leber* in ihrer Funktion schädigen, so daß die in der Leber stattfindende Transferrinbildung leidet und dadurch (nach Art eines Circulus vitiosus) das Mißverhältnis zwischen Eisenspiegel und Eisenbindungskapazität des Transferrins immer stärker wird.

Bei den Fällen von Hämochromatose, welche durch sehr häufige *Bluttransfusionen* ausgelöst sind[2], werden auf intravenösem Wege große Mengen von Eisen (als Hämoglobin) zugeführt unter Umgehung des dosierenden und regulierenden

Anmerkung. Als ein für die obigen Auffassungen sprechendes Experimentum *naturae* sei eine in der Freiburger Universitäts-Kinderklinik (Prof. KELLER) und in der Medizinischen Klinik Freiburg (Prof. HEILMEYER) beobachtete 6jährige Patientin erwähnt mit einer sonst wohl noch nie beobachteten *Atransferrinämie.* Der Fall gelangte erst während der Drucklegung zu unserer Kenntnis. Wir danken Herrn Prof. KELLER vielmals für die Mitteilung der Untersuchungsergebnisse. Immunbiologisch ließ sich bei dieser Patientin eine Herabsetzung des Transferrinspiegels im Plasma auf weniger als $1/_{128}$ des Normalen feststellen. In vitro zugesetztes Fe^{59} wanderte im elektrischen Feld zwischen β- und γ-Globulinen. Das Serumeisen betrug zwischen 5 und 10 γ-% (!); mit einer Gesamt-Bindungskapazität von 15 γ-% (ein anderes Laboratorium fand Eisenspiegel von 14 γ-% und eine Gesamtkapazität von 33 γ-%). (Weitere Daten s. S. 244.) Die Leber-Biopsie ergab: Exzessive Siderose der Leber bei periportaler Fibrose.

Es handelt sich hier also um eine Hämochromatose mit extra *niedrigem* (!) Eisenspiegel im Blute. Trotzdem ist dies nach den obigen Darlegungen völlig verständlich. Das pathogenetisch Primäre ist der (wohl angeborene) Transferrindefekt, dadurch fehlendes oder höchstens in Spuren vorhandenes spezifisches Transportmilieu für Eisen; dadurch Wegfall der III. Stufe des Transportgeschehens (vgl. S. 180) mit entsprechendem Error loci. Durch typische Fehlablagerungen in bestimmten Organen entsteht die Symptomatologie einer echten Hämochromatose!

Die von zahlreichen Autoren festgestellten Transferrintypen [neben dem normalen Transferrin (Transferrin C) werden bei einzelnen Angehörigen der weißen Rasse ein schneller wanderndes Transferrin B und bei Negern ein langsamer wanderndes Transferrin D beobachtet[3]] bei verschiedenen Menschen zeigen, wie stark genabhängig die Transferrinbildung vor sich geht. Damit ist auch ein solcher fast quantitativer Transferrindefekt genetisch gut vorstellbar. Die genetisch bedingte Doppelalbuminämie und Analbuminämie könnten bis zu einem gewissen Grade Parallelerscheinungen sein zur Doppeltransferrinämie und zur Atransferrinämie.

[1] LETTERER 1948, 1953.
[2] ZELTMACHER 1945, HUMPHREYS 1945, CHESNER 1946, SCHWARTZ 1947/48, MUIRHEAD 1949, WYATT 1950, FAVRE-GILLY 1953, SCHMIDT 1953, MORRIS 1958, KEIDERLING 1959.
[3] GIBLETT 1959, SMITHIES 1959.

Resorptionsvorganges im Darm. Deshalb ist auch die Möglichkeit einer Überlastung des Transferrins und einer Eisenfehlleitung im oben dargelegten Sinne
gegeben.

Das Gegenstück ist die bekannte Aderlaß*therapie*[1] der Hämochromatose.
Man kann sich vorstellen, daß dabei die großen Hämoglobinverluste (wöchent-
lich 500 cm³ Blut) das Abgabegefälle von Eisen in das Knochenmark so steigern,
daß die bei der Hämochromatose pathologische Prävalenz der Leber als Eisenspeicher vom Knochenmark überhöht wird und das abnorm locker am Transferrin
gebundene Eisen nun hauptsächlich vom Knochenmark absorbiert wird. Es erfolgt
dann ein rückläufiges Gleichgewicht zwischen Transportgut und Vehikel, ähnlich, wie wir es beim abheilenden Ikterus betreffs der Wiederabgabe des Bilirubins
vom Elastin an das Albuminvehikel kennengelernt hatten (vgl. S. 199). Es ist
dann auch verständlich, daß trotz der enormen Blutverluste bei der Aderlaß-
therapie der Hämochromatose kaum jemals Anämien zur Beobachtung kommen,
sofern nicht gleichzeitig ausgesprochene Blutkrankheiten vorhanden sind[2].

Genau entgegengesetzt ist die Transportlage bei der *Eisenmangelanämie*. Hier
finden wir eine ausgesprochene *Hyposiderinämie* und eine *Hypertransferrinämie*,
deren Ergebnis eine sehr vergrößerte latente Bindungskapazität des Transferrins
ist[3]. Besonders aus den Untersuchungen Pollycoves[4] mit Fe⁵⁹ wissen wir, daß
schon beim Gesunden nach intravenöser Injektion von Fe⁵⁹ das Knochenmark
die größte Avidität beim Abfangen des Eisens aufweist (Radioaktivität gemessen
am Kreuzbein). Die Speicherungsintensität in Leber und Milz folgt (innerhalb der
ersten 4 Tage) prozentual in sehr deutlichem quantitativem Abstand. Bei der
Eisenmangelanämie ist dieser Abstand noch wesentlich größer; Leber und Milz
sind an der Zuteilung des Eisens viel weniger beteiligt („höhere Abgabe-
schwelle"). Die peroralen und intravenösen Eisenbelastungskurven spiegeln diese
Transportverhältnisse des Eisens bei der Eisenmangelanämie sehr gut wieder:
nach peroraler Eisenzufuhr schneller und hoher Anstieg des Plasmaeisens mit
relativ langsamem Abfall; das entspricht einerseits der forcierten intestinalen
Eisenresorption und andererseits der verlangsamten Abgabe aus der Blutbahn
durch festere Haftung am weitgehend ungesättigten Transferrin. Nach intravenöser Injektion, wo also der Resorptionsfaktor wegfällt, tritt nur die festere
Haftung am Transferrin in Form der verlangsamten Abgabe des Eisens aus der
Blutbahn in Erscheinung. Es erscheint naheliegend, diese Befunde[4] mit der
Pathophysiologie der Eisenmangelanämie, gerade auch was die geringe Besetzung
der Eisenbindungskapazität des Transferrins und die damit einhergehende festere
Eisenhaftung am Transferrin betrifft, in Verbindung zu bringen. Die *Hebung
der Schwelle der Eisenabgabe vom Transferrin* wird dazu führen, daß das zirkulierende Eisen im wesentlichen *nur noch an die Orte höchster Avidität* abgegeben
wird; die Folge davon wird sein, daß das Knochenmark in erster Linie mit Eisen
versorgt wird und Einsparungen auf Kosten der Orte geringerer Affinität (Leber,
Milz, Fermente) gemacht werden. Es kommt zu einer *Konzentrierung der Eisenabgabe an das Knochenmark* im Interesse einer gesteigerten Erythropoese. Dies
würde also hier im Endeffekt dazu führen, daß vom Transportmilieu her die
Eisenzufuhr auf den Ort dringendsten Bedarfs konzentriert wird. In gleicher
Weise könnte auch die schnelle Hebung des Transferrinspiegels bei Ratten, die
man in größere Höhen versetzte, zu deuten sein (vgl. S. 203).

---

[1] Granick 1949, Finch 1950, Davis 1952, Houston 1953, Kalk 1953, Bothwell 1955.
[2] Beyers 1951, Houston 1953.
[3] Gisinger 1953, Konitzer 1955, Ramsay 1958.
[4] Pollycove 1957.   [5] Pollycove 1957, Lange 1958.

Es kommt gewissermaßen zu einer „Einblendung" und Ausrichtung des Transportgeschehens auf die Versorgung des Knochenmarks mit Eisen. Die Enzymprozesse werden darunter zu leiden haben; daher vielleicht die oft unerklärliche Schwäche der Patienten mit *latenter* Eisenmangelanämie.

Vergleichen wir noch einmal die funktionellen und klinischen Erscheinungen bei Hämochromatose und Eisenmangelanämie vom Gesichtspunkt des Eisentransportes. Bei der Hämochromatose: höchst belastete oder überbelastete Eisenbindungskapazität des Transferrins — ungeregelte Ausstreuung des Eisens im Organismus mit schweren multiplen Organschädigungen. — Bei der Eisenmangelanämie: sehr große freie Bindungskapazität des Transferrins — konzentrierter Eisentransport zum Knochenmark als dem Ort der Erythropoese[1].

HEILMEYER berichtet 1959 bei den von ihm beschriebenen und aus der Literatur zusammengestellten Fällen von erworbener und von hereditärer *sideroachrestischer Anämie* über hochgradige Hämosiderose und in 2 Fällen (von C. MAYER[2] und von CAROLI[3]) auch über echte Hämochromatose.

Die sideroachrestische Anämie kann toxisch (z. B. bei Bleivergiftung) oder auch durch Pyridoxinmangel oder genetisch bei gleichzeitigen Hämoglobinbildungsstörungen (Thalassämie) bedingt sein. Außerdem gibt es die Anaemia hypochromica sideroachrestica hereditaria[4] mit einem genetisch bedingten Mangel an einem Ferment, welches den Einbau des Eisens in das Häm bewirkt.

Bei den sideroachrestischen Anämien spricht nun nichts für eine „enthemmte Eisenresorption" im Darm; das Wesen der Krankheit liegt vielmehr im toxisch oder genetisch bedingten Mangel an Fermenten, welche den exakten Einbau des Eisens in das Häm-Molekül bewirken. Damit ist einerseits die durch Eisenmedikation inkurable Anämie erklärt; andererseits ist der hauptsächliche Abstromweg des Plasmaeisens zum Knochenmark zwecks Hämoglobinsynthese größtenteils blockiert; dies ließ sich nach intravenöser Applikation von Fe[59] deutlich zeigen: Die Radioaktivität im Knochenmark erwies sich — ganz im Gegensatz zur Norm! — als wesentlich geringer als die in der Leber. Mangels Abgabe des Eisens durch das sonst als Hauptabnehmer funktionierende Knochenmark kommt es zu einer Hypersiderinämie; wiederum paßt sich das Transferrin dieser erhöhten Eisenbelastung nicht an; das Transferrin ist abnorm stark besetzt[5]. Die Diskrepanz zwischen Hypersiderinämie und ungenügendem Transferrinschutz ist hier ebenfalls vorhanden, wenn auch nicht in dem Maße wie bei der Hämochromatose; der Faktor des besonders belasteten Pfortadergebiets kann hier wohl ebenfalls insofern eine Rolle spielen, als zu erwarten ist, daß die dauernde, durch Eiseneinbaustörung in das Häm bedingte Anämie an sich eine erhöhte Eisenresorption durch den Darm rein regulatorisch anfordert[5]. Der normalerweise dominierende Abflußweg des Plasmaeisens aus der Blutbahn besitzt mangels Hämoglobinbildung kein „Gefälle" und ist durch diese Verwertungssperre zum großen Teil ungangbar geworden. Dies führt zu einer Überlastung des Transportmilieus, insbesondere des Transferrins, und dadurch nach längeren Zeiträumen zu pathologischen Eisenablagerungen in Form von Hämosiderose, schließlich eventuell sogar zum Bild der Hämochromatose.

Eine analoge Pathogenese der Hämosiderinablagerung scheint auch bei der *perniziösen Anämie* vorzuliegen. Durch Mangel an Vitamin B_{12} ist der normale Hauptverbrauchsweg des Plasmaeisens weitgehend blockiert, hier allerdings nicht in der Phase des Eiseneinbaus in das Häm, sondern durch die mangelnde Ausreifung der roten Blutkörperchen; durch diesen Verwertungsstop kommt es —

---

[1] BENNHOLD 1960.   [2] C. MAYER, 1959.   [3] CAROLI 1959.
[4] GARBY 1957.   [5] HEILMEYER 1959.

gewissermaßen durch einen Rückstau des Eisens in die Blutbahn — zu einem
erhöhten Plasmaeisenspiegel bei relativ niedrigem Transferrinspiegel.

Pathogenetisch hat der *Morbus Wilson* aus der Sicht der Transportvorgänge mancherlei
Ähnlichkeit mit der Hämochromatose bei sideroachrestischer Anämie; auch bei ihm besteht
ein genetisch bedingter Mangel an einem Ferment, welches den Einbau eines Metalls (hier
Kupfer) in eine physiologisch wichtige Eiweiß-Metall-Verbindung bewerkstelligt. Dadurch
Verbrauchsstop des Kupfers und Insuffizienz des nun überlasteten spezifischen Transport-
milieus in Form einer besonders labilen Bindung des vermehrten Transportkupfers an Albumin.
(Näheres unter Transport des Kupfers S. 211.)

Aber auch auf einem anderen Stoffwechselabschnitt hat der Organismus
besondere Vorkehrungen getroffen, um Verlusten an Eisen vorzubeugen: der
Transport des Hämoglobins ist, wie vor allem Laurell u. Mitarb. 1947 zeigen
konnten, durch das im Plasma vorhandene *Haptoglobin* gegen Verluste, insbesondere durch die Niere, abgesichert. Der normale Spiegel des freien Hämoglobins im Plasma beträgt 1—3 mg-% ; das entspricht einem täglichen Plasma-
Hämoglobinumsatz von 3 g; dies bedeutet, daß etwa 50% des beim normalen
Zelluntergang entstehenden Hämoglobins in das Plasma einströmen. Freies
Hämoglobin mit seinem Molekulargewicht von nur 68000 passiert, wie wir aus
der Klinik und aus der Pathologie wissen, im freien Zustand die Glomerulummembran und tritt in den Primärharn über. Haptoglobin ist ein im elektrischen
Feld mit den α_2-Globulinen wanderndes Mucoproteid mit einem Molekulargewicht
von mindestens 85000 und einem Kohlenhydratgehalt bis 21% ; es ist in nur geringer
Konzentration im normalen Serum vorhanden (etwa 1% des gesamten Eiweißgehal-
tes). Es gibt mehrere Arten von Haptoglobinen mit verschiedenen Molekular-
gewichten; ihr jeweiliges Auftreten ist gen-bedingt[1]. Ihre spezifische Bindungsfähigkeit für Hämoglobin ist sehr groß[2]. Sobald Hämoglobin in die Blutbahn
gelangt, wird es von den Haptoglobinen gebunden, es entsteht ein hochmole-
kularer Komplex, der ein Molekulargewicht von mindestens 150000—310000 besitzt
und nicht mehr harnfähig ist. Analog dem Transferrin bestimmt man die Konzentration des Haptoglobins im Plasma aus seiner hämoglobinbindenden Kapazität
(HbK). Die Bindung geschieht über das Globin. Haptoglobin bindet kein Myoglobin und kein Haem. Ein anderes Serumprotein, welches in seiner Beweglichkeit wahrscheinlich den β-Globulinen näher steht, bindet sowohl Hämoglobin
als auch Myoglobin und Haem; seine Bindungsfähigkeit für Hämoglobin scheint
geringer zu sein als die der echten Haptoglobine. Die Bindung erfolgt hier an
der Haem-Gruppe; daher wurde es von Nyman[3] als „heme binding beta-protein"
bezeichnet. Dem Hämoglobin gegenüber scheint hier also eine Competition-
Situation vorzuliegen mit Vorrang der Haptoglobine; dem Myoglobin und dem
Haem gegenüber scheint dieser Eiweißkörper als Vehikel zu prävalieren[4]. Der
Haptoglobin-Hämoglobin-Komplex verschwindet ungespalten aus der Blutbahn,
hauptsächlich wohl in die Leber. So ist es zu erklären, daß bei größerer Hämoglobinzufuhr in das zirkulierende Blut — wenn die Haptoglobinnachlieferung nicht
mit der Hämoglobinzufuhr Schritt halten kann — alles Haptoglobin aus dem
Blute verschwindet. Dies findet sich z.B. bei verkürzter Lebensdauer der Erythrocyten und desgleichen bei hämolytischen Anämien. Der alsdann im Blut zirkulierende großmolekulare Hämoglobin-Haptoglobin-Komplex wird zum größten Teil
vom reticuloendothelialen System abgefangen und abgebaut; das restliche freie
Hämoglobin tritt — mangels des Kolloidschutzes durch das Haptoglobin — in
den Primärharn über und von dort zum Teil auch in den endgültigen Harn und
ist dann betreffs seines Eisenbestandteils verloren. Ein Teil wird vorher beim
Passieren der Tubuli mehr oder weniger stark verändert und führt in den Tubulus-

---

[1] Smithies 1959.   [2] Jayle 1955, Nyman 1959.   [3] Nyman 1959.   [4] Wheby 1960.

Epithelien zu Pigment- und Eiweißspeicherungen, welche wiederum zu sekundären Schädigungen dieser Zellen führen können (hämoglobinurische Nephrose nach ZOLLINGER[1]). — In diesen pathologischen Abläufen bei Hämochromatosen und hämoglobinurischen Nephrosen möchten wir ein besonders prägnantes klinisches Beispiel dafür sehen, wie aus einer Überlastung des Vehikelapparates (Transferrin bzw. Haptoglobin) das Transportgut einem Error loci unterliegt und dadurch an bestimmten Organen schwere Schäden auslöst.

Die Transportsicherung des Eisens durch Serumeiweißkörper geht schließlich noch weiter, indem das beim Hämoglobinabbau gebildete *Ferriprotoporphyrin*[2] auf dem Wege zur Leber, wo der Abbau weiter fortgesetzt wird, Bindungen an die Serumalbumine eingeht.

Bei der Verfolgung des Eisenstoffwechsels begegnen wir also vier verschiedenen Serumeiweiß-Vehikeln: dem Transferrin für den Transport des freien Eisens (als Aufbaumaterial, wo auch immer es gebraucht wird), dem Haptoglobin für den Transport des freien Hämoglobins zum Abbauort, dem „heme binding protein" für Transport von Myoglobin und Haem und schließlich dem Albumin für den Transport der Abbauprodukte Ferriprotoporphyrin und Hämatin. Diesen drei sonst recht verschiedenartigen Vehikeln ist die eine Funktion gemeinsam: Abschirmung gegen die Gefahr von Eisenfehlleitungen und -verlusten durch Error loci. Dem analogen Zweck dient das Ferritin als fixe Speicherform des Eisens.

Bindungen und Transport von Kupfer.

Die Wechselwirkung zwischen Cu und Serumalbumin ist mehrfach untersucht worden[3]. Für den Regelbereich niederer Cu-Konzentrationen ist sicher, daß 1 Cu^{++} 2 Protonen am Albumin ersetzt. Die weiteren Cu-Ionen reagieren 1:1 mit den Imidazolresten, ohne Sulfhydrylgruppen zu beteiligen[4]. Eine metallkatalytische Beeinflussung bei 10—20 Cu-Ionen beschrieb KLOTZ 1955. Auch Transferrin soll Cu binden[5].

Neben der nur lockeren Bindung an Serumalbumin ist Kupfer noch als Bestandteil des blauen *Coeruloplasmins* im Serum vorhanden. Das ist ein in der Leber gebildetes Protein mit Oxydaseeigenschaften. Elektrophoretisch zeigt es die Wanderungsgeschwindigkeit der α_2-Globuline. Im Mittel sind $34 \pm 4,0$ mg in 100 ml Serum enthalten. GITLIN studierte 1960 den Stoffwechsel des Coeruloplasmins[6]. Da das im Coeruloplasmin gebundene Kupfer nur eine indirekte Farbreaktion mit Diäthyldithiocarbamat gibt, während das albumingebundene direkt reagiert, ist die Unterscheidung der beiden Formen leicht geworden. Bei 10 gesunden Erwachsenen betrug das gesamte Serumkupfer $108\,\gamma \pm 9\%$ in 100 ml Serum; $5\,\gamma \pm 6\%$ reagierten direkt und $103\,\gamma \pm 11\%$ indirekt. Der Coeruloplasmingehalt war mit 34 ± 4 mg-% und die Oxydaseaktivität mit $3,9 \pm 0,7$ M O_2 je ml und Std normal[7]. Alle diese Werte waren im letzten Schwangerschaftsdrittel und bei chronischen Infektionen in sehr guter Korrelation zueinander erhöht und beim nephrotischen Syndrom[7], bei Neugeborenen[8] und bei Kindern mit idiopathischer Hypocuprämie[9] sowie bei Sprue[10] gleichfalls korreliert erniedrigt. Nur bei der *Wilsonschen Krankheit* (hepatolentikuläre Degeneration) hatten sie ihre Beziehungen zueinander verloren. Zahlreichen Untersuchern ist der *Kupferreichtum der Gewebe*, die *relative Hypocuprämie* (bezogen auf das Gesamtkupfer des Plasmas) und der *Mangel bzw. das Fehlen von Coeruloplasmin* bei dieser Krankheit aufgefallen. Man hat zunächst einen echten angeborenen Defekt an einem wichtigen Transport-

---

[1] ZOLLINGER 1952. [2] LAURELL 1959. [3] KLOTZ 1948b, SAROFF 1958. [4] LAL 1959.
[5] COHN 1948. [6] GITLIN 1960. [7] MARKOWITZ 1955, CARTWRIGHT 1960.
[8] SCHEINBERG 1956. [9] ZIPURSKY 1958. [10] BUTTERWORTH 1958.

14*

eiweiß[1] vermutet und die verminderte Bildung auch nachgewiesen[2]. Andererseits besteht aber keine lückenlose Beziehung zwischen dem verbliebenen Coeruloplasmingehalt und der Schwere der Krankheitserscheinungen, ja es sind sogar in ganz seltenen Fällen langjährige Beobachtungen von gesunden Personen bekannt geworden, die dauernd einen pathologisch erniedrigten Coeruloplasminspiegel besaßen und von echten Wilson-Patienten mit fast normalem Coeruloplasmingehalt[3].

Das peroral zugeführte Metall wird beim *gesunden Erwachsenen* unter Mitwirkung des sauren Magensaftes[4] im oberen Dünndarm[5] resorbiert und zu einem erheblichen Teil durch die Galle wieder in den Darm geleitet. Dieser *enterohepatische Kreislauf* des Kupfers verhindert eine Überschwemmung des Organismus und bewirkt, daß der Serumspiegel konstant und niedrig bleibt; er hat also bis zu einem gewissen Grade einen *Depot-* oder *Ventil-Effekt* mit mehrfachen Steuerungsmöglichkeiten. Dabei wird täglich eine gleichbleibend minimale Menge von 100—200 μg Cu im Urin ausgeschieden[6], während im Stuhl etwa 2 mg erscheinen[7]. Bei einer Zufuhr von etwas über 2 mg ist die Bilanz positiv; was darüber liegt, geht vorwiegend mit dem Kot ab. 8—40% des täglich aufgenommenen Kupfers werden nach Darby (1950) retiniert. Bei intravenöser Verabfolgung von Cu^{64} ist die Ausscheidung durch den Darm wesentlich geringer. Die Nieren beteiligen sich nur wenig mehr an der Eliminierung; der Blutspiegel steigt an. Er sinkt aber rasch innerhalb von 4 Std wieder ab. Während der folgenden 48 Std wird Kupfer in das Coeruloplasmin eingebaut, so daß auf die intravenöse Gabe von Radiokupfer hin in dieser Zeit im Blut ein Wiederanstieg der Radioaktivität erfolgt[8].

Patienten mit *hepatolentikulärer Degeneration* (Wilson) und fehlendem Coeruloplasmingehalt des Plasmas zeigen diesen zweiten Anstieg nicht. Offenbar kann das Kupfer nicht in das Eiweißmolekül eingebaut werden[9]. Durch Wegfall des mit dem α_2-Globulin wandernden Coeruloplasmins, welches normalerweise 90% des Gesamtkupfers im Plasma enthält, ist der Gesamtkupferspiegel erniedrigt auf etwa 60—26 μg%; es handelt sich dabei ausschließlich oder fast ausschließlich nur noch um locker am Albumin haftendes, mit Natriumdiäthyldithiocarbamat direkt reagierendes Transportkupfer, dessen Konzentration beim Gesunden nur 10—15 μg% beträgt. Das Kupfer im Coeruloplasmin ist demgegenüber fest in das Eiweißmolekül eingebaut und kann nicht dem eigentlichen, überall disponiblen Transportkupfer zugerechnet werden. Diese Vermehrung des Transportkupfers könnte rein *durch Verlegung des Hauptabstroms des Kupfers* z. B. in die Coeruloplasminsynthese bedingt sein, oder es könnte (eventuell auf regulativem Wege) der Coeruloplasminmangel eine *vermehrte Kupferresorption*, deren Vorhandensein aus den Untersuchungen von Cartwrigth[10] und Zimdahl[11] anzunehmen ist, auslösen. Das Mißverhältnis zwischen Albumin (als Vehikel) und Kupfer (als Transportgut) muß dann noch ungünstiger werden, wenn Hypalbuminämie auftritt. Das ist der Fall, wenn sich die zum Krankheitsbild gehörige Lebercirrhose ausbildet. Die übermäßige Resorption des Metalls im Dünndarmgebiet muß auch hier gerade im Pfortadergebiet das Transportmilieu auf dem direkten Wege zur Leber besonders belasten. Durch die Überlastung der Albumine mit Transportkupfer können Bindungsgefälle von Albumin an andere, sonst latent bleibende Haftpunkte untergeordneten Grades wirksam werden, wie wir es bei der Besprechung des Kernikterus im einzelnen darlegten. — *In den klinischen und anatomischen Befunden zeigen sich auffallend viele gemeinsame Züge zwischen Morbus Wilson und Hämochromatose*[12].

Analog sind die *Ablagerungsorte in Leber, Milz, Niere, Nebenniere.* Stärker betont ist beim Wilson die Ablagerung des Kupfers im *Stammhirn*, insbesondere im *Nucleus lenticularis*, wo ebenso wie in der Leber der Kupfergehalt das 10fache der Norm betragen kann[13]. Ferner findet sich die Kupferablagerung *in der Cornea als Kayser-Fleischerscher Cornealring*[14]. Genau wie bei der Hämochromatose entsprechen die klinischen Symptome exakt den so ganz heterogenen pathologischen Ablagerungsstätten des Metalls im Organismus. Beim Morbus Wilson ebenfalls: *Lebercirrhose, Adynamie, Eunuchoidismus,* eventuell (leichtere) Störungen des Zuckerstoffwechsels; hinzu kommen die schweren *Stammhirnschädigungen* nach Art eines *Morbus Parkinson* und die *Aminoacidurie,* welche auf sekundäre Tubulusschädigungen zurückgeführt wird. Auch andere Symptome, welche wir bei der Hämochromatose als Zeichen einer Überlastung des Transportmilieus deuteten[5], sind beim Morbus Wilson ähnlich: positive Kupferbilanz, trotz *ausgesprochener Hypercuprurie,* welche auf das 10—100fache der Norm

---

[1] Scheinberg 1952.   [2] Bearn 1953, Scheinberg 1955.
[3] Cartwright 1954, 1960; Bickel 1955.   [4] Bence 1933.   [5] Sachs 1943.
[6] Tompsett 1934, Chou 1935, Holt 1948.   [7] Chou 1935, Tompsett 1934.
[8] Cartwright 1955.   [9] Bearn 1954, Bush 1955, Jensen 1957.
[10] Carthwright 1954, Stokes 1955.   [11] Zimdahl 1954, Bush 1955.
[12] Bennhold 1960.   [13] Cartwright 1954.
[14] Literatur bei Heilmeyer, Bd. IV/2, S. 615 dieses Handbuches.

ansteigen kann (!). Auch hier möchten wir sie — analog der Hypersiderurie bei der Hämochromatose — *als klinisches Symptom einer Überlastung des Transportmilieus für das Metall auffassen*; als Folge davon vermehrter Übertritt des Kupfers in den Primärharn. Abweichend von den Feststellungen bei der Hämochromatose verhält sich der intravenöse Belastungstest; beim Morbus Wilson zeigt sich im Gegensatz zur Hämochromatose ein verlangsamtes Absinken des Kupferspiegels; dies betrifft allerdings hauptsächlich die ersten 15—30 min post injectionem[1]. Es ist wahrscheinlich, daß der initiale starke Absturz des Kupferspiegels beim Gesunden zu einem erheblichen Teil durch die normalerweise schnelle Aussonderung des locker am Albumin gebundenen Kupfers in die Leber zwecks Coeruloplasminsynthese bedingt ist, ein Faktor, der bei dem Wilson-Patienten in den meisten Fällen fehlt. — Nach dieser Konzeption haben wir es also *beim Morbus Wilson ebenfalls mit einer multilokulären Thesauropathie* zu tun[2]. Hier ist es das Kupfer, welches durch relative Insuffizienz der sonst die Transporte regelnden Serumeiweißvehikel im Gesamtorganismus weitgehend direktionslos ausgestreut wird; es bleibt dann an Orten im Organismus haften, deren Bindungsfähigkeit an sich so gering ist, daß sie sich den Albuminen gegenüber, welche nur in normalem Umfang mit Transportkupfer ausgelastet sind niemals hätte durchsetzen können. Die sonst latent bleibenden nachgeordneten Prädilektionsorte der Metallbindungen werden dadurch aktuell und manifest und verleihen durch die dort erfolgenden pathologischen Metallablagerungen den Krankheitsbildern ihre verhängnisvollen, vielfältigen Symptome.

Wenn diese zunächst als Arbeitshypothese aufgestellte Konzeption sich endgültig bestätigen sollte, dann wäre intravenöse Zufuhr von Albumin zwecks Ergänzung des überlasteten Vehikelapparates angezeigt.

Bindung und Transport von Jod
(unter Mitarbeit von Dr. E. KALLEE-Tübingen).

a) Anorganisches Jod.

Der Mensch nimmt täglich etwa 50 µg Jod hauptsächlich mit der Nahrung als Jodid auf[3]; inhaliert oder durch die Haut resorbiert werden normalerweise nur vernachlässigbar geringe Mengen. Das Jodid passiert die Darmwand rasch (5% der Dosis je min) und gelangt in das Blut und in die Flüssigkeitsräume des Körpers. Gemessen an NaJ^{131} erscheint in vitro nur sehr wenig an Albumin gebunden[4], und zwar höchstens 1—3%; selbst diese kleinen Mengen können in vitro durch J_2 verursacht sein, das infolge Bestrahlungsoxydation[5] aus NaJ^{131}-Lösungen frei wird.

Das Jodid verteilt sich zunächst gleichmäßig im Jodidraum, und dann fällt die Blutjodkonzentration etwa innerhalb 12 Std nahezu exponentiell ab[6]. Zwei Stunden nach intravenöser Injektion von NaJ^{131} beträgt die Radioaktivität durchspülter Rattenorgane nur etwa 1—6% der Serumradioaktivität[7]. Soweit das methodisch hinreichend interpretiert werden kann, entspricht dieses Verhalten des Jodids dem des Pseudohalogens Rhodanid und dem anderer Halogene. Der Schwund von Plasmajodid ist im übrigen hauptsächlich abhängig von der Ausscheidung durch die Nieren und von der Jodidaufnahme durch die Schilddrüse. Die Clearance-Leistung beider Organe ist in Abhängigkeit vom Blutjodidspiegel unterschiedlich[8].

Die Fähigkeit der Thyreoidea, Jodid zu konzentrieren, ist wohl außerordentlich groß, bei einem kritischen Plasmajodspiegel wird aber ein Gleichgewicht zwischen Jodaufnahme und Jodabgabe erreicht und ein Mehr an Jod nicht mehr aufgenommen.

Unter regelhaften Bedingungen konzentriert eine Rattenschilddrüse auf das 100 bis 300fache des Blutgehaltes[9]. Zwei Tage nach Verabreichung einer Testdosis von radioaktivem, trägerfreiem NaJ^{131} enthält die normale menschliche Schilddrüse größenordnungsmäßig etwa 10000mal mehr Radiojod pro Kubikzentimeter Gewebe als das Blutserum. Die euthyreote

---

[1] BEARN 1954, BUSH 1955, LANGE 1958.   [2] BENNHOLD 1960.
[3] GRAB 1959.   [4] MAURER 1952, BENNHOLD 1954, GEORGE 1959.
[5] BENNHOLD 1954.   [6] FELLINGER 1953.   [7] KALLEE 1954.
[8] POCHIN 1950, GERBAULET 1959.   [9] HESS 1952.

Schilddrüse nimmt etwa 0,2—10 μg Jodid pro Stunde auf[1]. Auch die Speicheldrüsen vermögen Jodid, entgegen dem Konzentrationsgefälle zum Blut, im Speichel zu konzentrieren[2], ebenso die Magendrüsen[3].

b) Organische Jodverbindungen.

Die Jodgier der Schilddrüse bewirkt unter regelhaften Bedingungen einen „Jodsog", dem das ungebundene[4] Jodid sehr rasch folgt[5]. In Abhängigkeit vom Aktivitätszustand des Organs wird „Hormonjod" gebildet und fortlaufend wieder in das Blut ausgeschüttet. Es liegt jetzt als organisches Jod vor, welches an die Bluteiweißkörper gebunden ist[6]. Diese *Hormonbindung* konzentriert sich normalerweise außer auf Albumin[7] vor allem auf eine noch unbekannte Substanz, die papierelektrophoretisch mit einer Beweglichkeit von α-Globulinen wandert[8]. Bei Seren von Menschen liegt diese α-Bande zwischen α_1- und α_2-Globulinen (= Inter-α-Globulin[9], [10]). Unter bestimmten Bedingungen soll beim Menschen auch eine Bindung an tryptophanreiches Präalbumin stattfinden[11]. Von anderen Autoren[12] wird eine Bindung von gereinigtem Thyroxin an reines Präalbumin bestritten. Eine weitere Bande geringeren Umfangs (etwa 10%) ist — besonders bei hohen in vitro-Zusätzen von J^{131}-Thyroxin — im β-Bereich anzutreffen[13].

Beim erwachsenen Kaninchen wandert die Hormonjod tragende α-Fraktion zwischen α_1-Globulin und Albumin[14], beim Kaninchenembryo (vom etwa 16. Trächtigkeitstage an) zwischen α_2- und β-Globulin[15], bei der erwachsenen Ratte in der Gegend von α_1-Globulin[16] und inter-α-Globulin[17]. Bei Hühnern und Enten wird Thyroxin nur an Albumin, und zwar locker, gebunden[18].

Die elektrophoretische Lokalisation der Thyroxinbindung ist abhängig vom Trägermedium und vom Puffer[19]. Immunoelektrophoretisch läßt sich eine Bindung von Thyroxin an Albumin, an ein α_2-Lipoproteid (= Inter-α-Globulin ?) und β-Lipoproteid demonstrieren[20]. Die Konzentration an Inter-α-Globulin, das auch „TBG" (= Thyroxin-bindendes Globulin) genannt wird[21], ist offenbar unabhängig von der Schilddrüsenfunktion[22].

Auch *Trijodthyronin* wird an inter-α-Globulin und Humanalbumin gebunden[23], allerdings wahrscheinlich weniger fest — also disponibler — als das Thyroxin[24]. Die Affinität des Trijodthyronins zum thyroxinbindenden Protein von Humanserum beträgt nur etwa 30% der Affinität des Thyroxins zum gleichen Protein[24].

Thyroxin[25] und Trijodthyronin werden in wäßriger Lösung von Filtrierpapier[26] und von Glasgeräten[27] reversibel absorbiert und besitzen in Abwesenheit bindungsfähiger Proteine eine elektrophoretische Beweglichkeit, die etwa den γ-Globulinen entspricht. Trijodthyronin kann — ebenso wie D-Thyroxin — J^{131}-L-Thyroxin aus der Bindung an Inter-α-Globulin verdrängen[27], wenn auch nur bei sehr hohen Zusätzen.

Das proteingebundene Hormonjod läßt sich zusammen mit den bindungsfähigen Proteinen durch Trichloressigsäure und durch anorganische Fällungsmittel (z. B. Zinkhydroxyd, Ammoniumsulfat u. a.) ausfällen[28]; ferner kann es mit Butanol, Methanol und anderen organischen

---

[1] Gerbaulet 1959.
[2] Fitting 1956, Gerbaulet 1956, Gabrielson 1956, Wase 1956, Gerbaulet 1957, Maurer 1957, Stein 1957.
[3] Foster 1955.　　[4] George 1959.　　[5] Wollman 1959, Halmi 1959.
[6] Salter 1947, Taurog 1948.　　[7] Gordon 1952, Maurer 1952.
[8] Gordon 1952, Maurer 1952, 1953.　　[9] Horst 1953.
[10] Larson 1952, Robbins 1952, Winzler 1952, Horst 1953, Bennhold 1954, Freinkel 1955.
[11] Hofmann-Credner 1957, Ingbar 1958, Tata 1959, Tanaka 1959.
[12] Gillich 1958, Lang 1959.
[13] Hofmann-Credner 1957, Gillich 1958, Vannotti 1959, Lohss 1960, Kallee 1960.
[14] Maurer 1953.　　[15] Osorio 1958, 1960, Myant 1959, 1960.
[16] Maurer 1952.　　[17] Kallee 1960.　　[18] Tata 1959.
[19] Tata 1960, Hamolsky 1960.　　[20] Munkner 1960, Clausen 1960, Lohss 1960.
[21] Albright 1955.　　[22] Gillich 1958, Lang 1960, Vannotti 1959.
[23] Albright 1953, Robbins 1955, Kallee 1958b.　　[24] Robbins 1960, Tata 1960.
[25] Freinkel 1955.　　[26] Kallee 1958b.　　[27] Robbins 1955.　　[28] Klein 1953.

Lösungsmitteln extrahiert werden[1]. Chromatographisch[2] besteht das in Butanol lösliche Hormonjod normalerweise fast ausschließlich aus Thyroxin[3]. Das Serumjodid kann an Anionenaustauscher adsorbiert und dadurch von Hormonjod abgetrennt werden[4].

Zwischen Erythrocyten und Plasmaproteinen stellen sich Trijodthyronin-Verteilungsgleichgewichte ein[5]; diese sind von der Schilddrüsenfunktion abhängig und können daher diagnostisch verwertet werden[6].

Nach *therapeutischen*, also größeren, J^{131}-Dosen tritt zusätzlich eine jodhaltige Fraktion im Serum auf, die mit der Beweglichkeit von α_1- bis einschließlich α_2-Globulin wandert[7] und in Butanol oder Methanol unlöslich ist[8]; vermutlich handelt es sich um Thyreoglobulin[9]. Nach Dosen von 5—10 mC J^{131} konnte bei 29 Patienten kein Thyreoglobulin im Serum nachgewiesen werden[10]. In vitro besitzt dieses Schilddrüseneiweiß kein Jodbindungsvermögen[11], wandert aber im elektrischen Feld im kompletten Bereich der α_1- und α_2-Globuline. Nicht nur bei der Strahlungsthyreoiditis, sondern auch bei der chronischen lymphatischen Strumitis („Hashimoto's disease") und bei manchen Schilddrüsencarcinomen[12] tritt Thyreoglobulin ins Blut über.

BENNHOLD (1954) beobachtete bei einer Patientin, die wegen eines Schilddrüsencarcinoms mit 15 mC J^{131} behandelt wurde, daß die Radioaktivität im Serum im Verlauf der ersten 8 Std nach peroraler Verabreichung zunächst ausschließlich im Albuminbereich zu finden war. Erst von der 12. Std ab trat auch eine radioaktive Bande im Inter-α-Bereich auf. Nach 48 Std war die Albuminbande zugunsten der inter-α-Bande fast ganz verschwunden. Ähnliche Befunde wurden inzwischen auch von anderen Autoren bei Schilddrüsencarcinomen[13], bei Myxödem[14] beim Lupus erythematodes[15] und bei Thyreotoxikosen[16] erhoben. Es handelt sich hier wahrscheinlich um ein Jodprotein, das kein Albumin ist, sondern lediglich elektrophoretisch mit der Beweglichkeit von Humanalbumin wandert[17]. Jedenfalls ist dessen Radioaktivität in Methanol-Eisessig nicht löslich, es kann sich also nicht um Thyroxin handeln[18].

Der normale Thyroxingehalt des Menschenserums (andere Species s. KATSH 1955) wird mit 4—6 μg/100 ml Serum angegeben[19]. Die Bindungskapazität des Inter-α-Globulins soll etwa 40—50 μg/100 ml betragen[20], nach anderen Autoren 20 μg%[21]. Oberhalb dieser ungefähren Grenze überwiegt in vitro die Thyroxinbindung an Albumin[22]. Da bei Hyperthyreosen vermehrt Thyroxin ins Blut gelangt, soll hier die Bindungsfähigkeit in vitro durch geringere Thyroxinzusätze überschritten werden als bei Hypothyreosen[20].

Jedoch wurde[23] in „Überwanderungselektrophoresen" nachgewiesen, daß bei hohen in vitro-Zusätzen von Thyroxin schon bei Normalen die Thyroxinbindungsfähigkeit des Inter-α-Globulins nur noch weniger stark ansteigt als die Albuminbindung, und daß die von anderen Autoren behaupteten spezifischen Bindungsunterschiede der Inter-α-Globuline bei Hypo- und Hyperthyreosen in den Fehlerbereich der Methode fallen. Die von TATA (1958) in Dialyseexperimenten oder mit Trichloressigsäurefällung ermittelten Thyroxin-Bindungskurven entsprechen Adsorptionsisothermen. Thyroxin läßt sich durch Veronal bei p_H 8,6 aus der Albuminbindung verdrängen; andererseits erhöht Tris-Puffer das Thyroxin-Bindungsvermögen von Plasmaproteinen, insbesondere von Präalbumin[24].

In der *Schwangerschaft* oder nach Behandlung mit Diäthylstilboestrol (30 mg täglich) steigt die Thyroxinbindungsfähigkeit der Serumproteine an[25]. Bei *Nephrosen*[26] kann durch die Proteinurie viel Hormonjod verlorengehen ($11 \pm 7\%$[27]), so daß die biologische Halbwertszeit des Thyroxins verkürzt wird[28] und daß durch den auftretenden Jodmangel[29] oft ein kompensatorischer Kropf und ein erniedrigter Grundumsatz[30] entsteht.

Bis zu einem Monat nach Ausbruch einer *Hepatitis epidemica* kann der Blut-Thyroxinspiegel in vivo erhöht sein[31], nicht dagegen bei Cirrhosen[32] oder anderen chronischen Leberkrankheiten[33].

---

[1] TAUROG 1948. [2] LARSON 1954. [3] WINZLER 1952.
[4] SCOTT 1954, ZIEVE 1955, FIELDS 1956, SILVER 1958.
[5] HAMOLSKY 1957, CHRISTENSEN 1960, HAMOLSKY 1960.
[6] URELES 1959. [7] ROBBINS 1952, TONG 1952. [8] MAURER 1952.
[9] ROBBINS 1952, MAURER 1953, HORST 1954. [10] KLEIN 1955. [11] HORST 1954.
[12] ROBBINS 1952, 1955, 1956, TATA 1956, OWEN 1956, WERNER 1957, VANNOTTI 1959.
[13] ROBBINS 1955, TATA 1956. [14] DE GROOT 1958. [15] ROBBINS 1957.
[16] LARSON 1954, CAMERON 1959. [17] TATA 1956, CAMERON 1959. [18] CAMERON 1959.
[19] VANNOTTI 1959, BEIERWALTES 1959, TANAKA 1959, HONETZ 1960. [20] ALBRIGHT 1955.
[21] VANNOTTI 1959, TANAKA 1959. [22] HORST 1954, ALBRIGHT 1955, VANNOTTI 1959.
[23] GILLICH 1958. [24] HAMOLSKY 1960. [25] DOWLING 1956. [26] ROBBINS 1957.
[27] KALANT 1959. [28] VANNOTTI 1959. [29] CRUCHAUD 1954. [30] RASMUSSEN 1956.
[31] KYDD 1951, SCAZZIGA 1955, D'ADDABBO 1958, BÉRAUD 1957, 1958, VANNOTTI 1959.
[32] MUELLER 1954. [33] D'ADDABBO 1958.

Vannotti (1959) versucht diese Erhöhung teilweise mit einer Vermehrung der Bindungskapazität des Serums zu erklären, da bei der Hepatitis das Albumin in vitro relativ weniger und das Inter-α-Globulin mehr Thyroxin bindet. Daneben ist bei der Hepatitis auch die enzymatische β-Glucuronidase (Eliminierung von Thyroxin durch die Leber)[1] und ferner die Permeabilität der Leberzellen[2] gestört, so daß eventuell schon dadurch der Anstieg des Thyroxinspiegels zu erklären wäre[3]. Für diese Annahme spricht vor allem auch das Fehlen von Thyroxinglucuronid in der Galle bei der Hepatitis epidemica[4]. Die relative Zunahme der Bindungsfähigkeit des Inter-α-Globulins im Verhältnis zur Albuminbindung in vitro kann vielleicht auch nur dadurch bedingt sein, daß bisher noch nicht identifizierte Substanzen im Blut auftreten, welche die Bindungsplätze des anionischen Schilddrüsenhormons Thyroxin am Albumin belegen[5]. Thyroxin läßt sich nämlich durch manche Anionen aus der Albuminbindung verdrängen, z. B. durch Bromthalein[5], Butazolidin[5], Dinitrophenol, Salizylsäure[6] und Na-Oleat[5], bei extrem hohen Zusätzen solcher Substanzen sogar aus der Bindung an inter-α-Globulin, während die geringfügige Bindung an β-Globulin offenbar unverändert bleibt. Jedoch beeinträchtigen diese Stoffe die übliche PBJ[131]-Bestimmung mit Trichloressigsäurefällung nicht, und auch nicht die Bindung von J[131]-Substanzen, die nach therapeutischen J[131]-Dosen im Serum auftreten[5]. Mit Gallensäuren, Bilirubin, Chloroquin, sowie mit Azorubin, Bromphenolblau und manchen anderen anionischen Farbstoffen war ein Verdrängungseffekt papierelektrophoretisch (p_H 8,6; Veronal-Puffer) nicht eindeutig nachzuweisen[3].

Bei *Analbuminämie* ist Thyroxin ausschließlich an inter-α-Globulin gebunden[7], bei einem euthyreoten Fall von *Inter-α-Globulin-Mangel*[8] vorwiegend an Albumin und Präalbumin. Beierwaltes (1959) berichtet über eine möglicherweise hereditäre *Vermehrung* der Thyroxin-Bindungsfähigkeit des Inter-α-Globulins.

Thyroxin und Trijodthyronin sind *innerhalb der Zellen* ziemlich gleichmäßig auf Mitochondrien, Mikrosomen und flüssiges Cytoplasma verteilt[9]. Diese Hormone werden teils an lösliche cytoplasmatische Proteine, teils an Strukturproteine von Mitochondrien und Mikrosomen reversibel gebunden[10].

In Verteilungsgleichgewichten zwischen löslichen, bindungsfähigen Proteinen und Zellorganellen ist die Adsorption der Schilddrüsenhormone abhängig vom Verhältnis der Proteinkonzentrationen beider Phasen. Die Bindungsgleichgewichte lassen sich nach Art einer Isotherme in Abhängigkeit von der Proteinkonzentration berechnen[11].

Da Thyroxin an Serumproteine[12] und an lösliche cytoplasmatische Proteine fester gebunden wird als Trijodthyronin, adsorbieren Lebermitochondrien in Verteilungsgleichgewichten weniger Thyroxin, aber mehr Trijodthyronin[13]. Damit hängt möglicherweise[14] zum Teil die unterschiedliche Schwundrate von intravenös injiziertem Thyroxin und von Trijodthyronin[15] zusammen.

Für die Vorstellungen über den Transport von Hormonjod ist vor allem ein embryologischer Befund[16] von Wichtigkeit: In den Kaninchenfetus tritt vor dem 16. Trächtigkeitstag kein J[131]-Thyroxin über, das dem Mutterkaninchen injiziert wurde. Erst etwa vom 20. Tag ab gelangt mütterliches Thyroxin in das Fetalblut. Von diesem Tage an tritt nämlich erstmals thyroxinbindendes Protein im Embryonalblut auf; dieses Protein unterscheidet sich deutlich vom mütterlichen thyroxinbindenden Protein: das mütterliche thyroxinbindende Protein wandert papierelektrophoretisch zwischen Albumin und $α_1$-Globulin, das fetale zwischen $α_2$ und $β$. Außerdem soll das fetale Protein eine höhere Affinität zu Thyroxin besitzen als das maternelle. Mit der absoluten Vermehrung der fetalen Bindungskapazität steigt auch die Thyroxinmenge an, die von der Mutter auf den Fetus übergeht. Es stellt sich also ein Verteilungsgleichgewicht zwischen Mutter und Embryo ein. Dabei wird Trijodthyronin vom Fetalblut rascher aufgenommen als Thyroxin, da Trijodthyronin an Serumproteine lockerer gebunden ist und deshalb

[1] Vannotti 1955.   [2] Eppinger 1920, 1949, Roholm 1942, Axenfeld 1942.
[3] Kallee 1960, 1961.   [4] Scazziga 1955.   [5] Kallee 1960a.
[6] Christensen 1960.   [7] Vannotti 1959, Beck 1959.   [8] Tanaka 1959.
[9] Lipner 1952.   [10] Freinkel 1957, Kallee 1958b, 1960b, Tata 1958.   [11] Kallee 1960b.
[12] Osorio 1960, Robbins 1960, Tata 1960.   [13] Kallee 1959, 1961.
[14] Kallee 1960b, Osorio 1960, Tata 1960, Lissitzky 1960.
[15] Rall 1953, Sterling 1954, Berson 1954.   [16] Osorio 1958, 1960, Myant 1959, 1960.

rascher als das fester gebundene Thyroxin[1] durch die Placentarschranke diffundieren kann. *Über die Thyroxinverteilung entscheiden also primär nicht dynamische Stoffwechselprozesse, sondern die physiko-chemische Art der Bindung[2] und die Anzahl der Bindungsplätze beiderseits einer Membran.*

Thyroxinbindende Zellproteine sind bisher im Muskel[3], in den Nieren[4] und in der Leber[5] nachgewiesen worden; sie scheinen selbst in Buttergelb-Hepatocarcinomen vorzukommen, wobei allerdings quantitative Vergleichsuntersuchungen mit normalem Gewebe derzeit noch nicht vorliegen[6].

Auch die adsorptive Bindung von Abkömmlingen und Homologen der Schilddrüsenhormone an Serumproteine ist teilweise bereits untersucht[7].

Wenn auch manche Details der Bindung von Schilddrüsenhormonen noch eines genaueren Studiums bedürfen, so tritt doch hier wie bei kaum einer anderen Substanz die überragende Bedeutung der reversiblen Adsorption an Proteine und die Rolle von Adsorptions-Verteilungsgleichgewichten für den Stofftransport zutage. Anorganisches Jodid wird an lösliche Proteine nicht gebunden; deshalb ist dieses Spurenelement jederzeit für eine Aufnahme und Wiederverwertung durch die Schilddrüse frei verfügbar. Der Transport von Schilddrüsenhormonen wird gewährleistet durch die Adsorptionsfähigkeit der mobilen Serumvehikel und der fixen Organproteine. Dadurch können Adsorptionsverteilungsgleichgewichte zwischen Blutbahn und Organen angenommen werden, welche einen Modellfall einer nahezu lückenlosen Transportkette darstellen könnten. Diese Kette könnte von den Serumproteinen über das flüssige Cytoplasma bis zu den Mitochondrien und Mikrosomen reichen. Infolgedessen ist die Annahme einer „aktiven Transportfunktion" der capillarseitigen Zellmembran für Schilddrüsenhormone ebenso wie für andere reversibel gebundene Substanzen[8] nicht unbedingt notwendig[9].

Bindung und Transport von Vitamin B$_{12}$.

Ganz besonders kompliziert und interessant sind die Transportvorgänge, welchen das Vitamin B$_{12}$ *(Castle's „extrinsic factor", Cobalamin)* zwischen der Aufnahme mit der Nahrung (aus Fleisch, Milch, Leber, Fischmehl) und der Verwertung im intracellulären Stoffwechsel (z.B. bei der Ausreifung der Erythrocyten) unterliegt. — Schon der Resorptionsvorgang im Magen-Darmtractus bedient sich eines initialen, komplizierten Transportmechanismus. Ohne besondere mitwirkende Faktoren kann B$_{12}$ im Darm nicht resorbiert werden. Es muß zunächst an ein Glykoproteid fixiert werden[10], welches im normalen Magensaft enthalten ist und welches dem *Castleschen intrinsic factor* (I.F.) entspricht. Der Eiweißcharakter ist durch die fehlende Ultrafiltrierbarkeit und durch die Angreifbarkeit durch Proteinasen erwiesen[11]. Im Magensaft von Patienten mit perniziöser Anämie fehlt dieser Eiweißkörper. Aber nur im Zustand der Bindung an dieses Eiweiß passiert B$_{12}$ die Darmschleimhaut.

Es besteht keine strenge Korrelation zwischen der Bindungskraft eines I.F.-Präparates und dem Resorptionseffekt für B$_{12}$ im Darmkanal. Erhitzen des normalen Magensaftes kann z.B. zu einem Verlust des Resorptionseffektes führen bei voll erhaltenem Bindungsvermögen seitens des I.F.-Eiweißkörpers[12]. Der vom Schweinemagen gewonnene I.F. *behindert* sogar die B$_{12}$-Resorption bei der intakten Ratte[13]. Für die Resorption ist wahrscheinlich die spezifische Bindungsfähigkeit *und* die bei der Isolierung intakt erhaltene kolloide Beschaffenheit des I.F. Voraussetzung; die Bindungsfähigkeit für B$_{12}$ ist wohl weniger

[1] Osorio 1960.   [2] Osorio 1960, Tata 1960.   [3] Tata 1958, Lissitzky 1959, 1960.
[4] Kallee 1958b, 1961, Lissitzky 1959.
[5] Freinkel 1957, Kallee 1958b, 1959, 1961, Lissitzky 1959.
[6] Kallee 1961.
[7] Larson 1955, Tanaka 1959, Tata 1960, Robbins 1960.
[8] Troschin 1958.   [9] Freinkel 1957, Kallee 1958a und b, 1960b, 1961.
[10] Latner 1953, Bishop 1955.   [11] Ternberg 1949, Pendl 1955, Gräsbeck 1956.
[12] Spray 1952.   [13] Williams 1957.

lädierbar. Hochgradig gereinigte I.F.-Präparate besitzen ein Molekulargewicht von 5000, 15000 und 40000[1]. Ob in den Resorptionsvorgang enzymatische Prozesse eingeschaltet sind[2] oder ob sich mit Hilfe der relativ kleinen Eiweißmoleküle ein rein kolloidaler Vorgang entsprechend den Beobachtungen an Ascites-Zellen oder in grober Analogie zu dem „embatischen Effekt" (vgl. S. 227) im Gelatinegel abspielt[3], kann noch nicht entschieden werden. Auch an Leberschnitten verstärkt ein Zusatz von I.F. in vitro die Aufnahme von B_{12}[4].

Bei über die Norm erhöhten Mengen von I.F. kann es auch zur Bremsung der B_{12}-Resorption kommen[5]. Die B_{12}-Resorption ist von den Mengenverhältnissen der reagierenden Substanzen abhängig[6]. Dies wird[7] als Zeichen eines gleichzeitigen Vorhandenseins von Inhibitorsubstanzen gedeutet; es könnte aber auch durch eine bei erheblich überschüssigem Trägerprotein eintretende abnorm feste Bindung bedingt sein[8] (vgl. S. 221), so daß dadurch die Ablösung vom Trägereiweiß nicht in normaler Weise und vielleicht auch nicht an normaler Stelle erfolgt. Die Bindung an ein Trägereiweiß (I.F.) ist somit *eine*, aber nicht die *einzige* Bedingung, welche die intestinale Resorption ermöglicht. Die Anwesenheit von Calcium scheint ein weiterer Faktor für die Wirksamkeit des I.F. zu sein[5]. — Die Abgabe des I.F. zusammen mit dem Magensaft wird vom Parasympathicus gesteuert. Der tägliche Bedarf an resorbiertem B_{12} beträgt angeblich 0,5—1,0 μg[9].

Gleichfalls von einem Glykoproteid wird im *zirkulierenden Plasma* das Vitamin B_{12} gebunden[10], dieses Trägereiweiß wandert im elektrischen Feld mit der Geschwindigkeit der α_1-Globuline[11] und hat ein Molekulargewicht von etwa 150000[12]. Das B_{12}-bindende Protein im Serum kann also nicht identisch sein mit dem niedrig molekularen I.F. und stellt außerdem nur einen sehr kleinen Anteil des α_1-Globulins dar. Von einigen noch nicht gesicherten Prämissen ausgehend (z.B., daß ein Molekül Eiweiß sich mit einem Molekül B_{12} verbindet) wird der Anteil des B_{12}-bindenden Proteins auf 0,003% der α_1-Globuline und auf 0,00016% des Gesamtserumeiweiß geschätzt[12]. — Die Angaben über den normalen B_{12}-Spiegel im menschlichen Serum schwanken zwischen 236 und 500 $\mu\mu$g/ml[13]. Die große Spanne der Werte ist zum Teil durch die verschiedenen Nachweismethoden (Euglena gracilis, Lactobacillus Leichmanii) bedingt. Das Trägerprotein hat wohl auch hier unter anderem die Funktion, B_{12}-Verlusten durch die Nierenglomeruli vorzubeugen (vgl. Eisen!)[14]. Freies B_{12} geht dank des niedrigen Molekulargewichts von etwa 1500 in den Harn über.

Zwei schwere Krankheiten gehen mit hochgradig verändertem B_{12}-Spiegel im Serum einher. Einerseits die *perniziöse Anämie* mit ihrem auf 32—37 $\mu\mu$g/ml *gesenkten B_{12}-Spiegel*, andererseits *die chronische myeloische Leukämie* mit ihrem auf 2150—5180 $\mu\mu$g/ml (sogar 11900 $\mu\mu$g/ml) erhöhten B_{12}-Spiegel[15]. Bei beiden werden entsprechende Konzentrationsänderungen der B_{12}-bindenden Proteine angenommen[16]. Klinisch findet sich bei beiden Erkrankungen als besonders auffälliges Symptom das massenhafte Auftreten unreifer Zellen im Blute und im Knochenmark (Megaloblasten einerseits und Myeloblasten andererseits).

Bei der perniziösen Anämie reifen die aus dem Knochenmark Perniciosa-Kranker angesetzten Kulturen von Megaloblasten nur dann zu Normoblasten heran, wenn dem Kulturmilieu außer Vitamin B_{12} auch Serum Gesunder (nicht Perniciosa-Kranker!) zugesetzt ist. Konzentrate von I.F. oder von B_{12}-bindenden Serumeiweißkörpern beschleunigen die Normoblastenreifung besonders deutlich, wenn der Megaloblastenkultur zunächst nur Serum einer perniziösen Anämie zugesetzt worden war[17]. Statt des Normalserums kann auch Folsäure, Folininsäure oder Magensaft Gesunder (mit seinem Gehalt an I.F.) verwandt werden.

[1] Clayton 1955.					[2] Clayton 1955, Latner 1958.					[3] Bennhold 1926, 1927, 1928.
[4] Miller 1957.					[5] Herbert 1959.					[6] Clayton 1955, Latner 1958.
[7] Williams 1957.					[8] Bennhold 1960.					[9] Darby 1958.
[10] Ross 1950, Pitney 1954.					[11] Pitney 1954, Beard 1954.					[12] Mendelsohn 1958.
[13] Erdmann-Oehlecker 1956, Dishkovich 1958, Christensen 1958, Cooper 1959, Halsted 1960.					[14] Schilling 1953, Heinrich 1954.
[15] Beard 1954, Mollin 1955, Erdmann-Oehlecker 1956.
[16] Pendl 1958, Miller 1959.					[17] Astaldi 1956, Pendl 1958.

Der niedrige B_{12}-Spiegel im Blut von Patienten mit perniziöser Anämie ist zweifellos bedingt durch die schwere intestinale Resorptionsstörung, welche durch den Mangel an I.F. im Magensaft bedingt ist; die Verminderung des B_{12}-bindenden Proteins im Plasma dieser Kranken könnte als Folge der geringeren Vehikel-Beanspruchung durch das verminderte Plasma-B_{12} aufgefaßt werden.

Bei der *chronischen myeloischen Leukämie* ist die analoge Frage schwieriger zu beantworten. Eine unmittelbare Ursache der sehr *starken Erhöhung des B_{12}-Spiegels* im Plasma ist unbekannt; Anhaltspunkte dafür, daß eine ungesteuerte erhöhte B_{12}-Resorption im Darm (etwa wie bei Hämochromatose-Kranken die Eisenresorption) eine Rolle spielen könnte, bestehen nicht[1]. Dabei scheint eine besonders große unbesetzte Bindungskapazität vorhanden zu sein[2]. Auch bei diesen Kranken ist B_{12} an ein mit der Geschwindigkeit der α_1-Globuline wanderndes Glykoproteid gebunden.

Nach intravenöser Injektion von radioaktivem Vitamin B_{12} zeigt sich bei Patienten mit chronischer myeloischer Leukämie ein sehr stark verlangsamter Schwund aus dem Blute (etwa auf $1/3$ des Normalen)[3] und eine stark herabgesetzte oder jedenfalls minimale[1] B_{12}-Ausscheidung mit dem Harn.

Interessanterweise fanden sich nach Röntgenbestrahlung der Milz Absinken des Blutspiegels und starke Abgabe durch die Nieren[4]. Untersuchungen über eine Beeinflussung des B_{12}-bindenden α_1-Globulins durch Milzbestrahlung stehen noch aus. Zwar sprechen der Glykoproteidcharakter, die gleiche anodische Wanderung im elektrischen Feld bei p_H 4,5 sowie gleiches Verhalten bei der Chromatographie mit Cellulose[5] für die qualitative Gleichartigkeit der B_{12}-bindenden Proteine bei Gesunden und bei diesen Leukämie-Kranken; dennoch ist die Möglichkeit nicht auszuschließen, daß es sich um einen nur ähnlichen Eiweißkörper mit zahlreicheren Haftplätzen für B_{12} handelt. Bei Leukämiepatienten wird dieser Eiweißkörper auch in Spuren mit dem Harn ausgeschieden[6]. — Mancherlei Unterschiede im physiologischen Verhalten des B_{12}-bindenden Proteins zeigen sich zwischen dem vom Gesunden und dem vom Leukämiker stammenden: das Letztere ist in seiner Bindungsfähigkeit resistenter gegen Erhitzen und gegen ein saures Milieu von p_H 3,6; auch ist das an Plasma von Leukämie-Patienten gebundene B_{12} geschützter gegen „die Freisetzung" und Verwertung durch Euglena gracilis[6] als das von Normalserum gebundene B_{12}.

Im Bereiche von Milz, Leber und Muskulatur fand sich normaler B_{12}-Gehalt[7]. Nelson fand bei Untersuchungen mit der Nadelbiopsie sogar abnorm niedrigen B_{12}-Gehalt in der Leber bei zwei Fällen von chronischer myeloischer Leukämie (30% unter der Norm)[8]. Aus der Unregelmäßigkeit der Schwundkurve hat man auf Mitwirken eines enterohepatischen Zirkels[9] oder auch auf eventuelle Ablagerungsstätten unbekannter Lokalisation geschlossen.

Die Differenz im B_{12}-Gehalt zwischen Gewebe und Plasma könnte an eine qualitative oder quantitative Veränderung des B_{12}-bindenden Proteins als pathogenetischen Faktor denken lassen.

Ob sich aus diesen Befunden vom Gesichtspunkt gestörter Transportfunktionen aus ein Hinweis auf die Pathogenese der chronisch-myeloischen Leukämie ableiten läßt, ist noch durchaus zweifelhaft. Es ist die Meinung vertreten worden, daß der erhöhte B_{12}-Spiegel vielmehr durch einen abnormen Stoffwechsel im Bereich des B_{12}-bindenden Proteins bedingt sein könnte[1, 5]. Es könnte aber die erhöhte Bindungskapazität auch zu einer Anreicherung des B_{12} im Blut führen und bei einem großen Überschuß an Trägerprotein die Haftfähigkeit am Vehikel erhöht sein, so daß die Abgabefähigkeit und Disponibilität des B_{12} vermindert wäre[10], wie es ja auch schon oben betreffs des Euglena-Testes erwähnt wurde.

Eine weitere Deutungsschwierigkeit läge dann aber darin, daß bei der chronisch-myeloischen Leukämie ja die Erythrocytenreifung meistens — allerdings nicht immer[4] — intakt bleibt, daß man also verschiedene Trägerproteine des B_{12} für die Reifung der Leukocyten und der Erythrocyten annehmen müßte.

Wenn auch zugegeben werden muß, daß an diesen letzten Gedankengängen vieles hypothetisch ist, so erscheint es doch in einem Kapitel, welches Transportfragen behandeln soll, gerechtfertigt, die erstaunliche Erhöhung des B_{12}-Spiegels (bis auf das 20—40fache des Normalen!) und die ebenso erstaunliche Vermehrung der entsprechenden Trägerproteine zusammen mit dem massenhaften Auftreten unreifer, weißer Blutzellen einmal unter dem Gesichtspunkt pathologischer Transportvorgänge zu betrachten.

---

[1] Halsted 1956, Weinstein 1960.   [2] Mollin 1956, Heinrich 1956, Miller 1957.
[3] Stevenson 1959.   [4] Heinrich 1954, Erdmann-Oehlecker 1956.
[5] Mendelsohn 1958.   [6] Miller 1959.   [7] Mollin 1955.   [8] Nelson 1958.
[9] Gräsbeck 1958.   [10] Bennhold 1960.

Transportformen der Lipide.

Obwohl den Fetten[1] der höchste Caloriengehalt unter unseren Nahrungsmitteln innewohnt, und sie deshalb eine wichtige Energiequelle für den Organismus darstellen, ist noch keineswegs erforscht, in welcher Weise diese nichtwasserlöslichen Stoffe in das wäßrige Milieu des Körpers einbezogen werden, und wie der Fetttransport dann abläuft. Die Gegenüberstellung von normaler Nahrungslipämie auf der einen Seite und pathologischer Fettembolie nach traumatischer Einschwemmung von körpereigenem Fett in das Blut auf der anderen Seite, macht nur einen Teil der Problematik des Fetttransportes deutlich: Die Emulgierung und die Stabilisierung der Fettemulsionen, die nur so toleriert werden. In den letzten Jahren ist gezeigt worden, daß die Lipide in einer Anzahl verschiedener Transportformen auftreten. Fredrickson und Gordon behandelten 1958 den „Fettsäurentransport" als Teil des Fettstoffwechsels.

Die wasserunlöslichen Fette sind aber nicht nur das Transportgut, das nach Zustand und Form durch seine Verbindung mit dem Proteinvehikel in Lösung bleibt und zirkuliert, sondern sie sind gleichzeitig selbst Vehikel für andere lipoidlösliche Stoffe. Die fettlöslichen Vitamine, Cholesterin und ein Teil der veresterten Fettsäuren sind im Lipidmaterial gelöst, welches seinerseits ein Teil der Protein-Fettverbindung ist.

Es ist hier nicht der Ort, auf die vielfältigen und umfangreichen Untersuchungen über die Fettverdauung und Resorption einzugehen[2], da bindende Aussagen, wieviel Triglyceride total hydrolisiert, wieviel nur in Di- oder Monoglyceride abgebaut[3] und wieviele unter Mithilfe von Phosphorlipiden bis zu Tröpfchen bestimmter Größenordnung dispergiert und auch so resorbiert werden, nicht gemacht werden können. Für jedes zugeführte Fett ist das Resultat von Spaltung und Aufnahme unterschiedlich[4]. Allgemein wird angenommen, daß die Hydrolyse der Triglyceride ein Stufenprozeß ist, daß die 2-Esterverbindung bedeutend widerstandsfähiger ist gegen die Spaltung, und daß der letzte Schritt vom Monoglycerid zum Glycerin irreversibel verläuft. Auch die Resyntheserate der Lipide in der Darmwand ist eine noch nicht zu übersehende Größe. Die Passage durch die Darmwand und die anschließende Weiterleitung erfolgt in Abhängigkeit von Sättigungsgrad und Kettenlänge der Fettsäuren. Während niedere Kettenlängen unmittelbar resorbiert werden und mit dem Pfortaderblut zur Leber strömen, finden sich die über 10 C-Atome langen und ganz besonders die ungesättigten Fettsäuren[4], die feinemulgierten Neutralfette und das Nahrungscholesterin nahezu vollständig (in veresterter Form) im Ductus thoracicus wieder[5]. Mit der Lymphe vermischt, ergießt sich die milchige Emulsion in das Blutgefäßsystem. Das feinemulgierte Fett der Chylomikronen, das stets einen proportionalen Teil Phosphorlipoide enthält[6], kann offenbar nur auf diesem Wege in das Blut gelangen. Nicht alle Blutlipide entstammen aber unmittelbar der Nahrung. Ein Teil der im Serum zirkulierenden endogenen Lipoproteide wird in der Leber gebildet und wenigstens zum Teil mit der Leberlymphe dem Kreislauf zugeführt[7]. Ein weiterer bedeutungsvoller Teil, die unveresterten Fettsäuren des Blutes, kommt hauptsächlich aus dem Fettgewebe.

Im Blut sind alle Serumlipide in einer stabilen Transportform unmittelbar oder mittelbar an Serumproteine gebunden. Das Cholesterin war das erste Lipid, für welches Bennhold 1931 auf Grund elektrophoretischer Untersuchungen eine Globulinbindung beschrieb, nachdem Macheboeuf 1929 auf die Wechselwirkungen zwischen Blutlipid und Bluteiweiß aufmerksam gemacht hatte.

Die *unveresterten Fettsäuren* sind insgesamt und praktisch vollständig an Proteine gebunden[8]. Die Bindungskonstanten nehmen mit der Kettenlänge zu[9].

---

[1] Shapiro 1957.

[2] Verzàr 1948, Frazer 1948, 1952, 1953, Bloom 1950, Favarger 1951, Mattson 1952, Peters 1953, Reise 1954, Fernandes 1955.

[3] Kuhrt 1952, Harris 1955.   [4] Fernandes 1955.

[5] Bloom 1951, Chaikoff 1952, Kiyasu 1952, Friedmann 1953.

[6] Albrink 1955.   [7] Forker 1952, Albrink 1955.

[8] Lecomte du Nouy 1926, Teresi 1952, Westphal 1953, Gordon 1955, Laurell 1955, Mora 1955, Goodman und Shafrir 1959.

[9] Teresi 1952, Goodman 1958.

Sie sind am größten für Serumalbumin, welches 3 Gruppen von Bindungsplätzen besitzt. In der ersten Gruppe üben 2 Plätze eine so starke Attraktion aus, daß sie bei den üblichen Präparationsmethoden zur Darstellung kristallisierten Albumins besetzt bleiben. Erst eine spezielle Entfettung des Albumins setzt sie frei[1]. Fünf weitere Plätze in der zweiten Gruppe haben eine kleinere Assoziationskonstante und etwa 20 Plätze in der dritten Gruppe vermitteln nur eine schwache Bindung. Die Prüfung der übrigen Proteine, Lipoproteide[2] und der Erythrocyten[3] ergab Bindungskonstanten, die eine Schätzung der Beteiligung der einzelnen Vehikel am Fettsäurentransport erlauben.

Im Verhältnis zum Albumin spielen die übrigen Vehikel in der Gesamtbilanz des Transportes der unveresterten Säuren nur eine untergeordnete Rolle. Drei Viertel der so zirkulierenden Fettsäuren bestehen aus Palmitat, welches nur zu 1% an den Erythrocytenhüllen und zu 0,5% an den Lipoproteiden niederer Dichte haftet. 0,01% ist ungebunden. Die Bindung an α_1-Lipoproteid ist noch nicht untersucht worden. Nach FREDRICKSON (1958) sollten sich die übrigen gewöhnlichen Fettsäuren nicht anders verhalten, was allerdings nicht ausschließt, daß ungewöhnliche und in geringer Menge vorkommende Fettsäuren stark abweichen können. Erhebliche Unterschiede in der Bindungsgeschwindigkeit von gesättigten und ungesättigten Fettsäuren an Albumin fand SOBOTA (1955) bei der Untersuchung der Freisetzung von Fettsäuremolekülen aus Filmen in Albuminlösung.

Die *unveresterten Fettsäuren* des Blutes sind die Fettfraktion, welche den schnellsten Veränderungen unterliegt[4]. Mit C^{14}-markierten Säuren gemessen, beträgt die Verweildauer im Blut nur wenige Minuten. Nach 1—3 min war C^{14}-Palmitat zur Hälfte verschwunden[5], oder pro Minute verliert das Plasma 0,09—1,5 mÄq langkettiger Fettsäuren. 10 Prozent der verabreichten Menge des markierten Carboxyl-C^{14} tauchte innerhalb einer Stunde in der Atemluft wieder auf[6]. Es kann demnach keinem Zweifel unterliegen, daß diese Fettsäuren einen erheblichen Beitrag zum Energiestoffwechsel leisten. Sie können auch nur zum geringsten Teil der Nahrung unmittelbar entstammen. Die im Chylus bestimmte Menge[7] reicht bei weitem nicht aus. Anders verhält es sich mit den kurzkettigen Fettsäuren, die ihren Weg ausschließlich vom Darm in das Portalblut nehmen. Sie spielen aber nur beim Kohlenhydrat und Cellulose verdauenden Wiederkäuer eine größere Rolle[8]. Die Bestimmung der arteriovenösen Differenz der verschiedenen Organe[9] und die in vitro-Untersuchung von Gewebe[10], zeigt daß das *Fettgewebe* die Hauptquelle der unveresterten langkettigen Fettsäuren ist. Es kann auch seinerseits Fettsäuren aufnehmen[11]. Alle Mechanismen, welche den Glucoseumsatz erhöhen (Glucoseinfusionen, Insulin, Glucagon u.a.), senken den Fettsäurespiegel[12], indem sie in noch nicht näher bekannter Weise die Fettsäurefreisetzung hemmen. Die Art der Einschleusung der Fettsäuren in das Blut und die Art der Lösung vom Albuminvehikel in den verschiedenen Geweben[13] ist noch nicht geklärt.

Die *veresterten Fettsäuren* liegen im Blutplasma zu 90% als Glycerin-, Cholesterin- oder Sphingosinester vor. Sie sind ein integraler Bestandteil der Plasma-Lipoproteide und der Chylomikronen. Obwohl große Fortschritte in der Charakterisierung der Lipoproteide gemacht wurden[14], ist eine Reindarstellung noch nicht gelungen. Auch mit den üblich gewordenen physikalischen Methoden lassen sich die Lipoproteide nicht scharf trennen und die Klassifizierung nach der elektro-

---

[1] GOODMAN 1957.
[2] GORDON 1956/57, LAURELL 1955, MORA 1955, GOODMAN und SHAFRIR 1959.
[3] GOODMAN 1958.   [4] HAVEL 1956, BIERMAN 1957, FREDRICKSON 1957/58, LAURELL 1957.
[5] HAVEL 1955.   [6] FREDRICKSON 1958.
[7] FREEMAN 1940, BORGSTRÖM 1956, SPITZER 1956.   [8] DOETSCH 1957, BALCH 1958.
[9] GORDON 1957.   [10] GORDON 1958, RESHEF 1958.   [11] STERN 1954, SHAPIRO 1957.
[12] DOLE 1956, GORDON 1956.   [13] GORDON 1957, MASORO 1957.
[14] ONCLEY 1953, GOFMAN 1954.

phoretischen Beweglichkeit in α_1-, α_2- und β-Lipoproteide läßt sich mit Hilfe der Ultrazentrifugierung oder der fraktionierten Fällung nicht vollkommen reproduzieren.

Die α_1-*Lipoproteide*, 3 Gewichtsprozent des Plasmaeiweißes, sind noch am besten von den übrigen zu differenzieren. Im Mittel bestehen sie aus 50% Protein, 25% Phosphatid, 20% Cholesterin und weniger als 10% Triglycerid[1]. Der hohe Proteingehalt macht sie zu den Lipoproteiden „hoher Dichte". De Lalla und Gofman beschreiben 1954 mindestens drei Klassen, die sich im wesentlichen durch verschiedenen Triglyceridgehalt unterscheiden. Molekulargewichte von $0,2 \cdot 10^6$[2], $1,75 \cdot 10^6$ und $4 \cdot 10^6$ wurden berichtet[3]. Die Proteinanteile besitzen eine N-endständige Asparaginsäure und ein C-endständiges Threonin[4]. Sie sind immunochemisch mit dem Protein der β-Lipoproteide nicht verwandt.

Die α_2-*Lipoproteide* lassen sich nur elektrophoretisch darstellen (Kunkel 1956) und gehören mit den β-Lipoproteiden zu den Lipoproteiden „niederer Dichte" (Tabelle 4). Etwa 5% des Plasmaeiweißes rechnen dazu. 75% des Gewichtes sind Lipide. Sowohl Ultrazentrifugierung als auch elektronenoptische Darstellung und chemische Analyse haben immer wieder gezeigt, daß es sich um Stoffe handelt, die nur innerhalb der bestimmten Untersuchungsmethode definiert werden können. Am empfindlichsten erwies sich die Abrahmung mit Hilfe der Ultrazentrifuge (Gofman 1949 und später).

Tabelle 4. *Chemische Zusammensetzung der β- und α_2-Lipoproteide nach* Gofman

Beweglichkeit . . .	β			α_2	
Dichte	1,063	1,019	0,99	0,96	
S_f-Wert	$S_f\,4$	$S_f\,12$	$S_f\,20$	$S_f\,400$	$S_f\,10000$
Gesamtcholesterin	30%	kontinuierlich abnehmend			5%
Cholesterinester .	75%	kontinuierlich abnehmend			0%
Phosphorlipoid . .	25%	kontinuierlich abnehmend			5%
Protein	25%	kontinuierlich abnehmend			5%
Glycerinester . . .	abwesend oder sehr wenig Prozent	kontinuierlich zunehmend			75—85%

Nach Einstellung des Serums durch NaBr-Zugabe auf die Dichte von 1,063[5] wird ultrazentrifugiert und ein Bild der sich entgegen der Schwerkraft abrahmenden Lipoproteide gewonnen. Gofman teilte in eine Reihe „S_f-Klassen" ein und definierte als S_f (= Flotierungs-Svedberg) die Sedimentationskonstante der Größenordnung von S_{20}. Eine etwas andere Definition mit -S gebrauchte Lewis[6]. Wie die Tabelle 4 zeigt, reicht die Dichteskala der Lipoproteide niederer Dichte von 1,063—0,96. Die β-*Lipoproteide* und die α_2-Lipoproteide überlappen stark im Gebiet von 1,019—0,99. Mit ansteigenden S_f-Werten nimmt der Protein-, Cholesterin-, Estercholesterin- und Phosphatidgehalt kontinuierlich ab und der Neutralfettgehalt zu. Es scheint dann von den leichtesten Lipoproteiden keinen scharfen Übergang zu den fast nur noch aus Neutralfett bestehenden Chylomikronen zu geben. Die verschiedene Größe und Gestalt der Moleküle wurde sowohl physikalisch als elektronenoptisch bestimmt[7]. In einer Reihe von Arbeiten ist dargelegt worden, wie die Lipoproteidsubfraktionen von Geschlecht, Alter, Konstitution und Ernährungszustand abhängen und wie sie sich bei den verschiedenen Krankheiten verändern[8]. Die Überprüfungen der komplizierten Methode[9] und die Bemühungen, mit Präcipitations-[10] und Elektrophoreseverfahren[11] zu den gleichen Ergebnissen zu kommen, sind zahlreich.

Genau so wenig wie bei den α_1-Lipoproteiden ist die Struktur der Proteinantiele der α_2- und β-Lipoproteide aufgeklärt. Es herrscht Einmütigkeit darüber, daß sich beide große Gruppen, die verschiedene Umsatzgeschwindigkeiten haben[12], sicher unterscheiden, und daß Unterschiede innerhalb der Gruppen wiederum „nicht groß" sein können[13]. Die Klassen S_f 0—20 besitzen eine N-endständige Glutaminsäure[14], die Dichteklassen um S_f 100

---

[1] Gofman 1954, Bragdon 1956.   [2] Oncley 1947.   [3] Hazelwood 1958.
[4] Shore 1957.   [5] Gofman 1950—1954, Lindgren 1951, Havel 1955.
[6] Lewis 1953.   [7] Oncley 1950, Prendergast 1951, Beischer 1954, Bing 1954.
[8] Gofman 1954.   [9] Gofman 1956.   [10] Lever 1951, Russ 1951.
[11] Durrum 1952, Kunkel 1952, Nikkilä 1953, Swahn 1953, Gross 1954, Ott 1954, Langan 1955, Schettler 1955.
[12] Volwiler 1955, Avigan 1957, Gitlin 1958.
[13] Korngold 1955, Levine 1955, Aladjem 1957.
[14] Avigan 1956, Shore 1957, Rodbell 1958.

dagegen wahrscheinlich Serin und Threonin[1]. Das Polypeptidende der Proteine, welche aus Chylomikronen abgelöst wurden[2], hat die gleiche N-endständige Aminosäure.

Die wenigen Daten über die Umsatzgeschwindigkeit der Lipoproteide müssen noch mit Vorsicht interpretiert werden, zumal beachtet werden muß, daß sich die Moleküle während der Untersuchungszeit verändern. J^{131}-markierte Proteinteile von α_1-Lipoproteid und S_f 3—9 β-Lipoproteid wurde bei Gesunden und Nephrotikern untersucht[3]. Das α_1-Lipoproteid hatte eine Umsatzhalbzeit von 4,4 und 4,8 Tagen bei zwei gesunden Personen, β-Lipoproteid von 3,1 und 3,4 Tagen. Danach verweilen die Proteinteile bedeutend länger als Fettsäuren oder Chylomikronen und sind entweder echte Vehikel oder sie entziehen das Lipoproteid dem raschen Umsatz. Die Entscheidung wird dann zu treffen sein, wenn die Umsatzzeiten von Protein und Fett getrennt bestimmbar sind.

Als *Chylomikronen* wird wegen der herrschenden Unsicherheit gegenüber den größten α_2- und β-Lipoproteiden am besten das fettige Material definiert, „welches sich von einem lipämischen Serum oder von Chylus innerhalb weniger Minuten hochtourig abzentrifugieren läßt"[4]. Die 0,5—1,5 μ großen Tröpfchen enthalten 85—90% Triglyceride, geringe Menge Phosphatide und Cholesterin, ganz geringe Mengen unveresterter Fettsäuren und nur 0,1 bis 0,2% Proteine[4]. Elektrophorese in Harnstoff ergab drei Fraktionen[5] mit Asparaginsäure am Aminosäureende in einer Fraktion und Serin in der Hauptfraktion. Inkubationsversuche mit Darmmucosa deuteten darauf hin, daß zumindest eine Komponente in der Darmwand selbst entsteht[6], während eine andere aus dem Blut zu kommen scheint. Ein in vivo markiertes Lipoproteid des Chylus verhielt sich im Blut als Lipoproteid „hoher Dichte"[7].

Die Chylomikronen kann man als die „Transportform der exogenen Fette" bezeichnen. Ähnlich den unveresterten Fettsäuren verschwinden sie rasch aus dem Blute[8]. Genau so wie bei der Infusion von Fettemulsionen hängt die Schwundrate von der verabfolgten Menge ab[9]. Da eine Hydrolyse schnell einsetzt, findet man Fettsäuren aus dem Triglyceridmaterial der Chylomikronen innerhalb von Minuten als albumingebundene Fettsäuren[10], dagegen erst nach Stunden in die Lipoproteide S_f 0—400 eingebaut. (Bei der hungernden Ratte war die Verteilung von C^{14} nach Injektionen markierten Palmitats oder von Chylomikronen in den Organen gleich.) Eine Ausnahme machte nur das Fettgewebe, welches nur durch die Chylomikronen markiert wurde![11] Große Mengen Chylomikronen nimmt die Leber auf und verbrennt sie[12], ein durch Protamin und Heparin beeinflußbarer Vorgang[13]. Bekannt ist das Eindringen in RES-Zellen, weniger bekannt das Passieren in Leber- und Thoracicuslymphe. Vielleicht ist es für die lipoidlöslichen Substanzen sogar einfacher durch die Endothelwand zu diffundieren als durch die wassergefüllten Capillaren[14]. Da das Proteinvehikel langsamer verschwindet als das zugehörige Triglycerid[1], bleibt vielleicht ein Teil des Proteinmoleküls im Blut zurück. Es ist aber zu berücksichtigen, daß ganze Teile des empfindlichen Komplexes abgelöst und ausgetauscht werden können[15].

Freie oder nur locker gebundene fettlösliche Stoffe müssen *Verteilungsgleichgewichte* anstreben. Freies Cholesterin geht leicht vom Plasma in Erythrocyten[16], von Chylomikronen in Lipoproteide hoher Dichte[9] und von diesen in Lipoproteide niederer Dichte über. Verestertes Cholesterin wird viel schlechter ausgetauscht. Auch Phosphatide wandern leicht von einem Lipoproteid in ein zweites, anders gestaltetes[17] und Triglyceride gehen von einer Klasse niederer Dichte unschwer in eine andere Klasse über[18]; sogar die von Erythrocyten gebildeten Triglyceride und Phosphatide werden in vitro von Lipoproteiden aufgenommen[19].

[1] RODBELL 1958.   [2] RODBELL 1958, 1958a.   [3] GITLIN 1958.
[4] BRAGDON 1958, RODBELL 1958.   [5] BRAGDON 1958.
[6] RODBELL und FREDRICKSON 1958.   [7] HAVEL 1958, SWANK 1958.
[8] WADDEL 1953, 1957.   [9] FREDRICKSON 1958.   [10] STEPHENSON 1958.
[11] BRAGDON und GORDON 1958.   [12] FRENCH 1956, MORRIS 1958.
[13] FREDRICKSON 1958, MORRIS 1958.   [14] RENKIN 1952.
[15] FREDRICKSON 1958, HAVEL 1958.   [16] HAGERMAN 1951.
[17] KUNKEL 1954, EDER 1957, McCANDLESS 1957, HAVEL 1957, OTT 1958.
[18] LINDGREN 1955.   [19] JAMES 1958.

Für Umbauvorgänge durch Enzyme kommen Transphosphatasen und die Lipoproteidlipase in Frage. Ausführlich studiert wurde die Umwandlung von Lipoproteidmolekülen hoher S_f-Klassen in niedere[1]. Sie ist besonders ergiebig nach Heparininjektion, wenn „Klärfaktor" freigesetzt wurde.

Trotz ausführlicher Untersuchungen (Übersicht bei BORGSTRÖM 1956, ROBINSON 1957) konnte die biologische Bedeutung des Kläreffektes (Clearing effect) aber noch nicht befriedigend dargelegt werden. 1943 zeigte HAHN, daß die Injektion von Heparin zur Zeit der Nahrungslipämie eine rasche Aufhellung des Serums und ein Verschwinden der Chylomikronen bewirkt. Heparin und andere Polyanionen (Polysaccharidschwefelsäure[2] oder Polymetaphosphate[3]) setzen aus Muskel, Lungen, Darm, Fett- und anderen Geweben, nicht aber aus Lebergewebe[4], eine von Pankreaslipase unterscheidbare[5] „Lipoproteidlipase"[6] frei, die die Triglyceride der Chylomikronen und der Lipoproteide hydrolisiert. Ohne Heparin ist diese Lipase nur ausnahmsweise zu finden gewesen und kann deshalb auch kein wesentlicher Teil der intravasalen Lipolyse sein. Es hat den Anschein, als ob das Enzym zu den lipatischen Gewebsfermenten gehört und durch zu hohe Heparinmengen freigesetzt wird.

Mit der Darstellung der Transportformen der Lipide ist nur ein Teil des Fetttransportes besprochen worden. Bildung und Verbrauch, Freisetzung und Speicherung von Lipid konnten in dem gesteckten Rahmen nicht behandelt werden. In einer abschließenden Bilanz steht der Umsatz an unveresterten Fettsäuren an erster Stelle, dann folgt der Umsatz an Triglyceridfettsäuren. Er ist 2—10mal größer als der Umsatz von Phosphatidfettsäuren und 20mal größer als der der Sterolesterfettsäuren[7]. Von ausschlaggebender Bedeutung für Aufnahme und Abgabe von Fettsäuren und für die Aufnahme von Triglyceriden ist die jeweilige Situation des Kohlenhydratstoffwechsels[8]. Allgemein kann gelten, daß Kohlenhydrate die Freisetzung von unveresterten Fettsäuren bremsen und damit den Blutspiegel senken[9]. Der rasche Transport über Albuminvehikel wird gedrosselt. Die Bildung von Lipoproteid und die Aufnahme von Chylomikronen ins Fettgewebe wird gefördert. Im Hunger (und bei Diabetes) werden Fettsäuren mobilisiert und albumingebunden verfügbar gemacht. Der Triglyceridspiegel ist hoch oder steigt an[10], weil bei genügend hohem Fettsäureangebot die Lipoproteidproduktion unbeeinflußt, die Aufnahme von Triglycerid in das Gewebe aber vermindert ist.

Bindung und Transport von Steroiden.

Durch neuere Forschungen sind auch die von den Sterinen abgeleiteten Hormone der Gonaden und der Nebennierenrinde auf ihre Bindungsfähigkeit an Plasmaeiweiß untersucht worden. Zunächst fiel auf, daß Testosteron, Progesteron und Oestradiol sowie die Nebennierenrindenhormone in isolierten Albuminlösungen viel besser in Lösung gehen als in eiweißfreiem Milieu. Die Steroidbindung an Albumin ließ sich ferner durch freie Elektrophorese nachweisen[11]. Progesteron und Oestradiol sowie Testosteron sind relativ fest an Albumin gebunden, Corticosteroide sehr viel schwächer. Die Bindungen von Oestradiol und von Testosteron sind abhängig vom p_H: beide steigen in ihrer Bindungskapazität von p_H 5,3—8,5 deutlich an; ähnliches gilt für Progesteron. Jenseits p_H 11 hört die Bindungsfähigkeit der Albumine für Testosteron auf.

DAUGHADAY hat in Gleichgewichtsdialysen mit markierten Corticosteroiden ein *corticosteroidbindendes Globulin* entdeckt[12]. Zusatz von 5 μg mit C^{14}-markierten Cortisols wurde bei $+4^\circ$ C mit 100 cm³ Plasma versetzt und dialysiert; es

---

[1] PIERCE 1954.   [2] ZINN 1952.   [3] HAVEL 1954.
[4] ANFINSEN 1952, JEFFRIES 1954.   [5] ROBINSON 1957.   [6] KORN 1955.
[7] PIBL 1950, HARPER 1953, LIPSKY 1955, BATES 1958.   [8] MAN 1956.
[9] LAURELL 1957, BRAGDON und GORDON 1958, FREDRICKSON 1958.
[10] WALKER 1953, BRAGDON 1954, AHRENS 1957, NICHOLS 1957, BRAGDON und GORDON 1958.
[11] WESTPHAL 1955, 1957.   [12] DAUGHADAY 1958.

ergab sich fast komplette Bindung dieses Steroids (nur 0,7—1,5% blieben ungebunden). Höhere Zusätze von Cortisol ergaben deutlichen Anstieg des freien Steroids. Corticosteron verhielt sich ähnlich, wurde jedoch nur schwächer gebunden. Bei Konzentrationen von mehr als 20—30 μg% Cortisol geht dieses auch Bindungen mit dem Albumin ein. Die Bindungen sind auffallend spezifisch; Aldosteron haftet z. B. weniger stark. Papierelektrophorese bei p_H 8,8 gab einen deutlichen Gipfel des mit C^{14} markierten Corticosteroids in der Gegend der α-Globuline, welche relativ reich an Hexosamin und Hexose sind[1], es wird vermutet, daß es sich um die Glykoproteide M1 und M2 handelt[2], welche möglicherweise dem thyroxinbindenden Eiweiß nahestehen. Im Plasma der Umbilikalvene fand sich 16,2%, im Liquor cerebrospinalis 93% (entsprechend seinem niedrigen Eiweißgehalt) ungebundenes Corticosteroid; Pleura- und Synovial-Flüssigkeit zeigte etwas höhere Bindungsfähigkeit den Corticosteroiden gegenüber. SLAUNWHITE und SANDBERG bezeichneten 1959 dieses hauptsächlich im α_1-Globulinbereich wandernde Corticosteroidbindende Protein als „Transcortin". Belastete man Plasma mit Zusätzen von 15—65 μg% Cortisol, dann konnten diese Autoren im Plasma von Schwangeren im letzten Drittel der Gravidität durch Ultrafiltration oder durch Dialyse eine außerordentliche Steigerung der Cortisol-Bindung nachweisen (sogar noch bei Zusätzen bis zu 250 μg%). Dieses war besonders interessant, weil schon bekannt war, daß im Blut von Schwangeren der Cortisol-Spiegel ansteigt[3]. Noch höheren Anstieg der Bindungskapazität für Cortisol fanden SANDBERG und SLAUNWHITE bei Patienten, welche wegen Prostatacarcinoms mit hohen Dosen Oestron behandelt waren[4]; der Anstieg begann bereits wenige Tage nach dem Anfang dieser Behandlung. Die Konzentration der Bindungsplätze des Transcortins wurde bei Normalpersonen auf $1,3 \times 10^{-7}$ M, bei Schwangeren auf $3,2 \times 10^{-7}$ M geschätzt. Entweder ist diese Erhöhung der Bindungskapazität durch einfache Vermehrung der normalen cortisolbindenden Globuline[4] oder durch das Auftreten eines unabhängigen andersartigen, stärker cortisolbindenden Globulins in der Blutbahn zu erklären[1]. Trotz des hohen Plasmaspiegels an Cortisol als Folge von Schwangerschaft[5, 6, 7] und von Oestron-Kuren[8, 9, 10] tritt merkwürdigerweise *kein* Cushing-Syndrom auf. Beides ist wohl mit größter Wahrscheinlichkeit auf die gleichzeitig auftretende gesteigerte Bindungsfähigkeit seitens der Cortisol-Vehikel zu erklären. Als Hormon wirkt nur das *freie* Steroid. An Albumin zeigt Cortisol nur eine sehr geringe Bindung, verglichen mit der Bindung an α_1-Globulin[11].

Forschungen von DOE (1960) am genuinen Plasma (also ohne in vitro-Zusätze von Cortisol als Bindungstest) haben klinisch sehr wichtige Befunde ergeben. Sie untersuchten 11 Normalfälle, 16 Schwangere, 30 Patienten mit Prostatacarcinom und längeren Diäthylstilboestrol-Kuren sowie 5 Fälle mit Cushing-Syndrom und ferner Patienten unmittelbar nach ACTH-Infusionen auf den Gehalt von freiem und gebundenem Cortisol im Plasma. Die Ergebnisse gibt umstehende Tabelle 5 wieder.

In allen Fällen geschah die Cortisol-Bindung hauptsächlich an das α_1-Globulin, in geringem Maße an das α_2- und nur in der Schwangerschaft in nennenswertem Maße auch an die β-Globuline. Diese Versuche zeigen somit eindrucksvoll, daß die spezifischen Trägerproteine im Plasma hier eine wesentliche Rolle bei der Entstehung — und bei der Verhütung — von endokrinen Erkrankungen spielen können. Die ACTH-Wirkung, welche direkt nach der Infusion nur das freie Cortisol ansteigen läßt, spricht dafür, daß die entsprechenden Trägerproteine erst eine gewisse Anlaufzeit brauchen, ehe sie bei plötzlicher Cortisol-Einschwemmung

---

[1] DAUGHADAY 1958.   [2] MEHL 1949.   [3] GEMZELL 1954.   [4] SANDBERG 1959.
[5] MIGEON 1956.   [6] COHEN 1958.   [7] MARTIN 1958.   [8] TALIAFERRO 1956.
[9] WALLACE 1957.   [10] DOE 1960.   [11] DAUGHADAY 1959.

Tabelle 5.

Diagnosen	Zahl der Fälle	Durchschnittswerte im genuinen Plasma		
		Gesamt-cortisol $\mu g\%$	An Eiweiß gebundenes Cortisol $\mu g\%$	freies Cortisol
Normale	11	17,2	16,3	0,9 $\mu g\%$
Schwangerschaft	16	45,9	39,0	7,3 $\mu g\%$
Prostatacarcinom (nach Diäthylstilboestrol) . . .	30	52,9	48,7	4,2 $\mu g\%$
Desgleichen vor ACTH-Infusion	1	62,1	54,3	7,8 $\mu g\%$
Desgleichen nach ACTH-Infusion (25 Einheiten) .		91,3	55,6	35,7 g%
Cushing-Syndrom	4	32,7	16,1	16,6 g%
Cushing-Syndrom (nach Lungencarcinom)	1	143,0	19,0	124,0 g%
Normalfälle nach Infusion von ACTH (25 Einheiten)				27,0 g%

für Transportaufgaben zur Verfügung stehen. Die übrigen Steroide (Progesteron, Testosteron, Oestriol) haften nur am Albumin; Oestron und Oestradiol scheinen ausschließlich mit Albumin-Bindungen einherzugehen, die zum Teil ziemlich fest sind[1].

Die Bindungen der Hormone an Plasma-Proteine verhindern weitgehend Hormonverluste durch die Niere. Die *Konjugate mit Glucuronsäure* und mit Schwefelsäure bedingen eine sehr viel weniger feste Bindung an die Eiweiß-Vehikel (analog den Ausscheidungsverhältnissen beim Bilirubin und Thyroxin); dadurch ist eine leichtere Glomerulumfiltration und eventuell auch Tubuluspassage möglich[2,3,4,5]. Für Tubulusbeteiligung bei der Ausscheidung von Cortisolglucuroniden spricht, daß die Clearance-Werte unter Gaben von Probenecid absanken[6]. Die Konjugierung mit Glucuronsäure und die dadurch bedingte Änderung der Bindungsfestigkeit an die Eiweißvehikel sind die Faktoren, welche diese Stoffe harnfähig machen.

Fremdvehikel.

Bindung und Transport durch Kollidon.

Seit der Entdeckung der Vehikelfunktion der Plasmaeiweißkörper war denkbar, daß auch körperfremde kolloidale Stoffe als Vehikel fungieren würden, wenn sie vom Organismus vertragen werden, eine Zeitlang im Kreislauf zirkulieren und andere Substanzen an sich binden können. Beim Studium von Blutersatzmitteln stießen Bennhold und Schubert 1944 auf einen solchen Stoff: das von Hecht und Weese 1943 eingeführte Kollidon. Andere derartige Substanzen sind bislang nicht gefunden worden; die quellungsfähigen, wasserbindenden Polysaccharide, die gleichfalls in der Schockbekämpfung und zum Blutflüssigkeitsersatz Verwendung finden (z.B. Dextran), sind keine Vehikel im allgemeinen Sinne, da sie außer zu Wasser keinerlei adsorptive Affinität zu anderen Stoffen aufweisen. Das Beispiel des Kollidons zeigt nun eindrucksvoll, in welcher Weise ein künstliches Vehikel in das Transportgeschehen des Körpers eingreifen und den Tropismus verschiedener, vorwiegend sogar körperfremder Stoffe zu ändern vermag[7].

Kollidon ist ein Polyvinylpyrrolidon (PVP) und kommt mit unterschiedlichem Polymerisationsgrad in den Handel. Die Vinylpyrrolidongruppe besitzt ein Molekulargewicht von 111 und eine zur Wechselwirkung befähigte, ladungstragende CONH-Konfiguration. Sicher spielen auch die Doppelbindungen im Molekül für die Kombinationsfreudigkeit der Verbindung eine Rolle. Vorläufig ist es aber noch nicht möglich, aus der Konstitution auf das Ausmaß der Bindungsfähigkeit zu schließen. Es muß nur registriert werden, daß die Skala der vom Kollidon gebundenen Stoffe erstaunlich groß ist und daß die Stärke der Bindung die des Serumalbumins in einzelnen Fällen sogar übersteigen kann. Gerade dieser Umstand macht

---

[1] Daughaday 1959.　　[2] Sandberg 1957.　　[3] Slaunwhite 1958.
[4] Bongiovanni 1955.　　[5] Daughaday 1958.　　[6] Daughaday 1956.
[7] Schubert 1951.

es zu einem neuartigen Therapeuticum. Große Hoffnungen knüpften sich an den Nachweis der Bindung von Diphtherie-, Botulinus-, Tetanus-, Shiga-, Kruse- und Flexnerruhrtoxinen, von Endotoxin des Bacterium coli und der Schlangengifte von Botrops, Kobra, Vipera ammodytes und Vipera mont. mer.[1].

Der Farbstoff Methylorange wurde von Kollidon stärker gebunden als von Serumalbumin $(1/r = 0{,}31 \cdot 10^{-4} \cdot 1/A + 1)^2$ (s. S. 193). Nicht nur im gegenseitigen Vergleich[3] schien die Bindungsfähigkeit häufig höher als die des Albumins; schon die ersten Untersuchungen 1944 und zahlreiche spätere (s. unten) zeigten, daß manche Teststoffe ihre Haftplätze an den Serumproteinen verlassen, um mit dem zugesetzten Kollidon Bindungen einzugehen. Kollidon gibt genau wie Serum einen ausgesprochenen „Embatischen Effekt"[4] bei Diffusionsversuchen mit grobdispersen Farbstoffen in Gelatine-Gel; d. h. erst nach Zusatz von Serum oder Kollidon diffundieren die grob dispersen sauren Farbstoffe (zusammen mit Serumeiweiß bzw. Kollidon) in die Gelatine hinein.

Da für die körperfremde, aber inerte Substanz kein Spaltungsmechanismus wirksam ist, wird sie unverändert im Harn ausgeschieden[5]. Harnfähig sind jedoch nur Moleküle bis zu einem Molekulargewicht von 40000—50000; was darüber liegt, wird gespeichert[6]. Aus diesem Grunde verwendet man zu therapeutischen Zwecken niedermolekulare Gemische (Periston N „Bayer" mittl. MG 12600).

Harnfähigkeit und Bindungsfähigkeit machen das PVP zu einem geeigneten Mittel, nichtharnfähige Stoffe über die Niere aus dem Organismus auszuschleusen[7]. Durch eine Kollidoninfusion kann sowohl vom Serumeiweiß gebundener Farbstoff abgelöst und ausgeschieden als auch in Speichern deponierter in die Blutbahn zurückgeholt und über die Niere eliminiert werden; Voraussetzung ist nur, daß der betreffende Stoff stärker von dem künstlichen Vehikel gebunden wird als von seinem natürlichen. Der Kontakt mit dem Kollidon bewirkt sofort, daß der von seinem ursprünglichen Vehikel schwächer gebundene Stoff so lange an das Kollidon hinüberwechselt, bis ein neues Gleichgewicht erreicht ist. So kommt eine „*Serum*"- oder sogar eine „*Gewebswäsche*" (SCHUBERT) zustande.

Die Ergiebigkeit der „Wäsche" ließ sich aus dem Übergewicht der PVP-Bindung vorbestimmen und ergab sich anschaulich aus in vitro-Untersuchungen des Serums. Als methodisch besonders geeignet erwiesen sich Elektrophoresen von Serum-Kollidongemischen. Bei der Wanderung im elektrischen Feld in der Tiselius-Apparatur trennen sich die einzelnen Eiweißkomponenten und andere Serumbestandteile voneinander ab. Kollidon mit einer sehr geringen elektrophoretischen Beweglichkeit erscheint — eine genügende Konzentration zum Nachweis vorausgesetzt — als leicht bestimmbarer Anteil. Da eine fest adsorbierte Substanz mit der Beweglichkeit des Adsorptionsmittels wandert, ist sehr leicht zu erkennen, wie durch die Kollidonzugabe ein ursprünglich am Protein haftender Stoff abgelöst wird und am Kollidon gebunden erscheint[8]. Als Beispiele wurden die beiden Farbstoffe Diaminrot 3 B und Diaminreinblau FF verwendet (Abb. 4 d, e).

Die vom PVP adsorbierten Stoffe verlassen, dem jeweiligen Bindungsgleichgewicht folgend, ihre bisherigen Bindungsstellen am Eiweiß und damit ihren natürlichen Weg im Organismus. Das Fremdvehikel zwingt sie in das ihm eigene Geleise, sei es, um als nunmehr nierenfähiger Komplex ausgeschieden zu werden, sei es, um mit dem Vehikel gespeichert[9] oder eventuell an einer anderen Stelle metabolisiert zu werden. So wird im Kaninchenversuch der fast ausschließlich *gallengängige* Farbstoff Diaminrot 3 B[10] auf eine Kollidoninfusion hin rasch *durch die Nieren* ausgeschieden und verschwindet aus der Galle, oder das an sich weder nieren- noch gallenfähige Trypanrot oder Diaminreinblau FF[11] erscheint alsdann im Harn. Selbst wenn der blaue Farbstoff gänzlich aus dem Blut verschwunden und in seine Speicher (vor allem das RES) gelangt war, bewirkte die nachträgliche Kollidongabe sein *Wieder-*

---

[1] SCHUBERT 1948, 1949, 1951, 1954.   [2] WEESE 1951.   [3] SPITZER 1956.
[4] BENNHOLD 1927.   [5] SCHUBERT 1950, WEESE 1951.
[6] FRESEN 1951.   [7] SCHUBERT 1948/49.   [8] SCHUBERT 1949, BENNHOLD 1950a.
[9] SCHUBERT 1951.   [10] SCHUBERT 1950.   [11] SCHUBERT und WERNER 1950.

erscheinen im Kreislauf und die Eliminierung mit dem Urin. Ähnliche Versuche gelangen mit Trypanblau beim Kaltblüter[1]. Dringt das kleinmolekulare Kolloid in die Zelle selbst ein, um dort den granulär gespeicherten Farbstoff zu mobilisieren? Verschiedene Beobachtungen könnten dies als möglich erscheinen lassen[2], z. B. der embatische Effekt in vitro und der histologisch kontrollierte Farbstoffschwund in vivo, nach intravenösen Injektionen von Periston N. Andererseits könnten auch die Speicher mit dem Serumeiweiß im Adsorptionsgleichgewicht stehen, und das Kollidon könnte eine diesen beiden überlegene Bindungsfähigkeit besitzen. Eine rasche Verschiebung an das neue wirksame Adsorbens im Blute wäre dann die Folge. Stellen sich der Ausscheidung des Kollidonfarbstoffkomplexes durch die Nieren keine weiteren Widerstände in den Weg, etwa in Form einer starken Rückresorption, dann kommt so über die Bindung an das Kollidon eine allmähliche Elution des Organismus zustande.

Zur Behandlung von Intoxikationen hat sich die Auswaschung mit Kollidon bewährt. Tierexperimente zeigten dabei, daß der möglichst rasche Einsatz des Elutionsmittels unumgänglich ist. Nur relativ kurze Zeit nach der Vergiftung mit Botulinus-, Tetanus- oder Diphtherie-Toxin war die Infusion von $^1/_5$ der Blutmenge lebensrettend[3]. Offenbar war für den positiven Auswascheffekt ein bestimmter Grad der Freiheit und Adsorbierbarkeit des Toxins notwendig. Eine in Gang gekommene Schädigung konnte nicht mehr unterbrochen werden. Leider gelang beim kranken Menschen der Nachweis der im Harn ausgeschleusten Bakteriengifte nicht in jedem Falle. Erst bei schweren toxischen Diphtherien, wobei sich die Kollidoninfusionen besonders gut, mitunter sogar lebensrettend bewährten[4], konnten ausgeschwemmte Toxine wiedergefunden werden[5]. Wertvolle Erfahrungen wurden auch bei der Behandlung schwerer Tetanusvergiftungen gewonnen[6] und die rettende Wirkung von Kollidoninfusionen immer wieder mitgeteilt[7].

Transport in die Zelle.

Aus dem vorbeifließenden Plasmastrom (Inhalt des linken Ventrikels) müßte im Gebiet des großen Kreislaufs jede Zelle auf eine wunderbare Art prüfen, welche Stoffe sie zur Aufnahme benötigt, müßte auswählen und aufnehmen oder ablehnen. Die Cellulartheorie Virchows hatte kein anderes Bild dafür als die Annahme einer besonderen „Vitalität". Das Vermögen einer Zelle kann aber nichts anderes sein als eine Summe von Eigenschaften, die aus ihrem Aufbau gegeben sind und die einer Analyse primär zugänglich sein müssen.

Die Menge der in die Zelle aufzunehmenden Stoffe richtet sich bei normalen Stoffen nach dem Angebot und nach dem Stoffwechselbedarf. Viele Substanzen diffundieren frei und breiten sich um und in die Zellen aus. Dem Eindringen durch Diffusion kann zwar durch die besondere Konstruktion der Außenbegrenzung oder durch aktive Zellarbeit vorgebeugt werden, jedoch ist auch diese Leistung nicht unerschöpflich, sondern z. B. abhängig von der extracellulären Konzentration. Andererseits werden sehr viele, obwohl nicht alle Stoffe aktiv unter Leistung von Arbeit aufgenommen, wobei der Ausdruck „aktiv" alle von der Zelle Energie fordernden Prozesse einschließt. Die Mechanismen, welche eine Zelle besonders befähigen, Stoffe aus dem Blut aufzunehmen, sind teilweise aus Modellversuchen oder durch Analogieschlüsse bisher nur sehr unvollkommen bekannt. Sie lassen sich recht grob als die Affinität der Zelle oder eines

---

[1] Schubert 1952.   [2] Schubert 1951.   [3] Schubert 1948/49, Krech 1953.
[4] Schubert 1948, Dieckhoff 1952, Ströder 1949.
[5] Dieckhoff 1952.   [6] Schubert 1949, Ströder 1951.
[7] Schubert 1954, 1956, Kindler 1952, Lübke 1954, Mühlhauer 1952, Groll 1952, Griesser 1956, Ramalhâo 1956.

primär wirksamen Zellbestandteiles ausdrücken. Unter Affinität soll aber nicht ein unbestimmtes Bedürfnis oder Vermögen verstanden werden, sondern die chemisch oder physikalisch-chemisch definierte Reaktionsfähigkeit der Zelle oder ihrer Bestandteile mit dem aufzunehmenden Material. Die Mechanismen der Aufnahme mögen außerordentlich vielfältig und im einzelnen undurchsichtig sein, prinzipiell sind sie jedoch einer einheitlichen Betrachtung zugänglich: einerseits handelt es sich um einfache Assoziationen mit den individuellen aktiven Stellen der Zellwand, die zu einem Auffüllen der Assoziationsflächen oder des Assoziationsraumes und dadurch zu einem Eindringen in die Zelle führen, andererseits um chemische bzw. fermentative Umsetzungen, welche die Aufnahme in die Zelle zur Folge haben (Lit. bei WILBRANDT 1956).

Da das linke Herz gut durchmischtes Blut fördert, findet sich *jede Körperzelle im Gebiet des großen Kreislaufs praktisch der gleichen Ernährungsflüssigkeit gegenüber*, die entweder spärlich oder reichlich — ganz entsprechend der regulierten Tätigkeit der Kreislauforgane — herangeführt wird. Die Stoffe treten in der extracellulären Flüssigkeit gleichmäßig an die Zellen heran. Dieses Herantreten geschieht aber nicht in einer unmittelbaren Art, nicht in Form einer regellosen Anschwemmung.

Sehr viele der im Blut zirkulierenden Stoffe sind, wie wir sahen, an Plasmaproteine gebunden und können, falls sie nicht ganz oder teilweise abgelöst werden, das Gefäßsystem nur dann verlassen, wenn auch das bindende Eiweiß austritt. Für ihre Abgabe an Zellen ist zuerst das Verhältnis von Haftfestigkeit am Protein zur Affinität der äußeren Zellgrenzfläche maßgebend. Dabei sind 4 Möglichkeiten denkbar:

1. Es stellt sich ein Bindungsgleichgewicht ein zwischen den adsorbierenden Zellgrenzen und den bindenden Plasmaproteinen.

2. Dieser Vorgang wird durch aktiven oder passiven Transport in die Zelle weiter gestaltet. Das kann dadurch gefördert werden, daß im Zellinnern Organellen sich befinden, welche sehr stark absorbierende Oberflächen besitzen und dadurch immer wieder ein Diffusionsgefälle in die Zelle hinein erzeugen (z. B. Mitochondrien s. S. 239). Dadurch wird die adsorbierende Zellgrenze frei, und es muß sich ein neues Gleichgewicht einstellen so lange, bis der gesamte bluteiweißgebundene Stoff oder wenigstens der größte Teil davon in die aufnehmende Zelle eingedrungen ist.

3. Das Trägereiweiß kann selbst in die Zelle eindringen und erst an eine Organelle wiederum durch konkurrierende Adsorption sein Transportgut abgeben (s. S. 239). Das Trägereiweiß selbst bleibt dabei intakt.

4. Das eingedrungene Trägerprotein wird in der Zelle abgebaut und erst dadurch der anhaftende Stoff in Freiheit gesetzt.

Extracapillärer Raum.

Nur an wenigen Orten im Körper gibt es einen unmittelbaren Kontakt zwischen Capillare und Zelle. Fast überall ist ein extracapillärer, extracellulärer Raum oft von großen Ausmaßen dazwischengeschaltet. 10—11% des Körpervolumens beträgt insgesamt der Raum, in welchen sich Beförderungsimpulse des Kreislaufsystems nur mittelbar fortsetzen können. Besonders groß ist seine Bedeutung für den Wasser- und Salzhaushalt, für die Regulierung des Blutvolumens und natürlich auch für die Diffusion; je weiter die Zelle von der Capillare entfernt liegt, um so ungünstiger sind zunächst einmal ihre Stoffwechselbedingungen.

Das Verständnis von Struktur und Funktion des extracapillären Raumes ist durch die chemische Analyse der *mesenchymalen Grundsubstanz* beträchtlich gefördert worden. In und durch diese „Matrix" des Interstitiums, die von Kollagen-, Reticulin- und elastischen Fasern durchzogen wird, findet der Stoffaustausch mit den Zellen statt. Der optisch homogene Inhalt des Bindegewebes ist ein Gemisch von Mucopolysacchariden wechselnden Polymerisationsgrades[1] sowie verschiedenen Wasser-, Protein- und Elektrolytgehaltes.

Rein volumenmäßig kann der interstitielle Raum durch Wassereinlagerung beträchtlich erweitert werden. Während in einzelnen Organen, z. B. in der Haut, die Funktion, Wasser aufnehmen zu können, ein Hilfs- und Entlastungsmechanismus ist, der eine enorme Kapazität besitzt, wirkt sich in anderen, parenchymatösen Organen, z. B. im Gehirn, ein Ödem sehr rasch stark beeinträchtigend aus. Bei ansteigendem Venendruck ist das subcutane Interstitium ein großes Flutbecken, welches mit einem Abfluß in die Körperhöhlen versehen, leicht zu eröffnen ist und durch Verminderung der zirkulierenden Blutmenge eine umfangreiche Kreislaufentlastung zustande kommen läßt, ohne daß ein tödliches Ödem der lebenswichtigen Organe entsteht.

Die Mucopolysaccharide, z. B. leicht lösliche Hyaluronsäure, schwerer extrahierbare Chondroitinschwefelsäuren, bestehen aus sich wiederholenden gleichen Grundeinheiten von Acetylglucosamin und Glucuronsäure bzw. Acetylgalaktosamin, Glucuronsäure und Sulfatresten (β-Heparin) oder sulfoniertem Glucosamin, Glucuronsäure und Sulfaten (α-Heparin) von verschiedenem Polymerisationsgrad[2]. So gut man jetzt diese Substanzen, die sich durch Hyaluronidase unterschiedlicher Herkunft aufspalten lassen, in vitro analysieren kann, so mangelhaft weiß man noch über ihren natürlichen Zustand im Gewebe Bescheid. Jede Änderung des Polymerisationsgrades ändert auch die Viscosität, das Wasserbindungsvermögen und die Bewegbarkeit von Ionen. Der Gehalt an Carboxyl- und Sulfatgruppen ordnet diese Stoffe den sog. Polyelektrolyten zu und verschafft ihnen Eigenschaften als *Ionenaustauscher*[3]. Da Bindungsfestigkeit und Bindungskapazität veränderlich sind, ist auch das Ausmaß der Ionenaufnahme und die Sättigung vom jeweiligen Zustand der Materie abhängig. So können Bedingungen entstehen, welche die Verteilung und Abdiffusion sonst stark gebundener Ionen erleichtern, so daß sich das Adsorbens entleert, ohne daß ein noch stärker gebundenes Ion als Verdränger aufgenommen werden muß. Die Rückverwandlung in den alten Zustand stellt die ursprüngliche Aktivität wieder her. Es ist leicht einzusehen, daß durch Anreicherung und Abgabe von Ionen eine Bewegung entsteht, welche ihrerseits wiederum auf andere physikochemische Zustände des interstitiellen Gewebes zurückwirkt. Schließlich sind Quellungsgrad, Viscosität, Vernetzungsgrad usw. alle von der Ionenstärke abhängig. Chondroitinschwefelsäure[4], besonders aber Hyaluronsäure[5] erwiesen sich als enorm empfindlich gegenüber Veränderungen der Ionenstärke des Natriums knapp unterhalb der Konzentration der physiologischen Kochsalzlösung. Bei Abnahme unter 0,15 molar nahmen Strömungsdoppelbrechung, Trübung und Sedimentationskonstante rasch stark zu, während eine Erhöhung des Salzes kaum einen Einfluß hatte. Dieser Effekt wurde als Aggregation oder als ein Aufrollen der polymeren Ketten gedeutet. Die sauren Gruppen reagieren bereitwillig mit basischen Eiweißkörpern. Besonders fest ist dabei die Bindung der Chondroitinschwefelsäure über die Sulfogruppen mit den Aminogruppen der Skleroproteine. Dadurch werden die Fasern fest in der Grundsubstanz des Bindegewebes verankert. Außerdem werden mit löslichen Proteinen salzartige Komplexe gebildet und verschiedene Fermentreaktionen, wie die Bildung des Thrombins, gehemmt.

Für den extravasculären Stofftransport sind *Wassergehalt* und *Wasserbewegung* durch das Interstitium und die Zellen entscheidend. Die Verschiebung und der Austausch von Wasser gehen sehr rasch vonstatten (s. S. 235), obwohl der wassererfüllte Raum im Körper sehr groß ist[6].

Mit der modernen Methode der Isotopenverdünnungstechnik kann er genau erfaßt werden. Die Verabfolgung von D_2O oder T_2O, welches sich im gesamten Körperwasser gleichmäßig

---

[1] Robb-Smith 1954.   [2] Meyer 1951, Gibian 1955.   [3] Mathews 1953, Gibian 1955.
[4] Blumberg 1955.   [5] Mathews 1953.   [6] Gamble 1950.

verteilt[1], gestattet leicht die Bestimmung des gesamten wassererfüllten Raumes und der Umsatzrate. 50—60% des Körpergewichts gesunder Männer und Frauen sind Wasser (Tabelle 5)[1]. Wenn man mit Hilfe der Antipyrinverdünnung den gleichen Raum bestimmt, dann fällt er 2—5% kleiner aus, weil sich das Antipyrin im proteingebundenen Wasser des Körpers nicht löst[2]. Diesen Raum könnte man in Analogie zu der allgemeinen kolloidchemischen Terminologie nach POLANY als den „nicht lösenden Raum" des menschlichen Körpers bezeichnen, der dann in der Größenordnung eines Liters läge. Da sich Inulin oder Thiosulfat nur im extracellulären Wasser ausbreiten, kann der wassererfüllte Raum weiter differenziert werden[2] (Tabelle 6a u. b). Die Werte aus beiden Methoden stimmen im großen und ganzen überein, obwohl Thiosulfat auch eine geringe Bindung mit dem Plasmaalbumin eingeht[3].

Tabelle 6a u. b. *Verteilungsraum des Körperwassers.*

a) nach GILDER 1954

b) nach IKKOS 1954

Substanz	Verteilungsraum Volumen in % des Körpergewichts (Mittelwerte)	Anzahl der untersuchten Personen	Wasser	Verteilungsraum			Anzahl der untersuchten Personen
				Prozent des Körpergewichts	Prozent des gesamten Körperwassers	Liter je m² Körperoberfläche	
Wasser	54,5 ± 6,6	22	extracelluläres .	14,8	29,9	5,5	
Natrium . . .	28,5	17		**15,2**	**30,5**	**5,7**	9
Blut	6,8 ± 0,9	22	intracelluläres .	34,9	70,1	13,0	
Blutplasma . .	4,0 ± 0,5	22		**34,6**	**69,5**	**12,9**	

Normaldruck = Berechnung aus dem Inulinraum, **Fettdruck** = Berechnung aus dem Thiosulfatraum.

Die Umsatzrate von Wasser beträgt nach HEVESY (1954) u. a.[4] 7,7 ± 1,2% je Tag und ist gleich für Männer und Frauen. Sie ist auch bei Schwangeren nicht anders und unterliegt nur durch die bekannte Diurese der Nachgeburtsperiode einer geringen Schwankung[5]. Herabgesetzt ist der Wasserumsatz, wenn sich Ödeme entwickeln und im Stadium der Präeklampsie. Für die Retention ist die Natriumanhäufung im Gewebe von großer Bedeutung; es ist aber sicher nicht nur die übermäßige Natriumzufuhr und Anreicherung, welche ein Ödem zur Folge haben, sondern auch eine erhöhte Depolymerisation der Bindegewebsmatrix, welche die Quellungsvorgänge im Interstitium erhöht. Bei Lebercirrhose mit Ascites waren stets das Körperwasser und das Körpernatrium vermehrt[6].

Mit Hilfe der Isotopenverdünnungstechnik läßt sich praktisch der „Verteilungsgrad" für jede beliebige in der Körperflüssigkeit gelöste Substanz ermitteln. Dabei hat sich gezeigt, daß die gefundenen Räume stark von dem des Wassers abweichen. Die allgemeinsten Stoffe, auch kleine Ionen, sind im Körper nicht gleich verteilt, sondern z. T. verdünnt, z. T. angereichert. Nimmt man für das Natrium eine Gleichverteilung in Höhe des Blutspiegels an, dann wird es nur in der Hälfte des vom Wasser erfüllten Raumes gefunden. Das intracelluläre Wasser ist beträchtlich natriumärmer als das Blut. Beim Kalium liegen die Verhältnisse bekanntlich umgekehrt; bei einem Blutspiegel von 0,16—0,2 g/l beträgt der mittlere Kaliumgehalt des Gesamtkörpers 1,5 g/kg. Dieses Verhalten findet seine Erklärung in der verschieden starken Affinität der gelösten Stoffe zu Proteinen, Kohlenhydraten o. a. hochpolymeren Substanzen und in der Eigenschaft bestimmter Zellen, unter Energieverbrauch Kalium zu konzentrieren.

Mit Erfolg sind die *Schwundraten markierter Substanzen*, die in verschiedener Weise in Körperhöhlen oder Gewebe appliziert worden waren, gemessen worden. Aus der Abwanderungsgeschwindigkeit oder der Gewebeclearance ließ sich ein Maß für die Haftfestigkeit im Gewebe finden und aus der Ungleichmäßigkeit des Abstroms ein Schluß ziehen auf die durchströmten Räume[7].

Wie zu erwarten war, verteilen sich markierte Serumproteine gleichmäßig über ein intra- und ein extracapilläres Stromgebiet. Beim Gesunden ist etwa 8 Std

---

[1] GILDER 1954, IKKOS 1954, HEVESY 1954.   [2] FRIIS-HANSEN 1951, PRENTICE 1952.
[3] SCHLOERB 1950.   [4] SCHEINBERG 1950.   [5] HUTCHINSON 1954.   [6] GILDER 1954.
[7] FLEXNER 1948, KETY 1948, EICHLER 1949, STONE 1949, HYMAN 1950, SWEET 1950, SCHWERMUND 1954, HORST 1955.

nach intravenöser Injektion einer Testmenge Albumin Gleichverteilung eingetreten; die Lymphe enthält dann die gleiche spezifische Radioaktivität wie das
Blutplasma[1] bzw. das Albumin[2]. In einen Ascites hinein dauert der Ausgleich
bedeutend länger[3]. Rasch dringen die Plasmaproteine und Lipoproteide in die
nicht vascularisierte Aorteninnenhaut ein[4].

Innerhalb der Körperzellen ist der Wassergehalt geringer als in der umgebenden
Flüssigkeit. Es ist daher Arbeit notwendig, um das Wasser aus der Zelle heraus-
zuschaffen. Sie wird von der lebendigen Zelle ununterbrochen geleistet. Bei
Vergiftungen der cellulären Fermentsysteme oder bei Sauerstoffmangel versagt
dieser aktive Wassertransport, der osmotische Druck sinkt, die Zelle bläht sich
auf und platzt.

Lymphe.

Ein Teil der extracellulären Flüssigkeit fließt in einem eigenen Capillar- und
Gefäßsystem als Lymphe. Die Beförderung erfolgt nur langsam, passiv, Klappen
verhindern ein Zurückströmen. Durch den Lymphstrom wird die Entwässerung
des Gewebes gefördert und die nicht mehr in die Capillaren zurückresorbierte
Flüssigkeit dem Kreislauf wieder zugeführt. Es werden aber auch von manchen
Organen gebildete Stoffe, insbesondere Lipoproteide, primär in die Lymphe
abgegeben, und auf diese Weise wird der portale Kreislauf umgangen.

Das *Lymphgefäßsystem* als Transportweg und die Lymphe als Transportmilieu sind in
ihrer Bedeutung lange Zeit unterschätzt. Die Lymphgefäße stellen ein Geflecht von Röhren
dar, deren peripherer *Ursprung in feinen, blind endigenden Säckchen besteht,* durch deren Wandungen außer Wasser und echt gelösten Substanzen auch großmolekulare und corpusculäre
Stoffe aufgenommen werden können wie z. B. Bakterien, Tusche, Quarzkörnchen, Geschwulstzellen und Eiweißkörper. Lymphgefäße finden sich ausschließlich in unmittelbarer Nachbarschaft des Bindegewebes, und zwar sowohl subepithelial im Bereich der inneren und äußeren
Körperoberfläche als auch im bindegewebigen Stützgerüst der Organparenchyme[5]. Alles,
was außerhalb dieses geschlossenen und in den Ductus thoracicus ausmündenden Lymphgefäßsystems im extravasculären Raum liegt, muß als den *Gewebsspalten* zugehörig betrachtet
werden; ihr Flüssigkeitsgehalt besteht nicht aus Lymphe, sondern aus Interstitialflüssigkeit.
Das Lymphgefäßsystem fehlt im Gehirn, im Knorpel, ebenso in allen Epithelien und dem rein
epithelialen Parenchym der großen Drüsen wie der Leber; auch die Disséschen Räume der
Leber gehören also nicht zum Lymphgefäßsystem.

Die Wandungen der größeren Lymphgefäße enthalten Muskelfasern. Für die *Fortbewegung
der Lymphe* spielt die Bewegung der in der Nachbarschaft gelegenen Organe (Muskulatur,
Thoraxkursion) eine große Rolle; ähnlich wie im Venensystem wird jede Druckwirkung aus
der Nachbarschaft auch im Lymphgefäßsystem durch Klappen abgefangen, so daß der Effekt
auf die Strömung sich nur in *einer* Richtung auswirken kann. Die Lymphzirkulation kann
nach Rusznyák[6] insuffizient werden 1. durch *mechanische* Behinderung (Filarien, Thromben,
Narben, Silicatkörner) und durch Lymphangiospasmen, 2. durch starke Erhöhung des
Venendrucks und dadurch bedingte Erschwerung der Entleerung des Ductus thoracicus in den
Angulus venosus *(hämodynamische Insuffizienz),* 3. durch Lähmung der für die Motorik so
wichtigen willkürlichen Muskulatur *(akinetische Insuffizienz),* 4. durch Dilatation der Lymphgefäße und dadurch entstehende Insuffizienz der Lymphgefäß-Klappen *(valvuläre Insuffizienz),*
5. durch vermehrte Transsudation in das Interstitium, z. B. bei Hyponkie oder venöser
Stauung, so daß die Transportkapazität des Lymphgefäßsystems überschritten ist und zur
normalen Drainage nicht mehr ausreicht *(dynamische oder relative Insuffizienz),* 6. wahrscheinlich auch durch Resorptionsbehinderung im Gebiet der resorbierenden Lymphgefäß-
membranen *(Resorptionsinsuffizienz).* Auch im Lymphgefäßsystem sollen die Eiweißkörper
eine *Vehikel*funktion[7] erfüllen.

Die Drainage- und Reinigungswirkung seitens des Lymphgefäßsystems gilt insbesondere
dem ihm anliegenden Bindegewebe. Das in der Lymphe enthaltene Wasser wird aus dem
Blutcapillarsystem auf der arteriolennahen Strecke in das Interstitium abgezweigt, wo einerseits der hämodynamische Druck noch höher ist als der onkotische und wo andererseits die
Gefäßwand bereits zart genug ist, um Wasser durchtreten zu lassen. Die so aus der Blutbahn

---

[1] Forker 1952.   [2] Sterling 1951, Wassermann 1951, Lewallen 1959.
[3] Schoenberger 1953, Berson 1954.   [4] Ott 1958, Meyer-Friedman 1959.
[5] Grau 1960.   [6] Rusznyák 1957, 1960.   [7] Földi 1957, 1960.

ausgetretene eiweißarme Flüssigkeit gelangt auf zwei Wegen zurück in die Blutbahn: 1. durch sofortige Rückresorption in den venolenwärts gelegenen Capillaranteil; 2. durch Übergang vom Interstitium in die langsam strömende Lymphe und mit ihr dann via Ductus thoracicus in die großen Venen. Der letztere Weg dient wohl normalerweise nur für einen kleinen Anteil als Rückflußstrecke in die Blutbahn. Unter pathologischen Umständen und bei besonderer Beanspruchung kann der Lymphweg jedoch zweifellos auch für die Zurückführung der interstitiellen Flüssigkeit in die Blutbahn — gewissermaßen als Reservestrombett mit langsamer Flüssigkeitsbewegung — von großer Wichtigkeit sein. In den peripheren Lymphgefäßen der Haut legt der Lymphstrom in 5 min eine Entfernung von 10—15 cm zurück[1].

Die Lymphmenge, die sich aus dem Ductus thoracicus dem Blut zumischt, wird auf wenige Kubikzentimeter je Minute (im Durchschnitt 0,5—2 cm^3) geschätzt, gegenüber der transcapillär abgegebenen Wassermenge von 20—30 cm^3 je Minute nur eine kleine Menge. Auf die Bedeutung der Lymphstagnation in der Lunge bei der Entstehung des Lungenödems und der stauungsbedingten Herz- und Lebernekrosen haben RUSZNYÁK[2] und seine Schule besonders hingewiesen.

Transportvorgänge an den Zellgrenzen.

Der passive Transport wird durch die physikalischen Größen der Filtration und Diffusion interpretiert. Leider ist es sehr schwierig, die einzelnen Meßgrößen so zu vereinheitlichen, daß genaue Angaben gewonnen werden können. Für den Transport bestimmter Stoffe wäre das von Wichtigkeit. Da aber sehr zahlreiche Faktoren aufeinander abgestimmt wirken, hat man sich gewöhnlich mit summarischen Angaben begnügt und ist damit auch der Versuchung entgangen, bestimmte Einzelgrößen zu überwerten.

Passiver Transport (Filtration und Diffusion).

Porengröße. Der mit einer Basalmembran und einem lockeren Belag von Adventitiazellen ausgestattete Endothelschlauch der Capillare besitzt keine mit dem Lichtmikroskop sichtbaren Stomata. Sollen Blutzellen austreten, dann ist ein direkter Angriff an oder zwischen den Endothelzellen mit Auflösung der Wand durch Hyaluronidase notwendig; ein nachfolgender Verschluß der Lücke stellt die Integrität des Gefäßes wieder her.

Im *Phasenkontrastverfahren* erscheint die Basalzone der Endothelzellen der Aorta zwar als löcheriger, syncytialer Verband; die lumennahen Zellschichten sind aber noch homogen und scharf begrenzt (hyaloplasmatische Deckplatte[3]). Es muß jedoch dahingestellt bleiben, ob sich diese an der Intima der Aorta erhobenen Befunde verallgemeinern lassen.

Elektronenmikroskopische Untersuchungen haben gezeigt, daß einzelne Elemente der Capillarwand der Glomerula eine poröse Struktur besitzen. So ist bekannt, daß sowohl das Capillarendothel wie auch die Deckzellen im Normalzustand keinen geschlossenen, lückenlosen Verband bilden. Es fehlt allerdings der Beweis dafür, daß diese Porenstruktur für die Filtration eine maßgebende Rolle spielt: die Durchmesser der *Endothelzellporen* sind mit 500—1000 Å[4] mehrfach größer als die Proteinmoleküle; die kleinsten gemessenen „*Schlitzporen*" *der Deckzellen* besitzen mit 70—100 Å[5] zwar eine ähnliche Größe wie die Proteine, doch sind diese Schlitzporen gerade bei denjenigen Krankheiten verschlossen und durch eine homogene Cytoplasmaschicht ersetzt, die mit einer starken Proteinurie und glomerulären Eiweißfiltration einhergehen[6]. In seinen ersten Untersuchungen fand HALL[7] auch in der *Basalmembran* eine Porenstruktur, doch sind diese Befunde später nicht bestätigt worden[8]. Die Basalmembran stellt vielmehr die einzige kontinuierliche Grenzschicht dar, durch die hindurch die Filtration stattfinden muß. In ihrer Zusammensetzung aus Mucoproteinen und fibrillären Untereinheiten[9]

---

[1] HUDACK 1933.　　[2] RUSZNYÁK 1955.　　[3] LINZBACH 1952,　　[4] RHODIN 1954, PEASE 1955.
[5] HALL 1953.　　[6] PIEL 1955, MILLER 1956, FARQUHAR 1957.　　[7] HALL 1953.
[8] RHODIN 1954, PEASE 1955, BARGMANN 1955, MILLER 1956.　　[9] RHODIN 1955.

besitzt sie einen Gel-ähnlichen Aufbau; es ist daher zu diskutieren, ob letzthin nicht das Maschenwerk des Gelnetzes für die Filtration maßgeblich ist und unter pathologischen Bedingungen in seiner Struktur und Durchlässigkeit verändert wird.

Es erscheint bisher noch nicht entschieden, wie mit den morphologischen Befunden die Theorie von Pappenheimer[1] in Einklang gebracht werden kann. Er fand, daß eine mathematisch definierbare Beziehung zwischen Filtration und Größe der Proteinmoleküle besteht und errechnete daraus „Poren" mit einem Halbmesser von etwa 35 Å. Die Gesamtfläche dieser „Poren" wurde auf $2\,^0/_{00}$ der Capillarfläche berechnet. In Muskelcapillaren sollen 2×10^9 Poren je cm^2 Capillarfläche vorhanden sein.

Die *Filtrationsgeschwindigkeit* ist abhängig von der effektiven *Filtrationsfläche*, dem effektiven *Filtrationsdruck* und der „*Permeabilität*"; die letztere entspricht der Beschaffenheit der Membran hinsichtlich Porengestalt, -größe, -länge, -zahl und aller anderen Faktoren, welche auf die Passage durch das Filter wirken können. Diese Permeabilität ist eine Größe, welche steten Veränderungen unterworfen sein muß. Schon die Dehnung allein verdünnt die Gefäßwand. Wenn eine Capillare ihren Radius von $3\,\mu$ auf $5\,\mu$ vergrößert, nimmt die Wanddicke etwa auf die Hälfte, nämlich von $0{,}94\,\mu$ auf $0{,}5\,\mu$ ab. Es ist geradezu undenkbar, daß solche Änderungen der Zellbeschaffenheit ohne Einfluß auf die Filtereigenschaften sein würden. Normalerweise herrscht beständig ein Spiel zwischen Erweiterung und Verengerung, welches als *Vasomotion* periodische Funktionsänderungen umfaßt[2]. Dabei — und nicht in einem allzu schematischen Modell einer fast starr gedachten Haarröhre — geht der Flüssigkeitsaus- und -einstrom vor sich. Die Messungen der Capillardruckhöhe von Landis (1932) haben so starke Unterschiede ergeben, daß man gezwungen ist anzunehmen, daß meistens in einem Teil der Capillaren reine Filtrationsprozesse ablaufen, während in benachbarten Gefäßen wiederum nur rückresorbiert wird. In der Haut ließen sich in recht nahe beieinander liegenden Capillaren beträchtliche Druckunterschiede messen. Das alte, fruchtbare Starlingsche Modell ist nur selten verwirklicht. Wahrscheinlich erfolgt in den langen Stromcapillaren des nutritiven Strombetts *sowohl* Flüssigkeitsein- wie -ausstrom, während in den Netzcapillaren filtriert oder rückresorbiert wird. Die muskulären Verschlußmechanismen an beiden Enden des Capillarsystems können leicht bewirken, daß die arterienwärts ankommenden Druckwellen im Haargefäß selbst zur Wirkung kommen oder vorher aufgebraucht werden. Um den effektiven Filtrationsdruck zu erhalten, muß von der Differenz der hydrostatischen intra- oder extracapillären Drucke die der osmotischen Drucke abgezogen werden. In den Wert der effektiven Filtrationsfläche geht auch die Strömungsgeschwindigkeit ein.

Die Vasomotion, die rhythmische Kaliberschwankung der Gefäße kann[3] nach Frequenz, Amplitude und der relativen Dauer der Kontraktionsphasen verstärkt oder herabgesetzt sein. Sie ist humoral gesteuert, erhält entscheidende Impulse aber auch auf nervalem Wege.

Um 2 Beispiele für die *absolute Größe des Flüssigkeitdurchtritts* durch Capillaren zu geben, seien die Versuche von Landis (1928) genannt, der am Froschmesenterium $56 \cdot 10^{-8}$ cm³/sec. je Quadratzentimeter Capillarfläche und Zentimeter Wasserdruckdifferenz fand, und von Pappenheimer (1948), der an der Katzenextremität $2{,}5 \cdot 10^{-8}$ bestimmte. Dazu mußte er eine Capillaroberfläche von 7000 cm² je 100 g annehmen. Die Filtrationsgeschwindigkeit war bei ihm proportional dem effektiven Filtrationsdruck. Bei einem Stauversuch am menschlichen Arm nimmt die Filtrationsgeschwindigkeit dagegen kontinuierlich ab, weil die extracapilläre hydrostatische und der kolloidosmotische Druck stärker zunehmen als der Venendruck. Der Versuch veranschaulicht lebhaft die Bedeutung der bei der Stauung unterbundenen Lymphströmung für den Flüssigkeitsaustritt aus den Capillaren.

Wenn die Filtration, das Produkt aus Filtrationsdruck und Filtrationsfläche, kleiner wird als die Resorption, das Produkt aus Resorptionsdruck und Re-

---

[1] Pappenheimer 1954.   [2] Chambers und Zweifach 1947, Nicoll 1946.
[3] Chambers 1947.

sorptionsfläche, dann fließt die filtrierte Flüssigkeit quantitativ in das Gefäß zurück. Einseitige Veränderungen dieser Größen müssen die extravasculäre Flüssigkeit vergrößern oder verkleinern. Einer Ansammlung wird vorgebeugt durch Bildung von *Lymphe*, welche in den allseits geschlossenen Lymphcapillaren zusammenströmt und gegen den Venenwinkel zu abfließt.

Farbstoffinjektionen in Gefäße und Mikroskopie mit hochauflösenden Systemen gestatten die *unmittelbare Verfolgung* von Flüssigkeitsströmen. Es gelingt mit dem Mikromanipulator, feinste Haargefäße zu punktieren und dann an bestimmten Stellen der Capillare eventuell das fontänenartige[1] Austreten von Farbstoffwolken zu beobachten. Auch der Weitertransport von Farbstoffen in die Lymphgefäße der Bindehaut ist verfolgt worden[2]. Als Etikette für den unter pathologischen Bedingungen sichtbaren Albuminaustritt dienten die albumingebundenen Farbstoffe Trypanblau[3] und Geigyblau[4]; Äskulin, welches zum größten Teil nicht an Eiweiß gebunden wird, zeigte durch seine Fluorescenz die Orte an, wo eiweißfreies Ultrafiltrat durchtreten kann.

Die *Diffusionsvorgänge* werden durch den Capillardruck nur indirekt beeinflußt. Bei einem erhöhten Druck wird das Gefäß ausgeweitet, und der Diffusionsweg nimmt ab; strömt dabei die intracapilläre Flüssigkeit rascher, dann kann auch die effektive Konzentration abnehmen. Anstelle der Druckdifferenz ist die Konzentrationsdifferenz wirksam, so daß die Diffusionsgeschwindigkeit von der effektiven Diffusionsfläche, der Differenz zwischen intra- und extracapillärer Konzentration und wiederum einem Faktor abhängig ist, der die Capillarwandeigenschaften repräsentiert. Auch hierfür wird der Ausdruck „Permeabilität" benutzt. Den Faktor der Wanddicke, nämlich den Diffusionsweg, aus der Permeabilität herauszulösen, ist wohl eine kaum gerechtfertigte Vereinfachung, da sich auch die Eigenschaften von Endothel- und Basalmembran je nach dem Dehnungsgrad ändern. Dabei ist es wiederum wahrscheinlich, daß bei einer Verdünnung der Wand nicht nur der Diffusionsweg abnimmt, sondern auch die restierende Permeabilität zunimmt, so daß die Abdiffusion mehr begünstigt wird, als es nur der Abnahme der Wanddicke entspricht. Gleichfalls begünstigt wird sie durch eine Vergrößerung der Diffusionsfläche bei optimaler Strömungsgeschwindigkeit.

Der Beitrag der Diffusion zu transcapillären Austauschvorgängen ist sehr groß. Insbesondere Untersuchungen mit Isotopen haben gezeigt, daß kleine Moleküle den Kreislauf außerordentlich rasch verlassen. Innerhalb einer Minute sind bereits 105% des Blutplasmawassers mit extravasculärem Wasser und 78% des Plasma-Natriums mit extravasculärem Natrium ausgetauscht[5]. Beide Stoffe treten also nicht im gleichen Verhältnisse aus, wie KROGH 1937 meinte. Es ist unwahrscheinlich, daß als Durchtrittsort ausschließlich die Intercellularsubstanz dient, welche ja nur 1% der Capillarwandfläche[6] bildet. Auch durch die Endothelzellen selbst müssen bestimmte Stoffe diffundieren können.

Über die Feinstruktur der Capillar- und Zellmembranen ist nur wenig bekannt. Schon die Filtration ist nicht nur vom Durchmesser und der Länge der Poren oder Kanäle abhängig. Wandpotential, Quellungsgrad, überhaupt die Materialbeschaffenheit wirken befördernd oder hemmend auf die Flüssigkeitsströmung. In noch viel größerem Maße ist der chemische Aufbau der Wand, die Verteilung lipophiler und hydrophiler Komponenten, ihr Wassergehalt, ihr Gehalt an Strukturproteinen usw. von Einfluß auf die in der Flüssigkeit gelösten Substanzen. Noch bevor man aktive, transportfördernde Stoffwechselvorgänge in Betracht zieht, hat man alle physikalisch-chemischen Faktoren zu berücksichtigen. Eine für den Transport höchst bedeutungsvolle Größe ist die *Adsorptionsfähigkeit*

---

[1] VOLLWILER 1955, BARGMANN 1955.   [2] KNÜSEL 1954.
[3] GOLDMANN 1909, PFUHL 1931, BARGMANN 1955.
[4] SAUTTER 1954.   [5] FLEXNER 1948.   [6] CHAMBERS 1947.

der Capillarwand für Ionen und Ionenkomplexe. Besteht an einer Stelle der Gefäßwand eine starke Affinität für einen bestimmten Stoff, dann wird er aus der anströmenden Flüssigkeit an die Wand fixiert, wenn er nur nahe genug angespült wurde. Die weitesten bindungsvermittelnden Kräfte reichen aber nur 10 mμ in das Gefäßlumen, das einen Durchmesser von 7000 mμ hat, hinein! Die meisten mit dem Blut ankommenden Stoffe könnten im gleichmäßigen Dahinfließen dabei nicht nahe genug an die Wand herangelangen, wenn nicht die turbulente Strömung und die Wasserbewegung senkrecht zur Wand das Herantreten begünstigen würde.

Um die Bedeutung der *Textur einer Membran* für ihre Durchdringbarkeit zu veranschaulichen, sei auf die klassische Permeabilitätslehre von biologischen Membranen verwiesen[1]. Die an Pflanzenzellen, Seeigeleiern, Erythrocyten o. a. geeigneten, großen Einzelzellen angestellten Versuche lassen sich aber nicht unmittelbar auf die Capillarwand übertragen, schon weil neben der Endothelzelle auch noch die Zwischenzellsubstanz vorhanden ist. Erstere ist nur bedingt mit anderen Zellen vergleichbar, und letztere ist überhaupt keine Zelle. Trotzdem sind seit jeher die Erkenntnisse über die Diffusion lipoidlöslicher Stoffe erfolgreich auf menschliche Verhältnisse übertragen und 1901 von Overton zur Narkosetheorie ausgebaut worden. Neuerdings wurde wieder experimentell bestätigt, daß die Passage von Drogen in den Liquor cerebrospinalis hauptsächlich durch die physikalischen Eigenschaften der Ionisation der Droge und der Lipoidlöslichkeit des undissoziierten Moleküls bestimmt ist. Für undissoziierte Stoffe ist die Lipoidlöslichkeit allein maßgebend und für ionisierte Stoffe das Verhalten des undissoziierten Anteils bei p$_H$ 7,4[2]. Für das Ausmaß des Übertritts in den Liquor cerebrospinalis spielt daneben natürlich die Bindung an Plasmaeiweiß eine Rolle.

Die ursprüngliche Lipoidtheorie von Overton[3] hat aber nicht in allen Fällen voll befriedigt, sondern mußte zur Lipoid-Porentheorie der Permeabilität erweitert werden[4]. Beim Studium der Penetration geeigneter Pflanzenzellmembranen von Chara ceratophylla stieg die Penetrationsfähigkeit für verschiedene Stoffe nicht nur mit dem Verteilungskoeffizienten der untersuchten Substanzen zwischen Olivenöl und Wasser, sondern auch mit der Abnahme der Molekularvolumina an. Allgemein galt stets, daß das Eindringen der Fettlöslichkeit parallel geht und durch nicht polare Gruppen (Alkyle, Halogene) vergrößert, durch polare (Hydroxyl, Amino, Carboxyl) eher verringert wird (Overtonsche Regel). Im besonderen Falle der Membran als kompliziert aufgebautem Mosaik lipophiler und hydrophiler Strukturen[5] diffundieren kleine, gut lipoidlösliche Stoffe aber schneller als größere, gleich gut lösliche. Das konnte nur als Behinderung der Diffusion durch die Gewebedichte der lipophilen Membranen gedeutet werden[6]. In gleicher Weise verhalten sich nichtdissoziierte schwache Säuren und Basen[7].

Austauschdiffusion. Durch Kombination von Adsorption und Diffusion kommt ein Penetrationsvorgang zustande, welcher mit dem Modell der Ionenaustauschchromatographie vergleichbar ist. Das adsorbierende Medium an der Wand strebt die Auffüllung nach allen Seiten hin an, und wenn seine Affinität zu einem haftfähigen Stoff groß ist, werden dabei wandeigene Moleküle abgegeben. Hat sich die Wand genügend stark angereichert, dann tritt auch nach der anderen Seite hin eine Abdiffusion ein. Sie wird begünstigt, wenn die Konzentration jenseits des Gefäßes gering ist, und wenn der nachfolgend adsorbierte Stoff nun seinerseits verdrängt wird. Die Austauschdiffusion selbst ist kein aktives Transportgeschehen, es ist aber wohl sehr häufig so, daß in der Zelle die Weiterleitung durch energiefordernde Stoffwechselprozesse gefördert wird. Indem neugebildete Adsorptionsgleichgewichte immer wieder gestört werden, wird das Durchtreten durch die Wand begünstigt. Durch dieses enge Miteinanderwirken von aktivem und passivem Transport ist das Ausmaß der Austauschdiffusion sehr schwer abzuschätzen[8].

Aktiver Transport.

Durch physikalische Vorgänge allein ist der Stoffdurchtritt durch die Capillaren nicht erklärt. Sehr häufig superponieren sich Transportmechanismen, welche einer aktiven, oft sehr komplizierten chemischen Leistung der Zellwände, insbesondere

---

[1] Brooks 1941, Davson 1943, Höber 1947.   [2] Brodie 1960.   [3] Overton 1899.
[4] Collander 1933.   [5] Schmidt 1939.   [6] Collander 1933, Ruhland 1925.
[7] Poijärvi 1928.   [8] Ussing 1949.

der Capillarzellwände entstammen. Heute wird das ganze System von passiver Durchlässigkeit und aktiven Verschiebungen gerne als das „Leck- und Pumpe-Prinzip" bezeichnet.

Lange hat man der Zellmembran einen vorwiegend passiven Charakter bei Stoffdurchtritten zugeschrieben. Ihre Siebeigenschaften, ihre durch einen wenig veränderlichen Aufbau gegebene Porengröße oder ihre Lösungseigenschaften, für bestimmte Stoffe z. B. für Lipoide, schienen das Maß für den Membran-Widerstand oder die eigentliche Permeabilität zu sein. Die Beobachtungen bei der Stoffaufnahme und Konzentrierung in Zellen, insbesondere in Erythrocyten haben der Membran aber einen weit bedeutenderen, aktiven Teil in der Zellmaschinerie zugewiesen. Wenn es bisher auch noch nicht gelungen ist, transportierende Fermente der Zellmembran zu isolieren, so ist an einem Fermente benötigenden Transport kein Zweifel mehr.

Der „*enzymatische Transport*" (WILBRANDT u. ROSENBERG 1951) läuft unabhängig von Konzentrationsgradienten durch die kombinierte Tätigkeit zweier Oberflächenfermente zu beiden Seiten der Membran ab. Das Substrat wird dabei in eine membranlösliche Transportform überführt, welche in einer besonderen Wechselwirkung zwischen Substrat und einem membraneigenen Träger („Carrier") besteht. Die Transportrichtung entspricht den natürlichen Diffusionstendenzen von Träger + Stoff. Im besonderen Falle des „thermodynamisch aktiven Transportes" folgt das Substrat so dem Träger, daß es von einem Ort niederen chemischen Potentials zu einem höheren gelangt (ROSENBERG 1948). Zu dieser Deutung haben im wesentlichen folgende Beobachtungen geführt: Die Erklärung durch Diffusion allein hat versagt, durch gleichzeitig penetrierende Substanzen kommen Verdrängungseffekte zustande, es besteht eine hohe strukturelle Spezifität, insbesondere Stereospezifität und Enzym-Effectoren (Inhibitoren oder Aktivatoren) sind wirksam. Außerdem machen die rechnerischen Ansätze der Reaktionsgenetik des Membrantransportes Fermentprozesse wahrscheinlich[1].

So wird der einfache Prozeß der CO_2-Diffusion durch die Carboanhydrase gesteuert[2]. Die Kaliumionenaufnahme durch biologische Membranen hindurch ist an die Anwesenheit von Cholinesterase gebunden[3], die wiederum dem Eindringen von Natrium entgegenwirkt. Noch besser erforscht ist der aktive Transport von Phosphationen und Glucose[4]. Die dabei mitwirkenden Fermente sind in das Proteingerüst der Zelle eingebaut und wirken als Carrier, indem sie einen reversiblen Komplex mit dem zu transportierenden Stoff bilden (LE FÈVRE 1951). So wird Phosphat in endergonischer Reaktion zu energiereichen Polyphosphaten[5] oder in Adenosintriphosphat[6] aufgebaut, welche dann durch Sekundärreaktionen in die eigentlichen transportablen Phosphorverbindungen umgewandelt werden. Da es sich dabei in erster Linie um Zucker-Phosphorsäure-Ester handelt, nimmt auch die Glucose an dem aktiven, transcapillären Transport teil[7].

Der Stoffdurchtritt durch die Capillarwand kann aktiv durch Reaktionen mit dem durchtretenden Substrat oder aber durch einen fermentativen Angriff an der Struktur der Wand beeinflußt werden.

Die Hyaluronidase und andere, die Kohlenhydratgruppen der Kittleisten (intercellular cement) beeinflussende Fermente gehören hierher[8], und eine Reihe von Hyaluronidaseinhibitoren werden zur therapeutischen Gefäßabdichtung benützt.

Außerdem wirken bestimmte Hormone auf die Capillarwand und die Elektrolytverteilung. Über den gefäßverengenden Effekt hinaus verhält sich Adrenalin capillarabdichtend, der Hyaluronidase entgegengesetzt. Auch die Nebennierenrinde drosselt die Schleusenfunktion der Capillarwand. Dabei soll den 11-Oxy-

---

[1] WILBRANDT 1956. [2] TOMASHEFSKI 1953, SHEPARD 1954. [3] HOLLAND 1950.
[4] SPIEGELMANN 1948, SACKS 1948, POPJAK 1950, ROTHSTEIN 1951. [5] ROTHSTEIN 1951.
[6] LINDBERG 1950. [7] LE FÈVRE 1948 und ROSENBERG 1956.
[8] ELSTER 1949, ZWEIFACH 1949.

steroiden[1] und dem Cortison[2] eher ein unmittelbarer Angriffsmodus zugrunde liegen als eine Hemmung der Hyaluronidase[3]. Die Capillardichtung wurde sogar so gleichmäßig gefunden, daß sie als Maß für eine verstärkte Aktivität des Hypophysen-Nebennierenrindensystems gebraucht werden könnte[4]. Eine sichere Wirksamkeit kommt auch den Sexualhormonen zu. Die Erhöhung der Capillardurchlässigkeit in der Schwangerschaft steht im Einklang mit dem Befund, daß sowohl Progesteron als auch Choriogonadotropin[5] die Permeabilität für Eiweiß und Farbstoffe steigern. Neben den klassischen Hormonen ist eine Vielzahl von Wirkstoffen des Gewebes (Gewebshormonen) bei der Steuerung des transcapillären Stoffdurchtritts beteiligt bzw. erhält unter pathologischen Bedingungen eine ausschlaggebende Bedeutung. Am besten bekannt ist der klassische Effekt des Histamins: Stase, Blutüberfüllung und Exsudation ins Interstitium. In Zusammenhang mit Schädigungen, Schocks oder Entzündungen ist es gelungen, das Auftreten permeabilitätssteigernder Stoffe nachzuweisen, die bisher aber nicht näher chemisch definiert werden konnten. Die sog. Entzündungsstoffe Menkins wie Leukotaxin, Exsudin u. a. sind Polypeptide oder Eiweißkörper hoher Wirksamkeit, die nur in sehr geringen Mengen auftreten und nur im biologischen Versuch getestet werden konnten.

Vitalspeicherung als Typus eines bis in die Zelle hineinreichenden Transportvorganges mit selektiven Ablagerungsplätzen.

Die Verfolgung von injizierten Farbstoffen stellt eine einfache und gute Möglichkeit dar, Transportphänomene bis in die Zelle hinein zu beobachten. Seit Einführung der Farbstoffe in experimentelle Arbeitsmethoden beschäftigt man sich mit Vitalfärbung und Vitalspeicherung (s. Band II/1 dieses Handbuches). Bei der Speicherung wird der Farbstoff in bestimmten Zellen angereichert und festgehalten. Allen, die solche Arbeiten ausführen, auch wenn sie ihren Blick vornehmlich auf das Ende des Geschehens, die Ablagerung, richten, mußte der Vorgang als ein Transport von Farbstoff erscheinen.

Die Zelle, welche begierig Farbstoff aufnimmt, um ihn zu speichern, kann ihn nur kraft einer besonders starken Bindung anziehen und festhalten. Über die hohe Affinität der Zelle hinaus ist zumeist außerdem ein ordnendes Prinzip wirksam, welches nicht in der vitalspeichernden Zelle selbst gesucht werden darf. Nur bei einem kontinuierlichen Angebot an Farbstoff ist zu erreichen, daß der Vorgang des Auffüllens optimal abläuft. Deshalb ist die Zufuhr zum Speicher dann am ergiebigsten, wenn das Speichergut durch Eiweißvehikel im Zirkulationssystem zunächst von zahlreichen anderen Zellgruppen zurückgehalten und der bestimmten Zelle mit der maximalen Affinität immer wieder angeboten wird.

Wie schon ausgeführt, setzen sich Speicher und Eiweißvehikel in ein Gleichgewicht, welches langsam und kontinuierlich gestört wird. Die Störquellen sind Verlust durch Zerstörung und Ausscheidung. Bei der Farbstoffinjektion werden die Eiweißvehikel belastet und tragen das gebundene Transportgut an die aufnahmefähigen Speicher heran. Dort geben sie es bis zur Auffüllung ab, d. h. so lange, bis sich ein Gleichgewicht eingestellt hat. Für leicht zu speichernde Substanzen liegt es ganz auf Seite der Speicherzellen, für nichtgespeicherte Stoffe läßt es einen größeren, an Eiweiß gebundenen oder auch freien, ganz ungebundenen Anteil zu. Dieser kann durch Diffusion oder aktive Aufnahme ohne erhebliche Konzentrationssteigerung in die Zelle eindringen, wird aber relativ rasch kontinuierlich verringert, wenn infolge Verbrauchs im Stoffwechsel oder Ausscheidung

---

[1] Menkin 1953.   [2] Robson 1952.   [3] Hechter 1950.
[4] Scarborough 1944, Wilhelm 1944, Kramar 1953, Menkin 1953, Moon 1952.
[5] Lurie 1950.

die Konzentration im Blut wieder abfällt. Es ist wieder eine Folge des Gleichgewichtes, daß auch die aufgefüllten Speicher langsam leerlaufen, weil sich die Farbstoffkonzentration im Plasma als Folge einer Eliminierung durch die Nierentubuli oder eines Verbrauchs an einer anderen Stelle des Stoffwechsels vermindert. — Daraus erhellt ohne weiteres, daß die Eiweißvehikel regulierend den fixen Speichern vorgeschaltet sind (vgl. Bilirubin S. 198).

Für die intracelluläre Farbstoffanreicherung sind präexistente Organellen, und zwar die *Mitochondrien*, notwendig, welche eine stärkere Farbstoffbindung aufweisen als die Eiweißvehikel. Ablagerungsorte, welche erst durch die Farbstoffe in der Zelle entstehen, konnten bisher nicht nachgewiesen werden (SEYBOLD 1956).

Die Mitochondrien (s. Band II/1 dieses Handbuches) zeigen in vivo und in vitro eine außerordentlich große Adsorptionsfähigkeit sowohl den sauren Farbstoffen (Trypanblau, Lithiumcarmin, Evansblue, Kongorot) als auch den basischen Farbstoffen (Brillantkresylviolett, Bismarckbraun, Neutralrot, Methylenblau, Janusgrün, Acridinorange) gegenüber[1]. Die Anlagerung an die isolierten Mitochondrien geschieht in vitro seitens der basischen Farbstoffe sehr viel schneller (mit signifikanten Unterschieden 10 bzw. 60 min nach Beginn der Farbstoffeinwirkung) als seitens der sauren Farbstoffe.

Durch adsorbierte Farbstoffe wird in der Warburg-Apparatur eine deutliche Herabsetzung des O_2-Verbrauches der Mitochondrien bewirkt. Die Intensität dieser Stoffwechselbremsung war bei Trypanblau am schwächsten und stieg über Lithiumcarmin, Methylenblau, Janusgrün, Neutralrot, Acridinorange an (SEYBOLD 1956).

Bei polarisationsmikroskopischer Betrachtung zeigen die Mitochondrien eine schwache Form- und Eigendoppelbrechung. Sie erfährt durch Zusatz von Farbstoffen keine Zunahme; Zusatz von Serum verstärkt sie nur gering. Setzt man dagegen den isolierten Mitochondrien Serum + Farbstoff (Kongorot, Evansblue) zu, so zeigt sich eine erhebliche Zunahme der Doppelbrechung, die auf eine besonders gerichtete, *strukturbedingte Einlagerung des Eiweißfarbstoffkomplexes in das Mitochondrienprotein* hinweist[2].

Daß auch das Vehikel zusammen mit seiner Last in bestimmte speichernde Zellen einzudringen vermag, zeigten die Versuche von BENNHOLD und SEYBOLD (1952) an der Molchniere. Bringt man durch die Bauchhöhle des Molchs Trypanblau in wäßriger Lösung direkt an die Epithelien der offenen Nephronen heran, dann wird es *fein*granulär gespeichert, und zwar mit dem Speicherungsmaximum in den *proximalen* Tubulusanteilen. Bringt man auf dem gleichen Wege Trypanblau in Molch- oder Menschenserum gelöst in die Tubuli hinein, dann wird der Farbstoff *grob*granulär (sagokornartig) gespeichert mit einem Ablagerungsmaximum im *distalen* Teil der Tubuli contorti I. Die KimmelstielFärbung ergab eiweißartige Blaufärbung der intracellulären „Sagokörner". Es konnte ferner nachgewiesen werden, daß bei der Speicherung von bestimmten Vitalfarbstoffen auch der Gehalt an Serumprotein in den speichernden Zellen und deren Mitochondrien signifikant ansteigt[3]. Allerdings mußte man in Betracht ziehen, daß bei dieser intracellulären Eiweißanreicherung, die durch Anhäufung radiomarkierten Serumproteins kenntlich gemacht wurde, möglicherweise eine durch den gespeicherten Farbstoff bedingte Bremsung der Stoffwechselprozesse und eine Verlangsamung der normalen Eiweißabbauvorgänge eine Rolle spielt.

Schließlich läßt sich histologisch mit der Methode der fluorescierenden Antikörper[4] in den Kupfferschen Sternzellen von Mensch, Ratte und Meerschweinchen Albumin und γ-Globulin, in den Leberzellen eine Spur von Albumin nachweisen[5]. Die Mitochondrienfraktion der Rattenleber enthielt in sehr geringen Mengen immunologisch nachweisbares Albumin[6]. Dieser Albumingehalt ist aber nicht ein wesentlicher Grund für das starke Farbstoffadsorptionsvermögen, zumal sich durch besondere Elutionsverfahren aus den isolierten Mitochondrien ein sehr viel stärker farbstoffbindender Eiweißkörper darstellen ließ[7]. Andere Versuche

---

[1] Literatur-Übersicht SEYBOLD 1956.   [2] MISSMAHL 1955.
[3] BENNHOLD 1953, 1955.   [4] COONS 1951.   [5] WOLLENSAK 1956.
[6] KALLEE 1954.   [7] KALLEE 1956.

zeigten auch, daß Serumproteine in nicht mehr auswaschbarer Menge aufgenommen wurden[1].

Am Beispiel der Vitalfärbung der Kupfferschen Zellen in der Rattenleber läßt sich der spezielle Transportvorgang in die Zelle hinein folgendermaßen analysieren:

1. Der ins Blut gelangte Farbstoff ist seiner Adsorptionsisotherme entsprechend am Plasmaprotein gebunden; d. h. er ist entweder praktisch ganz gebunden, wenn seine Affinität zu Eiweiß groß und seine Konzentration klein ist, oder nur zum Teil gebunden, besonders wenn seine Eiweißbindung schwach und seine Konzentration groß ist. Während der eiweißgebundene Farbstoff dem Weg des Eiweißes folgt, besetzt der freie Farbstoff alle adsorbierenden Medien und geht ein neues Gleichgewicht (auch mit dem eiweißgebundenen Anteil) ein.

2. Die intracellulär gelegenen Mitochondrien der speichernden Zellen zeigen eine intensive Bindungsfähigkeit den Farbstoffen gegenüber, welche aus der Blutbahn an Eiweiß gebunden oder auch nicht gebunden in das Zellinnere gelangen. Es besteht dadurch ständig ein Diffusionsgefälle in die Zelle hinein. Schließlich wird der Farbstoff in die Struktur der Mitochondrien eingelagert. Der Farbstoffgehalt des Blutes nimmt dadurch ab. Befand sich ein Teil des Farbstoffes zunächst an andere, weniger stark bindende Grenzflächen adsorbiert, dann wird er mit fallendem Blutspiegel von dort wieder abgelöst, um über die Vehikelbindung schließlich bis in den Speicher zu gelangen, vorausgesetzt, daß die Speicher in gleicher Weise aufnahmefähig bleiben.

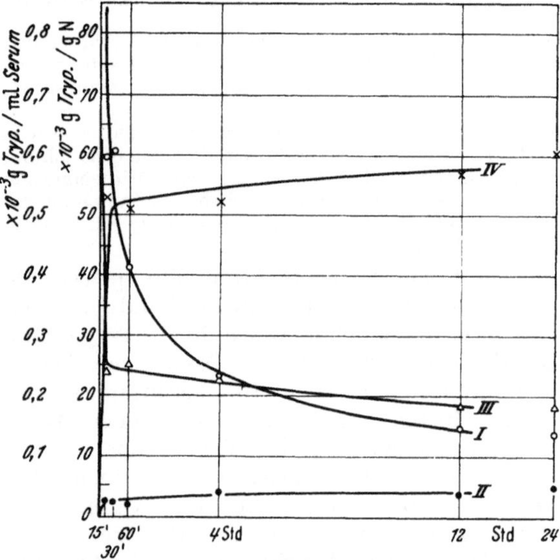

Abb. 6. Farbstoffgehalt von Mitochondrien und Serum. Vitalfärbung nach in vitro-Zusatz eines Farbstoffserums zu isolierten Mitochondrien. *I* Farbstoffabfall im Serum in vivo; *II* Vitalspeicherung durch die Mitochondrien; *III* Farbstoffabfall im Serum in vitro; *IV* Farbstoffadsorption der Mitochondrien in vitro. (Nach Wollensak 1955.)

Das enge funktionelle Zusammenwirken von Mitochondrien und Serumeiweiß zeigt sich auch darin, daß mit Farbstoffen in vitro beladene Mitochondrien in Elutionsversuchen auch stets Farbstoff nur an *die* Serumeiweißfraktion abgeben, welche den Farbstoff in vivo et in vitro bindet[2]. Die nebenstehenden Kurven[3] (Abb. 6) zeigen nach Trypanblauinjektion in vivo unter Nr. I den schnellen initialen Abfall des Farstoffgehaltes des Serums und unter Nr. II den gleichzeitig schnell ansteigenden Farbstoffgehalt der Mitochondrien nach einer Farbstoffgabe in vivo. Damit wird eine Transportbewegung wiedergegeben, wobei sich die Mitochondrien bis zu einem bestimmten Grade mit Farbstoff beladen. Die Kurven III und IV zeigen in vitro einen ähnlich schnellen initialen Austausch beim Zusammentreffen von Serum-Farbstoff mit isolierten Mitochondrien. Der hier dargestellte Farbstofftransport vom bindenden Albumin an die Lebermitochondrien ist der Grund für den raschen Farbstoffschwund aus dem Blute. Garrow hat 1959

---

[1] Bennhold 1953, 1955, Wollensak 1955.   [2] Seybold 1954.   [3] Wollensak 1955.

durch mehrfache Vorgaben alle evansbluebindenden Organellen abgesättigt; danach näherte sich die Schwundrate des blauen Azofarbstoffs mehr und mehr der Schwundgeschwindigkeit der transportierenden Albuminvehikel.

Inwieweit sich die Transporte mit oder ohne Vehikel in die Zelle hinein voneinander abgrenzen lassen, ist noch nicht bestimmbar. Man kann nur so viel sagen, daß die Vehikel einmal als schwimmende Speicher den Farbstoff in hoher Konzentration bis an die Zelle heranführen, wo dann auf Grund von Verteilungsgleichgewichten relativ große Mengen in das Innere der Zelle und an die Mitochondrien gelangen — daß sie aber andererseits auch bis in die Zelle selbst eindringen können, wie am Beispiel des Farbstoffimports in die Tubuli der Molchniere gezeigt werden konnte.

Die Defektpathoproteinämien als Beispiele von Transportinsuffizienzen und deren klinischer Folgen.

Wenn im Körper eine Plasmaeiweißfraktion völlig oder fast völlig fehlt, dann liegt eine Defektpathoproteinämie vor (BENNHOLD 1956/1960, RIVA 1960)*. Ist dieses Eiweiß dank seiner Fähigkeit, andere Stoffe an sich zu binden, ein Vehikel und damit Transportaufgaben unterworfen, dann muß das Fehlen desselben eine Transportstörung bewirken. Wie bereits bei der *Analbuminämie* (s. S. 198) angedeutet wurde, ist auch das vollkommene Fehlen einer bedeutenden Vehikelgruppe durch das Einspringen von Ersatzvehikeln und das Auftreten von Gegenregulationen kompensierbar; ohne solche Gegenmaßnahmen müßte eine Transportinsuffizienz resultieren, welche auf den von diesen Transporten abhängigen Gebieten zunehmend die Homöostase des Organismus beeinträchtigen könnte. Schwere krankhafte Organveränderungen können weitere Folgen sein. Wir müssen versuchen, aus solchen Organschädigungen Schlüsse zu ziehen auf den speziellen Funktionsausfall und auf sein Zustandekommen. Andererseits wird man bestrebt sein, die Kompensationsmechanismen aufzudecken und aus ihnen ebenfalls Hinweise auf die Funktionszusammenhänge abzuleiten. In diesem Sinne erweisen sich die Defektpathoproteinämien als Experimenta naturae und erhellen schlaglichtartig Transportmechanismen und Transportnotwendigkeiten.

Nicht alle Mangelzustände an bestimmten Eiweißanteilen des Plasmas haben Beziehung zu Transportstörungen. Die am längsten bekannte Afibrinogenämie[1] und die von BRUTON (1952) zuerst beschriebene A-γ-Globulinämie sind Störungen, welche als Gerinnungsausfall oder als Antikörpermangel[2] wirken und Krankheiten verursachen. Ähnlich können sich Defekte der β-2A- und β-2M-Globuline als Antikörpermangelsyndrom auswirken. Von einer direkten Transportstörung kann man dabei nicht sprechen.

---

* In einem unter Leitung von R. EMMRICH, Leipzig, auf dem 66. Kongreß der Deutschen Gesellschaft für innere Medizin 1960 stattgefundenen Podiumgespräch wurde auf Vorschlag von G. RIVA und unter Zustimmung von F. WUHRMANN und H. BENNHOLD folgende Bluteiweißnomenklatur empfohlen:

Elektrophoretisches Proteinogramm.

Normal	Pathologisch			
	Pathoproteinämie (alle elektrophoretischen Veränderungen)			
Euproteinämie	Defektpathoproteinämie	Anomalie (erblich)	Paraproteinämie (bes. bei Plasmocytom und Morbus Waldenström)	Dysproteinämie Rein quantitative Verschiebung der Eiweißfraktionen zueinander, ohne Rücksicht auf die klinischen Symptome

[1] RABE 1920.   [2] BARANDUN 1959.

Anders ist es beim Haptoglobinmangel infolge erhöhten Verbrauchs bei vermehrtem Anfall von Hämoglobin durch Hämolyse (s. S. 210). Das überschüssig anfallende Hämoglobin findet kein Vehikel und geht durch die Niere dem Körper verloren, wobei außerdem noch schwere Schädigungen der Tubuli entstehen können.

Die interessantesten Beispiele von Transportinsuffizienz zeigen sich bei den *angeborenen* Defektpathoproteinämien: der *Analbuminämie*, der *Atransferrinämie* und der *A-β-Lipoproteidämie*. Auch ein kompletter Mangel an thyroxinbindendem Globulin ist beschrieben worden[1], ohne daß allerdings Zeichen einer Jod- oder Thyroxintransportstörung und ohne daß überhaupt Krankheitssymptome vorlagen. Das ist nicht unverständlich, da das Schilddrüsenhormon auch an Albumin oder Präalbumin gebunden wird, also von vornherein ausreichend Ersatzvehikel zur Verfügung stehen. Sowohl 1-Thyroxin als auch Tetrajodthyreotropionsäure waren bei dem als euthyreot angesehenen 38jährigen Mann (Serumcholesterin 308 mg%, Grundumsatz —9%) an Albumin und an Präalbumin gebunden.

Die *Analbuminämie* wurde zuerst von Bennhold u. Mitarb. (1954) bei einem Geschwisterpaar beschrieben und ist seitdem nur bei drei weiteren Personen beobachtet worden[2]. Die relativ geringen Beschwerden und die Symptome der Träger dieser angeborenen und rezessiv erblichen Anomalie[3] gleichen sich in allen Fällen. Während die drei Männer durch den Albuminmangel keine Beeinträchtigung erfuhren, waren die beiden Frauen leichter ermüdbar, in ihrer Leistungsfähigkeit gehemmt und hatten prämenstruelle Knöchelödeme. Beide wurden mit Albumin behandelt. Die Männer sind schlank, die Frauen dagegen zeigen eine eigentümliche Fettansammlung der unteren Körperhälfte vom Typ der Dercumschen Fettsucht. Das von uns ausführlich untersuchte Geschwisterpaar bot die in der Tabelle 7 angeführten Befunde, welche zeigen, daß Albuminmangel mit einer allgemeinen Globulinvermehrung, einer Vermehrung der Glucoproteide, der Lipoproteide und der Blutlipide verbunden ist. Die Blutsenkungsgeschwindigkeit ist dadurch erhöht. Herabgesetzt sind Blutdruck, Capillardruck und kolloid-osmotischer Druck des Blutes. Der Schwund von Testfarbstoffen aus dem Blute ist beschleunigt (besonders deutlich beim Kongorot) und wird erst normal, wenn so viel Albumin zugeführt wird, daß ein nahezu normaler Albuminspiegel entsteht. Die Globulin-Vermehrung, die den Albuminmangel kompensiert, verschwindet sofort unter der Albumininfusion. Dann stellen sich rasch normale Globulinwerte und normale Lipidwerte ein. Das infundierte Serumalbumin verschwindet bei der Analbuminämie bedeutend langsamer aus dem Blute als bei Normalpersonen. Die Halbwertszeit des Albuminschwundes war auf 80—100 Tage (Norm 20 Tage) verlängert und differierte bei verschiedenen Untersuchungen[4]. Die Anomalie muß daher sowohl als eine Albumin-Bildungs- als auch als eine Albumin-Abbaustörung angesehen werden. Sie ist, wie sich auf Grund genauer immunochemischer Prüfungen ergab, auch nicht total[5]. Kleinste Albuminspuren (etwa 1/2000 der Norm) ließen sich im Serum nachweisen, und es gelang im National Health Institut in Bethesda die Inkorporierung von S^{35} in eigenproduziertes Albumin[6].

Im Transportbereich ist die Analbuminämie das Beispiel einer weitgehend kompensierten Vehikelinsuffizienz. Einerseits sind es Ersatzvehikel, welche für die fehlenden Albumine einspringen, andererseits regulative Umstellungen, welche den Proteinmangel und die damit verbundene Wassertransportstörung ausgleichen. Durch den Nachweis der Globulinbindung sonst albumingebundener Stoffe[7], der Lipoproteidbindung der sonst albumingebundenen Fettsäuren[8] sowie durch die Vermehrung der Globuline selbst sind die Ersatzmechanismen

---

[1] Tanaka 1959.   [2] Gordon 1959, Shetlar 1959, Beck 1959.   [3] Bennhold 1958.
[4] Bennhold 1959.   [5] Lohss 1960, Humphrey 1960.   [6] Ott 1961.   [7] Ott 1957.
[8] Gordon 1956.

klar geworden. Die Globuline sind infolge ihres hohen Molekulargewichtes aber nicht in der Lage, den sonst vom Albumin aufrechterhaltenen kolloid-osmotischen Druck oder mit anderen Worten die intravasale Wasserbindung voll zu garantieren. Im Zustand des Albuminmangels betrug der kolloid-osmotische Druck stets nur $^1/_3$—$^1/_2$ der Norm. Zum Ausgleich springen eine ganze Reihe von Regulationen ein: der Blutdruck, der Capillardruck und der osmotische Druck der extracapillären (gleichfalls albuminfreien) Flüssigkeit sind herabgesetzt. Darüber hinaus wird dem zu erwartenden pathologischen Wasserverlust durch die Nieren durch eine Drosselung der präglomerulären Arteriolen entgegengewirkt. Bei allen Clearance-Untersuchungen war die Filtrations-Fraktion stark erhöht, fast verdoppelt; die Nierendurchblutung war aber dafür herabgesetzt, fast halbiert[1]. Durch eine präglomeruläre Drosselung der Durchblutung der Niere wurde so einer zu starken Filtration von Wasser, welches osmotisch nicht genügend zurückgehalten werden kann, entgegengewirkt. Die Aldosteronausscheidung war

Tabelle 7. *Zusammenfassung der wichtigsten von der Norm abweichenden Befunde bei den beiden Geschwistern mit Analbuminämie.*

	Analbuminämie		Norm
	♀	♂	
Serumeiweiß	4,9	5,1	6,43 g%
Albumin	—	—	3,65 g%
α_1-Globulin	0,4	0,65	0,32 g%
α_2-Globulin	0,9	1,33	0,55 g%
β-Globulin	1,6	1,83	0,75 g%
γ-Globulin	2,0	1,22	1,16 g%
Fibrinogen	0,39	0,30	0,1—0,4 g%
Immunologische Bestimmung			
α_2-Makroglobulin	10,4	17,7	1,5—4,5%
Transferrin	11,2	14,4	3,0—6,5%
α_2-Lipoproteid	1,5	2,3	0,5—1,5%
β-Lipoproteid	15,3	19,8	4,0—14,0%
Präalbumin	unter der Nachweisgrenze	0,9	0,1—0,5%
BSG	60/90	40/65	5/12 mm n. W.
Proteingebundene Hexose	237	263	105—145 mg%
Hexosamin	180	226	85—110 mg%
Gesamtlipoide	1343		700—800 mg%
Cholesterin (gesamt)	372	430	160—210 mg%
Freies Cholesterin	33	33	33%
Serumcalcium	8,2	9,0	9,0—10,5 mg%
Perorale Eisenbelastung 4 Std-Wert	829	295	220 γ%
Cholinesterase	30	43	20%
Aldolase	25		8 E/m
Kongorotschwund	71	92	15—25%

dabei normal, jedoch war die Ausscheidung von Natrium und Chloridionen erhöht und beschleunigt. Auf eine Infusion einer relativ großen Kochsalzmenge hin antwortet die Analbuminämieniere in kompensierender Weise durch eine rasche Salzausscheidung ohne Aldosteronverminderung und wahrscheinlich auch unbeeinflußt durch das antidiuretische Prinzip[1, 2]. Der regulative Weg scheint dabei ein rein intrarenaler, onkotisch wirksamer Vorgang zu sein. — Wenn auch bei den durchgeführten Untersuchungen alle lebenswichtigen Funktionen der Albumine durch Ersatz- und Regulationsmechanismen in erstaunlicher Weise ausgeglichen erschienen, so zeigten doch andere Proben, z. B. die Untersuchung des Kongorotschwundes, daß die Bindung des körperfremden Farbstoffes im Blut herabgesetzt ist und dadurch der Farbstoff mit einer 3—4fachen Beschleunigung die Blutbahn verläßt. Aus diesem Grunde ist es auch möglich, daß noch andere Transportmechanismen nicht genügend abgesichert und nicht genügend geschützt sind. Insuffizienzerscheinungen könnten im höheren Alter da noch zur Beobachtung kommen.

Bei der *Atransferrinämie* liegt ein praktisch völliges Fehlen von Transferrin vor. An der Freiburger Universitäts-Kinderklinik (Prof. Dr. KELLER) wurde

---

[1] SCHEURLEN 1960.   [2] BENNHOLD 1960.

eine 6jährige Patientin beobachtet, die diese bislang noch nicht festgestellte Form einer Defektpathoproteinämie zeigte. Der Fall gelangte erst während der Drucklegung dieser Arbeit zu unserer Kenntnis*. Wir danken Herrn Prof. Keller und Herrn Prof. Heilmeyer vielmals für die Mitteilung der Untersuchungsergebnisse. Immunbiologisch ließ sich bei der Patientin eine Herabsetzung des Transferrinspiegels im Plasma auf weniger als 1/128 des Normalen feststellen. In vitro zugesetztes Fe^{59} wanderte im elektrischen Feld zwischen β- und γ-Globulinen. Das Serumeisen betrug zwischen 5 und 10 μg% ; mit einer Gesamtbindungskapazität von 15 μg% (ein anderes Laboratorium bestimmte einen Eisenspiegel von 14 μg% und eine Gesamtkapazität von 33 μg%). Außerdem wurden bestimmt: 4 bis 7,5 g% Hb, 2—4,12 Mill. Erythrocyten, eine Anisocytose und Poikilocytose, Reticulocyten zwischen 8 und 15 $^{0}/_{00}$. Im Knochenmark fand sich eine Steigerung der Erythropoese, 13% Sideroblasten waren vorhanden. Die Erythroblasten besaßen nur ein schmales, wie ausgefranst aussehendes Plasma.

Im Serum betrug der β-Globulinanteil nur 2,4 rel.%, der γ-Globulinanteil 27 rel.%. Im Anfangsteil der γ-Globuline fand sich ein deutlich abgrenzbares „Prä-γ-Globulin". Der Vergleich mit dem Radiogramm zeigte, daß hier die Eisenbindung lag. Die Abwanderung des Eisens aus dem Plasma war extrem beschleunigt und hatte eine Halbwertszeit von 5 min. Der Eiseneinbau in die Erythrocyten betrug bis zu 8 Tagen, maximal 126%. Die Eisenaufnahme in die Leber verlief rasch. Die Erythrocytenlebenszeit, t/2 für die Cr-Markierung: 24 Tage. Eine Leberbiopsie ergab eine *exzessive Siderose der Leber bei periportaler Fibrose*. Dem entsprach auch das Eiweißspektrum mit Takata von 60 mg%, Thymol von 4,0 MLE und einem Albumingehalt des Serums von 45%. Das Hautkolorit war graubräunlich, das Herz vergrößert, der Pulmonalbogen betont. Die Leber war 5 Qf unter dem Rippenbogen zu fühlen, derb. Die Milz war $1^{1}/_{2}$ Qf unter dem Rippenbogen mit manifester Resistenz palpierbar. Klinisch bot der beobachtete Fall also eine Hämochromatose mit extrem *niedrigem* (!) Eisenspiegel im Blute. Man kann ohne weiteres das pathogenetisch Primäre in der (möglicherweise angeborenen) Atransferrinämie sehen. Dadurch fehlt das Transportmilieu für Eisen oder ist höchstens in Spuren vorhanden. Die III. Stufe des Transportgeschehens (vgl. S. 180) ist weggefallen, und ein Error loci ist vorhanden mit Eisenablagerung speziell auch in der Leber, welche vom Resorptionsort direkt und ohne vorherige Durchmischung mit dem Gesamtblut zugängig ist. Die schweren Schädigungen des Leber-Parenchyms sind als Folgen der undosierten Eisenüberlastung der Leber anzusehen. Der niedrige Eisenspiegel ist bei Hämochromatosen etwas ganz Ungewöhnliches; er ist nur erklärbar durch das völlige Fehlen des spezifischen Transportmilieus, ebenso die extrem niedrige Halbwertszeit des injizierten Eisens. Beides spricht gegen die pathogenetische Bedeutung der wegen der Anämie mehrfach vorgenommenen Bluttransfusionen. Dieser Fall scheint die von uns früher aufgestellte Hypothese über die Pathogenese der Hämochromatose (durch Insuffizienz des Transportmilieus für Eisen, Bennhold 1960) voll zu bestätigen.

Die erste *A-β-Lipoproteidämie* wurde 1960 von Salt u. Mitarb. beschrieben. Es handelte sich dabei um ein 17 Monate altes Mädchen. Beide Eltern und ein Großelter hatten stark erniedrigte β-Lipoproteidwerte. Deshalb wurde bei dem Kind an einen autosomalen, rezessiven Erbgang gedacht. Der Defekt war mit Acanthocytose (Ausbildung von Stechapfelformen der Erythrocyten), Poikilocytose, Anisocytose und Fehlen der Geldrollenbildung, mit Steatorrhoe, bioptisch festgestellten Unregelmäßigkeiten im Zellbild der Dünndarmzotten und Ausbleiben der postprandialen Lipämie kombiniert. Die β-Lipoproteide fehlten bei dem Kind vollständig, und die α_1-Lipoproteide waren auf 80 mg% reduziert (als Normwerte

* Die ausführliche Publikation erscheint in der Dtsch. med. Wschr. 1961.

wurden 150—280 mg% genannt). Entsprechend lag auch der Serumcholesterinwert mit 22 mg%, der Serumphosphorlipidwert mit 45 mg% und der Gesamtlipidwert mit 80 mg% extrem niedrig. Carotinoide konnten überhaupt nicht nachgewiesen werden, und der Vitamin A-Gehalt war mindestens auf $^1/_5$ der Norm herabgesetzt.

Die Autoren brachten ihre Beobachtung mit der Beschreibung von vier weiteren Fällen von Acanthocytose und Hypocholesterinämie (37—60 mg%) in Zusammenhang, bei welchen zwar auf A-β-Lipoproteidämie nicht untersucht worden war, die aber durch die große Ähnlichkeit der Symptome als gleiche Krankheit imponierten. Bei allen vier Personen war *Konsanguinität* bei Eltern oder Großeltern vorhanden. Von größter Bedeutung waren Verlaufsbeobachtungen über mehrere Jahre[1], welche Schlüsse auf die Entwicklung, also auch auf die Folgen des β-Lipoproteidmangels, erlaubten. Alle Kranken, auch der von SALT beobachtete Fall, zeigten *cöliakieähnliche* Symptome: Durchfallperioden, Fettstühle und röntgenologisch weite Dünndarmlumina. Die älteren Patienten litten an einer *atypischen Retinitis pigmentosa* und an einer *Ataxie vom Typ Friedreich*[2]. Bei einem vom 13. bis 19. Lebensjahr beobachteten Knaben entwickelte sich in dieser Zeit die Retinitis, und es verstärkten sich die neurologischen Symptome[3].

Daraus ergab sich der naheliegende Schluß, daß die Progredienz des Leidens ihre Ursache in einem durch Transport- bzw. Vehikelinsuffizienz fortwirkenden spezifisch lokalisierten Mangelzustand haben kann. Ob der Mangel an Blutlipiden oder an in Lipiden gelösten Vitaminen und Wirkstoffen (etwa Vitamin A oder Carotinoid) bedeutungsvoller ist, das kann noch nicht näher bestimmt werden.

Besonders wichtig erscheint dieses Krankheitsbild insofern, als ähnlich der Wilsonschen Krankheit (s. S. 212) auch hier eine genetisch bedingte spezifische Transportinsuffizienz zu einer schweren, bisher unheilbaren, langsam sich entwickelnden Systemerkrankung führt. Dabei muß darauf hingewiesen werden, daß sich eine Transportinsuffizienz nicht stets in ungeordneter *Überschwemmung* bestimmter Organe und dadurch bedingter Schädigungen manifestieren muß; es ist auch durchaus denkbar, daß eine Insuffizienz eines spezifischen Transportmilieus einen gegenteiligen Effekt in Form einer *ungenügenden Versorgung* bestimmter Stellen mit lebenswichtigem Transportgut zur Folge hat.

Wenn sich in Untersuchungen, welche bereits begonnen wurden, diese Vorstellungen als experimentell stützbar erweisen sollten, dann wäre es gerechtfertigt zu versuchen, diesen Kranken durch Zufuhr von β-Lipoproteid zu helfen.

Zusammenfassung und Ausblick.

Im obigen Beitrag wurde versucht, alle *die* Organe und Substrate, welche speziell den extracellulären Transportvorgängen dienen, zu einer funktionellen Einheit, einer ,,Transportapparatur‘‘, zusammenzufassen. Das *Herz* steuert den Bewegungsvorgang, die *Lokomotion*, bei; die *Vasomotoren* regeln die grobe *Aufteilung* des *Minutenvolumens unter die einzelnen Organe*. Das *Blut als zirkulierendes Transportmilieu* stellt die *dritte Transportkomponente* dar; in ihm besitzen die Blutzellen und Blutplättchen sowie die Plasmaeiweißkörper für viele Transportvorgänge eine *große Bedeutung als Vehikel* oder mit anderen Worten als *lokale Abgaberegler*. Alle drei Elemente der Transportapparatur sind, wie darzulegen versucht wurde, mit einer großen Menge von Regulations- und Kompensationsmechanismen ausgestattet. Die *Grenzflächen der Zellen* und der *mikroskopischen Gewebselemente* spielen bei diesen Vorgängen als Abladerampe aus dem Transportmilieu heraus bzw. als Sitz von besonderen Aufnahmemechanismen in die Zelle hinein ebenfalls eine entscheidend wichtige Rolle. Die Vehikel kolloider Dimension sind stets Proteine, makromolekulare Stoffe, welche durch ihr von verschiedenen

[1] KORNZWEIG 1957, SINGER 1952, DRUEZ 1959.
[2] DRUEZ 1959, BASSEN 1950, JAMPEL 1958.   [3] JAMPEL 1958.

Faktoren abhängiges Bindungsvermögen die ins Blut gelangten Stoffe mindestens zum Teil an sich fesseln.

Die früheren so vielfältig festgestellten — und alljährlich neu gefundenen — Bindungen von Stoffen an Bluteiweißkörper müssen, wie uns scheint, in einem größeren Rahmen betrachtet werden. *Die Zahl der Einzelbeobachtungen ist so groß geworden, daß es erlaubt sein muß zu versuchen, sie unter einem einheitlichen Gesichtspunkt zu einer Theorie zusammenzufassen.* Es ist a priori höchst unwahrscheinlich, daß die Bindung so vieler lebenswichtiger Stoffe an die zirkulierenden Serumeiweißkörper als ein Zufallsbefund anzusehen ist, ohne daß Hinweise auf wichtige funktionelle Beziehungen abzuleiten wären. Immer klarer wird es, daß das Plasmaeiweiß einen begrenzenden Faktor bei der lokalen Abgabe von Stoffen aus der Blutbahn darstellt. Dabei besteht oft ein Gleichgewicht zwischen freiem und gebundenem Anteil dieser Stoffe im zirkulierenden Plasma.

Die Bindungsfestigkeit an Plasmaeiweiß kann im Rahmen des Transportmilieus abhängig sein von folgenden Faktoren:

1. Von der *Beschaffenheit des bindenden Eiweißes.*

2. Von der *Beschaffenheit der gebundenen Substanz.*

3. Von der *Menge der Substanz* pro Mol. des bindenden Eiweißkörpers; dabei ist bemerkenswert, daß in zahlreichen Fällen die Bindungsfestigkeit mit dem Betrag der nichtbesetzten Bindungskapazität zu- und abnimmt (z. B. Bilirubin, Farbstoffe).

4. Von einer *konkurrierenden Gleichgewichtsbindung an corpusculäre Blutbestandteile* (Erythrocyten, Thrombocyten) (z. B. bei Trijodthyronin, Atebrin und Fettsäuren).

5. Von einer *konkurrierenden Gleichgewichtsbindung an mehrere Plasmaeiweißfraktionen.* Dadurch können bei dem Transport bestimmter Stoffe gewissermaßen „Transportketten" entstehen zwischen schwächer und stärker bindenden Eiweißfraktionen; auch intracelluläre hochaktive Trägerproteine können bei der Herbeiführung dieses Adsorptionsgefälles eine Rolle spielen (Beispiel: Farbstofftransporte in die Zelle hinein bis zu den Mitochondrien bei Vitalfärbungsvorgängen).

6. Vom *Vorhandensein anderer kompetitiv ebenfalls am gleichen Eiweiß gebundener Stoffe,* welche gleiche Bindungsplätze besetzen und verdrängend wirken (z. B. Fettsäuren, Medikamente, Farbstoffe). *Auch zwischen Vehikeln selbst können Bindungskonkurrenzen* einem zu bindenden Stoff gegenüber bestehen, so zwischen verschiedenen Eiweißfraktionen gegenüber einem sauren Farbstoff oder zwischen einem Fremdvehikel, wie Kollidon und Albumin, gegenüber Diaminreinblau FF. — Solche Competition-Vorgänge können zu Kollisionen von Transportvorgängen und zu folgenschwerem error loci (z. B. beim Kernikterus der Frühgeburten) führen.

7. Vom p_H, *dem Redoxpotential und anderen das Gesamtmilieu beeinflussenden* physikalisch-chemischen *Faktoren.*

Zu Faktor 3 ist ergänzend hinzuzufügen:

Die Menge der zu transportierenden Substanz pro Mol. Vehikel-Eiweiß kann durch verschiedene biologische Situationen pathologisch verändert sein, z. B.:

I. Durch intravenöse oder perorale Zufuhr von *Fremdsubstanzen* (z. B. Farbstoffen oder Medikamenten).

II. Durch pathologisch veränderte *Resorptionsbedingungen* von im Körper heimischen Stoffen (z. B. pathologisch erhöht bei Hämochromatose, pathologisch erniedrigt bei der Eisenmangelanämie).

III. Durch Überschwemmung der Blutbahn mit körpereigenen Substanzen auf Grund von *Verwertungsstop* (z. B. Bilirubinretention durch Gallengangsverschluß; Eisenretention bei achrestischer Anämie durch Einbaustörung des Eisens in das Hämoglobin; durch die Unmöglichkeit, resorbiertes Kupfer in Coeruloplasmin einzubauen, und dadurch bedingten pathologischen Anstieg des Transportkupfers im Blut mit Überlastung der das Transportkupfer locker bindenden Albumine).

Die in auffallend hoher Konzentration zirkulierenden Serumproteine nehmen das zuströmende Transportgut auf, fesseln es weitgehend an die Blutbahn und befördern es geordnet, bis es an jeweils bestimmten Abhängeorten abgegeben wird. Die umfangreiche Aufzählung der an Serumeiweiß gebundenen Substanzen (Tabellen 2 und 5) gibt einen Einblick in die Vielfältigkeit der Bindungsmöglichkeiten. Wenn dem *Serumalbumin* infolge seiner spezifischen Eigenschaften die vielseitigste Bindungsfähigkeit zukommt, so können auch *Globuline* eine große Anzahl von Stoffen binden und einen Albuminmangel sogar kompensieren (vgl. Analbuminämie). Als Vehikel für Eisen, Vitamine, Hormone und Lipide spielen sie eine vorzügliche Rolle; ihre Bindungsfähigkeit hat im allgemeinen einen mehr spezifischen Charakter und bezieht sich oft auf kleine und kleinste Unterfraktionen (z. B. Trägerproteine für Thyroxin, Steroide, Vitamin B_{12}, Mangan).

Im biologischen Milieu der Körperflüssigkeiten ist die Bindung nur ein temporärer Vorgang, der durch Abhängung oder Verdrängung beendet wird. Es muß mit einer vielfach wechselnden Konkurrenz (competition) um Bindungsplätze gerechnet werden, derzufolge Bindungen geschwächt oder aufgehoben werden und Transportgut freigesetzt wird. Der Wechsel des Thyroxins in seinen Bindungsplätzen (S. 214, 216), die Verdrängung von Testfarbstoffen durch *Fettsäuren* sind Beispiele dafür.

Die *zirkulierenden Stoffdepots des Transportmilieus* stehen im Gleichgewicht *mit fixen Depots:* z. B. beim Transport des Sauerstoffs von den zirkulierenden Depots des Hämoglobins an Erythrocyten zum fixen Sauerstoffdepot in der Form des Myoglobins im Muskel; ferner beim Transport des Eisens als Beziehung: Transferrin → Ferritin (S. 204), beim Transport des Thyroxins von Schilddrüse → Interalphaglobulin (S. 214), beim Transport von Bilirubin oder von den Vitalfarbstoffen Trypanblau und Evansblue als Beziehung: Albumin-, α- und β-Globulin → reticuloendotheliale Zelle und Tubuluszelle der Niere. — Als besonders klassische Beispiele der Transportabhängigkeit von der Beschaffenheit der Blutvehikel seien noch einmal erwähnt: die Schädigung des Sauerstofftransports bei Kohlenoxyd- oder bei Methämoglobinvergiftung, ferner der beschleunigte Kongorotschwund bei den albuminarmen Nephrosen (S. 198) und bei den Fällen von familiärer Analbuminämie (S. 198, 242) und schließlich im Kaninchenversuch die Wirkung des Fremdvehikels Kollidon auf die Ausscheidung von sauren Farbstoffen (Diaminrot) in Form einer Umleitung von der Leber auf die Niere als Exkretionsorgane.

Die *Defektpathoproteinämien* (früher als „Defektdysproteinämien" bezeichnet) mit ihrem genetisch bedingten Fehlen bestimmter Bluteiweißkörper können als Experimenta naturae Wesentliches zur Klärung der Funktionen der Bluteiweißkörper beitragen. Am Beispiel der Analbuminämie und vor allem der Atransferrinämie und der A-β-Lipoproteidämie wird dies besonders klar. Sowohl die Kompensationsversuche des überlebenden Organismus als auch die manifesten Ausfälle sowie deren klinische Folgeerscheinungen können wichtige Hinweise geben. Viel mehr sollte man bei „Stoffwechselerkrankungen", bei „Systemerkrankungen" sowie bei „hereditär-degenerativen Erkrankungen" an spezifische Insuffizienzen des Transportmilieus als pathogenetische Ausgangspunkte oder als mitwirkende Faktoren „denken"! Subtilste weitere Auftrennung der Plasmaeiweißkörper und Gegenüberstellung der dabei gewonnenen Befunde mit bestimmten klinischen Syndromen könnten wichtige pathogenetische Aufschlüsse geben. Geregelter „Stoffwechsel" hat geregelte „Stofftransporte" (An- und Abtransport) zur Voraussetzung.

Die *α- und β-Globuline* gliedern sich funktionell in erstaunlich *viele Unterfraktionen* auf, welche nur in seltenen Fällen mit einfacher Elektrophorese faßbar sind; auch die Immunelektrophorese kann dabei im Stiche lassen, besonders sobald es sich um quantitative Auswertungen handelt. Denken wir nur an die minimalen Untergruppen des α_1-Globulins, welche das B_{12} und welche andererseits das Cortisol transportieren; im letzteren Falle entscheidet bei pathologisch erhöhtem Cortisol-Spiegel im Blute der Bestand an den spezifischen Trägerproteinen aus der α_1-Globulingruppe darüber, ob sich ein Morbus Cushing entwickelt oder nicht, da für den inkretorischen Effekt nur die Konzentration des *ungebundenen* Cortisols maßgebend ist.

Auch für die *Ausscheidungsvorgänge durch die Niere* spielen die Bindungen an spezifische Vehikel eine maßgebende Rolle; es sei nur auf Eisen, Kupfer, Bilirubin und Steroide hingewiesen. *Chelatbildungen der Metalle mit Äthylendiamintetraessigsäure (ADTE)* hebt den Bindungsschutz der Trägerproteine auf und führt zu Verlusten durch die Niere. Ähnlich ist es bei *Glucuronsäure-Konjugierung* des *Bilirubins*, des *Thyroxins* und *der Steroide;* das Konjugat haftet zwar meist noch locker an Eiweiß, ist aber jetzt durch die Niere abhängbar. So können die Eiweißvehikel des Blutes Entscheidendes beitragen zur Bildung der „Nierenschwelle". Die Schwundrate oder die biologische Halbwertzeit von Substanzen, welche dem Blute zugeführt wurden, kann erheblich mitbedingt sein durch den Grad der Bindung an das Transportmilieu; auch da ist die Analbuminämie mit ihren sonst gesunden Organbefunden, aber dem extrem beschleunigten Kongoschwund von großer Beweiskraft.

So wird das *zirkulierende Blut zu einem äquivalenten Gegenspieler des fixen, hochdifferenzierten Gewebes* und gewinnt eine Art „*funktioneller Struktur*" im *Transportgeschehen.* Aus einer reinen Hämodynamik, welche den eingeschwemmten Substanzen nur einen ziellosen, kreisförmig geschlossenen Bewegungsimpuls mitteilen kann, wird durch die Einschaltung der Eiweiß- (und Erythrocyten-) Vehikel ein echter Transportvorgang mit lokal dosierender Abgabe an den Capillar- und Zellgrenzen. Die große Anzahl von genetischen Faktoren, welche (nach neueren Forschungen) ihr Projektionsfeld im Transportmilieu (Erythrocyten, Hb, Thrombocyten, Plasmaeiweiß) finden, gibt diesen Überlegungen ein besonderes Gewicht

Literatur.
(Siehe auch Anhang zum Literaturverzeichnis, S. 274.)

Abderhalden, E., u. P. Möller: Untersuchungen über den Gehalt des Serums an Kupfer, Eisen und Mangan. Hoppe-Seylers Z. physiol. Chem. **176**, 95 (1928). — Achard, Ch.: Aperçu de la physiologie et de la pathologie général du système lacavoine. Paris 1924. — Adlersberg, D., E. Grishman and H. Sobotka: Uric acid partition in gout and in hepatic diseases. Arch. intern. Med. **70**, 101 (1942). — Ahrens, E. H., R. Blomstrand, J. Hinsch, W. Insull, T. T. Tsaltas and M. L. Peterson: The influence of dietary fats on serum-lipid levels in man. Lancet **1957**I, 1943. — Aidin, R., B. Corner and G. Tovey: Kernicterus and prematurity. Lancet **1950**I, 1153. — Aladjem, F., M. Liebermann and J. W. Gofman: Immunochemical studies on human plasma lipoproteins. J. exp. Med. **105**, 49 (1957). — Alberty, R. A.: A study of the variation of the average isoelectric points of several plasma proteins with ionic strength. J. phys. Colloid. Chem. **53**, 114 (1949). — Albright, E. C., F. C. Larson and W. P. Deiss: Single dimension chromatographic separation of thyroxine and triiodothyronine. Proc. Soc. exp. Biol. (N.Y.) **84**, 240 (1953). ~ Thyroxine binding capacity of serum alpha globulin in hypothyroid, euthyroid, and hyperthyroid subjects. J. clin. Invest. **34**, 44 (1955). — Albright, E. C., F. C. Larson, K. Tomita and H. A. Lardy: Enzymatic conversion of thyroxine and triiodothyronine to the corresponding acetic acid analogues. Endocrinology **59**, 232 (1956). — Albright, E. C., K. Tomita and F. C. Larson: In vitro metabolism of triiodothyronine. Endocrinology **64**, 208 (1959). — Albrink, M. J., W. W. L. Glenn, J. P. Peters and E. B. Man: The transport of lipoids in chyle. J. clin. Invest. **34**, 1467 (1955). — Albrink, M. J., E. B. Man and J. P. Peters: The relation of neutral fat to latescense of serum. J. clin. Invest. **34**, 147 (1955). — Allen, T. H., and P. D. Orahovats: Combination of toluidine dye isomers with plasma albumin. Amer. J. Physiol. **161**, 473 (1950). — Althausen, T. L., R. K. Doig, S. Weiden, R. Motteram, C. N. Turner and A. Moore: Hemochromatosis. Investigation of 23 cases, with special reference to etiology, nutrition, iron metabolism and studies of hepatic and pancreatic function. A.M.A. Arch. intern. Med. **88**, 553 (1951). — Altmann, R.: Ein bemerkenswerter Folinsäureeffekt, zugleich ein Beitrag zum Wirkungsmechanismus der Foline. Med. Mschr. **5**, 122 (1951). — Andersen, A. H.: On fixation of sulfathiazole, sulfapyridine, sulfanilamide a and p-aminobenzoic acid by plasma. Acta pharmacol. (Kbh.) **1**, 141 (1945). — Anfinsen,

C. B., E. Boyle and R. K. Brown: The role of heparin in lipoprotein metabolism. Science 115, 583 (1952). — Asher, Th.: Untersuchungen an isolierten Zell- und Gewebsbestandteilen von M. Behrens. II. Mitt. Isolierung und chemische Untersuchung des Haemosiderins in der Pferdemilz. Hoppe-Seylers Z. physiol. Chem. 220, 97 (1933). — Astaldi, G., and G. Cardinal: Cytology of B_{12} deficiency in vitro. 1. Europ. Symp. Hamburg, S. 361, 1956. — Augsberger, A.: Ultrafiltration und Kompensationsdialyse. Ein Beitrag zur Frage der Ionenbindung im Blutserum. Ergebn. Physiol. 24, 618 (1925). — Austen, F. K., M. E. Rubini, W. H. Meroney and J. Wolff: Salicylates and thyroid function. I. Depression of thyroid function. J. clin. Invest. 37, 1131 (1958). ~ II. The effect on the thyroid-pituitary interrelation. J. clin. Invest. 37, 1144 (1958). — Avigan, J.: The interaction between carcinogenic hydrocarbons and serum lipoproteins. Cancer Res. 19, 831 (1959). — Avigan, J., H. A. Eder and D. Steinberg: Metabolism of the protein moiety of rabbit serum lipoproteins. Proc. Soc. exp. Biol. (N.Y.) 95, 429 (1957). — Avigan, J., R. Redfield and D. Steinberg: N-terminal residues of serum-lipoproteins. Biochem. biophys. Acta 21, 557 (1956). — Axenfeld, H., u. K. Brass: Klinische und bioptische Untersuchungen über den sogenannten Icterus catarrhalis. Frankfurt. Z. Path. 57, 219 (1942).

Balch, D. A.: An estimate of the weights of volatile fatty acids produced in the rumen of lactating cows on a diet of hay and concentrates. Brit. J. Nutr. 12, 18 (1958). — Ballou, G. A., P. D. Boyer and J. M. Luck: The electrophoretic mobility of human serum albumin as affected by lower fatty acid salts. J. biol. Chem. 159, 111 (1945). — Banks, T. E., J. C. Boursnell and A. Wormall: Studies on mustardgas and related compounds. IV. Their action on proteins. Biochem. J. 40, 745 (1946). — Barac, G., et R. Roseman: Faits expérimentaux sur la stabilisation de la bilirubine par les protéines plasmatiques. J. Wash. Acad. Sci. 36, 296 (1949). — Barandun, S., H. Cottier, A. Hässig u. G. Riva: Das Antikörpermangelsyndrom. Basel u. Stuttgart: Benno Schwabe 1959. — Bargmann, W.: Morphologie der Kapillaren und des Intestitiums in „Kapillaren und Interstitium" von Bartelheimer und Küchmeister. Stuttgart: Georg Thieme 1955. — Barr, D. P., E. M. Russ and H. A. Eder: Protein-lipid relationship in human plasma. II. In atherosclerosis and related conditions. Amer. J. Med. 11, 480 (1951). — Barr, G.: A monograph of viscosity. London: Oxford University Press 1931. — Bassen, F. A., and A. L. Kornzweig: Malformation of the erythrocytes in a case of atypical retinitis pigmentosa. Blood 5, 381—387 (1950). — Basset, A. M., A. H. Coons and W. T. Salter: Proteinbound iodine in blood. V. Natural occuring and chemical behavior. Amer. J. med. Sci. 202, 516 (1941). — Bates, M. W.: Turnover rates of plasma lipids. Fed. Proc. 17, 186 (1958). — Bayliss, L. E.: In Frey-Wyssling, Deformation and flow in biological systems. Amsterdam 1952. — Beard, M. F., W. R. Pitney and E. H. Sanneman: Serum concentrations of vitamin B_{12} in patients suffering from leucemia. Blood 9, 789 (1954). — Bearn, A. G.: Genetic and biochemical aspect of Wilsons disease. Amer. J. Med. 15, 442 (1953). — Bearn, A. G., and H. G. Kunkel: Localisation of Cu^{64} in serum fractions following oral administration: An alteration in Wilson's disease. Proc. Soc. exp. Biol. (N.Y.) 85, 44 (1954). ~ Metabolic studies in Wilson's disease. J. Lab. clin. Med. 45, 623 (1955). — Bechhold, H.: Ultrafiltration. Biochem. Z. 6, 379 (1907). ~ Zur „Inneren Antisepsis". Hoppe-Seylers Z. physiol. Chem. 52, 117 (1907). ~ Kolloidstudien mit der Filtrationsmethode. Z. physik. Chem. 60, 257 (1907). — Beck, G. E., et T. Dorta: Un cas d'analbuminémie. Helv. med. Acta 26, 764 (1959). — Begemann, H., W. Keiderling u. F. Walter: Der Einfluß der Folsäure auf die Eisenresorption. Klin. Wschr. 31, 881 (1953). — Behrens, M., u. M. Taubert: Über die Beziehungen zwischen Hämosiderin und Ferritin. Hoppe-Seylers Z. physiol. Chem. 289, 116 (1952). — Beierwaltes, W. H., and J. Robbins: Familial increase in the thyroxine-binding sites in serum alpha Jlobulin. J. clin. Invest. 38, 1683 (1959). — Beischer, D. E.: Electron microscopy of human glasma lipoprotein separated by ultracentrifugation. Circulat. Res. 2, 164 (1954). — Bence, p.: Die Rolle des Kupfers in der Blutbildung. Z. klin. Med. 126, 173 (1933). — Bendien, W. M., u. J. Snapper: Untersuchungen über die Bindung der Serumkolloide mittels eiweißdurchlässiger Ultrafilter. Biochem. Z. 260, 105 (1933). ~ Weitere Untersuchungen über Bindung der Serumkolloide. Biochem. Z. 261, 1 (1933). — Bennhold, H.: Über die Ausscheidung intravenös einverleibten Congorotes bei den verschiedensten Erkrankungen, insbesondere bei Amyloidose. Dtsch. Arch. klin. Med. 142, 32 (1923). ~ Über die Adsorptionsfähigkeit der Serumkolloide tubulär Nierenkranker gegenüber Farbstoffen. Z. ges. exp. Med. 49, 71 (1926). ~ Über den Einfluß der Serumeiweißkörper auf die Diffusion saurer Farbstoffe in Gelatingele. Kolloid.-Z. 43, 328 (1927). ~ Über den Einfluß von Serumeiweiß auf Diffusionsvorgänge. Verh. dtsch. Ges. inn. Med. 15, 455 (1928). ~ Über die Funktion der Serumeiweißkörper im tierischen Organismus. Verh. dtsch. Ges. inn. Med. 41, 211 (1929). ~ Über die Anpassung der Serumeiweißkörper an die Transportnotwendigkeiten im kranken Organismus. Verh. dtsch. Ges. inn. Med. 42, 353 (1930). ~ Über die Bindung des Cholesterins an die Globuline; zugleich ein weiterer Beitrag zur Frage der Funktion der Serumeiweißkörper. Verh. dtsch. Ges. inn. Med. 43, 211 (1931). ~ Über die Vehikelfunktion der Serumeiweißkörper. Ergebn. inn. Med. Kinderheilk. 42, 273 (1932). ~ Ist das Blutplasma ein strömendes Eiweißdepot oder ein Transportorgan? Dtsch. med. Wschr.

1947, 401. ~ Die Rolle der Bluteiweißkörper im Regulationsgeschehen. Verh. dtsch. Ges. inn. Med. **59**, 195 (1953). ~ Die Serum-Elektrophorese in Klinik und Forschung: Möglichkeiten und Ausblicke. Med. Klin. **49**, 8 (1954). ~ Defektdysproteinaemien. Verh. dtsch. Ges. inn. Med. **61** (1955). ~ Störungen von Transportvorgängen als Ursachen von Krankheiten und von Krankheitssymptomen (dargestellt am Beispiel des Ikterus, der Hämochromatose und der Wilsonschen Krankheit sowie der Eisenmangelanämie). Klin. Wschr. **38**, 345 (1960). — Bennhold, H., and E. Kallee: Comporative studies on the halv-life of I^{131}-labeled albumine and nonradioactive human serum albumin in case of analbuminemia. J. clin. Invest. **38**, 863 (1959). — Bennhold, H., E. Kylin u. St. Rusznyák: Die Eiweißkörper des Blutplasmas. Dresden: Theodor Steinkopff 1938. — Bennhold, H., u. H. Ott: Über die Einordnung gefärbter Substanzen in das Gefüge der Plasmaeiweißkörper. Photographie u. Forsch. **5**, 12 (1952). ~ Die Globulinvehikel. Schweiz. med. Wschr. **82**, 475 (1952b). — Bennhold, H., H. Ott u. G. Scheurlen: Beitrag zur Frage der genbedingten Bluteiweißstörungen. Verh. dtsch. Ges. inn. Med. **64**, 280 (1958). — Bennhold, H., H. Ott u. M. Wiech: Über die Bindung leber- und nierengängiger Substanzen an die Serumeiweißkörper. Dtsch. med. Wschr. **1950a**, 11. ~ Unveröffentlichte Untersuchungen 1950b. — Bennhold, H., H. Peters u. E. Roth: Über einen Fall von kompletter Analbuminaemie ohne wesentliche klinische Krankheitszeichen. Verh. dtsch. Ges. inn. Med. **60**, 630 (1954). — Bennhold, H., u. R. Schubert: Untersuchung über die Möglichkeit einer Vehikelfunktion des Periston. Z. ges. exp. Med. **113**, 722 (1944). — Bennhold, H., u. G. Seybold: Der Aufnahmemechanismus plasmaeiweißgebundener Vitalfarbstoffe in speichernde Zellsysteme. Beitrag zur Frage der Durchgängigkeit der Zellmembran für Plasmaeiweiß. Z. ges. exp. Med. **118**, 407 (1952c). — Bennhold, H., G. Seybold u. E. Kallee: ^{131}J-Serumproteine und Farbstoffspeicherung. Z. Naturforsch. **10b**, 578 (1955). — Bennhold, H. H., u. P. G. Scheurlen: Analbuminaemie und deren Auswirkung auf die Nierenfunktion. Internat. Kongr. für Inn. Med., Basel, 1960. — Béraud, Th., J. Cruchaud et A. Vannotti: Influence du support protéique spécifique de la thyroxine sur la pénétration dans la cellule. Schweiz. med. Wschr. **88**, 105 (1958). — Béraud, Th., T. Dorta et A. Vannotti: Etude du metabolism de la diiodothyroxine en pathologie humaine. Schweiz. med. Wschr. **89**, 980 (1959). — Béraud, Th., et A. Vannotti: Au sujet de la déioduration in vitro de la thyroxine dans différent tissus chez le rat. Schweiz. med. Wschr. **87**, 56 (1957). ~ Liaison de la thyroxine aux protéines plasmatiques dans l'hépatite épidémique. Schweiz. med. Wschr. **87**, 996 (1957). — Bernhard, A., and J. J. Beaver: The electrodialysis of human blood serum. J. biol. Chem. **69**, 113 (1926). — Berson, S. A., and R. S. Yalow: The distribution of I^{131} — labeled human serum albumin introduced into ascitic fluid: Analysis of the kinetics of a three compartment catenary transfer system in man and speculations on possible sites of degradation. J. clin. Invest. **33**, 377 (1954). ~ Quantitative aspects of iodine metabolism. The exchangeable organic iodine pool, and the rates of thyroidal secretion, peripheral degradation and fecal excretion of endogenously synthesizied organically bound iodine. J. clin. Invest. **33**, 1533 (1954). — Betke, K.: In: Die physiologische Entwicklung des Kindes, von F. Linneweh, S. 172. Heidelberg: Springer 1959. — Beutner, R.: The binding power of serum for drugs tested by a new in vitro method. J. Pharmacol. exp. Ther. **25**, 365 (1925). — Beutner, R., and E. Heyden: The binding power of serum for alkaloids and the inhibition of this effect by homologous alcohols. A contribution to the theory of narcosis. J. Pharmacol. exp. Ther. **35**, 25 (1929). — Beyer, K. H., H. F. Russo and E. K. Tillwon: Carinamide its renal clearance and binding on plasmaprotein. Amer. J. Physiol. **159**, 181 (1949). — Beyers, M. R., and S. E. Gitlov: Metabolism of iron in hemochromatosis. Amer. J. clin. Path. **21**, 349 (1951). — Bickel, H.: Zur Biochemie der Wilsonschen Krankheit. Verh. dtsch. Ges. inn. Med. **1955**. — Bickel, H., H. E. Schultze, W. Grüter u. J. Göllner: Versuche zur Coeruloplasminsubstitution bei der hepatocerebralen Degeneration (Wilsonsche Krankheit). Klin. Wschr. **34**, 961 (1956). — Bieling, H. J., u. E. Bayer: Eisenaustausch zwischen Proteinen; Modellversuch zur Eisenresorption und Speicherung im Tierkörper. Naturwissenschaften **42**, 466 (1955). — Bierman, E. L., V. P. Dole and T. N. Roberts: An abnormality of nonesterified fatty acid metabolism in diabetes mellitus. Diabetes **6**, 475 (1957). — Bigger, J. W.: Inactivation of penicillin by serum. Lancet **1944II**, 400. — Billing, B. H., P. G. Cole and H. G. Lathe: The excretion of bilirubin as an ester glucuronide, giving the direct van den Bergh reaction. Biochem. J. **65**, 774 (1957). — Bing, R. J., A. Siegel, I. Ungar and M. Gilbert: Metabolism of the human heart. II. Studies on fat, ketone and amino acid metabolism. Amer. J. Med. **16**, 504 (1954). — Bischoff, F., and H. R. Pilhorn: The state and distribution of steroid hormones in biolog. systems. III. Solubility of testosterone, progresterone and α-estradiol in serum J. biol. Chem. **174**, 663 (1948). — Bischoff, F., and R. D. Stauffer: Orientation of circulating human estrogens by albumin. Amer. J. Physiol. **191**, 313 (1957). — Bishop, R. C., Milton Toporek, N. A. Nelson and F. H. Bethell: The relationship of binding power to intrinsic factor activity. J. Lab. clin. Med. **46**, 796 (1955). — Bjering, T., and E. Ollgaard: Studies in sulphate clearance. Acta med. scand. **102**, 55 (1939). — Blanc, W. A., and L. Johnson: Studies on kernicterus. Relationship with sulfonamide intoxication, report on kernicterus in rats with glucuronyl transferase deficiency and review of pathogenesis. J. Neuropath. exp. Neurol. 18, 165 (1959). — BLASIUS, R., u. W. SEITZ: Die Beeinflussung der elektrophoretischen Wanderungsgeschwindigkeit von Serumglobulin durch Zusatz von Heparin. Klin. Wschr. 1952, 905. BLOOM, B., I. L. CHAIKOFF and W. O. REINHARD: Intestinal lymph as pathway in transport of absorbet fatty acids of different chain lengths. Amer. J. Physiol. 166, 451 (1951). — BLOOM, B., I. L. CHAIKOFF, W. O. REINHARD and W. G. DAEUBEN: Participation of phosphorlipids in lymphatic transport of adsorbet fatty acids. J. biol. Chem. 189, 261 (1950). — BLUMBERG, B. S., G. OSTER and K. MEYER: Changes in the physical characteristics of the hyaluronat of ground substance with alteration in sodium chloride concentration. J. clin. Invest. 37, 1454 (1955). — BÖHME, W.: Über den aktiven Anteil des Herzens an der Förderung des Venenblutes. Ergebn. Physiol. 38, 251 (1936). —BOETTIGER, E. G.: The absorption of estriol by plasma proteins. J. cell. comp. Physiol. 28, 139 (1946). — BORGSTRÖM, B.: On the mechanism of intestinal fat absorption. II. Acta chem. scand. 5, 643 (1951). ~ III. Acta physiol. scand. 25, 140 (1952). ~ IV. Acta physiol. scand. 25, 291 (1952). — BORGSTRÖM, B., and N. TRYDING: Free fatty acid content of rat thoracic duct lymph during fat absorption. Acta physiol. scand. 37, 127 (1956). — BOTHWELL, T. H., B. C. ELLIS, H. VAN DOORN-WITTKAMPF and O. L. ABRAHAMS: Radioiron studies in hemochromatosis. The effect of repeated phlebotomies. J. Lab. clin. Med. 45, 167 (1955). — BOTHWELL, T. H., and C. A. FINCH: The intestine in iron metabolism: Its role in normal and abnormal states. Amer. J. dig. Dis. 2, 1451 (1957). — BOTHWELL, T. H., G. PIRZIO-BIROLI and C. A. FINCH: Iron absorption. I. Factors influencing absorption. J. Lab. clin. Med. 51, 24 (1958). — BOURS-NELL, J. C.: Some reactions of mustard gas with proteins. Biochem. Soc. Symp. 1948, No 2, 8. — BOURSNELL, J. C., W. G. DANGERFIELD and A. WORMALL: XI. Studies on Bayer 205 (germanin) and atrypol. III. Further observations on the method of determination and on the retention of this drug in the animal body. Biochem. J. 1939. — BOWEN, WILLET R., and W. J. WATERS: Bilirubin encephalopathie: Studies related to the site of inhibitory action of bilirubin on brain metabolism. Amer. J. Dis. Child. 93, 21 (1957). — BOWMAN, J. M., G. RAPMUND and R. C. HARRIS: Bilirubin levels in premature infants. Amer. J. Dis. Child. 93, 75 (1957). — BOXER, G. E., V. C. JELINEK and A. O. ADISON: Streptomycin: Clearance and binding to proteins. J. Pharmacol. exp. Ther. 97, 93 (1949). — BOYDEN, R., and V. R. POTTER: On the form of copper in bloodplasma. J. biol. Chem. 122, 285 (1937). — BOYER, P. D.: The prevention by caprylate of urea and guanidine denaturation of serum albumin. J. biol. Chem. 158, 715 (1945). — BOYER, P. D., G. A. BALLOU and J. M. LUCK: II. Stabilization against urea and guanidine denaturation. J. biol. Chem. 162, 199 (1946). ~ The combination of fatty acids and related compounds with serum albumin. The nature and extend of the combination. J. biol. Chem. 167, 407 (1947). — BOYER, P. D., F. G. LUM, G. A. BALLOU, J. M. LUCK and R. G. RICE: The combination of fatty acids and related compounds with serum albumin. I. Stabilization against heat denaturation. J. biol. Chem. 162, 181 (1946). — BRAGDON, J. H.: Hyperlipemia and atheromatosis in a hibernator, citeus columbianus. Circulat. Res. 2, 520 (1954). ~ $C^{14}O_2$ excretion after the intravenous administration of labeled chylomicrons in the rat. Arch. Biochem. 75, 528 (1958). — BRAGDON, J. H., and R. S. GORDON jr.: The distribution of C^{14} after the intravenous injection of labeled chylomicrons and unesterified fatty acids in the rat. J. clin. Invest. 37, 574 (1958). — BRAGDON, J. H., R. J. HAVEL and E. BOYLE: Human serum lipoproteins. I. Chemical composition of four fractions. J. Lab. clin. Med. 48, 36 (1956). — BRAUER, R. W., and L. R. PESOTTI: The mechanism of the extraction of bromsulfalein from bloodplasma by the liver. Fed. Proc. 7, 207 (1948). ~ The removal of bromsulphthalein from blood plasma by the liver of the rat. J. Pharmacol. exp. Ther. 97, 358 (1949). — BRAUER, R. W., L. R. PESOTTI and J. S. KREBS: The distribution and excretion of S^{35}-labeled sulfobromophthalein-sodium administered to dogs by continuous infusion. J. clin. Invest. 34, 35 (1955). — BRAUNSTEINER, H., E. GISINGER u. F. PAKESCH: Ferritin, Transferrin und Serumeisen. Klin. Wschr. 30, 394 (1952). — BREITINGER, H.: Über die Koffeinbindung an Serumproteine. Diss. Tübingen 1956. — BRENDSTRUP, P.: On the unsaturated copper binding capacity of blood serum. Scand. J. clin. Lab. Invest. 5, 18 (1953). — BRENNER, W.: Die Bedeutung des Kupfers in Biologie und Pathologie unter besonderer Berücksichtigung des wachsenden Organismus. Erg. inn. Med. Kinderheilk. 4, 806 (1953). — BRENTANO, C.: Klinische und experimentelle Untersuchungen über Haemolyse durch Gallensäure und ihre Hemmung durch Serum. Z. ges. exp. Med. 57, 234 (1927). — BRINKHOUS, K. M., H. P. SMITH, E. D. WARNER and W. H. SEEGERS: The inhibition of blood clotting. Amer. J. Physiol. 125, 683 (1938). — BRODIE, B. B., H. KURZ and L. S. SCHANKER: The importance of dissociation constant and lipid-solubility in influencing the passage of drugs into the cerebrospinal fluid. J. Pharmacol. exp. Ther. 130, 20 (1960). — BROOKS, S. C., and M. M. BROOKS: The permeability of living cells. Berlin: Gebrüder Bornträger 1941. — BRUGER, M.: The state of cholesterol and the nature of cholesterolprotein complex in path. body fluids. J. biol. Chem. 108, 463 (1935). — BRUNELLI, B.: Sulla „Functione veicolante“ delle proteine plasmatide. Arch. int. Pharmacodyn. 49, 262 (1934). — BRUTON, O. C.: Agammaglobulinemia. Pediatrics 9, 722 (1952). — BUCHER, K., u. H. EMMENEGGER: Über die Mischung des Blutes der Körpervenen im

Lungenkreislauf. Bull. schweiz. Akad. med. Wiss. 7, H. 5/6 (1951). ~ Besonderheiten der Lungendurchblutung. Arch. Kreisl.-Forsch. 18, 94 (1952). — Büchmann, P., u. G. Schenz: Haemochromatose und Eisenstoffwechsel. Zur Klinik und Pathogenese der Haemochromatose unter besonderer Berücksichtigung des Eisenstoffwechsels. Beih. z. Med. Wschr. 5 (1948). — Bueding, E.: Zit. nach Goldstein, The interactions of drugs and plasmaproteins. J. Pharmacol. exp. Ther. 95, 102 (1949). — Bueding, E., and J. Oliver-Gonzalez: Metabolism of schistosoma mansoni. Proc. 4. Int. Congr. of tropical medicine and malaria abstracts, pp. 80—81. Washington 1948. — Bull, H. B.: Adsorption of water vapor by proteins. J. Amer. chem. Soc. 66, 1499 (1944). — Burkhard, R. K., and F. A. Moore: Interactions of homologs of carcinogenics azodyes and bovine serum albumin. J. Amer. chem. Soc. 77, 6057 (1955). — Burr, W., C. Dunkelberg, J. C. McPherson and H. Tidwell: Blood levels of adsorbed labeled fat and chylomikronemia. J. biol. Chem. 210, 531 (1954). — Busck, G.: Die photobiologischen Sensibilisatoren und ihre Eiweißbindungen. Biochem. Z. 1, 425 (1906). — Bush, J. A., J. P. Mahoney, C. J. Gubler, G. E. Cartwright and M. M. Wintrobe: Studies on copper metabolism. XXI. The transfer of radiocopper between erythrocytes and plasma. J. Lab. clin. Med. 47, 898 (1956). — Bush, J. A., J. P. Mahoney, H. Markowitz, G. J. Gubler, G. E. Cartwright and M. M. Wintrobe: Studies on copper metabolism. XVI. Radioactiv copper studies with normal subjects and patients with hepatolenticular degeneration. J. clin. Invest. 34, 1766 (1955). — Butterworth jr., C. E., G. J. Gubler, G. E. Cartwright and M. M. Wintrobe: Studies on copper metabolism. XXVI. Plasma copper in patients with tropical sprue. Proc. Soc. exp. Biol. (N.Y.) 98, 594 (1958).

Cameron, Ch., and K. Fletcher: An iodine compound associated with albumin in the plasma of thyrotoxic patients. Nature (Lond.) 183, 116 (1959). — Cann, I. R.: Effect of binding of iron and other small molecules on protein structure. IV. Two electrophoretically distinguishable types of interaction at bovine serum albumin with acidic media. J. Amer. chem. Soc. 80, 4263 (1958). — Capell, D. F., H. E. Hutchinson and M. Jowett: Transfusional siderosis: The effect of excessive iron deficits on the tissue. J. Path. Bact. 74, 245 (1957). — Caroli, J. B., A. Bessis u. J. Bretton: Hämochromatose mit hypochromer Anämie und Fehlen von anormalem Hämoglobin. Elektronenmikroskopische Studie. — Caroll, B.: Use of dyestuffs for determining the activity of proteolytic enzymes. Science 111, 387 (1950). — Carter, C. E., and J. P. Greenstein: Protective effect of thymus nucleate on the heat coagulation of proteins. J. nat. Cancer Inst. 6, 219 (1946). — Cartwright, G. E., P. Black and M. M. Wintrobe: Chemical, clinical and immunological studies on the products of human plasma fraction XXXIX. J. clin. Invest. 28, 86 (1949). — Cartwright, G. E., J. A. Bush, H. Markowitz, J. P. Mahoney and C. J. Gubler: Further studies on the abnormalities in the metabolism of copper in Wilsons's disease. J. clin. Invest. 34, 925 (1955). — Cartwright, G. E., R. E. Hodges, C. J. Gubler, J. P. Mahoney, K. Daum, M. M. Wintrobe and W. B. Bean: Studies on copper metabolism. XIII. Hepatolenticular degeneration. J. clin. Invest. 33, 1487 (1954). — Cartwright, G. E., H. Markowitz, G. S. Shields and M. M. Wintrobe: Studies on copper metabolism. XXIX. A critical analysis of serum copper and ceruloplasmin concentrations in normal subjects, patients with Wilson's disease and relatives of patients with Wilson's disease. Amer. J. Med. 28, 555 (1960). — Casano, C., L. Baschieri u. P. Andreani: Bemerkungen über die Kropfentstehung bei übermäßig renaler Jodausscheidung. Rass. Fisiopat. clin. ter. 29, 253 (1957). — Chaikoff, I. L., B. Bloom, M. D. Siperstein, J. Y. Kiyasu, W. O. Reinhardt, W. G. Dauben and J. L. Wastham: C^{14}-cholesterol. The lymphatic transport of absorbed cholesterol $4 C^{14}$. J. biol. Chem. 194, 407 (1952). — Chalmers, J. G.: The role of soluble proteins in the elimination of carcinogens from the animal body. Proc. biochem. Soc. 1953, XIX. — Chambers, R., and B. W. Zweifach: Intercellular cement and capillary permeability. Physiol. Rev. 27, 436 (1947). — Chanutin, A., S. Ludewig and A. V. Masket: Studies on the calcium protein relationship with the aid of the ultracentrifuge. I. Observations on calcium caseinate solutions. J. biol. Chem. 143, 737 (1942). — Chargaff, E., M. Ziff and S. S. Cohen: Studies on the chemistry of blood coagulation. X. Observ. J. biol. Chem. 136, 257 (1940). — Chargaff, E., M. Ziff and D. H. Moore: Studies on the chemistry of blood coagulation. XII. Observ. J. biol. Chem. 139, 383 (1941). — Chernik, S., P. A. Svere and I. L. Chaikoff: The metabolism of arterial tissue. The formation in vitro of fatty acids and phospholipids by rat artery with C^{14} and P^{32} as indicators. J. biol. Chem. 179, 117 (1949). — Chesner, Ch.: Hemochromatosis, review of literature and presentation of a case without pigmentation or diabetes. J. Lab. clin. Med. 31, 1029 (1946).— Chinard, F. P.: Interaction of quarternary ammonium compounds and proteins. J. biol. chem. 176, 1439 (1948). — Chou, T., and W. H. Adolf: Copper metabolism in man. Biochem. J. 29, 476 (1935). — Christensen, H. P. O.: Vitamin B_{12}-inholdet i blodet; Metodik og diagnostik betydning vitamin B_{12} blood content. Ugeskr. Laeg. 120, 925 (1958). — Christensen, L. K.: Pituitary regulation of thyroid activity. Acta endocr. (Kbh.) 33, 111 (1960). ~ Triiodothyronine uptake by erythrocytes. Endocrinology 66, 138 (1960). ~ Free non-proteinbound serum thyroxine. Acta med. scand. 166, 133 (1960). — Claireaux, A. E.: Hemolytic disease of newborn. Clinical pathologic study of 157 cases nuclear jaundice

(Kernicterus). Arch. Dis. Childh. **25**, 61 (1950). — Clausen, J.: Immuno-Electrophoresis and autoradiography. In: Proteides of the biological fluids, Bd. VIII. Amsterdam: Elsevier 1960. (Im Druck.) — Clausen, J., and T. Munkner: Thyroid hormone binding proteins in human serum characterized by immuno-electrophoresis and auto-radiographic tracings. Proc. Soc. exp. Biol. (N.Y.) **104**, 40 (1960). — Clayton, C. G.: The absorption of radioactive B_{12} in normal and gastrectomized. J. Physiol. (Lond.) **129**, 56 (1955). — Cohen, M., M. Stiefel, W. J. Reddy and J. C. Laidlaw: The secretion and disposition of cortisol during pregnancy. J. clin. Endocr. **18**, 1076 (1958). — Cohen, S. S., and E. Chargaff: Studies of the chemistry of blood coagulation. IX. J. biol. Chem. **136**, 243 (1940). — Cohn, E. J.: The chemical spezifity of the interaction of diverse human plasmaproteins. Blood **3**, 471 (1948). — Cohn, E. J., and J. T. Edsall: Proteins, aminoacids a peptides as ions and dipolar ions, p. 686ff. New York: Reinhold Publ. Corporation 1943. — Cohn, E. J., F. R. N. Gurd, D. M. Surgenor, B. A. Barnes, R. K. Brown, G. Derouaux, J. M. Gillespie, F. W. Kahnt, W. F. Lever, C. H. Sinn, D. Mittelman, R. F. Mouton, K. Schmid and E. A. Uroma: A system for the separation of the components of human blood: Quantitative procedures for the separation of the protein components of human plasma. J. Amer. chem. Soc. **72**, 465 (1950). — Cohn, E. J., L. E. Strong, W. L. Hughes jr., D. J. Mulford, J. Ashworth, M. Melin and H. L. Taylor: Preparation and properties of serum a plasma proteins. IV. Separation into fractions. J. Amer. chem. Soc. **68**, 459 (1946). — Cohn, E. J., D. M. Surgenor, K. Schmid, W. H. Batchelor, H. C. Isliker and E. H. Alameri: The interaction of plasma proteins with heavy metals and with alkaline earth with specific anions and specific steroids, with specific polysaccharides and with the formed elements of the blood. Faraday Discuss. **13**, 176 (1953). — Collander, R., u. H. Bärlund: Permeabilitätsstudien an chara ceratophylla. II. Die Permeabilität für Nichtelektrolyte. Acta bot. fenn. **11** (1933). — Colvin, J. R.: Binding of anions by denaturated protein. Canad. J. Chem. **30**, 973 (1952). — Coolidge, T. B.: Chemistry of the van den Bergh reaction. J. biol. Chem. **132**, 119 (1940). — Coons, A. H., E. H. Leduc and N. H. Caplan: Localisation of antigen in tissue cells. J. exp. Med. **93**, 175 (1951). — Cooper, B. A.: Studies with a more rapid method of vitamin B_{12} assay utilizing euglena gracilis. J. clin. Path. **12**, 1959 (1959). — Copeland, B. E., and F. W. Sandermann: The Mg-binding property of the serum proteins. J. biol. Chem. **197**, 331 (1952). — Cremer, D.: Blutbildveränderungen bei experimenteller Eisenspeicherung. Z. ges. exp. Med. **107**, 467 (1940). — Crosby, W. H.: Metabolism of hemoglobin and bile pigment in hemolytic disease. Amer. J. Med. **18**, 112 (1955). — Cruchaud, S., C. Mahaim, B. R. Scazziga u. A. Vannotti: Fonction tyroidienne et néphrose lipoidique. Schweiz. med. Wschr. **84**, 478 (1954). — Cserna, S., u. S. Liebmann: Beitrag zur Lehre des Ikterus neonatorum. Klin. Wschr. **1923**, 2122.

D'Addabbo, A., F. Heni u. E. Kallee: Erfahrungen mit dem Radiojodtest bei einigen internen Krankheiten. Medizinische **1958**, 1212. — Dancis, J.: Aspects of bilirubin metabolism before and after birth. Pediatrics **24**, 980 (1959). — Darby, W. J.: Iron and copper. J. Amer. med. Ass. **142**, 1288 (1950). — Darby, W. J., E. B. Bridgforth, J. le Brocquy, S. L. Clark, J. D. de Oliveira, J. Kerany, W. J. McGantry and C. Perez: Vitamin B_{12} requirement of adult man. Amer. J. Med. **25**, 726 (1958). — Daughaday, W. H.: Binding of corticosteroids by plasma proteins. I. Dialysis equilibrium and renal clearence studies. II. Paper electrophoresis. J. clin. Invest. **35**, 1428, 1434 (1956). ~ Binding of corticosteroid by plasma proteins. J. clin. Invest. **37**, 511, 519 (1958). ~ Steroid protein interactions. Physiol. Rev. **38**, 885 (1959). — Davis, B. D.: Binding of sulfonamides by plasma proteins. Science **95**, 78 (1942). ~ Binding of sulfonamide drugs by plasma proteins. A factor in determining the distribution of drug in the body. J. clin. Invest. **22**, 753 (1943). ~ Physiological significance of the binding of molecules by plasma proteins. Amer. Scientist **34**, 611 (1946). — Davis, B. D., and R. J. Dubos: Interaction of serum albumin, free and estrified oleic acid and lipase in relation to cultivation of tbc. bac. Arch. Biochem. **11**, 201 (1946). ~ The binding of fatty acids by serum albumin, a protective growth factor in bacteriological medium. J. exp. Med. **86**, 215 (1947). — Davis jr., W. D., and W. R. Arrowsmith: The effect of repeated phlebotomies in hemochromatosis. J. Lab. clin. Med. **39**, 526 (1952). — Davson, H., and J. F. Danielli: The permeability of natural membranes. Cambridge: Cambridge University Press 1943. — Deiss, W. P., E. C. Albright and F. C. Larson: A study of the nature of the circulating thyroid hormone in euthyroid and hyperthyroid subjects by use of paper electrophoresis. J. clin. Invest. **31**, 1000 (1952). ~ Comparison of in vitro serum binding of thyroxin and thrijodthyronine. Proc. Soc. exp. Biol. (N.Y.) **84**, 513 (1953). — Derouax, G.: Liaison sulfamide-protéine et passage des sulfamides dans le liquide céphalorachidien. Acta biol. belg. **3**, 170 (1943). ~ Mesure de la diffusion générale du sulfathiazol, de la sulfapyridine et de la sulfacetamide. C. R. Soc. Biol. (Paris) **138**, 877 (1944). — Dewey, H. M., and A. Wormall: Studies on suramin. 5. The combination of the drug with the plasma proteins. Biochem. J. **40**, 119 (1946). ~ Studies on suramin. 6. Further observations on the determination of suramin in whole blood and serum. Biochem. J. **43**, 24 (1948). — Dieckhoff, J.: Behandlung der toxischen Dysenterie mit Periston N. Z. ges. inn. Med. **7**, 682 (1952). — Diemer, K., u. H. Bechtelsheimer: Zur Todesursache beim Morbus haemolyticus neonatorum. Z. Kinderheilk. **82**, 147 (1959). — Dishkovich, L.: Über den Stoffwechsel von Vitamin B_{12} bei Affektionen von Leber und Gallenwegen. Schweiz. med. Wschr. 88, 1087 (1958). — Doe, R. P., H. H. Zinneman, E. B. Flink and R. A. Ulstrom: Significance of the concentration of nonprotein-bound plasma cortisol in normal subjects, Cushing's syndrome pregnancy and during estrogen therapy. J. clin. Endocr. 20, 11 (1960). — Doetsch, R. N.: Ruminology — an interdisciplinary science. J. Dairy Sci. 40, 1204 (1957). — Doladilhe, M., et M. Mazille: In vitro, un seul constituant de l'édifice protéosérique fixe les matières colorantes. C.R. Soc. Biol. (Paris) 130, 128 (1939). — Dole, V. P.: Fractionation of plasma non esterified fatty acids. Proc. Soc. exp. Biol. (N.Y.) 93, 532 (1956). — Dow, P.: Brilliant vital red and T-1824: Comparative studies. Fed. Proc. 4, 16 (1945). — Dow, P., and R. W. Pickering: Behavior of dog serum dyed with brilliant vital red or Evans blue to precipitation with ethanol. Amer. J. Physiol. 161, 212 (1950). — Dowling, J. T., N. Freinkel and S. H. Ingbar: Thyroxine-binding by sera of pregnant women. J. clin. Endocr. 16, 280 (1956). ~ Thyroxine-binding by sera of prenant women, newborn infants, and women with spontaneous abortion. J. clin. Invest. 35, 1263 (1956). ~ Effect of diethylstilbestrol on the binding of thyroxine in serum. J. clin. Endocr. 16, 1491 (1956). — Drinker, N., A. A. Green and A. B. Hastings: Equilibria between calcium and purified globulins. J. biol. Chem. 131, 641 (1939). — Druez, G.: Un nouveau cas d'acanthocytose: dysmorphie érythrocytaire congénitale avec rétinite, troubles nerveux et stigmates dégénératifs. Rev. Hémat. 14, 3—11 (1959). — Duggan, E. L., and J. M. Luck: The combination of organic anions with serum albumin. IV. Stabilization against urea denaturation. J. biol. Chem. 172, 265 (1948). — Durrum, E. L., M. H. Paul and E. R. B. Smith: Lipid detection in paper electrophoresis. Science 116, 428 (1952). — Dutton, G. J.: Glucuronide synthesis in foetal liver and kidney. Lancet 1958 II, 49. — Dyke, H. B. van, N. A. Tupikowa, B. F. Chow and H. A. Walker: The pharmacological behavior of some derivates of sulfadiazine. J. Pharmacol. exp. Ther. 83, 203 (1945).

Eagle, H.: The inactivation of penicillins F, G, K and X by human and rabbit serum. J. exp. Med. 85, 141 (1947). ~ The variing blood levels afforded by penicillins F, G, K and X. J. exp. Med. 85, 163 (1947). ~ The therapeutic activity of penicillins F, G, K and X in experimental infections with pneumococcus I and streptococcus pyogenes. J. exp. Med. 85, 175 (1947). ~ The effect of human serum on the dilution bioassay of penicillin G, X and K. J. Bact. 56, 59 (1948). — Earle jr., D. P.: Rénal excretion of sulfamerazine. J. clin. Invest. 23, 914 (1944). — Earle jr., D. P., and B. B. Brodie: The renal excretion of caronamide. J. Pharmacol. exp. Ther. 91, 250 (1947). — Eder, H. A.: Lipoproteins of human serum. Amer. J. Med. 23, 269 (1957). — Eder, H. A., I. L. Beagdon and E. Boyle: The in vitro exachange of phosphorlipoid phosphorus between lipoproteins. Circulation 10, 603 (1954). — Eder, H. A., E. M. Russ, R. A. R. Pritchett, M. M. Wilber and D. P. Barr: Protein-lipid relationship in human plasma: In biliary cirrhosis, obstructive jaundice and acute hepatitis. J. clin. Invest. 34, 1147 (1955). — Edsall, J. T.: The plasma proteins and their fractionation. Advances in prot. chemistry 3, 384 (1947). — Eichler, O., E. Lindner u. K. Schmeiser: Untersuchungen des peripheren Kreislaufs mit radioaktiven Natrium. Klin. Wschr. 27, 480 (1949). — Eisfeld, G., u. H. Seefeld: Zum papierelektrophoretischen Verhalten der Paraaminosalicylsäure (PAS) und des Isonikotinsäurehydracids (INH) bei Anwesenheit von Serumeiweiß. Naturwissenschaften 41, 305 (1954). — Eisler, B., G. Rosdahl u. H. Theorell: Untersuchungen über die Zustandsform des Kupfers im Blutserum mit Hilfe der Kataphorese. Biochem. Z. 286, 435 (1936). — Elliot, H. C., and H. L. Holley: Serum sodium and potassium values in 400 normal human subjects determind by Beckman flame photometer. Fed. Proc. 10, 180 (1951). — Elsom, K. A., P. A. Bott and Z. H. Shiels: On the excretion of skiodan, diodrast and hippuran by the dog. Amer. J. Physiol. 115, 548 (1936). — Endicott, K. M., T. Gillman, G. Brecher, A. T. Ness, F. A. Clarke and E. R. Adamik. A study of histochemical iron using tracer methods. J. Lab. clin. Med. 34, 141 (1949). — Eppinger, H.: Permeabilitäts-Pathologie, S. 586. Wien: Springer 1949. ~ Hepatolienale Erkrankungen. Berlin: Springer 1920. ~ In Kraus u. Brugsch, Pathologie und Therapie, Bd. VI/2, S. 97. 1923. — Erdmann-Oehlecker, S.: Der Vitamin B_{12}-Stoffwechsel bei Hämoblastosen. 1. Europ. Symp. Hamburg 1956. Vitamin B_{12} und Intrinsic Factor, S. 250. 1957. — Esser, C.: Die Lokalisation tuberkulöser Lungenveränderungen beim Erwachsenen. Dtsch. med. Wschr. 80, 1835 (1955). — Everett, N. B., W. E. Garrett and B. S. Simmonds: Lymphatics in iron absorption and transport. Amer. J. Physiol. 178, 45 (1954).

Fairly, N. H., and R. J. Bromfield: Laboratory studies in malaria and blackwater fever. III. A new blood pigment and other observations. Trans. roy. Soc. trop. Med. Hyg. 28, 307 (1934). — Farah, A.: On the combination of some cardioactive glycosides with serum protens. J. Pharmacol. exp. Ther. 83, 143 (1945). — Favarger, P.: La résorption intestinale des aicides gras d'animal supérieur. Expos. ann. Biochem. méd. 13, 49 (1951). — Fawaz, G., and A. Farah: A study of the digitoxin binding power of serum and other proteins of the rabbit. J. Pharmacol. exp. Ther. 80, 193 (1944). — Federman, D. D., J. Robbins and J. E. Rall: Effect of methylesterone on thyroid function, thyroxine metabolism and thyroxine-binding protein. J. clin. Invest. 37, 1021 (1958). — Feldman, J. D.: Effect of oestrogen on thyroidal iodide trapping and conversion of inorganic ^{131}J to P.B.I.^{131}. Endocrinology 59,

289 (1956). ∼ Effect of estrogen on thyroidal and renal clearance of J^{131} in the rat. Amer. J. Physiol. 187, 369 (1956). ∼ Effect of estrogen on iodinated amino acids of the thyroid and serum. Amer. J. Physiol. 191, 301 (1957). — Fellinger, K.: Experimentelle Untersuchungen über den Einfluß des Bilirubins auf die Erythropoese. Z. exp. Med. 85, 369 (1932). — Fellinger, K., E. Mannheimer u. H. Vetter: Der Radiojod-Plasmatest. Wien. Z. inn. Med. 34, 359 (1953). — Ferguson, J. H.: The action of heparin, serum albumin (cristall) and salmine on blood clotting mechanismus. Amer. J. Physiol. 130, 759 (1940). — Fernandes, J., J. H. van der Kamer and H. A. Wejers: The absorption of fats studied in a child with chylothorax. J. clin. Invest. 34, 1026 (1955). — Fields, T., D. Kinnory, E. Kaplan, Y. Oester and E. Bowser: The determination of protein-bound iodine[131] with anion exchange resin column. J. Lab. clin. Med. 47, 333 (1956). —Fieser, L. F., and H. Heymann: Naphthoquinone antimalarials. XIX. Antirespiratory studie of protein binding. J. Pharmacol. exp. Ther. 94, 97 (1948). ∼ Naphthoquinone antimalarials. XXII. Antirespiratory activity. (Plasmod. lophurale.) J. biol. Chem. 176, 1363 (1948). — Figueroa, W. S., W. S. Adams, S. H. Bassett, L. Rosove and F. Davis: Effect of disodium calcium versenate on iron excretion in man. Amer. J. Med. 17, 101 (1954). — Finch, C. A.: Body iron exchange. J. clin. Invest. 38, 342 (1959). — Finch, C. A., M. Hegsted, T. D. Kinney, E. D. Thomas, C. E. Rath, D. Haskins, S. Finch and R. G. Fluharty: Iron metabolism and the pathophysiology of iron storage. Blood 5, 983 (1950). — Findlay, L., G. Higgens and M. W. Stanier: Icterus neonatorum: incidence and cause. Arch. Dis. Childh. 22, 65 (1947). — Fitting, W., u. K. Gerbaulet: Über das Jodkonzentrierungsvermögen der Speicheldrüsen (untersucht bei Patienten mit unterschiedlicher Schilddrüsenfunktion). In: Radioaktive Isotope in Klinik und Forschung, Bd. 2, S. 169. München u. Berlin: Urban & Schwarzenberg 1956. — Földi, M., L. Rusznyák u. G. Szabo: Die Rolle der Lymphzirkulation bei der Entstehung phlebohypertonischer Oedeme. Mag. belorv. Arch. 2, 332 (1949). — Földi, M.: Physiologie und Pathologie des Lymphkreislaufes. Verh. dtsch. Ges. inn. Med. 66 (1960). — Forker, L. L., and I. L. Chaikoff: Turnover of serum proteins in diabetes as studied with S 35 labeled proteins. J. biol. Chem. 196, 829 (1952). — Forker, L. L., I. L. Chaikoff and W. O. Reinhard: Circulation of plasma proteins: Their transport of lymph. J. biol. Chem. 197, 625 (1952). — Forrai, E., u. R. Sívó: Physikalisch-chemische Eigenschaften des Bilirubins in Körperflüssigkeiten. Biochem. Z. 189, 162 (1927). — Foster, W. C.: Tissue protein-bound radioactive iodide in rat stomach. Amer. J. Physiol. 183, 3 (1955). — Francis, G. E., and A. Wormall: The use of radioisotopes in the study of some metabolic and immunological reactions. Comm. XI. internat. Congr. of Pure and Appl. Chem., 1947, London. — Frazer, A. C.: The digestion and absorption of fat. Arch. Sci. physiol. 2, 15 (1948). ∼ Fat metabolism. Ann. Rev. Biochem. 21, 245 (1952). ∼ Normale und gestörte Fettresorption. Medizinische 1953, 1317. — Fredrickson, D. S., and R. S. Gordon jr.: Metabolism of albumin bound labeled fatty acid in man. J. clin. Invest. 36, 890 (1957). ∼ Transport of fatty acids. Physiol. Rev. 38, 585 (1958). — Fredrickson, D. S., R. S. Gordon jr., K. Ono and A. Cherkes: The metabolism of albumin bound C^{14}-labeled unesterified fatty acids in normal human subjects. J. clin. Invest. 37, 1504 (1958). — Frederickson, D. S., D. L. McCollester, R. Havel and K. Ono: Chemistry of lipides as related to atherosclerosis, p. 205. Edit. by I. H. Page. Springfield, Ill.: Ch. C. Thomas 1958. — Freeman, L. W., and V. Johnson: The hemolytic action of chyle. Amer. J. Physiol. 130, 723 (1940). — Freinkel, N., J. T. Dowling and S. H. Ingbar: The interaction of thyroxine with plasma proteins: Localization of thyroxine-binding protein in Cohn fractions of plasma. J. clin. Invest. 34, 1698 (1955). — Freinkel, N., S. H. Ingbar and J. T. Dowling: The influence of extracellular thyroxine-binding protein upon the accumulation of thyroxine by tissue slices. J. clin. Invest. 36, 25 (1957). — French, J. E., B. Morris and D. S. Robinson: In: Blood lipids and the clearing factor. (Third internat. Conf. on biochem. problems of lipids, July 1956.) Brussels Koninkl. Vlaam. Acad. Wetenschapen, p. 323, 1956.—Fresen, I., u. H. Weese: Das gewebliche Bild nach Infusion verschiedener Kollidonfraktionen (Periston N, Periston, hochvisköses Periston beim Tier). Beitr. path. Anat. 112, 44 (1952). — Frexner, L. B., D. B. Cowie and G. J. Vosburgh: Studies on capillary permeability with tracer substances. Cold Spr. Harb. Symp. quant. Biol. 13, 88 (1948). — Friedmann, M., S. O. Byers and E. Shibata: Observation concerning the production and excretion of cholesterol in mamals X. Factors affecting the absorption and fate of ingested cholesterol. J. exp. Med. 98, 107 (1953). — Friis-Hansen, B. J., M. Holiday, T. Stapleton and W. M. Wallace: Total body water in children. Pediatrics 7, 321 (1951). — Frisch, A.: Über familiäre Hämochromatose. Wien. Arch. klin. Med. 4, 149 (1922). — Fuller, A. T.: Antibacterial and chemical constitution in long chain aliphatic acides. Biochem. J. 36, 548 (1942).

Gabrielson, Z., and A. L. Kretchmar: Studies on the salivary secretion of iodide. J. clin. Encodr. 16, 1347 (1956). — Galimard, I. E.: Metabolisme du salicylate de sodium. III. Adsorption in vitro par le serum sanguin. Bull. Soc. Chim. biol. (Paris) 27, 206 (1945). — Gamble, J. L.: Extracellular fluid. Cambridge, Masachussetts: Harvard University Press 1950. — Garby, L, S. Sjölin and B. Vahlquist: Chronic refractory hypochromic anaemia with disturbed haemmetabolism. Brit. J. Haemat. 3, 55 (1957). — Gardner, I. A., and

J. Gainsborough: Studies on the cholesterol content of normal human plasma. II. The attraction of the plasmaproteins. Biochem. J. 21, 141 (1927). — Gardner, L. I.: Role of human plasma protein fractions IV and V in 17-ketosteroid transport. Bull. Johns Hopk. Hosp. 94, 105 (1954). — Garrow, J. S., and J. C. Waterloo: Observationes on evansblue dye as a tracer for human plasma albumin. Clin. Sci. 18, 35 (1959). — Gauer, O. H.: Wechselbeziehungen zwischen Herz- und Venensystem. Verh. dtsch. Ges. Kreisl.-Forsch. 1956, 61 ff. — Gauer, O. H., u. J. P. Henry: Klin. Wschr. 34, 356 (1956). — George, E. P., and W. Sollich: The adsorption of J^{131} iodide ions on plasma proteins. Austr. J. exp. Biol. med. Sci. 37, 289 (1959). — Gerbaulet, K., u. W. Fitting: Über das Jod-Konzentrierungs- und Sekretionsvermögen der Speicheldrüsen. (Untersucht mit Jod^{131} bei Patienten mit unterschiedlicher Schilddrüsenfunktion.) Klin. Wschr. 34, 120 (1956). — Gerbaulet, K., W. Fitting u. W. Maurer: Bestimmung der absoluten Jodidaufnahmen der menschlichen Schilddrüse bei unterschiedlicher Schilddrüsenfunktion. Minerva nucleare (Torino) 3, 156 (1959). ~ Über Messungen der quantitativen Jodid-Aufnahme der Schilddrüse und der Konzentration des Serum-Jodids. Klin. Wschr. 38, 474 (1960). — Gerbaulet, K., W. Fitting u. S. Rosenkaimer: Zum Sekretionsvermögen der Speicheldrüsen für anorganisches Serum-Jod. Klin. Wschr. 35, 576 (1957). — Gibian, H.: Der Beitrag des Chemikers zur Struktur und Funktionsaufklärung der mesenchymalen Grundsubstanz mit besonderer Bezugnahme auf die Hyaluronidase und ihre Substrate in „Kapillare und Interstitium". Von H. Bartelheimer u. H. Küchmeister. Stuttgart: Georg Thieme 1955. — Giblett, E. R., C. G. Hickman and O. Smithies: Serum transferrins. Nature (Lond.) 183, 1589 (1959). — Gildemeister, H.: Porphyrine und Serumeiweiß. Ein Beitrag zur Vehikelfunktion der Serumeiweißkörper. Z. ges. exp. Med. 102, 58 (1937). — Gilder, H., S. F. Redo, D. Barr and Ch. Gardner Child: Water distribution in normal subjects and in patients with Laenec's cirrhosis. J. clin. Invest. 33, 555 (1954). — Gillich, K. H.: Quantitative Bestimmung der Bindung von ^{131}-J-Thyroxin durch Serumeiweißkörper mit der Überwanderungselektrophorese. Z. ges. exp. Med. 130, 415 (1958). — Gillich, K. H., u. F. W. Aly: Die Präalbumin-Thyroxin- und Trijodthyroninbindung im Serum. Verh. dtsch. Ges. inn. Med. 66 (1960). — Gilligan, D. R.: Blood levels of sulfadiazine, sulfamerazine a sulfametharine in relation to binding in the plasma. J. Pharmacol. exp. Ther. 79, 320 (1943). — Gillman, T., and A. C. Ivy: A histological study of the participation of the intestinal epithelium, the reticuloendothelial system and the lymphatics in iron absorption and transport. Preliminary report. Gastroenterology 9, 169 (1947). — Gisinger, E.: Zum Wirkungsmechanismus der Ferrisaccharate. Wien. Z. inn. Med. 34, 223 (1953). — Gisinger, E.: Die Diagnose des Eisenmangels. Wien. Z. inn. Med. 34, 395 (1953). — Gitlin, D., D. G. Cornwall, D. Nagasato, J. L. Oncley, W. L. Hughes and C. Janeway: Studies on the metabolism of plasma proteins in the nephrotic syndrom. J. clin. Invest. 37, 172 (1958). — Gitlow, St. E., and M. R. Beyers: Metabolism of iron. I. Intravenous iron tolerance test in normal subjects and patients with hemochromatosis. J. Lab. clin. Med. 39, 337 (1952). — Gofman, J. W., O. DeLalla, F. Glazier, N. K. Freeman, F. T. Lindgren, A. V. Nichols, B. Strisower and A. Tamplin: The serum lipoprotein transport system in health, metabolic disorders, atherosclerosis and coronary heart disease. Plasma (Milano) 2, 413 (1954). — Gofman, J. W., F. Glazier, A. Tamplin, B. Strisower and O. de Lalla: Lipoproteins, coronary heart disease and atherosclerosis. Physiol. Rev. 34, 589 (1954). — Gofman, J. W., M. Hanig, H. B. Jones, M. A. Lauffer, E. J. Lawry, L. A. Lewis, G. V. Man, F. E. Moore, F. Olmstedt, J. F. Jaeger, E. C. Andrus, J. H. Barach, J. W. Beams, J. W. Fertig, J. H. Page, J. A. Shannon, F. J. Stare and P. D. White: Evaluation of serum lipoprotein and cholesterol measurements as prediction of clinical complications of atherosclerosis. Circulation 14, 691 (1956). — Gofman, J. W., H. B. Jones, F. T. Lindgren, T. P. Lyon, H. A. Elliot and N. Strisower: Blood lipids and human atherosclerosis. Circulation 2, 161 (1950). — Gofman, J. W., Fr. Lindgreen, H. Elliot, W. Mantz, J. Hewitt, B. Strisower and V. Herring: The role of lipids and lipoproteins in atherosclerosis. Science 111, 166, 186 (1950). — Goldbaum, L. R., and P. K. Smith: The binding of barbiturate by human and bovine serum albumin. Fed. Proc. 7, 222 (1948). — Goldeck, H., u. D. Remy: Über die Abwanderungsgeschwindigkeit des Eisens nach intravenösen Eisen III-Gaben. Klin. Wschr. 31, 608 (1953). — Goldman, D. S., J. L. Chaikoff, W. O. Reinhard, C. Entenman and W. G. Dauben: Site of formation of plasma phospholipides studies with C^{14} labeled palmitic acid. J. biol. Chem. 184, 727 (1950). — Goldmann, E. E.: Die äußere und innere Sekretion des gesunden und kranken Organismus im Lichte der vitalen Färbung. Beitr. klin. Chir. 64 (1909). — Goldring, W., R. W. Clark and H. W. Smith: The phenol red clearance in normal man. J. clin. Invest. 15, 221 (1936). — Goldstein, A.: Properties and behavior of human plasma cholinesterase. Zit. nach A. Goldstein, The interaction of drugs and proteins. J. Pharmacol. exp. Ther. 95, 102 (1949). — Gollwitzer-Meier, K.: Blutdruck und Organdurchblutung. Dtsch. Arch. klin. Med. 89, 167 (1942). — Goodman, D. S.: The preparation of human serum albumin free of longchain fatty acids. Science 125, 1296 (1957). ~ The interaction of human erythrocytes with long chain fatty anions. J. Amer. chem. Soc. 80, 3892 (1958). ~ The interaction of human erythrocytes with sodium palmitate. J. clin. Invest.

37, 1729 (1958). — GOODMAN, D. S., and E. SHAFRIR: The interaction of human low density lipoproteins with long chain fatty acid anions. J. Amer. chem. Soc. **81**, 364 (1959). — GORDON, A. H., J. GROSS, D. O'CONNOR and R. PITT-RIVERS: Nature of the circulating thyroid hormone-plasma protein complex. Nature (Lond.) **169**, 19 (1952). — GORDON jr., R. S.: Interaction between oleate and the lipoproteins of human serum. J. clin. Invest. **34**, 477 (1955). ~ Unesterified fatty acids in human blood plasma. II. The transport function of unesterified fatty acids. J. clin. Invest. **36**, 819 (1957). — GORDON jr., R. S., F. G. BARTTER and T. WALDMANN: Idiopathic hypoalbuminemias: Clinical staff conference at the NIH. Ann. intern. Med. **51**, 553 (1959). — GORDON jr., R. S., E. BOYLE, R. K. BROWN, A. CHERKES and C. B. ANFINSEN: The role of serum albumin in lipemia clearing reaction. Proc. Soc. exp. Biol. (N.Y.) **84**, 168 (1953). — GORDON jr., R. S., and A. CHERKES: Unesterified fatty acids in human blood plasma. J. clin. Invest. **35**, 206 (1956). ~ Production of unesterified fatty acids from isolated rat adipose tissue incubated in vitro. Proc. Soc. exp. Biol. (N.Y.) **97**, 150 (1958). — GOUDSMITH jr., A., M. H. POWER and J. L. BOLLMANN: The excretion of sulfates by the dog. Amer. J. Physiol. **125**, 506 (1939). — GRAB, W., u. K. OBERDISSE: Die medikamentöse Behandlung der Schilddrüsenerkrankungen. Stuttgart: Georg Thieme 1959. — GRÄSBECK, R.: Studies on the vitamin B_{12} binding principle and other biocolloids of human gastric juice. Acta med. scand. **154**, Suppl. 314 (1956). — GRÄSBECK, R., W. NYBERG and P. REIZENSTEIN: Biliary and fetal vitamin B_{12} excretion in man, an isotope study. Proc. Soc. exp. Biol. (N.Y.) **97**, 780 (1958). — GRAHAM, D. M., T. P. LYON, J. W. GOFMAN, M. D. JONES, A. YANKLEY, J. SIMONTON and S. WHITE: Blood lipids and human atherosclerosis II. The influence of heparin upon lipoprotein metabolism. Circulation **4**, 666 (1951). — GRANICK, S.: Ferritin increase of protein apoferritin in gastrointestinal mucosa as direct response to iron feeding. Funktion of ferritin in regulation of iron absorption. J. biol. Chem. **164**, 737 (1946) ~ Iron metabolism and hemochromatosis. Bull. N.Y. Acad. Med. **25**, 403 (1949). — GRANICK, S., and L. MICHAELIS: Ferritin and apoferritin. Science **95**, 439 (1942). — GRASER, V.: Klin. u. experiment. Untersuchungen über den Sulfathioharnstoff (Badional). Z. ges. inn. Med. **4**, 468 (1949). — GRASSMANN, W., K. HANNIG u. M. KNEDEL: Über ein Verfahren zur elektrophoretischen Bestimmung der Serumproteine auf Filtrierpapier. Dtsch. med. Wschr. **76**, 333 (1951). — GRAY, C. H., and R. A. KEKWICK: Bilirubin serum protein complexes and the van den Bergh reaction. Nature (Lond.) **161**, 274 (1948). — GREEN, A. A., L. A. LEWIS and J. H. PAGE: A method for the ultracentrifugal analysis of α- and β-Serumlipoproteins. Fed. Proc. **10**, 191 (1951). — GREENBERG, D. M.: The interaction between alkali earth cations, particularly calcium and proteins. Advanc. Protein Chem. **1**, 131 (1944). — GREENBERG, D. M., and L. GUNTHER: On the determination of diffusible and non-diffusible serum calcium. J. biol. chem. **85**, 491 (1930). — GREENWALT, T. J., et V. E. AYERS: 1. Vième Congr. Internat. d'Hématologie Paris 1954. 2. Calciumdisodium EDTA in transfusion hemosiderosis. J. clin. Path. **25**, 266 (1955). — GREGERSEN, M. J., and J. G. GIBSON: Conditions affecting the absorptions spectra of vital dyes in plasma. Amer. J. Physiol. **120**, 491 (1937). — GREGERSEN, M. J., and R. A. RAWSON: The disappearance of T-1824 and structurally related dyes compounds from the bloodstream. Amer. J. Physiol. **138**, 698 (1943). — GREGG, D. E.: Coronary circulation in health and disease. Philadelphia: Lea and Febiger 1950. — GRIESSER, G.: Über den Einfluß der Therapie auf die Prognose des Friedenstetanus. Arch. klin. Chir. **284**, 119 (1956). — GRODSKY, G. M., J. V. CARBONE and R. FANSKA: Enzymatic defect in metabolism of bilirubin in fetal and newborn rat. J. Proc. Soc. exp. Biol. (N.Y.) **97**, 291 (1957). — GROLL, F. X.: 69. Tagg. der Ges. für Chirurg., München, 1952. Zit. nach R. SCHUBERT 1954. — GROLLMANN, A.: Combination of phenol red and proteins. J. biol. Chem. **64**, 141 (1925). — GROOT, L. J. DE, S. POSTEL, J. LITVAK and J. B. STANBURY: Peptide-linked iodotyrosines and iodothyronines in the blood of a patient with congenital goiter. J. clin. Endocr. **18**, 158 (1958). — GROSS, J., and R. PITT-RIVERS: The identification of 3:5:3'-L-Triiodothyronine in human plasma. Lancet **1952 I**, 439. — GROSS, PH., u. H. WEICKER: Die Bedeutung des Lipoidelektrophoresediagrammes. Klin. Wschr. **32**, 509 (1954). — GUBLER, C. J., M. E. LAHEY, G. E. CARTWRIGHT and M. M. WINTROBE: Studies on copper metabolism. IX. The transportation of copper in blood. J. clin. Invest. **32**, 405 (1953). — GUTMANN, A. B., and E. B. GUTMANN: Relations of serumcalcium to serum albumin and globulins. J. clin. Invest. **16**, 903 (1937).

HAAN, J. DE: The renal function as judged by excretion of vital dye-stuffs. J. Physiol. (Lond.) **56**, 444 (1922). — HAAN, J. DE, u. S. VAN CREVELD: Über die Wechselbeziehung zwischen Blutplasma und Gewebsflüssigkeiten. I. Der Zuckergehalt und der gebundene Zucker. Biochem. Z. **123**, 190 (1921 b). ~ II. Durchlässigkeit für Fluorescin und Jodsalze. Biochem. Z. **124**, 172 (1921 a). — HAARMANN, W., A. HAGEMEISTER u. L. LENDLE: Über die Bindung von Digitalisglykosiden und Digitaloiden an die Eiweißstoffe des Blutserums. Naunyn-Schmiedeberg's Arch. exp. Path. Pharmak. **194**, 205 (1940). — HAARMANN, W., K. KORBMACHER u. L. LENDLE: Bedingungen der Bindung von Digitalisglykosiden an die Serumeiweißstoffe. Naunyn-Schmiedeberg's Arch. exp. Path. Pharmak. **194**, 229 (1940). — HAGERMAN, S. J., and R. G. GOULD: The in vitro interchange of cholesterol between plasma and red cells. Proc. Soc. exp. Biol. (N.Y.) **78**, 329 (1951). — HAGGARD, H. W.: An accurate method of determining small amounts of ethyl ether in air, blood and other fluids. J. biol. Chem. **55**, 131 (1923). — Hahn, P. F.: Abolishment of alimentary lipemia following injection of heparin. Science **98**, 19 (1943b). — Hahn, P. F., W. F. Bale, J. F. Ross, W. M. Balfour and G. H. Whipple: Radioactiv iron absorption by gastrointestinal tract. J. exp. Med. **78**, 169 (1943a). — Hahn, P. F., S. Granick, W. F. Bale and L. Michalis: Ferritin: Conversation of inorganic and hemoglobin iron into ferritin iron in animal body. Storage function of ferritin iron as shown by radioactive and magnetic measurements. J. biol. Chem. **150**, 407 (1943). — Hald, P. M.: The flame photometer for the measurement of sodium and potassium in biological materials. J. biol. Chem. **167**, 499 (1947). — Hall, B. V.: Studies of normal glomerular structure by electron microscopy. Proc. of fifth annual conference on the nephrotic syndrome 1953. — Halmi, N. S., and R. G. Stuelke: Comparison of thyreoidal and gastric iodine pump in rat. Endocrinology **64**, 103 (1959). — Halsted, J. A.: Serum and tissue concentration of vitamin B_{12} in certain pathologic states. New Engl. J. Med. **260**, 575 (1960). — Halsted, J. A., P. M. Lewis, E. E. Hoolboll, M. Gaster and M. E. Swendseid: An evolution of the fetal recovery method for determining intestinal absorption of cobalt[60] labeled vitamin B_{12}. J. Lab. clin. Med. **48**, 92 (1956). — Hamolsky, M. W., H. E. Ellison and A. S. Freedberg: The thyroid-hormone-plasma protein complex in man. I. Differences in different states of thyroid function. J. clin. Invest. **36**, 1486 (1957). — Hamolsky, M. W., D. B. Fischer and A. S. Freedberg: Further studies on the plasma protein-thyroid hormone complex. Endocrinology **66**, 780 (1960). — Hamolsky, M. W., M. Stein and A. S. Freedberg: The thyroid hormone-plasma protein complex in man. II. A new method for study of „uptake" of labeled hormonal components by human erythrocytes. J. clin. Endocr. **17**, 33 (1957). — Hardwicke, J.: Serum and urinary protein changes in the nephrotic syndrom. Proc. roy. Soc. Med. **47**, 832 (1954). — Harper, R. V., W. B. Neal and G. R. Hlavacek: Lipid synthesis and transport in the dog. Metabolism **2**, 69 (1953). — Harris, R. S., J. W. Chamberlein and J. H. Benedict: Digestion of neutral fat by human subjects. J. clin. Invest. **34**, 685 (1955). — Harris, R. S., J. F. Lucey and J. P. McLean: Kernicterus in premature infants associated with low concentrations of bilirubin in the plasma. Pediatrics **21**, 875 (1958). — Harvier, P., J. di Matthéo, R. Denil et J. Bescol-Liversac: Les manifestations cardiaque des cirrhoses pigmentaires. Ann. Méd. **51**, 101 (1950). — Haurowitz, F., F. DiMoira u. S. Tekman: Die Reaktion von nativem und denaturiertem Ovalbumin mit Congorot. J. Amer. chem. Soc. **74**, 2265 (1952). — Havel, R. J.: Early effects of fat ingestion on lipids and lipoproteins of serum in man. J. clin. Invest. **36**, 848 (1957). — Havel, R. J., and J. H. Bragdon: Heparin like aktivity of polymetaphosphate. Circulation **10**, 591 (1954). — Havel, R. J., and J. C. Clarke: Clin. Res. **6**, 264 (1958). — Havel, R. J., H. A. Eder and J. H. Bragdon: The distribution and chemical composition of ultracentrifugally separated lipoproteins in human serum. J. clin. Invest. **34**, 1345 (1955). — Havel, R. J., and D. S. Fredrickson: The metabolism of chylomicra. I. The removal of palmitic acid-1-C^{14} labeled chylomicra from dog plasma. J. clin. Invest. **35**, 1025 (1956). — Hayasida, A.: The „non-solvent space" of the serum and the chloride bound by the serum proteins. J. Biochem. (Tokyo) **18**, 107 (1933). — Hayman jr., J. M.: The excretion in organic sulfates. J. clin. Invest. **11**, 607 (1932). — Hazelwood, R. N.: The molecular weights and dimensions of some high density human serum lipoproteins. J. Amer. chem. Soc. **80**, 2152 (1958). — Hecht, G., u. H. Weese: Periston, ein neuer Blutflüssigkeitsersatz. Münch. med. Wschr. **1943**. — Hechter, O.: Mechanisms of spreading factor action. Ann. N.Y. Acad. Sci. **52**, 1028 (1950). — Hedinger, Ch.: Zur Pathologie des Hämochromatose-Syndroms. Helv. med. Acta **20**, Supp. 32 (1953). — Heidel, W.: Tagesrhythmische Serumeisen- und Eiweißschwankungen bei vegetativer Dystonie. Dtsch. Z. Verdau.- u. Stoffwechselkr. **15**, 62 (1955). — Heilmeyer, L.: Die Haemochromatose: Klinik, Eisenstoffwechsel und Pathogenese. Acta haemat. (Basel) **11**, 137 (1954). ~ Sideroachrestische Anaemien. Dtsch. med. Wschr. **39** (1959). — Heilmeyer, L., W. Keiderling u. F. Wöhler: Existiert bei der Eisenresorption im Dünndarm ein Mucosablock? Klin. Wschr. **35**, 690 (1957). — Heilmeyer, L., u. K. Plötner: Das Serumeisen und die Eisenmangelkrankheit. Jena: Fischer 1937. — Heim, F.: Änderung der Acetylcholinwirkung durch Adsorption an Eiweißkörper. Naunyn-Schmiedeberg's Arch. exp. Path. Pharmak. **192**, 276 (1939). — Heinemann, M.: Distribution of sulfonamides between cells and serum of human blood. J. clin. Invest. **22**, 29 (1943). — Heinrich, H. C., u. S. Erdmann-Oehlecker: Der Vitamin B_{12}-Stoffwechsel bei Hämoblastosen. II. Die Intravitale Bindung (Transport) der B_{12} Vitamine an die Serumproteinfraktionen bei Hämoblastosen. Clin. chim. Acta **1**, 311 (1956). — Heinrich, H. C., u. H. Lahann: Physiologie, Pathophysiologie und biochemischer Wirkungsmechanismus der B_{12}-Vitamine. Z. Vitam.-, Hormon- u. Fermentforsch. **5b**, 126 (1954). — Hemmeler, G.: Metabolism du fer. Paris: Masson et Co. 1951. — Henry, J. P., u. J. W. Pearce: J. Physiol. **131**, 572 (1956). — Henry, R. J., S. Berkmann and R. D. Housewright: Studies on streptomycin. II. Inactivation of streptomycin upon standing in certain culture media and human serum. J. Pharmacol. exp. Ther. **90**, 42 (1947). — Herbert, V.: Studies on the role of intrinsic factor in vitamin B_{12}, absorption, transport, and storage. Amer. J. clin. Nutr. **7**, 433 (1959). — Herbst, F. S. M., W. F. Lever,

M. E. Lyons and N. A. Hurley: Effects of heparin on the lipoproteins in hyperlipemia. An electrophoretic studie of the serum α- and β-lipoproteins after their separation by fractionation of the plasmaproteins or ultracentrifugal flotation. J. clin. Invest. **34**, 581 (1955). — Hering, H. E.: Carotissinusreflex. Dresden 1927. — Hess, B.: Zur Biochemie und Physiologie des Jodstoffwechsels. Ärztl. Wschr. **7**, 473 (1952). — Hess, W. R.: Regulierung des Blutkreislaufs. Leipzig 1930. ~ Das Zwischenhirn und die Regulation von Kreislauf und Atmung. Leipzig: Georg Thieme 1938. — Hevesy, G. v.: Eisenstoffwechsel. Teilbericht der 4. Tagg. der Nobelpreisträger vom 28. 6.—2. 7. 1954 in Lindau. — Hevesy, G. v., u. E. Hofer: Die Verweilzeit des Wassers im menschlichen Körper, untersucht mit Hilfe von „schwerem" Wasser als Indikator. Klin. Wschr. **27**, 1524 (1934). — Hewitt, L. F.: Combination of proteins with phthalein dyes. Biochem. J. **21**, 1305 (1927). — Heymann, H., and L. F. Fieser: Naphthoquinone antimalarials. XIX. Antirespiratory study of protein binding. J. Pharmacol. exp. Ther. **94**, 97 (1948). — Heymans, C., J. J. Bouckaert et P. Regniers: Le sinus carotidien et la zone homologue cardioartique. Paris 1933. — Hiatt, E. P., and V. Juhrie: Renal excretion of cinchona alkaloids a some quaternary base derivates, and their effect on renal hemodymanics. Fed. Proc. **5**, 46 (1946). — Hirschfelder, A. D., and H. N. Wright: Studies on the colloid chemistry of antisepsis and chemotherapy. II. Combination of antiseptic dyes with proteins. J. Pharmacol. exp. Ther. **38**, 411 (1930). — Hoch, F. L., and B. L. Vallee: Precipitation by trichloroacetic acid as a simplification in the determination of zinc in blood and its components. J. biol. Chem. **181**, 295 (1949). — Hoch, H., u. A. Chanutin: Einfluß von Antikoagulantien auf Serum und Plasma. J. biol. Chem. **197**, 503 (1952). — Höber, R.: Physikalische Chemie der Zellen und Gewebe. Bern: Stämpfli 1947. — Hoekstra, R. A.: Das Verhalten von Digitalisglykosiden in Blut und Gewebsflüssigkeit. Naunyn-Schmiedeberg's Arch. exp. Path. Pharmak. **162**, 649 (1931). — Hofmann-Credner, D.: Das Thyroxinbindungsvermögen des Serums als Diagnosticum bei Funktionsstörungen der subtotal-resezierten Schilddrüse. Klin. Wschr. **35**, 121 (1957). — Holland, W. C., and M. E. Greig: Studies on permeability. II. The effect of acetyl choline and physostigmine on the permeability to potassium of erythrocytes. Arch. Biochem. **26**, 151 (1950). — Holmberg, C. G.: Investigation on serum copper I. Nature of serum copper and its relation to the iron binding protein in human serum. Acta chem. scand. **1**, 744 (1947). Holmberg, C. G., and C. B. Laurell: Studies on capacity of serum to bind iron. Acta physiol. scand. **10**, 207 (1945). ~ Investigation on serum copper II. Isolation on copper containing protein and a description of some of its properties. Acta chem. scand. **2**, 550 (1948). ~ Investigation in serum copper III. Coeruloplasmin as an enzym. Acta chem. scand. **5**, 476 (1951). ~ Investigation in serum copper IV. Effect of different actions on the enzymatic activity of coeruloplasmin. Acta chem. scand. **5**, 921 (1951). — Holt, T., and F. H. Scoular: Iron and copper metabolism of young women on selfselected diets. J. Nutr. **35**, 717 (1948). — Honetz, N., u. R. Kotzaurek: Weitere Erfahrungen mit der Jodbestimmung im Blutserum nach Spitzy, Reese und Skrube. Klin. Wschr. **38**, 494 (1960). — Hopkins, Th., J. Eager and H. Eisenberg: Ultrafiltration studies on Ca and P on human serum proteins. Bull. Johns Hopk. Hosp. **91**, 1 (1952). — Horsfall, W. R.: Genetic control of some human serum β-globulins. Science **128**, 35 (1958). — Horst, W.: Transport und Bindung im Serum. Untersucht mit Papierelektrophorese und radioaktiven Indicatoren (Fe 55/59, Cu 64, Co 56/57, Mn 52, Ga 67, S 35, J 131). Klin. Wschr. **32**, 961 (1954). — Horst, W., E. Fischer, G. Hanken u. T. O. Lindenschmidt: Resultate der Gewebeclearancebestimmung am Menschen mit J[131] markiertem Jodid und J[131] markiertem Albumin (Proteinclearance) in „Kapillaren und Interstitium" von Bartelheimer u. Küchmeister. Stuttgart: Georg Thieme 1955. — Horst, W., u. H. Rösler: Der Transport des Hormonjods im menschlichen Serum untersucht mit Papierlektrophorese und Radiojod. (Zugleich ein Beitrag zur Frage der Existenz von sog. Zwischenfraktionen.) Klin. Wschr. **31**, 13 (1953). — Horst, W., u. K. H. Schäfer: Die Eisenbindung im Serum und in weiteren biologischen Flüssigkeiten, untersucht mit Papierelektrophorese und Radioeisen. Klin. Wschr. **31**, 791 (1953b). ~ Die Eisenbindung im Serum und in weiteren biologischen Flüssigkeiten, untersucht mit Papierelektrophorese und Radioeisen (Fe 59 und Fe 55). Zugleich eine neue Methode zur Beurteilung der Eisenbindungskapazität biologischer Flüssigkeiten. Klin. Wschr. **31**, 791 (1953c). — Horst, W., u. H. H. Schumacher: Papierelektrophoretische Untersuchungen von Schilddrüsenextrakten und Serum nach in vitro-Zusatz von Radiojodid, Radiomangan und Radiocobalt sowie nach in vivo-Gabe von Radiojodid. Klin. Wschr. **32**, 361 (1954a). — Horst, W., u. H. Schumacher: Papierelektrophoretische Untersuchungen von Schilddrüsenextrakten. Klin. Wschr. 32, 301 (1954b). — Houston, J. C.: Phlebotomy for hemochromatosis effect of removing 52 pints of blood in sixteen months. Lancet 1953 I, 766. — Huff, R. L., P. J. Elmlinger, J. F. Garcia, J. M. Oda, M. C. Cockrell and J. H. Lawrence: Ferrokinetics in normal persons and in patients having various erythropoetic disorders. J. clin. Invest. **30**, 1512 (1951). — Huggins, C., E. V. Jensen, M. A. Player and V. D. Hospelhorn: The binding of phenolsulfonephthalein by serum and by albumin isolated from serum in cancer. Cancer Res. **9**, 753 (1949). — Hughes jr., W. L.: An albumin fraction isolated from human plasma as a cristalline mercuric salt. J. Amer. chem. Soc. **69**, 1836 (1947). — Humphrey, J. H.: Serum albumin concentration in analbuminaemia and its immunological significance. Nature (Lond.) 187, 304 (1960). — HUMPHREY, J. H., and R. JAQUES: The histamin and serotonin content of the platelets and polymorphonuclear leucocytes of various species. J. Physiol. (Lond.) 124, 305 (1954). — HUNTER, M. J., and SP. L. COMMERFORD: Interaction of neutral amino acids with human serum albumin and γ-globulin. J. Amer. chem. Soc. 77, 4857 (1955). — HUTCHINSON, D. L., A. A. PLENTL and H. C. TAYLOR jr.: Total body water and the turnover in pregnancy studied with deuterium oxide as isotopic tracer. J. clin. Invest. 33, 235 (1954). — HYMAN, C., and S. J. RAPOPORT: Simultaneous multiple tissue clearances in measurement of transcapillary diffusion rates. Amer. J. Physiol. 163, 722 (1950).

IKKOS, D., R. LUFT and B. SJÖGREN: Body water and sodium in patients with acromegaly. J. clin. Invest. 33, 989 (1954). — INGBAR, S. H.: Prealbumin: A thyroxine-binding protein of human plasma. Endocrinology 63, 256 (1958).

JACKSON, E. L.: Zit. nach A. GOLDSTEIN. J. Pharmacol. exp. Ther. 95, 102 (1948). — JACQUES, L. B.: The reaction of heparin with proteins and complex bases. Biochem. J. 37, 189 (1943). — JAGER, B. V., and C. J. GUBLER: An immunologic study of the iron-binding protein. J. Immunol. 69, 311 (1952). — JAMES, A. T., J. E. LOVELOCK and J. B. M. WEBB: Zit. nach FREDRICKSON and GORDON 1958. Biochem. J. (1958). — JAMPEL, R. S., and H. F. FALLS: Atypical retinitis pigmentosa, acanthrocytosis, and heredodegenerative neuromuscular disease. A.M.A. Arch. Ophthal. 59, 818 (1958). — JANCSO, N. v.: Die Untersuchungen der Funktion des Retikuloendothels mit Durchströmungsversuchen. Z. ges. exp. Med. 64, 256 (1929). — JANDL, J. A., J. H. INMAN, R. L. SIMMONS and S. W. ALLEN: Transfer of iron from serum iron binding protein to human reticulocytes. J. clin. Invest. 38, 161 (1959). — JASINSKI, B.: Das Schicksal und die Verwertung intravenös verabreichten kolloidalen Eisens. Schweiz. med. Wschr. 84, 947 (1954). — JAYLE, M. F., and G. H. JEFFRIES: The sites at which plasma clearing activity is produced and destroyed in the rat. Quart. J. exp. Physiol. 39, 261 (1954). — JENSEN, W. N., H. KAMIN and N. C. DURHAM: Copper transport and excretion in normal subjects and in patients with Laenec's cirrhosis and Wilson's disease: a study with Cu^{64}. J. Lab. clin. Med. 49, 200 (1957). — JOHNSON, L. M.: The 25th Ross Pediatrics Research Conference 1957. — JOYCE, E. F., D. J. R. LAURENCE and V. H. REES: The dye binding capacity of human plasma determined fluorometrically and its relation to the determination of plasmaalbumin. J. clin. Path. 7, 326 (1954).

KALANT, N., W. C. McINTYRE and D. L. WILANSKY: Thyroid function in experimental nephrotic syndrome. Endocrinology 64, 333 (1959). — KALK, H.: Klinik der Hämochromatose. Verh. dtsch. Ges. Verdau.- u. Stoffwechselkr., 17. Tagg. Stuttgart: Georg Thieme 1954. — KALLEE, E.: Dye-binding ability of mitochondrial protein fractions. Arch. Biochem. 60, 265 (1956). ~ Bindung von Schilddrüsenhormonen an zytoplasmatische Leberproteine. Diskussionsbemerkung zu HELLAUER in: Radioaktive Isotope in Klinik und Forschung, Bd. III, S. 91. 1958 (b). ~ In vitro-Bindung von J^{131}-Thyroxin an Serumproteine von Euthyreosen, Hyper- und Hypothyreosen. Diskussionsbemerkung zu N. LANG u. K. H. GILLICH in: Radioaktive Isotope in Klinik und Forschung, Bd. IV. 1960 (a). ~ Binding ability of cytoplasmic proteins. II. Distribution equilibria of thyroid hormones, soluble proteins and liver mitochondria. In: Protides of the biological fluids, vol. 7, p. 161. Amsterdam: Elsevier Publ. Comp. 1960 (b). — KALLEE, E., F. LOHSS u. G. SEYBOLD: Albuminnachweis in Extrakten von Leberzellmitochondrien. Verh. dtsch. Ges. inn. Med. 60, 943 (1954). — KALLEE, E., u. W. OPPERMANN: Bindungsfähigkeit zytoplasmatischer Proteine. I. Farbstoffbindung. Z. Naturforsch. 13 b, 532 (1958) (a). — KALLEE, E., u. G. SEYBOLD: Über ^{131}J-signiertes Insulin. III. Verteilung im Rattenorganismus. Z. Naturforsch. 9 b, 307 (1954). — KAPPELER, R.: Familiäre Haemochromatose. Schweiz. med. Wschr. 86, 477 (1956). — KARUSH, F., and M. SONNENBERG: Interaction of homologus alkylsulfats with bovine serum albumin. J. Amer. chem. Soc. 71, 1369 (1949). ~ Heterogeneity of binding sites of bovine serum albumin. J. Amer. chem. Soc. 72, 2705 (1950). ~ The competitive interaction of organic anions with bovine serum albumin. J. Amer. chem. Soc. 72, 2714 (1950). ~ The interaction of optically isomeric dyes with human serum albumin. J. Amer. chem. Soc. 76, 5536 (1954). — KATSH, S., and E. WINDSOR: Unusual value for protein-bound iodine in the serum of the opossum. Science 121, 897 (1955). — KEHOE, R. A., J. CHOLAK and R. V. STORY: Spectrochemical study of normal ranges of concentration of certain trace metals in biologic materials. J. Nutr. 19, 579 (1940). — KEIDERLING, W.: Über die Kupferproteinbindung im Blutplasma. Klin. Wschr. 28 (1950). ~ Eisenstoffwechsel. Beiträge zur Forschung und Klinik. Stuttgart: Georg Thieme 1959. — KEILIN, J.: Reaction of human serum albumin with haematin and haem. Nature (Lond.) 154, 120 (1944). — KELLER, W.: 59. Tagg. der Dtsch. Ges. für Kinderheilk. 26. 9. 1960. — KELLEY, F. J., A. H. SVEDBERG and V. C. HARP jr.: The transfer of radioactive mercury across a membrane produced by the application of cantharides to skin of man. J. clin. Invest. 23, 988 (1950). — KINDLER: Zit. nach R. SCHUBERT 1954. — KIYASU, J. Y., B. BLOOM and I. L. CHAIKOFF: The portal transport of absorbed fatty acids. J. biol. Chem. 199, 415 (1952). — KLATSKIN, G., and L. J. BUNGAROLS: Bilirubin-protein linkages in serum and their relationship to the van den Bergh reaction. J. clin. Invest. 35, 537 (1956). — KLEIN, E.: Der Jodgehalt der einzelnen Bluteiweißkörper. Z. ges. exp. Med. 121, 44 (1953). —

KLEIN, E., u. F. H. FRANKEN: Das elektrophoretische Lipoproteinspektrum des Serums nach Heparineinwirkung und bei Leberkrankheiten. Dtsch. med. Wschr. 1955, 44. — KLEIN, E., u. H. BRÜGEL: Der Einbau von J^{131} in die Hormonjodfraktionen des Blutes. Nachweis von Hormonabbauprodukten. Z. klin. Med. 153, 126 (1955). — KLEINSCHMIDT, H.: Icterus neonatorum gravis. Klin. Wschr. 9, 2133 (1951). — KLEMPERER, H. G.: Uncoupling of oxidative phosphorylation in rat liver mitochondria by thyroxine. triiodothyronine and related substances. Biochem. J. 60, 122 (1955). — KLOPSTOCK, F.: Über den Einfluß von Heparin und Germanin auf Immunreaktionen. Z. Immun-Forsch. 75, 348 (1932). — KLOTZ, J. M.: Spectrophotometric investigation of the interactions of proteins with organic ions. J. Amer. chem. Soc. 68, 2299 (1946a). ~ The application of the law of mass action to binding by proteins. Interaction with calcium. Arch. Biochem. 9, 109 (1946c). ~ Zit. nach A. GOLDSTEIN, J. Pharmacol. exp. Ther. 95, 102 (1949). ~ The nature of some ion-protein complexes. Cold Spr. Harb. Symp. quant. Biol. 14, 97 (1950b). — KLOTZ, J. M., and H. G. CURME: The thermodynamics of metalloprotein combinations. Copper with bovine serum albumin. J. Amer. chem. Soc. 70, 939 (1948b). — KLOTZ, J. M., J. L. FALLER and J. M. URQUHART: Spectra of copper complexes with some proteins, amino acids and related substances. J. phys. colloid Chem. 54, 18 (1950a). — KLOTZ, J. M., and J. B. MELCHIOR: Some aspects of the action of sulfonamides I. Binding of S^{35} labeled sulfonamide by Echerichia coli. Arch. Biochem. 21, 35 (1949). — KLOTZ, J. M., A. H. SCHLESINGER and F. TIETZE: Comparison of the binding ability of hemocyanin and serumalbumin for organic ions. Biol. Bull. 94, 40 (1948c). KLOTZ, J. M., and J. M. URQUHART: The combination of adenine, adenosine and adenylicacids with serum albumin. J. biol. Chem. 173, 21 (1948a). — KLOTZ, J. M., J. M. URQUHART, RH. A. KLOTZ and J. AYERS: Slow intramolecular changes in copper complex of serum album^{in}. The role of neighboring groups in protein reaction. J. Amer. chem. Soc. 77, 1919 (1955)· — KLOTZ, J. M., and F. M. WALKER: The binding of organic ions by proteins, charge and p_H effects. J. Amer. chem. Soc. 69, 1609 (1947). — KLOTZ, J. M., F. M. WALKER and R. B. PIVAN: The binding of organic ions by proteins. J. Amer. chem. Soc. 68, 1486 (1946b). KNEDEL, M.: Quantitative Glycoproteidbestimmung in isolierten Serumeiweißfraktionen. Verh. dtsch. Ges. inn. Med. 61, 277 (1955). — KNÜSEL, O.: Sichtbarmachung von Lymphgefäßen in der Augenbindehaut. Ophthalmologica (Basel) 127, 298 (1954). — KOCIAN, V.: Über die Schutzwirkung des Germanins (Bayer 205) auf die Koagulation der Bluteiweißstoffe. Naunyn-Schmiedeberg's Arch. exp. Path. Pharmak. 182, 313 (1936). — KÖIW, E., G. WALLENIUS und A. GRÖNWALL: Färbung der papierelektrophoretisch getrennten Serumpolysaccharide auf Filtrierpapier. Scand. J. clin. Lab. Invest. 4, 47 (1952). — KOELLE, G. B.: Protection of cholinesterase against irreversible inactivation by di-isopropyl fluorophosphate in vitro. J. Pharmacol. exp. Ther. 88, 232 (1946). — KONITZER, K.: Resorption, Transport und Speicherung des Eisens. Z. ges. inn. Med. 8, 333 (1953). — KONITZER, K., E. ENDELL u. G. THIEME: Die Bedeutung der Bestimmung der Eisenbindungsfähigkeit des Serums für die differentialdiagnostische Unterscheidung der einzelnen Hyposideraemieformen und für die Kontrolle der Eisenspeicher unter therapeutischer Eisenzufuhr. Z. ges. inn. Med. 10, 801 (1955). — KORN, E. D.: Clearing factor and heparin-activated lipoprotein lipase. J. biol. Chem. 215, 1 (1955). — KORNGOLD, L., and R. LIPARI: Immunochemical studies of human betaplasmaprotein. Science 121, 170 (1955). — KRAMÁR, J.: Stress and capillary resistance. Amer. J. Physiol. 175, 69 (1953). — KRAMÁR, J., and M. SIMAY-KRAMÁR: The effect of adrenalectomy, surgical trauma, and ether anesthesia upon the capillary resistance of the albino rat. Amer. J. Physiol. 175, 69 (1953). — KRECH, U.: Die unspezifische Bindung und Inaktivierung bakterieller Toxine in vivo und in vitro. Z. Immun.-Forsch. 109, 177 (1952). — KROGH, A.: Introductory paper: Animal membranes. Trans. Faraday Soc. 33, 912 (1937). — KÜHNAU, J.: Steuerungsmechanismen für den Stoffaustausch durch die Kapillarwand in „Kapillaren und Interstitium" von BARTELHEIMER u. KÜCHMEISTER. Stuttgart: Georg Thieme 1955. — KUHRT, N. H., E. A. WELCH, W. P. BLUM, E. S. PERRY, W. H. WEBER and E. S. NASSET: Isolation and identification of monoglycerides in the intestinal contents of human. J. Amer. biol. chem. Soc. 29, 271 (1952). — KUNKEL, H. G., and A. G. BEARN: Phospholipid studies of different serum lipoproteins employing P^{32}. Proc. Soc. exp. Biol. (N.Y.) 86, 887 (1954). — KUNKEL, H. G., and R. J. SLATER: Lipoprotein patterns of serum obtained by zone electrophoresis. J. clin. Invest. 31, 677 (1952). — KUNKEL, H. G., and R. TRAUTMAN: The α_2-liproteins of human serum. Correlation of ultrazentrifugal and electrophoretic properties. J. clin. Invest. 35, 641 (1956). — KYDD, D. M., and E. B. MAN: Precipitable iodine of serum (SPI) in disorder of the liver. J. clin. Invest. 30, 874 (1951).

LAFERRE, MAVIC, NUN u. AUBRY: Zit. nach LÖHR u. REINWEIN, Dtsch. Arch. klin. Med. 200, 53 (1952). — LAL, H.: Hydrogen ion eguilibria and the interaction of Cu^{II} and Co^{II} with bovine serum albumin. J. Amer. chem. Soc. 81, 844 (1959). — LANDIS, E. M.: Capillary pressure and capillary permeability. Physiol. Rev. 14, 404 (1934). — LANDIS, E. M., u. J. GIBBON: In A. KROG, E. M. LANDIS and A. H. TURNER, The movement of fluid through the human capillary wall in relation to venous pressure and to the colloid osmotic pressure of the blood. J. clin. Invest. 11, 63 (1932). — LANG, N.: Quantitative Untersuchungen mit Überwanderungselektrophorese über die Bindungskapazität von Plasmaproteinen. In:

Protides of the biological fluids, vol. 6, p. 68. Amsterdam: Elsevier Publ. Comp. 1959. — Lang, N., u. K. H. Gillich: In vitro-Bindung von J^{131}-Thyroxin an Serumproteine von Euthyreosen, Hyper- und Hypothyreosen. In: Radioaktive Isotope in Klinik und Forschung, Bd. 4. München: Urban & Schwarzenberg 1960. — Langan, Th. A., E. L. Durrum and W. P. Jencks: Paper electrophoresis as an quantitative method: Measurement of alfa and beta lipoprotein-cholesterol. J. clin. Invest. 34, 1427 (1955). — Lange, J.: Eisen, Kupfer und Eiweiß am Beispiel der Leberkrankheiten. Stuttgart: Georg Thieme 1958. — Langmuir, I.: The constitution and fundamental properties of solids and lipids. Part. I. J. Amer. chem. Soc. 38, 2221 (1916). ~ Part. II. J. Amer. chem. Soc. 39, 1848 (1917). — Laporta, M.: Circa l'adsorbimento dei sali biliari sulle proteine del siero. Arch. clin. Sci. Biol. 26, 15 (1940). — Larson, F., W. P. Deiss and E. C. Albright: Localization of protein bound radioactive iodine by filter paper electrphoresis. Science 115, 626 (1952). — Larson, F. C., and E. C. Albright: The specificity of thyroxine binding by serum alpha globulin. Endocrinology 56, 737 (1955). — Larson, F. C., W. P. Deiss and E. C. Albrigh: Radiochromatographic identification of thyroxin in an alpha globulin fraction of serum separated by starch zone electrophoresis. J. clin. Invest. 33, 230 (1954). — Lathe, G. H.: „Bilirubin" and „conjugated bilirubin". Lancet 1956 II, 683. — Latner, A. L.: Intrinsic factor and vitamin B_{12} absorption. Brit. med. J. 1958 II, 278. — Latner, A. L., and C. C. Ungley: Electrophoresis of human gastric juice in relation to Castle's intrinsic factor. Brit. med. J. 1953 I, 467. — Laurell, C. B.: Studies on transportation and metabolism of iron in body with special reference of iron binding component in human plasma. Acta physiol. scand. 14, 1 (1947). ~ Studies on the transportation and metabolism of iron in the body. Acta physiol. scand. 14, Suppl. 46 (1947). — Laurell, C. B., and B. Ingelman: The iron binding protein of swine serum. Acta chem. scand. 1, 770 (1947). — Laurell, S.: The effect of free fatty acids on the migration rates of lipoproteins in paperelectrophoresis. Scand. J. clin. Lab. Invest. 7, 28 (1955). ~ Turnover rate of unesterified fatty acids in human plasma. Acta physiol. scand. 41, 158 (1957). — Lawrence, R. D.: Hemochromatosis in three families and in a woman. Lancet 1949 I, 736. — Leblond, C. P.: Recent progres in hormon research. Advanc. biol. med. Phys. 1, 353 (1948). — Lecomte du Nouy, P.: Surface equilibria of biological organic colloids, p. 155. New York: Chem. Catalog Co. 1926. ~ Sur la capacité d'adsorption des protéines du serum vis-à-vis des sels biliaires. C. R. Soc. Biol. (Paris) 99, 1097 (1928). — Le Fèvre, P. G.: Evidence of active transfer of certain nonelectrolytes across the human red cell membrane. J. gen. Physiol. 31, 505 (1948). ~ Active transport the human erythrocyte: Evidence from comparative kinetics and competition among monosaccharides. J. gen. Physiol. 34, 515 (1951). — Lein, A.: The binding of thyroxine, diiodotyrosine and triiodothyronine by bovine serum proteins. J. Amer. chem. Soc. 75, 19 (1953). — Lendle, L., u. P. Pusch: Über die Bindung der Digitaliskörper an die Eiweißstoffe des Blutes. Naunyn-Schmiedeberg's Arch. exp. Path. Pharmak. 177, 550 (1935). — Letterer, E.: Speicherungskrankheiten. Dtsch. med. Wschr. 73, 147 (1948). ~ Diskussionsbemerkung zum Vortrag von H. Kalk. Verh. Dtsch. Ges. Verdau.- u. Stoffwechselkr. Stuttgart: Georg Thieme 1953. — Leupold, F., H. Frank u. H. Büttner: Über proteingebundenes Acetalphosphatid im Blut. Hoppe-Seylers Z. physiol. Chem. 296, 55 (1954). — Lever, W. F., F. R. N. Gurd, E. Uroma, R. K. Brown, K. Schmid and E. Schultz: Chemical clinical and immunological studies on the products on human plasma fractionation XL. Quantitative separation and determination of the protein components in small amounts of normal human plasma. J. clin. Invest. 30, 99 (1951). — Lever, W. F., P. A. J. Smith and N. A. Hurley: Idiopathic hyperlipemia and primary, hypercholesteremic xanthomatosis. II. and III. J. invest. Derm. 22, 53, 71 (1954). ~ IV. and V. Arch. Derm. Syph. (Chicago) 77, 150, 158 (1955). — Levine, L., D. L. Kauffman and R. K. Brown: The antigenic similiarity of human low density lipoproteins. J. exp. Med. 102, 105 (1955). — Levine, R., W. Q. Wolfson and R. Lenel: Concentration and transport of true urate in the plasma of the azotemic chicken. Amer. J. Physiol. 151, 186 (1947). — Lewallen, Ch. G., M. Berman and J. E. Rall: Studies on iodoalbumin metabolism. J. clin. Invest. 38, 66 (1959). — Lewis, L. A., and J. H. Page: Electrophoretic and ultracentrifugal analysis of serum lipoprotein of normal, nephrotic and hypertensive persons. Circulation 7, 707 (1953). — Lindberg, O.: Exp. Cell Res. 1, 105 (1950). — Lindgren, F. T., H. A. Elliot and J. W. Gofman: The ultracentrifugal characterization and isolation of human blood lipid and lipoproteins with applications to the study of atherosclerosis. J. phys. Coll. Chem. 55, 80 (1951). — Lindgren, F. T., N. K. Freeman and D. M. Graham: In vitro lipoprotein transformation. Circulation 6, 474 (1952). — Lindgren, F. T., A. V. Nichols and N. K. Freeman: Physical and chemical composition studies on the lipoproteins of fasting and heparinized human serum. J. physic. Chem. 59, 930 (1955). Lintzel, W.: Verhalten intravenös injizierten Eisens im Organismus. Ärztl. Forsch. 7 (I), 134 (1953). — Lintzel, W., u. T. Radeff: Über die Wirkung der Luftverdünnung auf Tiere. 2. Mitt. Pflügers Arch. ges. Physiol. 224, 451 (1930). — Linzbach, A. J.: Vergleichende phasenmikroskopische Untersuchung am Deckepithel der Leberkapsel und am Aortenendothel. Z. Zellforsch. 37, 554 (1952). — Lipner, H. J., S. B. Barker and T. Winnick: The distribution of thyroxine in rat liver cell fractions. Endocrinology 51, 406 (1952). —

Lipsky, S. R., J. S. McGuire jr., P. K. Bondy and E. B. Man: The rates of synthesis and the transport of plasma fatty acid fractions in man. J. clin. Invest. 34, 1760 (1955). — Lissitzky, S.: Considerations actuelles sur le metabolisme peripherique des hormones thyroidiennes. Atti dell' VIII. Congr. Nazionale della Società Italiana die Endocrinologia. Simposio su gli ipertiroidismi. Napoli, 7, 1959. — Lissitzky, S., M. Roques et M. T. Bénévent: Combinaison protéine cellulaire-thyroxine et désiodation de l'hormone. C. R. Soc. Biol. (Paris) 153, 803 (1959). — Löffler, W., Ch. Wunderly u. F. Wuhrmann: Bilirubin und Albumin. Schweiz. med. Wschr. 79, 595 (1949). — Löhr, K., u. H. Reinwein: Konkordantes Auftreten von Lebercirrhose und Diabetes mell. (Haemochromatose) bei eineiigen Zwillingen. 1. Dtsch. Arch. klin. Med. 200, 53 (1952). ~ 2. Dtsch. Arch. klin. Med. 202, 767 (1956). (Nachtrag zu 1.) — Lohss, F., and E. Kallee: Immunological detection of the binding of Fe^{59} ascorbinate, I^{131}-thyroxine and I^{131}-insulin to serum proteins. In: Protides of the biological fluids, vol. 8. Amsterdam: Elsevier Publ. Comp. 1960. — Lohss, F., u. H. Ott: Immunbiologische Untersuchungen zum Nachweis von Albuminspuren im Analbuminämieserum. Dtsch. Arch. klin. Med. 206, 426 (1960). — Loiseleur, J., et R. Colliard: Sur l'adsorption des polypeptides par les protéides du plasma sanguin. C. Rend. Acad. Sci. (Paris) 205, 261 (1937). — Lonti, R., P. R. Morrison, H. Edelhoch and J. T. Edsall: Light scattering in solutions of serum albumin and β-globulin. Presented at Amer. Chem. Soc., Div. Biolog. Chem. 31. VIII. 1948. — Luck and Welsh: Nicht publizierte Untersuchungen, zit. in J. M. Luck, The combination of fatty acid anions with protein. Discuss. Faraday Soc. 1949, 44. — Luck, J. M.: The combination of fatty acid anions with proteins. Discuss. Faraday Soc. 6, 44 (1949). — Luck, J. M., and A. S. Schmit: The combination of serum albumin with organic compounds. Stanf. med. Bull. 6, 133 (1948). — Ludewig, S., A. Chanutin and A. V. Masket: Studies on the calciumprotein relationship with the aid of the ultrazentrifuge. II. Observ. J. biol. Chem. 143, 753 (1942). — Lübke: Zit. nach R. Schubert 1954. — Lüthy, F.: Liquor cerebrospinalis. In Handbuch der inneren Medizin, 4. Aufl., Bd. V/1. Berlin: Springer 1953. — Lundquist, F.: Renal tubular secretion of sulfonamides and p-aminobenzoic acid. Acta pharmacol. (Kbh.) 1, 307 (1945). — Lurie, M. B.: Mechanism affecting spread in tuberculosis. Ann. N. Y. Acad. Sci. 52, 1074 (1950). — Lybeck, H.: Electrophoretic studies on free and protein bound I^{131} in the serum. Acta med. scand. 158, Suppl., 327 (1957).

Macheboeuf, M.: Etat des lipides dans la matière vivante. Paris 1937. — Macheboeuf, M.: Récherches sur les phosphoaminolipides et les stérides du sérum et du plasma sanguins. Bull. Soc. Chim. biol. (Paris) 11, 268 (1929). — Macheboeuf, M., et M. Viscontini: Etudes des combinaisons entre protéides et cuivre prenant naissance en milieu alcalin. C. R. Acad. Sci. (Paris) 218, 977 (1944). — Malinow, U. R., and W. Korzon: An experimental method for obtaining an ultrafiltrate of the blood. J. Lab. clin. Med. 32, 461 (1947). — Malloy, H. T., and K. A. Evelyn: The determination of bilirubin with the photoelectric colorimeter. J. biol. Chem. 119, 481 (1937). — Malloy, H. T., and L. Lowenstein: Canad. med. Ass. J. 42, 122 (1940). — Man, E. B., and M. J. Albrink: Serumlipids in different phases of carbohydrat metabolism. Yale J. Biol. Med. 29, 316 (1956). — Mann, T., and D. Keilin: Haemocuprein and hepatocuprein, copperprotein compounds of blood and liver in mammals. Proc. roy. Soc. 126, 330 (1938). — Marble, A., and R. M. Smith: Studies of iron metabolism in a case of hemochromatosis. Ann. intern. Med. 12, 1592 (1939). — Markowitz, H., C. J. Gubler, J. P. Maloney, G. E. Cartwright and M. M. Wintrobe: Studies on copper metabolism. XIV. Copper, coeruloplasmin and oxydase activity in serum of normal human subjects, pregnant woman, and patients with infection, hepaticolenticular degeneration and the nephrotic syndrom. J. clin. Invest. 34, 1498 (1955). — Marshall jr., E. K.: The secretion of phenol red by the mammalian kidney. Amer. J. Physiol. 99, 77 (1931). — Marshall jr., E. K., and J. L. Vickers: The mechanism of the elimination of phenolsulfonphthalein by the kidney a proof of secretion by the convoluted tubules. Bull. Johns Hopk. Hosp. 34, 1 (1923). — Martin, J. D., and J. H. Mills: Effect of pregnancy on adreanl steroid metabolism. Clin. Sci. 17, 137 (1958). — Martin, N. H.: Bilirubin-serumprotein complexes. Biochem. J. 42, No 1 Proceed., XI (1948). ~ Preparation and properties of serum and plasma proteins. XXI. Interaction with bilirubin. J. Amer. chem. Soc. 71, 1230 (1949). — Martin, N. H., and D. J. Perkins: The interaction of serum albumin with calcium. Biochem. J. 47, 323 (1950). — Masoro, E. J., and J. M. Felts: Role of carbohydrate metabolism in fatty acid oxydation. Fed. Proc. 16, 85 (1957). — Mathews, M. B.: Chondroitin sulfaric acid a linear polyelectrolyt. Arch. Biochem. 43, 181 (1953). — Mattson, F. H., J. H. Benedict, J. B. Martin and L. W. Beck: Intermediates formed during the digestion of triglycerides. J. Nutr. 48, 335 (1952). — Maurer, W.: Zur Frage der Transportfunktion einzelner Serum-Eiweiß-Fraktionen für Phosphatide. Klin. Wschr. 1953 c, 325. ~ Ergebnisse der medizinischen Grundlagenforschung mit radioaktiven Isotopen. Dtsch. med. J. 8, 324 (1957). — Maurer, W., u. E. R. Müller: Zur Frage der Transportfunktion einzelner Serum-Eiweiß-Fraktionen für die organischen Jodverbindungen des Serums. Biochem. Z. 324, 325 (1953). ~ Untersuchung der Transportfunktion einzelner Serum-Eiweiß-Fraktionen für Phosphatide nach einer neuen papierelektrophoretischen Methode. Biochem. Z. 324, 255 (1953 b). — Maurer, W., u. L. Reichenbach: Über die Bindung des organischen Jods im Serum an einzelne Serum-Eiweißfraktionen. Natur-

264   H. BENNHOLD und H. OTT: Der Stofftransport.

wissenschaften **39**, 261 (1952). — MAYER, C.: Zit. nach HEILMAYER: Die sideroachrestischen Anämien. Dtsch. med. Wschr. **84**, 39 (1959). — MAYER, M., H. ZEISS, G. GIEMSA u. J. HALBERKANN: Weitere Beobachtungen über das Verhalten des Trypanosomenheilmittels „Bayer 205" im Blut. Arch. Schiffs- u. Tropenhyg. **26**, 140 (1922). — MAZUR, A., S. GREEN and A. CARLETON: Mechanism of plasm iron incorporation into hepatic ferritin. J. biol. Chem. **235**, 595 (1960). — McCALLUM, A. B.: On the demonstration of the presence of iron chromatin by microchemical methods. Proc. roy. Soc. B **50**, 277 (1891/92). — McCANDLESS, E. L., and D. B. ZILVERSMIT: Disappearance of I^{131}-labeled lymph triglycerides and phosphatides from blood of dogs. Fed. Proc. **16**, 85 (1957). — McCONNEL, K. P., and B. J. COOPER: Distribution of selenium in serumproteins and red blood cells J. biol. Chem. **183**, 459 (1950). — McLEAN, F. C., and A. B. HASTINGS: The state of calcium in the fluids of the body. I. The conditions affecting ionization of calcium. J. biol. Chem. **108**, 285 (1935). — MEHL, J. W., F. GOLDEN and R. S. WINZLER: Mucoproteins of human plasma. IV. Electrophoretic demonstration of mucoprotein in serum on p_H 4—5. Proc. Soc. exp. Biol. (N.Y.) **72**, 110 (1949). — MELLANDER, O.: Kataphoretische Untersuchung über die Bindungsverhältnisse des Cholesterins im Blutserum. Biochem. Z. **277**, 305 (1935). — MELLON, E. F., A. H. KERN and S. R. HOOVER: Water absorption of proteins. J. Amer. chem. Soc. **71**, 827 (1949). — MENDELSOHN, R., D. M. WATKIN, A. P. HORBETT and J. L. FAHEY: Identification of the vitamin B_{12}-binding protein in the serum of normals and patients with chronic myelotic leucemia. Blood **13**, 740 (1958). — MENKIN, V.: Newer concepts of inflammation. Springfield: Ch. C. Thomas 1950. ~ Further studies on mechanism of increased capillary permeability in inflammation with the aid of cortisone and ACTH. Exp. biol. Med. **77**, 592 (1951). ~ The significance of the accumulation of cortisone in an inflammed area. Brit. J. exp. Path. **34**, 412 (1953). — MEYER, H. H.: Der Liquor. Untersuchung und Diagnostik. Berlin-Göttingen-Heidelberg: Springer 1953. — MEYER, K.: Mucoids and glycoproteins. Advances in protein chemistry, vol. 2, p. 249. New York: Academic Press 1945. — MEYER, K., and M. RAPPORT: The mucopolysaccharides of the ground substance of connective tissue. Science **113**, 596 (1951). — MEYER-FRIEDMANN, S., O. BYERS, L. FELTON and P. CADY: Localization and retention of I^{131} from fed triolein in the atherosclerotic infiltration of rabbit aortas. J. clin. Invest. **38**, 539 (1959). — MIGEON, C. J., H. PRYTOWSKY, M. M. GRUMBACH and M. C. BYRON: Placental passage of 17-hydroxycorticosteroids. Comparison of the levels in maternal and fetal plasma and effect of ACTH and hydrocortisone administration. J. clin. Invest. **35**, 488 (1956). — MILLER, A., H. F. CORBUS and J. F. SULLIVAN: The plasma disappearence, excretion and tissue distribution of $cobalt^{60}$ labeled vitamin B_{12} in normal subjects and patients with chronic myelogenous leucemia. J. clin. Invest. **36**, 18 (1957). — MILLER, A., and J. SULLIVAN: Electrophoretic studies of the vitamin B_{12} binding protein of normal and chronic myelogenous leucemia serum. J. clin. Invest. **38**, 2135 (1959). — MILLER, E. C., and J. A. MILLER: Zit. nach H. A. COOK, Tissue proteins and carcinogenesis. II. Electrophoretic studies on serum proteins. J. biol. Chem. **177**, 373 (1949). — MISCHEL, W.: Die anorganischen Bestandteile der Placenta. VI. Mitt. Der Gesamt- und Gewebseisengehalt der reifen und unreifen, normalen und pathologischen menschlichen Placenta. Arch. Gynäk. **190**, 638 (1958). — MISSMAHL, H. P.: Bisher unveröffentlichte Untersuchungen über die Mitochondrienstruktur. 1955. — MOHRING, D.: Über die Bindung von Phenylbutazone an Albumine. Ärztl. Forsch. **12**, 66 (1958). — MOLLIN, D. L., W. R. PITNEY, S. J. BAKER and J. E. BRADLEY: The plasma clearence and urinary excretion of parenterally administered ^{58}Co-B_{12}. Blood **11**, 31 (1956). — MOLLIN, D. L., and G. I. M. ROSS: Serum vitamin B_{12} concentrating in leucaemia and in some other haematological conditions. Brit. J. Haemat. **1**, 155 (1955). ~ Vitamin B_{12} und Intrinsic Factor, i, 1957. Europäisches Symposion über Vitamin B_{12} und Intrinsic Factor, Hamburg 1956, S. 413. Stuttgart: Ferdinand Enke. — MOON, H., and G. A. TERSHAKOVEE: Influence of cortisone upon acute inflammation. Proc. Soc. exp. Biol. (N. Y.) **79**, 63 (1952). — MOORE, B., and H. E. ROAF: On certain physical and chemical properties of solutions of chloroform in water, saline, serum and hemoglobin. 1th Comm. Proc. roy. Soc. B **73**, 382 (1904). ~ On certain physical and chemical properties of solutions of chloroform and other anaesthetics. 2nd Comm. Proc. roy. Soc. B **77**, 86 (1905). — MORA, R. R., P. REBEYROTTE et J. POLONOVSKI: Influences des substances tensioactives sur la mobilitée éléctrophoretique des lipoprotéines plasmatiques. Bull. Soc. Chim. biol. **37**, 957 (1955). — MORCZEK, A.: Untersuchungen über den Eisenstoffwechsel. I. Mitt. Die renale Eisenausscheidung unter physiologischen Verhältnissen. Dtsch. Z. Verdau.- u. Stoffwechselkr. **10**, 148 (1950). ~ II. Mitt. Die renale Eisenausscheidung bei verschiedenen Krankheiten. Dtsch. Z. Verdau.- u. Stoffwechselkr. **12**, 14 (1952). — MORRIS, B., and J. FRENCH: The uptake and metabolism of C^{14}-labeled chylomicron fat by the isolated perfused liver of the rat. Quart. J. exp. Physiol. **43**, 180 (1958). — MÜHLBAUER, H.: Zit. nach R. SCHUBERT 1954. — MÜLLER, A.: Abhandlungen zur Mechanik der Flüssigkeiten mit besonderer Berücksichtigung der Haemodynamik. Abhandlung II: Strömen in Röhren. 5. Teil. Anwendungen über einige der durch Versuche mit heterogenen Flüssigkeiten erworbenen Kenntnisse auf den Kreislauf. Arch. Kreisl.-Forsch. **10**, 326 (1942). — MÜLLER, E. R.: Zur Frage der Bindung des Calciums im Serum (Papierelektrophorese von Ca^{45}-markierten

Seren). Naturwissenschaften 40, 442 (1953). — MUELLER, R., C. C. BRAUSCH, E. Z. HIRSCH, R. S. BENUA and B. M. DOBYNS: Uptake of radioactive iodine in the thyroid of patients with impaired liver function. J. clin. Endocr. 14, 1287 (1954). — MUIRHEAD, E. E., G. BRASS, F. JONES and J. M. HILL: Iron overload (hemosiderosis) aggravated by blood transfusion. Arch. intern. Med. 83, 477 (1949). — MUMENTHALER, A.: Zur Frage der Strömungsverhältnisse im Pfortaderkreislauf. Schweiz. Z. allg. Path. 16, Nr 2 (1953). — MUNKNER, T.: Diskussionsbemerkung zu N. LANG u. K. H. GILLICH in Radioaktive Isotope in Klinik und Forschung, Bd. 4. München: Urban & Schwarzenberg 1960. — MUNN, J. I., N. H. WALTERS and H. C. DUDLEY, PHD: Urinary excretion of gallium by man and animals. J. Lab. clin. Med. 37, 676 (1951). — MYANT, N. B.: The passage of thyroxine and triiodothyronine from mother to foetus in pregnant rabbits, with a note on the concentration of protein-bound iodine in foetal serum. J. Physiol. (Lond.) 142, 329 (1958). — MYANT, N. B., and C. OSORIO: Serum proteins, including thyroxine-binding proteins, in maternal and foetal rabbits. J. Physiol. (Lond.) 146, 344 (1959). ~ The passage of thyroxine-binding substances between mother and foetus in pregnant rabbits. J. Physiol. (Lond.) 151, 66 (1960).

NAPP, J. H., u. J. PLOTZ: Die Bedeutung der Leber für die Genese des Ikterus neonatorum. Arch. Gynäk. 176, 781 (1949). — NERGAARD, K. V.: Bestimmung des molekular gelösten Silbers und seines Ionisationsgrades in Gegenwart von kolloidem Silber bei einigen therapeutischen Silberpräparaten mit Angaben einer potentiometrischen Methode. Naunyn-Schmiedeberg's Arch. exp. Path. Pharmak. 100, 162 (1923). ~ Experimentelles zur intravenösen Silbertherapie. III. Mitteilung. Silbereiweißverbindungen. Naunyn-Schmiedeberg's Arch. exp. Path. Pharmak. 108, 295 (1924). — NEUHAUSEN and E. K. MARSHAL: An electrochemical study of the condition of several electrolytes in the blood. J. biol. Chem. 53, 365 (1922). — NEUWEILER: Über das Vorkommen von Vitamin C im foetalen und Neugeborenen-Darm. Z. Vitaminforsch. 14, 32 (1943). — NICHOLS, A. V., V. DOBBIN and J. W. GOFMAN: Influence of dietary factors upon human serum lipoprotein concentration. Geriatrics 12, 7 (1957). — NICOLL, P. A., u. R. L. WEBB: Blood circulation in the subcutaneous tissue of the living Bat's wing. Ann. N.Y. Acad. Sci. 46, 697 (1946). — NIKKILÄ, E.: Studies on the lipid-protein relationship in normal and pathological sera and the effect of heparin on serum lipoproteins. Scand. J. clin. Lab. Invest. 5, Suppl. 8 (1953). — NYMAN, M.: Serum Haptoglobin. Scand. J. clin. Lab. invest. Suppl. 39 (1959).

ODELL, G. B.: Society for pediatric research. A.M.A. J. Dis. Child. 96, 419 (1958). ~ Studies in kernicterus. I. The protein binding of bilirubin. J. clin. Invest. 38, 823 (1959). — OEFF, K.: Papierelektrophoretische Untersuchung der Bindung von radioaktivem Biliselektan an Serumalbumin. Naunyn-Schmiedeberg's Arch. exp. Path. Pharamak. 222, 523 (1954). — OLIVER, J., and E. DOUGLAS: Biologic reactions of arsphenamin. V. Its reactions with plasmaproteins and certain hydrophilic colloids. Arch. Derm. Syph. (Chicago) 7, 778 (1923). — ONCLEY, J. L., and F. R. N. GURD in: Blood cells and plasmaproteins, their state in nature, Hrsg. J. K. TULLIS. New York, N.Y.: Academic Press 1953. — ONCLEY, J. L., F. R. N. GURD and M. MELIN: Preparations and properties of serum and plasma proteins. XXV. Composition and properties of human serum-β-lipoprotein. J. Amer. chem. Soc. 72, 458 (1950). — ONCLEY, J. L., G. SCATCHARD and A. BROWN: Physical-chemical characteristics of certains of the proteins of normal human plasma. J. physic. Chem. 51, 184 (1947). — OPPÉ, TH. E.: Hyperbilirubinaemia in premature infants. Lancet 1960 I, 922. — OPPENHEIMER, E.: Zur Frage der Fixation der Digitaliskörper im tierischen Organismus und deren Verhalten zum Blut. Biochem. Z. 55, 134 (1913). — OPPERMANN, W., u. H. OTT: Azorubinbindung an Humanserumalbumin. Hoppe-Seylers Z. physiol. Chem. 308, 43 (1957). — ORCUTT, F. S., and M. H. SEEVERS: The solubility coefficients of cyclopropane for water, oils and human blood. J. Pharmacol. exp. Ther. 59, 206 (1937). — ORTH, J.: Über das Vorkommen von Bilirubinkrystallen bei neugeborenen Kindern. Virchows Arch. path. Anat. 63, 447 (1875). — OSORIO, C., and N. B. MYANT: Thyroxine-binding protein in the serum of rabbit foetuses. Nature (Lond.) 182, 866 (1958). ~ The passage of thyroid hormone from mother to foetus and its relation to foetal development. Brit. med. Bull. 16, 159 (1960). — OTT, H.: Unveröffentlichte Untersuchungen mit Farbstoffen. 1952. ~ Gibt es Paraalbumine? Ärztl. Forsch. 6 (I), 177 (1952a). ~ Über die Bindung kolloidaler Partikel an die Plasmaproteine. Z. ges. exp. Med. 122, 346 (1953). ~ Über Serumalbumin-Bindung und Ausscheidung der Gallekontrastmittel Biliselektan und Biligrafin und der Nierenkontrastmittel Uroselektan und Urografin beim Kaninchen. Bisher unveröffentlicht. 1956. ~ Das Blutserum bei Analbuminaemie. Weitere Untersuchungen über die Serumfraktionen, das Farbstoffbindungsvermögen und den kolloidosmotischen Druck. Z. ges. exp. Med. 128, 340 (1957). ~ Austausch von P^{32} zwischen markierten und unmarkierten Serumlipoproteiden in vitro. Z. Naturforsch. 13b, (1958). — OTT, H., u. E. KALLEE: Azorubinverdrängung vom Serumalbumin. Kolloid-Z. 127, 40 (1952). — OTT, H., u. FR. LOHSS: Die Serumproteine und Serumlipoproteide der Aortenintima. Verh. dtsch. Ges. inn. Med. 64, 620 (1958). — OTT, H., FR. LOHSS u. J. GERGELY: Der Nachweis von Serumlipoproteiden in der Aortenintima. Klin. Wschr. 36, 383 (1958). — OTT, H., u. E. ROTH: Fettfärbung der Serumlipoproteide am Filtrierpapier. Klin. Wschr. 1954, 1099. — OTT, H., u. C. SEEGER: Untersuchungen zur Frage der Germaninbindung an die Serumproteine. Z. ges. exp. Med. **125**, 455 (1955). — Otto, G.: Bindungsvorgänge zwischen aromatischen Körpern und der Eiweißfaser. Leder **4**, 193 1953). ~ Die Wechselwirkung von Hautsubstanz mit aromatischen Gerb-, Farb- und Hilfstoffen. Leder **6**, 207 (1955). — Overkamp, H.: Über die Serumeisenerniedrigung bei Infektionskrankheiten. Klin. Wschr. **31**, 53 (1953). — Overton, E.: Vjschr. naturforsch. Ges. Zürich **44**, 88 (1899). ~ Studien über die Narkose. Jena: Gustav Fischer 1901. — Owen, Ch. A., u. W. McConahey: Zit. nach Vannotti, Fed. Proc. **15**, 140 (1956).

Paget, M., et C. Vittu: Recherche de l'existence d'une combinaison serum-paraaminophénylsulfonamide par l'étude de réfraction. C. R. Soc. Biol. (Paris) **104**, 227 (1946). — Pak, C.: Versuche über den Übertritt chemischer Substanzen aus der Gefäßbahn in das Gewebe. Naunyn-Schmiedeberg's Arch. exp. Path. Pharmak. **111**, 42 (1926). — Pappenheimer, J. R., E. M. Renkin and L. Borrero: Filtration and molecular diffusion from the capillary in muscle, with deductions concerning the number and dimensions of ultramicroscopic openings in the capillary walls. Proc. XVIII. Internat. physiol. Congr., Copenhagen, p. 384, 1950. ~ Passage of molecule, through the capillary walls. Physiol. Rev. **33**, 387 (1953). — Patek jr., A. J., and R. G. Minot: Bile pigment and regeneration hemoglobin. The effect of bile pigment in cases of chronic hypochrome anemia. Amer. J. med. Sci. **188**, 206 (1934). — Patzer, H.: Die Pathogenese des Ikterus gravis neonatorum. Leipzig: Georg Thieme 1953. — Pauli, W., u. M. Schön: Untersuchungen an elektrolytfreien, wasserlöslichen Proteinen. III. Mitt., Salzeiweißverbindungen ($ZnCl_2$). Biochem. Z. **153**, 253 (1924). — Pauli, W., u. E. Valko: Kolloidchemie der Eiweißkörper. Dresden: Theodor Steinkopff 1933. — Pearson, P. B., and H. R. Catchpole: Correlated studies of the position of calcium and inorganic phosphorus in the blood sera of equidae. Amer. J. Physiol. **115**, 90 (1936). — Pedersen, K. O., u. J. Waldenstroem: Studien über das Bilirubin in Blut und Galle mit Hilfe von Elektrophorese und Ultrazentrifugierung. Hoppe-Seylers Z. physiol. Chem. **245**, 152 (1937). — Pendl, J., u. W. Franz: Vitamin B_{12}-Gehalt und Vitamin B_{12}-Bindungsvermögen im Magensaft bei perniciöser Anämie und anderen Erkrankungen. Acta haemat. (Basel) **13**, 207 (1955). ~ Transformation of megaloblasts to normablasts by cultivating human bone marrow in presence of vitamin B_{12} and vitamin B_{12} binding protein. Nature (Lond.) **181**, 488 (1958). ~ Vitamin B_{12} mit Vitamin B_{12} bindendem Protein als antianämisch wirksames Prinzip. Hoppe-Seyler's Z. physiol. Chem. **313**, 259 (1958). — Peters, Th., and Chr. B. Anfinsen: Production of radioactive serum albumin by liver slices. J. biol. Chem. **182**, 171 (1950). ~ Net production of serum albumin by liver slices. J. biol. Chem. **186**, 805 (1950). — Peterson, R. E., J. B. Wyngaarden, S. L. Guerra, B. B. Brodie and J. J. Bunim: The physiological disposition and metabolic fate of hydrocortison in man. J. clin. Invest. **34**, 177a (1955). — Pezold, F. A.: Über die Bindung von Phenoltetrabromphthalein-dinatriumsulfonat an Humanserum im Hinblick auf den „Bromsulfaleintest". Z. ges. exp. Med. **121**, 700 (1953). — Pfaff, W., u. W. Herold: Grundlagen einer neuen Therapieforschung der Tuberkulose. Leipzig 1937. — Pfuhl, W.: Untersuchungen über die Fixierung der vitalen Trypanblauspeicherung. Z. Zellforsch. **13**, 783 (1931). — Pibl, A., and K. Bloch: The relatives rates of metabolism of neutral fat and phospholipides in various tissues of the rat. J. biol. Chem. **183**, 431 (1950). — Pierce, F. T.: The interconversion of serum lipoproteins in vivo. Metabolism **3**, 142 (1954). — Pitney, W. R., M. F. Beard and E. J. van Loon: Observations on the bound form of vitamin B_{12} in human serum. J. biol. Chem. **207**, 143 (1954). — Pitts, R. F.: The excretion of phenol red by the chicken. J. cell. comp. Physiol. **11**, 99 (1938). — Plattner, F.: Zur Frage der Ausscheidung saurer Farbstoffe durch die Leber. Arch. ges. Physiol. **206**, 91 (1924). — Plückthun, H.: Physiologische Entwicklung des Kindes, S. 316. Hrsg. F. Linneweh. Berlin: Springer 1959. — Pochin, E. E.: Investigation of thyroid function and disease with radioactive iodine. Lancet **1950**, 41. ~ Second phase of the iodine cycle: Retention in the thyroid. Lancet **1950**, 84. — Poijärvi, L. A. P.: Über die Basenpermeabilität pflanzlicher Zellen. Acta bot. fenn. **4**, 2 (1928). — Pollicove, M.: Funktionen, Verteilung und Eigenschaften der Eisenverbindungen im menschlichen Körper. In Thannhauser, Lehrbuch des Stoffwechsels und der Stoffwechselkrankheiten, von Dr. N. Zöllner. Stuttgart: Georg Thieme 1957. — Popják, G.: Mechanism of absorption of inorganic phosphate from blood by tissue cells. Nature (Lond.) **166**, 184 (1950). — Prasad, A. S., E. B. Flink and H. H. Zinneman: The base binding property of the serum proteins with respect to magnesium. J. Lab. clin. Med. **54**, 355 (1959). — Prentice, T. C., N. J. Berlin, W. Sini, G. M. Hyde, R. J. Parson, E. E. Joiner and J. H. Lawrence: Studies of total body water with tritium. J. clin. Invest. **31**, 412 (1952). — Putnam, F. W.: The interactions of proteins and synthetic detergents. Advanc. Protein Chem. **4**, 79 (1948). — Putnam, F. W., and H. Neurath: Complex formation between synthetic detergents and proteins. J. biol. Chem. **150**, 263 (1943). ~ Interaction between proteins and synthetic detergents: II. Electrophoretic analysis of serum albumin and sodium dodecylsulfat mixtures. J. biol. Chem. **159**, 195 (1945).

Quick, A. J.: The normal antithrombin of the blood and its relation to heparin. Amer. J. Physiol. **123**, 712 (1938).

RAKOFF, A. E., K. E. PASCHKIS and A. CANTAROW: Conjugated estrogens in human pregnancy serum. Amer. J. Obstet. Gynec. **46**, 856 (1943). — RALL, J. E., O. H. PEARSON, M. B. LIPSETT and R. W. RAWSON: Metabolic effects in man of the acetic-acid analogues of thyroxine and triiodothyronine. J. clin. Endocr. **16**, 1290 (1956). — RALL, J. E., J. ROBBINS, D. BECKER and R. W. RAWSON: The metabolism of labeled l-tri-iodothyronine, l-thyroxine and d-thyroxine. J. clin. Invest. **32**, 596 (1953). — RAMALHÂO, J.: Portugal méd. **40**, 96 (1956). — RAMSAY, W. N. M.: Plasma iron. In: Advances in clinical chemistry, p. 1—39. New York: Academic Press 1958. — RASMUSSEN, H.: Thyroxine metabolism in the nephrotic syndrome. J. clin. Invest. **35**, 792 (1956). — RATH, C. E., and C. A. FINCH: Sternal marrow hemosiderin. A method for the determination of avaiable iron stores in man. J. Lab. clin. Med. **33**, 81 (1948). ~ Chemical, clinical a immunological studies on the products of human plasma fractionation. XXXVIII. Serum iron transport. Measurement of ironbinding capacity of serum of man. J. clin. Invest. **28**, 79 (1949). — RAWLINS, L. M. C., and C. L. A. SCHMIDT: The mode of combination between certain dyes and gelatin granules. J. biol. Chem. **88**, 271 (1930). — RAWSON, R. A.: The binding of T-1824 and structurally related diazo dyes by the plasmaproteins. Amer. J. Physiol. **138**, 708 (1943). — REIN, H.: Physiologie des Menschen. Berlin: Springer 1955. — REINDELL, H., u. L. DELIUS: Klinische Beobachtungen über die Haemodynamik beim gesunden Menschen. Dtsch. Arch. klin. Med. **193**, 639 (1948). — REINHOLD, J. G., H. F. FLIPPIN, A. H. DOMM u. L. POLLACK: Bindung von Sulfonamiden an Proteine. J. Amer. med. Ass. **207**, 413 (1944). — REISE, R.: Some recent studies on fat digestion and absorption. J. Amer. biol. chem. Soc. **31**, 292 (1954). — REMINGTON, J. W.: Volume quantitation of the aortic pressure pulse. Fed. Proc. **11**, 750 (1952). — REMY, D.: Der Eisenstoffwechsel bei der Haemochromatose. Dtsch. med. Wschr. **79**, 1042 (1954). — RENKIN, E. M.: Capillary permeability to lipid soluble molecules. Amer. J. Physiol. **168**, 538 (1952). — RESHEF, L., E. SHAFRIR and B. SHAPIRO: In vitro release of unesterfied fatty acids by adipose tissue. Metabolism **7**, 723 (1958). — RICHARDS, A. N., and A. M. WALKER: Quantitative studies of the glomerular elimination of phenol red and indigocarmine in frogs. J. biol. Chem. **87**, 479 (1930). — RIGGS, D. S.: Serum protein-bound iodine as a diagnostic aid. Trans. Amer. study goiter **1947**, 137. ~ Zit. nach A. GOLDSTEIN, J. Pharmacol. exp. Ther. **95**, 102 (1949). — RIVA, G.: Die klinische Bedeutung des Serumeiweißbildes. Verh. dtsch. Ges. inn. Med. **66**, 291 (1960). — ROBBINS, J.: Reverse-flow zone electrophoresis. A method for determining the thyroxine-binding capacity of serum protein. Arch. Biochem. **63**, 461 (1956). — ROBBINS, J., and J. H. NELSON: Thyroxinbinding by serum protein in pregnancy and in the newborn. J. clin. Invest. **37**, 153 (1958). — ROBBINS, J., and J. E. RALL: Zone electrophoresis in filter paper of serum I^{131} after radioiodide administration. Proc. Soc. exp. Biol. (N.Y.) **81**, 530 (1952). ~ Thyroxinebinding capacity of serum in normal man. J. clin. Invest. **34**, 1324 (1953). ~ Effects of triiodothyronine and other thyroxine analogues on thyroxine-binding in human serum. J. clin. Invest. **34**, 1331 (1955). ~ Proteins associated with the thyroid hormones. Physiol. Rev. **40**, 415 (1960). — ROBBINS, J., J. E. RALL, D. V. BECKER and R. W. RAWSON: The nature of the serum iodine after large dosis of I^{131}. J. clin. Endocr. **12**, 856 (1952). — ROBBINS, J., J. E. RALL and M. L. PETERMANN: Proteinbinding of thyroxin in normal and nephrotic serum. J. clin. Invest. **33**, 959 (1954). ~ Thyroxine-binding by serum and urine proteins in nephrosis. Qualitative aspects. J. clin. Invest. **36**, 1333 (1957). — ROBBINS, J., J. E. RALL and R. W. RAWSON: A new serum iodine component in patients with functional carcinoma of the thyroid. J. clin. Endocr. **15**, 1315 (1955). — ROBB-SMITH, A. M. T.: The significance of connective tissue. Lectures on the scientific basis of medicine, vol. 2. London 1954. — ROBERTS, A., and C. M. SZEGO: The nature of circulating extrogen: Lipoproteinbound estrogen in human plasma. Endocrinology **39**, 183 (1946). — ROBINSON, D. S., and J. E. FRENCH: The heparin clearing reaction and fat transport. Quart. J. exp. Physiol. **42**, 151 (1957). — ROBINSON, H. W., and C. G. HOGDEN: The influence of serumproteins on the spectrophotometric absorption curve of phenol red in a phosphate puffer mixture. J. biol. Chem. **137**, 239 (1941). — ROBSON, H. N., and J. J. R. DUTHIE: Capillary resistance and adrenocortical activity. Brit. med. J. **1950**II, 971. ~ Further observations on capillary resistance and adrenocortical activity. Brit. med. J. **1952**I, 994. — RODBELL, M.: N-Terminal amino acid and lipid composition of lipoproteins from chyle and plasma. Science **127**, 701 (1958). — RODBELL, M., and D. S. FREDRICKSON: Nature and function of chylomicron proteins. Fed. Proc. **17**, 298 (1958). — ROHOLM, K., u. P. IVERSEN: Zit nach EPPINGER 1949, Acta path. microbiol. scand. **16**, 427 (1942). — RONA, P., F. HAUROWITZ u. H. PETOW: Beitrag zur Frage der Ionenverteilung im Blutserum. II. Biochem. Z. **149**, 391 (1924). — RONA, P., u. D. TAKAHASHI: Über das Verhalten des Calziums im Serum und über den Gehalt der Blutkörperchen an Calzium. Biochem. Z. **31**, 336 (1911). — ROSENBERG, TH., B. VESTERGAARD-BEGIND u. W. WILBRANDT: Modellversuche zur Trägerhypothese von Zuckertransporten. Helv. physiol. Acta **14**, 334 (1956). — ROSENBERG, TH., and W. WILBRANDT: Encymatic processes in cell membrane penetration. Rev. Cytol. **1**, 65 (1952). — ROSENFELD, M.: Zit. nach E. J. COHN, Blood **3**, 471 (1948). — ROSENFELD, M., and D. M. SURGENOR: Methemalbumin: Interaction between human serum albumin and ferriprotoporphyrin. IX.

J. biol. Chem. **183**, 663 (1950). — Rosenthal, F.: Die Bedeutung des Elastins beim Ikterus. Klin. Wschr. **41**, 1909 (1930). — Rosenthal, S. M.: The liberation of adsorbed substances from proteins a function of the bile salts. I. Preliminary report. J. Pharmacol. exp. Ther. **25**, 449 (1925). ~ The liberation of adsorbed substances from proteins. II. Affect of addition of sodium oleate to whole blood upon the non protein nitrogen in blood filtrates. J. biol. Chem. **70**, 129 (1926a). ~ Studies upon the combining power of proteins with rose bengal. J. Pharmacol. exp. Ther. **29**, 521 (1926). — Rosenthal, S. M., and E. C. White: Studies in hepatic function VI. A and B. The behavior and value of phthalein dyes. J. Pharmacol. exp. Ther. **24**, 265 (1924). — Ross, G. I. M.: Vitamin B_{12} assay in body fluids. Nature (Lond.) **166**, 270 (1950). — Rossier, P. H., A. Bühlmann u. K. Wiesinger: Physiologie und Pathophysiologie der Atmung. Berlin-Göttingen-Heidelberg: Springer 1956. — Rothlin, E.: The glucoside binding action of different fractions of human serum and plasma proteins. Unpublished. Zit. bei A. Goldstein, J. Pharmacol. exp. Ther. **95**, 102 (1949). — Rothstein, A., and R. Meyer: The relationship of the cell surface to metabolism. I. Phosphatases in the cell surface of binding yeast cells. J. cell. comp. Physiol. **32**, 77 (1948). ~ IV. The chemical nature of uranium complexing groups of the cell surface. J. cell. comp. Physiol. **38**, 245 (1951). — Rübsam, C.: Die Wirkung der Sauerstofftherapie auf das arterielle Blut. Inaug.-Diss. Zürich 1942. — Ruhland, W., u. C. Hoffmann: Planta (Berl.) **1**, 1 (1925). — Russ, E. M., H. A. Eder and D. P. Barr: Protein-lipid relationship in human plasma. I. In normal individuals. Amer. J. Med. **11**, 468 (1951). — Rusznyák, J., M. Földi u. Gg. Szabo: Physiologische und pathologische Bedeutung des Lymphkreislaufs. Schweiz. med. Wschr. **85**, 1037 (1955). ~ Physiologie und Pathologie des Lymphkreislaufs. Budapest 1955. Deutsche Ausgabe Jena: Gustav Fischer 1957.

Sachs, A., V. E. Levine, C. F. Hill and R. Hughes: Copper and iron in human blood. A.M.A. Arch. intern. Med. **71**, 489 (1943). — Sacks, J.: Mechanism of phosphate transfer across all membranes. Cold Spr. Harb. Symp. quant. Biol. **13**, 180 (1948). — Salt, H. B., O. H. Wolff, J. K. Lloyd, A. S. Fosbrooke, A. H. Cameron and D. V. Hubble: On having no beta-lipoprotein. A syndrome comprising A-β-lipoproteinaemia, acanthocythosis, and steatorrhea. Lancet **1960**, 325. — Salter, W. T.: Zit. nach Maurer u. Reichenbach, West. J. Surg. **55**, 15 (1947). — Salter, W. T., W. F. White and A. E. McKay: The lymphatic congregance of thyroid hormone. Fed. Proc. **5**, 90 (1946). — Samson, J. W., u. H. Götz: Körpereiweiß und Arzneimittelallergie. Z. ges. exp. Med. **52**, 121 (1926). — Sandberg, A. A., and W. R. Slaunwhite jr.: Transcortin, a corticosteroid-binding protein of plasma. II. Levels in various conditions and the effects of estrogens. J. clin. Invest. **38**, 1290 (1959). — Sandberg, A. A., W. R. Slaunwhite jr. and H. N. Antoniades: The binding of steroids and steroid conjugates to human plasma proteins. Recent Progr. Hormone Res. **13**, 209 (1957). — Saroff, H. A., and W. L. Choate: Reversible aggregation of serum albumin in the reaction with copper. II. Arch. biochem. Biophys. **74**, 245 (1958). — Saroff, H. A., and H. J. Mark: Zit. nach A. Goldstein, J. Pharmacol. exp. Ther. **95**, 102 (1949). — Sass-Kortsack, A., M. Chernia, D. W. Geiger and R. J. Slater: Observations on ceruloplasmin in Wilson's disease. J. clin. Invest. **38**, 1672 (1959). — Sautter, H., H. Hager u. R. Seitz: Experimentelle Vitalforschung des Augenhintergrundes. Albrecht v. Gräfes Arch. Ophthal. **155**, 115 (1954). — Scarborough, H.: Edinb. med. J. **51**, 335 (1944). — Scatchard, G.: The attraction of proteins for smal molecules and ions. Ann. N. Y. Acad. Sci. **1949**. — Scatchard, G., A. C. Batchelder and A. Brown: Preparation and proteries of serum and plasmaproteins. VI. Osmotic equilibria in solution of serum albumin and sodium chloride. J. Amer. chem. Soc. **68**, 2320 (1946). — Scatchard, G., and E. S. Black: The effect of salts on the isoionic and isoelectric points of proteins. J. phys. Colloid Chem. **53**, 88 (1949a). — Scatchard, G., I. H. Scheinberg and S. H. Armstrong jr.: Physikal chemistry of protein solutions IV. The combination of human serum albumin with the chloride ion, S. 535. V. The combination of human serum albumin with thiocyanate ion, S. 540. J. Amer. chem. Soc. **71** (1949b). — Scatchard, G., I. H. Scheinberg and S. H. Armstrong jr.: Physical chemistry of protein solution. I. The chlorideion. II. Combination with thiocyanateion. J. Amer. chem. Soc. **72**, 535 (1950). — Scazziga, B. R., Th. Béraud et A. V. Vannotti: Etude du métabolisme hépatobiliaire de l'hormone thyroïidiease chez l'homme á l'aide de l'iode 131. Schweiz. med. Wschr. **85**, 1019 (1955). ~ La fonction thyroidienne dans l'ictère par obstruction. Schweiz. med. Wschr. **86**, 875 (1956). — Schade, A. L., and L. Caroline: An iron-binding component in human blood plasma. Science **104**, 340 (1946). — Schade, A. L., R. W. Reinhard and H. Levy: Carbon dioxide and oxygen in complex formation with iron and siderophilin, the iron binding component of human plasma. Arch. Biochem. **20**, 170 (1949). — Schade, H.: Die physikalische Chemie in der inneren Medizin. Dresden: Theodor Steinkopff 1923. — Schäfer, K. H., u. J. Boenecke: Vegetative Steuerung des Eisenstoffwechsels. Naunyn-Schmiedeberg's Arch. exp. Path. Pharmak. **207**, 666 (1949). — Scheinberg, I. H.: Relation of coeruloplasmin and plasma copper to hepatolenticular degeneration (Wilson's disease). In: Neurochemistry von S. R. Korey and Nurnberger, p. 52. London 1956. — Scheinberg, I. H., and D. Gitlin: Deficiency of coeruloplasmin in patients with hepatolenticular degeneration (Wilson's disease). Science **116**, 484 (1952). —

Scheinberg, J. H., D. T. Dubin and R. S. Harris: The survival of normal coeruloplasmin in patients with hepatolenticular degeneration (Wilson's disease). J. clin. Invest. 34, 961 (1955). — Scheinberg, J. H., and H. J. Kowalski: The binding of thiocyanate to albumin in normal human serum and defibrinated blood with rel. to „thiocyanate space". J. clin. Invest. 29, 475 (1950). — Scherman, R., B. B. Brodie, B. B. Levy, J. Axelrod, V. Hollander and J. M. Steele: The use of antipyrine in the measurement of total body water in man. J. biol. Chem. 179, 31 (1949). — Schettler, G.: Lipidosen. In Handbuch der inneren Medizin, Bd. VII/2. Berlin: Springer 1955. — Scheurlen, P. G., u. D. Klaus: Flüssigkeitshaushalt und Volumenregulation bei extremem Serumalbuminmangel (Analbuminämie). I. Mitt. Hämodynamische Regulation. Klin. Wschr. 1960, 123. ~ II. Mitt. Renale Wasser- und Elektrolytausscheidung. Klin. Wschr. 1960, 1075. — Schilling, R. F.: Intrinsic factor studies. II. The effect of gastric juice on the urinary excretion of radioactivity after the oral administration of radioactive vitamin B_{12}. J. Lab. clin. Med. 42, 860 (1953). — Schloerb, P. R., B. J. Frics-Hansen, I. S. Edelmons, A. K. Salomon and F. D. Moore: The measurement of total body water in the human subject by deuterium oxide dilution. J. clin. Invest. 29, 2196 (1950). — Schmid, K.: Preparation and properties of serum and plasma proteins. XXIX. Separation from human plasma of polysaccharides, peptides and proteins of low molecular weight. Crystallization of an acid glycoprotein. J. Amer. chem. Soc. 75, 60 (1953). ~ Isolation of a group of alpha$_2$-glycoproteins from human plasma. J. Amer. chem. Soc. 77, 742 (1955). — Schmid, R.: Direct reacting bilirubin, bilirubin glucoronide in serum, bile and urine. Science 124, 76 (1956). — Schmidt, C. L. A.: The chemistry of amino acids and proteins. Springfield: Ch. C. Thomas 1944. — Schmidt, K. E. A.: Sekundäre hämochromatotische Lebercirrhose durch Bluttransfusionen bei chronischer Erythroblastenphthise. Folia haemat. 72, 94 (1953). — Schmidt, W. J.: Der molekulare Bau der Zelle. Nova Acta Leopoldina (Halle) 7, 1 (1939). — Schmorl, G.: Zur Kenntnis des Ikterus neonatorum, insbesondere der dabei auftretenden Gehirnveränderungen. Verh. dtsch. path. Ges. 6—8, 109 (1903/04). — Schneider, W., G. Böwing u. R. Schaich: Die Behandlung hypochromer Anämien mit einem intramuskulär injizierbaren Eisenpräparat. Medizinische 2, 2234 (1959). — Schoenberger, J. A., G. Kroll, A. Sakamoto and R. M. Kark: Investigation of the permeability factor in ascites and edema using albumin tagged with I^{131}. Gastroenterology 22, 607 (1952). ~ Endothelial permeability in man studied with albumin-J^{131} injected intravenously or intraperitoneally. J. clin. Invest. 82, 601 (1953). — Schönholzer, G.: Die Bindung von Prontosil an die Bluteiweißkörper. Klin. Wschr. 1940, 790. — Schubert, R.: Verhalten wasserlöslicher Vitamine gegenüber den Serumeiweißkörpern mit besonderer Berücksichtigung des Transportproblems. Z. Vitaminforsch. 19, 119 (1947). ~ Neue Wege der Entgiftung durch Infusion niedermolekularer Kollidonfraktionen. Dtsch. med. Wschr. 1948, 551. ~ Serumsanierung mit künstlichen Kolloiden. Nicht nierenfähige Stoffe permeieren mit Kollidon die Niere. Dtsch. med. Wschr. 1949, 1489. ~ Einfluß von Kollidon auf Tetanustoxin. Ärztl. Forsch. 16, 425 (1949). ~ Können nicht nierenfähige Stoffe durch Bindung an künstliche nierenfähige Kolloide über die Niere zur Ausscheidung gebracht werden? I. Mitt. Versuche mit Trypanrot M bei intravenöser Kolloidgabe. Z. Klin. Med. 145, 608 (1949). ~ II. Mitt. Versuche mit Trypanrot M bei intraperitonealer und subcutaner Kolloidgabe. Z. Klin. Med. 145, 637 (1949). ~ Serum- und Gewebswäsche mit künstlichen Kolloiden; Möglichkeiten eines neuartigen Therapieprinzips. Verh. dtsch. Ges. inn. Med. 303 (1949). ~ A new means of detoxicating the body by replacing the bileliver system by the kidneys as organs of excretion of substances bound to artificial colloids. Rev. Gastroenterol. 17, 165 (1950). ~ Die Anwendung von Periston N zur Serum- und Zellwäsche und ihre klinische Bedeutung. Dtsch. med. Wschr. 1951, 1487. ~ Ergebnisse einer neuartigen Therapie des schweren Tetanus mit niedermolekularem PVP. Dtsch. med. Wschr. 1954, 179. ~ Experimentelle und klinische Erfahrungen mit der Osmotherapie und Onkotherapie. Naturwissenschaften 1956, H. 5; Fest-Zeitschr. zum 70. Geburtstag von Prof. Bürger. ~ Larvierte Formen des Tetanus in der Inneren Medizin und ihre Behandlungsmöglichkeit. Arch. klin. Chir. 184, 116 (1956). — Schubert, R., u. G. Seybold: Entfernung granulär gespeicherter Stoffe aus gewissen Zellsystemen durch Kollidon verschiedenen Molekulargewichts. Ärztl. Forsch. 6, 2 (1952). — Schubert, R., u. H. Werner: Serum- und Gewebssanierung durch Kollidon (Versuche am Kaninchen mit Diaminreinblau FF). Z. ges. inn. Med. 1950a, 9/10, 286. — Schulten, H.: Über die Harnbildung in der Froschniere. III. Ausscheidung von Säurefarbstoffen durch die überlebende Froschniere. Arch. ges. Physiol. 208, 1 (1925). — Schulz, G. V.: Über den makromolekularen Stoffwechsel der Organismen. Naturwissenschaften 37, 196, 223 (1950). — Schulze, G.: Über die Sulfonamid-Bindungsfähigkeit des Blutes. Verh. dtsch. Ges. inn. Med. 1955. — Schwartz, St. O., and S. Blumenthal: Exogenous hemochromatosis. J. Lab. clin. Med. 32, 1928 (1947). ~ Exogenous hemochromatosis resulting from blood transfusions. Blood 3, 617 (1948). — Schwermund, H. J., H. A. Künkel u. H. Küchmeister: Gewebeclearance-Untersuchungen mit Na^{24} beim Schwangerschaftsoedem. Klin. Wschr. 1954, 33. — Schwiegk, H.: Der Lungenentlastungsreflex. Pflüg. Arch. ges. Physiol. 236, 206 (1935). — Schwietzer, C. H.: Eiweißmangel als ätiologisches Moment der Hämochromatose. Dtsch. med. Wschr. 1952,

17. ~ Die Zustandsformen des Eisens in der Leber. Vorträge u. Diskussionsbemerkungen des Leber-Kolloquiums in Bad Bertrich vom 17.—18. 4. 1953. — SCOTT, K. G., and W. A. REILLY: Use of anionic exchange resin for determination of protein-bound I^{131} in human plasma. Metabolism 3, 506 (1954). — SEI, S.: Über das Verhalten von Lösungen einiger Bismutyltartrate bzw. deren Mischungen mit Blutserum bei der Ultrafiltration. Arch. Derm. Syph. (Berl.) 146, 48 (1924). — SEYBOLD, G.: Die Bedeutung der Plasmaproteine und Mitochondrien für die Vitalspeicherung: Modellversuch für Transport und Stoffaustausch. Habil.-Schr. Tübingen 1956. Medizinische 1958, 1232. — SEYBOLD, G., u. E. KALLEE: Farbstoffbindungs-Studien an Mitochondrien. I. Z. Naturforsch. 9b, H. 3 (1954). — SHANNON, J. A.: The excretion of phenol red by the dog. Amer. J. Physiol. 113, 602 (1935). — SHAPIRO, B., I. CHOWERS and G. ROSE: Fatty acid uptake and esterification in adipose tissue. Biochim. biophys. Acta 23, 115 (1957). — SHELDON, J. H.: Hemochromatosis. London: Oxford University Press 1935. — SHEPARD, R. H.: Interference with release of CO_2 from pulmonary capillary blood after inhibition of carbonic anhydrase. Fed. Proc. 13, 135 (1954). — SHEPARD, R. H., and E. H. WOOD: Oxygen content of pulmonary artery blood in man during various phases of the respiratory and cardiac cycle. Fed. Proc. 13, 135 (1954). — SHETLAR, M. R., R. W. PAYNE, G. STIDWORTHY and D. MOCK: Absence of serum albumin associated with rheumatoid arthritis. Ann. intern. Med. 51, 1379 (1959). — SHORE, B.: C- and N-terminal amino acids of human serum lipoproteins. Arch. Biochem. 71, 1 (1957). — SIENGALE-WICZ, S. S., and A. J. CLARK: A note on the passage of trypanblue from the blood stream into body fluids. J. Pharmacol. exp. Ther. 24, 301 (1924). — SILVER, S.: Blood plasma levels of radioactive iodine-131 in the diagnosis of hyperthyroidism. Advanc. clin. Chem. 1, 111 (1958). — SILVERMANN, W. A., D. H. ANDERSON, W. A. BLANC and D. N. CROZIER: A difference in mortality rate and incidence of kernicterus among premature infants alloted to two prophylactic antibacterial regimens. Pediatrics 18, 614 (1956). — SIMON, N.: Radioactive gold in filter paper electrophoresis patterns of plasma. Science 119, 95 (1954). — SINGER, K., B. FISHER and M. A. PERLSTEIN: Acanthrocytosis; a genetic erythrocytic malformation. Blood 7, 577—591 (1952). — SIROTA, J. H., and A. SALTZMAN: The renal clearance and plasmaprotein binding of aureomycin in man. J. Pharmacol. exp. Ther. 100, 210 (1950). — SJÖSTRAND, F.: The regulation of the blood distribution in man. Acta physiol. scand. 26, 312 (1952). — SLAUNWHITE jr., W. R., and A. A. SANDBERG: Binding of urinary conjugated steroids to serum albumin: A new method of extraction. Endocrinology 62, 283 (1958). ~ Transcortin: a corticosteroid-binding protein of plasma. J. clin. Invest. 38, 384 (1959). — SMITH, CL. A.: Physiology of the newborn infant. Blackwell scientific publications. Oxford 1959. — SMITH, H. W., N. FINKELSTEIN, L. ALIMINOSA, B. CRAWFORD and M. GRABER: The renal clearance of substituted hippuric acid derivates and other aromatic acids in dog and man. J. clin. Invest. 24, 388 (1945). — SMITH, M. D., and I. M. PANNACCIULLI: Absorption of inorganic iron from graded doses: its significances in relation to iron absorption tests and the „mucosabloc" theory. Brit. J. Haemat. 4, 428 (1958). — SMITH, P. K., H. L. GLEASON, C. G. STOLL and S. OGORZALEK: Studies on the pharmacology of salicylates. J. Pharmacol. exp. Ther. 87, 237 (1946). — SMITH, R. M., D. A. JOSLYN, O. M. GRUHZIT, J. W. McLEAN jr., M. A. PENNER and J. EHRLICH: Chloromycetin: Biologic studies. J. Bact. 55, 425 (1948). — SMITH, W. W., and H. W. SMITH: Protein binding of phenol red, diodrast and other substances in plasma. J. biol. chem. 124, 107 (1938). — SMITHIES, O.: Third allele at serum β-globulin locus in humans. Nature (Lond.) 181/2, 1203 (1958). ~ Zone electrophoresis in starch gels and its application to studies of serum proteins. Advanc. protein Chem. 14, 1959. — SMITHIES, O., and O. HILLER: The genetic control of transferrins in humans. Biochem. J. 72, 121 (1959). — SOLOMON, A. K.: Equations for tracer experiments. J. clin. Invest. 28, 1297 (1949). — SPIEGELMAN, S., M. D. KAMEN and M. GUSSMAN: Phosphate metabolism and the dissociation of anaerobic glycolysis from synthesis in the presence of sodium azide. Arch. Biochem. 18, 409 (1948). — SPINKS, A.: Persistance in the blood-stream of some compounds related to suramin. Biochem. J. 44, 109 (1948). — SPITZER, J. J.: In: Blood lipids and the clearing factor. Third. Internat. Conf., Brussles, 1956. Koninkl. Vlaam. Acad. Wetenschap. 3, 243 (1956). — SPITZER, R. H., and H. J. McDONALD: Binding of organic anions by bovine plasma albumin compared with the binding properties of PVP. Clin. chim. Acta 1, 545 (1956). — SPRAY, G. H.: The effect of heap on the microbiological and antianaemic properties of human gastric juice mixed with vitamin B_{12}. Biochem. J. 50, 587 (1952). — SQUIRE, J. R.: The nephrotic syndrom. Brit. med. J. 1953, 1389. — STARLING, E. H.: Linacre lecture on law of the heart. Cambridge 1915. — STARY, Z., H. BODUS, S. G. LISIE u. F. BATIYOK: Über die Polysaccharide des Blutserums und die bei der Lungentuberkulose auftretenden Typen der Polysaccharidämie. Klin. Wschr. 1953, 399. — STAUFF, J., u. R. DUDEN: Zugänglichkeit der Disulfitgruppen im Rinderalbumin. Biochem. Z. 331, 10 (1958). — STEIN, J. A., Y. FEIGE and A. HOCHMAN: Salivary excretion of I^{131} in various thyroid states. J. Lab. clin. Med. 49, 843 (1957). — STEINHARD, J.: Participation of anions in the combination of proteins with acids. Ann. N. Y. Acad. Sci. 41, 287 (1941). — STENHAGEN, E., and T. TEORELL: Electrophoretic properties of thymonucleid acid. Trans. Faraday Soc. 35, 743

(1939). — Stephenson, J. L., u. D. S. Fredrickson: Zit. nach Fredrickson u. Gordon, Physiol. Rev. 38, 585 (1958). — Sterling, K.: The turnover rate of serum albumin in man as measured by J^{131} tagged albumin. J. clin. Invest. 30, 1228 (1951). — Sterling, K., and R. B. Chodos: Radiothyroxine turnover studies in myxedema, thyrotoxicosis, and hypermetabolism without endocrine disease. J. clin. Invest. 35, 806 (1956). — Sterling, K., J. C. Lashof and F. B. Man: Disappearance from serum of J^{131}-labeled l-thyroxine and l-triiodothyronine in euthyroid subjects. J. clin. Invest. 33, 1031 (1954). — Stern, I., and B. Shapiro: The transport of lipids into adipose tissue. Metabolism 3, 539 (1954). — Stern, P., R. Kosak u. A. Misirlija: Beitrag zur Frage der Eisenresorption. Experientia (Basel) 10, 247 (1954). — Stevenson, T. D., and M. F. Beard: Serum vitamin B_{12} content in liver disease. New Engl. J. Med. 260, 206 (1959). — Stiefel, G. E., u. B. Jasinski: Kolloidale Eisenverbindungen und ihr Transport im Blut. Schweiz. med. Wschr. 84, 946 (1954). — Stokes, J. B., A. B. Beck, D. H. Curnow, J. G. Topliss and E. G. Saint: Aspects of copper metabolism in Wilson's disease. Austr. Ann. Med. 4, 36 (1955). — Stone, P. W., and W. B. Müller: Mobilization of radioactive sodium from the gastrocnemius muscle of the dog. Proc. Soc. exp. biol. (N. Y.) 71, 529 (1949). — Storm van Leeuwen, W.: On the influence of colloids on the action of non colloidal drugs. I. J. Pharmacol. exp. Ther. 17, 1 (1921). ~ On sensitiveness to drugs in animals and man. J. Pharmacol. exp. Ther. 24, 13 (1924). ~ A possible explanation for certain cases of hypersensitiveness to drugs in man. J. Pharmacol. exp. Ther. 24, 25 (1924). — Storm van Leeuwen, W., u. H. Drzimal: Über die Bindungsfähigkeit des Blutes für Salizylsäure im Zusammenhang mit Überempfindlichkeit gegen Salizyl. Naunyn-Schmiedeberg's Arch. exp. Path. Pharmak. 102, 218 (1924). — Storm van Leeuwen, W., and A. Szent Györgyi: On the influence of colloids on the action of noncolloidal drugs. III. J. Pharmacol. exp. Ther. 18, 271 (1921). — Stricks, W., and J. M. Kolthoff: Polarographic determination of the molecular weight of serum albumin by its effect on the diffusion current of methyl orange. J. Amer. chem. Soc. 71, 1519 (1949). — Ströder, J.: Zit. nach R. Schubert, Die Anwendung von Periston zur Serum- und Zellwäsche und ihre klinische Bedeutung. Dtsch. med. Wschr. 1951. — Ströder, J., u. Th. Hockerts: Die Peristonbehandlung der toxischen Diphtherie des Kindes. Dtsch. med. Wschr. 1949, 282. — Surgenor, D. M., L. E. Strong, H. L. Taylor, R. S. Gordon jr. and D. M. Gieson: Preparation and proterties of serum and plasma proteins. XX. The separation of cholinesterase, mucoprotein and metalcombining protein into subfractions of human plasma. J. Amer. chem. Soc. 71, 1223 (1949). — Suter, H.: Strömen des Blutes in Kapillaren, z. T. Ergänzungen zu den Abhandlungen zur Mechanik der Flüssigkeiten. Arch. Kreisl.-Forsch. 10, 339 (1942). — Swahn, B.: A method for localization and determination of serum lipids after electrophoretical separation on filter paper. Scand. J. clin. Lab. Invest. 4, 98 (1952). ~ Studies in blood lipids. Scand. J. clin. Lab. Invest. 5, 9 (1953). — Swank, R. L., and J. H. Fellman: Plasmaproteins and fat transport in dogs. Amer. J. Physiol. 192, 318 (1958). — Sweet, W. H., B. Selverstone, S. Soloway and D. Stetten: Studies of flow, formation and absorption of cerebrospinal fluid. Surg. Forum 376 (1950). — Szego, C. M., and S. Roberts: The nature of circulating estrogen. Proc. Soc. exp. Biol. (N.Y.) 61, 161 (1946). ~ Nature of protein-bound estrogen formed in vitro. Fed. Proc. 14, 150 (1955).

Taggart, J. V., and D. P. Earle jr.: Zit. by B. D. Davis, The binding of chemotherapeutic agents to proteins and its effect on their distribution and activity. Chapter in: Evaluation of chemotherapeutic agents. New York: Acad. of Med. Columbia University Press 1948. — Talafant, Ed.: Properties and composition of the bile pigment giving a direct diazo reaction. Nature (Lond.) 178, 312 (1956). — Taliaferro, J., R. Cobey and L. Leone: Effect of diethylstilbestrol on plasma 17-hydroxycorticosteroid levels in humans. Proc. Soc. exp. Biol. (N.Y.) 92, 742 (1956). — Tanaka, Sh., and P. Starr: Clinical observations on serum globulin thyroxine-binding capacity, using a simplified technique. J. clin. Endocr. 19, 84 (1959). ~ A euthyroid man without thyroxine-binding globulin. J. clin. Endocr. 19, 485 (1959). ~ The binding of thyroxine analogues by human serum protein. Acta endocr. (Kbh.) 31, 161 (1959). — Tata, J. R.: A cellular thyroxine-binding protein fraction. Biochem. biophys. Acta 28, 91 (1958). ~ Prealbumin as a complex in the alpha-globulin fraction in human serum. Nature (Lond.) 183, 877 (1959). ~ Transport of thyroid hormones. Brit. med. Bull. 16, 142 (1960). — Tata, J. R., J. E. Rall and R. W. Rawson: Studies on an iodinated protein in the serum of subjects with cancer of the thyroid. J. clin. Endocr. 16, 1554 (1956). — Tata, J. R., and C. J. Shellabarger: Zit. nach Tata 1960, Biochem. J. 72, 608 (1959). — Taurog, A., F. N. Briggs and I. L. Chaikoff: I^{131}-labeled l-thyroxine. I. An unidentified excretion product in bile. J. biol. Chem. 191, 29 (1951). — Taurog, A., and I. L. Chaikoff: The nature of the circulating thyroid hormone. J. biol. Chem. 176, 639 (1948). — Taurog, A., J. D. Wheat and I. L. Chaikoff: Nature of the I^{131} compounds appearing in the thyroid vein, after injection of iodine I^{131}. Endocrinology 58, 121 (1956). — Tayeau, F., et E. Rolland: Le pouvoir adsorbant des protéines vis-à-vis des sels biliaires. Bull. Soc. Chim. biol. 29, 108 (1947). — Taylor, F. H. L., and A. G. Young: Biochemic studies on mercury compounds. I. The effect of acids, bases, salts and blood serum on the diffusion of mercury compounds in vitro. J. Pharmacol. exp. Ther. **38**, 217 (1930). — Teppermann, J., N. Rakilten, G. Valley and E. W. Lyon: Inactivation of penicillin G and K by liver and kidney. Science **105**, 18 (1947). — Teresi, J. D., and J. M. Luck: The combination of organic anions with serum albumin. VI. Quantitative studies by equilibrium dialysis. J. biol. Chem. **174**, 653 (1948). ~ VII. The protein sites involved in the combination. J. Amer. chem. Soc. **72**, 3972 (1950). ~ VIII. Fatty acid salts. J. biol. Chem. **194**, 823 (1952). — Ternberg, J. L., and R. E. Eakin: Erythein and apoerythein and their relation to the antipernicious anemia principle. J. Amer. Chem. **71**, 3858 (1949). — Thedering jr., F.: Bindung des Transporteisens an die Plasmaproteine. Verh. dtsch. Ges. inn. Med. **55**, 310 (1949). — Thedering, F.: Die Bindung des Serumeisens an die Plasmaproteine. Acta haemat. (Basel) **3**, 210 (1950). — Theorell, H.: Studien über die Plasmalipoide des Blutes. Biochem. Z. **223**, 1, (1930). — Thimann, K. V., and J. Rothschild: Zit. bei A. Goldstein, J. Pharmacol. exp. Ther. **95**, 102 (1949). — Tietze, K. H.: Über die Strömungsgeschwindigkeit des Blutes. Leipzig: Georg Thieme 1954. — Tomashefski, J. F., R. T. Clark and H. I. Chinn: Effect of a carbonic anhydrase inhibitor (Diamox) on respiratory gas transport. Fed. Proc. **12**, 144 (1953). — Tompsett, R., S. Schultz and W. McDermott: Relation of protein binding to the pharmacology and antibacterial activity of penicillins X, G, F, K. J. Bact. **53**, 581 (1947). — Tompsett, S. L.: The copper content of blood. Biochem. J. **28**, 1544 (1934). ~ The excretion of copper in urine and faeces and its relation to the copper content of the diet. Biochem. J. **28**, 2088 (1934). — Tong, W., A. Taurog and I. L. Chaikoff: Nature of plasma iodine following destruction of the rat thyroid with I^{131}. J. biol. Chem. **195**, 407 (1952). — Town, B. W., E. D. Wills, E. J. Wilson and A. Wormall: Studies on suramin. VIII. The action of the drug on enzymes and other proteins. Biochem. J. **47**, 149 (1950). — Troschin, A. S.: Das Problem der Zellpermeabilität. Jena: VEB Gustav Fischer 1958.

Ureles, A. I., and M. Murray: The erythrocyte uptake of I^{131}-labeled l-triiodothyronine as a measure of thyroid function. J. Lab. clin. Med. **54**, 178 (1959). — Ussing, H. H.: Permeability. Physiol. Rev. **29**, 127 (1949). — Uzman, L. L.: The intrahepatic distribution of copper in relation to the pathogenesis of hepatolenticular degeneration. Arch. Path. (Chicago) **64**, 464 (1957).

Vahlquist, B.: Das Serumeisen. Acta paediat. (Uppsala) **28**, Suppl. 5 (1941). — Vallee, B. L., and J. G. Gibson: The zinc content of normal human whole blood, plasma, leucocytes, and erythrocytes. J. biol. Chem. **176**, 445 (1948). — Vannotti, A.: A propos de l'hypothyréose. Helv. med. Acta **26**, 545 (1959). ~ Die Schilddrüsenhormone. Verh. dtsch. Ges. inn. Med. **66** (1960). — Vannotti, A., et Th. Béraud: Rôle du foie dans la regulation périphérique de la fonction thyroidienne. Bull. Acad. suisse Sci. Méd. **14**, 214 (1955). ~ Functional relationships between the liver, the thyroxine-binding protein of serum, and the thyroid. J. clin Endocr. **19**, 466 (1959). ~ Transport plasmatique des hormones thyroidiennes. Expos. ann. Biochim. **21**, 57 (1959). — Vannotti, A., Th. Béraud et J. Cruchaud: Influence du support protéique spécifique de la thyroxine sur la pénétration dans la cellule. Schweiz. med. Wschr. **5**, 88 (1958). — Velick, S. F.: The interaction of enzymes with smal ions. I. An electrophoretic and equilibrium dialysis of aldolase in phosphate and acetate buffers. J. phys. Colloid. Chem. **53**, 135 (1949). — Verzár, F.: Fat absorption and transport. Influence of internal secretion on them. Arch. Sci. physiol. **2**, 43 (1948). — Virchow, R.: Die Zellularpathologie. August Hirschwald 1858. — Vollwiler, P.: Sichtbarmachung des Stoffdurchtritts durch die Kapillaren. In: Kapillaren und Intersitium von Bartelheimer u. Küchmeister. Stuttgart: Georg Thieme 1955. — Volwiler, W., P. D. Goldsworth, M. P. Martin, P. A. Wood, I. R. Mackay and K. Fremont-Smith: Biosynthetic determination with radioactive sulfur of turnover rates of various plasma proteins in normal and cirrhotic man. J. clin. Invest. **34**, 1126 (1955).

Waddel, W. R., and R. P. Geyer: Effect of insulin on clearance of emulsified fat from the blood in depancreatized dogs. Proc. Soc. exp. Biol. (N.Y.) **96**, 251 (1957). — Waddel, W. R., R. P. Geyer, E. Clarke and F. J. Stare: Role of various organs in the removal of emulsified fat from the blood stream. Amer. J. Physiol. **175**, 299 (1953). — Wagner, R.: Probleme und Beispiele biologischer Regelung. Stuttgart: Georg Thieme 1954. — Waldenström, J.: Om järn och järnterapie. Malmö 1944. — Walker, W. J., E. Y. Lawry, D. E. Love, G. V. Man, S. A. Levine and F. J. Store: Effect of weight reduction and caloric balance on serum lipoprotein and cholesterol levels. Amer. J. Med. **14**, 654 (1953). — Wallace, E. Z., M. J. Silverberg and A. C. Carter: Effect of ethinylestradiol on plasma 17-hydroxycorticosteroids, ACTH responsiveness and hydrocortisone clearance in man. Proc. Soc. exp. Biol. (N.Y.) **95**, 805 (1957). — Wallenius, G.: A note on serum iron transportation. Scand. J. clin. Lab. Invest. **4**, 24 (1952). — Wase, A. W., and Y. S. L. Feng: Some salivary-thyroid gland relationships. Acta endocr. (Kbh.) **23**, 413 (1956). — Wassermann, K., and H. S. Mayerson: Exchange of albumin between plasma and lymph. Amer. J. Physiol. **165**, 15 (1951); **171**, 218 (1952). — Way, E. L., P. K. Smith, D. L. Howie, R. Weiss and R. Swanson: The absorption, distribution, excretion and fate of p-aminosalicylic acid. J. Pharmacol. exp. Ther. **83**, 368 (1948). — Weber, G., and D. J. R. Lawrence: Fluorescent indicators of adsorption in aqueous solution and on the solid phase. Biochem. J. **56**, XXXI

(1954). — WEBER, H. H.: Massenwirkungsgesetz und Kolloide. Biochem. Z. 189, 381 (1927). ~ Die Bjerrumsche Zwitterionentheorie und die Hydration der Eiweißkörper. Biochem. Z. 218, 1 (1930). — WEBER, H. H., u. I. H. VERSMOLD: Untersuchungen an Eiweißsystemen. Nichtlösender Raum und Bindung von Nichtelektrolyten in Eieralbuminlösungen. Biochem. Z. 34, 61 (1931). — WEESE, H., u. W. SCHOLTAN: Pharmakologie des Periston N. Dtsch. med. Wschr. 1951, 1492. — WEGENER, H.: Über 2 Fälle von familiärer Haemochromatose. Z. klin. Med. 107, 113 (1928). — WEICKER, H.: Das Verhalten der Serumlipoproteine bei Leberparenchymschädigungen und ihre Bedeutung für die verschiedenen Ikterusformen. Ärztl. Wschr. 1955, 1057. — WEINSTEIN, B. J., and D. M. WATKIN: $Co^{54}B_{12}$ absorption, plasma transport and excretion. J. clin. Invest. 39, 11 (1960). — WEITZEL, G.: Chemie und Physiologie biogener Zinkverbindungen. Angew. Chem. 68, 566 (1956). — WERNER, S. C., R. J. BLOCK and R. M. MANDL: Zit. nach VANNOTTI (POLONOVSKI) 1957, J. clin. Endocr. 17, 1141 (1957). — WERTHEIMER: Zit. bei B. FISCHER WASELS: Grundsätzliches über Funktionsstörungen der Kreislaufperipherie. Verh. dtsch. Ges. Kreisl.-Forsch. 11, 205 (1938). — WESTPHAL, U.: Interaction between hydrocortison-4-C^{14} or progesterone-4-C^{14} and serumalbumin as demonstrated by ultracentrifugation and electrophoresis. Endocrinology 57, 456 (1955). ~ Spectrophotometric demonstration of interaction between proteins and ketosteroid hormones. Fed. Proc. 15, 382 (1956). ~ Steroidprotein interactions III. Spectrophotometric demonstration of interaction between proteins and progesterone, desoxycorticosterone and cortisol. Arch. Biochem. 66, 71 (1957). — WESTPHAL, U., R. DE ARMOUT, S. G. PRIEST and J. F. STETS: Azorubinbinding capacity and protein composition of serum of rats subjected to tourniquet shock and to treatment with carbon tetrachloride. J. clin. Invest. 31, 1064 (1952). — WESTPHAL, U., u. P. GEDIGK: Über das Verhältnis von direktem zu indirektem Bilirubin. Hoppe-Seylers Z. physiol. Chem. 284, 274 (1949). — WESTPHAL, U., P. GEDIGK u. F. MEYER: Über eine chromatographische Methode zur Charakterisierung von Serumeiweiß. Hoppe-Seylers Z. physiol. Chem. 285, 36 (1950). — WESTPHAL, U., H. OTT u. P. GEDIGK: An welche Komponenten der Serumproteine ist das Bilirubin gebunden. Hoppe-Seylers Z. physiol. Chem. 285, 200 (1950). — WESTPHAL, U., J. F. STETS and S. G. PRIEST: Influence of fatty acids and related anions on the azorubin binding capacity of serum albumin. Arch. Biochem. 43, 463 (1953). — WETTERER, E., u. H. PIEPER: Über die Gesamtelastizität des arteriellen Windkessels und ein experimentelles Verfahren zu ihrer Bestimmung am lebenden Tier. Z. Biol. 106, 23 (1953). — WIDENBAUER, F.: Über eiweißgebundenes Calcium im Blutserum. Klin. Wschr. 1943, 63, 320. — WILBRANDT, W., S. FREI and TH. ROSENBERG: The kinetics of glucose transport through the human red cellmembrane. Exp. Cell. Res. 1956. — WILBRANDT, W., u. TH. ROSENBERG: Die Kinetik des enzymatischen Transportes. Helv. physiol. pharmacol. Acta 9, 86 (1951). — WILHELM, C. M.: Fasting and realimentation with high carbohydrate or high protein diets on capilary resistance and eosinophiles of normal. Fed. Proc. 13, 165 (1954). — WILLIAMS, W. L., B. F. CHOW, L. ELLENBOGEN and K. OKUDA: Intrinsic factor preparations which augmented and inhibited absorption of vitamin B_{12} in healthy individuals. 1. Europ. Symp. Hamburg 1956. Vitamin B_{12} and Intrinsic factor p. 456, 1957. — WILSON, J., and A. WORMALL: Studies on suramin (Bayer 205). VII. The combination of the drug with proteins. Biochem. J. 45, 224 (1949). — WINZLER, R. J., and S. R. NOTRICA: Association of thyroxine with plasma proteins. Fed. Proc. 11, 312 (1952). — WITH, T. K.: Spectral adsorption of bilirubin measurements in pure aqueous solutions and in solutions containing human serum. Acta physiol. scand. 10, 172 (1945). — WÖHLER, F.: Zur Physiologie und Pathologie des Speichereisen. III. Mitt. Über den intermediaren Eisenstoffwechsel der Plazenta. Dtsch. med. Wschr. 80, 30 (1955). — WÖHLER, F., K. J. BIELIG u. W. KEIDERLING: Eisenstoffwechsel. Stuttgart: Georg Thieme 1959. — WÖHLER, F., L. HEILMEYER, D. EMRICH u. SHIN HO KANG: Zur Funktion des Ferritins bei der Eisenresorption. Naunyn-Schmiedeberg's Arch. exp. Path. Pharmak. 230, 107 (1957). — WÖHLISCH, E., u. V. KÖHLER: Zur Frage der gerinnungsphysiologischen Bedeutung der Serumproteine. Naturwissenschaften 28, 550 (1940). — WOLFF, H. P.: Untersuchungen zur Pathophysiologie des Zinkstoffwechsels. Klin. Wschr. 34, 417 (1956). — WOLFF, H. P., N. LANG u. M. KNEDEL: Untersuchungen mit Cu^{64} über die Bindung des Kupfers an Serumeiweißkörper. Z. ges. exp. Med. 125, 359 (1955). ~ Hemopoetic active metals as bound by different serum protein fractions. Rev. belge Path. 24, 98 (1955). — WOLFSON, W. Q.: Zit. bei A. GOLDSTEIN, J. Pharmacol. exp. Ther. 95, 102 (1949). — WOLFSON, W. Q., C. COHN, R. LEVINE and B. HUDDLEYTUN: The transport and excretion of uric acid in man. III. Physiolog. significance. Amer. J. Med. 4, 774 (1948). — WOLFSON, W. Q., R. LEVINE and M. TINSLEY: The transport and excretion of uric acid in man. I. True uric acid in normal fluid. J. clin. Invest. 26, 991 (1947). — WOLLENSAK, J., E. KALLEE u. G. SEYBOLD: Farbstoffbindungs-Studien an Mitochondrien II. Z. Naturforsch. 10b, 582 (1955). — WOLLENSAK, J., u. G. SEYBOLD: Serum-Protein-Nachweis durch fluoreszierende Antikörper in Leber und Niere. Z. Naturforsch. 12b, 147 (1957). — WOLLHEIM, E.: Zur Funktion der suprapapillären Gefäßplexus in der Haut. Klin. Wschr. 1927, 2134. — WOLLMAN, S. H., and F. E. REED: Transport of radioiodine between thyroid gland and blood in mice and rats. Amer. J. Physiol. 64, 113 (1959). — WUHRMANN. F., u. B. JASINSKI:

Untersuchungen über die Bindung des Eisens an das Serumglobulin β_1 mit Hilfe des Radioeisens Fe[59] und dessen klinische Bedeutung. Schweiz. med. Wschr. 1953, 611. — Wunderly, Ch.: Über Modellversuche mit Plasmaproteinen als Elutionsmittel. Ärztl. Forsch. 4, I 29 (1950a). ~ Über die Kolloidelution durch Serumproteine, Bence-Jones Protein und Galle. Naturwissenschaften 37, 454 (1950b). ~ Die Lösung von Buttergelb in Serum. Science 117, 248 (1953a). — Wunderly, Ch., u. F. A. Pezold: Über die Bindung von Fettfarbstoffen an die einzelnen Serumproteinfraktionen. Z. ges. exp. Med. 120, 613 (1953b). — Wyatt, J. P., H. K. Mighton and V. Moragues: Transfusional siderosis. Amer. J. Path. 26, 883 (1950).

Yoshikawa, H.: Studies on the biochemistry of copper. II. Jap. J. Med. Sci., Trans. II 4, 219, 231 (1939).

Zeltmacher, K., and M. Bevans: Aplastic anemia and its assotiation with hemochromatosis. Arch. intern. Med. 75, 395 (1945). — Zetterström, R.: Die physiologische Entwicklung des Kindes, hersgeg. von H. Linneweh. Berlin: Springer 1959. — Zieve, L., W. C. Vogel and A. L. Schultz: Determination of protein-bound radioiodine with an anion exchange resin. J. Lab. clin. Med. 47, 663 (1956). — Ziff, M., and E. Chargaff: Studies on the chemistry of blood coagulation. XI. Action of heparin. J. biol. Chem. 136, 689 (1940). — Zilversmit, D. B., M. L. Shore and R. F. Ackerman: The origin of aortic phosphorlipid in rabbit atheromatosis. Circulation 9, 581 (1954). — Zimdahl, W. I., I. Hyman and W. F. Stafford: The effect of drug upon the copper metabolism in hepatolenticular degeneration and in normal subjects. J. Lab. clin. Med. 43, 774 (1954). — Zinn, W. J., J. B. Field and G. G. Griffith: Effect of heparin and treburon in postprandial hyperlipemia. Proc. Soc. exp. Biol. (N.Y.) 80, 276 (1952). — Zipursky, A., H. Dempsey, H. Markowitz, G. E. Cartwright and M. M. Wintrobe: Studies on copper metabolism. XXIV. Hypocupremia in infancy. Amer. J. Dis. Child. 96, 148 (1958).

Anhang.

Aber, G. M., and D. S. Rowe: The binding of haematin by serum proteins. Brit. J. Haemat. 6, 160 (1960). — Bargmann, W., A. Knoop u. Th. H. Schiebler: Histologische, cytochemische und elektronenmikroskopische Untersuchungen am Nephron mit Berücksichtigung der Mitochondrien. Z. Zellforsch. 42, 386 (1955). — Bongiovanni, A. M., and W. R. Eberlein: Determination, recovery, identification and renal clearance of conjugated adrenal corticoide in human peripheral blood. Proc. Soc. exp. Biol. (N.Y.) 89, 281 (1955). — Burkhard, R. K., and F. A. Moore: Interactions of homologs of carcinogenics azodyes and bovine serum albumin. J. Amer. chem. Soc. 77, 6057 (1955). — Cotzias, G. C., and A. J. Bertinchamps: Transmanganin, the specific manganese-carrying protein of human plasma. J. clin. Invest. 39, 979 (1960). — Cremer, H. D., u. A. Tiselius: Elektrophorese von Eiweiß in Filtrierpapier. Biochem. Z. 320, 273 (1950). — Dieckhoff, J.: Internat. Kongr. Leipzig 1950. Zit. nach Schubert, Dtsch. med. Wschr. 76, 1487 (1951). — Elster, S. K., M. E. Freeman and A. Dorfman: Effect of hyaluronidase on the passage of fluid and of T-1824 through the capillary wall. Amer. J. Physiol. 156, 429 (1949). — Farquhar, M. G., R. L. Vernier and R. A. Good: The application of electron microscopy in pathology: study of renal biopsy tissues. Schweiz. med. Wschr. 87, 50 (1957). — Favre-Gilly, J., R. Lejeure u. L. Revol: Transfusion-Haemosiderose. Internat. Haem. Kongr. Amsterdam 1953. — Fisher, E. R., and S. Tishermann: The association of idiopathic hemochromatosis and excessiv iron overload. A.M.A. Arch. Path. 69, 683 (1960). — Friedberg, C. K.: Diseases of the heart. Philadelphia and London 1956. — Gemzell, C. A.: Variations in plasma levels of 17-hydroxycorticosteroids in mother and infant following parturition. Acta endocr. (Kbh.) 17, 100 (1954). — Grabar, P., et C. A. Williams: Methode permettant l'étude conjugée des propriétés électrophoretiques et immuno chimiques d'un mélange des proteines application en sérum sanguin. Biochim. biophys. Acta 10, 193 (1953). — Grassmann, W. u. K. Hannig: Ein einfaches Verfahren zur Analyse der Serumproteine und anderer Proteingemische. Naturwissenschaften 37, 397 (1950). — Grau, H.: Prinzipielles und Vergleichendes über das Lymphgefäßsystem. Verh. Dtsch. Ges. inn. Medizin 1960. — Heilmeyer, L., W. Keller, O. Vivell, K. Betke, F. Wöhler, W. Keiderling u. H. E. Schultz: Dtsch. med. Wschr. (1961, im Druck). — Hochrein, M., u. J. Keller: Untersuchungen am Koronarsystem. Naunyn-Schmiedeberg's Arch. exp. Path. Pharmak. 159, 300 (1931). — Hudack, S. S., and P. D. McMaster: The lymphatic participation in human cutaneous phenomena. J. exp. Med. 57, 751 (1933). — Jayle, M. F., et G. Boussier: Les séromucoides du sang, leurs rélations avec mucoproteines de la substance fondamentale du tissue conjonctif. Expos. ann. Biochim. méd. 17, 157 (1955). — Kallee, E.: Zur Natur der Azorubinbindung an Serumalbumin. Hoppe-Seylers Z. physiol. Chem. 290, 207 (1952). ~ Die reversible Bindung von Schilddrüsenhormonen und anionischen Farbstoffen an Proteine und ihre Bedeutung für Permeabilitätsvorgänge an den Zellgrenzen. Habilitationsschrift Tübingen 1961. — Kallee, E. u. E. Roth: Ein Beitrag zum papierelektrophoretischen Nachweis des Farbstoffbindungsvermögens. Z. Naturforsch. 8b, 34 (1953). — Kety, S. S., and C. F. Schmidt: Nitrousoxide method for quantitative determination of cerebral blood flow in man; heory, procedure and normal values. J. clin. Invest. 27, 476 (1948). — Klamerth, O.:

Zur Frage der Histaminbindung an Plasmaproteine. Biochem. Z. **327**, 39 (1955). — KLEPZIG, H.: Untersuchungen über die Arbeitsweise des menschlichen Herzens bei vermehrter Belastung. Arch. Kreisl.-Forsch. **23**, 96 (1955). — KORNZWEIG, A. L., and F. A. BASSEN: Retinitis pigmentosa acanthrozytosis and heredogenerative neuromuscular disease. A.M.A. Arch. Ophthal. **58**, 183 (1957). — LAURELL, C. B.: Serumproteine und Eisentransport. Beiträge zur Forschung und Klinik von W. KEIDERLING. Stuttgart: Georg Thieme 1959. — LISSITZKY, S., M. ROQUES et M.-TH. BÉNÉVENT: Désiodations enzymatique des hormones thyroïdiennes. Propriétés de la thyroxine-désiodase et signification physiologique. In: Radioaktive Isotope in Klinik und Forschung, Bd. 4, S. 301 u. 315. 1960. — MILLER, F., u. A BOHLE: Vergleichende licht- und elektronenmikroskopische Untersuchungen an der Basalmembran der Glomerulumkapillaren der Maus bei experimentellem Nierenamyloid. Klin. Wschr. **34**, 1204 (1956). — MORRIS, J. E.: The transport of uric acid in serum. Ann. J. med. Sci. **235**, 1029, 43 (1958). — NELSON, R. S., and V. M. DOCTOR: The vitamin B_{12} content of human liver as determined by bio-assay of needle biopsic material. Ann. intern. Med. **49**, 1361 (1958). NEWBOULD, B. B., and R. KILPATRICK: Long-acting sulphonamides and protein-binding. Lancet **1960 I**, 886. — OEFF, K., S. RUST, E. SCHWARZ u. H. E. WEISE: Frage der Bindung von Penicillin an Serumeiweißkörper. Klin. Wschr. **33**, 419 (1955). — OTT, H.: Unveröffentlichte Untersuchung 1951. ~ Albuminbildung bei Analbuminämie. Verh. Dtsch. Ges. Inn. Med. 1961. — PAPPENHEIMER, J. R.: Über die Permeabilität der Glomerulummembran. Klin. Wschr. **33**, 362 (1954). — PEASE, D. C.: Fine structures of the kidney seen by electron microscopy. J. Histochem. Cytochem. **3**, 295 (1955). — PERLICK, E.: Antikoagulantien. Leipzig: VEB Thieme 1960. — PETERSON, R. E., and J. D. MANN: Transport of radioactive iron in interstitial lymph. Amer. J. Physiol. **169**, 763 (1952). — PIEL, C. F., L. DONG, F. W. S. MODERN, J. R. GOODMAN and R. MOORE: The glomerulus in experimental renal disease in rats as observed by light and electron microscopy. J. exp. Med. **102**, 573 (1955). — PRENDERGAST, J. J., and D. M. TEAGNE: Electron micrograph of plasma lipoprotein molecule. Circulation **4**, 23 (1951). — RHODIN, J.: Correlation of ultrastructural organization and function in normal and experimentally changed proximal convoluted tubule cells of the mouse kidney. Thesis Stockholm 1954. ~ Electron microscopy of the glomerular capillary wall. Exp. Cell. Res. **8**, 572 (1955). — RUSZNYÁK, J.: Die Insuffizienz des Lymphgefäßsystems. Verh. Dtsch. Gesell. für Inn. Med. 1960. — SANO, I., Y. KAKIMOTO u. K. TANIGUCHI: Binding and transport of serotonin in rabbit blood platelets and action of reserpine. Amer. J. Physiol. **195**, 495 (1958). — SCATCHARD, G., J. S. COLEMAN and A. L. SHEN: Physical chemistry of protein solutions. VII. The binding of some small anious to serum albumin. J. Amer. chem. Soc. **79**, 17 (1957). — SCHADE, A. L.: Persönliche Mitteilung 1960. — SCHEURLEN, P. G.: Untersuchungen über die Beziehung zwischen Urin- und Serumeiweiß. Ein Beitrag zur Frage der glomerulären Eiweißfiltration. Habilit.-Schrift Tübingen 1961. — SCHUMACHER, H.: Experimentelle Untersuchungen über die Adsorption von Bluteiweißfraktionen an Quarz- und andere Mineralpartikel. Beitr. Silikose-Forsch. **41**, 19 (1956). — SIMPSON, S. A., J. F. TAIT, A. WETTSTEIN, R. NEHER, J. v. EUW u. T. REICHSTEIN: Isolierung eines neuen kristallisierten Hormons aus Nebennieren mit besonders hoher Wirksamkeit auf den Mineralstoffwechsel. Experientia (Basel) **10**, 132 (1954). — SKOUGE, E.: Klinische und experimentelle Untersuchungen über das Serumeisen. Skrifter utg. av det norske videnskaps-Akad. Oslo 1939. — SMITH, D. T., R. S. ABERNATHY, G. B. SMITH jr. and ST. BONDURANT: The apical localization of reinfection pulmonary tuberculosis. I. The stream flowtheory. Amer. Rev. Tuberc. **70**, 547 (1954). — TISELIUS, A.: Die wandernde Grenze als Methode zur Untersuchung der Elektrophorese von Proteinen. Nova Acta Reg. Soc. Sci. Upsaliensis 4, 7, Nr 4 (1930). Diss. Upsala 1930. — TURBA, F., u. H. FRENKEL: Elektrophorese von Proteinen in Filterpapier. Naturwissenschaften **37**, 93 (1950). — TURNBULL, A., and E. R. GIBLETT: The binding and transport of iron by transferrin variants. J. Lab. clin. Med. **57**, 3, 450 (1960). — UDENFRIEND, S., H. WEISSBACH and C. T. CLARK: The estimation of 5 HT (serotonin) in biological tissue. J. biol. Chem. **215**, 337 (1955). — WALLER, H. D., G. W. LÖHR, F. GRIGNANI u. R. GROSS: Über den Energiestoffwechsel normaler menschlicher Thrombozyten. Throm. diath. haemorrhag. **3**, 520 (1959). — WALSER, M.: Protein-binding of inorganic phosphate in plasma of normal subjects and patients with renal disease. J. clin. Invest. **39**, 501 (1960). — WEIL-MALHERBE, H., and A. D. BONA: Association of adrenaline and noradrenaline with blood platelets. Biochem. J. **70**, 14 (1958). — WHEBY, K. S., O'N. BARRETT and W. H. CROSBY: Serum protein binding of myoglobin, hemoglobin and hematin. Blood **16**, 5 (1960). — WIGGERS, C. J.: Interplay of coronary vascular resistance and myocardial compression in regulating coronary flow. Circulat. Res. **2**, 271 (1954). — WOLLENSAK, J., u. G. SEYBOLD: Untersuchungen über die Bildungsstätten von Myelomproteinen bzw. γ-Globulinen. Z. Naturforsch. **11 b**, 588 (1956). — WOODWORTH, R. C.: Rate of dissociation the iron siderophilin complex determined by means of an immunological technique. Abstr. 136th Meeting Amer. Chem. Soc. Atlantic Cy. 13. 9. 1959. — ZOLLINGER, H. U.: Anurie bei Chromoproteinurie. (Hämolyseniere, Crushniere.) Stuttgart: Georg Thieme 1952.—ZUCKER, M. B. Serotonin (5-Hydroxytryptamin). Fortschritte der Hämatologie, Bd. II. Stuttgart: Georg Thieme 1961. — ZWEIFACH, B. W., and R. CHAMBERS: Action of hyaluronidase extracts on capillary wall. Ann. Acad. Sci. **52**, 1047 (1950).

Funktionelle Orthologie der Atmung.
Die Lungenbelüftung und der alveolare Gasaustausch.

Von

Ulrich C. Luft, Albuquerque (New-Mexico).

Mit 7 Abbildungen.

Einleitung.

Die Atmung umfaßt im weiteren biologischen Sinne alle Vorgänge, welche zum oxydativen Stoffwechsel der lebenden Zelle mittelbar oder unmittelbar beitragen. Im Warmblüterorganismus gehört dazu eine ganze Kette eng ineinandergreifender Funktionen. Zunächst der Gasaustausch der Zelle mit dem sie umgebenden Gewebe und dem Blut, ferner der Gastransport durch den Blutkreislauf, der Gaswechsel zwischen dem Pulmonalblut und dem Gasraum der Lunge und schließlich die ständige Erneuerung der Lungenluft mit Außenluft. All diese Vorgänge sind im gesunden Individuum fein aufeinander abgestimmt und werden je nach den Bedürfnissen des Gesamtstoffwechsels oder der Umweltbedingungen mittels chemischer, physikalisch-nervöser und hormonaler Regulationen gesteuert. In pathologischen Zuständen, welche dieses oder jenes Glied dieser Funktionskette beeinträchtigen, ist in gewissen Grenzen ein Ausgleich möglich durch kompensatorische Mehrleistung anderer Glieder. Im allgemeinen wird dies jedoch nicht ohne Einschränkung der Belastungsbreite der Atemfunktionen möglich sein[1].

Der vorliegende Abschnitt beschränkt sich auf diejenigen Vorgänge, die als *äußere Atmung* bezeichnet werden, nämlich die Lungenbelüftung, der Gasaustausch in der Lunge und die beteiligten Steuermechanismen. Die mit der äußeren Atmung verbundene Bewegung gilt seit dem Altertum als eines der elementarsten Kennzeichen animalischen Lebens (animus = der Hauch). Die Beobachtung und Messung der Lungenbelüftung und des Gaswechsels gewährt nicht allein einen Einblick in den Funktionszustand der Atmungsorgane, sondern erlaubt darüber hinaus weitgehende Rückschlüsse auf den Blutkreislauf und den Gesamtstoffwechsel.

Untersuchungsmethoden: Messungen der Atemfunktionen, auf deren Methodik im einzelnen hier nicht eingegangen werden soll[1], erstrecken sich auf Bestimmungen von 1. Volumen, 2. Druck, 3. Strömungsgeschwindigkeit, 4. Zusammensetzung der Atemgase an verschiedenen Orten in oder außerhalb des Körpers und zu verschiedenen Phasen des Atemcyclus. Gasvolumina, sofern sie eine Belüftungsgröße darstellen, werden auf den Barometerdruck der Umgebung, auf Körpertemperatur und volle Wasserdampfsättigung bezogen, während Gaswechselgrößen (Sauerstoff und Kohlensäure) zwecks direkter Umrechnung in Energieeinheiten auf physikalische Standardbedingungen (760 mm Hg, 0^0 C, trocken) korrigiert zu werden pflegen.

---

[1] Rossier, Bühlmann und Wiesinger 1958, Anthony 1937, Comroe 1950, Bartels, Bücherl, Hertz, Rodenwald und Schwab 1959.

I. Die Lungenbelüftung.

Volumenänderungen des Brustraums.

1. Bewegungsformen der Atmung.

Die fortwährende Erneuerung der Luft in den Alveolen der Lunge wird aufrechterhalten durch rhythmische Volumenänderungen des Brustkorbes, die unmittelbar auf die Lungen übertragen werden und abwechselnd eine Verdünnung und Verdichtung der Lungengase hervorrufen. Jede Ebbe und Flut der Luft setzt sich solange fort, bis in allen Teilen der Lunge Druckgleichheit mit der umgebenden Atmosphäre wieder hergestellt ist.

Die Ausdehnung des Brustkorbes bei der Einatmung ist stets mit einem aktiven Aufwand an Muskelkraft verbunden, während die Ausatmung in Ruhe fast ausschließlich auf der Auslösung der bei der Einatmung gespeicherten Lage- und Spannungsenergie beruht. Die inspiratorische Ausdehnung des Brustkorbes geschieht zwar in allen drei Dimensionen; Größe und Richtung der Bewegung ist jedoch in verschiedenen Brustkorbabschnitten keineswegs gleichartig.

Bei ruhiger Atmung sind vor dem Röntgenschirm die folgenden Hauptbewegungen erkennbar (Abb. 1):

a) Der Brustraum verändert sich in caudaler Richtung auf Kosten des Abdominalraumes infolge Abflachung der Zwerchfellkuppel und Entfaltung des Phrenicocostalwinkels.

b) Die Hebung sämtlicher Rippen, vor allem aber der oberen

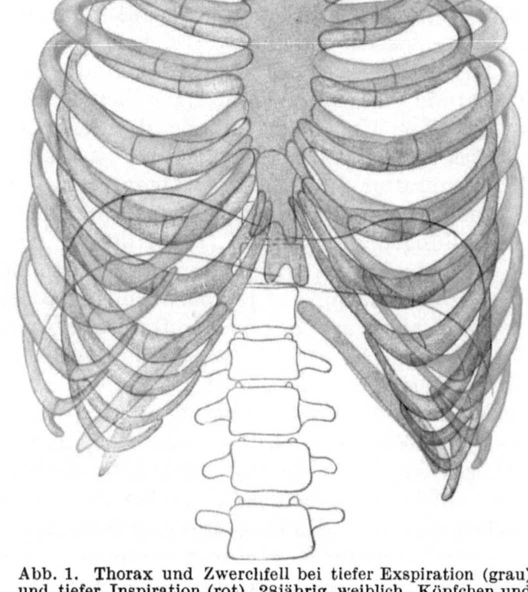

Abb. 1. Thorax und Zwerchfell bei tiefer Exspiration (grau) und tiefer Inspiration (rot), 28jährig, weiblich. Köpfchen und Hals der 1. Rippe decken sich nicht infolge der inspiratorischen Streckung der Wirbelsäule. Nach Röntgenstereoaufnahmen von Prof. A. HASSELWANDER (aus BRAUS-ELZE, Bd. 1, 3. Aufl.).

5—6 Paare bewirkt vorwiegend eine Ausdehnung des Thorax in der Sagittalebene, wobei die gleiche Bewegung auf Grund der Kegelform der oberen Brustpartie auch eine geringe frontale Erweiterung dieses Bereiches herbeiführt.

c) Die Bewegung der unteren Rippen dagegen führt fast ausschließlich zu einer Ausdehnung in der Frontalebene (Flankenatmung) infolge der besonderen Stellung und Mechanik ihrer Rippen-Wirbelgelenke.

Nach vorherrschender Ansicht[1] ist „der normale Hauptfaktor der aktiven Inspiration das Zwerchfell". Der relative Anteil der Rippenbewegung und der Zwerchfellbewegung ist individuell und je nach der Atmungsintensität sehr verschieden. Nach HUTCHINSON (1849) überwiegt beim Manne die Zwerchfellatmung

---

[1] ROHRER 1925.

und bei weiblichen Individuen die Costalatmung. Bei der Zwerchfellbewegung sind die Muskeln des Brustkorbes zumindest durch Fixierung der Rippen mitbeteiligt. Ohne dies würde eine Verkürzung des Zwerchfellmuskels eine Verengerung der unteren Brustöffnung herbeiführen. Umgekehrt führt die Vergrößerung der unteren Thoraxöffnung durch die Flankenatmung zu einer rein passiven Anspannung des Zwerchfelles. Als sicherstes Zeichen der aktiven Beteiligung des Zwerchfelles ist die inspiratorische Vorwölbung des Abdomens anzusehen, die zu Beginn der Einatmung am deutlichsten ist. Bei forcierter Einatmung, an der die costale Komponente wieder größeren Anteil nimmt, kann es schließlich zu einem Einsinken des Abdomens kommen durch passive Streckung der Bauchwände. Bei kraftvoller Ausatmung spielt die „Bauchpresse" zweifellos eine wesentliche Rolle zumal bei erhöhten Atemwiderständen. Die Tatsache, daß ein- oder gar beiderseitige Lähmung des Zwerchfelles ohne wesentliche Beeinträchtigung des Atemvolumens ertragen wird, spricht weniger gegen die Bedeutung dieses Muskels für den normalen Atemvorgang als für die vielseitige Anpassungsfähigkeit des Bewegungsapparates der Atmung. In diesem Zusammenhang ist es von Interesse, daß es gelingt, bei Fällen von zentraler Atemlähmung durch rhythmische Reizung der Phrenicusnerven eine ausreichende Lungenbelüftung aufrechtzuerhalten[1].

Bei erhöhten Anforderungen an die Atmung, sei es durch physiologische Steigerung des Energieumsatzes bei Arbeit, bei Atembehinderung oder aus krankhaften Ursachen, können die Atembewegungen in Ausmaß und Kraftentwicklung um ein Vielfaches der Ruheatmung verstärkt werden, wobei auch die Exspiration einen stark aktiven Charakter annimmt. Für die anatomischen Einzelheiten der Kinetik normaler und gesteigerter Atemtätigkeit sei auf die Darstellungen von BRAUS (1921) und v. HAYEK (1953) verwiesen.

Eine qualitative Beurteilung des Zustandes der Atemtätigkeit läßt sich aus der Gesamthaltung, der Beobachtung der Rumpfwandbewegungen und der Atemfrequenz ableiten. Ruhige rhythmische Atmung in entspannter Haltung wird als *Eupnoe* bezeichnet. *Dyspnoe* dagegen kennzeichnet eine angestrengte gesteigerte Atemform, die zumeist mit dem subjektiven Empfinden der Atemnot verbunden ist. Eine hochgradige Form der Dyspnoe, die häufig bei Versagen des rechten Herzens zu beobachten ist und durch Aufrichtung des Oberkörpers eine gewisse Erleichterung erfährt, führt den Namen *Orthopnoe*. Atemstillstand kann auf Fehlen *adäquater* Reize beruhen (Apnoe), oder aber durch Atemlähmung verursacht sein. Hierbei unterscheidet man die schlaffe Lähmung, *Asphyxie*, von der Lähmung in Einatmungsstellung, *Apneusis*. Die Bezeichnungen *Hyperpnoe* und *Hypopnoe*, welche schlechthin Vermehrung oder Verminderung der Atmung andeuten, sind nicht gleichbedeutend mit *Hyperventilation* bzw. *Hypoventilation*. Letztere beziehen sich streng gesehen auf das Verhältnis der Lungenbelüftung zu den Erfordernissen des Gasstoffwechsels. In der Erörterung der Atemregulation wird hierauf näher einzugehen sein.

2. Die Belüftungsgröße.

Genaueren Einblick in den Belüftungserfolg der Atembewegungen ergeben Messungen der geförderten Gasmengen. Hierzu ist es erforderlich, einerseits das Fassungsvermögen der Lungen in verschiedenen Atemlagen zu bestimmen, andererseits die jeweils mit einem Atemzug oder in der Zeiteinheit bewegte Luftmenge mit dieser in Beziehung zu setzen.

Die folgende Unterteilung des Lungenvolumens, die für klinische Funktionsprüfungen geeignet ist, bezieht sich auf die Ruhelage der Atmung und auf die beiden Grenzlagen der aktiven Atemexkursionen (Abb. 2 links).

---

[1] JAMIN 1921, WHITTENBERGER 1949.

a) *Ruhekapazität* (Normalkapazität, engl. Functional Residual Capacity): Dies ist der Gasgehalt der Lunge bei Entspannung aller Atemmuskeln und völligem Ausgleich aller statischen Kräfte entsprechend der normalen Exspirationslage. Sie beträgt durchschnittlich 2,5 Liter[1] und gibt Auskunft über die Größe des Mischgefäßes für den Gasaustausch in der Ruhelage.

b) Die *Vitalkapazität* ist das Volumen, welches ausgehend von äußerster Einatemstellung bis zur vollständigen Ausatmung aus der Lunge gefördert wird und ist lediglich ein Maß für die „Blasebalgfunktion" des Atemapparates. Normaler Durchschnittswert 4,5 Liter.

c) Die *Gesamtkapazität*, durchschnittlich 6,0 Liter, ergibt sich aus der Vitalkapazität und dem nach vollständiger Ausatmung in der Lunge verbleibenden *Residualvolumen* (durchschnittlich 1,5 Liter). Von der Atemruhelage ausgehend

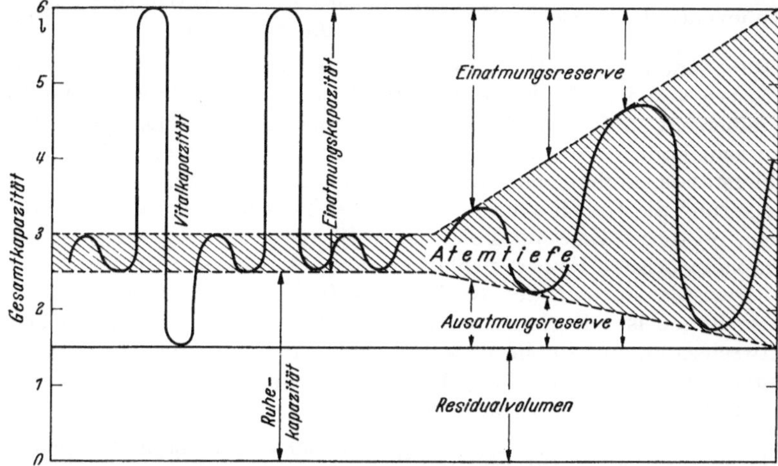

Abb. 2. Die funktionelle Unterteilung des Lungenraumes. Die als Kapazität bezeichneten Volumina sind statische Meßwerte des Fassungsvermögens. Auf der rechten Seite ist dargestellt, in welcher Weise das Fassungsvermögen bei verschiedener Atemtiefe beansprucht wird.

läßt sich die Vitalkapazität noch in die *Einatmungskapazität* und die *Ausatmungskapazität* unterteilen.

Während die genannte Unterteilung Atemlagen betrifft, die aus meßtechnischen Gründen statisch sind und sich gegenseitig überschneiden, werden zur Beurteilung dynamischer Zustände neuerdings Bezeichnungen vorgeschlagen[2], welche der wechselnden Inanspruchnahme des verfügbaren Lungenvolumens je nach der *Atemtiefe* gerecht werden. Die *Atemtiefe* kann von einem Ruhewert von etwa 0,5 Liter bei schwerer Arbeit bis zu 3,0 Liter anwachsen. Die mittlere Lungenfüllung, die aus dem Flächenintegral der Volumen-Zeitkurve gewonnen werden kann, muß dabei beträchtlich anwachsen, da die *Einatemreserve* bedeutend größer ist als die *Ausatemreserve*. Dieser Umstand ist, wie später dargetan wird, sowohl aus energetischen Gründen als auch hinsichtlich der verfügbaren respiratorischen Oberfläche günstig.

Das *Minutenvolumen* der Ventilation ergibt sich aus der Atemtiefe und der Frequenz (in Ruhe 10—14 je Minute) als 6—7 Liter. Zweifellos ist das Minutenvolumen das wichtigste Kriterium für den Funktionszustand der Atmungsorgane. Die Bestimmung nicht nur der Ruheventilation, sondern auch des Atemgrenzwertes[3, 4] sollte bei Funktionsprüfungen die statische Messung der Lungen-

---

[1] HURTADO 1933.   [2] PAPPENHEIMER 1950.   [3] HERMANNSEN 1933.   [4] GRAY 1950.

volumina ergänzen. Der Atemgrenzwert ist die höchste Lungenbelüftung, welche bei angestrengtester willkürlicher Atmung geleistet werden kann. Für gesunde junge Männer (20—25 Jahre) wurde im Durchschnitt 167 Liter je Minute und bei Frauen der gleichen Altersstufe 116 Liter je Minute für den Atemgrenzwert gefunden[1]. Dieses willkürliche Ventilationsmaximum ist beträchtlich größer als es bei intensivster Muskelarbeit zu finden ist (etwa 120 Liter je Minute)[2]. Aus der Differenz zwischen dem Atemgrenzwert und der jeweiligen Ventilation ergibt sich die *Ventilationsreserve*[3]. Bezogen auf den Atemgrenzwert bedeutet die Ventilationsreserve denjenigen Anteil der gesamten Ventilationskapazität, der nicht beansprucht wird und somit im Falle funktioneller Belastung noch zur Verfügung steht.

Zum Beispiel:

$$\text{Ruheventilationsreserve } \% = \frac{\text{Atemgrenzwert} - \text{Ruheventilation}}{\text{Atemgrenzwert}} \cdot 100.$$

An 100 Studenten im Alter von 20—25 Jahren ergab sich eine Ruheventilationsreserve von 95%[3]. Es ist ersichtlich, daß ein Verlust der Ventilationsreserve einerseits auf eine Beschränkung der Ventilationskapazität zurückzuführen sein kann — etwa durch Störungen der Atemmechanik oder erhöhte Atemwiderstände, andererseits auf eine Erhöhung des Atemvolumens. Ist eine Atemsteigerung die Ursache der verminderten Ventilationsreserve, so erhebt sich die Frage, ob dieser Zustand Folge einer Stoffwechselsteigerung ist, oder aber eine kompensatorische Hyperventilation darstellt, wie sie z. B. bei Stoffwechselacidose, gewissen Formen der Kreislaufinsuffizienz oder einfachem Sauerstoffmangel zu finden ist. Im letzteren Falle ist die Atemsteigerung größer als dem Gasstoffwechsel entspricht, im ersteren nicht. Auskunft über diese Beziehungen erhält man durch die Ermittlung des *Ventilationsäquivalents für Sauerstoff*[4] aus dem Minutenvolumen der Atmung und dem Sauerstoffverbrauch je Minute

$$\text{Ventilationsäquivalent für Sauerstoff} = \frac{\text{Gesamtatemvolumen (Liter/min)}}{\text{Sauerstoffverbrauch (cm}^3\text{/min)}} \cdot 100.$$

Bei gesunden Individuen ist dieses Verhältnis in Ruhe und bei Stoffwechselsteigerungen durch Muskeltätigkeit bis zu schwerer Arbeit wenig verändert und beträgt durchschnittlich 2,5. Bei kompensatorischer Hyperventilation dagegen werden bedeutend höhere Werte erreicht.

II. Die Atemkräfte.

A. Statische Zustände.

In jeder einzelnen, der insgesamt auf 300 Millionen geschätzten[5] Lungenalveolen und in den zuführenden Wegen setzt sich der pneumatische Druck der Luft mit der Oberflächenspannung der feuchten Wände und den elastischen Kräften des umgebenden Parenchyms ins Gleichgewicht. Dieses wabenartige System, bestehend aus einem pneumatischen und einem elastischen Medium, bietet hervorragende Bedingungen für eine rasche und gleichmäßige Fortleitung von Kräften. Der innere Kräfteausgleich wird weiterhin begünstigt durch das verschiebliche Anhaften der Lunge an der Brustwand und an den oberen Brustorganen. An jeder Berührungsfläche mit ihrer Umgebung hat die Lunge in den *zwei Dimensionen* derselben Ebene große Bewegungsfreiheit, die durch den feinen Film der Intrapleuralflüssigkeit gefördert wird. In der *dritten Dimension* ist sie

---

[1] GRAY 1950. [2] ÅSTRAND 1952. [3] MATHESON 1950.
[4] ANTHONY 1937. [5] v. HAYEK 1953.

infolge der Undehnbarkeit (Inkompressibilität) gerade dieses Mediums absolut an die Bewegungen der äußeren Thoraxwand gebunden. Auf Grund dieser mechanischen Verhältnisse werden nur senkrecht zur Oberfläche angreifende Kraftkomponenten auf die gegenüberliegende Wand übertragen. Eine Lösung der Pleurablätter ist nur möglich im Falle des Eindringens eines elastischen Mediums in den Pleuraspalt (z. B. Pneumothorax). Ohne dies ist eine Trennung nur im Falle eines „Zerreißens" des Flüssigkeitsfilms denkbar, wozu[1] bei Körpertemperatur eine Kraft von mehr als 3600 Torr. (mm Hg/cm²) erforderlich wäre. Die Schicht der Intrapleuralflüssigkeit ist so dünn, daß in ihr die Wandadhäsion die Schwerkraft überwiegt und so eine hydrostatische Druckschichtung ausschließt.

Hinsichtlich ihrer Einwirkung auf die Brusthöhlenwandung läßt sich die Lunge in mancher Beziehung mit einem homogenen elastischen Medium vergleichen, bei dem die Summe aller inneren Kräfte auf die Flächeneinheit der Oberfläche zusammenwirkt und sich hier wiederum mit den von außen herantretenden Kräften in Beziehung setzt. In diesem Kräftespiel befinden sich die elastischen Kräfte der Lunge in Gegenspannung zu denen der Brustwand einschließlich des Zwerchfelles. Die Bauchdecken hingegen sind durch Vermittlung des im wesentlichen inkompressiblen Bauchhöhleninhalts elastische Gegenspieler des Zwerchfelles und somit der Lungenspannung gleichgerichtet.

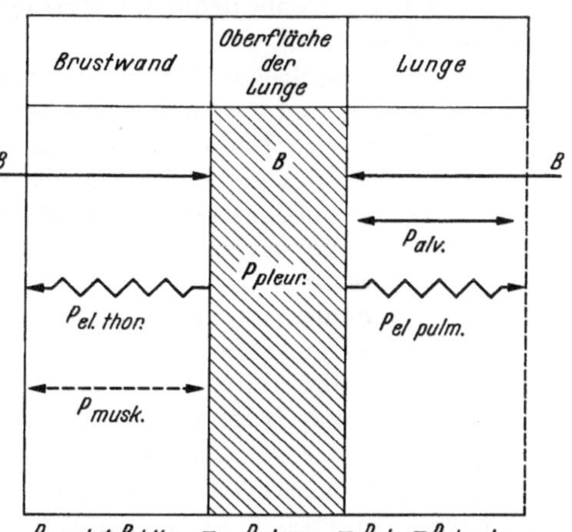

$$p_{musk.} + p_{el. thor.} = p_{pleur.} = p_{alv.} - p_{el. pulm.}$$

Abb. 3. An der Lungenoberfläche setzen sich alle statischen und dynamischen Kräfte der Atmung ins Gleichgewicht. p_{musk} = Muskelkräfte; $p_{el\,thor}$ = elastische Kräfte des Thorax; p_{pleur} = Pleuradruck, p_{alv} = Alveolardruck als Differenz zum Barometerdruck (B); $p_{el\,pulm}$ = elastische Kräfte der Lunge.

Dabei wirkt das Gewicht des Bauchhöhleninhalts je nach der Körperlage mehr oder weniger stark auf die Zwerchfellspannung ein.

In jeder Ruhelage stehen die statischen Kräfte an der Lungenoberfläche in einem Gleichgewicht, dessen Resultante die Summe aus dem Pleuradruck und dem Atmosphärendruck darstellt (Abb. 3). Nach ROHRER (1925) ist

$$B + p_{el\,thor} + p_{musk} = B + p_{pleur} = B + p_{alv} - p_{el\,pulm} \tag{1}$$

Worin: B = Barometerdruck

$p_{el\,thor}$ = elastische Spannung der Brusthöhle,

p_{musk} = aktive Kraft der Atemmuskeln

p_{pleur} = Pleuraldruck als Differenz zum Barometerdruck

p_{alv} = Alveolardruck als Differenz zum Barometerdruck

$p_{el\,pulm}$ = elastische Spannung der Lunge.

Durch Abzug des Barometerdruckes läßt sich diese Beziehung vereinfachen auf

$$p_{el\,thor} + p_{musk} = p_{pleur} = p_{alv} - p_{el\,pulm} \tag{2}$$

Nun ist für jede passive Dehnungslage der Lunge ($p_{musk} = 0$)

$$p_{el\,thor} + p_{el\,pulm} = p_{alv} \tag{3}$$

oder

$$p_{alv} - p_{pleur} = p_{el\,pulm} \cdot \tag{4}$$

---

[1] BURNS 1945.

Aus dieser Darstellung der Kräfteverhältnisse an der Lungenoberfläche läßt sich hinsichtlich praktischer Messungen folgendes schließen: Bei vollständiger Muskelentspannung ergibt der Alveolardruck für jede passive Dehnungslage die Resultante aller statischen Kräfte (Entspannungsdruck) und ermöglicht es, die passive Druck-Volumen-Charakteristik des Atmungsapparates zu beschreiben [Gl. (3), Abb. 4]. Die Messung des Pleuradruckes bei offenen Atemwegen ($p_\text{alv} = 0$) ergibt die elastische Spannung der Lungen [Gl. (4)]. Die klassischen Messungen von DONDERS (1853) wurden allerdings so vorgenommen, daß er an der Leiche Luft in den Pleuraraum eindringen ließ ($p_\text{el thor} = 0$), [Gl. (3)] und aus dem Alveolardruck die Retraktionskraft der Lunge bestimmte (im Durchschnitt 6 mm Hg).

An der elastischen Spannung der Lunge haben zweifellos die elastischen Fasern, deren dichtes Netz vor allem in der Bronchiolenwandung und in den Alveolarsepten zu finden ist, großen Anteil. NEERGARD (1929) hat darauf hingewiesen, daß neben der Gewebselastizität auch die Oberflächenspannung der die Alveolen auskleidenden Flüssigkeitshaut mit ihrem äußerst kleinen Krümmungsradius die Alveolen zu verkleinern bestrebt sei und zur Retraktionskraft beitrage. Am isolierten Organ konnte er und neuerdings v. HAYEK (1952) u. a.[1] dies experimentell veranschaulichen. Ob diesen Kräften auch in der menschlichen Lunge eine größere Bedeutung beizumessen ist als der eigentlichen Gewebselastizität, bleibt weiterer Klärung vorbehalten, die insbesondere hinsichtlich des Emphysems von Interesse ist.

Während der Alveolardruck in jeder beliebigen passiven Dehnungslage die Summe der elastischen Spannung der Lunge einerseits und der Brustwand andererseits ergibt, kann man durch gleichzeitige Messung des Pleuradruckes die Lungenspannung ermitteln und somit auch die elastische Spannung der Thoraxwand getrennt wiedergeben.

$$p_\text{el thor} = p_\text{alv} - p_\text{el pulm} \cdot \tag{5}$$

In Abb. 4 ist für den ganzen Bereich der Vitalkapazität die Entspannungsdruckkurve mit ihren beiden Komponenten eingetragen. Am Ende normaler Ausatmung entspricht der Entspannungsdruck dem Barometerdruck. Lungenspannung und Thoraxspannung sind hier gleich groß und einander entgegengerichtet. Es ist ersichtlich, daß ein Nachlassen der Lungenspannung (z. B. Emphysem) zwangsläufig durch das Überwiegen der Thoraxspannung zu einer Verschiebung der Ruhegleichgewichtslage und einer Vergrößerung der Ruhekapazität führen muß. Im gleichen Sinne bewirkt die Eröffnung der Brusthöhle, bei der beide Komponenten den Druck Null annehmen (Pneumothorax) nicht nur einen Kollaps der Lungen, sondern auch eine Ausdehnung des Brustkorbes.

Die *Lungenspannungskurve* nimmt wahrscheinlich über den physiologischen Dehnungsbereich einen nahezu linearen Verlauf[2]. Die S-förmige Gestalt der Entspannungsdruckkurve wird demnach vor allem von dem Verhalten der Thoraxspannung in verschiedenen Dehnungslagen bestimmt. Im Bereich ruhiger Atmung ist die Entspannungsdruckkurve ebenfalls geradlinig mit einer Neigung entsprechend 100 cm³ Volumenänderung für 1 mm Hg. Änderungen der Körperhaltung verändern die statischen Kräftebeziehungen in deutlicher Weise. Beim Übergang von aufrecht sitzender Stellung in die Rückenlage wird z. B. infolge Verminderung des Gewichtszuges der abdominalen Organe das Lungenvolumen bei normaler Ausatmung (Ruhekapazität) um 13% der Vitalkapazität herabgesetzt[3].

---

[1] KILCHES 1940, WICK 1952.   [2] CLOETTA 1913, NEERGARD 1927.   [3] RAHN 1946.

Die Darstellung der Kräftebeziehungen in den passiven Dehnungslagen läßt sich durch Hinzuziehen der aktiven Kräfte (p_{musk}) in Gl. (2) z. B. für den Grenzfall äußersten inspiratorischen und exspiratorischen Kraftaufwandes für den gesamten Dehnungsbereich ergänzen. Es ergeben sich charakteristische Druck-Volumenkonturen (Abb. 4) nach der Art eines Spannungs-Dehnungsdiagramms der Technik[1], [2]. Der höchste positive Druck, durchschnittlich 107 mm Hg, wird ausgehend von äußerster Einatemstellung aufgebracht und führt durch Kompression zu einer Verkleinerung des Lungenraumes. Auf der Seite negativen Druckes wird das Maximum (— 85 mm Hg) ausgehend von der tiefsten Ausatmung erreicht, begleitet von einer geringen Volumenzunahme. Die von den

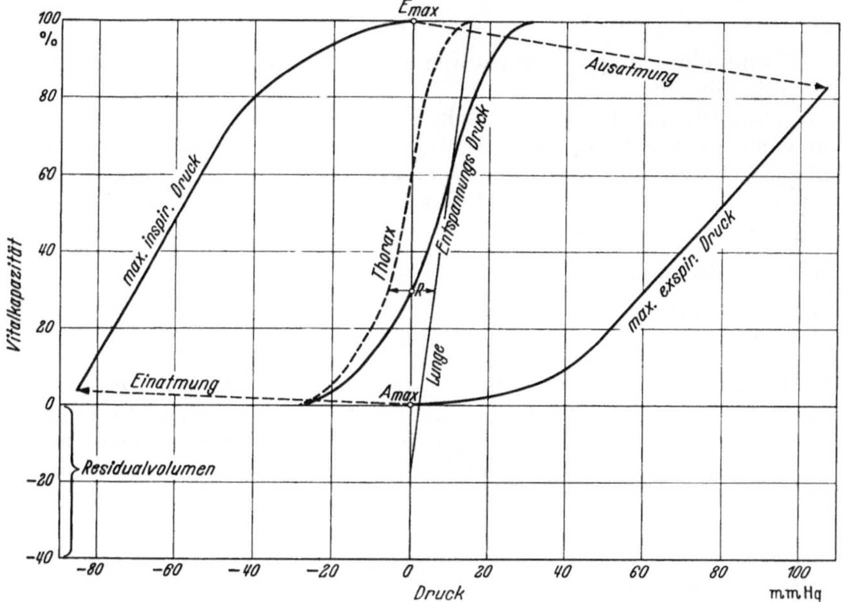

Abb. 4. Das Druck-Volumendiagramm der Lunge und Brustwand. Der Entspannungsdruck ist die Resultante aus der elastischen Spannung des Thorax und der der Lunge. In der normalen Ausatemstellung (R) sind Lungen- und Thoraxspannung gleich und entgegengerichtet. Die äußeren Konturlinien verbinden Druck und Volumen bei maximaler exspiratorischer und inspiratorischer Muskelanstrengung je nach der Ausgangslage. A_{max} ist maximale Ausatemstellung und E_{max} äußerste Einatemstellung. (Nach Rohrer 1925 und Rahn 1946.)

Konturlinien für maximalen Einatmungs- und Ausatmungsdruck umgrenzte Fläche erfaßt somit alle Druck-Volumenbeziehungen, die dem Atmungsorgan zur Verfügung stehen. Nur ein äußerst kleiner Teil dieses Funktionsbereichs wird im Verlauf der normalen Atemarbeit in Anspruch genommen.

B. Dynamische Zustände.

Um die für den Gasaustausch notwendige ständige Erneuerung der Luft im Alveolarraum aufrechtzuerhalten, ist eine Luftbewegung erforderlich, die sowohl hinsichtlich ihrer Richtung als auch ihrer Geschwindigkeit wechselt. Dieser Bewegung setzen sich Widerstände verschiedener Art und Größe entgegen, die von den Triebkräften der Atmung, sowohl muskulärer als elastischer Natur überwunden werden müssen.

Eine quantitative Darstellung der einzelnen Faktoren der Atemdynamik beim Menschen ist uns vorerst versagt wegen der begrenzten Möglichkeit direkter Messung der wichtigsten Faktoren wie Alveolardruck und Pleuradruck am intakten

Rahn 1946. [2] Rohrer 1925.

Organismus. Die folgende Übersicht beschränkt sich darauf, die einzelnen Komponenten miteinander in Beziehung zu bringen und auf Grund von Messungen an Tieren oder indirekten Daten in ihrer Größenordnung abzuschätzen. Dabei wird auf die grundlegenden Arbeiten von ROHRER (1925), FLEISCH (1934) und FENN (1951) für eingehende Behandlung verwiesen.

1. Die Strömungswiderstände.

Auf ein System enger Röhren, wie es die Atemwege darstellen, sollte zunächst das HAGEN-POISEUILLEsche Gesetz Anwendung finden:

$$v = p \cdot \frac{r^4 \cdot \pi \cdot t}{l \cdot \eta \cdot 8}$$

v = Stromvolumen, p = Druckdifferenz, r = Radius, l = Länge, η = Viscosität, t = Zeiteinheit.

Das geförderte Stromvolumen steht im direkten Verhältnis zur Druckdifferenz und der vierten Potenz des Radius. Dies vergegenwärtigt die Bedeutung physiologischer und pathologischer Veränderungen des Querschnitts der Luftwege. Länge des Systems und die Viscosität des strömenden Mediums sind dem Stromvolumen reziprok. Löst man diese Gleichung für den Alveolardruck (p_{alv}) und faßt die Rohrwiderstände $\left(\dfrac{l}{r^4}\right)$ als w_1 und die unveränderlichen $\left(\dfrac{8}{\pi}\right)$ als k_1 zusammen, so ergibt sich

$$p_{\mathrm{alv}} = k_1 \cdot w_1 \cdot \eta \cdot v.$$

Nun behält diese Gesetzmäßigkeit nur solange Gültigkeit, wie die Voraussetzungen für „laminare Strömung" gegeben sind. Beim Überschreiten kritischer Strömungsgeschwindigkeit geht diese Parallelströmung in turbulente Strömung über. Dieser Grenzfall läßt sich unter Berücksichtigung der REYNOLDSschen Zahl abschätzen

$V_{kr} = 1160 \cdot v \cdot \pi \cdot r$
V_{kr} = kritische Volumgeschwindigkeit in cm³/sec
  r = Radius in cm
  v = kinematische Zähigkeit der Atemluft = 0,168 cm²/sec.

In einem glattwandigen Rohr vom Durchmesser der Trachea (2 cm) würde demnach turbulente Strömung bei einer Volumgeschwindigkeit von mehr als 600 cm³/sec oder 36 Liter/min auftreten. Dies liegt durchaus im Bereich normaler Atembewegungen. Aber auch ohne die kritische Geschwindigkeit zu überschreiten, kann der Übergang von einer Strömungsform in die andere vor sich gehen, nämlich dort, wo sprungweise Änderungen des Stromquerschnitts und der Strömungsrichtung eintreten. Auch hier kommt es zu Wirbelbildungen, die den Strömungswiderstand erheblich vermehren. Der zur Überwindung derartiger Extrawiderstände (w_2) notwendige Druck wächst mit dem Quadrat der Strömungsgeschwindigkeit (V) und ist von der Dichte (ϱ) abhängig

$$p_{\mathrm{alv}} = k_2 \cdot w_2 \cdot \varrho \cdot V^2.$$

Da auch bei ruhiger Atmung beide Strömungsformen nebeneinander in verschiedenen Teilen des Atmungsweges vorkommen, ist folgende additive Beziehung anzunehmen[1]

$$p_{\mathrm{alv}} = k_1 \cdot W_1 \cdot \eta \cdot V + k_2 \cdot w_2 \cdot \varrho \cdot V^2$$
$$(p \text{ in cm}^3 \text{ H}_2\text{O}, \quad V \text{ in Liter/sec}).$$

---

[1] ROHRER 1915.

Auf Grund anatomischer Messungen der einzelnen Längen- und Querschnittsverhältnisse in allen Teilen der Atemwege hat ROHRER berechnet, daß die Anteile des Rohrwiderstandes und der Extrawiderstände etwa gleich groß sind:

$$p_{\mathrm{alv}} = 0{,}79\ V + 0{,}80\ V^2.$$

dabei entfielen auf den Bereich oberhalb der Trachea

$$p = 0{,}43\ \mathrm{V} + 0{,}71\ \mathrm{V}^2$$

und auf die darunter liegenden Abschnitte

$$p = 0{,}36\ \mathrm{V} + 0{,}09\ \mathrm{V}^2.$$

Die Turbulenzwiderstände wären demnach fast ausschließlich in den oberen Luftwegen zu suchen. Bei gesteigerter Lungenventilation muß allerdings auch in den unteren Abschnitten mit einem starken Anwachsen dieses Faktors gerechnet werden. Bei geringerer Dichte der Atemgase, wie sie in großen Höhen zu finden ist, oder bei der Atmung eines Gemisches von geringerem spezifischem Gewicht als Luft (z. B. Sauerstoff und Helium[1]) läßt sich für gleiche Stromvolumina eine Erleichterung der Atmung nachweisen, die zweifellos auf eine Verminderung der Atemwiderstände infolge turbulenter Strömungen zurückzuführen ist, da nur in diesem Faktor die Dichte eingeht.

Über die Druck-Strömungsbeziehungen in den menschlichen Atemwegen liegen wegen methodischer Schwierigkeiten nur wenige Meßwerte vor. Vor allem bietet die Ermittlung des dynamischen Alveolardruckes erhebliche Schwierigkeiten. Durch periodische kurze (0,1 sec) Unterbrechungen der inspiratorischen und exspiratorischen Strömung läßt sich im Verlauf der Atembewegung ein momentaner Druckausgleich erzielen, der dem mittleren Alveolardruck entsprechen soll[2]. Die auf diesem Wege in Verbindung mit pneumotachographischer Messung des Volumens erhaltenen Werte stimmen erstaunlich gut mit der Strömungsgleichung von ROHRER (1915) überein, wenn auch die Atemwiderstände am Lebenden etwas größer zu sein scheinen. So erhielten OTIS und PROCTOR (1948) im Durchschnitt einen Alveolardruck von 1,8 cm Wassersäule für 0,5 Liter/sec.

2. Trägheits- und Deformationswiderstände.

Bei der Atembewegung entstehen Trägheitskräfte, die von der Masse und Beschleunigung der beteiligten Organe bestimmt sind. Auch bei angestrengtester Atemtätigkeit kommt ihnen gegenüber den Strömungswiderständen wahrscheinlich eine sehr untergeordnete Bedeutung zu. Auch die Reibungswiderstände an der Lungenoberfläche bei ihrer Verschiebung gegenüber der Brustwand und den übrigen Organen ist äußerst gering. Dahingegen sind die inneren Reibungswiderstände, welche bei der Deformierung der Lunge, der Brustwand und der angrenzenden Organe entstehen, nicht zu vernachlässigen. Sie sind nach Angaben von WIRZ (1923) von der gleichen Größenordnung wie die Strömungswiderstände in den Luftwegen und ändern sich ebenfalls mit der Strömungsform.

3. Die Strömungsgeschwindigkeit.

Die fortlaufende Aufzeichnung der Strömungsgeschwindigkeit mit dem Pneumotachographen[3] gestattet es zu jedem Zeitpunkt des Atemcyclus, das Verhältnis von Atemkraft zu Atemwiderstand zu verfolgen (Abb. 5). Gegenüber der spirometrisch gewonnenen Volumenkurve, die eine Integration darstellt, liefert das *Pneumotachogramm* die dazugehörige Differentialkurve. An ihr lassen

---

[1] OTIS 1945.　　[2] NEERGARD 1927, VUILLEUMIER 1944.　　[3] FLEISCH 1925.

sich die Phasenwechselpunkte mit großer Genauigkeit bestimmen. Bei ruhiger Atmung liegt die Höchstgeschwindigkeit der Inspiration um 600 cm³/sec, die der Exspiration um 500 cm³/sec. Bei größerer Atemtiefe hingegen wird die Strömungsgeschwindigkeit der Exspiration größer als bei der Inspiration. So konnten bei schwerer körperlicher Arbeit exspiratorische Spitzengeschwindigkeiten von 7700 cm³/sec beobachtet werden, während bei der Inspiration nur 4830 gemessen wurden. Bei Hustenstößen sollen für Bruchteile von Sekunden Strömungen von 20 Liter/sec auftreten können[1]. Es ist oft darauf hingewiesen worden, daß das Pneumotachogramm für jedes Individuum Eigenheiten der Form aufweist, die vergleichbar der Charakteristik des Ganges oder der Handschrift die Individualität der nervös-mechanischen Koordinationen verdeutlicht. Bei pathologischen Zuständen der Atmungsorgane sind bezeichnende Veränderungen des Pneumotachogramms vorhanden ebenso wie bei Störungen in der Atemregulation.

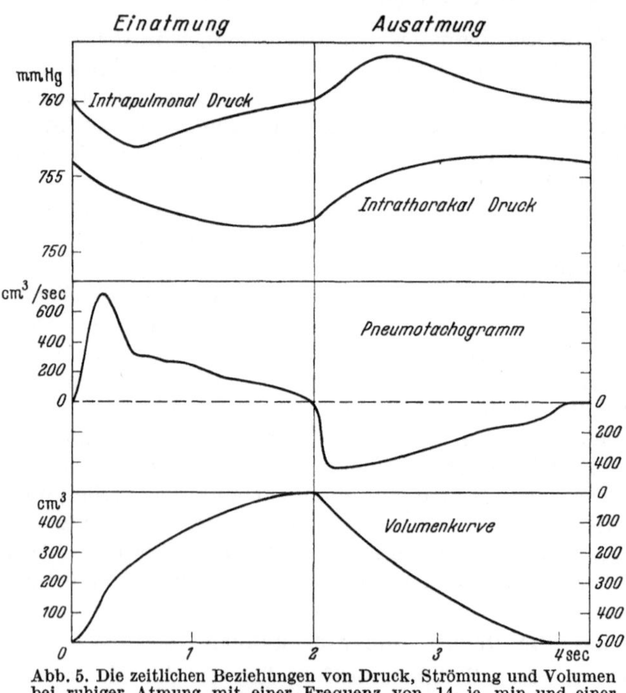

Abb. 5. Die zeitlichen Beziehungen von Druck, Strömung und Volumen bei ruhiger Atmung mit einer Frequenz von 14 je min und einer Atemtiefe von 0,5 Liter.

Innerhalb der Luftwege ist nach Berechnungen Rohrers (1915), die allerdings unter Annahme einer Laminarströmung und konstantem Druck gemacht wurden, die Höchstgeschwindigkeit an der Glottis zu suchen Unterhalb der Trachea finden sich mehrere sprunghafte Verengerungen der Strombahn, so in den großen Bronchien und wiederum auf dem Wege zu jedem Lobulus. An diesen Stellen sind Stromgeschwindigkeitsspitzen zu erwarten, die wohl auskultatorische Phänomene hervorrufen und bei Beförderungen von Sekretmassen durch Husten wirksam werden. Änderungen der Dehnungslage der Lunge, wie sie normalerweise im Laufe der Atmung auftreten, beeinflussen die Strömungsverhältnisse in dem Sinne, daß in erhöhter Dehnungslage (Inspiration) die Widerstände geringer sind als im unteren Dehnungsbereich (Exspiration)[2].

4. Die Atemarbeit.

Die Arbeit der Atembewegung als Volumänderung gegen die Summe aller Widerstände läßt sich als Fläche in einem Koordinatensystem wiedergeben, dessen Abszisse Druck und dessen Ordinate Volumen darstellen (Abb. 6). Die Arbeit für eine gegebene Volumenzunahme (Inspiration) erfordert zunächst die Kraft, um den statischen Widerstand der Lunge und des Brust-

---

[1] Fleisch 1934.   [2] Maloney 1950.

korbes zu überwinden. Diese ist definiert durch den entsprechenden Abschnitt der Entspannungsdruckkurve (Abb. 4), die in Abb. 6 der Geraden R—I entspricht. Das Dreieck R—I—V charakterisiert den statischen Anteil der Arbeit allein. Der zusätzliche Kraftaufwand zur Überwindung der dynamischen Widerstände, welche durch Strömung, Deformation, Reibung und Trägheit erwachsen, ist in der Fläche zwischen der Geraden R—I und der inspiratorischen Schleife enthalten. Im Moment des Phasenwechsels (I) steht zur Exspiration die gewonnene elastische Energie zur Verfügung. Bei normaler ruhiger Atmung ist diese mehr als ausreichend, um die dynamischen Widerstände zu überwinden, die von der exspiratorischen Schleife und der Linie I—R umrissen sind. Ein derartiges Arbeitsdiagramm der Atmung wird gewonnen, indem eine Versuchsperson bei Ausschaltung aller aktiven Atemkräfte in einer „eisernen Lunge" beatmet wird und die Luftbewegung mittels eines Tachographen registriert wird[1]. Die Druckdifferenz zwischen dem Inneren des Respirators und dem Munde der Versuchsperson ersetzt die Atemkräfte und kann so fortlaufend zur Luftbewegung in Beziehung gesetzt werden. Die gleichzeitige Registrierung des intrathorakalen Druckes erlaubt eine isolierte Darstellung der statisch-elastischen und der dynamischen Widerstände. Bei ruhiger Atmung werden etwa $^2/_3$ der Gesamtarbeit zur Dehnung des Brust-

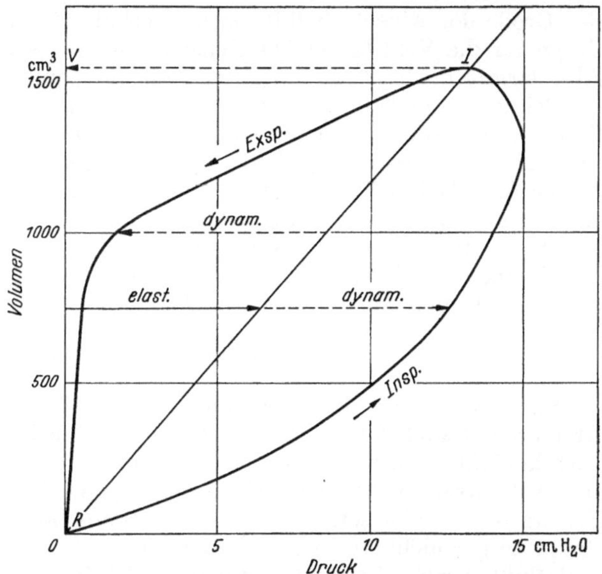

Abb. 6. Das Arbeitsdiagramm eines tieferen Atemzuges (nach OTIS 1950). Die Arbeit gegen den elastischen Widerstand der Lunge und des Brustkorbes bei der Einatmung entspricht dem Dreieck R—I—V. Zur Überwindung der dynamischen Widerstände ist die Arbeit gleich der Fläche zwischen der inspiratorischen Schleife und der Geraden I—R.

korbes und der Lunge benötigt, der Rest entfällt auf Strömungs- und Reibungswiderstände. Aus der Betrachtung des Arbeitsdiagramms ist ersichtlich, daß bei Vergrößerung der Atemtiefe die elastische Arbeit anwächst, während erhöhte Frequenz bei gleichem Minutenvolumen den dynamischen Anteil vergrößert. Die Ökonomie der Atemarbeit wird daher von der zweckmäßigen Abstimmung beider Komponenten abhängig sein, die der Atemregulation obliegt.

Bei einer durchschnittlichen Atemtiefe von 500 cm³ und einer Frequenz um 15 je Minute beträgt die *mechanische Leistung* des Atemapparates 0,5 mkg/min. Selbst unter Anrechnung eines verhältnismäßig niedrigen Wirkungsgrades von nur 5%[1] beläuft sich der Energieverbrauch der Atmung in Ruhe mit 35 kcal je Tag nur auf rund 1—2% des Gesamtumsatzes. Bei erhöhten Anforderungen an die Atmung wächst die Atemarbeit nicht proportional der Belüftungsgröße, sondern in Form einer Parabel an und kann bei maximaler Leistung auf über 200 mkg/min ansteigen.

---

[1] OTIS 1950.

III. Die Alveolarluft.

Die Lunge ist das Mischgefäß der Atemgase. Auf der einen Seite wird dem Lungenraum vom Blute fortlaufend Sauerstoff entnommen und Kohlensäure zugeführt; demgegenüber verläuft der Austausch mit der Umwelt nicht kontinuierlich, wie es in einem festen Gefäß mit getrenntem Zu- und Abfluß denkbar wäre, sondern durch rhythmische Volumenänderungen mit wechselnder Strömungsrichtung nach Art eines Blasebalgs. Auf Grund dessen ist die Zusammensetzung der Alveolarluft andauernd Schwankungen unterworfen, die den Atembewegungen synchron sind und in ihrer Amplitude von der Atemtiefe abhängen. Der Mittelwert, um den sich diese Schwankungen abspielen, wird bestimmt von der Größe der Alveolarbelüftung im Verhältnis zum Gaswechsel mit dem Blut. Je größer die Ventilation bei gleichem Gaswechsel, desto mehr nähert sich die Alveolarluft in ihrer Qualität der Außenluft und umgekehrt.

Bei der Betrachtung der *alveolaren Ventilation* ist zu berücksichtigen, daß ein Teil der mit jedem Atemzug eingeatmeten Luft in den Atemwegen zurückbleibt und daher am Gaswechsel nicht teilnimmt. Umgekehrt bleibt eine entsprechende Menge Alveolarluft bei der Ausatmung zurück und muß zu Beginn des folgenden Atemcyclus in den Alveolarraum zurückkehren. Die Größe des *respiratorischen Totraumes* (V_{Dx}) läßt sich aus der Atemtiefe (V_t) berechnen, wenn der Raumanteil eines der Atemgase (x) in der Einatmungsluft (F_{Ix}), in der Alveolarluft (F_{Ax}) und in der Ausatmungsluft (F_{Ex}) bekannt ist[1].

$$V_{Dx} = \frac{F_{Ex} - F_{Ax}}{F_{Ix} - F_{Ax}} \cdot V_t.$$

Haldane (1915) hatte angenommen, daß der Totraum proportional der Atemtiefe anwächst und hatte dies auf eine Ausdehnung der unteren Atemwege zurückgeführt. Obwohl diese Ansicht nicht unwidersprochen blieb[2], hat sich erst auf Grund vielseitiger Untersuchungen mit verschiedenen Methoden die Erkenntnis durchgesetzt, daß der anatomische Totraum von Atemtiefe und -frequenz gar nicht und von der Dehnungslage der Lunge nur in geringem Maße beeinflußt wird[3]. Dagegen kann der effektive Totraum, d. h. derjenige Anteil eines Atemzuges der nicht am Gasaustausch teilnimmt, je nach der Atemdynamik und der Blutverteilung in der Lunge, größer und sogar kleiner sein als der anatomische Totraum[2, 4]. Ist der Totraum bekannt, so läßt sich die alveolare Ventilation, je nach der Atemtiefe und der Frequenz berechnen:

Alveolarventilation = Gesamtventilation — Totraum · Frequenz.

Ist z. B. die Gesamtventilation 6 Liter/min bei einer Frequenz von 12 und der Totraum 150 cm³, so beträgt die alveolare Ventilation 4,8 Liter/min. Wird dagegen dasselbe Gesamtvolumen geatmet, aber bei der doppelten Frequenz, so ergibt sich bei gleichbleibendem Totraum eine alveolare Ventilation von nur 2,4 Liter/min. Obwohl offenbar bei langsamer, tiefer Atmung ein größerer Teil der Gesamtventilation der Alveolarbelüftung zugute kommt, können dadurch andererseits übermäßige Schwankungen in der Zusammensetzung der Lungengase und im Blut auftreten. Die Einhaltung einer optimalen Beziehung zwischen Amplitude und Frequenz ist demnach nicht nur hinsichtlich der Atemmechanik (s. oben) von besonderer Bedeutung.

In Anbetracht der anatomischen Struktur der Lunge, die aus vielen Millionen einzelner Funktionseinheiten besteht, erscheint es fraglich, ob die relativ kleine Gasmenge, die mit jedem Atemzug der Ruhekapazität beigemischt wird, allen

---

[1] Bohr 1890.   [2] Krogh, Lindhard 1917, Grosse-Brockhoff und Schoedel 1936.
[3] Bateman 1950, Pappenheimer 1952, Hatch 1953.   [4] Fishman 1954.

Teilen gleichmäßig zugute kommt. Obwohl anzunehmen ist, daß innerhalb der einzelnen Alveolen durch Diffusion und Wirbel ein rascher Ausgleich stattfindet[1] und eine Schichtung der Gase vermieden wird, ist es durchaus denkbar, daß regionale Unterschiede in der Luftversorgung auf Grund ungleichmäßiger Dehnbarkeit gegeben sind. Dies ist sicherlich in manchen pathologischen Zuständen der Fall[2]. Als weitere Ursache einer ungleichmäßigen Verteilung der Atemluft, kommen zeitliche Differenzen in der Entfaltung verschiedener Lungenbezirke in Betracht, die dazu führen können, daß die zuerst versorgten Teile der Lunge einen größeren Anteil der Totraumluft erhalten[3]. Die Ansicht ENGELHARDTs (1939), daß normalerweise ein beträchtlicher Teil der Alveolen überhaupt nicht am Luftwechsel teilnimmt, ist einer weiteren Nachprüfung wert. Die Mehrzahl der bisherigen Untersuchungen spricht dafür, daß bei gesunden Personen[4] zumal bei größerer Atemtiefe[5] die alveolare Durchmischung derjenigen in einem idealen, ungekammerten System sehr nahe kommt. Um so größere Bedeutung hat für die Beurteilung der pulmonalen Mischungsverhältnisse bei krankhaften Prozessen die Bestimmung der Auswaschungszeit für Stickstoff[6] beim Übergang von Luft- zu Sauerstoffatmung gewonnen.

Der für die Atemregulation bedeutungsvolle mittlere *Kohlensäuregehalt der Alveolarluft* ($F_{A\,CO_2}$) steht in direktem Verhältnis zur Kohlensäureabgabe ($\dot{V}_{A\,CO_2}$) und ist umgekehrt proportional der alveolaren Ventilation ($\dot{V}_A$)

$$F_{A\,CO_2} = \frac{\dot{V}_{A\,CO_2}}{\dot{V}_A}.$$

Die in einer gegebenen Zeit ausgeschiedene Kohlensäure kommt im allgemeinen dem aufgenommenen Sauerstoff nicht gleich, sondern steht — je nach der Qualität der chemischen Umsetzungen im Körper — im Verhältnis $CO_2/O_2 = 0{,}7$ bis $1{,}0$ (respiratorischer Quotient). Es ist zu beachten, daß dieses Austauschverhältnis in der Lunge nur dann mit dem metabolischen respiratorischen Quotienten identisch ist, wenn Atmung und Kreislauf sich mit den Stoffwechselvorgängen im Gleichgewicht befinden. Strenggenommen ist dies nur im absoluten Ruhenüchternzustand der Fall, nicht dagegen, wenn die Atemtätigkeit dem Stoffwechselgeschehen vorauseilt oder ihm nachsteht (z. B. Arbeitsbelastung, Sauerstoffmangel, Dekompression).

Die Veränderung im *Sauerstoffgehalt der Alveolarluft* ($F_{A\,O_2}$) gegenüber dem der Inspirationsluft ($F_{I\,O_2}$) und seine Beziehung zur alveolaren Kohlensäure ($F_{A\,CO_2}$) läßt sich wie folgt ableiten[7]

$$\frac{F_{A\,CO_2}}{F_{I\,O_2} - F_{A\,O_2}} = R \quad \text{(resp. Quot.)} \tag{1}$$

oder

$$F_{I\,O_2} - F_{A\,O_2} = F_{A\,CO_2} \cdot \frac{1}{R} \tag{2}$$

und

$$F_{A\,O_2} = F_{I\,O_2} - F_{A\,CO_2} \cdot \frac{1}{R} \tag{3}$$

Wird nun mehr Sauerstoff aufgenommen als Kohlensäure abgegeben, so kommt es zu einer Verminderung des Gasgehaltes der Lunge, die jedoch fortlaufend durch nachströmende Luft ausgeglichen wird. Die Menge der hinzukommenden Luft entspricht der Differenz:

$$(F_{I\,O_2} - F_{A\,O_2}) - F_{A\,CO_2}.$$

---

[1] MUNDT 1940, RAUWERDA 1946.   [2] ROELSEN 1937.   [3] FOWLER 1949.
[4] COMROE 1951.   [5] ARMITAGE 1949.   [6] COURNAND 1941.
[7] SCHOEDEL 1937, BENZINGER 1938, FENN 1946, GRAY 1950.

Dies wird durch Substitution aus Gl. (2):

$$F_{A\,CO_2} \cdot \frac{1}{R} - F_{A\,CO_2} \quad \text{oder} \quad F_{A\,CO_2}\left(\frac{1}{R} - 1\right).$$

Der alveolare Sauerstoff wird dabei um den Sauerstoffanteil der nachströmenden Inspirationsluft vermehrt

$$F_{A\,CO_2}\left(\frac{1}{R} - 1\right) \cdot F_{I\,O_2}.$$

Dieser Ausdruck wird in Gl. (3) eingesetzt

$$F_{A\,O_2} + F_{A\,CO_2}\left(\frac{1}{R} - 1\right) F_{I\,O_2} = F_{I\,O_2} - F_{A\,CO_2} \cdot \frac{1}{R}. \tag{4}$$

Durch Auflösung für den alveolaren Sauerstoff erhält man schließlich

$$F_{A\,O_2} = F_{I\,O_2} - F_{A\,CO_2}\left[F_{I\,O_2} + \frac{1 - F_{I\,O_2}}{R}\right]. \tag{5}$$

Ist der respiratorische Quotient gleich 1,0, so fällt der Ausdruck in der Klammer der letzten Gleichung fort, ebenso falls reiner Sauerstoff eingeatmet wird.

Der für die Gasdiffusion wirksame Teildruck eines beliebigen Atemgases ($P_{A\,x}$) ergibt sich aus dem Barometerdruck (B) und dem trockenen Volumenanteil des Gases ($F_{A\,x}$) unter Berücksichtigung voller Wasserdampfsättigung bei Körpertemperatur (Wasserdampfdruck = 47 mm Hg) in der allgemeinen Form

$$P_{A\,x} = (B - 47)\,F_{A\,x}.$$

In der folgenden Tabelle sind Durchschnittswerte angegeben für die Raumanteile und Teildrucke der Atemgase auf ihrem Wege durch das Atemorgan (Ruhezustand in Meereshöhe, $B - 47 = 713$ mm Hg).

Gas	Inspiration		Alveolar		Exspiration	
	F_I	P_I mm Hg	F_A	P_A mm Hg	F_E	P_E mm Hg
O_2	0,2094	149	0,140	100	0,161	115
CO_2	0,0004	—	0,056	40	0,039	28
N_2	0,7902	564	0,804	573	0,800	570

Die Zunahme des Stickstoffanteils bei der Passage durch die Lunge ist darauf zurückzuführen, daß die gleiche Anzahl Stickstoffmoleküle in dem kleineren Alveolar- und Exspirationsvolumen (RQ: 0,8) einen relativ größeren Raum einnimmt.

Trägt man in einem Koordinatensystem (Abb. 7), dessen Abszisse den Sauerstoffteildruck und dessen Ordinate den Kohlensäureteildruck der Alveolarluft darstellen, einen gemessenen oder berechneten Alveolarpunkt ein, so wird damit dieser Wert sowohl hinsichtlich des respiratorischen Quotienten als auch der alveolaren Ventilation charakterisiert. In dieser Darstellung[1], die unter Verwendung der Alveolargleichung (Gl. 5) konstruiert wird, liegen alle Punkte mit gleichem respiratorischem Quotienten auf Geraden, die vom Punkt der inspiratorischen Sauerstoff- und Kohlensäurespannung ausstrahlen. Bei Änderungen des Barometerdruckes verschiebt sich dieser Punkt und damit das Strahlenbündel längs der Abszisse. Die Geraden des parallelen Liniensystems dagegen verbinden alle Punkte mit dem gleichen alveolaren Ventilationsäquivalent für Sauerstoff

$$\text{Alveolares Ventilationsäquivalent } O_2 = \frac{\text{Alveolare Ventilation (Liter/min)}}{\text{Sauerstoffaufnahme (cm}^3\text{/min)}} \cdot 100.$$

---

[1] Fenn 1946.

Mit Hilfe dieses Diagramms kann man sich ohne umständliche Berechnungen die Beziehungen der Atemgase zur Belüftung und zum Gaswechsel allein auf Grund gegebener Alveolarluftproben rasch veranschaulichen.

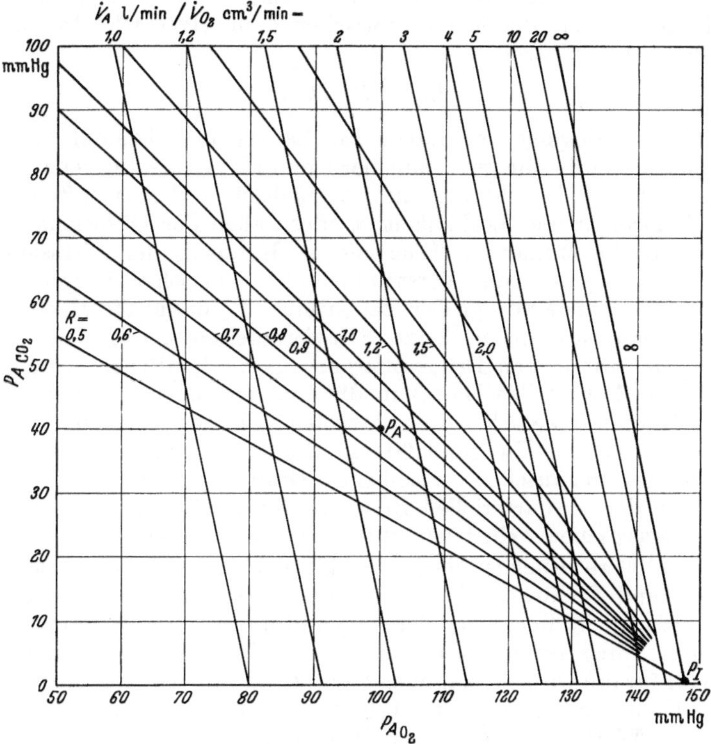

Abb. 7. Der Teildruck des Sauerstoffs (Abszisse) und der Kohlensäure (Ordinate) und ihre Beziehungen zum respiratorischen Quotienten (R) und dem alveolaren Ventilationsäquivalent für Sauerstoff. P_a Alveolarpunkt; P_I Inspirationspunkt.

IV. Der Gasaustausch.

Bei der Atmung begegnen sich die Inspirationsluft mit hohem Sauerstoff- und niedrigem Kohlensäuredruck und das venöse Mischblut mit niedrigem Sauerstoff- und hohem Kohlensäuredruck an der Austauschfläche der Lunge mit dem Erfolg eines fast vollständigen Druckausgleiches der beiden Stoffwechselgase, aus dem einerseits das arterielle Blut, andererseits die Alveolarluft hervorgeht. Die Erfahrung, daß auch bei Steigerung des Stoffwechsels auf das Zehnfache des Ruhewertes der Gaswechsel bei schwerer Arbeit den Anforderungen zu genügen vermag, vergegenwärtigt die hohe Leistungsfähigkeit der Atemfunktion, zu der eine Reihe verschiedener Faktoren beitragen.

Die *respiratorische Oberfläche* der Lunge, an der die Gase in unmittelbarer Berührung mit den Pulmonalcapillaren stehen, kann nur annähernd geschätzt werden. Nach v. HAYEK (1953) soll sie je nach der Dehnungslage der Lunge bei höchster Inspiration etwa 100 m² und bei tiefster Exspiration 30 m² betragen. Demnach stünden bei ruhiger Atmung 50—60 m² zur Verfügung. Der *Diffusionsweg*, den die Gasmoleküle zurücklegen müssen, wäre im ungünstigsten Falle vom Mittelpunkt einer annähernd kugelförmigen Alveole bis zur Capillarwand $100\,\mu$ und durch diese hindurch weitere $2\,\mu$.

Nach dem Gesetz der Diffusion steht die in der Minute ins Blut passierende Sauerstoffmenge ($\dot{V}_{O_2}$) im direkten Verhältnis zur wirksamen Druckdifferenz zwischen Alveolarluft und Blut ($\varDelta \bar{P}$) und der Diffusionsfähigkeit (D_{O_2}) der Alveolarmembran. Letztere ist hier nicht im rein anatomischen Sinne gedacht, sondern als die Summe der Medien zwischen dem Alveolarhohlraum und dem Hämoglobin in den Blutzellen

$$\dot{V}_{O_2} = \bar{P} \cdot D_{O_2}.$$

Die Diffusionsfähigkeit der Lunge für Sauerstoff[1] bedeutet also diejenige Sauerstoffmenge (cm^3), die in 1 min je 1 mm Hg Druckdifferenz diffundiert. In diesem Begriff sind nicht nur die physikalischen Eigenschaften des Gases, wie Molekulargewicht und Löslichkeit, sondern auch der Diffusionsweg und die Diffusionsoberfläche enthalten. Eine genaue Kenntnis der Diffusionsfähigkeit der Lunge wäre sowohl zum Verständnis physiologischer Vorgänge als auch pathologischer Zustände von großer Bedeutung. Während die Messung der aufgenommenen Sauerstoffmenge keine Schwierigkeiten bereitet, ist die exakte Bestimmung der wirksamen Druckdifferenz aus methodischen Gründen problematisch. Beim Eintritt des Blutes in die Lungencapillare beträgt das Druckgefälle für Sauerstoff zwischen den Alveolen (100 mm Hg) und dem venösen Mischblut (etwa 40 mm Hg) rund 60 mm Hg. Nach neuerer Kenntnis[2] ist die am Ende des Gasaustausches verbleibende Druckdifferenz zwischen alveolarem Sauerstoff und dem des arteriellen Blutes 2—8 mm Hg, also bedeutend weniger als nach der klassischen Arbeit von Bock und Mitarbeitern (1929) angenommen wurde. Das mittlere Druckgefälle ($\varDelta \bar{P}$) läßt sich nicht als arithmetisches Mittel der Anfangs- und Enddruckdifferenz ermitteln. Da das Druckgefälle längs der Lungencapillare nicht linear, sondern asymptotisch verläuft, muß die mittlere Druckdifferenz integriert werden. Auf diesem Wege erhielten Lilienthal und Riley (1946) für die Diffusionsfähigkeit der Lunge im Durchschnitt 21 cm^3/mm Hg/min in Ruhe und 60cm^3/mm Hg/min bei Arbeit. In der Größenordnung stimmen diese Werte mit denen von M. Krogh (1915), die Kohlenmonoxyd als Diffusionsgas verwandte, überein.

V. Die Beziehungen zwischen Durchblutung und Belüftung.

Unter gewöhnlichen Umständen ist die Blutmenge, die in der Zeiteinheit die Lunge durchströmt, der Belüftung des Alveolarraumes angeglichen. Nach Untersuchungen von Roughton (1945) befinden sich insgesamt jeweils 60 cm^3 Blut zur gleichen Zeit in den Lungencapillaren und sind dort für etwas weniger als 1 sec dem Gasaustausch ausgesetzt. Bei körperlicher Anstrengung erhöht sich die Blutmenge in den Capillaren durch Erweiterung des Strombettes auf 90 bis 100 cm^3. Gleichzeitig ist die Strömungsgeschwindigkeit erhöht, so daß die Verweildauer in den Capillaren nur etwa $1/_3$ sec beträgt. Es ist durchaus denkbar, daß bei weiterer Verkürzung der Verweildauer der Sauerstoffaustausch unvollständig wird.

Abgesehen von der allgemeinen Kreislaufinsuffizienz und spezieller Einschränkungen des Lungenkreislaufs durch Anomalien des Herzgefäßsystems kann eine Störung der normalen Belüftungs-Durchblutungsbeziehungen dadurch zustande kommen, daß ein Teil des Lungenblutes ohne mit den Atemgasen in Berührung gekommen zu sein, die Lunge wieder verläßt. In einem gewissen Ausmaß ist dieses vielleicht auch im Gesunden der Fall. Nach der Anlage des Lungengefäß-

---

[1] Bohr 1909, Barcroft 1927.
[2] Roughton 1944, Comroe 1944, Lilienthal 1946, Gladston 1947.

netzes[1] ist es denkbar, daß bis zu 15% des Pulmonalblutes durch arteriovenöse Anastomosen dem Gasaustausch entgehen können. Die großen individuellen Unterschiede in der normalen alveolar-arteriellen Sauerstoffdruckdifferenz sind vielleicht hierauf zurückzuführen. Im gleichen Sinne ist die Durchblutung von Lungenbezirken, die entweder atelektatisch oder von der Belüftung zeitweise ausgeschlossen sind hinsichtlich des Gasaustausches als Kreislaufkurzschluß zu bewerten. Andererseits ist eine starke Belüftung weniger durchbluteter Lungenabschnitte unzweckmäßig, da sich dies nur im Sinne einer Vergrößerung des respiratorischen Totraumes auswirkt. So scheint die Erhaltung eines Gleichgewichts zwischen Belüftung einerseits und Durchblutung andererseits in einer möglichst großen Anzahl von Alveolen eine wichtige Voraussetzung für die normale Atemfunktion darzustellen.

Wahrscheinlich wird dieses Gleichgewicht über den Sauerstoffdruck der Alveolarluft gesteuert. Verminderung des alveolaren Sauerstoffdruckes erhöht den Strömungswiderstand der Lungengefäße[2]. Da es sich dabei anscheinend um eine lokale Steuerung abgegrenzter Lungenbezirke handelt, wird auf diese Weise die Durchblutung von Alveolen mit niederem Sauerstoffdruck herabgesetzt und das Blut den besser belüfteten Lungenabschnitten zugeleitet[3].

Literatur.

ANTHONY, A. J.: Funktionsprüfung der Atmung. Leipzig: Johann Ambrosius Barth 1937. — ARMITAGE, G. H., and W. M. ARNOTT: Air distribution in the lung during hyperventilation. J. of Physiol. 109, 70 (1949). — ÅSTRAND, P. O.: Experimental studies of physical working capacity. Copenhagen: Munksgard 1952. — ATWELL, R. J., J. B. HICKAM, W. W. PRYOR and E. B. PAGE: Reduction of blood flow through the hypoxic lung. Amer. J. Physiol. 166, 37 (1951).

BARCROFT, J.: Die Atmungsfunktion des Blutes, Teil I. Berlin: Springer 1927. — BARTELS, H., E. BÜCHERL, C. W. HERTZ, G. RODEWALD und M. SCHWAB: Lungenfunktionsprüfungen. Methoden und Beispiele klinischer Anwendung. Berlin-Göttingen-Heidelberg: Springer 1959. — BATEMAN, J. B.: Studies of lung volume. J. Appl. Physiol. 3, 143 (1950) — BENZINGER, TH.: Untersuchungen über die Atmung und den Stoffwechsel. Erg. Physiol. 40, 1 (1938). — BIRATH, G.: Lung volume and ventilation efficiency. Acta med. scand. (Stockh.) Suppl. 154 (1944). — BOCK, A. V., D. B. DILL, H. T. EDWARDS, L. J. HENDERSON and J. H. TALBOTT: The partial pressure of oxygen and carbon dioxide in alveolar air and arterial blood. J. of Physiol. 68, 277 (1929). — BOHR, C.: Über die Lungenatmung. Skand. Arch. Physiol. (Berl. u. Lpz.) 2, 236 (1890). ~ Über die spezifische Tätigkeit der Lunge bei der respiratorischen Gasaufnahme. Skand. Arch. Physiol. (Berl. u. Lpz.) 22, 221 (1909). — BRAUS-ELZE: Anatomie des Menschen, Bd. I. Berlin: Springer 1921. — BURNS: Zit. nach LOVATT-EVANS, Principals of human physiology, 9. Aufl. London: J. a. A. Churchill 1945.

CLOETTA, M.: Untersuchungen über die Elastizität der Lunge. Pflügers Arch. 152, 339 (1913). — COMROE, J. H.: Methods in medical research, Bd. II. Chicago: Yearbook Publishers 1950. — COMROE, J. H., and R. D. DRIPPS: The oxygen tension of arterial blood and alveolar air. Amer. J. Physiol. 142, 700 (1944). — COMROE, J. H., and W. S. FOWLER: Detection of uneven alveolar ventilation. Amer. J. Med. 10, 408 (1951). — COURNAND, A.: Some aspects of the pulmonary circulation in normal man and in chronic cardiopulmonary diseases. Circulation (New York) 2, 647 (1950). — COURNAND, A., E. BALDWIN, R. C. DARLING and D. W. RICHARDS: Studies on intrapulmonary mixing. J. Clin. Invest. 20, 681 (1941). — COURNAND, A., and D. W. RICHARDS: Pulmonary insufficiency. I. Amer. Rev. Tbc. 44, 26 (1941).

DONDERS: Beiträge zur Mechanik der Respiration und Zirkulation. Z. rat. Med. 3, 1853).— DUBOIS, A. B., A. G. BRITT and W. O. FENN: Alveolar carbon dioxide during the respiratory cycle. J. Appl. Physiol. 4, 535 (1952).

ENGELHARDT, A.: Über den Verlauf der Entlüftung der Lunge bei reiner Sauerstoffatmung. Z. Biol. 99, 596 (1939). — EULER, U. v., u. G. LILJESTRAND: Observations on the pulmonary arterial blood pressure in the cat. Acta physiol. scand. (Stockh.) 12, 301 (1946).

FENN, W. O.: Mechanics of respiration. Amer. J. Med. 10, 77 (1951). — FENN, W. O., H. RAHN and A. B. OTIS: A theoretical study of the composition of alveolar air at altitude. Amer. J. Physiol. 140, 637 (1946). — FISHMAN, A. P.: Studies in man of the volume of the

[1] v. HAYEK 1953.
[2] v. EULER und LILJESTRAND 1946, COURNAND 1950, WESTCOTT u. a. 1951.
[3] RAHN und BAHNSON 1950, ATWELL u. a. 1951, PETERS und ROOS 1952.

respiratory deadspace and the composition of the alveolar gas. J. Clin. Invest. **33**, 469 (1954). — FLEISCH, A.: Die Pneumotachographie. In ABDERHALDENS Handbuch der biologischen Arbeitsmethode, Abt. V, Teil 8. 1925. ~ Neuere Ergebnisse über die Mechanik der Atmungsbewegungen. Erg. Physiol. **36**, 249 (1934). — FOWLER, W. S.: Uneven pulmonary ventilation. J. Appl. Physiol. **2**, 283 (1949).

GLADSTON, M., and A. C. WOLLACK: Oxygen and carbon dioxide tension of alveolar air and arterial blood. Amer. J. Physiol. **151**, 276 (1947). — GRAY, J. S.: Pulmonary ventilation and its regulation. Springfield, Illinois: Ch. C. Thomas 1950. — GRAY, J. S., D. R. BARNUM, H. W. MATHESON and S. N. SPIES: Ventilatory function tests I. Voluntary ventilation capacity. J. Clin. Invest. **29**, 677 (1949). — GROSSE-BROCKHOFF, F., u. W. SCHOEDEL: Der effektive schädliche Raum. Pflügers Arch. **238**, 213 (1936).

HALDANE, J. S.: The variations in the effective dead space in breathing. Am. J. Physiol. **38**, 20 (1915). — HATCH, TH., K. M. COOK and P. E. PALM: Respiratory deadspace. J. Appl. Physiol. **5**, 341 (1953). — HAYEK, H. V.: Über die Veränderlichkeit der Oberflächenspannung in den Alveolen und ihre Bedeutung für die Retraktionskraft der Lungen. Arch. exper. Path. u. Pharmakol. **214**, 266 (1952). ~ Die menschliche Lunge. Berlin: Springer 1953. — HERMANNSEN, J.: Maximale Ventilationsgröße (Atemgrenzwert). Z. exper. Med. **90**, 130 (1933). — HURTADO, A., and C. BOLLER: Studies of total pulmonary capacity. J. Clin. Invest. **12**, 793 (1933). — HUTCHINSON: Von der Kapazität der Lunge. Braunschweig: F. Vieweg & Sohn 1849.

JAMIN, F.: Zwerchfell und Atmung. In GROEDEL, Röntgendiagnostik, 3. Aufl. München 1921.

KILCHES, R.: Zur Frage der Retraktionskraft der Lunge. Klin. Wschr. **1940**, 695. — KROGH, A., and J. LINDHARD: Das Volumen des Totraumes der Atmung. J. of Physiol. **51**, 59 (1917). — KROGH, M.: Diffusion of gases through the lungs of man. J. of Physiol. **49**, 271 (1915).

LILIENTHAL, J. L., R. L. RILEY, D. D. PROEMMEL and R. E. FRANKE: Analysis of oxygen pressure gradient from alveolar air to arterial blood. Amer. J. Physiol. **147**, 199 (1946).

MALONEY, J. V., A. B. OTIS, W. O. FENN and J. L. WHITTENBERGER: The effect of positive pressure breathing on air flow resistance. J. Clin. Invest. **29**, 832 (1950). — MATHESON, H. W., and J. S. GRAY: Ventilatory function tests III. J. Clin. Invest. **29**, 688 (1950). — MUNDT, E., W. SCHOEDEL u. H. SCHWARZ: Über die Gleichmäßigkeit der Lungenbelüftung. Pflügers Arch. **244**, 99 (1940).

NEERGARD, K. V.: Neue Auffassungen über Atemmechanik. Z. exper. Med. **66**, 373 (1929). — NEERGARD, K. V., u. W. WIRZ: Über eine Methode zur Messung der Lungenelastizität. Z. klin. Med. **105**, 35 (1927).

OTIS, A. B., and W. C. BEMBOWER: Effect of gas density on resistance to respiratory gas flow in man. J. Appl. Physiol. **2**, 300 (1945). — OTIS, A. B., W. O. FENN and H. RAHN: Mechanics of breathing in man. J. Appl. Physiol. **2**, 592 (1950). — OTIS, A. B., and D. F. PROCTOR: Measurements of alveolar pressure. Amer. J. Physiol. **152**, 106 (1948).

PAPPENHEIMER, J. R.: Standardization of definitions and symbols in respiratory physiology. Federat. Proc. **9**, 602 (1950). — PAPPENHEIMER, J. R., A. D. FISHMAN and L. M. BORRERO: New experimental methods for determination of effective alveolar gas composition. J. Appl. Physiol. **4**, 855 (1952). — PETERS, R. M., and A. ROOS: Effect of unilateral nitrogen breathing upon pulmonary blood flow. Amer. J. Physiol. **171**, 250 (1952).

RAHN, H., and H. T. BAHNSON: Federat. Proc. **9**, 102 (1950). — RAHN, H., A. B. OTIS, L. E. CHADWICK and W. O. FENN: The pressure valume diagram of the thorax and lung. Amer. J. Physiol. **146**, 161 (1946). — RAUWERDA, P. E.: Unequal ventilation of different parts of the lung. Diss. Universität Groningen 1946. — ROELSEN, E.: Fraktionierte Alveolarluftanalyse. Diss. Copenhagen 1937. ~ Composition of alveolar air. Acta med. scand. (Stockh.) **98**, 141 (1939). — ROHRER, F.: Die Strömungswiderstände in den menschlichen Atemwegen. Pflügers Arch. **162**, 225 (1915). ~ Handbuch der normalen und pathologischen Physiologie, Bd. II, B/1. 1925. — ROSSIER, P. H., A. BÜHLMANN u. K. WIESINGER: Physiologie und Pathophysiologie der Atmung, 2. Aufl. Berlin-Göttingen-Heidelberg: Springer 1958. — ROUGHTON, F. J. W.: The average time spent by the blood in the human lung capillary. Amer. J. Physiol. **143**, 621 (1945). — ROUGHTON, F. J. W., R. C. DARLING and W. S. ROOT: Determination of oxygen capacity, content and pressure. Amer. J. Physiol. **142**, 708 (1944).

SCHOEDEL, W.: Die Alveolarluft. Erg. Physiol. **39**, 54 (1937).

VUILLEUMIER, P.: Über eine Methode zur Messung des intraalveolären Druckes und der Strömungswiderstände in den Atemwegen des Menschen. Z. klin. Med. **143**, 698 (1944).

WESTCOTT, R. N., N. O. FOWLER, R. C. SCOTT, V. D. HAUENSTEIN and J. McGUIRE: Anoxia and human pulmonary vascular resistance. J. Clin. Invest. **30**, 957 (1951). — WHITTENBERGER, J. L., S. J. SARNOFF and E. HARDENBERGH: Electrophrenic respiration. J. Clin. Invest. **28**, 124 (1949). — WICK, H.: Änderung der Lungenelastizität durch Kohlensäure. Arch. internat. pharmacodynamie **1952**. — WIRZ, K.: Das Verhalten des Druckes im Pleuraraum. Pflügers Arch. **199**, 1 (1923).

Die Atmungsregulation*.

Von

WOLF SCHOEDEL-Göttingen.

Mit 18 Abbildungen.

Atmungsregulation wäre ein recht komplexer Begriff, wenn darunter alle
regulatorischen Vorgänge fielen, die — wie es dem heutigen Gebrauch des Wortes
Atmung in der Physiologie entspricht — etwas mit der Regulation der Sauerstoffversorgung des Gewebes oder der des Kohlensäureabtransportes zu tun haben.
Üblicherweise wendet man ihn nur für die Regulation der Lungenbelüftung an.
Die Erfolgsorgane sind die quergestreifte „äußere" Atmungsmuskulatur, die
glatte Muskulatur der Lunge und der Luftwege und die Lungen- und Bronchialgefäße. Die Vorgänge an den Blutgefäßen und der glatten Muskulatur werden
besser in anderem Zusammenhang besprochen, so daß hier die regulatorischen
Vorgänge, die sich auf die äußeren Atemmuskeln auswirken, ganz im Vordergrund stehen.

Die Atmung sollte so eingestellt sein, daß das Blut in der Lunge optimal
arterialisiert wird. Das bedeutet, daß das Hämoglobin möglichst vollkommen mit
Sauerstoff aufgesättigt und der Kohlensäuredruck und die H-Ionen-Konzentration
auf einen optimalen Wert eingestellt werden. Die Atemarbeit sollte dabei möglichst klein gehalten sein, wobei es in erster Linie auf die richtige Einstellung der
Atemfrequenz und der Atemform ankommt. Die Einstellung der Atmung wird
häufig dadurch gestört, daß die Atemmuskulatur zu anderen Funktionen benötigt
wird, etwa wenn sie zu andersartiger Muskeltätigkeit herangezogen wird, oder
wenn der Atemstrom dem Sprechen oder Singen dient.

Der Vorgang der Atmungsregulation läßt sich sehr kurz folgendermaßen
beschreiben: Das Atemzentrum erhält nervöse oder über das Blut chemische
Antriebe aus der Peripherie. Das Ausmaß dieser Antriebe bestimmt den Ausfluß
der Erregungen zu den Erfolgsorganen, in erster Linie also zu den quergestreiften
Atemmuskeln. Die Abb. 1 gibt eine Übersicht über die wichtigsten afferenten
und efferenten Bahnen des im Rautenhirn gelegenen Atemzentrums. Dazu
kommen Einwirkungen durch Stoffe, die mit dem Blut an das Atemzentrum
herangebracht werden. Das Atemzentrum steht in den allermeisten Fällen gleichzeitig unter verschiedenen Antrieben. Die Kohlensäure des Blutes spielt dabei
recht häufig, aber durchaus nicht immer eine entscheidende Rolle. Sie wird von
manchen Autoren als adäquater Reiz der Atmung bezeichnet, ein Ausdruck,
dessen Wert bezweifelt werden kann.

Um die Verständigung zwischen den Naturwissenschaftlern zu erleichtern, bemühen sich
Mediziner und Biologen, auf die biologischen Regulationsvorgänge die Sprache der Regelungstechnik anzuwenden[1]. Es ist fraglich, ob dabei in jedem Fall der Biologie ihr Recht geschieht.
Physikalische und technische Systeme sind meistenteils gut abgrenzbar. Damit sind auch der
Regelkreis und seine Teile meist gut definiert. In der Physiologie ist die Abgrenzung des zu
betrachtenden Systems meist recht schwierig. Auch sind die Regelkreise häufig so miteinander „vermascht", daß es mühevoller Auseinandersetzungen bedarf, welche biologische

---

* Die Bearbeitung dieses Beitrages wurde am 8. 6. 1959 abgeschlossen.
[1] WAGNER 1954.

Regelung im einzelnen Fall betrachtet werden soll. In jedem Falle sollte man aber in der Regulationsphysiologie folgende Begriffe auseinanderhalten[1]:

1. Regelung. Der Wirkungsablauf ist geschlossen. Die Regelgröße wirkt auf den Regler, der Regler wirkt auf die Regelgröße zurück. Beispiel: Regelung des Kohlensäuredrucks im arteriellen Blut. Der Kohlensäuredruck im arteriellen Blut ist die Regelgröße. Veränderungen des arteriellen Kohlensäuredruckes wirken auf den Regler, den nervösen Apparat für die

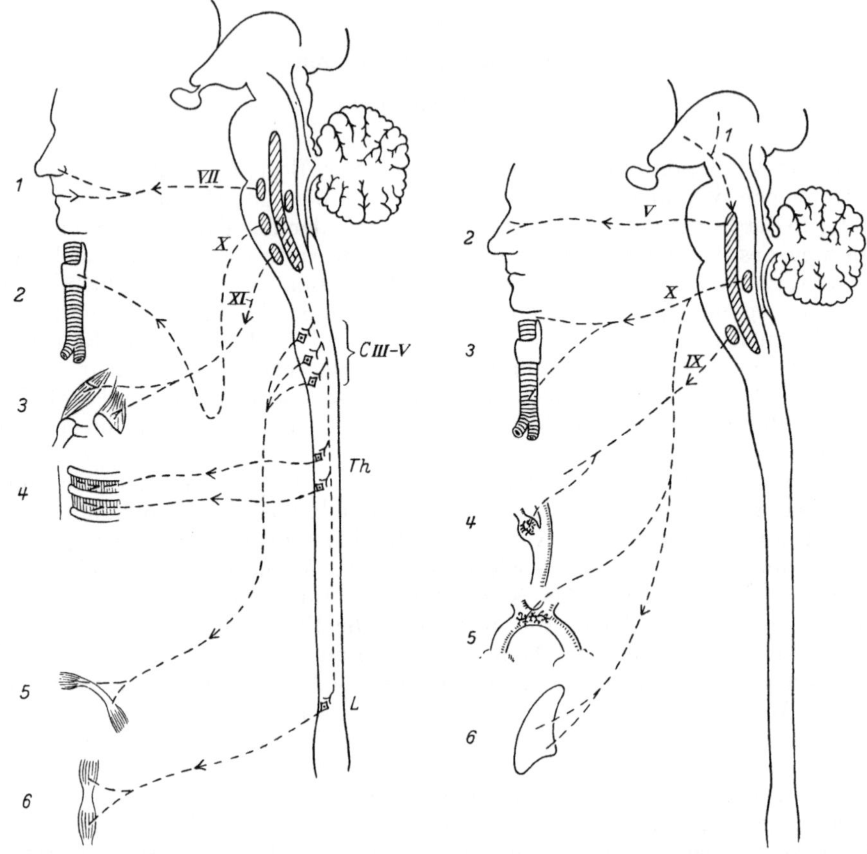

Abb. 1. Die wichtigsten afferenten und efferenten Bahnen des Atemzentrums. Efferente Bahnen (linkes Bild): *1* zu Nase und Mund; *2* zum Kehlkopf; *3* zur Halsmuskulatur; *4* zu den Intercostalmuskeln; *5* zum Zwerchfell; *6* zur Bauchmuskulatur. Afferente Bahnen (rechtes Bild): *1* von höheren Hirnabschnitten; *2* aus dem Trigeminusgebiet; *3* aus den oberen Luftwegen; *4* vom Carotis sinus; *5* vom Aortenbogen; *6* aus der Lunge. (In Anlehnung an H. F. Rein, Einführung in die Physiologie des Menschen, 10. Aufl. Berlin-Göttingen-Heidelberg 1949.)

Atmungsregelung ein. Dadurch wird die Lungenbelüftung geändert und die Einstellung der Regelgröße bestimmt.

2. Steuerung. Der Wirkungsablauf ist offen. Das gesteuerte System wirkt nicht auf das steuernde System zurück. Beispiel: Willkürliche Beeinflussung der Atmung von der Großhirnrinde aus.

3. Regulation oder Einstellung sind übergeordnete Begriffe, bei denen noch nicht festgelegt ist, ob es sich um Regelung oder um Steuerung handelt.

Die Angleichung an die Sprache der Regeltechniker führt zu einer teilweise ungewohnten Ausdrucksweise. Die äußere Atmung dient der Arterialisierung des Blutes. Im Sinne des Regeltechnikers geregelt wird dementsprechend diese Größe, d. h. Kohlensäuredruck, Sauerstoffdruck und p_H des arteriellen Blutes. Dagegen ist das Atemzeitvolumen als Stellgröße ein Teil des Reglers. Es ist nicht geregelt, sondern es regelt[2].

---

[1] Oppelt 1954.   [2] Winterstein 1953.

A. Die Einstellung des Atemvolumens.

I. Regelung der Arterialisierung.

1. Regelung des Kohlensäuredruckes.

Fordert man eine Versuchsperson auf, willkürlich ihre Atmung einzuschränken, so beobachtet man eine verstärkte Ausnutzung der Atemluft (Abb. 2). Atmet die Versuchsperson dann wieder „unwillkürlich", so steigt das Atemzeitvolumen zunächst über die Norm an und sinkt allmählich auf den Ausgangswert. Dabei geht es sehr weitgehend dem Kohlensäuregehalt der Ausatmungsluft parallel. Die Sauerstoffausnützung sinkt während der Mehratmungsphase unter die Norm, verhält sich also völlig anders wie das Atemvolumen. Unter den gegebenen Bedingungen ist man berechtigt anzunehmen, daß der alveolare und arterielle Kohlensäuredruck der Kohlensäurekonzentration in der Ausatmungsluft weitgehend parallel

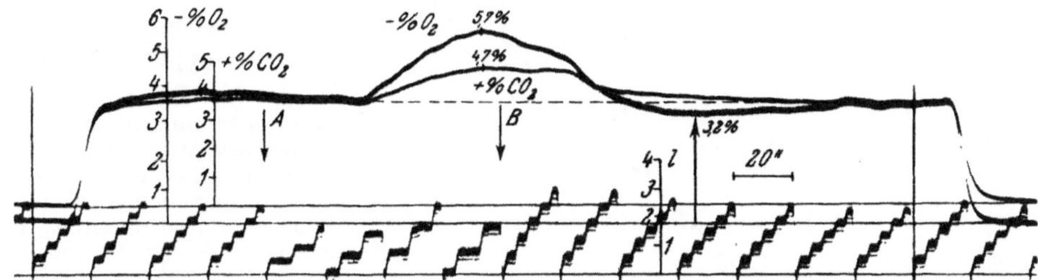

Abb. 2. Auswirkungen einer kurzdauernden willkürlichen Hypoventilation. Registrierung von Kohlensäuregehalt und Sauerstoffverarmung der Ausatmungsluft und des Atemvolumens (unterste treppenförmige Kurve, wobei jede Stufe einem Atemzug entspricht). Von A bis B wird willkürlich die Atmung eingeschränkt, wobei es zur stärkeren „Ausnutzung" der Atemluft kommt. Sobald bei B wieder unwillkürlich geatmet wird, steigt das Atemvolumen vorübergehend über den Ausgangswert an. Dabei zeigt es eine deutliche Beziehung zum Kohlensäuregehalt der Ausatmungsluft, nicht aber zum Sauerstoffgehalt. Die Regelung erfolgt in diesem Falle über die Kohlensäure. (Aus H. F. REIN, Einführung in die Physiologie des Menschen, 10. Aufl. Berlin-Göttingen-Heidelberg 1949.)

verläuft. Aus der Parallelität von Atemzeitvolumen und Kohlensäuregehalt kann man danach schließen, daß das Atemzeitvolumen so eingestellt wird, daß dadurch der arterielle Kohlensäuredruck geregelt wird. Dagegen besteht anscheinend in diesem Falle keine Regelung des arteriellen Sauerstoffdruckes.

Aus dem parallelen Verlauf von Atemzeitvolumen und arteriellem Kohlensäuredruck ist oft geschlossen worden, daß über das Atemzeitvolumen speziell der arterielle Kohlensäuredruck geregelt wird, damit umgekehrt der arterielle Kohlensäuredruck in erster Linie die Einstellung des Atemzeitvolumens bestimmt. Es könnte sich dabei um einen Proportionalregler handeln: Jede Erhöhung des arteriellen Kohlensäuredruckes führt über Meßwerk und Regler zu einer Steigerung des Atemzeitvolumens. Die erhöhte Ventilation läßt den alveolaren und arteriellen Kohlensäuredruck gegen den Sollwert hin abfallen, ohne daß dieser Wert vollkommen wieder erreicht wird. Bei der Proportionalregelung ist eine feste Beziehung zwischen Atemzeitvolumen und arteriellem Kohlensäuredruck zu erwarten. Dem erhöhten Kohlensäuredruck entspricht ein vergrößertes Atemvolumen, einem verminderten Kohlensäuredruck ein Absinken der Ventilation.

Abb. 3 zeigt die Beziehung zwischen dem alveolaren Kohlensäuredruck und der alveolaren Ventilation. Eine Steigerung des Kohlensäuredruckes von 40 mm Hg (Normalwert) auf 42,5 mm Hg genügt bereits, um die Ventilation zu verdoppeln[1]. Steigert man durch Zusatz von Kohlensäure zur Einatmungsluft den alveolaren Kohlensäuredruck auf 65 mm Hg, so kann man die Ventilation gegenüber dem Ruhewert etwa verzehnfachen. Diese Steigerung ist immer noch geringer als die bei Muskeltätigkeit. NIELSEN (1936) konnte durch Zusatz von CO_2 zur Einatmungsluft nur ein Atemvolumen von 60 Liter/min erreichen,

---

[1] HALDANE und PRIESTLEY 1905.

während die gleiche Versuchsperson bei Muskeltätigkeit 120 Liter/min atmete. Sinkt der alveolare Kohlensäuredruck unter 34 mm Hg, so hört von der Kohlensäureseite aus jeder Antrieb der Atmung auf. Es gibt also eine Schwelle für die Kohlensäureregelung[1]. Das Fortbestehen der Atmung hängt dann allein von anderen Antrieben, etwa von der Sauerstoffregelung ab.

Im Unterschied zum Sauerstoffmangel, der seine atmungssteigernde Wirkung über die peripheren Chemoreceptoren entfaltet, wirkt die Kohlensäure in erster Linie direkt auf das Atemzentrum. Nach Entnervung der Glomera an den Carotiden und der Aorta ist die Wirkung der Kohlensäure auf die Atmung kaum vermindert. Auch liegt der Kohlensäuredruck, mit dem man am isoliert durchströmten Glomus caroticum eine Atmungssteigerung erreicht, sehr hoch[2].

Es ist nicht unbedenklich, die Einstellung des Atemzeitvolumens auf eine einfache Proportionalregelung des arteriellen Kohlensäuredruckes zurückzuführen. Es sei auf folgende Punkte hingewiesen:

1. Bei einem Proportionalregler für den arteriellen Kohlensäuredruck sollte das Meßwerk die Regelgröße „arterieller Kohlensäuredruck" direkt messen. Für die Erregung der für die Atmung verantwortlichen Chemoreceptoren sind aber die chemischen Bedingungen im umgebenden Gewebe verantwortlich, die von denen im arteriellen Blute abweichen können (s. S. 301).

2. Der Regler ist durch Einflüsse, die von anderen Systemen ausgehen und kurz- oder langdauernd einwirken, „verstellbar". Sie führen dazu, daß die Beziehungen zwischen arteriellem

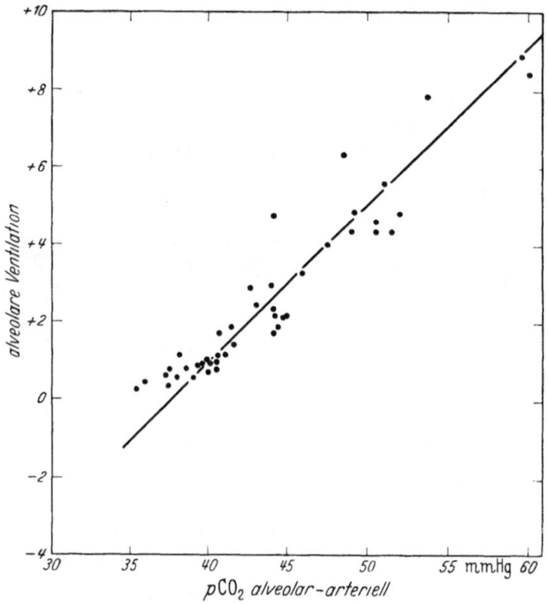

Abb. 3. Beziehung zwischen der alveolaren Ventilation (in „Normaleinheiten") und dem alveolaren bzw. arteriellen Kohlensäuredruck. Die eingezeichneten Punkte sind Mittelwerte von 10 Versuchspersonen, an denen 200 Einzelbestimmungen vorgenommen wurden. (Nach GRAY 1949.)

Kohlensäuredruck und Atemzeitvolumen sich ändern. Der Regler kann sogar völlig ausgeschaltet werden, etwa dann, wenn die Atemmuskulatur zu anderweitiger körperlicher Tätigkeit herangezogen wird. So läuft der Hundert-Meter-Läufer zumindest den ersten Teil seiner Strecke bei stillgestellter Atmung.

3. Die Lungenatmung dient der Arterialisierung des Blutes. Sie soll so eingestellt sein, daß der richtige Kohlensäuredruck, die volle Sauerstoffsättigung und die richtige H-Ionenkonzentration im arteriellen Blut zustande kommen. Es handelt sich also um 3 Stoffe, deren Konzentration gemessen wird und die die Funktion des Reglers beeinflussen. Solange eine feste Beziehung in der Änderung der 3 Konzentrationen im arteriellen Blut besteht, wie das weitgehend für Änderungen der Stoffwechselintensität gilt, kann es gleichgültig sein, durch welchen Stoff die Atmung eingestellt wird. Die Regelung bleibt trotzdem in Ordnung. Es gibt aber genügend Fälle, wo nur die Konzentration von einem oder zwei der 3 Stoffe verändert wird. Dann ist entscheidend, in welchem Ausmaß jeder der Stoffe an der Einstellung des Atemzeitvolumens beteiligt ist. Die Größe der Ventilation hängt dann von einem neuen Gleichgewicht aller 3 Stoffe im arteriellen Blut und ihrer Rückwirkung auf das Atemvolumen ab. So wird die atemsteigernde Wirkung des Sauerstoffmangels dadurch gedämpft, daß die erhöhte Atmung Kohlensäuredruck und H-Ionenkonzentration senkt. Möglichkeiten eines Antriebs der Atmung durch verschiedene „Regelvorgänge" zeigt Tabelle 1. Für die Atmungssteigerung bei Kohlensäurezusatz zur Einatmungsluft und bei Acidose wäre danach die

---

[1] NIELSEN und SMITH 1952, HALL 1953.　　[2] GOLLWITZER-MEIER und LERCHE 1940.

Steigerung des arteriellen Kohlensäuredruckes, bzw. der H-Ionenkonzentration verantwortlich zu machen. Die Atmungssteigerung im Sauerstoffmangel ist dagegen auf die Senkung des arteriellen Sauerstoffdruckes zurückzuführen. Schließlich kommt für die Mehratmung bei mäßiger Muskeltätigkeit keine der drei angeführten Veränderungen des arteriellen Blutes in Frage. Es greifen andere Faktoren von außen in die Regelkreise ein.

Tabelle 1. *Verhalten des arteriellen CO_2- und O_2-Druckes und der arteriellen H-Ionenkonzentration bei verschiedenen Formen der Hyperpnoe. (Nach* GRAY *1949.)*

Bedingungen	Maximale Ventilation Liter/min	Änderungen im arteriellen Blut		
		p_{O_2}	p_{CO_2}	H-Ionenkonz.
Anoxie.	12	gesenkt	gesenkt	gesenkt
CO_2-Einatmung	70	gesteigert	gesteigert	gesteigert
Acidose bei Stoffwechsel-störungen	35	gesteigert	gesenkt	gesteigert
Mäßige Muskeltätigkeit	50	unverändert	unverändert	unverändert
Schwere Muskeltätigkeit . . .	120	unverändert	gesenkt	gesteigert

4. Je nach den atemmechanischen Bedingungen ist das Stellglied des Reglers verschieden wirkungsvoll. Die gleiche Zahl von Impulsen, die vom Atemzentrum ausgesandt wird, hat nicht in jedem Falle den gleichen ventilatorischen Effekt. So wird etwa bei einem erhöhten Strömungswiderstand in den Luftwegen eine stärkere Aktivierung der Atemmuskulatur nötig sein, um ein hinreichendes Atemzeitvolumen zu erreichen. Der erhöhte Antrieb kann durch einen erhöhten arteriellen Kohlensäuredruck erreicht werden. Wir finden also bei schlechten atemmechanischen Bedingungen einen erhöhten arteriellen Kohlensäuredruck für ein entsprechendes Atemzeitvolumen.

2. Die Chemoreceptoren.

Seit der Entdeckung durch HEYMANS und HEYMANS (1924, 1927) wissen wir, daß ein Teil der Chemoreception für die Einstellung der Atmung gar nicht im Atemzentrum selbst, sondern in peripheren Receptoren zustande kommt. Man muß also zwei Arten des chemischen Antriebs der Atmung unterscheiden, den zentral-chemischen und den reflex-chemischen. Im ersten Falle findet die Chemoreception im Atemzentrum selbst statt, im zweiten Falle in peripher gelegenen Chemoreceptoren, von denen aus die Erregungen über afferente Bahnen das Atemzentrum erreichen.

Die wichtigsten peripheren Chemoreceptoren sind die in der Nachbarschaft des Aortenbogens und der Carotissinus (s. Abb. 4). Diese „branchiogene Reflexzone" gehört zu dem phylogenetisch älteren System der Atmungsregulation, das besonders auf Änderungen des Sauerstoffdruckes anspricht[1].

Neue Untersuchungen von LOESCHCKE u. Mitarb. (1958) machen es wahrscheinlich, daß die Atmung zusätzlich von Receptoren im Boden des vierten Hirnventrikels angetrieben wird.

Häufig ist behauptet worden, daß die Atmung auch noch von anderen Stellen her durch spezifische Chemoreceptoren gesteuert würde. So hat man besonders solche Receptoren im Bereich der Lunge vermutet[2], ohne daß hinreichende Beweise für diese Annahme erbracht werden konnten. Auch eine chemische Kontrolle vom Darmgebiet aus wurde diskutiert[3].

In jedem Falle sollte man unterscheiden, ob es sich um eine Atmungsänderung handelt, die auf eine Erregung spezifischer Receptoren durch die Regelgrößen Kohlensäure, Sauerstoff und H-Ionen zurückzuführen ist, oder ob irgendwelche Receptoren oder Schmerznerven durch andersartige Stoffe erregt werden. Auch in letzterem Falle kann es zu Änderungen der Atmung kommen. Hierher gehören die Atmungsänderungen, die nach Gaben von Veratrin-Derivaten beobachtet werden, wobei Receptoren im Herzen und in der Lunge erregt werden[4].

---

[1] KROGH 1941, Lit. bei WINTERSTEIN 1955.   [2] PI-SUÑER 1947.
[3] BEAN 1952.   [4] DAWES und COMROE 1954.

Durch operative Ausschaltung der peripheren Chemoreceptoren kann man das verschiedenartige Ansprechen des zentral-chemischen und reflex-chemischen Systems zeigen[1] (Abb. 5). Das zentral-chemische System spricht besonders auf Steigerung des arteriellen Kohlensäuredruckes an. Dagegen führt eine Senkung des arteriellen Sauerstoffdruckes zu einer Depression der zentralen Erregung. Für die Steigerung der Atmung bei Sauerstoffmangel sind besonders die peripheren Chemoreceptoren verantwortlich. Abnahme des p_H erregt das Zentrum. Bei einem starken Grad von Acidose kommt es aber auch zur Erregung der peripheren Receptoren (Abb. 6).

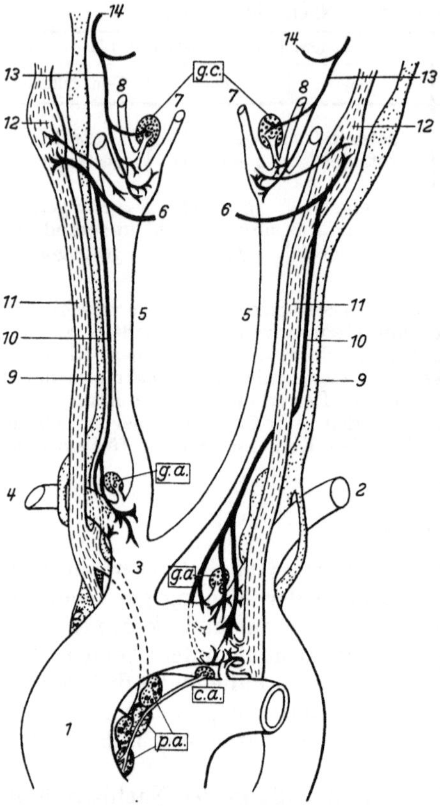

Abb. 7 zeigt die Beziehung zwischen dem arteriellen Sauerstoffdruck und der Zahl der Impulse, die in der Zeiteinheit von den Chemoreceptoren im Carotissinus ausgesandt werden[2]. Im Gegensatz zu älteren Untersuchungen[3] fand sich ein starkes Ansteigen der Impulsfrequenz, sobald der Sauerstoffdruck unter 110 Torr absank. Da er normalerweise bei 100 Torr liegt, müssen sich die peripheren Chemoreceptoren dann bereits im Zustand der Erregung befinden.

Abgesehen von der verschiedenen Ansprechbarkeit auf den CO_2- und den O_2-Druck gibt es noch weitere Unterschiede zwischen der zentral-chemischen und reflex-chemischen Regelung. Das jüngere zentral-chemische System hat die besseren Regeleigenschaften, das ältere ist resistenter gegen jede Art von Schädigungen. Das jüngere System wird schon durch kleine Änderungen im Blutchemismus angestoßen, das ältere ist besonders geeignet, in Notfällen die Regelung zu übernehmen, währen des unter orthologischen Bedingungen eine zwar deutlich nachweisbare, aber geringere Rolle spielt. Eine gute Regeleigenschaft des zentralen Systems ist besonders das Ansprechen auf sehr kleine Änderungen des Kohlensäuredruckes (s. S. 297). Die peripheren Chemoreceptoren sind diesem Reize gegenüber sehr viel weniger empfindlich[4]. Die peripher-chemische Steuerung zeigt den weiteren Nachteil, daß auf ihren Antrieb hin ungünstige Atemformen auftreten[5]. Die Resistenz der über die peripheren Chemoreceptoren wirkenden Regelung zeigt sich besonders bei Schädigung des Atemzentrums durch Narkotica. In diesem Falle wird die Atmung häufig allein

Abb. 4. Zur Lage und zur Innervation der peripheren Chemoreceptoren. Für die Chemoreception von Bedeutung: (*g.c.*) Glomera carotica; (*c.a.*) Corpusculum aorticum; (*p.a.*) Paraganglion aorticum supracardiale; (*g.a.*) Glomera aortica (Bedeutung für die Chemoreception angezweifelt). *1* Aorta; *2* A. subclavia sin.; *3* Truncus brachiocephalicus; *4* A. subclavia dextr.; *5* A. carotis comm.; *6* Sinus carotici; *7* A. carotis int.; *8* A. occipitalis; *9* N. sympathici; *10* Rami aortici n. vagi (N. depressores); *11* N. vagi; *12* Ggl. jugularia; *13* Rami carotici n. glossopharyngici; *14* N. glossopharyngici. (Nach DE CASTRO 1951.)

---

[1] SCHMIDT und COMROE 1940.   [2] WITZLEB und Mitarbeiter 1955.
[3] EULER, LILJESTRAND und ZOTTERMAN 1939.   [4] GOLLWITZER-MEIER und LERCHE 1940.
[5] BENZINGER, OPITZ und SCHOEDEL 1938, TSCHIRGI 1946.

über die peripheren Chemoreceptoren in Gang gehalten, wobei der Antrieb in erster Linie über den Sauerstoffmangel erfolgt[1].

Die Receptoren im Boden des 4. Ventrikels sprechen besonders auf Änderungen der H-Ionen-Konzentration an. Auch pharmakologisch reagieren sie

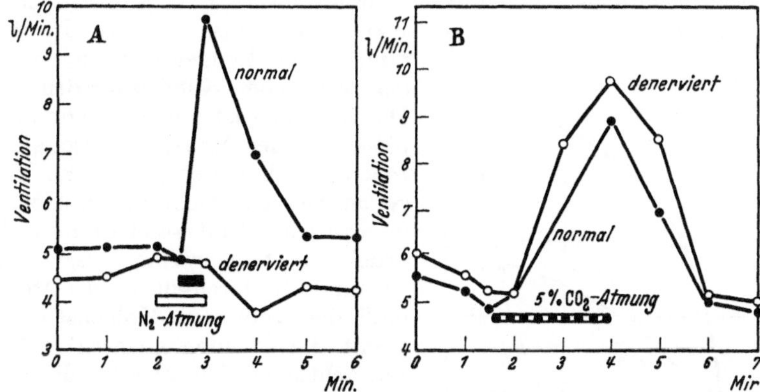

Abb. 5. Wirkung von Sauerstoffmangel (*A*) und Kohlensäureatmung (*B*) vor und nach Denervierung der peripheren Chemoreceptoren. Beachte die Atmungshemmung auf Stickstoffatmung nach Denervierung und die Unabhängigkeit der Atmungssteigerung auf Kohlensäure von der Intaktheit der peripheren Chemoreceptoren. (Nach GEMMILL und REEVES 1933.)

anders als die peripheren Chemoreceptoren im Bereich der großen Arterien. So werden sie durch Lobelin und Kaliumcyanid gehemmt, während diese Stoffe auf die peripheren Receptoren erregend wirken[2].

Das unterschiedliche Verhalten der zentralen und peripheren Chemoreceptoren auf Anreicherung von Kohlensäure und auf Sauerstoffmangel braucht nicht

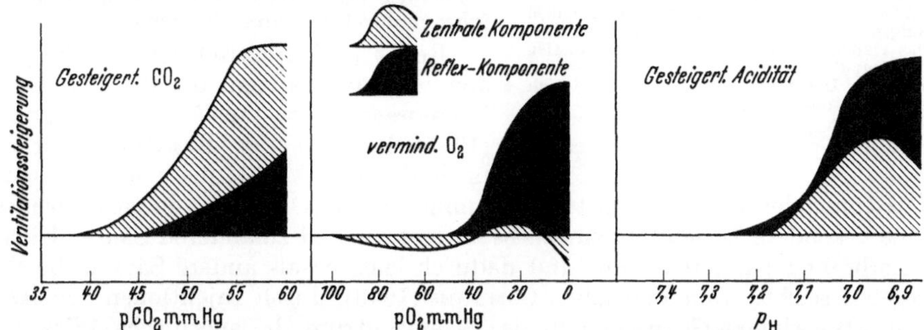

Abb. 6. Zentraler und reflektorischer Anteil der Atmungssteigerung durch Kohlensäure, Sauerstoffmangel und H-Ionenkonzentration. Abszissen: Kohlensäuredruck, Sauerstoffdruck und pH. Ordinate: Ventilationssteigerung bzw. Verminderung (SCHMIDT 1956).

unbedingt auf grundsätzlichen Unterschieden im Auslösungsvorgang der Erregung zu beruhen. Es kann auch durch ein anderes Verhältnis der Durchblutung der umgebenden Gewebe zu ihrem Stoffwechsel und durch verschiedene Diffusionsbedingungen für die erregenden Stoffe im Bereich der Receptoren hervorgerufen sein. Bei den peripheren Receptoren ist die Durchblutung so hoch, daß praktisch durch den Stoffwechsel der Receptoren die Blutbeschaffenheit nicht verändert wird. Damit wird die Reizung der Receptoren allein abhängig von der Beschaffenheit des arteriellen Blutes. Dagegen wird im Atemzentrum das Milieu sowohl von

---

[1] BENZINGER, OPITZ und SCHOEDEL 1938, COMROE und SCHMIDT 1938, KRAMER 1941, ÅSTRÖM 1952.

[2] LOESCHCKE und Mitarbeiter 1958.

der Beschaffenheit des arteriellen Blutes als auch vom lokalen Stoffwechsel bestimmt. Der arterielle Kohlensäuredruck ist also nicht unbedingt dem Kohlensäuredruck im Atemzentrum gleichzusetzen. Ist die Kohlensäurebildung im Zentrum gesteigert oder der Abtransport aus dem Zentrum durch verschlechterte Kohlensäurebindungsfähigkeit des Blutes erschwert, so vergrößern sich die Unterschiede zwischen arteriellem und zentralem Kohlensäuredruck. In diesem Falle nimmt die Lungenbelüftung zu, während der arterielle Kohlensäuredruck absinkt[1]. Die Regelung ist abhängig von den Verhältnissen an der Meßstelle, also am Orte der zentralen Chemoreception. Es wird strenggenommen gar nicht der Kohlensäuredruck im arteriellen Blut, sondern der Kohlensäuredruck im Atemzentrum geregelt. Auch eine verminderte Durchblutung des Atemzentrums muß den zentralen Kohlensäuredruck und damit die Atmung steigern[2]. Die gleichen Betrachtungen, die hier für die Kohlensäure angestellt wurden, gelten für die H-Ionenkonzentration[3].

LANDGREEN und NEIL (1951) vertreten die Auffassung, daß unter bestimmten Bedingungen auch der Gewebsstoffwechsel der peripheren Chemoreceptoren für den Antrieb der Atmung von Bedeutung ist. Nach Aderlässen konstringieren die zuführenden Arteriolen, so daß die Durchblutung stark gedrosselt ist. Das veränderte Verhältnis von Gewebsstoffwechsel und Durchblutung senkt den Sauerstoffdruck im Gewebe der Chemoreceptoren und führt dadurch zu ihrer Erregung.

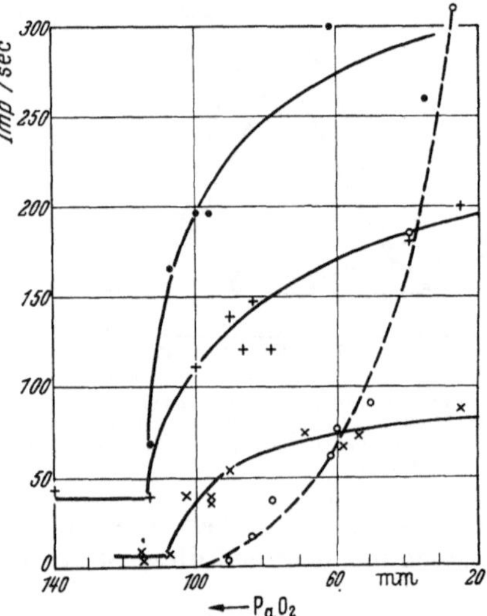

Abb. 7. Beziehung zwischen dem arteriellen Sauerstoffdruck und der Zahl der Impulse, die in der Zeiteinheit von den Chemoreceptoren im Carotis sinus ausgesandt werden. Alle drei aufgenommenen Kurven zeigen grundsätzlich das gleiche Verhalten. Der steilste Anstieg der Impulsfrequenz liegt zwischen 120 und 80 Torr. Die gestrichelte Kurve ergibt sich aus den von v. EULER, LILJESTRAND und ZOTTERMAN angegebenen Werten (WITZLEB u. Mitarb. 1955).

Recht problematisch ist die Frage nach den Grundvorgängen, die die Erregung der Chemoreceptoren auslösen. WINTERSTEIN (1955) hält an der Reaktionstheorie fest, nach der das Verhältnis von H-Ionen und OH-Ionen den Erregungszustand bestimmt. Dem CO_2 kommt danach nur insofern eine besondere Bedeutung zu, als es im Unterschied zu anderen Säuren leicht alle Membranen passieren kann und dadurch leichter als andere Säuren die Receptoren erreicht. Den Versuchen COMROEs (1943), durch Injektionen von Kohlensäure-Bicarbonat-Gemischen in das Atemzentrum die spezifische Wirkung des HCO_3-Ions auf die Receptoren nachzuweisen, erkennt WINTERSTEIN keine Beweiskraft zu. Auch die Frage, ob die Erregung der Chemoreceptoren an die Freisetzung von Acetylcholin gebunden ist, ist umstritten[4].

3. Die gleichzeitige Regelung des Kohlensäuredruckes, des Sauerstoffdruckes und der H-Ionen-Konzentration im arteriellen Blut.

Würden die drei genannten Größen sich in jedem Falle bei Umstellungen im Organismus gleichsinnig verändern, so genügte eine sehr einfache Regelung der Arterialisierung des Blutes. Sie könnte etwa allein über den arteriellen Kohlensäuredruck erfolgen. Es besteht aber häufig keine Parallelität im Verhalten der drei geregelten Größen bei den verschiedenen Arten von Belastungen, denen der

[1] LOESCHCKE 1949. [2] SCHMIDT 1956.
[3] WINTERSTEIN 1921, 1923, GESELL 1925. [4] WINTERSTEIN 1955.

Organismus ausgesetzt ist. Deshalb müssen alle drei geregelten Größen getrennt gemessen werden, und der Regler muß so funktionieren, daß er der Regelung aller drei Größen möglichst gerecht wird. Vereinfacht kann man sich vorstellen, daß unter normalen Bedingungen das Atemzentrum den arteriellen Kohlensäuredruck, die peripheren Chemoreceptoren in der Nähe der großen Arterien den arteriellen Sauerstoffdruck und die Receptoren im Boden des 3. Ventrikels die H-Ionen-Konzentration messen. In Wahrheit liegen die Verhältnisse insofern komplizierter, als die Erregung jeder der Receptorenarten von der Konzentration aller drei Stoffe abhängig ist, wobei aber jeweils einer der Stoffe einen überwiegenden Einfluß hat.

Zur Beurteilung der gleichzeitigen Einwirkung von Kohlensäuredruck, Sauerstoffdruck und H-Ionenkonzentration fand GRAY (1946, 1949) folgenden Ausdruck:

$$VR_{H, pCO_2, pO_2} = 0,22\,H + 0,262\,pCO_2 - 18 + 2,118 \cdot 10^{-8}(104 - pO_2)^{4,9}$$

(VR_H, p_{CO_2}, p_{O_2} ist die durch Sauerstoff- und Kohlensäuredruck sowie durch pH beeinflußte alveolare Ventilation in Normaleinheiten. p_{CO_2} und p_{O_2} sind Kohlensäure- und Sauerstoffdruck des arteriellen Blutes in mm Hg. H ist die H-Ionenkonzentration des arteriellen Blutes, ausgedrückt in 10^{-8} Mol je Liter. Danach entspricht pH $7,0 = 100$ H, und der Normalwert des arteriellen Blutes mit einem pH von 7,41 entspricht 38,9 H). Die Gesamtwirkung wird also als Summe der 3 Teilwirkungen aufgefaßt.

Die von GRAY gefundene Beziehung erlaubt für jeden Zustand des arteriellen Blutes das Atemvolumen abzuschätzen. Die Abb. 8 und 9 bringen dazu graphische Darstellungen. Abb. 8 läßt erkennen, daß bei stoffwechselbedingten Änderungen des pH die Ventilationsänderungen sehr viel stärker ausfallen würden, wenn nicht die Kohlensäure diesem Effekt entgegenwirkte. Ähnlich wird die atmungssteigernde Wirkung des Sauerstoffmangels weitgehend durch Gegenwirkungen von seiten der Kohlensäure und der H-Ionenkonzentration gehemmt (Abb. 9).

Bei den praktischen und teilweise auch theoretischen Gewinnen, die GRAYS Untersuchungen gebracht haben, ist nur schade, daß er nicht die Grenzen angibt, in denen seine Berechnungen allein Gültigkeit haben können. Wahrscheinlich war es auch nicht sehr glücklich, daß er den Ausdruck ,,Mehrfaktorentheorie'' der Atmungsregulation (multiple factor theory) einführte, wobei es sich ja in Wirklichkeit um eine ,,Summandentheorie'' handelt. Im übrigen sagt GRAYS ,,Theorie'' nichts aus über Angriffspunkte der Reize und Vorgänge im Zentrum, sondern

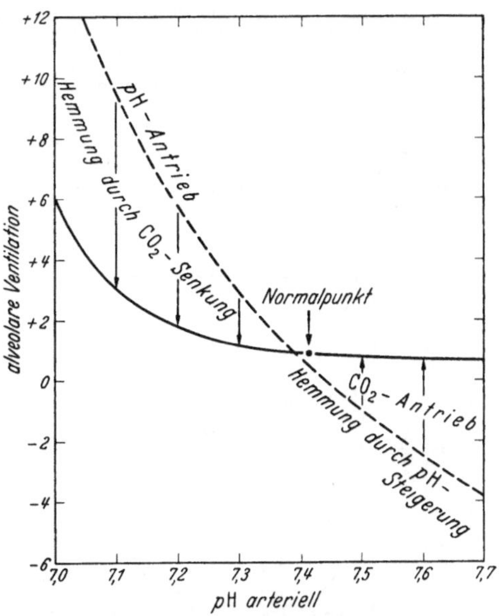

Abb. 8. Beziehung zwischen dem arteriellen pH und der alveolaren Ventilation (ausgedrückt in Einheiten der ,,normalen'' alveolaren Ventilation). Die ausgezogene Kurve entspricht den experimentell gefundenen Werten, die gestrichelte Linie den Werten, die zu erwarten wären, wenn nicht die veränderte Kohlensäurespannung der pH-Änderung entgegenwirkte. (Nach GRAY 1949.)

sie beschränkt sich auf die Aufstellung von Beziehungen zwischen dem Zustand des arteriellen Blutes und der Lungenventilation, also dem Anfangs- und Endpunkt der Reaktionskette bzw. zwischen Regelgrößen und Stellgröße des Regelkreises.

Will man einen genaueren Überblick über den gleichzeitigen Einfluß von alveolarem Kohlensäure- und Sauerstoffdruck auf die Einstellung der Atmung gewinnen, so muß man im Experiment jeweils eine der beiden Größen konstant halten und die andere variieren. Das gelingt durch die Verwendung geeigneter Gasgemische für die Beatmung der Versuchspersonen[1]. Abb. 10 und 11 zeigen

---

[1] CORMACK und Mitarbeiter 1957, LOESCHCKE und GERTZ 1958.

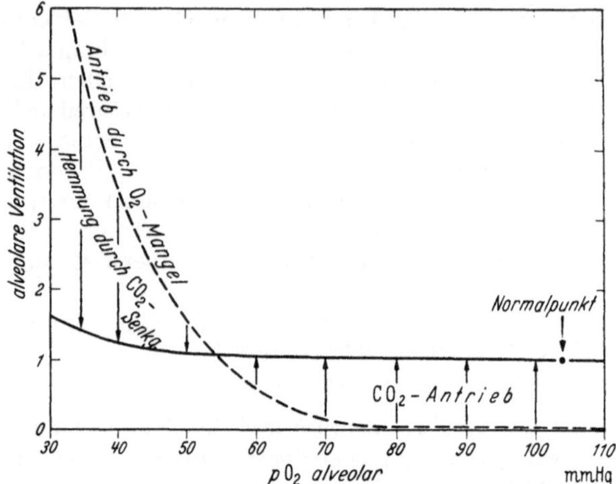

Abb. 9. Beziehung zwischen dem alveolaren Sauerstoffdruck und der alveolaren Ventilation (ausgedrückt in Einheiten der „normalen" alveolaren Ventilation). Die ausgezogene Kurve entspricht den experimentell gefundenen Werten, die gestrichelte Kurve den Werten, die zu erwarten wären, wenn nicht der veränderte Kohlensäuredruck und die veränderte H-Ionenkonzentration die Wirkung des Sauerstoffmangels beeinflußte. (Nach GRAY 1949.)

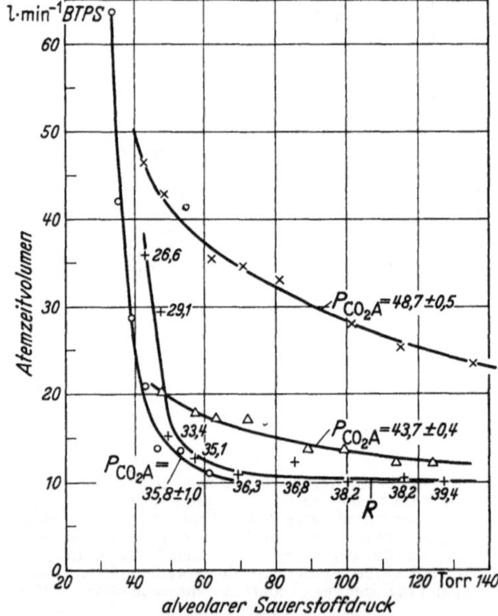

Abb. 10. Abhängigkeit des Atemzeitvolumens vom alveolaren Sauerstoffdruck bei Versuchsperson La. Drei Kurven mit reguliertem CO_2-Druck (35,8, 43,7 und 48,7 Torr) und ein Rückatmungsversuch ohne CO_2-Regulierung (R), bei dem die alveolaren Kohlensäuredrucke durch Zahlen angegeben sind (LOESCHCKE und GERTZ 1958).

die Ergebnisse solcher Untersuchungen. Daraus läßt sich folgendes ableiten:

1. Die Kohlensäure liefert nur einen sehr schwachen Antrieb für die Atmung, wenn der alveolare Kohlensäuredruck unterhalb 35 Torr liegt.

2. Der Einfluß des Sauerstoffdruckes ist gering, solange der alveolare Sauerstoffdruck über 100 Torr liegt. Das ist insofern eigentümlich, als die peripheren Chemoreceptoren schon sehr zahlreiche Impulse aussenden, wenn der arterielle Sauerstoffdruck unter 110 Torr absinkt (s. S. 300). Anscheinend kommt dabei eine Atmungssteigerung kaum zustande, weil der dadurch bedingte Kohlensäureverlust gleichzeitig den Kohlensäureantrieb vermindert.

3. Der Verlauf der Kurven (Abb. 10 und 11) macht es bis zu einem gewissen Grade wahrscheinlich, daß die Ruheatmung der Versuchspersonen nur zu einem Teil über die Kohlensäure und den Sauerstoffmangel angetrieben wird. Man könnte daran denken, daß die spontane Aktivität des Atemzentrums hierbei von Bedeutung ist (s. S. 317). Es könnte sich aber auch um zusätzliche Antriebe des Atemzentrums handeln, wobei an Einwirkungen der H-Ionenkonzentration auf Chemoreceptoren im Boden des 4. Ventrikels zu denken ist[1].

4. Oberhalb der CO_2-Schwelle ist der CO_2-Antrieb um so größer, je niedriger der Sauerstoffdruck ist[2]. Die einfache Annahme GRAYs, daß sich die beiden Antriebe einfach addieren, hat also streng genommen keine Gültigkeit.

Bei Atmung reinen Sauerstoffs findet man einen geringgradigen Anstieg des Atemzeitvolumens. Er beruht auf dem erschwerten Kohlensäureabtransport aus dem Atemzentrum bei hochgradiger Sauerstoffsättigung des Hb[3].

---

[1] LOESCHCKE und Mitarbeiter 1958. [2] NIELSEN und SMITH 1952.
[3] SHOCK und SOLEY 1940, HECK 1942, HECK und LOESCHCKE 1942; Literatur bei BAKER und HITCHCOCK 1957.

II. Beeinflussung der Atmung von anderen Systemen.

Die Größe der Lungenbelüftung wird in erster Linie von der Beschaffenheit des arteriellen Blutes bestimmt und sie wirkt andererseits auf die Beschaffenheit des arteriellen Blutes zurück. So weit handelt es sich also um eine Regelung. Aber die Einstellung der Ventilation hängt nicht allein von diesen Regelvorgängen ab. Häufig wird die Atmung von außen durch andere Systeme beeinflußt. Wenn aber von anderen Systemen her in den Ablauf der Atmung eingegriffen wird, so werden die Regelungsvorgänge eine Gegenwirkung entwickeln. Ein Beispiel hierfür zeigt Abb. 2. Die von der Großhirnrinde ausgelöste willkürliche Steigerung der Atmung senkt den Kohlensäuredruck. Dies führt zur nachträglichen Senkung des Atemvolumens. Die Regelung sorgt dafür, daß die Normalwerte wieder eingestellt werden. Wird die Atmung von außen beeinflußt, so wird dadurch die Zusammensetzung des arteriellen Blutes verändert. Das führt zur Auslösung von Regelvorgängen, die auch bei Fortbestehen des äußeren Einflusses ihn abschwächen.

Anscheinend kann durch Erregung fast sämtlicher peripherer Receptoren wie auch durch Veränderungen im Erregungsablauf des Zentralnervensystems an irgendeiner Stelle außerhalb des Atemzentrums die Atmung beeinflußt werden. Die Erregungsänderung muß nur stark genug sein, daß sie in ihrer Ausstrahlung das Atemzentrum erreicht. Die Atmungsänderungen betreffen dabei freilich recht häufig in stärkerem Maße die Atemform als das Atemvolumen. Häufig sind die Änderungen auch recht kurzdauernd und beeinflussen nur einen oder nur wenige Atemzüge. Bei Erregungen, die von peripheren Receptoren ausgehen, handelt es sich häufig nicht um direkte Einwirkungen auf das Atemzentrum, sondern es werden zunächst höhere Zentren beeinflußt, die dann auf das Atemzentrum rückwirken.

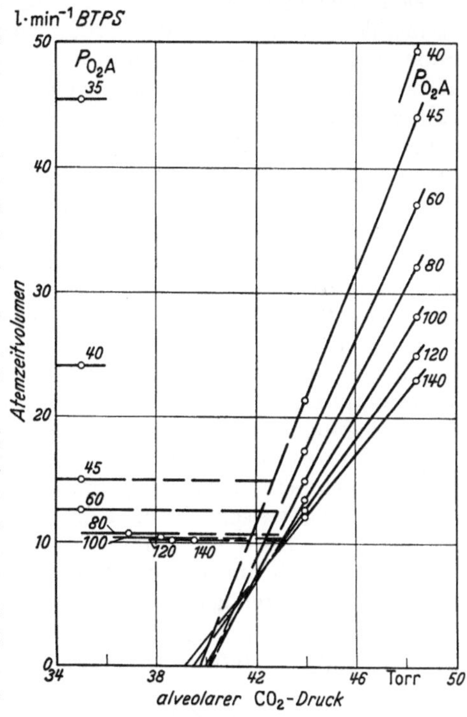

Abb. 11. Abhängigkeit des Atemzeitvolumens vom alveolaren CO₂-Druck für variable Sauerstoffdrucke bei Versuchsperson La. Die horizontale Linienziehung im Bereich niedriger alveolarer CO₂-Drucke ist willkürlich. Die experimentellen Daten sind auch mit Linien verträglich, die mit höheren CO₂-Drucken flach ansteigen (LOESCHCKE und GERTZ 1958).

Recht starke und für die Größe des Atemvolumens wichtige Einflüsse gehen vom Hypothalamus aus[1]. Von einer ganzen Reihe von Rindenfeldern, besonders im Bereich des Stirnhirns, läßt sich die Atmung verändern[2]. Dabei handelt es sich weniger um Einflüsse, die die Atmung für längere Zeit hemmen oder fördern, sondern um Schaltungen, die die Atmung mit anderen motorischen Vorgängen koordinieren, wie das im hohen Maß beim Sprechen, aber auch bei Bewegungen des Rumpfes und der Extremitäten notwendig ist. Im allgemeinen geht ein erhöhter Erregungszustand des Zentralnervensystems mit

---

[1] HESS 1948.
[2] SMITH 1938, SPEAKMAN und BABKIN 1949, HESS u. a. 1951.

einer gesteigerten Atmung einher. Bei psychischer Erregung findet man ein erhöhtes Atemvolumen und einen verminderten alveolaren Kohlensäuredruck. In der Nacht ist der alveolare Kohlensäuredruck erhöht. Dabei ist die Änderung der Atmung nicht allein durch den Übergang vom Wachen zum Schlafen bedingt[1], sie folgt auch bestimmten Tagesrhythmen[2].

Die Atmung kann von außen her nicht nur im fördernden, sondern auch im hemmenden Sinne beeinflußt werden. Insbesondere kann sie stillgelegt werden, bis sich auch hier wieder die Regelung von den Blutgasen her durchsetzt. Der Atemstillstand kann von der Großhirnrinde ausgelöst werden, etwa im Zustand erhöhter Aufmerksamkeit oder bei bestimmten motorischen Leistungen. Ein charakteristisches Beispiel hierfür ist das meist vollkommene Fehlen der Atmung während eines 100 m-Laufes. Verständlich sind die Atemstillstände, die von den Receptoren der Luftwege ausgelöst werden. Die Lunge wird auf diese Weise vor dem Eindringen schädlicher Stoffe geschützt. In enger Beziehung zu diesen reflektorischen Atemstillständen stehen Schutzreflexe wie Husten und Niesen, bei denen an Stelle des geregelten Atemvorganges eine ganz andere Form der Betätigung der Atemmuskulatur tritt. In ihrer physiologischen Bedeutung noch völlig undurchsichtig sind Atemstillstände, die von Receptoren in der Lunge und in der Herzmuskulatur ihren Ursprung nehmen. Bisher ist es nur gelungen, diese Reflexe durch körperfremde Stoffe (Veratrine, Amidine) auszulösen[3]. Tauchende Tiere können die Atmung sehr lange anhalten. Ihr Atemzentrum ist wenig empfindlich gegen Kohlensäure und wohl auch gegen Sauerstoffmangel[4]. Die Stillegung der Atmung während des Tauchens wird aber auch durch Reflexe unterstützt, die an den Öffnungen der Atemwege, d. h. an Mund und Nase, ihren Ausgang nehmen. Derartige Reflexe lassen sich eigentümlicherweise auch beim Menschen nachweisen. Taucht eine Versuchsperson das Gesicht in ein Waschbecken, so kann sie die Atmung sehr viel länger anhalten, als das sonst möglich ist. Es muß sich um hemmende Einflüsse handeln, die über den Trigeminus das Atemzentrum erreichen[5].

Von besonderer Bedeutung sind Einflüsse auf die Atmung von seiten des Blutkreislaufs (S. 306), der Temperaturregulation (S. 307) und der Motorik (S. 307).

1. Kreislauf und Atmungsregulation.

Wenn man unter Atmung, wie das heute meist in der Physiologie geschieht, die Gewebsatmung versteht, dann wird der Blutkreislauf zu einem Teil des Atmungsapparates. Dies zeigt die enge Verknüpfung der beiden Funktionen. Jeder Steigerung des Herzzeitvolumens sollte eine solche des Atemzeitvolumens entsprechen. Sehr weitgehend wird die Parallelität dadurch gewahrt, daß die Zentren der beiden Funktionen durch die gleichen Vorgänge angetrieben werden[6]. Dies gilt für die zentrale Wirkung des arteriellen Kohlensäuredruckes und die Wirkung des arteriellen Sauerstoffdruckes auf die peripheren Chemoreceptoren. Auch die Pressoreceptoren im Thoraxraum und am Carotissinus wirken auf den Kreislauf und die Atmung gleichzeitig ein[7]. Die von den Pressoreceptoren ausgelösten Reflexe erklären zum Teil das Verhalten der Atmung bei Kreislaufkrankheiten. Für die Atmungssteigerung bei Muskeltätigkeit dürften sie von untergeordneter Bedeutung sein[8].

<hr>

[1] Literatur bei WINTERSTEIN 1955, ROBIN u. a. 1958.
[2] MILLS 1953.   [3] DAWES und COMROE 1954.
[4] IRVING 1939.   [5] EBBECKE 1944.   [6] REIN 1935.
[7] DAWES und COMROE 1954, AVIADO und SCHMIDT 1955.   [8] AVIADO u. a. 1951.

2. Temperaturregulation und Atmung.

Bei einer Reihe von Tieren, besonders beim Hund, ist Steigerung der Atmung ein wichtiger Vorgang der Temperaturregulation. Beim Hecheln wird in erster Linie die Atemfrequenz gesteigert und die Atemtiefe eher herabgesetzt. Die Folge ist eine relativ niedrige alveoläre Ventilation bei hohem Atemzeitvolumen. Dadurch ist die Ausnützung der Atemluft gering, und der Organismus verliert verhältnismäßig wenig von seinem Kohlensäurevorrat. Das Hecheln wird vom Temperaturregulationszentrum im Hypothalamus ausgelöst, das über Schaltstellen in der Brücke das Atemzentrum beeinflußt[1].

Auch beim Menschen ist bei Hyperthermie das Atemvolumen gesteigert und der alveolare Kohlensäuredruck vermindert[2]. Diese Veränderungen dürften zum Teil über das Temperaturregulationszentrum zustande kommen. Von dieser Wirkung sind andere thermische Einflüsse auf die Atmung abzutrennen. So wirkt starke Kälte oder Wärme unter Umständen über die Erregung der Schmerznerven von der Körperoberfläche. Beim Fieber beruhen die Atmungsänderungen teils auf Umstellungen im hypothalamischen Temperaturregulationszentrum, teils sind sie Folge der erhöhten Gewebsatmung.

3. Muskeltätigkeit und Atmungsregulation.

Abb. 12 zeigt die Beziehung zwischen Sauerstoffverbrauch und Atemzeitvolumen bei Muskeltätigkeit des Menschen. Solange die Arbeiten nicht sehr schwer sind, ist das Atemzeitvolumen dem Sauerstoffverbrauch proportional. Ähnliche Beziehungen zwischen den beiden Größen finden sich auch am trainierten Hund. Sie finden sich auch dann, wenn die Muskeltätigkeit bei Mensch oder Tier durch elektrische Reizung hervorgerufen wurde. Im letzteren Falle bleiben sie auch bestehen, wenn das Tier narkotisiert ist. Steigert man im Tierversuch den Stoffwechsel durch Dinitrophenol, so findet man ebenfalls die gleichen Beziehungen[3].

Es liegt die Annahme nahe, daß bei erhöhtem Gewebsstoffwechsel das Blut in der Lunge nicht mehr hinreichend arterialisiert wird, und daß auf diesem Wege die Steigerung der Atmung zustande kommt. In der Tat findet man bei leichter Muskeltätigkeit häufig einen Anstieg des arteriellen Kohlensäuredruckes. Bei sehr schwerer Muskeltätigkeit steigt nicht selten die arterielle H-Ionen-Konzentration an. In nicht ganz wenigen Fällen findet man auch eine Senkung des arteriellen Sauerstoffdruckes. Andererseits kann besonders bei mäßiger Arbeit häufig keiner der „geregelten" Faktoren im arteriellen Blut für die Mehratmung verantwortlich gemacht werden. In den seltensten Fällen reicht jedenfalls das Ausmaß der Veränderung der „geregelten" Größen aus, um die sehr großen Steigerungen des Atemzeitvolumens zu erklären. Es müssen weitere antreibende Faktoren an der Steigerung des Atemzeitvolumens bei Muskeltätigkeit beteiligt sein. Es gibt sehr viele Faktoren, die dafür verantwortlich gemacht werden. Wahrscheinlich handelt es sich nicht um eine einzige Antriebsart. Es dürften recht verschiedene Antriebe sein, die je nach der Art der Muskeltätigkeit einzeln oder meistens kombiniert wirksam werden[4].

Fast jeder Vorgang, der die Atmung antreibt, kann auch an der Arbeitshyperpnoe beteiligt sein. SCHMIDT (1955) bespricht eingehend die vielen Faktoren, die an der Mehratmung bei Muskeltätigkeit beteiligt sein können. Hier sei nur kurz auf folgende Punkte eingegangen:

---

[1] HICSTAND und RANDALL 1942, HESS und STOLL 1944.
[2] CUNNINGHAM und O'RIORDAN 1957; Literatur bei WINTERSTEIN 1955.
[3] RAMSAY 1959.   [4] GRAY 1949, GRODINS 1950, SCHMIDT 1956.

1. Zentraler Antrieb von der Großhirnrinde her. KROGH u. LINDHARD äußerten bereits 1913 die Ansicht, daß das Atemzentrum bei Muskeltätigkeit von der Großhirnrinde her im Sinne einer Mitinnervation angetrieben werden könnte. Das sollte besonders im Beginn der Muskeltätigkeit von Bedeutung sein. Seitdem ist eine Reihe von Arbeiten erschienen, in denen eine Steigerung der Atmung bei elektrischer Reizung von Rindenfeldern gezeigt wurde. Dabei weichen jedoch im allgemeinen die Atemformen sehr stark von denen ab, die bei Muskeltätigkeit beobachtet werden. Wenn es gelänge, durch eine entsprechende elektrische Reizung im Bereich der Großhirnrinde eine Atmung zu erzeugen, die der Arbeits-hyperpnoe ihrer Form nach gleicht, so würde dies sehr für die Hypothese des zentralen Antriebs sprechen. Die Hypothese paßt gut in unsere heutigen Vorstellungen über die Funktion des Zentralnervensystems. Sie hat eine Parallele zur Kreislaufphysiologie, wo man ebenfalls an eine Umstellung des Kreislaufs im Beginn der Arbeit von der Großhirnrinde aus denken muß. Eine Stütze der Hypothese vom zentralen Antrieb stellen neuere Untersuchungen mit leichter Curaresierung der Versuchspersonen dar[1]: Der erhöhte motorische Antrieb, der in diesem Falle für die Leistung einer Beinarbeit von der Versuchsperson aufgebracht werden mußte, führte auch zu einem stärkeren Antrieb der Atmung als vor der Curaresierung. Zentral-motorischer Antrieb der Skeletmuskulatur und Atmungssteigerung gingen also parallel. Gegen die Bedeutung des zentralen Antriebs sprechen bis zu einem gewissen Grade Untersuchungen mit elektrischer Reizung der Beinmuskulatur, bei der im ganzen Verlauf der Muskeltätigkeit, also auch im Beginn und am Ende, die Atmung sich völlig gleich verhielt wie bei der willkürlichen Muskelarbeit[2].

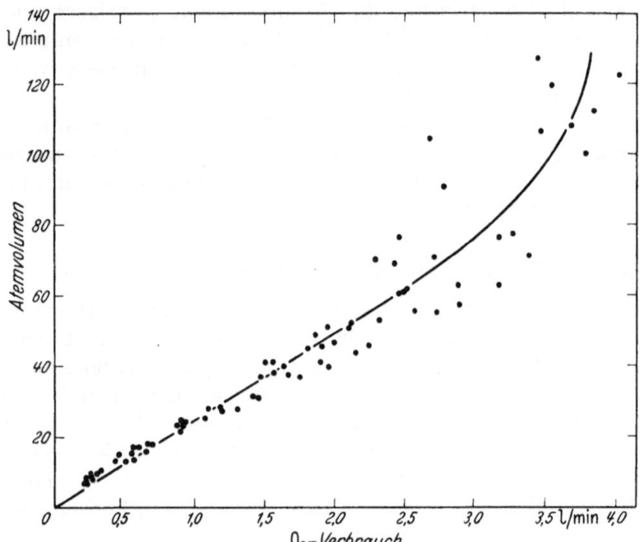

Abb. 12. Beziehung zwischen Atemvolumen und Sauerstoffverbrauch bei Beinarbeit (Gehen, Rennen, Radfahren). 611 Beobachtungen an 86 Versuchspersonen. (Nach GRODINS 1950.)

2. Antriebe, die vom Bewegungsapparat ausgehen. Dafür sprechen folgende Experimente.

a) Bringt man die Beinmuskulatur von Versuchspersonen durch elektrische Reizung in Tätigkeit, so erhält man die gleiche Atmungssteigerung wie bei Spontanbewegung[3].

b) Unterbindet man bei willkürlicher Muskeltätigkeit Blutzustrom und Blutabstrom zu den arbeitenden Extremitäten der Versuchsperson, so erhält man die gleiche Atmungssteigerung wie bei freigegebener Durchblutung[4].

Diese Befunde wurden durch Tierexperimente gestützt.

---

[1] OCHWADT und Mitarbeiter 1959.   [2] ASMUSSEN und NIELSEN 1948.
[3] ASMUSSEN, NIELSEN, WIETH-PEDERSEN 1943, ASMUSSEN und NIELSEN 1948.
[4] ASMUSSEN, CHRISTENSEN und NIELSEN 1943.

c) Bei kreuzweiser Kopfdurchblutung löst das Atemzentrum, das nur nervös mit der arbeitenden Muskulatur in Verbindung steht, die gleiche Atmungssteigerung aus wie im Kontrollversuch[1].

Gegen alle diese Versuche läßt sich der Einwand erheben, daß durch den experimentellen Eingriff der elektrischen Reizung oder durch unzureichende Blutversorgung unspezifische Receptoren oder Schmerznerven erregt werden, die die Atmung antreiben, ohne daß dieser Antrieb unter normalen Bedingungen von Bedeutung wäre. Jedoch ist die gute Übereinstimmung im Ausmaß der Atmungssteigerung in allen diesen Experimenten auffallend.

Die angeführten Untersuchungen lassen es unwahrscheinlich erscheinen, daß spezifische chemische Stoffe, die aus der tätigen Muskulatur stammen und das Atemzentrum mit dem Blut erreichen, die Atmung steigern. ASMUSSEN und NIELSEN (1946, 1950) nehmen freilich an, daß bei sehr schwerer Muskeltätigkeit von der Muskulatur auch spezifisch atmungssteigernde Stoffe in das Blut abgegeben werden. Im allgemeinen denkt man aber an nervöse Impulse, die von Chemoreceptoren oder Mechanoreceptoren ausgehen. Für letztere spricht die Atmungssteigerung, die bei passiver Bewegung der Gliedmaßen beobachtet wird. Dabei bleibt es freilich zweifelhaft, ob der Antrieb ausreichend ist, um auch nur einen beachtlichen Anteil für die Arbeitsmehratmung zu liefern, und ob es sich nicht auch bei diesen Experimenten teilweise um Erregung von Schmerznerven handelt. Bei den für die Atmungssteigerung verantwortlichen Mechanoreceptoren soll es sich nicht um solche in den Muskeln und in den Sehnen handeln, sie sollen vielmehr in den Gelenken liegen[2].

3. Antriebe, die durch Druckänderungen im Gefäßsystem zustande kommen. Ein recht großer Teil der Receptoren des Blutkreislaufs beeinflußt gleichzeitig die Atmung[3]. Das gilt besonders für die Receptoren im arteriellen Bereich. Arterielle Drucksenkungen lösen Atmungssteigerungen aus. An diesem Vorgang sind nicht nur die Pressoreceptoren, sondern auch die Chemoreceptoren im Bereich des Carotissinus und des Aortenbogens beteiligt. In den freilich sehr seltenen Fällen, in denen bei Muskeltätigkeit der arterielle Druck absinkt, wird also auf dem Weg über die arteriellen Receptoren die Atmung angetrieben werden. Vielleicht sind die Receptoren im Niederdrucksystem des Blutkreislaufs für die Einstellung der Atmung bei Muskeltätigkeit von größerer Bedeutung. Hier führt im allgemeinen ein Anstieg des Druckes und der Blutfüllung zu einer Atmungssteigerung über die langsam adaptierenden Dehnungsreceptoren der Lunge[4]. Die stärkere Blutfüllung der Lungengefäße bei Muskeltätigkeit könnte recht häufig einen zusätzlichen Antrieb für die Atmung ergeben[5].

4. Antriebe über Temperaturänderungen. Bei körperlicher Arbeit steigt nicht nur die Gewebstemperatur im arbeitenden Muskel[6], sondern auch die Rectaltemperatur[7] an. Die Temperaturanstiege sind aber im allgemeinen zu gering, als daß sie für das Zustandekommen einer Arbeitshyperpnoe von entscheidender Bedeutung sein könnten[8].

Wir müssen annehmen, daß fast in jedem Falle nicht ein einzelner Faktor, sondern viele Faktoren für das Zustandekommen der Arbeitshyperpnoe verantwortlich sind. Dabei kann die Art der Faktoren und ihre Bedeutung von Fall zu Fall je nach der Form der Muskeltätigkeit verschieden sein. Das macht eine quantitative Lösung des Problems der Arbeitshyperpnoe fast unmöglich.

---

[1] KAO 1956.   [2] COMROE und SCHMIDT 1943.
[3] AVIADO und SCHMIDT 1955.   [4] COSTANTIN 1959.
[5] MITCHELL und Mitarbeiter 1958.   [6] MORGAN und Mitarbeiter 1955.
[7] NIELSEN 1938.   [8] GRODINS 1950.

III. Die Anpassung der Lungenatmung an veränderte Bedingungen.

Man bezeichnet gern als Einstellung einen rasch verlaufenden, als Anpassung einen langsam verlaufenden regulatorischen Vorgang. Der klassische Fall der Anpassung der Lungenbelüftung ist der an langdauernden Sauerstoffmangel. Wie bei der Einstellung so kommt es auch bei der Anpassung darauf an, eine möglichst gute Arterialisierung des Blutes zu erreichen. Im Sauerstoffmangel sollte also durch eine Atmungssteigerung die Sauerstoffsättigung des arteriellen Blutes trotz des erniedrigten Sauerstoffdruckes der Einatmungsluft hochgehalten werden, ohne daß es dabei zu zu starken Kohlensäureverlusten und Verschiebungen der H-Ionen-Konzentration käme. Anpassungsvorgänge der Lungenatmung müssen besonders für den Bereich der Pathophysiologie eine große Bedeutung haben. Manche Autoren sprechen davon, daß sich die Empfindlichkeit des Atemzentrums unter solchen Bedingungen verändert. Es sind häufig die gleichen Autoren, die der Kohlensäure unter den Atemreizen eine besondere Stellung einräumen, indem sie sie als den adäquaten Atemreiz bezeichnen. Wenn wir heute im allgemeinen die Kohlensäure als einen zwar sehr wichtigen, aber doch nur einen von vielen Antrieben für die Atmung ansehen, so ist damit in stärkerem Maße zu prüfen, wie weitgehend andere Antriebe in solchen Fällen verändert sind. Prüft man die Empfindlichkeit des Atemzentrums gegen Kohlensäure, indem man planmäßig den Kohlensäuredruck verändert und dabei den Anstieg der Ventilation mißt, so findet man, daß sie häufig in gleichem Sinne wie der Ventilationsgrad verändert ist. Dabei kann es sich aber darum handeln, daß sehr häufig die Atmungsantriebe sich nicht einfach addieren, sondern daß der Gesamteffekt größer ist als die Summe der Einzelantriebe (s. S. 304). Eine Änderung der Erregbarkeit des Atemzentrums gegen Kohlensäure sagt aus diesem Grunde nicht allzuviel über den Mechanismus der Atmungsanpassung aus. Wahrscheinlich gibt es sehr viele Ursachen, die zu einer langdauernden veränderten Atmungseinstellung führen. Hier sei besonders auf zwei Faktoren hingewiesen: 1. die Veränderung in den atemmechanischen Bedingungen, 2. Verschiebungen im Säure-Basengleichgewicht.

In Krankheitsfällen sind sehr häufig die *atemmechanischen Bedingungen* verändert. Häufig sind Fälle mit erhöhtem Atemwiderstand. Das kann den elastischen oder viscösen Gewebswiderstand oder auch den Strömungswiderstand in den Luftwegen betreffen. Bei erhöhtem Atemwiderstand liefert eine bestimmte Anzahl von Impulsen, die vom Atemzentrum ausgesandt werden, eine kleinere Ventilation. Der dadurch bedingte Anstieg des Kohlensäuredrucks treibt das Atemzentrum an, es stellt sich ein neues Gleichgewicht der Regelung ein, bei dem der Kohlensäuredruck gegenüber der Norm leicht erhöht, das Atemzeitvolumen leicht vermindert ist. Solche Änderungen in der Regelung zeigen sich sehr deutlich, wenn man bei Versuchspersonen im Experiment zusätzliche Widerstände in die Luftwege einschaltet. Neben Änderungen der Atemfrequenz und der Atemlage findet sich eine Zunahme des alveolaren Kohlensäuredruckes und eine Abnahme des Atemzeitvolumens[1]. Die Veränderungen des Atemzeitvolumens und der Alveolarluft durch die Einschaltung zusätzlicher Atemwiderstände werden besonders groß bei Muskeltätigkeit. Die nötige Ventilationsleistung kann dann nicht mehr aufgebracht werden, und die Atmung wird insuffizient. Wenn in Krankheitsfällen der Atemwiderstand über lange Zeiten gesteigert ist, so werden die Verhältnisse noch dadurch kompliziert, daß die langdauernde Hypoventilation zu einem Anstieg der Bicarbonatkonzentration führt, und daß dadurch die anfänglich bestehende, durch die Kohlensäure bedingte respiratorische Acidose gemildert oder aufgehoben wird (s. S. 312).

---

[1] Zechman und Mitarbeiter 1957.

Veränderungen des Atemwiderstandes sind für die Einstellung der Atmung bei den meisten Lungenerkrankungen von Bedeutung. Das gilt besonders für das Emphysem[1]. Es ist fraglich, wieweit atemmechanische Faktoren bei Kreislaufstörungen für die Einstellung der Atmung eine Rolle spielen. Jede Blutanschoppung in der Lunge steigert ihren elastischen Widerstand[2]. Wahrscheinlich sind aber hier reflektorische Einflüsse, die von Receptoren in der Nachbarschaft der Lungengefäße und des Herzens ausgehen, von größerer Wichtigkeit[3].

Auch eine Zunahme der Totraumventilation auf Kosten der alveolaren Ventilation muß die Einstellung der Atmung beeinflussen. Die Totraumventilation nimmt relativ zur Gesamtventilation zu, wenn die Atemtiefe vermindert ist, oder wenn die Beziehung von Durchlüftung und Durchblutung einzelner Lungenabschnitte gestört ist. Beide Vorgänge können bei der Atmungseinstellung des Emphysematikers von Bedeutung sein[4]. Dabei sind Kohlensäuredruck und Atemzeitvolumen gesteigert, die alveolare Ventilation aber vermindert.

Für jeden Anpassungsvorgang der Atmung ist der *Säure-Basen-Haushalt* von entscheidender Bedeutung. Steigt bei gleichbleibender Kohlensäurebildung die Ventilation an, so wird im Übermaß Kohlensäure verloren, wir haben das Bild der respiratorischen Alkalose. Daraufhin sorgt die Niere durch erhöhte Alkaliausscheidung für eine Verminderung des Bicarbonats. Die H-Ionen-Konzentration wird dadurch wieder weitgehend normalisiert. Umgekehrt führt eine verminderte Atmung bei gleichbleibender Kohlensäurebildung zu einer respiratorischen Acidose. Auch sie wird von der Niere durch vermehrte Säureausscheidung und Alkalieinsparung weitgehend kompensiert.

Das einfachste Beispiel einer *respiratorischen Alkalose* sind die Veränderungen bei langdauernder Hyperventilation in einer „Eisernen Lunge"[5], das bekannteste Beispiel bieten die Verhältnisse bei der Höhenanpassung. In letzterem Falle erklärt sich die gesteigerte Ventilation in erster Linie durch den Antrieb der Atmung über die peripheren Chemoreceptoren. Ungeklärt ist die Ursache der weiteren Atmungssteigerung bei längerem Höhenaufenthalt[6].

Sehr viel komplizierter liegen die Verhältnisse bei arterieller Hypoxie unter pathologischen Bedingungen. Hierbei ist im allgemeinen nicht nur die Sauerstoffaufnahme, sondern auch die Kohlensäureabgabe gestört. Patienten, deren arterielle Hypoxie durch einen Rechts-Links-Shunt bedingt ist, haben, bezogen auf den arteriellen Kohlensäure- und Sauerstoffdruck und die arterielle H-Ionen-Konzentration, eine auffallend geringe Ventilation[7]. Bei normalem Kohlensäuredruck findet man eine anscheinend metabolisch bedingte Acidose. Es ist unklar, warum in diesem Falle die Acidose und der verminderte arterielle Sauerstoffdruck die Atmung weniger antreiben als bei der Höhenanpassung. Dabei ist diese Art der Atmungseinstellung u. U. für den Organismus günstig, weil im Falle des Kurzschlusses eine weitere Atmungssteigerung die arterielle Sauerstoffsättigung nicht verbessern kann, die Acidose andererseits die Abgabe von Sauerstoff aus dem Blut ins Gewebe der Körperperipherie begünstigt. Bei sehr lang dauerndem Sauerstoffmangel scheinen Anpassungsvorgänge im Gewebe — verbesserte Capillarisierung und veränderter Fermentbesatz — gegenüber den anderen Anpassungsfaktoren immer stärker in den Vordergrund zu treten[8]. Das könnte

---

[1] CHERNIACK und SNIDAL 1956, PRYOR und Mitarbeiter 1957.
[2] FRANK und Mitarbeiter 1957.   [3] AVIADO und SCHMIDT 1955.
[4] ULMER 1956.   [5] BROWN 1953.
[6] DEJOURS, GIRARD, LABROUSSE u. TEILLAC 1959.
[7] MÜRTZ und NEUHAUS 1954, HUSSON und OTIS 1957.   [8] OPITZ und LÜBBERS 1957.

auch erklären, daß Menschen, die jahrelang in großen Höhen leben, wieder eine geringere Ventilation haben als solche, die nur einige Monate an diese Höhe angepaßt sind[1].

Eine einfache Form einer *respiratorischen Acidose* entwickelt sich, wenn gesunde Versuchspersonen sich längere Zeit in einer mit Kohlensäure angereicherten Umgebung befinden. Die Kompensation der Acidose durch Anstieg des Blutbicarbonats vermindert den von der H-Ionen-Konzentration abhängigen Atemantrieb und führt auf diese Weise zu einem weiteren Ansteigen des arteriellen Kohlensäuredruckes[2].

Komplizierter liegen die Verhältnisse unter pathologischen Bedingungen. Sehr viele Arbeiten beschäftigen sich mit der Einstellung der Atmung beim Emphysem[3]. Dabei scheint die erhöhte Atemarbeit die primäre Ursache der Atmungsumstellung zu sein[4]. Die Beantwortung der zentralen Impulse durch den peripheren Atmungsapparat wird unzureichend, so daß der Kohlensäuredruck ansteigt. Bei länger bestehender respiratorischer Acidose steigt die Bicarbonatkonzentration des Blutes an, wodurch die Ventilation weiter abnimmt. Schließlich kann ein sehr stark erhöhter Kohlensäuredruck eine narkotische Wirkung auf das Atemzentrum entfalten. Auch eine Schädigung des Atemzentrums durch einen erhöhten intrakraniellen Druck kann bei langdauernder respiratorischer Acidose von Bedeutung sein. Wenn der Antrieb der Atmung durch die Kohlensäure so stark verschlechtert ist, dann gewinnt der Sauerstoffmangel für die Einstellung der Atmung um so größere Bedeutung. In solchen Fällen beobachtet man ein Versagen der Atmung, wenn die Patienten mit Sauerstoff beatmet werden[5].

Andere Anpassungsvorgänge der Lungenbelüftung sind auf Veränderungen im *Hormongleichgewicht* zurückzuführen. Das gilt für die gesteigerte Atmung in der Schwangerschaft[6]. Für die Beatmung des Foeten über die Placenta ist dies nicht bedeutungslos. Zwar wird dadurch die Sauerstoffversorgung des Foetus kaum verbessert, dagegen wird der Kohlensäureabtransport erleichtert. Die Ventilationssteigerung der Schwangerschaft beruht im allgemeinen nicht auf einer Acidose, wie früher angenommen wurde, sondern auf atmungssteigernden Wirkungen der weiblichen Sexualhormone. Es läßt sich auch eine Änderung der Erregbarkeit des Atemzentrums während des Cyclus feststellen, wobei die Erregbarkeit der Konzentration der weiblichen Sexualhormone im Blut parallel geht. Von den Steroidhormonen kommt weiterhin dem Cortison eine atmungssteigernde Wirkung zu. Bei Testosteron läßt sie sich nicht mit Sicherheit feststellen. Ob die Steroidhormone direkt am Atemzentrum oder über andere Abschnitte des Zentralnervensystems die Atmungssteigerungen hervorrufen, ist nicht entschieden.

Auch Schilddrüsenhormon steigert die Erregbarkeit des Atemzentrums. Die gleiche Wirkung läßt sich durch thyreotropes Hormon erreichen[7]. Bei schilddrüsenlosen Kaninchen ist die Erregbarkeit herabgesetzt, während sie nach Entfernung der Milz gesteigert sein soll[8]. Ein erhöhter Gehalt des Blutes an Schilddrüsenhormon geht regelmäßig mit einem erhöhten Erregungszustand des Zentralnervensystems einher, und das erklärt allein schon die gesteigerte Atmung. Es kann dabei aber auch der erhöhte Stoffwechsel im Atemzentrum selbst von Bedeutung sein.

---

[1] CHIODI 1957.   [2] SCHÄFER 1949.
[3] JULICH 1953, ALEXANDER und Mitarbeiter 1955, FISHMAN und Mitarbeiter 1955, SCHWAB 1957.
[4] TENNEY 1954, CHERNIACK und SNIDAL 1956.
[5] Literatur bei MATTHES und ULMER 1955.
LOESCHCKE 1954.   [7] SPIELMANN 1934.   [8] FELDER 1934.

B. Der nervöse Apparat der Atmungsregulation und die Einstellung der Atemform.

I. Begriff und Aufbau des Atemzentrums.

Als ein Zentrum kann man einen Teil des Zentralnervensystems bezeichnen der für das Zustandekommen eines zentral-nervösen Vorgangs eine ausschlag, gebende Bedeutung hat. Der Begriff des Zentrums ist damit rein funktionell gefaßt und nicht an eine bestimmte anatomische Struktur gebunden. Danach gehören zum Atemzentrum alle Abschnitte des Zentralnervensystems, die an der Funktion der Lungenatmung maßgeblich beteiligt sind. Das sind besonders Gebiete im Rückenmark, im Rautenhirn und in der Brücke. Selbstverständlich

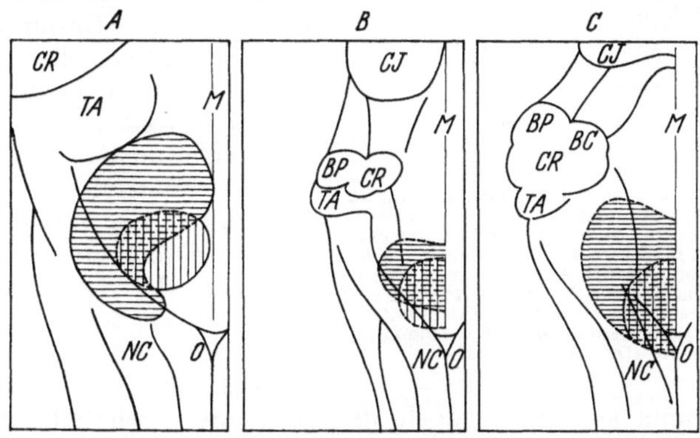

Abb. 13. Schematische Darstellung der Lage des inspiratorischen (senkrecht schraffiert) und exspiratorischen (horizontal schraffiert) bulbären Atmungszentrums bei Affe (*A*), Katze (*B*) und Schaf (*C*), nach Untersuchungen mit zentraler elektrischer Reizung; *BC* Brachium conjunctivum; *BP* Brachium pontis; *CJ* Colliculus inferior; *CR* Corpus restiforme; *M* Medianlinie; *NC* Nucleus cuneatus; *O* Obex; *TA* Tuberculum acusticum (OBERHOLZER 1957).

kann aber noch von sehr vielen anderen Abschnitten des Zentralnervensystems aus die Atmung beeinflußt werden. Man sollte auch nicht vergessen, daß die Atemmuskulatur als Skeletmuskulatur ein Teil des motorischen Systems ist, und daß deshalb die zentral-nervösen Abschnitte, die für die Funktion der Lungenatmung verantwortlich sind, mit anderen motorischen Gebieten des Zentralnervensystems in engstem Kontakt stehen müssen. In diesem Sinne ist das Atemzentrum nur ein weiter spezialisierter Abschnitt des größeren motorischen Systems, das sich über den gesamten Bereich der Substantia reticularis erstreckt[1].

Von der Funktion her ergibt sich folgende Einteilung:

1. Das *spinale Atemzentrum im Rückenmark*, das beim erwachsenen Säuger im allgemeinen nicht in Funktion ist. Es ermöglicht nur eine schnappende Atmung.

2. Das *Atemzentrum im engeren Sinne*, das *in der Substantia reticularis* der *Medulla oblongata* gelegen ist. Es zerfällt in einen inspiratorischen und einen exspiratorischen Teil[2]. Da meistens die Ausatmung ein passiver Vorgang ist, der durch elastische Kräfte bedingt ist, und nur in extremen Fällen die Exspirationsmuskulatur aktiv eingesetzt wird, ist das Exspirationszentrum fast ausschließlich ein Hemmungszentrum der Inspiration[3].

3. *Gebiete, von denen* aus die *Atmung moduliert wird*. Hierzu gehören besonders die intrazentralen Schaltstellen atmungswirksamer Afferenzen in der Nachbarschaft des eigentlichen Atemzentrums. Von besonderer Bedeutung sind die

---

[1] HOFF und BRECKENRIDGE 1955.   [2] Literatur bei PITTS 1946.   [3] CAMPBELL 1958.

Schaltstellen des Vagus[1]. Hierhin gehört aber auch das pneumotaktische Zentrum im oberen Teil der Brücke, das für die Umschaltung von der Inspiration auf die Exspiration von Bedeutung ist (s. S. 318)[2].

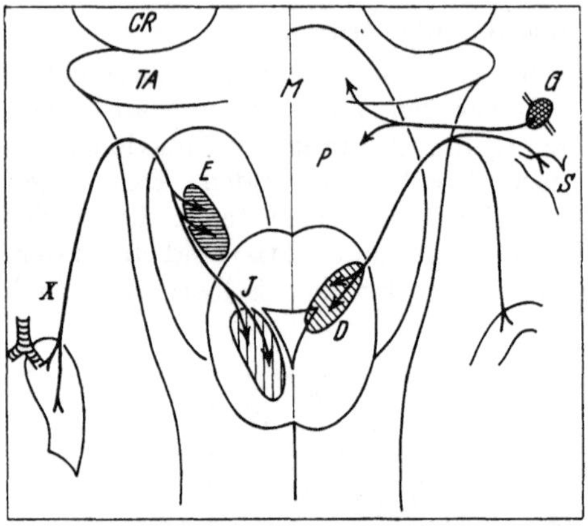

4. *Stellen*, die die *Atmung* mit anderen zentralnervösen Funktionen *koordinieren.* Hierhin gehören besonders Hypothalamus und Großhirnrinde (s. S. 305). Diese Gebiete sollte man nicht dem Atemzentrum zurechnen.

Abb. 13 zeigt die Lage des Inspirations- und Exspirationszentrums, wie sie nach Versuchen mit elektrischer Reizung anzunehmen ist[3]. Es muß freilich betont werden, daß Versuche mit Ableitungen der Aktionsströme von atmungssynchron tätigen Zellelementen nur teilweise die Reizexperimente bestätigen und daß deshalb an der Lokalisation und der Trennbarkeit der beiden Halbzentren gezweifelt wird[4]. Für eine Abtrennbarkeit des Inspirations- und Exspirationszentrums sprechen jedoch die getrennten Schaltstellen für in- und exspiratorische Atmungsreflexe vagalen Ursprungs, deren Lage in Abb. 14 dargestellt ist[5].

Abb. 14. Bulbäre Lage der Schaltstellen für vagale Atmungsreflexe (*X*) links und für aortale, eventuell sinusale Depressorreflexe (*S*) rechts. Verlauf der entsprechenden afferenten Fasern im Solitärbündel. Vermutlicher Verlauf der Fasern aus dem Glomus caroticum (*G*). Lage der medullären Atmungszentren (*E* exspiratorisch, *J* inspiratorisch) sowie der Kreislaufzentren (*D* depressorisch, *P* pressorisch). Übrige Bezeichnungen wie in Abb. 13 (OBERHOLZER 1957).

II. Die afferenten Bahnen des Atemzentrums.

In Abb. 1 (S. 296) sind die wichtigsten afferenten Bahnen des Atemzentrums aufgezeichnet. Über einen großen Teil dieser Bahnen laufen Impulse, die das Atemzentrum hemmen oder fördern und damit das Atemzeitvolumen verkleinern oder vergrößern. Über andere Bahnen laufen Impulse, die das Atemzentrum über die jeweilige Atemlage orientieren. Diese Reafferenzen gehen in erster Linie von Receptoren aus, die in Lunge und Pleura gelegen sind und deren Fasern über den Lungenvagus verlaufen. Es spielen hier aber auch Reflexe von den oberen Luftwegen[6], von der Thoraxwand[7] und vom Zwerchfell[8] hinein. Diese Reafferenzen sind für die Modulierung der Atemform von besonderer Bedeutung.

Bläst man im Tierversuch von den Luftwegen aus eine Lunge auf, so kommt es reflektorisch zur Ausatmung. Saugt man auf dem gleichen Wege Luft aus der Lunge ab, so daß sie sich verkleinert, wird reflektorisch eine Inspirationsbewegung ausgelöst[9]. Ausschaltung der Vagi führt zum Erlöschen dieser Reflexe. Ähnliche Erscheinungen findet man bei vielen motorischen Vorgängen. Der Bewegungsablauf wirkt auf das motorische Zentrum zurück. Es sind reafferente Bahnen vorhanden, die die Auswirkungen der motorischen Innervation an das Zentrum zurückmelden[10]. Die Reflexe dienen dabei der Feineinstellung der Atembewegungen. Sie sind häufig als „Selbststeuerung der Atmung" bezeichnet worden. Die Mechanoreceptoren, von denen diese Reflexe ausgehen, sind auffallend empfindlich

---

[1] Literatur bei WYSS 1954, OBERHOLZER 1957.   [2] TANG 1953.
[3] PITTS 1946, Literatur bei OBERHOLZER 1957.
[4] v. BAUMGARTEN und Mitarbeiter 1956, 1957.   [5] OBERHOLZER 1957.
[6] BUCHER 1952, WIDDICOMBE 1954.   [7] FLEISCH 1934, BUCHER 1952.   [8] DOLIVO 1946.
[9] HERING 1868, BREUER 1868.   [10] SHERRINGTON 1906, v. HOLST 1950.

gegen eine große Reihe chemischer Substanzen, durch die sie sowohl erregt als auch gelähmt werden können[1]. Chemische Einflüsse führen dadurch zu eigentümlichen Änderungen der Atemform wie kurzdauernden Atemstillständen, vertiefter Atmung oder auch sehr frequenter Atmung. Die Receptoren liegen teils den Bronchien, teils der visceralen Pleura benachbart[2].

Die über die Vagi vermittelten Rückwirkungen auf die Atmung sind vierfach: inspirationsfördernde Wirkungen, exspirationsfördernde Wirkungen, Wirkungen auf die Umschaltung von einer Atemphase auf die andere und Wirkungen auf die Atemlage.

1. *Inspirationsfördernde Wirkungen.* a) Zusammenfallen der Lunge führt zu einer Inspirationsbewegung[3]. Der Reflex wird von Receptoren ausgelöst, die durch Entspannung der Lunge erregt werden[4]. Er tritt nur bei forcierter Ausatmung auf.

b) Bei vertiefter Einatmung kommt es mit wachsender Lungendehnung zu einem Anstieg der motorischen Impulse zu den Atemmuskeln. Sie dienen dazu,

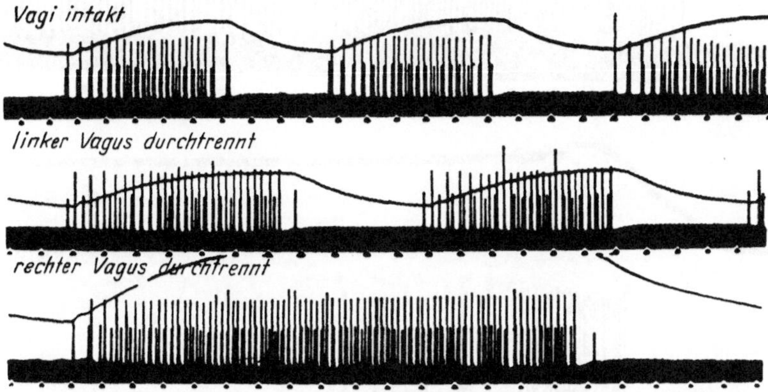

Abb. 15. Verlangsamung und Vertiefung der Atmung nach Vagusdurchschneidung. Oberste Kurve: Atembewegung (Inspiration nach oben). Mittlere Kurve: Aktionsströme zweier motorischer Phrenicusfasern. Untere Kurve: Zeit in 0,2 sec. (Nach PITTS 1942.)

den wachsenden Gewebswiderstand zu überwinden. Der zusätzliche Antrieb erfolgt reflektorisch über den Vagus. Die Receptoren für diese Reflexe sprechen auf stärkere Dehnung des Lungengewebes an und adaptieren sehr stark, so daß die Impulse nur sehr kurze Zeit anhalten[5].

2. *Die exspirationsfördernde Wirkung* beruht auf Dehnungsreceptoren, die wenig adaptieren und mit wachsender Lungendehnung höhere Impulszahlen aussenden. Diese Impulse hemmen das Inspirationszentrum und treiben das Exspirationszentrum an.

3. Die Wirkung auf die *Umschaltung von einer Atemphase auf die andere* ist wohl mit der oben angeführten exspirationsfördernden Wirkung langsam adaptierender Dehnungsreceptoren identisch. Sie zeigt sich am deutlichsten durch ihren Wegfall nach Vagotomie, die zu einer vertieften und verlangsamten Atmung führt. Es fallen durch die Vagusausschaltung steuernde Einflüsse aus, die für eine rechtzeitige Umschaltung Sorge tragen (s. Abb. 15).

4. Nicht oder sehr langsam adaptierende Dehnungsreceptoren steuern den *Tonus der Einatmungsmuskulatur* und damit *die Atemlage*[6].

[1] DAWES und COMROE 1954.   [2] Literatur bei LILJESTRAND 1958.
[3] HERING 1868, BREUER 1868.
[4] ADRIAN 1933, LARRABEE und KNOWLTON 1946, KNOWLTON und LARRABEE 1946.
[5] KNOWLTON und LARRABEE 1946.   [6] HESS 1941, SOMMER 1941, HESS und WYSS 1936.

Die sehr verwirrenden Befunde, die bei den zahlreichen Untersuchungen der Vaguswirkung auf die Atmung erhoben wurden, lassen sich besonders auf folgendes zurückführen:

1. Es müssen verschiedene Arten von Mechanoreceptoren in der Lunge angenommen werden. Der größere Teil der afferenten Vagusfasern zeigt Aktionsströme bei Dehnung der Lunge, ein kleinerer Teil bei Entspannung[1]. Es sind

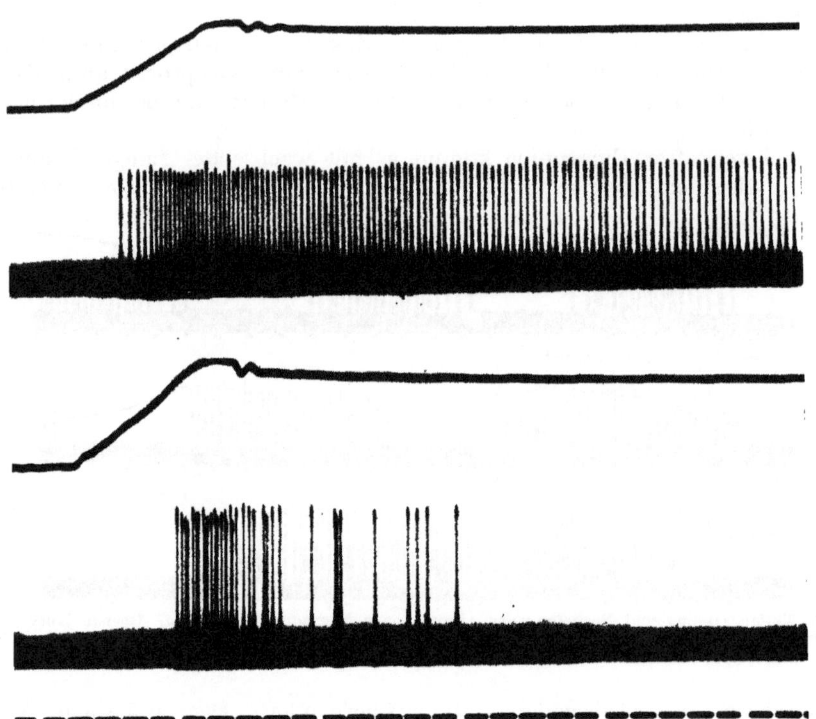

Abb. 16. Aktionsströme von einzelnen Vagusfasern, die ihre Impulse von langsam und rasch adaptierenden Lungenreceptoren erhalten. Versuch an einer Katze mit eröffnetem Thorax. Die Atempumpe wurde kurz vor den Registrierungen angehalten, während der Registrierung wurde die Lunge aufgeblasen. Die obere Kurve gibt den intratrachealen Druck an, ganz unten Registrierung der Zeit (0,1 sec). Oben: der langsam adaptierende Receptor sendet Impulse, solange die Lunge gebläht bleibt. Unten: der rasch adaptierende Receptor sendet nur einen kurzen Impulsstoß aus (KNOWLTON u. LARRABEE 1946).

2 Gruppen von Dehnungsreceptoren zu unterscheiden, die durch Verschiedenheit der Adaptation gegen den Dehnungsreiz und dementsprechend verschiedenen Wirkungen auf das Zentrum gekennzeichnet sind[2] (Abb. 16).

2. Von gleichen Receptoren können verschiedene Wirkungen auf das Zentrum ausgeübt werden. So haben anscheinend die Dehnungsreceptoren einen inspirationshemmenden Einfluß bei hoher Erregungsfrequenz, dagegen einen inspirationsfördernden bei niedriger Frequenz[3]. Weiterhin wirken die von der Peripherie ausgesandten Impulse verschieden auf das Zentrum je nach der Atemphase, in der sie eintreffen und der gleichzeitigen Einwirkung von Impulsen aus anderen Receptoren[4].

---

[1] BEIN und HELMICH 1949.
[2] LARRABEE und KNOWLTON 1946, KNOWLTON und LARRABEE 1946.
[3] WYSS 1947b.   [4] SOMMER 1941, LUEKEN und TIMM 1947, WYSS 1947a.

3. Während die eigentliche Steuerung der Atemform von Receptoren ausgelöst wird, die durch Dehnung oder Entspannung des Lungengewebes erregt werden, verlaufen über den Lungenvagus afferente Fasern, deren Receptoren wahrscheinlich in der Nähe der kleineren Lungengefäße liegen. Sie haben eine Bedeutung für die Entstehung der frequenten und flachen Atmung bei multipler Lungenembolie[1]. Sie haben eher eine allgemein erregende Wirkung auf die Atmung (ähnlich wie sie bei Erregung von Schmerznerven beobachtet wird), als daß sie typisch die Atemform beeinflussen.

III. Die efferenten Bahnen des Atemzentrums.

Vom Atemzentrum ziehen die Bahnen der Atemmotorik im zentralen Abschnitt des Seitenstranges und im lateralen Abschnitt des Vorderstranges im Rückenmark abwärts zu den Vorderhornzellen der Atemmuskeln. Die meisten Fasern verlaufen ungekreuzt und innervieren die motorischen Vorderhornzellen der gleichen Seite. Es gibt aber auch sich kreuzende Fasern, besonders für die Zwerchfellinnervation[2]. Weiterhin verlaufen vom Atemzentrum aus Fasern über den 5., 7., 9., 10., 11. und 12. Hirnnerven zur Innervation quergestreifter Muskulatur an Hals, Mund, Nase, Pharynx, Larynx und Zunge, sowie zu der glatten Muskulatur der Luftwege. Alle diese Muskeln werden bei starker Atmung innerviert, während bei ruhiger Atmung nur die Inspirationsmuskeln, Pharynx, Larynx und die glatten Muskeln des Bronchialbaums Impulse erhalten[3].

IV. Die Funktionen des Atemzentrums.

Das Atemzentrum erhält nervöse und über das Blut chemische Antriebe aus der Peripherie. Die Größe des Antriebs bestimmt die Zahl der zu den Erfolgsorganen ausgesandten Erregungen und damit die Größe des Atemvolumens. Das Atemzentrum bestimmt aber weiterhin die Art, wie dieses Atemvolumen gefördert wird, d. h. Tiefe und Form jedes einzelnen Atemzuges, Frequenz der Atmung und Atemlage. Im Atemzentrum werden die von den verschiedensten Stellen her einströmenden Erregungen gesammelt und in geordneter Form an die Erfolgsorgane weitergegeben.

Von einem Verständnis des Erregungsablaufs in den medullären Zentren sind wir noch sehr weit entfernt. Man muß daran denken, daß speziellen Zellen oder Zellgruppen auch besondere Funktionen als Oscillatoren, Modulatoren, Integratoren und Schrittmachern zukommen[4]. Jedoch reichen die bisherigen Ergebnisse nicht aus, solche speziell funktionierenden Zellgruppen zu lokalisieren und ihr Zusammenwirken zu verstehen. Folgende Fragen seien im einzelnen besprochen:

1. Der Ursprung der Erregung.

Wahrscheinlich besitzen Zellen des Inspirationszentrums die Fähigkeit der automatischen Erregungsbildung[5]. Sie wird durch chemische und nervöse Einflüsse der verschiedensten Art gefördert und gehemmt. Kompliziert wird die Frage nach dem Ursprung der Erregung durch Befunde, die daran denken lassen, daß die Chemoreception an besondere Zellen des Atemzentrums gebunden ist. Bei Narkose ist die Empfindlichkeit des Atemzentrums gegen Kohlensäure stark herabgesetzt, während der reflektorische Antrieb der Atmung kaum beeinflußt wird (s. S. 300). Nun kann man sich vorstellen, daß an der gleichen Zelle die Chemoreception durch die Narkose gestört wird, während der synaptische Antrieb

---

[1] Whitteridge 1950.   [2] Rosenbaum und Renshaw 1949.   [3] Pitts 1940.
[4] Brodie und Borison 1957.   [5] Hoff und Breckenridge 1955, Schmidt 1956.

unverändert bleibt[1]. Es gibt aber Befunde, nach denen bestimmte Bezirke des Rautenhirns zwar chemosensibel, für die reflektorische Erregungsübertragung aber ohne Bedeutung sind[2].

2. Die Ursache der Periodizität der Atmung.

Unter bestimmten experimentellen Bedingungen beobachtet man eine Dauerkontraktion der Inspirationsmuskulatur, die als Apneusis bezeichnet wird. Manchmal ist der Inspirationskrampf durch Exspirationsphasen unterbrochen. Man spricht dann von einer apneustischen Atmung.

Der Abb. 17 liegt folgender Versuch zugrunde: Bei einer Katze wurde der Hirnstamm in Höhe der Brückenarme durchtrennt. Die Atmung blieb zunächst weitgehend unverändert.

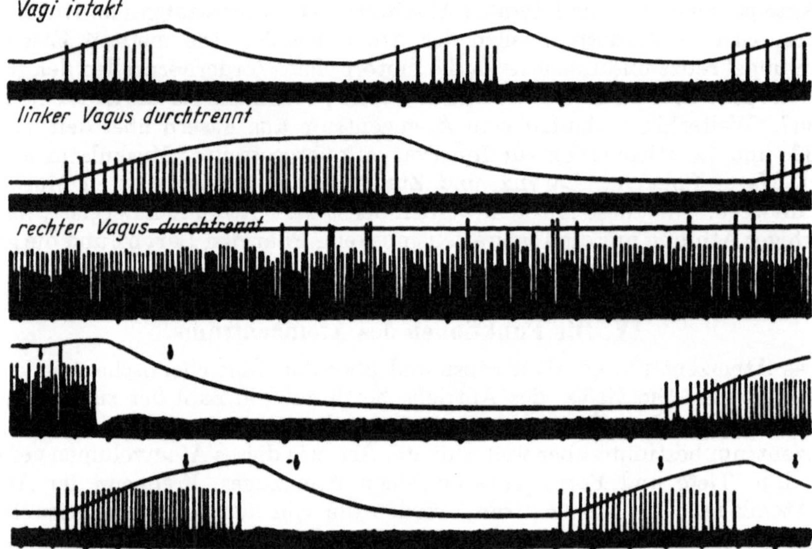

Abb. 17. Erzeugung eines inspiratorischen Atemkrampfes (Apneusis) durch Vagusdurchschneidung nach vorheriger Ausschaltung des in der Brücke gelegenen pneumotaxic center und Wiederherstellung der rhythmischen Atmung durch Reizung des zentralen Vagusendes. Obere Kurve: Atembewegungen (Inspiration nach oben). Mittlere Kurve: Aktionsströme zweier motorischer Phrenicusfasern. Untere Kurve: Zeit in 0,2 sec. In den beiden unteren Zeilen wird das zentrale Ende eines Vagus jeweils zwischen 2 Pfeilen elektrisch gereizt. (Nach Pitts 1942.)

Ausschaltung des linken Vagus verlängerte die Inspiration. Ausschaltung des zweiten Vagus löste den Zustand der Apneusis aus. Schließlich wurde durch Reizung des zentralen Stumpfes eines Vagus die rhythmische Atmung wiederhergestellt[3].

Nach derartigen Versuchen gewinnt man den Eindruck, daß das Atemzentrum äußerer Einflüsse bedarf, die in bestimmten zeitlichen Abständen das Inspirationszentrum hemmen und so die Atemperiodik bedingen[4]. In erster Linie läuft die Umschaltung über die afferenten Lungenvagi. Sind im Tierexperiment die Lungenvagi ausgeschaltet, so kann die Atemperiodik durch die Funktion des pneumotaktischen Zentrums aufrechterhalten bleiben. Es handelt sich dabei um ein ziemlich eng umschriebenes Gebiet im oberen Abschnitt der Brücke[5]. Die Tachypnoe bei Hyperthermie ist an ein intaktes pneumotaktisches Zentrum gebunden[6].

[1] Winterstein 1955.
[2] v. Euler und Söderberg 1952, Liljestrand 1953, Literatur bei Liljestrand 1958.
[3] Pitts 1942.
[4] Marckwald 1887, Stella 1938, Pitts und Mitarbeiter 1939b, Lumsden 1923.
[5] Literatur bei Liljestrand 1958.   [6] Hicstand und Randall 1942.

Früher nahm man an, daß der überwiegende Einfluß des Inspirationszentrums immer zur Apneusis oder zur apneustischen Atmung führen müsse, wenn das Atemzentrum nicht von außen durch Vaguswirkungen oder durch Einwirkungen des pneumotaktischen Zentrums gehemmt würde, daß es also äußerer Einflüsse auf das medulläre Zentrum bedürfte, um die Atemperiodik zu erhalten[1]. Dagegen zeigen neuere Untersuchungen, daß das medulläre Zentrum von sich aus die Atemperiodik erzeugen kann[2]. Es genügen die reziproken Hemmungen zwischen Inspirations- und Exspirationszentrum. Wie Versuche mit elektrischer Reizung zeigen, führt die Erregung des Exspirationszentrums zur Hemmung des Inspirationszentrums und umgekehrt[3]. Ein dauerndes Überwiegen des Inspirationszentrums kommt erst durch den Einfluß des sog. apneustischen Zentrums im caudalen Teil der Brücke zustande. HOFF u. BRECKENRIDGE nehmen an, daß es sich dabei nur um einen Teil des ausgedehnten motorischen Gebietes in der Substantia reticularis handelt, die ganz allgemein Kontraktionsvorgänge der

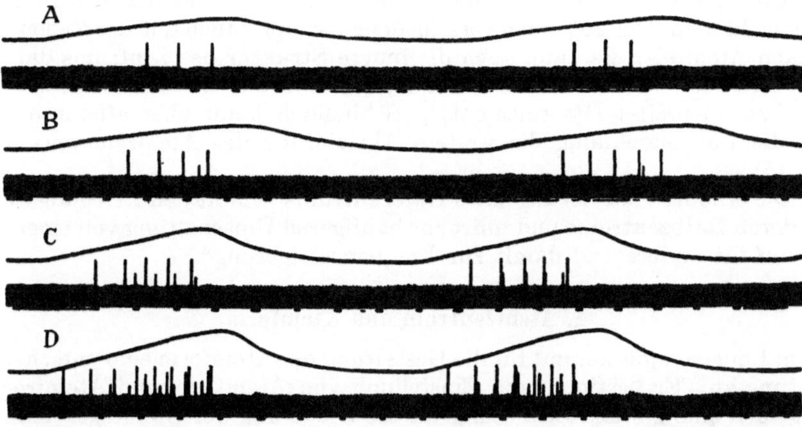

Abb. 18. Aktionsströme dreier motorischer Fasern des N. phrenicus bei Einwirkung verschiedener Kohlensäurekonzentrationen. Durch Rückatmung reichert sich die Kohlensäure in der Atemluft des Versuchstieres an (Registrierungen *A—D*). Oberste Kurve: Atembewegungen (Inspiration nach oben). Mittlere Kurve: Aktionsströme dreier motorischer Phrenicusfasern, die durch die verschiedene Höhe der Ausschläge voneinander zu unterscheiden sind. Untere Kurve: Zeit in 0,2 sec. Mit wachsender Kohlensäurekonzentration nehmen für die einzelne Faser Frequenz und Dauer der Erregung zu. Die zweite und dritte motorische Einheit kommt erst bei höheren Konzentrationen ins Spiel (Recruitment). (Nach PITTS 1951.)

quergestreiften Muskulatur erleichtert. Apneusis tritt in den meisten Versuchen nach Durchtrennung des Hirnstammes gleichzeitig mit dem Bild der Enthirnungsstarre auf. Es wird damit zu einem Teilsymptom für den Ausfall übergeordneter motorischer Gebiete[4]. Die Wirkungen, die vom pneumotaktischen Zentrum ausgehen, beruhen wahrscheinlich darauf, daß sie das apneustische Zentrum hemmen.

3. Der Vorgang der Atmungssteigerung.

Er ist am besten an den Aktionsströmen der Atemmuskeln oder ihrer motorischen Nerven zu verfolgen. Abb. 18 zeigt die Aktionsströme von drei motorischen Fasern des N. phrenicus bei normaler und bei durch Kohlensäurezusatz gesteigerter Atmung. Zunächst ist nur ein Neuron in Tätigkeit (Aktionsströme des gleichen Neurons lassen sich aus der gleichen Größe der Amplitude erkennen!). Bei verstärkter Atmung laufen über zwei, später über alle drei Nervenfasern Erregungswellen. Dabei nehmen die zeitlichen Abstände der Erregungswellen auf

---

[1] PITTS 1946.　　[2] HOFF und BRECKENRIDGE 1949, 1955.　　[3] PITTS 1946.
[4] BRECKENRIDGE und HOFF 1953.

der einzelnen Faser ab. Schließlich nimmt die Inspirationsdauer, d. h. die Zeit, über die inspiratorische Impulse zu beobachten sind, zu. Danach gibt es folgende Möglichkeiten, die Atemtiefe zu steigern:

a) Erhöhte Impulsfrequenz der einzelnen motorischen Einheit, b) längere Dauer des Erregungsstoßes, c) erhöhte Zahl der tätigen Einheiten[1]. Hinzu kommt der Einsatz weiterer Atemmuskeln und Atemhilfsmuskeln und die Aktivierung der Exspirationsmuskulatur. Schließlich kann das Atemzeitvolumen nicht nur durch Erhöhung der Atemtiefe, sondern auch durch häufigeres Umschalten von einer Atemphase auf die andere und damit durch die Erhöhung der Atemfrequenz gesteigert werden.

Der Atmungssteigerung liegen wahrscheinlich folgende Vorgänge im Atemzentrum zugrunde.

a) Die einzelne Zelle wird durch die verschiedenen chemischen oder nervösen Einflüsse stärker angetrieben und sendet eine größere Zahl von Erregungen aus[2].

b) Eine größere Zahl von Zellen gerät in den Zustand der Erregung. Das beruht wohl zum Teil auf einer verschiedenen Empfindlichkeit der Zellen gegenüber dem Atemreiz. Es kann auch die innere Struktur des Zentrums dafür verantwortlich sein, wobei sich der Erregungszustand auf eine immer größere Zahl von Zellen ausbreitet (Recruitment)[3]. Schließlich kann über afferente Vagusfasern die Lungendehnung die weitere Aktivierung des Atemzentrums fördern (s. S. 315).

c) Die erhöhte Aktivierung eines Halbzentrums hemmt den Erregungszustand des anderen Halbzentrums und führt zur häufigeren Umschaltung von einer Atemphase auf die andere und damit zur Frequenzsteigerung[4].

4. Atemzentrum und Atemform.

Dem Lungenvagus kommt für die Gestaltung der Atemform eine entscheidende Bedeutung zu. Er bestimmt die Einstellung von Atemtiefe und Atemfrequenz. Er hat auch eine gewisse Bedeutung für die Steuerung der Atemlage. Man muß sich vorstellen, daß wie die gesamte Skeletmuskulatur auch die Atemmuskulatur einen Dauertonus besitzt. Die Stärke dieses Dauertonus bestimmt die Atemlage. Dabei wird vom Atemzentrum aus je nach der Atemphase wechselweise der Tonus der Inspirations- und Exspirationsmuskulatur erhöht oder abgeschwächt. Das gilt besonders für die Inspirationsmuskeln und davon wieder ganz besonders für das Zwerchfell. Die Einstellung des Zwerchfelltonus verläuft aber über den Lungenvagus[5]. Nach neuen elektromyographischen Untersuchungen ist freilich der Dauertonus der Atemmuskulatur recht gering, so daß man seine Bedeutung für die Einstellung der Atemlage nicht überschätzen darf[6]. Die Atemlage wird wahrscheinlich mehr durch atemmechanische Bedingungen, wie Elastizität des Lungengewebes und Strömungswiderstand in den Luftwegen, als durch die Tonisierung der Atemmuskulatur bestimmt.

Besondere Atemformen findet man bei gestörter Funktion des Atemzentrums. Auf die apneustische Atmung wurde schon S. 318 eingegangen. Häufig ist ein Atemtyp, der als Alles-oder-Nichts-Atmung bezeichnet wird. Bei jedem Atemzug ist die Kontraktion der Inspirationsmuskulatur samt der zugehörigen Hilfsmuskulatur maximal. Die Atmung besteht aus gleichmäßig tiefen Atemzügen. Nur die Atemfrequenz variiert. Die Atmung kann dabei rhythmisch oder arrhythmisch sein. Im Tierexperiment findet man diesen Zustand besonders häufig bei

---

[1] Adrian und Bronk 1928, Bronk und Ferguson 1935.
[2] Gesell 1940, Gesell und Hansen 1945.   [3] Gesell 1940.   [4] Pitts 1946.
[5] Hess 1941, Hoff und Breckenridge 1955.   [6] Campbell 1958.

tiefer Barbituratnarkose, wobei gleichzeitig die Empfindlichkeit des Atemzentrums gegen Kohlensäure herabgesetzt oder sogar aufgehoben ist. Man hat den Eindruck, daß der Ausfall der zentralen Chemoreception gleichzeitig die Fähigkeit des Atemzentrums aufhebt, die Atmung zu modulieren. Eine Alles-oder-Nichts-Atmung findet man auch, wenn nach Ausschaltung des medullären Zentrums eine spinale Atmung fortbesteht. Sie wird aber auch bei Störungen in höheren motorischen Gebieten beobachtet. Die „Schnappatmung" hat anscheinend nichts mit Störungen im Bereich des Vagussystems zu tun. Manches spricht dafür, daß abgesehen von den modulierenden Einflüssen, die der Vagus auf die Atmung ausübt, im Atemzentrum selbst Modulatoren vorhanden sind, die die Alles-oder-Nichts-Atmung in die Eupnoe umwandeln. Auffallend bleibt dabei, daß die reflexgetriebene Atmung zur Alles-oder-Nichts-Atmung neigt, während die zentral-chemisch getriebene Atmung modulationsfähig ist.

Literatur.

ADRIAN, E. D.: Afferent impulses in the vagus and their effect on respiration. J. of Physiol. **79**, 332 (1933). — ADRIAN, E. D., and D. W. BRONK: The discharge of impulses in motor nerve fibers. Impulses in single fibers of the phrenic nerves. J. of Physiol. **66**, 81 (1928). — ALEXANDER, J. H., J. R. WEST, J. A. WOOD and D. W. RICHARDS: Analysis of the respiratory response to carbon dioxide inhalation in varying clinical states of hypercapnia, anoxia, and acid-base derangement. J. Clin. Invest. **34**, 511 (1955). — ASMUSSEN, E.: Blood pyruvate and ventilation in heavy work. Acta physiol. scand. (Stockh.) **20**, 133 (1950). — ASMUSSEN, E., E. H. CHRISTENSEN and M. NIELSEN: Humoral or nervous control of respiration during muscular work? Acta physiol. scand. (Stockh.) **6**, 161 (1943). — ASMUSSEN, E., u. M. NIELSEN: Studies on the regulation of respiration in heavy work. Acta physiol. scand. (Stockh.) **12**, 171 (1946). ~ Studies on the initial changes in respiration at the transition from rest to work and from work to rest. Acta physiol. scand. (Stockh.) **16**, 271 (1948). ~ The effect of auto-transfusion of „Work-Blood" on the pulmonary ventilation. Acta physiol. scand. (Stockh.) **20**, 79 (1950). — ASMUSSEN, E., M. NIELSEN and G. WIETH-PEDERSEN: Cortical or reflex control of respiration during muscular work? Acta physiol. scand. (Stockh.) **6**, 168 (1943). — ÅSTRÖM, A.: On the action of combined carbon dioxide excess and oxygen deficiency in the regulation of breathing. Acta physiol. scand. (Stockh.) **27**, Suppl., 98 (1952). — AVIADO, D. M., T. H. LI, W. KADOW, C. F. SCHMIDT, G. L. TURNBULL, G. W. PESKIN, M. E. HESS and A. J. WEISS: Respiratory and circulatory reflexes from the perfused heart and pulmonary circulation of the dog. Amer. J. Physiol. **165**, 261 (1951). — AVIADO, D. M., and C. F. SCHMIDT: Reflexes from stretch receptors in blood vessels, heart and lungs. Physiologic. Rev. **35**, 247 (1955).

BAKER, S. P., and F. A. HITCHCOCK: Immediate effects of inhalation of 100% oxygen at one atmosphere on ventilation volume, carbon dioxide output, oxygen consumption and respiratory rate in man. J. Appl. Physiol. **10**, 363 (1957). — BAUMGARTEN, R. v.: Koordinationsformen einzelner Ganglienzellen der rhombencephalen Atemzentren. Pflügers Arch. **262**, 573 (1956). — BAUMGARTEN, R. v., A. v. BAUMGARTEN u. K. P. SCHÄFER: Beitrag zur Lokalisationsfrage bulboreticulärer respiratorischer Neurone der Katze. Pflügers Arch. **264**, 217 (1957). — BEAN, J. W.: Intestine in reflex chemical control of breathing. Amer. J. Physiol. **171**, 522 (1952). — BEIN, H. J., u. H. HELMICH: Über afferente Vagusfasern. Helvet. physiol. Acta **7**, C 40 (1949). — BENZINGER, TH., E. OPITZ u. W. SCHOEDEL: Atmungserregung durch Sauerstoffmangel. Pflügers Arch. **241**, 71 (1938). — BRECKENRIDGE, C. G., and H. E. HOFF: Ischemic and anoxic dissolution of the supramedullary control of respiration. Amer. J. Physiol. **175**, 449 (1953). — BREUER, J.: Die Selbststeuerung der Atmung durch den Nervus vagus. Akad. Sitzber. Wien, Abt. 2, **58**, 909 (1868). — BRODIE, D. A., and H. L. BORISON: Evidence for a medullary inspiratory pacemaker: Functional concept of control regulation of respiration. Amer. J. Physiol. **188**, 347 (1957). — BRONK, D. W., and L. K. FERGUSON: The nervous control of intercostal respiration. Amer. J. Physiol. **110**, 700 (1935). — BROWN, E. B.: Physiological effects of hyperventilation. Physiologic. Rev. **33**, 445 (1953). — BUCHER, K.: Elektrische Aktivität des isolierten, künstlich durchströmten Medulla oblongata-Präparates. Helvet. physiol. Acta **3**, C 34 (1945). ~ Reflektorische Beeinflußbarkeit der Lungenatmung. Wien 1952.

CAMPBELL, E. J. M.: The respiratory muscles and the mechanics of breathing. London 1958. — CASTRO, E. DE: Sur la structure de la synapse dans les chemorecepteurs: Leur mécanisme d'excitation et rôle dans la circulation sanguine locale. Acta physiol. scand. (Stockh.)

22, 14 (1951). — CHERNIACK, R. M., and D. P. SNIDAL: The effect of obstruction to breathing on the ventilatory response to CO_2. J. Clin. Invest. 35, 1286 (1956). — CHIODI, H.: Respiratory adaptions to chronic high altitude hypoxia. J. Appl. Physiol. 10, 81 (1957). — COMROE, J. H.: The effects of direct chemical and electrical stimulation of the respiratory center in the cat. Amer. J. Physiol. 139, 490 (1943). —COMROE, J. H., and C. F. SCHMIDT: The part played by reflexes from the carotid body in the chemical regulation of respiration on the dog. Amer. J. Physiol. 121, 75 (1938). ~ Reflexes from the limbs as a factor in the hyperpnea of muscular exercise. Amer. J. Physiol. 138, 536 (1943). — CORMACK, S., D. J. C. CUNNINGHAM and J. B. L. GEE: The effect of carbon dioxide on the respiratory response to want of oxygen in man. Quart. J. Exper. Physiol. 42, 303 (1957). — COSTANTIN, L. L.: Effect of pulmonary congestion on vagal afferent activity. Amer. J. Physiol. 196, 49 (1959). —CUNNINGHAM, D. J. C., and J. L. H. O'RIORDAN: The effect of a rise in the temperature of the body in the respiratory response to carbon dioxide at rest. Quart. J. Exper. Physiol. 42, 329 (1957).

DAWES, G. S., and J. H. COMROE: Chemoreflexes from the heart and lungs. Physiologic. Rev. 34, 167 (1954). — DEJOURS, P., F. GIRARD, Y. LABROUSSE et A. TEILLAC: Étude de la régulation de la ventilation de repos chez l'homme en haute altitude. Rev. franç. Ét. clin. biol. 4, 115 (1959). — DIRKEN, S., and M. N. J. WOLDRING: Unit activity in bulbar respiratory centre. J. of Neurophysiol. 14, 211 (1951). — DOLIVO, M.: Impulsions afférentes dans les racines anterieures du nerf phrénique. Helvet. physiol. Acta 4, 199 (1946).

EBBECKE, U.: Der Gesichtsreflex des Trigeminus als Wärmeschutzreflex des Kopfes. Klin. Wschr. 1944, 141. — EULER, C. v., and U. SÖDERBERG: Medullary chemosensitive receptors. J. of Physiol. 118, 545 (1952a). ~ Slow potentials in the respiratory centres. J. of Physiol. 118, 555 (1952b). — EULER, U. S. v., G. LILJESTRAND and Y. ZOTTERMAN: The excitation mechanism of the chemoreceptors. Skand. Arch. Physiol. (Berl. u. Lpz.) 83, 132 (1939).

FELDER, J.: Untersuchungen über die Erregbarkeit des Atemzentrums in Abhängigkeit von Schilddrüse und Milz. Z. exper. Med. 94, 384 (1934). — FISHMAN, A. P., P. SAMET and A. COURNAND: Ventilatory drive in chronic pulmonary emphysema. Amer. J. Med. 19, 533 (1955). — FLEISCH, A.: Neuere Ergebnisse über Mechanik und propiozetive Steuerung der Atmungsbewegung. Erg. Physiol. 36, 249 (1934). — FRANK, N. R., H. A. LYONS, A. A. SIEBENS and T. F. NEALON: Pulmonary compliance in patients with cardiac disease. Amer. J. Med. 22, 516 (1957).

GEMMILL, C. L., and D. L. REEVES: The effect of anoxemia in normal dogs before and after denervation of the carotid sinuses. Amer. J. Physiol. 105, 487 (1933). — GESELL, R.: The chemical regulation of respiration. Physiologic. Rev. 5, 551 (1925). ~ A neurophysiological interpretation of the respiratory act. Erg. Physiol. 43, 477 (1940). — GESELL, R., J. BRICKER and C. MAGEE: Structural and functional organization of the central mechanism controlling breathing. Amer. J. Physiol. 117, 423 (1936). — GESELL, R., and E. T. HANSEN: Anticholinesterase activity as a biological instrument of nervous integration. Amer. J. Physiol. 144, 126 (1945). — GOLLWITZER-MEIER, K., u. E. LERCHE: Reflektorischer und zentraler Anteil der Kohlensäurewirkung auf die Atmung. Pflügers Arch. 244, 145 (1940). — GRAY, J. S.: The multiple factor theory of the control of respiratory ventilation. Science (Lancaster, Pa.) 103, 739 (1946). ~ Pulmonary ventilation and its physiological regulation. Springfield, Ill. 1949. — GRODINS, F. S.: Analysis of factors concerned in regulation of breathing in exercise. Physiologic. Rev. 30, 220 (1950).

HALDANE, J. S., and J. G. PRIESTLY: The regulation of the lung-ventilation. J. of Physiol. 32, 225 (1905). — HALL, F. G.: Carbon dioxide and respiratory regulation at altitude. J. Appl. Physiol. 5, 603 (1953). — HECK, E.: Wirkung hoher Sauerstoffdrucke auf die Atmung. Luftfahrtmed. 6, 105 (1942). — HECK, E., u. H. H. LOESCHCKE: Wirkung hoher Sauerstoffdrucke auf die Atmung. II. Mitteilung. Die Lage der die Atmung regulierenden Zellgebiete im arteriovenösen Kohlensäuredruckgefälle. Luftfahrtmed. 6, 114 (1942). — HERING, E.: Die Selbststeuerung der Atmung durch den Nervus vagus. Akad. Sitzber. Wien 57, 672 (1868). HESS, W. R.: Weitere Beobachtungen über den tonischen Vaguseinfluß bei verschiedenem konstanten Lungenvolumen. Pflügers Arch. 244, 360 (1941). ~ Die funktionelle Organisation des vegetativen Nervensystems. Basel 1948. — HESS, W. R., K. AKERD u. D. A. McDONALD: Beziehungen des Stirnhirnes zum vegetativen System. Helvet. physiol. Acta 9, 101 (1951). — HESS, W. R., u. W. A. STOLL: Experimenteller Beitrag betreffend die Regulierung der Körpertemperatur. Helvet. physiol. Acta 2, 461 (1944). — HESS, W. R., u. O. A. M. WYSS: Die Analyse der physikalischen Atmungsregulierung an Hand der Aktionsstrombilder des Phrenicus. Pflügers Arch. 237, 761 (1936). — HEYMANS, J. F., et C. HEYMANS: Sur les modifications directes et sur la regulation reflexe de l'activité du centre respiratoire de la tête isolée du chien. Arch. internat. Pharmacodynamie 33, 273 (1927). — HICSTAND, W. A., and W. C. RANDALL: Influence of proprioceptive vagal afferents on panting and accessory panting movements in mammals and birds. Amer. J. Physiol. 138, 12 (1942). — HOFF, H. E., and C. G. BRECKENRIDGE: The medullary origin of respiratory periodicity in the dog. Amer. J.

Physiol. **158**, 157 (1949). ~ The neurogenesis of respiration. FULTON's Textbook of Physiology, 17. Aufl., S. 843. 1955. — HOLST, E. v.: Das Reafferenzprinzip: Wechselwirkungen zwischen Zentralnervensystem und Peripherie. Naturwiss. **37**, 464 (1950). — HUSSON, G., and A. B. OTIS: Adaptive value of respiratory adjustments to shunt hypoxia and to altitude hypoxia. J. Clin. Invest. **36**, 270 (1957).

IRVING, L.: Respiration in diving mammals. Physiologic. Rev. **19**, 112 (1939).

JULICH, H.: Über die Dyspnoe bei Herzkranken und Emphysematikern und einige Fragen des Gastransportes. Z. exper. Med. **121**, 131 (1953).

KAO, F. F.: Regulation of respiration during muscular activity. Amer. J. Physiol. **185**, 145 (1956). — KNOWLTON, G. C., and M. G. LARRABEE: An unitary analysis of pulmonary volume receptors. Amer. J. Physiol. **147**, 100 (1946). — KRAMER, K.: Zur Theorie der Atemregulierung im Sauerstoffmangel. Pflügers Arch. **244**, 592 (1941). — KROGH, A.: The comparative physiology of respiratory mechanism. Philadelphia 1941. — KROGH, A., and J. LINDHARD: The regulation of respiration and circulation during the initial stages of muscular work. J. of Physiol. **47**, 112 (1913).

LANDGREEN, S., and E. NEIL: Chemoreceptor impulse activity following haemorrhage. Acta physiol. scand. (Stockh.) **23**, 158 (1951). — LARRABEE, M. G., and G. C. KNOWLTON: Excitation and inhibition of phrenic motoneurones by inflation of the lungs. Amer. J. Physiol. **147**, 90 (1946). — LILJESTRAND, Å.: Respiratory reactions elicited from the medulla oblongata of the cat. Acta physiol. scand. (Stockh.) **29**, Supp. 106, 321 (1953). ~ Neural control of respiration. Physiologic. Rev. **38**, 691 (1958). — LOESCHCKE, H. H.: Über Reiz und Erregbarkeit der zentralen Atmungsregulation. Klin. Wschr. **1949**, 761. ~ Über die Wirkung von Steroidhormonen auf die Lungenbelüftung. Klin. Wschr. **1954**, 441. — LOESCHCKE, H. H., u. K. H. GERTZ: Einfluß des O_2-Druckes in der Einatmungsluft auf die Atemtätigkeit des Menschen, geprüft unter Konstanthaltung des alveolaren CO_2-Druckes. Pflügers Arch. **267**, 460 (1958). — LOESCHCKE, H. H., u. H. P. KOEPCHEN: Über das Verhalten der Atmung und des arteriellen Druckes bei Einbringen von Veratridin, Lobelin und Cyanid in den Liquor cerebrospinalis. Pflügers Arch. **266**, 586 (1958). ~ Beeinflussung von Atmung und Vasomotorik durch Einbringen von Novocain in den Liquorraum. Pflügers Arch. **266**, 611 (1958). ~ Versuch zur Lokalisation des Angriffsortes der Atmungs- und Kreislaufwirkung von Novocain im Liquor cerebrospinalis. Pflügers Arch. **266**, 628 (1958). — LOESCHCKE, H. H., H. P. KOEPCHEN u. K. H. GERTZ: Über den Einfluß von Wasserstoffionenkonzentration und CO_2-Druck im Liquor cerebrospinalis auf die Atmung. Pflügers Arch. **266**, 569 (1958). — LOESCHCKE, H. H., U. C. LUFT u. E. OPITZ: Höhenanpassung am Jungfraujoch. Luftfahrtmed. **7**, 218 (1942). — LUEKEN, B., u. C. TIMM: Über die Erregbarkeit des Atemzentrums in den einzelnen Phasen des Atemzyklus. Pflügers Arch. **249**, 241 (1947). — LUFT, U. C.: Die Höhenanpassung. Erg. Physiol. **44**, 256 (1941). — LUMSDEN, T.: Observations on the respiratory centres in the cat. J. of Physiol. **57**, 153 (1923); **58**, 81 (1924).

MARCKWALD, M.: Die Atembewegungen und deren Innervation beim Kaninchen. Z. Biol. **23**, 149 (1887). — MATTHES, K., u. W. ULMER: Untersuchungen zur Analyse der Sauerstoffwirkung bei Patienten mit arterieller Hypoxämie. Dtsch. Arch. klin. Med. **202**, 548 (1955). — MILLS, J. N.: Changes in alveolar carbon dioxide tension by night and during sleep. J. of Physiol. **122**, 66 (1953). — MITCHELL, J. H., B. J. SPROULE and C. B. CHAPMAN: Factors influencing respiration during heavy exercise. J. Clin. Invest. **37**, 1693 (1958). — MORGAN, D. P., F. KAO, T. P. K. LIM and F. S. GRODINS: Temperature and respiratory responses in exercise. Amer. J. Physiol. **183**, 454 (1955). — MÜRTZ, R., u. G. NEUHAUS: Über die Erregbarkeit des Atemzentrums bei Patienten mit Morbus caeruleus. Klin. Wschr. **1954**, 847.

NIELSEN, M.: Die Regulation der Körpertemperatur bei Muskelarbeit. Skand. Arch. Physiol. (Berl. u. Lpz.) **79**, 193 (1938). — NIELSEN, M., and H. SMITH: Studies on the regulation of respiration in acute hypoxia. Acta physiol. scand. (Stockh.) **24**, 293 (1952).

OBERHOLZER, R. J. H.: Zentren für Atmung und Kreislauf in der Medulla oblongata. Klin. Wschr. **1957**, 448. — OCHWADT, B., E. BÜCHERL, H. KREUZER u. H. H. LOESCHCKE: Beeinflussung der Atemsteigerung bei Muskelarbeit durch partiellen neuromuskulären Block (Tubocurarin). Pflügers Arch. **269**, 613—621 (1959). — OPITZ, E.: Über akute Hypoxie. Erg. Physiol. **44**, 315 (1941). — OPITZ, E., u. D. LÜBBERS: Allgemeine Physiologie der Zell- und Gewebsatmung. Handbuch der allgemeinen Pathologie, Bd. 4/2. 1957. — OPPELT, W.: Unser Normblatt. Regulationsbegriffe und Aufgabe der Regelung. Regulationstechnik **2**, 26 (1954). ~ Din **19**, 226 (1954).

PI-SUÑER, A.: The regulation of the respiratory movements by peripheral chemo-receptors. Physiologic. Rev. **27**, 1 (1947). — PITTS, R. F.: The respiratory center and its descending pathways. J. Comp. Neur. **72**, 605 (1940). ~ The function of components of the respiratory complex. J. of Neurophysiol. **5**, 403 (1942). ~ Organisation of the respiratory center. Physiologic. Rev. **26**, 609 (1946). — PITTS, R. F., H. W. MAGOUN and S. W. RANSON: Localization of the medullary respiratory rhythmicity. Amer. J. Physiol. **126**, 673 (1939). — PRYOR, W. W., J. B. HICKAM, H. O. SICKER and E. B. PAGE: Effect of circulatory changes on the pulmonary compliance of normal subjects and patients with mitral stenosis. Circulation 15, 721 (1957).

Rahn, H., H. T. Bahnson, J. F. Munworthy and J. M. Hagen: Adaption to high altitude. J. Appl. Physiol. 6, 154 (1953). — Rahn, H., and A. B. Otis: Man's respiratory response during and after acclimatization to high altitude. Amer. J. Physiol. 157, 445 (1949). — Ramsay, A. G.: Effects of metabolism and anesthesia on pulmonary ventilation. J. appl. Physiol. 14, 102 (1959). — Rein, H. F.: Die physiologische Verknüpfung von Atmung und Kreislauf. Fortbild. lehrg. Nauheim 1935. — Rickenbach, K., u. H. Meessen: Vergleichende reizphysiologische und anatomische Untersuchungen der reflektorischen Atemzentren der Medulla oblongata des Kaninchens. Acta anat. (Basel) 12, 135 (1951). — Riley, R. L., and C. S. Houston: Composition of alveolar air and volume ofpul monary ventilation during long exposure to high altitude. J. Appl. Physiol. 3, 526 (1951). — Robin, E. D., R. D. Whaley, Ch. H. Crump and D. M. Travis: Alveolar gas tensions, pulmonary ventilation and blood pH during physiologic sleep in normal subjects. J. clin. Invest. 37, 981 (1958). — Rosenbaum, H., and B. Renshaw: Descending respiratory pathways in the cervical spinal cord. Amer. J. Physiol. 157, 460 (1949).

Schäfer, K. E.: Atmung und Säure-Basengleichgewicht bei langdauerndem Aufenthalt in 3% CO_2. Pflügers Arch. 251, 689 (1949). — Schmidt, C. F.: The respiration. In Bards, Medical physiology. St. Louis 1956. — Schmidt, C. F., and J. H. Comroe: Function of the carotid and aortic bodies. Physiologic. Rev. 20, 115 (1940). — Schwab, M.: Zur Behandlung des Lungenemphysems mit chronischer respiratorischer Acidose. Klin. Wschr. 1957, 157. — Sherrington, C. S.: The integrative action of the nervous system. London 1906. — Shock, N. W., and M. H. Soley: Effekt of oxygen tension of inspired air on the respiratory response of normal subjects to carbon dioxide. Amer. J. Physiol. 130, 777 (1940). — Smith, W. K.: The representation of respiratory movements in the cerebral cortex. J. of Neurophysiol. 1, 55 (1938). — Sommer, J.: Über Atemreflexe (Vagus-Zwerchfellreflexe). Z. Biol. 100, 162 (1941). — Speakman, T. J., and B. P. Babkin: Effect of cortical stimulation on respiratory rate. Amer. J. Physiol. 159, 239 (1949). — Spielmann, R.: Abhängigkeit der Erregbarkeit des Atemzentrums von der Schilddrüse. Z. exper. Med. 94, 378 (1934). — Stella, G.: On the mechanism of production and the physiological significance of „apneusis". J. of Physiol. 93, 10 (1938).

Tang, P. C.: Localization of the pneumotaxic center in the cat. Amer. J. Physiol. 172, 645 (1953). — Tenney, S. M.: Ventilatory response to carbon dioxide in pulmonary emphysema. J. Appl. Physiol. 6, 477 (1954). — Tschirgi, R. D.: Carotid receptors essential in the gasping of the isolated rat head. Proc. Soc. Exper. Biol. a. Med. 63, 397 (1946).

Ulmer, W.: Untersuchungen über die effektive Ventilationsleistung bei Emphysematikern. Verh. dtsch. Ges. inn. Med. 62, 68 (1956).

Wagner, R.: Probleme und Beispiele biologischer Regelung. Stuttgart: 1954. — Whitteridge, D.: Multiple embolisme of the lung and rapid shallow breathing. Physiologic. Rev. 30, 475 (1950). — Widdicombe, J. G.: Respiratory reflexes excited by inflation of the lungs. J. of Physiol. 123, 105 (1954). — Winterstein, H.: Die Reaktionstheorie der Atmungsregulation. Pflügers Arch. 187, 293 (1921). ~ Atmungsregulation und Reaktionsregulation. Naturwiss. 28, 625 (1923). ~ Die Atmung als chemischer Regulator. Naturwiss. 40, 427 (1953). ~ Die chemische Steuerung der Atmung. Erg. Physiol. 48, 328 (1955). ~ Die Hendersonsche Gleichung und die Reaktionstheorie. Klin. Wschr. 1958, 356. — Winterstein, H., u. N. Gökhan: Ammoniumchlorid-Acidose und Reaktionstheorie der Atmungsregulation. Arch. Internat. Pharmacodynamic 93, 212 (1953). — Witzleb, E., H. Bartels, H. Budde u. M. Mochizucki: Der Einfluß des arteriellen O_2-Drucks auf die chemoreceptorischen Aktionspotentiale in Carotissinusnerven. Pflügers Arch. 261, 211 (1955). — Woldring, S., and M. N. J. Dirken: Site and extension of bulbar respiratory centre. J. of Neurophysiol. 14, 227 (1951). — Wyss, O. A. M.: Respiratory effects from stimulation of the afferent vagus nerve in the monkey. J. of Neurophysiol. 10, 315 (1947a). ~ Reflex reversal as determined by the frequency of afferent stimulation. Arch. néerl. Physiol. 28, 44 (1947b). ~ Respiratory centre and reflex control of breathing. Helvet. physiol. Acta 12, Suppl. 10, 5—35 (1954).

Zechman, F., F. G. Hall and W. E. Hull: Effects of graded resistance to tracheal air flow in man. J. Appl. Physiol. 10, 356 (1957).

Funktionelle Pathologie der Atmung.

Von

H. W. KNIPPING und **W. BOLT** (Köln).

Unter Mitwirkung von

H. VALENTIN und **H. VENRATH**

Mit 46 Abbildungen.

I. Funktionelle Pathologie der Atmung.

Einleitung.

Die funktionelle Pathologie erstrebt die Aufdeckung der Mechanismen krankhafter Funktionsstörungen durch naturwissenschaftliche Analyse des Krankheitsgeschehens.

Atmung oder Respiration bedeutet Gasaustausch zwischen Organismus und Umgebung, insbesondere Aufnahme von Sauerstoff und Abgabe von Kohlendioxyd. In der Physiologie unterscheidet man die *äußere Atmung* (Lungenatmung = Gasaustausch zwischen Außenluft bzw. Alveolarluft und dem Blut in den Lungencapillaren) und die *innere Atmung* (Gewebsatmung = Gasaustausch zwischen Blut und peripherer Zelle bzw. Zellbestandteilen).

Hieraus ergibt sich eine generelle *Unterteilung der Atemfunktionsstörungen* in:
Störungen der äußeren Atmung:

a) Störungen der Ventilation bzw. der Atemmechanik,
b) Störungen der Perfusion,
c) Störungen der Diffusion und
Störungen der inneren Atmung.

Die *klinische Funktionsdiagnostik der Atmung* hat seit den Pionierleistungen BRAUERs und seiner Schüler eine besondere praktische Bedeutung erlangt. Sie ergänzt wirkungsvoll die eigentliche nosologische Diagnostik mit dem Ziel, die oft komplexe Natur funktioneller Störungen aufzudecken, sowie den Umfang vorhandener Leistungseinschränkungen festzulegen durch quantitative Erfassung der Leistungsgrenzen des kardio-pulmonalen Systems. Neben praktisch-internistischen Fragestellungen handelt es sich vornehmlich um solche der Arbeits- und Sporttherapie, der Gutachtenmedizin und der Thoraxchirurgie[1].

Die allgemein-ärztliche Untersuchung, deren grundsätzliche Bedeutung nicht besonders betont zu werden braucht, geht in allen Fällen der funktionsdiagnostischen Prüfung voran.

Ein umfangreiches Krankengut der *Lungenklinik* und der *Infektionsklinik* (Tuberkulose, Emphysem, Silikose, Bronchialcarcinom, Pneumonie, Poliomyelitis) und viele *Herzkranke* mit Lungenkomplikationen sind in den letzten 2 Jahrzehnten mit neu erarbeiteten funktionsanalytischen Methoden untersucht worden. Diese klinischen Ergebnisse sind ein wesentliches Kernstück einer funktionellen Pathologie der Atmung. Das Tierexperiment hat erst in der jüngsten Zeit begonnen, für die Pathophysiologie der Atmung fruchtbar zu sein, vor allem, nachdem es gelang, an größeren Tieren Pneumonien, kavernöse Lungentuberkulosen

---

[1] KNIPPING, BOLT, VALENTIN und VENRATH 1955, 1960.

usw. zu setzen und Bedingungen zu schaffen, welche in etwa mit den in der Klinik beobachteten vergleichbar sind[1].

Zuerst hat sich die *Silikoseklinik* über die alte, nur die Ätiologie dieser Krankheit, die Lokalisation und weniger die funktionellen Beziehungen berücksichtigende Form der Routineuntersuchung hinaus bemüht. Im Mittelpunkt stand bisher neben der einfachen ärztlichen Untersuchung vor allem die Röntgenuntersuchung zur Aufdeckung der morphologischen Charakteristika. Die Erfordernisse der Sozialversicherung und die wirtschaftliche Belastung durch die Entschädigung der vielen Silikotiker erzwangen bei dieser Erkrankung in den vergangenen Jahren ein sorgfältiges Durcharbeiten der Funktionsprobleme, um im Einzelfall zu einer objektiven Beurteilung der funktionellen Situation zu kommen.

Die bei dieser Krankheit gewonnenen Erkenntnisse und entsprechende neue Methoden kamen späterhin der sich stark entwickelnden Lungenchirurgie zugute. Weitere Fortschritte der Lungenchirurgie werden maßgeblich von der Vertiefung der funktionellen Pathologie der Atmung und der Durchbildung neuer funktionsanalytischer Methoden getragen sein.

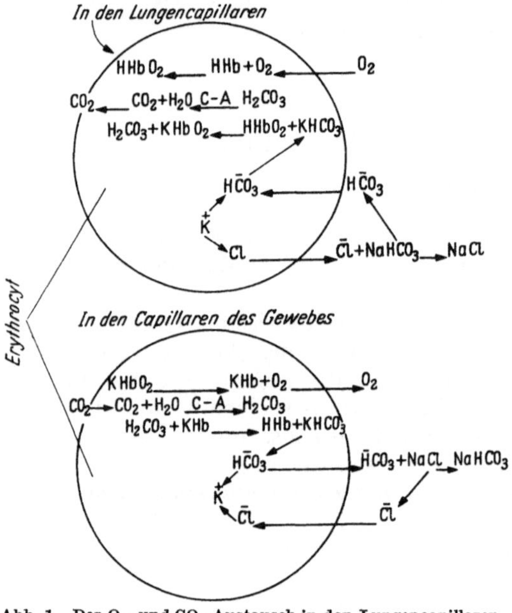

Ein Beispiel mag das verdeutlichen. Der „trend" der operativen Behandlung der Lungentuberkulose und soweit möglich auch des Bronchialcarcinoms geht neuerdings dahin, selektiv und funktionsschonend vorzugehen, d. h. funktionstüchtiges Gewebe und möglichst viele Segmente zu erhalten. Damit kommen wir zu dem schwierigsten und zur Zeit erst partiell gelösten Teil der funktionsanalytischen quantitativen Technik, zu einer *regionalen Funktionsdiagnostik*, auf deren Ergebnisse noch eingegangen wird.

Schließlich erforderte die Weiterentwicklung der Herzchirurgie eine Ausweitung unserer Kenntnisse von der funktionellen Pathologie der Stauungslunge (speziell der Diffusionsstörungen bei chronischen Stauungslungen), und von den Veränderungen des Lungenkreislaufs bei angeborenen und erworbenen Vitien. Hier sind neue und leistungsfähige Methoden unter dem Druck dieser Erfordernisse entstanden.

Abb. 1. Der O_2- und CO_2-Austausch in den Lungencapillaren und den Capillaren des großen Kreislaufs.

Interessante und für die funktionelle Pathologie der Atmung bedeutungsvolle Ergebnisse brachten schließlich die Funktionsstudien bei der *Poliomyelitis*, die hier nur angedeutet werden können.

Demgegenüber ist die Bearbeitung der *funktionellen Pathologie der inneren Atmung* noch ganz im Beginn. Angesichts solch wichtiger Teilprobleme wie der serösen Entzündung und der durch letztere (ebenso wie auch durch das Ödem generell) bedingten Störungen der inneren Atmung ist unser methodisches Rüstzeug noch unvollkommen. Hier handelt es sich zum Teil auch um Diffusionsstörungen, wenn wir den Gasaustausch zwischen Blut und Zelle als Ganzes betrachten und die Atmung der Zellteile ausnehmen. Vielfach sind es die gleichen *Diffusionsfragen*, wie sie bei den Diffusionsstörungen in der Lunge abgehandelt werden, quasi mit umgekehrten Vorzeichen. Große praktische Bedeutung hat dieser Diffusionskomplex im Rahmen der funktionellen Beziehungen zwischen Training, Capillarisierung, Diffusionsfläche und Diffusionsweg erlangt. Diese Detailfragen können, ebenso wie die Atmung der Zellbestandteile — soll nicht der Rahmen dieses Kapitels völlig gesprengt werden —, nur ganz am Rande erörtert werden. Denn gerade das Gebiet der Atmung der Zellbestandteile

---

[1] CEYHAN, JUNG und VARLIK 1951.

(die Atmungsfermente und die spezielle chemische Problematik der Zellatmung, die Gifte der Zellatmung) hat einen riesigen Umfang angenommen.

KARL NEUBERG entwickelte als einer der ersten eine ganz neue chemische Methodik für diese besondere Zielsetzung. Er führte das 2,4-Dinitrophenylhydrazin in die Analyse des chemischen Ablaufes der Aerobiose und der Anaerobiose ein. Die Auftrennung der Hydrazone durch eutektische Schmelzen, Hochvakuumsublimation, Chromatographie usw. (wir verweisen auf die Arbeiten von P. und M. LIPP und von MATTHIESSEN aus unserem Arbeitskreis) ist noch nicht abgeschlossen. Es zeigte sich, daß die Carbonylkörper der C_2- und der C_3-Stufe auch an der äußeren Atmung teilhaben.

Von überragender Bedeutung für unsere Kenntnisse des Chemismus der inneren Atmung sind die Arbeiten von WARBURG. Durch sie ist ein gänzlich neues Rüstzeug mit hoher Präzision entstanden [1]. Methoden und Ergebnisse dieser beiden neuen Arbeitsrichtungen mit im wesentlichen chemischen Grundlagen und Aspekten und einer fast unübersehbaren Fülle neuerer Arbeiten (vorzüglich die bedeutenden Arbeiten von KREBS), welche im weiteren Sinne zur funktionellen Pathologie der inneren Atmung zu rechnen wären, würden ein eigenes Handbuch füllen. Sie werden hier nur einleitend berührt, aber nicht im einzelnen behandelt. Wir verweisen auf die speziellen Kapitel in diesem Handbuch (II. Band, 1. Teil).

Der Schwerpunkt des nachfolgenden Kapitels soll demnach mehr auf dem pulmonalen Sektor der funktionellen Pathologie der Atmung liegen. Der O_2- und CO_2-Austausch in den Lungencapillaren und in den Capillaren des Gewebes sei in Abb. 1 schematisch wiedergegeben. Methoden und Problematik der funktionellen Pathologie der Atmung überschneiden sich vielfältig mit denen der Physiologie und können im folgenden Kapitel mit wenigen Ausnahmen nicht ganz übergangen werden.

II. Die Stellung der Lunge im Rahmen einiger wichtiger Funktionssysteme.

Die Funktion der Lunge besteht vor allem in der Arterialisierung des venösen Mischblutes, d. h. in der Aufnahme von Sauerstoff und der Ausscheidung von Kohlendioxyd.

So einfach, wie sich die Aufgabe der Lunge definieren läßt, so schwierig gestaltet sich die Erfassung des funktionellen Gesamtkomplexes und der Details der äußeren Atmung, besonders unter pathischen Bedingungen. Der Grund hierfür liegt in der Tatsache, daß die Lunge nur eines der wesentlichen Glieder in dem lebenswichtigen Funktionssystem Atmung, Blut, Herz und Kreislauf darstellt. Die Funktion der Lunge wird vom Chemismus des Blutes, der Arbeitsweise des Herzens, der Regulation des Kreislaufs und vor allem von den Anforderungen des Körperstoffwechsels beeinflußt bzw. bestimmt. Hierzu kommen unter pathologischen Bedingungen die Einwirkungen durch Krankheiten der Lunge und anderer Organsysteme.

Erstaunlich ist die große Anpassungsfähigkeit in allen Teilvorgängen während Belastung und unter pathologischen Verhältnissen. Auf Einzelheiten der normalen Funktion der Atmung wird an anderer Stelle eingegangen [2]. Hier soll lediglich zum besseren Verständnis der nachfolgenden Abschnitte die Stellung der Lunge im Rahmen des Gaswechsels, im Zusammenhang mit der Atmungsfunktion des Blutes und des Kreislaufsystems, im Hinblick auf den Säure-Basenhaushalt und in Abhängigkeit vom Atemzentrum kurz dargestellt werden.

---

[1] LANG 1952, RONA und KNIPPING 1926, Prakticum der physiologischen Chemie, Bd. III.
[2] U. C. LUFT 1961 (dieses Handbuch).

1. Der Gasstoffwechsel.

Beim Gasstoffwechsel im Rahmen der äußeren Atmung lassen sich zwei Teilvorgänge unterscheiden, deren treibende Kräfte die physikalischen Prozesse der Konvektion und der Diffusion sind. Durch die Atembewegungen (Ventilation) wird die Außenluft in die Alveolen eingesaugt und wieder ausgeschieden (Konvektion). Der Sauerstoff gelangt durch Diffusion in das Blut. Das arterialisierte Blut wird durch den Kreislauf zu den Gewebscapillaren transportiert. Für die Kohlensäureabgabe gilt das gleiche Prinzip in umgekehrter Richtung.

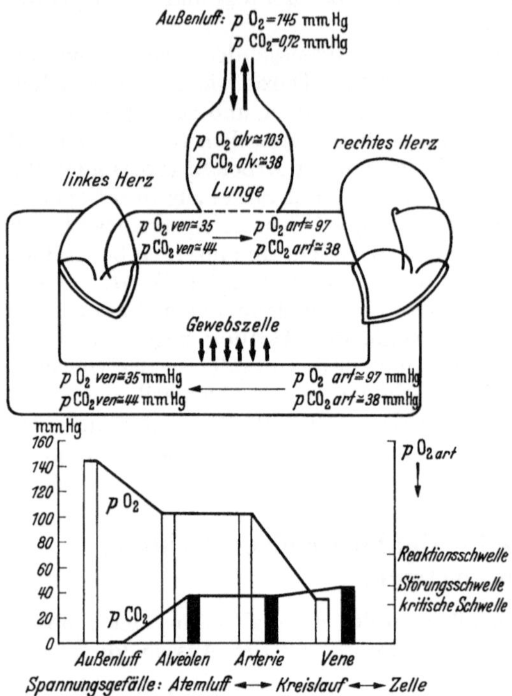

Abb. 2. Sauerstoffspannung (PO_2) und Kohlendioxydspannung (PCO_2) in der Außenluft, in der Alveolarluft und im Blut (schematisch) in Ruhe.

Die schematischen Abb. 2, 3a—d und 4 zeigen die quantitative Seite des Gasaustausches. In Abb. 2 sind die Sauerstoff- und Kohlendioxydspannungen in der Außenluft, der Alveolarluft und im Blut unter Ruhebedingungen aufgeführt. Abb. 3 bringt die Sauerstoffspannung und Sauerstoffsättigung des Blutes während eines Atemcyclus zur Darstellung, und zwar a) bei Normalverhältnissen in Ruhe, b) bei Verschiebung infolge einer arteriellen Sauerstoffsättigung von 80% ohne Eintreten kompensatorischer Maßnahmen, c) den gleichen Zustand wie b), aber mit Kompensation durch Herzminutenvolumen-Anstieg, d) bei Kompensation durch p_H-Verschiebung zur sauren Seite hin. Aus Abb. 4 können die Normalwerte der Atmung, des Gasstoffwechsels und der Drucke in Herz und Kreislauf entnommen werden.

Bei einem Atemminutenvolumen von 6—10 Litern und durchschnittlich 15 Atemzügen sowie einem Totraum von 140 cm³ werden die Lungen mit 4 bis 8 Liter Außenluft durchspült. Hieraus werden in Ruhe rund 300 cm³ Sauerstoff aufgenommen. Ein Großteil der in der Außenluft enthaltenen Sauerstoffmenge wird also nicht verwendet, und zwar fast zwei Drittel.

Der Gasaustausch von der Alveolarluft ins Blut erfolgt, wie schon angedeutet, durch *Diffusion*.

Die Ficksche *Gleichung*:

$$\frac{dn}{dt} = DF\,\frac{dc}{dx}$$

zeigt, daß die je Zeiteinheit diffundierende Gasmenge (dn/dt) von dem Diffusionskoeffizienten (D), der Diffusionsfläche (F) und dem Konzentrationsgefälle (dc/dx) abhängig ist. Die Alveolaroberfläche der Gesamtlunge wird mit 60—150 m² angegeben. Die Gasaustauschfläche, d. h. die Kontaktfläche der Capillaren in der Lunge, soll um 90 m² liegen. Dieser Wert dürfte bei Sauerstoffmangel und Arbeit erheblich schwanken und mit zunehmendem Alter kleiner werden. Der Faktor (dc/dx) bedeutet das mittlere Druckgefälle zwischen dem O_2-Druck in der Alveolarluft und in der Capillare über die Strecke (dx); (dx) ist der Weg des Moleküls aus der Gasphase der Alveolarluft über das Alveolarepithel, die Gefäßwand, das Serum bis in die Erythrocyten und an das Hämoglobin.

2. Die Atmungsfunktion des Blutes.

Die Atmungsfunktion des Blutes ist ein Teil seiner allgemeinen Transportaufgabe. Bei dieser speziellen Funktion schafft es den Sauerstoff von der Lunge zu den Geweben, nimmt dort die Kohlensäure auf und bringt sie zur Lunge. In der Lunge und der Peripherie wird das Blut in den ausgedehnten Capillarnetzen zu einem feinen Film ausgebreitet, der nur durch eine dünne Membran

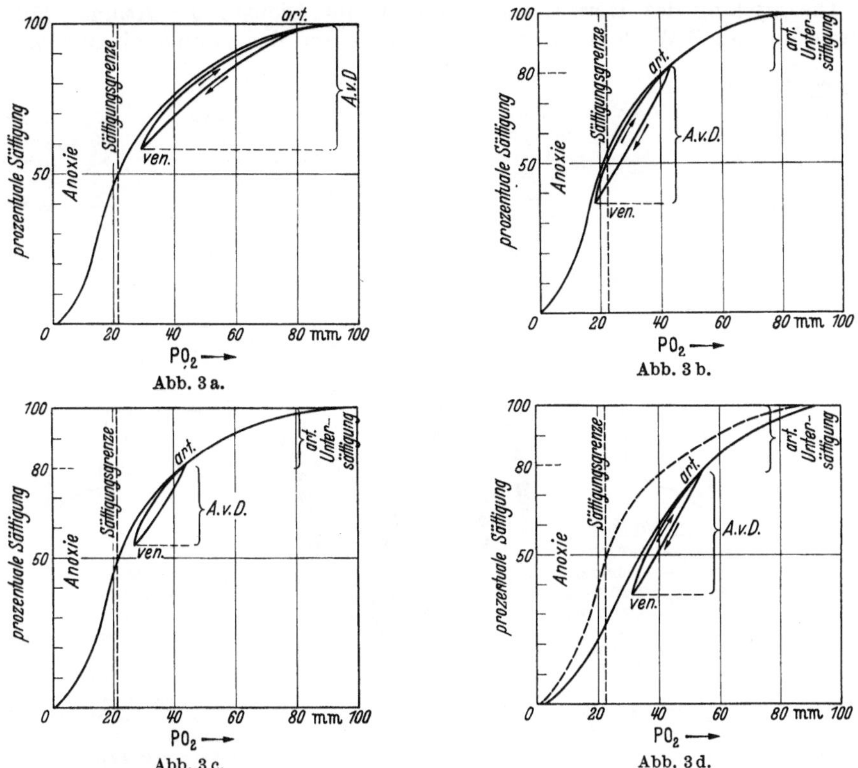

Abb. 3a.

Abb. 3b.

Abb. 3c.

Abb. 3d.

Abb. 3a. Schematische Darstellung des Sauerstoffaustausches in Gewebe und Lunge. Arterielle O_2-Sättigung 98%, Sättigung des venösen Mischblutes 58%. Die Sättigungsgrenze liegt bei 23 mm O_2.

Abb. 3b. Dieselben Vorgänge wie in Abb. 3a bei einer arteriellen Untersättigung von 20%. Bei unverändertem O_2-Bedarf der Gewebe und gleichbleibender AVD kommt es neben der arteriellen Untersättigung zu einer chemischen Sauerstoffschuld im Gewebe, da die Sättigungsgrenze unterschritten wird.

Abb. 3c. Kompensationsmechanismen (I), durch Verkleinerung der AVD als Folge einer Herzminutenvolumenzunahme bei gleichbleibender arterieller O_2-Untersättigung und unverändertem O_2-Bedarf des Gewebes.

Abb. 3d. Kompensationsmechanismen (II). Durch Säuerung des Gewebes wandert die O_2-Dissoziationskurve nach rechts. Dadurch O_2-Spannungsgewinn. Bei unveränderter AVD und gleicher arterieller Untersättigung kommt es nicht zu einer chemischen Sauerstoffschuld.

von den umgebenden Körperzellen getrennt ist. Aufnahme und Abgabe der Gase erfolgt nach den allgemeinen physikalischen Gesetzen.

Die Bindung des Sauerstoffs an das Bluthämoglobin ist reversibel. Der normale Hämoglobingehalt schwankt zwischen 12 und 16,3 g-%. Blut kann maximal 18,8—21,9 Vol.-% Sauerstoff binden. Werden Blutproben verschiedenen Sauerstoffpartialdrucken ausgesetzt und trägt man als Ordinate die prozentuale Sättigung und als Abszisse den zugehörigen Partialdruck in ein Koordinatensystem ein, so erhält man als charakteristische Kurve für das Gleichgewicht zwischen Oxyhämoglobin und sauerstofffreiem Hämoglobin die *Sauerstoffdissoziationskurve.*

Abb. 5a zeigt die normalen Variationen der O_2 Dissoziationskurve des menschlichen Blutes, Abb. 5b den Einfluß der Wasserstoffionenkonzentration, Abb. 5c den Einfluß der Kohlendioxydspannung. In Abb. 7 ist die Dissoziationskurve des Kohlendioxyds dargestellt.

3. Herz und Kreislauf im Dienste der Atmung.

Die Stellung des Herz-Kreislaufsystems im Dienste der Atmung läßt sich durch folgende 3 Werte definieren: Den Druck und das Volumen in den einzelnen

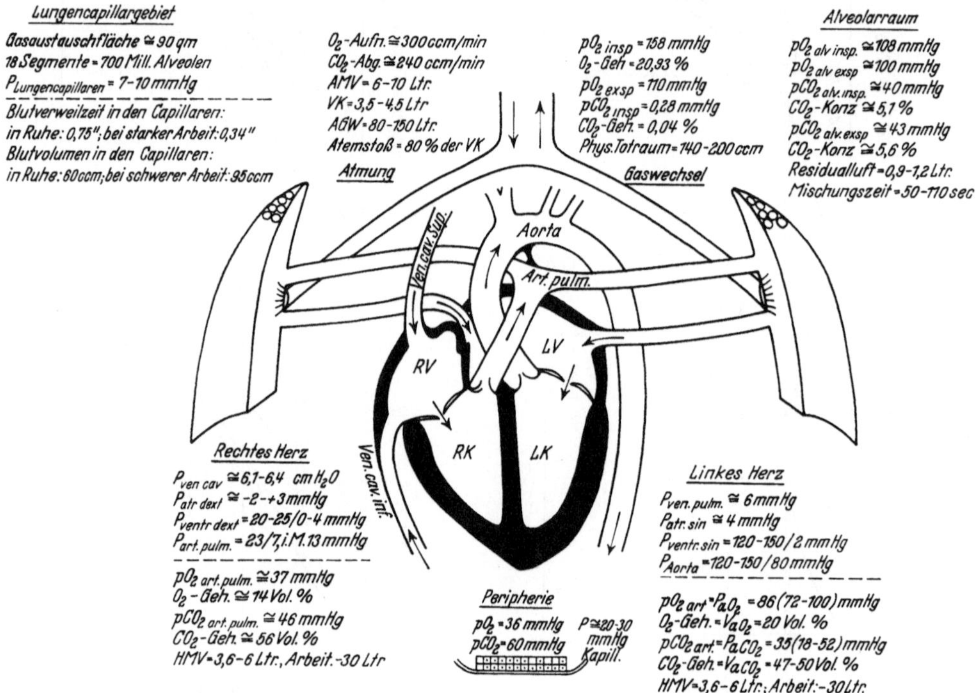

Abb. 4. Die Normalwerte der Atmung, des Gasstoffwechsels und der Drucke im Kreislauf (schematisch).

Kreislaufabschnitten und Herzhöhlen sowie das Fördervolumen des Herzens. In Abb. 4 sind die normalen Druckwerte aufgeführt. Sie können bei den verschiedenen Krankheiten der Lunge und besonders des linken Herzens erheblich ansteigen und zu Störungen der äußeren Atmung führen. Abb. 6 zeigt die Änderung der Blutvolumina bei den verschiedenen Versagenszuständen von Herz und Kreislauf. Insbesondere bei der Linksinsuffizienz des Herzens spielen die Lungenstauung und die sekundäre respiratorische Insuffizienz eine wichtige Rolle. Das Fassungsvermögen der Lunge soll normalerweise zwischen 500 cm³ und 1500 cm³ Blut liegen [1].

Das Fördervolumen des Herzens beträgt in Ruhe 3,6—6,0, im Durchschnitt 5 Liter/min. Hierdurch werden bei normaler O_2-Aufnahme und O_2-Kapazität etwa 1000 cm³ Sauerstoff je min transportiert. Ein Drittel wird in der Lunge neu aufgenommen. Unter schwerer Arbeit kann die Durchblutung der Lunge auf fast 30 Liter ansteigen und die maximale Sauerstoffaufnahme Werte von 3 bis

----

[1] Cournand 1941.

5 Liter/min erreichen. Die Steigerung des Herzzeitvolumens und die vermehrte Ausschöpfung des venösen Mischblutes ermöglichen diese Vita maxima-Größe.

Der Einfluß der Herzminutenvolumenzunahme auf den Gasaustausch in Lunge und Gewebe ist in Abb. 3c dargestellt.

4. Das Säure-Basen-Gleichgewicht und seine normalen und krankhaften Variationen.

Das p_H des Arterienblutes schwankt zwischen 7,39 und 7,44. Die Normalwerte des Plasmabicarbonats des venösen Mischblutes betragen zwischen 53 und 75 Vol.-% CO_2. Das freie CO_2, das etwa $1/20$ davon ausmacht, liegt zwischen 2,5 und 3,5 Vol.-%. Die Maximalschwankungsbreite des Blut-p_H bewegt sich zwischen 7,0 und 7,8. Extremere Werte sind mit dem Leben kaum vereinbar. Das p_H des venösen Mischblutes liegt etwa 0,02 tiefer als das des arteriellen Blutes. Die Erythrocyten sind etwa 0,08—0,14 saurer als das Plasma. Abb. 5b zeigt den Einfluß der Wasserstoffionenkonzentration auf die Sauerstoff-Dissoziationskurve.

In Abb. 7 sind das Säure-Basengleichgewicht des Arterienblutes in Beziehung zur Kohlendioxydspannungskurve sowie die normalen und pathologischen Variationen dargestellt. Alkalose und Acidose spielen in diesem Zusammenhang eine besondere Rolle.

Um wenige Begriffe der Stoffwechselphysiologie ist so viel Verwirrung entstanden wie um die Definition der Acidose und Alkalose. Die Bezeichnung *Acidose* wurde von NAUNYN in die medizinische Terminologie eingeführt. Er verstand darunter die normale Produktion saurer Stoffwechselbestandteile im Organismus. Der Begriff wurde später von VAN SLYKE und CULLEN übernommen. Sie bezeichneten einen Abfall der *Alkalireserve des Blutes* ($= CO_2$-Bindungsfähigkeit des Blutes in Vol.-% bei einer CO_2-Spannung von 40 mm Hg) als Acidose und einen Anstieg über die Norm als Alkalose. Die Größe der Alkalireserve ist abhängig von dem Bicarbonatgehalt des Plasmas nach Abpufferung der fixen Säuren im Blut, also von dem für die CO_3H-Bindung noch übrig bleibenden Bicarbonatgehalt. Eine Verminderung besagt daher, daß ein Anstieg von fixen Säuren vorhanden ist oder daß der Bicarbonatgehalt des Blutes reduziert ist. Die Kompensationsmechanismen,

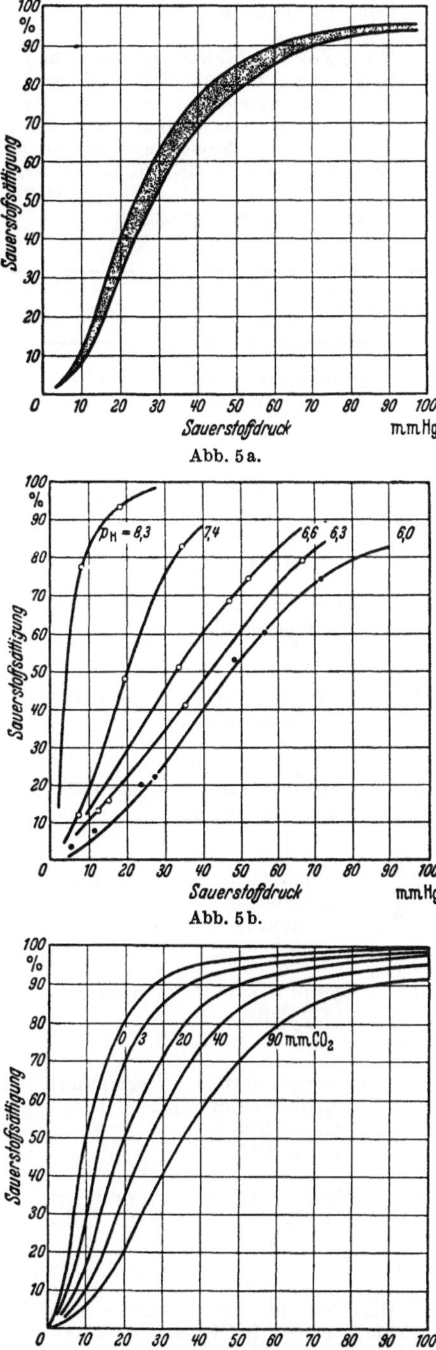

Abb. 5a.

Abb. 5b.

Abb. 5c.

Abb. 5. a Normale Variation der O_2-Dissoziationskurve von Blut. b Einfluß der Wasserstoffionenkonzentration. c Einfluß der CO_2-Spannung auf die O_2-Dissoziationskurve von Hämoglobin.

über die der Organismus verfügt, um sein p_H normal zu halten, sind groß. Sie gehen aus Tabelle 1 hervor.

Beide Zustandsbilder zeigen also keine reale Säuerung oder Alkalisierung des Blutes an.

Van Slyke unterscheidet 9 Säure-Basen-Zustandsbilder, ein normales Gleichgewicht und 8 pathologische bzw. anormale. Er vermeidet die Bezeichnung Alkalose und Acidose und spricht von Alkalidefizit oder CO_2-Erhöhung und Alkaliüberschuß oder CO_2-Defizit. Es geht aus dieser Bezeichnung hervor, daß das wesentlichste Agens zur Aufrechterhaltung des normalen p_H beim Gesunden der CO_2-Gehalt bzw. die CO_2-Spannung des Blutes ist. Es besagt, daß das Verhältnis $H_2CO_3/NaHCO_3$ entweder erhöht oder erniedrigt ist, entsprechend der Steigerung oder Senkung des p_H.

Tabelle 1.

	Zustandsbild Gruppe	p_H	Ursache	Kompensation und klinisches Vorkommen
1	Dekompensierter Alkaliüberschuß I	erhöht	Bicarbonataufnahme vermehrt, HCl-Verlust	Artefiziell (Ulcustherapie) langdauerndes Erbrechen. Festhalten von Säure
2	Dekompensiertes CO_2-Defizit „Gasalkalose" II u. III	erhöht	CO_2-Verlust (Hyperventilation)	Bicarbonatausscheidung oder Säureretention (Niere)
3	Kompensierter Alkaliüberschuß IV	normal	wie bei I, nicht so ausgeprägt	siehe bei I
4	Kompensierter CO_2-Überschuß IV	normal	CO_2-Anstieg	Emphysem
5	Normales Säure-Basen-Gleichgewicht V	normal	—	—
6	Kompensiertes Alkalidefizit (Acidose!) VI	normal	abnorme Produktion fixer Säuren Alkaliverlust	Bicarbonatausscheidung reduziert, Säureabgabe erhöht. Diabetes, Nephritis
7	Kompensiertes CO_2-Defizit VI	normal	wie bei 2	siehe 2
8	Dekompensierter CO_2-Überschuß „Gasacidose" VII u. VIII	vermindert	mangelhafte Ventilation	Pneumonie, Bronchusverschluß, (Shunt) M-Wirkung. Alkalianstieg
9	Dekompensiertes Alkalidefizit IX	vermindert	Plasmabicarbonatgehalt vermindert, Alkalireserve unter 20,0	Alkalianstieg, Säureabgabe in den Nieren. Hyperventilation, Diabetes, Nephritis

Wie sehr die Bezeichnungen Acidose und Alkalose irreführen können, mögen einige Beispiele zeigen. In II der Abb. 7 hat eine vermehrte CO_2-Abrauchung in gewissem Umfang eine kompensatorische Verminderung des Bicarbonates zur Folge gehabt. Die Verminderung der Alkalireserve, die dem parallel geht, würde daher als Acidose bezeichnet, obgleich das Blut alkalischer ist als normal. Bei VII der gleichen Abbildung ist andererseits das Blut weniger alkalisch als normal, obgleich eine gewisse kompensatorische Erhöhung der Alkalireserve vorliegt. Der Begriff Alkalose würde, wenn man ihn im vorliegenden Fall benutzt, eine irrige Vorstellung vom wahren Säure-Basen-Gleichgewicht geben.

Das British Medical Research Council hat vor einiger Zeit eine Regelung dahingehend vorgeschlagen, daß jede Minderung des Blut-p_H als *Acidämie* zu bezeichnen ist, jede p_H-Er-

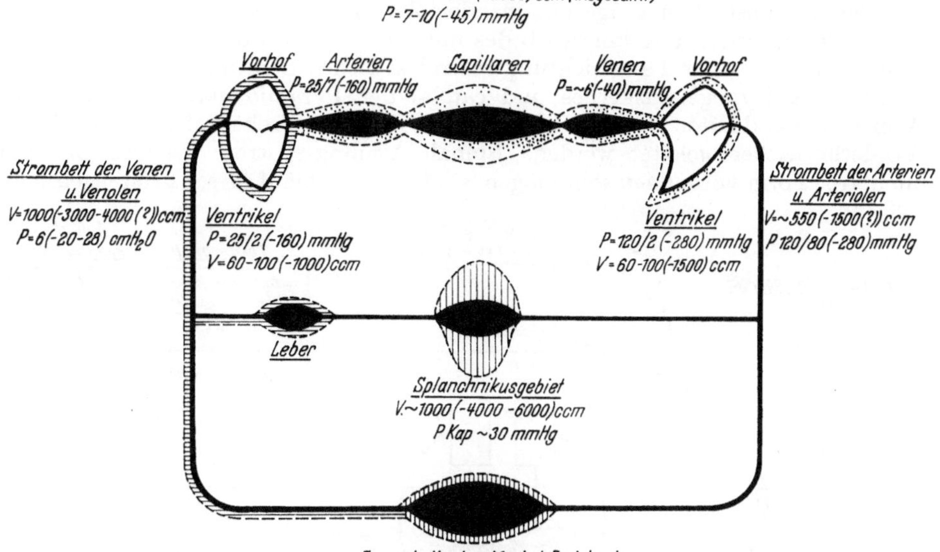

Abb. 6. Druck (P) und Volumen (V) in den einzelnen Kreislaufabschnitten bei den verschiedenen Kreislaufzuständen.

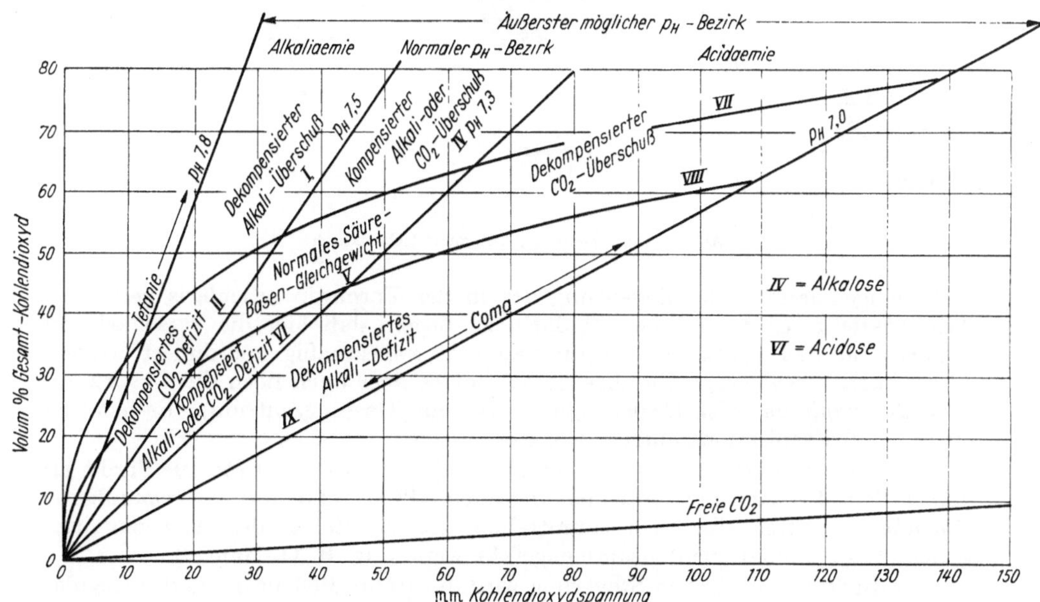

Abb. 7. Das Säure-Basengleichgewicht des Arterienblutes in Beziehung zur Kohlendioxydspannungskurve. (Nach v. SLYKE und STRAUB.)

höhung als *Alkaliämie*. Verminderungen der Alkalireserve bei normalem p_H werden demnach als *Acidose* bezeichnet, Erhöhungen der Alkalireserve bei normalem p_H als *Alkalose*.

5. Die Regulation der Atmung.

Als *Atemzentrum* wird anatomisch meist eine Zellgruppe in der Gegend der Formatio reticularis angegeben.

Die als Substrat in Frage kommenden Zellen befinden sich in einem Bezirk, der in der Querrichtung innerhalb des mittleren Drittels der Medulla oblongata liegt und sich in der Längsrichtung rostral zwischen dem mittleren und oberen Drittel des Hypoglossuskernes und caudal der Pyramidenkreuzung erstreckt. Von hier aus dürften *die efferenten Atmungsimpulse* direkt auf die motorischen Vorderhornzellen geleitet werden. Spinale Atmungszentren, die zwar in rudimentärer Form vorhanden sein mögen, sind in den Ablauf dieser Efferenzen nicht

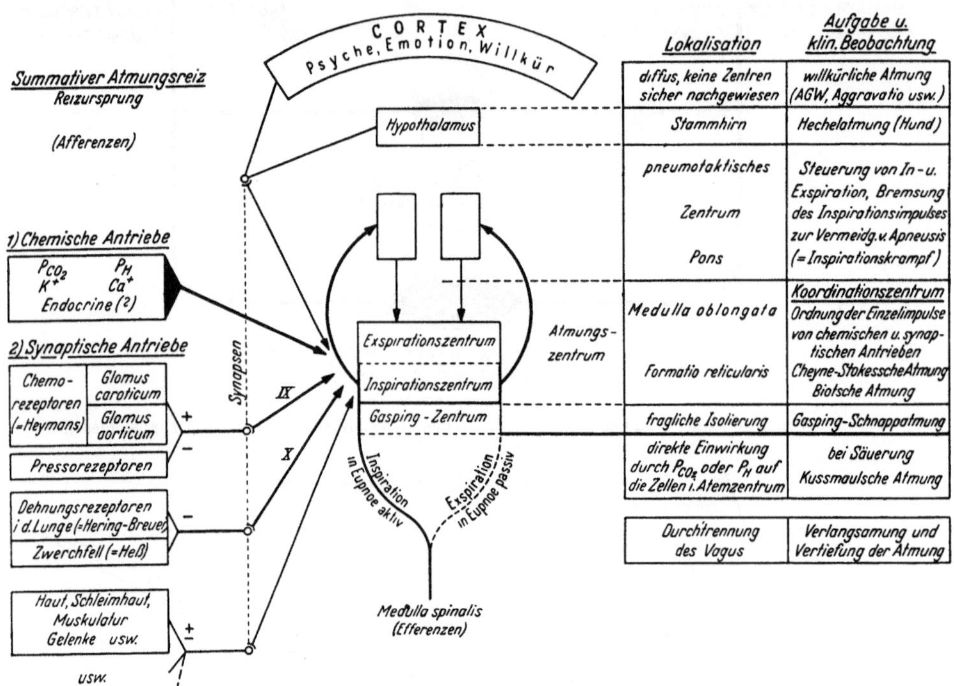

Abb. 8. Die Steuerung der Atmung (schematisch).

mehr eingeschaltet. Die Bedeutung des in der Formatio reticularis gelegenen Atmungszentrums scheint einmal darin zu liegen, daß hier die verschiedenen Impulse für den peripheren Atmungsapparat zweckmäßig koordiniert werden *(Koordinationszentrum)*. Gleichzeitig scheint es aber auch noch die *Ursprungsstätte des respiratorischen Grundrhythmus* zu sein (Gaspingzentrum). Es hat sich ein In- und Exspirationszentrum isolieren lassen.

Die Regulation der Atmung erfolgt über: a) *chemische Antriebe*, die direkt an den Zellen des Atmungszentrums angreifen (PCO_2 und p_H); b) *synaptische Antriebe*, worunter alle nicht unmittelbar auf die Zellen des Atemzentrums gerichteten Stimulationen zusammengefaßt werden (z. B. O_2-Mangel).

Der direkten chemischen Steuerung wird die größte Bedeutung in der Regulation der Atmung beigemessen. Entscheidend sind dabei die mittlere PCO_2 und das p_H im Atemzentrum selbst. Normalerweise liegt die PCO_2 um 40 mm Hg, das p_H um 7,40. Eine weitere Rolle spielt die Durchblutung dieses Gebietes und seine Umgebungstemperatur (Fieberhyperventilation?).

Die synaptischen Antriebe werden demgegenüber vielfach als Modulatoren der Atmung aufgefaßt. Die wichtigsten Antriebe dieser Art sind schematisch in Abb. 8 dargestellt.

Um einen Einblick in *die komplexe funktionelle Organisation der Atmung* zu erhalten, seien drei Mechanismen kurz im Zusammenhang diskutiert.

Der *chemisch-nervale Mechanismus* stellt gewissermaßen den Basisreiz für das Atmungszentrum selbst dar. Die Agentien, PCO_2 und p_H, wirken direkt auf die Zellen des Atmungszentrums, bzw. auch synaptisch über die Chemorezeptoren. Sie bewirken die Inspiration. In Ruhe bei Eupnoe, wo die Schwankungen der arteriellen Blut-p_H- und Gaszusammensetzung durch das große Puffervolumen des Blutes sehr gering sind, ist dieser chemische Reiz weitgehend konstant. Infolge des inspiratorischen Dauer- oder Basisreizes — die inspiratorischen Neurone im Atmungszentrum sind empfindlicher als die exspiratorischen — würde ein Inspirationskrampf = Apneusis resultieren. Dieser tritt im Tierversuch auch ein, wenn die Hemmungsimpulse über den Vagus oder das pneumotaktische Zentrum im Pons wegfallen.

In der Eupnoe erzeugt die Inspiration durch Hemmungsimpulse von den *Dehnungsrezeptoren* in der Lunge (Afferenzen via Nn. vagi) und durch Aktivierung des *pneumotaktischen Zentrums* eine Umschaltung zur Exspiration. Zu einer Reizung des Exspirationszentrums kommt es allerdings in der Eupnoe nicht, sondern lediglich zu einer Hemmung der inspiratorischen Impulse, so

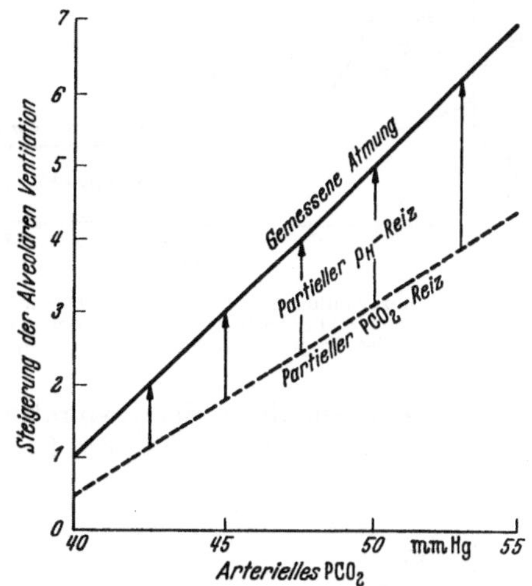

Abb. 9. Einfluß von CO_2 auf die Atmung. Eine Darstellung des additiven Effektes von p_H und CO_2-Reiz. (Nach J. S. GRAY: Pulmonary Ventil. 1949.)

daß die Exspiration passiv erfolgt. Am Ende der Exspiration erfolgt Reaktivierung des Inspirationszentrums und erneute Einatmung.

Ist das Atmungszentrum hypoxisch geschädigt, oder ist durch Alkalisierung des Blutes infolge Hyperventilation der chemische Basisreiz zur Inspiration reduziert oder aufgehoben, so schalten sich synaptische Antriebe ein, die normalerweise schlummern (z. B. der O_2-Mangel über die Chemorezeptoren). Das typische Beispiel in der Klinik ist die CHEYNE-STOKESsche Atmung.

Fällt die vagale und pneumotaktische Bremsung des Inspirationszentrums fort, so überwiegt letzteres. Die Atmung sistiert in Apneusis. Ist die Hemmung zu gering, so kann sich zentral ausgelöst ein asthmoider Zustand entwickeln.

Bei Hyperventilation wird auch das Exspirationszentrum eingeschaltet. Die vorhergehende Stärke des Inspirationsreizes entscheidet über die anschließende Reizstärke des Exspirationszentrums. Ein klinisches Beispiel für eine große Atmung mit ausgeprägter in- und exspiratorischer Aktivität ist die KUSSMAULsche Atmung, die meist durch Säuerung des Blutes verursacht ist.

Geht infolge Durchschneidung beider Nn. vagi die Vagushemmung verloren, so wird die Atmung tiefer und langsamer. Die Umschaltung zur Exspiration erfolgt dann dominierend vom pneumotaktischen Zentrum aus.

Einige für die funktionelle Pathologie der Atmung wichtige prinzipielle Beispiele für eine kompensatorische Steigerung des Atemminutenvolumens seien hier angeführt:

a) *CO_2-Atmung.* Enthält die Einatmungsluft z. B. 5% CO_2 (das entspricht einer PCO_2 von etwa 38 mm Hg), so müßte bei einem Ausgangswert der $PCO_{2\,alv.}$ von 40 mm Hg letztere auf 78 mm Hg ansteigen. Diese hohen CO_2-Werte haben bereits narkotischen Effekt. Das p_H des arteriellen Blutes würde auf 7,21 absinken (Acidämie). Durch den Anstieg des Atemminutenvolumens um 268% erfährt die $PCO_{2\,alv.}$ lediglich eine Erhöhung auf 47,7 mm Hg, d. h. sie liegt nur 9,7 mm über dem $PCO_{2\,in}$-Wert. Diese Steigerung der Atmung ist verursacht durch die *Summation* zweier, atmungssteigernder Agentien, durch die Hypercarbie und die Acidämie ($p_H = 7,33$). Das Atemäquivalent steigt auf 9,2 an (Abb. 9).

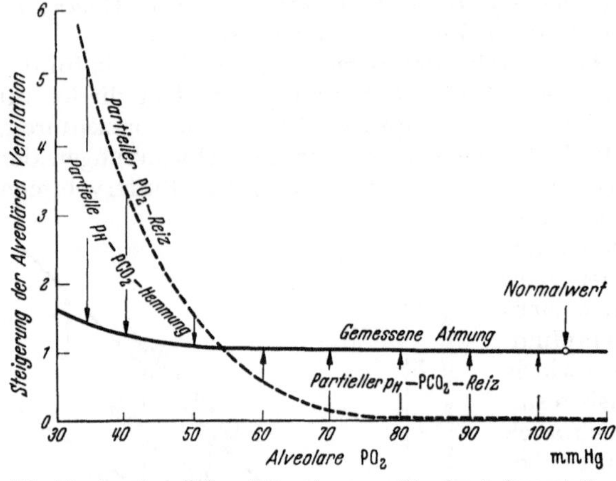

Abb. 10. Anoxieeinfluß auf die Atmung. Die durch Sauerstoffmangel erzeugte Hyperventilation wird durch CO_2-Verlust und Anstieg des p_H gehemmt. (Nach J. S. Gray.)

b) *Anoxie (Höheneffekt).* Die Kompensationsmaßnahmen bei der Anoxie in der Inspirationsluft dienen dazu, die arterielle O_2-Untersättigung zu bessern. Der durch O_2-Mangel verursachte Hyperventilationseffekt wird durch den CO_2-Verlust und die dadurch auftretende Alkaliämie gestoppt, so daß nur ein Anstieg des Atemäquivalentes auf 4,2 erfolgt. Würde die Hyperventilation nicht eintreten, so fiele die $PO_{2\,alv.}$ rasch auf bedrohliche Werte ab. Die Höhengrenze der Menschen liegt etwa bei 6700 m. Sie würde ohne die anoxisch bedingte Hyperventilation nur bei 4800 m liegen (Abb. 10).

c) *Stoffwechsel-bedingte Störungen des Säure-Basengleichgewichtes.* Ein Anstieg von fixen Säuren im Blut (z. B. bei Diabetes mellitus, im Coma hepaticum, bei Niereninsuffizienz, Herzinsuffizienz, besonders bei der Rechtsinsuffizienz, usw.) bedingt eine Senkung des p_H. Sinkt das p_H auf 7,2 ab, so steigt die Atmung um 100% an. Dadurch fällt die PCO_2 auf etwa 20 mm Hg ab. Das Atemäquivalent für Sauerstoff steigt auf 5,0 an. Ohne diese kompensatorische AMV-Steigerung würde die PCO_2 40 mm Hg bleiben und das p_H des arteriellen Blutes auf 7,05 absinken. Damit wäre die Coma-Grenze erreicht (Abb. 11).

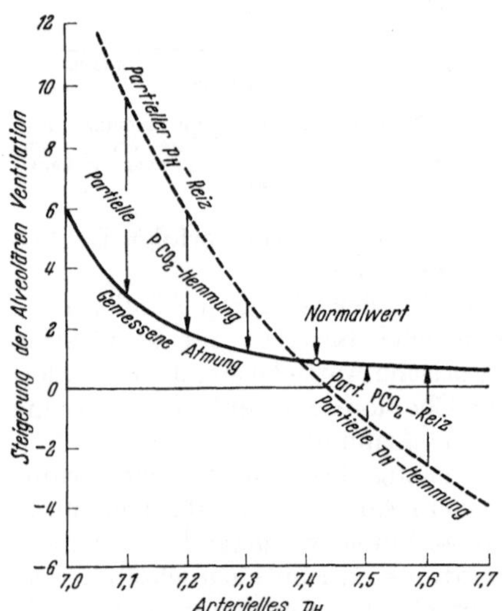

Abb. 11. Stoffwechselbedingte Säuerung des Blutes. Der Hyperventilationsreiz wird durch CO_2-Verlust gebremst. (Nach J. S. Gray.)

III. Methoden zur Untersuchung des Gasaustausches in der Lunge.

Die Methoden zur Untersuchung des Gasaustausches in der Lunge sind zahlreich und haben in der Physiologie, funktionellen Pathologie und Klinik erhebliches

Interesse gefunden. Entsprechend den bei Lungenkrankheiten auftretenden Kardinalsymptomen „Dyspnoe" und „Cyanose" können wir im wesentlichen zwei Gruppen von Untersuchungsverfahren unterscheiden:

a) Bei der ersten Gruppe handelt es sich um spirographische Methoden sowie Pneumometrie, Pneumotachographie und andere. Hierbei werden die Lungenvolumina, die Atmung in Ruhe und bei Arbeit, der Gasstoffwechsel, die Grenzwerte des Gasstoffwechsels unter den Bedingungen der Vita maxima, die Geschwindigkeit des Luftstromes, die Höhe der maximalen Exspirationsstärke und vieles andere quantitativ ermittelt.

b) Die zweite Gruppe umfaßt die gasanalytischen Methoden. Hiermit werden die Gaskonzentrationen in der Lungenluft und im arteriellen oder venösen Blut bestimmt.

c) In einem dritten Abschnitt seien spezielle neue Methoden, wie die selektive Angiographie der Lungengefäße von BOLT und die quantitative Bestimmung der Diffusionsstörung nach RILEY und COURNAND wiedergegeben.

Die spirographischen Verfahren erlauben Aussagen über Ventilationsstörungen und indirekt über Störungen des Gasaustausches. Sie haben den Vorzug, kurzfristig und den Patienten wenig strapazierend durchführbar zu sein. Unter diesen Gesichtspunkten haben sie in der Klinik zur Lungenfunktionsprüfung weite Verbreitung erlangt. Vor allem erhält man mit ihnen die letztlich entscheidenden maximalen Bruttowerte des Gasaustausches.

Die gasanalytischen Verfahren können andererseits Störungen des Gasaustausches durch ihre Folgen im Arterienblut und nur indirekt Ventilationsstörungen aufdecken. Fast immer sind Arterienpunktionen, Herzkatheterung u. a. notwendig. Außerdem sind die Analysen zum Teil umständlich und zeitraubend und setzen ein hochdifferenziertes Laboratorium in einer großen Klinik oder ein Speziallaboratorium voraus.

Die indirekten, den Patienten wenig tangierenden spirographischen Untersuchungsverfahren werden bevorzugt, wenn eine Funktionsdiagnose unterbaut werden soll, ein krankhafter Mechanismus gedeutet werden muß oder der Schweregrad bzw. die noch erhaltene Leistungsbreite unter Arbeit interessiert. Die mehr direkten, eingreifenderen gasanalytischen Methoden werden angewandt, um eine Funktionsdiagnose zu erhärten, die Beurteilung der Lunge vor einer Thoraxoperation zu ergänzen oder grundsätzliche wissenschaftliche Fragestellungen zu klären.

Beide Gruppen von Methoden zur Untersuchung des Gasaustausches in der Lunge konkurieren nicht, sondern ergänzen sich. Beide haben das Ziel, die respiratorische oder pulmonale Insuffizienz aufzudecken und ihre Größe sowie ihren Mechanismus zu erfassen.

1. Spirographie.
a) Spirographische Lungenfunktionsprüfung in Ruhe.

Die Lungenvolumina, die Atmung und der Gasstoffwechsel können mit offenen und mit geschlossenen Meßsystemen bestimmt werden.

Besonders bewährt hat sich bei der spirographischen Lungenfunktionsprüfung in Ruhe der kleine Spirograph nach KNIPPING. Es ist ein geschlossener Kreislauf-Stoffwechselapparat mit Spirometerglocke, Pumpe und Motor, Kalilauge-Waschflasche oder Natronkalk-Behälter und Wechsellaufkymographen. Die Atemfunktionsgrößen werden volumetrisch bestimmt. Ähnlich arbeitet der Spirograph nach KROGH.

Offene Systeme werden bei der DOUGLAS-Sack-Methode, dem TISSOT-Spirometer und der wärmeelektrischen Messung der Atemgase angewandt.

Bei der spirographischen Lungenfunktionsprüfung werden die Sauerstoffaufnahme (O_2-Aufnahme), das Atemvolumen (AV), das Atemminutenvolumen (AMV), die Atemfrequenz (AF), die Vitalkapazität (VK), Komplementärvolumen und Reservevolumen, der Atemstoß (AST), der Atemgrenzwert (AGW), eventuell die inspiratorische oder exspiratorische Apnoepause sowie der respiratorische Quotient (RQ) ermittelt.

Die Ventilationsmessung wird zunächst unter Luftatmung, dann unter Saueroffatmung durchgeführt. Eine O_2-Mehraufnahme unter Sauerstoffatmung in uhe von mehr als 40 cm³/min wird als spirographisches O_2-Defizit bewertet.

Das Auftreten dieser Defizite ist als pathologisch anzusehen. Spirogramme hierzu s. Abb. 15 [1].

Bei Bestimmung des Sauerstoffverbrauches und der Kohlensäureabgabe kann der *respiratorische Quotient* ermittelt und damit der Energieumsatz sowie bei Arbeitsversuchen der Wirkungsgrad körperlicher Arbeit berechnet werden.

Hat man außer dem exspiratorischen den alveolären oder arteriellen Kohlensäuredruck ermittelt, so können der *Totraum* nach der Bohrschen Formel und zusammen mit dem Atemminutenvolumen die alveoläre bzw. die Totraum-Ventilation berechnet werden.

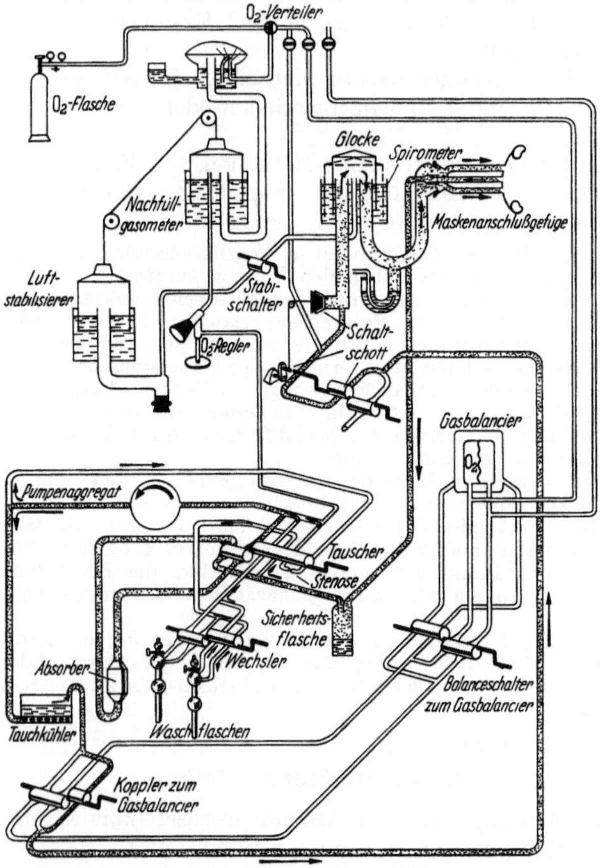

Unter *Ventilationsäquivalent* versteht man den Luftwechsel in Liter/100 cm³ O_2-Verbrauch. Der Ausnutzungskoeffizient für O_2 ist der reziproke Wert, d. h. Kubikzentimeter O_2-Aufnahme/Liter AMV.

Folgende Abweichungen der einzelnen Größen dieser spirographischen Lungenfunktionsprüfungen haben in der funktionellen Pathologie der Atmung besondere Bedeutung erlangt:

Steigerungen des *Atemminutenvolumens* um mehr als $^1/_2$ des Sollwertes müssen bei längerer Beobachtung als pathologisch angesehen werden und weisen auf eine respiratorische Ruheinsuffizienz hin. Der *Atemzeitquotient* zeigt bei Bronchostenose, Asthma bronchiale und Emphysem eine Verlängerung der Exspirationsdauer. Senkungen der *Vitalkapazität* unter 1,5 Liter sind als Kontraindikationen für Lungenresektionen aufzufassen. Das gleiche gilt für Einschränkungen des *Atemgrenzwertes* auf 25—30 Liter/min. Als Mindestwert der Atemreserven bei der Indikationsstellung zu thoraxchirurgischen Eingriffen muß das 4fache des Ruheatemminutenvolumens verlangt werden. Die Werte des Atemstoßes liegen bei Erkrankungen mit Erschwerung der Exspiration (Emphysem, Asthma bronchiale, chronische Bronchitis usw.) um 60% und niedriger.

Abb. 12. Schemazeichnung eines Kombinations-Spirographen nach Knipping. Es werden wahlweise Grundumsatzbestimmungen und Arbeitsuntersuchungen ermöglicht.

b) Die Bestimmung des Residualvolumens und der Mischungszeit.

Mit Hilfe von Fremdgasmethoden (Wasserstoff, Helium) wird nach einem Vorschlag von Knipping (1924) die Größe des Residualvolumens und der Mischungszeit wärmeelektrisch bestimmt.

Hierbei muß eine automatische Meßkammer nach dem diaferometrischen Prinzip in den Nebenschluß eines Spirographen nach Knipping geschaltet werden. Dann gibt man eine bekannte Menge Fremdgas in das System. Aus der gemessenen Konzentrationsänderung zwischen dem vorher bestimmten Inhalt des Apparates und diesem plus Thoraxinhalt bei

---

[1] Knipping 1932, Uhlenbruck 1930, Rossier 1948, Valentin und Venrath 1948.

Exspirationsstellung läßt sich das Residualvolumen berechnen. Wasserstoff und Luft haben ein unterschiedliches Wärmeleitvermögen, wodurch sich Widerstandsänderungen im Meßgerät ergeben, die zur Konzentrationsbestimmung des Fremdgases dienen[1].

Als *Residualvolumen* wird die nach extremer Ausatmung im Thorax restierende Luftmenge bezeichnet. Das Residualvolumen beträgt normalerweise zwischen 20 und 30% der Totalkapazität. Da der absolute Wert keine sichere Aussage erlaubt, wird zweckmäßig das *Residualvolumen in Prozenten der Totalkapazität* angegeben. Zur Beurteilung des schwer abschätzbaren Lungenemphysems mit seinen Folgen für das rechte Herz hat diese Relation praktische Bedeutung erlangt. Werte über 35% bis 48—50% sind als mäßig bis mittelschwer pathologisch anzusehen. Weitere Steigerungen zeigen eine schwere respiratorische Insuffizienz auf der Basis eines Emphysems an.

Die Mischungszeit gibt die Dauer an, bis zu der sich die Spannung eines Fremdgases (Helium, Wasserstoff) zwischen dem Thoraxvolumen (Residualvolumen und Reservevolumen) und dem Kreislaufsystem ausgeglichen hat.

Die Mischungszeit bei Gesunden schwankt zwischen 50 und 110 sec in Ruhe (Pumpenleistung 24 Liter/min, Systeminhalt 10 Liter). Unter Arbeit ist sie schon nach wenigen Atemzügen bei Normalpersonen abgeschlossen.

Verlängerungen der Mischungszeit über 2 min weisen unter anderem in Richtung eines Emphysems oder einer erheblichen Bronchostenose.

Zur Untersuchung der intrapulmonalen Gasmischungsverhältnisse ist auch die Atmung von reinem Sauerstoff über 7 min empfohlen worden. Bei dieser Methode der Stickstoffentmischung nach CHRISTIE wird hiernach eine Alveolarluftprobe durch forcierte Ausatmung entnommen und auf ihren Stickstoffgehalt analysiert. COURNAND und Mitarbeiter[2] haben hiermit die intrapulmonale Gasmischung einem eingehenden Studium unterzogen. Bei Emphysematikern entstehen deutliche Differenzen, welche auf eine ungleiche Ventilation der verschiedenen Lungenpartien hinweisen.

Einen anderen Weg zum Studium der pulmonalen Gasmischung sind SCHERRER und Mitarbeiter gegangen.

In einem ersten Untersuchungsgang wird hierbei mit Helium wie üblich das Residualvolumen bestimmt und damit die pulmonale Gasmischung im gesamten Alveolarraum gemessen. Die Ergebnisse trägt man in ein Diagramm mit logarithmischer Ordinate (= die abfallenden Heliumkonzentrationen) und mit linearer Abszisse (= die ventilierten Atemminutenvolumina) ein. Außerdem kontrolliert man oxymetrisch die Sauerstoffsättigung des arteriellen Blutes beim Übergang von reiner O_2-Atmung auf Zimmerluft- bzw. O_2-Mangel-Atmung. Hierdurch wird die pulmonale Gasmischung nur im durchbluteten, gasaustauschenden Alveolarraum geprüft. In analoger Weise muß man diese Desaturationskurve zu einem O_2-Mischdiagramm verarbeiten und in das gleiche semilogarithmische Koordinatensystem eintragen.

Im Normalfall wird die Lunge annähernd gleichmäßig belüftet. O_2-Desaturationsdiagramm und Heliummischdiagramm verlaufen übereinstimmend steil und geradlinig. Beim Asthma bronchiale findet man im Heliummischdiagramm einen flacheren Abfall und ein deutliches Abweichen vom geradlinigen Verlauf. Das O_2-Mischdiagramm zeigt ein übereinstimmendes Verhalten, da alle geblähten Lungenalveolen gleichmäßig durchströmt werden. Auch beim chronisch substantiellen Lungenemphysem ergibt sich ein Heliummischdiagramm, wie vorher geschildert, aber das O_2-Mischdiagramm verläuft steiler, weil beim Emphysem die schlecht ventilierten Alveolarräume infolge von Septenschwund kaum oder gar nicht durchblutet werden (vgl. Abb. 24).

c) Bronchospirographie.

Dieses Verfahren erlaubt die getrennte Spirographie beider Lungen. Es wird nur fakultativ angewandt, wenn eine funktionelle Differenzierung beider Lungenhälften notwendig wird (z. B. zur präoperativen Beurteilung vor Lungenresektionen, vor Kollapstherapie).

Als absolute Kontraindikationen in der Anwendung der Bronchospirographie sind ulcerierende Tracheo-Bronchial-Tuberkulose und frische Hämoptysen bis zu 3 Wochen nach

---

[1] Einzelheiten BOLT, VALENTIN und VENRATH 1951.
[2] COURNAND, BALDWIN, DARLING und RICHARDS 1941.

der Blutung anzusehen. Relative Gegenanzeigen sind der Verschluß des linken Hauptbronchus beim Bronchialcarcinom und schwere Tuberkulosen mit Intoxikationserscheinungen.

Normalerweise betragen die einzelnen Atemgrößen der rechten Lunge 55—60% des Gesamtwertes. Bei der *isolierten Frühkaverne* ist die Funktion der erkrankten Seite kaum erkennbar verändert. Bestehen dagegen *Pleuraverwachsungen oder Verschwartungen*, so nimmt die respiratorische Funktionsbreite beträchtlich ab. Beim *intrapleuralen Pneumothorax* sinken Sauerstoffaufnahme und Atemminutenvolumen gleichsinnig entsprechend dem Ausmaß des Kollapses ab. Die Beeinträchtigung der Zwerchfellatmung durch *Phrenicuslähmung* bedingt eine erhebliche funktionelle Reduzierung auf der betroffenen Lungenseite. Die Ausschaltung des Nervus phrenicus kann für den Lungenkranken eine funktionelle Katastrophe bedeuten[1]. Nach *partiellen Lungenresektionen* ist entscheidend, daß die Atemmotorik intakt bleibt. Dementsprechend wird eine Zwerchfelldrainage wegen der in der Regel durch Verwachsung eintretenden Beeinträchtigung der Zwerchfellfunktion abgelehnt. Bleibt die Motilität des Zwerchfells erhalten, so ist 3—4 Monate nach einer Segmentresektion keine Minderung der Lungenfunktion gegenüber der kontralateralen gesunden Seite bronchospirographisch nachweisbar.

Zusammenfassend kann festgestellt werden, daß die spirographische Lungenfunktionsprüfung bei Lungenkrankheiten wertvolle Aufschlüsse über die Lungenfunktion vermittelt. Sichere Aussagen sind immer über die Ventilationsverhältnisse möglich, indirekte Hinweise erhält man über Störungen des Gaswechsels. Die Lungenvolumina sollten bei allen pulmonalen Erkrankungen spirographisch bestimmt werden, denn weder die allgemein-ärztliche Untersuchung noch das Röntgenbild ermöglichen exakte Aussagen. Es ist zu beachten, daß oft nicht die einzelne Größe bindende Schlüsse zuläßt, sondern erst die Kombination der Ergebnisse das richtige funktionelle Bild ergibt.

Als allgemeiner Maßstab zur Begutachtung mag dienen, daß Unterschreitungen der jeweiligen Sollwerte bei der spirographischen Lungenfunktionsprüfung bis zu einem Drittel als „mäßige Einschränkung" (EV = 30—50%), bis zu zwei Drittel als „erheblich bis schwer" (EV = 50—70%) und oberhalb dieser Grenze als „für körperliche Arbeiten im täglichen Leben nicht tauglich" zu beurteilen sind.

Zu beachten ist weiterhin, daß die Lungenvolumina bei Mundstückatmung um rund 10% kleiner sind als bei Maskenatmung, da eine mäßige Stenose bei ersterer vorliegt. Auch die Körperhaltung spielt bei Ermittlung dieser Werte eine Rolle; so sind diese im Stehen um rund 10% größer als im Liegen.

Abschließend mag noch zum Thema Spirographie betont sein, daß sie wichtige Aussagen fortlaufend zu erheben gestattet, ohne daß punktiert oder irgend etwas appliziert werden muß. Dies scheint deshalb beachtlich, weil die moderne Funktions- und auch Kontrast-Diagnostik die Kranken zu sehr beansprucht (Arterienpunktion, Bronchographie, Herzkatheterung usw.). Man muß sehr sparsam mit diesen Dingen sein, damit in schwierigen Entscheidungen derartige Eingriffe nicht versagt werden, zumal sich in der Bevölkerung eine grundsätzlich ablehnende Haltung zu entwickeln beginnt. Die Funktionswerte sind aber für eine exakte funktionelle Betrachtungsweise unbedingt notwendig. Auf die letztere kann in prinzipiellen Fragestellungen nicht verzichtet werden.

2. Pneumotachographie und Pneumometrie.

Der Atemwiderstand der Luftwege ist nach dem Ohmschen Gesetz dem Alveolardruck direkt und der Strömungsgeschwindigkeit umgekehrt proportional. Dementsprechend wurde zunächst die Strömungsgeschwindigkeit der Luft bei Normalatmung mit dem von Fleisch eingeführten Pneumotachographen und der Alveolardruck durch Bestimmung des intrapleuralen Druckes, unter Addition der Retraktionskraft der Lunge, gemessen und so der Atemwiderstand bestimmt.

---

[1] Bolt 1953.

Der *Pneumotachograph nach* FLEISCH (1925) stellt im wesentlichen eine Differential-stromuhr dar. Er dient ausschließlich zur Messung der Geschwindigkeit von strömender Luft. Das Auftreten von Turbulenz wird durch die Aufteilung des gesamten zu messenden Luftstromes auf eine größere Zahl von engen parallelen Einzelröhren vermieden. Die zwischen 2 Punkten der Röhren auftretenden Druckdifferenzen sind den Strömungsgeschwindigkeiten direkt proportional.

HOCHREIN (1928) benutzt zur Pneumotachographie das Staublendenprinzip nach VEN-TURI. Hierbei entstehen wesentlich größere Druckdifferenzen, weil diese mit zunehmender Stromstärke nicht linear, sondern quadratisch ansteigen. Diese Tatsache soll den Wert des Verfahrens einschränken.

Späterhin wurde die unliebsame Pleurapunktion umgangen und der Alveolar-druck nach der Methode von VUILLEUMIER durch sinnreiche kurzdauernde Unterbrechungen des Atemstromes gemessen. Nach diesem Prinzip wird mittels der *Pneumometrie* nach HADORN (1943) die maximale Strömungsgeschwindig-keit der Luft während einer möglichst kräftigen, ausgiebigen und raschen Exspiration bestimmt.

Die Normalwerte liegen bei gesunden, erwachsenen Männern zwischen 7 und 12 Liter je sec., bei Frauen zwischen 6,5 und 8 Liter/sec. Unter *Arbeitsbelastungen* erfahren sie sowohl bei Gesunden wie auch unter pathologischen Verhältnissen eine Erhöhung.

Die *Abnahme des Pneumometerwertes* ist ein charakteristisches *Zeichen des Lungen-Emphysems und der bronchialasthmatischen Zustände.* Hieraus kann beim Emphysem auf einen erhöhten exspiratorischen Widerstand geschlossen werden. Eine Klärung der Streitfrage, ob diese Widerstandsvermehrung durch eine Stenose der Bronchioli oder durch Thorax- und Lungenstarre zustande kommt, ist aber noch nicht möglich.

3. Die Isotopen-Thorakographie mit Xenon[133].

Da die Bronchospirographie für den Patienten unangenehm und belastend ist und eine detaillierte Aussage der ventilatorischen Verhältnisse über eine Lungenseite hinaus nicht ermöglicht, wurde an der Kölner Klinik auf Vorschlag von KNIPPING der Weg beschritten, durch Einatmung künstlich radioaktiver isotoper Gase Einblick in die regionäre Ventilation zu erhalten[1].

Voraussetzungen, die an das Isotop gestellt werden müssen, sind, daß es bei Außen-temperatur gasförmig, chemisch indifferent und inhalierbar ist, sowie einen Gammastrahler darstellt. Nach *experimentellen Vorversuchen* mit Jod[131]-Alkyl hat sich das Edelgas Xenon[133] bewährt. Es wird praktisch kaum vom Körper aufgenommen. Die inhalierte Dosis kann somit hoch gewählt werden.

Mit Hilfe von Gammazählrohren wird die Aktivität über den verschiedenen Lungenteilen fortlaufend gemessen. Der radioaktive Effekt wird integriert als Kurve direkt aufgeschrieben. Die Abb. 13 und 14 zeigen so gewonnene Radiothorakogramme eines gesunden Mannes und einer Patientin mit linksseitiger, teilweise nicht ausdehnbarer Lunge (inexpendable lung) nach Pneumothoraxbehandlung wegen Lungentuberkulose. Einzelheiten finden sich in den Legenden.

Es ist mit Hilfe der Isotopenthorakographie erstmalig gelungen, die regionale Ventilation einzelner Lungenbezirke ohne spirographische Volumenregistrierung aufzunehmen. Durch diese Methode fällt jede Belästigung für den Patienten fort und jede methodisch verursachte Veränderung. Kontraindikationen, wie sie für die Bronchospirographie gegeben sind, bestehen bei diesem Untersuchungs-verfahren nicht. Die Strahlenexposition des Patienten kann minimal gehalten werden, d. h. geringer als bei einer üblichen Röntgendurchleuchtung.

4. Ergospirographie.

Zur quantitativen Beurteilung pulmonaler, aber auch kardio-zirkulatorischer Arbeitsinsuffizienzen hat sich seit Jahren die Ergospirographie nach KNIPPING (1929) praktisch bewährt.

---

[1] KNIPPING, BOLT, VENRATH, VALENTIN, LUDES und ENDLER 1957.

Bei diesen Arbeitsuntersuchungen wird eine ergospirographische Apparatur mit Sauer-stoff-Stabilisator und Luft-Sauerstoff-Balancegefäß benötigt. Es handelt sich um eine Stoffwechselapparatur mit geschlossenem und ventilfreiem Kreislaufsystem. Eine unblutige, direkt fortlaufende, beliebig lange Registrierung der Gaswechselwerte und gleichzeitig der Lungenvolumina wird ermöglicht, während der Proband eine genau meß- und reproduzierbare Drehkurbelarbeit am Wirbelstromergometer in verschiedenen Belastungsstufen verrichtet.

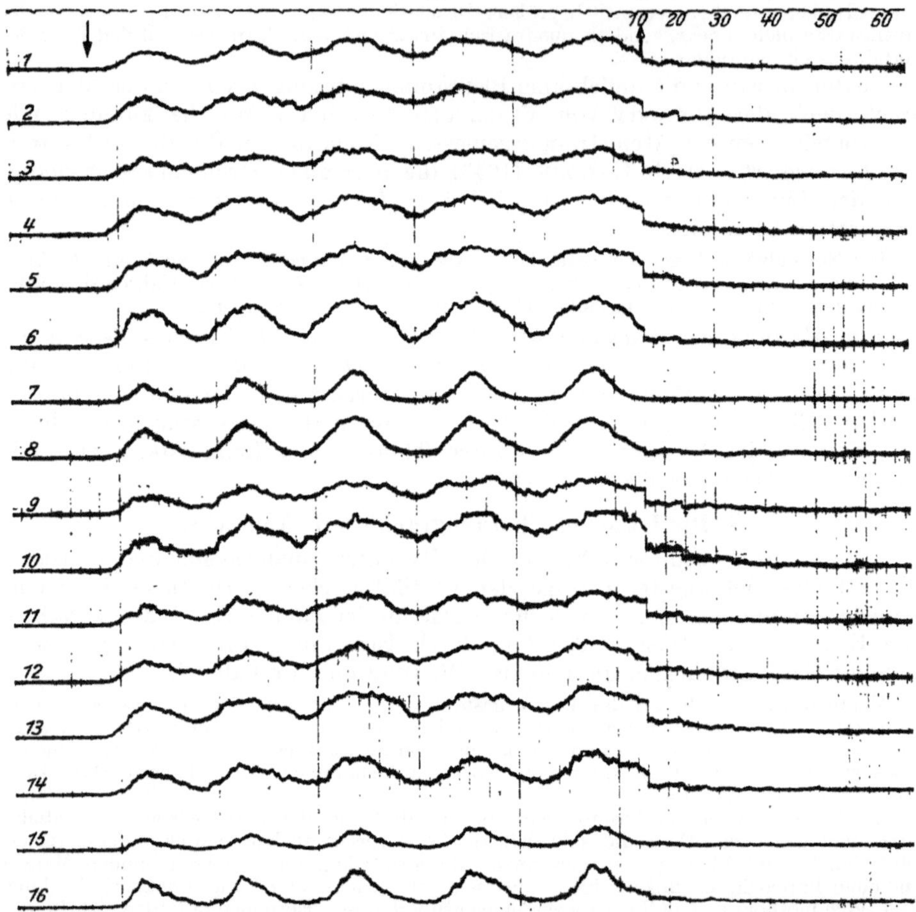

Abb. 13. Isotopenthorakogramm eines gesunden, 30 Jahre alten Mannes. Der Abwärtspfeil zeigt den Beginn der Aktivitätsatmung an. Die Zählrohre sind von 1—16 durchnumeriert, 1—8 = rechte, 9—16 = linke Thoraxseite. Man sieht deutlich die respiratorischen Schwankungen des Aktivitätsgehaltes über allen Lungenpartien. Durch die Auf- und Abwärtsbewegungen des Zwerchfells findet in Exspiration keine Einstrahlung von Aktivität in die Zählrohre 7—8 und 15—16 statt. Dadurch kehren die Kurven exspiratorisch bis praktisch zum Nullwert zurück. Die Streustrahlung ist sehr gering. Die Kurvenausschläge sind über symmetrischen Lungenteilen nahezu gleich groß.

Als einzig mögliche normale Belastungsart, welche auch den Anforderungen des täglichen Lebens am ehesten entspricht, hat sich die genau reproduzier- und meßbare körper-liche, dynamische Arbeit bewährt. Im Knippingschen Arbeitskreis werden seit vielen Jahren Drehkurbelergometer verwendet. Über Untersuchungen der Atmung unter Verwendung von Fahrradergometern haben Krogh, E. A. Müller, Fleisch und Sigrist, Karnell und Lanooy berichtet. Auch das Laufband nach Benedict ist in diesem Zusammenhang von Interesse[1].

Der Proband wird angehalten, über 10—12 min eine quantitativ dosierbare, konstante dynamische Drehkurbelarbeit zu leisten. Nach der Arbeitsanlaufzeit wird ein steady state von Atmung und Sauerstoffaufnahme erreicht. Während dieses Zeitraumes wird von Luft-auf Sauerstoffatmung umgeschaltet.

---

[1] Knipping, Bolt, Valentin und Venrath 1955, 1960.

Eine Reihe weiterer Übungstests, wie der MASTER-Test, der JAMES-Test, das Treppensteigen, die Kniebeugen usw., haben sich durch die individuelle Variation des Körpergewichtes, die unterschiedliche Exaktheit der Übungsausführung usw. als weniger geeignet zur Prüfung der Ursache einer Arbeitsdyspnoe erwiesen.

Bei einer geklagten Arbeitsdyspnoe werden im Belastungsversuch folgende Kriterien geprüft:

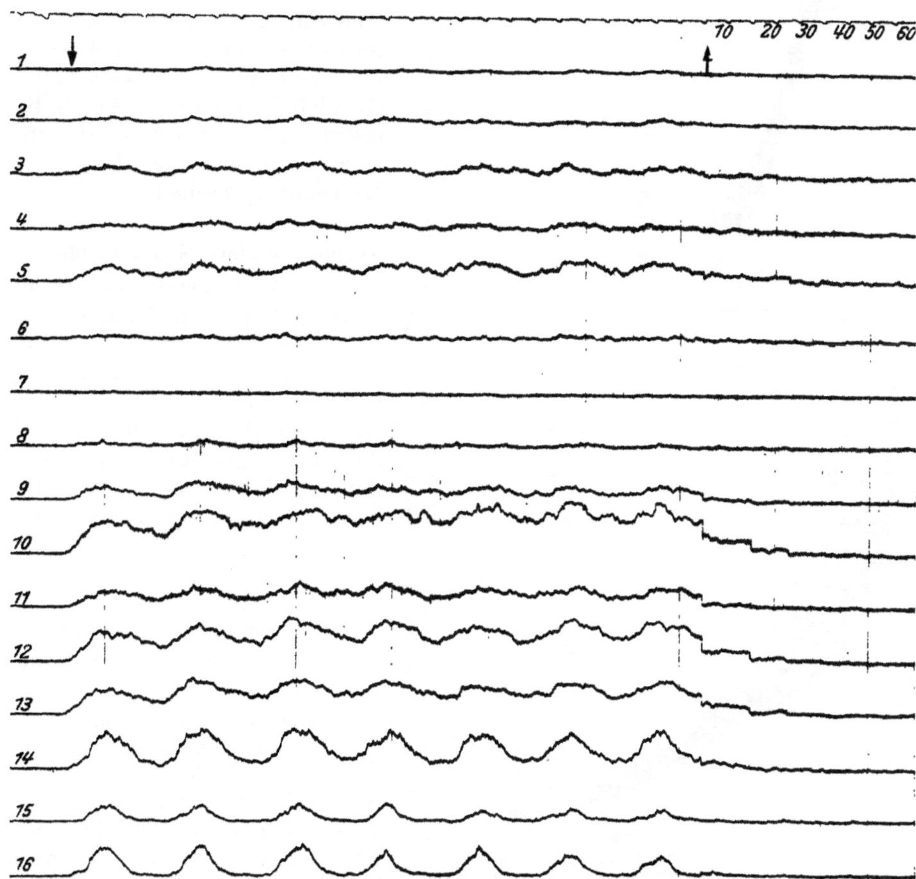

Abb. 14. Isotopenthorakogramm eines 28 Jahre alten Mannes mit einer „inexpendable lung" nach Pneumothorax rechts. Die Beatmung der rechten Lunge ist bis auf ein Minimum reduziert, während die Kurven, die über der linken Lunge gewonnen sind (9—16) praktisch normale Verläufe zeigen.

a) Das spirographische Sauerstoffdefizit.

Das spirographische Sauerstoffdefizit, welches von UHLENBRUCK mit Hilfe des KNIPPING-Spirographen zuerst beobachtet und von unserem Arbeitskreis in die klinische Funktionsanalyse eingeführt wurde, ist ein Phänomen, das in leichten und mittelschweren Belastungsstufen bei Gesunden nie beobachtet wird. Es umfaßt die Sauerstoffmehraufnahme nach Übergang von Luft- auf Sauerstoff-Atmung in Ruhe oder bei Arbeit im steady state. Nur Lungen- und sekundär respiratorisch insuffiziente Herzkranke zeigen von nicht mehr adäquaten Belastungsstufen ab diese Erscheinung (s. Abb. 15). Das spirographische Sauerstoffdefizit gibt quantitativ über den Sauerstoffmangel des Organismus und qualitativ über die Sauerstoffsättigung des arteriellen Blutes Auskunft.

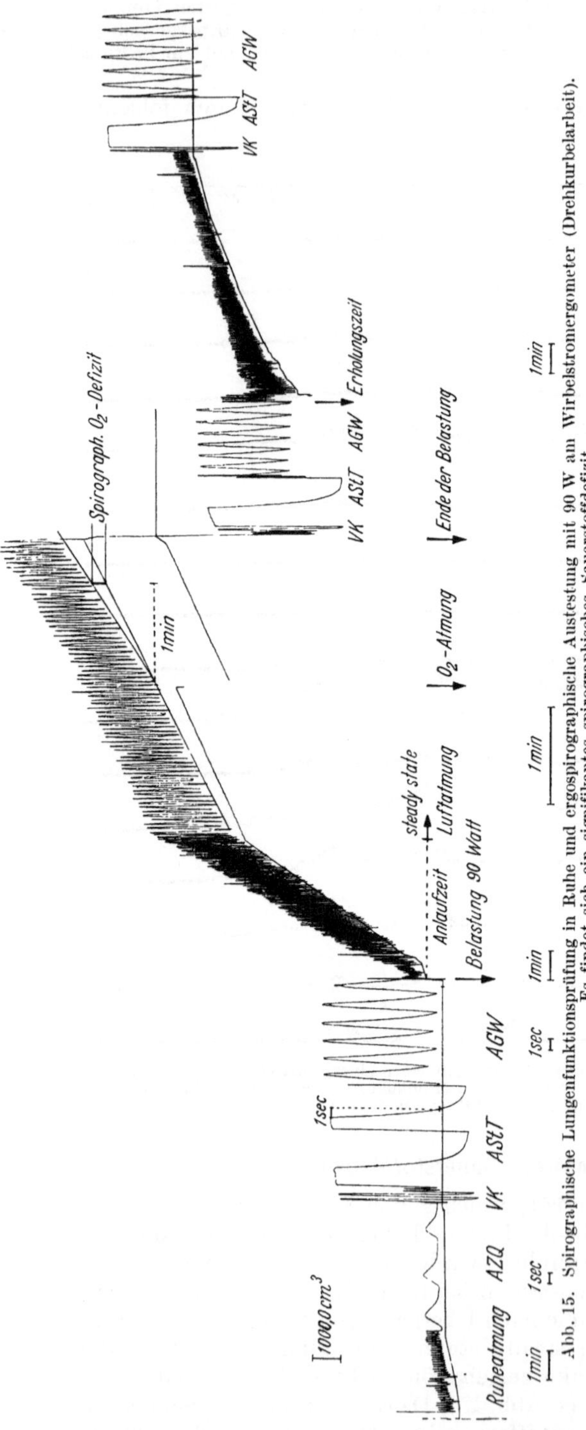

Abb. 15. Spirographische Lungenfunktionsprüfung in Ruhe und ergospirographische Austestung mit 90 W am Wirbelstromergometer (Drehkurbelarbeit). Es findet sich ein signifikantes spirographisches Sauerstoffdefizit.

Dieses Phänomen kann direkt durch die Beobachtung von Cyanose, indirekt durch Arterienpunktionen und Blutgasanalysen sowie die oxymetrische Technik bestätigt werden.

Als pathologisch bewertet werden nur Sauerstoffmehraufnahmen von 100 cm³ je min und mehr im steady state. Die Arbeitsstufe, bei der ein spirographisches Sauerstoffdefizit auftritt, wird als Belastungsgrenze bei Arbeitsinsuffizienz von Atmung, Herz und Kreislauf angesehen.

b) Das kaschierte Sauerstoffdefizit.

Das kaschierte[1] oder kompensierte[2] Sauerstoffdefizit wird dann angenommen, wenn sich im steady state die Arbeitsatmung bei Umschaltung von Luft- auf Sauerstoff-Atmung um mehr als 20% beruhigt. Meist findet sich dann in der nächst höheren Belastungsstufe ein spirographisches Sauerstoffdefizit.

c) Die Senkung des Atemäquivalentwertes.

Der Atemäquivalentwert unter Arbeit im steady state wird nach der Formel: Atemäquivalentwert $= \dfrac{\text{AMV (in Liter)} \times 100}{O_2\text{-Aufnahme/min (cm}^3)}$ berechnet[3]. Er liegt normalerweise zwischen 1,8 und 4,0. Ein Abfall von mehr als 1,0 nach Umschaltung auf O_2-Atmung weist auf eine respiratorische Arbeitsinsuffizienz hin. Der reziproke Wert der Gleichung ergibt den Ausnutzungskoeffizienten für Sauerstoff[4]. Die Normalwerte betragen zwischen 37 und 45 cm³. Hierbei ist der Anstieg von mehr als 7 cm³ als krankhaft zu werten.

d) Erhöhung der Arbeitsventilation.

Eine Erhöhung der Arbeitsventilation von mehr als 50%

---

[1] Knipping 1938.   [2] Zorn 1940.   [3] Anthony 1937.   [4] Herbst 1928.

über den Normalwert im steady state und keine Beruhigung der Atmung nach Umschaltung auf Sauerstoff muß als Zeichen einer respiratorischen Insuffizienz oder einer hochgradigen Arbeitsentwöhnung angesehen werden.

e) Die maximale Sauerstoffaufnahme.

Die maximale Sauerstoffaufnahme ist der höchste Minutenwert des O_2-Aufnahmevermögens bei von Minute zu Minute gesteigerter Arbeitsbelastung am Drehkurbelergometer. Die Pulszahl sofort nach der Arbeit soll mindestens 150/min erreichen. Sie gibt Aufschluß darüber, ob bei Arbeitsabbruch, der wegen

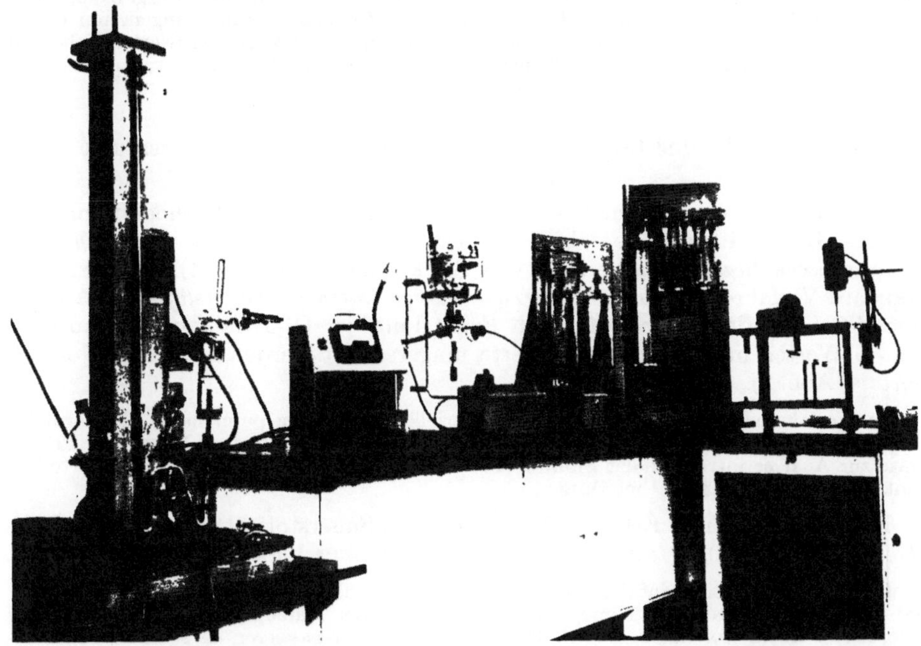

Abb. 16. Arbeitsraum für die Gasanalyse mit (von links nach rechts) a VAN SLYKE-Apparat, b pH-Meßgerät, c Scholander-Gerät, d Hämoreflektor nach BRINKMAN, e Gasmischgerät, f HALDANE-Apparat, g Gerät zur O_2- und CO_2-Spannungs-Bestimmung nach RILEY, PROEMMEL und FRANKE.

Nichtmehrkönnens, Dyspnoe, Herzklopfen und anderer Ursachen eintritt, eine Auslastung erfolgt ist. Bei intakter Herz-Kreislauffunktion und normalem Blutchemismus erhalten wir durch die Bestimmung der maximalen Sauerstoffaufnahme einen für die Klinik ausreichenden quantitativen Einblick in die unter steigender Arbeitsbelastung mögliche Sauerstofflieferung an die Peripherie und damit in die reduzierte Leistungsbreite bei Lungenkrankheiten[1].

Zusammenfassend ist festzustellen, daß sich die *Arbeitsbelastung*, zum Teil bis zur Vita maxima, zur Aufdeckung der reduzierten Leistungsgrenze von Atmung, Herz und Kreislauf bei der respiratorischen Arbeitsinsuffizienz in der Klinik, der Begutachtungs-, Sport- und Arbeitsmedizin bewährt hat. Die *ergospirographische Untersuchung* bei quantitativ dosierter Arbeitsbelastung hat den Vorteil gegenüber anderen Methoden, ein indirektes und wenig eingreifendes Verfahren zu sein. Die Methode kann wesentlich zur Erfassung und Beurteilung von Frühschäden an Lungen und Herz beitragen und eine vieldeutige Arbeitsdyspnoe oft aufklären.

---

[1] VALENTIN 1956.

5. Gasanalytische Methoden zur Beurteilung der Lungenfunktion.

Neben den spirographischen Methoden sind *die Blut- und Atemgasanalysen* von Wichtigkeit. Während in der Klinik, der Begutachtungs-, Sport- und Arbeitsmedizin, besonders aber zur Früherfassung respiratorischer oder kardialer Insuffizienzen unter Arbeitsbelastung die indirekten, wenig eingreifenden und zeitsparenden spirographischen Verfahren größere Bedeutung erlangt haben, stehen im Funktions-Großlabor die Arterienpunktion sowie die Herzkatheterung und die nachfolgende Gasanalyse mehr im Vordergrund.

Bei der Interpretation der Funktion der Lungen aus den arteriellen Blutgasen muß beachtet werden, daß das *arterielle Blut* ein Gemisch der verschiedensten Lungenblut-Fraktionen darstellt und nur im Hinblick auf die Konsequenzen für den Gesamtorganismus ausgewertet werden kann. Die Einwirkung regional-funktioneller Veränderungen, um die es sich jedoch in der Lungenpathologie meist handelt, ist nicht mit wünschenswerter Sicherheit zu erschließen. Außerdem gestatten die meisten gasanalytischen Verfahren nur, einen momentanen funktionellen Querschnitt zu erfassen.

a) Sauerstoff- und CO_2-Gehalt, Sauerstoff-Kapazität und prozentuale O_2-Sättigung des Blutes.

Zur Analyse des Gasgehaltes des Blutes stehen mehrere Methoden zur Verfügung. Eine zeitraubende, aber sehr exakte Methode ist *die chemische und manometrische Blutgasanalyse nach* van Slyke und Neill (1924). Sie stellt das Standard-Verfahren dar und liefert zuverlässige *Daten des Sauerstoff- und Kohlendioxyd-Gehaltes* des Blutes, die nach Ermittlung der O_2-Totalkapazität aus den Vol.-%-Werten in Sättigungs-%-Werte umgerechnet werden können. (Normalwerte s. Abb. 2).

Das Verfahren findet zur Erfassung einer arteriellen Hypoxämie pulmonalen oder kardialen Ursprungs und zur Bestimmung des Herzminutenvolumens nach dem Fickschen Prinzip sowie zur Analyse intrakardialer Shunts Verwendung. Voraussetzung sind immer Arterienpunktionen und die Herzkatheterung.

Eine kontinuierliche Erfassung der arteriellen Sauerstoffsättigung ist durch *die photoelektrische Oxymetrie nach* Kramer (1934, 1935) und Matthes (1934) möglich.

Das Verfahren basiert auf der Tatsache, daß Lichtstrahlen des roten Spektralbereiches — 600—700 mμ — durch Oxyhämoglobin und reduziertes Hämoglobin verschieden stark absorbiert werden. Oxyhämoglobin läßt rotes Licht stärker passieren als reduziertes Hämoglobin. Allgemein werden heute Zweifarbmethoden verwendet. Man unterscheidet Transmissions- (Ohrläppchen, Fingerbeere) und Reflektions-Verfahren (Stirn, Cyclop).

Während der Narkose bei thoraxchirurgischen Eingriffen erlauben die oxymetrischen Methoden z. B. eine relative Kontrolle der O_2-Sättigung des Blutes. Auch bei Sauerstoffmangelbelastungen in Ruhe erwies sich die Oxymetrie als wertvoll. Hingegen ließen sich bei Arbeitsbelastungen nur in vereinzelten Fällen und dann nur qualitative Aussagen über die Sauerstoffsättigung des Arterienblutes machen.

Zahlreiche zur Gasanalyse anfallende Blutproben werden heute photometrisch mit Hilfe des Hämoreflektors auf O_2-Kapazität und prozentuale O_2-Sättigung untersucht.

b) Sauerstoff- und CO_2-Spannungen im Blut.

In der funktionellen Pathologie der Atmung interessieren sowohl der Gehalt als auch die Spannung der Blutgase, insbesondere des Arterienblutes und des venösen Mischblutes. Verschiedene Verfahren sind zur Lösung folgender Probleme angewandt worden:

a) Tritt der Sauerstoff durch Diffusion oder durch Sekretion aus der Alveole in das Blut über ?

b) Wie groß ist der alveolo-arterielle Sauerstoffdruckgradient ?

c) Bei welchen Krankheitszuständen tritt eine Pneumonose nach Brauer auf ?

Ein indirektes Verfahren besteht darin, aus der *Analyse der Sauerstoffsättigung über die Dissoziationskurve auf die Sauerstoffspannung* zu schließen[1]. Erhebliche Fehlermöglichkeiten beeinträchtigen dieses Verfahren, da die Dissoziationskurve im Bereich der besonders interessierenden arteriellen Sauerstoffsättigung bereits derart flach verläuft, daß geringe Fehler in der Sättigungsbestimmung zu großen Differenzen in der Spannungsablesung führen.

Eine weitere methodische Möglichkeit besteht in der Untersuchung der Zusammensetzung einer *Gasblase, die mit Blut zum Gasaustausch gelangt* ist. Mit dem *Mikroanalysator von* KROGH (1908) können Gasblasen von einigen Kubikmillimetern Größe mit einer Genauigkeit von $\pm 2\%$ analysiert werden. Die zu untersuchende Gasblase wird in eine Capillare gesaugt, und ihre Länge wird vor und nach Absorption von Kohlensäure und Sauerstoff gemessen. — Im Jahre 1934 hat F. MEYER die Methode weiter ausgebaut und zur Bestimmung der Gewebe-, Blut- und Alveolarluftspannung angewandt.

Weitere Verbesserungen erfuhr diese Methode durch SCHOLANDER sowie RILEY, PROEMMEL und FRANKE.

Als weiteres Verfahren wurde die *polarographische Methode zur Messung der Sauerstoffspannung* im Plasma aus vollständig gesättigtem Blut von BERGGREN herangezogen. Hierbei benutzt man die im Plasma gelöste O_2-Menge zur Spannungsbestimmung. Polarographisch läßt sie sich mit einer Genauigkeit von $\pm 1\%$ bestimmen. WIESINGER (1950) führte den Ausbau für unvollständig gesättigtes Blut durch. Beim gesunden Menschen in Ruhe soll eine alveolo-arterielle Sauerstoffspannungsdifferenz von durchschnittlich $8 \pm 1{,}6$ mm Hg bestehen.

BARTELS und RODEWALD (1952) haben zur Bestimmung der Sauerstoffspannung ein „*Hämoxytensiometer*" entwickelt. Sie haben die bisherige ampèrometrische Analyse mit der Quecksilbertropfelektrode in eine *potentiometrische Analyse* umgewandelt. Hierdurch läßt sich die Reduktion des Sauerstoffs an der Elektrodenoberfläche auf ein Minimum beschränken. Dieses elektrochemische Verfahren gestattet, den Sauerstoffdruck im Blut zwischen 10 und 500 mm Hg PO_2 mit einer Genauigkeit von $\pm 2\%$ zu bestimmen. Es muß jedoch für jedes Blut durch Tonometrieren mit bekanntem Sauerstoffdruck eine Eichkurve mit 3 Eichpunkten aufgestellt werden.

Die arterielle Sauerstoffspannung ist zur Beurteilung der Lungenfunktion herangezogen worden. Der Ruhewert des Arterienblutes soll eine exakte Aussage über die intakte Funktion des Gasaustausches erlauben. Normalerweise beträgt die Sauerstoffspannung im Arterienblut in Ruhe 86 ± 6 mm Hg mit Schwankungen zwischen 70 und 100 mm Hg. Der Wert von 70 mm Hg wird als Grenze angesehen und eine Sauerstoffspannung unter 65 mm Hg als pathologisch betrachtet. Arbeitsbelastungen haben keinen signifikanten Einfluß auf die arterielle Sauerstoffspannung, da die Hyperventilation diese Werte konstant halten soll[2].

Bei Absinken der Sauerstoffspannung im arteriellen Blut unter die „*Reaktionsschwelle*" von 60—70 mm Hg kommt es zunächst zu einer Aktivierung von Atmung und Kreislauf sowie der Zellfunktionen im Zentralnervensystem. Der chronische Sauerstoffmangel wird durch erhöhte Capillarisierung im Gewebe auszugleichen versucht[3]. Bei Erreichen eines „*kritischen Wertes*" von 35 mm Hg, was einer arteriellen Sauerstoffsättigung von rund 50% entspricht, treten Lähmungen der Zellfunktionen, besonders an den Ganglienzellen der Großhirnrinde auf[4]. So konnten im akuten Hypoxie-Versuch bei einer arteriellen Sauerstoffspannung von 45—40 mm Hg bereits Gedächtnisschwäche, Apnoe, psychische Depression oder Euphorie beobachtet werden. In der Klinik sieht man bei schweren respiratorischen Ruheinsuffizienzen (Poliomyelitis, Tuberkulose, Silikose usw.) oft Desorientiertheit, schlafähnliche Zustände und anderes.

„*Hypoxie*" findet sich bei Absinken der Sauerstoffspannung unter die Norm, doch nicht unter den „kritischen Wert". Bei weiterem Absinken bis auf Werte, bei denen die Gewebsatmung aus Mangel an Sauerstoff eingeschränkt wird, spricht man von „*Anoxie*"[4].

c) Bestimmung des Gasgehaltes der Exspirationsluft.

Die Bestimmung des Gasgehaltes der Exspirationsluft hat in der Klinik keine entscheidende Bedeutung erlangt, in speziellen Fragestellungen ist sie nützlich.

Fortlaufende Analysen ermöglichen der REINsche Gaswechselschreiber, das Diaferometer nach NOYONS und der Massenspektrograph. Für den Routinebetrieb sind diese Verfahren zu störanfällig. Die fortlaufende Sauerstoffbestimmung wird unter Ausnutzung der paramagnetischen Eigenschaften des Sauerstoffs erreicht. Für die fortlaufende Kohlendioxyd-Anzeige kann der Infrarotabsorptionsschreiber[5] als schnell registrierendes Gerät verwendet werden.

---

[1] BARCROFT 1925.   [2] BJÖRK 1953.   [3] KROGH 1929.   [4] OPITZ und SCHNEIDER 1950.
[5] K. F. LUFT 1943, PFUND und Mitarbeiter 1947, R. C. FOWLER 1949, GÖPFERT und FREY 1954.

d) Bestimmung des alveolären Sauerstoffdruckes und des physiologischen Totraumes.

Die *direkte Untersuchung der Alveolarluft* und weiterhin die Bestimmung des Totraumes stellt besondere Anforderungen an den Patienten und bereitet methodische Schwierigkeiten. Dies dürfte der Grund sein, daß diese Werte in der Klinik zunächst keine praktische Bedeutung erlangt haben. Außerdem ist es fraglich, ob die Alveolarluft als homogenes Medium überhaupt existiert.

Aus diesen Gründen ist die Methode von HALDANE und PRIESTLEY nur bedingt anwendbar. Die automatische Alveolarluft-Sammelanordnung von RAHN liefert bei Ruheatmung mit anderen Methoden übereinstimmende Werte, bei Arbeit liegen die Resultate tiefer, und bei unregelmäßiger Atmung ist sie nicht brauchbar. In den ersten beiden Fällen wurden mit dem Alveolarstufenverfahren nach KNIPPING befriedigende Ergebnisse erhalten.

Die *Berechnung des alveolären Sauerstoffdruckes über das arterielle Blut* wurde zuerst von ENGHOFF durchgeführt und später von ROSSIER bzw. RILEY ausgebaut.

Hierbei werden das p_H, die Sauerstoffsättigung und -Kapazität sowie der CO_2-Gehalt des Arterienblutes bestimmt. Aus diesen Größen läßt sich dann mit der HENDERSON-HASSELBALCHschen Formel die Kohlensäurespannung im Alveolarraum berechnen, unter der Voraussetzung gleicher Spannung in Lungenarterie und Alveole.

Zur Ermittlung des physiologischen Totraumes werden außerdem am Spirographen das Atemminutenvolumen, die Sauerstoffaufnahme und die Kohlensäureabgabe ermittelt. Bei bekannter CO_2-Spannung und -Ausscheidung je Minute läßt sich die *alveoläre Ventilation* nach folgender Formel berechnen:

$$\text{Alveoläre Ventilation} = \frac{CO_2\text{-Gehalt} \times k}{pCO_2} \; ; \; \text{Phys. Totraum} = \frac{\text{AMV—Alv. Vent.}}{\text{Atemfrequenz}} \; .$$

Zur Bestimmung der alveolären Sauerstoffspannung ging man von der Überlegung aus, daß die mittlere alveoläre O_2-Spannung am Ende der Exspiration gleich dem Sauerstoffdruck der Inspirationsluft minus demjenigen Teil an Sauerstoff ist, der je Zeiteinheit im Körper verschwindet. Die Formel lautet

$$pO_2\,\text{alv.} = \frac{20{,}93\,(P-49{,}5)}{100} - \frac{\text{art. } pCO_2}{RQ} \; .$$

RILEY und Mitarbeiter gelangten auf anderen Wegen zu einer ähnlichen Formel. Die indirekt ermittelten alveolären Gasspannungen bezeichnen sie als *effektive Spannungen*. Diese müssen kontinuierlich und gleichförmig in allen funktionierenden Alveolen herrschen, um den Gasaustausch zwischen Alveolen und Blut während einer Serie von Atemzügen zu gestatten.

e) p_H-Messung.

Da die p_H-Verschiebung im Blut im allgemeinen sehr gering ist, kommen für die exakte Messung nur hochempfindliche Apparate in Frage. Von den bekannten p_H-Meßverfahren ist das *elektrometrische* im klinischen Labor verbreitet.

Im Prinzip beruht es auf der Tatsache, daß eine in die Untersuchungslösung, in diesem Falle arterielles Blut, tauchende geeignete Elektrodenkette eine vom p_H-Wert abhängige elektrische Spannung abgibt. die somit ein Maß für den p_H-Wert darstellt. Verschiedene Elektrodenketten und Eichlösungen werden für die einzelnen Bereiche verwendet.

Auch *eine nomographische Ermittlung des p_H-Wertes im Serum* ist möglich.

Die Kenntnis der O_2-Kapazität bei bekanntem CO_2-Gehalt und definierter CO_2Spannung erlaubt, auf dem Nomogramm von HENDERSON den Drehpunkt der CO_2-Dissoziationskurve festzulegen. Für die CO_2-Spannung von 20, 40, und 60 mm Hg kann man den zugehörigen CO_2-Gehalt ermitteln. Die Resultate ergeben doppelt logarithmisch aufgetragen eine Grade. Über letztere erhält man den dem arteriellen CO_2-Gehalt zugehörigen CO_2-Druck. Mit diesem Resultat sowie der O_2-Kapazität und der prozentualen O_2-Sättigung rechnet man den CO_2-Gehalt des Blutes auf den des Serums um und subtrahiert die physikalisch gelöste Kohlensäuremenge ($P_{CO_2} \times 0{,}0671$). Unter Verwendung der HENDERSON-HASSELBALCH-Gleichung

$$p_H{}^s = 6{,}10 + \log \frac{CO_2\text{-Gehalt} - CO_2 \text{ gelöst}}{CO_2 \text{ gelöst}}$$

erhält man das p_H des Serums.

f) Berechnung der Kurzschlußdurchblutung der Lunge.

Zur Bestimmung der Kurzschlußdurchblutung der Lunge steht heute ein kompliziertes indirektes Verfahren zur Verfügung, welches von RILEY und COURNAND, OPITZ und BARTELS u. a. ausgearbeitet wurde. Die Berechnung der Kurzschlußdurchblutung fußt auf der Annahme, daß bei Diffusionsstörungen keine nennenswerte Differenz der O_2-Drucke zwischen Alveolarluft und Lungencapillarblut mehr besteht, wenn ein 40% O_2 enthaltendes Gasgemisch eingeatmet wird.

Methodisch wird so vorgegangen, daß der Proband zunächst über 30 min aus einem Spirographen ein Gasgemisch mit etwa 40% Sauerstoff atmet. Dann werden die notwendigen Gas- und Blutproben durch Arterienpunktion und Alveolarluftentnahme gewonnen. Im einzelnen bestimmt man die Sauerstoffspannung der Alveolarluft und des arteriellen Blutes, den O_2-Gehalt und die O_2-Kapazität des letzteren, den CO_2-Gehalt und die CO_2-Spannung des arteriellen Blutes, sowie die Alkalireserve und das p_H.

Durch Herzkatheterung erhält man venöses Mischblut und bestimmt dessen O_2-Gehalt und den p_H-Wert.

Die Differenz zwischen dem O_2-Gehalt des Lungencapillarblutes und demjenigen des arteriellen Blutes wird unter den gewählten Bedingungen auf venöse Beimischung zurückgeführt. Diese Differenz ist außer von der Menge auch vom Reduktionsgrad des venösen Mischblutes abhängig. Der Anteil der Kurzschlußblutmenge (Q_{sh}) an der Lungendurchblutung (Q_l) kann nach folgender Gleichung berechnet werden:

$$\frac{Q_{sh}}{Q_l} = \frac{C_{c'O_2} - C_{aO_2}}{C_{aO_2} - C_{\bar{v}O_2}}.$$

Der Zähler der rechten Seite dieser Gleichung (O_2-Gehalt des Lungencapillarblutes minus demjenigen des Arterienblutes) ist nicht direkt zu ermitteln, da schon kleinste Differenzen in der Bestimmung des O_2-Gehaltes große Verfälschungen der Shuntblutmenge bewirken können.

Man geht daher einen Umweg und bestimmt den dem Lungencapillargasdruck entsprechenden O_2-Druck in der Alveolarluft. Die O_2-Sättigung wird dann beim gleichen p_H auf einer Standarddissoziationskurve abgelesen, wobei zunächst letztere um den physikalisch gelösten O_2-Gehalt erhöht werden muß. Unter Benutzung der gemessenen O_2-Kapazität errechnet man einen Wert für den O_2-Gehalt des Lungencapillarblutes[1].

Um den arteriellen O_2-Druck zu erhalten, verfährt man in gleicher Weise unter Zurhilfenahme des O_2-Gehaltes des arteriellen Blutes. Damit ist aber auch die Differenz im Zähler der obigen Gleichung gegeben.

Zwischen dem alveolären und arteriellen O_2-Druck besteht bei Luftatmung normalerweise eine kurzschlußbedingte Differenz von 5—10 mm Hg. Beim Gesunden muß man mit 2—4% Kurzschlußblut rechnen.

g) Berechnung der Diffusionskapazität der Lunge.

Zur Berechnung der Diffusionskapazität der Lunge müssen die gleichen Verfahren durchgeführt werden, wie sie zur Ermittlung der Kurzschlußdurchblutung der Lunge geschildert wurden. In diesem Fall ist aber dem Probanden Luftatmung anzubieten.

Folgende Größen werden bestimmt: Die Sauerstoffspannung der Alveolarluft und des Lungencapillarblutes, sowie der O_2-Gehalt des arteriellen und des gemischt-venösen Blutes. Nach der Formel von KROGH erhält man einen Wert für die mittlere O_2-Druckdifferenz zwischen Alveolarluft und Blut in der Lunge ($\overline{\Delta p}$) und daraus mit dem spirographisch ermittelten O_2-Verbrauch die Diffusionskapazität:

$$D_{O_2} = \frac{O_2\text{-Verbrauch/cm}^3/\text{min}}{\overline{\Delta p}\ \text{mm Hg}}.$$

Die O_2-Diffusionskapazität ist diejenige Menge O_2, die in der Minute durch die gesamte Lungenoberfläche je Millimeter Hg mittlerer Druckdifferenz ($\overline{\Delta p}$) aufgenommen wird.

---

[1] OPITZ und BARTELS 1955.

Der Normalwert beträgt bei Luftatmung etwa 20 cm³ O_2/min/mm Hg $\overline{\Delta p}$. Bei Arbeit und Hypoxie nimmt diese Zahl zu.

Wenn der Sauerstoffdruck des Lungencapillarblutes um mehr als 5 mm Hg niedriger liegt als die O_2-Spannung der Alveolarluft, kann angenommen werden, daß eine Diffusionsstörung vorliegt. Die Berechnung der Diffusionskapazität erlaubt Schlüsse über das Ausmaß dieser Störung und gibt Aufklärung über die Anpassungsfähigkeit der Lunge.

Aus diesem Grunde werden diese Bestimmungen auch bei 12—14% O_2 in der Inspirationsluft durchgeführt. Die arterielle O_2-Spannung ist hierbei durch Verminderung des Kurzschlußblutmengen-Einflusses nahezu gleich der O_2-Spannung des Lungencapillarblutes.

Eine bei diesen Hypoxieversuchen ermittelte Zunahme der Diffusionskapazität von etwa 50% gegenüber der bei Luftatmung muß als normal angesehen werden.

Im Hypoxieversuch wird bei einer Diffusionsstörung durch die Vergrößerung des Druckgefälles eine Verbesserung der Diffusionsbedingungen eintreten, bei vergrößertem Kurzschlußblutanteil dagegen die alveolo-arterielle Differenz erheblich zunehmen.

Unter Hypoxiebedingungen findet sich bei Diffusionsstörungen eine größere alveoloarterielle Differenz. Liegt eine Kurzschlußstörung vor, so wird die bei Luftatmung abnorm erhöhte alveolo-arterielle Differenz unter Hypoxie in den Bereich der Norm absinken. Ursache ist der charakteristische Verlauf der O_2-Dissoziationskurve.

Nach neueren Untersuchungen findet sich eine vergrößerte alveolo-arterielle Differenz in folgenden Fällen:

a) Bei vielen Lungenerkrankungen und nach manchen operativen Eingriffen ist damit zu rechnen, daß die Lungenbelüftung ungleichmäßig geworden ist. Dies führt dann zu einer Erhöhung des Wertes. b) Auch durch Verschlechterung der Diffusionsbedingung infolge von Epithelverdickungen, Exsudaten usw. kann diese bedingt sein. c) Vor allem aber kann die Diffusionsfläche zu klein werden.

Zusammenfassend ist festzustellen, daß es eine alles umfassende Funktionsprüfung der Atmung nicht gibt. Eine Reihe von spirographischen Methoden können in der Klinik generell angewandt werden. Andere Verfahren sind nur von Fall zu Fall einzusetzen und haben ein spezielles gasanalytisches Laboratorium zur Voraussetzung. Entscheidend ist immer die Zumutbarkeit für den Patienten und die zu bearbeitende Fragestellung.

6. Spezielle Methoden.

a) Diffusionsmessung in den Lungen.

Zur Messung der Diffusionsverhältnisse in den Lungen sind nur solche Gase brauchbar, welche im Blut in wesentlich größerer Menge absorbiert werden als in der alveolo-capillären Membran. Bis heute sind nur 2 Gase bekannt, die diese Voraussetzungen in idealer Weise erfüllen, und zwar der Sauerstoff (O_2) und das Kohlenmonoxyd (CO). Beide verdanken ihre große „Löslichkeit" im Blut der chemischen Bindung an das Hämoglobin. Die mit beiden Gasen erhaltenen Diffusionswerte können direkt miteinander korreliert werden, wenn man den CO-Wert mit 1,23 multipliziert.

Für die Diffusionsmessung in den Lungen mittels O_2 oder CO ist von Bedeutung, daß die Bestimmung des Membrangradienten nur dann exakt erfolgen kann, wenn die Sättigung des Hämoglobins im arteriellen Blut nicht vollständig ist, also ein Spannungsgefälle durch die laufende O_2-Bindung an das Hämoglobin des Blutes zwischen Alveolarluft und Lungencapillarblut aufrecht erhalten bleibt. Sobald das nicht mehr der Fall ist — bei Sauerstoff im horizontalen Bereich der O_2-Dissoziationskurve — sind die Membrangradienten nicht mehr bestimmbar. Das gleiche trifft zu, wenn man zuviel CO dem Atemgas zumischt (mehr als 0,2—0,4%). Bereits eine CO-Spannung von 0,46 mm Hg würde die gleiche Hb-Sättigung zur Folge haben wie eine Sauerstoffspannung von 100 mm Hg bzw. 14 Vol.-% O_2, wenn nicht die trennende alveolo-capilläre Membran zwischen Alveolarluft und Blut existierte[1]. Das heißt aber, daß der Eintritt des Kohlenmonoxyd in das Blut in den gewählten Spannungsbereichen allein von dessen Diffusionsfähigkeit durch die Alveolarmembran abhängt. Das gilt um den Faktor 210 weniger für Sauerstoff, da die Affinität von CO zum Hämoglobin 210mal größer ist als die des Sauerstoffs.

---

[1] Comroe 1955.

Wie bereits ausgeführt, ergibt sich die Diffusionskapazität der Gesamtlunge aus der Gasaufnahme als Minutenwert und der alveolo-capillären Gasspannungsdifferenz. Für den Sauerstoff lautet die Formel (s. S. 349):

$$\text{DKap O}_2 = \frac{\text{O}_2\text{-Aufnahme je Minute}}{\text{alveolo-capilläre PO}_2\text{-Differenz}}.$$

Die *Bestimmung der Sauerstoffaufnahme* erfolgt spirographisch. Durch Verbinden der Fußpunkte der Atmungskurven läßt sich die Sauerstoffaufnahme leicht und direkt berechnen.

Die *Bestimmung der mittleren Alveolarluft* stößt in der Klinik auf technische Schwierigkeiten.

Die Methode von HALDANE und PRIESTLEY setzt soviel verstehende Mitarbeit des Patienten voraus, insbesondere seinen guten Willen, daß sie im Routinebetrieb nicht anwendbar ist. Bei der von RAHN angegebenen Methode wird automatisch Alveolarluft abgesaugt. Die damit erhaltenen Alveolarluftwerte sind recht gut und brauchbar, wenn die Atmung regelmäßig ist.

VENRATH[1] hat eine ähnliche Methode an der Kölner Medizinischen Universitätsklinik ausgearbeitet. Es wird automatisch aus einem Spezialmundstück die letzte Phase der Exspirationsluft abgesaugt. Aus diesem Wert, der Sauerstoffaufnahme je Minute, der Größe der funktionellen Residualkapazität und des Atemvolumens sowie aus dem Atemzeitquotienten ist mit Hilfe einer mathematischen Relation die mittlere Alveolarluft berechenbar. Im Detail wird auf die Originalveröffentlichung verwiesen.

ENGHOFF später auch ROSSIER und RILEY berechnen die mittlere Alveolarluft aus der *CO₂-Spannung des arteriellen Blutes*, indem sie letztere entweder direkt bestimmen oder über das p_H des Serums berechnen[2]. Die CO_2-Spannung des arteriellen Blutes wird gleich der der Alveolarluft gesetzt. Die Methode ist dann gut, wenn die venöse Kurzschlußkomponente des Blutes in den Lungen klein ist und nicht ins Gewicht fällt. Bei größeren Shunt-Volumina liegt der im arteriellen Blut ermittelte CO_2-Spannungswert zu hoch. Entsprechend ist der bestimmte Totraum zu groß.

Die *indirekte Bestimmung der mittleren Alveolarluft* mit Hilfe der BOHRschen Formel — bei theoretischer Annahme der Größe des Totraumes der Luftwege oder dessen Berechnung nach der LINDHARDschen Formel — birgt nicht die befürchteten großen Fehlerquellen in sich, da der Totraum eine auch unter Arbeit und Hyperventilation weitgehend konstante Größe ist[3].

$$\text{TR} = \text{AV} \cdot \left(\frac{\text{O}_2\text{ex} - \text{O}_2\text{alv}}{\text{O}_2\text{in} - \text{O}_2\text{alv}} \right).$$

Ein Annahmefehler des physiologischen Totraumes von $\pm 10\%$ bedingt einen Fehler in der Bestimmung der mittleren alveolaren Sauerstoffspannung von $\pm 1,8$ mm Hg.

Die Bestimmung der Gasverhältnisse im Lungencapillarblut. Lungencapillarblut, woraus die Gasverhältnisse für die Bestimmung der alveolo-capillären Sauerstoffspannungsdifferenz ermittelt werden könnten, ist im Experiment nicht zu gewinnen. Das mittels Herzkatheter abgesaugte Capillarblut ist nicht verwertbar, da venöse Zuflüsse, doppelter Hin- und Rückstrom des Blutes in den Lungencapillaren und Zumischung von Lungengewebsflüssigkeit im Detail nicht übersehbar sind. Bei Normalluftatmung kann arterielles Blut nicht an Stelle von Lungencapillarblut genommen werden, da die capilläre Sauerstoffspannung infolge der normalen venösen Zumischung abfällt. Eine nur geringgradige venöse Zumischung macht sich im hohen Sättigungsbereich entsprechend dem Verlauf der Dissoziationskurve auf die Spannungsverhältnisse im arteriellen Blut stark bemerkbar. *Der Einfluß dieser venösen Zumischungskomponente wird aber mit zunehmendem Sauerstoffmangel in der Inspirationsluft kleiner*[4], da die

---

[1] VENRATH, Habilitationsschrift 1956. [2] ENGHOFF 1938, ROSSIER 1946, RILEY 1946.
[3] FOWLER u. a. 1948, PAPPENHEIMER u. a. 1952/53, VENRATH 1956.
[4] LILIENTHAL, RILEY u. a. 1946.

Sauerstoffdissoziationskurve bei einer Sättigung von etwa 80—85% bereits ziemlich steil verläuft (s. Abb. 17 a).

So wirkt sich z. B. eine venöse Zumischung von 10% des Herzminutenvolumens in Form einer 5%igen Sättigungsminderung auf das arterielle Blut aus. Bei Normalluftatmung beträgt die dadurch verursachte Spannungsdifferenz zwischen capillärem und arteriellem Blut 19 mm Hg (s. Abb. 17 a). Im Sauerstoffmangel bei 80—85% Sättigung des arteriellen Blutes, entsprechend einem Sauerstoffgehalt in der Inspirationsluft von 12—14 Vol.-%, ist die Sättigungsdifferenz bei gleichbleibender venöser Zumischung von 10% des HMV (letzteres ebenfalls unverändert) konstant 5%, die Spannungsdifferenz aber nur mehr 1,2 mm Hg.

Das heißt mit anderen Worten: im Sauerstoffmangel wird der venöse Zumischungsgradient so klein, daß er schließlich entfällt. Hinzu kommt, daß der Membrangradient aus oben ausgeführten Gründen in dem Umfang ansteigt, wie

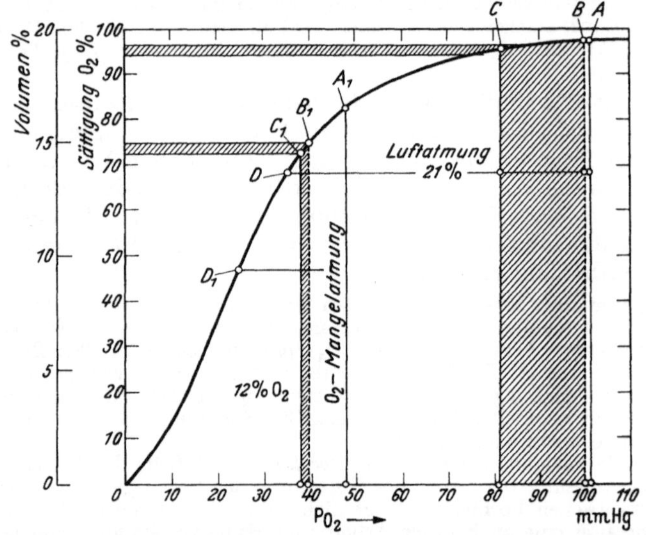

Abb. 17a. Das Verhalten des venösen Zumischungsgradienten und des Membrangradienten bei Atmen atmosphärischer Luft und eines Sauerstoffmangelgemisches von 12 Vol.-% O₂ in N₂. Die venöse Zumischung ist mit 10% des Herzminutenvolumens sehr groß angenommen. Bei Luftatmung zeigt A die O₂-Sättigung und -Spannung des Arterienblutes (auf eine O₂-Dissoziationskurve nach Dill u. a. aufgetragen) bei der Annahme, daß ein vollständiger Spannungsausgleich zwischen Alveolarluft und Lungencapillarblut einträte und die venöse Zumischung gleich Null wäre. In B ist die Spannungsminderung wiedergegeben, die durch unvollständigen Spannungsausgleich zwischen Alveolarluft und Capillarblut bedingt ist. Sie ist sehr klein, macht sich auf die O₂-Sättigung dadurch nicht meßbar bemerkbar. Die Sättigungs- und Spannungsminderung infolge einer venösen Zumischung von 10% des HMV ist in C wiedergegeben. D stellt die Spannungs- und Sättigungswerte des venösen Mischblutes dar. Somit entsprechen A—C der alveolo-arteriellen O₂-Spannungsdifferenz (= Δ PO₂) und C—D der arteriovenösen Differenz. — Bei Sauerstoffmangelatmung sinkt der Einfluß des Shunt auf die Sättigungs- und Spannungsminderung im Arterienblut deutlich ab, während die Membrankomponente an Bedeutung wesentlich gewinnt. Die Differenz zwischen A₁ und B₁ gibt den Membrangradienten wieder, die Spanne zwischen B₁ und C₁ den venösen Zumischungsgradienten. Der Einfluß des venösen Zumischungsgradienten auf die Blutgasverhältnisse ist schraffiert dargestellt.

der venöse Zumischungsgradient abfällt[1]. Somit ist es möglich, im Sauerstoffmangel an Stelle des Lungencapillarblutes peripheres arterielles Blut zur Bestimmung der alveolo-capillären Sauerstoffspannungsdifferenz zu verwenden.

Die Registrierung von Atmung und O₂-Aufnahme am Spirographen erfolgt nach Knipping (s. oben), die Bestimmung des O₂-Gehaltes der verschiedenen Luftproben wird entweder im Haldane-Apparat vorgenommen oder bei bekanntem Ausgangs-O₂-Gehalt in der Systemluft (z. B. bei Füllung des Apparates mit Außenluft von 20,9 Vol.-% O₂) und bekanntem Systemvolumen rechnerisch ermittelt unter Abzug der jeweils aufgenommenen O₂-Menge. Zur Messung der Blutgase und Gasspannungen im Blut s. S. 346.

Sind arterielle Punktionen bei Kranken kontraindiziert, so kann die O₂-Sättigung im arteriellen Blut oxymetrisch laufend registriert werden.

---

[1] Krogh 1915.

Zum Ausschluß von Ventilationsstörungen geht der Messung der Diffusion grundsätzlich eine Lungenfunktionsprüfung in der an unserer Klinik geübten Form (s. oben) voraus. Es ist ebenfalls zweckmäßig, vor allen Diffusionsmessungen *Verteilungsstörungen* mit Hilfe der De- bzw. Resaturations- und Mischungskurven auszuschließen.

Zur *Messung der Diffusionsverhältnisse* in den Lungen wird der Patient in Exspiration an den mit einem bekannten Volumen Außenluft gefüllten Spirographen angeschlossen. Durch die laufende Entnahme von Sauerstoff atmet sich der Patient gleichsam „auf Höhe", d. h. der O_2-Partialdruck nimmt kontinuierlich ab. Gleichzeitig wird fortlaufend oxymetrisch die arterielle O_2-Sättigung registriert. Entsprechend der Minderung der O_2-Spannung in der Systemluft sinkt die arterielle O_2-Sättigung kontinuierlich ab. Spirographisch und oxymetrisch zum gleichen Zeitpunkt erhaltene Werte lassen sich leicht tabellarisch oder in Kurven miteinander koordinieren. Erreicht die O_2-Sättigung im arteriellen Blut 80—85%, so wird stabilisiert und je nach Notwendigkeit die Zusammensetzung der mittleren Alveolarluft bestimmt und arterielles Blut zur Blutgasanalyse und PO_2-Bestimmung entnommen.

Die *Kohlenmonoxyd-Methode* ist namentlich in skandinavischen Ländern[1] zur Bestimmung der Diffusionskapazität verwendet worden. Zwei Methoden haben sich eingebürgert:

1. Die Diffusionskapazitätsmessung mittels der *Ein-Atemzug-CO-Methode*. Aus einem Beutel wird ein Luftgemisch geatmet, welches unter anderem 0,3% CO und 10% Helium enthält. Das Residualvolumen muß bekannt sein. Nach maximaler Exspiration wird aus dem Beutel das Gasgemisch tief eingeatmet, auf der Höhe der Inspiration die Luft angehalten und nach gemessener Zeit wieder ausgeatmet. Die Ausatmungsluft wird auf ihren Helium- und CO-Gehalt untersucht. Die Diffusionskapazität der Lungen läßt sich dann nach der KROGHschen Formel errechnen[2].

2. Bei der *CO-Steady state-Methode* wird die alveoläre CO-Spannung nach etwa 5—10 minütiger CO-Gasgemisch-Atmung bestimmt und die Rate an CO ermittelt, die je Zeiteinheit in der Lunge verschwindet. Es wird dabei die Tatsache ausgenutzt, daß der Durchtritt von CO nur von der Diffusionsfähigkeit durch die alveolo-capilläre Membran begrenzt wird[3].

b) Bestimmung der Atemmechanik.

In den letzten Jahren wurden die Untersuchungen von ROHRER[4] und VUILLEUMIER[5] sowie von v. NEERGAARD[6] und BUYTENDIJK[7] über die Atemmechanik erneut aufgegriffen mit dem besonderen Aspekt, die subjektiven Beschwerden des Patienten bei der *Dyspnoe* einer objektiven Messung zugänglich zu machen. Die Prüfung der Atemmechanik dient zur Messung der Widerstände, die sich den Atembewegungen in der Lunge und im Thorax entgegensetzen.

Methodisch basiert sie auf der gleichzeitigen spirographischen oder pneumotachographischen Registrierung der Atmung und des intrathorakalen Druckes. Um Pleurapunktionen zu umgehen, die bei der direkten Messung des Pleuradruckes notwendig wären, wird heute im allgemeinen der intraoesophageale Druck bestimmt (BUYTENDIJK[7]). Er wird dem intrapleuralen Druck gleichgestellt.

Der intrapleurale Druck setzt sich zu jedem Zeitpunkt des Atemcyclus aus 3 Komponenten zusammen: Aus dem elastischen Retraktionsdruck der Lungen in Abhängigkeit vom Lungenvolumen, aus dem Reibungsdruck der Gase in den Luftwegen, dann aber auch aus der Stoffreibung (Deformierung) im Lungengewebe und schließlich aus dem Trägheitsdruck, das ist die Kraft, die notwendig ist, Luftstrom und Gewebsverschiebung zu beschleunigen. Letzterer spielt bei ruhiger Atmung keine Rolle, wird aber mit Größerwerden der Atmung immer bedeutender. Somit ist der elastische Retraktionsdruck (P_{el}) eine Funktion des Lungenvolumens ($P_{el} = \frac{1}{C} \cdot V$), der Reibungsdruck ($P_{reib}$) eine Funktion der Atemstromstärke ($P_{reib} = R \cdot V/t_2$) und der Trägheitsdruck ($P_{träg} = T \cdot V/t_2$) eine Funktion der Beschleunigung von Atemstrom und Gewebsverschiebung.

---

[1] KROGH und LINDHARD 1913, 1914.   [2] FORSTER u. a. 1954.
[3] PACE 1946, KRUHØFER 1954.   [4] ROHRER 1915.   [5] VUILLEUMIER 1944.
[6] v. NEERGAARD 1929.   [7] BUYTENDIJK 1949.

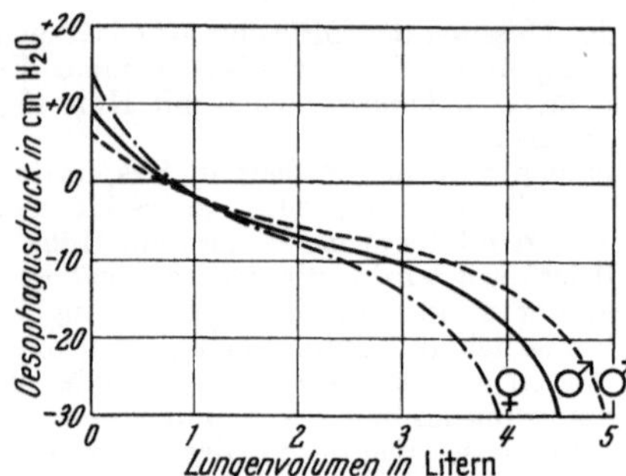

Abb. 17b. Volumen-Druckbeziehungen der Lunge unter statischen Bedingungen.

Bei Vernachlässigung des Trägheitsdruckes würde sich der Oesophagusdruck errechnen aus

$$P_{oe} = \frac{1}{C} \cdot V + R \cdot V/t.$$

Werden bei Atemstillstand, Atemstromstärke und Reibungsdruck O, so ist der Oesophagusdruck dem elastischen Retraktionsdruck der Lunge gleich und damit direkt abhängig vom Lungenvolumen.

$$P_{oe} = \frac{1}{C} \cdot V.$$

Unter statischen Bedingungen ergeben sich für jede Lunge typische Kurven, wovon einige in Abb. 17b dargestellt sind.

Die Compliance (C) schwankt beim Gesunden in Abhängigkeit vom Alter zwischen 0,055—0,22 Liter/cm H_2O. Der große Streubereich, welchen bereits der Gesunde aufweist, zeigt an, daß eine hohe statische Compliance nur mit Vorbehalt als Ausdruck eines Elastizitätsverlustes oder eine niedrige, nicht zwangsläufig im Sinne einer Lungenstarre gedeutet werden kann[1].

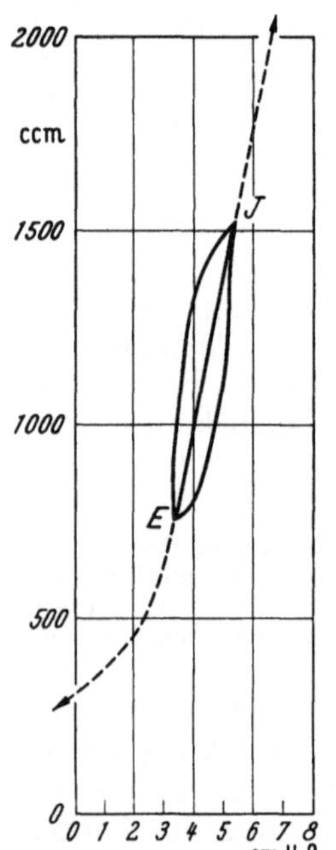

Abb. 17c. Arbeitsdiagramm der Atmung. Die schleifenförmige Kurve gibt das kinetische Druck-Volumendiagramm der Atmung wieder.

Mit tiefer Inspiration knickt die Kurve des statischen Druckvolumendiagrammes von anfänglich nahezu geradem Verlauf ab, was besagt, daß bei extremer Inspiration eine erhöhte Atemarbeit verrichtet werden muß. Das Pendant findet sich bei maximaler Exspiration, wobei die Pleuradrucke positiv werden.

Je ausgeprägter der Elastizitätsverlust der Lungen ist, z. B. beim Emphysem, um so größer ist das Lungenvolumen, bei dem von negativen Drucken ausgehend, der Nullwert erreicht wird.

Dem gegenüber zeigt das kinetische Druckvolumendiagramm das Verhalten von Druck und Volumen über den Atemcyclus hin. Zu gleichen Zeitpunkten werden das spirographisch gemessene Volumen der Atmung und der Druck im Oesophagus gemessen und entweder mechanisch oder zeichnerisch miteinander in Beziehung gebracht. Das kinetische Druckvolumendiagramm hat Schleifenform. Die Schleife wird bei zunehmendem Reibungswiderstand weiter und würde der statischen Druckvolumenbeziehung kongruent verlaufen, wenn der Reibungswiderstand Null wäre. Da aber in der Bewegungsphase immer Reibungswiderstände zu überwinden sind, weicht die Verbindungslinie aller Meßpunkte bogenförmig von dieser Geraden ab. Die ober- und unterhalb der Schleifendiagonale gelegenen Flächen sind oft nicht gleich groß, da inspiratorischer und exspiratorischer Reibungswiderstand nicht gleich groß sind. In den Umschlagpunkten von Inspiration zur Exspiration und umgekehrt, sind Strömungs- und Reibungswiderstand gleich Null. Entsprechend liegen sie auf der Kurve des statischen Druckvolumendiagrammes (Abb. 17c).

---

[1] Venrath 1959.

Die Diagonale zwischen E und I ist somit ein Teil der statischen Elastizitätskurve.

Beim Lungengesunden liegen E und I immer auf der Elastizitätskurve, gleichgültig, ob er ruhig und tief oder frequent und flach atmet. Die Schleifendiagonale bleibt der statischen Druckvolumenbeziehung treu. Sie weichen aber deutlich ab, wenn akut ein Bronchospasmus auftritt.

Die Fläche des Druckvolumendiagrammes stellt die *Atemarbeit* dar und wird durch planimetrische Integration gewonnen. Sie ist beim Emphysem und beim

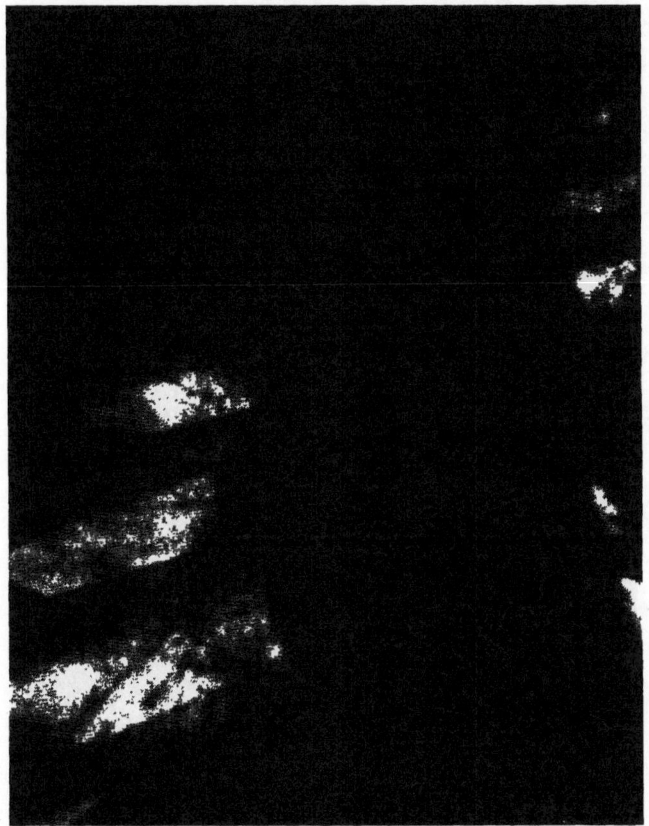

Abb. 18. Hochgradiges Emphysem. Die selektive Angiographie zeigt außerordentlich enggestellte Verzweigungen der A. pulmonalis, die einen gestreckten, besenreiserartigen Verlauf nehmen. Die Kontrastmittelpassage durch diese engen Arterienverzweigungen in der Lungenperipherie ist stark verlangsamt.

Asthma bronchiale vergrößert und kann einen objektiven Wert für die Schwere der Atmungsarbeit geben ohne aber zwangsläufig etwas über die subjektiv empfundene Dyspnoe zu sagen.

c) Selektive Lungenangiographie.

Für die funktionellen Pathologie der Lungenkrankheiten ist neben der Kenntnis der Ventilation die Kenntnis der *Lungendurchblutung* wichtig, da zwischen der alveolären Ventilation und der Lungendurchblutung enge Wechselbeziehungen bestehen. Die instruktiven Tierversuche von v. EULER, LILJESTRAND und NISELL lassen auch für den Menschen die Möglichkeit einer Selbststeuerung des Verhältnisses von Lungenbelüftung zu Lungendurchblutung in dem Sinne annehmen, daß eine Herabsetzung der alveolären O_2-Spannung zu einer regulatorischen Drosselung der Durchblutung der Verzweigungen der A. pulmonalis führt.

Venrath, Rotthoff, Valentin und Bolt konnten darüber hinaus nachweisen, daß auch umgekehrt eine *Drosselung der Durchblutung* eine *Verkleinerung der Atmung* herbeiführt, die erkennbar wird, wenn im Experiment nach Blockierung eines Astes der A. pulmonalis durch einen aufblasbaren Herzkatheter genügend lange bronchospirographisch kontrolliert wird.

Durch die Sondierung der einzelnen Segmentäste der A. pulmonalis mit der Forssmannschen Herzsonde und die von Bolt und Mitarbeitern entwickelte

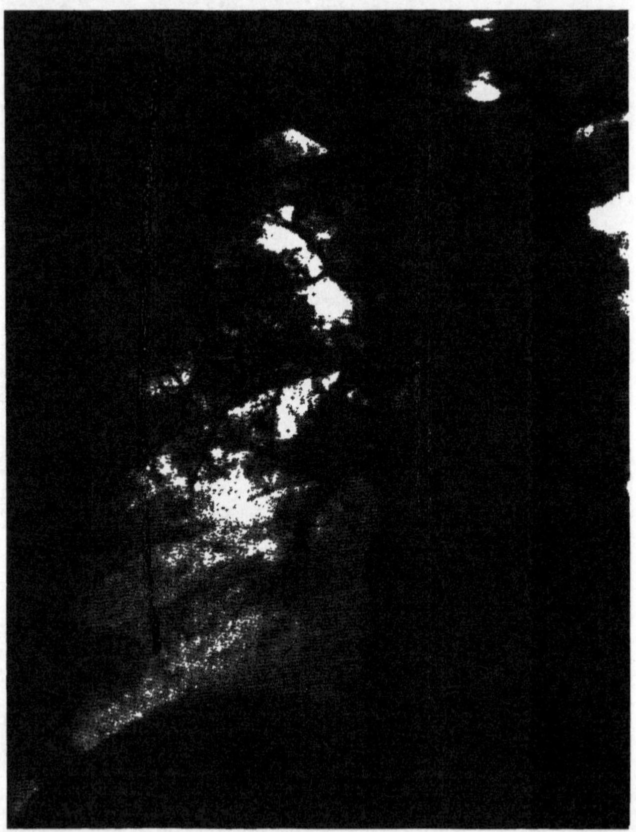

Abb. 19. Kleinkavernisierte Spitzenoberfeldtuberkulose rechts. Im Bereiche der Kavernisierung des apikalen-medialen und apikalen-posterioren Oberlappensegmentes sind die Arterienverzweigungen deutlich enggestellt. Sie nehmen, im Gegensatz zur Abb. 18 (Emphysem) jedoch mehr ihren natürlichen, etwas geschlängelten Verlauf ein. Vor Erreichen der Lungenperipherie bricht die Gefäßfüllung im kavernisierten Bereich infolge endangitischer Prozesse ab. Das pectorale Segment des rechten Oberlappens zeigt eine Engstellung der Arterienäste, jedoch nicht die Gefäßabbrüche wie in den beiden apikalen Oberlappensegmenten.

selektive Angiographie der Lungengefäße konnte die funktionelle Analyse bis zur Größenordnung der einzelnen Lungensegmente und Subsegmente erweitert werden. Besondere praktische Bedeutung hat diese Methode in der prä- und postoperativen Beurteilung bei Lungenresektionen, Dekortikationen und bei dem selektiven Lungenkollaps erlangt[1]. Zur exakten klinischen Beurteilung einer sekundären Pulmonalsklerose bei Mitralstenosen und bei kongenitalen Herz-

---

[1] Bolt, Knipping und Rink 1953, Bolt, Forssmann und Rink 1953, 1957.

fehlern ist dies die einzige brauchbare Methode, die Fehlindikationen zur operativen Behandlung vermeiden läßt.

Nach Einführung eines Herzkatheters von der Cubitalvene her durch das rechte Herz in das zu explorierende Lungensegment werden in den betreffenden Ast der A. pulmonalis durch den Katheter kleine Mengen Kontrastmittel injiziert (5—10 cm³ eines trijodierten Röntgenkontrastmittels, z. B. Urografin 76%). Während der Injektion geschossene Röntgenaufnahmen geben ein klares Bild der Gefäßversorgung in den einzelnen Lungensegmenten, und zwar des arteriellen Schenkels, der capillaren Phase und des venösen Rückflusses aus

Abb. 20. Hilusnahes Bronchialcarcinom links mit Teilstenose des zum apikalen-posterioren Oberlappensegment führenden Bronchus. Ummauerung der aus diesem Segment rückführenden Pulmonalvenen durch Metastasen in der Nähe des linken Vorhofs. Infolge der durch die Bronchusstenose gegebenen Hypoventilation des apikalen-posterioren Oberlappensegmentes sind die zugehörigen Verzweigungen der A. pulmonalis bis zur Lungenperipherie hin enggestellt. Der Arterienverlauf ist normal. Hilusnah ist der venöse Rückfluß durch Carcinommetastasen gedrosselt und kommt als kelchförmiger Kontrastmittelschatten vor dem Herzen zur Darstellung. Die venösen Rückflüsse aus den betroffenen Subsegmenten sind enggestellt. Deutliche arterielle und venöse Verzögerung der Kontrastmittelpassage.

dem Segment. Röntgenkinematographische Serienaufnahmen lassen die zeitlichen Verhältnisse einwandfrei objektiv erfassen.

Abb. 18—21 zeigen verschiedene Formen funktioneller und organischer Durchblutungsstörungen bei Patienten mit Emphysem, kavernöser Lungentuberkulose, partieller Bronchostenose infolge eines Bronchialcarcinoms und bei „funktionell toter Lunge"[1].

Die selektive Angiographie der Lungengefäße ermöglicht, wie aus den Beispielen hervorgeht, eine mit keiner anderen Methode erreichbare regionale

---

[1] BOLT 1953.

funktionelle Analyse der Durchblutung und indirekt auch der Ventilation der einzelnen Lungensegmente, entsprechend den von v. Euler und Liljestrand aufgedeckten Wechselbeziehungen zwischen Ventilation und Perfusion.

Als Pendant zur selektiven Lungenangiographie gestattet die neuerdings entwickelte Isotopenthorakographie (s. S. 341) die regionale Analyse der Ventilation.

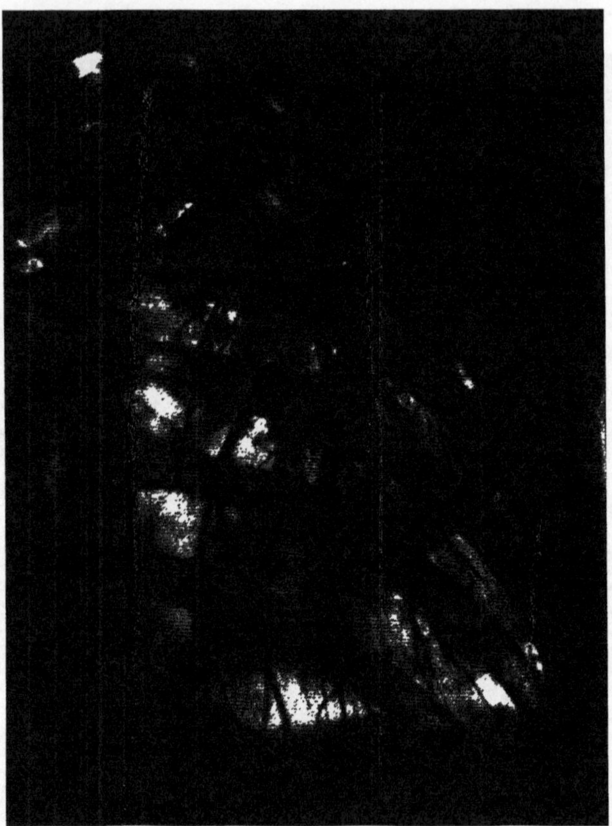

Abb. 21. Zustand nach spezifischem Empyem bei kavernöser Oberfeldtuberkulose links. Starke Raffung des Stammes der A. pulmonalis apikalwärts. Die Oberlappenäste der A. pulmonalis sind weitgehend blockiert. Im Unterlappen: Atrophisches Gefäßsystem mit Schwund der Gefäßperipherie und nahezu völliger Drosselung der Durchblutung bei „funktionell toter Lunge".

IV. Definition der respiratorischen Insuffizienz und Einteilungsprinzipien.

Die Aufgabe der Lungen ist einfach und klar definierbar: *Arterialisierung des venösen Blutes.* Sauerstoff wird in das Blut aufgenommen, CO_2 wird in die Alveolarluft abgegeben.

Voraussetzung für einen normalen Gasaustausch in den Lungen sind:

1. Eine genügende Ventilation der Alveolen.
2. Ein adäquater Blutstrom durch die Lungencapillaren.
3. Eine diffusible Membran zwischen Blut und Alveole.

Störungen eines oder mehrerer dieser Faktoren (Ventilations-, Perfusions- und Diffusionsstörungen) können zur *respiratorischen Insuffizienz* führen.

Die Wortprägung „respiratorische Insuffizienz" geht auf BRAUER und KNIP-PING zurück, die darunter definitionsgemäß solche Zustandsbilder verstehen, bei denen die Atmung nicht mehr genügt, um das arterielle Blut mit Sauerstoff zu sättigen und soweit von CO_2 zu befreien, daß die Zusammensetzung des Blutes den Bedürfnissen des Organismus entsprechend reguliert ist.

In den Jahren 1924—1930 haben BRAUER und Mitarbeiter den Begriff respiratorische Insuffizienz in die klinische Alltagsarbeit übernommen und die 1. Einteilung der verschiedenen Formen vom klinischen Standpunkt aus vorgeschlagen. Sie trennen die zentral bedingte respiratorische Insuffizienz von der pulmonal- und aerogen bedingten Insuffizienz ab.

Nachdem sich die funktionelle Betrachtungsweise in der Lungenklinik zunehmend durchgesetzt hat, sind eine Reihe von Einteilungen vorgeschlagen worden.

Einteilungsprinzipien.

Im Vordergrund steht ohne Frage eine *pathologisch-anatomisch* orientierte Einteilung. Sie wird, insbesondere in morphologischer Hinsicht, immer maßgeblich bleiben (vgl. die entsprechenden pathologisch-anatomischen Kapitel in diesem Handbuch). Aber die Klinik bedarf daneben der *funktionellen Aufgliederung* des Insuffizienzgeschehens. Man kann die respiratorische Insuffizienz nach der *Schwere des Insuffizienzbildes* unterteilen. WINTRICH trennte bereits 1854 die absolute Atmungsinsuffizienz (als mit dem Leben unvereinbar) von der relativen. BRAUER und KNIPPING (1932)[1] haben zuerst von *Ruhe-* und *Arbeitsinsuffizienz* gesprochen. Diese Einteilung trägt mehr summarischen Charakter. Die klinische Praxis erfordert allerdings eine Cäsur, sowohl von der analytischen Seite aus wie auch für die Therapie. Da die Leistungsbreite der Atmung normalerweise etwa das 10—20fache der Ruhebeanspruchung umfaßt, ist zur Aufdeckung von Frühschäden, die im Bereich der Arbeitsinsuffizienz liegen, vielfach die *Untersuchung unter Belastung* erforderlich[2].

Weiterhin kann nach den *Auswirkungen* der respiratorischen Insuffizienz auf die *Gaszusammensetzung des arteriellen Blutes* unterschieden werden. Das Blut ist letztlich das Erfolgsorgan bzw. der Spiegel der Respiration.

So hat ROSSIER eine *Globalinsuffizienz*, eine *Partialinsuffizienz* und den *vasculären Kurzschluß* unterschieden.

Bei der Globalinsuffizienz ist im arteriellen Blut eine Erniedrigung der Sauerstoffspannung bei erhöhter CO_2-Spannung nachweisbar, bei der Partialinsuffizienz infolge Mischung von hypo- und hyperventiliertem Blut meist eine Abnahme von Sauerstoff- und CO_2-Spannung. Der vasculäre Kurzschluß stellt gewissermaßen den Extremfall der Partialinsuffizienz dar. Die Blutgasbefunde ähneln denen bei Partialinsuffizienz.

Um *quantitative Aussagen* über die Respirationsverhältnisse in den Lungen im Einzelfall aus den Blutgasen machen zu können, genügen die arterielle CO_2- und Sauerstoffspannung nicht. Da eine Unterarterialisierung — durch Partialinsuffizienz oder vasculären Kurzschluß — infolge kompensatorischen Eingreifens des Kreislaufs (s. S. 367) unter Umständen beträchtlich modifiziert werden kann, sind die Kenntnis der Ausnutzung des venösen Mischblutes, die Größe des HMV und die Blutmenge für eine verbindliche Aussage eine Voraussetzung[3]. Das ist in Ruhe oft schon schwierig zu bestimmen, unter Arbeit im Routinebetrieb unmöglich.

Die größten Chancen, sich in der Praxis durchzusetzen, hat eine Gliederung nach dem *Charakter* bzw. der *Ätiologie* der funktionellen Störung, die im Endeffekt, wenn auch in zum Teil schwer faßbaren Dimensionen, die Arterialisierung des Blutes in Mitleidenschaft zieht. Alle Formen können als *regionale* bzw. *partielle* oder als *totale Störungen* auftreten.

I. Respiratorische Ruhe- und Arbeitsinsuffizienz.

1. Ventilationsstörungen.

a) Einschränkung der Ventilationsbewegungen,

---

[1] BRAUER und KNIPPING 1932. [2] KNIPPING, BOLT, VALENTIN und VENRATH 1955, 1960.
[3] VENRATH, LECHTENBÖRGER, VALENTIN und BOLT 1955.

b) Stenosen der Luftwege,

c) Mischstörungen,

d) Vergrößerung des funktionellen Totraumes; Pendelatmung.

2. Perfusionsstörungen (vasculärer Kurzschluß).

a) Abnorme intrapulmonale und intrakardiale „Shunt"verbindungen,

b) Durchblutung nicht beatmeter Lungenteile.

3. Diffusionsstörungen.

a) Primär pulmonal bedingte Diffusionsstörungen,

b) primär kardial bedingte Diffusionsstörungen.

II. Ruhe- bzw. Arbeitsinsuffizienz des linken oder des rechten Herzens mit sekundärer respiratorischer Insuffizienz.

In ähnlicher Weise ist die klare und klinisch brauchbare Gliederung orientiert, welche Richards, Baldwin und Cournand 1948 gegeben haben. Unter dem Oberbegriff: *Pulmonale Insuffizienz* trennen sie eine *ventilatorische* Insuffizienz (mechanisch bedingt mit dem Hauptsymptom Dyspnoe) von einer *respiratorischen* Insuffizienz (physikochemisch bedingt mit dem Hauptsymptom Cyanose).

Schließlich müssen noch — unabhängig von den bisher aufgeführten Einteilungen — vom generellen oder totalen Insuffizienzgeschehen streng *regionale funktionelle Insuffizienzvorgänge* abgetrennt werden. Die Entwicklung der Thoraxchirurgie in Richtung des gezielten Kollapses oder der Segmentresektion (in der Tuberkuloseklinik ganz besonders) verlangt mit Nachdruck eine stärkere Berücksichtigung, aber auch eine bessere Erfassung der *regionalen Durchblutung und Ventilation*[1].

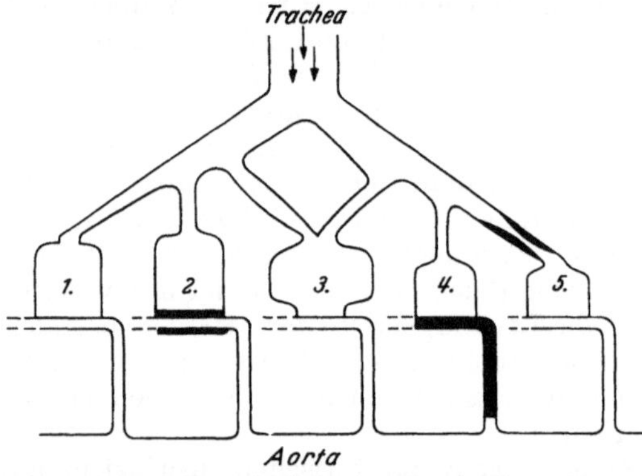

Abb. 22. Schematische Darstellung der Gaswechselstörungen in der Lunge. 1. Normales Zustandsbild, Beatmung und Durchblutung im Gleichgewicht. 2. Diffusionserschwerung durch Verdichtung der trennenden Membran zwischen Alveole und Blut. 3. Ventilationsstörung z. B. Emphysem, TR-Vergrößerung, Durchmischungsstörung. 4. Beatmete, nicht durchblutete Alveole. Diese Alveole ist ein funktioneller Totraum. 5. Intrapulmonaler Kurzschluß (Shunt). Die Beatmung der Alveole ist blockiert, die Durchblutung normal. Es fließt also unarterialisiertes Blut zum linken Herzen und in die Aorta.

So übersichtlich die normalen Zusammenhänge auch immer sein mögen, so verwirrend sind vielfach die *pathologischen Variationen*, vor allem dann, wenn man sie vom *funktionellen Standpunkt* aus betrachtet, da man selten ihrer Ätiologie nach reine Insuffizienzformen vorfindet. Die Abwägung der einzelnen Faktoren in ihrer Auswirkung auf die Funktionsminderung ist oft nicht leicht. Trotzdem gelang es in den letzten Jahren, nahezu das ganze Gebiet der respiratorischen Insuffizienz quantitativ zu durchdringen.

V. Die wichtigsten funktionell pathologischen Störungsmechanismen.

Die respiratorische Ruhe- und Arbeitsinsuffizienz. Die Abgrenzung von Ruhe- und Arbeitsinsuffizienzen hat sich bei der Funktionsdiagnostik der Herz- und Lungenkrankheiten als zweckmäßig erwiesen. Als *respiratorische Ruheinsuffizienz* werden die Zustandsbilder bezeichnet, bei denen bereits in Ruhe klinische Sym-

---

[1] Bolt 1953, Knipping und Bolt, Valentin, Venrath, Ludes und Endler 1955, 1958, 1961.

ptome der ungenügenden Atmung nachweisbar sind. Diese Zeichen sind insbesondere *Dyspnoe und Cyanose*. Objektiv belegt wird das Bild der respiratorischen Ruheinsuffizienz durch eine Minderung des Atemgrenzwertes (AGW) auf weniger als das Doppelte des Ruheatemminutenvolumens (= untere Grenze der extremen Arbeitsinsuffizienz)[1, 2]. Eine arterielle Cyanose tritt dann auf, wenn die O_2-Sättigung des Arterienblutes unter 90% absinkt. Kardiale Faktoren sowie Shuntverbindungen in den Lungen sind dabei auszuschließen. Im arteriellen Blut ist neben der ungenügenden O_2-Sättigung bei bestimmten Formen der respiratorischen Insuffizienz eine Erhöhung der CO_2-Spannung nachweisbar. Alle aufgeführten Störungen können schließlich zur Ruheinsuffizienz führen.

Jede Form der respiratorischen Ruheinsuffizienz hat ihre typischen Symptome, die sich von denen der *Arbeitsinsuffizienzen* lediglich dadurch unterscheiden, daß die Abweichungen von der Norm extremer sind. Ihr Unterschied liegt also im Graduellen. Die Skala der respiratorischen Arbeitsinsuffizienz beginnt gleich hinter dem Normalstatus und geht fließend über in die Ruheinsuffizienz als letzte Szene des letzten Aktes des Insuffizienzgeschehens[3].

1. Die Ventilationsstörungen.

Die Gruppe der Ventilationsstörungen ist die größte der 3 Untergruppen der respiratorischen Insuffizienz. Zur *Funktionsdiagnostik* dieser praktisch bedeutendsten Gruppe sei ausgeführt, daß sie im wesentlichen durch die *spirographischen Methoden* auch in ihren Unterformen quantitativ charakterisierbar ist.

Die Registrierung der Ruheatmung, der Lungenvolumina (Vitalkapazität, Residualvolumen, Totalkapazität), der Lungenfunktionswerte (Mischungszeit, Atemstoßwert, Atemgrenzwert und Atemzeitquotient) und die Belastungsuntersuchungen mit Austestung der Leistungsgrenze sowie die Untersuchung des Einflusses von O_2-Spannungsänderungen auf Atmung und O_2-Aufnahme in Ruhe und im steady state der Belastung erlauben meist eine erschöpfende Funktionsdiagnostik und Analyse. Nur in Ausnahmefällen ist es notwendig, blutgasanalytische Untersuchungen zur Ergänzung heranzuziehen.

Nach *ätiologischen Gesichtspunkten* haben wir[4] die Ventilationsstörungen unterteilt in:

a) Zentrale und periphere Atembehinderung.

Einschränkungen der Ventilationsbewegungen können *zentralen* Ursprungs sein (Abstumpfung der Zentren, Barbitursäure-, Morphiumvergiftungen usw., bulbäre und spinale Lähmungen der Atemmuskulatur, Zustand nach Phrenikuslähmung, Myasthenia gravis) oder *peripher* bedingt sein (nach großen Thorakoplastiken, ausgedehnten Lungenresektionen, bei Kyphoskoliose, ausgedehnten Pleuraverschwartungen, multiplen Rippenfrakturen, raumbeengenden Prozessen in den Pleurahöhlen sowie Exsudationen, Stenosen der Trachea usw.).

Charakteristisch für diese Gruppe ist die kontinuierliche Abnahme der Ventilationsbewegung (Abb. 23). Je kleiner das Atemminutenvolumen wird, desto stärker wirkt sich der den Alveolen vorgeschaltete physiologischen Totraum der Luftwege aus. Sinkt das Atemminutenvolumen schließlich auf das Volumen des Totraumes ab, so erfolgt ein Gasaustausch mit der Alveolarluft nur noch mittels Diffusion, selbst bei hohen Atemfrequenzen, bei denen das Atemminutenvolumen als Produkt aus Atemvolumen und Atemfrequenz noch normal, ja sogar gegenüber der Norm vergrößert sein kann. Folge dieser ungenügenden alveolären Ventilation ist ein Absinken der arteriellen Sauerstoffsättigung und -Spannung und ein entsprechender Anstieg des CO_2-Gehaltes[5]. O_2-Atmung kann zwar zu einer Normalisierung der Sauerstoffwerte im arteriellen Blut führen, die Abgabe des Kohlendioxyds wird aber dadurch nicht verbessert. Sauerstoffatmung ist daher nur von vorübergehendem Wert,

[1] REGLI und WYSS 1954.
[2] BOLT, W.: Emphysem (Hämodynamik). Beitr. Klin. Tbk. 111, 1954.
[3] KNIPPING 1935.   [4] KNIPPING, BOLT, VALENTIN und VENRATH 1953.
[5] BOLT, VALENTIN und VENRATH 1951.

362 H. W. KNIPPING und W. BOLT: Funktionelle Pathologie der Atmung.

in manchen Fällen sogar kontraindiziert[1]. Man kann versuchen, durch Einlegen einer Trachealsonde bis zur Bifurkation der Trachea und O_2-Insufflation das Totraumvolumen zu verkleinern[2]. Die ideale Behandlungsmethode der zentralen Formen ist aber die *künstliche Beatmung* entweder in der Eisernen Lunge oder die Intratrachealbeatmung. Auch der Pulmotor hat sich bei flüchtigen Formen bewährt.

Die *Behandlung der peripheren Formen* ist dominierend symptomatisch: Schmerzbeseitigung oder Ruhigstellung bei Rippenfrakturen und bei akuten trockenen Pleuritiden, Absaugen des Ergusses bei massiven Pleuraexsudationen, so daß sich die kollabierte Lunge wieder ausdehnen kann und die Gasaustauschfläche dadurch größer wird. Das gleiche gilt für den Spontan- oder Überdruckpneumothorax. Stenosen in der Trachea sind zu beseitigen. Im akuten Status wird man gerne bei diesen Krankheitsbildern zur O_2-Atmung greifen. Man muß sich aber bewußt sein, daß sie sich nur auf die Sauerstoffsättigung auswirkt, nicht aber die Abgabe des Kohlendioxyds fördert. Daher ist der Erfolg nur ein vorübergehender (s. oben).

Ventilationsbehinderungen im Gefolge thoraxchirurgischer Eingriffe sind im akuten postoperativen Stadium vielfach bereits durch entsprechende Lagerung des Patienten günstig zu beeinflussen. Die Anwendung des Sauerstoffzeltes wird in manchen Fällen notwendig sein. Man muß sich aber auch hier bewußt sein, daß die CO_2-Aufstockung im Blut dadurch nicht günstig beeinflußt wird. Frühzeitig einsetzende aktive und passive Atmungsübungen, vielleicht schon präoperativ

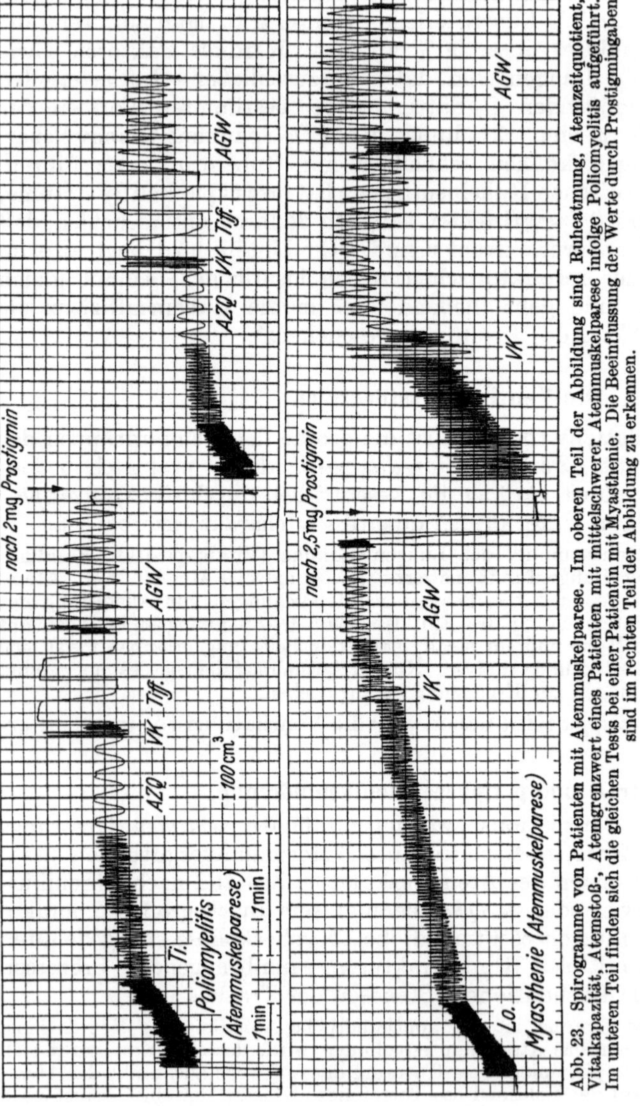

Abb. 23. Spirogramme von Patienten mit Atemmuskelparese. Im oberen Teil der Abbildung sind Ruheatmung, Atemzeitquotient, Vitalkapazität, Atemstoß-, Atemgrenzwert eines Patienten mit mittelschwerer Atemmuskelparese infolge Poliomyelitis aufgeführt. Im unteren Teil finden sich die gleichen Tests bei einer Patientin mit Myasthenie. Die Beeinflussung der Werte durch Prostigmingaben sind im rechten Teil der Abbildung zu erkennen.

beginnend, sind vielfach von günstigem Einfluß, ebenfalls peinlichste Bronchialtoilette. Im Notfall wird man auch hier eine intratracheale künstliche Beatmung durchführen müssen[3]. Lange bestehende *Kyphoskoliosen*, die schließlich respiratorisch dekompensieren, leiten in ihrem Funktionsbild bereits zur Gruppe c (Mischstörungen) über. Es handelt sich bei Kyphoskoliosen und ebenfalls bei den Thoraxstarren infolge BECHTEREWscher Erkrankung um Zustandsbilder, welche sich über Jahre hin langsam entwickeln. Das Atmungszentrum ist infolge der respiratorischen Leistungsminderung häufig gegen Kohlendioxyd so weit abgestumpft, daß die Anoxie die Atmungsleitung über die Chemorezeptoren im Glomus caroticum übernommen hat. Nimmt man nun durch Sauerstoffatmung den Hypoxiereiz, so

---

[1] DONALD und PATON 1955.   [2] BRAUER 1932.   [3] BJÖRK und HILTY 1954.

schläft das Atemzentrum ein, und der Patient stirbt infolge extremer Hypercarbie. Auch Diamox ist in solchen Fällen nicht immer indiziert. Künstliche Beatmung, insbesondere O_2-Überdruckbeatmung wirkt sich vielfach günstig auf den Gesamtzustand des Patienten aus. Als Folge der künstlichen Hyperventilation kommt es nicht nur zu einer Normalisierung der arteriellen O_2-Sättigung, sondern ebenfalls zu einem vermehrten Abrauchen des Kohlendioxyds und zu einem Abfall der oft extrem hoch angestiegenen Alkalireserve. Diese Therapie ist unter Umständen mit Diamox günstig zu unterstützen. So gelingt es häufig, das Atmungszentrum wieder gegen Kohlendioxyd und das p_H des Blutes zu sensibilisieren. Die Patienten fühlen sich nach einer längeren künstlichen Hyperventilation oft wochenlang wohl.

Bei der Funktionsaustestung der zentralen Atemlähmungen findet sich eine Minderung aller Lungenfunktionswerte. Vitalkapazität und Atemgrenzwert sind oft extrem reduziert, u. U. letzterer bis auf das Atemminutenvolumen. Das Atemvolumen ist klein, die Atemfrequenz meist sehr hoch. Der Atemstoßwert ist regelrecht, da keine stenosierenden Prozesse im Bronchialbaum vorliegen. Das Residualvolumen ist ebenfalls normal, die Mischungszeit entsprechend der schlechten alveolären Ventilation verlängert. Im arteriellen Blut finden sich eine Abnahme der O_2-Sättigung und -Spannung und ein entsprechender Anstieg des CO_2-Gehaltes und der CO_2-Spannung.

Bei den peripher bedingten Formen ist das funktionelle Bild nicht so einheitlich. Bei raumbeengenden Prozessen im Thorax werden ebenfalls die Lungenfunktionswerte und das Ruheatemvolumen zunehmend kleiner. Das Residualvolumen nimmt ab. Bei den Kyphoskoliosen oder bei den Thoraxstarren infolge BECHTEREWscher Krankheit und auch bei ausgedehnten Pleuraverschwartungen kann es zur sekundären Überblähung der Lungen kommen. Entsprechend ist das Residualvolumen vergrößert, die Mischungszeit im Sinne der Blählunge verändert (s. Gruppe c). Die Blutgaswerte sind den Veränderungen bei den zentralen Formen ähnlich. Die Auswirkungen auf den kleinen Kreislauf können im Detail nicht aufgeführt werden (sie werden an anderer Stelle des Handbuchs behandelt).

b) Stenosen der Luftwege.

In diese Gruppe gehören alle stenosierenden Prozesse *distal der Bifurkation der Trachea*, wie Stenosen infolge von Sekretanhäufung in den großen Bronchien, die Bronchustuberkulose, das Bronchialcarcinom und -adenom, Fremdkörper im Bronchialbaum und auch, gewissermaßen als diffuse Stenose (mit Übergang zur nächsten Gruppe c), das Asthma bronchiale und die spastische Bronchitis.

Es ist zweckmäßig, diese Gruppe in lokalisierte und diffuse Stenosen im Bronchialbaum einzuteilen. In die Gruppe der lokalisierten Stenosen gehört die Bronchustuberkulose, das Bronchialcarcinom, das Bronchialadenom usw. Morphologisch kommt es zur isolierten Einengung des Lumens eines einzelnen Bronchus, welche sich bronchoskopisch und bronchographisch nachweisen läßt. Während die Ventilation der übrigen Lunge normal ist, ist die Beatmung des distal von der Bronchostenose liegenden Lungenteils entsprechend der Einengung des Bronchiallumens reduziert. Das Ausmaß der verminderten Ventilation hängt dabei nicht nur von der Einengung des Lumens ab, sondern auch von der Größe des hypoventilierten Lungenbezirks. Auch ein nicht vollständiger Verschluß eines kleineren Bronchus kann den zugehörigen Lungenteil infolge Turbulenzströmung an der Stenosestelle bereits funktionell von der Ventilation ausschalten. Das ist zu berücksichtigen, wenn sich Diskrepanzen zwischen Funktionsaustestung und bronchographischer Darstellung zeigen.

Die Funktionsbefunde ergeben sich aus der Ungleichmäßigkeit der Ventilation beider Lungenpartien. Der distal von der Stenose liegende Lungenteil wird noch beatmet, aber schlechter als die übrige Lunge. Die Vitalkapazität, die ja bei langsamer maximaler In- und Exspiration gemessen wird, ist meist noch normal, während der Atemgrenzwert bereits deutlich reduziert sein kann. Der Atemstoß zeigt eine Abknickung im Kurvenverlauf, die dadurch bedingt ist, daß die normalventilierten Lungenpartien einen regelrechten Atemstoßwert ergeben, während der metastenotische Bezirk nur verlangsamt sein Luftvolumen durch den stenosierten Bronchus pressen kann. Am deutlichsten wird diese Funktionsbeeinflussung, wenn man Vitalkapazität und Atemgrenzwert in Relation zueinander setzt, wie es im *Ventilationsleistungsindex* geschieht[1]. Der VLJ drückt das Verhältnis von Ist-Atemgrenzwert in Prozent des Sollatemgrenzwerts zu Ist-Vitalkapazität in Prozent der Soll-Vitalkapazität aus. Es wird also eine Zeit-Volumengröße (AGW) zu einer durch die Zeit unbeeinflußten Volumengröße (VK) in Beziehung gesetzt. Normalerweise beträgt dieser Wert 1. Je ausgedehnter und ausgeprägter die Stenose ist, um so kleiner wird dieser Wert sein. Bei vollständigem Verschluß des Bronchus wird er sich wieder 1 nähern.

Vor einigen Jahren wurde von Gaensler[1] in den USA ein röntgenologisch nachweisbares Phänomen zur Diagnostik von stenosierenden Bronchusprozessen beschrieben: Das „*Air trapping-Phänomen*". Läßt man einen Gesunden unter

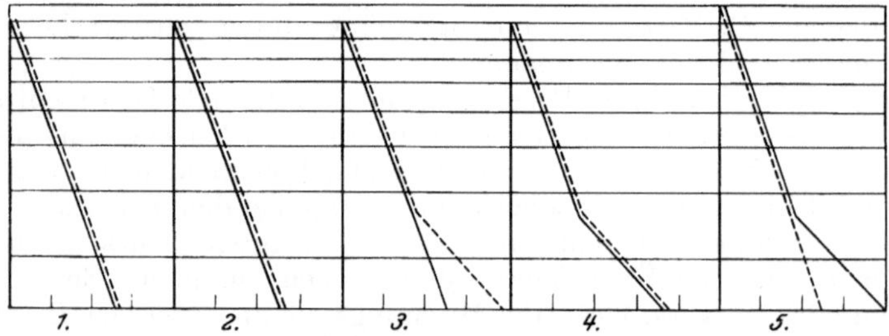

Abb. 24. Die Ermittlung des Verteilungsgradienten aus der Mischungs-, Desaturations- und Resaturationskurve (schematisch). 1. Gesunder. — 2. Rechts-Links-Shunt bei normaler Ventilation. — 3. Perfusion normal, Ventilation unterschiedlich in den einzelnen Lungenpartien. — 4. Perfusion und Ventilation in einzelnen Lungenpartien gleichsinnig unterschiedlich. — 5. Rechts-Links-Shunt bei normaler Ventilation. Die Werte der Beispiele 1—4 sind mit Hilfe der Desaturation, in Beispiel 5 mit der Resaturation gewonnen. Die Kurven sind auf halblogarithmisches Papier aufgetragen, auf der X-Achse die Atemzüge, auf der Y-Achse die Mischvolumina in den Lungen.

Durchleuchtungskontrolle rasch ausatmen, so nimmt entsprechend der Minderung des Luftgehaltes in den Lungen die Durchlässigkeit für Röntgenstrahlen ab. Das heißt, die Lunge wird bei rascher Exspiration gleichmäßig dunkler. Atmet dagegen ein Patient mit einer partiellen Bronchostenose nach maximaler Inspiration forciert aus, so wird — wie bereits beschrieben — im stenosierten Bezirk das Luftvolumen länger zurückgehalten als in der gesunden Lunge. Man findet dann röntgenologisch, daß der stenosierte Bezirk länger hell bleibt als die übrige Lunge. Wir konnten in der Klinik dieses Phänomen mehrfach beobachten.

Durch Bestimmung der Mischungsverhältnisse eines Fremdgases in den Lungen ist es möglich, einen quantitativen Einblick in die Ventilationsverhältnisse der einzelnen Lungenpartien zu erhalten. Registriert man bei der Bestimmung des Residualvolumens gleichzeitig die *Durchmischung des Fremdgases* (H_2, He) nach der oben beschriebenen Methode, so läßt sich aus der Durchmischungskurve ablesen, ob alle Partien der Lungen gleichmäßig ventiliert worden sind. Bei halblogarithmischer Darstellung der Mischungskurve werden diese Verhältnisse noch viel deutlicher (Abb. 24). Es ist dann meist möglich, quantitative Angaben über die Volumina der verschieden ventilierten Lungenpartien zu machen.

Bei diffusen Bronchostenosen sind die beschriebenen Veränderungen nicht so exakt analysierbar. Funktionell sind diese Krankheitsbilder zweckmäßigerweise in die Gruppe c (Mischstörungen) einzuordnen.

---

[1] Gaensler 1950, Lechtenbörger, Valentin und Venrath 1951.

c) Mischstörungen in den Lungen.

Zu den Mischstörungen gehören, wie bereits oben gesagt, das unter b aufgeführte Asthma bronchiale, namentlich im schweren asthmatischen Anfall, dann aber als der Hauptvertreter der respiratorischen Insuffizienz schlechthin das *Lungenemphysem* in den verschiedenen Formen. Auch beim Emphysem können lokal stenosierende Faktoren eine Rolle spielen.

Pathologisch-anatomisch[1] findet sich beim chronischen substantiellen Emphysem ein Zusammenfließen mehrerer Alveolarsäckchen mit Schwund der die Alveolen voneinander abtrennenden Septen und eine Rarifizierung der elastischen Fasern. Es kommt schließlich zu einer so weitgehenden Zerstörung des Lungengewebes, daß ganze Lobuli zu großen Emphysemblasen (Emphysema bullosum) konfluieren können. Dieser extremen Erweiterung der Alveolarsäckchen gegenüber ändert sich das Lumen der Alveolargänge nicht entsprechend. Die Folge davon ist ein Mißverhältnis von Alveolengröße und -weite des Bronchiolus respiratorius, was im Sinne einer Stenose interpretiert werden kann. Zudem mündet der Bronchus in den ektatischen Alveolarsack nicht mehr zentral, sondern infolge asymmetrischer Überdehnung, oft nahezu tangential, so daß es bei forcierter Ausatmung zu einem Lippenpfeifenphänomen kommen kann. Diese Veränderungen sind meist nicht einheitlich in den Lungen ausgeprägt (Rand- und Spitzenemphysem usw.). Vielfach stellt sich ein Mißverhältnis von Durchblutung und Ventilation ein, da die Rarifizierung der Lungencapillaren den Alveolarwandveränderungen nicht immer parallel geht. Dadurch geht die sonst in allen Lungenpartien weitgehend konstante Relation: Durchblutung zu Ventilation verloren. Es kommt zu *Störungen im Verteilungsgradienten.*

Diese unterschiedliche Ventilation und Perfusion der einzelnen Lungenpartien (Störungen des Verteilungsgradienten) läßt sich summarisch erfassen. Methodisch beruht dieses Verfahren auf der *gleichzeitigen* Bestimmung der Mischkurve in den Lungen mittels Fremdgasen und der oxymetrischen Registrierung von Auf- oder Absättigungskurven im arteriellen Blut. Die *Desaturationskurve* erhält man, wenn der Patient nach Atmen von Außenluft auf ein Sauerstoffmangelgemisch von 12—14 Vol.-% O_2 umgeschaltet wird, die *Resaturationskurve*, wenn er primär ein Sauerstoffmangelgemisch von 12—14 Vol.-% atmet und anschließend auf Luftatmung umgeschaltet wird. Die Sauerstoffsättigung wird — wie oben bereits gesagt — kontinuierlich oxymetrisch registriert. Man erhält auf diese Weise 2 Kurven, die sich bei halblogarithmischer Darstellung normalerweise mit den *Mischungskurven* in den Lungen decken. Die gleichzeitige Bestimmung von Mischkurven in den Lungen und Debzw. Resaturationskurven im arteriellen Blut erscheint uns deshalb besonders zweckmäßig, da unregelmäßiges Atmen sich auf beide Werte gleichsinnig auswirkt und somit eine häufig nur approximativ mögliche Korrektur vermieden werden kann. Korrekturen sind aber notwendig, wenn beide Kurven in verschiedenen Untersuchungsgängen gewonnen wurden, da die Ventilation nicht immer gleich ist. Abweichungen der Sauerstoffauf- oder absättigungskurve von der Mischkurve sprechen für ungleichmäßige Ventilation oder Perfusion. Beim Gesunden fallen Mischkurve und Sauerstoffsättigungskurve zusammen, da Mischung, Aufbzw. Absättigung annähernd vergleichbare Vorgänge sind.

Während die Fremdgasmischkurve das rein ventilatorische Bild der Gasverteilung in den Lungen — unabhängig von ihrer Durchblutung — wiedergibt, zeigt das oxymetrische Diagramm bei der Desaturation das Bild der ventilatorischen Durchmischung ausschließlich in den durchbluteten Lungenbezirken. Letztlich kann das arterielle Blut nur Sättigungsänderungen widerspiegeln, die in den durchbluteten Lungenteilen stattfinden. Der Verlauf der Desaturationskurve wird außerdem von der mengenmäßigen Verteilung des Blutes in den differierend ventilierten Lungenteilen beeinflußt. Wir fanden in unseren Untersuchungen folgende Verlaufsmöglichkeiten beider Kurven:

1. Mischungs- und Desaturationskurve sind bei gleichmäßiger Ventilation und Durchblutung kongruent.

2. Ist die Ventilation gleichmäßig und ausreichend und die Durchblutung ungleichmäßig (auch bei Shuntdurchblutung), so verlaufen beide Kurven wie beim Gesunden.

3. Werden schlecht ventilierte Lungenpartien nicht durchblutet, passiert das gesamte Herzminutenvolumen gut ventilierte Alveolen, so verläuft die Fremdgasmischkurve geknickt, während die Desaturationskurve normal ist.

4. Ist die Ventilation eines Lungenteiles reduziert, bei regelrechter Durchblutung, so verlaufen Fremdgasmischkurve und Desaturationskurve beide kongruent geknickt.

Die Resaturationskurven erlauben daneben einen Einblick in Kurzschlußverbindungen im Herzen oder in der Lunge, gleichgültig welchen Umfanges sie sind. Sind die Ventilations- und Durchblutungsverhältnisse in den Lungen normal, besteht aber ein Rechts-Links-Shunt,

---

[1] BEITZKE 1928.

so verläuft die Fremdgasmischkurve normal, die Resaturationskurve dagegen geknickt. Die Resaturationszeit ist verlängert (s. Abb. 24).

Die funktionellen Veränderungen, welche man beim Lungenemphysem findet, erklären sich aus den pathologisch-anatomischen Gegebenheiten. Entsprechend der Schwere der Veränderungen sind die Atemreserven vermindert (infolge Abnahme des Atemgrenzwertes), der Atemstoßwert ist oft extrem eingeschränkt, während das Residualvolumen eine entsprechende Zunahme zeigt und die Mischungszeit in den Lungen verlängert ist. Die Vitalkapazität kann noch lange Zeit normal oder wenigstens weitgehend normal sein. Hat der Emphysematiker Zeit genug, langsam seine überblähten Alveolen leer zu atmen, so kann noch eine normale Vitalkapazität resultieren. — Die ungleichmäßige Ventilation der verschiedenen Lungenpartien zeigt sich am deutlichsten bei halblogarithmischer Darstellung der Mischungskurve. Es finden sich oft 2—3 Knickungen in der Kurve, welche anzeigen, daß 2 oder 3 unterschiedlich ventilierte Lungengebiete vorliegen. Im arteriellen Blut spiegelt sich die ungenügende alveoläre Durchmischung in Form einer O_2-Untersättigung und CO_2-Überladung wider.

Ganz im Vordergrund stehen also beim substantiellen Emphysem *Ventilationsstörungen*. Zu *echten Diffusionsstörungen in den Lungen kommt es beim reinen Emphysem nicht*, da der Diffusionsweg in der intakten Capillare morphologisch nicht verändert ist. Die *Kontaktzeit* des Blutes in den Lungencapillaren mit der Alveolarluft kann abnehmen, da infolge der Rarifizierungserscheinungen am Lungencapillarbett die Durchströmung des Blutes in den restierenden Capillaren beschleunigt sein kann. Diese Veränderungen lassen sich aber nicht zwanglos als „Diffusionsstörung" interpretieren, sondern sind besser als „Perfusions- oder Kontaktstörungen" zu bezeichnen.

Die Leistungsfähigkeit dieser Patienten hängt weitgehend von der Schwere der Veränderungen und den sekundären Erscheinungen am Herzen (Cor pulmonale usw.) ab.

d) Vergrößerung des funktionellen Totraums der Luftwege.

Es handelt sich um relativ seltene Krankheitsbilder mit großen ventilierten, aber nicht oder kaum durchbluteten Cysten, wie die angeborene Cystenlunge, ausgedehnte Bronchiektasen, multiple Embolisierung in den Lungen, wodurch normal ventilierte Lungenpartien von der Durchblutung ausgeschaltet werden. Diese Gruppe weist eine Vergrößerung der Luftquote auf, die bei jedem Atemzug nicht mit dem Blut in Gasaustausch tritt, d. h. unausgenutzt verlorengeht. Spirographisch findet man eine vergrößerte Ruhe- und Arbeitsatmung mit entsprechend großem Atemäquivalent[1]. Eine Vergrößerung des funktionellen Totraumes ist für den Gesunden eine Frage der Atemökonomie, für den Atmungsinsuffizienten ist seine Größe aber unter Umständen von vitaler Bedeutung. Der Gesunde ist ohne weiteres in der Lage, seinen schädlichen Raum — auch bei künstlicher Vergrößerung in bestimmten Grenzen — zu überatmen. Wird aber das Atemvolumen durch Elastizitätsverlust der Lungen, Starre des Thorax, Parese der Atemmuskulatur usw. verkleinert, so ist der Kranke schließlich nicht mehr in der Lage, seinen Totraum — auch wenn er nicht vergrößert ist — zu hyperventilieren. Es bietet sich das Zustandsbild, wie es bereits in Gruppe a beschrieben worden ist. Die Therapie richtet sich nach der Ursache der Störung.

e) Pendelatmung.

Die Pendelatmung wurde erstmals von Brauer[2] und Mitarbeitern unmittelbar nach Thorakoplastik beobachtet und in ihrem Funktionsmechanismus geklärt.

---

[1] Knipping und Moncrieff 1932, Anthony 1937.   [2] Brauer 1932.

Sie beruht darauf, daß während der Exspiration bei beweglichem Mediastinum ein Teil des Atemvolumens in die kontralaterale, funktionell gestörte Lunge entweicht und inspiratorisch in die gesunde Lunge zurückventiliert wird. Auch beim Pneumothorax — namentlich beim offenen Pneumothorax — oder nach der ersten Pneuanlage wird vielfach eine leichte Cyanose beobachtet, die auf Pendelatmung zurückzuführen ist. Sie hört sofort auf, wenn man jede Lunge getrennt atmen läßt, z. B. bei der Bronchospirographie. Auch die Cyanose verschwindet, wenn sie auf Pendelatmung beruhte.

Die Lungenfunktionswerte sind entsprechend reduziert. Im arteriellen Blut findet man eine verminderte Sauerstoffsättigung bei erhöhter CO_2-Spannung.

2. Perfusionsstörungen (vasculärer Kurzschluß).

Fließt venöses Blut unarterialisiert zum Lungencapillarblut, so spricht man von einem „vasculären Kurzschluß". Dieser Befund ist nicht immer als pathologisch zu bewerten, da auch beim Gesunden etwa 3—5% des Herzminutenvolumens in den Lungen kurzgeschlossen fließen. Der „physiologische Shunt" kommt über folgende Gefäßverbindungen zustande:

a) Als Shuntverbindung von der A. pulmonalis über Capillaren nicht beatmeter Alveolen[1] zur V. pulmonalis.
b) Durch Zumischung venösen Blutes der Vv. bronchiales zu den Vv. pulmonales.
c) Über die Thebesischen Venen zum linken Herzen.

Jede Zumischung venösen Blutes zum Lungencapillarblut wirkt sich in Form eines arteriellen Sättigungs- und Spannungsabfalles für Sauerstoff und in einer Erhöhung des CO_2-Gehaltes und der CO_2-Spannung aus und ist die Ursache dafür, daß das arterielle Blut nicht 100%ig mit Sauerstoff gesättigt ist und die arterielle PO_2 nicht mit derjenigen der Alveolarluft identisch ist.

Der physiologische Shunt spielt in der Klinik keine Rolle. Inwieweit er eine funktionelle Bedeutung besitzt, ist nicht bekannt. Lediglich bei der Bestimmung des Diffusionsgradienten wirkt er sich störend aus (s. S. 349).

Für die Klinik wird der venöse Kurzschluß erst dann von Interesse, wenn er einen größeren Umfang annimmt, z. B. bei intrapulmonalen arterio-venösen Aneurysmen[2], (wie bei Morbus Osler), bei Durchblutung von Lungenteilen, welche nicht beatmet werden, oder bei intrakardialen Rechts-Links-Shunts. (Auf die intrakardialen Shuntverbindungen soll hier nicht eingegangen werden, da sie in den entsprechenden Kreislaufkapiteln behandelt werden.) Das quantitative Ausmaß der Shuntzumischung, welches sich klinisch als Cyanose verschiedenen Schweregrades zeigt, läßt sich *nur aus dem arteriellen Blut nachweisen*, bei gleichzeitiger Kenntnis der Gaszusammensetzung des venösen Mischblutes und der Größe des Herzminutenvolumens. Die Gasanalyse des arteriellen Blutes allein genügt nicht und gibt uns auch keinen Maßstab für die Leistungsfähigkeit der Patienten[3].

Das geht aus dem Folgenden hervor.

Globaler Sauerstoffmangel, wie wir ihn z. B. beim Aufstieg in große Höhen, bei zentral oder peripher ausgelöster Hyperventilation, bei exzessiver Vergrößerung des Totraumes der Atemwege usw. finden, führt zu einer Senkung der arteriellen Sauerstoffsättigung und Spannung. Sind Diffusionsstörungen in den Lungen ausgeschlossen, so gehen alveoläre und arterielle Sauerstoffspannung weitgehend parallel. Unterschreitet die arterielle Sauerstoffsättigung die Reaktionsschwelle des Kreislaufzentrums, so steigt das Herzminutenvolumen an und verhindert dadurch eine zu tiefe Ausschöpfung des venösen Blutes, ohne

---

[1] GIESE 1961 (dieses Handbuch).
[2] Siehe DIENEMANN 1955.   [3] MILLER, FOWLER und HELMHOLZ 1953.

allerdings die arteriellen Blutgaswerte zu beeinflussen. Letztere sind in den vorliegenden Fällen allein von den Gasverhältnissen im Alveolarraum abhängig und erfahren durch Herzminutenvolumensteigerung keine Besserung.

Bei *partiellem Sauerstoffmangel* oder bei Kurzschlußverbindungen in den Lungen liegen die Verhältnisse dagegen grundsätzlich anders. Die kompensatorische Herzminutenvolumenzunahme bewirkt bei diesen Zustandsbildern (partielle Ventilations- oder Diffusionsstörungen, alle Rechts-Links-Shunts oder arterio-venöse Anastomosen in den Lungen) nicht nur eine Minderung der venösen Ausschöpfung des Blutes, sondern darüber hinaus eine eindeutig nachweisbare Zunahme der arteriellen Sauerstoffsättigung und -Spannung. Daher ist es notwendig, um etwas Quantitatives über das Ausmaß einer venösen Zumischung zu sagen, die venöse Ausschöpfung zu kennen und die Größe des Herzminutenvolumens[1].

Mit Hilfe der selektiven Angiographie der Lungengefäße[2] (s. S. 355) bei gleichzeitig durchgeführten Blutgasuntersuchungen haben wir gefunden, daß intrapulmonale vasculäre Kurzschlüsse bei chronischen Lungenerkrankungen nicht die Rolle spielen, die ihnen oft in der Literatur zugemessen wird. Bei akuten Lungenerkrankungen ist die Bedeutung des vasculären Kurzschlusses ebenfalls überschätzt worden. Die selektive Angiographie der Lungengefäße ergab eindeutig, daß bei regionaler Reduktion der Beatmung, ähnlich wie beim Gesunden, ebenfalls die Durchblutung mehr oder weniger stark vermindert ist.

Spirographisch finden wir bei größeren Rechts-Links-Shunts gleich welcher Ätiologie eine Erhöhung des Atemminutenvolumens bei Verminderung der alveolären CO_2-Spannung gegenüber der arteriellen und — das ist wichtig — keinen Beruhigungseffekt von Sauerstoffatmung auf das vergrößerte Atemminutenvolumen. Entsprechend ist das Atemäquivalent groß und ändert sich unter Sauerstoffatmung nicht[3].

3. Diffusionsstörungen.

Die *Diffusion der Gase* von der Alveolarluft ins Blut und umgekehrt gehorcht — soweit heute bekannt — physikalischen Gesetzen. Der Austausch erfolgt im allgemeinen so vollständig, daß Spannungsdifferenzen von Sauerstoff und CO_2 zwischen Alveolarluft und Capillarblut unter Normalbedingungen nicht nachweisbar sind. Erst bei einer Verlängerung des Diffusionsweges (Verdickung der Alveolarwand, Ödem usw.) zeigen sich Störungen im Spannungsausgleich für Sauerstoff als eine oft deutlich meßbare O_2-Spannungsdifferenz zwischen Lungencapillarblut und Alveolarluft.

In der Hamburger Medizinischen Klinik hat Brauer in den 20er Jahren den Begriff der *Pneumonose* konzipiert. Er deutete die tiefe Cyanose schwerster Grippeformen bei einer Epidemie als Diffusionsstörung. In der Folge wurde auf breiterer Basis die Frage der Diffusion in den Lungen überprüft[4]. Wenn auch schwere Diffusionsstörungen verhältnismäßig selten vorkommen und innerhalb der Formen der respiratorischen Insuffizienz nur einen geringen Anteil an den arteriellen Cyanosen haben, so muß doch an der Brauerschen Konzeption der Pneumonose festgehalten werden[5].

Der Ätiologie nach können wir die Diffusionsstörungen in 2 Gruppen trennen:

1. Die primär pulmonal bedingten Fibrosen,

2. die (primär kardial bedingten) Lungenveränderungen infolge akuter oder chronischer Lungenstauung.

Die Gruppe der primären Lungenfibrosen umfaßt den diffusen Lungen-Boeck, die Sklerodermie mit Lungenbeteiligung, Zustände nach miliarer Metastasierung von malignen Tumoren (Teratomen, Sarkomen, Carcinomen), die Berylliumlunge, die Asbestose der Lungen, Lungen-

[1] Venrath, Lechtenbörger, Valentin und Bolt 1955.   [2] Bolt 1953.
[3] Landen 1954.   [4] Knipping 1933.   [5] Knipping 1935, Schoen und Derra 1930.

schädigungen nach Phosgen- oder SO_2-Inhalation, Zustandsbilder nach ausgeheilter Miliar-tuberkulose u. a. Die Schwere der Diffusionsstörungen geht dem Ausmaß der Veränderungen parallel.

Ähnliche Befunde sind bei den primär kardial bedingten Lungenfibrosen (den Stauungslungen) zu erheben. Die funktionellen Veränderungen sind am verständlichsten, wenn man sich das pathologisch-anatomische Bild kurz vor Augen führt.

Die Stauungslunge zeigt histologisch eine Erweiterung und Schlängelung der Capillaren mit Verdickung ihrer Wandung, namentlich des Grundhäutchens und eine Zunahme des

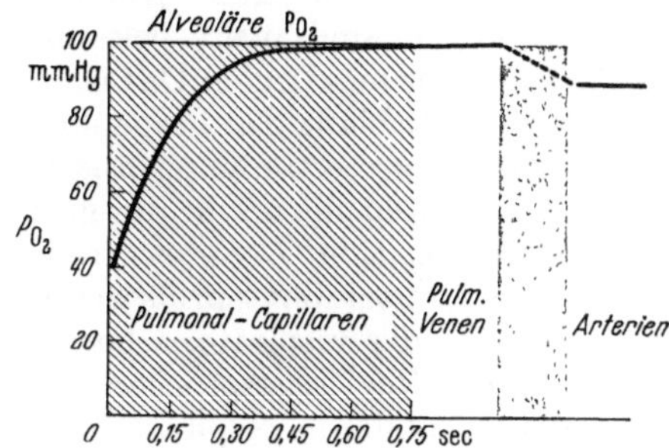

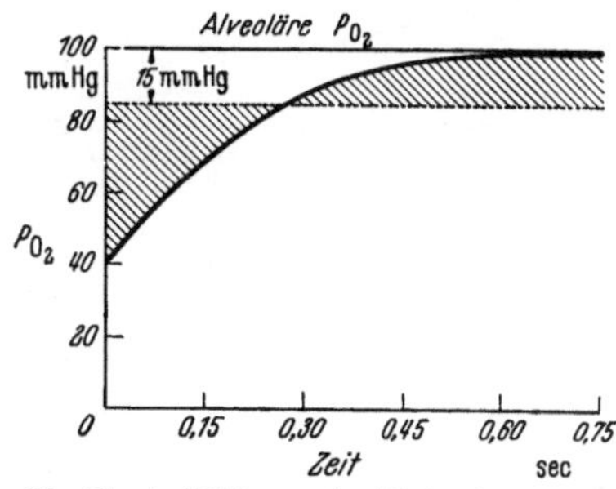

Abb. 26. Die Aufsättigung des Blutes in den Lungen-capillaren bei Außenluftatmung ($= 20{,}9$ Vol.-% O_2). Die Kontaktzeit reicht bei der hohen Sauerstoff-spannung in der Alveolarluft für einen vollständigen Spannungsausgleich aus. (Nach COMORE).

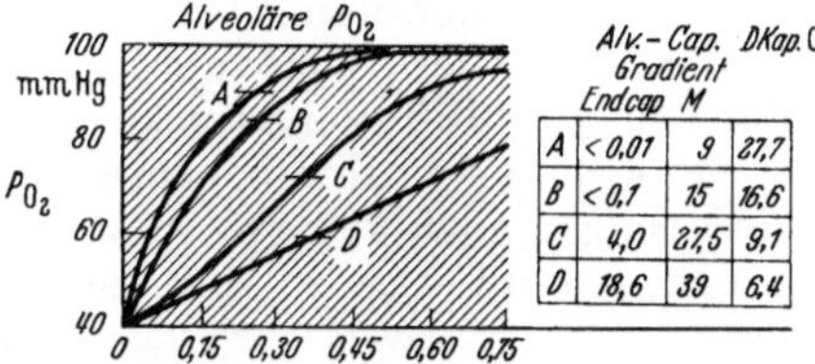

Abb. 25. Die Aufsättigung des Lungencapillarblutes mit Sauerstoff in Abhängigkeit von der Diffusions-kapazität des Sauerstoffes in der Lunge (oberer Teil = Normalverhältnisse). — Die alveoläre Sauerstoff-spannung beträgt jeweils 100 mm Hg, der Endcapillar-druck 99,99; 99,9; 96 bzw. 81,4 mm Hg entsprechend den Zustandsbildern A, B, C und D. Obgleich der end-capilläre Sauerstoffdruck bei A und B nicht bestimm-bar ist, läßt er sich doch annäherungsweise berechnen (s. Text). Die Sättigung des Blutes am Ende der Capillare ist bei A, B und C normal bzw. weitgehend normal, obwohl die Diffusionskapazität unterschiedlich ist. Nur in D ist die Sättigung des Blutes reduziert und zeigt bereits deutlich die Diffusionserschwerung an. Wird aber die Kontaktzeit des Blutes mit der Alveolarluft kürzer, z. B. unter Belastung, so wird auch in B und C eine arterielle Sauerstoffuntersättigung nachweisbar. (Nach COMORE u. a.)

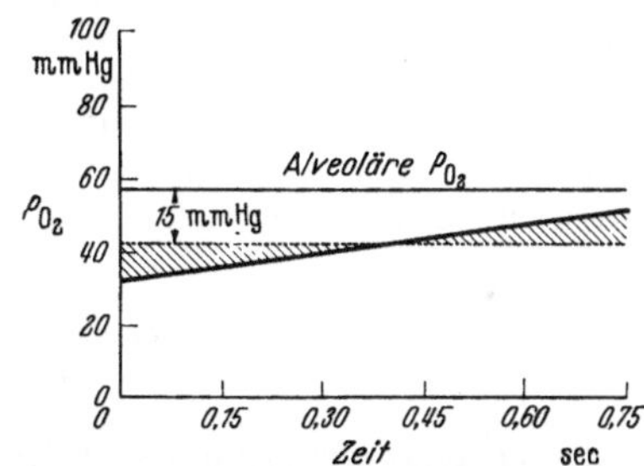

Abb. 27. Bei Sauerstoffmangelatmung (12 % O_2 in N_2) ist die Anfangsspannung des Sauerstoffs in der Alveolar-luft bedeutend niedriger, entsprechend langsamer erfolgt der Gasaustausch. Obgleich der mittlere alveolocapilläre Spannungsgradient der gleiche ist wie bei Luftatmung (s. oben), erfolgt kein vollständiger Spannungsausgleich zwischen Alveolarluft und Lungen-capillarblut. Am Ende der Capillare ist noch eine deutliche Spannungs- und Sättigungsdifferenz nach-weisbar. Die Kontaktzeit in der Lunge ist die gleiche wie in obiger Darstellung. (Nach COMORE.)

interstitiellen Bindegewebes mit ödematöser Durchtränkung entsprechend dem Schwere-grad der Stauung[1]. Dadurch werden das Grundhäutchen der Capillaren und die Basal-membran der Alveolen voneinander abgedrängt. Der Diffusionsweg des Sauerstoffs von der Alveole ins Blut wird länger.

Während zunächst die Kontaktzeit in den Lungen noch ausreicht, um eine vollständige Sättigung des Blutes während des Durchflusses durch die Capillaren zu garantieren, genügt sie schließlich trotz wahrscheinlicher Verlängerung gegenüber der Norm nicht mehr. Die Ursache ist ein Anstieg des Membrangradienten, die Folge eine der Veränderung parallel gehende zunehmende Sauerstoffuntersättigung.

Auch bei Patienten mit vergrößertem Lungendurchfluß infolge kongenitaler Mißbildungen am Herzen und an den Gefäßen (Ductus arteriosus Botalli, Morbus Roger, Vorhof- und Ventrikelseptumdefekt u. a.) fanden wir eine Erschwerung der Diffusion gegenüber der

---

[1] Zu JEDDELOH 1931, PARKER und WEISS 1936.

Norm, wenn es infolge des lang dauernden erhöhten Lungendurchflusses zu vorzeitigen Aufbraucherscheinungen an den Lungencapillaren gekommen war. Letzteres hängt weitgehend von der Größe des Shuntvolumens ab. Die Veränderungen an den Lungenarterien sind für die Diffusion von sekundärer Bedeutung. Pulmonalsklerosen können z. B. normale Diffusionsverhältnisse aufweisen.

Geht man über die Bestimmung des Membrangradienten in Ruhe hinaus und ermittelt ihn unter Belastung, so findet man, daß die maximale Diffusionskapazität in den Lungen (s. S. 349, 350) bereits jenseits des 25. Lebensjahres langsam abzufallen beginnt[1]. Morphologische Veränderungen, welche diese Abnahme erklären können, sind nicht bekannt[2]. Die Abnahme der maximalen Diffusionskapazität im Alter läßt den Fragenkomplex der Diffusionsbestimmung aus der Welt der Raritäten hinaus in die große summarische Position: *Geriatrie* treten. Während das Altersemphysem als wesentlichste Ursache der respiratorischen Insuffizienz im Alter angesprochen wird (neben den sekundären respiratorischen Insuffizienzen infolge alter Linksfehler des Herzens), stellt die Abnahme der maximalen Diffusionskapazität infolge von Alters-Ab- oder -Umbauprozessen im Bereiche der Diffusionsstrecke eine bisher vernachlässigte Komponente dar.

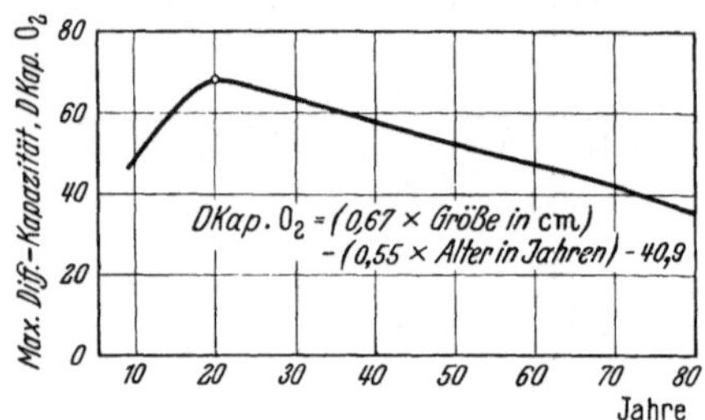

Abb. 28. Die maximale Diffusionskapazität während des Lebens. Mit dem Alter nimmt sie deutlich ab. Sie errechnet sich nach der Rileyschen Formel: DKapO₂ = 0,67 × Größe in cm − 0,55 × Alter i. J. − 40,9. Es liegen bereits in den Ausgangswerten der maximalen Diffusionskapazität starke individuelle Unterschiede vor, und auch im Alter sind die Änderungen stark unterschiedlich, wie ja der Altersprozeß überhaupt individuell verläuft. Es ist möglich, daß sich die Veränderungen an den Lungencapillaren ähnlich entwickeln wie die an anderen Organen.

Wenn die dadurch bedingten Funktionsminderungen auch keine so schweren Ausmaße erreichen werden, daß Ruheinsuffizienzen resultieren, so sind sie für Arbeitsinsuffizienzen sicherlich von Bedeutung.

VI. Klinische Beispiele.
1. Emphysem.

Auf eine Klassifizierung des Emphysems nach seiner Pathogenese und seinen pathologisch-anatomischen Charakteristika sei hier verzichtet. Es wird auf das entsprechende pathologisch-anatomische Kapitel in diesem Handbuch verwiesen.

Zum funktionellen Bild des Emphysems mag vorweg folgendes bemerkt werden: Die hohen Grade von respiratorischer Ruhe- oder Arbeitsinsuffizienz bei alten Leuten sind oft nur zum Teil durch das Emphysem selbst bedingt. Große funktionelle Einbußen sind auf das Konto eines starren Thorax, eines Trainingsverlustes und unter Umständen einer Atrophie der Atemmuskulatur zu setzen.

Beim Emphysem sind die Störungen des Verhältnisses von alveolärer Belüftung zu alveolärer Durchblutung komplexer Natur. Der Effekt der funktionellen Störungen kann Modifikationen erfahren, je nachdem *die Totraumvergrößerung, die Stenose der Luftwege* oder *die Drosselung der Durchblutung* der Capillaren als Störungsmechanismen mehr im Vordergrund stehen. Im Prinzip werden sich beim Emphysem alle drei genannten Mechanismen nachweisen lassen (vgl. die schematische Übersicht über die pathologischen Variationen der alveolären und capillären Sauerstoffspannung Abb. 25—27). In ausgeprägten Fällen findet man eine Kombination der funktionellen Folgen einer alveolären Hypoventilation und eines Capillarschwundes. Bei der resultierenden Hypertonie

---

[1] Lilienthal 1931, Riley 1946, Krogh 1915 u. a.
[2] Goebel (persönliche Mitteilung) 1956.

im arteriellen Schenkel des Lungenkreislaufs ergibt sich nach dem Strömungsgesetz des Kreislaufs von WEZLER-SINN und — im Bereich höherer Drucke — nach dem Poiseuilleschen Gesetz eine Strömungsbeschleunigung in den noch verbliebenen Lungencapillaren und damit eine verringerte Kontaktzeit zwischen Blut und Alveolargasen. In fortgeschrittenen Stadien des Emphysems können so die blutgasanalytischen Befunde dieser Perfusionsstörung denen ähneln, die bei echten Membrandiffusionsstörungen (z. B. bei der Pneumonose BRAUERs) zu finden sind (vgl. schematische Abb. 25).

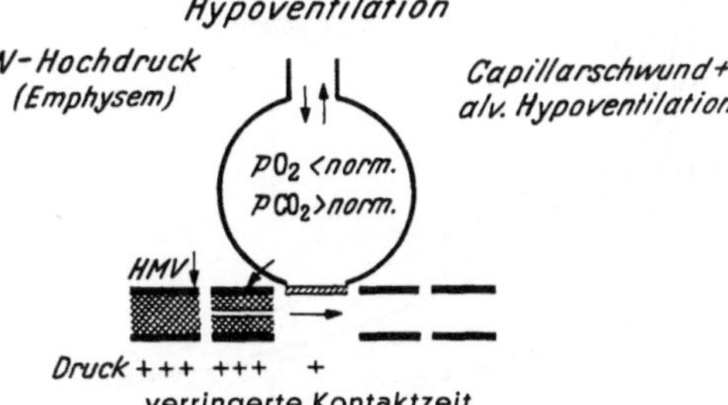

Abb. 29. Schematische Darstellung der ursächlichen Faktoren des Widerstandshochdrucks beim Emphysem (Capillarschwund + alveoläre Hypoventilation).

Funktionelle Klassifizierung des Emphysems.

Da eine Einteilung des Emphysems in Schweregrade etwa nur nach dem röntgenologischen Befund meist unzulänglich ist, wurden zur Charakterisierung des Umfanges der Störungen funktionelle Kriterien herangezogen.

BALDWIN, COURNAND und RICHARDS[1] geben eine *funktionelle Einteilung des Emphysems* in 4 Gruppen. Danach lassen sich folgende Kriterien nach Belastung herausstellen:

Gruppe 1. Arterielle Sauerstoffsättigung über 92,0% nach einer leichten Belastung in Form des standard exercise test. Keine Retention bei der CO_2-Ausscheidung. Es besteht eine Ventilationsstörung im Sinne einer leistungsbegrenzenden Verkleinerung der Atemreserven, die zu einer respiratorischen Arbeitsinsuffizienz mit dem Symptom der Dyspnoe führt.

Gruppe 2. Arterielle Sauerstoffsättigung unter 92,0% nach Belastung, arterielle Kohlendioxydspannung unter 48 mm Hg.

Gruppe 3. Arterielle Sauerstoffsättigung unter 92,0%, arterielle Kohlendioxydspannung über 48 mm Hg.

In Gruppe 2 und 3 ist die Einschränkung der ventilatorischen Funktion ausgesprochener als in Gruppe 1.

Gruppe 4. Zusätzlich zur respiratorischen Insuffizienz besteht eine kardiale Rechtsinsuffizienz. Das Ausmaß der ventilatorischen und alveolo-respiratorischen Insuffizienz ist bei großen Variationen ähnlich der bei Gruppe 2 und 3. Infolge Abstumpfung der cerebralen Zentren findet sich in dieser Gruppe oft keine sonst übliche Hyperventilation. Dieses Syndrom wurde zuerst von KNIPPING-LEWIS-MONCRIEFF[2] und KNIPPING beschrieben. Bei solchen Patienten kann das Ausmaß der Acidose und der Hypoxämie erheblich sein.

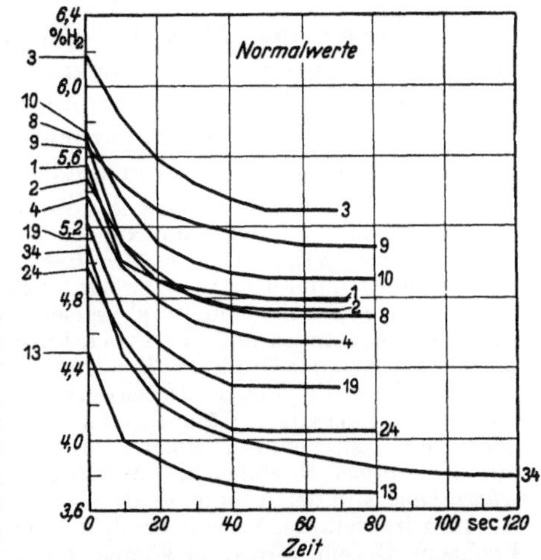

Abb. 30. Mischungszeiten bei Gesunden. Das Ende der Mischungszeit ist erreicht, sobald die Mischungskurve parallel der Zeitachse verläuft.

Diese Klassifizierung setzt einen erheblichen methodischen Aufwand voraus. Für die Routinepraxis kann folgende, einfachere, auf der Bestimmung des Residualvolumens basierende Einteilung empfohlen werden[3].

Normal: . . . . Residualvolumen = bis 25% der Totalkapazität
Gruppe 1: Leichtes Emphysem . . . . . Residualvolumen = 25—35% der Totalkapazität
Gruppe 2: Mittelgradiges Emphysem . . Residualvolumen = 35—45% der Totalkapazität
Gruppe 3: Fortgeschrittenes Emphysem . Residualvolumen = 45—55% der Totalkapazität
Gruppe 4: Schweres Emphysem . . . . Residualvolumen = über 55% der Totalkapazität

---

[1] BALDWIN, COURNAND und RICHARDS 1949.   [2] KNIPPING, LEWIS und MONCRIEFF 1931.
[3] COURNAND 1941, MOTLEY 1950, BOLT 1953.

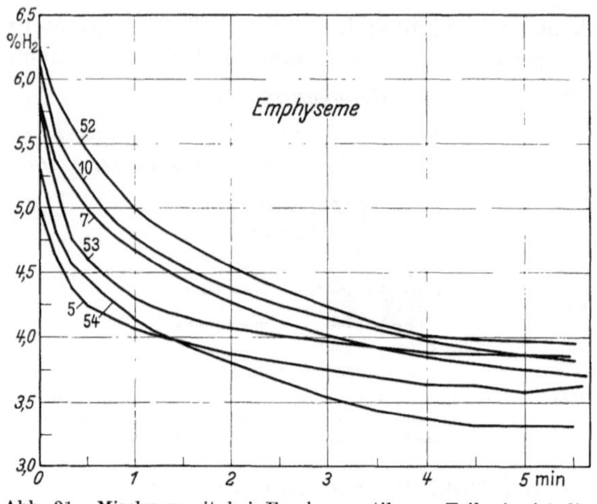

Abb. 31. Mischungszeit bei Emphysematikern. Teilweise ist die Mischungszeit nach 5 min noch nicht abgeschlossen.

Zur praktischen Beurteilung der beim Emphysem bestehenden *Durchmischungsstörung* hat sich die Wasserstoffmethode unter Benutzung der automatisch-registrierenden wärmeelektrischen Meßkammer nach KNIPPING bewährt (s. S. 338). Nach Anschluß an einen Spirographen, in dessen System geringe H_2-Mengen gegeben wurden, zeigt sich beim Emphysematiker die H_2-Mischzeit entsprechend dem Grade des Emphysems gegenüber der Norm verlängert (s. Abb. 30 und 31).

Da die Mischzeitkurven beim Normalen einer e-Funktion entsprechen, ist es zweckmäßig, die Kurven in einem semi-logarithmischen Koordinaten·system als Gerade zur Darstellung zu bringen. Veränderungen der Mischzeit infolge von Emphysem oder Asthma bronchiale sind dann durch Abwinkelung dieser Mischzeitkurven deutlich erkennbar.

a) Lungenkreislauf beim Emphysem.

Die Fragen der *Wechselbeziehungen von Atmung und Kreislauf* sollen am Beispiel des Emphysems besonders hervorgehoben werden; ist doch das Emphysem — sei es primär oder sekundär entstanden — wegen der respiratorischen wie der zirkulatorischen Funktionsminderung in der Klinik der Lungenkrankheiten oft von ernst zu nehmendem Gewicht.

1. Drucke im rechten Herzen und in der A. pulmonalis[1]. Bei leichtem, auch bei mittelgradigem Emphysem liegen die Ruhedruckwerte in der Regel im Rahmen der Norm. Signifikante *Drucksteigerungen im rechten Herzen und in der A. pulmonalis* zeigen sich in diesen Fällen bereits unter leichterer Arbeit. Drucke von 30—60 mm Hg in Ruhe finden sich bei fortgeschrittenen schweren Emphysemen. Während ein Parallelismus zwischen dem Grade des Röntgenbefundes und der Drucksteigerung durchaus nicht immer besteht, ergeben sich jedoch zwischen der Größe des *Residualvolumens* und der Druckerhöhung im kleinen Kreislauf eindeutigere Beziehungen. Druckwerte über 60 mm Hg in Ruhe werden beim Emphysem nur selten beobachtet. Hämodynamisch handelt es sich vorwiegend um einen Widerstandshochdruck, seltener um einen Kombinationshochdruck (Widerstandshochdruck + Herzminutenvolumen-Hochdruck). Auffällig sind beim Emphysem *große respiratorische Druckschwankungen* in der A. pulmonalis.

Tritt im weiteren Verlauf bei dekompensierendem *Cor pulmonale chronicum* eine kardiale Rechtsinsuffizienz hinzu, so können die systolischen Maximaldrucke in der A. pulmonalis und im rechten Ventrikel entsprechend der versagenden vis a tergo eine Abnahme erfahren, die jedoch mit einer signifikanten Druckzunahme im rechten Vorhof und in den großen Körpervenen verbunden ist[2].

Hervorzuheben ist, daß eine Hypertonie der Lungenstrombahn nicht ohne weiteres bei schweren Silikosen und Tuberkulosen anzutreffen ist, sondern daß das *sekundäre Begleitemphysem* als ursächlicher Faktor oft im Vordergrund steht.

2. Herzminutenvolumen. In einem Teil der Fälle von ausgesprochenem Emphysem ist eine *Steigerung des Herzminutenvolumens* nachweisbar[3]. Diese Herzminutenvolumenzunahme läßt sich als eine kompensatorische Maßnahme bei Hypoxämie erklären.

Im *akuten O_2-Mangelversuch* ist mit großer Regelmäßigkeit bei einer arteriellen Sauerstoffsättigung von 82—85% eine Reaktionsschwelle festzustellen, nach deren Überschreiten eine Herzminutenvolumensteigerung nachweisbar ist[4]. Durch diese Herzminutenvolumen-

[1] COURNAND 1950, BOLT 1953.   [2] BOLT 1955.
[3] COURNAND 1950.   [4] OPITZ und SCHNEIDER 1950.

steigerung kommt es bei der akuten experimentellen Hypoxie zu einer Verkleinerung der arteriovenösen Sauerstoffdifferenz und der venösen Ausschöpfung. Unter Sauerstoffatmung normalisieren sich die arterielle Sauerstoffsättigung und das Herzminutenvolumen. Dieser Effekt ist in einem Teil der Fälle auch bei der chronischen Hypoxie des mittelschweren bis fortgeschrittenen Emphysems nachweisbar.

3. Der periphere Gefäßwiderstand der Lungenstrombahn, der analog dem Ohmschen Gesetz nach der Formel $W = Pm/i$ berechnet wird ($Pm =$ mittlerer Blutdruck, $i =$ Herzsekundenvolumen), weist bei den verschiedenen Graden von Emphysem und besonderen Arbeitsbedingungen eine Erhöhung auf, deren Ausmaß einen Schluß auf die Schwere des Emphysems zuläßt.

Die *selektive Angiographie der Lungenstrombahn*[1] zeigt in Fällen von stärker entwickeltem Emphysem mit erhöhtem Lungengefäßwiderstand eine auffallende Engstellung der Segmentäste der A. pulmonalis mit Streckung des Gefäßverlaufs, oft mit deutlicher Rarifizierung der kleineren Verzweigungen im Bereiche der Lungenperipherie (s. Abb. 18).

Die Tierversuche von v. EULER und Mitarbeitern[2] lassen auch für den Menschen eine Selbststeuerung des Verhaltens von Belüftung der Lunge zu deren Durchblutung annehmen in dem Sinne, daß eine Herabsetzung der alveolaren Sauerstoffspannung regulatorisch zu einer Vasoconstriction der Lungenarterien und Arteriolen führt. Diese Engstellung erfolgt nicht reflektorisch, da sie auch an

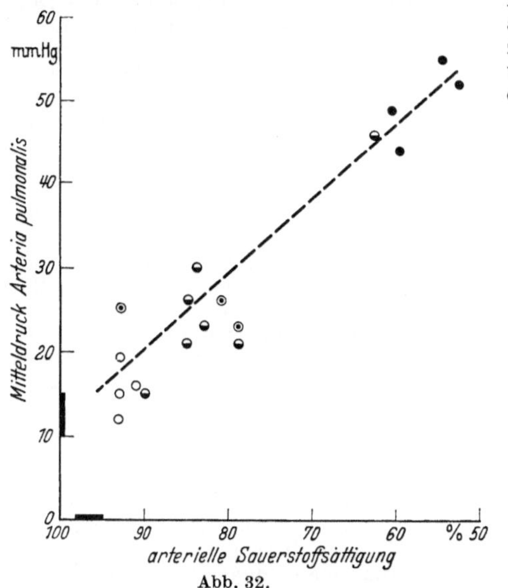

Abb. 32.

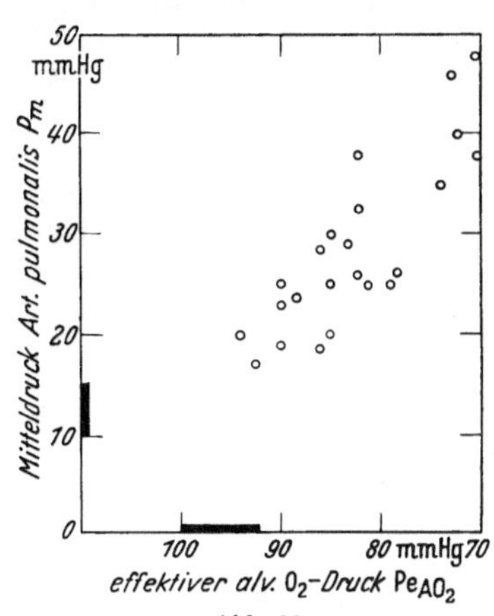

Abb. 33.

Abb. 32 und 33. Darstellung der Abhängigkeit von Mitteldruck in der A. pulmonalis [und arterieller Sauerstoffsättigung nach COURNAND (32) und Mitteldruck in der A. pulmonalis und effektivem alveolärem O_2-Druck nach BÜHLMANN (33).

der denervierten Lunge nachweisbar ist. Beobachtungen von COURNAND über das Verhalten des Druckes in der A. pulmonalis beim Menschen sprechen in gleichem Sinne. Nach BOLT und KNIPPING spielt beim Menschen neben der Hypoxie die *Hyperkapnie* eine ähnliche Rolle.

Eine Erhöhung des Gefäßwiderstandes der Lungenstrombahn und eine Druckerhöhung in der A. pulmonalis bei Lungentuberkulose und Silikose wird nach BOLT und ZORN maßgeblich durch das begleitende Emphysem bedingt.

4. Korrelationen. Betrachtet man auf Grund der Befunde beim Emphysem die wechselseitigen Beziehungen zwischen *arterieller Sauerstoffsättigung, Mitteldruck in der A. pulmonalis, Herzminutenvolumen* und *Blutvolumen* im einzelnen, so lassen sich, wie Arbeiten der Cournand-Gruppe ergaben, folgende Abhängigkeiten herausstellen, die in den wiedergegebenen Diagrammen zum Ausdruck kommen.

Abb. 32 gibt die Abhängigkeit des *Mitteldruckes in der A. pulmonalis von der arteriellen Sauerstoffsättigung* beim chronischen Lungenemphysem wieder.

Die Normalbereiche sind an der Ordinate und an der Abszisse in Form von Balken eingetragen. Bei arteriellen Sauerstoffsättigungen zwischen 60 und 50% können die arteriellen Mitteldrucke bis über 50 mm Hg ansteigen, d. h. die Druckbelastung des rechten Herzens beträgt hierbei das 4—5fache der Norm. BÜHLMANN[3] setzte die arterielle O_2-Spannung und den Mitteldruck in der A. pulmonalis beim Emphysem in Beziehung (Abb. 33). Nach GROSSE-

---

[1] BOLT 1951.   [2] v. EULER und LILJESTRAND 1949.   [3] BÜHLMANN 1954.

Brockhoff[1] und Bolt ist die Frage noch nicht zu entscheiden, ob in der Beziehung zwischen Erhöhung des Mitteldrucks in der A. pulmonalis und Sauerstoffmangel die arterielle O_2-Untersättigung oder die herabgesetzte alveoläre O_2-Spannung als kausal anzusehen ist, oder ob es sich um Ausdrucksformen eines übergeordneten Prinzips handelt.

Die Entscheidung dieser Frage wird insofern noch erschwert, als akute Experimente nicht unbedingt für chronische Zustände beweiskräftig sind. Da ein großer Teil der Patienten mit C. p. eine Hypertension des Lungenkreislaufs ohne O_2-Untersättigung aufweist, wie aus den gezeigten Diagrammen zu entnehmen ist, ist darüber hinaus sicher, daß der organisch bedingten Widerstandserhöhung in der Lungenstrombahn besondere Bedeutung zukommt.

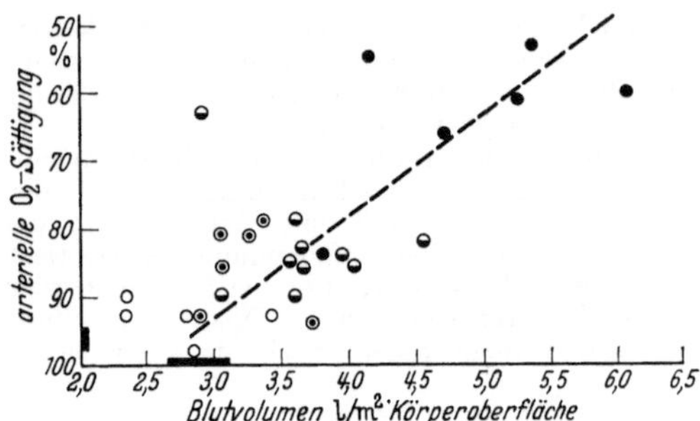
Abb. 34. Abhängigkeit von arterieller O_2-Sättigung und Blutvolumen/m² Körperoberfläche bei Emphysem (Cournand).

Abb. 34 läßt beim chronischen Emphysem zwischen *arterieller Sauerstoffsättigung* und *Blutvolumen* (berechnet auf einen Quadratmeter Körperoberfläche, eine weitgehende lineare Abhängigkeit erkennen. Bei Rückgang der arteriellen Sauerstoffsättigung kann der Anstieg des Blutvolumens das Doppelte des Normalvolumens betragen. Diese *Blutmengenzunahme* ist für die Größe des *Herzminutenvolumens* beim chronischen Emphysem von besonderer Bedeutung, wie aus Abb. 35 hervorgeht. Es besteht eine auffallende Beziehung zwischen dem beim chronischen Emphysem oft erhöht gefundenen Herzminutenvolumen und der Vergrößerung der Blutmenge.

Im allgemeinen sind in *Gruppe 1* der Emphyseme[2], die keine signifikante O_2-Untersättigung erkennen läßt und einen Hämatokrit um 40 besitzt, Herzminutenvolumen und Blutvolumen normal. In der *2. und 3. Gruppe* mit arterieller O_2-Untersättigung und einem mittleren Hämatokrit zwischen 49 und 51 sind sowohl Herzminutenvolumen als auch Blutvolumen erhöht. Schließlich sind in der *4. Gruppe* mit starker arterieller Untersättigung und einem mittleren Hämatokrit von 64 Blutvolumen und Herzminutenvolumen deutlich vergrößert. Es handelt sich bei diesen Zuständen um eine *kardiale Dekompensation mit hohem Herzminutenvolumen*[3], dem high cardiac output failure der angloamerikanischen Autoren[4].

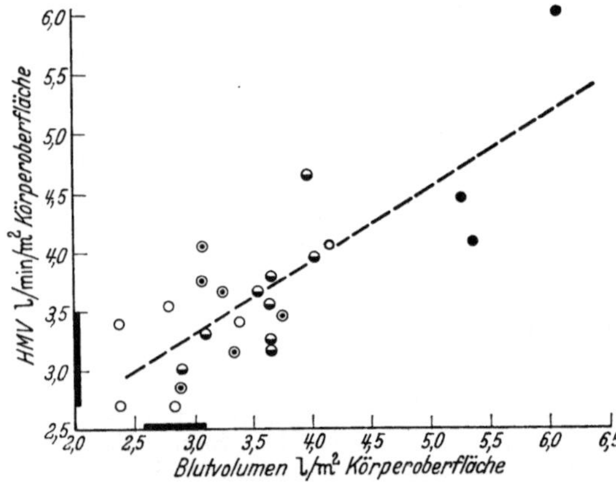
Abb. 35. Abhängigkeit von Herzminutenvolumen und Blutvolumen bei Emphysem.

b) Folgen für das rechte Herz.

Die emphysembedingten hämodynamischen Veränderungen im Bereiche der Lungenstrombahn haben zwangsläufig intensive Rückwirkungen auf das vorgeschaltete rechte Herz im Sinne der Entwicklung eines *Cor pulmonale chronicum* und im Finalstadium als *kardiale Rechtsinsuffizienz*[5].

Die Folgen des Emphysems für die Hämodynamik des kleinen Kreislaufs und des rechten Herzens und die dabei auftretenden maßgeblichen Störungsmechanismen lassen sich in den Schemata (Abb. 36 und 37) zusammenfassen.

---

[1] Grosse-Brockhoff 1952.   [2] Baldwin, Cournand und Richards 1948.
[3] Vgl. F. Meyer 1941.
[4] Richards 1948, McMichael und Sharpey-Schafer 1944.
[5] Ferrer, Harvey, Cathcart, Webster, Richards und Cournand 1950, Bolt, Valentin und Venrath 1950.

c) Folgen für den großen Kreislauf.

Die Hypoxie, besonders die akute, führt, wie RAAB, HEYMANS u. a. tierexperimentell zeigten, und wie aus Untersuchungen bei *Poliomyelitiskranken mit*

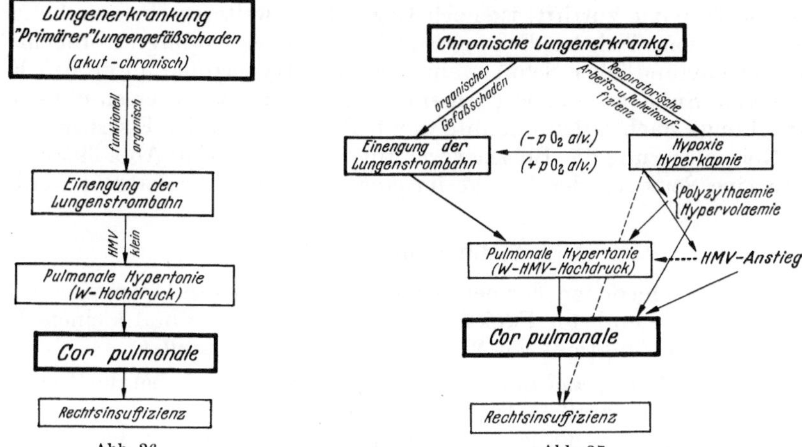

Abb. 36.   Abb. 37.

Abb. 36. Die Entstehung des Cor pulmonale als Folge eines „primären" Lungengefäßschadens (schematische Übersicht).

Abb. 37. Schematische Übersicht über die ursächliche Verknüpfung von Hypoxie, Hyperkapnie, Einengung der Lungenstrombahn und Cor pulmonale.

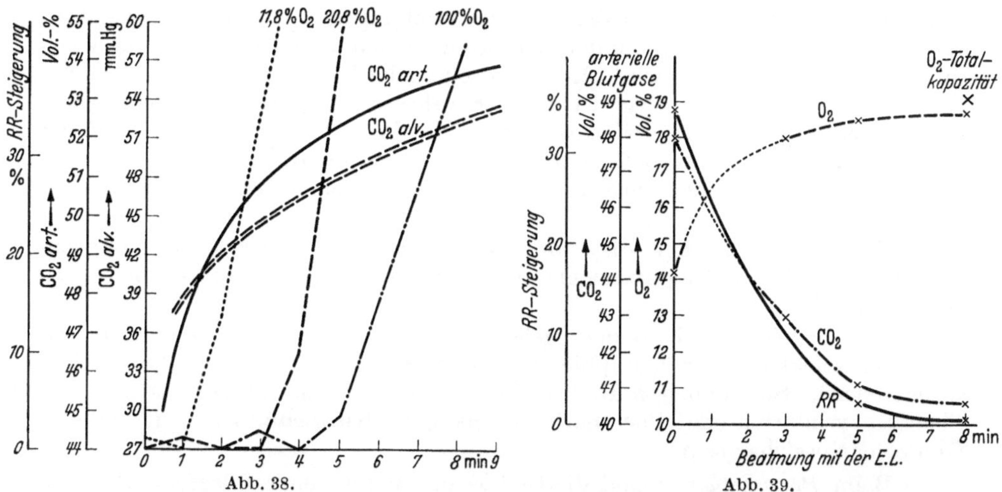

Abb. 38.   Abb. 39.

Abb. 38. Reizschwellenuntersuchungen der Kreislaufzentren durch CO_2-Rückatmung bei Atemmuskellähmung. Konstante künstliche Beatmung in der Eisernen Lunge. Verhalten der Blutdrucksteigerung im CO_2-Rückatmungsversuch bei Sauerstoffmangel (11,8% in der Einatmungsluft), bei normalem O_2-Gehalt der Atemluft (20,8%) und bei Sauerstoffatmung. [Einzelheiten: s. BOLT-VALENTIN-VENRATH, Dtsch. Arch. klin. Med. **198**, 474 (1951).]

Abb. 39. Subchronische Hypoxie und Hyperkapnie (Atemmuskellähmung bei Poliomyelitis). Verhalten des Blutdrucks im großen Kreislauf und der arteriellen Blutgaswerte vor und nach Beginn einer richtig dosierten künstlichen Beatmung mit der Eisernen Lunge. Mit der Regularisierung der arteriellen CO_2- und O_2-Werte tritt eine Normalisierung des vorher erhöhten arteriellen Blutdrucks ein. (Vgl. BOLT-VALENTIN-VENRATH: Die Medizinische **1953**, Nr. 5.)

Atemmuskellähmung[1] hervorgeht, über die Chemoreceptoren zu einem zusätzlichen Antrieb der Atem- und Kreislaufzentren (neben der Kohlensäure) und in

---

[1] BOLT, VALENTIN und VENRATH 1951.

deren Gefolge zu einer *Blutdrucksteigerung im großen Kreislauf* (Abb. 38). Befunde bei Poliomyelitiskranken zeigen, daß der Entstehungsmechanismus des Hochdrucks durch Sauerstoffmangel und Hyperkapnie nicht nur für die *akute* Hypoxie, sondern auch sicher für die *subchronische* Hypoxie gilt. Wieweit das für die chronische Hypoxie zutrifft, ist noch Gegenstand weiterer Untersuchungen.

Die bei einem Teil der *Emphysematiker*, besonders während bronchialspastischer oder entzündlicher Schübe, anzutreffende Hypertonie im großen Kreislauf ist in diesem Sinne zu erklären. In einzelnen Fällen von Altersemphysem (große schlaffe Lunge nach Giese) konnte durch Beatmung in der Eisernen Lunge und durch Normalisierung der Blutgasverhältnisse analog den in Abb. 39 abgebildeten Kurven eine Senkung der Drucke im *großen* Kreislauf beobachtet werden[1].

2. Lungentuberkulose.

Bei den verschiedenen Formen der Lungentuberkulose lassen sich auf Grund kombiniert durchgeführter Funktionsanalysen von Lunge und kleinem Kreislauf generell folgende funktionellen Störungsbefunde herausstellen:

a) Lungenbelüftung und Lungendurchblutung gehen auch bei der Lungentuberkulose in der Regel parallel. Tuberkulöse Veränderungen des Lungenparenchyms ziehen in den meisten Fällen eine adäquate Herabsetzung der Lungendurchblutung von der A. pulmonalis aus nach sich[2], wie eindeutig durch Kombination von Blutgasanalyse sowie selektiver Angiographie der Lungengefäße und Isotopenthorakographie gezeigt werden konnte. Dabei ist zunächst eine regulatorisch erfolgende Selbststeuerung entsprechend den tierexperimentellen Befunden von v. Euler[3] anzunehmen, nach denen durch Senkung der alveolären Sauerstoffspannung und durch Erhöhung der alveolären Kohlendioxydspannung eine Vasoconstriction hervorgerufen wird. Eine Drosselung der Durchblutung der A. pulmonalis auf reflektorischem Wege ist weniger wahrscheinlich, da die Engerstellung der Gefäße auch bei denervierter Lunge statthat. Im weiteren Verlauf der Tuberkulose treten dann pathologisch-anatomische Veränderungen der Gefäßwand im Sinne einer Endangitis hinzu, die bis zum völligen Verschluß der Gefäße führen kann.

b) Demzufolge ist der *vasculäre intrapulmonale Kurzschluß* via Lungencapillaren in der Pathophysiologie der Lungentuberkulose meist nicht von Bedeutung.

Jedoch ließen sich besonders gelagerte Ausnahmen beobachten und mit Hilfe der selektiven Angiographie der Lungengefäße und der Blutgasanalyse sicherstellen[4]. So können z. B. bei Pleuraschwarten als Folgezustände nach Pleuritis exsudativa oder Pneumothorax bisweilen Kurzschlußzustände mäßigen Grades nachweisbar sein[5].

c) Beim *Pneumothorax* sind die Gefäße in der Lungenperipherie weitgehend entsprechend der Größe des Kollapses gedrosselt. Ähnliche Befunde wie mit der selektiven Lungenangiographie wurden mit der Angiokardiopneumographie von de Carvalho, Löffler und Steinberg und Mitarbeitern erhoben. Im gleichen Sinne sprechen oxymetrische Befunde von Matthes[6], der bei einseitigem Pneumothorax normale O_2-Sättigungswerte fand, was er auf eine proportionale Einschränkung der Lungenfunktion in der Kollapslunge zurückführte.

Der Pneumothorax bedeutet hinsichtlich der Gesamt-Leistungsbreite eine relativ große Funktionseinbuße, da auf der entsprechenden Lungenseite die im

---

[1] Bolt 1954.   [2] Bolt 1953, Bolt und Rink 1951, Bolt und Zorn 1951.
[3] v. Euler und Liljestrand 1949.   [4] Bolt 1951.   [5] Rink 1955.   [6] Matthes 1951.

Lungenmantel liegende Masse der Alveolen in toto vom Kollaps betroffen wird und nicht nur das erkrankte Gebiet selektiv ausgeschaltet wird.

d) Die *Pneumolyse mit extrapleuralem Pneumothorax* hat sich als das funktionell schonendste Kollapsverfahren bewährt, da die erkrankten Bezirke weitgehend selektiv ausgeschaltet werden können. Die nicht vom Kollaps betroffenen Lungensegmente der Seite mit extrapleuralem Pneumothorax weisen bei normaler

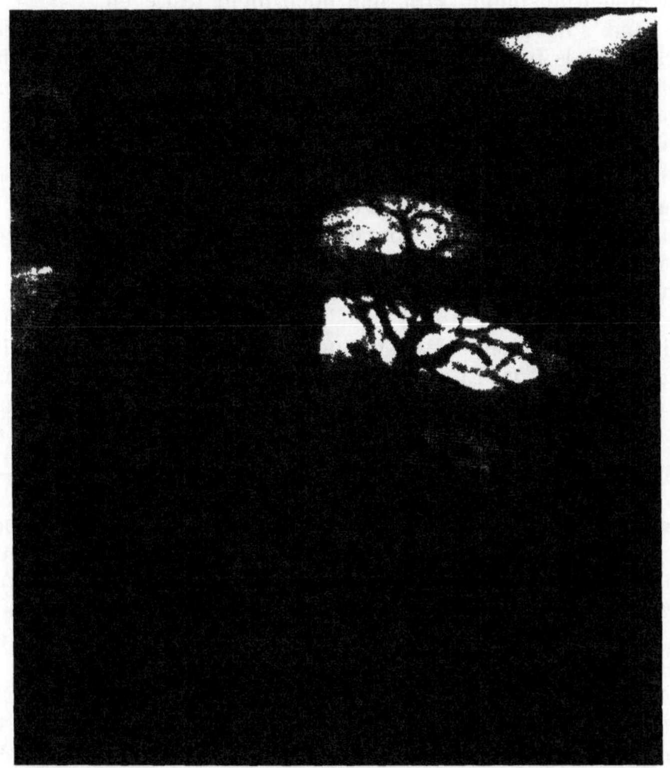

Abb. 40. Zustand nach Lobektomie der Lingula und des linken Lungen-Unterlappens. Dehnung des verbliebenen linken Lungen-Oberlappens.

Belüftung eine normale Durchblutung auf. Die spirographischen Befunde von GAENSLER und STRIEDER entsprechen den Beobachtungen von GAUBATZ, BOLT, KNIPPING, RINK u. a.[1]

e) Die *Thorakoplastik* bewirkt eine mehr oder weniger starke funktionelle Einbuße durch starren Kollaps. Unter einer guten Thorakoplastik ist das Lungengefäßsystem weitestgehend dem Umfang des operativ gesetzten Kollapses entsprechend gedrosselt.

Bei schlechter Thorakoplastik mit Nischenbildung[2] können Symptome eines vasculären Kurzschlusses nachweisbar sein. Die Gefahr der Skoliose mit Emphysembildung der kontralateralen Lunge trägt dazu bei, daß das durchschnittliche Lebensalter der Plastikträger 10 Jahre unter dem Bevölkerungsdurchschnitt liegt.

f) Hinsichtlich der Funktionsbeurteilung der postoperativen Zustände nach *Lobektomie* und *Pneumektomie* sei auf die Untersuchungen von COURNAND und Mitarbeitern, ROSSIER und BOLT-STANISCHEFF-ZORN und BOLT-WEDEKIND ver-

[1] GAENSLER und STRIEDER 1950, GAUBATZ 1938.   [2] PETZOLD 1942.

wiesen. Die Frage der Verhütung ernster Spätfolgen, insbesondere des Emphysems der Restlunge, ist noch nicht voll befriedigend gelöst. Es zeigte sich in den ersten 2 Jahren nach durchgeführter Lobektomie eine Dehnung der restlichen verbliebenen Lungensegmente auf der operierten Seite, denen die für das Emphysem charakteristische Atrophie fehlte (s. Abb. 40). Wieweit sich aus dieser Lungendehnung später ein Emphysem mit den S. 371 ff. beschriebenen funktionellen Folgen ausbildet, läßt sich noch nicht festlegen.

Der Lob- und Pneumektomie gegenüber beansprucht die *Segmentresektion* in der Tuberkulose als funktionsschonendes Resektionsverfahren erhöhtes Interesse. Hier ist die *selektive Angiographie* der Lungengefäße und in der weiteren Entwicklung die *Isotopenthorakographie* zur präoperativen Funktionsbeurteilung der einzelnen Lungensegmente von wesentlicher Bedeutung[1].

g) Die mit Hilfe der Herzsondierung gemessenen *Drucke in der A. pulmonalis und im rechten Ventrikel* sind bei der Tuberkulose in Ruhe vielfach *nicht* erhöht. Druckerhöhungen unter Arbeit können prognostisch hinsichtlich der Frage eines sich entwickelnden Cor pulmonale wertvolle Hinweise geben. Deutliche Druckerhöhungen fanden sich beim sekundären Emphysem.

Zwischen den *Drucken im großen und im kleinen Kreislauf* und Druckschwankungen in diesen Systemen bestehen auch bei der Tuberkulose keine gesetzmäßigen Beziehungen[2]. v. Euler und Liljestrand zeigten tierexperimentell, daß der Sinusentlastungsreflex die Lungengefäße nicht merklich beeinflußt.

h) Zum *Cor pulmonale chronicum:* Berblinger fand nur in einem Teil seiner autoptischen Kontrollen bei Lungentuberkulose eine Hypertrophie des rechten Herzens.

Als Voraussetzung zur Ausbildung eines Cor pulmonale chronicum bei Lungentuberkulose gehört a) eine *Hypertonie der Lungenstrombahn*, die nur in einem Teil der Fälle, besonders bei Begleitemphysem (vgl. auch S. 372), besteht; b) eine *Reaktionsbereitschaft des Herzmuskels zur Hypertrophie*. Bei marantischen Formen der Lungentuberkulose ist diese Reaktionsbereitschaft des Herzmuskels nicht gegeben.

i) Nach Cournand, Richards, Mayer, Bolt u. a. bedeutet die *Ausschaltung des N. phrenicus* für die betroffene Lungenseite eine entscheidende Funktionseinschränkung mit erheblichen Rückwirkungen auf die respiratorischen Funktionsgrößen (insbesondere auf die Ventilationsgrößen), und auf den kleinen Kreislauf. Ist die kontralaterale Lungenseite funktionell intakt, werden diese Folgen in Ruhe und unter kleinen Belastungsstufen kaschiert, mit Hilfe der Bronchospirographie und der selektiven Angiographie der Lungengefäße sind sie jedoch in ihrem wahren Umfang aufzudecken[3].

Kommt es im weiteren Verlauf zu Erkrankung auch der kontralateralen Seite, so ist man im Falle der Notwendigkeit kollapstherapeutischer Maßnahmen oft in unheilvoller Weise blockiert. Bolt steht auf dem gleichen Standpunkt wie Rossier, daß die Phrenicus-Exhairese einer funktionellen Katastrophe gleichkommen kann.

k) Zur „*funktionellen Pathologie der Alveole*" bei Lungentuberkulose: Bei den geübten Operationsverfahren muß es eines der Prinzipien sein, möglichst *funktionsschonend* vorzugehen. In diesem Sinne sind der *selektive Kollaps* und die *Segmentresektion* von besonderer Bedeutung.

Wenn man nun in seinen Berechnungen von der *Voraussetzung der Gleichheit der Ventilation der Alveolen* ausgeht, so ist das höchstens im Hinblick auf den

---

[1] Bolt 1952, Bolt und Rink 1958.   [2] Bolt und Zorn 1951.
[3] Sadoul und Mitarbeiter 1954, Bolt, Rink Valentin und Venrath 1954.

Gesamtorganismus gestattet. Für die gezielten therapeutischen Bemühungen, bei denen es mehr auf die Funktion der einzelnen Lungensegmente ankommt, hilft es nicht weiter, wenn die Alveolen als Kollektiv in den Kreis der funktionellen Betrachtungen gezogen werden. Eine *ideale Alveolarluft* gibt es bei den Lungenkranken nicht und ebenso keine *ideale „alveoläre Ventilation"*. Diese unter vereinfachenden Voraussetzungen angenommenen Begriffe stellen für die aktuelle operative Therapie nur ein interessantes, mehr theoretisches Kalkül dar.

Das ist der Grund, weswegen die Knippingsche Schule neben der Anwendung der *Bronchospirographie* bewußt die *selektive Angiographie der Lungengefäße* entwickelte und sich intensiv um die *Isotopenthorakographie* bemühte, um bei der Lungentuberkulose zu einer Funktionsanalyse des kleinen Kreislaufs und der Lungenfunktion zu kommen im Sinne einer *regionalen Aussage. Die therapeutischen Belange der Kollapstherapie wie auch der Resektionsverfahren stehen dabei im Vordergrund des Interesses.*

3. Silikose.

Die Störungen der Atemfunktion gehen bei der Silikose in der Regel der kardialen Insuffizienz voran. Ein zwangsläufiger Parallelismus zwischen Ausdehnung der Silikose und Einschränkung der Lungenfunktion ist nicht gegeben[1]. Im einzelnen zeigt die funktionsanalytische Prüfung der Atmung bei Silikose der verschiedenen Schweregrade folgendes:

a) Atemminutenvolumen.

Bei einem Teil der Kranken kommt es im Verlauf der Silikose zum Auftreten einer Hyperventilation[2], die von ROSSIER und BUCHER (1947) auf eine mit dem Fortschreiten der Silikose einhergehende Vergrößerung des funktionellen Totraumes zurückgeführt wird, während sich die alveoläre Ventilation in den verschiedenen Stadien fast immer als normal erweist. So fanden z. B. die Schweizer Autoren eine durchschnittliche Steigerung des Atemminutenvolumens in Ruhe von 31% bei Silikose I, von 54% bei Silikose II und von 62% bei Silikose III. Die Vergrößerung des funktionellen Totraums erklärt zu einem Teil die Dyspnoe bei fortgeschrittener Silikose. ZORN[1] stellte hingegen im Ruhrbergbau fest, daß bei *unkomplizierten* Silikosen des röntgenologisch I. und II. Stadiums die O_2-*Aufnahme* unter Ruhe und Arbeit durchweg der Norm entsprach, und daß ebenfalls die Atemminutenvolumina im allgemeinen normal waren.

Die Hyperventilation erreicht bei *schweren* Silikoseformen bereits in Ruhe oft ein beachtliches Ausmaß. Unter körperlicher Belastung steigt das Atemminutenvolumen wesentlich rascher an als bei Gesunden und nähert sich entsprechend der Leistungseinschränkung mehr oder weniger bald dem reduzierten Atemgrenzwert[3].

b) Atemgrenzwert.

Die Abnahme des Atemgrenzwertes erfolgt im allgemeinen etwa mit dem Schweregrad der Silikose. Dementsprechend sind die funktionellen Reserven der Lunge durch die silikotischen Prozesse und ihre Folgeerscheinungen vermindert. Eine ähnliche Herabsetzung wie der Atemgrenzwert erfährt auch der Atemstoßwert.

---

[1] ROELSEN und BAY 1940, ZORN 1940, 1943, MINET, FONTAN und BONDUELLE 1947, BALDWIN, COURNAND und RICHARDS 1949, BOLT 1950, ROSSIER und BÜHLMANN 1950, LACHNIT 1950, MOTLEY, GORDON, LANG und THEODOS 1950, SPAIN 1950.
[2] BÖHME 1939.   [3] BOLT, VALENTIN und VENRATH 1954.

Sichere Anhaltspunkte für ein gehäuftes Vorkommen einer *spastischen Bronchitis*, deren Bedeutung bei der Silikose Rossier und Bühlmann (1950) hervorheben, konnte Zorn bei den verschiedenen Silikoseformen auf Grund eingehender Studien über die Wirkung von Suprarenin, Dolantin, Polamidon und vergleichsweise von physiologischer Kochsalzlösung nicht gewinnen.

c) Vitalkapazität.

Hingegen ist die Vitalkapazität auch in schwereren Silikosefällen oft relativ wenig reduziert. Rossier und Bucher (1947) fanden so z. B. die *Vitalkapazität* im Durchschnitt bei Silikose I = 6%, bei Silikose II = 8%, bei Silikose III = 16% vermindert, jedoch den *Atemgrenzwert* bei Silikose I = 9%, bei Silikose II = 27%, bei Silikose III = 44% herabgesetzt. Die stärkere Einschränkung des Atemgrenzwertes im Vergleich zu der weniger betroffenen Vitalkapazität beruht im wesentlichen auf dem Elastizitätsverlust der Lunge, weniger auf Bronchialspasmen, die sich durch den Adrenalinversuch erfassen lassen.

Reichmann, Zorn und Bolt[1] konnten eine Beeinträchtigung der Lungenfunktion insbesondere bei der Silikose I. und II. Grades in diesem Ausmaß nicht bestätigen. Im allgemeinen werden erst bei Silikose III. Grades Störungen der ventilatorischen Größen manifest, wenngleich sie auch hier keine festen Beziehungen zeigen. Entscheidend für die Funktionseinschränkung der Atmung ist im wesentlichen das Ausmaß des bei der Silikose jeweils vorhandenen Begleitemphysems.

d) Spiroergometrische Befunde.

Die Bedeutung der Spiroergometrie für die quantitative Beurteilung der Funktion von Atmung und Kreislauf bei der Silikose geht aus den Ergebnissen von Reichmann und Zorn, Bolt, Valentin, Venrath[1] an einem umfangreichen Beobachtungsgut hervor: Die leichtgradigen Silikosen zeigen gegenüber den Normalwerten keine signifikanten Veränderungen. Die reine mittelgradige Silikose bedingt bei mittleren Arbeitsbelastungen bis 90 Watt (Drehkurbelergometer nach dem Wirbelstromprinzip) noch keine respiratorische Insuffizienz und keine Störungen der Gesamtsauerstoffaufnahme. Bei schweren Silikosen verursachen Oberfeldschwielen relativ geringe Insuffizienzerscheinungen, Schwielen im Mittelfeld bereits deutliche Ausfälle und Unterfeldprozesse erhebliche Insuffizienzen. Bei den schwersten Formen ist der Grad der Leistungsminderung mehr von dem sekundären Begleitemphysem als von Größe und Sitz der Schwielenbildung abhängig. Böhme[2] konnte die Resultate in den wesentlichen Punkten bestätigen. Allerdings fand er bei II.-gradiger und III.-gradiger Silikose häufiger ein spirographisches O_2-Defizit als Zorn. Nach allgemeiner Auffassung ist eine erhebliche Beeinträchtigung der Leistungsfähigkeit von Atmung und Kreislauf dann anzunehmen, wenn der Erkrankte nicht mehr in der Lage ist, eine Leistung von 100 Watt (am Wirbelstromergometer) über 10 min ohne spirographisches Sauerstoffdefizit auszuführen.

e) Blutgasanalytische Befunde.

Bruce (1942) gab für die Sauerstoffsättigung im arteriellen Blut bei Silikose folgende Mittelwerte an:

Silikose I: 95,7% (94,1—97,7),
Silikose II: 94,3% (93,2—95,5),
Silikose III: 93,7% (90,4—97,3).

---

[1] Reichmann 1940, 1950 und Zorn 1940, 1943, 1950, Bolt 1949, Valentin und Venrath 1955.
[2] Böhme 1943, 1950.

Obgleich das Beobachtungsgut von BRUCE Fälle mit hochgradiger Dyspnoe enthielt, fanden sich nur mäßige Untersättigungen. Die von JÉQUIER-DOGE und LOB (1945) bei 14 Silikosekranken bestimmte arterielle Sauerstoffsättigung lag nur zweimal unter 96%; sie betrug bei diesen Patienten, die allerdings Komplikationen aufwiesen (Tuberkulose, Thoraxdeformierung und Pleuraschwarten), 94,1% bzw. 91,3%. ROSSIER beobachtete 1950 eine unwesentliche Erniedrigung der arteriellen Sauerstoffsättigung bei Silikose II (94,8%), jedoch nicht selten eine deutliche Untersättigung in den Spätstadien der Krankheit (91%). Nach BOLT (1951) sind die arteriellen Blutsauerstoff- und Kohlendioxydwerte selbst bei schweren Silikosen in Ruhe oft weitgehend normal, sofern kein schwereres komplizierendes Emphysem vorhanden ist. FRIEHOFF und KARRASCH (1954)[1] fanden eine höhere Korrelation zwischen der Erniedrigung der *arteriellen O_2-Spannung und -Sättigung* und dem Ausmaß des Begleitemphysems als zwischen der Erniedrigung dieser Werte und dem röntgenologischen Grad der Silikose.

f) Verhalten von Lungenkreislauf und Herz bei der Silikose.

Mit Fortschreiten der Silikose kommt es neben der Einschränkung der respiratorischen Funktionsbreite zu einer zunehmenden Belastung des rechten Herzens. Die Konsequenzen der vorgeschrittenen Silikose für Herz und Kreislauf sind folgende:

Durch eine *Widerstandserhöhung in der Lungenstrombahn,* sei es infolge reaktiver Wandveränderungen, Einengung und Verödung der Lungengefäße in emphysematös veränderten silikotischen Lungenbezirken, oder sei es durch Lageveränderungen des Herzens und der großen Gefäße infolge schrumpfender Schwielen, wird das rechte Herz zunehmend belastet. Die Funktionsbeeinträchtigung des Lungenkreislaufs resultiert einmal aus den Störungen des alveolären Gasaustausches, entsprechend dem v. Euler-Liljestrand-Effekt, zum anderen aus dem organischen Verlust an Capillarfläche.

Toxische Einflüsse infolge begleitender Sekundärinfektionen können eine zusätzliche Beanspruchung des kardiozirkulatorischen Systems mit sich bringen. Bei der fortgeschrittenen Silikose steht die Insuffizienz des Cor pulmonale am Ende der Entwicklung. Als entscheidender Faktor für die Entstehung der kardialen Rechtsinsuffizienz ist meist das Lungenemphysem anzusprechen (s. Abb. 36, 37).

Von BOLT und ZORN (1950) bei Silikotikern durchgeführte *Herzkatheterungen* haben die Kenntnis über die *Druckverhältnisse im rechten Herzen und in der A. pulmonalis* wesentlich erweitert. Diese Untersuchungen ergaben, daß die *Druckerhöhung im kleinen Kreislauf bei der Silikose im allgemeinen erst sehr spät auftritt.* Bei reinen Silikosen, selbst III. Grades, konnte nicht immer eine Drucksteigerung im rechten Ventrikel und in der A. pulmonalis festgestellt werden, wohl aber fast immer dann, wenn gleichzeitig ein substantielles Emphysem vorlag. Hier wurden teilweise Werte von 50 mm Hg und in einem Fall von Silikose II mit erheblichem Emphysem sogar eine Drucksteigerung auf 70 mm Hg gemessen. GAULTIER und MAURICE (1947) fanden bei 15 Staublungenkranken keine verwertbare Erhöhung der mittleren Drucke in der rechten Herzkammer, obwohl einige der Untersuchten unter starker Dyspnoe litten. Im dekompensierten Stadium des chronischen Cor pulmonale sind die Ventrikeldrucke nach BOLT und ZORN bei deutlich erhöhten Vorhofdrucken unter Umständen erniedrigt. Bei Silikotuberkulosen ohne Emphysem und ohne ausgedehnte silikotuberkulöse Mischschwielen in den Lungenfeldern fanden sich keine Druckerhöhungen. Nach BOLT und ZORN (1950) handelt es sich bei der Hypertonie

---

[1] FRIEHOFF und KARRASCH 1954.

im kleinen Kreislauf der emphysematösen Silikosekranken teils um einen Widerstandshochdruck bei einem Herzminutenvolumen in normalen Grenzen, teils aber
auch um einen kombinierten Herzminutenvolumen-Hochdruck. Gleichzeitige
EKG-Kontrollen erbrachten nur in 18 von 25 Fällen mit einwandfreier Drucksteigerung im rechten Ventrikel einen Rechtstyp.

Obgleich bei der Silikose die respiratorische Insuffizienz meist vor der kardialen
auftritt, kann auch das Umgekehrte vorkommen, wenn silikotische Schwielen
eine verstärkte Druck- oder Zugwirkung auf das Herz ausüben und dadurch
mechanisch die Leistung des Herzens beeinträchtigen[1].

Bei der kardialen Insuffizienz ergibt sich trotz ausreichender Atemreserven unter in-
äquater Arbeit ein Zurückbleiben der O_2-Aufnahme hinter den Normalwerten bei meist
hohen Herzschlagfrequenzen[2]. In Diagrammen zeigt die O_2-Aufnahmekurve unter steigender
Belastung nach Überschreiten der adäquaten Leistungsgrenze ein Abknicken. Das Atemminutenvolumen steigt in der Regel über die Norm. Sowohl die Anlaufzeit der O_2-Werte
bis zum steady state als auch die Erholungszeit sind bei der kardialen Insuffizienz verlängert.
Die vergrößerte Sauerstoffschuld nach Arbeit kann bei kardialer Insuffizienz im Gegensatz
zum spirographischen Sauerstoffdefizit der respiratorischen Insuffizienz durch O_2-Spannungs-
erhöhung nicht beeinflußt werden.

Intrapulmonale Kurzschlußzustände von funktionellem Gewicht konnten Bolt
und Zorn (1950) bei der schweren Silikose nicht nachweisen. Das Ausbleiben
der Kurzschlußhypoxämie ließ sich mit Hilfe der selektiven Angiographie der
Lungengefäße durch das Fehlen von funktionstüchtigen bzw. durchgängigen
Blutgefäßen in den großen silikotischen Schwielen einwandfrei erklären.

4. Intrakardialer Kurzschluß.

Intrakardiale Kurzschlüsse, die zu einer *arteriellen O_2-Untersättigung* im großen
Kreislauf führen (Rechts-Links-Shunt), finden sich bei folgenden kongenitalen
Vitien: *Fallotsche Tetralogie* (hoher Ventrikelseptumdefekt, überreitende Aorta,
Pulmonalstenose, Hypertrophie des rechten Ventrikels), *Fallotsche Pentalogie*
(hoher Ventrikelseptumdefekt, Vorhofseptumdefekt, überreitende Aorta, Pulmo-
nalstenose, Hypertrophie des rechten Ventrikels), *Fallotsche Trilogie* (Vorhofsep-
tumdefekt, Pulmonalstenose, Hypertrophie des rechten Ventrikels), *Eisenmenger-
Komplex* (hoher Ventrikelseptumdefekt, Hypertrophie des rechten Ventrikels),
Truncus arteriosus communis.

Ein Rechts-Links-Shunt bei Vorhofseptumdefekt hat eine sekundäre Pulmonalsklerose mit einer Hypertonie im Lungenkreislauf und einer Überbelastung des
rechten Ventrikels als Voraussetzung. Dementsprechend wird dieser Rechts-Links-
Shunt als intrakardialer Kurzschluß nur in fortgeschrittenen Stadien zu finden
sein. Eine dem intrakardialen Rechts-Links-Kurzschluß ähnliche Situation findet
sich bei persistierendem Ductus arteriosus Botalli, wenn es infolge der sekundären
Veränderungen in der Lungenstrombahn zu einer Hypertonie des Lungenkreislaufs und damit zu einer Shuntumkehr gekommen ist. Blutgasanalytisch finden
sich Kriterien, die unter dem Kapitel: Intrapulmonaler Kurzschluß (s. unten)
besprochen werden. Die Indikation zu einer operativen Therapie richtet sich nach
der Art der bestehenden Anomalie und nach dem Umfang der entstandenen
funktionellen Störungen.

Über eine respiratorische Besonderheit bei kongenitalen Vitien hat Landen
berichtet. Der Grad der Cyanose, an der die Mischstörung des Blutes den Hauptanteil hat, wird zusätzlich durch *Diffusionsstörungen in der Lunge* im Sinne
einer Pneumose[3] beeinflußt.

---

[1] Zorn 1950.   [2] Bolt 1950.   [3] Landen 1954, Meessen 1951.

5. Intrapulmonaler Kurzschluß.

Das Zustandsbild des ausgeprägten *intrapulmonalen vasculären Kurzschlusses* ist nach den Darlegungen auf S. 376 keineswegs häufig, da im allgemeinen in Lungenbezirken mit herabgesetzter Ventilation auch die Durchblutung gedrosselt ist. Störungen dieses gegenseitigen Verhältnisses von Belüftung zu Durchblutung im Sinne eines vasculären Kurzschlusses können bei inkomplettem Pneumothorax, bei starrem Kollaps unter Verschwartungen und auch bei schlechten Thorakoplastiken mit Nischenbildungen eintreten.

Als therapeutische Maßnahme bei starrem Kollaps unter Verschwartungen mit vasculären Kurzschlüssen kann die *Dekortikation* indiziert sein, durch die eine Wiederherstellung der normalen Lungenfunktion in geeigneten Fällen möglich ist. Ob unter einem starren Kollaps ein noch funktionstüchtiges Lungengewebe vorhanden ist, läßt sich präoperativ nur durch die selektive Angiographie der Lungengefäße entscheiden. Findet sich angiographisch unter dem Kollaps ein bis zur Peripherie der Lunge hin noch intaktes Gefäßsystem, so kann bei Wiederentfaltung der Lunge in diesen Bereichen mit einer ausreichenden Lungenfunktion gerechnet werden [1].

Massive *arteriovenöse Lungenaneurysmen* findet man gelegentlich beim *Morbus Osler der Lunge.* In diesen Fällen zwingen die Folgen des intrapulmonalen vasculären Kurzschlusses zur operativen Entfernung. Abb. 41 gibt ein selektives Angiogramm der A. pulmonalis bei Morbus Osler wieder.

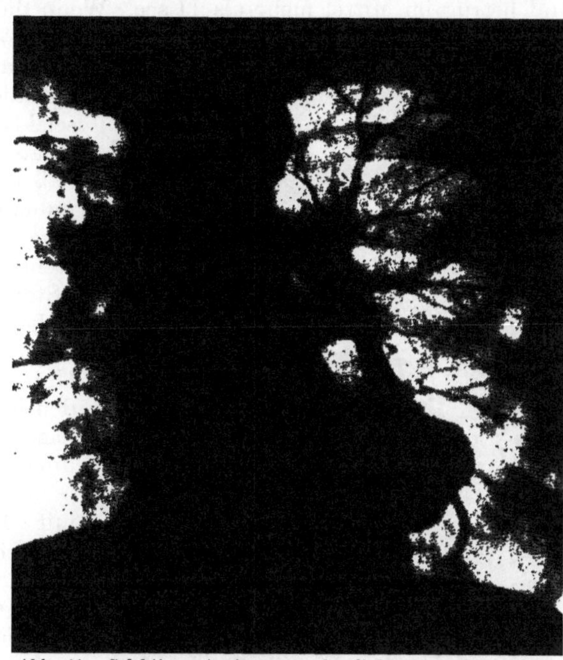

Abb. 41. Selektives Angiogramm der linken A. pulmonalis bei einem arteriovenösen Aneurysma im Bereiche des linken Lungenunterlappens (Morbus Osler). (Aus: BOLT-KNIPPING-RINK: Probleme des kleinen Kreislauf bei Herz- und Lungenkrankheiten; 2. Weltkongreß für Kardiologie, Washington September 1954.)

Nach den Untersuchungen von ZORN und BOLT sind bei *Silikose* nennenswerte intrapulmonale Kurzschlüsse selten, da in den verschwielten Bezirken auch die Lungengefäße untergegangen sind (s. S. 382).

6. Diffusionsstörungen bei Stauungslungen.

Als Beispiele der Diffusionsstörungen chronischer Stauungslungen sollen hier die Befunde wiedergegeben werden, die bei Patienten mit *Mitralstenose* erhoben worden sind. Diese Zustandsbilder sind heute von besonderer Aktualität, da hämodynamisch eine Normalisierung durch die Valvulotomie vielfach erreicht werden kann. In diesem Zusammenhang sollen die *prä- und postoperativ* erhobenen Diffusionsbefunde im Detail besprochen werden.

Einheitlich findet sich bei allen Patienten mit Mitralstenose eine der Schwere der Erkrankung entsprechende *Erhöhung der alveolo-arteriellen Sauerstoffspannungsdifferenz,* die wir nach der oben beschriebenen Methode ermittelten (s. S. 350).

---

[1] BOLT und RINK 1952.

Daneben ist die *Kontaktzeit des Blutes* in den Lungencapillaren im allgemeinen deutlich verlängert.

Auf eine Verlängerung der Kontaktzeit des Blutes in den Lungencapillaren läßt sich indirekt aus der *Lungencapillarzeit (LCT)* schließen, die wir oxymetrisch bestimmen. Die LCT ist die Zeit, welche das Blut benötigt, um von der Lungencapillare zur Capillare der Stirnhaut zu gelangen. Sie beträgt normalerwiese 5—7 sec[1].

Die LCT war bei 28 untersuchten Mitralstenose-Patienten deutlich verlängert und betrug im Mittel mehr als 11 sec. Wenn die LCT auch den ganzen Kreislaufschenkel von der Lungencapillare bis zur Capillare der Stirnhaut umfaßt,

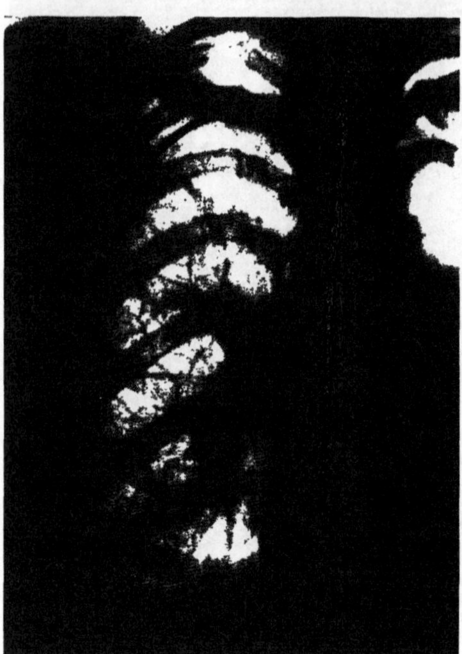

so erlaubt sie doch indirekte Schlüsse auf die Kontaktzeit. Mit Hilfe der selektiven Angiographie der Lungengefäße nach Bolt konnten wir zeigen, daß das via Herzkatheter in die A. pulmonalis injizierte Kontrastmittel langsamer fließt und im Capillarsee stehenbleibt. Es zeigen sich sog. „Sternchenbildungen", die wir als Folge einer capillären Stase ansprechen (Abb. 42). Auch radiozirkulographische Untersuchungen mit $Na^{24}Cl$ zeigen deutlich eine Verzögerung der Blutpassage (Abb. 43), rechtes Herz — linkes Herz.

Zinsser und Johnson konnten mit Hilfe der Angiokardiographie ähnliche Befunde erheben.

Die Diffusionsverhältnisse vor und nach der Valvulotomie wurden bei 9 Patienten untersucht. Vor der Operation ist die LCT — wie bereits gesagt — deutlich verlängert und normalisiert sich nach der Operation bei allen Patienten. Sie beträgt postoperativ im Mittel 7,4 sec. Dagegen nimmt die alveolo-arterielle Sauerstoffspannungsdifferenz, die präoperativ zwar mit im Durchschnitt 17,5 mm

Abb. 42. Selektives Angiogramm der A. pulmonalis dextra bei einer Patientin mit Mitralstenose. Die Aufnahme ist 4 sec nach Injektion des Kontrastmittels in die A. pulmonalis (via Herzkatheter) geschossen. Man sieht „Sternchenbildungen" infolge Stagnierens des Kontrastmittels in den feinsten peripheren Arterienverzweigungen.

Hg deutlich vergrößert ist, außer in 2 Fällen postoperativ zum Teil beträchtlich zu und steigt im Mittel auf 25,2 mm an. Das heißt, *einer hämodynamischen Besserung der Durchflußverhältnisse in den Lungen nach Valvulotomie steht eine deutliche Senkung der Diffusionskapazität in den Alveolen gegenüber* (Abb. 44). Damit ist aber der hämodynamische Erfolg einer Klappensprengung von fraglichem Wert, wenn sie von einer so wesentlichen Verschlechterung der Diffusionsverhältnisse begleitet ist. Letzteres kann eine Erklärung für manchen operativen „Versager" sein, bei dem alle sonstigen Untersuchungsergebnisse im Sinne einer Besserung sprechen, der Patient sich aber schlechter fühlt als vor der Operation.

Wir sind heute noch nicht in der Lage, aus den präoperativ ermittelten Werten einen bindenden Schluß auf die postoperativ zu erwartenden Resultate zu ziehen. Auch die Frage, inwieweit die morphologischen Veränderungen an den Lungencapillaren nach Sprengung der Mitralklappe reversibel sind, kann

---

[1] Hollmann 1957 (persönl. Mitteilung).

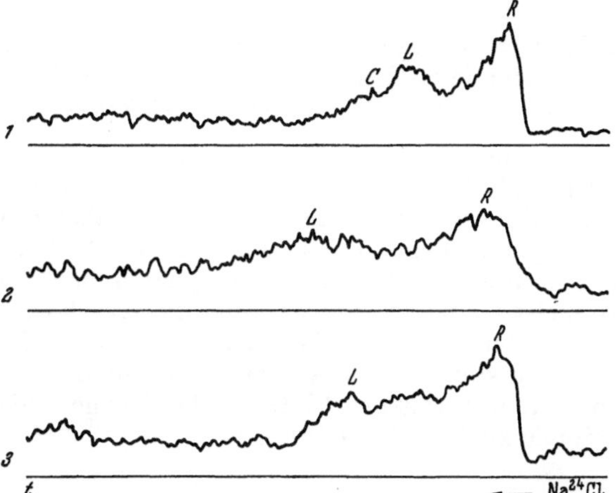

Abb. 43. Radiozirkulogramme bei (1) einem gesunden Mann und (2 und 3) bei Patientinnen mit Mitralstenose. Injektionen von 0,01—0,02 mC Na²⁴Cl in eine Vena cubitalis. Etwa 3—4 sec nach der Injektion registriert ein über dem Herzen gegenüber Streustrahlen abgeschirmter Szintillationszähler zunächst einen steilen Anstieg der Aktivität. Na²⁴Cl passiert das rechte Herz. Mit dem Abströmen der Aktivität in die Lungen sinkt sie über dem Herzen deutlich ab und steigt mit Rückfluß des Na²⁴Cl in das linke Herz wieder an (die Kurven sind entsprechend der Pfeilrichtung von rechts nach links zu lesen). Der Gipfel 2, in der Abbildung mit L markiert, ist infolge der Verdünnung der aktiven Substanz mit Blut nicht mehr so hoch wie der R-Gipfel (R = Aktivität über dem rechten Herzen). Die kleine C-Zacke im abfallenden L-Kurvenschenkel ist vermutlich auf das Einströmen aktiven Blutes in die Coronararterie zurückzuführen. Ein C-Gipfel ist in Kurve 2 und 3 nicht sicher auszumachen. In den Kurven 2 und 3 sind die R-L-Zeiten deutlich verlängert und insbesondere der L-Gipfel verbreitert und abgeflacht gegenüber Kurve 1. Ursache dafür ist das verzögerte Einströmen des Blutes in das linke Herz und das längere Verweilen des Blutes im linken Vorhof.

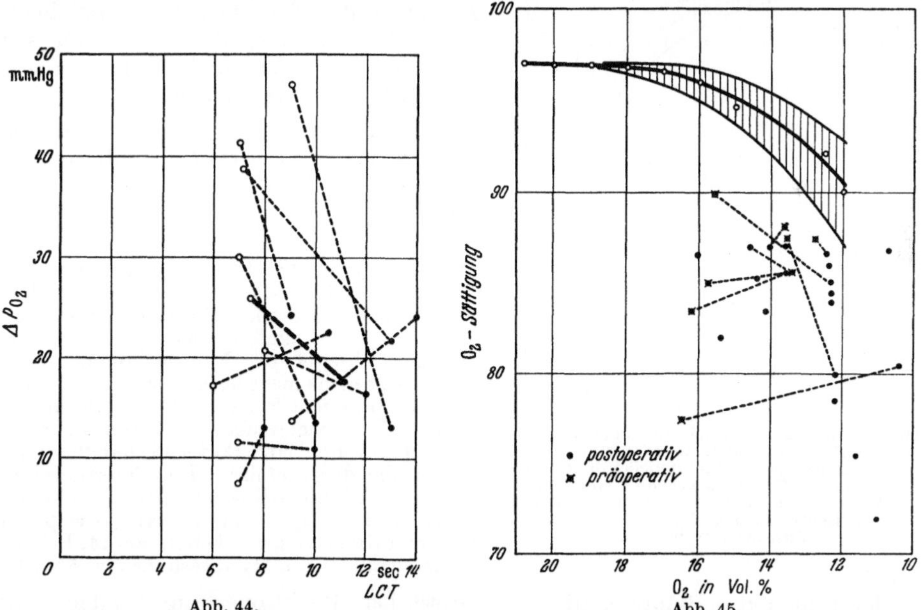

Abb. 44. Abb. 45.

Abb. 44. Das Verhalten der Lungen-Capillarzeit (LCT) und der alveolo-arteriellen Sauerstoffspannungsdifferenz (ΔPO₂) nach Valvulotomie der Mitralis wegen einer Mitralstenose. Der prä- und postoperative Wert sind mit einer gestrichelten Linie verbunden. Der präoperative Wert ist als voller Kreis, der postoperative als offener Kreis in der Abbildung dargestellt. Die betonten Kreise und die Verbindungslinie zwischen ihnen stellen die Mittelwerte von 9 Untersuchungen dar.

Abb. 45. Die Sauerstoffsättigung des arteriellen Blutes in Beziehung zum Sauerstoffgehalt in der Inspirationsluft während des Rückatmungsversuches. Die Mittelwerte von 30 Bestimmungen bei Gesunden mit der entsprechenden Streubreite (±σM) sind aufgeführt. Die größer werdende Streubreite findet ihre Erklärung in der unterschiedlichen Empfindlichkeit des Atemzentrums gegenüber Sauerstoffmangel. In die Normalwertkurven sind die Endwerte von O₂ insp. und O₂-Sättigung im Arterienblut von Patienten mit Mitralstenose eingetragen. Die Werte liegen zum Teil beträchtlich außerhalb der Streubreite der Norm. Die prä- und postoperativ beim gleichen Patienten ermittelten Werte sind durch punktierte Linien verbunden.

noch nicht beantwortet werden. Bei laufenden Kontrollen der Diffusionskapazität nach Valvulotomie fand sich nach 4—6 Wochen eine geringe Besserung
der Diffusionsverhältnisse gegenüber dem ersten postoperativen Wert.

Zusammenfassen kann man die Befunde, die bei Patienten mit Mitralstenose
allgemein vor und nach Valvulotomie erhoben worden sind, dahingehend, daß in
allen Fällen eine der Schwere des Krankheitsbildes parallel gehende Störung der
Diffusion in den Lungen vorliegt. Die LCT ist in allen Fällen verlängert. Nach
der Operation zeigt sich als Zeichen der hämodynamischen Besserung eine Verkürzung der LCT meist bis zur Norm, während die alveolo-arterielle Sauerstoffspannungsdifferenz vielfach zum Teil beträchtlich ansteigt. Diesen Anstieg der
alveolo-arteriellen Sauerstoffspannungsdifferenz möchten wir insbesondere auf
die Verkürzung der Kontaktzeit des Blutes in den Lungen mit der Alveolarluft
nach der Valvulotomie zurückführen (Abb. 44).

7. Diffusionsstörungen bei Lungenfibrosen.

Aus der Gruppe der *primären Lungenfibrosen* sei der diffuse Morbus Boeck
aufgeführt. Alle Patienten mit Boeckschem Sarkoid der Lungen zeigen eine
deutliche Erschwerung der Diffusion, die den röntgenologischen Veränderungen
nicht immer parallel geht. Das Diffusions-
bild ist nahezu identisch mit dem der
Stauungslungen bei Mitralstenose. Da die
Kontaktzeit in den Lungen aber bei diesen
Erkrankungen normal ist, machen sich
Diffusionsstörungen bereits früher bemerkbar als bei der Stauungslunge.

Von AUSTRIAN, RILEY u. a. sowie WILLIAMS
und STONE[1] wurde eine rasche Beeinflussung der
Diffusion in den Lungen bei Morbus Boeck durch
Cortison und *ACTH* gefunden. Diese Diffusions-
besserung ist wesentlich früher nachweisbar als
eine röntgenologische Änderung des Befundes.
Da aber nicht in allen Fällen mit einer günstigen
Reaktion der Krankheit auf Cortison gerechnet
werden kann, da es vielmehr im Gegenteil nicht
selten zu einer akuten Verschlechterung und
zum Fortschreiten der Fibrose kommt — die
dann meist nicht mehr aufhaltbar ist —, ist eine
laufende funktionelle Kontrolle mit Beginn der
Cortison-Therapie zweckmäßig. Bei einem unserer
Patienten wurde eine Cortisonbehandlung mit
200 mg/die durchgeführt. Die Funktionswerte
zeigen eine deutliche Besserung. Die alveolo-arterielle Sauerstoffspannungsdifferenz, die primär
44,5 mm Hg betrug, war bereits am 14. Behand-
lungstag auf 22 mm Hg abgesunken (s. Abb. 46).

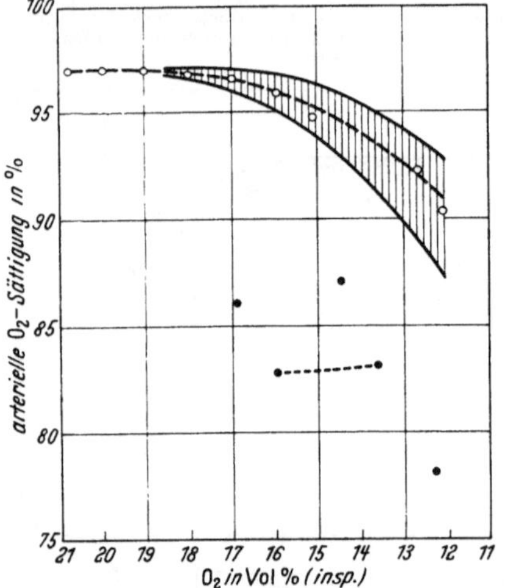

Abb. 46. In Analogie zu Abb. 45 sind die Normal-
wertdarstellungen benutzt. In sie sind die O₂ Insp.
und O₂-Sättigungswerte des arteriellen Blutes von
Patienten mit diffusem Lungenboeck eingetragen.
Die Werte eines Patienten vor und während
einer Cortisonbehandlung sind durch eine Linie
miteinander verbunden.

Faßt man die Befunde, die bei fibrotischen Reaktionen am Bindegewebs-
apparat der Lungen gefunden wurden, kurz zusammen, so zeigt sich auch hier
eine der Schwere der Veränderungen parallelgehende Vergrößerung der alveolo-
arteriellen Sauerstoffspannungsdifferenz. Der Effekt einer Morbus Boeck-Be-
handlung mit Cortison oder ACTH läßt sich leicht funktionell kontrollieren. Es
findet sich bereits eine Beeinflussung der Diffusion, lange bevor röntgenologische
Änderungen nachweisbar werden.

---

[1] AUSTRIAN und Mitarbeiter 1951, RILEY und Mitarbeiter 1952, WILLIAMS 1953, STONE 1953.

Literatur.

ALBRECHT, H., H. VALENTIN u. H. VENRATH: Über die Atmung und das Herzminutenvolumen bei Arbeit und Sport, sowie die Herzleistung. Z. exper. Med. **122**, 356—368 (1953). — ALEXANDER, R. S., and M. M. REYDMAN: Simple test of pulmonary function employing the oximeter. J. Thorac. Surg. **25**, 95 (1953). — ALLERÖDER, H., u. H. C. LANDEN: Über den störenden Einfluß äußerer Faktoren im Belastungsversuch bei Herzkranken. Zbl. inn. Med. **63**, 273 (1942). — ALTSCHULTE, M. D.: Physiology in diseases of the heart and lungs. Harvard University Monograph in Medicine, No 10. Cambridge: Harvard University Press 1949. — ANDERSON, L. L., J. C. BELL and S. G. BLOUNT jr.: An evaluation of factors affecting the alveolar-arterial oxygen tension gradient in chronic pulmonary disease. Amer. Rev. Tbc. **69**, 71 (1954). — ANTHONY, A. J.: Untersuchungen über Lungenvolumina und Lungenventilation. Dtsch. Arch. klin. Med. **167**, 129 (1930). ~ Funktionsprüfung der Atmung. Leipzig: Johann Ambrosius Barth 1937. — ANTHONY, A. J., u. R. HANSEN: Lungenventilation und Atmung in der Schwangerschaft. Z. Geburtsh. **105**, 183—196 (1933). — ANTHONY, A. J., u. W. LENT: Untersuchungen über die Wirkung erhöhter Atemwiderstände. Z. exper. Med. **109**, 624 (1941). — ANTHONY, A. J., u. R. ROHLAND: Ein Spirograph mit automatischer Regelung des Sauerstoffgehaltes. Z. exper. Med. **106**, 555—560 (1939). — ARMITAGE, G. H., and W. M. ARNOTT: Air distribution in lungs during hyperventilation. J. of Physiol. **1949**, 70—80. — ARNAUD, J., P. TULOU et R. MÉRIGOT: L'exploration de la fonction respiratoire: physiologie, méthode d'exploration, indications et résultats. Paris: Masson & Cie. 1947. 318 S. — ARNOTT, W. M.: Order and disorder in pulmonary function. Brit. Med. J. **1955**, No 4934, 279—284, 342—348. — ASLETT, E. A., P. D. HART and J. McMICHAEL: Lung volume and its subdivisions in normal males. Proc. Roy. Soc. Lond. **126**, 502 (1939). — AUB, J. C., and E. F. DuBOIS: Basal metabolism of old men. Arch. Int. Med. **19**, 823 (1917). — AUSTRIAN, R. u. Mitarb.: Clinical and physiologic features of some types of pulmonary diseases with impairment of alveolar-capillary diffusion: syndrome of „alveolar-capillary block". Amer. J. Med. **11**, 667 (1951).

BAHNSON, H. T.: Effect of brief period of voluntarily increased pulmonary pressure upon vital capacity. J. Appl. Physiol. **5**, 273—276 (1952). — BALCHUM, O. J., S. A. HARTMAN, N. B. SLONIM, S. H. DRESSLER and A. RAVIN: Permeability of douglas-type bag to respiratory gases. J. Labor. a. Clin. Med. **41**, 268—280 (1953). — BALDWIN, E. DE F., A. COURNAND and D. W. RICHARDS jr.: Pulmonary insufficiency. I. Physiological classification. clinical methods of analysis, standard values in normal subjects. Medicine **27**, 243 (1948). ~ II. A study of thirty-nine cases of pulmonary fibrosis. Medicine **28**, 1 (1949). ~ III. A study of 122 cases of chronic pulmonary emphysema. Medicine **28**, 201 (1949). — BALDWIN, E. DE F., K. A. HARDEN, D. G. GREENE, A. COURNAND and D. W. RICHARDS jr.: Pulmonary insufficiency. IV. A study of 16 cases of large pulmonary air cyts or bullae. Medicine **29**, 169—194 (1950). — BANSI, H. W.: Arbeitsstoffwechsel und Kreislauf bei endokrinen Erkrankungen. Dtsch. med. Wschr. **1929**, 347. — BARACH, A. L., and M. N. WOODWELL: Studies in oxygen therapy with determinations of blood gases. Arch. Int. Med. **28**, 367 (1921). — BARCROFT, J.: The respiratory function of the blood. Part I. The diffusion of O_2 through pulmonary epithelium. Vol. I, p 63—74. Cambridge: University Press 1925. ~ Features in the architecture of physiological function. Cambridge: University Press 1934. — BARTELS, H.: Potentiometrische Bestimmung des Sauerstoffdruckes im Vollblut mit der Quecksilbertropfelektrode. Pflügers Arch. **254**, 107 (1951). — BARTELS, H., R. BEER, E. FLEISCHER, H. J. HOFFHEINZ, J. KRALL, J. WENNER u. J. WITT: Bestimmung von Kurzschlußdurchblutung und Diffusionskapazität der Lunge bei Gesunden und Lungenkranken. Pflügers Arch. **261**, 99—132 (1955). — BARTELS, H., R. BEER, E. FLEISCHER u. G. RODEWALD: Methoden zur Untersuchung des Gasaustausches in der Lunge. Klin. Wschr. **1955**, 969. — BARTELS, H., R. BEER, H.-P. KOEPCHEN, J. WENNER u. J. WITT: Messung der alveolo-arteriellen O_2-Druckdifferenz mit verschiedenen Methoden am Menschen bei Ruhe und Arbeit. Pflügers Arch. **261**, 133—151 (1955). — BARTELS, H., u. G. RODEWALD: Die arterielle Sauerstoffspannung, die alveolo-arterielle Sauerstoffspannungsdifferenz und weitere atmungsphysiologische Daten gesunder Männer. Pflügers Arch. **256**, 113 (1952). ~ Die alveolo-arterielle Sauerstoffspannungsdifferenz und das Problem des Gasaustausches in der menschlichen Lunge. Pflügers Arch. **258**, 163—176 (1953). ~ Die alveolär-arterielle Sauerstoffdruckdifferenz und das Problem des Gasaustausches in der menschlichen Lunge. Pflügers Arch. **258**, 163 (1954). — BARTELS, H., G. RODEWALD u. E. OPITZ: Untersuchungen zum Problem des Gasaustausches in der Lunge. Klin. Wschr. **1953**, 1020. — BARTELS, J., J. W. SEVERINGHAUS, R. E. FORSTER, W. A. BRISCOE and D. V. BATES: The respiratory dead space measured by single breath analysis of oxygen, carbon dioxide, nitrogen and helium. J. Clin Invest. **33**, 41—48 (1954). — BATEMAN, J. B.: Studies of lung volume and intrapulmonary mixing. Nitrogen clearance curves. J. Appl. Physiol. **3**, 143 (1950). — BATES, D. V.: Uptake of CO in health and emphysema. Clin. Sci. **11**, 21—32 (1952). — BATES, D. V., and R. V. CHRISTIE: Intrapulmonary mixing of helium in health and in emphysema. Clin. Sci. 9, 17—29 (1950). — Bates, D. V., W. S. Fowler, R. E. Forster and B. van Lingen: Uniformity of alveolar ventilation at different lung volumes. J. Appl. Physiol. 6, 598—602 (1954). — Beale, H. D., I. W. Schiller, M. H. Halperin, W. Franklin and F. C. Lowell: Delirium and coma precipitated by oxygen in bronchial asthma complicated by respiratory acidosis. New England J. Med. 244, 710 (1951). Beer, E. G.: Clinical evaluation of pulmonary function tests. Current Res. Anesth. a. Analges. 32, 411 (1953). — Beitzke, H.: Atmungsorgane. In Aschoffs Pathologische Anatomie, Bd. II, S. 312. 1923. — Bence, A. E., A. Lanari y E. J. Rodriguez: Relación entre el volumen del aire insuflado en la camera pleural y la disminución del volumen pulmonar: estudio broncoespirométrico. Medicina (Buenos Aires) 8, 16 (1948). — Benedict, F. G., R. C. Lee u. F. Strieck: Influence of breathing oxygen-rich atmospheres on human respiratory exchange during severe muscular work and recovery from work. Arb.physiol. 8, 266—303 (1934). — Berggren, S. M.: The oxygen deficit of arterial blood caused by nonventilating parts of the lung. Acta physiol. scand. (Stockh.) Suppl. 11 (1942). — Birath, G.: Lung volume and ventilation efficiency. Acta med. scand. (Stockh.) Suppl. 154, 1—125 (1944). ~ Simultaneous samples of alveolar air from each lung and parts thereof: preliminary report of method using bronchial catheterization. Amer. Rev. Tbc. 55, 444 (1947). — Bjerknes, W., u. P. F. Scholander: Method for continual airbreathing in closed-circuit apparatus. Skand. Arch. Physiol. (Berl. u. Lpz.) 79, 164—168 (1938). — Björk, V. O.: Cardio-pulmonary functions tests. J. Thorac. Surg. 26, 67 (1953). — Björk, V. O., and J. H. Hilty: The arterial oxygen and carbon dioxide tension during the postoperative period in cases of pulmonary resection an thoracoplastics. J. Thorac. Surg. 27, 455 (1954). — Björk, V. O., P. A. Michas and L. G. Uggla: The arterial oxygen tension at rest and during effort as a lung function test. J. Thorac. Surg. 25, 558 (1953). — Björk, V. O., and E. F. Salen: The blood flow through an atelectatic lung. J. Thorac. Surg. 20, 933 (1950). — Björkman, S.: Bronchospirometrie: Eine klinische Methode, die Funktion der menschlichen Lungen getrennt und gleichzeitig zu untersuchen. Acta med. scand. (Stockh.) Suppl. 56, 1 (1934). ~ Anwendbarkeit der Acetylenmethode bei pathologischen Zuständen in den Lungen. Eine bronchospirometrische Studie. Beitr. Klin. Tbk. 88, 519 (1936). — Björkman, S., u. E. Carlens: Lung function during rest and exercise in lung diseases: bronchospirometric study. Acta med. scand. (Stockh.) 40, Suppl. 259, 63 (1951). — Blickenstorfer, E.: Der Totraum und seine Berechnung. Schweiz. Z. Tbk. 4, Suppl. 1, 49 (1947). — Bloomer, W. E.: Respiratory function and its clinical evaluation. In G. E. Lindskog and A. A. Liebow, Thoracic Surgery and Related Pathology, p. 109—139. New York: Appleton-Century-Crofts 1953. — Blount jr., S. G., M. C. McCord, L. L. Anderson and S. Komesu: Analysis of alveolar-arterial oxygen pressure gradient in mitral stenosis. J. Labor. a. Clin. Med. 42, 108 (1953). — Böhme, A.: Die Anwendung der Ergometrie zur Prüfung der Leistungsfähigkeit, besonders bei der Silikose. Reichsarbeitsbl. 23, 87 (1943). — Bohr, Ch.: Über die Lungenatmung. Skand. Arch. Physiol. (Berl. u. Lpz.) 2, 236—268 (1890). ~ Specific activity of lungs in respiratory gas uptake and its relation to gas diffusion through the alveolar wall. Skand. Arch. Physiol. (Berl. u. Lpz.) 22, 221 (1909). — Bøje, O.: Der CO_2-Gehalt des arteriellen Blutes während Muskelarbeit beim Menschen. Skand. Arch. Physiol. (Berl. u. Lpz.) 71, 61—72 (1934). — Bolt, W.: Funktionsprüfung bei Staublungenerkrankungen. In Jötten-Gärtner, Die Staublungenerkrankungen, S. 34—43. Darmstadt 1950. ~ Zum Lungenkreislauf unter Berücksichtigung der Lungenfunktionsprüfung. Beitr. Klin. Tbk. 110, 39 (1953). ~ Selektive Lungenangiographie. 12. Vortragsreihe der Augsburger Fortbildungstage für praktische Medizin, S. 44, 1953. ~ Emphysem (Haemodynamik). Beitr. Klin. Tbk. 111, 266—286 (1954). ~ Pathologische Physiologie des Cor pulmonale. Verh. dtsch. Ges. Kreislaufforsch. 21, 196—217 (1955). ~ Klinische Funktionsdiagnostik der Atmungsstörungen. In Klinische Funktionsdiagnostik, herausgeg. von H. Küchmeister. Stuttgart: Georg Thieme 1956, 2. Aufl. 1958. — Bolt, W., W. Forssmann u. H. Rink: Technik und praktische Bedeutung der Herzkatheterung für die funktionelle Diagnostik und die Therapie von Herz- und Lungenerkrankungen. Med. Klin. 1953, 1614. ~ Selektive Lungenangiographie. Stuttgart; Georg Thieme 1957. — Bolt, W., u. H. W. Knipping: Probleme des kleinen Kreislaufs bei Herz- und Lungenkrankheiten. 2. Weltkongr. für Kardiologie, Washington 1954, S. 484. Medizinische 1955, 480—482. — Bolt, W., H. W. Knipping u. H. Ludes: Zur präoperativen Herzdiagnostik unter Berücksichtigung der Isotopenchemie. Verh. Dtsch. Ges. Kreislaufforschg. 20, 102—110 (1954). — Bolt, W., H. W. Knipping u. H. Rink: Münch. med. Wschr. 95, 421 (1953). ~ 2. Weltkongreß für Kardiologie, Washingotn, Sept. 1954. Medizinische 1955, 480. — Bolt, W., H. W. Knipping, H. Valentin u. H. Venrath: Respiratorische Ruhe- und Arbeitsinsuffizienz. Die Gruppierung der verschiedenen Formen und die Abgrenzung von der kardialen Insuffizienz unter besonderer Berücksichtigung der Lungentuberkulose. Beitr. Klin. Tbk. 108, 394—405 (1953). ~ Physiologie der Atmung. In Arnold, Lehrbuch der Sportmedizin. Leipzig 1956. — Bolt, W., D. Michel, H. Valentin u. H. Venrath: Über die Druckverhältnisse im kleinen Kreislauf, rechten Herzen und in den dem Herzen vorgelagerten Venen unter den Bedingungen der Bürgerschen Preßdruckprobe. Z. Kreislaufforsch. **44**, 261 (1955). — BOLT, W., u. H. RINK: Selektive Angiographie der Lungengefäße bei Tuberkulose. Schweiz. Z. Tbk. **8**, 380 (1951). ~ Selective angiography of pulmonary vessels in pulmonary tuberculosis. XII. Conf. de l'Union Internat. contre la Tuberculose, Rio deJaneiro, 24.—27. August 1952, S. 592. ~ Thoraxchirurgie **5**, 379 (1958). — BOLT, W., H. RINK, H. VALENTIN u. H. VENRATH: Bronchospirographie. Beitr. Klin. Tbk. **111**, 317—334 (1954). — BOLT, W., G. ROTTHOFF, H. VALENTIN u. H. VENRATH: Zum Mechanismus der Lungenstauung bei der Arbeit linksinsuffizienter Herzkranker. Münch. med. Wschr. **1952**, 16. — BOLT, W., K. T. SCHILD, H. VALENTIN u. H. VENRATH: Zur Frage der intrapulmonalen Oxydation und der Gültigkeit des Fickschen Prinzips. Z. Kreislaufforsch. **43**, 840 (1954). — BOLT, W., A. STANISCHEFF u. O. ZORN: Die selektive Angiographie der Lungengefäße. Münch. med. Wschr. **1951**, 303. — BOLT, W., H. VALENTIN u. H. VENRATH: Beitrag zur Stenosenbeurteilung in der Lungenklinik. Beitr. Klin. Tbk. **104**, 450—454 (1951). ~ Beitrag zur Frage der Korundschmelzerlunge. Bundesarbeitsbl. **1954**, H. 2. — BOLT, W., u. H. VENRATH: Functional analysis with special reference to surgical treatment of mitral stenosis. Vortr. a. d. I. europäischen Kongr. für Cardiologie, London 1952. Z. Kreislaufforsch. **41**, 942 (1952). — BOLT, W., u. O. ZORN: Verh. dtsch. Ges. inn. Med. **56**, 179 (1950). ~ Intrakardiale Druckmessungen bei Silicose. Beitr. klin. Tuberk. **105**, 100 (1951). ~ Z. ges. inn. Med. **6**, 729 (1951). — BOOTHBY, W. M., H. LUNDIN and H. F. HELMHOLZ jr.: Gaseous nitrogen elimination test to determine pulmonary effiency. Proc. Soc. Exper. Biol. a. Med. **67**, 558 (1948). — BOUTOURLINE-YOUNG, H. J., and J. L. WHITTENBERGER: Use of artificial respiration in pulmonary emphysema accompanied by high carbon dioxide levels. J. Clin. Invest. **30**, 838 (1951). — BRAUER, L.: Die respiratorische Insuffizienz. Verh. dtsch. Ges. inn. Med. **44**, 120 (1932). ~ Gasanalytische Herzfunktionsprüfung. Verh. dtsch. Ges. inn. Med. **50**, 78 (1938). — BRAUER, L., u. H. W. KNIPPING: Zur respiratorischen Insuffizienz. Beitr. Klin. Tbk. **101**, 424 (1948). ~ Über das sogenannte spirographische Defizit und einige Bemerkungen zur arteriellen Blutgasanalyse in der Herz- und Lungenklinik. Med. Klin. **1949**, 1429—1433. — BRAUN, P.: L'exploration fonctionnelle des poumons séparés par bronchospirometrie. Nancy: Société d' Impressions Typographiques 1951. — BREBION, G., et H. MAGNE: L'espace mort et le volume totale de l'appareil respiratoire. Ann. de Physiol. **13**, 65—92 (1937). — BRETSCHGE, H. J.: Die Geschwindigkeitskurve der menschlichen Atemluft (Pneumotachogramm). Arch. ges. Physiol. **210**, 134 (1925). — BRINKMAN, R., u. W. G. ZIJLSTRA: Determination and continuous registration of the percentage oxygen saturation in clinical conditions. Arch. chir. neerl. **1**, 177 (1949). — BRISCOE, W. A.: The assessment of the ventilatory function of the lungs in normal and emphysematous subjects. Thèse Oxford, 108 p, décembre 1950. ~ Further studies on the intrapulmonary mixing of helium in normal and emphysematous subjects. Clin. Sci. **11**, 45—58 (1952). — BRISCOE, W. A., M. R. BECKLAKE and T. F. ROSE: Intrapulmonary mixing of helium in normal and emphysematous subjects. Clin. Sci. **10**, 37—51 (1951). — BRONFIN, G. J., S. H. DRESSLER and A. RAVIN: Apparatus for exercising patient in recumbent position. J. Labor. a. Clin. Med. **35**, 317 (1950). — BROWN jr., C. C., D. L. FRY and R. V. EBERT: Mechanics of pulmonary ventilation in patients with heart disease. Amer. J. Med. **27**, 438 (1954). — BROWN, L. M., and J. H. COMROE jr.: Blood pO_2 derived from measurements of O_2 physically dissolved in blood. In Methods in Medical Research, vol. 2, edit. by J. H. COMROE jr. Chicago: Yearbook Publ. 1950. — BRUCE, R. A., F. W. LOVEJOY, G. B. BORTHERS and T. VELASQUEZ: Observation on causes of dyspnea in chronic pulmonary granulomatosis in beryllium workers. Amer. Rev. Tbk. **59**, 364—390 (1949). — BRUCE, R. A. u. Mitarb.: Normal respiratory and circulatory pathways of adaptation in exercise. J. Clin. Invest. **28**, 1423 (1949). — BRUCE, T.: Die Silikose als Berufskrankheit in Schweden. Stockholm 1942. — BUDELMANN, G.: Die Beeinflussung der Vitalkapazität der Lunge durch Wickelung der Extremitäten. Klin. Wschr. **1937**, 1711. — BÜHLMANN, A.: Oxymetrie, Arbeitsversuche und Bestimmung der Arbeitsfähigkeit. Schweiz. med. Wschr. **1951**, 374. — BÜHLMANN, A., C. MAIER, M. HEGGLIN, R. KÄLIN u. F. SCHAUB: Zur Pathogenese der arteriellen pulmonalen Hypertonie mit besonderer Berücksichtigung des Cor pulmonale beim Emphysem. Cardiologia (Basel) **24**, 96 (1954). — BÜHLMANN, A., C. MAIER u. P. H. ROSSIER: Zur Ätiologie und Therapie des Cor pulmonale. Schweiz. med. Wschr. **1954**, 587. — BUYTENDIJK, H. J.: Oesophagusdruk en longelasticiteit. Groningen: Electrische Drukkerij 1949.

CAIN, C. C., and A. B. OTIS: Some physiological effects resulting from added resistance to respiration. J. Aviation Med. **20**, 149—160 (1949). — CARA, M.: Correlation entre les taux proposés par l'expert dans la silicose et les données de l'exploration ventilatoire. Journées Lorraines de la Silicose Nancy-Merlebach (12.—13. déc. 1950), pp. 39—43. ~ Bases physiques pour un essai d'évaluation des taux d'incapacités respiratoires. Arch. Mal. profess. **6**, 613—624 (1950). ~ Bases physiques pour un essai de mécanique ventilatoire avec application à la cinésithérapie. Poumon (Paris) **9**, 371 (1951). ~ Diagnostic fonctionnel de l'emphysème pulmonaire. J. franç. Méd. et Chir. thorac. **8**, 35 (1954). — CARA, M., et D. JOUASSET: La ventilation maxima peut etre atteinte au cours du rebreathing. C. r. Soc. Biol. Paris **1953**. — CARA, M., et P. SADOUL: Essai de sémiologie spirographique appliqué à la pneumologie.

Poumon (Paris) **1953**, 295. — Carlens, E.: A new flexible double-lumen catheter for broncho-spirometry. J. Thorac. Surg. **18**, 742—746 (1949). — Carlens, E., H. E. Hanson and B. Nordenström: Temporary unilateral occlusion of pulmonary artery: new method of determining separate lung function and of radiologic examination. J. Thorac. Surg. **22**, 527 (1951). — Carroll, D., J. E. Cohn and R. L. Riley: Pulmonary function in mitral valvular disease: distribution and diffusion characteristics in resting patients. J. Clin. Invest. **32**, 510 (1953). — Carvalho, Lopo de: Angiopneumography in the study of the pharmaco-dynamic properties of certain drugs. Dis. Chest **25**, 121 (1954). — Caswell, A., I. Milne and R. H. Taplin: The oxygen resaturation curve, a measure of cardiopulmonary function. Canad. Med. Assoc. J. **70**, 176—179 (1954). — Caughey jr., J. L.: Analysis of breathing pattern. Amer. Rev. Tbc. **48**, 382 (1943). — Ceyhan, S., H. Jung u. A. Varlik: Studien über die experimentelle Pneumonie. Med. Welt **20**, 1484 (1951). — Christensen, E. H.: Beiträge zur Physiologie schwerer körperlicher Arbeit. Arb.physiol. **4**, 128, 154, 175; **5**, 463 (1931). — Christiansen, J., C. G. Douglas and J. B. S. Haldane: The absorption and dissociation of carbon dioxide by human blood. J. of Physiol. **48**, 244 (1914). — Christie, R. V.: Lung volume and its subdivisions. J. Clin. Invest. **11**, 1099—1118 (1932). ~ Dyspnoea in relation to visco-elastic properties of lung. Proc. Roy. Soc. Med. **46**, 381 (1953). — Christie, R. V., and C. A. Macintosh: The measurement of the intrapleural pressure in man and its significance. J. Clin. Invest. **13**, 279—294 (1934). — Clark jr., L. C., R. Wolf, D. Granger and Z. Taylor: Continuous recording of blood O_2 tensions by polarography. J. Appl. Physiol. **6**, 189 (1953). — Clement, Mc, J. H., A. R. Renzetti, A. Himmelstein and A. Cournand: Cardiopulmonary function in the pulmonary form of Boeck's sarcoid and its modifikation by cortisone therapy. Amer. Rev. Tbc. **67**, 154 (1953). — Cobb, S., D. J. Blodgett, K. B. Olson and A. Strana-han: Determination of total lung capacity in disease from routine chest roentgenograms. Amer. J. Med. **16**, 39 (1954). — Cohen, A. G., and A. Geffen: Roentgenographic methods in pulmonary disease. Amer. J. Med. **10**, 375 (1951). — Cohn, J. E., D. G. Carroll, B. W. Armstrong, R. H. Shepard and R. L. Riley: Maximal diffusing capacity of the lung in normal male subjects of different ages. J. Appl. Physiol. **6**, 588—597 (1954). — Comroe jr., J. H.: Methods in medical research. Year book publ., vol. 2, p. 74. 1950. ~ The value of pulmonary function tests in the diagnosis of pulmonary disease. Trans. Stud. Coll. Physicians Philadelphia **18**, 49 (1950). ~ Interpretation of commonly used pulmonary function tests. Amer. J. Med. **10**, 356 (1951). — The functions of the lung. Harvey Lect. **48**, 110—144 (1952/53). — Comroe jr., J. H., and S. Botelho: Unreliability of cyanosis in recognition of arterial anoxemia. Amer. J. Med. Sci. **214**, 1 (1947). — Comroe jr., J. H., and R. D. Dripps: Oxygen tension of arterial blood and alveolar air in normal human subjects. Amer. J. Physiol. **142**, 700—707 (1944). ~ The physiological basis for oxygen therapy. Springfield, Ill.: Ch. C Thomas 1950. — Comroe jr., J. H., R. E. Forster, A. B. DuBois, W. A. Briscoe and E. Carlens: The lung; clinical physiology and pulmonary function tests. Chicago: Yearbook Publ. 1955. — Comroe jr., J. H., and W. S. Fowler: Lung function studies. VI. Detection of uneven alveolar ventilation during single breath of oxygen. Amer. J. Med. **10**, 408 (1951). — Comroe jr., J. H., and E. H. Wood: Measurement of the oxygen saturation of blood by filter photometers (oximeters). In J. H. Comroe jr. (edit.), Methods in Medical Research, vol. 2, pp. 144—159. — Consolazio, C. F., R. E. Johnson, and E. Marek: Metabolic methods. St. Louis: C. V. Mosby Comp. 1951. — Coster, A. de, et H. Denolin: Les aspects physiopathologiques de l'insuffisance respiratoire. Acta tbc. belg. **44**, 464 (1953). — Cour-nand, A.: Cardio-pulmonary function in chronic diseasis. Harvey Lect. **1952**. — Cour-nand, A., E. de F. Baldwin, R. C. Darling and D. W. Richards jr.: Studies on intra-pulmonary mixture of gases: IV. Significance of pulmonary emptying rate, J. Clin. Invest. **20**, 681—689 (1941). — Cournand, A., J. Lequime et P. Régniers: L'insuffisance cardiaque chronique. Etudes physiopathologiques. Rapport au 27. Congr. de Médecine, Bruxelles, 1951. Paris: Masson & Cie. 1952. 262 p. — Cournand, A., and D. W. Richards jr.: Pulmonary insufficiency. I. Discussion of a classification and presentation of clinical tests. Amer. Rev. Tbc. **44**, 26 (1941). — Cournand, A., D. W. Richards jr. and R. C. Darling: Graphic tracings of respiration in study of pulmonary disease. Amer. Rev. Tbc. **40**, 487—516 (1939). — Cournand, A., R. L. Riley, A. Himmelstein and R. Austrian: Pulmonary circulation and alveolar ventilation-perfusion relationships after pneumonectomy. J. Thorac. Surg. **19**, 80 (1950). — Croce, P.: New catheter for bronchospirometry which combines advantages of double lumen and single lumen catheters. J. Thorac. Surg. **27**, 187 (1954). — Curry, J. J., and F. C. Lowell: Measurement of vital capacity in asthmatic subjects receiving histamine and acetyl-beta-methyl choline: clinical study. J. Allergy **19**, 9 (1948). Curti, P. C., G. Cohen, B. Castleman, J. G. Scanell, A. L. Friedlich and G. S. Myers: Respiratory and circulatory studies of patients with mitral stenosis. Circulation (New York) **8**, 893 (1953).

Darling, R. C., A. Cournand and D. W. Richards jr.: III. An open circuit for measuring residual air. J. Clin. Invest. **19**, 609—618 (1940). ~ Studies on intrapulmonary mixture of gases: V. Forms of inadequate ventilation in normal and emphysematous lungs, analyzed by means of breathing pure oxygen. J. Clin. Invest. **23**, 55—67 (1944). — DAUTREBANDE, L.: Les échanges respiratoires. Press. Univ. de France, vol. 1. 1930. 448 p. ∼ L'Aerosologie, vol. 1. London: J. B. Baillière & Fils 1950. 340 p. — DAVENPORT, H.: The ABC of acid base chemistry. Chicago: University of Chicago Press 1950. — DAYMAN, H.: Mechanics of airflow in health and in emphysema. J. Clin. Invest. **30**, 1175 (1951). — DECHOUX, J.: La pneumoconiose des mineurs de fer du bassin de Lorraine. Thèse Nancy 1954. 170 p. — DEJOURS, P., and H. RAHN: Residual volume measurements, by the gas expansion method, and nitrogen dilution method. J. Appl. Physiol. **5**, 445 (1953). — DENOLIN, H.: L'exploration de la fonction cardio-pulmonaire au cours de l'effort. Acta clin. belg. **7**, 229 (1952). ∼ Le coeur pulmonaire chronique en médicine interne. Verh. dtsch. Ges. Kreislaufforsch. **21** (1955). — DENOLIN, H., and A. deCOSTER: Les méthodes d'investigation de la fonction pulmonaire et leurs applications. Acta tbc. belg. **43**, 245—292 (1952). — DEXTER, L., J. W. DOW, F. W. HAYNES, J. L. WHITTENBERGER, B. G. FERRIS, W. T. GOSDALE and H. K. HELLEMS: Studies of the pulmonary circulation in man at rest. J. Clin. Invest. **29**, 602 (1951). — DIENEMANN, G.: Das arterio-venöse Lungenaneurysma bei Morbus Osler. Münch. med. Wschr. **97**, 818—820 (1955). — DIRKEN, M. N. J., and H. HEEMSTRA: Adaption of lung circulation to ventilation. Quart. J. Exper. Physiol. **34**, 213—226 (1948). — DONALD, K. W.: Definition and assessment of respiratory function. Brit. Med. J. **1**, 415—422 (1953). — DONALD, K. W., and R. V. CHRISTIE: Respiratory reponse to carbon dioxide and anoxia in emphysema. Clin. Sci. **8**, 33 (1945). ∼ New method of clinical spirometry. Clin. Sci. **8**, 21 (1949). — DONALD, K. W., and W. D. M. PATON: Gases administered in artificial respiration with particular reference to the use of carbon dioxide. A report to the medical research council by its committee for research on breathing apparatus for protection against dangerous fumes and gases. Brit. Med. J. **1955**, No 4909, 313—318. — DONALD, K. W., A. RENZETTI, R. L. RILEY and A. COURNAND: Analysis of factors affecting concentrations of oxygen and CO_2 in gas and blood of lungs: results. J. Appl. Physiol. **4**, 497 (1952). — DOTTER, C. T., and D. S. LUKAS: Acute cor pulmonale: experimental study utilizing special cardiac catheter. Amer. J. Physiol. **164**, 254 (1951). — DOUGLAS, J. C., and O. G. EDHOLM: Measurement of saturation time and saturation tension with Millikan oximeter, in subjects with normal pulmonary function. J. Appl. Physiol. **2**, 307 (1949). — DRABKIN, D. L., and C. F. SCHMIDT: Spectrophotometric studies. XII. Observation of circulating blood in vivo, and direct determination of saturation of hemoglobin in arterial blood. J. of Biol. Chem. **157**, 69 (1945). — DRIPPS, R. D., and J. H. COMROE jr.: Respiratory and circulatory response of normal men to inhalation of 7.6 and 10.4 per cent CO_2 with comparison of maximal ventilation produced by severe muscular exercise, inhalation of CO_2 and maximal voluntary hyperventilation. Amer. J. Physiol. **149**, 43 (1947). — DRUTEL, P., et J. DECHOUX: Un test spirographique de la perméabilité bronchique: le rapport de la capacité pulmonaire utilisable à l'effort avec la capacité vitale. J. franç. Méd. et Chir. thorac. **6**, 517—542 (1952). — D'SILVA, J. L., and D. MENDEL: Maximum breathing capacity test. Thorax (Lond.) **5**, 325—332 (1950). — DU BOIS, D., and E. F. DuBOIS: Clinical calorimetry. X. Formula to estimate approximate surface area if height and weight be known. Arch. Int. Med. **17**, 863 (1916). — DU BOIS, A. B., A. G. BRITT and W. O. FENN: Alveolar CO_2 during the respiratory cycle. J. Appl. Physiol. **4**, 535 (1952). — DU BOIS, A. B., W. O. FENN and A. G. BRITT: CO_2-dissiciation curve of lung tissue. J. Appl. Physiol. **5**, 13 (1952). — DU BOIS, A. B., and B. B. ROSS: New method for recording of pressure-volume diagram of chest and lungs by means of cathode ray oscillograph. AF Techn. Rep., U.S. Air Force No 6528, August, 1951, p 202. — DU BOIS, E. F.: Physiology of respiration. U.S. Nav. Med. Bull. **26**, 1—16, 247—270 (1928).

ELAM, J. O., J. L. EHRENHAFT, W. N. ELAM jr. and H. L. WHITE: Photo-electric measurements of arterial O_2 saturation dynamics in man for study of cardiopulmonary function. Federat. Proc. **8**, 40 (1949). — ELIASCH, H.: The pulmonary circulation at rest and on effort in mitral stenosis. Scand. J. Clin. a. Labor. Invest. **4**, Suppl. 4 (1952). — ENGELHARDT, A.: Der verschiedene Kohlensäuregehalt einzelner Lungenabschnitte. Z. Biol. **101**, 21 (1942). — ENGHOFF, H.: Zur Frage des schädlichen Raumes bei der Atmung. Skand. Arch. Physiol. (Berl. u. Lpz.) **63**, 15 (1932). ∼ Volumen inefficax: Bemerkungen zur Frage des schädlichen Raumes. Uppsala Läkör. Förh. **44**, 191—218 (1938). ∼ Der Barospirograph, ein portativer Apparat für Respirations-, Zirkulations- und Gaswechseluntersuchungen. Skand. Arch. Physiol. (Berl. u. Lpz.) **81**, 91 (1939). — EULER, U. S. v.: Physiologie des Lungenkreislaufs. Verh. dtsch. Ges. Kreislaufforschg. **17**, 8—16 (1951). — EULER, U. S. v., u. G. LILJESTRAND: Observation on the pulmonary arterial blood pressure in the cat. Acta physiol. scand. (Stockh.) **12**, 301 (1947).

FACQUET, J., J. M. LEMOIN, P. ALHOMME et J. LEFEBVIE: La mesure de la pression auriculaire gauche par voie transbrochique. Arch. Mal. Coeur **8**, 741 (1952). — FELIX, K.: Die Atmungsfunktion des Blutes. Aus Physiologische Chemie von FLASCHENTRÄGER u. LEHNARTZ, Bd. 2, Teil 1. Berlin: Springer 1954. — FENN, W. O.: Mechanics of respiration. Amer. J. Med. **10**, 77—90 (1951). — FENN, W. O., A. B. OTIS and H. RAHN: Studies in respiratory physiology. Chemistry and mechanics of pulmonary ventilation. AF Techn. Rep., U. S. Air Force No 6528, August, 1951. — Fenn, W. O., H. Rahn and A. B. Otis: A theoretical study of the composition of the alveolar air at altitude. Amer. J. Physiol. 146, 637 (1946). ~ Respiratory system. Annual Rev. Physiol. 1950, 179. — Ferrer, M. I., R. M. Harvey, R. T. Cathcart, C. A. Webster, D. W. Richards jr. and A. Cournand: Digoxin in chronic cor pulmonale. Circulation 1, 161 (1950). — Ferris jr., B. G., J. E. Affeldt, H. A. Kriete and J. L. Whittenberger: Pulmonary function in patients with pulmonary disease treated with ACTH. Arch. Industr. Hyg. 3, 603 (1951). — Ferris jr., B. G., H. A. Kriete and B. C. Kriete: Alveolar-arterial oxygen difference. A comparison of two methods. J. Appl. Physiol. 3, 519 (1951). — Ferris jr., B. G., J. Mead, J. L. Whittenberger and G. A. Saxton jr.: Pulmonary function in convalescent poliomyelitic patients. III. Compliance of lungs and thorax. New England J. Med. 247, 390 (1952). — Filley, G. F., E. Gay and G. W. Wright: The accuracy of direct determinations of oxygen and carbondioxyde tensions in human blood in vitro. J. Clin. Invest. 33, 510 (1954). — Filley, G. F., F. Gregoire and G. W. Wright: Alveolar and arterial oxygen tensions and the significance of the alveolar-arterial oxygen tension difference in normal men. J. Clin. Invest. 33, 517 (1954). — Filley, G. F., D. J. McIntosh and G. W. Wright: Carbon monoxyde uptake and pulmonary diffusing capacity in normal subjects at rest and during exercise. J. Clin. Invest. 33, 530 (1954). — Fishman, A. P.: Studies in man of the volume of the respiratory dead space and the composition of the alveolar gas. J. Clin. Invest. 33, 469 (1954). — Fleisch, A.: Der Pneumotachograph: Ein Apparat zur Geschwindigkeitsregistrierung der Atemluft. Pflügers Arch. 209, 713 (1925). ~ Die Pneumotachographie. In Handbuch der biologischen Arbeitsmethoden, Bd. V, S. 8. Berlin 1935. ~ Le métabographe. Helvet. physiol. Acta 1953, 361. ~ Nouvelles méthodes d'étude des échanges gazeux et de la fonction pulmonaire. Basel: Benno Schwabe & Co. 1954. — Folkow, B., and J. R. Pappenheimer: Proportion of the respiratory dead space contained within the lungs. Federat. Proc. 13, 45 (1954). — Forbes, W. H., F. Sargent and F. J. W. Roughton: Rate of carbon monoxide uptake by normal man. Amer. J. Physiol. 143, 594—608 (1945). — Forssander, C. A.: Some observations on testing of pulmonary function. Dis. Chest 22, 626 (1952). — Forssmann, W.: Geschichtliche Entwicklung und Methodik der Herzkatheterung; ihr Anwendungsgebiet unter besonderer Berücksichtigung der Lungenerkrankungen. Langenbecks Arch. u. Dtsch. Z. Chir. 279, 450—473 (1954). — Forster, R. E., W. S. Fowler and D. V. Bates: Consideration on uptake of carbon monoxide by lungs. J. Clin. Invest. 33, 1128—1134 (1954). — Forster, R. E., W. S. Fowler, D. V. Bates and B. van Lingen: The absorption of CO by the lungs during brath-holding. J. Clin. Invest. 33, 1135—1145 (1945). — Foss, P. O.: Sclerodermi med lungefibrose. Nord. Med. 52, 917—919 (1954). — Fowler, R. C.: Rev. Sci. Instrum. 20, 175 (1949). — Fowler, W. S.: The respiratory dead space. Amer. J. Physiol. 154, 405—416 (1948). ~ Uneven pulmonary ventilation. J. Appl. Physiol. 2, 283—299 (1949). ~ In: Methods in Medical Research, vol. 2. Chicago: Yearbook Publ. 1950. ~ Lung function studies. V. Respiratory dead space in old age and in pulmonary emphysema. J. Clin. Invest. 29, 1439 (1950). ~ Intrapulmonary distribution of inspired gas. Physiologic. Rev. 32, 1—20 (1952). — Fowler, W. S., and J. H. Comroe jr.: Lung function studies. I. Rate of increase of arterial oxygen saturation during inhalation of 100 per cent O_2. J. Clin. Invest. 27, 327 (1948). — Fowler, W. S., E. R. Cornish and S. S. Kety: Measurement of alveolar ventilatory components. Amer. J. Med. Sci. 220, 112 (1950). ~ Analysis of alveolar ventilation by pulmonary N_2 clearance curves. J. Clin. Invest. 31, 40—50 (1952). — Frank, H., u. J. Seusing: Über die alveolär-arterielle Sauerstoffdruckdifferenz unter Sauerstoffmangelatmung. Dtsch. Arch. klin. Med. 201, 242 (1954). — Friehoff, F., u. K. Karrasch: Das Verhalten von Sauerstoffdruck und Sauerstoffsättigung bei chronischen Lungenerkrankungen unter Berücksichtigung der Silikose. Beitr. Silikoseforsch. 26, 78 (1954). — Fry, D. L., R. V. Ebert, W. W. Stead and C. C. Brown: Mechanics of pulmonary ventilation in normal subjects and in patients with emphysema. Amer. J. Med. 16, 80 (1954). — Fry, D. L., W. W. Stead, R. V. Ebert, R. I. Lubin and H. S. Wells: Measurement of intraesophageal pressure and its relationship to intrathoracic pressure. J. Labor. a. Clin. Med. 40, 664 (1952). — Furusawa, K.: Muscular exercise, lactic acid, and supply and utilization of oxygen. Proc. Roy. Soc. Lond., Ser. B 99, 155 (1926).

Gaensler, E. A.: Ventilatory tests in bronchial asthma, evaluation of vital capacity and maximum breathing capacity. J. Allergy 21, 232 (1950). ~ Air velocity index: a numeral expression of the functionally effective portion of ventilation. Amer. Rev. Tbc. 62, 17 (1950). ~ Analysis of the ventilation defect by timed capacity measurement. Amer. Rev. Tbc. 64, 256 (1951). ~ Analysis and critique of pulmonary function studies. Bull. New England Med. Cent. 13, 49 (1951). ~ Instrument for dynamic vital capacity measurements. Science (Lancaster, Pa.) 114, 444 (1951). ~ Bronchospirometry. I. Review of literature. J. Labor. Clin. Med. 39, 917 (1952). ~ Clinical pulmonary physiology. J. Med. (New England) 252, 177, 221 (1955). — Gaensler, E. A., and D. W. Cugell: Bronchospirometry. IV. Ambient-air and oxygen-recording bronchospirometry. J. Labor. a. Clin. Med. 40, 410—430

(1952). ~ Bronchospirometry. V. Differentiel volume determination. J. Labor. a. Clin. Med. 40, 558 (1952). — GAENSLER, E. A., J. V. MALONEY jr. and V. O. BJÖRK: Bronchospirometry. II. Experimental observations and theoretical considerations of resistance breathing. J. Labor. a. Clin. Med. 39, 935—953 (1952). — GAENSLER, E. A., W. E. PATTON and N. R. FRANK: Bronchospirometry. VII. Indications. J. Labor. a. Clin. Med. 41, 456 (1953). — GAENSLER, E. A., D. F. RAYL and D. M. DONNELLY: Breath holding test in pulmonary insufficiency: evaluation of 1,000 studies. Surg. etc. 92, 81—90 (1951). — GAENSLER, E. A., and J. W. STRIEDER: Pulmonary function before and after extrapleural pneumothorax. A comparison with other forms of collapse and resection. J. Thorac. Surg. 20, 774 (1950). — GAENSLER, E. A., and T. R. WATSON jr.: Bronchospirometry. III. Complications, contraindications, technique, and interpretation. J. Labor. a. Clin. Med. 40, 223 (1952). — GAENSLER, E. A., T. R. WATSON jr. and W. E. PATTON: Bronchospirometry. VI. Results of 1,089 examinations. J. Labor. a. Clin. Med. 41, 436 (1953). — GALDSTON, M., S. WEISENFELD, B. BENJAMIN and M. B. ROSENBLUTH: Effect of ACTH in chronic lung disease: study of five patients. Amer. J. Med. 10, 166 (1951). — GAUBATZ, E.: Über Funktionsprüfungen vor und nach operativer Kollapstherapie. Beitr. Klin. Tbk. 88, 730 (1936). ~ In HEIN-KREMER-SCHMIDT, Kollapstherapie der Lungentuberkulose. Leipzig: Georg Thieme 1938. — GAULTIER, M., et P. MAURICE: Bull. Soc. méd. Hôp. Paris 63, 836 (1947). — GEBAUER, P. W.: Catheter for bronchospirometry. J. Thorac. Surg. 8, 674 (1939). — GEORG, J.: Apparatus and methods for estimation of pulmonary function. Scand. J. Clin. a. Labor. Invest. 1, 239—244 (1949). — GILMORE, H. R., M. HAMILTON, H. KOPELMAN and L. SOMMER: The ear oxymeter. Its use clinically and the determination of cardiac output. Brit. Heart J. 16, 301—310 (1954). — GILSON, J. C., and P. HUGH-JONES: Measurement of total lung volume and breathing capacity. Clin. Sci. 7, 185 (1949). — GIRARD, J., P. LOUYOT, P. SADOUL et J. P. GRILLIAT: La ventilation pulmonaire des spondylosiques. Rev. du Rheumatisme 18, 679 (1951). — GLASER, E. M., and J. McMICHEAL: Effect of venesection on capacity of lungs. Lancet 1940, 230. — GÖPFERT, H., u. R. FREY: Ein schnellanzeigendes Meßgerät für die Kohlensäure in der Ausatmungsluft. Arch. klin. Chir. 279, 803 (1954). — GOGGIO, A. F.: Abnormal physiology of chronic pulmonary emphysema. New England J. Med. 231, 672 (1944). — GORALEWSKI, G.: Zentralnervensystem und Anoxämie. Arb.physiol. 9, 94—118 (1935). — GORDON, J., and E. S. WELLES: Decortication in pulmonary tuberculosis including studies of respiratory physiology. J. Thorac. Surg. 18, 337 (1949). — GRAY, J. S.: Pulmonary ventilation and its physiological regulation. Springfield, Ill.: Ch. C. Thomas 1950. 82 p. — GRAY, J. S., D. R. BARNUM, H. W. MATHESON and S. N. SPIES: Ventilatory function tests. I. Voluntary ventilation capacity. J. Clin. Invest. 29, 677 (1950). — GRAY, J. S., and E. L. GREEN: Measurement of voluntary ventilation capacity. Federat. Proc. 5, 35 (1946). — GRÉHARD, M.: L'espace mort respiratoire et la determination. J. Anat. et Physiol. (Paris) 1, 523 (1864). — GREIFENSTEIN, F. E., R. M. KING, S. S. LATCH and J. H. COMROE jr.: Pulmonary function studies in healthy men and women 50 years and older. J. Appl. Physiol. 4, 641 (1952). — GROSSE-BROCKHOFF, F.: Hämodynamik des Lungenkreislaufes. Tuberkulosearzt 6, 38 (1952). — GROSSE-BROCKHOFF, F., u. W. SCHOEDEL: Eine Apparatur zur Untersuchung der Veränderungen der alveolaren Exspirationsluft in der Ausatmungszeit. Pflügers Arch. 238, 204 (1936).

HADORN, W.: Untersuchungen über das Lungenemphysem. Ein neues Pneumometer zur Messung der maximalen Exspirationsstärke (Exspirationsstoß). Helvet. med. Acta 10, 81 (1943). ~ Die Pneumometrie als klinische Methode zur quantitativen Beurteilung bronchostenotischer Zustände. Bull. schweiz. Akad. med. Wiss. 7, 39 (1951). — HALDANE, J. B. S.: Methods of air analysis. London: Chas. Griffin 1920. — HALDANE, J. B. S., and J. B. PRIESTLEY: Respiration, p. 427. New Haven: Yale University Press 1935. — HALL, P. W.: Effects of anoxia on postarteriolar pulmonary vascular resistance. Circulation Res. 1, 238 (1953). — HANSEN, E.: Über die Sauerstoffschuld bei körperlicher Arbeit. Arb.physiol. 8, 151 (1934). — HANSON, H. E.: Temporary unilateral occlusion of the pulmonary artery-in man. Acta chir. scand. (Stockh.) Suppl. 187, 1—55 (1954). — HARVEY, R. M., and M. I. FERRER: Pulmonary circulation: Its relation to normal and altered dynamics. Dis. Chest 25, 3, 247 (1954). — HAYEK, H. v.: Die menschliche Lunge. Berlin: Springer 1952. — HAYMAN, L. D., and R. E. HUNT: Pulmonary fibrosis in generalized scleroderma. Dis. Chest 21, 705—708 (1951). — HEBESTREIT, H.: Der Verlauf der Erholung nach körperlicher Arbeit. Arch. ges. Physiol. 222, 738 (1929). — HELLEMS, H. K., F. W. HAYNES and L. DEXTER: Pulmonary „capillary" pressure in man. J. Appl. Physiol. 2, 24—29 (1949). — HENDERSON, L. J.: Blood: A study in general physiology. New Haven: Yale University Press 1928. — HENDERSON, Y., F. P. CHILLINGWORTH and J. L. WHITNEY: Respiratory dead space. Amer. J. Physiol. 38, 1—19 (1915). — HENDERSON, Y., and H. W. HAGGARD: Circulation and its measurement. Amer. J. Physiol. 73, 193 (1925). — HERBST, R.: Der Gasstoffwechsel als Maß der körperlichen Leistungsfähigkeit. Dtsch. Arch. klin. Med. 162, 33, 129, 257 (1928). — HERMANNSEN, J.: Untersuchungen über die maximale Ventilationsgröße. Z. exper. Med. 90, 130 (1933). ~ Die ergometrische Methode als Funktionsprüfung für Herz und Lunge. Beitr. Klin. Tbk.

92, 395 (1938). — Hermannsen, J., u. P. van Uytvanck: Einige Untersuchungen über die Kreislauf- und Lungenleistung bei schwerer Arbeit. Z. exper. Med. **88**, 279 (1933). — Herrald, F. J. C., and J. McMichael: Determinations of lung volume. Simple constant volume modification of Christie's method. Proc. Roy. Soc. Lond., Ser. B **126**, 491 (1939). — Herxheimer, H., u. R. Kost: Untersuchungen über den Arbeitssauerstoffverbrauch bei Basedowkranken. Z. klin. Med. **110**, 37 (1929). — Heyden, R.: Respiratory function in laryngectomized patients. Acta oto-laryng. (Stockh.) Suppl. **85**, 1 (1950). — Heyrovsky, J.: Polarographisches Praktikum. Berlin: Springer 1948. — Hick, F. K.: Partial pressure of oxygen in arterial blood of patients: description of aerotonometer method. Proc. Soc. Exper. Biol. a. Med. **33**, 582 (1936). — Hill, A. V., C. N. H. Long and H. Lupton: Muscular exercise, lactic acid, and supply and utilization of oxygen. Proc. Roy. Soc. Lond. Ser. B **96**, 348, 455 (1924); **97**, 84, 155 (1924). — Hirdes, J. J., u. G. van Veen: Spirometric lung function investigations. II. Form of expiration curve under normal and pathological conditions. Acta tbc. scand. (København.) **26**, 264 (1952). — Hitchcock, F. u. Mitarb.: Volume and composition of air expelled from lungs during explosive decompression. Federat. Proc. **5**, 48 (1946). — Hochrein, M.: Über Pneumotachographie. Pflügers Arch. **219**, 753 (1928). — Hochrein, M., u. I. Schleicher: Die Funktion des kardiopulmonalen Systems. Med. Klin. **1953**, 765. — Hugh-Jones, P.: Tests nouveaux dans l'exploration du poumon silicotique. Arch. Mal. profess. **10**, 430 (1949). — Hurley, L.: Clinical pulmonary physiology. II. Detection of early lung function changes in industrial exposure. Industr. Med. a. Surg. **22**, 262—267 (1953). — Hurtado, A., and W. Fray: Studies of pulmonary capacity and its subdivisions; correlation with physical and radiological measurements. J. Clin. Invest. **12**, 807 (1933). — Hurtado, A., W. Fray, N. L. Kaltreider and W. D. W. Brooks: Studies of total pulmonary capacity and its subdivisions. J. Clin. Invest. **13**, 149 (1934). — Hutchinson, J.: On capacity of lungs and on respiratory functions, with view of establishing precise and easy method of detecting disease by spirometer. Trans. Med.-Chir. Soc. Lond. **29**, 137—252 (1846).

Jacobaeus, H. C., P. Frenckner u. S. Björkman: Some attempts at determining volume and function of each lung separately. Acta med. scand. (Stockh.) **79**, 174 (1932). — Jansen, K., H. W. Knipping u. K. Stromberger: Klinische Untersuchungen über Atmung und Blutgase. Beitr. Klin. Tbk. **80**, 304—374 (1932). — Jaquet, A.: Zur Mechanik der Atembewegungen. Arch. exper. Path. u. Pharmakol. Suppl. **59**, 309 (1908). — Jeddeloh, B. zu: Untersuchungen über die Histologie der Stauungslungen. Gleichzeitig ein Beitrag zur normalen Histologie der Lunge. Beitr. path. Anat. **86**, 387 (1931). — Jéquier-Doge, E.: A propos du déficit-oxygène. Schweiz. med. Wschr. **1950**, 13. — Jéquier-Doge, E., u. M. Lob: Schweiz. med. Wschr. **75**, 283 (1945). — Joergensen, H.: Die Bestimmung der Wasserstoffionenkonzentration. Dresden u. Leipzig: Theodor Steinkopff 1943. — Jordi, A.: Untersuchungen zum Studium des Trainiertseins. Arb. physiol. **7**, 1 (1933).

Kaltreider, N. L., and W. S. McCann: Respiratory response during exercice in pulmonary fibrosis and emphysema. J. Clin. Invest. **16**, 23 (1937). — Kaltreider, N. L., W. W. Fray and H. V. Z. Hyde: Effect of age on total pulmonary capacity and its subdivisions. Amer. Rev. Tbc. **37**, 662 (1938). — Kapferer, J. M.: Der nutzbare Anteil der Vitalkapazität. Thoraxchirurgie **1**, 547 (1954). — Kennedy, M. C. S.: Demonstration of bronchial spasm, by means of spirometric tracings of the vital capacity and the maximum breathing capacity. Tagg des Silikose-Forschungs-Instituts Bochum, 28. 9. 1949. ~ A practical measure of the maximum ventilatory capacity, in health and disease. Thorax (Lond.) **8**, 72 (1953). — Kjerulf-Jensen, K., u. P. Kruhøfer: The lung diffusion coefficient for carbon monoxide in patients with lung disorders, as determined by C^{14}. Acta med. scand. (Stockh.) **150**, 395 (1954). — Klein, O., u. W. Nonnenbruch: Die Funktionsprüfung der Lunge durch Histamin. Z. klin. Med. **125**, 29 (1933). — Knipping, H. W.: Ein einfacher Apparat zur exakten Gasstoffwechseluntersuchung in der Klinik und ärztlichen Praxis. Münch. med. Wschr. **1924**, 553. ~ Über die Möglichkeiten einer rationellen Stickoxydulnarkose. Z. physiol. Chem. **137**, 287 (1924). ~ Über die Bestimmung der Kohlensäurespannung in der Alveolarluft. Z. physiol. Chem. **141**, 1 (1924). ~ Beitrag zur gasanalytischen Technik in der Medizin. Z. exper. Med. **53**, 1 (1926); **66**, 517 (1929). ~ Dyspnoe. Beitr. Klin. Tbk. **82**, 133 (1933). ~ Die Pneumonose. Erg. inn. Med. **48**, 249—260 (1935). ~ Über die respiratorische Insuffizienz. Klin. Wschr. **1935**, 406—409. ~ Über die Funktionsprüfung von Atmung und Kreislauf. Beitr. Klin. Tbk. **88**, 503 (1936). ~ Über die respiratorische Insuffizienz. Beitr. Klin. Tbk. **89**, 95 (1937). ~ Das Verhalten des gesunden und des kranken Körpers unter Arbeit: Ergebnisse der ergometrischen Untersuchung in der Klinik. Klin. Wschr. **1938**, 1097. — Knipping, H. W., W. Bolt, H. Valentin u. H. Venrath: Untersuchung und Beurteilung des Herzkranken. Stuttgart: F. Enke 1955, 1960. ~ Spanische Ausgabe: Exploración clínica y valoración funcional del cardiópata. Editorial Científico-Medica. Barcelona, Madrid, Lisboa, Rio de Janeiro 1959. ~ Normale und pathologische Physiologie der Atmung. In Handbuch der Thoraxchirurgie. Heidelberg: Springer 1957. — Knipping, H. W., W. Bolt, H. Venrath, H. Valentin, H. Ludes u. P. Endler: Eine neue Methode zur Prüfung der Herz- und

Lungenfunktion. Dtsch. med. Wschr. 1955, 1146. — KNIPPING, H. W., W. H. LEWIS and A. MONCRIEFF: Beitr. klin. Tuberk. 79, 1 (1931). — KNIPPING, H. W., H. LUDES, H. VALENTIN u. H. VENRATH: Beitrag zur Differenzierung der Insuffizienz des linken, des rechten Herzens und der Lungen nebst Bemerkungen zur Herzsondierung und zum Defizitproblem. Med. Klin. 1953, 161. — KNIPPING, H. W., and A. MONCRIEFF: The ventilation equivalent for oxygen. Quart. J. Med. 1, 17 (1932). — KNIPPING, H. W., u. H. VALENTIN: Funktionsprüfungen der Atmung. Im Handbuch der Tuberkulose von HEIN, KLEINSCHMIDT. UEHLINGER. 1962. — KOCH, A., u. B. SCHMIDT: Sauerstoffaufnahme und Atemumfang bei körperlicher Arbeit und ihre Bedeutung für die Funktionsprüfung von Herz und Lunge bei Gesunden und Kranken. Z. exper. Med. 112, 612 (1943). — KOLTHOFF, I. M., and J. J. LINGANE: Polarography. New York: Interscience 1952. — KOSSMANN, C. E., and S. A. BRILLER: Oxigram as measure of cardiorespiratory reserve. Proc. Soc. Exper. Biol. a. Med. 65, 63 (1947). — KRAMER, K.: Bestimmung des Sauerstoffgehaltes und der Hämoglobinkonzentration in Hämoglobinlösungen und hämolytischem Blut auf lichtelektrischem Wege. Z. Biol. 95, 126 (1934). ~ Ein Verfahren zur fortlaufenden Messung des Sauerstoffgehaltes im strömenden Blut an uneröffneten Gefäßen. Z. Biol. 96, 61 (1935). — KRAMER, K., J. O. ELAM, G. A. SAXTON and W. N. ELAM: Development of photoelectric methods determination oxygen saturation, hemoglobin and dyes in blood. I. The influence of oxygen saturation and erythrocyte concentration of whole blood. Rapport de l' USAF School of Aviation Medicine Randolph Field-Texas, October 1950. — KRAMER, K., D. E. TIMMONS and H. MAYNE: Development of photoelectric methods determining oxygen saturation, hemoglobin and dyes in blood. II. A photoelectric hypoxia warning device. Rapport de l' USAF School of Aviation Medicine Randolph Field-Texas, Sept. 1950. — KRIETE, B. C., B. G. FERRIS jr. and L. E. KRUGER: Pulmonary mechanics in patients with poliomyelitis involving muscles of respiration. Clin. Res. Proc. 2, 74 (1954). — KROGH, A.: Some new methods for tonometric determination of gastension in fluids. Skand. Arch. Physiol. (Berl. u. Lpz.) 20, 259 (1908). ~ Bicycle ergometer and respiration apparatus for experimental study of muscular work. Skandinav. Arch. Physiol. (Berl. u. Lpz.) 30, 375 (1913). ~ Anatomie und Physiologie der Capillaren. Berlin 1929. — KROGH, A., u. M. KROGH: On the tension of gases in the arterial blood. Skand. Arch. Physiol. (Berl. u. Lpz.) 23, 179 (1910). — KROGH, A., and J. LINDHARD: Regulation of respiration and circulation during initial stages of muscular work. J. of Physiol. 47, 112 (1913). ~ On average composition of alveolar air and its variations during respiratory cycle. J. of Physiol. 47, 431 (1914). ~ The volume of dead space is breathing and the mixing of gases in the lungs of man. J. of Physiol. 51, 59—90 (1917). — KROGH, M.: Diffusion of gases through lungs of man. J. of Physiol. 49, 271 (1915). — KRUHØFER, P.: Studies on the lung diffusion coefficient for carbon monoxide in normal human subjects by means of $C^{14}O$. Acta physiol. scand. (Stockh.) 32, 106 (1954).

LACHNIT, V.: Wien. Z. inn. Med. 31, 227 (1950). — LAGERLÖF, H., and L. WERKÖ: Studies on the circulation of blood in man. Scand. J. Clin. a. Labor. Invest. 1, 147 (1949). — LAMBERTSON, C. J. u. Mitarb.: Comparison of relationship of respiratory minute volume to pCO_2 and p_H of arterial and internal jugular blood in normal man during hyperventilation produced by low concentrations of CO_2 at 1 atmosphere and by O_2 at 3.0 atmospheres. J. Appl. Physiol. 5, 803 (1953). — LAMPE, R.: Über die Bestimmung der venösen Sauerstoff- und Kohlensäurespannung. Z. exper. Med. 101, 2 (1937). — LANDEN, H. C.: Die funktionelle Beurteilung des Lungen- und Herzkranken. Darmstadt: Dr. Dietrich Steinkopff 1954. — LANG, K.: Der intermediäre Stoffwechsel. Lehrbuch der Physiologie, herausgeg. von W. TRENDELENBURG u. E. SCHÜTZ. Berlin-Göttingen-Heidelberg: Springer 1952. — LARMI, R. K. I.: Spirometric and gas analytic studies in pulmonary insufficiency at rest and during graduated exercise. Scand. J. Clin. a. Labor. Invest. 6, Suppl. 12 (1954). — LASSEN, H. C. A., A. COURNAND and D. O. RICHARDS jr.: Distribution of respiratory gases in closed breathing circuit. I. In normal subjects. J. Clin. Invest. 16, 1 (1937). — LAVENNE, F., O. L. WADE, P. HUGH-JONES et J. C. GILSON: Prédiction du volume pulmonaire résiduel à partir de mesuration thoraciques et radiologiques. J. franç. Méd. et Chir. thor. 8, 1 (1954). — LECHTENBÖRGER, H., H. VALENTIN u. H. VENRATH: Beitrag zur Beurteilung von Bronchialstenosen in der Klinik der Bronchialtumoren. Z. ges. exp. Med. 117, 638 (1951). — LECHTENBÖRGER, H., H. VALENTIN, H. VENRATH, G. FRUHMANN, I. S. ÖZSOY, H. STEINFORT, TH. SCHMITZ u. H. GRIESEMANN: Der Gasstoffwechsel bei akutem Atemstillstand. Thoraxchirurgie 2, H. 3 (1954). — LEHMANN, G.: Die Wasserstoffionenmessung. Leipzig: Johann Ambrosius Barth 1948. — LEINER, G. C.: Spirometric and bronchospiremetric studies in pneumothorax. Amer. Rev. Tbc. 50, 267 (1944). — LESLIE, A.: Inspiratory-expiratory vital capacity test of pulmonary function. Amer. J. Med. 13, 809 (1952). — LIEBENOW, R.: Spätwirkungen erschöpfender Muskelarbeit auf den Sauerstoffverbrauch. IV. Mitteilung: Der Verlauf der Erholungskurve unmittelbar nach der Anstrengung. Z. exper. Med. 59, 49 (1928). — LILIENTHAL jr., J. L., R. L. RILEY, D. D. PROEMMEL and R. E. FRANKE: Experimental analysis in man of oxygen pressure gradient from alveolar air to arterial blood during rest and exercise at sea level and at altitude.

Amer. J. Physiol. **147**, 199 (1946). — Lilly, J. C.: Studies on mixing of gases within respiratory system with new type nitrogen meter. Federat. Proc. **5**, 64 (1946). ~ Respiratory system: Methods; gas analysis (O. Glaser). Medical Physics, vol. 2, p. 845. Chicago: Year Book Publ. 1950. ~ Flow meter for recording respiratory flow of human subjects. In Methods in Medical Research. Edit. by J. H. Comroe jr., vol. 2. Chicago: Year Book Publ. 1950. — Lilly, J. C., V. Legallais and R. Cherry: Variable capacitor for measurement of pressure and mechanical displacements: theoretical analysis and its experimental evaluation. J. Appl. Physiol. 18, 613 (1947). — Lindgren, I., J. Mead, E. A. Gaensler and J. I. Whittenberger: Pulmonary mechanics in emphysema. Clin. Res. Proc. **1**, 115 (1953). — Lindhard, J.: The dead space in breathing. Proc. Physiol. Soc. Lond. **1944**, 44. — Lob, M.: Contrôle oxymétrique du déficit oxygéne. Schweiz. med. Wschr. **1950**, 99. — Loeschcke, H. H.: Über den Gasaustausch in der Lunge unter normalen und pathologischen Bedingungen. Arch. physik. Ther. **6**, 69 (1954). ~ Über den Gasaustausch in der Lunge. Klin. Wschr. **1954**, 145—153. — Loeschcke, H. H., E. Opitz u. W. Schoedel: Eine Methode zur fortlaufenden automatischen Registrierung des alveolaren Sauerstoff- und Kohlensäuregehaltes. Arch. Physiol. **243**, 126 (1939). — Luft, K. F.: Z. techn. Physik **24**, 97 (1943). — Lundsgaard, C., and D. D. van Slyke: Studies of lung volume. I. Relation between thorax size and lung volume in normal adults. J. of Exper. Med. **27**, 65 (1918). ~ Cyanosis. Medicine **2**, 1 (1923).

Malamos, A.: Klinische Prüfung der Leistungsfähigkeit der Lungen im Stufenverfahren. Klin. Wschr. **1939**, 468. — Malmström, G., u. P. A. Michas: Oxygen and carbon dioxide partial pressures in blood from the systemic circulation and the pulmonary capillaries. Acta med. scand. (Stockh.) **145**, 91 (1953). — Maloney jr., J. V., W. S. Derrick, J. L. Whittenberger and J. P. Isaacs: Method for measurement of pulmonary ventilation during anesthesia. Anesthesiology **13**, 571 (1952). — Marsh, K.: Double lumen catheter for bronchospirometry. J. Thorac. Surg. **25**, 495 (1953). — Martin, C. J., F. Cline jr. and H. Marshall: Lobar alveolar gas concentrations: effect of body position. J. Clin. Invest. **32**, 617 (1953). — Master, A. M.: Physiological basis of medicine. A Lecture. Postgraduate Course, Amer. Coll. of Physicans, Chicago, June 1948. ~ The two-step exercise electrocardiogram — A preliminary follow-up study of 200 cases. Bull. New York Acad. Med. **27**, 383 (1951). — Matheson, H. W., and J. S. Gray: Ventilatory function tests. III. Resting ventilation, metabolism, and derived measures. J. Clin. Invest. **29**, 688 (1950). — Matheson, H. W., S. N. Spies, J. S. Gray and D. R. Barnum: Ventilatory function tests. II. Factors affecting the voluntary ventilation capacity. J. Clin. Invest. **29**, 682 (1950). — Mathieu, L., J. P. Grilliat et P. Pillot: Variations de l'air résiduel au cours du rétrécissement mitral. Arch. Mal. Cœur **45**, 341 (1953). ~ Les modifications du volume pulmonaire résiduel lors de la décompensation cardiaque des emphysémateux. Arch. Mal Cœur **45**, 539 (1953). — Matthes, K.: Über den Einfluß der Atmung auf die Sauerstoffsättigung des Arterienblutes. Arch. exper. Path. u. Pharmakol. **176**, 683 (1934). ~ Untersuchungen über die Sauerstoffsättigung des menschlichen Arterienblutes. Arch. exper. Path. u. Pharmakol. **179**, 698 (1935). ~ Über die Regulation von Kreislauf und Atmung im Dienste des respiratorischen Gaswechsels. Erg. inn. Med. **53**, 169 (1937). ~ Kreislaufuntersuchungen am Menschen mit fortlaufend registrierenden Methoden. Stuttgart: Georg Thieme 1951. ~ Patho-Physiologie des Lungenkreislaufs. Arch. physik. Ther. **6**, 80 (1954). — Maurath, J.: Pathophysiologie der Atmung in der Lungenchirurgie. Stuttgart: Georg Thieme 1955. — McMichael, J.: Rapid method of determining lung capacity. Clin. Sci. **4**, 167 (1939). ~ Hyperpnea in heart failure. Clin. Sci. **4**, 19 (1939). — McMichael, J., and E. P. Sharpey-Schafer: The action of intravenous Digoxin in man. Quart. J. Med. **13**, 123 (1944). — Mead, J., N. R. Frank, I. Lindgren, E. A. Gaensler and J. L. Whittenberger: Technic for measurement of pulmonary compliance and resistance: its application to normal patients and patients with mitral stenosis. Clin. Res. Proc. **1**, 116 (1953). — Mead, J., and J. L. Whittenberger: Physical properties of human lungs measured during spontaneous respiration. J. Appl. Physiol. **5**, 779 (1953). ~ Evaluation of airway interruption technique as a method for measuring pulmonary air flow resistance. J. Appl. Physiol. **6**, 408 (1954). — Meakins, J. C., and H. W. Davies: Respiratory function in disease. Edinburgh: Oliver & Boyd 1925. — Meakins, J., and C. N. H. Long: Oxygen consumption, oxygen debt and lactic acid in circulatory failure. J. Clin. Invest. **4**, 273 (1927). — Meessen, H.: Zur pathologischen Anatomie des Lungenkreislaufs. Verh. dtsch. Ges. Kreisl.-forsch. **17**, 25 (1951). — Meneely, G. R., and N. L. Kaltreider: Volume of lung determined by helium dilution: Description of method and comparison with other procedures. J. Clin. Invest. **28**, 129 (1949). — Meyer, F.: Über die Messung des Sauerstoffdrucks im Gewebe und die relative Anoxie der Kreislaufkranken. Klin. Wschr. **1935**, 627. ~ Eine neue Definition der Herzschwäche. Klin. Wschr. **20**, 468 (1941). — Miller, F., A. Hemingway, R. L. Varco and A. O. C. Nier: Alveolar ventilation studies using mass spectrometer. Proc. Soc. Exper. Biol. a. Med. **74**, 13 (1950). — Miller, R. D., W. S. Fowler and H. F. Helmholz jr.: The relationship of arterial hyoxemia to disability and to cor pulmonale with congestive failure in patients with chronic pulmonary emphysema. Proc. Staff Meet. Mayo Clin.

28, 737 (1953). — MILLS, J. N.: Influence upon vital capacity of procedures calculated to alter volume of blood in lungs. J. of Physiol. 110, 207 (1949). — MINET, J., M. FONTAN et A. BONDUELLE: Presse méd. (Paris) 55, 389 (1947). — MONTGOMERY, H., and O. HORWITZ: Oxygen tension of tissues by polarographic method. I. Introduction. Oxygen tension and blood flow of skin of human extremities. J. Clin. Invest. 29, 1120 (1950). — MOTLEY, H. L.: Pulmonary function studies in bituminous coal miners. West Virginia Med. J. 46, 8 (1950). ~ Use of pulmonary function tests for disability appraisal: including evaluation standards in chronic pulmonary disease. Dis. Chest 24, 378—389 (1953). — MOTLEY, H. L., B. GORDON, L. P. LANG and P. A. THEODOS: Arch. industr. Hyg. 1, 133 (1950). — MOTLEY, H. L., L. P. LANG and B. GORDON: Pulmonary emphysema and ventilation measurements in one hundred anthracite coal miners with respiratory complaints. Amer. Rev. Tbc. 59, 270 (1949). ~ Studies of the respiratory gas exchanges in one hundred anthracite coal miners with pulmonary complaints. Amer. Rev. Tbc. 61, 201 (1950). — MOTLEY, H. L., and J. F. TOMASHEFSKI: Effect of high and low oxygen levels and intermittent positive pressure breathing on oxygen transport in lungs in pulmonary fibrosis and emphysema. J. Appl. Physiol. 3, 189 (1950). — MUNDT, E., W. SCHOEDEL, u. H. SCHWARZ: Über die Gleichmäßigkeit der Lungenbelüftung. Arch. ges. Physiol. 244, 99 (1940).

NEERGAARD, K. v.: Neue Auffassung über einen Grundbegriff der Atemmechanik. Z. exper. Med. 66, 373 (1929). — NEERGARD, K. v., u. K. WIRZ: Über eine Methode zur Messung der Lungenelastizität am lebenden Menschen, insbesondere beim Emphysem. Z. klin. Med. 105, 35 (1927). — NISELL, O.: The influence of blood gases on the pulmonary vessels of the cat. Acta physiol. scand. (Stockh.) 23, 85 (1951). — NOELPP-ESCHENHAGEN, B. NOELPP, K. LOTTERBACH u. G. FORSTER: Untersuchungen zur Genese der Dyspnoe. Z. exper. Med. 123, 258 (1954). — NORDENSTRÖM, B.: Temporary unilateral occlusion of pulmonary artery. Method of roentgen examination of pulmonary vessels. Acta radiol. (Stockh.) Suppl. 108, 1 (1954). — NYLIN, G.: Clinical tests of function of heart. Acta med. scand. (Stockh.) Suppl. 52, 1 (1933).

OLIVIER, H. R., and P. DRUTEL: Méthode de dépistage des petites insuffisances de la ventilation pulmonaire. Soc. Biol. 22, 1 (1949). — OPITZ, E., u. H. BARTELS: Gasanalyse. In HOPPE-SEYLER/THIERFELDER, Handbuch der physiologisch-pathologisch-chemischen Analyse, Bd. II, S. 183. Berlin: Springer 1955. — OPITZ, E., u. M. SCHNEIDER: Über die Sauerstoffversorgung des Gehirns und den Mechanismus von Mangelwirkungen. Erg. Physiol. 46, 126 (1950). — ORNSTEIN, G. G.: Measurement of function of lungs. Dis. Chest 15, 280—302 (1949). — ORSÒS, R.: Gerüstsystem der Lunge. Beitr. Klin. Tbk. 87 (1936). — OSHER, W. J.: Change of vital capacity with assumption of supine position. Amer. J. Physiol. 161, 352—357 (1950). — OTIS, A. B., and W. C. BEMBOWER: Effect of gas density on resistance to respiratory gas flow in man. J. Appl. Physiol. 2, 300 (1949). — OTIS, A. B., W. O. FENN and H. RAHN: Mechanics of breathing in man. J. Appl. Physiol. 2, 592 (1950).

PACE, N., W. V. CONSOLAZIO, A. W. WHITE jr. and A. R. BEHNKE: Formulation of the principal factors affecting the rate of uptake of carbon monoxide by man. Amer. J. Physiol. 147, 352 (1946). — PAINE, J. R.: Clinical measurement of pulmonary elasticity. Comparison of methods of CHRISTIE and MCINTOSH and of NEERGARD and WIRZ. J. Thorac. Surg. 99, 550 (1940). — PAPPENHEIMER, I. R., A. P. FISHMAN and L. M. BORRERO: New experimental methods of determination of effective alveolar gas composition in respiratory dead space in the anaesthetized and man. J. of Physiol. 4, 855 (1952/53). — PAPPENHEIMER, I. R. u. Mitarb.: Standardization of definitions and symbols in respiratory physiology. Federat. Proc. 9, 602 (1950). — PARKER jr., F., and S. WEISS: The nature and significance of the structural changes in the lungs in mitral stenosis. Amer. J. Path. 12, 573 (1936). — PASARGIK-LIAN, M.: Über die Methoden R. MARGARIAS und H. W. KNIPPINGS beim Studium der Atemfunktion. Experimentelle Untersuchungen bei der Silicose und der Lungentuberkulose. Beitr. Klin. Tbk. 110, 351 (1953). — PEIN, H. v.: Die Messung des Gasstoffwechsels bei Belastungen als Herzfunktionsprüfung. Z. klin. Med. 132, 227 (1937). — PETERS, J. P., and D. D. v. SLYKE: Quantitative clinical chemistry. Baltimore: Williams & Wilkins company 1932. — PETZOLD, G.: Die Beurteilung der Lungenfunktionsprüfung für die Klinik der Lungentuberkulose. Beitr. klin. Tbc. 98, 552 (1942). — PFUND, H. H., and W. G. FASTIE: J. opt. Soc. Amer. 37, 762 (1947). — PINNER, M., G. C. LEINER and W. A. ZAVOD: Bronchospirometry. III. Functional capacity of normal lungs, severely damaged lungs, lungs with strictly parenchymal lesions, thoracoplasty lungs, and reexpanded pneumothorax lungs. J. Thorac. Surg. 11, 241 (1942). — POISEUILLE, J. M.: Recherches expérimentales sur le mouvement des liquides dans les tubes de très-petits diamètres. Ann. Chim. et Physiol. 7, 50—74 (1843). — POPOVIĆ, I., u. P. LALEVIĆ: Spirometric evaluation of respiratory function. Medicinski Glasnik 8, 195 (1954). — PROCTOR, D. F., and J. B. HARDY: Studies of respiratory air flow. I. Significance of normal pneumotachogram. Bull. Johns Hopkins Hosp. 85, 253 (1949).

RADFORD jr., E. P., B. G. FERRIS and B. C. KRIETE: Clinical use of nomogram to estimate proper ventilation during artificial respiration. New England J. Med. 251, 877 (1954). —

Rahn, H.: A concept of mean alveolar air and the ventilation-blood flow relationships during pulmonary gas exchange. Amer. J. Physiol. 158, 21 (1949). — Rahn, H., and H. T. Bahnson: Simultaneous determination of bloodflow through each lung. Federat. Proc. 9, 102 (1950). — Rahn, H., W. O. Fenn and A. B. Otis: Daily variations of vital capacity, residual air and expiratory reserve, including a study of the residual air method. J. Appl. Physiol. 1, 725 (1949). — Rahn, H., H. L. Motley, A. B. Otis and W. O. Fenn: Method for the continuous analysis of alveolar air. J. Aviation Med. 17, 173 (1946). — Rahn, H., and A. B. Otis: Alveolar air during simulated flights to high altitudes. Amer. J. Physiol. 150, 202 (1947). ~ Continuous analysis of alveolar gas composition during work hyperpnea, hypercapnia and anoxia. J. Appl. Physiol. 1, 717 (1949). — Rahn, H., A. B. Otis, L. E. Chadwick and W. O. Fenn: Pressure-volume diagram of thorax and lung. Amer. J. Physiol. 146, 161 (1946). — Ramser, O.: Über den Wirkungsgrad verschiedener Broncholytika bei Asthma bronchiale. Helvet. med. Acta 20, 86 (1953). — Rauwerda, P. E.: Unequal ventilation of different parts of lung and determination of cardiac output. Groningen: Groningen University 1946. — Regli, J., u. F. Wyss: Die Ursachen der Dyspnoe. Praxis (Bern) 1954, 514—516. — Reichert, P., and H. Roth: Ventilograph: Improved recording ventilometer and its application. J. Labor. a. Clin. Med. 25, 1091—1096 (1940). — Reichmann, V.: Verh. dtsch. Ges. Kreislaufforsch. 13, 66 (1940). ~ Beitr. Silikoseforsch. Bochum, H. 7, 1 (1950). — Richards jr., D. W.: Respiratory system: External respiration. In O. Glaser, Medical Physics, vol. II, p. 836. Chicago: Year Book Publ. 1950. ~ Nature of cardiac and of pulmonary dyspnea. Circulation (New York) 7, 15 (1953). — Riley, R. L.: Pulmonary gas exchange. Amer. J. Med. 10, 210 (1951). — Riley, R. L., and A. Cournand: „Ideal" alveolar air und the analysis of ventilations perfusion relationship in the lungs. J. Appl. Physiol. 1, 811, 825 (1949). ~ Analysis of factors affecting partial pressures of oxygen and carbon dioxide in gas and blood of lungs: Theory. J. Appl. Physiol. 4, 77 (1951). — Riley, R. L., A. Cournand and K. W. Donald: Analysis of factors affecting partial pressures of O_2 and CO_2 in gas and blood of lungs: I. Theory, II. Methods. J. Appl. Physiol. 4, 77—101, 102—120 (1951). — Riley, R. L., A. Himmelstein, H. L. Motley and A. Cournand: Studies of the pulmonary circulation at rest and during exercise in normal individuals and in patients with chronic pulmonary disease. Amer. J. Physiol. 152, 372 (1948). — Riley, R. L., J. L. Lilienthal jr., D. D. Proemmel and R. E. Franke: On the determination of the physiological effective pressures of oxygen and carbon dioxide in alveolar air. Amer. J. Physiol. 147, 191 (1946). — Riley, R. L. u. Mitarb.: On determination of physiologically effective pressures of O_2 and CO_2 in alveolar air. Amer. J. Physiol. 147, 191 (1946). — Riley, R. L., D. D. Proemmel and R. E. Franke: Direct method for determination of O_2 and CO_2 tensions in blood. J. of Biol. Chem. 161, 621 (1945). — Riley, R. L., M. C. Riley and H. D. McHill: Diffuse pulmonary sarcoidosis. Diffusing capacity during exercise and other lung function studies in relation to ACTH therapy. Bull. Johns Hopkins Hosp. 91, 345 (1952). — Riley, R. L., R. H. Shepard, J. E. Cohn, D. G. Caroll and B. W. Armstrong: Maximal diffusing capacity of the lungs. J. Appl. Physiol. 6, 573 (1954). — Rinck, H., H. Venrath, H. Valentin u. Th. Schmitz: Diffusionsstörungen in den Lungen bei alten Insuffizienzen des linken Herzens und bei der Mitralstenose, nebst einigen Bemerkungen zur Operation der Mitralfehler. Thoraxchirurgie 1, 403 (1954). — Rink, H.: Lungenfunktion und Lungenchirurgie. Eine lungenangiographische Untersuchung. Z. Tbk. 106, 11—30 (1955). — Robertson, J. S., W. E. Siri and H. B. Jones: Lung ventilation patterns determined by analysis of nitrogen elimination rates: Use of mass spectrometer as continuous gas analyzer. J. Clin. Invest. 29, 577 (1950). — Robinson, S.: Experimental studies of physical fitness relation to age. Arb. physiol. 10, 251 (1938). — Roelsen, E.: Composition of alveolar air investigated by fractional sampling. Acta med. scand. (Stockh.(98, 141 (1939). — Roelsen, E., u. N. Bay: Acta med. scand. 103, 55 (1940). — Rössel, W., L. Wullen, H. Valentin u. H. Venrath: Atmung und Sauerstoffaufnahme des gesunden Menschen bei dosierter Arbeit während artifizieller Insulinhypoglykämie. Z. klin. Med. 152, 552—559 (1955). — Rohrer, F.: Der Zusammenhang der Atemkräfte und ihre Abhängigkeit vom Dehnungszustand der Atmungsorgane. Arch. ges. Physiol. 165, 419 (1916). ~ Physiologie der Atembewegung. In Handbuch der normalen und pathologischen Physiologie, Bd. II. Berlin 1925. — Rona, P., u. H. W. Knipping: Praktikum der physiologischen Chemie, Bd. IV. 1926. — Roos, A., and J. A. Rich: Spectrophotometric determination of oxyhemoglobin saturation and oxygen content of blood. J. Labor. a. Clin. Med. 40, 431 (1952). — Ross, A., and H. Black: Direct determination of partial and total tensions of respiratory gases in blood. Amer. J. Physiol. 160, 163 (1950). — Rossier, P. H.: Lungenkreislauf und Lungenfunktion. Verh. dtsch. Ges. Kreislaufforsch. (17. Tagg) 1951, 67. ~ Zur Physiopathologie der Atmung. Beitr. Klin. Tbk. 110, 13 (1953). — Rossier, P. H., u. E. Blickenstorfer: Espace mort et hyperventilation. Helvet. med. Acta 13, 328 (1946). — Rossier, P. H., u. H. Bucher: Z. Unfallmed. Zürich 40, 159 (1947). — Rossier, P. H., u. A. Bühlmann: Vjschr. naturforsch. Ges. Zürich 95, Beih. 2/3, 51 (1950). — Rossier, P. H., A. Bühlmann u. P. Luchsinger: Bemerkungen über Diffusionsstörungen der Lunge. Schweiz. med. Wschr. 1954, 25. — Rossier, P. H., A. Bühlmann u. H. R. Müller: Expace mort respiratoire et clearance alvéolaire. Schweiz.

med. Wschr. 1953, 577. — Rossier, P. H., and K. Wiesinger: Fonction pulmonaire et physio-pathologie. Rev. Tbc. 12, 461 (1948). — Roth, P.: Modifications of apparatus and improved technique adaptable to Benedict type of respiratory apparatus. Boston Med. J. 186, 457—498 (1922). — Rothstein, E., F. B. Landis and B. G. Narodick: Broncho-spirometry in lateral decubitus position. J. Thorac. Surg. 19, 821 (1950). — Roughton, F. J. W.: Average time spent by blood in human lung capillary and its relation to rates of CO uptake and elimination in man. Amer. J. Physiol. 143, 621 (1945). — Roughton, F. J. W., R. C. Darling and W. S. Root: Factors affecting determination of oxygen capacity, content and pressure in human arterial blood. Amer. J. Physiol. 142, 708 (1944). — Ruff, S., u. H. Strughold: Grundriß der Luftfahrtmedizin. Leipzig 1939. — Ruyssen, L.: L'examen de la fonction respiratoire dans l'expertise des silicotiques. Rev. méd. Nancy 76, 147 (1951). — Ryan, J. M., and J. B. Hickam: Alveolar-arterial oxygen pressure gradient in anemia. J. Clin. Invest. 31, 188 (1952).

Sadoul, P.: Exploration de la fonction pulmonaire dans les pneumoconioses. XXVII. Congr. Internat. de Médecine du Travail Strassbourg 1954. — Sadoul, P., et J. P. Grilliat: Bronchospirométrie. II. Les volumes pulmonaires, la ventilation minute. Poumon (Paris) 10 (1954). — Santenoise, D.: L'exploration biochimique des centres respiratoires. Exposés annuels de Biochimie, 12. sér., p. 223. Paris: Masson & Cie. 1950. — Sarnoff, S. J., E. A. Gaensler and J. V. Maloney jr.: Electrophrenic respiration. IV. Effectiveness of contralateral ventilation during activity of one phrenic nerve. J. Thorac. Surg. 19, 929 (1950). — Scherrer, M.: Das Studium der intrapulmonalen Gasmischung zur Beurteilung der ungleichmäßigen Ventilation und Perfusion der Lungen. Acta davosiana 14, 7 (1955). — Schmidt, C. F.: The reflex regulation of respiration, in Maclead's physiology in modern medicinie, 9. edit. St. Louis: C. V. Mosby & Comp. 1941. — Schmidt, F., N. v. d. Broek, and M. Scherrer: Respiratory function tests and their clinical application. Tubercle 36, 328 (1955). — Schmidt, H.: Die essentielle Hypertonie des Lungenkreislaufes und deren Beziehung zur sogenannten Pulmonalsklerose. Arch. Kreislaufforsch. 19, 91 (1953). — Schneider, M., u. W. Schoedel: Neuere Methoden der Spirographie und Spirometrie. In Handbuch der biologischen Arbeitsmethoden, Abt. IV, Teil 13, S. 835. 1937. — Schoedel, W.: Alveolarluft. Erg. Physiol. 39, 450—488 (1937). — Schoen, R., u. E. Derra: Untersuchungen über die Bedeutung der Cyanose als klinisches Symptom. — Cyanose durch chronische Stauung im Lungenkreislauf, besonders bei Mitralstenosen. Dtsch. Arch. klin. Med. 168, 52, 176 (1930). — Scholander, P. F.: Analyser for accurate estimations of respiratory gases in one-half cubic centimeters samples. J. of Biol. Chem. 167, 235 (1947). — Scholander, P. F., S. C. Flemister and L. Irving: Microgasometric estimation of blood gases. J. of Biol. Chem. 169, 173 (1947). — Scholander, P. F., and F. J. W. Roughton: Microgasometric estimation of blood gases. J. of Biol. Chem. 148, 573 (1943). — Segal, M. S., and M. J. Dulfano: Chronic pulmonary emphysema: Physiopathology and treatment. New York: Grune & Stratton 1953. — Selzer, A.: Chronic cyanosis. Amer. J. Med. 10, 334 (1951). — Shock, N. W., and A. B. Hastings: Studies of acid-base balance of blood. I. Microtechnic for determination of acid-base balance of blood. J. of Biol. Chem. 104, 565 (1934). — Shuford, W. H., W. B. Seaman and A. Goldman: Pulmonary manifestation of scleroderma. A. M. A. Arch. Int. Med. 92, 85—97 (1953). — Siebeck, R.: Über den Gasaustausch zwischen der Außenluft und den Alveolen. III. Die Lungenventilation beim Emphysem. Dtsch. Arch. klin. Med. 102, 390 (1911). — Silverman, L.: Respiratory air flow characteristics and their relation to certain lung conditions occurring in industry. J. Industr. Hyg. a. Toxicol. 28, 183 (1946). — Silverman, L., R. C. Lee and C. K. Drinker: New method for studying breathing, with observations upon normal and abnormal subjects. J. Clin. Invest. 23, 907 (1944). — Silverman, L., G. Lee, R. Plotkin, L. A. Sawyer and A. R. Yancey: Air flow measurements on human subjects with and without respiratory resistance at several work rates. Arch. Industr. Hyg. a. Occup. Med. 3, 461 (1951). — Simonin, P., P. Drutel et J. Dechoux: L'insuffisance ventilatoire dans la silicose pulmonaire. Etude spirographique. Arch. Mal. profess. 14, 461 (1953). — Simonin, P., J. Girard, J. P. Grilliat u. Mitarb. Etude spirographique de l'emphysème bronchique. Semaine Hôp. 30, 367 (1954). — Simonin, P., J. Girard, P. Sadoul u. Mitarb.: Place de la spirographie dans l'étude de la fonction respiratoire. Semaine Hop. 30, 351 (1954). — Simonson, E., and N. Enzer: Physiology of muscular exercise and fatigue in disease. Medicine 21, 345 (1942). — Singer, R. B., and A. B. Hastings: Improved clinical method for estimation of disturbances of acid-base balance of human blood. Medicine 27, 223 (1948). — Sjöstrand, T.: Über die Bedeutung der Lungen als Blutdepot beim Menschen. Acta physiol. scand. (Stockh.) 2, 231—248 (1941). — Slyke, D. D. van, and J. M. Neill: Determination of gases in blood and other solutions by vacuum extraction and manometric measurement. J. of Biol. Chem. 61, 523 (1924). — Slyke, D. D. van, and J. Sendroy jr.: Studies of gas and electrolyte equilibria in blood. XV. Line charts for graphic calculations by Henderson-Hasselbalch equation, and for calculating plasma carbon dioxide content from whole blood content. J. of Biol. Chem. 79, 781 (1928). — Sonne, C.: On movements in lungs during respiration: Survey of problems and description of apparatus. Acta med. scand. (Stockh.) **105**, 313—328 (1940). — Spain, M. D.: Ann. intern. Med. **33**, 1150 (1950). — Stead, W. W., D. L. Fry and R. V. Ebert: Elastic properties of lung in normal man and in patients with chronic pulmonary emphysema. J. Labor. a. Clin. Med. **40**, 674 (1952). — Steinmann, E. P.: Zur Frage der Bronchospirometrie. Praxis (Bern) **1949**, 799. — Stewart, C. A.: Vital capacity of lungs of children in health and disease. Amer. J. Dis. Childr. **24**, 451—496 (1922). — Stone, D. J., A. Schwartz, J. A. Feldman, F. J. Lovelock and D. Denolin: Pulmonary function in sarcoidosis. Results with cortisone therapy. Amer. J. Med. **15**, 468 (1953). — Stroud, R. C., and H. Rahn: Effect of O_2 and CO_2 tension upon resistance of pulmonary blood vessels. Amer. J. Physiol. **172**, 211 (1953). — Sutton, F. C., J. A. Britton and J. G. Carr: Estimation of cardiopulmonary functional capacity by means of oxygen debt studies. Amer. Heart J. **20**, 423 (1940).

Taylor, C.: Some properties of maximal and submaximal exercise with reference to physiological variation and measurement of exercise tolerance. Amer. J. Physiol. **142**, 200 (1944). — Tenney, S. M.: Ventilatory response to carbon dioxide in pulmonary emphysema. J. Appl. Physiol. **6**, 477 (1954). — Tietz, N.: Herzleistungsquotient und Arbeitsökonomie sowie Lungenvolumina bei Sportlern von 35—70 Jahren. Diss. Köln 1954. — Tiffeneau, R., et P. Drutel: Facteurs alvéolaires et bronchiques des insuffisances de la ventilation pulmonaire. Semaine Hôp. **28**, 1717 (1952). ~ L'épreuve du cycle respiratoire maximum pour l'étude spirographique de la ventilation pulmonaire. Presse méd. **1952**, 640. — Tiffeneau, R., et A. Pinelli: Régulation bronchique de la ventilation pulmonaire. J. franç. Méd. et Chir. thorac. **2**, 221 (1948). ~ La capacité pulmonaire utilisable à l'effort; test pour l'exploration de la fonction ventilatoire pulmonaire. 10. Congr. Nat. Tub. Strasbourg, Mai 1948. — Toussaint, C.: Technique de la mesure de l'air résiduel fonctionnel. Acta med. belg. **3**, 189 (1953).

Uhlenbruck, P.: Beobachtungen zur rechtsventrikulären Herzinsuffizienz. Dtsch. Arch. klin. Med. **163**, 220 (1929). ~ Über die Wirksamkeit der Sauerstoffatmung. Z. exper. Med. **74**, 1 (1930).

Valentin, H.: Der Insuffizienzbegriff in der Herzklinik und die Abgrenzung der Arbeitsinsuffizienz unter besonderer Berücksichtigung klinischer Beurteilungsfragen. Habil.-Schr. Köln 1956. — Valentin, H., u. H. Venrath: Beitrag zur Arterienpunktion in der Lungen- und Herzklinik. Beitr. Klin. Tbk. **101**, 430 (1948). ~ Über das spirographische und das arterielle Sauerstoffdefizit in der Herz- und Lungenklinik. Ärztl. Forsch. **6**, 431 (1952). ~ Die Differenzierung der respiratorischen Arbeitsinsuffizienz von der kardialen Arbeitsinsuffizienz unter besonderer Berücksichtigung der Links- und Rechtsinsuffizienz des Herzens. Beitr. Klin. Tbk. **107**, 35 (1952). ~ Die Spiro-Ergometrie nach Brauer und Knipping. Ein objektiver und quantitativer Test für die Beurteilung der Leistungsfähigkeit des Herzens und der Lungen. Acta med. scand. (Stockh.) **211**, 90 (1952). ~ Aus der Praxis der Herz- und Lungenbegutachtung. Ärztl. Wschr. **1953**, 969. ~ Zur Klinik und Beurteilung der Silikose. Münch. med. Wschr. **1954**, 404. ~ Einige Bemerkungen zu den Herzfunktionsprüfungen im Bereiche der Vita maxima. Münch. med. Wschr. **1955**, 695—698. — Valentin, H., H. Venrath, J. Balodimos u. G. Giovannelli: Die maximale Sauerstoffaufnahme. Z. Kreislaufforsch. **44**, 770 (1955). — Valenzuela, C. u. Mitarb.: Structural changes in intrapulmonary arteries exposed to systemic pressures from birth. Arch. of Path. **57**, 1, 51 (1954). — Veen, G. van, N. G. M. Orie u. J. J. Hirdes: Spirometric lungfunctions investigations. I. A rapid constant volume method for the determination of the fonctional residual air. Acta tbc. scand. (København) **26**, 251 (1952). — Venrath, H.: Die respiratorische Insuffizienz unter besonderer Berücksichtigung der Diffusionsstörungen. Köln 1956. ~ Die Pathophysiologie der Atmung. In Goetze, Lehrbuch der Pathophysiologie. Jena: Gustav Fischer 1959. — Venrath, H., H. Lechtenbörger, H. Valentin u. W. Bolt: Das Verhalten von Atmung und Kreislauf bei uni- und bilateraler Sauerstoffmangelatmung. Ein Beitrag zur Kompensation akuter Hypoxie durch Kreislaufumstellung. Z. Kreislaufforsch. **44**, 544 (1955). — Venrath, H., G. Rotthoff, H. Valentin u. W. Bolt: Bronchospirographische Untersuchungen bei Durchblutungsstörungen im kleinen Kreislauf. Beitr. Klin. Tbk. **107**, 291 (1952). — Venrath, H., H. Valentin u. W. Hollmann: Anwendung und Grenzen der Oxymetrie in der Herz- und Lungenklinik. Ärztl. Wschr. **1955**, 526. — Völker, R.: In Joetten-Gaertner, Funktionsprüfung bei Staublungen-Erkrankungen. Wissenschaftl. Forschungsreihe Bd. 60, S. 55. Darmstadt: Dr. Dietrich Steinkopff 1950. — Vuilleumier, P.: Über eine Methode zur Messung des intraalveolären Drucks und der Strömungswiderstände in den Atemwegen des Menschen. Z. klin. Med. **143**, 698 (1944).

Wachtler, F., u. K. Grabenwöger: Interstitielle Lungenfibrose bei Sklerodermie. Wien. med. Wschr. **1952**, 456. — Wahlund, H.: Dertermination of physical working capacity: Physiological and clinical study with special reference to standardization of cardio-pulmonary functional tests. Acta med. scand. (Stockh.) Suppl. **215**, 1 (1948). — Warring jr., F. C.: Ventilatory function. Experience with simple practical procedure for its evaluation in patients with pulmonary tuberculosis. Amer. Rev. Tbk. **51**, 432 (1945). ~ Ventilatory function: Its evaluation in patients with pulmonary tuberculosis. Amer. Rev. Tbc. **51**, 432—454 (1945). — WELCH, G. E. u. Mitarb.: Comparison of new step test with treadmill test for evaluation of cardiorespiratory working capacity. Amer. J. Med. Sci. **223**, 607 (1952). — WEST, J. R. u. Mitarb.: Effects of cortisone and ACTH in cases of chronic pulmonary disease with impairment of alveolarcapillary diffusion. Amer. J. Med. **10**, 156 (1951). — WEST, J. R., E. DE F. BALDWIN, A. COURNAND and D. W. RICHARDS: Physiopathologic aspects of chronic pulmonary emphysema. Amer. J. Med. **10**, 481 (1951). — WHITEFIELD, A. G., J. A. H. WATERHOUSE and W. M. ARNOTT: Subdivisions of lung volume: Normal standards. Brit. J. Soc. Med. **4**, 1—25 (1950). ~ Total lung volume and its subdivisions: Study in physiological norms. II. Effect of posture. Brit. J. Soc. Med. **4**, 86—97 (1950). — WHITTENBERGER, J. L.: Lung volume and air flow characteristics in asthma. In: Somatic and Psychiatric Treatment of Asthma, p. 50—61. Edit. by H. A. ABRAMSON. Baltimore: Williams & Wilkins 1951. ~ Resuscitation and other uses of artificial respiration. New England J. Med. **251**, 775, 816 (1954). — WIDLUND, G.: Cardio-pulmonal function during pregnancy. Acta obstetr. scand. (Stockh.) Suppl. **25**, 1 (1945). — WIESINGER, K.: Patho-physiologische Differenzierung durch den Sauerstoffversuch. Helvet. med. Acta **14**, 407 (1947). ~ Die polarographische Messung der Sauerstoffspannung im Blut und ihre klinische Anwendung zur Beurteilung der Lungenfunktion. Bull. schweiz. Akad. med. Wiss. **7** (1948). ~ Patho-Physiologie der Atmung. Schweiz. Z. Tbk. Suppl. **1**, 26 (1948). ~ Zur polarographischen Bestimmung der Sauerstoffspannung im ungesättigten Blut. Helvet. physiol. Acta **6**, c 13—c 72 (1948). — WIGGERS, C. J.: Physiology in health and disease. Philadelphia: Lea a. Febiger 1949. — WILLIAMS jr., M. H.: Pulmonary function in Boeck sarcoid. J. Clin. Invest. **32**, 909—913 (1953). ~ Pulmonary function studies in mitral stenosis before and after commissurotomy. J. Clin. Invest. **32**, 1049 (1953). — WILLMON, T. L., and A. R. BEHNKE: Residual lung volume determinations by methods of helium substitution and volume expansion. Amer. J. Physiol. **153**, 138 (1948).— WILSON, R. H., R. V. EBERT, C. W. BORDEN, R. T. PEARSON, R. S. JOHNSON, A. FALK and M. E. DEMPSEY: The determination of blood flow through nonventilated portions of the normal and diseased lung. Amer. Rev. Tbc. **68**, 177 (1953). — WILSON, R. H., R. L. EVANS, R. S. JOHNSON and M. E. DEMPSEY: An estimation of the effective alveolar respiratory surface and other pulmonary facts in normal persons. Amer. Rev. Tbc. **70** (1954). — WILSON, R. H., W. HOSETH and M. E. DEMPSEY: Effects decreasing respiratory minute volume in patients with severe chronic pulmonary emphysema with specific reference to oxygen, morphine and barbiturates. Amer. J. Med. **17**, 464 (1954). — WINTRICH: Zit. nach A. J. ANTHONY u. H. VENRATH, Funktionsprüfung der Atmung, 2. Aufl. (im Druck). — WOLFE, W. A., and L. D. CARLSON: Studies of pulmonary capacity and mixing with nitrogen meter. J. Clin. Invest. **29**, 1568 (1950). — WOOD, E. H.: Normal oxygen saturation of arterial blood during inhalation of air and oxygen. J. Appl. Physiol. **1**, 567 (1949). ~ Oymetrie. Med. Physics **2**, 664 (1950). — WORTH, G., u. E. SCHILLER: Die Pneumokoniosen. Köln: Staufen-Verlag 1954. — WORTH, G., H. VALENTIN, L. GASTHAUS, H. HOFFMANN u. H. VENRATH: Bewirkt die Staubinhalation bei Bergarbeitern eine akute respiratorische Insuffizienz? Arch. Gewerbepath. **14**, 37—57 (1955). ~ Über den unmittelbaren Einfluß der Staubinhalation auf die Lungenfunktion bei Bergarbeitern. Münch. med. Wschr. **1955**, 732—733. — WRIGHT, G. W.: Disability evaluation in industrial pulmonary disease. J. Amer. Med. Assoc. **141**, 1218—1222 (1949). ~ Functional abnormalities of industrial pulmonary fibrosis. Arch. of Industr. Health. **11**, 196—203 (1955). — WRIGHT, G. W., and G. F. FILLEY: Pulmonary fibrosis and respiratory function. Amer. J. Med. **10**, 642 (1951). — WRIGHT, G. W., and E. MICHELSON: Bronchospirometry. In Methods in Medical Research, vol. 2. Edit. by J. H. COMROE jr. Chicago: Year Book Publ. 1950. — WRIGHT, G. W. u. Mitarb.: Observations concerning pathological physiology underlying disease granulomatosis occurring in beryllium workers. Symposium on Military Physiology (Digest Ser. No 4) 1947, p. 135. — WYSS, F.: Untersuchungen mit einem neuen Pneumometer. Hevet. med. Acta **17**, 516 (1950). — WYSS, F., u. W. HADORN: Die Pneumometrie. Fortschr. Allergielehre **3**, 290 (1952). — WYSS, F., u. F. SCHMIDT: Beruht die bronchialasthmatische Dyspnoe auf einer Bronchialstenose? Schweiz. med. Wschr. **1951**, 916.

ZAEPER, G.: Über die Bedeutung und Verwertung arbeitsphysiologischer Erkenntnisse in der Klinik der Lungen- und Kreislaufkranken. Dtsch. Arch. klin. Med. **186**, 1(1940). — ZAVOD, W. A.: Bronchospirography. I. Description of catheter and technique of intubation. J. Thorac. Surg. **10**, 27 (1940). — ZIEGLER, E. E.: New measurement of oxygen absorbing power. Med. Ann. District of Columbia **2**, 225 (1933).— ZIJLSTRA, W. G.: Clinical oximetry (fundamentals and applications). Thèse d'Utrecht 1951, 134 S. — ZORN, O.: Die quantitative Lungen- und Kreislauffunktionsprüfung bei Bergarbeitern (unter besonderem Einschluß der Silikose). Beitr. Klin. Tbk. **94**, 544 (1940). ~ Klin. Wschr. **22**, 618 (1943). ~ Funktionsprüfungen von Atmung und Kreislauf mittels der Spiroergometrie nach BRAUER-KNIPPING. Beitr. Silikoseforsch. **1950**, H. 7, 21. — ZUIDEMA, P., u. M. SCHERRER: Beitrag zur funktionellen Diagnostik des chronisch substantiellen Lungenemphysems. Schweiz. Z. Tbk. **12**, 215 (1955).

Die allgemeine Pathologie der äußeren Atmung.

Von

W. Giese-Münster (Westf.).

Mit 87 Abbildungen.

Zur äußeren Atmung gehören alle Vorgänge, die den Gasaustausch zwischen Luft und Blut in der Lunge möglich machen. Die Luft wird durch die Atembewegungen des Thorax-Lungensystems in die Lungen eingesogen, über das luftleitende Röhrensystem der Bronchien in der Lunge verteilt und den Alveolarräumen zugeführt. In diesen erfolgt der Gasaustausch mit dem Blut, das die Capillaren der Alveolarwand durchströmt und hier in engen Kontakt mit der Alveolarluft tritt. Aufnahme des Sauerstoffs in das Blut und Abgabe der Kohlensäure an die Alveolarluft sind die wesentlichen, für die Erhaltung des Lebens notwendigen Funktionen der äußeren Atmung, während unter innerer Atmung der Gasaustausch in den Geweben und der Transport der Gase mit dem Blut verstanden wird.

Die allgemeine Pathologie der äußeren Atmung befaßt sich mit den Störungen dieser Vorgänge, die sich einteilen lassen in Störungen der Luftbewegung, der intrapulmonalen Luftverteilung, der Gasdiffusion durch die alveolo-capilläre Membran und der Lungendurchblutung, soweit sie zum Gasaustausch in Beziehung steht.

Die Betrachtung dieser Probleme vom morphologischen Standpunkt aus bedeutet eine Beschränkung, da zwar die Vielfalt der geweblichen Veränderungen im Respirationstrakt erkennbar ist, die damit verbundenen Funktionsstörungen in der Regel jedoch nur in einer groben Annäherung abgeschätzt werden können.

Krankhafte Prozesse in der Lunge, in den zuleitenden Luftwegen oder im pulmonalen Gefäßsystem mindern die großen Funktionsreserven des respiratorischen Systems und führen oft zur respiratorischen Insuffizienz. Diese liegt dann vor, wenn im Blut, das die Lunge durchströmt hat, kein ausreichender Gasaustausch erfolgt ist. Sie begegnet uns in ihrer leichten Form als relative oder latente Insuffizienz, wenn der Gasaustausch den Anforderungen bei körperlicher Arbeit nicht mehr genügt (Arbeitsinsuffizienz), und als manifeste Insuffizienz, wenn Sauerstoffuntersättigung oder Kohlensäureüberladung des Blutes auch in körperlicher Ruhe bestehen (Ruheinsuffizienz).

Die Darstellung der Beziehungen zwischen Pathomorphologie und Pathophysiologie der Atemorgane ist Absicht und Ziel dieses Beitrags.

A. Bewegungsstörungen des Thorax-Lungensystems.

I. Anatomische und funktionelle Vorbemerkungen.

a) Die Lunge als elastischer Hohlkörper.

Die Lunge befindet sich als Organ des Luftwechsels in einem dauernden Spannungszustand, der mit der Atembewegung in den Grenzen der Vitalkapazität schwankt. Das Lungenvolumen wird unter normalen Verhältnissen von den Änderungen der Thoraxweite bestimmt, beide Größen sind voneinander abhängig.

Auch in maximaler Exspirationsstellung bleibt die Lunge in einem elastischen Spannungszustand. Wenn der negative Druck im Thoraxraum fortfällt, dann retrahiert sich die Lunge bis zum Ausgleich aller elastischen Kräfte des Lungenkörpers. Diesen Zustand bezeichnen wir als Lungenkollaps. Das nach völliger Exspiration bei der Entspannung noch entweichende Luftvolumen ist die Kollapsluft, der in der Lunge zurückbleibende Rest die Minimalluft. Die Kollapsluft beträgt im Mittel 700—800 ml, die Minimalluft etwa 800 ml. Kollapsluft und Minimalluft sind Anteile der Residualluft, für die Mittelwerte von 1500—1800 ml angegeben werden. In der Leichenlunge ist diese Menge etwas größer, da der Thorax im Tode nicht in völliger Exspirationsstellung, sondern in einer Mittellage stehen bleibt.

Die Kräfte, die mit der inspiratorischen Atembewegung durch die elastische Spannung der Lunge im Thoraxraum erzeugt werden, sind ein wesentlicher Faktor der exspiratorischen Bewegung und damit entscheidend für das Ausmaß des Luftwechsels. Die Atembewegungen sind weitgehend durch das Spiel elastischer Kräfte bedingt, das bei ruhiger Atmung durch nur geringe, vorwiegend inspiratorisch wirkende Muskelkräfte unter Verschiebung der Gleichgewichtslage unterhalten wird[1]. Die Lunge durchläuft dabei entsprechend dem Atemcyclus eine mehr passive und eine mehr aktive Phase, sie ist bewegtes und sich bewegendes Organ. Während der Inspiration wird sie, zwangsläufig der Erweiterung des Brustraumes folgend, passiv gedehnt. Dabei wachsen ähnlich einer unter Spannung geratenden Feder ihre elastischen Kräfte und der Widerstand gegen weitere Dehnung bis zum Umschlag in die Gegenphase ständig an. Die Exspiration ist als die aktive Phase der mechanischen Lungenleistung anzusehen und ganz wesentlich durch die auf die Verkleinerung des Lungenvolumens gerichteten Kräfte der Lunge bestimmt. Bei ruhiger Atmung pendeln die wenig ausgiebigen Verschiebungen um eine Mittellage, in der die elastischen Kräfte der Lunge einerseits und die der Wände des Brustraums andererseits im Gleichgewicht sind. Nach dem Tode verschiebt sich die Mittellage in Richtung der Exspirationsstellung infolge des Fortfalls des Tonus der Inspirationsmuskulatur[2].

1. Begriffsbestimmung der Elastizität.

Eine allgemein anerkannte Definition der Elastizität in der Anwendung auf biologische Fragestellungen ist bisher noch nicht erreicht. Deshalb ist es notwendig, die hier unter Elastizität verstandenen Begriffe näher zu erläutern, da sich in der Literatur unterschiedliche Interpretationen und daraus folgende Mißverständnisse gezeigt haben.

In der Definition der Elastizität lassen sich bestimmte Eigenschaften elastischer Körper in den Vordergrund stellen:

1. Wählt man *den Widerstand*, den der Körper einer verformenden Kraft entgegensetzt, indem er eine elastische Spannung entwickelt, dann kommt man zum Begriff des *Elastizitätsmoduls.*

2. Geht man von der elastischen *Dehnbarkeit* aus, die im Verhältnis zu einer verformenden Kraft eintritt, dann kommt man zum Begriff der *Dehnungszahl* (compliance der amerikanischen Literatur, im deutschen Schrifttum teilweise auch als Komplianz übernommen).

3. Stellt man die *Verformbarkeit* und das *Maß ihrer Rückbildung* in den Mittelpunkt der Definition, dann kommt man zum Begriff der *elastischen Vollkommenheit.*

---

[1] HOFBAUER 1909, 1921, 1925, v. HAYEK 1953, ROSSIER und Mitarbeiter 1956, 1958, LOTTENBACH und Mitarbeiter 1956, PIRCHER 1957, MINKOWSKI und BITTORF 1912.
[2] GAD 1879, BÖNNIGER 1909.

Die strenge Definition der Elastizität ist aus dem Widerstand hergeleitet, den ein Körper als elastische Spannung gegen eine auf ihn einwirkende verformende Kraft entwickelt; sie führt zum Begriff des Elastizitätsmoduls. Vielfach wird statt dessen jedoch der Kehrwert des Elastizitätsmoduls zur Charakterisierung eines Stoffes als sog. Dehnungszahl herangezogen. Hoch dehnbare Stoffe haben danach einen kleinen Modul und umgekehrt. Dabei wird in jedem Fall das Vorliegen elastischer Vollkommenheit vorausgesetzt, d. h. die praktisch momentane und vollständige Rückbildung der Verformung nach Beendigung der Belastung. Sie pflegt im allgemeinen nur innerhalb kleiner Verformungsgrenzen gegeben zu sein. Daß aber hoher Modul und hohe elastische Vollkommenheit durchaus nicht übereinzustimmen brauchen, beweisen gerade die im Sprachgebrauch als hochelastisch bezeichneten Stoffe von der Elastizität vulkanisierten Kautschuks. Sie sind hochdehnbar, haben also einen kleinen Modul und besitzen dabei eine besonders hohe elastische Vollkommenheit; sie können große Verformungen erleiden und diese wieder ausgleichen. Der Unterschied wird im biologischen Bereich aus dem Verhalten der kollagenen und elastischen Fasern deutlich; erstere sind bei hohem Modul bis zu einer Dehnung von 5% der Ausgangslänge, letztere bis zu etwa 50% vollkommen, bis zu 100% Dehnung fast vollkommen elastisch[1]; die elastische Vollkommenheit ist jedoch bei gleicher bezogener Spannung gleich, nur das rückbildbare Dehnungsausmaß differiert[2]. Es ist also sehr wohl auch eine Definition der Elastizität aus dem Maß an reversibler Verformbarkeit möglich. Dieses Prinzip ist bei der sog. technischen Definition von Föppl (1919) angewandt, der unter Elastizität die Fähigkeit versteht, Formänderungsarbeit in nutzbarer Weise vorübergehend zu speichern.

Die letztgenannte Definition, die schon früh von Ranke (1925), Redenz (1927) u. a. gebraucht worden ist und Eingang in das neue Schrifttum gefunden hat[3], erweist sich bei der Betrachtung biologischer Probleme als besonders fruchtbar. So wird man die biologische Bedeutung der elastischen Eigenschaften einer Aortenwand nicht so sehr in ihrer Widerstandsfähigkeit gegen die systolische Druckbelastung zu betrachten, als vielmehr in ihrer Windkesselfunktion zu sehen haben. Ähnlich liegen die Verhältnisse bei der Lunge, deren Retraktionskraft durch die Dehnung während der Inspirationsphase erhöht wird, um dann in der für die Thorax- und Atemmuskulatur vorwiegend passiven Gegenphase exspiratorisch wirksam zu werden.

Gegenüber dieser Ausweitung des klassischen Elastizitätsbegriffes ist jedoch immer wieder gefordert worden, auf den ursprünglichen Begriff des Elastizitätsmoduls zurückzugehen. Danach wäre das schon immer als elastisch bezeichnete Gewebe, speziell auf Grund der besonderen physikalischen Eigenschaften der elastischen Fasern, weniger elastisch als ein kollagenes Gewebe, weil es entsprechend seiner Dehnbarkeit einen kleineren Elastizitätsmodul besitzt. Dies hat auch Triepel (1902) hervorgehoben und weiter bemerkt, daß alle Gewebe bis zu gewissen Belastungsgrenzen elastisch seien, wenn man Elastizität als Fähigkeit zum Wiederausgleich einer erlittenen Verformung definiere; allerdings könnten gerade elastische Fasern sehr große Formveränderungen ausgleichen. Darin liegt aber neben der hohen Dehnbarkeit und dem schnellen Ablauf der elastischen Nachwirkung[4] die charakteristische Eigenschaft, die — wie Redenz (1927) näher ausführt — das hohe Maß an Speicherungsfähigkeit von umkehrbarer Formänderungsarbeit schon bei der Einwirkung relativ kleiner Kräfte ermöglicht. Die alleinige Zugrundelegung des Moduls, der die letztgenannten Eigenschaften nicht erfassen kann, würde also nur zur Einführung eines neuen Begriffes zwingen, um der Bedeutung des elastischen Gewebes gerecht zu werden. Föppl (1919) hat dafür „Ergophilie" und „ergophile Faser" vorgeschlagen, eine sehr treffende Bezeichnung, die sich aber nicht eingebürgert hat. Daher wird im folgenden von Elastizität, elastischer Faser und elastischem Gewebe im Sinne der technischen Definition als Fähigkeit zur Speicherung umkehrbarer Formänderungsarbeit, also im Sinne von Ergophilie, gesprochen.

Da es sich bei der Lunge um einen elastischen Hohlkörper handelt, führt die Beanspruchung zu Volumenänderungen. Man bestimmt als statische Werte die Volumendehnbarkeit (compliance) bzw. deren von manchen Autoren bevorzugten Kehrwert, die Volumenelastizität (elastance). Die mit dem Grad der Dehnung wechselnden Druck-Volumenbeziehungen werden durch die Änderungen der in den verschiedenen Dehnungslagen gültigen Volumenelastizitätsmoduln genauer erfaßt. Der Grad an elastischer Vollkommenheit wird aus dem dynamischen

---

[1] Redenz 1927, v. Schweinitz 1959.   [2] Ranke 1925.
[3] Lottenbach und Mitarbeiter 1956.   [4] Standenath 1928.

Ablauf der Retraktion auf das Ausgangsvolumen und durch Messung etwa auftretender irreversibler Dehnungsrückstände (Hysterese) erkennbar[1]. (Näheres in den folgenden Abschnitten.)

2. Beziehungen zwischen Druck, Volumen und Retraktionskraft (statische Elastizitätswerte).

α) Messungen an der Leichenlunge im Thorax.

Die elastischen Eigenschaften der Lunge sind an der Leichenlunge meßbar. DONDERS (1853, 1859) hat mit einem in die Trachea eingebundenen Manometer den Druck bestimmt, der bei der Eröffnung des Thorax entsteht, und einen Wert von 6 mm Hg gefunden. PERLS (1869) und LOESCHCKE (1928) haben die Messungen mit der gleichen Methode forgesetzt, sind aber nicht zu verwertbaren Ergebnissen gekommen, weil die nicht bestimmbare Ausgangslage der Lunge variiert, etwa bestehende Pleuraverwachsungen den Kollaps behindern und die so häufigen Schleimfüllungen der Bronchien die Meßwerte stark beeinflussen[2].

H. MÜLLER (1922) hat bei Messung des Pleuradruckes an der Leiche ähnliche Werte für den sog. Donderschen Druck der Lunge gefunden, die der Retraktionskraft der Lunge am leichenstarren Thorax entsprechen. Die Fehlerquellen sind die gleichen wie bei den früheren Untersuchungen.

Elastometrische Untersuchungen an der Pleurafläche der geblähten Lunge[3] haben keine sicheren Ergebnisse erbracht.

β) Messungen an der isolierten Leichenlunge.

An der isolierten Leichenlunge haben WINTRICH (1854), LIEBERMEISTER (1907), BÖNNIGER (1909), ROMANOFF (1910/11)[4] diese Messungen fortgesetzt und wesentlich erweitert. Sie füllten die Lunge durch Unterdruck auf und erhielten aus der Variation der zugefüllten Luftmenge Volumen/Druckkurven. Diese zeigen, daß die Retraktionskraft der Lunge mit zunehmender Dehnung anwächst. Die Kurven haben einen leicht S-förmigen Verlauf. Bei maximalem Inspirationsvolumen liegt der Druck etwa bei 22 cm Wasser.

Untersuchungen an der Tierlunge zeigen im Grunde ähnliche Verhältnisse[5]. HARTUNG (1957, 1958, 1959) hat in systematischer Fort-

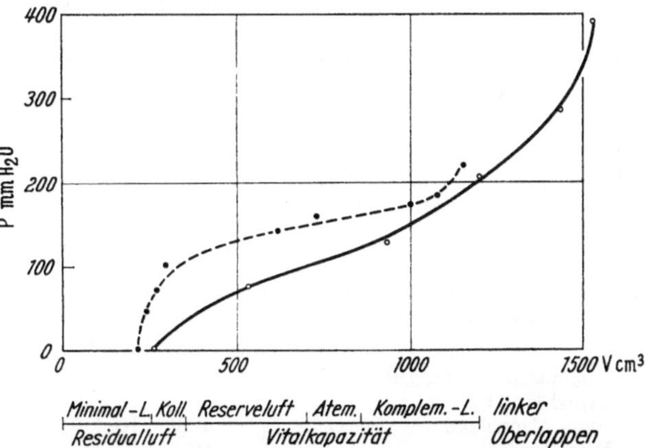

Abb. 1. Druck-Volumendiagramm von dem linken Lungenoberlappen eines 15jährigen Mannes. Die gestrichelte Kurve ist nach Werten von LIEBERMEISTER von der Lunge eines Hingerichteten gezeichnet. Darunter als Vergleich die Volumengrenzen des Lebenden. (Aus HARTUNG 1957.)

führung dieser Versuche die Lungen statt der Füllung im Unterdruck vom Bronchus her aufgebläht und die Messungen bis zur Grenze der Dehnbarkeit fortgesetzt. Jenseits des maximalen Inspirationsvolumens nimmt der Druck im Verhältnis zum Volumen wesentlich stärker zu, die Kurve steigt steil an. Bei

---

[1] Über klinische Messungen s. bei PAINE 1940, LOTTENBACH und Mitarbeiter 1956.
[2] LOESCHCKE 1928, DEAN und VISSCHER 1941.   [3] THIES 1932.
[4] Methodik s. bei LOESCHCKE 1924.   [5] CLOETTA 1913, LAWTON und KING 1949.

einem Druck von 35 cm Wasser wird die Pleura für Luft durchlässig, bei etwa
40 cm Wasserdruck zerreißt das Lungengefüge. Die Kurve gibt das jeweilige
Verhältnis von Druck und Volumen an, man bezeichnet sie als Lungencharakteristik (Abb. 1). Aus ihr kann man den Volumenelastizitätsmodul errechnen.
Hartung (1957) gibt dafür folgende Ableitung:

Für einen elastischen Hohlkörper ist als Maß seiner Elastizität bei Volumbeanspruchung
die Beziehung zwischen Volum- und Druckänderung charakteristisch (1). Dieses Verhältnis
hat Ranke (1925) als Volumelastizität E' (Elastance) bezeichnet, da es außer von der Elastizität des Wandmaterials auch vom Ausgangsvolumen abhängig und somit für vergleichende
Untersuchung von Körpern verschiedenen Ausgangsvolumens nicht brauchbar ist. Will man
den allgemein vergleichbaren Volumelastizitätsmodul ermitteln, so muß das Ausgangsvolumen in die Gleichung eingehen. Dies kann nach v. Neergaard (1927) durch Multiplikation mit dem jeweiligen Gesamtvolumen, in dem das Ausgangsvolumen enthalten ist, geschehen (2); das Gesamtvolumen V ist als Mittelwert der zur Berechnung herangezogenen
Grenzvolumina V_1 und V_2 zu bilden; die manometrisch ermittelten Drucke sind in dyn/cm²
umzurechnen.

$$(1) \qquad E' = \frac{dp}{dV} \left[\frac{\mathrm{dyn}}{\mathrm{cm^5}} \right]$$

$$(2) \qquad E' \cdot V = \varkappa = \frac{dp}{dV} \cdot V \left[\frac{\mathrm{dyn}}{\mathrm{cm^2}} \right].$$

Rossier u. Mitarb. (1958) schlagen eine Multiplikation mit dem Kollapsvolumen vor.
Diese ist für Leichenlungenmessungen weniger gut geeignet, weil das Kollapsvolumen starken
Schwankungen unterliegt und von den zu untersuchenden elastischen Qualitäten wesentlich
bestimmt wird.

Tabelle 1. *Elastizitätswerte der vollelastischen jugendlichen Leichenlunge im Vergleich zu
klinischen Meßwerten.*

	Jugendliche normale Leichenlungen (mittleres Alter 22 Jahre)	Klinische Vergleichswerte
Statische Retraktionskraft (Lungenzug) (Exspiration-Inspiration)	—2 bis —12 cm HOH	etwa —6 cm HOH statischer Mitteldruck
„Komplianz", gesamter Bereich der Vitalkapazität (Mittel)	0,22 Liter/cm HOH	0,23 Liter/cm HOH Dayman 0,21 Liter/cm HOH Mead u. Mitarb. (Emphysematiker, bei ruhiger Atmung)
„Elastance", gesamter Bereich der Vitalkapazität (Mittel)	4,5 cm HOH/Liter (Donders: 4,5 cm HOH/Liter)	4,3 cm HOH/Liter Dayman 7,7 cm HOH/Liter v. Neergaard
Volumelastizitätsmodul ($\Delta p/\Delta V \times V_m$) Inspirationslage Mittellage Exspirationslage	$42,9 \times 10^3$ $18,0 \times 10^3$ $11,9 \times 10^3$ $\left.\right\}\frac{\mathrm{dyn}}{\mathrm{cm^2}}$	liegen nicht vor
Tiffeneau-Test, 2-Sekundenwert aus Vitalkapazitätsauffüllung	46%	$> 90\%$ (1-Sekundenwert $> 70\%$)
Maximale Atemstromstärke in der 1. sec aus Vitalkapazitätsauf-füllung	bis 1,25 Liter/sec	etwa 2—4 Liter/sec
Hysteretischer Dehnungsrest nach mehrfacher Vitalkapazitätsauf-füllung (Akkommodations-breite)	$< 3\%$	(Vorübergehende Restluftver-mehrung nach starken Belastungen des Atem-apparates bekannt)

Zur näheren Charakterisierung der Werte s. Legende zu Tabelle 2, S. 426.

Der Volumelastizitätsmodul läßt sich praktisch also aus den meßbaren Druck- und Volumänderungen berechnen.

$$(2a) \qquad \varkappa_{V_1-V_2} \simeq \frac{p_2-p_1}{V_2-V_1} \cdot \frac{V_1+V_2}{2} \left[\frac{\text{dyn}}{\text{cm}^2} \right].$$

Sein Wert wird um so genauer, je kleiner die gemessenen Änderungen gewählt werden.

Die an Leichenlungen ermittelten statischen Meßwerte der Elastizität stimmen überein mit den Ergebnissen klinischer Messungen am Lebenden. Die Retraktionskraft der Leichenlunge läßt sich auch durch Bestimmung des Retraktionszuges im Rezipienten, analog einer intrapleuralen Druckmessung, ermitteln. Die Werte decken sich im Bereich der Vitalkapazität mit den klinischen Druckwerten im Pleuraspalt (Tabelle 1).

3. Die Retraktionsleistung (dynamische Elastizitätswerte).

Die Bestimmung der Retraktionskraft durch Messung statischer Werte ist die Voraussetzung für das Verständnis physiologischer und pathologischer Vorgänge bei der Atmung. Der Ablauf der Atmung läßt sich an der isolierten Leichenlunge in analoger Weise messend verfolgen wie beim Lebenden[1].

Als Modell dient die Bestimmung des maximalen Exspirationsstoßes, die nach früheren Untersuchungen von VOLHARD (1909, 1921) und RAITHER (1912) als sog. Tiffeneau-Test[2] in der Klinik eine wesentliche diagnostische Bedeutung erlangt hat.

Mit diesem Test wird der nutzbare Anteil der Vitalkapazität in der Weise ermittelt, daß die Versuchsperson nach maximaler Inspiration mit aller Kraft soviel und so schnell als möglich ausatmet. Dabei werden das geatmete Luftvolumen und die Ausatmungszeit bestimmt. In der Klinik wird den Berechnungen der maximalen Ventilationsfähigkeit (Atemgrenzwert) das Ausatmungsvolumen in der ersten Sekunde zugrunde gelegt.

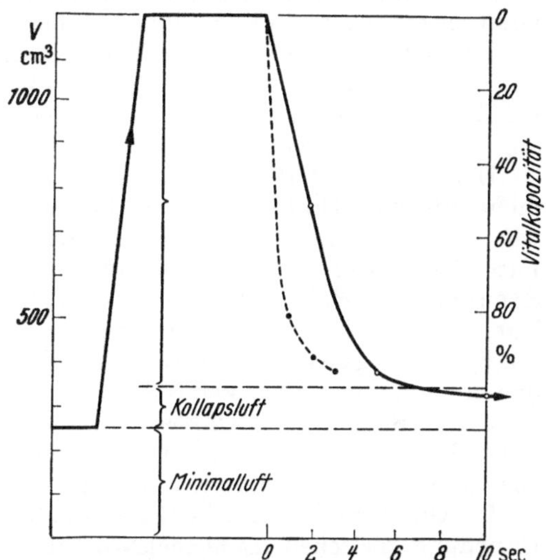

Abb. 2. Retraktion der Leichenlunge aus einer Auffüllung in der Größe der Vitalkapazität; die freie Retraktion beginnt bei der Zeit 0 sec. Die gesonderte Prozentskala entspricht der für den klinischen Tiffenau-Test üblichen Darstellungsweise; gestrichelt: klinische Sollwerte. (Nach HARTUNG 1957.)

Auch die Leichenlunge bläst mit Hilfe ihrer elastischen Retraktionskraft die hineingegebene Luft aus. Da die aktiven muskulären Exspirationskräfte in dieser Versuchsanordnung ausgeschaltet sind, kann auf diese Weise der allein auf Elastizität der Lunge beruhende Anteil der exspiratorischen Funktion festgestellt werden[3]. Die normale Lunge des jugendlichen Erwachsenen bläst in 2 sec etwa 50% der bis zur Grenze der Vitalkapazität aufgefüllten Luft aus, nach 6 sec ist die untere Grenze der Vitalkapazität erreicht (Abb. 2). Die Druckdifferenz zwischen diesen Grenzen beträgt etwa 20 cm Wasser. Die allgemeinen Retraktionsleistungswerte in der Dimension erg/sec können aus der Änderung des Druckes oder des Volumens im Verhältnis zur Zeit errechnet werden[4].

---

[1] GIESE 1956, HARTUNG 1957.
[2] TIFFENEAU 1957, TIFFENEAU und Mitarbeiter 1948, 1952, KAPFERER 1954 u. a.
[3] GIESE 1956, HARTUNG 1957.   [4] Formel bei HARTUNG 1957.

4. Die elastische Unvollkommenheit der Lunge.

Die elastische Funktion der Lunge beruht auf ihrem elastischen Fasersystem. Die einzelnen elastischen Fasern bilden ein ineinandergreifendes Netzwerk[1]. Die Dehnbarkeit dieses Systems hängt von der Elastizität der Einzelfasern ab, die an der Lunge noch nicht bestimmt ist. Wir greifen deshalb auf die Messungen der Elastizität isolierter elastischer Fasern zurück, die Redenz (1927) am Nackenband des Rindes durchgeführt hat.

Die elastische Faser ist danach um 100—140% dehnbar. Diese hohe Dehnbarkeit läßt auf einen geringen Dehnungswiderstand schließen, der Elastizitätsmodul ist also klein. Für die Dehnung der elastischen Fasern braucht nur eine geringe Kraft aufgewandt zu werden, die bei Entspannung und Retraktion der Faser frei wird. Die Retraktion ist bei Dehnung bis zu 50% vollkommen, bei Dehnungen bis zu 100% nahezu vollkommen. Wöhlisch u. du Mesnil de Rochemont (1927) haben den Elastizitätskoeffizienten berechnet und die gummielastische Dehnbarkeit der elastischen Fasern nachgewiesen.

Die elastische Faser ist also in hohem Maße dehnbar und zeigt innerhalb weiter Grenzen große elastische Vollkommenheit. Sie besitzt einen kleinen Elastizitätsmodul, hat dagegen nach der Föpplschen (1919) Definition einen hohen Grad von Elastizität. Sie kann eine Formänderungsarbeit mit großen Deformationen bei Einwirkung kleiner Kräfte aufnehmen und die so gespeicherte Arbeit während der Retraktion abgeben.

Die elastische Faser hat nur eine geringe Biegungsfestigkeit, sie kann deshalb nicht mit einer Stahlfeder verglichen werden, sondern verhält sich auf Biegung wie ein Kautschukstab[2]. Mit direkten Messungen an der isolierten elastischen Faser haben Petersen[2] und Redenz (1927) die für die Lunge von Orsós (1907), Sternberg (1925) und Loeschcke (1928) entwickelten Anschauungen widerlegt, daß das elastische Fasersystem der Lunge als wenig dehnbares und hochgradig biegungsfestes, stahlfederartiges Material nur einen Schutz gegen Überdehnung darstelle, aber keine Retraktionskraft entwickele.

Die Auffassung von Orsós (1907) und Loeschcke (1928) sowie von Sternberg (1925) scheint aus einer ungenauen Trennung der Begriffe Dehnbarkeit und Elastizitätsmodul entstanden zu sein.

Im Gegensatz zu Orsós (1907, 1936) muß betont werden, daß eine kausale Beziehung zwischen Lungenelastizität und elastischen Fasern besteht. *Die elastischen Fasern sind das tragende Element der Lungenelastizität.*

Die Biegungselastizität gewinnt dann Bedeutung, wenn die Lunge kollabiert ist. Wenn man am kollabierten Lungengewebe durch Fingerdruck eine Delle setzt, dann gleicht sich diese in kurzer Zeit aus. Dieser Ausgleich der durch Druck gesetzten Verformung ist Ausdruck einer Biegungselastizität, die erst an der entspannten und verkürzten Faser in Erscheinung tritt.

Nach eigenen neuen Untersuchungen steht die elastische Funktion der Lunge im Sinne von Tendeloo (1910, 1925, 1929) u. a. außer Zweifel[3].

In den Geweben, die wie die Lunge aus mehreren Faserarten aufgebaut sind, stehen den Messungen an isolierten Fasern große methodische Schwierigkeiten entgegen. Für die Elastica interna der Blutgefäße gibt Redenz (1927) eine Dehnbarkeit des Fasernetzes bis zu 20% an; sie liegt wahrscheinlich höher, läßt sich darüber hinaus aber nicht messen, weil das eingespannte Fasernetz bei dieser Methode an den Fixationspunkten ausreißt.

Tendeloo u. Mitarb[4]. haben Messungen an Lungenstreifen durchgeführt. Die aus verschiedenen Lungenlappen entnommenen, 40—50 mm langen, 10 mm breiten und 5 mm dicken Streifen, die sämtlich von Pleura überzogen waren, wurden einer Längsdehnung von 10%

---

[1] Orsós 1907, 1936.   [2] Petersen, 1927, 1935, Redenz 1927.
[3] Ebenso auch Christie 1934, McIlroy und Christie 1952.
[4] Tendeloo, Hennemann und Metz 1929, Metz 1930.

über 5 min Dauer unterworfen und auf die Fähigkeit zur Rückbildung der Dehnung untersucht. Die Dehnbarkeit wurde auch unter abgestufter Belastung gemessen[1]. Die Ergebnisse (s. S. 405) stehen hinsichtlich der elastischen Vollkommenheit des Lungengewebes mit den Volummessungen[2] in guter Übereinstimmung, während sich bei den statischen Werten, also der Dehnbarkeit, gegenüber der Volumbelastung der intakten Lunge prinzipielle Abweichungen ergeben. Diese Diskrepanz wird bei einem Vergleich der Versuchsanordnung verständlich. Die Streifenmessung kann jeweils nur einzelne Belastungsrichtungen herausgreifen. Dabei wird zwangsläufig die Materialkomponente mit geringerer Dehnbarkeit, sei es Pleura bei pleuraparallelen Streifen, sei es der Bronchial- und Gefäßbaum bei hiluswärts geschnittenen Streifen, dominieren müssen, um so mehr, als die Streifen von vornherein unter einer durch die Dehnungsvorrichtung gegebenen Vorspannung stehen. Die den physiologischen Verhältnissen besser angepaßte Volumdehnung trifft dagegen die mechanisch unterschiedlichen Bauelemente in ihrer charakteristischen Textur und beansprucht in den für die Atmung gegebenen Dehnungsgrenzen vor allem das elastische Fasersystem, während die Bauelemente von höherem Dehnungswiderstand erst an der Grenze der Vitalkapazitätsfüllung in Streckung übergehen und zu dem nun deutlich stärkeren, schließlich unproportional starken Modulanstieg führen.

Aus den bisher vorliegenden Messungen an der Lunge ergibt sich also, daß neben den elastischen Fasern auch kollagene und reticuläre Fasern sowie Bronchien und Blutgefäße durch ihre andersartigen elastischen Eigenschaften die Meßergebnisse beeinflussen.

α) Die elastische Nachwirkung.

Bei den bisher angeführten Messungen hat der für die Lungenfunktion so wichtige Zeitfaktor nur zum Teil Berücksichtigung gefunden. Wenn man auch annehmen darf, daß die Beanspruchung der einzelnen elastischen Fasern in der Lunge nicht über die Grenze der vollkommenen Rückbildungsfähigkeit hinausgeht, so haben die Befunde an der Lunge in ihrer Gesamtheit doch ergeben, daß schon bei Auffüllungen im Bereich der Vitalkapazität eine Nachdehnung erkennbar wird, wenn man den Ausgleich des elastischen Spannungszustandes abwartet. Der mit dem Ende der Zufüllung erreichte Druck sinkt nach Spannungsausgleich innerhalb von Sekunden um wenige Millimeter Wasser ab.

Bei der Entspannung erfolgt die Rückbildung der elastischen Verformung exponentiell. In einer ersten schnellen Phase wird das Kollapsvolumen aus der oberen Grenze der Vitalkapazität unter starkem Druckabfall in etwa 6 sec nahezu erreicht. Dann folgt eine etwa bis 10 min dauernde langsame Phase, in der durch elastische Nachwirkung noch eine zusätzliche geringfügige Retraktion nachfolgt, mit der schließlich die Grenze der elastischen Vollkommenheit erreicht wird. Nachdehnung und Nachkontraktion sind damit Ausdruck einer Trägheit der elastischen Fasern. Diese ist so gering, daß sie im Ablauf des normalen Atemcyclus nicht zur Geltung kommt.

β) Hysterese.

Neben der elastischen Nachwirkung muß auch die Hysterese Berücksichtigung finden. Diese ist als endgültiger Verlust von aufgewandter Dehnungsarbeit definiert. Sie äußert sich als Dehnungsrückstand. In der Lunge wirkt sich der Dehnungsrückstand des elastischen Fasersystems als eine Vermehrung des Kollapsvolumens aus. Den durch Dehnungsrückstand vermehrten Anteil des Kollapsvolumens kann man als Hysteresevolumen bezeichnen.

Im Versuch an der Leichenlunge wächst der Dehnungsrückstand mit der Vergrößerung des zugefüllten Volumens, also mit der Erhöhung der elastischen Beanspruchung. Das von TENDELOO (1910) aufgestellte Gesetz, nach dem die Dauer der elastischen Nachwirkung durch das Produkt von Dehnungsgrad und

---

[1] METZ 1930.   [2] HARTUNG 1957, 1958.

Dehnungsdauer bestimmt wird, findet somit auch bei der Volumdehnung der Leichenlunge eine Bestätigung. An der normalen jugendlichen Lunge liegt das Hysteresevolumen bei einmaliger Belastung bis zur Grenze der Vitalkapazität unter 3% der Vitalkapazität. Die Hysterese wird auf Änderung der Molekularstruktur des elastischen Fasersystems zurückgeführt. Es ist anzunehmen, daß diese sich in der Leichenlunge stärker auswirkt als beim Lebenden, bei dem sie erfahrungsgemäß reversibel ist[1]. Der im Experiment erst durch mehrfache Dehnung und Entdehnung zu erreichende Zustand der Akkommodation ist bei der lebenden Lunge von vornherein gegeben. Daß auch an der lebenden Lunge nach stärkeren Belastungen vorübergehende hysteretische Restdehnungen vorkommen können, scheinen klinische Beobachtungen[2] nahezulegen. Über diesen Mechanismus lassen sich jedenfalls vorübergehende Erhöhungen der Atemmittellage und Vermehrungen der Restluft nach schwerer körperlicher Arbeit erklären.

5. Die Homogenität der Lunge.

In den bisherigen Erörterungen wurde die Lunge als homogener Körper betrachtet, in dem praktisch eine Koeffizienz von Dehnung und elastischen Kräften besteht[3]. Dagegen hat Liebermeister (1922) aus einem Vergleich der Pleuradehnung über Ober- und Unterlappen bei Aufblähung der Lunge geschlossen, daß der Oberlappen weniger dehnbar sei. Tendeloo (1910) und Orsós (1912) weisen ebenfalls auf eine unterschiedliche Dehnung der Lunge im Ober- und Unterlappen hin. Orsós (1912) erläutert dies am Modell mit einer durchlöcherten Gummiplatte. v. Hayek (1953) weist dagegen nach, daß die Lunge in jedem Dehnungsgrad ihre Form behält, eine Beobachtung, die wir an eigenen Dehnungsversuchen bestätigen können. Der Ausgleich unterschiedlicher Weiteänderungen des Thorax wird durch innere Verschiebung in der Lunge ausgeglichen, Lappenspalten und Septen wirken als Gleitvorrichtungen[4]. Druckwellen pflanzen sich in der geblähten Lunge in allen Richtungen schnell und gleichmäßig fort[5].

Wir müssen also davon ausgehen, daß die normale Leichenlunge ein homogener elastischer Hohlkörper ist.

6. Die Oberflächenkräfte in ihrer Beziehung zur Elastizität.

v. Neergaard (1929) hat die Retraktion der Lunge auf die Oberflächenspannung an den Grenzflächen zwischen der Alveolarluft und der die Alveolarwand benetzenden Flüssigkeit zurückgeführt. Nach seinen Untersuchungen an Schweine- und Hundelungen soll mehr als die Hälfte der Retraktionskraft auf der Oberflächenspannung beruhen. Der passiv elastische Kollaps der Lunge soll für gewöhnlich nur 25%, höchstens aber 30% der gesamten Retraktionskraft der Lunge erreichen. Die Oberflächenspannung kann sich mit der verschiedenen H-Ionenkonzentration ändern, die sich aus dem Wechsel der CO_2-Spannung ergibt; Kohlensäureeinwirkung auf die überlebende Lunge vergrößert das Lungenvolumen um das Fünffache[6]. Kläsi (1886) hat in seiner Epitheltheorie des Emphysems schon entsprechende Gedanken geäußert.

Den Einfluß von Flüssigkeiten mit verschiedener Oberflächenspannung auf die Retraktion der Lunge hat v. Hayek (1952) untersucht. Meerschweinchen-

---

[1] Literatur bei Giese 1956 und Hartung 1957.
[2] Bohr 1907, Liebermeister 1908, Wacholder 1928.
[3] Wirz 1923, Rohrer 1925.   [4] v. Hayek 1953, Schall 1931.
[5] Liebermeister 1922, v. Neergaard 1930, Lottenbach und Mitarbeiter 1956.
[6] Wick 1952.

lungen, die mit 2 cm³ Luft aufgefüllt werden, entleeren diese Luft nach Benetzung mit Tannin vollständig, während eine mit gallensaurem Natrium benetzte Lunge noch doppelt so groß bleibt wie im Kollapszustand.

Welchen Anteil die Oberflächenkräfte an der Lungenretraktion im Atemvorgang haben, ist daraus noch nicht zu ersehen. Es wird vermutet, daß die der Oberflächenwirkung zugeschriebenen Kräfte in den Versuchen v. NEERGAARDs doch auf der Funktion der elastischen Fasersysteme beruhen. KILCHES (1940) konnte in Nachprüfungen die Auffassung v. NEERGAARDs nicht bestätigen. Lungen, die intrathorakal mit Flüssigkeit aufgefüllt werden, entfalten ebenso wie luftgefüllte Lungen eine Retraktionskraft, die bis zum Kollapszustand führt. Damit kann die beim Emphysem nachgewiesene verringerte Retraktionskraft der Lungen nicht auf einer Abnahme der Oberflächenkräfte beruhen. Ähnliche Bedenken äußerte K. ALTMANN (1955).

7. Zusammenfassung.

Überblickt man die in den vorstehenden Abschnitten diskutierten Untersuchungsergebnisse und Überlegungen, so kommt man zu dem Ergebnis, daß die Lunge als elastischer Hohlkörper angesehen werden kann, der nach physikalischen Gesetzen analysierbar ist. Nach den mit HARTUNG durchgeführten Untersuchungen an der Leichenlunge können folgende für die Analyse der Lungenfunktion unter krankhaften Verhältnissen wichtigen Ergebnisse herausgestellt werden, die aus Messungen normaler Lungen des 3. Lebensjahrzehnts (Durchschnittsalter 22,5 Jahre) gewonnen worden sind:

Wenn man Luft in die Lunge einfüllt, entsteht ein Widerstand, der sich als intrapulmonaler Druckanstieg äußert. Aus dem Verhältnis des eingefüllten Luftvolumens zum intrapulmonalen Druck ergibt sich eine S-förmige Volumendruckkurve, die sog. Lungencharakteristik. Der im regelhaften Auffüllungsbereich liegende Anteil dieser Kurve verläuft nahezu gradlinig. Der Widerstand (elastance) entspricht bei Einfüllung von 1 Liter Luft einem Druck von 4,5 cm Wasser und deckt sich mit neuen klinischen Meßwerten. Mit einem Druck von 1 cm Wasser kann man im Bereich der Vitalkapazität 0,22 Liter Luft in die Lunge einfüllen. Auch dieser Wert entspricht klinischen Messungen der Lungendehnbarkeit (compliance, Komplianz).

Mit steigender Zufüllmenge müssen relativ höhere Drucke angewandt werden, da der Dehnungswiderstand mit zunehmender Dehnung anwächst.

Das Maß für das Anwachsen dieses Widerstandes geben die Elastizitätsmoduln, die wegen des S-förmigen Verlaufs der Volumendruckkurve in den verschiedenen Dehnungsbereichen variieren. Für die wenig gedehnte Lunge der Exspirationsphase sind sie klein, für die stark gedehnte Lunge der tiefen Inspiration groß. Sie sind indirekt ein Maß der aufzuwendenden Atemarbeit.

Die Retraktionskraft, die eine isolierte Leichenlunge entwickelt, liegt zwischen minus 2 cm in der Exspiration und minus 12 cm H_2O in der Inspiration. Sie nimmt im regelhaften Auffüllungsbereich linear mit der Dehnung zu und entspricht den klinischen Meßwerten des Pleuradruckes, der ein Maß des elastischen Lungenzuges an der Thoraxwand ist.

Die freie Retraktion der isolierten, auf Vitalkapazität aufgefüllten Lunge erfolgt in einer ersten Phase (bis zu 6 sec) rasch, in einer zweiten Phase (bis zu 10 min) langsam. Die Retraktionskurve gibt Auskunft über das Ausmaß der elastischen Retraktionsleistung in den einzelnen Phasen der Exspiration.

In der Ruheatmung wird ein kleines Luftvolumen bei niedriger Atemfrequenz so gut wie vollständig allein durch die elastische Retraktion der Lunge entleert.

Im Tiffeneau-Test (Atemstoß-Test) sinkt dieser Anteil auf etwa 50%, der Rest entfällt auf die Tätigkeit der Exspirationsmuskulatur. So behält die Lungenelastizität auch in der forcierten Atmung einen bedeutenden und wie aus der Pathologie des Emphysems gezeigt werden kann, entscheidenden Einfluß auf den Ablauf der Exspiration.

Die Lunge allein entwickelt bei der Retraktion aus der Auffüllung bis zur Grenze der Vitalkapazität eine Atemstromstärke bis zu 1,25 Liter/sec in der ersten Sekunde.

Die Rückbildung der Dehnung wird durch elastische Nachwirkung verzögert und kann durch Hysterese unvollkommen werden. In der normalen Leichenlunge ist die Hysterese so gering, daß nach einer Minute kein Restvolumen mehr meßbar ist.

Die vorstehenden Werte sind unmittelbar mit den Meßergebnissen am Lebenden zu vergleichen und stimmen mit diesen weitgehend überein. Sie zeigen, daß aus den Messungen an der Leichenlunge Rückschlüsse auf die ventilatorische Lungenfunktion während des Lebens möglich sind und daß umgekehrt der allein auf Elastizität beruhende Anteil an der Lungenbewegung aus den klinischen Meßwerten ablesbar ist.

b) Lungenstruktur und Elastizität.

Das im vorstehenden Abschnitt erörterte Verhalten der Lunge als elastischer Hohlkörper ist in der dem Atemvorgang nachgebildeten Bewegung an das Vorhandensein elastischer Strukturen gebunden, die auch nach dem Tode ihre Wirkung in dem vorgezeichneten Rahmen entfalten. Es ist durch eine Materialprüfung des toten Gewebes ermittelt.

Die Lunge erfüllt ihre mechanische Funktion mit Hilfe der in ihrem Gerüst enthaltenen und zu einem Geflecht verbundenen Fasern[1]. *Sie ist ein elastisches Organ.*

1. Die Faserarten in ihrer Beziehung zur Elastizität.

Für die funktionelle Betrachtung der Lungenmechanik teilen wir die in diesem Geflecht vorkommenden und das Lungengerüst bildenden Fasern in 3 Gruppen:

1. die elastischen Fasern;
2. die Reticulumfasern und die kollagenen Fasern;
3. die glatten Muskelfasern.

Die elastischen Fasern stellen den Hauptanteil am Fasergerüst der Lungen. Sie bilden ein endlos in sich zusammenhängendes Netzwerk, dessen Konstruktionsplan Orsós (1907) beschrieben hat. Er unterscheidet ein Netzsystem aus groben Fasern, das die Fortsetzung der Bronchien bildet, sich genetisch aus diesen ableitet und bis zum Ende der Alveolargänge verfolgt werden kann. Dieses grobe Fasersystem bildet die durch Ausstülpung der Alveolen siebartig durchlöcherte Wand des Arbor alveolaris. Die Fasern sind vorwiegend zirkulär und spiralig, aber auch in der Längsrichtung angeordnet und bilden um die Zugänge zu den Alveolen verdickte Eingangsringe. Aus diesem Netzwerk grober Fasern spalten sich feine elastische Fasern ab, die in den Alveolarwänden zwischen den Blutcapillaren verlaufen und in einem zweiten Netzwerk Faserkörbe um die Alveolen bilden. Die feinen elastischen Fasern hängen mit den Blutcapillaren zusammen und werden von diesen abgeleitet[2]. Mit den elastischen Fasern stehen die Reticulumfasern in Verbindung, deren Fibrillen sich am Aufbau der elastischen

---

[1] Policard 1955, v. Gehlen 1941, v. Hayek 1953, Felix 1928, F. K. Fischer 1952, Giese 1956, 1957.
[2] Orsós 1907.

Fasern beteiligen und durch Einlagerung des Elastins maskiert werden[1]. Die
Reticulumfasern sind nur wenig dehnbar[2] und haben einen hohen Elastizitätsmodul[3]. Sie setzen sich aus Elementarfibrillen von 200 Å Dicke zusammen.

Kollagene Fasern, die elektronenoptisch durch eine deutliche Querstreifung
mit einer Periode von 650 Å Dicke gekennzeichnet sind[4], werden in dem Faser-
korb, der die Alveolarwand umspinnt, nicht gefunden[5], sind aber in den zentralen
Abschnitten des Arbor alveolaris als Fortsetzung der fibro-elastischen Schicht
der Bronchialwand reichlich vorhanden und verlieren sich in den Eingangsringen
um die Alveolen. Sie sind das wesentliche Bauelement der Lobularsepten und
finden sich auch zwischen den Acini.

Kollagene Fasern sind kaum dehnbar, ihre Dehnungsgrenze liegt unter
maximaler Belastung bei 20%. Im entspannten elastischen System sind sie
gewellt, im gedehnten gestreckt.

Die glatten Muskelfasern im Acinusbereich sind als Verlängerung der Bronchialmuskulatur zu denken. Sie bilden die Wand des Arbor alveolaris, der das
Gangsystem des Acinus darstellt. Die Muskelfasern sind im Stiel des Acinus am
stärksten entwickelt, verlieren sich allmählich nach Aufteilung des Alveolar-
bäumchens in die Alveolargänge und sind in den Infundibula kaum noch vorhanden. Die spiralig verlaufenden Muskelfasern überkreuzen sich wie Scheren-
gitter um die Alveolargänge. Sie bilden einen Bestandteil der Eingangsringe der
Alveolen, überbrücken in geradem Verlauf gelegentlich mehrere Alveolen[6] und
gehen in die elastischen Fasern über, die ihnen als Sehnen dienen[7]. In den Eingangsringen der Alveolen, die im Schnittpräparat die Alveolarknöpfchen bilden,
liegen in der Kuppe des Knöpfchens die elastischen Faserbündel, darunter die
Muskelfasern und unter diesen die kollagenen Fasern. Der Alveolenboden ist frei
von Muskelfasern. In den Septen und im subpleuralen Gewebe werden nur
einzelne Muskelfasern gefunden.

Den Nachweis von glatten Muskelfasern in der Lunge hat bereits REISSEISEN (1822)
geführt. In der Folgezeit ging die Diskussion um die Frage, ob auch in den Alveolarwänden
Muskelfasern vorkommen, wie es MOLESCHOTT (1860) annahm. Zahlreiche Nachuntersucher
bestätigten den Befund[8], andere lehnten ihn ab[9]. BALTISBERGER (1921) hat dann die Lungenmuskulatur in ihrem Verlauf bis ins einzelne beschrieben und festgestellt, daß in der Alveolarwand selbst keine glatten Muskelfasern vorkommen. Alle späteren Untersucher bestätigen
mit geringen Abweichungen die von BALTISBERGER gefundene Anordnung der Muskelfasern
in den Eingangsringen der Alveolen und in den Alveolargängen, lehnen aber das Vorkommen
von glatten Muskelfasern im Interstitium für die normale Lunge ab[10].

Umstritten blieb die Frage, ob die in der von BALTISBERGER untersuchten Lunge sehr
kräftig ausgebildete Muskulatur einen Normalzustand darstelle. Heute kann auf Grund
zahlreicher Nachuntersuchungen[11] als sichergestellt gelten, daß es sich bei dem von BALTIS-
BERGER untersuchten Fall um eine pathologische Überentwicklung der Muskulatur in der
Lunge gehandelt hat. Die Stärke der Lungenmuskulatur unterliegt beträchtlichen individuellen Schwankungen, die ORSÓS (1907) als Hyper- und Oligomyose bezeichnet[12]. Im ganzen
gesehen entfällt auf die Muskelfasern nur ein geringer Anteil am Fasersystem des Acinus.

---

[1] GIESE und GIESEKING 1957.

[2] LENGYEL 1932.

[3] PLENK 1927, MÄRK 1943

[4] WOLPERS 1943, GRASSMANN 1956, HOFFMANN und KÜHN 1956, KUHNKE 1958.

[5] GIESE und GIESEKING 1957.

[6] BALTISBERGER 1921, v. HAYEK 1950, 1953.

[7] v. EBNER 1902, v. GEHLEN 1940.

[8] J. GERLACH 1849, L. GERLACH 1876, HIRSCHMANN 1866, RINDFLEISCH 1886, 1872, PISO-
BORME 1860.

[9] KÖLLIKER 1881, SCHULZE 1871, EBERTH 1878.

[10] v. HAYEK 1950, 1953, v. MÖLLENDORFF 1941, ENGEL 1948, BEHRENS 1950, A. KAUFMANN
1952 u. a.

[11] W. S. MILLER 1947, ENGEL 1948, v. HAYEK 1950, A. KAUFMANN 1952, WURM 1954 u. a.

[12] Bestätigt von A. KAUFMANN 1952.

2. Die Lungentextur.

Elastisches Fasernetz, kollagene und reticuläre Fasern, sowie glatte Muskulatur sind in sich und untereinander geflechtartig verbunden. Sie bilden eine geordnete Textur des Lungengewebes. Diese hat, ähnlich wie die Webart eines Stoffes, Einfluß auf die Dehnbarkeit und geht so in den Begriff der Elastizität der Lunge als Ganzes ein.

α) Die Dehnbarkeitsgrenze.

Die obere Grenze der Dehnbarkeit einer normalen Leichenlunge liegt bei einem Druck von 40 cm H_2O und einem Lungenvolumen, das über die Vitalkapazität hinaus noch einmal um etwa 2000 cm³ vermehrt werden kann. Jenseits dieses Druckes und Volumens wird die Lunge undicht und zerreißt schließlich, die Luft entweicht in das Gewebe und durch die Pleura nach außen. Die Grenze der Dehnbarkeit liegt also oberhalb der Vitalkapazität und wird erst bei einem Druck erreicht, der den maximalen Inspirationsdruck von 20 cm H_2O um das Doppelte übersteigt. Daraus folgt, daß diese Grenze durch forcierte Inspiration nicht erreicht werden kann, weil die maximalen negativen Pleuradrucke etwa bei 30 cm H_2O liegen. Dagegen können höhere intrathorakale Drucksteigerungen durch maximale Anspannung der Exspirationsmuskulatur beim Husten und hinter Bronchialstenosen entstehen oder durch atmosphärischen Überdruck erreicht und bei Explosionen auch überschritten werden. Interstitielles Emphysem aus inneren Lungenzerreißungen und Pleuraeinrisse sind die Folgen.

Die äußere Eigenform der Lunge[1], die dem Thoraxraum angepaßt ist, bleibt auch nach Aufhören der Zugspannung im Kollaps erhalten. Bei Überdehnung runden sich die Randkonturen der Lunge ab, ungleichmäßig gedehnte Teile werden gegeneinander verschoben, wobei die Segment- und Interlobularsepten ebenso wie die Lappenspalten als Gleitvorrichtungen dienen. Atelektasen können von der Brustwand abgelöst und von geblähtem Gewebe überlagert werden. Die in Pleura und Septen sehr reichlich entwickelten kollagenen Fasern setzen der Ausdehnungsfähigkeit der Lunge als Ganzes ihre Grenze. Mit der Anspannung der kollagenen Fasern ist der starke Anstieg der Druckvolumenkurve und damit auch des Elastizitätsmoduls erklärt. Dieser Anstieg tritt erst oberhalb der Grenze der Vitalkapazität ein (s. Abb. 1, S. 405).

β) Der Acinus als kleinste Funktionseinheit des respiratorischen Systems.

Der im wesentlichen durch die Pleura und ihre hiluswärts einstrahlenden Septen bedingten äußeren Lungenform steht die innere Eigenform der Lunge gegenüber. Diese ist nach den Verzweigungen des Bronchialbaumes gegliedert und in Funktionseinheiten aufgeteilt, in deren Mittelpunkt vom Ventilationsmechanismus her gesehen der Acinus steht. Der Acinus wird verschieden definiert. Folgende Abgrenzungen sind vorgeschlagen worden:

1. Verzweigungsgebiet des Bronchiolus terminalis[2].
2. Verzweigungsgebiet des Bronchiolus respiratorius 1. Ordnung[3].
3. Verzweigungsgebiet des Bronchiolus respiratorius 2. Ordnung[4].
4. Verzweigungsgebiet des Bronchiolus respiratorius 3. Ordnung[5].
5. Ductus alveolaris[6].

---

[1] Liebermeister 1922, v. Hayek 1940.
[2] Loeschcke 1921, Braus 1934, Maximow und Bloom 1948, Policard 1955, Giese 1957, Engel 1958.
[3] Husten 1921, Aschoff 1935.   [4] v. Hayek 1953.
[5] Laguesse 1899, Beitzke 1923.   [6] Grethmann 1935.

Hier wird unter Acinus der Lungenabschnitt verstanden, der an einem Bronchiolus terminalis hängt. Dieser anatomisch leicht abgrenzbare Abschnitt reagiert bei Ventilationsstörungen als Einheit, die ganze Lunge kann aus solchen kleinen Einzel-Lungen zusammengesetzt gedacht werden[1]. Die alte Bezeichnung Acinus[2] hat in Verbindung mit zahlreichen pathologischen Prozessen eine gut umgrenzte Bedeutung gewonnen[3] und wird anderen vorgeschlagenen, übrigens auch verschieden definierten Namen wie Pneumonon[4] usw. vorgezogen. MILLER hat die Verzweigung eines Bronchiolus terminalis als Lobulus bezeichnet und damit die Verwirrung noch größer gemacht. Die Acini umfassen das gesamte respiratorische Parenchym der Lunge. Sie gliedern sich in den Arbor alveolaris[5], der das aus den Bronchioli respiratorii und Ductus alveolares bestehende Gangsystem bildet und in die Alveolen übergeht.

Die Dehnungsgrenze wird von den kollagenen und reticulären Fasern bestimmt, die aus dem gewellten Zustand in den gestreckten überführt werden. Die Streckung erfolgt mit der Inspiration, die bewegende Kraft ist die Inspirationsmuskulatur, durch die auch die elastischen Fasern in Spannung gesetzt werden.

Mit der exspiratorischen Entspannung werden die kollagenen Fasern wieder gewellt, im Kollaps ist die völlige Entspannung und die größtmögliche Verkürzung sowohl der elastischen als auch der kollagenen Fasern erreicht. Mit der Kompression wird nur noch eine Verlagerung, Verschiebung und Stauchung der Fasern erzielt, die durch die elastischen Fasern nach Aufhören des Druckes ausgeglichen werden können. Komprimierte kleine Lungenstückchen entfalten sich im Wasser bis zum Kollapsvolumen. Insofern wirkt das elastische Fasernetz nach Art von Spiralfedern.

Da der Acinus als Ganzes keine geschlossene Außenhaut besitzt — interacinös verlaufen nur spärliche kollagene Fasern —, setzt nahezu die gesamte Zug- und Druckspannung an den intraacinösen Faserstrukturen, also an der inneren Acinustextur an. Innerhalb des Acinus verteilt sich bei der Ruheatmung die Zugspannung gleichmäßig auf alle Anteile des Acinus, wirkt sich aber zunächst an den Alveolen mit ihren zarten Faserkörben aus.

Bei vertiefter Atmung und bei Volumen pulmonum auctum verschiebt sich die Größenrelation zwischen Gangsystem und Alveolen insofern, als jetzt der Arbor alveolaris einen größeren Anteil an dem vermehrten Volumen gewinnt. Bronchioli respiratorii und Alveolargänge werden zu makroskopisch erkennbaren, 0,2—0,3 mm weiten Röhrchen, während die Alveolen unter Erweiterung der Eingangsringe sich abflachen. Die Alveolen gewinnen an Breite, verlieren aber an Tiefe. Diese Verschiebung in der Größenrelation des Gangraumes zum Alveolarraum wird im Flächenbild des Querschnittes durch einen Alveolargang deutlich (Abb. 3 und 4). v. HAYEK (1953) schätzt den Flächenanteil eines Ganges auf ein Viertel (25—30%), den Anteil der zugehörigen Alveolen auf drei Viertel eines Querschnittes durch den Alveolargang mit seinen Alveolen. Im Volumen auctum beansprucht der Alveolargang über die Hälfte des Radius dieses Gebietes, im Lungenkollaps, auch bei Kontraktion der Gangmuskulatur, wird er zu einem schmalen Schlitz, hat also nur noch einen geringen Anteil am Flächenquerschnitt, während die Alveolen sich nicht im gleichen Verhältnis verkleinern. Die Bronchioli respiratorii verhalten sich gleichsinnig.

Die mit der Atmung eintretende Spannung und Entspannung des elastischen Lungengerüstes wirkt sich also auf die Gänge und Alveolen verschieden aus. Die Gänge werden mit der Inspiration zylindrisch erweitert, die Alveolen von Bechern zu Schalen umgeformt.

---

[1] BRAUS 1934, ENGEL 1950, 1958. [2] RINDFLEISCH 1886.
[3] ASCHOFF 1935, GIESE 1957. [4] LETTERER 1959. [5] F. E. SCHULZE 1871.

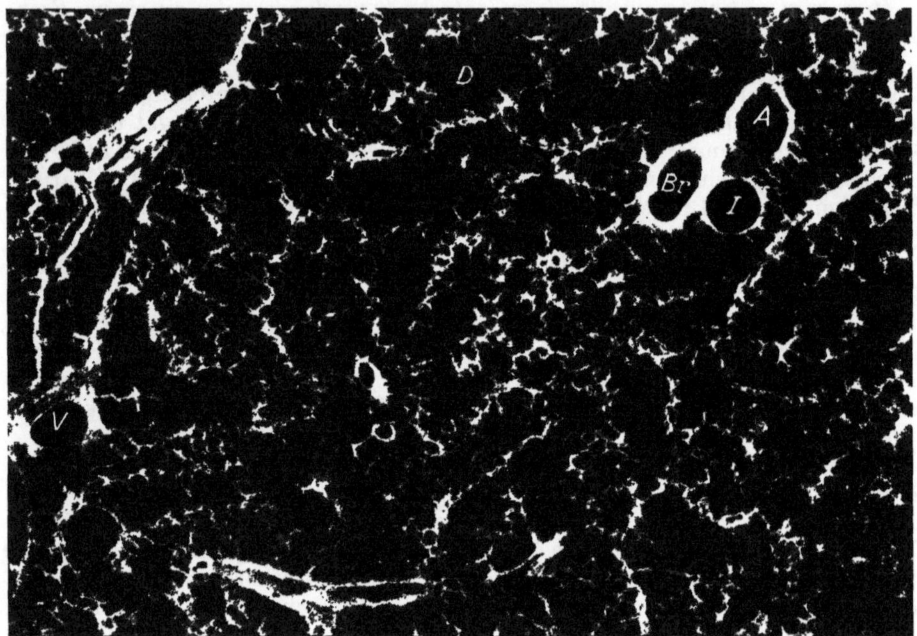

Abb. 3. Volumen pulmonum auctum. Lungenschnittfläche makroskopisch in der Aufsicht. Vergr. 10fach. Durchschnitt durch einen Acinus. Rechts oben Arteria terminalis (*A*), Bronchiolus terminalis (*Br*) und Bronchiolus respiratorius I. Die Ductus alveolares (*D*) erscheinen als schwarze Löcher und Gänge. Dazwischen das feinmaschige Wabenwerk der Alveolen. *V* periacinöse Vene.

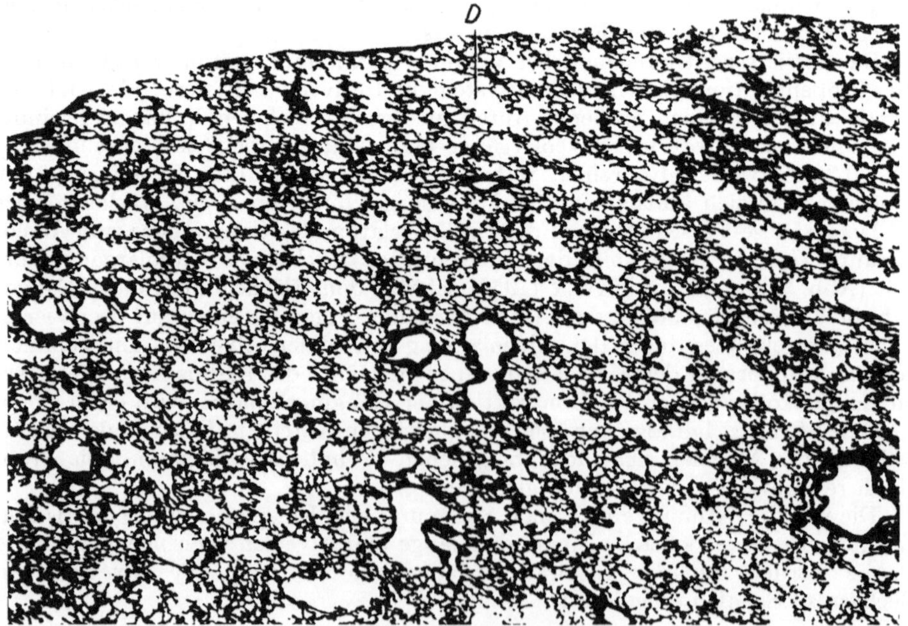

Abb. 4. Volumen pulmonum auctum. Histologischer Schnitt des gleichen Falles wie Abb. 3, ebenfalls bei 10facher Vergrößerung. Weite Ductus alveolares (*D*).

Die inspiratorische Dehnung des Acinus kann man sich zweiphasisch denken. In der ersten Phase wird der Alveolarraum vertieft und vergrößert, in der zweiten Phase das Gangsystem zylindrisch erweitert.

In dem kräftigen elastischen Fasersystem der Gänge des Arbor alveolaris und in den zarten elastischen Faserkörben der Alveolen entsteht mit der inspiratorischen Dehnung die elastische Spannung, mit deren Hilfe die Luft aus den Acini wieder ausgetrieben wird. Die elastische Retraktion des Acinus in der Exspirationsphase ist auf den Bronchus-Gefäßstiel in der Achse des Acinus ausgerichtet. Dort liegen auch die Bezugspunkte des elastischen Fasersystems[1].

γ) Die Lunge als myoelastisches, innerviertes System.

In dieses nach Regeln der Mechanik auch am toten Organ auflösbare Kräftespiel sind die glatten Muskelfasern eingeschaltet, denen besonders von klinischer Seite ein so wesentlicher Anteil an der Atemmechanik beigemessen wird, daß die Lunge als ein myoelastisches System[2] aufgefaßt wird. Dabei verschiebt sich der in den vorstehenden Abschnitten besprochene Anteil der elastischen Fasern an der Lungenfunktion bei manchen Autoren so weit, daß die Lungenmuskulatur schließlich als der wesentliche Faktor in der Atemmechanik betrachtet wird[3].

LOESCHCKE (1928), auf dessen Formulierung oft besonders auch in der klinischen Literatur[4] zurückgegriffen wird und die deshalb hier wiederholt sei, sagt dazu: „Wir kommen damit zu der Vorstellung, daß alle Versuche, eine Parallele zwischen Lungenelastizität und elastischen Fasern herzustellen, von vornherein verfehlt waren, eben weil die elastische Faser gar nicht der Bestandteil in der Lunge ist, der die Retraktion derselben bei Entspannung bedingt. Wir müssen die contractile Substanz in der Wandung der Lungenacini und in der Muskulatur der Alveolargänge suchen. Das sie umspinnende elastische Fasernetz geht dank seiner Anordnung in Spiralen und dank der Verknüpfung seiner Einzelelemente in der von ORSÓS geschilderten Art bei der Inspiration mit, bis es bei maximaler Inspiration vollständig gespannt nun eine stärkere Lungendehnung unmöglich macht, es wird von der contractilen Substanz nachher wieder mitgenommen und in die Ruhestellung gebracht, wie sie dem Exspirationsstadium entspricht, sie wird, falls die Lunge bei Eröffnung des Brustkorbs oder durch raumfordernde intrathorakale Prozesse entspannt wird, schließlich durch die sich stärker kontrahierenden Wandungen des Acinus gezwungen, sich zu schlängeln und so Formen anzunehmen, wie wir sie bei der kontrahierten Arterie kennen. Natürlich kann bei dieser Auffassung der Funktion der elastischen Fasern ein etwaiger Ausfall oder eine Unterbrechung des elastischen Systems nicht gleichgültig sein, sondern es werden die betroffenen Teile des Acinus schutzlos der Überdehnung preisgegeben, ebenso wie der Ausfall der elastischen Elemente der Gefäßwand diese der aneurysmatischen Ausstülpung durch den Blutdruck preisgibt.“

Inzwischen ist zur Genüge erwiesen, daß elastische Fasern dehnbar und retraktionsfähig sind und im Lungengefüge eine erhebliche Retraktionskraft entwickeln. Eine Wellung der elastischen Fasern in der entspannten Lunge hat sich nicht bestätigt, sie kommt nur in narbigen Lungenindurationen, besonders bei der elastischen Lungencirrhose alter Atelektasen vor und beruht hier auf der narbigen Schrumpfung des neugebildeten kollagenen Fasergewebes. Insofern bedarf die Formulierung LOESCHCKEs[5] einer Revision.

Es kann aber nicht bestritten werden, daß die Lungenmuskulatur in den Atemmechanismus als aktiv contractiles und innerviertes Element eingreift. Zur Diskussion steht heute die Frage, in welcher Form und in welchem Maße dies geschieht.

Die gemeinsam mit elastischen Faserzügen aus dem Bronchiolus terminalis auf den Arbor alveolaris sich fortsetzenden Muskelfasern umgreifen in flachen oder steilen Spiralen die Alveolargänge und werden bei Kontraktion in jedem Falle das Gangsystem verkürzen und auch einengen. Die Auffassung v. GEHLENs, daß

---

[1] GIESE 1956.
[2] v. GEHLEN 1940, LÖFFLER 1956, O. A. M. WYSS 1952, VERZÁR 1933, R. SCHOEN 1936.
[3] STURM 1948, 1951.   [4] LÖFFLER 1956.   [5] LOESCHKE 1928.

die Muskelfasern, die tangential an den elastischen Fasern der Alveolareingangsringe angreifen, diese erweitern, läßt sich aus den anatomischen Befunden nicht
belegen, es muß vielmehr v. Hayek zugestimmt werden, der Kontraktionszu-
stände der Muskulatur mit entsprechender Verengerung der Lichtung zeigt. Ob
diese Muskelfasern die Aufgabe haben, dem Lungengewebe eine Stabilität zu verleihen[1] und der Deformierung der Alveolen bei der Inspiration entgegenzuwirken[2],
ist noch zweifelhaft, eigene Dehnungs- und Kollapsversuche am Lungengewebe
sprechen nicht dafür, sondern lassen den Schluß zu, daß die Anordnung und
gegenseitige Verbindung der elastischen Fasern diese Funktion erfüllen. In Deh-

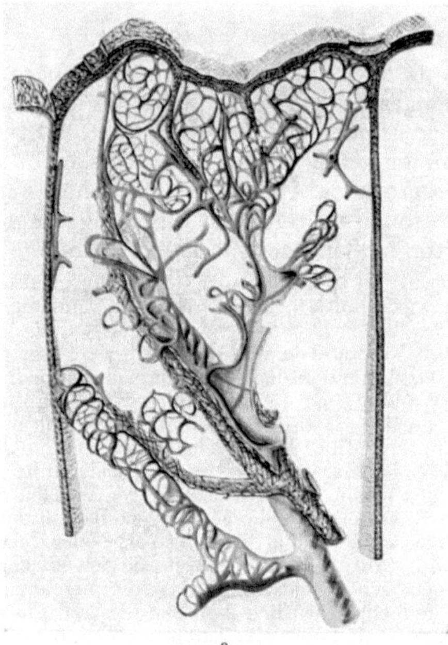

nungs- und Druckversuchen an
dicken Lungenschnitten läßt
sich jedenfalls zeigen, daß Alveolargänge und Alveolen selbst
dort, wo sie angeschnitten sind,
immer ihrer ursprünglichen
Form zustreben und diese auch
nach wiederholter Kompression und Dehnung beibehalten.

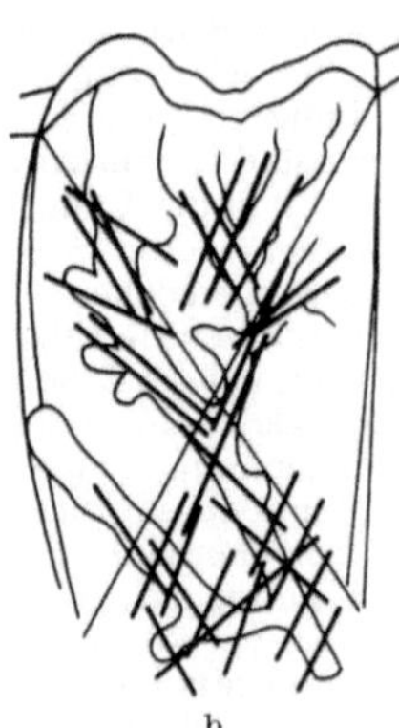

Abb. 5a u. b. a Halbschematische Darstellung des myoelastischen Systems in einem Acinus. Hellblau elastische
Fasern, orangerot Muskelfasern, karmin Arterien, violett Venen. b Hauptspannungsrichtungen im Acinus.
(Aus v. Gehlen 1940.)

Nach v. Gehlen (1940) ist die glatte Muskulatur wesentlich bei der Regulation der Spannung im allgemeinen elastischen System der Lunge und damit an
der Anpassungsfähigkeit der Lunge an die verschiedenen Dehnungslagen beteiligt (Abb. 5). Sie hält also einen Tonus aufrecht. Ob dieser, wie Luisada
(1934) meint, antagonistisch zur quergestreiften Muskulatur des Thorax wirkt,
ist dabei noch zweifelhaft. Eine Mitwirkung der Muskelfasern bei jedem Atemzug
ist unwahrscheinlich, weil die glatte Muskulatur nur träge reagiert. An der Bronchialmuskulatur treten Tonusänderungen ebenfalls nur sehr langsam auf[3].

Rhythmische Schwankungen in der Lungengröße, die Luisada (1934) an
Katzenlungen fand, könnten mit der Tätigkeit der glatten Muskulatur im Acinus,
die sich dann aber gleichsinnig zur Bronchialmuskulatur verhalten müßte, erklärt werden.

Ebensowenig wie die Beziehungen zwischen Lungentonus und glatter Muskulatur als geklärt gelten können, ist über die Lungenkontraktion etwas Abschließen-
des zu sagen.

---

[1] Engel, 1948, Policard 1955.   [2] Aschoff 1935.   [3] Trendelenburg 1912, 1913.

REINHARDT (1934, 1935, 1941) beobachtete an der Kaninchenlunge im Unterdruck bei mechanischen Reizungen der Pleura bis 1 mm tiefe Furchen und Dellen, die sich histologisch als kegelförmige Atelektasen mit einem verschlossenen Bronchiolus terminalis an der Spitze des Kegels erwiesen. Die Dellen treten in einer Sekunde oder in Bruchteilen davon auf und lassen sich durch quantitativ verschieden starke Reizung nicht abstufen. Sie lösen sich nur langsam. REINHARDT (1934) erklärt die Dellenbildung als Folge einer Verkürzung der Muskulatur des Ductus alveolaris und durch Verschluß sowie gleichzeitige Verkürzung des Bronchiolus terminalis. Im Rande dieses Herdes sind die Alveolen erweitert.

Beim Menschen sind diese Dellenbildungen nach mechanischer Pleurareizung ebenfalls beobachtet worden[1]. Die Alveolen um den kontrahierten Alveolargang werden teils erweitert, teil in die Länge gezogen[2], sie können auch kollabiert sein[3].

Die sich aus dem Dellenphänomen ergebenden Beziehungen zur Entstehung größerer Atelektasen, insbesondere zum akuten massiven Lungenkollaps, werden gesondert besprochen.

Mit der Pleurareizung entsteht gleichzeitig eine Strömungsverlangsamung in den erweiterten Capillaren (peristatische Hyperämie), ausgelöst durch die außerhalb der Delle liegende kontrahierte Arteriole[4].

Die Kontraktilität der glatten Muskulatur im Acinus und ihre Fähigkeit zur Verringerung des Lungenvolumens in einem umschriebenen Lungenbezirk kann nach dem Ergebnis dieser Versuche nicht bezweifelt werden. Kontraktion und Tonus stehen unter dem Einfluß des auch in der Lunge reich entwickelten autonomen Nervensystems[5]. REINHARDT (1934) faßt die zur Dellenbildung führende Kontraktionsatelektase als einen pleuro-pulmonalen Reflex auf. Wieweit solche Reaktionen der Lunge auch von anderen Orten her ausgelöst werden können, ist noch nicht ausreichend geklärt. Vom anatomischen Standpunkt aus ist immer wieder darauf hinzuweisen, daß bei allen Eingriffen am autonomen Nervensystem nicht nur die glatte Muskulatur der Lunge und der Bronchien, sondern auch das Gefäßsystem[6] und die Schleimhäute beeinflußt werden, die mit Weiteänderungen der Capillaren und Obstruktionsmechanismen der Bronchien oder mit Ödem die Versuchsergebnisse entscheidend beeinflussen[7].

Zusammenfassend läßt sich sagen, daß die Lunge als elastischer Hohlkörper durch das eingebaute System glatter Muskelfasern einen des Wechsels fähigen Tonus erhält. Die glatten Muskelfasern greifen als Spannvorrichtungen in das Gefüge der nur passiv wirkenden elastischen, kollagenen und reticulären Fasersysteme ein. Sie gewinnen dadurch Einfluß auf das Lungenvolumen, das sie durch Erschlaffung vergrößern, durch Kontraktion verkleinern können.

c) Die Beziehungen zwischen Lunge und Thorax.

Die meisten der für die Pathogenese von Ventilationsstörungen entscheidenden Faktoren liegen in der Lunge selbst und können daher am isolierten Organ studiert werden. Im Organismus bildet die Lunge mit dem Thorax eine funktionelle Einheit. Alle klinischen Untersuchungen erfassen die globalen Werte des elastischen Thorax-Lungensystems. Dabei ist unter der Bezeichnung Thorax dessen Knochen- und Bandapparat zu verstehen, zu dem das Zwerchfell, die Atemmuskulatur und das halbstarre Mediastinum kommen. Einfluß auf die Thoraxbewegung hat auch der Bauchraum, insbesondere dessen muskulärer Wandapparat. Änderungen der Thoraxweite oder der Zwerchfellfunktion und zum Teil auch der

---

[1] NIEDNER 1950, v. HAYEK 1952, GRAY und GRODINS 1951, Literatur bei v. HAYEK 1953.
[2] BRONKHORST und DIJKSTRA 1940.   [3] REINHARDT 1934, v. HAYEK 1953.
[4] HEUCK und FLACH 1953, HEUCK 1959.
[5] BAYER 1925, TAKINO 1933, SUNDER-PLASSMANN 1938, FEYRTER 1938, FRÖHLICH 1949, MAGNENAT 1951, SCHOENMACKERS 1950, HOFF 1952, Literatur bei KEHLER 1953.
[6] Neue Versuche von LESCHKE 1952, 1953, 1956.   [7] HEUCK und FLACH 1953, HEUCK 1959.

muskulären Bauchwand sind in verschiedenen grundlegenden Emphysemtheorien, auf die später eingegangen wird, besonders beachtet worden.

Der knöcherne Thorax bildet die feste äußere Wandung des der Respiration
dienenden Brustraumes, bietet der Atemmuskulatur ihre Ansatzfläche und
bestimmt Form und Volumen der darin ausgespannten Lunge. Er stellt ein elastisches System dar, das mit Hilfe der Atemmuskulatur die Atembewegungen ausführt und weitgehend als Gegenspieler der elastischen Retraktionskraft der
Lunge wirkt[1].

In neueren Untersuchungen[2] konnten bei passiver Beatmung unter Ausschaltung der muskulären Kräfte sog. Relaxationsdiagramme für das Thorax-
Lungensystem gewonnen werden (Abb. 6). Die intrapulmonalen Drucke liegen
dabei innerhalb der Volumgrenzen der Vitalkapazität zwischen — 30 mm Hg exspiratorisch und + 40 mm Hg inspiratorisch; die Ruhelage des Systems bei Null-Druck findet sich bei einer Auffüllung von etwa 35% der Vitalkapazität. Diese unmittelbar gemessene Kurve ist eine Resultante der Druckkurven von Thorax und Lunge, die in ihrer vermutlichen Richtung ebenfalls eingetragen sind. Die eigenen Meßwerte an der isolierten Leichenlunge (s. S. 406) zeigen, daß eine gute Übereinstimmung mit der angenommenen Relaxationsdruckkurve der Lunge besteht. Ihre elastische Ruhelage liegt noch unterhalb der Exspirationsgrenze der Vitalkapazität und entspricht dem Kollapsvolumen;

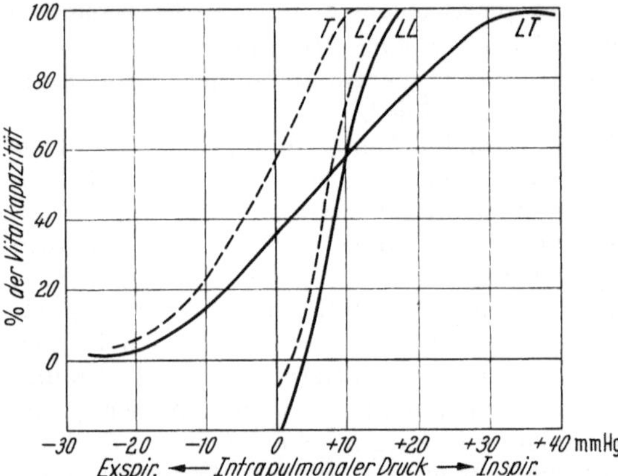

Abb. 6. Relaxationsdruckkurve von Lunge und Thorax von 14 gesunden Versuchspersonen. Passive Beatmung unter Registrierung des Volumens in Prozent der Vitalkapazität und des zugehörigen Exspirations- bzw. Inspirationsdruckes. *LT* Relaxationsdruckkurve des Thorax-Lungensystems; *L* vermutliche Relaxationsdruckkurve der Lunge; *T* vermutliche Relaxationsdruckkurve des Thorax (Skelet und Muskulatur); *LL* an der Leiche gemessene Volum-Druckkurve der Lunge. (Unter Benutzung der Darstellung von Rahn, Otis, Chadwick u. Fenn 1946.)

in jeder Respirationslage des Thorax besteht also noch ein elastischer Lungenzug, der nahezu linear mit der Auffüllung anwächst. Die elastische Ruhelage
des Thorax findet sich dagegen bei einer Auffüllung von 60% der Vitalkapazität,
sie kennzeichnet zugleich den Umschlagspunkt, von dem ab die Eigenelastizität
des Thorax einer weiteren Inspiration entgegenzuwirken beginnt, sich nunmehr
also der Lungenretraktionskraft hinzuaddiert und den inspiratorischen Muskelkräften einen weiteren zusätzlichen Widerstand entgegenstellt.

Die elastische Ruhelage des Thorax-Lungensystems ist für die Einstellung
der Atemmittellage entscheidend; um sie herum pendeln, in Gang gesetzt durch
relativ geringe, vorwiegend inspiratorisch wirksame Muskelkräfte, die Atemausschläge, die bei Ruheatmung durchschnittlich ein Luftvolumen von 500 ml
bewegen (Abb. 7). Änderungen der Elastizität der Lunge einerseits, des Thorax
andererseits führen zu Verschiebungen der Atemmittellage und somit zu Änderungen der Größe von Komplementär- und Reserveluft, vielfach auch des Residualluftvolumens. Im Tode wird die Atemmittellage wegen des Fortfalles des
Grundtonus der Atemmuskulatur in Richtung der Exspirationsstellung verschoben[3].

---

[1] Felix 1920, v. Hayek 1953, Töndury 1956, Uehlinger 1960, Hartung 1960.
[2] Rahn und Mitarbeiter 1946.   [3] Gad 1879.

Es wird weiterhin auch verständlich, daß maximale Ventilationsleistungen, z. B. bei der Atemgrenzwertbestimmung, zumeist nicht unter voller Ausschöpfung der Vitalkapazität, die in ihren Grenzlagen bedeutende Kräfte zur Überwindung der elastischen Widerstände erfordern würde, sondern unter individuell wechselnder Einstellung eines ökonomischeren Kompromisses zwischen Atemvolumen und Atemfrequenz bewältigt werden[1].

Die Atembewegungen des knöchernen Thorax, u. a. von KEITH (1909) eingehend untersucht, führen zu einer ungleichmäßigen Erweiterung seiner einzelnen Abschnitte. So kommt es vor allem zu einer Vergrößerung des Tiefendurchmessers in seiner sternalen Partie, während die Wirbelsäule praktisch einen Fixpunkt aller Atembewegungen bildet. Zudem werden etwa 60% des Atemvolumens durch das Zwerchfell bewegt, dessen inspiratorischer Zug vornehmlich in den basalen Lungenteilen wirksam wird. Die gesunde Lunge vermag sich aber diesen ungleichmäßigen Weiteänderungen, die primär ihre basalen und vorderen Anteile treffen, so anzupassen, daß eine gleichmäßige Belüftung zustande kommt. Die zunächst auf theoretische Überlegungen gestützte Konzeption ROHRERs (1925), daß die Lunge einen ideal-elastischen Körper mit weitgehender Homogenität seiner Teile darstelle, hat sich vielfach bestätigt und ist ziemlich allgemein anerkannt[2]. Örtliche Druck- und Span-

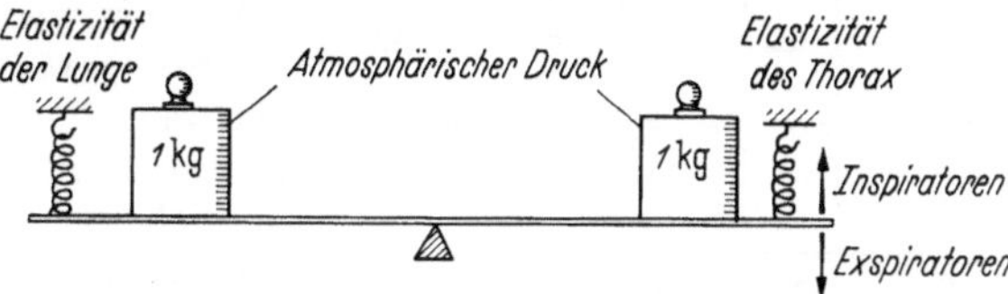

Abb. 7. Kräfteverhältnis im Thorax-Lungensystem, dargestellt am Beispiel einer federgebremsten Waage. (Aus v. HAYEK 1953.)

nungsdifferenzen werden praktisch momentan und vollständig ausgeglichen[3]. Die relativ weniger dehnbaren Spannungssysteme der pleuralen Septen übertragen die inspiratorischen Dehnungsspannungen gleichmäßig auf das Lungengewebe und werden von den mit den Bronchien und Gefäßen vom Hilus ausstrahlenden Spannungssystemen (système fibreux de tension, POLICARD 1955) aufgefangen und auf die zentralen Lobuli übertragen, so daß trotz der insgesamt weniger ausgiebigen Atembewegungen im Lungenkern mit seiner Massierung von Bronchien und Gefäßen eine annähernd gleich ergiebige Belüftung der zentral gelegenen respiratorischen Endabschnitte resultiert. Die Gleitflächen der Pleura ermöglichen eine schnelle Verschieblichkeit der Lungenlappen untereinander und tragen somit ebenfalls wesentlich zu der Gleichmäßigkeit der Atemexkursionen der Lunge bei. Alle krankhaften Prozesse in der Lunge, Pleuraverwachsungen, herdförmige Narbenbezirke u. dgl., heben die Homogenität auf.

Der Pleuraspalt ist Schnittpunkt aller im dynamischen Wechsel der Atembewegungen auftretenden Kräfte (Abb. 8). Die statischen Drucke (p_{el}), wie sie den Druck-Volumkurven entsprechen (s. Abb. 1 und 6), werden bei den Atembewegungen durch zusätzliche dynamische Drucke überlagert. Nur in den inspiratorischen und exspiratorischen Endpunkten (J und E) herrschen wegen des vorübergehenden Atmungsstillstandes statische Drucke. Während der Atembewegungen treten, insbesondere durch die Strömungswiderstände, in geringem Maße auch durch den Gewebsdeformationswiderstand und Trägheitskräfte bedingte, zusätzliche Drucke auf (p_R insp. + p_R exsp.). Dadurch entsteht das charakteristische schleifenförmige Druck-Volumdiagramm des Atemcyclus mit den tatsächlich gemessenen dynamischen Pleuradrucken (p_{pl} insp. + p_{pl} exsp.). Zwischen dem inspiratorischen (J) und dem exspiratorischen (E) Endpunkt, in denen wegen des vorübergehenden Atemstillstandes statischer und dynamischer Pleuradruck zusammenfallen, verläuft die (statische) Elastizitätsachse (E—J). Die Strecke J—E' kennzeichnet den mit der angenommenen Volumzunahme

---

[1] HEINE, BENESCH und HERTZ 1953.
[2] LOTTENBACH und Mitarbeiter 1956, ROSSIER und Mitarbeiter 1956, 1958, v. HAYEK 1953 u. a.
[3] LIEBERMEISTER 1922, v. NEERGAARD 1927.

E—E' verbundenen elastischen Druckzuwachs, die Höhe von p_{el} den jeweiligen statisch-elastischen Druckanteil, dem sich während der Atembewegungen die zusätzlichen, von der Atemgeschwindigkeit stark abhängigen Widerstände p_R jeweils hinzuaddieren, so daß für den tatsächlichen Druckverlauf während des Atemcyclus die (ausgezogenen) Schleifen mit den Einzeldrucken p_{pl} insp. und p_{pl} exsp. zustande kommen.

Die Atemschleifen sind aus dem Atemvolumen und dem Pleuradruck, der zumeist intraoesophageal gemessen wird, bestimmbar. Sie können bei Lungenerkrankungen beträchtliche Abweichungen zeigen. Eine Elastizitätseinbuße der Lunge führt z. B. zu einer Verlagerung der Elastizitätsachse auf ein geringeres Druckniveau, intrabronchiale Stenosen lassen die Strömungswiderstände beträchtlich anwachsen, die dann durch erhöhte Muskelarbeit überwunden werden müssen. Unter der Bedingung, daß p_R exspiratorisch größer wird als p_{el}, ist auch exspiratorisch Muskelarbeit zu leisten; zugleich ist damit eine Vorbedingung für vorübergehende positive Intrapleuraldruckwellen gegeben, die durch dynamische Bronchostenosen (sog. air trapping) eine weitere Exspirationshemmung bewirken und blasenbildend wirksam werden können (s. S. 533)[1].

Ein Rückschluß auf die gestörten Beziehungen zwischen Lunge und Thorax und auf die veränderte Atemarbeit ist durch die anatomischen Befunde an der isolierten Lunge, insbesondere durch die Elastizitätsmessungen möglich. Bei der Interpretation der klinischen Thorax-Lungendiagramme wird man von den anatomischen Meßwerten ausgehen müssen, die sich in den statischen Meßpunkten der exspiratorischen und inspiratorischen Ruhestellung mit denen der Klinik unmittelbar decken. Für die pathologischen Verhältnisse mit ihren oft komplexen Funktionsstörungen geben sie die Möglichkeit zur Abgrenzung des Lungenanteils und damit eine anatomische Basis für die Diskussion.

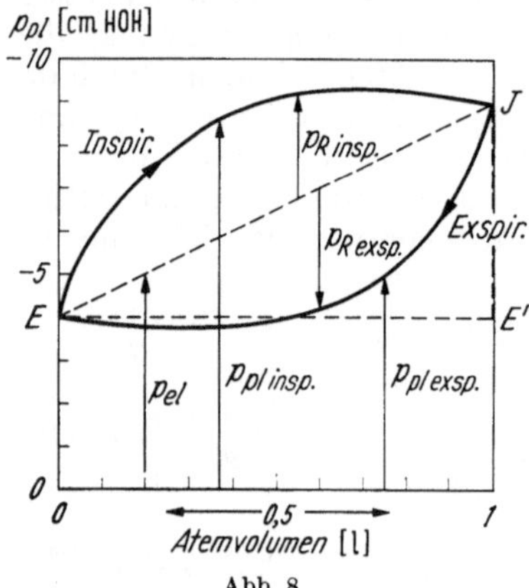

Abb. 8.
Schematische Darstellung des Pleuradruckverlaufes während eines Atemcyclus. Siehe Text. (Umgezeichnet nach Pircher 1957.)

II. Pulmonogene Störungen der Ventilation.

So gut wie alle Lungenerkrankungen führen zu Störungen der elastischen Eigenschaften des Lungenkörpers, die teils als globale Änderungen der Dehnbarkeit, teils in Form örtlicher Störungen der Homogenität in Erscheinung treten und beträchtliche Folgen für die Belüftung der Lunge haben. Sie lassen sich bei Elastizitätsmessungen in verschiedene mechanische Grundformen einteilen[2].

Im Typus der *schlaffen Lunge* findet sich eine Minderung aller geprüften elastischen Qualitäten. Die Lunge wird stärker dehnbar, ihr Volumelastizitätsmodul sinkt ab. Die Retraktionsleistung ist vermindert, die hysteretischen Dehnungsrückstände wachsen an. Die Minimalluft ist vermehrt. Diese Entwicklung liegt in physiologischen Grenzen, solange sie die Alterskurve der Lungenelastizität nicht überschreitet. Sie führt die Lunge durchschnittlich im 6. Lebensjahrzehnt an die kritische Grenze des diffusen senilen Emphysems. Ihre Homogenität bleibt in der Regel erhalten. Wir finden die schlaffe Lunge aber auch als Folge anhaltender Überdehnung bei einem Mißverhältnis zwischen Thoraxweite und Lungengröße.

---

[1] Wegen weiterer Einzelheiten, insbesondere hinsichtlich der energetischen Konsequenzen, wird auf die Darstellungen von Rohrer (1925), Lottenbach und Mitarbeiter (1956), Rossier und Mitarbeiter (1956, 1958) und auf den pathophysiologischen Teil in diesem Handbuch verwiesen.

[2] Hartung 1958, 1959, Giese 1960.

Die schlaffe Lunge ist leicht und blaß, ihr Gewebsanteil reduziert, der Luftgehalt vermehrt. Sie kollabiert auch bei freien Luftwegen nur unvollständig.

Das Hauptkennzeichen der *starren Lunge* ist die geringe Dehnbarkeit und der stark erhöhte Volumelastizitätsmodul. Die übrigen elastischen Funktionen sind innerhalb des geringen Dehnungsausmaßes zumeist intakt. Die Lunge ist nur unvollkommen belüftet, ihre Minimalluft verringert. Zur starren Lunge gehören alle Zustände von Gerüstfibrose und Lungencirrhose. Ist diese diffus, wie bei chronischer Stauungslunge, dann bleibt die Homogenität der Lunge weitgehend erhalten. Ist sie wie bei Strahlenfibrose, Sklerodermie u. a. auf größere oder kleinere Lungenabschnitte beschränkt, dann mischen sich gut und schlecht ventilierte Lungenteile, die Lunge wird inhomogen.

In der *Narbenlunge* ist die Homogenität nicht nur durch die eingestreuten Narbenfelder, sondern auch durch die Verziehung des Lungengerüstes behindert. Die Störfelder der Ventilation liegen in den Narben und in ihrer Umgebung. Vernarbte Miliartuberkulosen, kleinknotige Silikosen und zahlreiche andere vernarbende Lungenprozesse sind Beispiele aus dieser großen, in ihren Erscheinungsformen sehr vielgestaltigen Gruppe. Die Dehnbarkeit ist mäßig eingeschränkt, die Retraktionsleistung herabgesetzt. Die Dehnungsrückstände sind vermehrt.

Die *gefesselte Lunge* wird durch Pleuraschwarten nach chronischen Ergüssen oder Pneumothorax in ihrer Exkursion behindert, sie ist wenig dehnbar, faßt nur ein kleines Luftvolumen und hinkt gegenüber der gesunden Lunge bei der Ventilation nach. Die Elastizität der Lunge selbst ist dabei, solange keine Lungenfibrose oder atelektatische Induration komplizierend hinzutritt, kaum eingeschränkt. Die Lunge kann nach Entfesselung durch Dekortikation wieder funktionsfähig werden.

Bei der in zu engem Thoraxraum *eingesperrten Lunge* liegen die Verhältnisse ähnlich.

Mischungen und Überschneidungen dieser Typen kommen oft vor. Besondere Bedeutung gewinnen dabei die begleitenden Veränderungen an den kleinen Bronchien und Bronchiolen, die beim Altersemphysem funktionell, bei allen Fibrosen durch Narben eingeengt oder verschlossen sein können. Ihre Folgen sind Verteilungsstörungen und Herdemphyseme oder Atelektasen, die unter den Erkrankungen der Luftwege besprochen werden.

Die Grundformen der hier aufgestellten Typen lassen sich bei kombinierter histomechanischer und histologischer Untersuchung in der Regel einwandfrei herausschälen.

a) Die schlaffe atonische Lunge.

Die Elastizität der Lunge ist Voraussetzung für den normalen Ablauf der Ventilationsbewegung. In der Inspirationsphase ist die Dehnbarkeit, in der Exspirationsphase die Retraktionskraft der Lunge und die Vollkommenheit ihrer elastischen Rückbildung entscheidend. Diese Eigenschaften sind im Laufe des Lebens nicht konstant. Die elastischen Fasern als die wesentlichen Träger der elastischen Funktion des Lungenkörpers unterliegen wie alle anderen Organe und Gewebe der Alterung. Sie durchlaufen eine Phase der Reifung, eine Phase der Funktionshöhe und eine Phase der Rückbildung. Diese Phasen lassen sich in ähnlicher Weise an dem eingehend untersuchten Gefäßsystem nachweisen, eine Parallele, auf die für die Lunge besonders TENDELOO (1929) hingewiesen hat[1].

---

[1] ASCHOFF 1908, REUTERWALL 1922, THOMA 1889, 1920, JORES 1924, RANKE 1925, U. METZ 1949, SIMON und MEYER u. a.

1. Die Alterslunge.

Für die Lunge wurde ein solches Verhalten schon seit langem vermutet. Die älteren Untersuchungen mit globaler Messung des Retraktionsdruckes der nach Eröffnung des Thorax zusammensinkenden Lunge[1], auch in Kombination mit Messung des Intrapleuraldruckes[2], sind praktisch an zahlreichen methodischen Fehlermöglichkeiten gescheitert. Dagegen haben schon Tendeloo u. Mitarb.[3] an herausgeschnittenen Lungenstreifen eine Alterskurve der Lungenelastizität hinsichtlich der elastischen Vollkommenheit ermittelt, die von einem niedrigen Ausgangswert beim Neugeborenen bis zu einem Gipfel im 3. Lebensjahrzehnt ansteigt, um schon im 4. Jahrzehnt wieder abzusinken (Abb. 9). Die Streifenmessungen sind ebenfalls mit einer großen Zahl von methodischen Fehlern behaftet, ihre Ergebnisse haben daher nicht die Beachtung gefunden, die sie in der

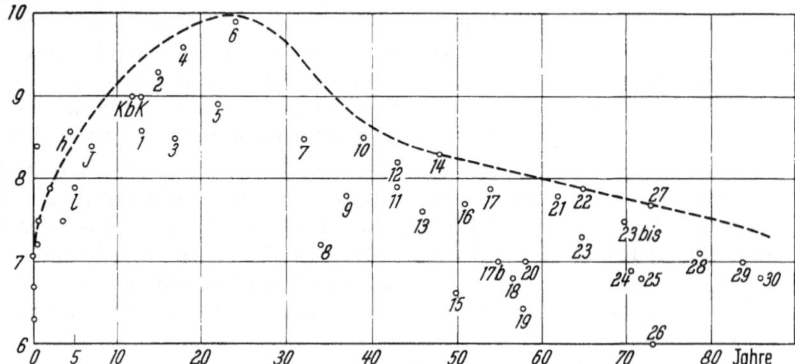

Abb. 9. Die Alterskurve der Lungenelastizität nach Tendeloo, Hennemann und Metz 1929. Abszisse: Lebensalter in Jahren; Ordinate: Maß der elastischen Vollkommenheit der Rückbildung einer 10%igen Dehnung von Lungenstreifen, die Zahl 10 kennzeichnet eine vollständige Rückbildung auf das Ausgangsvolumen, die Zahl 8 einen Dehnungsrest von 20% usw.

Pathogenese der mit der Lungenelastizität zusammenhängenden Ventilationsstörungen verdienen. In den eigenen Untersuchungen konnten die Ergebnisse von Tendeloo u. Mitarb. (1929) bestätigt und erweitert werden[4].

Das Maximum aller elastischen Qualitäten fand sich ebenfalls im jugendlichen Erwachsenenalter, mit zunehmendem Alter ergab sich eine individuellen Schwankungen unterworfene Abnahme der Werte, die im Typus der schlaffen Lunge endet und kontinuierlich in das diffuse senile Emphysem übergehen kann (Abb. 10).

Mit zunehmendem Alter läßt sich in allen Bereichen der Vitalkapazität eine vermehrte Dehnbarkeit (Komplianz 0,3 Liter/cm HOH; Elastance 3,3 cm HOH/Liter) mit erniedrigten Volumelastizitätsmoduln nachweisen (s. Tabelle 2). Die statische Retraktionskraft ist mit einem Mittelwert von −5 cm HOH mäßig erniedrigt. Die Retraktion ist deutlich verzögert (Wert des Tiffeneau-Testes 37%, s. Abb. 17, S. 432) und die maximale Ausatmungsstromstärke entsprechend vermindert.

Eine wesentliche Erhöhung des Minimalluftanteiles an den vergrößerten Kollapsvolumina liegt noch nicht vor. Eine genauere Aufgliederung in verschiedene Altersbereiche hat gezeigt, daß dieser Abfall der elastischen Werte mit zunehmendem Alter kontinuierlich erfolgt[5]. Neben der zeitlichen Verzögerung des Retraktionsvorganges tritt an der Alterslunge auch die Hysterese mit mittleren Dehnungsresten von 7,5% deutlich in Erscheinung.

Diesem Funktionswandel entspricht kein morphologisch faßbarer Befund am Fasersystem. Die elastischen Fasern reifen etwa vom 4. Schwangerschaftsmonat an in dem embryonalen Mesenchym der Lunge aus; sie bilden zunächst das grobe

---

[1] Donders 1853, Perls 1869, Loeschcke 1928.   [2] H. Müller 1922.
[3] Tendeloo, Hennemann und Metz 1929, G. A. Metz 1930.
[4] Giese 1956.   [5] Hartung 1958.

Faserwerk des Gangsystems und erscheinen erst spät in den im 7. Monat aussprossenden Alveolen. In der postfetalen Entwicklung setzt sich die Faserneubildung fort, solange die Lunge wächst[1]. Das bei Neugeborenen noch sehr zellreiche Mesenchym differenziert sich schließlich so weit, daß die elastischen Fasern den Hauptanteil des Lungengewebes bilden. Das respiratorisch wirksame Elasticagerüst gelangt erst mit einsetzender Funktion zu voller Ausreifung[2]. Im Alter ist die einsetzende Atrophie zwar global an einem allmählichen Gewichtsrückgang zu erkennen[3], die Gewebsstruktur bietet aber in der Regel keine Änderungen, aus denen man auf einen funktionellen Elastizitätsverlust schließen könnte. Insbesondere wird am elastischen Fasersystem mit den üblichen Färbungen weder eine Reduktion, noch ein Zerfall einzelner Fasern, noch eine Auflösung des Netzgefüges gefunden[4].

Das Volumen der Alterslunge ist gegenüber dem der gesunden jugendlichen Lunge im Kollapszustand durch Zunahme der Minimalluft vergrößert. Es liegt nahe, diese Volumenzunahme auf die im Laufe des Lebens nicht mehr voll ausgleichbaren hysteretischen Dehnungsrückstände zu beziehen[5]. Die Erscheinungen elastischer Unvollkommenheit sind an der Alterslunge zwar sehr deutlich ausgeprägt. Über die Ermüdbarkeit der elastischen Strukturen ist aber einstweilen noch zu wenig bekannt, als daß man das von TENDELOO am Kautschukmodell und an der Aorta, von WENZEL (1950) an der Haut geprüfte Gesetz der Abhängigkeit der unvollkommenen elastischen Nachwirkung von dem Produkt aus Dehnungsausmaß und Dehnungsdauer ohne weiteres auf die lebende Lunge übertragen könnte. Mit der Volumenvermehrung ist eine Erweiterung der Acini, besonders des Arbor alveolaris, verbunden.

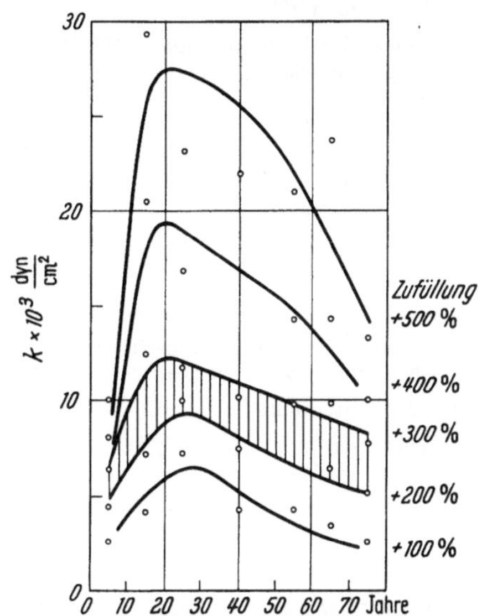

Abb. 10. Altersdiagramm der Volumelastizitätsmoduln ($\varkappa$) bei steigender Auffüllung; das gestrichelte Kurvenstück entspricht der Atemmittellage. Der Kurvenverlauf stellt das Ansteigen und Absinken des elastischen Widerstandes dar. (Aus HARTUNG 1958.)

Es entsteht ein Volumen pulmonum auctum, das auf einer senilen Ektasie der Lunge beruht, die wegen ihrer Einpassung in den Thoraxraum nicht einer volummäßigen Altersinvolution verfallen kann[6]. Die Lunge wird im Alter größer, obwohl sie an Substanz verliert. Dieser Zustand geht morphologisch fließend in das senile Emphysem über, wie sich auch die elastischen Funktionswerte des senilen Emphysems und der nicht emphysematischen Alterslunge nur graduell unterscheiden.

Die Minderung der ventilatorischen Funktion einer gealterten Lunge können wir als Folge des Elastizitätsverlustes ansehen. Ihr morphologischer Ausdruck ist Erschlaffung und Erweiterung der Lufträume, besonders des Gangsystems im Acinus, ihr physiologischer die abgeschwächte und verzögerte Retraktion mit Vergrößerung des Restvolumens, Verschiebung der Atemmittellage nach der Inspirationsseite und Abnahme der Atemstromstärke[7].

---

[1] ENGEL 1950. [2] KOESTLIN 1849, SUDSUKI 1899, LINSER 1900, v. HAYEK 1953.
[3] ROESSLE und ROULET 1932. [4] TENDELOO 1910, LOESCHCKE 1928, GIESE 1956 u. a.
[5] TENDELOO 1929. [6] L. MÜLLER 1929, GIESE 1959.
[7] Vgl. auch S. 148/149 Diffusionskapazität der Alterslunge.

Tabelle 2. *Elastizität der Leichenlunge im Alter und bei senilem Emphysem**.

	Normale Lungen, mittleres Alter 22 Jahre	Normale Lungen, mittleres Alter 56 Jahre	Senile Emphyseme, mittleres Alter 68 Jahre
1. Kollapsvolumen ml	1615	1810	2665
2. Minimalluftanteil am Kollapsvolumen %	45,2	45,6	52,7
3. Mittlerer elastischer Widerstand gegen Dehnung (Elastance) cm HOH/Liter .	4,5	3,3	2,0
4. Mittlere Dehnbarkeit (Komplianz) Liter/cm HOH	0,22	0,30	0,50
5. Volumelastizitätsmoduln $\times 10^3$ dyn/cm^2 Inspirationslage	42,9	26,0	13,0
Mittellage	18,0	16,5	9,0
Exspirationslage	11,9	8,8	6,3
6. Statische Retraktionskraft (Lungenzug) cm HOH Inspirationslage	−12	−8,5	−5,5
Exspirationslage	−2	−1,5	−0,5
7. Tiffeneau-Test, Zweisekundenwert %	46	37	24
8. Maximale Atemstromstärke Liter/sec	1,1	0,9	0,6
9. Hysteretischer Dehnungsrückstand (Akkommodationsbreite) %	<3	7,5	10,0
10. „Totraumeffekt"	⌀	⌀	⌀
Bemerkungen	5 ♂, 3 ♀ mittleres Alter 22 Jahre Entsprechend Gruppe I nach Cournand	4 ♂, 8 ♀ mittleres Alter 56 Jahre Entsprechend Gruppe III nach Cournand	6 ♂, 3 ♀ im Mittel 68 Jahre

* Die Werte wurden nach Messungen am Oberlappen für die gesamte Lunge umgerechnet und sind für den Vergleich mit klinischen Messungen im Bereich der Vitalkapazität, d. h. im Normalauffüllungsbereich, angegeben. Methodik und Originalwerte bei Hartung 1957 und 1958/59.

1. Kollapsvolumen in elastischer Ruhelage mit dem Druck Null, gemessen im Überlaufgefäß.

2. Zur Berechnung des Minimalluftanteiles wurde das „Nicht-Luftvolumen" nach Bönniger durch Division des Gewichtes durch 1,06, das vermutliche spezifische Gewicht des Lungengewebes, ermittelt und vom gesamten Kollapsvolumen abgezogen.

3. Druckzuwachs in Zentimeter Wassersäule pro Liter Volumdehnung, errechnet als Mittelwert im gesamten physiologischen Auffüllungsbereich der Vitalkapazität; entspricht der Lage der „Elastizitätsachse" in diesem Bereich.

4. Volumzunahme in Liter bei Erhöhung des Einfülldruckes um 1 cm Wassersäule; Kehrwert von 3.

5. Volumelastizitätsmoduln ($\Delta p / \Delta V \times V_m$), berechnet für Auffüllungen in Höhe der Inspirations- und Exspirationsstellung und in Atemmittellage.

6. Zugkraft in Zentimeter Wassersäule der sich im Rezipienten gegen Luft frei retrahierenden Lunge; angegeben für die Inspirations- und Exspirationsstellung.

7. Durch elastische Retraktion der Leichenlunge mit schleimfreiem Bronchialbaum ausgeblasene Luftmenge, prozentual bezogen auf die = 100 % gesetzte, in Höhe einer der Vitalkapazität entsprechenden Auffüllung gehaltene Auffüllmenge; entspricht dem klinischen Atemstoßtest nach Tiffeneau.

8. Durch elastische Retraktion der Leichenlunge bewirkte maximale Atemstromstärke während der 1. Sekunde der freien Retraktion; errechnet aus dem Tiffeneau-Test.

9. Irreversible, auf Hysterese beruhende Restvolumina über das Ausgangsvolumen nach wiederholten Volumdehnungen, prozentual bezogen auf die in Höhe einer der Vitalkapazität entsprechenden Auffüllung gehaltene Auffüllmenge. Kennzeichnet zugleich die Akkommodationsbreite.

10. Ein positiver Totraumeffekt besagt, daß in ventilationsgestörten Lungenbezirken als Teil des ventilatorischen Totraumes praktisch nicht oder kaum bewegte Luft festgehalten wird, was bei den Versuchen unmittelbar beobachtet werden und an dem Verlauf der hierdurch verfälschten Hysteresekurven erkannt werden kann. Dieser Totraum ist mit dem sog. funktionellen Totraum der Physiologie und Pathophysiologie nicht identisch (s. auch S. 472).

2. Das Altersemphysem.

Die Atmungsstörungen beim Emphysem sind in ihrer Form und Ausprägung abhängig von den Mechanismen, die die Lungenblähung ausgelöst haben. Wir unterscheiden für die Funktionsanalyse im Hinblick auf die Elastizität das *genuine konstitutionelle Emphysem*, bei dem die Homogenität der Lunge erhalten bleibt, von den *sekundären Emphysemen*, die in der Mehrzahl herdförmig sind, zur Inhomogenität der Lunge führen und durch Bronchusobstruktion, Narbenzug, örtliche Überdehnung des Lungengewebes oder ähnliche Vorgänge ausgelöst werden[1].

α) Morphologische Befunde.

Das *genuine* konstitutionelle *oder senile* Emphysem ist ein diffuses Emphysem, als dessen Hauptkriterien Dehnung, Atrophie und Anämie der Lunge gelten[2]. Dabei kommt es zu einem langsam fortschreitenden Umbau des Respirationsraumes mit irreversibler Erweiterung der Alveolen tragenden Lufträume. Dieser Umbau scheidet das Emphysem vom Volumen pulmonum auctum mit seiner korrespondierenden, stets reversiblen Vergrößerung der Alveolen und der Alveolargänge.

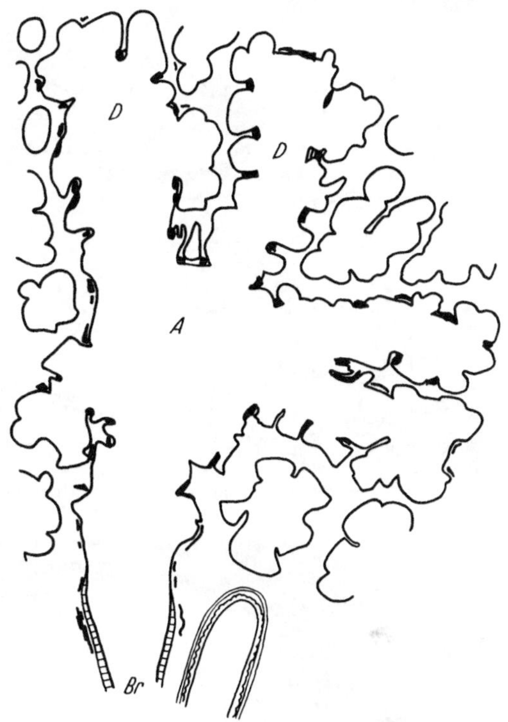

Abb. 11. Schematische Darstellung eines Schnittes durch den Stiel eines Acinus bei leichtem Emphysem. Auseinanderrücken der Teilungssporne der Bronchioli respiratorii und Bildung eines Atrium (*A*). Erweiterung der Ductus alveolares (*D*). Bronchiolus terminalis (*Br*).

Beim chronischen diffusen Emphysem beginnt der Umbau mit einer Erweiterung des Gangsystems im Acinus. Im Bereich der dicht aufeinanderfolgenden Teilungen der Bronchioli respiratorii I bis III bildet sich ein Atrium dadurch, daß die Teilungssporne der Bronchioli respiratorii auseinanderrücken. Das Atrium geht in die schlauchartigen Alveolargänge über, deren Alveolen muldenförmig abgeflacht und schließlich ganz verstrichen sind. Die Emphysemlunge zeigt in dieser Entwicklungsphase im histologischen Schnitt nicht das gleichmäßige Gitternetz der Alveolen, sondern weite Gänge, zwischen denen nur spärliche Reste flacher Alveolen liegen (Abb. 11—13). Im Raumbild eines Alveolarganges fehlen die etagenförmig oder nach Art eines Kabinenganges angeordneten Alveolen, in das schlauch- oder sackförmige Gebilde ragen nur stummelförmige Reste von Alveolarsepten hinein (s. Abb. 60, S. 552). Dem makroskopischen Bild des diffusen bläschenförmigen, sog. substantiellen Emphysems entspricht in diesem Zustand histologisch die sehr gleichmäßige grobwabige Gangstruktur. Dadurch, daß alle Acini, zum mindesten in einer Lungenregion,

---

[1] Giese 1959, 1960.
[2] Laennec 1826, Virchow 1856, 1888, Loeschcke 1928, Lauche 1956.

sich gleichmäßig verändern, werden die Segment- und Lobularsepten gleichmäßig in Spannung versetzt und verlaufen geradlinig (Abb. 14).

Das grobe elastische Fasersystem des Arbor alveolaris ist auseinandergerückt, aber in seiner Anordnung erhalten, das feine Elasticanetz der Alveolen zwischen den Gangfasern

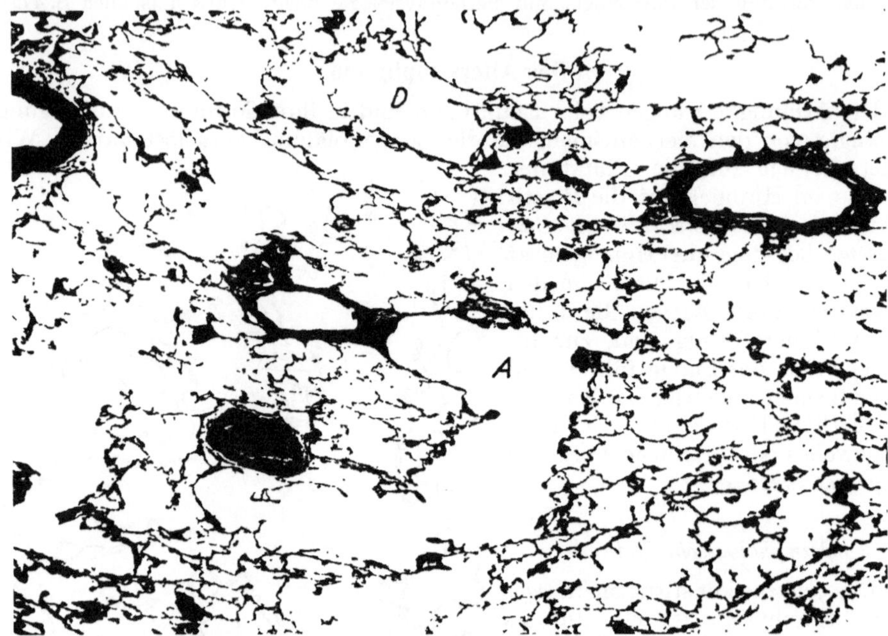

Abb. 12. Seniles Emphysem mit Bildung von Atrien (*A*) und Erweiterung der Ductus alveolares (*D*).
S.-Nr. 1433/55.

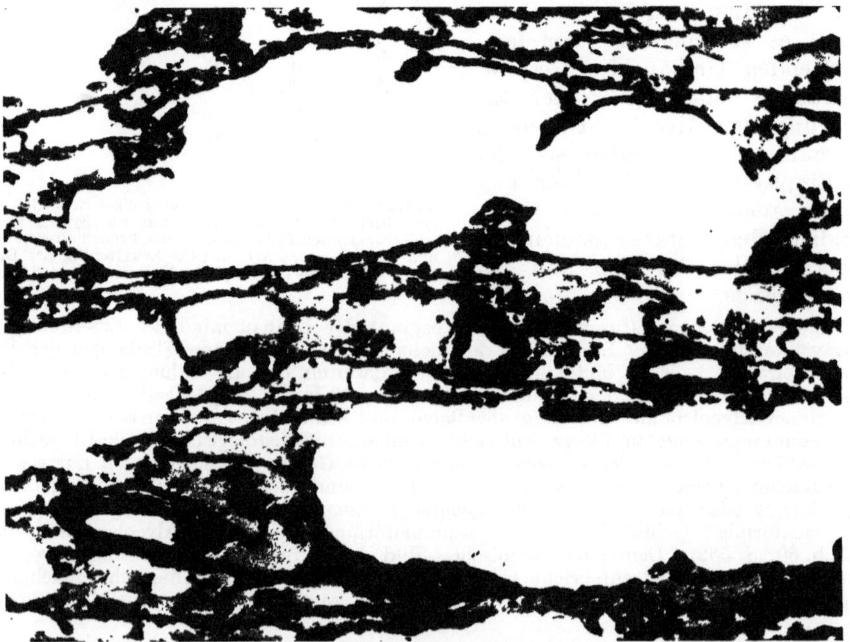

Abb. 13. Erweiterte Alveolargänge mit Schwund der Alveolar-Struktur durch Verstreichen der Alveolarsepten.
Seniles Emphysem. S.-Nr. 1433/55.

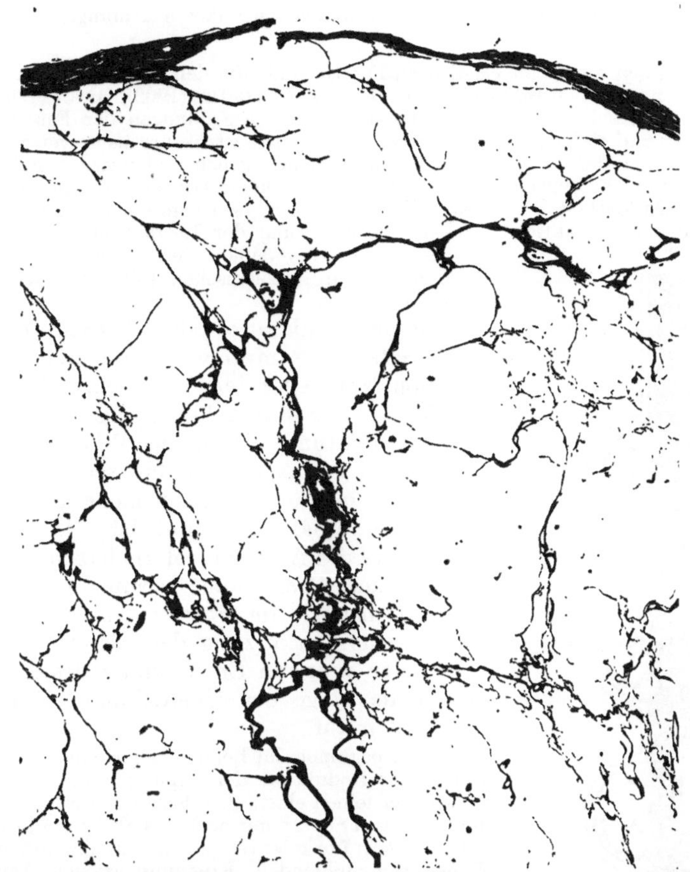

Abb. 14. Diffuses senil-atrophisches weit fortgeschrittenes Emphysem. Völliger Schwund der Alveolarstruktur. Das Lungengerüst wird nur noch von den stark gedehnten Acinussepten gebildet. Weite dünnwandige Bronchioli terminales. 79jähriger Mann. S.-Nr. 391/56. Vergr. 7:1.

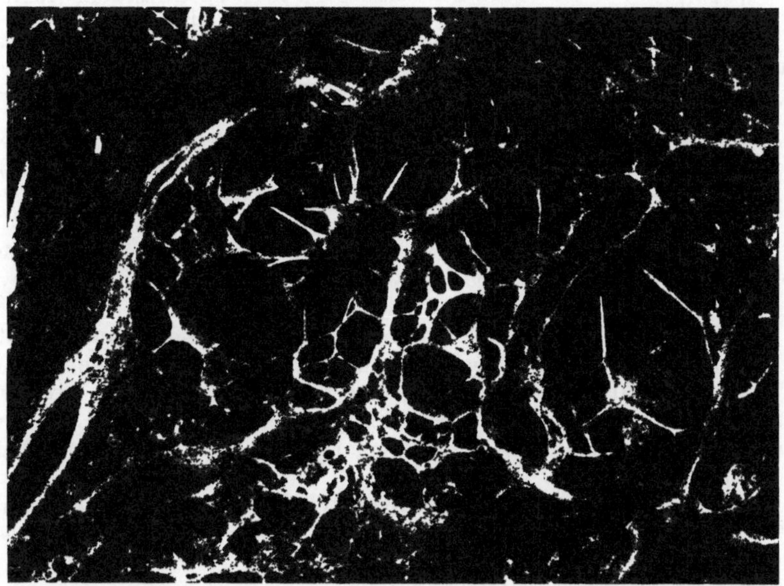

Abb. 15. Fortgeschrittenes Emphysem. Gitterförmiges Fasernetz nach Ausbau der Alveolarsepten. Fensterung der Acinussepten über erweiterten Kohnschen Poren. Vergr. 12:1.

ausgespannt. An den einzelnen elastischen Fasern sind mit den üblichen Färbungen keine Unterschiede vom normalen Bild zu finden[1]. Die von Eppinger (1902), Orsós (1907), Russakoff (1909) u. a. beschriebenen Aufsplitterungen und Aufrollungen der Fasern sind erst bei ausgedehnter und tiefgreifender Zerstörung der Lungenstruktur, insbesondere beim Narbenemphysem vorhanden. Ebenso ist auch an den kollagenen und reticulären Fasern oder an den spärlichen, nicht hypertrophierten Muskelfasern keine Degeneration zu erkennen. Die mit physikalischen Methoden bei diesem Grad des Emphysems stets nachweisbare und meßbare Abnahme der Retraktionskraft, die Verlängerung der Retraktionszeit und die Vergrößerung des irreversiblen Dehnungsrückstandes (Hysterese) haben im histologischen Bild der Faserstrukturen kein Äquivalent.

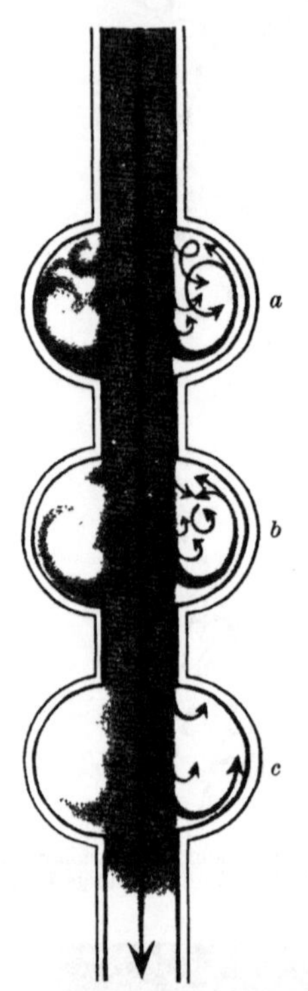

Abb. 16. Einmischung einer gefärbten Flüssigkeit in ein wassergefülltes Glasmodell eines Alveolarganges.
a Bereits vorgeschrittene Durchmischung; *b* bevorzugte Wandströmung, beginnende Durchmischung im Zentrum; *c* beginnende Einmischung. Pfeile: Strömungsrichtungen.

Die Gefügedilatation oder Distension des Acinus[2] ist bereits ein Symptom der unzureichenden Retraktionsfähigkeit seines elastischen Fasersystems. Sie hat in der Entwicklung des Emphysems insofern Bedeutung, als mit der Bildung des Atrium die bei der Inspiration entstehende elastische Spannung im Acinus nicht mehr auf den Bronchiolus terminalis gerichtet ist. Die peripheren Abschnitte des Arbor alveolaris haben ihre Bezugspunkte zum Bronchiolus terminalis verloren, die Retraktionskraft im Fasersystem des Acinus bewirkt keine Verkürzung des Acinus.

In der weiteren Entwicklung des Emphysems treten als Folge der Überdehnung Fensterungen der Septen auf.

Diese beginnen im Bereich der Kohnschen Poren, die sich unter Reduktion der Capillaren und Schwund des Netzes der feinen elastischen Fasern vergrößern, bis in den intraacinösen Septen nur noch das Skelet der groben elastischen Fasern übrig ist (Abb. 15). Aus den auf die gleiche Weise sich bildenden Kommunikationen benachbarter Acini entstehen schließlich immer größer werdende Blasen, die an mehrere Bronchioli terminales angeschlossen sind. Die Verschmelzung der Acini hat Loeschcke (1921, 1928) am Ausgußpräparat gezeigt. Die Lobularsepten bleiben lange erhalten, sie sind mit ihrem kollagenen Fasernetz resistent gegen Dehnung und bilden Scheidewände, wenn im ganzen Lobularraum nur noch spärliche Faserzüge nach Art eines Spinnennetzes ausgespannt sind.

Der Gewebsschwund ist ein wesentliches Merkmal des Emphysems. Beitzke (1923, 1925) hat gezeigt, daß nicht nur das Acinusgefüge umgebaut wird, sondern daß auch die Bronchioli terminales trompetenartig erweitert werden. Diese Erweiterung schreitet mit Zunahme des Emphysems hilipetal fort, die Bronchialwand wird in die Wand der Emphysemblasen einbezogen.

Mit der trompetenartigen Erweiterung der Bronchioli terminales fällt der Bronchusabschnitt fort, durch dessen Enge die Inspirationsluft wie durch eine Düse in den weiten Acinus einströmt, hier an den Gangsepten und Alveolareingangsringen gebrochen und in den Alveolen umhergewirbelt wird. Die Durchmischung der Luft im Acinus, also der Alveolarluft im klinischen Sinne, ist durch diesen Umbau gestört[3].

Nach eigenen Untersuchungen fließt Luft oder Wasser in einem Glasmodell, das dem normalen Alveolargang mit den zugehörigen Alveolen nachgebildet ist, bei der Inspiration

---

[1] Sudsuki 1899, Tendeloo 1910, Loeschcke 1928.
[2] Giese 1956.   [3] Dreser 1922, Beitzke 1925.

mit einem laminaren Zentralstrom ein. An den distalen Kanten der Alveolareingangsringe bricht sich der Strom, wird unter Wirbelbildungen in die Alveolen zurückgeworfen und füllt den Alveolarraum in turbulenter rückläufiger Strömung aus (Abb. 16).

Der emphysematöse, intraacinös beginnende Umbau endet in einem Schwund des respiratorischen Parenchyms mit seinem Fasersystem und in einer Verkürzung des in seinen Endverzweigungen abgebauten Bronchialbaumes. Er entspricht einer progressiven Lungendystrophie.

Im fortgeschrittenen senilen Emphysem entwickeln sich vorwiegend in den Lungenrändern und in den Oberlappen Luftblasen mit den Merkmalen des bronchostenotischen Emphysems. Diese blasige Überformung des primär-dystrophischen Emphysems ist Folge einer Kompression der kleinen Bronchien und Bronchiolen während der Exspiration.

Die Emphysembronchitis, die in den Endzuständen des senilen Emphysems selten vermißt wird, ist ebenfalls eine Folge (Komplikationsbronchitis), die bronchostenotische Effekte auslöst.

Über den Einfluß des Emphysems auf die Blutströmung und auf das Gefäßbett der Endstrombahn siehe in den Abschnitten Perfusions- und Diffusionsstörungen.

β) Elastizitätsmessungen bei Altersemphysem.

An der isolierten Emphysemlunge lassen sich in ähnlicher Weise wie bei der normalen Lunge nach der dort beschriebenen Methode Elastizitätsmessungen durchführen und mit diesen vergleichen.

Eine Abnahme der Lungenelastizität bei Emphysem ist schon aus den Ergebnissen von TENDELOO u. Mitarb. (1929) wahrscheinlich gemacht worden. Der von G. A. METZ (1930) aus Messungen an Lungenstreifen gezogene Schluß, daß die Emphysemlunge geringer dehnbar sei, beruht auf Unzulänglichkeiten der Streifenmessung und kann nicht mehr aufrecht erhalten werden. Genauere Werte haben erst die mit HARTUNG (1958) durchgeführten Messungen ergeben.

Bei den senilen Emphysemen ist der Typus der schlaffen Lunge noch wesentlich stärker ausgeprägt als bei der Alterslunge (s. Tabelle 2, S. 426). Die Grenzen zu dieser sind aber fließend, die Gruppe der senilen Emphyseme, deren Werte gesondert dargestellt sind, wurde daher nach morphologischen Kriterien vor Durchführung der Elastizitätsmessungen abgetrennt. Die Dehnbarkeit ist sehr beträchtlich erhöht (Komplianz 0,5 Liter/cm HOH; Elastance 2,0 cm HOH/Liter), die Volumelastizitätsmoduln sind im Bereich der Vitalkapazitätsfüllung etwa auf die Hälfte des Wertes der normalen jugendlichen Leichenlunge herabgesetzt. Eine gleiche Fülldruckzunahme ruft also eine über doppelt so große Volumzunahme der Lunge hervor. Die statische Retraktionskraft ist mit einem Mittelwert von — 2,5 cm HOH ebenfalls auf die Hälfte abgesunken. Die Einbuße an elastischer Retraktionsfähigkeit wird auch in dem stärker verzögerten Ablauf des Retraktionsvorganges erkennbar (Tiffeneau-Test Wert 24% ; Abb. 17), die maximale Ausatmungsstromstärke ist somit ebenfalls etwa um die Hälfte vermindert. Während an normalen jugendlichen Leichenlungen das elastische Fasergewebe und die Lunge als Ganzes ein hohes Maß an elastischer Vollkommenheit besitzen, werden an den senil-emphysematischen Lungen die Erscheinungen elastischer Unvollkommenheit nicht nur an dem verzögerten Retraktionsablauf, sondern auch an irreversiblen hysteretischen Dehnungsresten von im Mittel 10% sehr deutlich. Der Minimalluftanteil am Kollapsvolumen ist auf 52,7% erhöht.

v. NEERGAARD (1930) fand bei gesunden Versuchspersonen eine Druckzunahme von 14,5 cm H_2O je Liter Volumdehnung einer Lunge, beim Emphysematiker dagegen nur 6 cm H_2O/Liter. Der normale statische Mitteldruck von —5,6 cm H_2O sank auf —3,2 cm H_2O ab.

Dayman (1951) ermittelte in ähnlicher Weise, ebenfalls durch statische Oesophagusdruckmessungen bei gestufter Exspiration, einen Lungenzugskoeffizienten in cm H_2O/ 100 ml Volumänderung, der etwa der Volumelastizität entspricht (Tabelle 2). Die Werte lagen bei 10 Emphysematikern im Mittel etwas höher (0,56) gegenüber den Lungengesunden (0,43). Diese Erhöhung ist jedoch nur eine scheinbare, da bei den Emphysematikern die Atemmittellage wesentlich höher ist. So finden sich die statischen Oesophagusdrucke im Bereich der funktionellen Residualkapazität normal bei $-6{,}02$ cm H_2O, bei Emphysematikern sind sie dagegen auf $-3{,}65$ cm H_2O vermindert. Der Quotient aus Residualluft/Totalkapazität, normal bei 25,1, ist bei den Emphysematikern auf 57,1 erhöht. Dayman (1951) selbst hat daher aus seinen Werten auf einen tatsächlich bestehenden, aber durch die Verschiebung der Atemmittellage kompensierten Elastizitätsverlust der Emphysemlunge geschlossen.

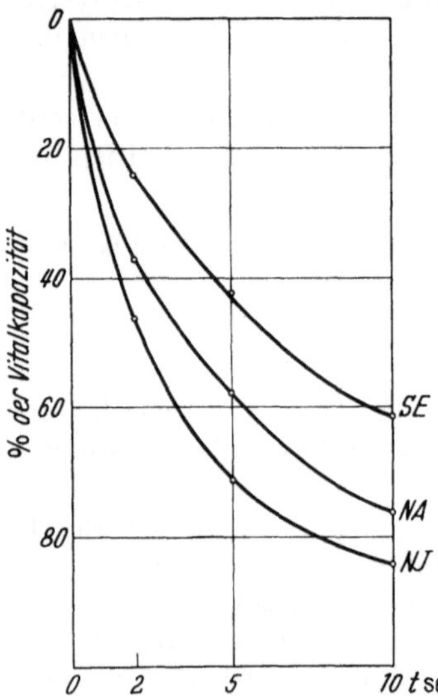

Abb. 17. Retraktionskurven (Tiffeneau-Test) nach Untersuchungen an Leichenlungen. Vergleich normaler Lungen aus verschiedenen Lebensaltern. *NJ* Jugendliche Altersgruppe (Durchschnitt 22 Jahre); *NA* höheres Lebensalter (Durchschnitt 56 Jahre); *SE* seniles Emphysem (Durchschnitt 68 Jahre).

Faßt man diese Ergebnisse der Messungen an der isolierten Leichenlunge zusammen, so ergibt sich, daß auch die Emphysemlunge noch eine Restelastizität besitzt. Sie zeigt ebenso wie die normale Lunge noch eine etwa lineare Druck-Volumrelation, die Druckzunahme ist aber im Verhältnis zum Auffüllungsgrad wesentlich geringer; das gleiche gilt für die Retraktionskraft, die bis auf ein Drittel absinken kann. Entscheidend für die mechanische Lungenleistung wird aber die sehr erhebliche Verzögerung des Retraktionsablaufes. Die Emphysemlunge kann im Ablauf des zeitlich eng begrenzten Atemcyclus nur einen sehr kleinen Teil ihrer noch erhaltenen Elastizität für die Exspiration nutzbar machen. Die elastischen Kräfte der Emphysemlunge haben auch beim Lebenden nur geringen Teil an den Atembewegungen.

γ) Die funktionelle Bedeutung des Elastizitätsverlustes für die Lungenventilation.

Mit dem Nachlassen der Lungenelastizität geht eine Vergrößerung des Respirationsraumes und eine Verminderung der Respirationskraft Hand in Hand.

Die Vergrößerung des Ventilationsraumes, die sich anatomisch nicht nur in einer Erweiterung, sondern auch im progressiven Umbau des Acinus zu einem ungegliederten, schließlich auch gefensterten Hohlraum äußert, wird in ihrem Beginn ausgeglichen durch eine erhöhte Atemmittellage. Durch die vermehrte Dehnung der Lunge wird die noch vorhandene Elastizität für die Ventilation ausgenutzt, der Luftwechsel findet im Bereich der Komplementärluft statt, die Residualluft ist vermehrt[1]. Mit der Vergrößerung des Lungenvolumens geht eine Erweiterung des Thoraxraumes einher, die schließlich in dem faßförmigen, in der Inspirationsstellung verharrenden starren Thorax endet. Die Thoraxerweiterung folgt dem Verlust der Lungenelastizität nach, sie ist sozusagen Ausdruck des Elastizitätsschwundes und steht in einer festen Relation dazu. Diese Auffassung ist besonders von Tendeloo (1910) und Hofbauer (1921) vertreten und der Loeschckeschen Ansicht von der primären Thoraxstarre entgegengesetzt worden.

In den ungenügend ventilierten Räumen sinkt der Sauerstoffpartialdruck, die Kohlensäure wird angereichert, die Luft wird schlecht durchmischt. Während

---

[1] Hurtado und Mitarbeiter 1933—1935, Anthony 1937 (Literatur), Baldwin und Mitarbeiter 1949, Lottenbach 1956 (Literatur).

sich das Lungenvolumen mit der Schwere des Emphysems zunehmend vergrößert, sinkt im gleichen Verhältnis dazu der nutzbare Anteil des Atemvolumens, also der mit der Ventilation ausgetauschte Anteil der Luft ab. Der Atemgrenzwert ist beim Emphysem auf 25—30 Liter (gegenüber bis 125 Liter in der Norm) eingeschränkt[1], der Alveolarraum wird hypoventiliert, es kommt zu Untersättigung mit Sauerstoff und zur Vermehrung der Kohlensäure im Lungenblut, die insuffiziente Ventilation führt zur Globalinsuffizienz, die der Kliniker aus den Blutwerten (O_2, CO_2, Acidose) erschließt. Die Einschränkung des Gasaustausches wegen der Reduktion von Lungencapillaren wird bei den Störungen der Diffusion und Zirkulation besprochen.

Die verringerte Respirationskraft wird in einer Abschwächung und Verlängerung der Exspirationsphase erkennbar. Die Exspiration ist gestört, weil die elastische Retraktionskraft, mit deren Hilfe ein wesentlicher Teil der exspiratorischen Atemarbeit geleistet wird, nicht in genügendem Maße zur Verfügung steht. Dafür tritt in zunehmendem Maße die Exspirationsmuskulatur ein, die verminderte Elastizität wird durch Muskelkraft ersetzt, der Pleuradruck wird positiv. Die Luft wird nicht mehr durch die statischen Elastizitätskräfte der Lunge ausgeblasen, sondern durch die Exspirationsmuskulatur ausgepreßt. Die Atemarbeit ist dabei vermehrt[2]. Der positiv werdende Druck im Pleuraraum wirkt sich auf die Weite der Bronchien aus. Aus bronchographischen Untersuchungen[3] ist bekannt, daß Bronchien und Trachea bei intrathorakaler Drucksteigerung komprimiert werden. Der gleiche Vorgang wird auch für das Emphysem angenommen. Er führt in der Exspirationsphase zu einer Einengung der knorpelfreien Endabschnitte der Bronchiolen und erschwert, vielleicht über einen Ventilmechanismus, das Ausströmen der Luft. Dieser funktionelle Faktor ist anatomisch im histologischen Schnitt nicht faßbar, dort werden die Endabschnitte der Bronchien stets weit gefunden, weil die Kompression mit dem Druckausgleich zwischen Alveolarluft und Außenluft aufhört. Sein Nachweis im Versuch an der Leichenlunge steht noch aus. Dieses Gefangenbleiben der Luft, in der amerikanischen Literatur als *air trapping* bezeichnet, erklärt, warum der schwache Atemstrom des Emphysematikers auch durch maximale Anspannung der Exspirationsmuskulatur nicht verstärkt werden kann. Anatomisch ist der Ventilmechanismus aus dem Verlust der Innengliederung des Acinus beim Emphysem verständlich, weil mit dem Schwund der Bronchioli respiratorii auch die Fasersysteme verlorengehen, mit denen der Bronchiolus terminalis an seinen peripheren Haltepunkten fixiert ist. Aus den Ventilstenosen entsteht eine ungleichmäßige Durchlüftung (ventilatorische Verteilungsstörung), die, wenn sie sich am Blut auswirkt, als Partialinsuffizienz bezeichnet wird. An den vorderen Lungenrändern sind die Folgen der intrathorakalen Drucksteigerung besonders deutlich.

Für das genuine konstitutionelle Altersemphysem werden damit aus den morphologischen Befunden und den vorgelegten Meßwerten *folgende Schlüsse* gezogen:

Die Erweiterung der Lunge beim Altersemphysem ist Folge der Elastizitätsabnahme. Die Abnahme der Elastizität beruht auf einer Alterung der elastischen Fasersysteme, die morphologisch an der Einzelfaser nicht erkennbar ist. Sie ist Ursache für die Gefügedilatation im Acinus und für den progressiven Schwund des respiratorischen Parenchyms. Sie äußert sich in einer Verzögerung der Retraktion und im Auftreten irreversibler hysteretischer Dehnungsrückstände.

Im konstitutionellen Emphysem kommen die bereits in jeder Alterslunge meßbaren Minderungen der elastischen Funktion vermehrt zum Ausdruck. Die

---

[1] Rossier 1956, Knobloch und Hilscher 1958, Hamm 1958.
[2] Rossier 1956, McIlroy und Christie 1954 u. a.
[3] Stutz 1948, Di Rienzo 1949, Wyss 1955, H. H. Weber 1959 u. a.

Funktionsminderung in der Lunge läuft gleichsinnig zur Abnahme der elastischen Funktion der Aorta[1]. Ihre Folgen sind eine Verzögerung der Retraktion, eine Minderung der Retraktionskraft und ein Auftreten irreversibler Dehnungsrückstände, die durch zusätzliche Inanspruchnahme der Atemmuskulatur nicht voll ersetzt werden können.

Das genuine konstitutionelle Emphysem, dessen Hauptvertreter das senile Emphysem ist, fügt sich damit in den Rahmen der Aufbrauchkrankheiten ein. Es wird im hohen Alter nur selten vermißt[2]. Ein vor dem Senium auftretendes konstitutionelles Emphysem wird als Zeichen vorzeitiger Alterung aufgefaßt[3].

b) Die starre fibrotische Lunge.

Während bei der atrophischen Alterslunge und beim Altersemphysem der Verlust an Lungenelastizität zu einer Erschlaffung der Lunge mit einer Vermehrung der Restluft, Erhöhung der Dehnbarkeit, Erniedrigung des Dehnungswiderstandes und Absinken der Retraktionskraft führt, liegen die Verhältnisse bei der Lungenfibrose umgekehrt. Durch die zunehmende Vermehrung des Fasergewebes wird die Lunge fester und schließlich in eine starre Lunge umgewandelt, die sowohl der inspiratorischen Dehnung als auch dem exspiratorischen Lungenkollaps vermehrten Widerstand entgegensetzt. Die Exkursionsbreite der fibrotischen Lunge ist eingeengt, die Spitzen der Atemkurve sind abgeschnitten[4]. Die Vitalkapazität ist eingeschränkt, Reserveluft steht wegen der verminderten Dehnbarkeit nicht zur Verfügung. Die Komplementärluft kann nicht voll ausgenutzt werden. Bei vielen Fibrosen finden sich auch Stenosen und Obliteration der kleinen Bronchien mit nachfolgender ungleichmäßiger Verteilung der Atemluft (Verteilungsstörung) und herdförmiges Emphysem, durch das die Lunge wabig umgewandelt wird. Zu der globalen, die Gesamtkapazität der Lunge erfassenden und zu der differentialen, als Verteilungsstörung sich äußernden Einschränkung der Ventilation tritt stets noch eine Erschwerung der Diffusion, die sich aus der Verdickung der Alveolarsepten erklärt, und in schweren Fällen auch eine Behinderung der Perfusion durch Verödung von Lungencapillaren.

Den Funktionsstörungen bei der fibrotisch starren Lunge liegen also zahlreiche verschiedenartige Vorgänge zugrunde, die schon in den Frühstadien des fibrosierenden Prozesses ineinandergreifen und die Analyse des Einzelfalles komplizieren. Die Belastung des kleinen Kreislaufs mit dem Cor pulmonale als Endzustand tritt bei dieser komplexen Störung der Ventilation, der Verteilung, der Diffusion und der Perfusion früher und nachhaltiger in Erscheinung als beim diffusen, atrophischen Emphysem. Die fibrosierenden Prozesse sind selten diffus über alle Lungenteile gleichmäßig ausgedehnt (Stauungsinduration), häufiger herdförmig (Tuberkulose, Morbus Boeck, Silikose, interstitielle Pneumonie u. a.).

1. Mechanische Eigenschaften der fibrotischen Lunge.

α) Gewebswiderstand bei Lungenfibrose.

Die fibrotische Lunge setzt den Verformungen, denen sie bei den Ventilationsbewegungen ausgesetzt ist, einen erhöhten Gesamtwiderstand entgegen. Die elastischen Widerstände lassen sich als statische Werte in den verschiedenen Dehnungsphasen messen. Zu diesen treten die nur in der Bewegung faßbaren viscösen Widerstände, die sich aus den später zu besprechenden (S. 468) Strömungswiderständen und dem Gewebsdeformationswiderstand („tissue viscance")

---

[1] Tendeloo 1910, 1929, Jores 1924, dort weitere Literatur, Simon und W. W. Meyer 1958.
[2] Keck 1955.   [3] Bürger 1954.   [4] Uehlinger 1957.

zusammensetzen. Auf die Bedeutung der Gewebsdeformationswiderstände haben bereits ROHRER (1925) sowie v. NEERGAARD u. WIRZ (1927) hingewiesen. Sie beruhen vor allem auf inneren Reibungswiderständen, während der Trägheitswiderstand gegen Bewegungsänderungen praktisch vernachlässigt werden kann. Die viscösen Widerstände sind methodisch nur schwer von einander zu trennen. Man schätzt, daß beim Menschen von der totalen inspiratorisch zu leistenden Arbeit

    63,3% gegen elastische Widerstände,

    28,0% gegen Strömungswiderstände und

    8,7% gegen den Gewebsdeformationswiderstand

verbraucht werden[1].

Die Gesamtwiderstände wachsen bei pathologischen Prozessen erheblich an und vermindern dadurch den Nutzeffekt der Atemarbeit. Untersuchungen bei Emphysem und Asthma bronchiale haben noch keine ausreichende Klärung über die Höhe der zusätzlichen Widerstände, bei denen vor allem die Strömungswiderstände in den Vordergrund treten, erbringen können[2]. Bei den Lungenfibrosen besteht eine Vermehrung der elastischen Widerstände, aber auch des Gewebsdeformationswiderstandes. Sie beruht auf Störungen der Lungentextur durch Fibrosierung des Acinusgerüstes und auf Sklerose der Lobular- und Segmentsepten, die nach v. HAYEK (1953) die Funktion von Gleitflächen haben, weiter auf Verdickung der bindegewebigen Umhüllung der Bronchien und Gefäße. Ob und inwieweit kollagenes, präkollagenes und reticuläres Gewebe in der Lunge durch die bei der Inspiration entfaltete Zugwirkung gedehnt werden kann, ist noch nicht gemessen. Die gleiche Frage stellt sich für die Pleura bei der Erörterung der Folgen von Pleuraschwarten.

β) Elastizitätsmessungen an fibrotischen Lungen.

Der Einfluß der Lungenfibrose auf die Globalelastizität kann an der Leichenlunge bestimmt werden (Tabelle 3; weitere Einzelwerte HARTUNG 1959). Der elastische Widerstand (Elastance) ist stark erhöht (5,3 cm HOH/Liter im Bereich der unteren Hälfte der Vitalkapazitätsfüllung bei Stauungslungen, 12,0 cm HOH/Liter im gleichen Bereich bei Sklerodermie und 9,1 cm HOH/Liter bei vernarbter Miliartuberkulose; 10,3 cm HOH/Liter im gesamten Vitalkapazitätsbereich bei M. Boeck). Die Dehnbarkeit ist also stark eingeschränkt, wie die entsprechenden Werte der Komplianz unmittelbar zeigen (0,19 Liter/cm HOH in der unteren Hälfte der Vitalkapazitätsfüllung bei den Stauungslungen, 0,08 Liter/cm HOH im gleichen Bereich bei Sklerodermie und 0,11 Liter/cm HOH bei vernarbter Miliartuberkulose; 0,09 Liter/cm HOH im gesamten Vitalkapazitätsbereich bei M. Boeck gegenüber 0,22 Liter/cm HOH bei normalen jugendlichen Lungen und 0,50 Liter/cm HOH bei senilem Emphysem). Die in den verschiedenen Auffüllungsbereichen gültigen Volumelastizitätsmoduln zeigen schon innerhalb des Vitalkapazitätsbereiches einen unproportional starken Anstieg, der bei normalen Lungen erst außerhalb des im Thorax möglichen Dehnungsausmaßes durch den Endwiderstand der angespannten Pleura hervorgerufen wird. So fand sich bei den Stauungslungen ein Modul von $91,0 \times 10^3$ dyn/cm² (entsprechend etwa 93 cm HOH), von $89,0 \times 10^3$ dyn/cm² (entsprechend etwa 91 cm HOH) bei der vernarbten Miliartuberkulose, von über 100×10^3 dyn/cm² bei Sklerodermie bereits in einer der Atemmittellage entsprechenden Auffüllungshöhe und ein Modul von $107,8 \times 10^3$ dyn/cm² (entsprechend etwa 105 cm HOH) bei M. Boeck in inspiratorischer Auffüllungshöhe gegenüber $42,9 \times 10^3$ dyn/cm² (entsprechend etwa 44 cm HOH) bei der inspiratorisch gedehnten normalen und nur $13,0 \times 10^3$ dyn/cm² (entsprechend etwa 13 cm HOH) in der senil-emphysematischen Lunge. Die volle Inspirationsauffüllung ist bei diesen starren Lungen nicht mehr möglich, sie haben bis zur Hälfte ihrer Vitalkapazität eingebüßt. Weil die Ausdehnungsfähigkeit eingeschränkt ist, spricht man von *restriktiver ventilatorischer Insuffizienz*.

Die Retraktionsfähigkeit kann bei den fibrotischen Lungen zumindest gegenüber den Emphysemlungen noch relativ gut erhalten sein (Tiffeneau-Test mit Zweisekundenwerten von 36% bei den Stauungslungen, von 38% bei vernarbter Miliartuberkulose, über 30% bei

---

[1] OTIS, FENN und RAHN 1950.   [2] LOTTENBACH, NOELPP-ESCHENHAGEN und NOELPP 1956.

Tabelle 3. *Elastizität von Leichenlungen bei verschiedenen krankhaften Prozessen (Gerüststarre, Pleuraschwarte und Narbenemphysem).*

	Normale jugendliche Lungen	Stauungslungen	Lunge bei Sklerodermie	Lunge mit vernarbter Miliartuberkulose	Lunge bei M. Boeck**	Pleuraschwarte (gefesselte Lunge)	Restlunge nach Pneumektomie
1. Kollapsvolumen ml	1615	2300	1600	2050	2200	1890	1800
2. Minimalluftanteil am Kollapsvolumen %	45,2	29,4	21,7	35,4	34,1	26,8	39,6
3. Mittlerer elastischer Widerstand gegen Dehnung (Elastance) cm HOH/Liter .	4,5	5,3*	12,0*	9,1*	10,3	15,6***	4,8****
4. Mittlere Dehnbarkeit (Komplianz) Liter/cm HOH	0,22	0,19*	0,08*	0,11*	0,09	0,06***	0,21****
5. Volumelastizitätsmoduln $\times 10^3$ dyn/cm²							
Inspirationslage	42,9	Ø	Ø	Ø	107,8	Ø	>100
Mittellage.	18,0	91,0	>100	89,0	14,0	Ø	24,0
Exspirationslage	11,9	11,9	25,2	22,4	4,2	54,2	Ø
6. Statische Retraktionskraft (Lungenzug) cm HOH							
Inspirationslage	−12 } −5*		} −4*	} −7*	−10	Ø } − 3****	
Exspirationslage	−2				−1	−6,5***	
7. Tiffeneau-Test Zweisekundenwert % . . .	46	36	>30	38	19	42	24
8. Maximale Atemstromstärke Liter/sec	1,1	0,5*	?	0,5*	0,5	0,3***	0,3****
9. Hysteretischer Dehnungsrückstand (Akkommodationsbreite)	<3	5*	4*	6*	24	>10***	12****
10. „Totraumeffekt"	Ø	Ø	Ø	Ø	+	Ø	Ø

Erläuterung zu dieser Tabelle s. Legende zu Tabelle 2, S. 25.

    * Nur halbe Vitalkapazitätsauffüllung möglich.
  ** Ausgesprochenes Narbenemphysem.
 *** Nur ein Viertel der Vitalkapazitätsauffüllung möglich.
**** Nur halbe Vitalkapazitätsauffüllung in Mittellage bezogen auf Gesamtlunge.

Sklerodermie). Sie wird aber stark eingeschränkt, wenn nennenswerte Grade von Narbenemphysem mit den fibrosierenden Prozessen verbunden sind wie in dem Fall von M. Boeck (Tiffeneau-Wert 19%). Die maximalen Atemstromstärken sind jedoch entsprechend der absolut eingeschränkten Füllungsgrade durchschnittlich auf die Hälfte der Normwerte herabgesetzt. Die statische Retraktionskraft liegt innerhalb der verminderten Ventilationsbreite in regelrechter Höhe. Erscheinungen elastischer Unvollkommenheit treten nicht besonders hervor, weil auch die kollagenen Anteile bei gleichen bezogenen Spannungen eine relativ hohe elastische Vollkommenheit zeigen (Ranke 1925). Es fanden sich irreversible Dehnungsrückstände von 5% bei den Stauungslungen, von 6% bei der vernarbten Miliartuberkulose und von 4% bei Sklerodermie, dagegen von 24% bei dem mit Narbenemphysem verbundenen Fall von M. Boeck.

Der Minimalluftgehalt ist bei den fibrotischen Lungen meist auf Kosten der vermehrten Gerüstsubstanz herabgesetzt, sofern nicht ein erhebliches, insbesondere bronchostenotischbullöses Emphysem besteht. Bei den Stauungslungen spielt auch der stark vermehrte Blutgehalt eine wesentliche Rolle (29,4% Minimalluftanteil am Kollapsvolumen). Eine grobe Abschätzung des Gewebs- und Blutanteiles ist möglich, wenn man entsprechend Clösges (1949) den Quotienten von Minimalluft/Gewebevolumen (Nicht-Luftvolumen) bildet. Er betrug 0,41 bei den Stauungslungen, 0,55 bei vernarbter Miliartuberkulose, 0,52 bei M. Boeck.

0,28 bei Sklerodermie (mit gleichzeitig starkem urämischem Lungenödem) gegenüber 0,82 bei normalen Lungen und über 1,0 liegenden Werten für Emphysemlungen.

Die vorstehenden Meßwerte an starren Lungen beziehen sich auf Fälle von Stauungslungen, Sklerodermie, M. Boeck und vernarbter Miliartuberkulose. Allen untersuchten Fibrosen ist gemeinsam die starke Erhöhung des elastischen Widerstandes mit der Folge verminderter Dehnbarkeit. Die elastische Retraktionsfähigkeit ist nur in geringen Grenzen eingeschränkt, solange nicht Emphysem komplizierend hinzugetreten ist. Die Minimalluft der fibrotischen Lunge ist vermindert.

Lungenfibrose und Lungenemphysem haben ähnliche Folgen für die Ventilationsfähigkeit und Atmungsökonomie, obwohl sie in der Relation von Lungengewicht zum Luftgehalt und in ihrer unterschiedlichen Dehnbarkeit extreme Gegensätze darstellen. Bei den Lungenfibrosen bedeutet ein hinzutretendes Narbenemphysem eine besonders schwere Komplikation für die Ventilationsfunktionen.

Im Gegensatz zu den vorwiegend diffusen Gerüstsklerosen (z. B. bei Stauungslungen) ergibt sich bei den ausgesprochen herdförmigen Fibrosen als gemeinsames mechanisches Prinzip eine *statische Inhomogenität* daraus, daß fibrosierte, wenig dehnbare Abschnitte und schwielenfreie Lungenbezirke mit erhaltener Elastizität unmittelbar benachbart sind. Die funktionelle Folge ist eine inhomogene Belüftung (s. unter Verteilungsstörungen S. 458), während das Gesamtmaß an Fibrose die Einschränkung der globalen Ventilationsvolumina bestimmt. Das morphologische Substrat der differentialen Dehnbarkeitsunterschiede (Modulsprünge) ist die Verzerrung der Lungentextur bei fokalem Emphysem.

2. Vorwiegend diffuse Gerüstsklerosen.

Das beste Beispiel dieser Gruppe ist die häufige Stauungsinduration. Jede chronische Lungenstauung führt zu einer Verfestigung des Lungengerüstes. Die chronische Stauungslunge sinkt im eröffneten Thorax weniger zurück als eine normale Lunge, sie fühlt sich fester an und fällt nach der Herausnahme nicht zusammen. Blutstauung in den Lungen vergrößert das Gesamtvolumen der kollabierten Lunge, setzt die Lungenelastizität herab und schränkt die Beweglichkeit des Organs ein. Die Minimalluft ist vermindert, weil die Alveolarräume durch Capillarerweiterung eingeengt sind (angiektatische Alveolarkompression, GIAMPALMO u. SCHOENMACKERS 1952, s. auch S. 561).

Als Ursache dieser stets diffusen, oft erheblichen Lungenstarre kommen in Betracht: die stärkere Blutfüllung der Blutgefäße und die Gefäßsklerose, das interstitielle Ödem und die Vermehrung des interstitiellen Fasergewebes. Der intravasale Druck wirkt sich wegen des großen Gefäßreichtums der Lunge ebenfalls auf die Lungenfestigkeit aus. Blutreiche Lungenteile fühlen sich bei jedem Dehnungszustand etwas fester an als blutarme. In der Ventilationsbewegung der Lunge äußert sich die vermehrte Festigkeit als erhöhter Gewebswiderstand (s. Tabelle 3, S. 436). Ähnliche Folgen kann interstitielles Ödem durch Aufquellung der Alveolarwände und der gröberen Septen haben. Die verminderte Dehnbarkeit (Komplianz) der Stauungslunge ist auch von klinischer Seite gemessen worden[1].

Bei chronischer Stauung tritt zu dem erhöhten Innendruck eine Erstarrung der Gefäßwand, die besonders im Bereich der kleinen Arterien und Arteriolen von Bedeutung sein kann.

---

[1] v. BASCH 1888, CHRISTIE und MEAKINS 1934, FRANK und Mitarbeiter 1952, MARSHALL und Mitarbeiter 1954, HAYWARD und KNOTT 1955.

Wesentlicher ist die Vermehrung des interstitiellen Fasergewebes in den Alveolarsepten, die am Gefäßstiel der Acini so groß werden kann, daß ganze Alveolargruppen nur noch geringe Ventilationsbewegungen ausführen. An diesen Stellen werden die abgestoßenen Alveolarepithelien nicht mehr entleert und sammeln sich zu Haufen an, die auch im Röntgenbild als Verschattung erkennbar werden. Die cyanotische und braune Induration ist im fortgeschrittenen Zustand fast stets mit einem Randemphysem und einer Stauungsbronchitis kombiniert, die durch Sekretstauung eine Verteilungsstörung mit herdförmigen Atelektasen auslösen kann. Die Ventilationsstörungen spielen in der gesamten Atmungsfunktion der Stauungslunge neben den Folgen der gestörten Zirkulation nur eine untergeordnete Rolle[1].

3. Herdförmige Lungenfibrosen.

Die Folgen interstitieller Pneumonie und Fibrose sind abhängig von der Ausbreitung des entzündlichen Exsudates, der nachfolgenden Zellproliferation und dem Ausmaß der Kollagenisierung des Fasergerüstes[2].

α) Interlobuläre Fibrose.

Die interlobuläre Fibrose, die in den groben Septen zwischen den Segmenten und Subsegmenten, weniger zwischen den Lobuli aus interstitieller, oft pleurogener Pneumonie entsteht und auf dem Durchschnitt durch die Lunge als schachbrettartige Felderung des Lungengewebes erkennbar ist, schränkt die Exkursionsfähigkeit des respiratorischen Parenchyms ein. In reinen Formen dieser interstitiellen Fibrose bleibt die Bindegewebswucherung auf die groben Septen beschränkt und der Gasaustausch sowie der Luftwechsel in den Acini unbehindert. Dehnt sich die Fibrose auch auf die feinen Septen und auf die peribronchialen Lymphbahnen aus, dann kommt es zu einer weitgehenden Lungenstarre. Die fortgeschrittenen Stadien der Lymphangiosis carcinomatosa sind ein Beispiel dafür. Rossier hat in einem Fall von Lungenkarzinose eine Einschränkung der Vitalkapazität um etwa $1/3$ gefunden[3]. Sehr oft spielen hier aber auch Stenosen der kleinen Bronchien und damit Verteilungsstörungen hinein.

β) Die intralobulären und peribronchiolären Fibrosen.

Eine wesentlich stärkere Einschränkung der Lungenfunktion ergibt sich bei den interstitiellen Fibrosen der Alveolarsepten und des peribronchiolären Bindegewebes. Dazu gehören die progressive interstitielle Lungenfibrose[4], die Lungencirrhose[5], die Lymphangiosis reticularis[6], die muskuläre Cirrhose[7] (Abb. 18), die Strahlenfibrose[8], die Fibrosen bei Sklerodermie, Restzustände interstitieller Pneumonien und anderes[9].

Die progressive Lungenfibrose, der nach den Mitteilungen von Hamman und Rich (1935, 1944) sowie von Meessen (1949) vermehrte Beachtung geschenkt wird, ist ätiologisch noch wenig geklärt. Für zahlreiche Fälle ist eine Virusinfektion wahrscheinlich gemacht[10]. Pokorny (1955) hat bei Menschen gehäufte Fibrosen nach Behandlung maligner Hypertonien mit blutdrucksenkenden Mitteln, insbesondere mit Hexamethonin beobachtet und erklärt die Fibrose durch Störung der enzymatischen Fibrinolyse des im Interstitium sich bildenden Exsudats. Im Tierversuch wurden gleichartige Fibrosen bei der Ratte nach intratrachealer

---

[1] Weiteres über Stauungslungen siehe unter Diffusionsstörungen, die bei der Atmungsfunktion der Stauungslunge ganz im Vordergrund stehen.
[2] Giese 1959, 1960.   [3] Rossier, Bühlmann und Wiesinger 1958.
[4] Hamman und Rich 1935, 1944.   [5] Rindfleisch 1897, Meessen 1949.
[6] v. Hansemann 1915.   [7] v. Stössel 1937.   [8] Teschendorf 1938, Zuppinger 1956.
[9] Uehlinger und Schoch 1957 (Literatur), Hegglin 1956 (Literatur), Giese 1959 (Literatur).
[10] Hamman und Rich 1935, 1944, Meessen 1949, Haemmerli 1955, Vaněk 1954.

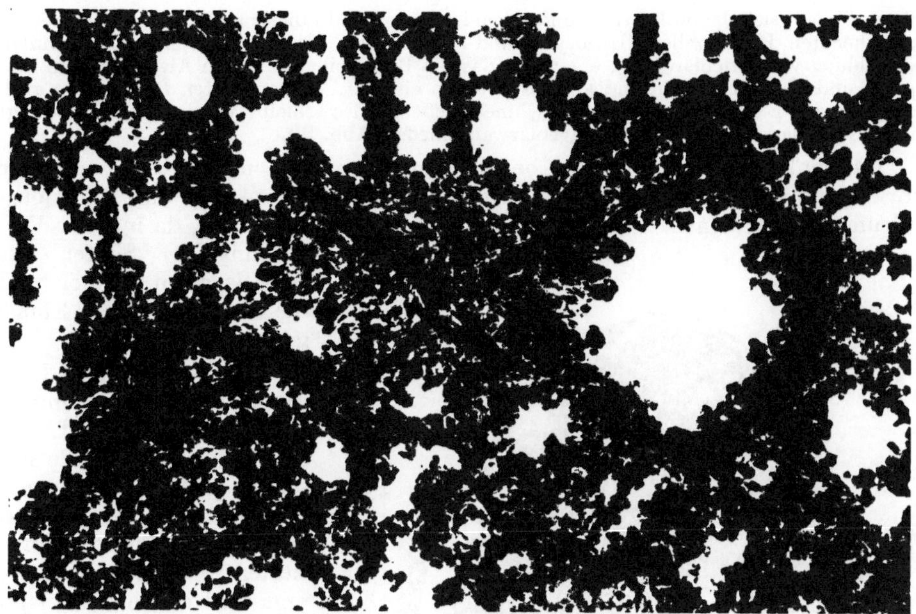

Abb. 18. Muskuläre Lungencirrhose bei chronischer Lungenstauung. Scherengitterartige Muskelzüge, enge Alveolen, dicke Alveolarwände. S.-Nr. 610/57.

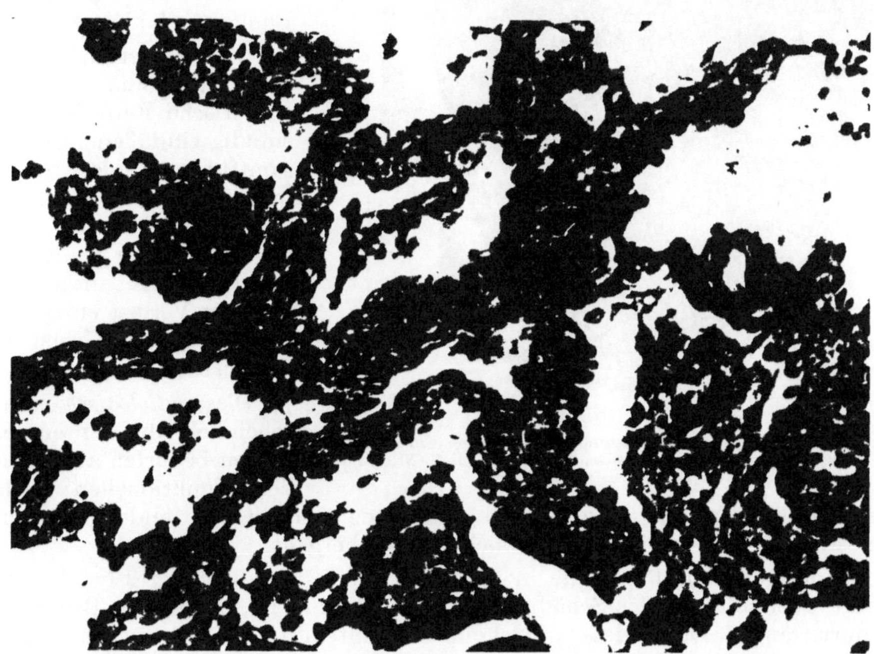

Abb. 19. Progressive Lungenfibrose. Frühstadium mit Fibrinabscheidung und Hyalinisierung in den zellreichen Alveolarsepten. Bereits deutliche Faservermehrung und Verkleinerung der Alveolarräume. Verringerte Ventilation. J.-Nr. 895/57. Vergr. 200fach.

Injektion von Histamin erzeugt[1]. Die progressive interstitielle Fibrose beginnt mit initialem Ödem und Fibrinabscheidung im Zwischengewebe der Alveolarsepten. An die exsudative

---

[1] Uspenskij 1952.

Phase schließt sich die infiltrativ proliferierende Phase an. In dieser erscheinen in den Septen Lymphocyten, Plasmazellen, Histiocyten und Fibroblasten. Es kommt zu einer ausgedehnten Neubildung von reticulärem Fasergewebe, das die Blutcapillaren in den Alveolarsepten umspinnt und die Bronchiolen und kleinen Arterien einhüllt. In der akuten Phase kann auch serofibrinöses Exsudat in die Alveolen hineinfließen. Dieses bleibt aber gering und schlägt sich in hyalinen Bändern auf der Alveolarwand nieder (Abb. 19).

Die funktionellen Störungen beruhen in der akuten und subakuten Phase vorwiegend auf alveolo-capillärem Block[1], sind in der Hauptsache also Diffusionsstörungen. Die Ventilation ist aber auch bereits eingeschränkt, da mit der Verdickung der Septen der Alveolarraum kleiner und die Dehnbarkeit der Lunge geringer wird.

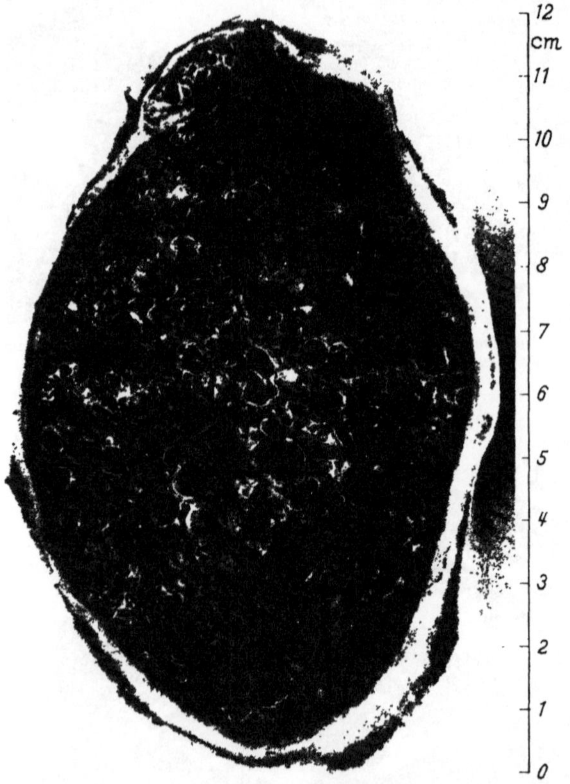

Im chronischen Stadium der interstitiellen Lungenfibrose wird die Lunge durch die zunehmende Faserentwicklung weitgehend immobilisiert. Das kollagene Fasergewebe der fibrosierten Septen schrumpft und wird durch den inspiratorischen Zug nicht mehr dehnbar. Die fibrotische Lunge wird kleiner.

Die fibrosierten Lungenabschnitte können ihre ventilatorische Funktion vollständig einbüßen. Die Gesamtfunktion der Lunge wird erst dann in stärkerem Maße beeinträchtigt, wenn die Fibrose über große Lungenabschnitte ausgedehnt ist. Der Verlust entspricht dann etwa der Größe des fibrotischen Bezirkes.

Diese *ätiologisch* wahrscheinlich differenten Fibrosen bedürfen auch nach der funktionellen Seite einer Aufgliederung in eine Gruppe, die ohne und in eine andere, die mit Stenose und Obliteration der Bronchiolen einhergeht.

Abb. 20. Wabenlunge als Endzustand einer progressiven Lungenfibrose. Breite Bindegewebszüge zwischen den Blasen. S.-Nr. 404/58.

Bei der Strahlenfibrose, die in ähnlicher Weise wie die progressive Fibrose abläuft, aber stets auf das Schädigungsfeld beschränkt ist, bleiben die Bronchien frei durchgängig. Der Endzustand ist eine reine interstitielle Lungenschrumpfung.

Bei vielen Fällen der progressiven Lungenfibrosen bildet sich zusätzlich ein kleinblasiges Lungenemphysem aus, das der Lunge die charakteristische gebuckelte Oberfläche und die wabige Schnittfläche gibt (Abb. 20 und 21). Nachuntersuchungen haben uns gezeigt, daß bei Wabenlungen regelmäßig auch Obliteration und Fibrose der Bronchiolen gefunden werden, so wie das bereits Meessen (1949) in seinen Fällen abgebildet hat.

---

[1] Austrian, McClement, Renzetti, Donald, Riley und Cournand 1951.

Das Emphysem, das eine Lungenfibrose besonders in ihren Spätzuständen begleitet, ist also Ausdruck und Folge einer Bronchusbeteiligung (bronchiolostenotisches Emphysem). Bei dieser Kombination von Fibrose und bronchiolostenotischem Emphysem bleibt die Lunge groß, aus der wabigen Umwandlung wird mitunter ein großblasiges Emphysem.

In der Funktionsstörung wird die Schrumpfung durch den zusätzlichen Totraum überlagert. Die klinischen Volummeßwerte bedürfen deshalb in jedem Fall einer entsprechenden Analyse und Interpretation.

Eines besonderen Hinweises bedürfen die Verkalkungen des Lungengerüstes bei allgemeiner Calcinosis und Kalkmetastase im Verlauf von Osteodystrophia fibrosa generalisata und

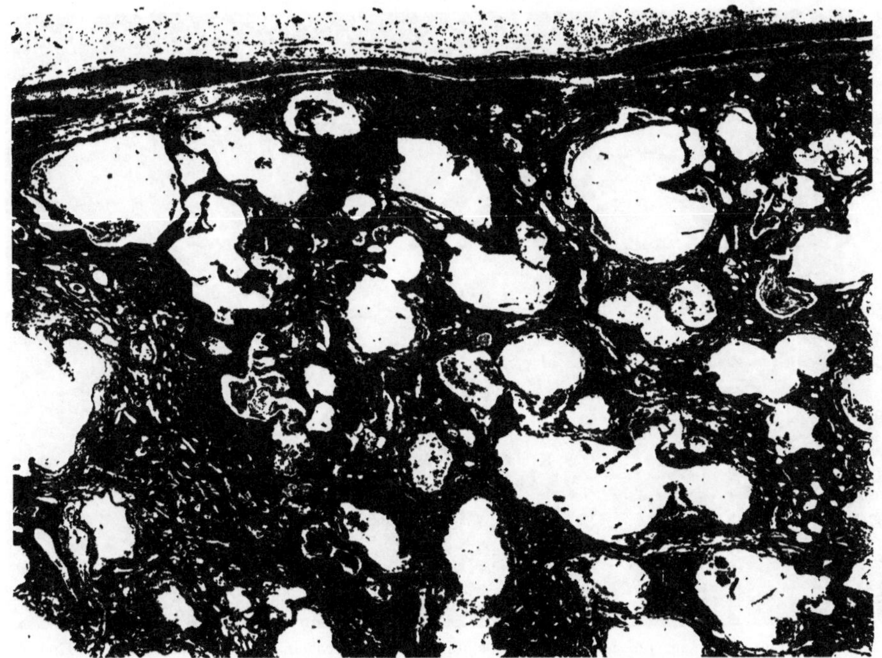

Abb. 21. Fortgeschrittene interstitielle Lungenfibrose mit kleinblasigem Emphysem. Lungenstarre. Fast völliger Alveolarverlust. S.-Nr. 404/58. Vergr. 7:1.

ähnlichen Prozessen. Hier entsteht eine besonders ausgeprägte Lungenstarre bei erhaltener Alveolarstruktur. Die Auswirkung dieser Form der Lungenstarre auf die Ventilation bedarf noch der Analyse. Wahrscheinlich wirken die verkalkten Lungenabschnitte als funktioneller Totraum.

γ) Die herdförmigen Fibrosen bei granulomatösen Lungenprozessen.

Bei allen granulomatösen Lungenprozessen, die sich im Interstitium abspielen, kommt es zu örtlichem Umbau des Lungengewebes und während der narbigen Ausheilung zu Schrumpfungsherden, die manchmal nur geringe, oft aber erhebliche Verzerrungen der Lungenstruktur zur Folge haben[1]. Die abheilende Miliartuberkulose, die ausgebreitete kleinknotige Silikose, die Boecksche Krankheit und auch manche Formen bronchogener und abortiver hämatogener Streuungen bei Tuberkulose sind Beispiele dafür. Sie enden alle in einer Einschränkung der Ventilation, die auch dann schon erheblich sein kann, wenn die Schwielenbildung nur kleinherdig, oft erst mikroskopisch erkennbar ist. Jede

[1] UEHLINGER 1956 (Literatur), 1958, FRESEN 1958, GIESE 1959 (Literatur).

Narbe stört die Homogenität der Lunge. Die Narbenherde sind als Bezirke ge-
minderter oder aufgehobener Funktion in das Lungengewebe eingestreut. Sie
stören die Ventilation dadurch, daß sie die inspiratorische Entfaltung ihrer Umgebung behindern oder häufiger noch den Luftwechsel durch Obliteration anliegender oder eingeschlossener Bronchiolen unterbrechen. Die zugehörigen
Acini und Lobuli werden dabei in der Regel kollateral von den Nachbaracini
oder -lobuli über erweiterte Kohnsche Poren belüftet.

Die Inhomogenität der Lunge äußert sich bei der Ventilation darin, daß der
Luftwechsel in der Umgebung der Narben wegen des Umweges über die Kohnschen Poren verzögert und vermindert ist. Miliare und submiliare Narben liegen

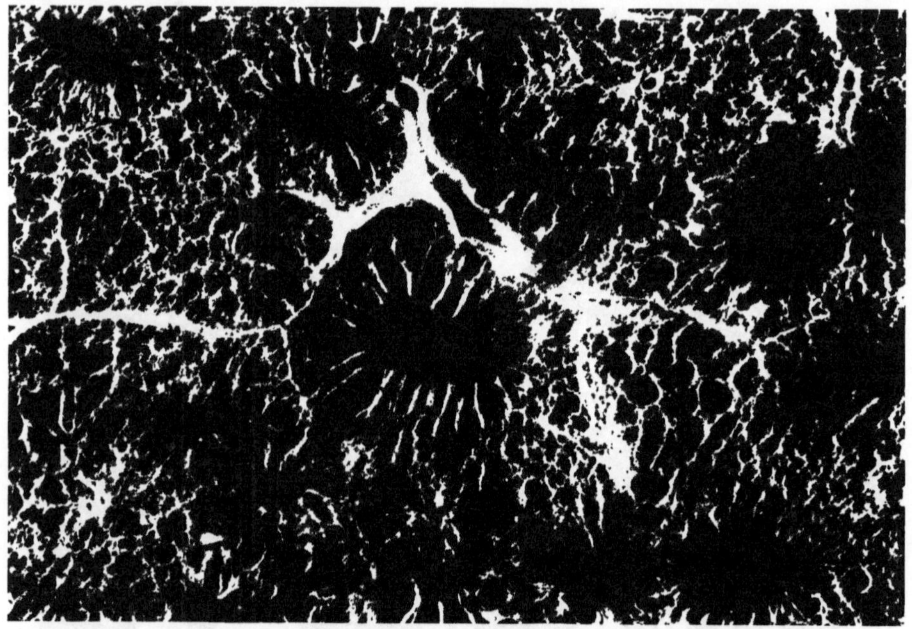

Abb. 22. Traktionsemphysem um multiple centrolobuläre und centroacinäre anthrakosilikotische Knötchen.
Faserstrukturen auf die geschrumpften Knötchen ausgerichtet. Daneben diffuses Emphysem mit stark erweiterten
Alveolargängen. S.-Nr. 626/58. Vergr. 4:1.

fast stets centrolobulär, größere in der Mitte der Praelobuli oder Subsegmente.
Bei der Schrumpfung dieser Narben werden die Wände der anliegenden Alveolen
und Alveolargänge gedehnt, während die interlobulären Septen nur selten, die
gröberen Septen zwischen Subsegmenten und Segmenten fast nie verzogen
werden, sie behalten ihren geradlinigen Verlauf. Bläht man eine Lunge mit miliaren
Narben stark auf, so liegen die Narben wie Spinnen in einem Netz, das zwischen
den erhaltenen Septen ausgespannt ist (Abb. 22 und 23).

Der verzögerte Luftwechsel in den perinodulär geblähten Alveolen hat eine
schlechte Durchmischung der Luft zur Folge, die vorwiegend durch die Störung
der exspiratorischen Entleerung der perinodulären Alveolargruppen bedingt ist.
Diese verzögerte Entleerung ist in klinischer Untersuchung an der Knickung der
Atemstromkurve, an der Leichenlunge an dem verzögerten oder ausbleibenden
Kollaps der perinodulären Abschnitte erkennbar. Das Lungenvolumen ist dabei
fast immer vergrößert, die Residualluft vermehrt.

Diese Vermehrung des ventilatorischen Totraumes wird auch bei der Untersuchung des Retraktionsablaufes an der isolierten Leichenlunge meßbar. Die

Retraktion erfolgt nicht nur stark verlangsamt, sondern auch in hohem Maße unvollständig (Restluftvolumina über 20% der eingefüllten Luftmenge, vielfach noch höher). Im Gegensatz zu den allein auf elastischer Unvollkommenheit beruhenden hysteretischen Dehnungsresten, die mit zunehmend stärkerer Auffüllung anwachsen, bleiben schon nach niedrigen Auffüllungsgraden hohe Restluftmengen zurück, die in emphysematös umgewandelten Lungenabschnitten festgehalten werden. Einen solchen „Totraumeffekt" zeigen unter den angeführten Beispielen der Fall von M. Boeck (s. Tabelle 3, S. 436), bei dem ein ausgesprochenes Narbenemphysem bestand, und alle bronchostenotischen bullösen

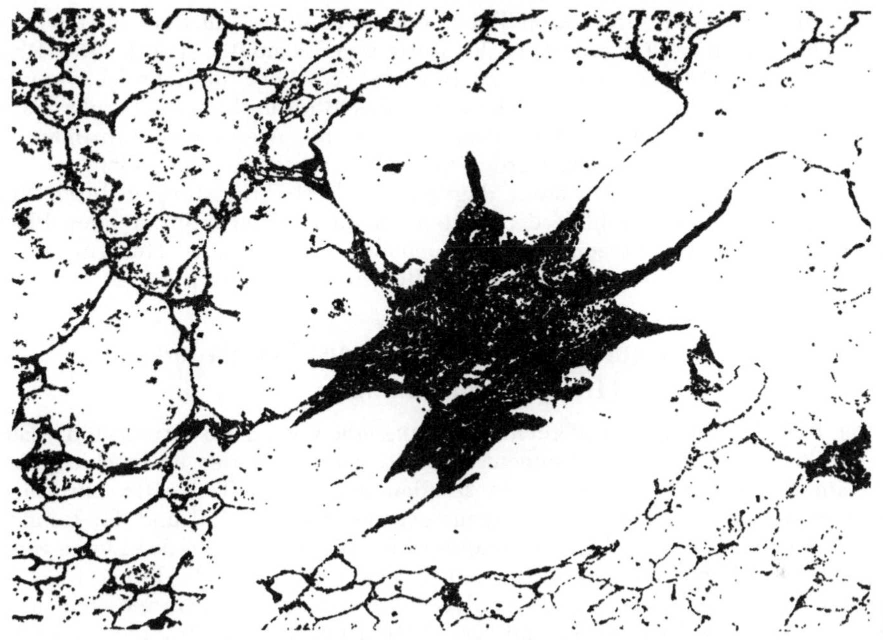

Abb. 23. Perinoduläres Emphysem bei Anthrako-Silikose. E.-Nr. 1409/55.

Emphyseme (s. Tabelle 7, S. 536); nähere Angaben bei der Diskussion des Totraumes (S. 471).

In den Endzuständen ist die Lunge sehr oft wabig umgewandelt, ähnlich wie bei bronchiolostenotischem Emphysem, das die diffuse interstitielle Fibrose begleitet.

4. Infiltrative alveoläre Verfestigungen.

Pneumonische Prozesse im Alveolarraum verdrängen die Luft und füllen die Alveolen mit Exsudat. Bei der lobären Pneumonie sind die Acini durch das Exsudat bis zu maximaler Inspirationsstellung gedehnt. Aus den toxisch geschädigten Capillaren strömt Plasma bis zum Druckausgleich in die Alveolen. Da die Bronchien im Anfang des pneumonischen Prozesses noch durchgängig sind, macht der pneumonische Abschnitt Inspirationsbewegungen mit und erzeugt einen negativen Druck. Mit der Gerinnung des Exsudates erlischt die Ventilationsbewegung und sistiert in der Inspirationsstellung. Die auf der Höhe der Hepatisation stets zu findende Blutleere der Capillaren beruht wahrscheinlich weniger auf der Konstriktion der Arteriolen als auf der intraalveolären Druckwirkung, da auch der venöse Capillarschenkel blutleer ist.

Der pneumonische Lappen fällt nicht nur für die Ventilation aus, sondern nimmt durch die Fixierung in maximaler Inspiration so viel Thoraxraum in Anspruch, daß die inspiratorische Entfaltung der anderen Lappen dieser Thoraxseite hochgradig eingeschränkt ist. Der Luftgehalt des Unterlappens entspricht bei einer Oberlappenpneumonie kaum mehr als der Kollapsluft. Die Ventilationseinschränkung bei Lobärpneumonien muß als eine Summierung von pneumonischer Infiltration, gestörter Entfaltung der Nachbarlappen und Folgen der gleichzeitigen Pleuritis aufgefaßt werden. Sie wird Ursache der Cyanose, die teilweise auch auf funktionellem Kurzschluß beruht, weil das Lungenblut nicht ausreichend ventilierte Lungenabschnitte durchströmt.

Bei der chronischen alveolären Pneumonie wird dieser Zustand im pneumonischen Bereich durch Organisation des fibrinösen Exsudates fixiert. Der Blutdurchfluß durch den nicht ventilierten Teil wird reduziert, die Netzcapillaren der Alveolarwände veröden. Die Verminderung des Blutdurchflusses beruht wahrscheinlich auf dem v. Eulerschen Prinzip (s. unter Atelektase). Intimaproliferationen der kleinen Arterien werden dabei fast regelmäßig gefunden.

Bei den Herdpneumonien steht dagegen die Verteilungsstörung durch Verschluß der Bronchien sowohl in der akuten, als auch in der indurierenden Phase im Vordergrund. Atelektasen durch Bronchialobstruktion oder Herdemphysem durch kollaterale Ventilation sind häufige Begleiterscheinungen.

III. Die pleurogenen Störungen der Ventilation.
(Die gefesselte Lunge.)

Der freie Pleuraspalt ermöglicht die Lungenbewegung im Brustraum. Eine gleichmäßige Dehnung aller Lungenabschnitte ist wegen der unterschiedlichen Wirksamkeit der an der Lunge ansetzenden dehnenden Teilkräfte nur durch die gleitende Verschieblichkeit der Lunge gegen die Brustwand und der Lungenlappen untereinander möglich. Die cranio-caudale Verschiebung der Lunge gegen die Brustwand hängt von der Exkursion des Zwerchfells ab, die Lunge folgt bei der Inspiration dem Zug des Zwerchfells. Der untere Lungenrand verschiebt sich bei maximaler Inspiration und Exspiration um mehrere Intercostalbreiten, kranialwärts wird die Verschiebung kleiner, im Spitzengebiet ist sie nur noch gering. Die transversale Verschiebung der Lunge gegen die Thoraxwand ist ebenfalls an den basalen Lungenteilen wesentlich stärker als an den kranialen, sie bleibt in ihrer absoluten Größe für alle Lungenteile hinter der cranio-caudalen Verschiebung zurück.

Noch geringer ist die Verschiebung der einzelnen Lungenlappen gegeneinander in den Lappenspalten. Sie gewinnt an Bedeutung, wenn benachbarte Lungenlappen ungleichmäßig belüftet sind (z. B. bei Lappenatelektase, Pneumonie oder Bronchitis). Den intrapulmonalen Septen schreibt v. Hayek (1953) die Funktion von Verschiebeschichten zu.

Die Pleuritis hinterläßt fast regelmäßig Verdickungen oder Verwachsungen der Pleurablätter, von deren Ausdehnung und Lokalisation es abhängt, ob und in welchem Grade die Lungenbewegung gestört ist (Klinische Übersicht bei Jaccard 1956). In der Lokalisation der Pleuraverwachsungen unterscheiden wir seit den Untersuchungen von Aschoff (1923) Verwachsungen zwischen Lunge und Brustwand, zwischen den Lungenlappen und zwischen Brustwandflächen.

Pleuraverwachsungen findet man in etwa einem Drittel aller Sektionen[1]. Am häufigsten sind sie im Spitzenbereich, dort oft schwielig. Dann folgen Verwach-

---

[1] Dina und Cussini 1956.

sungen im costo-vertebralen Raum und am Zwerchfell, hier oft doppelseitig, und zuletzt costale Adhäsionen, die oft locker sind und sich zu langen Fäden ausziehen.

Die Ventilationsstörungen bei Pleuraverwachsungen lassen sich zurückführen auf:

1. Fixierung der Lunge an der Brustwand,
2. Verdickung, Raffung oder Schwartenbildung der Pleura,
3. Behinderung der Thorax- und Zwerchfellbewegung.

Diese Folgen der Pleuritis sind sehr oft kombiniert und können zu schweren Einbußen der Lungenfunktion führen[1], die klinisch mit der Spirographie und Blutgasanalyse bereits eingehend untersucht worden sind[2]. Ausgangspunkt dieser Untersuchungen sind die oft sehr erheblichen Funktionseinschränkungen der Lunge nach Pneumothorax gewesen[3]. WERNLI-HAESSIG (1950) fand nach Pneumothorax in 40% geringfügige, in 60% grobe Pleuraveränderungen und Komplikationen.

Die Vitalkapazität ist nach komplikationslosem intrapleuralem Pneumothorax im Durchschnitt etwa um 23%, bei hinzutretenden Komplikationen um 56% reduziert[4]. Die Stärke der Einbuße hängt zum größten Teil von den Pleuraveränderungen, zum geringen Teil von intrapulmonalen Fibrosen ab. HERTZ[5] fand in einem Fall eine Reduktion der Vitalkapazität auf 900 ml. Die Atemmittellage ist oft erhöht, die Residualluft dadurch vermehrt (Abb. 24). Die eingeschränkte Vitalkapazität kann durch erhöhte Atemfrequenz soweit ausgeglichen werden, daß der Atem-

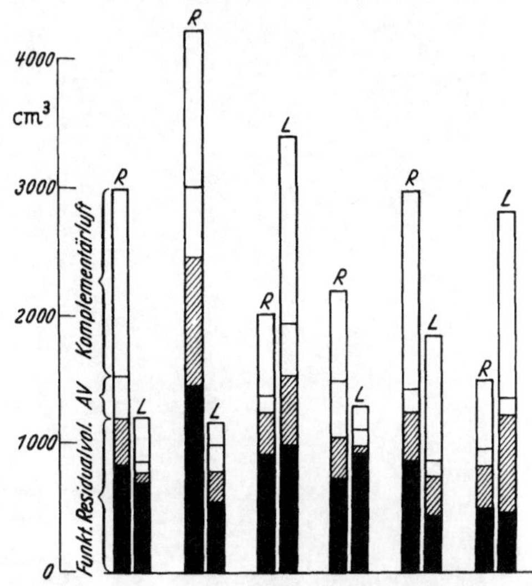

Abb. 24. Lungenvolumina (einschließlich Residualvolumen) jeder Lungenseite bei 6 Patienten mit Pleuraschwarte. *R* rechte, *L* linke Lunge. Die ganzen Säulen geben die Totalkapazität jeder Lungenseite wieder, die schwarzen Anteile das Residualvolumen, die schraffierten die Reserveluft, zusammen also die sog. funktionelle Residualkapazität. Darüber befinden sich abgeteilt Atemvolumen und Komplementärluft. Die Schwartenseite ist immer diejenige mit der kleineren Totalkapazität. (Aus HERTZ 1957.)

grenzwert nur wenig verringert ist[4]. Bei starker Einschränkung der Ventilation kommt es schließlich zu erheblichem Absinken der Sauerstoffsättigung im Arterienblut.

Eine untersuchte, durch Pleuraschwarte gefesselte Lunge zeigt (s. Tabelle 3, S. 436 und Abb. 25) den höchsten gemessenen Dehnungswiderstand, sie kann nur bis zu einem Viertel der normalen Vitalkapazitätsfüllung gedehnt werden. Innerhalb dieses geringen Dehnungsausmaßes ist die globale Dehnbarkeit gering (Elastance 15,6 cm HOH/Liter; Komplianz 0,06 Liter/cm HOH); der Volumelastizitätsmodul beträgt in exspiratorischer Atemlage bereits 54,2 × 10³ dyn/cm² (entsprechend etwa 55 cm HOH). Die Retraktion läuft regelrecht schnell ab (Zweisekundenwert des Tiffeneau-Tests 42%), die maximale Atemstromstärke ist jedoch wegen der geringen Auffüllungsmenge mit 0,3 Liter/sec extrem vermindert. Die hysteretischen Dehnungsrückstände liegen unter 10% der eingefüllten Luftmenge. Die statische Retraktionskraft ist mit −6,5 cm HOH in exspiratorischer Atemlage groß, der Minimalluftanteil am gesamten Kollapsvolumen mit 26,8% gering.

Damit zeigt sich auch hier die Möglichkeit eines Vergleiches der anatomischen und klinischen Meßwerte. Die restriktive Form der ventilatorischen Insuffizienz

---

[1] UEHLINGER 1960.   [2] HEIN 1950, SCHERRER 1956, HERTZ 1953—57, ZÖLLNER 1958 u. a.
[3] Übersicht HEIN, KREMER und SCHMIDT 1938.   [4] SCHERRER 1956.   [5] HERTZ 1953.

beruht im Falle einer Pleuraschwarte auf anatomischen Gegebenheiten, nämlich auf der geringen Dehnbarkeit des zusätzlich entwickelten kollagenen Fasergewebes, und ist hierdurch ohne Zuhilfenahme weiterer funktioneller Mechanismen erklärt.

Die Fixierung der Lunge an die Brustwand bleibt ohne erkennbare Einschränkung der Funktion, wenn die Verwachsungen locker und herdförmig sind. Die so häufigen Spitzenverwachsungen behindern die Lungenbewegung kaum, Adhäsionen an der vorderen Brustwand werden durch Anpassungsvorgänge in der Lunge selbst vollständig ausgeglichen.

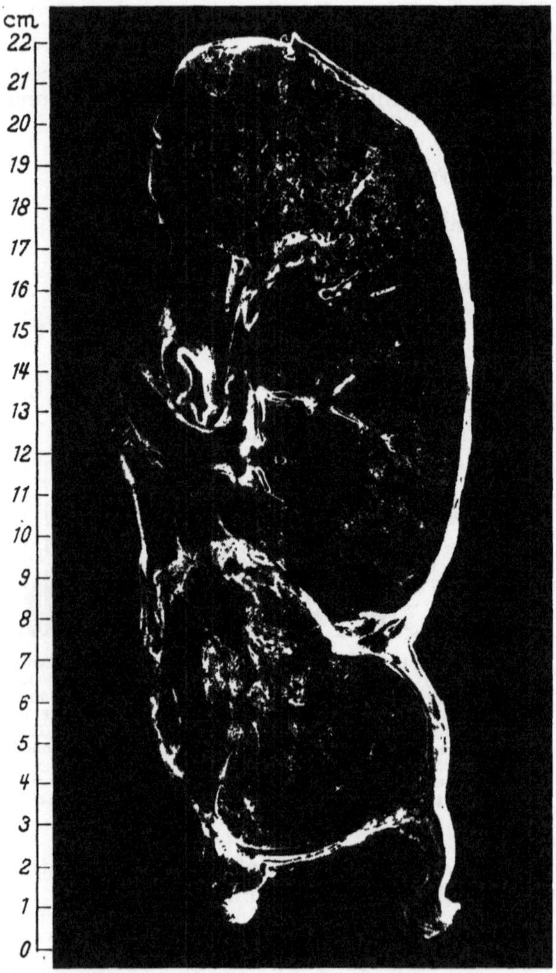

Wird die Lunge nach lange bestehenden, basalen Pleuraergüssen hochgedrängt, dann legt sich der untere Lungenrand der seitlichen Brustwand an und wächst hier fest. In der Regel erfolgt diese Adhäsion oberhalb des verödeten Zwerchfellsinus. Nach Resorption des Ergusses bleibt die Lunge hier hängen, die corticale Lungenschicht ist nicht mehr entfaltbar. Dem Zwerchfell folgt nur der Lungenkern und der innere Teil des Lungenmantels.

Der Sinus phrenico-costalis wird durch Verwachsungen der Lungenbasis und des unteren Lungenrandes oft abgedeckt[1]. Das geschieht vorwiegend bei trockener Pleuritis oder kleinen Exsudaten, die nicht in den Sinusraum hinabsteigen. Der untere Lungenrand wird dabei ringförmig an der Thoraxwand fixiert. Verklebungen im Sinusraum können dabei ausbleiben.

Abb. 25. Durch Pleuraschwarten gefesselte Lunge. Einrollung des unteren Lappenrandes. Verödung des Zwerchfellsinus. Verschiebezonen innerhalb der Pleuraschwarte. S.-Nr. 69/58. (Aus Hartung 1959.)

Nach größeren pleuritischen Ergüssen, ebenso nach Pneumothorax, der von Erguß begleitet ist, und nach langdauernden Stauungstranssudaten verödet der Sinusraum und fällt so als Komplementärraum aus. Der Sinusraum hat seine größte Tiefe zwischen Mammillar- und Axillarlinie, er mißt hier im Durchschnitt 9—11,5 cm in der Exspirationsstellung des in toto gehärteten Leichenthorax. Nach vorn und hinten flacht er sich ab und erreicht hinten etwa 6 cm, vorn etwa 3—4 cm.

---

[1] Aschoff 1923.

Deutlicher wird die Einschränkung der Lungenbewegung, wenn sich nach länger bestehendem großem Erguß oder Pneumothorax über der mehr oder minder kollabierten Lunge eine mantelartige Bindegewebsschicht bildet. Diese hüllt die Lunge vollständig ein und verhindert bei Resorption des Ergusses oder beim Auflassen des Pneumothorax ihre Entfaltung. Unter der visceralen Schwarte ist die Pleura gerafft und oft eingefaltet. Der untere Lungenrand klappt in der Atelektase mitunter um und wird durch Verwachsungen an der seitlichen Brustwand, seltener an der Unterfläche fixiert. Die verschiedenen Formen dieser Faltung haben SCHÜMMELFEDER (1956) und GIESE (1957) beschrieben. Auch am vorderen Lungenrand kommen solche Umklappungen vor. In ihrem Bereich bleibt die Lunge nach der Entfaltung atelektatisch (Abb. 26).

Durch die bindegewebige Fixierung der Falten werden große Teile des Lungenmantels wenig oder überhaupt nicht mehr dehnbar. Die Lunge ist in diesen Verwachsungen gefesselt, der Zustand wird im amerikanischen Schrifttum als unexpandable lung bezeichnet[1].

Die Einbuße an Funktion ist bei dieser Form der Verwachsungen erheblich. Beim Aufblasen der Leichenlunge steigt der Widerstand plötzlich stark an, wenn die Schwarte unter Spannung gesetzt wird[2]. Hernienartige Vorwölbungen von emphysematösem Lungengewebe[3] an Stelle geringer Pleurafibrose können sich ausbilden und mehren sich, wenn im Laufe der Zeit Lockerungen und strangförmige oder plattenartige Auflösungen der Pleuraschwarte infolge des ständigen inspiratorischen Dehnungszuges eintreten[4]. In diesen Endzuständen finden sich überdehnte und emphysematöse Lungenabschnitte neben Atelektasen. Ventilstenosen der Bronchien erklären sich aus Abknickungen bei inneren Verziehungen

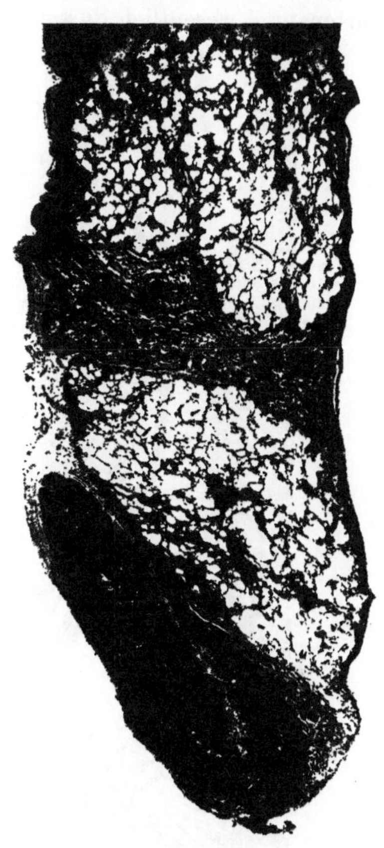

Abb. 26. Streifenatelektase und Umklappung des atelektatischen unteren Lungenrandes unter Pleuraschwarte nach chronischem Pleuraerguß. S.-Nr.144/57.

der Lungenstruktur. Die mantelförmigen Pleurafibrosen sind mitunter auch von intrapulmonalen Fibrosen begleitet, die sich subpleural in einer schmalen Schicht ausbreiten. Das neugebildete Bindegewebe liegt teils interstitiell, teils intraalveolär. Das Spitzengebiet der Lunge ist eine bevorzugte Lokalisation dieser Form der Mantelfibrose, selten sind großflächige Fibrosen der mittleren und unteren Lungenabschnitte. Ihre Folgeerscheinungen decken sich mit denen der visceralen Pleuraschwarten.

Bei länger bestehenden Verwachsungen können sich, ausgelöst durch die inspiratorische Lungenbewegung, Anpassungsvorgänge in der Weise heraus-

<hr>

[1] FARBER 1939, 1941, 1942, MULVIHILL und KLOPSTOCK 1948.
[2] HARTUNG 1959.   [3] ASCHOFF 1923.   [4] DELORME 1894, LILIENTHAL 1915.

bilden, daß sich entweder innerhalb der pleuralen Verwachsungen oder in der Lunge selbst neue Verschiebeschichten bilden (Abb. 27). Die sekundäre pleurale Verschiebeschicht entsteht zwischen dem costalen und pleuralen Anteil der Pleuraschwarte dadurch, daß die kollagenen Faserzüge in der Dehnungszone sich lockern und zu einem weiträumigen, oft gefäßreichen Maschenwerk umbilden. Die Exkursionsbreite kann mehrere Zentimeter erreichen. In der Regel ist der pleurale Schwartenanteil wesentlich dicker als der pulmonale. In der Grenzzone bleiben

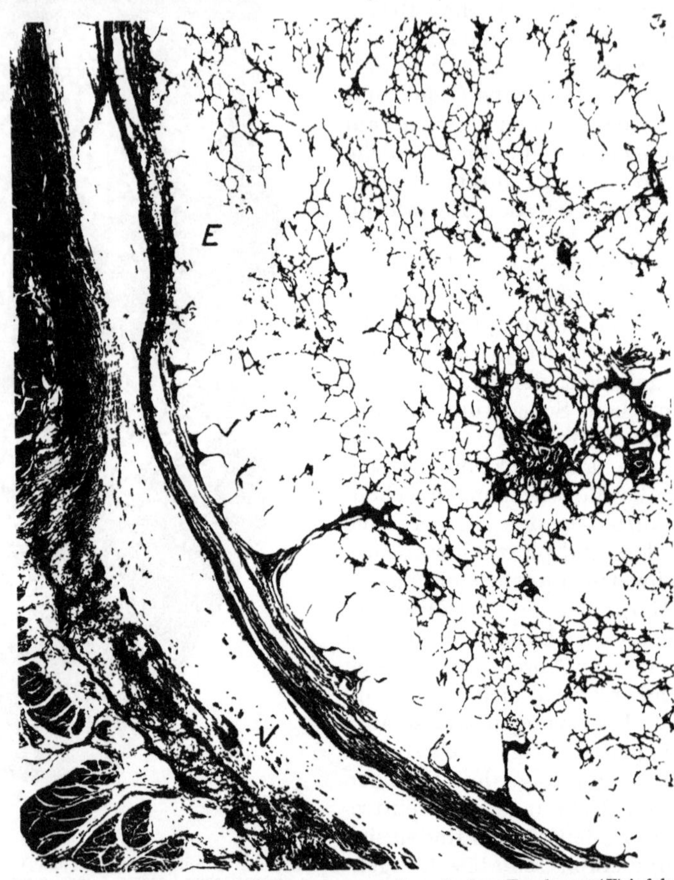

Abb. 27. Gefesselte Lunge. Intrapulmonale Dehnungszone mit corticalem Emphysem(*E*) infolge respiratorischer Verschiebung der Lunge gegen die Pleuraschwarte. Verschiebeschicht (*V*) in der Pleuraschwarte. S.-Nr. 69/58. Vergr. 7,5:1.

schmale Restergüsse oft sehr lange erhalten. In dicken Pleuraschwarten entstehen zuweilen mehrere Verschiebeschichten, in denen sich die Schwiele auseinanderblättern läßt[1].

Bleibt die Schwartenlösung aus, dann entsteht in der Lunge selbst subpleural eine Zone mit überdehnten Alveolar- und Acinussepten und corticalem Überdehnungsemphysem. Der Zug des Zwerchfells konzentriert sich anscheinend auf die subpleurale Schicht, die in Dauerspannung gehalten wird und so durch Überdehnung ihre elastischen Eigenschaften verliert.

Die in Pleuraschwarten eingehüllte Lunge kann operativ durch Dekortikation von ihren Fesseln befreit werden. Mit der Entfernung der costalen und der

---

[1] Giese 1959.

pulmonalen Schwarten gewinnt die Lunge einen wesentlichen Anteil ihrer ursprünglichen Dehnbarkeit wieder, solange keine nennenswerten intrapulmonalen Fibrosen entstanden sind. Die von der Schwarte befreite Lunge legt sich der Thoraxwand an und verwächst mit dieser.

Die Ergebnisse der operativen Lösung hinsichtlich der Lungenfunktion hängen in hohem Maße von dem Grad intrapulmonaler Fibrose und von der reaktiven Einschränkung der Lungenstrombahn ab. Jede über viele Jahre (in der Klinik rechnet man im Durchschnitt mit mehr als 4 Jahren) bestehende Atelektase ist durch intrapulmonale Fibrosen und Reduktion der Perfusion kompliziert[1].

Da intrapulmonale Fibrosen und Verödungen der Blutgefäße irreversibel sind, kann die Lungenfunktion durch Dekortikation in diesen Fällen nicht gebessert werden.

IV. Die thorakogenen Störungen der Ventilation. (Die Thoraxstarre.)

a) Der enge starre Thorax.

Bei starker *Verschwielung der costalen Pleura* nach chronischer fibrinöser Pleuritis oder Pleuraempyem ist die Exkursionsbreite des Thorax sehr stark eingeschränkt. Das schrumpfende Narbengewebe, dessen Ausläufer oft in die Intercostalmuskulatur hineinreichen, verkürzt die Intercostalräume, zieht die Rippen dachziegelartig übereinander und versteift die ganze Thoraxwand. Im Mediastinalbereich ist die Schwielenbildung zwar geringer, es kommt aber auch hier zu weitgehender Sklerosierung und Schrumpfung. Das Zwerchfell ist stets in die Schwielenbildung mit einbezogen. Durch den Narbenzug wird der Thoraxraum stark verkleinert, das Mediastinum auf die kranke Seite herübergezogen und die Wirbelsäule skoliotisch[2].

Dieser schwielig fixierte Thorax führt nur geringe Atembewegungen aus. Inspiration und Exspiration sind in gleicher Weise eingeengt, Verluste der Vitalkapazität um mehr als die Hälfte häufig. Bronchospirometrische Messungen am Lebenden sind vor allem bei Tuberkulosen angestellt worden[3]. Sie zeigen, daß bei Fixierung des Zwerchfells und der unteren Thoraxabschnitte wesentlich stärkere Einbußen an Vitalkapazität zu erwarten sind als bei Starre der oberen Thoraxabschnitte.

An der *Leiche* ist die Einengung des Thoraxraumes meßbar, während die Einschränkung der durch die aktive Kraft der Inspirationsmuskulatur noch erzielbaren Bewegung sich nicht abschätzen läßt. Für die Lungenventilation und damit für die funktionelle Leistung der Lunge ist aber nicht so sehr die absolute Größe des Thorax als vielmehr das Ausmaß der Lungenbewegung entscheidend. Lungenteile, in denen kein ausreichender Luftwechsel stattfindet, sind zusätzlicher Totraum.

Bei der künstlichen Verkleinerung des Thoraxraumes durch *Thorakoplastik* ist die Vitalkapazität bei oberer Plastik um etwa ein Drittel, bei unterer um etwa zwei Drittel vermindert[4]. Der Atemgrenzwert ist bei Spitzenplastik um 15%, nach oberer Teilplastik um 30% und bei Totalplastik um 40% verringert[5]. Anatomische Befunde hat AUERBACH (1941) mitgeteilt.

In dieser *eingesperrten Lunge* sind die Residualluft und der funktionelle Totraum aus den gleichen Gründen vergrößert wie bei costaler Pleuraschwarte.

---

[1] BUCHER und GLOOR 1953, HERTZ 1957, COURNAND 1950, TANNER 1956, ROSSIER, BÜHLMANN und WIESINGER 1956.

[2] PUTSCHAR 1937, HOFBAUER 1921, 1925.

[3] SCHERRER 1956, HERTZ 1953, TANNER 1956, VOGEL 1959.

[4] SCHERRER 1956.   [5] GAUBATZ 1936 u. a.

Bei Totalplastik wird als Folge dieser Ventilationsstörung das Blut in 25—30%
der Fälle nicht mehr genügend mit Sauerstoff gesättigt[1].

Die Deformierung des Thoraxraumes bei *Kyphoskoliose* hat ähnliche Folgeerscheinungen. Während die Thoraxerweiterung auf der konkaven Seite der
Wirbelsäulenkrümmung Überdehnung und Emphysem auslöst, entsteht auf
der konvexen Seite eine Thoraxeinengung und teilweise auch völlige Starre, in
deren Bereich die Lunge nur unvollständig oder überhaupt nicht ventiliert wird.
Bei der Kyphoskoliose wird der Thorax teilweise in Form der starren Dilatation
und teilweise durch Verkürzung und Verkleinerung des Thoraxraumes immobilisiert.

Uehlinger (1956) macht darauf aufmerksam, daß der Thoraxstarre, die erst
in den späteren Phasen der Krankheit durch Blockierung von Wirbelkörpern und
durch knöcherne Brücken zwischen den enggestellten Rippen eintritt, eine vorwiegend funktionell bestimmte Phase vorausläuft, die durch gegensinnige Verschiebung der Atemmittellage in den Brustkorbhälften bedingt ist. Bei Mittellage der Lungenentfaltung steht der Thorax auf der konvexen Seite der Wirbelsäulenkrümmung in Inspirationsstellung. Dadurch wird auf der konvexen Seite
die Inspirationsbewegung, auf der konkaven Seite die exspiratorische Bewegung
vorzeitig gehemmt. Der Atemgrenzwert liegt deshalb tiefer als nach der Vitalkapazität zu erwarten wäre.

Messungen von Chapman u. Mitarb. (1939) haben eine Herabsetzung des
Mittelwertes der Vitalkapazität bei 6 Kyphoskoliotikern auf 1577 cm³ (Schwankung zwischen 700 und 2250 cm³) gegenüber 3973 cm³ bei Vergleichsfällen ergeben.
Die Vitalkapazität beträgt in diesen Fällen nur noch 35—53% der Totalkapazität
der Lunge (normale Werte 67—69%). Die Residualluft ist ähnlich bei der Lungenstarre und der gefesselten Lunge beträchtlich erhöht, der funktionelle Totraum
damit vergrößert[2].

Die Einschränkung der atmenden Lungenfläche wird durch eine höhere
Atemfrequenz und ein größeres Minutenvolumen ausgeglichen. Wird die respiratorische Leistung unzureichend, dann sinkt die Sauerstoffsättigung des Blutes
und die Kohlensäurewerte steigen an. In Endzuständen bildet sich eine pulmonale,
durch reflektorische Engstellung der kleinen Lungenarterien ausgelöste Hypertonie mit Hypertrophie des rechten Herzens. Die Sauerstoffsättigung des Blutes
bleibt lange im Rahmen normaler Werte, weil schlecht ventilierte Lungenteile
auch weniger von Blut durchströmt werden (s. auch unter Atelektasen S. 497
und bei Perfusionsstörungen S. 596).

Ähnlich wie Kyphoskoliosen wirken auch die heute nur selten vorkommenden
schweren rachitischen Verformungen des Thorax, die alle mit einer Verkleinerung
und Einschränkung der Thoraxbewegung einhergehen[3].

Bei der Trichterbrust ist die untere Thoraxapertur eingeengt. Infolge der
Verkürzung des Zwerchfells wird der untere Teil des Sternums eingezogen[4].
Die Verkürzung des sagittalen Thoraxdurchmessers wirkt sich anscheinend weniger
auf die Lungenkapazität als auf die Funktion des verlagerten Herzens aus. Bär
u. Mitarb. (1958) fanden jedenfalls keine alveoläre Hypoventilation und keine
nennenswerte Einschränkung der Atemreserven. Dagegen wurde regelmäßig
eine Druckerhöhung im rechten Vorhof und ein diastolischer Druckablauf im
rechten Ventrikel wie bei der konstriktiven Perikarditis festgestellt.

---

[1] Rossier und Mitarbeiter 1956, 1958.
[2] Schaub, Bühlmann, Kälin und Wegmann 1954, Uehlinger 1956, 1960.
[3] M. B. Schmidt 1929.
[4] Hofbauer 1921, 1925, Putschar 1937, Rossier, Bühlmann und Wiesinger 1956.

b) Der weite starre Thorax.

1. Die primäre Thoraxerweiterung.

Thoraxerweiterung und Lungengröße stehen in festen Relationen zueinander. Jede Erweiterung des Thoraxraumes ist zwangsläufig mit einer Vermehrung des Lungenvolumens gekoppelt. Bei einem konstitutionell großen Thorax ist auch die Lunge im allgemeinen groß angelegt. Von einer Thoraxerweiterung spricht man nur dann, wenn die Stellung des Thorax sich aus der normalen Mittellage heraus nach der Inspirationsseite verschoben hat. Die Verschiebung kann während einer Phase angestrengter Atmung als regulativer Ausgleich eintreten, zeitlich begrenzt und reversibel sein. Die Lunge folgt der Erweiterung des Thorax und gerät in den Zustand des Volumen pulmonum auctum, das durch korrespondierende Erweiterung der Alveolen und der respiratorischen Bronchiolen gekennzeichnet ist. Diese Zustände sollte man nicht als Emphysem bezeichnen, bei dem die normale Lungenstruktur durch Distension der Acini und Schwund der Alveolen — im chronischen Emphysem irreversibel — gestört ist.

Neben der funktionellen reversiblen Thoraxerweiterung spielt die chronische irreversible, anatomisch fixierte Erweiterung des Thorax die größere Rolle in der Pathologie der Lungenventilation. Aus der Erfahrung, daß ein faßförmig erweiterter, mitunter starrer Thorax nicht selten beim chronischen Emphysem gefunden wird, sind zwei Theorien entwickelt worden, in denen die Thoraxerweiterung als Ursache des Emphysems angesehen wird.

W. A. FREUND (1906, 1911—1913) geht davon aus, daß die asbestartige *Degeneration der Rippenknorpel* vorwiegend im Bereich der 1., 2. und 3. Rippe zu einer Verlängerung der Rippen und dadurch zu einer Verschiebung des Thorax in die Inspirationsstellung führe, die mitunter nur einseitig ausgebildet sei. Die Verlängerung der Rippen und nachfolgende Verkalkung ziehe eine Erstarrung des Thorax nach sich, die als allgemein starre Dilatation vorkomme. Die untere Thoraxapertur ist in diesem starren Thorax erweitert, das Zwerchfell abgeflacht und gedehnt, der Sinus phrenicocostalis entfaltet. Die Thoraxerweiterung soll nach FREUND (1906) chondrogen sein.

LOESCHCKE (1928) stellt dagegen die Wirbelsäule in den Mittelpunkt. Im Modell und in einer großen Zahl von Thoraxschnitten weist er nach, daß mit der *kyphotischen Krümmung der Wirbelsäule* auch eine Erweiterung des Thorax eintritt, deren Form von der Lokalisation der Wirbelsäulenkrümmung abhängig ist (Abb. 28). Durch die Abknickung wird der Thorax in einen oberen inspiratorischen und in einen unteren exspiratorischen Abschnitt zerlegt. Je tiefer die Krümmung sitzt, um so stärker ist die inspiratorische Dehnung des Thorax. Im Rahmen dieser Erweiterung passen sich Rippen und Gelenkflächen durch Umbau der Thoraxerweiterung an und erlauben eine über die normalen Grenzen hinausgehende Thoraxdehnung. Der fronto-dorsale Durchmesser des kyphotischen Thorax ist besonders im Kyphosebereich vergrößert, die Rippen verlaufen horizontal, der Thorax ist seitlich abgeplattet. Die Atembewegung des in dieser Stellung durch Verkalkung erstarrten Thorax erfolgt durch Hebung und Senkung des ganzen Thorax, eine seitliche Erweiterung ist nicht möglich.

Die Funktion des Zwerchfells ist dadurch eingeschränkt, daß der ventrale Ansatzpunkt mit der kyphotisch bedingten Verkürzung des cranio-caudalen Durchmessers tiefer tritt und die Bauchmuskulatur entspannt wird. Die Hubhöhe des Zwerchfells ist verringert. Die Lunge paßt sich der Verformung des Thorax an. Im normalen Thorax hat sie bei seitlicher Betrachtung eine deutliche Kegelform. Im kyphotischen Thorax wird die Lungenkuppe abgerundet, ihr höchster Punkt wandert bei hochsitzender Kyphose nach dorsal, bei tiefer Kyphose nach ventral. Die Kegelform der Lunge geht verloren. Der größte fronto-dorsale Durchmesser liegt unterhalb des Angulus sterni. Caudalwärts laufen die Randlinien der Lunge in der Seitenansicht parallel oder konvergieren sogar. Der Oberlappen wird dabei stark vergrößert, die abgerundeten vorderen Lungenränder schieben sich in den zwischen Herz und Sternum erweiterten Raum und überdecken den Herzbeutel.

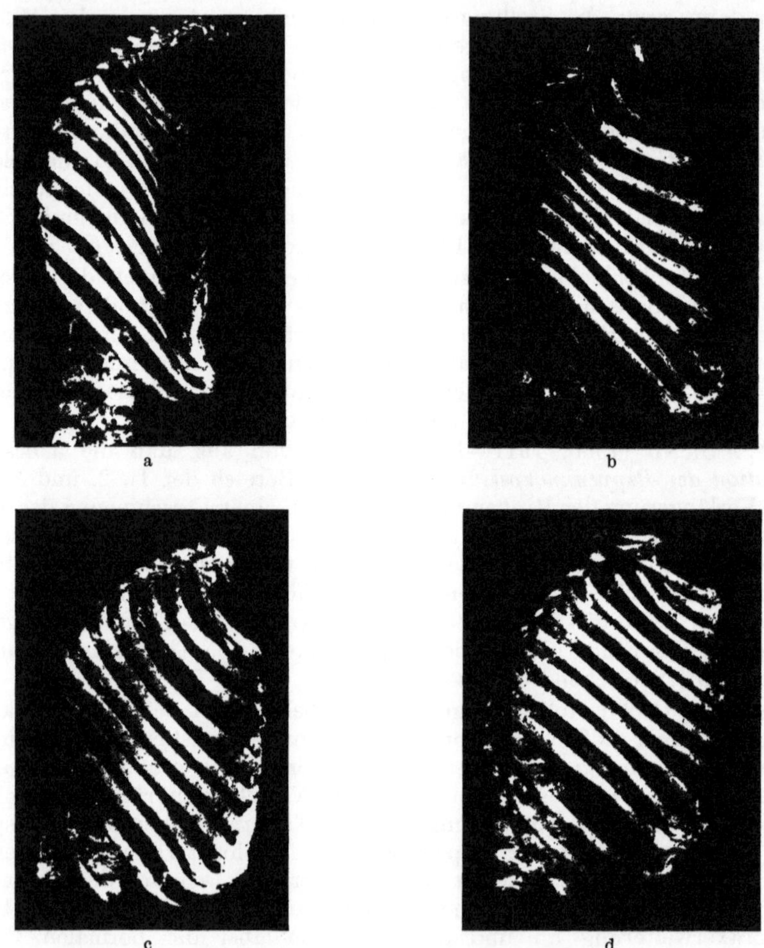

Abb. 28a—d. Abhängigkeit der Thoraxerweiterung von der Lokalisation der Kyphose. a Kyphose in Höhe des 4. Brustwirbels. b Kyphose in Höhe des 6. Brustwirbels. c Kyphose in Höhe des 7.—8. Brustwirbels. d Kyphose in Höhe des 9.—10. Brustwirbels. (Aus Loeschcke 1928.)

Das Emphysem bei Kyphose findet Loeschcke (1928) vorwiegend in den Lungenteilen lokalisiert, die in den vergrößerten Anteilen des Thoraxraumes liegen und auf diese begrenzt sind, während die Lungenteile im nicht vergrößerten Thoraxteil kein Emphysem aufweisen. Er bezeichnet die vergrößerten Anteile als Dehnungszonen und führt das Emphysem auf die thorakogene Überdehnung des Lungengewebes zurück.

Nach Loeschcke (1928) besteht eine prinzipielle Übereinstimmung zwischen dem starr dilatierten Thorax von Freund (1906) und dem Kyphosethorax, er erklärt beide für identisch. Beide Formen decken sich mit den von klinischer Seite[1] gegebenen Merkmalen des typischen Emphysemthorax.

Den Einwänden, daß die Erweiterung des Thorax auch sekundäre Folge eines primären Elastizitätsverlustes der Lunge sein könne, begegnet er mit dem Hinweis auf die Verhältnisse bei der Kyphoskoliose und bei traumatischen oder tuberkulösen Wirbelsäulenveränderungen.

Bei der *Kyphoskoliose* entsteht auf der konkaven Seite eine Dehnungszone im oberen Thoraxabschnitt und auf der konvexen Seite eine Dehnungszone im unteren Thoraxanteil. Die übrigen Thoraxabschnitte werden dagegen erheblich verkleinert. Die Dehnung gleicht die Verkleinerung nicht völlig aus, das Volumen des Thorax ist bei der Kyphoskoliose erheblich verringert, die Vitalkapazität herabgesetzt; sie beträgt nach CHAPMAN u. Mitarb. (1939) 35—53% gegenüber 67—69% der Vitalkapazität im normalen Thorax. Die Residualluft ist relativ erhöht und damit der funktionelle Totraum erheblich vergrößert. Die Atmung spielt sich auf einem erhöhten Füllungsniveau, also bei erhöhter Atemmittellage ab. Damit ist die respiratorische Leistungsbreite weiter stark eingeengt. Sie wird durch die Raumveränderung bestimmt, die in einer Verkürzung der Längsachse, Asymmetrie der Brustkorbhälften und Asymmetrie des Zwerchfellstandes besteht. Auf der konvexen Seite wird die Inspiration, auf der konkaven Seite die Exspiration vorzeitig gehemmt[2]. Überdehnungszonen treten in den erweiterten Thoraxabschnitten auf. Über die Störungen der Ventilation bei ankylosierender Spondylitis berichten D'SILVA u. Mitarb. (1953).

Gleichartige Dehnungszonen bilden sich bei Deformierungen der Wirbelsäule nach Wirbeltuberkulose, Trauma oder Osteomalacie. In solchen Fällen hat LOESCHCKE (1928) schon bei Jugendlichen großblasiges Emphysem der Dehnungszone gefunden.

Die vorgelegten Beispiele sind ein ausreichender Beweis für die These von LOESCHCKE, *daß chronische Überdehnung der Lunge zum Emphysem führt.* In den Dehnungszonen verliert die Lunge ihre elastischen Eigenschaften. Vergleichende Messungen überdehnter und nichtüberdehnter Teile derselben Lunge stehen noch aus, sie sind notwendig, wenn man dem Einwand begegnen will, daß Emphysem in der Überdehnungszone nur die vermehrte Auswirkung eines primären allgemeinen Elastizitätsschwundes der Lunge sei.

Nach den bisherigen Ergebnissen darf man als genügend gesichert ansehen, daß eine andauernde Überdehnung der elastischen Fasersysteme der Lunge zur Minderung der elastischen Eigenschaften des Lungengewebes führt, denn wo Emphysem, d. h. eine irreversible Distension des Acinus mit Schwund der Alveolarstruktur entsteht, da schwindet auch die Elastizität. Wir müssen also dem in unseren Untersuchungen gemessenen primären Elastizitätsschwund einen sekundären Verlust an Elastizität an die Seite stellen.

Mit diesem Problem hat sich schon TENDELOO (1910, 1925) beschäftigt und am Kautschukstab gezeigt, daß Dehnungsgrad und Dehnungsdauer die elastische Vollkommenheit beeinflussen. Die Dehnbarkeit eines Kautschukstabes nimmt bei wiederholter Belastung zu. Bei Überdehnung wird die Rückbildung der Verformung infolge Hysterese unvollkommen. Ob dieses Prinzip auf die Lunge übertragen werden kann, ist noch offen, da entsprechende Untersuchungen ausstehen.

Auch die Frage der unterschiedlichen Ventilation von Oberlappen und Unterlappen ist viel diskutiert worden. Sie geht aus der Beobachtung hervor, daß costaler und Zwerchfelltypus der Atmung sich häufig unterscheiden lassen. Die

---

[1] ROHRER 1916, HOFBAUER 1921, 1925.   [2] UEHLINGER 1956, 1960.

Ansicht, daß bei Frauen der costale Typus vorherrsche, wird neuerdings in Zweifel gezogen[1]. Im Rahmen der Emphysempathogenese steht hier die Frage zur Erörterung, ob ähnlich wie bei den thorakogenen Dehnungszonen Loeschckes auch solche funktionellen Mehrbelastungen von Einfluß auf die Lokalisation von Emphysemen sind. Tendeloo (1910, 1929) unterscheidet kraniales und caudales Emphysem.

Die unterschiedliche Dehnung kranialer und caudaler Lungenabschnitte erschließt Heckmann (1951) aus Änderungen der Helligkeit im Röntgenbild, erklärt sie aber nicht durch costalen oder diaphragmalen Atemtypus, sondern durch regionale Tonuserhöhungen der Bronchialmuskulatur, in deren Folge regional begrenzte Hypoventilation eintreten soll.

2. Die sekundäre Thoraxerweiterung.

Bei der primären Thoraxerweiterung sind Veränderungen am Thoraxskelet die Ursache für die Vergrößerung des Thoraxraumes.

Es ergibt sich die Frage, ob eine Thoraxerweiterung auch sekundär als Folge pathologischer Vergrößerung des Lungenvolumens eintreten kann. Solche Überlegungen müssen angestellt werden, wenn man anerkennt, daß die Lunge im Zuge der Alterung an Elastizität verliert, einen Teil ihrer Retraktionsfähigkeit einbüßt und sich nun unter Vergrößerung der Residualluft auf eine höhere Atemmittellage einstellt[2].

Die notwendige Folge ist eine Weiterstellung des Thorax, die teils durch den Fortfall oder die Verringerung des elastischen Lungenzuges, teils als regulative Anpassung an die höhere Atemmittellage zu erklären ist. Wenn mit zunehmender senil-emphysematischer Erschlaffung der Lunge die Atemmittellage an die Grenze der Thoraxkapazität rückt, werden die Atemexkursionen immer kleiner. Die Erstarrung des Skelets fixiert durch fortschreitende altersbedingte Verknöcherung des Knorpels oder durch arthritische und arthrotische Versteifungen der costovertebralen Gelenke schließlich den Altersthorax in der Inspirationsstellung.

Loeschcke (1928) hat sich bereits mit der Frage auseinandergesetzt, wie sich Formänderung des Thoraxraumes und Emphysem zeitlich und kausal fügen. Er kommt zu der Auffassung, daß weitaus der größte Teil der Emphyseme auf der Grundlage einer durch Thoraxdeformitäten, meist Kyphosen bedingten starren Dilatation des Thorax entsteht.

Wir möchten auf Grund der eigenen Untersuchung annehmen, daß in der ganz überwiegenden Zahl der Emphyseme das Primat bei der primären Elastizitätseinbuße der Lunge liegt. Die Thoraxdeformierung der Alterskyphose modifiziert die Intensität des Emphysems in den Dehnungszonen. Überdies werden seniles Emphysem und Alterskyphose in der Regel zusammenfallen, es sind koordinierte Faktoren im Rahmen allgemeiner Alterungsvorgänge. Den von Freund (1906) in den Vordergrund gestellten degenerativen Veränderungen der Rippenknorpel möchten wir in der Genese des Emphysems keine Bedeutung beimessen, sondern sie als sekundäre Vorgänge im Rahmen der kyphotischen oder emphysematösen Umbauvorgänge des Thorax ansehen.

Auch Böhmig (1928/29) lehnt einen Zusammenhang zwischen Lungenerkrankungen und Rippenknorpelveränderungen ab. Er hat nachgewiesen, daß Verknöcherungen in den Knorpeln der 1. Rippe unregelmäßig und frühzeitig auftreten, und hat auf weitere kataplastische Veränderungen aufmerksam gemacht, welche die übrigen Rippen weniger durchgängig erfassen und ohne Rückwirkung auf die Lunge bleiben. W. H. Schultze (1914) kam bei seinen Untersuchungen

---

[1] Campbell 1958.   [2] Hartung 1960.

an der 1. Rippe ebenfalls zu einem negativen Ergebnis, während sich v. HANSEMANN (1916) und JUNGMANN (1909) für die Freundsche Theorie ausgesprochen haben.

Die Frage, ob es eine anhaltende Weiterstellung des Thorax durch erhöhten Tonus der Inspirationsmuskulatur gibt, ist von HOFBAUER (1921), TENDELOO (1929) und R. SCHOEN (1936) diskutiert und bejaht worden. CAMPBELL (1958) schließt sich dieser Auffassung an. Er kommt auf Grund elektromyographischer Studien an der Atemmuskulatur zu dem Ergebnis, daß die Atemmittellage bei Relaxation der Atemmuskulatur um etwa 200—300 ml absinkt und während verstärkter Ventilation um 300—500 ml ansteigt. Er bestätigt damit frühere Untersuchungen[1]. FLEISCH und LEHNER fanden die Erhöhung der Atemmittellage nur bei physischer Belastung, nicht bei chemischer Reizung des Atemzentrums.

3. Folgen der Thoraxstarre für die Ventilation.

Erstarrt der Thorax in Inspirationsstellung durch Kyphose der Brustwirbelsäule[2], durch Verkalkung der Rippenknorpel[3] oder durch Verknöcherung der Intercostalgelenke bei Bechterewscher Krankheit, dann wird auch der weite Thorax trotz seiner hohen Totalkapazität nur ein geringes Atemvolumen vorwiegend mit Hilfe des Zwerchfells bewältigen. Der Atemgrenzwert ist klein, die Residualluft wächst beträchtlich an und ist Ausdruck des vergrößerten funktionellen Totraumes, in dem die Mischungszeit verlängert ist.

Der primäre Verlust an Lungenelastizität wird durch eine regulative Erweiterung des Thoraxraumes ausgeglichen und die Atemmittellage allmählich nach oben verschoben. Bei ausgesprochenem senil-atrophischem Emphysem ist das Fassungsvermögen des Thorax bis zu seiner äußersten Grenze ausgenutzt. Der Thorax wird durch die Atemmuskulatur in der Inspirationsstellung mehr oder minder fixiert festgehalten. Die zunächst funktionelle Thoraxstarre kann schließlich durch sekundäre Veränderungen am Thoraxskelet organisch fixiert werden. Die Folgen für die Ventilation sind dann die gleichen wie bei der primären Thoraxstarre.

An der Leiche ist die fixierte Thoraxerweiterung am Tiefstand des Zwerchfells, an den weiten Zwischenrippenräumen und an der Größe der Thoraxmaße (Umfang und Durchmesser) erkennbar. Thoraxweite und Emphysem sind dabei voneinander abhängig und entsprechen sich in ihrem Größenverhältnis.

Vergleicht man die Ventilationsstörungen bei engem und bei weitem starrem Thorax, so kommt man zu folgendem Ergebnis:

Der enge starre Thorax:
  Atemexkursion klein, nahe der Exspirationslage.
  Lunge klein mit Übergängen zum Kollaps und zur Atelektase.
  Totalkapazität und Vitalkapazität klein.
  Residualluft absolut klein, relativ groß zum Atemvolumen.
Der weite starre Thorax:
  Atemexkursion klein, nahe der Inspirationslage.
  Lunge groß, Volumen pulmonum auctum mit Übergängen in alle Stadien des atrophischen Emphysems.
  Totalkapazität sehr groß, Vitalkapazität klein.
  Residualluft absolut und relativ groß.

Beiden Formen der Thoraxstarre gemeinsam ist ein kleines Atemvolumen. Dieses verliert sich in der großen Residualluftmenge des weiten Thorax. Der weite Thorax ist dadurch in seiner Funktion noch schlechter gestellt als der enge.

---

[1] FLEISCH und LEHNER 1949, GREENE und HEEREN 1936, GREENE und SWANSON 1938.
[2] LOESCHCKE 1928.   [3] FREUND 1906.

V. Das Mißverhältnis zwischen Thorax und Lungengröße.
(Die zu kleine Lunge.)

Ein Mißverhältnis in der Größe von Thorax und Lunge kann dadurch bedingt sein, daß die Lunge für den normalen Thorax relativ oder absolut zu klein ist. Als Ursache der zu kleinen Lunge kommen in Betracht:

1. Angeborene Lungendefekte und Fehlbildungen,
2. Zustände nach Lungenresektion,
3. dauernde Funktionsverluste großer Lungenabschnitte durch Atelektase, Induration u. a.

In diesen Fällen stellt sich die Frage, auf welchem Wege der funktionelle Ausgleich erfolgt, inwieweit er durch regulative Anpassung möglich ist, und ob plastische Regulationen mit Hypertrophie und Hyperplasie von Lungengewebe eintreten.

a) Lungenwachstum und Thoraxgröße.

Das Größenverhältnis von Lunge und Thorax ist vom Lebensalter abhängig. Beim Feten füllt die nichtbeatmete Lunge den Thoraxraum völlig aus. Der Thorax scheint am Ende der Fetalzeit für die rasch wachsende Lunge zu klein zu sein. Die bei Feten der letzten Schwangerschaftsmonate und bei Säuglingen in den ersten Lebensmonaten häufigen Rippeneindrücke an der Lungenoberfläche, die in den cranio-dorsalen Teilen stärker ausgeprägt zu sein pflegen als in den caudalen, deutet Engel (1950) als Zeichen eines Mißverhältnisses der Größe von Thorax und Lunge. Dieses besteht auch noch beim Säugling.

Der Thorax wächst in den ersten Lebensmonaten sehr rasch und eilt der Lunge im Wachstum voraus. Dadurch wird die Lunge stärker entfaltet. Die Rippen stehen beim Säugling fast horizontal. Sie beginnen sich erst im 6.—7. Monat zu senken. Vor dieser Zeit gibt es beim Säugling kaum eine thorakale Atmung, der Säugling atmet mit dem Zwerchfell. Er hat nur kleine Atemreserven und lebt in einem Zustand relativer respiratorischer Insuffizienz[1].

Vom 2. Lebensjahr ab verlangsamt sich das Wachstumstempo des Thorax. Der Thorax gewinnt gegenüber der Lunge trotzdem zunehmend an Raum, weil das Zwerchfell absteigt. Das Zwerchfell steht im 12. Lebensjahr etwa um 2 Wirbelkörper tiefer als beim Neugeborenen[1].

Im weiteren Wachstum nimmt das Lungenvolumen sehr viel stärker zu als die Körperlänge. Die Vitalkapazität vergrößert sich von 1 Liter bei 100 cm Körperlänge auf 5 Liter bei 180 cm Körperlänge, die Totalkapazität in der gleichen Zeit von 1,5 auf 6 Liter[2]. Mit der Vermehrung des Volumens läuft parallel eine Zunahme des Lungengewichtes[3] und eine vermehrte Dehnbarkeit. In dieser Wachstumsperiode gewinnt die Lunge ihre Atemreserven, die im 3. Lebensjahrzehnt am höchsten sind[4] (s. auch S. 548).

Bei angeborenen einseitigen Lungendefekten oder Hypoplasien ist die Weiterentwicklung des Thorax im allgemeinen nur wenig gestört. Der leere Raum wird durch Verlagerung der Thoraxorgane eingenommen und durch Hochstand des Zwerchfells verkleinert. Die andere Lunge wird größer und tritt kompensatorisch für die hypoplastische Lunge ein.

Das Problem der Lungenvergrößerung in der Wachstumsperiode ist von Engel (1950) eingehend erörtert worden. Er unterscheidet zwei Perioden des Lungenwachstums. In der ersten Periode, die etwa bis zum 4. Lebensjahr reicht,

---

[1] Engel 1950.   [2] Helliesen und Mitarbeiter 1958.   [3] Rössle und Roulet 1932.
[4] Weitere Literatur über Physiologie der Kinderlunge bei Engström und Mitarbeitern 1957, Cook und Mitarbeitern 1957, Berglund und Karlberg 1956, Deming und Hanner 1936

erfolgt die Vergrößerung durch Bildung neuer Acini und durch Auswachsen noch nicht ausdifferenzierter Acini. In der zweiten Periode wächst die Lunge nur noch durch Vergrößerung der Acini. Eine Gesamtübersicht über die Veränderungen der Lungenproportionen im Laufe des Lebens hat Hieronymi (1960) gegeben.

Auch bei der Ratte sind Wachstumsschübe festgestellt worden[1]. Starke Wachstumstendenzen zeigen sich zum Ende des 2. Drittels der Jugendzeit und danach wieder in der Reifungsperiode. Das Wachstum der Lunge erfolgt in den einzelnen Lappen bei der Ratte gleichmäßig.

Beim Menschen ergeben sich Verschiebungen in der Alveolenweite wegen verschiedener Wachstumstendenzen des Thorax in oberen und unteren Abschnitten (s. S. 549, Haas 1958).

b) Angeborene Defekte und Hypoplasien.

Bei angeborenen einseitigen Lungendefekten treffen bereits intrauterin und auch extrauterin verstärkte Wachstumsimpulse auf eine noch in der Entwicklung stehende Lunge. Es kommt zu einer zusätzlichen Bildung und vermehrten Ausdifferenzierung neuer Acini, es erfolgt also echtes Lungenwachstum. Ob diese Hyperplasie den Defekt auf der anderen Seite vollkommen ausgleicht, ist zweifelhaft, wahrscheinlich tritt noch eine Hypertrophie durch relative Vergrößerung der Lufträume und vermehrte Capillarisierung ihrer Wände hinzu.

c) Die Restlunge.

Anders liegen die Verhältnisse, wenn von einer vollentwickelten Lunge große Anteile, etwa Segmente, Lappen oder ein ganzer Lungenflügel durch operative Eingriffe entfernt werden, oder wenn Lungengewebe durch Atelektase und Schrumpfung für die Atmungsfunktion ausfällt. Die Verkleinerung atelektatischer Lungenabschnitte kann so hochgradig sein, daß Segmente zu dünnen Streifen und Platten ausgezogen werden und Lungenlappen, etwa der Mittellappen, zu nußgroßen fibrösen Gebilden zusammenschrumpfen. Durch die Schrumpfung wird Thoraxraum frei, der ebenso wie nach Resektionen von dem restlichen Lungengewebe eingenommen und vollständig ausgefüllt wird.

Das Verhalten der *Restlunge* rückt bei der hier aufgeworfenen Frage der Größenbeziehungen zwischen Thorax und Lunge in den Mittelpunkt der Betrachtung.

Morphologisch steht die ausgleichende Vergrößerung der verbliebenen beatmeten Lungenteile im Vordergrund. Bei Pneumektomie ist das Volumen der zurückgebliebenen Lunge stark vergrößert, der vordere Rand abgerundet und das Mediastinum nach der leeren Thoraxseite hin verschoben. Nach den bisher vorliegenden Beobachtungen, die erst über wenige Jahre reichen, hält sich die Lungenvergrößerung in mäßigen Grenzen und erreicht nicht die Werte wie bei primärer Lungenfehlbildung, etwa bei Agenesie einer Lunge. Der akuten Überdehnung der Lunge wirkt die Fibrosierung der Pleura nach der Pneumektomie und die mitunter angeschlossene Thorakoplastik entgegen.

Bei Lobektomien schiebt sich die Restlunge in den leeren Pleuraraum hinein. Nach Entfernung des Oberlappens legt sich die Spitze des Unterlappens in die Pleurakuppel und paßt sich der Thoraxform an (Abb. 29). Nach Resektion des Unterlappens dehnt sich der Oberlappen bis zum Zwerchfell aus. Bei Segmentresektionen und Keilexcisionen sind die Verschiebungen nur gering. Geschrumpfte Segmentatelektasen werden von benachbartem Lungengewebe überlappt, sie sind von der Oberfläche nur an der Einziehung der Pleura erkennbar[2]. Der

---

[1] Thierfelder 1958, Rufer 1958, Clemens 1955.   [2] Wurm 1954.

geschrumpfte Mittellappen wird von Oberlappen und Unterlappen völlig überdeckt und hängt als kleine fibröse Appendix an der Lungenwurzel. Bei Pleuraverwachsungen entstehen zipfelige und zeltdachförmige Ausziehungen der Atelektasen. Atelektatische Oberlappen pflegen durch Pleuraverwachsungen in der Pleurakuppel fixiert zu sein.

Das Verhalten der Restlunge nach dauerndem Funktionsausfall von Lungengewebe ist in der älteren Literatur von verschiedenen Autoren[1] diskutiert worden.

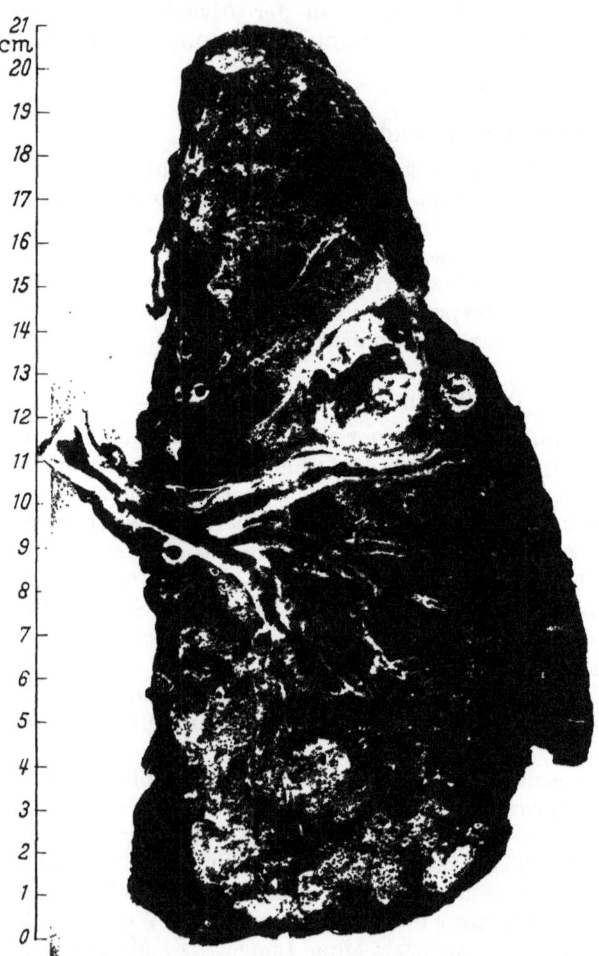

CHIARI (1914) nimmt nach Obduktionsbefunden beim Menschen eine wahre Hyperplasie der Lunge mit Vermehrung und Vergrößerung der Alveolen an, wenn die andere durch Schrumpfungen, Mißbildungen und dergleichen für die Funktion ausgefallen ist. DA FANO (1912), HELLIN (1906), KAWAMURA (1914), NISSEN (1927) u. a. sehen dagegen nur eine Hypertrophie der Restlunge mit Vergrößerung und vermehrter Capillarisierung der Alveolen ohne Vermehrung ihrer Zahl. DA FANO und KAWAMURA beschreiben eine Zunahme der Blutgefäße in der Alveolarwand mit Vermehrung der elastischen Fasern der Restlunge nach Exstirpation einer ganzen Lunge. Dieser Hypertrophie, die im zweiten Monat nach der Exstirpation deutlich wird, geht eine Phase der akuten Blähung vom Typus des Volumen auctum voraus. TIEMANN (1936) hat an Ratten ein Lungenwachstum durch Vermehrung der Alveolen gesehen, NÜRMBERGER (1939) nach sportlichem Training.

Die relativ kurzfristigen Trainingsversuche sprechen mehr für ein Volumen pulmonum auctum, das auch beim Menschen nach vermehrter körperlicher Arbeit beobachtet wird.

Abb. 29. Dem Thoraxraum angepaßte Restlunge nach Oberlappenresektion vor 1½ Jahren. Die Lungenspitze wird jetzt vom Mittellappen gebildet. Neuer kavernisierter Rundherd im 6. Segment. Volumen pulmonum auctum. 16jährig ♀. E.-Nr. 9712/56.

Beim Menschen erfolgt die Vergrößerung der Restlunge zunächst durch gleichmäßige Dehnung aller Teile. Bronchien, Alveolargänge und Alveolen werden weit gestellt, es entsteht ein Volumen pulmonum auctum. Die Atemmittellage dieser Lungenteile ist nach der inspiratorischen Seite verschoben und kann bei Lobektomien und ausgiebigen Resektionen ihre obere Grenze erreichen oder sogar überschreiten. Die Residualluft ist dadurch erheblich vermehrt, der funktionelle Totraum mit der zunehmenden

---

[1] PONFICK 1870, SCHUCHARDT 1885, HAASLER 1892, DA FANO 1912, CHIARI 1914.

Erweiterung aller Lufträume vergrößert. Bei starker Dehnung der Restlunge werden schließlich mit der maximalen Erweiterung der Alveolargänge auch die Alveolen abgeflacht und die Alveolarsepten verkürzt.

Im histologischen Bild ist die Dehnung der Restlunge, die makroskopisch aus der Vermehrung des Gesamtvolumens und aus der Relation zur Größe des Thoraxraumes gut abzuschätzen ist, oft nicht eindeutig erkennbar, solange noch kein Emphysem entwickelt ist.

Ob eine andauernde Überdehnung, die funktionell bereits einem Emphysem nahe kommt, in ein echtes Emphysem übergeht, ist heute noch nicht eindeutig entschieden. TANNER (1956) hat den Dehnungsfaktor berechnet, der sich nach Resektion der Hälfte des Lungengewebes für die Restlunge ergibt, und der normalen Lunge gegenüber gestellt. Setzt man den Umfang einer Alveole, die als Würfel oder als Kugel gedacht sei, in der Atemmittellage gleich 1, dann verlängert sich der Umfang bei maximaler Inspiration von 1 auf 1,2, d. h. um ein Fünftel.

Nimmt man an, die Hälfte des Lungengewebes sei reseziert und die Restlunge müsse sich auf das Doppelte ausdehnen, dann ergibt sich in der Atemmittellage eine Verlängerung von 1 auf 1,26 oder um ein Viertel, in maximaler Inspiration bei Annahme einer Gesamtdehnung der Restlunge auf 300% eine Verlängerung auf 1,44.

Aus den Erfahrungen bei anderweitigen pathologischen Prozessen, die mit starken Lungenschrumpfungen einhergehen, müssen wir schließen, daß auch in diesen Fällen eine anhaltende Überdehnung des Lungengewebes zu Minderung und Verlust der Elastizität führt, daß also echtes Emphysem sich dort entwickelt, wo diese Überdehnung über die Inspirationsgrenze hinaus für längere Zeit anhält. Da der Dehnungswiderstand in den vorderen Lungenabschnitten geringer ist als im Lungenkern, entwickelt sich das Überdehnungsemphysem vorwiegend am vorderen Lungenrand.

TANNER (1956) schätzt die Gefahr eines kompensatorischen Emphysems der Restlunge nach Operation nur gering ein.

In welcher Zeitspanne aus dem initialen Volumen pulmonum auctum mit noch erhaltener elastischer Lungenfunktion ein Emphysem mit Elastizitätsschwund wird, ist für den Menschen noch nicht untersucht.

Die Ergebnisse der Tierversuche sind nur in beschränktem Maße verwendbar, weil die Versuchsdauer meist zu kurz ist und bei Tieren noch ein Lungenwachstum als Ausgleich eintritt. NISSEN (1927) hat bereits nach 3—4 Monaten blasiges kompensatorisches Lungenemphysem gesehen, DA FANO (1912) ebenso auch KAWAMURA (1914) beschrieben eine Zunahme der Blutgefäße in der Alveolarwand mit Vermehrung der elastischen Fasern der Restlunge nach Exstirpation einer ganzen Lunge. Dieser Hypertrophie, die im zweiten Monat nach der Exstirpation deutlich wird, geht eine Phase der akuten Blähung vom Typus des Volumen pulmonum auctum voraus.

Die Schlüsse, die aus Lungenresektionen im Tierversuch zur Frage des Emphysems und der Lungenhypertrophie gezogen sind, lassen sich nur schwer verwerten, da bis in die neuere Zeit hinein, besonders in den Hundeversuchen die Differenzierung zwischen Volumen pulmonum auctum und Emphysem nicht klar durchgeführt ist[1].

Die Funktion der Restlunge nach operativer Entfernung von Lungenlappen und Segmenten oder nach Ektomie einer ganzen Lunge ist von klinischer Seite in jüngster Zeit oft untersucht worden[2]. Das Ergebnis dieser Untersuchungen ist, daß bei unkompliziertem Operationsverlauf Vitalkapazität und Atemgrenzwert entsprechend der Größe der ausgeführten Resektion absinken. Bei Pneumektomie

---

[1] NISSEN 1927, DA FANO 1912, BREMER 1936/37, RIENHOFF 1936/37, LONGACRE und Mitarbeiter 1937, 1940, NEUHOF und NABATOFF 1948 (Literatur), KESSLER 1956, BORELLI und ESPOSITO 1952, SCHILLING und Mitarbeiter 1956.

[2] LESTER und Mitarbeiter 1941/42, MAIER und COURNAND 1943, COURNAND und BERRY 1942, BOLT und Mitarbeiter 1953/54, GNÜCHTEL und Mitarbeiter 1955.

ist die Vitalkapazität auf etwa die Hälfte der Norm abgesunken (—58% des Sollwertes), ebenso bei Resektion mehrerer Lappen (—50% des Sollwertes). Bei
Lobektomie eines Unterlappens oder eines Oberlappens beträgt die Reduktion
43 bzw. 42%, bei Segmentresektionen etwa 31% des Sollwertes. Teilresektionen,
die zur Entfernung von tuberkulösen Rundherden oder isolierten Kavernen angewandt werden, mindern die Lungenkapazität nur etwa um 16%[1]. Die Sauerstoffsättigung des Blutes ist auch bei Pneumektomien in der Regel nicht vermindert, erst bei Arbeitsbelastung wirkt sich die nun zu kleine Austauschfläche
durch zu geringe Diffusionskapazität aus[2]. Bei körperlicher Belastung kommt es
auch zu einem Anstieg des Pulmonalarteriendruckes, während in Ruhe noch
normale Werte gemessen werden[3].

Messungen an der Leichenlunge liegen bisher nur in einem Fall vor[4]. Die Elastizitätsmessungen an der linken Restlunge eines 43jährigen Mannes 2 Jahre nach rechtsseitiger
Pneumektomie wegen Tuberkulose mit angeschlossener Adaptationsplastik ergaben annähernd normale Werte (Tabelle 3, S. 436). Als Zeichen der kompensatorischen Hypertrophie
sind Gewicht (1030 g) und Kollapsvolumen (1800 ml) groß. Der prozentual niedrige Minimalluftanteil von 39,6% am absolut großen Kollapsvolumen erklärt sich in diesem Falle aus dem
bestehenden Ödem. Die Auffüllbarkeit entspricht der für *eine* Lunge gewöhnlichen Breite
der Vitalkapazität, die Gesamtvitalkapazität ist also etwa auf die Hälfte herabgesetzt und
bezogen auf Gesamtlungenverhältnisse wegen der vergrößerten Ausgangsvolumina in inspiratorischer Richtung zu einer erhöhten Mittellage verschoben. Innerhalb dieses eingeschränkten Vitalkapazitätsbereiches entspricht die globale Dehnbarkeit der Norm (Komplianz
0,21 Liter/cm HOH; Elastance 4,8 cm HOH/Liter). Der Volumelastizitätsmodul ist in der
Atemmittellage gering erhöht (24,0 × 10³ dyn/cm², entsprechend etwa 25 cm HOH), die
statische Retraktionskraft mit —3 cm HOH gering erniedrigt. Die Retraktionsfähigkeit
findet sich stärker eingeschränkt, vor allem zeitlich verzögert (Zweisekundenwert des Tiffeneau-Tests 24%), die maximale Atemstromstärke deswegen, vor allem aber wegen der auf die
Hälfte verminderten Vitalkapazität mit 0,3 Liter/ sec stark herabgesetzt. Die hysteretischen
Dehnungsrückstände betragen bei negativem Totraumeffekt 12% der Auffüllungsmenge, sind
also deutlich vermehrt.

Ein Emphysem liegt nach diesen Werten nicht vor, sondern nur ein chronisches Volumen
pulmonum auctum. Histologisch bestanden daneben eine geringe interstitielle Fibrose,
eine katarrhalische Bronchitis und ein Lungenödem, keine wesentlichen tuberkulösen Herdbildungen. Diese Veränderungen erklären sowohl die eher verminderte Gesamtdehnbarkeit,
als auch zumindest teilweise die Einschränkung der Retraktionsfähigkeit. Der Tod war
infolge Herzinsuffizienz bei Cor pulmonale eingetreten.

Die bereits von Chiari *(1914) erörterte Frage der kompensatorischen Lungenhyperplasie muß heute, angewandt auf die Resektionsbehandlung, dahin beantwortet
werden, daß ein echtes Wachstum der Restlunge beim Menschen nach Abschluß der
Wachstumsperiode bisher nicht erwiesen und daß die Lungenvergrößerung in einer
ersten Anpassungsphase ein Volumen pulmonum auctum ist. Aus diesem kann
nach langjährigem Bestehen in einer zweiten Phase allmählich durch Elastizitätsschwund ein irreversibles Emphysem werden. Diese Auffassung deckt sich mit der
Ansicht von* Beitzke *(1909).*

Operationsmethoden, bei denen an die Resektion eine Thoraxverkleinerung
durch Thorakoplastik oder ähnliche Eingriffe angeschlossen wird, wirken zwar
der Entwicklung des kompensatorischen Emphysems entgegen, engen aber auch
gleichzeitig die Kapazität der Restlunge und die Entfaltung ihrer Reserven ein[5].

VI. Diaphragmatogene Ventilationsstörungen.

Die Vergrößerung des Thoraxraumes bei der Inspiration beruht zu einem
sehr wesentlichen Teil auf der Bewegung des Zwerchfells, die in den dorsalen

---

[1] Zahlen nach A. und J. Mockenhaupt 1957, ähnlich auch bei Rossier, Bühlmann und
Wiesinger 1956.
[2] Rossier und Bühlmann 1956.   [3] Grosse-Brockhoff 1957.   [4] Hartung 1959.
[5] Literatur bei Rodewald 1957, Schostok und Stiller 1956/57, Hertz 1957 u. a.

Teilen am größten ist. Die Grundeinstellung des Zwerchfells wird außer vom Tonus auch von den im Thorax und im Bauchraum herrschenden Drucken bestimmt[1]. Die tonischen Reflexe laufen über den Lungenvagus[2].

Tritt das Zwerchfell durch Kontraktion tiefer, dann wirkt sich der inspiratorische Zug vorwiegend auf die unteren Lungenabschnitte aus. Das Zwerchfell erweitert bei seiner Kontraktion die untere Thoraxapertur[3]. Etwa 60% des Inspirationsvolumens entfallen auf den Zug des sich kontrahierenden Zwerchfells. Der Anteil des Zwerchfells an der Inspiration ist vom Atemtypus abhängig, beim costalen Typ ist er kleiner als beim diaphragmalen Typus. Beim Stehen überwiegt die Zwerchfellatmung, beim Liegen die costale Atmung[4]. Bei ruhiger Atmung erfolgt die Inspiration ganz überwiegend durch die Zwerchfellbewegung. Nach den elektromyographischen Untersuchungen von CAMPBELL (1958) ist das Zwerchfell in der Ruheatmung bei manchen Menschen der einzig bewegte Muskel aus der Gruppe der Inspirationsmuskulatur. Bei tiefer Inspiration leistet es die Hauptarbeit. Mit der Kontraktion des Zwerchfells wird das Centrum tendineum in der Ruheatmung etwa um 1,5 cm, bei angestrengter Atmung bis zu 7 cm gesenkt[5]. Das Volumen der Lunge nimmt in der Ruheatmung um etwa 350 ml pro cm vertikaler Zwerchfellbewegung zu[6]. Diese Volumenzunahme wird auch als Ventilationseffekt bezeichnet.

Bei Ausfall einer Lungenseite kann eine Kompensation durch verstärkte Zwerchfellaktion auf der Gegenseite erfolgen[7].

a) Zwerchfellhochstand.

Bei Hochstand des Zwerchfells kommt es nach bronchographischen Untersuchungen[8] nicht zu einer gleichmäßigen Retraktion der ganzen Lunge, sondern zu einem Kollaps der dem Zwerchfell benachbarten unteren Lungenabschnitte. Die Ursachen des Zwerchfellhochstandes können in der Lunge liegen und durch Verkleinerung der Lungen infolge Fibrose, Infiltration usw. bedingt sein oder vom Bauchraum her durch peritoneale Reizung bei Oberbauchprozessen, besonders bei Cholecystitis, ausgelöst sein.

Die Hochdrängung des Zwerchfelles kann auch bei abdominaler Fettsucht so erheblich sein, daß die Lunge hypoventiliert wird. Häufige Folgen sind Sauerstoffuntersättigung und Kohlensäureanreicherung im Blut, gelegentlich auch Drucksteigerungen im kleinen Kreislauf. Klinisch sind dabei Zustände von Somnolenz als Folge der Hyperkapnie beobachtet worden. Diesen Atmungsstörungen bei Fettsucht ist in neuerer Zeit größere Aufmerksamkeit geschenkt worden[9]. BURWELL u. Mitarb. (1956) verwandten dafür die Bezeichnung *Pickwick-Syndrom.* Sie beziehen sich auf die Schilderung von DICKENS, der in seinen „Posthumous Papers of the Pickwick Club" einen solchen Kranken beschreibt als „a fat and red faced boy in a state of somnolence"[10].

Künstliche Erweiterung des Thoraxraumes im Tierexperiment wird durch reflektorischen Zwerchfellhochstand ausgeglichen, ein Emphysem konnte auf diesem Wege beim Hund nach 12 Wochen nicht erzeugt werden, ebenso auch nicht durch künstlich fixierten Zwerchfelltiefstand und auch nicht durch Ausschaltung der exspiratorisch tätigen Atemmuskulatur (NISSEN 1927).

---

[1] WINKLER 1903, FELIX 1928, POLGAR 1949 u. a.
[2] TER BRAAK und NIEKERK 1935.　　　[3] TENDELOO 1910.　　　[4] HERXHEIMER 1948.
[5] Ältere Literatur bei MINKOWSKI 1912, EPPINGER 1911, HITZENBERGER 1927, SPUEHLER 1956.
[6] WADE 1954.　　　[7] HEINE und HELL 1953, K.-H. WEBER 1958.
[8] MEYLER und HUIZINGA 1950.　　　[9] ROSSIER, BÜHLMANN und WIESINGER 1958.
[10] SANEN 1958 (Literatur).

b) Zwerchfelltiefstand.

Ein Tiefstand des Zwerchfells gehört zum Emphysem, zum Asthma bronchiale und zu Stenosen der oberen Luftwege. Das Tiefertreten des Zwerchfells bei Emphysem faßt Loeschcke (1913, 1928) als wesentliche Folge des nachlassenden Retraktionszuges der Lunge auf, während er einen Einfluß des Elastizitätsverlustes der Lunge auf die Ausweitung der knöchernen Thoraxwand in Abrede stellt. Das tiefstehende und abgeflachte Zwerchfell führt nur geringe vertikale Bewegungen aus und kann nicht mehr zur Erweiterung der unteren Thoraxapertur beitragen. Der Ausfall des Zwerchfells kann nur durch die Anspannung der Atemhilfsmuskulatur ausgeglichen werden.

Das Gewicht des Zwerchfells steht unter normalen Verhältnissen in einer festen Relation zum Gewicht der übrigen Körpermuskulatur und zum Gewicht des Herzens[1]. Im Kindesalter ist das Zwerchfellgewicht relativ groß, beim Neugeborenen fünfmal so hoch wie beim Erwachsenen. Das entspricht dem rein abdominalen Atemtypus des Kleinkindes. Eine relative Erhöhung des Zwerchfellgewichtes findet sich weiter bei Herzhypertrophie und bei Pleuraverwachsungen. Bei Abmagerung nimmt das Zwerchfellgewicht nicht in gleichem Maße ab wie die übrige Körpermuskulatur. Eine reine senile Atrophie des Zwerchfells ist wahrscheinlich vorhanden, tritt aber erst relativ spät auf und findet sich stets bei seniler Thoraxstarre. Ebenso liegt das Zwerchfellgewicht bei senilem Emphysem unter dem Mittelwert.

c) Zwerchfellähmung.

Die Bewegung des gelähmten Zwerchfells ist eine Resultante der Druck- und Zugkräfte, die einerseits vom Bauchraum und von der Lunge her, andererseits von der unteren Thoraxapertur ausgeübt werden. Diese Kräfte wirken gegensinnig: Lungenzug und positiver Druck im Bauchraum drängen das Zwerchfell nach oben, die inspiratorische Weitung der unteren Thoraxapertur flacht das Zwerchfell ab.

Das gelähmte, nicht durch Schwarten oder Verwachsungen fixierte Zwerchfell steht bei ruhiger Atmung fast still oder führt nur geringe paradoxe Bewegungen aus. Selten kommt es zu leichten Verschiebungen im Sinne der Atembewegungen[2]. Bei tiefer Inspiration folgt es dem vermehrten Lungenzug und steigt nach oben. Die Luft der unteren Lungenteile wird dabei einerseits in die kranialen Lungenabschnitte verlagert, die der inspiratorischen Dehnung des Thorax folgen, andererseits aber auch in die Lunge der Gegenseite eingesogen, weil nur auf dieser Seite ein ausreichender negativer Druck bei der Inspiration zustande kommt (Abb. 30).

Bei der Exspiration sinkt das gelähmte Zwerchfell mit der Abnahme des Pleuradruckes abwärts. Dadurch vergrößert sich der Thoraxraum, die Lunge wird in den caudalen Abschnitten entfaltet und nimmt einen Teil von der Exspirationsluft der anderen Seite auf. Diese Verschiebung der Lungenluft in die gelähmte Thoraxseite und der Austausch mit der gesunden Seite wird als Pendelatmung bezeichnet. Aus der geringen Zufuhr von Frischluft in die gelähmte Seite erklärt sich der starke Funktionsverlust der Lunge bei der Zwerchfelllähmung.

Die Pendelatmung kommt nur bei vollständig gelähmtem und frei beweglichem Zwerchfell zustande. Sie wird beim fixierten Zwerchfell und in der Regel auch bei temporärer Zwerchfellausschaltung durch Phrenicusquetschung vermißt[3]. Bei Relaxatio diaphragmatica, bei der die Muskelfasern des Zwerchfells vollständig oder bis auf geringe Reste verschwunden sind, ist das Zwerchfell zu

---

[1] Fromme 1916.   [2] Campbell 1958.   [3] Hertz 1957.

einer dünnen bindegewebigen Membran ausgezogen, in die zuweilen Fett eingelagert ist[1]. Die Folgen sind ähnlich wie bei der totalen Zwerchfellähmung.

Bei angeborenen oder erworbenen Zwerchfellhernien sind die Ventilationsstörungen von der Größe der Hernien abhängig. Angeborene oder erworbene
Zwerchfelldefekte gewinnen ihre Bedeutung für die Atmung dadurch, daß durch
die Lücken im Zwerchfell Inhalt der Bauchhöhle in den Thoraxraum eintritt.
Magen, Darmanteile, Milz und Leber können durch die Lücke in den Thorax
verlagert werden und diesen weitgehend ausfüllen. Die Lunge wird dabei komprimiert und das Mediastinum mit der zunehmenden Luftfüllung des Darmes verdrängt. Kinder mit solchen großen angeborenen Defekten sterben in der Regel
am 1. oder 2. Lebenstag an Erstickung. Die kongenitalen Defekte und Hernien
liegen ganz überwiegend auf der linken Seite[2].

Bei entzündlichen Prozessen wird das Zwerchfell reflektorisch ruhiggestellt.
Dabei ist es für die Funktion des Zwerchfells von untergeordneter Bedeutung,

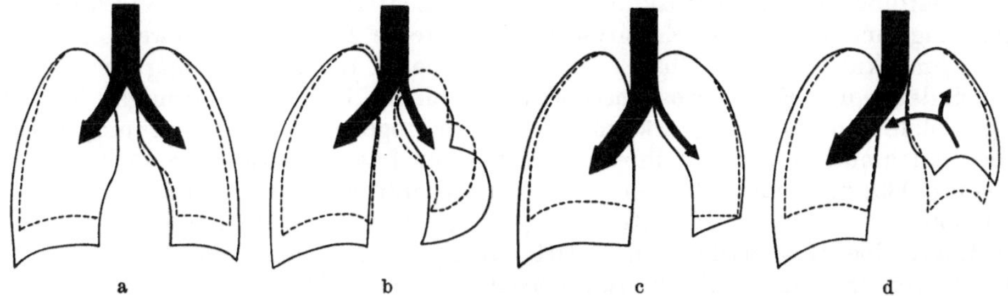

Abb. 30 a—d. Schematische Darstellung der Ventilation bei normalen und pathologischen Verhältnissen. Die
gestrichelten Linien stellen die Lungenumrisse nach der Exspiration, die ausgezogenen nach der Inspiration dar.
Die Pfeile sollen Stärke und Richtung des geatmeten Luftvolumens während der Inspiration demonstrieren.
a Normale Verhältnisse. b Pneumothorax. c Pleuraschwarte. d Komplette Phrenicuslähmung. (Aus HERTZ 1957.)

ob die Entzündung sich im Zwerchfell selbst abspielt, etwa als Myositis des Zwerchfells bei der Bornholmer-Krankheit als Folge einer Infektion mit Coxsackie-Virus,
oder ob eine basale Pleuritis oder eine subphrenische Peritonitis die Zwerchfell-
reizung auslöst. Die Belüftung der basalen Lungenabschnitte ist dabei herabgesetzt, basale Atelektasen, auch Streifenatelektasen kommen oft vor.

Wird das Zwerchfell durch schwielige Verwachsungen oder therapeutisch durch
Phrenicusausschaltung stillgelegt, dann ist die Totalkapazität der Lunge stark
herabgesetzt und die Residualluft vermehrt. Es treten ähnliche Folgen ein wie
bei der Thoraxstarre. Die Lungenventilation kann bei Zwerchfellähmung allein
auf weniger als die Hälfte der gesunden Seite absinken[3].

d) Bauchmuskulatur.

Das Zwerchfell ist ausgespannt zwischen Räumen unterschiedlichen Druckes,
die es mit seiner Kontraktilität beeinflussen kann. Selbst bei maximaler Inspiration sind seine Muskelkräfte nicht voll eingesetzt, sie treten erst gegen stark
erhöhte Intraabdominaldrucke ein[4]. Beim Husten und Niesen wirkt es als Regulator der Expulsionskraft des gesteigerten Intraabdominaldruckes[5]. Dabei zeigt
sich eine gewisse Abhängigkeit der Zwerchfellfunktion von der Tätigkeit der
Bauchmuskulatur.

Die Bauchmuskulatur ist ein wesentlicher Bestandteil der Atemhilfsmuskulatur. Mit ihrer Kontraktion steigert sie den intraabdominalen Druck und senkt

---

NEUMANN 1933, FELIX 1953, ASSMANN 1950.   [2] GRUBER 1953.
[3] ROSSIER und BÜHLMANN 1956.   [4] CAMPBELL 1958.   [5] CORYLLOS 1937.

mit ihren schräg verlaufenden Anteilen die Rippen. Alle willkürlichen Atembewegungen und die hohen Drucke beim Husten und Niesen beruhen auf einer Anspannung der Bauchdeckenmuskulatur. Bei Ruheatmung oder einer nur mäßig verstärkten Atmung sind dagegen keine Kontraktionen in der Bauchmuskulatur nachweisbar, sie treten erst bei Ventilationsvolumina über 10 Liter je Minute gegen Ende der Exspiration auf und führen bei Ventilationsvolumina über 70—90 Liter/min zu deutlichen Steigerungen des intraabdominalen Druckes[1]. Bei Stenoseatmung treten die Bauchmuskeln erst dann in Funktion, wenn die Widerstände höher als 10 cm Wassersäule liegen.

Bei Erschlaffung der Bauchmuskulatur sinken die Baucheingeweide ab und üben einen vermehrten Zug auf das Zwerchfell aus. Damit werden gleichzeitig die elastischen Kräfte der Lunge vermehrt beansprucht. Bei voll erhaltener Lungenelastizität kommt es dabei zu einer Einziehung der oberen Bauchabschnitte. Bei Emphysem ist die Elastizitätseinbuße der Lunge häufig mit einer Erschlaffung der Bauchmuskulatur vergesellschaftet[2]. Selbst bei angestrengter Atmung sind bei vielen Emphysematikern keine Exspirationsbewegungen der Bauchmuskulatur feststellbar[1]. An der Leiche ist die Erschlaffung der Bauchmuskulatur mit Enteroptose besonders an einem U- oder V-förmigen Verlauf des Colon transversum zu erkennen[3]. In den eingehenden Untersuchungen über die Bauchmuskulatur und ihre Beziehung zur Lage der Eingeweide hat Linzbach (1939) bei seinen Studien über die Enteroptose eine Gewichtsabnahme und Atrophie der Bauchmuskulatur festgestellt. Die Atrophie ist konstitutionell bedingt, eine Muskelschädigung tritt häufig hinzu. Diese kann z. B. in einer Überdehnung während der Schwangerschaft liegen[4]. Die Häufigkeit der Bauchmuskelerschlaffung bei Frauen, die oft schon im jugendlichen Alter eintritt, spricht dafür, daß eine pathogenetische Beziehung zwischen Emphysem und Enteroptose schon aus diesem Grunde nicht besteht.

VII. Die raumfordernden Prozesse im Thorax.

Alle im Thorax ablaufenden Prozesse, die Raum beanspruchen, müssen eine Rückwirkung auf die Belüftung der Lunge haben, weil sie die Entfaltung der Lunge stören[5]. Sie können intrapulmonal, intrapleural oder extrapleural lokalisiert sein. Das Lungenvolumen wird um die Größe des intrathorakalen raumfordernden Prozesses reduziert. Die Störung der Lungenfunktion ist damit in erster Linie von der Größe des raumfordernden Prozesses abhängig. Behinderte Lungenentfaltung, Lungenkollaps und Kompression sind verschiedene Grade der Störung, die alle in Atelektase enden.

a) Der Pneumothorax.

Luft, die in den geschlossenen Thoraxraum eingeführt wird, verteilt sich gleichmäßig über die ganze Lunge und hebt diese von der Thoraxwand ab. Der Pleuradruck bleibt dabei negativ, wenn keine Pleuraverwachsungen bestehen. Daraus folgt, daß die Ablösung durch die elastische Retraktion der Lunge vor sich geht. Ist die eingefüllte Luftmenge klein, dann entwickelt sich ein mantelförmiger Pneumothorax. Unter diesem verkleinert sich die Lunge gleichmäßig in allen ihren Teilen, indem sie sich auf den Hilus retrahiert. Die Verkleinerung ist etwas geringer als das eingefüllte Luftvolumen, weil sich der Thorax

---

[1] Campbell 1958.   [2] Parow 1950, 1953.
[3] Walker und Kuprijanoff 1923, zit. nach Linzbach 1939.
[4] Strauss 1927.   [5] Jaccard 1956 (Literatur), Mülly 1956.

gleichzeitig reflektorisch erweitert. Bei Pneumothorax nimmt der Brustkorb Inspirationsstellung ein und vergrößert damit sein Fassungsvermögen um 2—3 Liter, ebenso auch bei Lungenkollaps. Deshalb sind Atemvolumen und Residualluft bei Pneumothorax in der Ruheatmung nur wenig eingeschränkt[1]. Solange der intrapleurale Druck negativ bleibt, tritt das Zwerchfell nur wenig tiefer und wird erst bei positiven Drucken nach der Bauchhöhle vorgewölbt.

Das Mediastinum ist in der Ruhelage nach der gesunden Seite verzogen, weil dort der Druck stärker negativ ist, als auf der Pneumothoraxseite. In der Inspirationsbewegung wächst der negative Pleuradruck auf der Pneumothoraxseite stärker an als auf der gesunden Seite, weil der elastische Dehnungswiderstand der kollabierten Lunge geringer ist als in der entfalteten Lunge. In der Exspiration sinkt er rasch ab. Das Mediastinum wandert deshalb gegen Ende der Inspirationsphase zur Pneumothoraxseite und mit Beginn der Exspirationsphase zur gesunden Seite zurück. Diese Pendelbewegung des Mediastinums kann so stark sein, daß die Lunge der Pneumothoraxseite ventiliert wird[2].

Bei positivem Pleuradruck kann das Mediastinum erheblich verschoben sein und sich im vorderen Anteil sowie im hinteren unteren Abschnitt retrokardial hernienartig zur gesunden Seite hin ausbuchten.

Beim offenen Pneumothorax pendelt die Luft im Pleuraraum durch das Loch in der Thoraxwand (äußerer offener Pneumothorax) oder in der Lunge (innerer offener Pneumothorax) mit der Atmung hin und her, es besteht kein negativer Druck. Das Mediastinum wird deshalb bei der Inspiration nach der gesunden, bei der Exspiration nach der Pneumothoraxseite hin bewegt. Dieser Vorgang, den man als Mediastinalflattern bezeichnet, kann die Ventilation der gesunden Seite so erschweren, daß Erstickung eintritt.

Der Ventilpneumothorax macht mit seinem stark positiven Pleuradruck die stärkste Mediastinalverschiebung zur gesunden Seite und behindert durch die Kompression der großen Hohlvenen den Blutrückfluß zum Herzen. Das Mediastinum wird durch diesen Überdruck festgestellt und macht keine Ventilationsbewegungen mit.

Der therapeutische Pneumothorax hat eine Entspannung der Lunge zum Ziel, die bei Druckausgleich im Pleuraraum eintritt. Die Lunge kollabiert. Wird der Pleuradruck positiv, dann tritt zu dem Kollaps noch die Kompression der Lunge. Bei einfachem Lungenkollaps wird die Lunge nicht völlig luftleer, sie behält die Restluft und wird auch noch schwach ventiliert. Die Verkleinerung der Lunge beruht im wesentlichen auf der elastischen Retraktion der Acini. Dabei werden die Alveolen sehr stark verkleinert, während die Alveolargänge und die Bronchioli respiratorii relativ weit bleiben. Auf dem Schnitt durch die kollabierte Lunge ist makroskopisch bei Lupenvergrößerung das System der Alveolargänge noch deutlich erkennbar. Ebenso ist auch die Weite der Bronchien nur wenig reduziert. Die im Gangsystem befindliche Luft ist für den Gasaustausch nicht nutzbar. Sie ist funktionell Totraum — Luft. Der Luftwechsel ist wegen der minimalen Ventilationsbewegung der Kollapslunge so gering, daß die Alveolarluft nicht mehr genügend mit frischer Luft durchmischt wird[3] (Mischstörung) und das Lungenblut nicht genügend Sauerstoff aufnimmt[4] (Partialinsuffizienz).

Die Funktionsstörung bei Pneumothorax besteht also in einer Verminderung des Atemvolumens, die sich in einer Sauerstoffuntersättigung des Blutes auswirkt. Der Anteil der Pneumothoraxlunge am Gasaustausch und an der Ventilation beträgt nur noch etwa 30%[5].

---

[1] ANTHONY 1937. [2] SARNOFF 1950. [3] KNIPPING und BOLT, dieser Handbuchband.
[4] ROSSIER und BÜHLMANN 1956. [5] BJÖRKMAN 1934.

Aus anatomischen Untersuchungen ist bekannt, daß die durch Erguß oder Pneumothorax komprimierte Lunge blaß aussieht, also blutarm ist, während bei einfachem Lungenkollaps Hyperämie der Lunge besteht[1].

Messungen mit dem Herzkatheter haben ergeben, daß der Blutdurchfluß durch die Kollapslunge gedrosselt ist. Die Drosselung wird mit einer reflektorischen Engstellung der Arteriolen erklärt, die nach dem von Eulerschen Prinzip durch die Hypoventilation der Alveolen in der kollabierten Lunge ausgelöst sein kann. Nach eigenen Untersuchungen[2] kann aber der Lungenkollaps auch auf rein mechanischem Wege den Blutdurchfluß durch die Gefäße im Kollapsbereich erschweren (Abb. 31). Durchströmungsversuche an der Leichenlunge bei konstantem Druck zeigen, daß die Durchflußmengen mit zunehmender Dehnung

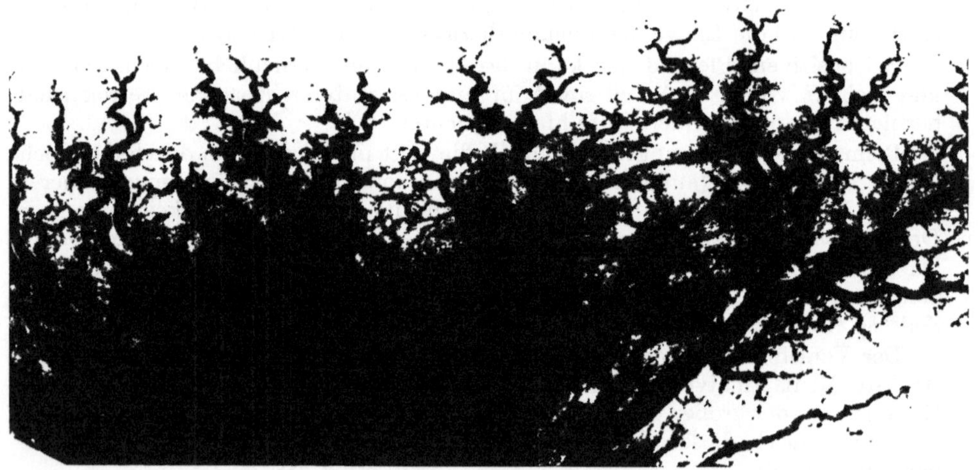

Abb. 31. Chronische Kompressionsatelektase des Unterlappens im Angiogramm der Leichenlunge. Korkzieherartige Schlängelung der Prälobular- und Lobulararterien. Kein venöser Rückfluß wegen des erhöhten Strömungswiderstandes in der Endstrombahn der Lunge.

größer werden. In der Kollapslunge ist der Strömungswiderstand am größten. Diese Messungen stimmen im Prinzip mit den von Altmann (1954) am Rattenthorax gewonnenen Ergebnissen überein (s. auch unter Perfusion, S. 585 u. 594).

Bei einem über lange Jahre geführten Pneumothorax wird dieser Zustand der funktionellen Minderdurchblutung der Lunge dadurch fixiert, daß die Lichtung der kleinen Arterien durch Intimaproliferation eingeengt wird. Daraus erklärt sich, daß nach Auflassen des Pneumothorax die Durchblutung reduziert und damit die Sauerstoffaufnahme trotz ausreichender Ventilation gering bleibt[3].

b) Der Pleuraerguß.

Beim Pleuraerguß durchläuft die Lunge, ähnlich wie beim Pneumothorax, Phasen der Entspannung bis zum Kollaps und bei positivem Pleuradruck auch der Kompression. Während beim Pneumothorax der positive Druck und damit die Kompression der Lunge nur unter besonderen Voraussetzungen (z. B. beim Spannungspneumothorax oder nach zu großen Zufüllmengen bei therapeutischem Pneumothorax) erfolgt, tritt beim Erguß die Kompression bereits früher in

---

[1] Westenhöfer 1928, 1935.   [2] Hartung und Delfmann 1960.
[3] Rossier und Mitarbeiter 1956, 1958.

Erscheinung, da der hydrostatische Druck des im Pleuraraum vorhandenen Ergusses sich nicht gleichmäßig verteilt, sondern in den abhängigen Abschnitten des Pleuraraumes, dort wo sich die größere Menge der Flüssigkeit ansammelt, am stärksten einwirkt.

Hier steigt der intrapleurale Druck auf positive Werte, während er oberhalb des Ergusses negativ bleibt. Daraus folgt, daß die Einschränkung der Ventilation im wesentlichen auf den Ort der Einwirkung des Ergusses beschränkt bleibt. Die Atelektasezone zeigt auch an der herausgenommenen Leichenlunge Stand und Größe des Ergusses an. Oberhalb der Ergußzone wird die Lunge eher vermehrt belüftet, da der Thorax, ähnlich wie bei Pneumothorax, auch bei Erguß reflektorisch weitergestellt wird.

Bei Pleuraerguß wird die Lunge im Bereich des positiven Pleuradruckes komprimiert, sie wird luftleer und blaß. Die Kompressionszone liegt regelmäßig am hiluswärts verschobenen unteren Lungenrand und rückt mit Ansteigen des Ergusses entsprechend der Ellis-Damoiseauschen Linie cranialwärts. Tritt bei freien Pleuraergüssen unter Lagewechsel eine Verschiebung der Flüssigkeit ein, dann wandert auch die Kompressionszone. Bei Ergüssen, die durch Verklebung oder Verwachsungen der Pleura fixiert sind, ist die Atelektasezone entsprechend begrenzt.

Nach kurzdauernden eiweißarmen Ergüssen bleibt die Lunge voll entfaltbar. Eine gleichmäßige Entfaltung tritt an der Leichenlunge in der Regel aber erst ein, wenn die Luft unter Anwendung eines Druckes eingeblasen wird, der etwa einer tiefen Inspiration entspricht. Bei geringen Drucken kommt es nur zur Auffüllung der noch beatmeten Lungenabschnitte. In den vollständig kollabierten und luftleeren Lungenabschnitten liegt zwischen den Alveolarwänden eine schmale Flüssigkeitsschicht. Diese bewirkt eine Capillaradhäsion der Alveolarwände, die beim Einblasen von Luft erst durch Anwendung eines höheren Druckes gesprengt werden muß.

Nach chronischen und fibrinreichen Ergüssen bleiben stets Daueratelektasen zurück, die teils auf Verschwartung der Pleura, teils auf Fibrose und Atelektase des Lungengewebes beruhen. Nach Pleuraempyemen werden Pleuraschwarten und Daueratelektasen nie vermißt.

c) Intrathorakale Tumoren.

Intrathorakale Tumoren stören die Lungenentfaltung nur im Bereich der direkten Druckwirkung, solange keine Bronchusabknickung hinzutritt. Die Auswirkung kleiner Tumoren ist für die Lungenfunktion in ihrer Gesamtheit ohne Bedeutung, Riesentumoren können ebenso wie große Ergüsse die Lunge hochgradig komprimieren. Regelmäßig kommt es dabei auch zu Abknickung und Stenosen der Bronchien. Bei intrapulmonalen Prozessen hängt der Grad der Ventilationsstörung ebenfalls von der Größe des Tumors und von der begleitenden Lungenkompression ab.

B. Störungen im luftleitenden System.

Die Atemluft wird den Alveolarräumen durch die Luftwege mit der Inspiration zugeführt und mit der Exspiration abgegeben. Die Luftwege bilden ein kompliziertes System aus Räumen, Kammern und Röhren mit weiten und engen Abschnitten. In diesen wird die eingeatmete Luft mit Wasserdampf gesättigt und so weit vorgewärmt, daß in den tiefen Luftwegen Körpertemperatur von etwa 37^0 C herrscht.

Die oberen Luftwege sind ein weites, kommunizierendes Raumsystem, das von Nase, Mundhöhle und Pharynx gebildet wird und bis zum Kehlkopf reicht.

Das Röhrensystem der unteren Luftwege beginnt im Kehlkopf, dessen Weite durch die Stellung der Stimmbänder variiert wird. Hier liegt auch die engste Stelle im ganzen System, an der die Luftströmung durch Glottisschluß völlig blockiert werden kann.

Alle Störungen des Luftwechsels, die durch Veränderungen in den oberen Luftwegen und in der Trachea ausgelöst werden, wirken sich an beiden Lungen gleichmäßig aus. Unterhalb der Carina sitzende Veränderungen führen zu Störungen der Luftverteilung in den Lungen. Wir unterscheiden deshalb globale Störungen der Ventilation, bei denen beide Lungen gleichmäßig beteiligt sind, und partielle Störungen der Luftverteilung (ventilatorische Verteilungs- oder Distributionsstörungen), die sich auf mehr oder minder zahlreiche, wechselnd große Abschnitte einer oder beider Lungen auswirken[1].

Im Mittelpunkt der Pathophysiologie des luftleitenden Systems stehen Änderung und Behinderung der Luftströmung, im Mittelpunkt der allgemeinen Pathologie ihre Ursachen und ihre Folgen für die Lungenbelüftung.

I. Anatomische und funktionelle Vorbemerkungen.

a) Die Luftströmung in den Atemwegen.

Unter normalen Verhältnissen herrscht im Röhrensystem der Luftwege Parallelströmung. Die Grenze der kritischen Strömungsgeschwindigkeit mit Auftreten von Wirbelströmung (Turbulenz) wird nur bei Hustenstößen erreicht[2]. Die Druckdifferenz zwischen Anfang und Ende des Röhrensystems, Weite und Länge der Röhren, Viscosität des strömenden Mediums, in diesem Falle der Luft, und Strömungscharakter sind entscheidend für die Strömungsleistung. Extrawiderstände[3] durch Wechsel des Röhrenquerschnittes und der Strömungsrichtung bedingen weitere Druckdifferenzen, die bei ruhiger Atmung unbedeutend sind, bei forcierter Atmung aber berücksichtigt werden müssen[4]. Der Hauptanteil des Druckgefälles zwischen Außenluft und Alveolarluft entfällt bei ruhiger Atmung auf die Rohrwiderstände. Diese sind etwa zur Hälfte in den Nasengängen und zur Hälfte im intrapulmonalen Röhrensystem, besonders in den Bronchiolen lokalisiert. Die Extrawiderstände liegen zu $^9/_{10}$ in den oberen Luftwegen bis zur Glottis, wobei $^2/_3$ durch die Glottisenge und etwa $^1/_3$ durch den Querschnittwechsel in Nase und Pharynx bedingt sind. Nur $^1/_{10}$ der Extrawiderstände liegt in den unteren Luftwegen[5] (vgl. Tabelle 4).

Tabelle 4. *Strömungswiderstände in den menschlichen Atemwegen.* (Nach Rohrer 1915.)

	Rohrwiderstände %	Extrawiderstände %
Obere Luftwege, gesamt	54	89,1
Nase und Pharynx	52,06	22,2
Glottis	1,2	66,9
Trachea	0,74	—
Broncholobuläres System, gesamt	46	10,9
Bronchialweg (Mittel)	13,4	10,15
Läppchen (Mittel)	32,6	0,75

Die Strömungsgeschwindigkeit ist am größten in der Glottis und nimmt bis zu den Bronchiolen stark ab. Sie ist von der Atemtiefe abhängig und erreicht beim Hustenstoß ihren höchsten Wert (Abb. 32, s. auch S. 514).

---

[1] Giese 1960.   [2] Rohrer 1915, Wyss und Hadorn 1952.   [3] Rohrer 1925.
[4] Wyss und Hadorn 1952, Gray und Grodins 1951.   [5] Nach Rohrer 1915.

Der Strömungswiderstand, der sich aus der Atemstromstärke und aus der Druckdifferenz zwischen Alveolarluft und Außenluft berechnen läßt (resistance), bleibt bei ruhiger Atmung in der ganzen Atemphase etwa gleich[1]. Bei angestrengter Ausatmung steigt er aber deutlich an und kann im Exspirationsstoß bei Pneumometrie um das Doppelte und mehr anwachsen[2]. Daraus wird geschlossen, daß der erhöhte intrathorakale Druck, der zur Erzeugung der größeren Stromstärke notwendig ist, das Röhrensystem einengt und so die Zunahme des Strömungswiderstandes in der Exspiration erzeugt[3].

Die Strömung in den Luftwegen folgt ganz allgemein dem Hagen-Poiseuilleschen Gesetz. Danach ist das geförderte Volumen proportional der Druckdifferenz und der 4. Potenz des den Rohrquerschnitt bestimmenden Radius. Es ist umgekehrt proportional der Rohrlänge sowie der hier als konstant zu betrachtenden Viscosität des strömenden Mediums. Diese Beziehung gilt nur für Parallelströmung; bei Turbulenz treten Extrawiderstände durch Wirbelbildungen bei plötzlichen Sprüngen der Lichtungsweite oder Änderungen der Strömungsrichtung auf. Bei den Widerständen aus turbulenter Strömung stehen Druckdifferenz und gefördertes Volumen in einem quadratischen Verhältnis.

ROHRER (1915, 1925) hat diese Beziehungen an Hand von Modellversuchen und Messungen an der kollabierten Leichenlunge unter Berücksichtigung der praktisch bestehenden Konstanz einiger der in die Gleichung eingehenden Größen zu einer einfachen Summenformel zusammengefaßt, sie lautet:

$$p = 0.8 \times V + 0.8 \times V^2 \text{ (cm H}_2\text{O)}.$$

Diese Formel von ROHRER, deren aus Leichenlungenmessungen gewonnene Faktoren nicht unmittelbar auf die Verhältnisse beim Lebenden übertragbar sind, erfuhr nach den Messungen von v. NEERGAARD[4] eine Modifikation. Die Widerstände wurden beim Lebenden insgesamt höher gefunden. Weiter ergab sich eine Differenz zwischen der Inspiration und der Exspiration; für letztere wurden wegen der geringeren Lichtungsweiten im Rohrsystem höhere Werte gemessen. Eine

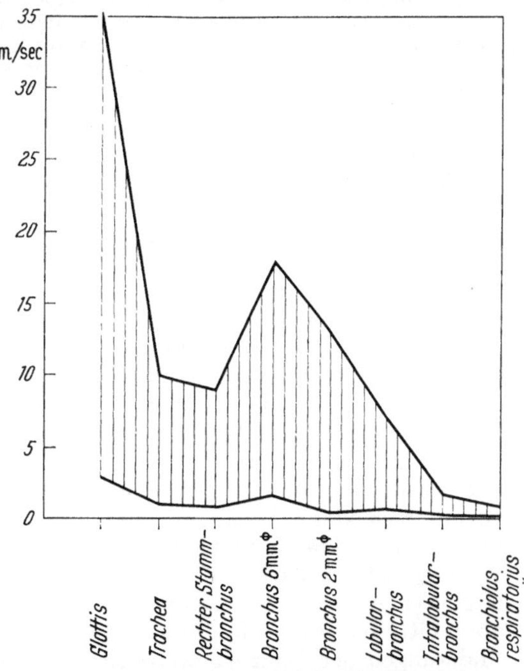

Abb. 32. Strömungsgeschwindigkeiten im Tracheobronchialbaum, aufgezeichnet nach den Meßwerten von ROHRER (1915). Schwankungsbreite zwischen Ruheatmung = untere Linie und maximaler Atmung = obere Linie.

solche Differenz wurde in neuerer Zeit nicht bestätigt[5]. Bei Strömungsvolumina über 2 Liter/sec nehmen die Strömungswiderstände für die Exspiration stärker zu als für die Inspiration[6]. Dieser Befund wird mit einer Kompression der Bronchien durch die stark vermehrten intrapulmonalen Drucke erklärt[7].

In röntgenographischen Untersuchungen[8] konnte gezeigt werden, daß die Amplituden der Weiten- und Längenänderungen im Bronchialbaum von zentral nach peripher zunehmen. Während an der Trachea die Radien bei tiefer Atmung nur um etwa 6%, an den großen Bronchien nur wenig mehr zunehmen, betragen die inspiratorischen Durchmesservergrößerungen

---

[1] WYSS und SCHMID 1951.

[2] HADORN 1942, 1943, HADORN und Mitarbeiter 1951, WYSS und HADORN 1952, BUHR 1958.

[3] WYSS 1955 (Literatur).

[4] Druckdifferenz zwischen statischem und dynamischem Pleuradruck bzw. Verschlußdruck und pneumotachographisch bestimmter Strömungsgeschwindigkeit, v. NEERGAARD und WIRZ 1927.

[5] OTIS und PROCTOR 1948, OTIS, FENN und RAHN 1950, SHELDON und OTIS 1951.

[6] MEAD und WHITTENBERGER 1953.　　　[7] WYSS und REGLI 1954.

[8] STUTZ 1950, STUTZ und VIETEN 1955 (dort weitere Literatur).

an den kleineren Bronchien bis zu 100%, besonders in den dorsalen Teilen der Unterlappen-
basis. Diese starken Kaliberschwankungen bringen es mit sich, daß die größten Änderungen
der Widerstände im Bereich der kleinen Bronchien angenommen werden müssen[1]. Wenn
die Rohrlänge und etwa auftretende Extrawiderstände gegenüber dem in der 4. Potenz
auftretenden und somit überragend wichtigen Radius vernachlässigt werden, dann gilt für
jeweils zwischen zwei Aufteilungen liegende Abschnitte des Röhrensystems die vereinfachte
Strömungsformel $w = \dfrac{1}{r^4}$; sie ändert sich zwischen In-und Exspiration entsprechend der
Radiusänderung $r_{insp.} \leftrightarrow r_{exsp.}$. Der Quotient aus den Widerständen in den Endstellungen
der maximalen Inspirations- und Exspirationslage kann dann als Maß für die inspiratorische
Widerstandsminderung gelten. Er beträgt nach Stutz für die Trachea nur 1,24, für die kleinen
Bronchien mit einer Radiusänderung von 100% dagegen 16; in den letzteren nimmt also
der Strömungswiderstand bei tiefer Einatmung um das 16fache ab.

Die bronchographischen Messungen der Radien, die bis zu den Bronchien 8.—9. Ordnung
möglich waren, haben weiterhin gezeigt, daß die Lichtungen des natürlichen Tracheobronchialbaumes peripherwärts stärker abnehmen als in einem den theoretischen Berechnungen zugrunde liegenden „idealisierten" Röhrensystem, in dem der Strömungswiderstand im Gesamtquerschnitt aller gleichgeordneten Röhrenabschnitte überall gleich ist. Die Widerstände
nehmen dagegen von der Trachea in Richtung der kleinen Bronchien laufend zu, ihr Maximum
liegt in der Peripherie, wahrscheinlich im Bereich der Bronchioli terminales. Die Differenz
zwischen den einzelnen Rohrabschnitten ist dabei so beträchtlich, daß sie trotz der inspiratorisch wesentlich stärkeren Widerstandsverminderung in der stark dehnbaren Peripherie auch
noch in maximaler Inspirationsstellung, wenn auch in geringerem Maße als in der Exspirationsstellung, erhalten bleibt. Daß im übrigen auch die hier vernachlässigten absoluten Rohr-
längen für Widerstandsdifferenzen zwischen Lungenmantel und Lungenkern wirksam werden,
hat Rohrer (1915, 1925) hervorgehoben und auf bestimmte Lokalisationstypen des Emphysems angewandt (s. S. 526).

Aus dieser allgemeinen Betrachtung ergibt sich ferner, daß lokale Beschrän-
kungen der Bronchialbewegungen unter krankhaften Verhältnissen erhebliche
dynamische Konsequenzen haben werden. So können z. B. basale Pleuraschwarten, paradoxe Zwerchfellbewegungen bei Phrenicuslähmung, Interlobärver-
wachsungen und andere Zustände, die die normalen respiratorischen Bewegungen
der Gesamtlunge und die Verschieblichkeit ihrer Lappen gegeneinander behindern,
zu unterschiedlichen Längen- und Lichtungsweiteänderungen und zu Verschiebungen der Abgangswinkel in einzelnen Bronchialprovinzen führen (H. H.
Weber 1936, Orsós 1913) und durch unterschiedliche Änderungen des Strömungswiderstandes eine lokal unterschiedliche Belüftung der abhängigen Lungenabschnitte bewirken. In ähnlicher Weise müssen Parenchymprozesse mit lokalen
Änderungen der Lungengewebselastizität im Sinne der statischen und dynamischen Inhomogenität wirksam werden, da sie die gleichmäßige Übertragung der
respiratorischen Amplitude der Thorax- und Zwerchfellbewegungen auf die Bron-
chiallumina stören. Änderungen der respiratorischen Weiten im Bronchialsystem
sind schließlich auch bei infiltrativen und indurativen Prozessen in der Bronchialschleimhaut oder im Peribronchium zu erwarten. Über die aktiven Änderungen
der Lichtungsweiten durch Tonusänderungen der Bronchialmuskulatur s. S. 510.

Vergrößerte Widerstände im Röhrensystem, die etwa durch Stenosen und
erhöhte Strömungsgeschwindigkeiten entstehen, setzen reflektorisch durch
Änderung des Atemtypus und Anspannung der Hilfsmuskulatur dynamische
Kräfte in Funktion und verschieben die Dehnungslage der Lunge in die inspiratorische Richtung[2].

Die vermehrte Spannung der Atemmuskulatur ist Folge von Widerstands-
reflexen, die wahrscheinlich über den Nervus phrenicus zum Atemzentrum laufen
und von dort her durch vermehrte Impulse die inspiratorische Kraft der Atemmuskulatur verstärken oder bei Wegfall der Stenose entspannend wirken[3].

---

[1] Stutz und Vieten 1955.   [2] W. R. Hess 1931.

[3] R. Schoen und Hempel 1933, Hempel 1933, Fleisch 1934, Campbell 1958, vgl. auch
Schoedel in diesem Handbuch.

Bei Erhöhung der Atemwiderstände durch Kanülen steigt die Atemarbeit, die unter normalen Verhältnissen in der Ruhe 2—3% des Stoffwechsels beansprucht, auf 6—9%[1].

Die Ausatmungskräfte sind nach neueren Untersuchungen[2] größer als die Inspirationskräfte. Die maximalen Drucke, die bei Exspiration gegen ein geschlossenes Manometer erzeugt werden können, betragen im Mittel 114 mm Hg, die inspiratorischen nur 65,7 mm Hg[3].

Neben dem Strömungswiderstand ist auch der Gewebswiderstand zu berücksichtigen. McIlroy u. Christie (1952) trennen an Leichenlungen Reibungs- und Strömungswiderstand. Der durchschnittliche Gewebsdeformationswiderstand beträgt nach diesen Messungen 30—40% des gesamten Widerstandes in der Atembewegung.

b) Der Totraum.

In der Lungenphysiologie unterscheidet man einen anatomischen und einen funktionellen Totraum. Die Luftmenge, die sich im Nasen-Rachenraum, im Kehlkopf, in der Trachea, in den Bronchien und in den Bronchiolen befindet, nimmt nicht unmittelbar am Gasaustausch teil, da durch die Schleimhäute keine direkte Gasdiffusion in das Blut erfolgt. Dieser Raum wird als Totraum oder als schädlicher Raum bezeichnet.

α) Der anatomische Totraum.

Seine Größe ist statisch durch Ausgießen der Luftwege mit Wasser[4] oder mit Gips[5] an Tier- und Menschenlungen gemessen worden. Die Menge der Luft, die diesen anatomisch definierten, von der Atemöffnung bis zu den Bronchioli terminales reichenden Raum ausfüllt, ist nicht konstant, sondern wechselt mit den respiratorischen Bewegungen der Lunge. Die Schwankungen beruhen darauf, daß die dehnbaren Teile dieses Röhrensystems, nämlich Trachea, Bronchien und Bronchiolen mit der Inspiration weiter und mit der Exspiration enger gestellt, bei positiven Pleuradrucken, etwa bei Hustenstoß, sogar komprimiert werden[6]. Die Abhängigkeit des im Totraum vorhandenen Luftvolumens von der Lungenentfaltung hat Rohrer (1915) festgestellt, dessen Werte heute allgemein anerkannt werden (Tabelle 5).

Die respiratorischen Weiteänderungen sind bronchoskopisch[7] und röntgenstereoskopisch[8] gemessen worden. Die durchschnittlichen Werte sind:

Tabelle 5. *Anatomischer Totraum* (nach Rohrer).

Entfaltungsgrad der Lunge	Anatomischer Totraum ml
Kollaps	150
Totale Exspiration	180
Normale Exspiration	220
Normale Inspiration	230
Totale Inspiration	260

Trachea inspiratorisch . . . . . . 18,2 mm
exspiratorisch . . . . . . 16,9 mm
rechter Bronchus inspiratorisch . . 17,0 mm
exspiratorisch . . 14,2 mm
linker Bronchus inspiratorisch . . . 13,0 mm
exspiratorisch . . . 11,2 mm

Stutz (1949) gibt als Durchmesser der Trachea 15—20 mm an.

Bei Hustenstößen wird die Trachea stark seitlich komprimiert und die Hinterwand eingedellt. Bei Jugendlichen kann die Lichtung der Trachea auf diese Weise bis auf ein Zehntel verringert werden[6].

Ebenso treten auch an den kleinen Bronchien und Bronchiolen erhebliche Schwankungen in der Weite auf, die vom Entfaltungszustand der Lunge und

---

[1] Anthony und Lent 1941, Lent 1941, Anthony, Lent und Müller 1941, Bühlmann 1949 (dort ältere Literatur).
[2] Rahn, Otis, Chadwick und Fenn 1946, MacLeod 1935.   [3] Wyss 1955.   [4] Bohr 1891.
[5] Loewy 1894.   [6] Stutz 1949, di Rienzo.   [7] Brünings 1910.   [8] Brückner 1952.

vom intrathorakalen Druck abhängig sind[1]. Am geringsten sind die passiven Änderungen der Lichtungsweite an den Bronchiolen, an denen sich wegen der muskelstarken Wandung die Eigenbewegung mit Konstriktion und Dilatation deutlich bemerkbar macht. Die Fasersysteme sind in den Bronchiolen spiralig angeordnet.

Der Kehlkopf steigt während der Exspiration um $1/_2$—$1^1/_2$ Wirbelkörper höher, die Längendifferenz der Trachea zwischen Inspiration und Exspiration beträgt etwa 1,5—2,5 cm.

β) Der funktionelle Totraum.

Der anatomisch definierte Totraum füllt sich in der Inspiration mit atmosphärischer Luft und enthält am Ende der Exspiration Alveolarluft, die Sauerstoff und Kohlensäure mit dem Blut ausgetauscht hat.

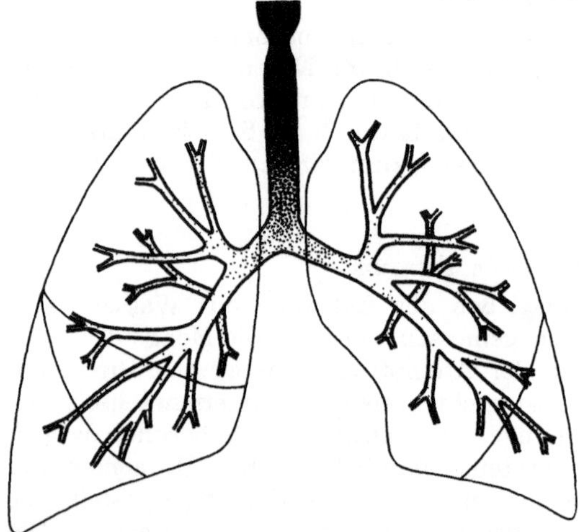

Abb. 33. Gliederung des funktionellen Totraumes. Atemluft im Tracheobronchialbaum am Beginn der Exspiration. Schwarz absoluter Totraum mit atmosphärischer Luft; grau relativer Totraum mit Mischluft; weiß Alveolarluft nach erfolgtem Gasaustausch.

Die funktionelle Auswirkung des anatomischen Totraumes bei der Atmung entspricht nicht unmittelbar seinem Volumen. Die Teilung in Totraumluft und Alveolarluft ist eine Abstraktion. Der größte Teil der Luftwege ist vielmehr von Mischluft ausgefüllt, die hinsichtlich ihrer Gasspannungen zwischen der Außenluft und der Alveolarluft steht. Die unterschiedlichen Gasspannungen der einzelnen Luftportionen gleichen sich in den Atemwegen durch Diffusion und zusätzlich durch mechanische Mischung infolge pulssynchroner Schwankungen des intrapulmonalen Druckes teilweise aus[2].

Die ausgeatmete Luft läßt sich bei fortlaufender Messung der Gaszusammensetzung mit schnell anzeigenden Gasanalysatoren in 3 Anteile aufgliedern (Abb. 33):

1. Den Anteil aus atmosphärischer Luft (absoluter Totraum). Dieser stammt aus den oberen Luftwegen, in denen die Gaszusammensetzung bis in die Trachea hinein bei ruhiger Atmung unverändert bleibt. Seine Größe beträgt 40—80 ml[3] im Mittel 44,2 ml[4].

2. Den Mischluftanteil (relativer Totraumanteil). Dieser füllt im Beginn der Exspiration den Bronchialbaum und Teile der Trachea aus. Er beträgt im Mittel 249 ml[4]. Bei vorübergehendem Atemstillstand nimmt die Größe des absoluten Totraumes infolge der genannten Mischungsvorgänge innerhalb der Luftsäule relativ schnell ab. Die Größe des gemessenen Mischluftanteiles macht es wahrscheinlich, daß auch die Luft in den Gängen des Arbor alveolaris in ihrer Gaszusammensetzung noch nicht vollkommen der Alveolarluft entspricht[5]. Er liegt

---

[1] Stutz 1949, di Rienzo.   [2] Bartels und Mitarbeiter 1954, Ulmer 1959.
[3] Fowler 1950.   [4] Ulmer und Lechner 1959.
[5] Haldane 1927, Henderson und Mitarbeiter 1915, Ulmer und Lechner 1959.

in seiner Gaskonzentration zwischen der atmosphärischen Luft und der Alveolarluft. Er nähert sich in der fortschreitenden Exspiration der Zusammensetzung der Alveolarluft.

3. Die Alveolarluft. Als Alveolarluft wird der Anteil der Atemluft bezeichnet, in dem ein Gasaustausch mit dem Blut erfolgt und ein Gleichgewicht zwischen den Gasen der Luft und des Blutes der Lungencapillaren entstanden ist. Ihre Menge ist abhängig von der Tiefe der Exspiration, also in weiten Grenzen variabel, während der absolute Totraum und der Mischluftanteil nur geringen Schwankungen unterliegen. Am Ende der Exspiration ist der gesamte anatomische Totraum mit Alveolarluft gefüllt. Diese wird im Beginn der Inspiration erneut in die Alveolen eingeatmet.

Der funktionelle Totraum wird auf 3 Wegen gemessen:

1. Aus der Differenz zwischen den Werten der Gaszusammensetzung in der Ein- und Ausatmungsluft durch Bestimmung des Sauerstoffs oder der Kohlensäure[1]. Die Berechnung erfolgt nach der Formel von BOHR (1909).

$$\text{Totraum} = \frac{a-e}{a-i} \times V,$$

wobei a die Gaskonzentration in den Alveolen, e die Gaskonzentration in der Exspirationsluft, i die Gaskonzentration in der Inspirationsluft ist.

2. Mit den Fremdgasmethoden, bei denen statt Luft Wasserstoff[2], Stickstoff, Helium oder ein anderes Gas eingeatmet wird.

3. Durch die Bestimmung des Ventilationseffektes, gemessen an der Kohlensäurekonzentration in der Alveolarluft[3] bzw. in der aus der Kohlensäurespannung im arteriellen Blut erschlossenen „idealen" Alveolarluft[4].

Mit diesen verschiedenen Methoden wird der Totraum unterschiedlich groß bestimmt; die Differenzen treten besonders bei verstärkter Ventilation unter Arbeitsbelastung hervor. In die ursprünglich anatomische Definition wird ein funktionelles Moment, der effektive Gasaustausch, neu und zusätzlich hineingetragen. Der funktionelle Totraum hat seine räumlichen Eigenschaften damit weitgehend verloren. Der von den Fremdgasmethoden erfaßte „ventilatorische Totraum" steht noch am ehesten mit dem anatomisch erfaßbaren in Übereinstimmung.

In der Ruheatmung decken sich die Werte für den anatomischen und funktionellen Totraum, der mit 140—150 cm³ bestimmt wurde, annähernd, doch können sie nicht unmittelbar miteinander verglichen werden[5].

Die Bestimmung des funktionellen Totraumes durch Untersuchung des Auswaschungseffektes der CO_2 aus dem Blut (CO_2-Clearance) hat eine besondere klinische Bedeutung. Sie integriert alle wesentlichen Faktoren der Ventilation, der Perfusion und der Diffusion[6]. Die Größe des funktionellen Totraumes ist also abhängig:

a) von der Größe des anatomisch erfaßbaren Totraumes,

b) von der Gleichmäßigkeit der Frischlufteinmischung in die Alveolarluft,

c) von dem Verhältnis zwischen Belüftung und Durchblutung,

d) von der Intensität des Gasaustausches, also von der Größe der Kontaktfläche, der Dauer der Kontaktzeit und von der Permeabilität der Grenzflächen.

Von der Gesamtventilation werden unter normalen Verhältnissen etwa $^2/_3$ bis $^3/_4$ der geatmeten Luft zur Belüftung der Alveolarräume verwandt, während

---

[1] HALDANE und PRIESTLEY 1905.   [2] SIEBECK 1910/11.
[3] AITKEN und Mitarbeiter 1927, GROSSE-BROCKHOFF und SCHOEDEL 1937.
[4] ENGHOFF 1938, ROSSIER und Mitarbeiter 1953, 1956, 1958, RILEY und Mitarbeiter 1946.
[5] ENGHOFF 1932, ULMER und STAMMBERGER 1959.   [6] GOEBEL 1959.

der Rest im Totraum bewegt wird, ohne am Gasaustausch teilzunehmen. Die Atmung ist um so ökonomischer, je kleiner der Totraum ist. Ein großer funktioneller Totraum vermehrt die Luftmenge, die zur Bewältigung des erforderlichen Gasaustausches bei der Ventilation bewegt werden muß. Das Atemäquivalent, d. h. die im Verhältnis zur O_2-Aufnahme zu ventilierende Luftmenge, steigt an. Bei oberflächlicher schneller Atmung, dem Hecheln, ist der Nutzeffekt besonders gering, weil die Luft vorwiegend im anatomischen Totraum bewegt wird.

Eine Residuallufterhöhung allein bewirkt bei Lungengesunden noch keine Vergrößerung des funktionellen und absoluten Totraumes, weil die intrapulmonalen Mischungsvorgänge umso wirksamer werden, je weiter zur Peripherie hin die Grenze des Totraumes verschoben wird[1]. Diese Anpassung des Austauscheffektes an ein erhöhtes Alveolarvolumen bei gesteigerter Ventilation hat eine korrespondierende Vergrößerung der Austauschfläche zur Voraussetzung, die bei dem Volumen pulmonum auctum des Lungengesunden gegeben ist. Bei Emphysem dagegen ist eine entsprechende Kontaktflächenvergrößerung infolge des Gliederungsverlustes der terminalen Lufträume nicht möglich. Die übermäßige Erweiterung der Alveolarräume mit Erhöhung des Residualluftvolumens wirkt sich bei Emphysematikern in einer erheblichen Zunahme des funktionellen und des absoluten Totraumes aus.

Eine wesentliche Vergrößerung des funktionellen Totraumes tritt auch dann ein, wenn belüftete, aber nicht durchblutete Lungenabschnitte ohne Austauscheffekt ventiliert werden. Dabei können sich deutliche Differenzen zwischen Totraumbestimmungen aus den alveolären und aus den arteriellen CO_2-Spannungen ergeben[2]. In diesen Fällen mit alveolär-arteriellen CO_2-Spannungsdifferenzen wird nach Folkow u. Pappenheimer (1956) in der Patho-Physiologie von „Paralleltotraum" gesprochen.

II. Stenosen der oberen Luftwege und der Trachea.

Fast alle Erkrankungen der oberen Luftwege und der Trachea, die Einfluß auf die äußere Atmung haben, engen die Gänge, Kammern, Höhlen und Röhren ein, durch die Luft bei der Ein- und Ausatmung hindurchtritt. Sie stören die Luftströmung in diesem Teil des luftleitenden Systems und ändern die Größe des Totraumes.

Erweiterungen dieser Räume, etwa durch Laryngo- und Tracheocelen, durch Verbindungen der Nasen- und Mundhöhle bei Gaumenspalte oder durch ungewöhnliche Größe der Nebenhöhlen vermehren zwar den Totraum, spielen aber in der Pathophysiologie der äußeren Atmung eine nur geringe Rolle. Ebenso hat die Verkürzung des Atemweges, etwa bei Mundatmung oder nach Tracheotomien, für die Belüftung der Lunge keine große Bedeutung, da sie den Luftwechsel eher erleichtert als erschwert. Die Ausschaltung der Nase als Vorwärmkammer und als Filter bei der Mundatmung und die Umgehung der gesamten oberen Luftwege bei der Tracheotomie haben aber Nebenwirkungen, die sich in der Neigung zu Infektionen und chronischen Katarrhen der tiefen Luftwege äußern und so erst indirekt auf die Lungenventilation Einfluß gewinnen.

So beschränkt sich die allgemeine Pathologie der äußeren Atmung in diesem Bereich fast ausschließlich auf den Effekt der Stenosierung, sie ist eine Pathologie der Stenosen.

Aus den sehr wechselnden anatomischen Verhältnissen in dem System der oberen Luftwege ergibt sich eine Fülle von Möglichkeiten, unter denen Stenosen

---

[1] Herberg, Reichel u. Ulmer 1960.   [2] Forster 1957, Ulmer u. Stammberger 1959.

entstehen. Sie können hier nicht im einzelnen besprochen werden, ebenso nicht die zahlreichen Variationen ihrer Morphologie[1].

Dagegen sollen hier bereits einige Formen der Stenosen erwähnt werden, deren Unterscheidung für das Verständnis ihres Einflusses auf die Luftströmung von Bedeutung ist.

Wir unterscheiden starre Stenosen, weiche Stenosen und Ventilstenosen.

Die starre Stenose behindert Inspiration und Exspiration in gleicher Weise.

Die Wirkung einer weichen Stenose ist abhängig von den Druckverhältnissen im Röhrensystem und in seiner Umgebung. Innendruck und Außendruck wirken dabei gegensinnig. Ein positiver Außendruck verengt, ein positiver Innendruck erweitert die Lichtung. Umgekehrt tritt bei negativem Innendruck durch Ansaugen oder Kollaps eine Stenose, bei negativem Außendruck eine Erweiterung ein. Wegen der intrathorakalen und extrathorakalen Druckdifferenz kollabiert eine malacische Trachea im extrathorakalen Anteil, erweitert sich aber im endothorakalen Abschnitt. Weiche extrathorakale Stenosen behindern die Inspiration, endothorakale die Exspiration.

Die Ventilstenose unterbricht die Luftströmung in einer Richtung, an den oberen Luftwegen gewöhnlich inspiratorisch, in der Lunge teilweise auch exspiratorisch.

a) Störungen der Nasenatmung.

Die Luft tritt bei der Inspiration durch die Nasen- oder Mundöffnung in die Luftwege ein. Beide Wege können getrennt oder gemeinsam benutzt werden. Der Nasenweg, der durch die Nasenscheidewand in zwei symmetrische Hälften getrennt ist, beginnt mit den Nasenöffnungen, die durch ein Knorpelgerüst offengehalten werden. Dieses wird von den Flügeln des knorpeligen Septums und den Cartilagines alares majores gebildet, die durch Sehnen verbunden und gegeneinander beweglich sind. Die Nasenöffnung kann durch Muskeln in den Nasenflügeln verengt oder erweitert werden. Bei Inspiration werden die Nasenflügel etwas eingezogen, durch leichten Druck oberhalb der Nasenflügel im Bereich der Nasenklappe völlig verschlossen[2].

Die bei Ruheatmung nur geringe Bewegung verstärkt sich bei angestrengter Inspiration zum Nasenflügelatmen, etwa bei Pneumonie oder bei anderen Respirationsstörungen, die in der Lunge liegen. Die zusätzliche Erweiterung der Nasenlöcher bleibt aber nur gering und hat keinen nennenswerten Nutzen für die Lungenbelüftung[3].

Beim Tier liegen die Verhältnisse anders. So können z. B. Robben und Tauchvögel ihre Nasenöffnungen völlig schließen. Bei Pferden führen Lähmungen der Nüstern zur Erstickung[4].

Das Druckgefälle, das bei Inspiration zwischen Nasenöffnung und Alveolen in diesem etwa 50 cm langen Luftweg entsteht, beträgt etwa 8—10 cm H_2O, der Druckunterschied zwischen Nasenvorhof und Atmosphäre nur etwa 3 mm H_2O[5].

Der Weg, den der Luftstrom bei der Inspiration zum Rachen nimmt, ist von dem Bau der Nase abhängig. In den weiten Nasenhöhlen steigt der Luftstrom in symmetrischen Bögen bis zum Nasendach an, biegt hier um und fließt zwischen mittlerer und oberer Nasenmuschel durch die Choanen in den Rachenraum ein. Bei der Ausatmung nimmt er etwa den gleichen Weg. Nur in diesem Abschnitt der Nasenhöhlen wird die Luft bei der Atmung ständig bewegt, in den unteren, oberen und seitlichen Teilen der Nasenhöhle steht sie fast ruhig[6]. Für den Verlauf

[1] Literatur bei HELLMANN und SIEGMUND 1931, LUCHSINGER 1956, GIESE 1959.
[2] MINK 1907, v. SKRAMLIK 1925, MARX 1949 u. a.   [3] MARX 1949.
[4] CLAUDE BERNARD, zit. nach MINK 1907.   [5] MINK 1907.   [6] v. SKRAMLIK 1925.

des Inspirationsstromes in der Nase ist der Winkel von entscheidender Bedeutung, den die Ebene der Nasenöffnungen und der Oberlippe miteinander bilden, während der Verlauf des Exspirationsstromes von der Gestalt des Rachenraumes und der Lage der Choanen beeinflußt wird[1].

Nach Eintritt der Luft aus dem engen Naseneingang in die weite Nasenhöhle bilden sich zwei große gegenläufige Wirbel. Diese entstehen an den Köpfen der mittleren und unteren Nasenmuscheln, die sich dem Einatmungsstrom als Hindernis entgegenstellen. An diesen Stellen schlägt sich Staub der Einatmungsluft bevorzugt nieder. Die Wirbelbildungen sind für die Reinigung der Luft von großer Bedeutung[2]. Die Druckdifferenz zwischen Außenluft und Nasenrachenraum beträgt bei der Einatmung 2,5—4 cm H_2O. Bei schnuppernder Atembewegung werden die Wirbelbildungen vermehrt und führen zu einer stärkeren Durchmischung der Luft[3]. Abweichungen im Bau der Nase, besonders die Stellung des Nasenseptums ändern den Verlauf der Stromlinien[4].

Zusätzliche Hindernisse, etwa Nasenpolypen, vermehren die Wirbelbildung. Auch bei abnormer Weite der Nasenhöhle treten zusätzliche Wirbelbildungen auf, die so groß sein können, daß sie fast die ganze Nase ausfüllen und die laminare Parallelströmung vernichten[5].

Die Nasennebenhöhlen werden durch Diffusion oder durch Nebenströmungen belüftet, die am Ende der Inspirationsphase entstehen[6]. In der Inspiration wird infolge des negativen Druckes im Nasen-Rachenraum Luft aus den Nebenhöhlen angesaugt, in der Exspiration strömt die Luft wieder ein. Die Druckschwankungen sind bei angestrengter Atmung sehr erheblich[7].

Jede Einengung erschwert die Atmung durch Erhöhung der Widerstände[8]. Häufigste Ursachen dafür sind Schleimhautschwellungen, die schon durch vermehrte Füllung der Blutgefäße in den Schwellkörpern der Muscheln wirksam werden[6], im Verlaufe entzündlicher oder allergischer Reaktionen durch Schleimhautödem aber erhebliche Grade erreichen können. Bei gleichzeitiger vermehrter Schleimsekretion kommt es zu mehr oder minder völliger Verlegung der Atemwege. Ebenso führen Schleimhautpolypen, Tumoren, Cysten, Fremdkörper, traumatische Deformierungen u. ä., oft auch fibrinöses oder schleimigeitriges Exsudat zur Stenose oder völligen Verlegung. Jede vorübergehende oder dauernde Erschwerung der Luftströmung in der Nase erfordert eine vermehrte Atemarbeit und führt bereits bei geringen Graden zu einer hilfsweisen oder vollständigen Umschaltung auf die Mundatmung.

b) Die Mundatmung.

Die Mundatmung wird auch bei freien Nasenwegen zeitweilig in Anspruch genommen, wenn das erforderliche Atemvolumen z. B. bei schwerer körperlicher Arbeit sehr groß wird[9]. Dann wächst der inspiratorische Widerstand im Nasenweg so stark an, daß die Atemarbeit unökonomisch wird.

Die Mundatmung ist phylogenetisch spät erworben und erst bei den Primaten nachweisbar. Bei allen übrigen Säugern ist ein Ausgleich einer gestörten Nasenatmung durch den Mundweg nicht möglich. Eine Tamponade der Nasenhöhle führt bei Kaninchen zu schwerer Stenoseatmung und zum Tod nach 4—8 Tagen[10]. Auch Meerschweinchen, denen die Nase zugenäht oder zugebunden wird[11], sterben innerhalb eines Tages an Erstickung.

---

[1] Danziger 1896, Hellmann 1927, van Dishoeck 1937.   [2] G. Lehmann 1938.
[3] Franke 1893.   [4] Danziger 1896.
[5] Scheideler 1939, Tonndorf 1939, Marx 1949 (Literatur).
[6] Mink 1915.   [7] Döderlein 1932, Wessely 1921, Henrici 1907, Marx 1949 (Literatur).
[8] Burchhardt 1905.   [9] Matthes 1941.   [10] Sandmann 1885.
[11] Marx 1949, Hofbauer 1921.

Marx (1949) erklärt die Erstickung mit dem Bau des Nasenrachenraumes. Bei diesen Tieren reicht die Epiglottis so hoch in den Epipharynx, daß sie sich der Hinterwand des weichen Gaumens anlegt (z. B. beim Pferd, Hund und auch noch beim Orang). Dadurch entsteht ein kontinuierlicher Luftweg, der durch die Muskulatur des Gaumenbogens gegen die Mundhöhle völlig abgeschlossen werden kann. Der Speiseweg geht neben der Epiglottis durch die Fauces in den Schlund, diese Tiere können gleichzeitig atmen und schlucken.

Bei den Primaten berühren sich weicher Gaumen und Epiglottis nicht mehr. Die Nahrung wird über den Kehldeckel in den Schlund befördert.

Beim Säugling und Kleinkind steht die Epiglottis noch hoch. Das Neugeborene atmet ausschließlich durch die Nase und erlernt die Mundatmung erst im Laufe des ersten Lebensjahres[1]. Es kann gleichzeitig atmen und trinken.

Beim Erwachsenen ist der obere Atemweg bei der Mundatmung kürzer und weiter als bei der Nasenatmung. Die Atemwiderstände sind geringer. Nur wenn sich die Zunge im Schlafe dem Gaumen anlegt, entsteht vermehrter Widerstand.

Nebenerscheinungen der Mundatmung sind geringere Anfeuchtung und Vorwärmung der Atemluft und der Fortfall der Luftreinigung von Staubteilchen[2]. Für die eigentliche Atmungsfunktion haben diese Störungen keine Bedeutung.

c) Die Pharynxstenosen.

Im Pharynx vereinigen sich Nasenweg und Mundweg des Luftstromes. Die Luft, die bei Nasenatmung durch die beiden Choanen in den Epipharynx eintritt, strömt unter Freilassung eines Mittelstreifens seitlich und an der Hinterwand des Pharynx zum Kehlkopf. Beide Ströme vereinigen sich erst im Bereich der Stimmlippen.

Der Epipharynx kann durch Anpressen des Gaumenweges an die Rachenwand verschlossen werden. Dadurch wird der Luftstrom in die Mundhöhle gelenkt, wobei die Zungenwurzel gesenkt und das Gaumensegel gehoben wird.

Bei der Nasenatmung legen sich Gaumensegel und Gaumenbögen durch Kontraktion ihrer Muskeln und durch Anlegung an die Zunge so fest aneinander, daß der Zugang zur Mundhöhle fast vollständig verlegt wird.

Ein gleichzeitiger Verschluß der Zugänge zur Nase und zur Mundhöhle entsteht beim Niesen.

Diese Verschlußfunktionen sind bei Lähmungen der Pharynxmuskulatur, insbesondere des Gaumensegels, gestört. Ihre Auswirkungen auf die Lungenventilation sind ohne besondere Bedeutung. Verkleinerung des Pharynx durch Schleimhautschwellungen, Tonsillenvergrößerungen, Tumoren u. a. können diesen Raum so einengen, daß Stenoseatmung eintritt. Die Folgen für die Lungenventilation sind die gleichen wie bei Stenosen des Kehlkopfes und der Trachea (s. S. 481).

d) Die Kehlkopfstenosen.

Mit dem Kehlkopf beginnt das tracheobronchiale Röhrensystem, das ebenso wie die Lunge mit dem ersten Atemzug in einen elastischen Spannungszustand gesetzt wird. Der Kehlkopf ist durch Muskeln am Pharynx und am Zungenbein fixiert. Beim Schlucken wird er um etwa 3 cm gehoben. Beim Heben und Senken des Kopfes bewegt er sich gleichsinnig mit. Diese Bewegung überträgt sich auch auf die Trachea, deren Bifurkation sich bei Kopfbewegungen über 1 cm heben und senken kann[3]. Infolge des elastischen Lungenzuges tritt der Kehlkopf bei der Inspiration etwas tiefer[4].

---

[1] van Gilse 1936.   [2] Perwitzschky 1928, G. Lehmann 1938.
[3] v. Hayek 1953.   [4] Mink 1916, 1918.

Der Kehlkopf wird durch die Stimmbänder geöffnet und geschlossen. Bei der Inspiration wird die Stimmritze erweitert, bei der Exspiration verengert. In ihrem Bereich liegt die engste Stelle des luftleitenden Systems, hier entstehen die größten Strömungswiderstände.

1. Die akuten Kehlkopfstenosen.

Zahlreiche Ursachen können eine rasch entstehende Stenose im Bereich des Kehlkopfes auslösen. Sie können funktionell und organisch bedingt sein.

Durch lokale Reizung von der Schleimhaut her kann die Glottis reflektorisch wie bei der Schluckbewegung fest verschlossen werden. Der Reflex wird ausgelöst durch Fremdkörper und reizende Gase (Chlor, Ammoniak, Salzsäuredämpfe, Kampfgase usw.). Auch Luft, die unter erhöhtem Druck in die oberen Luftwege eingeblasen wird, löst diesen Reflex aus. Ein Glottisverschluß entsteht schließlich auch beim Pressen.

Unter den funktionellen Stenosen sind auch Lähmungen der Kehlkopfmuskulatur zu erwähnen. Eine doppelseitige Recurrenslähmung, die z. B. nach Strumaoperationen eintritt, engt die Glottis durch mediane oder paramediane Stellung der Stimmbänder zu einem schmalen Spalt ein. Damit entsteht im Augenblick des Eintritts der Lähmung eine schwere Dyspnoe, die ohne Therapie zur Erstickung führt. Auch einseitige Recurrenslähmung kann durch Medianstellung des Stimmbandes der gelähmten Seite ein beträchtliches Hindernis für die Atmung sein.

Organische Stenosen können bedingt sein durch Schleimhautschwellungen der Epiglottis und der aryepiglottischen Falten, durch phlegmonöse Laryngitis, durch Fibrinauflagerungen bei Kehlkopfdiphtherie und durch Verletzungen des Kehlkopfes. Obturationen durch aspirierte Fremdkörper sind nicht selten.

Das akute Larynxödem, das im Rahmen eines Quinckeschen Ödems als allergischer Vorgang sich in wenigen Stunden entwickelt, bei Entzündungen des Kehlkopfes und seiner Umgebung entsteht, als kollaterales Ödem Affektionen des Mundbodens und Tumoren des Hypopharynx begleitet oder durch andere Vorgänge ausgelöst wird, engt den Aditus laryngis ein. Die Stenose wirkt sich vorwiegend inspiratorisch aus, da die zu Wassersäcken angeschwollenen Schleimhautfalten inspiratorisch angesogen werden und sich auf die Stimmritze legen. Dabei entsteht zunächst ein inspiratorischer, mit zunehmender Schwellung auch ein exspiratorischer Stridor. Die Atmungshilfsmuskulatur wird in Tätigkeit gesetzt, Supraclaviculargruben, Jugulum, Intercostalräume und Epigastrium sind eingezogen. Der Druck im Thoraxraum erreicht seinen tiefsten negativen Wert. Tritt der Tod an Erstickung ein, dann findet man eine luftarme, dunkelrote Lunge, deren Gefäße sich mit Blut vollgesogen haben. Die Luftarmut erklärt sich aus der raschen Absorption der Luft in den Lungen. Die Absorption fehlt bei plötzlichem reflektorischem Atemstillstand, etwa bei dem Bolustod, bei akutem Atemstillstand durch Reizung des Nervus laryngeus superior im Würgegriff und beim Laryngospasmus der Kinder. Deshalb sind die Lungen in diesen Fällen von plötzlichem Erstickungstod stets groß, oft sogar deutlich gebläht.

2. Die chronischen Kehlkopfstenosen.

Die chronischen Kehlkopfstenosen beruhen sehr häufig auf narbigen Strikturen, die nach entzündlichen Prozessen, z. B. nach Syphilis und Tuberkulose, nach Kehlkopfverletzungen, etwa durch Druck der Intubationskanüle, nach Osteochondritis des Kehlkopfskelets und ähnlichen Vorgängen entstehen. Unter den Tumoren, die durch Obturation zur Erstickungsursache werden, steht das

Larynxcarcinom an erster Stelle. Die seltenen Fehlbildungen spielen nur eine untergeordnete Rolle. Schleimcysten und Tumoren können ähnlich wie das Glottisödem mitunter einen inspiratorischen Ventilmechanismus auslösen. Wie bei der akuten Stenose steht auch hier die Erschwerung der Inspiration ganz im Vordergrund. Auch hochgradige Einengungen der Kehlkopflichtung sind noch mit dem Leben vereinbar, wenn sie langsam entstehen.

Über Folgeerscheinungen der Kehlkopfstenosen an den Lungen siehe unter Trachealstenosen.

e) Die Trachealstenosen und ihre Formen.

Weite und Form der Trachea unterliegen erheblichen Schwankungen. Die Enden der hinten offenen Knorpelspangen der Trachea werden durch quer-verlaufende Muskelbündel zu Ringen geschlossen. Die Kontraktion der Muskeln verengt die Lichtung der Trachea um etwa ein Viertel ihres Umfanges und ver-ringert auf diese Weise den anatomischen Totraum[1]. Bei der Atmung verhalten sich intra- und extrathorakale Anteile der Trachea gegensinnig. Bei der Inspi-ration wird der intrathorakale Anteil durch den negativen Druck im Thorax-raum gedehnt, bei der Exspiration enger gestellt, beim Hustenstoß sogar kompri-miert. Die Atmungsschwankungen in der Weite des extrathorakalen Anteils sind nur gering.

Die engste Stelle der Trachea ist der Ringknorpel. Weitere physiologische Engen[2] werden durch die normale Schilddrüse, durch den Druck des Aorten-bogens oberhalb des linken Hauptbronchus und durch die Arteria anonyma her-vorgerufen. Diese Gefäße können schon beim Kinde deutliche Furchen an der Trachea hinterlassen[3].

Die akute Trachealstenose hat ähnliche Folgen wie die akute Verlegung des Kehlkopfes. Häufigste Ursachen sind aspirierte Fremdkörper, fibrinöse Laryngo-tracheitis bei Diphtherie, Druckwirkungen der Schilddrüse bei Blutungen in substernalen Strumaknoten und ähnliches[4].

Bei der chronischen Stenose der Trachea zeigen die Folgeerscheinungen Variationen, die im wesentlichen von der Art der Stenose abhängig sind. Folgende Gruppen lassen sich unterscheiden:

1. Der intratracheale Tumor,
2. die Kompression der Trachea,
3. die Tracheomalacie,
4. die starre Trachealstenose.

1. *Intratracheale Tumoren* sind selten. Die intratracheale Struma, die als glatter Tumor breitbasig der lateralen Trachealwand aufsitzt, hängt entweder mit der an normaler Stelle liegenden Schilddrüse zusammen[5] oder hat sich aus einer Keimversprengung entwickelt. Mit der Pubertät pflegt ein stärkeres Wachs-tum einzusetzen und dadurch Stenoseerscheinungen hervorzurufen, die sich während der Menses oder in der Schwangerschaft durch Schwellung der Schild-drüse verstärken.

Adenome durchsetzen gleichzeitig die Trachealwand, ebenso auch Fibrome und Chondrome, die vom Trachealknorpel ausgehen. Auch die seltenen Plasmo-cytome gehören hierher. Die Trachealcarcinome wachsen mehr diffus infil-trierend, mitunter aber auch polypös.

Da sich die Trachea mit der Inspiration erweitert und bei der Exspiration komprimiert wird, wirkt sich die Tumorstenose zunächst in der Exspirationsphase

---

[1] v. HAYEK 1948, HESS 1931, REIN 1947.   [2] FRÄNKEL 1913.
[3] SIMMONDS 1904, FRÄNKEL 1913, Literatur bei HART 1928.
[4] Literatur bei HASLINGER 1929, ESCHER 1956.   [5] PENDL 1947, THORÉN 1947.

aus und zeigt sich bei leichter Stenose durch ein pfeifendes Geräusch, bei starker Stenose durch Stridor an. Bei starker Stenose stellt sich Stridor auch bei der Inspiration und schließlich Dyspnoe ein. Mit der Erschwerung der Exspiration kommt es zu einer Lungenblähung mit Erhöhung der Mittellage und Vermehrung der Residualluft. Das verlängerte Exspirium schließt sich ohne Atempause der erschwerten Inspiration an[1]. Die Atemfrequenz sinkt ab und vermindert dadurch die funktionelle Totraumventilation[2].

2. Die *Kompression der Trachea* erfolgt durch Strumen, Vergrößerungen des Thymus, Mediastinaltumoren, Aneurysmen der großen Arterien oder durch Gefäßanomalien, seltener durch entzündliche Prozesse, unter denen besonders die Lymphknotenschwellungen hervorzuheben sind.

Die Struma congenita ist in Kropfländern eine nicht seltene Ursache des Erstickungstodes bei Neugeborenen. Die diffus vergrößerte Schilddrüse umklammert die bei Neugeborenen noch weiche Trachea so stark, daß Erstickung eintritt. Der Knotenkropf des Erwachsenen dellt die Trachea bis auf einen schmalen Schlitz seitlich ein. Der substernale Strumaknoten komprimiert sie in sagittaler Richtung. Auch bei der Thymushyperplasie des Kleinkindes werden Stenoseerscheinungen mit sagittaler Abplattung der Trachea gefunden. Ähnlich wirken Mediastinaltumoren bei Lymphogranulomatose, Thymustumoren und Teratome des Mediastinums. Der Aortenbogen zeichnet sich bei Neugeborenen durch Abflachung der Trachealknorpel dicht oberhalb der Bifurkation ab. Syphilitische Aneurysmen des Erwachsenen können die Trachea verdrängen, sie komprimieren und in ihre Lichtung einbrechen.

Das Kleinkind ist durch Stenosierung der Trachea wegen der Enge des Rohres, seiner weichen Wandung und der leichten Ermüdbarkeit der Atemmuskulatur besonders gefährdet[3].

3. Bei allen genannten Prozessen, besonders aber bei Strumen, hat der anhaltende Druck auf die Trachea eine *Erweichung der Trachealknorpel* zur Folge. Die Trachealwand wird dadurch zu einer bindegewebig elastischen Haut, die dem inspiratorischen Zug und dem exspiratorischen Druck leicht nachgibt. Wenn der Trachea nach chirurgischer Entfernung eines Kropfes der feste Halt genommen wird, wirkt sich die Tracheomalacie in der Inspirationsphase als Stenose aus, da der inspiratorische Sog die ihres stützenden Knorpels beraubte Trachealwand aneinanderlegt. Tracheomalacien des endothorakalen Abschnittes, die nach klinischen Beobachtungen[4] in den letzten Jahren häufiger im Anschluß an Tuberkulosen der tracheobronchialen Lymphknoten beobachtet worden sind, weiten sich in der Inspiration unter dem negativen Druck im Thoraxraum stärker aus und fallen in der Exspiration zusammen. Nur ausgedehnte Erweichungen machen exspiratorische Stenoseerscheinungen.

4. Die *starre Stenose* findet sich am häufigsten als Alterssäbelscheidentrachea ausgebildet, bei der die Trachea seitlich stark eingeengt ist. Die an Trachealausgüssen studierten Formänderungen beginnen etwa mit dem 50. Lebensjahr, selten schon früher. Die stärkste Verengung liegt in der Regel im intrathorakalen Anteil, also vorwiegend in der unteren Hälfte oder im unteren Drittel[5]. Durch Verkalkung der Knorpel ist die Trachea in dieser Stellung, die der Trachealkompression in der Exspirationsphase entspricht, fixiert. Die Kombination mit Altersemphysem ist dabei fast regelmäßig festzustellen. Ob diese Prozesse als

---

[1] Steinmann 1949, Fleisch 1934, Bühlmann 1949.   [2] Rossier u. Mitarbeiter 1958.
[3] Escher 1956.   [4] Tanner 1957, Herzog und Nissen 1954, Herzog 1959.
[5] Simmonds 1897, 1904, 1905, Fränkel 1913, Oppikofer 1913, Hart 1928, dort weitere Literatur.

regelhafte Alternsvorgänge parallel laufen oder ursächlich miteinander verknüpft sind, ist noch nicht geklärt (Abb. 34).

Bei der Tracheopathia osteoplastica wird das Trachealrohr durch knöcherne
und knorpelige Wucherungen zwischen den Trachealknorpeln in eine starre enge
Röhre umgewandelt, deren Lichtung aber noch so groß bleibt, daß nennenswerte
Ventilationsstörungen dabei nicht eintreten. Das deckt sich mit der klinischen
Erfahrung, daß Kranke mit Einengungen der Trachea, die nur noch $^1/_5$ des

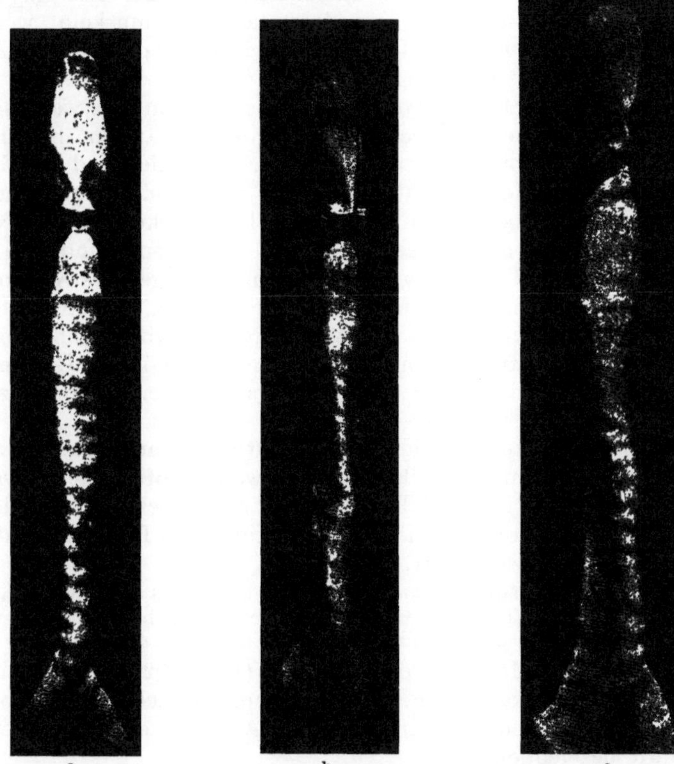

a   b   c

Abb. 34 a—c. Verschiedene Formen der Alterssäbelscheidentrachea. Seitliche Kompression des intrathorakalen
Abschnittes. Gipsausgüsse. (Aus SIMMONDS 1905.)

Tracheallumens offen lassen, in der Ruhe beschwerdefrei sind und nur eine
Arbeitsdyspnoe zeigen[1].

Andere Ursachen der starren Stenose der Trachea sind narbige Veränderungen,
die vorzugsweise nach Tracheotomien eintreten, wenn durch den Druck der
Kanüle Usuren der Schleimhaut mit nachfolgenden Granulationen oder Erweichungen der Knorpelringe sich eingestellt haben. Strikturen nach Syphilis
oder nach Tuberkulose, die früher häufig gesehen wurden, sind heute nur noch
selten zu beobachten.

f) Die Folgen von Stenosen der oberen Luftwege.

Bei Stenosen in den oberen Luftwegen ist die Atemfrequenz herabgesetzt, die
Atmung vertieft und verlängert[2].

[1] ESCHER 1956.
[2] MORAWITZ und SIEBECK 1909, SIEBECK 1909, FORSCHBACH und BITTORF 1910, BÜHLMANN
1949 (Literatur).

Bei inspiratorischer Stenoseatmung, die durch Ventilstenosen im Kehlkopf oder in der Trachea ausgelöst wird, bleibt das Atemvolumen klein, die funktionelle Residualluft ist vermindert, die Atemmittellage etwas erniedrigt[1].

Bei exspiratorischen Stenosen wird die Atemmittellage nach der Inspirationsseite verschoben und der Thoraxraum weit gestellt. Die Residualluft ist erhöht. Die Erhöhung der Atemmittellage verstärkt die passiv-elastischen Retraktionskräfte des Thorax-Lungensystems in einem für die Überwindung gering bis mäßig erhöhter Strömungswiderstände ausreichenden Maße. Die exspiratorisch wirksame Atemhilfsmuskulatur, insbesondere die Bauchmuskeln, werden erst oberhalb eines exspiratorischen Zusatzwiderstandes von 10 cm H_2O, bei Anaesthesie erst oberhalb von 20 cm H_2O eingesetzt[2].

Bei überwiegend inspiratorischen Stenosen der oberen Luftwege sind beide Lungen klein und blutreich. Durch den erhöhten negativen intrathorakalen Druck werden die Blutcapillaren stärker gefüllt. Tritt der Tod an Erstickung ein, dann enthalten die kleinen blutreichen und schweren Lungen auch Ödem, das als Folge des erhöhten negativen intrathorakalen Druckes und hypoxämischer Schädigung der Capillaren aufzufassen ist. Bei Neugeborenen und Kleinkindern, die bei Struma congenita, Thymushyperplasie, Fehlbildungen des Kehlkopfes und ähnlichen Leiden in eine inspiratorische Asphyxie geraten, werden die Lungen so luftarm, daß nur noch kleine Teile davon positive Schwimmprobe zeigen. Die maximalen und krampfhaften Inspirationsbewegungen können Deformierungen des Thorax und beim kindlichen Thorax sogar Rippenfrakturen zur Folge haben[3].

Bei exspiratorischen Stenosen der oberen Luftwege staut sich die Luft in den Lungen[4]. Die im Röntgenbild hellen Lungen werden oft als emphysematisch bezeichnet. Diese vermehrte Luftfüllung ist aber reversibel und entspricht einem Volumen pulmonum auctum. Ob daraus ein chronisches Lungenemphysem hervorgehen kann, ist noch zweifelhaft.

Nissen (1927) hat bei experimenteller Trachealstenose nach 3—6 Monaten an Hunden, Kaninchen und Katzen eine oft hochgradige Lungenüberblähung, besonders in den mediastinalen Lungenrändern mit Übergängen in herdförmiges Emphysem gesehen.

Nissen teilt damit die Meinung von Tendeloo (1910, 1929), daß Emphysem aus Überdehnung entstehen kann. „Permanent inspiratorische Expansion" nennt er den Zustand, den wir heute als Erhöhung der Atemmittellage mit Vermehrung der Residualluft bezeichnen.

Simmonds (1904, 1905) hat einen kausalen Zusammenhang zwischen Stenose und Emphysem angenommen. Fränkel (1913), Oppikofer (1913), Loeschcke (1928) konnten sich davon nicht überzeugen. Loeschcke (1928) lehnt einen Zusammenhang zwischen Emphysem und Trachealstenose überhaupt ab und hält die Fälle, in denen vermehrter Luftgehalt der Lunge bei Trachealstenose gefunden wird, für ein Volumen pulmonum auctum, das man vom eigentlichen Emphysem unterscheiden müsse.

III. Stenosen und Verschlüsse der großen und mittleren Bronchien.

a) Anatomische und funktionelle Vorbemerkungen.

Während bei Stenosen der oberen Luftwege und der Trachea bis zur Carina die Ventilation beider Lungen in gleicher Weise gestört ist und vollständige Verschlüsse (totale oder komplette Stenosen nach Escher 1956, Haefliger u. Mark 1956) durch Erstickung zum Tode führen, bleiben die Folgen von Stenosen

---

[1] Lent 1941.   [2] Campbell 1958.   [3] Escher 1956.
[4] Harris und Chillingworth 1919, Pfanner 1920.

jenseits der Carina auf wechselnd große Abschnitte einer oder beider Lungen beschränkt. Neben einfachen Einengungen der Bronchuslichtung (Partialstenosen) sind auch vollständige Okklusionen großer Bronchien mit dem Leben vereinbar. Die überaus häufigen Verschlüsse einzelner kleiner Bronchien bleiben oft symptomlos. Stenosen und Okklusionen großer Bronchien haben als führende Symptome Emphysem oder Atelektase. Beide Zustände können aufeinanderfolgen oder bei multiplen Bronchusstenosen nebeneinander bestehen. Die Bronchiektasie ist ein häufiges Begleitsymptom[1].

Die örtlichen Folgen sind abhängig von dem Kaliber des betroffenen Bronchus und von der Art der Stenose, während die allgemeinen Auswirkungen der Bronchusstenose auf die gesamte Lungenfunktion von der Ausdehnung des Prozesses bestimmt werden.

1. Der Bau der Bronchialwand.

Man unterscheidet nach dem Kaliber große, mittlere und kleine Bronchien.

Die großen Bronchien, zu denen die beiden Hauptbronchien und die des Unterlappens gehören, haben einen ähnlichen Bau wie die Trachea. Die Tunica fibrocartilaginea schließt in ihre vorwiegend in Längsrichtung verlaufenden elastischen und kollagenen Faserzüge halbringförmige Knorpel ein, die durch Längsbalken und Faserknorpel miteinander in Verbindung stehen und sehr unregelmäßige Formen haben[2]. Die kollagenen und elastischen Faserzüge strahlen in das Perichondrium der Knorpel ein.

In den mittleren Bronchien werden die Knorpel kleiner und lösen sich in unregelmäßig geformte Knorpelplättchen auf, an den kleinen Bronchien gibt es bei weiterer Reduktion der Knorpelplättchen bereits größere knorpelfreie Abschnitte. Die Teilungsstellen in die Bronchiolen enthalten in der Gabelung die sog. Reiterknorpel.

Die biegungssteifen elastischen Knorpel der Bronchialwand halten die Bronchiallichtung offen und haben ähnliche statische Funktionen wie die Trachealknorpel. Die vorwiegend in Längsrichtung verlaufenden Fasersysteme der Bronchien werden durch die inspiratorische Dehnung der Lunge unter Längsspannung gesetzt. Die fibrocartilaginöse Schicht ist an der Bifurkation am stärksten ausgebildet, sie ist in den großen Bronchialästen ebenso wie in der Trachea nur wenig dehnbar. Hilifugal wird die Tunica fibrocartilaginea immer dünner und damit stärker dehnbar. Sie verliert mit der Reduktion der Bronchialknorpel an Biegungsfestigkeit und gibt so leichter einem von außen auf die Röhren einwirkenden Druck nach. Nach bronchographischer Untersuchung nehmen die Bronchien einen spiraligen Verlauf[3]. H. H. Weber (1936) spricht von Torsion. Die Spiralen werden bei der Inspiration am stärksten im Bereich der mittleren Bronchien gestreckt.

In der Hülle der Fibrocartilaginea steckt die Ringmuskulatur als innen anliegende weitere Schicht. Sie beginnt in der Trachea als Spannmuskel zwischen den Enden der Trachealknorpel und verbindet in den großen Bronchien die Knorpelplättchen. Von den mittleren Bronchien ab geht sie in eine selbständige Schicht über, die sich von der Fibrocartilaginea löst und eine hilifugal immer stärker werdende Haut bildet, die an den kleinen Bronchien und Bronchiolen zum Hauptbestandteil der Wand wird. Gegen die verhältnismäßig starre Fibrocartilaginea ist sie durch eine lockere gefäßreiche Verschiebeschicht abgegrenzt. Die zirkulär laufenden Muskelfasern sind in den großen Bronchien durch elastische

---

[1] Churchill 1953, Literatur bei Kartagener 1956.
[2] Policard und Galy 1945, v. Hayek 1953, (Literatur).
[3] Huizinga 1937, Hudson und Jarre 1929.

Sehnen[1] an der Innenseite der Bronchialknorpel befestigt, an den mittleren Bronchien nur durch einzelne Muskelzüge mit den Knorpeln verbunden. In den kleinen Bronchien verlaufen die Muskelfasern spiralig und überkreuzen sich in Schraubentouren. In den Bronchioli terminales ist die Muskelschicht am stärksten, distalwärts splittert sie sich im Arbor alveolaris auf und endet in den Alveolargängen als Spannfasern des elastischen Gefüges im Acinus.

Die Muskelschicht verengt bei Kontraktion die Bronchiallichtung. In den großen und mittleren Bronchien wird dabei der Abstand der Muskelschicht von der Fibrocartilaginea größer, teilweise tritt auch eine Verschiebung der Knorpel gegeneinander auf. In den Bronchiolen wird die Muskelschicht durch Kontraktion dicker, die Lichtung gleichfalls eng.

Die aktive Änderung der Lichtungsweite wirkt sich auf die Schleimhaut aus. Bei weitgestelltem Lumen ist die Innenfläche glatt, bei kontrahierter Lichtung in Falten gelegt. Der Durchmesser der kleinen Bronchien kann dadurch nach v. Hayek (1948) etwa auf die Hälfte verkleinert werden.

Den passiven Einwirkungen des wechselnden intrathorakalen Druckes sind diese Bronchusabschnitte ebenfalls ausgesetzt. Die elastischen Fasern der angrenzenden Alveolen stehen im Bereich der Bronchiolen direkt mit der Muskelwand in Verbindung und üben auf diese eine Zugwirkung aus, die in der Inspiration stärker ist als in der Exspiration.

Die Bewegungen der Bronchien im Lungengewebe werden durch das lockere Peribronchium möglich, das als Verschiebeschicht funktioniert und neben Bronchialarterien und Nervenstämmen auch lymphatisches Gewebe enthält[2].

2. Die Bronchien in der Atembewegung.

Bei der Atembewegung wird der Bronchialbaum durch Spreizung aufgefächert[3]. Nach bronchographischen Untersuchungen[4] hängen die Winkelbewegungen der Bronchien von der Richtung des inspiratorischen Zuges ab. Neben der durch Querdehnung bedingten Spreizung kommen auch Verkleinerungen der Winkel vor, wenn der Längszug größer ist als der Querzug. Die Bronchien werden bei Inspiration vorwiegend in vertikaler Richtung, oft in erheblichem Ausmaß verlagert[5]. Die Verlagerung ist von der Zugrichtung abhängig.

Die inspiratorische Verlängerung des Tracheobronchialbaumes ist beträchtlich; an der Trachea beträgt sie etwa 1,5 cm. Die kleinen Unterlappenbronchien nehmen zwischen tiefer Exspiration und Inspiration um 78% an Länge zu[6].

Die Verlängerung erfolgt durch eine Streckung der spiralig verlaufenden Bronchien und durch Dehnung des myoelastischen Fasersystems[7]. Sie ist an den kleinen Bronchien stärker als an den mittleren und größeren Bronchien.

Mit der Dehnung kommt es zu erheblichen respiratorischen Kaliberschwankungen. An der Trachea beträgt die inspiratorische Erweiterung des Querschnitts 12%, an den großen Bronchien etwas mehr. An den kleinen Bronchien vergrößern sich die Durchmesser inspiratorisch auf das Doppelte, die Querschnitte auf das Vierfache[8]. Die respiratorischen Schwankungen in Länge und Weite der Bronchien sind am stärksten in den am besten belüfteten Lungenteilen. Sie stehen also in enger Beziehung zum Grad der Lungendehnung.

Die inspiratorische Erweiterung und die exspiratorische Einengung der Bronchien werden als druckabhängige passive Vorgänge aufgefaßt und sind Folge der Druckdifferenzen, die in der Atembewegung zwischen Lungengewebe und

---

[1] v. Ebner 1902.   [2] Policard 1938, Policard und Galy 1945, v. Hayek 1948, 1953.
[3] Orsós 1913, Macklin 1925.   [4] Stutz 1949.   [5] Huizinga 1937, Weber 1936.
[6] Stutz 1950.   [7] Miller 1950, v. Hayek 1953.   [8] v. Hayek 1953.

Bronchien entstehen[1]. Die Annahme aktiver respiratorischer Eigenbewegungen der Bronchien mit einem Tonuswechsel der Bronchialmuskulatur, die LUISADA (1934) aus der Elektrobronchographie geschlossen hat, wird seit den Untersuchungen von SCHRIEVER (1933), BRONKHORST u. DIJKSTRA (1940), ELLIS u. LIVINGTON (1935) als Fehldeutung angesehen.

Die von HENLE (1844) angenommene Bronchialperistaltik schien auf Grund zahlreicher bronchographischer Untersuchungen ausreichend gesichert zu sein[2].

Diese Annahme wird heute auf Grund anderer Untersuchungen abgelehnt[3]. H. H. WEBER (1959) mißt der Bronchialmuskulatur eine aktive Rolle bei der Expectoration zu. Nach WEBER soll es bei gesunden Personen im Hustenstoß auch zu keiner druckpassiven Verengung der Luftwege kommen. Die bronchographischen Untersuchungen seien zu dieser Frage nicht beweisend, weil es unter dem Reiz des Kontrastmittels zu einer Bronchuskontraktion mit Erhöhung des bronchialen Strömungswiderstandes und Ausbildung eines dem Aspirationsmechanismus ähnlichen akuten Bronchographie-Emphysems komme.

Bei Bronchographien mit öligen Substanzen werden die Bronchien reflektorisch eng gestellt und zeigen bei starker Reizung fadendünne Einschnürungen[4]. Diese Wirkung wird auf Reizung der hellen Zellen in der Bronchialschleimhaut bezogen[5]. Die Bronchialmuskulatur verhält sich wie ein Tonusmuskel[4], der nervösen, hormonalen und anderen Einflüssen unterliegt und die Bronchiallichtung eng oder weit stellen kann.

3. Ventilatorische Verteilungsstörung und Inhomogenität der Lunge.

Die von ROHRER (1925) stammende Auffassung von der Homogenität der normalen Lunge (s. S. 410) ist allgemein anerkannt. Die alveolentragenden respiratorischen Endabschnitte werden gleichmäßig belüftet. Das Maß ihrer Belüftung wird durch die Dehnbarkeit der Wände (Komplianz) einerseits, durch die Strömungswiderstände in den luftzuführenden Atemwegen (Resistance) andererseits bestimmt. Die anatomischen Unterschiede zwischen im Lungenmantel und im Lungenkern gelegenen Läppchen (erstere haben infolge des längeren Bronchialweges etwa doppelt so große Strömungswiderstände[6]) sind durch die im Lungenmantel größere Dehnbarkeit so auskompensiert, daß sich für alle Endabschnitte ein gleiches Produkt aus Dehnbarkeit und Strömungswiderstand ergibt. Die Dimension dieses Produktes ist die Zeit (sog. Zeitkonstante, MEAD, LINDGREN u. GAENSLER 1955):

$$\frac{\text{lit}}{\text{cm HOH}} \; (\text{Komplianz}) \times \frac{\frac{\text{cm HOH}}{\text{lit}}}{\text{sec}} \; (\text{Resistance}) = \text{sec}.$$

Man kann Homogenität also als einen Zustand definieren, bei dem in allen Lungenabschnitten gleiche Zeitkonstanten bestehen.

Es zeigt sich aber schon bei Lungengesunden, daß im Bereich sehr hoher Atemfrequenzen zwischen 50—60/min die Strömungswiderstände in den pleuranahen Lungenabschnitten mit langem Bronchialweg stärker anwachsen und als

---

[1] STUTZ und VIETEN 1955, HUIZINGA 1952, WESTERMARK 1938.

[2] REINBERG 1925, MACKLIN 1925, 1929, BRAUER und LOREY 1928, POPOVIC 1929, HUDSON und JARRE 1929, BULLOWA und GOTTLIEB 1931, MAYEDA 1931, MOUNIER-KUHN und LÉVY 1931, PARADE 1934, KAUTZKY 1936, DI RIENZO 1949.

[3] STUTZ und VIETEN 1955 (Literatur), DUKEN 1927, GORDONOFF und SCHEINFINKEL 1936, HUIZINGA 1937, POHL 1937, MEYER und ROLFS 1939, HÖRSTER 1941, TORELLI und VALLI 1948, FLEISCHNER 1949, STUTZ 1950, TANNER 1957 (Literatur).

[4] STUTZ und VIETEN 1955.

[5] FRÖHLICH 1949, BÜCHNER und FRÖHLICH 1948, FEYRTER 1938, 1954.

[6] ROHRER 1915, 1925.

Folge ihrer relativ geringeren Belüftung einen mäßigen Anstieg der dynamischen elastischen (effektiven) Widerstände bewirken[1]. Bei Kindern ist diese frequenzgebundene Widerstandsdifferenz wegen ihrer geringeren Bronchialweite größer als bei Erwachsenen[2]. Schon Rohrer (1915) hatte auf die Sonderstellung der besonders in der Spitze und an den vorderen Rändern gelegenen Lungenabschnitte aus seinen anatomischen Untersuchungen an Leichenlungen geschlossen, sie am Lebenden aber noch nicht nachweisen können. In der Lungenpathologie treten derartige Störungen in wesentlich stärkerem Maße hervor.

Fast alle Lungenerkrankungen heben die Homogenität der Lunge auf. Die Untersuchung der elastischen Widerstände unter statischen Bedingungen oder bei sehr langsamen Atemfrequenzen ergibt weitgehend von den Strömungswiderständen unabhängige Summenwerte der statischen Einzelelastizitäten, die als Typus der schlaffen, der starren und der Narbenlungen mit *statischer Inhomogenität* bereits (auf S. 437) besprochen und mit entsprechenden klinischen Befunden verglichen sind. Im Ablauf der normalen oder gesteigerten Atmung rücken die unterschiedlichen Strömungswiderstände gegenüber den statischen Dehnbarkeitsdifferenzen im Sinne einer *dynamischen Inhomogenität* in den Vordergrund.

Messungen der dynamischen Pleuradrucke unter gleichzeitiger Registrierung der Volumina haben den zunächst überraschenden Befund einer Erhöhung der Gesamtdehnungswiderstände der Emphysemlunge ergeben. So fand Christie (1934) die Dehnbarkeit der Emphysemlunge bei kleinen Pendelluftvolumina vermindert, bei großen Inspirationsvolumina schien die Lunge in einen Bereich der Überdehnung (overdistension) zu gelangen, wobei die lineare Beziehung zwischen Dehnung und Druck verlorenging. Erst später[3] wurde es deutlich, daß die dynamischen Pleuradruckmessungen nicht wie statische Meßwerte behandelt werden können (s. dazu weiter bei Lottenbach 1956), weil sie sich in Abhängigkeit von der Atemfrequenz ändern. Rossier (1956) hat darauf hingewiesen, daß dieses „elastische Paradoxon" erhöhter Widerstände bei klinisch bedeutsamem Emphysem mit bronchialen Wegsamkeitsstörungen auf der globalen Messung zahlreicher momentan unterschiedlicher Blähungszustände beruht. Es verschwindet bei Atemstillstand, d. h. unter statischen Bedingungen, und läßt dann die tatsächlich bestehende Elastizitätsminderung der Emphysemlunge hervortreten. Die Bedeutung gerade der bronchialen Strömungswiderstände für die Gesamtwiderstände (effektive Elastance bzw. Komplianz) geht auch aus den Messungen bei experimentellem Meerschweinchenasthma hervor[4]. Dabei wurden ebenfalls stark erhöhte globale elastische Widerstände gefunden.

Das elastische Paradoxon läßt sich an der isolierten Leichenlunge mit verschleimtem Bronchialbaum unmittelbar beobachten[5]. Bei schneller Aufblähung werden zunächst nur die schleimfreien Lungenabschnitte stark gebläht, wobei es zu einem unproportional starken Druckanstieg bei relativ kleinen Einfüllungsvolumina kommt. Dadurch wird bei Bezug auf den gesamten, wegen der Bronchialverschlüsse aber unvollständig belüfteten Lungenlappen ein erhöhter elastischer Gesamtwiderstand vorgetäuscht. Allmählich tritt dann vor allem durch kollateralen Luftübergang eine gleichmäßigere Luftverteilung ein, der erhöhte Druck sinkt dabei auf normale oder unternormale Werte ab und nähert sich den für statische Messung gültigen Drucken. Dieser Versuch zeigt nicht nur die durch die Inhomogenität veränderten dynamischen Druckabläufe während der Atembewegung, sondern läßt auch unmittelbar die mit partieller Bronchus-

---

[1] Otis und Mitarbeiter 1956 u. a.   [2] Helliesen und Mitarbeiter 1958.
[3] Christie und Mitarbeiter 1954.   [4] Noelpp und Noelpp-Eschenhagen 1952, 1956.
[5] Hartung 1957.

verlegung verbundene Ungleichmäßigkeit der Belüftung (ventilatorische Verteilungsstörung) erkennen.

Die quantitativen Aspekte der Stenosewirkung im luftleitenden System sind in Anlehnung an ROHRER (1925) am einfachen Lungenmodell mit zwei den gleichen Dehnungsdrucken unterworfenen, gleich großen Gummiballons mit identischer Wandelastizität untersucht worden[1]. Die aus ROSSIER u. Mitarb. (1958) entnommene Abb. 35 zeigt die Versuchsanordnung. Ohne Stenose addieren sich die Einzelwiderstände der mittels eines Y-förmigen Rohres mit der Außenluft verbundenen Ballons. Das gleiche gilt trotz einseitiger Stenose auch bei langsamer Beatmung des Modells. Bei gesteigerter Blähungsfrequenz wirkt sich der höhere Strömungswiderstand in der stenosierten Zuleitung dadurch aus, daß in den stenosefreien Ballon mehr Luft einfließt. Der stenosierte Ballon bläht sich weniger stark und hinkt gleichzeitig hinsichtlich Blähung und Entleerung nach (Abb. 36). In diesem Stadium macht sich der Dehnungswiderstand des stenosefreien Ballons am Gesamtwiderstand des Modells bereits stärker geltend. Bei sehr schneller Belüftungsfrequenz nähert sich der effektive Widerstand des Gesamtsystems den doppelt so hohen Werten für nur einen Ballon. Umgekehrt sinkt der Gesamtströmungswiderstand bei hohen Frequenzen ab, weil der erhöhte Teilwiderstand in der stenosierten Leitung zunehmend an Einfluß verliert. Die durch die Phasenverschiebung von Blähung und Entleerung hervorgerufenen Druckdifferenzen führen weiterhin zum Auftreten von Pendelluft zwischen dem stenosierten und stenosefreien Ballon.

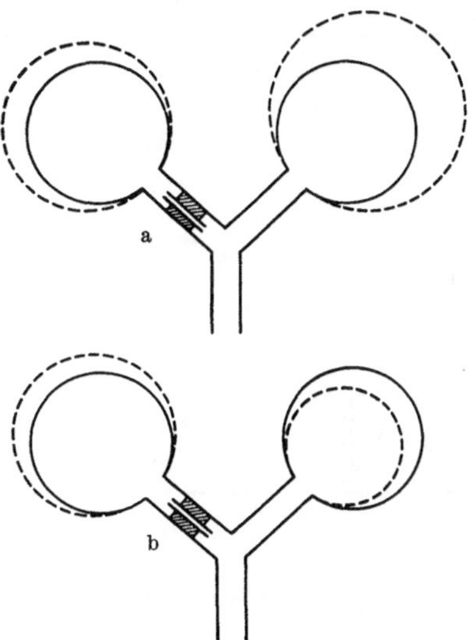

Abb. 35a u. b. Lungenmodell. Einseitige Stenosierung. a Blähungsdifferenz der beiden Ballons am Ende der Inspiration. b Blähungsdifferenz am Ende der Exspiration. (Aus ROSSIER-BÜHLMANN-WIESINGER 1958.)

Diese auf einfache mechanische Gesetzmäßigkeiten zurückführbaren Verhältnisse gelten auch in der Lunge, die aus zahllosen derartigen Ballons, den Acini als den kleinsten respiratorischen Einheiten, zusammengesetzt ist. Hier tritt die Inhomogenität aber nicht nur als Folge von krankhaften Lungenprozessen auf, sie kann auch selbst zur Ursache weiterer Parenchymveränderungen werden und einen Circulus vitiosus für die Ventilationsfunktion in Gang setzen. Dies gilt insbesondere für Stenosen im Bronchialsystem, bei denen u. U. auch Mediastinalwandern wegen der unterschiedlichen Teildrucke beobachtet werden kann[2]. Die gestörte Dynamik im Ablauf der Atembewegungen kann durch Minderbelüftung in Atelektase, durch lokale Überdehnung in herdförmigem Emphysem enden.

Für die Gesamtatemfunktion ergibt sich als Folge der ungleichmäßigen Belüftung der Lunge eine Störung der Relation zwischen Ventilation und Perfusion (s. S. 608). Alle stärkeren Grade von ventilatorischer Verteilungsstörung gehen mit einer verminderten Arterialisierung des Lungenblutes im Sinne der klinischen Distributionsstörung[3] bzw. Partialinsuffizienz[4] einher, weil sich die Durch-

---

[1] OTIS und Mitarbeiter 1956, RAU und Mitarbeiter 1957.
[2] HASLINGER und HITZENBERGER 1926.
[3] COURNAND und RICHARDS 1941, BALDWIN, COURNAND und RICHARDS 1948.
[4] ROSSIER, BÜHLMANN und WIESINGER 1956, 1958.

blutung den wechselnden Ventilationsverhältnissen nicht vollkommen anpassen kann. Hinzu kommt die Störung der Ökonomie der Ventilationsbewegungen, weil gegen die erhöhten Widerstände eine erhöhte Atemarbeit unter Einsatz der Atemhilfsmuskulatur geleistet werden muß[1] (s. S. 468).

In der Klinik können die auf Verteilungsstörung beruhenden Belüftungsdifferenzen mit der Isotopen-Thorakographie jetzt unmittelbar sichtbar gemacht werden[2].

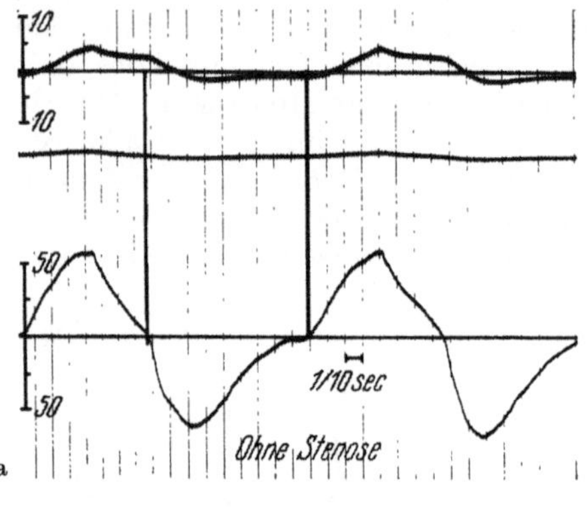

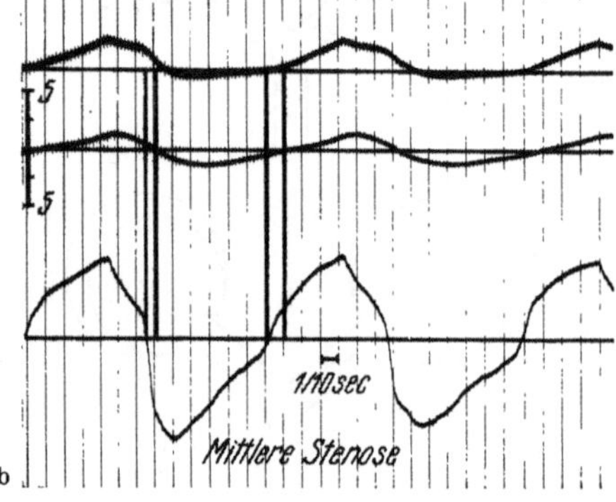

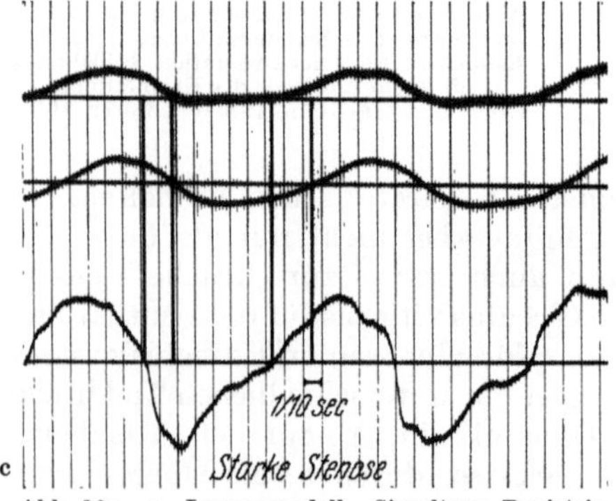

Abb. 36 a—c. Lungenmodell. Simultane Registrierung des Gesamtdruckes, des Differentialdruckes (cm Wasser) und der Strömungsgeschwindigkeit der Luft (cm³ pro ¹/₁₀ sec.). a Beidseits freie Zuleitung. b Leichte einseitige Stenose. c Schwere einseitige Stenose. Der Differentialdruck zwischen beiden Ballons zeigt das Maß der ungleichen Blähung der beiden Ballons, die senkrechten Linien, durch die 0-Punkte von Fluß und Druck gezogen, zeigen die Phasenverschiebung. (Aus Rossier-Bühlmann-Wiesinger 1958.)

b) Arten und Ursachen der Stenosen.

Die Vorgänge, die mit Stenosen und Verschlüssen von Bronchien einhergehen, lassen sich nach morphologischen Gesichtspunkten gliedern und zurückführen auf:

1. Kompression der Bronchien,
2. Deformierung der Wand durch intramurale Prozesse,
3. intrabronchiale Obstruktion oder Obturation der Lichtung.

Eine ähnliche Einteilung hat bereits v. Schrötter (1896) durchgeführt. Tanner (1957) hat diese Einteilung übernommen und dazu als 4. Form die bei Tuberkulose häufige periphere Stenose angefügt, die wir an dieser Stelle noch nicht berücksichtigen, sondern unter den Bronchiolostenosen behandeln.

Ein anderes Prinzip der Einteilung wählt Ch. Jackson (1945, 1950), das auch Escher (1956) anwendet. Jackson stellt den funktionellen Mechanismus an der Stenosestelle in den Vordergrund und teilt ein in:

1. Das halboffene Ventil oder die partielle Obstruktion,
2. die Ventilstenose,
3. die Totalstenose.

Dabei wird der bei partieller Stenose so häufige Ventilmechanismus besonders berücksichtigt.

Huizinga (1951) geht schließlich von der Belüftung der poststenotischen Lungenabschnitte aus und kommt dabei zur Einteilung in zwei Hauptgruppen:

1. Die Unterbelüftung und schließlich die Atelektase der poststenotischen Lungenabschnitte bei inspiratorisch wirkenden Stenosen.

---

[1] Hartung 1960.   [2] Venrath 1957, Bolt 1960.

2. Die Luftretention und das Emphysem hinter der exspirationshemmenden Stenose.

Misch- und Übergangsformen zwischen beiden Zuständen kommen vor[1].

Diesen Gliederungen liegen verschiedene Betrachtungsweisen des Problems zugrunde: in der ersten Einteilung die Morphogenese der Stenosen, in der zweiten die Mechanik der Luftströmung an der Stenosestelle und in der dritten Einteilung die Störung des Luftwechsels hinter der Stenose.

Alle Betrachtungsweisen sind für das volle Verständnis der bronchostenotisch bedingten Ventilationsstörung notwendig.

1. Die Kompressionsstenosen.

Bei der Kompressionsstenose großer und mittlerer Bronchien erfolgt die Druckwirkung stets herdförmig und ist auf einen mehr oder minder kleinen Bronchusabschnitt beschränkt, in dem die Bronchialwand nach innen vorgewölbt und die Lichtung abgeplattet oder sichelförmig eingedellt wird. Lange andauernder Druck bringt die Knorpel zur Atrophie.

Am häufigsten wird dieser Druck von den vergrößerten bronchopulmonalen Lymphknoten ausgeübt, deren hilusnahe Lokalisation an den Hauptbronchien und besonders an den Abgangsstellen der Lappen- und Segmentbronchien die Prädilektionsorte bezeichnet, an denen solche Stenosen entstehen. Die Vergrößerung der Lymphknoten beruht in erster Linie auf Tuberkulose, im Kindesalter so gut wie ausschließlich auf der Lymphknotenverkäsung in der Primärinfektionsphase.

Beim Kinde kann schon eine mäßige Lymphknotenvergrößerung das relativ weiche Knorpelskelet der Bronchus- und Trachealwand eindellen und die kleine Lichtung so weit verlegen, daß eine Atelektase eintritt. Diese ist am häufigsten auf ein Segment, seltener auf einen Lappen oder auf ein Subsegment ausgedehnt.

Die früher als Epituberkulose[2] bezeichneten flüchtigen Lungenverschattungen im Verlauf einer Primärtuberkulose hat Rössle (1936) als Atelektase durch den Druck der vergrößerten tuberkulösen Hiluslymphknoten aufgedeckt[3]. Die Atelektasezone fällt dabei fast regelmäßig mit dem Sitz des Primärherdes in der Lunge zusammen.

Beim Erwachsenen tritt die Tuberkulose als Ursache der Bronchuskompression in den Hintergrund, weil die Zahl der Primärinfekte in diesem Alter geringer wird und die Lymphknotenvergrößerungen bei postprimären Tuberkulosen in mäßigen Grenzen bleiben.

Über die Lokalisation der Bronchusstenosen nach lymphadenogener und endobronchialer Bronchustuberkulose geben Haefliger u. Mark (1956) eine Skizze, aus der die Begrenzung der stenotischen Prozesse auf die hilusnahen Bronchusabschnitte deutlich wird (Abb. 37).

Häufiger kommen beim Erwachsenen Tumormetastasen, leukämische Prozesse, Lymphogranulomatose, auch Boecksche Krankheit u. a. als Ursache der Lymphknotenvergrößerung in Betracht.

2. Die Bronchitis deformans.

Deformierungen der Bronchialwand sind in der Regel Begleiterscheinungen oder Folge von entzündlichen Prozessen in der Bronchialwand, seltener von Tumoren oder von primären degenerativen Veränderungen.

Die Bronchitis deformans wurde ursprünglich von Schmorl (1925) als Folge anthrakotischer Veränderungen der bronchopulmonalen Lymphknoten aufgefaßt. Heute können wir als ihre häufigste Ursache die Tuberkulose und die Silikose der

---

[1] Escher 1956.
[2] Eliasberg und Neuland 1920, 1921.
[3] Sors 1952, Literatur bei Häfliger und Mark 1956, Görgényi-Göttche und Kassay 1958.

bronchopulmonalen Lymphknoten ansehen[1]. Bei den lymphadenogenen Bronchialwandschäden unterscheiden wir die Frühschäden, die den floriden Primärkomplex begleiten, von den Spätschäden, die mit Exacerbationsperioden der Tuberkulose im höheren Lebensalter zusammenfallen[2].

Bei der progressiven Lymphknotentuberkulose der Primärinfektionsperiode greift die käsige Nekrose auf die anliegende Bronchialwand über, zerstört diese und bricht in die Bronchiallichtung ein. Durch die Perforationsöffnung wird käsig-nekrotisches Material der Lymphknoten und der Bronchialwand entleert und nekrotischer Knorpel abgestoßen. Der Restzustand sind Lymphknotenfisteln und ulceröse Wandprozesse, nach deren Rückbildung Narben zurückbleiben. Diese sind sternförmig, flach oder wulstartig. Neben trichterförmigen

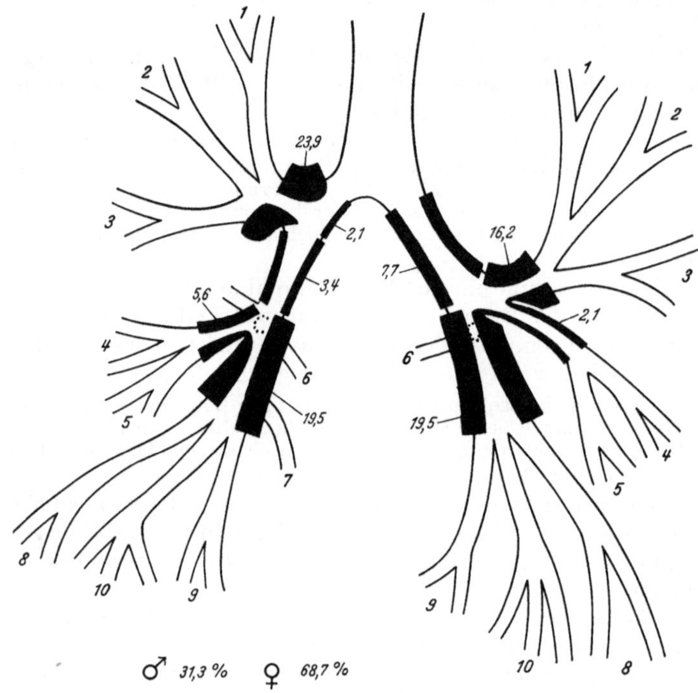

Abb. 37. Lokalisation und Häufigkeit lymphadenogener Bronchusstenosen. (Aus HAEFLIGER u. MARK 1956.)

Einziehungen entstehen auch leistenartige Vorsprünge. Die schrumpfenden flachen Narben raffen die Bronchialwand. Große Wanddefekte [PH. SCHWARTZ (1948) beschreibt Ulcerationen von 2—3 cm Ausdehnung] werden bindegewebig überbrückt.

Diese aus anatomischen Untersuchungen[3] seit langem bekannten, in neuerer Zeit von SCHWARTZ (1948, 1956) studierten Begleiterscheinungen der Primärtuberkulose sind mehr in das klinische Interesse gerückt, seit sie mit der Bronchoskopie erfaßt werden können, da sie ganz überwiegend in den großen Bronchialästen bis zur Verzweigung der Segmentbronchien liegen[4] (s. auch Abb. 37).

<hr>

[1] GIESE 1933, DI BIASI 1933, WÄTJEN 1944, BOHN 1950, NICOD 1952, 1953, HERZOG und CONRAD 1955 u. a.
[2] UEHLINGER 1942, 1950, 1953, P. A. FISCHER 1955, KÖNN 1953, H. I. WYSS 1956.
[3] GHON 1912, BEITZKE 1953, RANKE 1916 u. a.   [4] Literatur bei TANNER 1957.

Die Häufigkeit der Frühschäden wird im Obduktionsgut mit etwa 7—20% angegeben[1].

Die lymphonodulären Bronchialwandschäden des höheren Lebensalters entwickeln sich am häufigsten aus einer chronisch indurierenden Lymphknotentuberkulose. Diese entsteht durch Exacerbationen aus Residuen des Primärinfektes, neigt zu schleichendem progredientem Verlauf und bleibt selten nur auf eine Lymphknotengruppe beschränkt. Im Verlauf dieser vorwiegend produktiven Tuberkulose verbacken die Lymphknoten mit der Bronchialwand und den angrenzenden Blutgefäßen. Das Granulationsgewebe wächst in die Bronchialwand ein und zerstört diese. Die Einbruchstellen sind durch das mitgeführte anthrakotische Pigment schwarz gefärbt. Durch Aufbrüche können käsige Nekrosen und Kalkkonkremente in die Bronchuslichtung entleert werden. Mit der narbigen Schrumpfung entstehen ähnlich wie bei der Frühperforation der Herde des frischen Primärkomplexes Deformierungen der Bronchialwand, die meist multipel sind und sich durch die schwarze Pigmentierung von den Frühperforationen unterscheiden.

Die schrumpfenden Narben ziehen die Bronchialknorpel zusammen, bilden Wülste und Spangen und stenosieren die Lichtung[2].

Die Häufigkeit der narbigen Spätschäden wird im Sektionsgut mit 4,2—4,5%[3] bzw. mit 25%[4] angegeben. Sie liegen wie die Frühperforationen zwischen Carina und Aufteilungen der Hauptbronchien in die Segmentbronchien, zuweilen auch in der Trachea. Ähnliche Deformierungen entstehen auch bei Siliko-Tuberkulose und bei der reinen Silikose der bronchopulmonalen Lymphknoten[5]. Lymphonoduläre Kompression der Bronchien durch die großen schwieligen Lymphknotenpakete und schwielige Wanddeformierungen gehen hier oft ineinander über. Diese vorwiegend an den Segment- und Subsegmentbronchien liegenden Stenosen sind auch bronchoskopisch erfaßbar.

Narbige Stenosen der großen und mittleren Bronchien können auch aus endobronchialer Schleimhauttuberkulose hervorgehen, die auf die tiefen Wandschichten übergreift und ausgedehnte Wandzerstörungen nach sich zieht[6].

Verschiedene Autoren[7] haben an Resektionspräparaten die bei ulceröser Tuberkulose fast regelmäßig vorkommenden begleitenden Bronchustuberkulosen genauer untersucht und besonders auf die fibroplastischen Formen aufmerksam gemacht, die zu schwieliger Umbildung der Bronchuswand, zu Stenosen und zu völliger Obliteration der Bronchuslichtung führen können. Die fibroplastische Reaktion kann auch unspezifische Begleiterscheinung der Tuberkulose sein. Von den lymphonodulären Formen unterscheidet sie sich durch die Ausdehnung auf größere Bronchusabschnitte. Die Destruktion ist dabei oft so stark, daß alle spezifischen Wandelemente des Bronchus verlorengehen. Bei Obliteration bleibt nur ein Narbenfeld übrig, das zuweilen Reste von Bronchialknorpel oder von Schleimdrüsen einschließt.

Ähnlich wie bei der Tuberkulose können auch anderweitige infektiöse Prozesse zur Zerstörung der Bronchialwand und zu narbiger Stenose führen. Unter diesen sind besonders die strickleiterartigen Narben nach Bronchialsyphilis und die schweren Wanddestruktionen nach Fremdkörperaspiration zu nennen.

---

[1] Literatur bei GOHN 1912, UEHLINGER 1953, SCHWARTZ 1953, 1956, TANNER 1957, KÖNN 1953, BRECKLINGHAUS 1955 u. a.

[2] Literatur bei SCHMORL 1925, GEY 1925, ARNSTEIN 1934, GIESE 1933, 1960, FLEISCHNER 1934, 1936.

[3] ARNSTEIN 1934, KÖNN 1953, P. A. FISCHER 1955.

[4] SCHWARTZ 1953, 1956, H. I. WYSS 1956.   [5] GERSTEL 1933, DI BIASI 1933.

[6] TOUSSAINT-FRANCX und TOUSSAINT 1955.

[7] MASSHOFF 1955 sowie TOUSSAINT-FRANCX und TOUSSAINT 1955 u. a.

3. Die Obstruktionsstenosen.

Verstopfungen der Bronchiallichtungen können durch zahlreiche Mechanismen hervorgerufen werden, die sich in drei Gruppen ordnen lassen.

Der *akute Verschluß* ist am häufigsten Folge einer Fremdkörperaspiration[1]. Die erste Reaktion auf die plötzliche Verlegung eines Lappen- oder Segmentbronchus besteht in lokalen und reflektorischen Reizerscheinungen mit Atemnot,

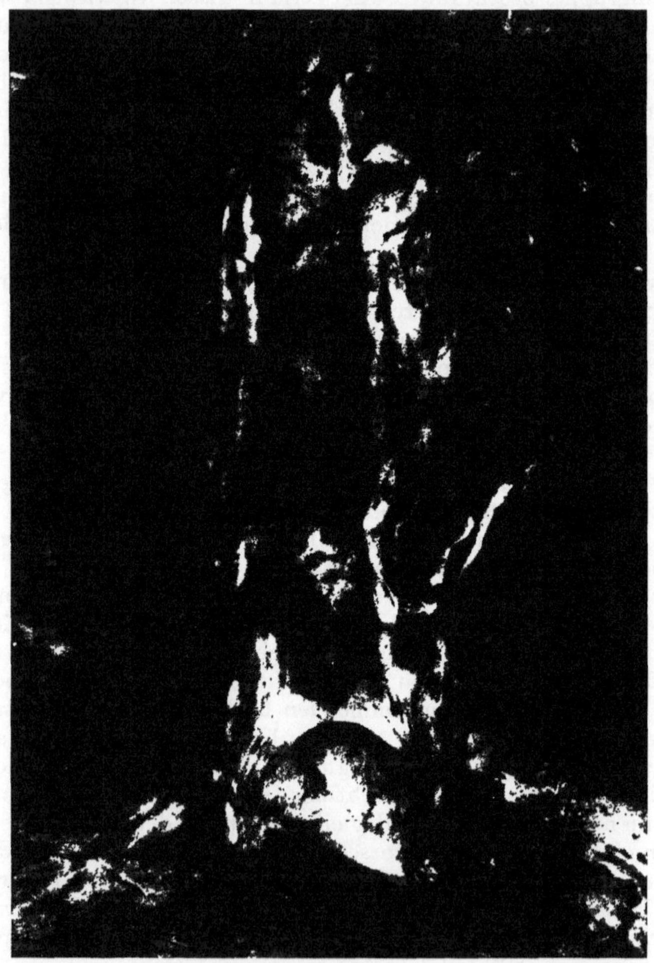

Abb. 38. Polypöses pendelndes Carcinoid des Oberlappenbronchus. Ventilmechanismus. Hypoventilation des zugehörigen Lungenabschnittes. Kr. 1773/53.

Erstickungserscheinungen und Hustenanfällen. In der späteren Phase sind die Folgeerscheinungen wesentlich von der Form und Größe des Fremdkörpers mitbestimmt. Der glatte eingeklemmte Fremdkörper unterbricht die Ventilation, der bewegliche und unregelmäßige macht eine Partialstenose. Nach langer Verweildauer treten sekundäre entzündliche Veränderungen mit Abscedierung hinzu, die die primären Ventilationsstörungen völlig überlagern.

Die *langsam zunehmende*, örtlich begrenzte *Obturation* entsteht bei Tumoren, die aus der Bronchialwand in die Bronchuslichtung vorwachsen. Symptomatik

---

[1] Heller 1914.

und Folgeerscheinungen werden auch hier ähnlich wie bei der Fremdkörperaspiration bestimmt von der Form der Tumoren, von der Geschwindigkeit ihres
Wachstums und von ihrem Sitz.

Unter den gutartigen Tumoren sind das flache, breitbasig der Wand aufsitzende und in
ihr verwurzelte Adenom und der gestielte, im Luftstrom beweglich flottierende Schleimhaut-
polyp die Haupttypen der obstruierenden Tumoren, die beide mit ihrem sehr langsamen
Wachstum die Folgen chronischer circumskripter Stenosen in den großen und mittleren
Bronchien in voller Breite zur Entwicklung kommen lassen (Abb. 38). Ihre Hauptlokalisation
sind die Hauptbronchien und die proximalen Teile der Segmentbronchien. Bei den breit-
basigen Formen der Adenome ist die Beweglichkeit der Bronchialwand an dieser Stelle eingeschränkt oder aufgehoben, bei den polypösen Adenomen kaum beeinträchtigt.

Bei den Carcinomen tritt dagegen die Starre der Wand wegen der diffusen Tumorinfil-
tration aller Schichten schon früh in Erscheinung. Die Bronchusobstruktion durch das
intracaniculäre Tumorwachstum erfolgt ebenfalls in relativ kurzer Zeit.

Die gutartigen und bösartigen intracaniculären Tumoren sind damit Beispiele für die Abhängigkeit der Folgeerscheinungen von dem Tempo der Stenose-
bildung.

Die dritte Gruppe bilden die Zustände, bei denen durch exsudative Entzündung der Schleimhaut, teilweise auch schon durch starke *Schleimhautschwellung*
Einengungen und Obstruktionen der Lichtung eintreten. Diese Prozesse sind
fast nie auf kleine Bronchusabschnitte beschränkt, sondern in der Regel auf
größere Teile der Lunge, mitunter auf den gesamten Tracheobronchialbaum ausgedehnt. Dazu gehört die descendierende Schleimhautdiphtherie, deren fibrinöse
Pseudomembranen die Lichtung der Trachea und der großen Bronchien stark
stenosieren, mittlere und kleine Bronchien vollständig verlegen.

Bei Bronchitis caseosa sind die Bronchien kleiner Lungenabschnitte, oft nur
eines Segmentes, mit Exsudat verstopft. Schleimobstruktionen finden sich
häufig in den kleinen Bronchien und Bronchiolen[1].

c) Die funktionelle Bedeutung der Stenosen.

Die Folgen von Bronchusstenosen für die Lungenbelüftung sind abhängig vom
Typus der Stenosen (Tabelle 6, S. 497).

1. Die starre Bronchusstenose.

Die Ursachen starrer Stenosen in großen und mittleren Bronchien sind vielfach. Im Vordergrund stehen herdförmige Narben, die sich im Anschluß an Entzündungen der Bronchialwand bilden. Auch hier steht die Tuberkulose an erster
Stelle, die entweder über eine lymphadenogene Bronchialwandschädigung in
einer lokalen, auf einen engen Bezirk beschränkten strahligen, wulst- oder leisten-
förmigen Narbe endet, in deren Bereich die Lichtung des Bronchus eingeengt ist,
oder die bei endobronchialer Ausbreitung auch größere Strecken der Bronchialwand in schwieliges Gewebe umwandelt. Die konzentrischen oder exzentrischen
Stenosen können die Lichtung trichter- oder röhrenförmig umwandeln oder auch
ringförmig angeordnet sein[2]. Den gleichen Effekt haben Verschwielungen des
Hilusgebietes etwa im Verlauf einer Silikose, bei der die Bronchien eingemauert,
in das Schwielengewebe einbezogen und durch Übereinanderschiebung der
Knorpelplättchen stenosiert werden (Abb. 39). In der Enge faltet sich die
Schleimhaut, die Bronchuslichtung sieht auf dem Durchschnitt sternförmig aus.
Diese Stenosen liegen fast alle im Abschnitt zwischen Bifurkation und Abgängen
der Segmentbronchien.

---

[1] Literatur bei GIESE 1954, 1960.
[2] GALY und PÉROL 1952, HUZLY und BÖHM 1954, 1955 u. a.

Die multiplen, auf große Strecken der Bronchien ausgedehnten, strickleiterartigen Narben der Syphilis sind heute selten, ebenso die Bronchitis osteoplastica[1]. Weiter gehören dazu die Bronchialwandadenome und -carcinome.

In der Klinik gilt die Regel, daß diese Stenosen erst bemerkbar werden, wenn die Bronchuslichtung bis auf ein Drittel eingeengt ist[2]. Störungen der Ventilation sind aber schon bei geringen Graden der Stenose vorhanden. Der Strömungswiderstand ist im Bereich der Stenose zunächst inspiratorisch erhöht, da die normale Erweiterung des Bronchus ausbleibt. Die starre Stenose behindert die Inspiration stärker als die Exspiration.

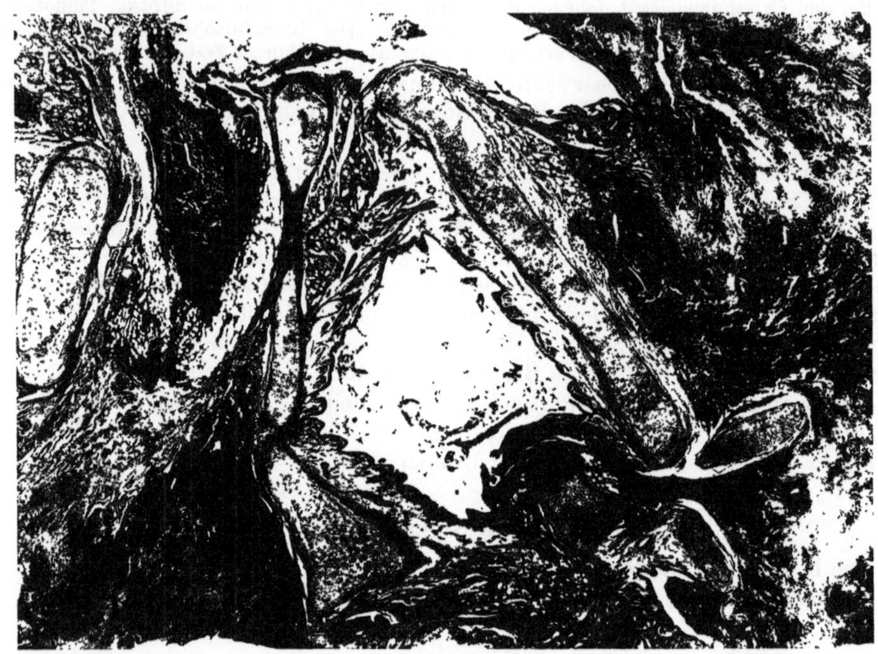

Abb. 39. Starre Bronchostenose bei Bronchitis deformans. Silikotische peribronchiale Verschwielung mit Auflösung von Knorpeln und Vordringen des Schwielengewebes in die Bronchuslichtung. S.-Nr. 280/58. Vergr. 9fach.

Der poststenotische Abschnitt füllt sich bei der Inspiration schlechter und langsamer als die Nachbargebiete. Bei der Exspiration verzögert sich die Entleerung in entsprechender Weise, die Ausatmung ist noch nicht beendet, wenn die nächste Inspiration beginnt, der poststenotische Abschnitt hinkt im Atemcyclus nach. Der intraalveoläre Druck bleibt in der Exspiration höher als in der Nachbarschaft. Die Druckdifferenz hat eine leichte Dehnung des poststenotischen Abschnittes im Beginn der Exspirationsphase zur Folge[3]. Die poststenotische Luftretention in der Exspirationsphase ist mitunter im Röntgenbild an dem Ausbleiben der respiratorischen Verdunkelung der Lunge zu erkennen (sog. „air trapping-Phänomen"[4]).

Bei leichten Stenosen bleibt es bei dieser Einschränkung des Luftwechsels, bei schweren Stenosen sind verschiedene Folgeerscheinungen möglich.

---

[1] Hempel 1957.   [2] Haslinger 1929.
[3] Rohrer 1925, siehe auch unter Verteilungsstörungen S. 485.
[4] Fry und Mitarbeiter 1954, Stead und Mitarbeiter 1952, Dayman 1951, Mead und Mitarbeiter 1955.

Regelmäßig bildet sich eine poststenotische Bronchiektasie, die durch Sekret-stauung bedingt ist. Entzündliche Veränderungen können dabei völlig fehlen, wenn keine Infektion hinzutritt. Der leukocytenarme Schleim dickt sich ein, füllt die Bronchien bis in die kleinen Verzweigungen aus und macht aus der Stenose einen vollständigen Verschluß mit nachfolgender Atelektase.

In anderen Fällen erweitern sich auch die Acini. Das poststenotische Segment gewinnt dabei ein wabiges Aussehen, das sich vom genuinen Emphysem durch dicke Septen unterscheidet (Abb. 40). Die erweiterten Bronchiolen enden in dickwandigen, teilweise miteinander kommunizierenden Blindsäcken. Ein Gasaustausch findet in diesen Waben nicht mehr statt, der post-stenotische Abschnitt ist anato-misch und physiologisch Totraum. Die alveolären wabigen Bronchi-ektasen, die auf das Vorhandensein gutartiger Bronchialwandtumoren hinweisen, sind auch durch Broncho-graphie darstellbar[1].

Die Sekretstauungen fördern In-fektionen. In Schüben rezidivie-rende Bronchitiden und Pneumo-nien modifizieren die Vorgänge im poststenotischen Abschnitt in ähn-licher Weise wie bei vollständiger Bronchusokklusion. Die poststeno-tischen Lungenentzündungen wer-den auch als Obturationspneumo-nien bezeichnet.

2. Die Ventilstenose.

Manche partiellen oder inkom-pletten Stenosen der großen und mittleren Bronchien sind dadurch charakterisiert, daß die Stenose wie ein Ventil wirkt und Luft-strömung nur in einer Richtung zuläßt.

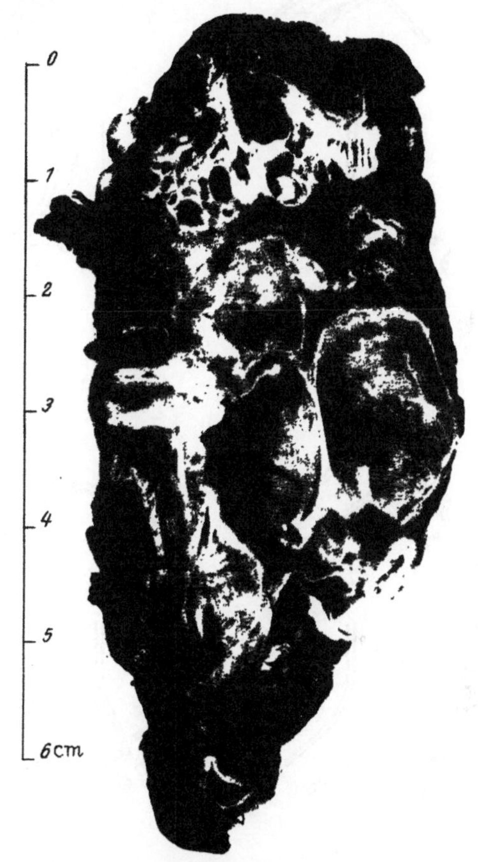

Abb. 40. Großwabige Bronchiektasie des 2. Segments bei narbigem Verschluß des Segmentbronchus nach Bronchial-wandtuberkulose. 50jährige Frau. (Aus HARTUNG 1958.)

In der älteren Literatur ist vor allem RIBBERT (1916) zu nennen, der das Emphysem als Folge einer Ventilstenose in den kleinen Bronchien angesehen hat.

Von der Klinik ist diese Frage in neuerer Zeit aufgegriffen und sowohl für das Emphysem als auch für die Stenose größerer Bronchien eingehend untersucht und diskutiert worden[2].

Das Schema der Ventilstenosen von JACKSON ist in die meisten Darstellungen der Bronchusstenosen eingegangen[3]. Es wird, erweitert um die weiche Stenose, beistehend wiedergegeben (Abb. 41 und Tabelle 6).

---

[1] ESSER 1949, STUTZ und VIETEN 1955.
[2] CH. JACKSON 1945, SOULAS und MOUNIER-KUHN 1949, HUIZINGA 1951, LOTTENBACH 1956 u. a.
[3] HAEFLIGER und MARK 1956.

Für die Entwicklung des Ventilmechanismus gibt es mehrere Möglichkeiten, die einerseits aus der Form des stenosierenden Prozesses, andererseits aus der Bewegung des Bronchus in der Ventilation ihre Erklärung finden:

1. Die *exspiratorische Strömungsunterbrechung* ist die häufigste Art der Ventilwirkung. Jede Stenose, die nicht starr ist, bei der die Bronchialwand also noch der inspiratorischen Dehnung folgen kann, wird in der Inspiration weiter, in der Exspiration enger. Die exspiratorische Entspannung der Bronchuswand läßt damit die Stenose stärker zur Geltung kommen und hochgradige Stenosen schließlich in einen exspiratorischen Verschluß übergehen.

Breitbasige Bronchialwandadenome, in die Lichtung einwachsende Carcinome, Narben mit septenartigen Vorsprüngen, einseitige Eindellungen des Bronchus und Abknickung der Bronchien können dieses Ergebnis haben.

Bei völliger Unterbrechung des Rückstromes ist die Luft hinter der Stenose gefangen, bei leckem Ventil strömt ein kleiner Teil der Luft aus.

In jedem Fall wird der poststenotische Teil in der Exspirationsphase unter positiven Druck gesetzt. Dadurch erweitern sich poststenotisches Gangsystem und Alveolen gleichmäßig. Aus der Überblähung dieses Lungenabschnittes kann bei langdauerndem Ventilmechanismus schließlich ein Emphysem werden, das sich je nach Lokalisation der Stenose über einen Lappen, ein Segment oder ein Subsegment ausbreiten kann. Mittellappen und Lingula sind bevorzugte Lokalisationen.

Die Erfahrung zeigt, daß stärkere positive Drucke im poststenotischen Bereich nur selten bestehen bleiben. Mit der zunehmenden Blähung eines Segmentes läßt die elastische Retraktionskraft nach, der Überdruck herrscht schließlich

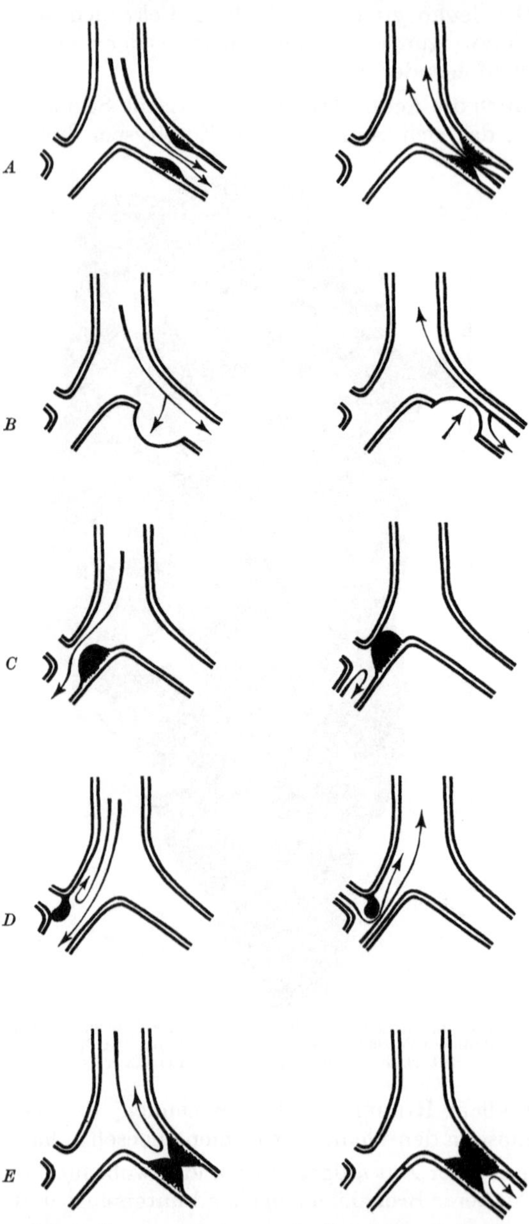

Abb. 41. Typen von Stenosen großer Bronchien nach Jackson, umgezeichnet und erweitert. *A* Starre Stenose, halboffenes Ventil; *B* weiche Stenose, Bronchomalacie; *C* exspiratorisch wirksames Ventil; *D* inspiratorisch wirksames Ventil; *E* komplette Stenose.

nur im Beginn der Exspirationsphase. Die Dehnung der Septen schafft weiterhin durch Erweiterung der Kohnschen Poren ein Ventil, durch das ein Ausgleich des Überdruckes erfolgen kann, wenn die Stenose in Segmentbronchien oder in

Tabelle 6. *Folgen von Bronchusstenosen.*

A. Starre Stenose, halboffenes Ventil	Selten Emphysem, häufiger Atelektase durch zusätzlichen Schleimverschluß, poststenotische Bronchiektasie
B. Weiche Stenose, Bronchomalacie	Unvollständige Exspiration, Emphysem
C. Exspiratorisch wirksame Ventilstenose	Emphysem
D. Inspiratorisch wirksame Ventilstenose	Hypoventilation durch Lufteinstrom in der Exspiration, Atelektase
E. Vollständiger inspiratorischer und exspiratorischer Verschluß	Atelektase

kleineren Einheiten liegen. Der Mittellappen kann bei Ventilstenose des Bronchus wabig umgebaut werden. Große Blasen bilden sich fast nur bei Stenosen kleinerer Bronchusäste.

Ursachen exspiratorischer Ventilstenosen können aber auch Bronchomalacien sein, die sich entweder über große Teile des Bronchialbaumes erstrecken oder auf kleine Abschnitte beschränkt sein können. Die generalisierten Bronchomalacien beruhen auf degenerativen Veränderungen und völligem Schwund des Knorpels, die herdförmigen auf Zerstörung des Knorpels im Rahmen entzündlicher Wandprozesse. Sie sind nicht selten Restzustände lymphadenogener Bronchialwandschäden. Schließlich kann jede chronische tiefgreifende Bronchitis, besonders die ulceröse Form, Bronchialknorpel zum Schwinden bringen.

Die Ventilwirkung bei den Bronchomalacien entsteht dadurch, daß der weiche Bronchusabschnitt während der Inspiration angesogen wird. Dabei legen sich die Bronchialwände aneinander und bilden so ein Ventil, das den Eintritt der Luft behindert oder unterbricht[1].

2. Die *inspiratorische Strömungsunterbrechung* bei Ventilstenosen ist verhältnismäßig selten. Ihre Folge ist eine rasch eintretende Atelektase, wenn das Ventil vollkommen schließt, eine Hypoventilation, wenn es undicht ist. Ursachen sind gestielte endobronchiale Tumoren, die sich als polypöse Pfröpfe in der Inspiration vor benachbarte Bronchusabgänge legen, Schleimpfröpfe und Fremdkörper sowie starke polypöse Schleimhautschwellungen.

Im Typ d (Abb. 41) der Ventilstenose ist die Belüftung des Segmentbronchus in der Inspiration blockiert. In der Exspiration kommt es nach Öffnung des Ventils zu einer Luftstauung hinter dem pendelnden Tumor und zum Lufteinstrom in den Segmentbronchus.

d) Der Bronchusverschluß.

Dem völligen Verschluß eines großen oder mittleren Bronchus folgt im Regelfall eine Atelektase des zugehörigen Lungenabschnittes. Der Bronchusverschluß ist gleichzeitig auch die häufigste Ursache von Atelektasen. Die allgemeine Pathologie der Ventilationsstörungen bei Bronchusverschluß ist damit in ihren wesentlichen Teilen die Lehre von den Atelektasen.

1. Die Atelektase.

Unter den experimentellen Studien über die Folgen von Bronchialverschlüssen haben neben den Untersuchungen von TRAUBE (1846), der den Zusammenhang von Bronchialverschluß und Atelektase erkannte, vor allem die Versuche von

---

[1] POHL 1951, LEMOINE und GARAIX 1953, HERZOG und NISSEN 1954, WYSS 1955, KIENER und Mitarbeiter 1957.

Lichtheim (1879) Bedeutung gewonnen. Lichtheim verschloß Haupt- oder Lappenbronchien durch Laminariastifte oder durch Unterbindung und sah danach im Verlauf von 24—28 Std im zugehörigen Bereich eine Atelektase, in den übrigen Lungenabschnitten Emphysem, gelegentlich mit Spontanpneumothorax eintreten.

Das Verschwinden der Luft hinter dem Bronchialverschluß erklärt er durch Absorption der Gase in das Blut. Die Absorptions- oder Resorptionsgeschwindigkeit ist für die einzelnen Bestandteile der atmosphärischen Luft verschieden.

Die gesamte Luft wird in Versuchen am Kaninchen in 2—4 Std resorbiert. Füllt man dagegen in eine Lunge mit Bronchialverschluß Kohlensäure ein, so ist diese bereits nach 30 min verschwunden. Sauerstoff braucht zur Resorption etwa 1 Std, während die Resorption von Stickstoff mehr als 3 Std dauert und oft 6—9 Std nach Versuchsbeginn noch nicht abgeschlossen ist.

Bei Anwendung künstlicher Beatmung mit sauerstoffreichen Gasgemischen entsteht die Atelektase rascher als bei Atmung von atmosphärischer Luft. Nach 10—15 min ist bereits eine massive Atelektase des Unter- oder Mittellappens bei Blockade des zugehörigen Bronchus eingetreten[1].

Die Resorption der Gase erfolgt in das strömende Blut[2]. Die Atelektase tritt nur bei intakter Blutzirkulation ein. Sie bleibt aus, wenn die Perfusion dieser Lungenabschnitte durch Unterbindung der Blutgefäße oder durch Abklemmung der Lungenarterien unterbrochen wird. Ihre Bildung wird durch Novocain-Blockade des Nervensystems nicht beeinflußt[3].

Bei Unterbindung eines Lappenbronchus am Hund verschwindet die Luft zunächst aus den zentralen Abschnitten des Lappens. Diese werden schon nach 2 Std luftleer, während die peripheren Anteile noch bis zu 4 Std Luft enthalten. Nach dieser Zeit ist die Luftresorption im allgemeinen beendet[4].

Peripher von der Unterbindungsstelle sammelt sich in den Bronchien Sekret, das etwa 3 Tage nach der Unterbindung makroskopisch sichtbar wird[5]. Es besteht aus Schleim, abgestoßenen Epithelien und einer wechselnden Menge von Leukocyten. Bis zum 14. Tag vermehrt sich die Sekretmenge, bleibt aber von da ab etwa gleich groß. Die Leukocyten und Epithelien verfetten und zerfallen, gleichzeitig erscheinen im Sekret Cholesterinkristalle. Bei Durchtrennung der den Bronchus begleitenden Nerven ist die Sekretmenge vermehrt, die Eiterung stärker. Die Sekretansammlung bleibt auf die knorpeltragenden Bronchien beschränkt, die Bronchiolen werden nicht ausgeweitet. Nur bei stärkerer Eiterung gelangen Leukocyten auch in die Alveolen.

Im weiteren Verlauf kommt es zu ampullenartigen Erweiterungen der Bronchien mit Sklerosierung der Wand und Abbau des Bronchialknorpels, gleichzeitig auch zu Wandverdickungen der Arterien durch Intimaproliferation.

Beim Kaninchen entsteht häufig ein Pleuraempyem[6], besonders wenn gleichzeitig die Arteria bronchialis unterbunden wird[4].

Das atelektatische Lungengewebe erfährt nach der Luftresorption eine fortschreitende Verkleinerung. Nissen (1923) findet in seinen Versuchen 2 Formen der Schrumpfung:

Bei leukocytenarmem Bronchussekret bleiben die Alveolen, abgesehen von spärlicher Desquamation der Alveolarepithelien, leer, das interstitielle Fasergewebe proliferiert, wobei die Zellvermehrung vom adventitiellen Gewebe der Gefäße und Bronchien ausgeht.

Bei überwiegend eitrigem Bronchialsekret erscheinen auch in den Alveolen vom 4.—5. Tag an reichlich Leukocyten oder vorwiegend abgestoßene Alveolar-

---

[1] Colombo, Beatrice und Rulla 1952.   [2] Henderson 1929, Coryllos 1930.
[3] Eisenreich 1953.   [4] Nissen 1923.
[5] Nissen 1923, Lichtheim 1879, Coryllos 1929, Churchill 1953.   [6] Lichtheim 1879.

epithelien. Eine fortschreitende Wucherung des peribronchialen und interlobulären Bindegewebes schließt sich an.

In beiden Formen der interstitiellen Fibrose bleiben die Alveolen und die Pleura fast unbeteiligt.

Ähnliche Formen der Lungenschrumpfung haben SAUERBRUCH u. BRUNS (1911) auch bei Unterbindung der Arteria pulmonalis gesehen.

Die Atelektase kann nach den Erfahrungen im Experiment bereits eintreten, wenn die Bronchuslichtung durch einen endobronchialen Prozeß auf $^1/_3$ verengt wird[1]. Dabei treten aber sekundäre Infektionen wesentlich häufiger ein als bei Kompression oder Unterbindung des Bronchus. Diese Atelektasen sind wegen der bei Infektionen rasch nachfolgenden zusätzlichen Lungenfibrose fast stets irreversibel. Wenn bei völligem Bronchusverschluß die in älteren Versuchen häufigen Infektionen des Atelektasebereiches vermieden werden, dann bleibt die Lunge über lange Jahre unverändert und entfaltbar.

2. Die kollaterale Ventilation.

In neuen Versuchen haben HAAG u. EISENREICH (1956) nach Unterbindung von Segmentbronchien bei Hunden keine totale Atelektase des zugehörigen Gebietes, sondern vielmehr eine Blähung mit Übergang in ein Emphysem gefunden. Sie erklären diese unerwartete Folge durch kollaterale Ventilation, d. h. durch Einstrom von Luft aus der Nachbarschaft in das von der Belüftung durch den zugehörigen Bronchus ausgeschlossene Gebiet. Auch aus Befunden am Menschen ergibt sich, daß selbst bei den ausgedehnten Bronchialobstruktionen, die im Verlaufe käsiger Bronchitis auftreten, das Lungengewebe noch belüftet ist (Abb. 42).

Diese kollaterale Ventilation ist nur dort möglich, wo präformierte Verbindungen zu den Nachbarabschnitten vorhanden sind. Die Lungenlappen sind in der Regel durch die zum Hilus einschneidende Pleura völlig voneinander getrennt. Deshalb wird kollaterale Ventilation nicht bei Verschluß eines Lappenbronchus beobachtet. Die Lungensegmente sind dagegen durch vielfach gefensterte Septen begrenzt, benachbarte Segmente schieben sich ineinander. Die Grenzlinien verlaufen dadurch unregelmäßig[2]. In den Fenstern berühren sich Lobuli und Acini verschiedener Segmente ohne eine zusätzliche Scheidewand. Über die Kohnschen Poren ist ein Luftaustausch möglich.

Als kollaterale Respiration bezeichnet VAN ALLEN (1932) den Luftaustausch zwischen Lungenabschnitten, die von verschiedenen Bronchi oder Bronchioli versorgt werden. Von dem Bestehen solcher Verbindungen kann man sich durch Aufblasen einer kollabierten Leichenlunge überzeugen. Die in einen Segmentbronchus eingeblasene Luft dehnt zuerst das zugehörige Segment und springt dann an vielen Stellen auf die Nachbarsegmente über, die schließlich vollständig entfaltet werden. Es bedarf aber stets eines größeren Druckes, um diese kollaterale Belüftung in Gang zu setzen. Sie ist also von einer ausreichenden Atemtiefe abhängig.

Die Alveolarporen, die auch in der normalen Lunge vorkommen[3], haben nach v. HAYEK (1953) einen Durchmesser von 10—15 μ. Reticuläre und elastische Fasern bilden in der Alveolarwand ein lockeres Netzwerk, in dem die Netzcapillaren liegen. Die Innenfläche der Alveolarwand ist mit Alveolarepithelien bedeckt, deren zarte Fortsätze kontinuierlich den Alveolarboden bedecken. Im Bereich der Alveolarporen ziehen diese Fortsätze von einer Alveole in die andere. Durch

---

[1] BIANCALANA und COLOMBO 1952.
[2] v. HAYEK 1953, WEBER 1951, TÖNDURY 1956, LERNER 1952, BOYDEN und SCANELL 1948.
[3] KOHN 1893, v. HANSEMANN 1895, STÖHR 1903, PETERSEN 1935, MACKLIN 1935.

Ablösungen von Epithelzellen, die teilweise pflockartig in der Alveolarwand sitzen, sollen auch sekundäre Poren entstehen können[1].

Die Existenz dieser Poren, auf deren Bedeutung für pathologische Vorgänge Kohn (1893) aufmerksam gemacht hat, läßt sich durch die Brückenbildungen des Fibrins bei Pneumonie, ebenso auch durch Zapfen aus Carcinomzellen nachweisen, die bei Krebspneumonie an der gleichen Stelle wie das Fibrin über vorgebildete Wandlücken in Nachbaralveolen des gleichen oder auch des benachbarten Acinus

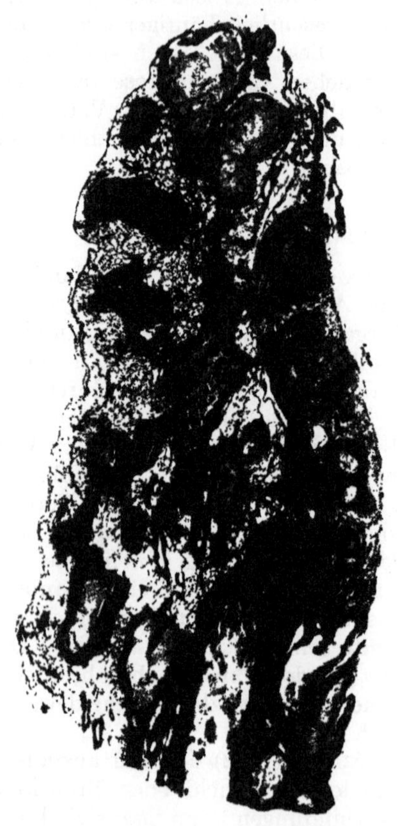

Abb. 42. Kollaterale Ventilation der Lunge bei ausgedehnter alter käsiger Bronchitis mit Obstruktion von Segment- und Subsegmentbronchien. J.-Nr. 6969/56.

gelangen. Für die kollaterale Ventilation sind nur die Poren zwischen benachbarten Acini von Bedeutung, die beim Menschen ohne besondere Septen aneinanderstoßen. Ebenso sind auch die Interlobulärsepten, die beim Hund fehlen, beim Menschen nicht überall vorhanden, so daß auch ein Austausch von Lobulus zu Lobulus möglich ist. Diese interlobuläre Kommunikation ist die entscheidende Voraussetzung für eine kollaterale Ventilation zwischen Lungensegmenten.

Die Beobachtungen van Allens (1932) am Hund haben Baarsma u. Dirken (1948) für den Menschen bestätigt. Atelektasen entstehen erst dann, wenn mehrere benachbarte Segmentbronchien verstopft sind[2]. Unter Histamineinfluß hört bei Hunden diese kollaterale Ventilation auf[3].

Die kollaterale Atmung soll bis zu 70% des normalen Luftgehaltes in den verschlossenen Bezirk bringen. Die auf diesem Umweg zugeführte Luft ist reicher an Sauerstoff und ärmer an Kohlensäure als die Exspirationsluft, sie hat also auch für den Gasaustausch Bedeutung[4].

In den Versuchen von Haag u. Eisenreich (1956) lagen die zur vollständigen Kollateralbelüftung notwendigen Drucke um 2—6 cm H_2O höher als die Druckwerte für die Lappenblähung bei intakter Bronchialatmung. Die kollaterale Entlüftung blieb dagegen am offenen Thorax merkbar zurück.

In den kollateral ventilierten Abschnitten bleibt also mehr Residualluft zurück als in den Nachbargebieten. Diese vermehrte Residualluft hält die kollateral ventilierten Teile unter vermehrter Dauerspannung, die nach früheren Ausführungen über die Folgen dauernder Überdehnung des Lungengewebes geeignet ist, ein Emphysem auszulösen. Mit dieser Vorstellung decken sich auch die Beobachtungen von Haag u. Eisenreich (1956), die in ihren Versuchen bereits ein halbes Jahr nach Bronchusunterbindung ein Emphysem mit Schwund der Alveolarsepten entstehen sahen.

---

[1] v. Hayek 1953, Engel 1950.   [2] Middeldorpf 1933.   [3] Lindskog und Alley 1948.
[4] Biancalana und Colombo 1952.

Der Nutzeffekt der kollateralen Ventilation für den Gasaustausch kann in diesen Fällen also nur·gering sein[1]. Oft wird sie gerade zum Ausgleich des resorbierten Luftanteils ausreichen[2].

3. Formen und Ausdehnung der Atelektasen.

Beim Menschen sind die Folgen einer Bronchusblockade ähnlich wie im Tierversuch. Auch hier steht die Atelektase im Mittelpunkt. Die Ausdehnung der Atelektase wird bestimmt von dem Sitz des Verschlusses und der Größe seines Versorgungsbereiches[3]. Die Störungen der Atmung stehen in annähernder Relation zur Größe der Atelektase. Sie äußern sich 1. auf der Ventilationsseite durch vermehrte Dehnung des restlichen Lungengewebes, 2. in der Diffusion durch Einschränkung der atmenden Fläche und 3. auf der Blutseite dadurch, daß in der anfangs *roten Atelektase* Blut ohne Gasaustausch durch das unbelüftete Gewebe hindurchfließt und als „funktionelles Kurzschlußblut" in den großen Kreislauf gelangt, während in der chronischen *blassen Atelektase* die Perfusion gedrosselt, die Menge des funktionellen Kurzschlußblutes verringert und der Strömungswiderstand in der Lunge erhöht wird (s. S. 596).

Die in ihrer Symptomatik stark variierenden Folgeerscheinungen der Bronchialverschlüsse werden in der Klinik teilweise als besondere Krankheitsbilder abgegrenzt, z. B. Mittellappensyndrom, Lingulasyndrom, Plattenatelektase[4]. Auch hier ergibt sich die Notwendigkeit einer Gliederung, die nach dem Sitz der Stenose im Bronchialbaum durchgeführt wird.

α) *Verschluß eines Hauptbronchus.*

Ursachen eines akuten vollständigen Verschlusses eines Hauptbronchus sind in der Regel Fremdkörperaspirationen, seltener Tumoren, gelegentlich auch ein traumatischer Bronchusabriß[5].

Als Folge der plötzlichen Unterbrechung des Luftstromes entsteht ebenso wie im Tierversuch ein vollständiger Kollaps der ganzen Lunge. Mit der Resorption der Luft, die in wenigen Stunden, mitunter schon nach einer Stunde abgeschlossen sein kann, verkleinert sich die Lunge in kurzer Zeit bis zur völligen Atelektase[6]. Das Lungengewebe ist wegen der Capillarerweiterung blutreich, feucht, milzähnlich. Die Bezeichnung Splenisation[7] oder rote Atelektase kennzeichnet diesen Zustand. Die starke Durchfeuchtung der Lunge beruht auf einer Transsudation in die Alveolen, die oft recht beträchtlich sein kann[8].

Der Thoraxraum der Verschlußseite wird eng gestellt, die Respirationsbewegung ist fast aufgehoben. Das Zwerchfell steigt hoch, das Mediastinum wird nach der Atelektasenseite verzogen. Diese Verziehung wird in der Inspirationsphase stärker. Der inspiratorische Sog ist wahrscheinlich Ursache der Blutanschoppung und des Ödems in der atelektatischen Lunge. Dieses kann ähnlich wie bei den zentralen Formen verminderter Lungenventilation so vorherrschen, daß LEOPOLD (1924) und CH. JACKSON u. LEE (1925) von drowned lung, ertrunkener Lunge, sprechen. E. KAUFMANN (1931) führt die Ansammlung des Transsudates darauf zurück, daß die vermehrte Flüssigkeit in der Atelektasezone nicht abgeatmet werden kann.

---

[1] CHURCHILL 1953, WURM 1954.   [2] PEROMET 1950.
[3] Literatur bei ALEXANDER 1951, LÖFFLER 1956, GIESE 1959.
[4] UEHLINGER und SCHOCH 1957 (Literatur), HEUCK 1959, HEINE 1960.
[5] W. KOCH 1930, LÖFFLER und NAGER 1941, ESCHER 1956, KRAUSS 1958,
[6] ESCHER 1956 u. a.   [7] E. KAUFMANN 1931.
[8] JORES 1906, ANGLADE 1935, SPAIN 1954 u. a.

Die andere Lunge wird vermehrt ventiliert und gebläht, es entsteht ein kontralaterales akutes Volumen auctum. Nach Abklingen der akuten neuralen Reizerscheinungen mit Krampfhusten, Dyspnoe und Erstickungserscheinungen stellt sich häufig die Ventilation auf die veränderten Atmungsbedingungen ein, die Dyspnoe verschwindet und ist jedenfalls in der Ruhe nicht vorhanden, wenn die ventilierte Lunge noch voll leistungsfähig ist. Bestehen Pleuraverwachsungen, Emphysem oder andere Prozesse, die eine ausreichende Ventilation verhindern, dann bleibt die Dyspnoe auch in der Ruhe bestehen.

Der Lungenkreislauf paßt sich ebenfalls rasch den veränderten Bedingungen an[1]. Das Blut wird in die beatmete Lunge umgelenkt, der Zufluß zur atelektatischen Lunge reflektorisch gedrosselt. Dadurch verringert sich der Anteil des nicht arterialisierten Blutes (Shunt-Blutes), die anfängliche Cyanose geht zurück.

Wird der Verschluß durch Extraktion des Fremdkörpers oder durch chirurgische Versorgung des Bronchusabrisses beseitigt, dann entfaltet sich die Lunge wieder, das Ödem wird rasch resorbiert.

Bleibt der Verschluß bestehen, dann entwickelt sich als Folge des chronischen totalen Verschlusses eine Daueratelektase. In dieser wird der Blutzufluß gedrosselt, die Endstrombahn der Lunge enggestellt. Die anfängliche Stauung und Anschoppung des Blutes erfährt eine deutliche Reduktion, es kommt zur blassen Atelektase. Die sehr kleine Lunge ist grau, von zäher Konsistenz. Das Blut, das die atelektatische Lunge noch durchströmt, wird nicht arterialisiert und erscheint als venöse Beimischung im linken Herzen. Die Bronchien werden durch angestautes Sekret erweitert.

Bei Fremdkörperaspirationen treten fast regelmäßig entzündliche Erscheinungen hinzu, die durch begleitende oder nachfolgende Infektion bedingt sind. Diese können auf die nächste Umgebung des Fremdkörpers beschränkt bleiben, zu Wanddestruktion des Bronchus führen oder sich auch auf das Lungengewebe ausdehnen und hier eine abscedierende Pneumonie auslösen.

Aus der akuten Überblähung der anderen Lunge wird häufig ein kompensatorisches Emphysem. Das Restlungenproblem stellt sich hier in ähnlicher Weise wie nach Pneumektomie.

β) Verschluß eines Lappenbronchus.

Jeder Lappen ist eine in sich geschlossene Einheit mit eigenem Bronchus, eigenem Gefäßstiel und eigener Abgrenzung durch die Pleura, die in den Fissurae interlobares bis zum Hilus einschneidet. Nur bei Variationen dieser Fissuren, die mitunter nicht bis zum Hilus reichen, gehen Nachbarlappen im Hilusbereich ohne Abgrenzung ineinander über. In diesen Fällen ist eine kollaterale Belüftung auch zwischen Lappen möglich.

Akute Obstruktion eines Lappenbronchus hat ähnliche Folgen wie der Verschluß eines Hauptbronchus. Auch hier stehen die Fremdkörperaspirationen an erster Stelle. Dazu kommen aber auch Kompressionen durch extrabronchiale Prozesse, Verstopfungen mit Sekret oder Tumorgewebe und schließlich auch Abknickung durch narbige Verziehungen oder durch Verlagerungen des Mediastinums.

Lappenatelektasen werden nicht mit gleicher Häufigkeit in allen Lungenteilen gefunden. Fremdkörperobstruktionen liegen vorwiegend in den Unterlappen. Verschlüsse aus anderer Ursache werden vorwiegend in den Oberlappen oder im Mittellappen gefunden.

Im Mittellappen manifestiert sich die Atelektase unter dem klinisch wohlumrissenen Bild des Mittellappensyndroms[2].

---

[1] Coryllos und Birnbaum 1929, de Toeuf und Conard 1953 u. a.
[2] Graham, Burford und Mayer 1948, Uehlinger und Schoch 1957.

Unter den Ursachen dieses in seiner Häufigkeit erst durch die Bronchologie deutlich gewordenen Prozesses[1] steht die Tuberkulose der bronchopulmonalen Lymphknoten an erster Stelle. Der Mittellappenbronchus wird an seiner Abgangsstelle aus dem Stammbronchus von Lymphknoten umscheidet, die ihn bis zur Teilung in die Segmentbronchien begleiten[2].

Wenn diese Lymphknoten im Rahmen des Primärkomplexes anschwellen, verkäsen, mit der Bronchialwand verbacken und schließlich sogar in den Bronchus einbrechen, dann entsteht die Atelektase mehr oder minder plötzlich, oft nach vorausgegangener Überblähung. Bei Kompression der Lichtung auf etwa ein Drittel können zusätzliche Schleimhautschwellung oder schleimiges Bronchialsekret den endgültigen, dann oft rasch wieder reversiblen Verschluß herbeiführen. Dieser Mechanismus ist vor allem dann anzunehmen, wenn anatomisch am Resektionspräparat kein vollständiger Verschluß mehr nachgewiesen werden kann. Unspezifische Schwellungen der Lymphknoten[3], Tumormetastasen und andere Lymphknotenprozesse können den gleichen Effekt haben.

Ob neben der Lage der peribronchialen Lymphknoten auch noch topographische Besonderheiten des Mittellappenbronchus als Ursache der Atelektase eine Rolle spielen, ist zweifelhaft. Der Mittellappenbronchus geht nach bifurkationsähnlicher Teilung unter Bildung einer hohen Carina aus dem Stammbronchus (Zwischenbronchus, STUTZ [1949/50]) ab, verläuft zunächst auf einer Strecke von 0,5—1 cm fast parallel zu diesem, biegt dann nach ventral um und teilt sich in die beiden Segmentbronchien. Dieses 2—3 cm lange Stück des Bronchus soll eine schwache Wand haben. Präparatorisch läßt sich diese Annahme nicht sicher belegen. Der Hauptgrund für die Häufigkeit von Stenosen in diesem Bereich, die nach Röntgenuntersuchungen etwa 1—1,5 cm vom Stammbronchus entfernt sitzen[4], ist die Lokalisation der Lymphknotenveränderungen an dieser Stelle.

Durch zunehmende Schrumpfung wird der Mittellappen mitunter bis zu Nußgröße verkleinert und sitzt als pyramidenförmiger, von dem belüfteten Lungengewebe der Nachbarschaft überdeckter Bürzel dem Hilus auf.

Die zunächst reflektorisch eng gestellten Äste der Pulmonalarterie werden durch Proliferation der Intima bis auf kleine Restlichtungen stenosiert (s. auch unter Zirkulationsstörungen, Abb. 82, S. 598).

Zum Mittellappensyndrom gehören außer der Atelektase auch Bronchiektasen, chronische Pneumonie und Abscedierungen. Diese komplizieren die Atelektase und sind die Hauptursache dafür, daß sich die Atelektase nach Lösung des Bronchusverschlusses nicht zurückbildet. Die Endzustände mit interstitieller Fibrose, Karnifikation und Bronchiektasie sind von einer primären Pneumonie dieses Lungenabschnittes oft nicht zu unterscheiden[5].

In den Atelektasen nach tuberkulösen Lymphknotenperforationen entwickeln sich zusätzlich auch noch Aspirationstuberkulosen, die dann das Bild der sog. „unreinen Atelektase" bieten, die RÖSSLE (1936) für den Lymphknotendurchbruch in Oberlappenbronchien beschrieben hat.

Der Mittellappen ist das beste und praktisch wichtigste Beispiel für die obstruktive Lappenatelektase. Die Obstruktion anderer Lappenbronchien hat grundsätzlich die gleichen Folgen. Vollständige Lappenatelektasen finden sich nur noch an den Oberlappen, in den Unterlappenbronchien ist ein vollständiger Verschluß wegen der zahlreichen, über eine größere Strecke verteilten Astabgänge nur selten. Deswegen treten völlige Lappenatelektasen bei zentral

---

[1] STUTZ 1949/50, ESSER 1950, BROCK 1950, SCHULZE 1956, TANNER 1957 u. a.
[2] SUKIENNIKOW 1903, BROCK 1950, ENGEL 1950, v. HAYEK 1953, TÖNDURY 1956 u. a.
[3] HUZLY und BÖHM 1955, BIANCALANA 1952, weitere Literatur bei STUTZ und VIETEN 1955.
[4] STUTZ 1949/50. [5] WURM 1954.

sitzenden Bronchialcarcinomen erst in den späten Stadien auf, wenn der wachsende Tumor den Lappen- oder Stammbronchus völlig obturiert hat.

Häufiger kommt es in diesen Lappen zu Verschlüssen von Segmentbronchien. Diese können solitär oder multipel sein. Gelegentlich umfaßt ein Atelektase-bezirk zwei benachbarte Segmente.

Das Beispiel dafür ist das Lingula-Syndrom.

Ähnlich wie der Mittellappen bei den Lappenatelektasen nimmt die Lingula bei den Segmentatelektasen eine bevorzugte Stellung ein. Sie entspricht topo-graphisch dem Mittellappen, ohne dessen pleurale Abgrenzung zu haben. Beide Segmente der Lingula reagieren in der Regel gemeinsam. Die gegenüber dem Mit-tellappen geringere Häufigkeit von Atelektasen der Lingula hat ihren Grund darin, daß die bronchopulmonalen Lymphknoten dieses Bereichs weniger oft tuberkulös affiziert sind.

Auch der Selektivkollaps tuberkulös befallener Lungenlappen unter Pneumo-thoraxtherapie beruht nach Heine (1960) auf Bronchostenosen, die sich so aus-wirken, daß die Entlüftung des erkrankten Lappens bei Anlage des Pneumothorax zunächst gegenüber den sich sofort retrahierenden gesunden Lungenteilen ver-zögert eintritt. Der später besonders stark und oft irreversibel eintretende Kollaps der erkrankten Partien entsteht erst allmählich. Heine unterscheidet dabei einen hilusnahen monostenotischen Prozeß, der auch durch Torsion des absinken-den Lappens bedingt sein kann, von den polystenotischen Verschlüssen kleiner Bronchien, die insbesondere bei der unreinen Atelektase mit ausgedehnter Be-herdung des erkrankten Lappens vorliegen.

γ) Verschluß eines Segmentbronchus.

Verschlüsse von Segmentbronchien sind häufig. An ihren Abgangsstellen aus den Lappenbronchien liegen bronchopulmonale Lymphknoten, die ebenso wie an den Lappenbronchien durch Schwellung und Vergrößerung die Bronchus-lichtung deformieren und schließlich auch komprimieren können. An den Teilungswinkeln sind Lymphknotenperforationen und daraus hervorgehende lymphadenogene Bronchialwandschäden mit narbiger Verziehung keine Selten-heit. Ebenso sind Bronchialwandadenome, Polypen und andere gutartige Ge-schwülste wie auch Lungencarcinome oft an dieser Stelle lokalisiert. Schleim-hautschwellungen spielen wegen der engeren Lichtung hier bereits eine größere Rolle als zusätzlicher Faktor bei stenosierenden Bronchusprozessen. Chronische Bronchitis und Bronchiektasen breiten sich vorzugsweise in den Segment- und Subsegmentbronchien aus.

Die Lungensegmente (Sublobi), die heute eine große klinische Bedeutung erlangt haben, sind Unterabschnitte der Lappen. Sie haben einen eigenen axial liegenden Bronchus- und Arterienstiel[1]. Ihre Bindegewebssepten teilen sie mit dem Nachbar-segment, ebenso auch die Lungenvenen, die randständig in intersegmentalen Septen verlaufen und Blut aus zwei Nachbarsegmenten aufnehmen. Nur aus den Segmenten der Lingula, des Oberlappens und aus dem 6. Segment des Unter-lappens fließt das Blut vorwiegend in eine zugehörige eigene Vene zurück[2].

Die Lage der inter- und intrasegmentalen Septen fällt also mit dem Verlauf der Venen zusammen und wird bei der chirurgischen Isolierung von Segmenten und Subsegmenten als Leitweg gewählt[3]. Von Churchill u. Belsey (1939) und Churchill (1949, 1953) stammt der Vorschlag, die Lungensegmente als chirur-gische Einheiten zu betrachten.

---

[1] Kramer und Glass 1932, Backmann 1937, Brock 1940, Huizinga und Mitarbeiter 1940, 1949, v. Hayek 1953, Töndury 1954, 1956.
[2] Töndury 1956. [3] Zenker und Mitarbeiter 1954.

Die Septen sind locker gebaut, vielfach gefenstert und bilden damit keine durchgehende Scheidewand zwischen den Segmenten. Die Untereinheiten der Segmente berühren sich vielmehr an zahlreichen Stellen unmittelbar.

Die Segmente teilen sich weiter in Subsegmente, Praelobuli und Lobuli, an denen sich das gleiche Bauprinzip mit axialer Lage von Arterie, Bronchus und randständigen, mehreren Subsegmenten oder Lobuli zugeordneten Venen wiederholt[1].

Die septale Begrenzung der Lobuli ist im Lungenmantel deutlich, in den Läppchen des Lungenkerns nur durch spärliche Faservermehrung um die Venen angedeutet. So ist es zu verstehen, daß Läppchen und damit auch Acini und Alveolen verschiedener Segmente und Subsegmente in den Lücken der Septen unmittelbar aneinander stoßen und über Kohnsche Poren ihre Luft austauschen können.

Das Hauptsymptom des Verschlusses eines Segmentbronchus ist die Atelektase. Segmentatelektasen sind nach den klinischen Erfahrungen der letzten Jahre so häufig, daß man sie, wie LÖFFLER (1956) sagt, in ihrer Bedeutung für die Klinik der Lungenaffektionen vor allem in topischer Hinsicht kaum überschätzen kann. Sie werden mit der Röntgenuntersuchung erfaßt, die eine genaue topographische Zuordnung erlaubt und auch über ihre Häufigkeit Auskunft gibt. Sie stellen sich als verkleinerte Segmente dar, die bei länger bestehender Atelektase stark schrumpfen und durch Blähung des Nachbargewebes überlagert werden.

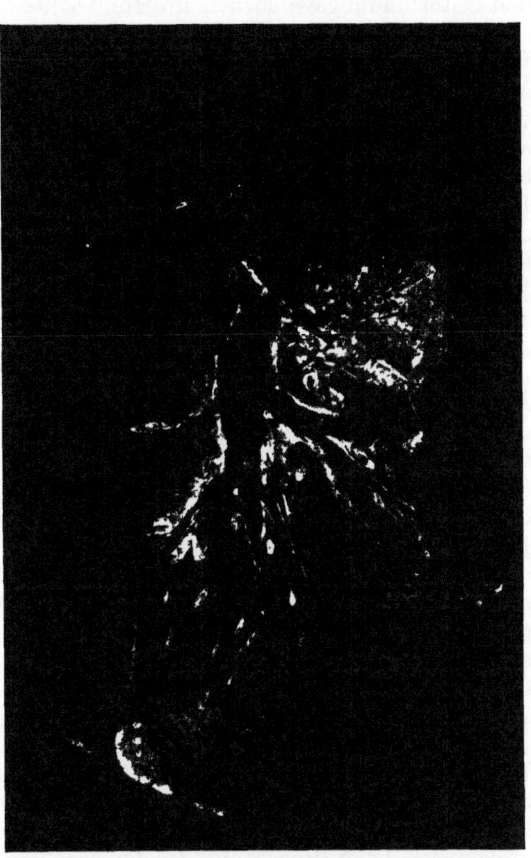

Abb. 43. Segmentatelektase mit Induration und Bronchiektasen bei tuberkulöser Narbenstenose des 3. Segmentbronchus. S.-Nr. 37/53.

Im makroskopischen Lungenpräparat fallen die akuten Segmentatelektasen durch Einsenkung und dunkle Verfärbung der Pleura auf. Sind die Nachbarsegmente gebläht, dann zeichnen sich die Grenzen der Atelektasezone auch auf der Pleura scharf ab. Auf der Schnittfläche der Lungen bilden die Segmentatelektasen dunkle Keile, die mit ihrer Spitze hiluswärts gerichtet sind. Frische Atelektasen mit starkem Ödem sind nur schwer von pneumonischer Infiltration zu unterscheiden, da die Verkleinerung unbeträchtlich ist[2]. Da die Segmente untereinander verzahnt sind, läuft die Begrenzung dieser Atelektasezone unregelmäßig, oft gezackt.

Chronische Segmentatelektasen werden infolge Drosselung der Perfusion blaß. Bronchiektasen durch Schleimstauung und nachfolgende Infektionen kommen darin häufig vor (Abb. 43).

---

[1] GIESE 1957c, JUNGHANSS 1958.   [2] RAHN 1959.

Über alten Atelektasen, die mit fibröser Umwandlung und starker Schrumpfung einhergehen, ist die Pleura tief eingezogen, die Atelektase durch geblähtes Lungengewebe der Nachbarschaft überlappt[1]. Solche Narben sind oft nur durch topographische Orientierung vom Bronchialbaum her als Segmentatelektasen zu identifizieren.

Nicht alle Verschlüsse von Segmentbronchien enden in der Atelektase. Nach den Unterbindungsversuchen am Hund sollte man annehmen, daß die Atelektasen eher ausbleiben, da van Allen (1932) sowie Haag u. Eisenreich (1956) in ihren Fällen stets eine poststenotische kollaterale Belüftung gefunden haben. Beim Menschen gehören vollständige Belüftungen bei akuten kompletten Bronchusverschlüssen zu den Seltenheiten. Wahrscheinlich liegt der Grund dafür in dem abweichenden anatomischen Bau. Hund, Kaninchen und andere Versuchstiere haben keine Segmentsepten. Diese sind beim Schwein dagegen stark ausgebildet[2]. Eine ausreichende kollaterale Ventilation kommt beim Menschen offenbar erst dann zustande, wenn die Köhnschen Poren erweitert sind. Die Bahnung der kollateralen Belüftung hat eine Erhöhung des intrabronchialen Druckes zur Voraussetzung, die besonders dann zu erwarten ist, wenn kein völliger Verschluß, sondern zunächst eine Ventilstenose bestanden hat.

Wie hoch der Druck sein muß, der die kollaterale Ventilation in Gang setzt, ist schwer zu bestimmen. An Blähungsversuchen total oder partiell kollabierter Leichenlungen läßt sich zeigen, daß die unter leichtem Druck einströmende Luft nicht alle Lungenteile gleichmäßig entfaltet, sondern von Läppchen zu Läppchen springt. Der dünne Flüssigkeitsfilm auf der Wand der kollabierten Alveolen und Alveolargänge wirkt als Adhäsionskraft, die durch intraalveolären Druck oder durch den Sog des negativen Pleuradruckes überwunden werden muß[3]. Der für die Öffnung der Alveolen eines völlig luftleeren Lungenabschnittes notwendige Druck ist noch nicht näher bestimmt. In einer eigenen Messung bei akutem massiven Lungenkollaps lag der Eröffnungsdruck bei 10 cm H_2O[4]. Für die Entfaltung einer luftleeren Lunge ist zur Überwindung der Adhäsionskraft stets ein höherer Druck notwendig als bei einer Lunge, die noch Minimalluft enthält. Nach Beobachtungen bei Thoraxoperationen sind Drucke von 10 bis 30 cm H_2O zur vollständigen Wiederbelüftung erforderlich[5].

Bei der intravital entstandenen Atelektase liegen die Verhältnisse ähnlich. Die in der entfalteten Lunge 10—15 μ weiten Kohnschen Poren sind in der Atelektase so eng, daß sie von dem Flüssigkeitsfilm überdeckt werden. Wahrscheinlich liegt hierin der Grund für die nur seltene kollaterale Belüftung der Segmentatelektasen beim Menschen. In den wenigen Fällen, in denen es nach akuter, durch Bronchusverschluß ausgelöster Segmentatelektase doch zu kollateraler Belüftung kommt, dehnt sich diese selten über das ganze Segment aus, sondern bleibt auf seine Randabschnitte beschränkt. Die Erfahrungen am Sektionstisch decken sich insoweit mit denen der Klinik, aus denen hervorgeht, daß die Folge eines akuten totalen Bronchusverschlusses eine Atelektase ist und daß diese nur selten sekundär kollateral ventiliert wird.

4. Der massive Lungenkollaps.

Unter den Atelektasen großer Lungenabschnitte, oft auch einer ganzen Lunge, ist in diesem Zusammenhang der akute massive Lungenkollaps zu nennen, der plötzlich eintritt, oft fieberhaft verläuft und mit Schmerzen, Dyspnoe und Cyanose einhergeht[6]. Die Atelektase ist in der Regel einseitig. Doppelseitige, mehr kleinherdige Atelektasen haben aber ähnliche Entstehungsmechanismen. Bei

---

[1] Wurm 1954.   [2] Töndury 1956.
[3] v. Neergaard 1929, Lenggenhager 1952, Heckmann 1951.   [4] Hartung 1959.
[5] Heine 1960.   [6] Pasteur 1908, Churchill 1925, Löffler 1956 (Literatur).

einseitigen Atelektasen wird der gleichseitige Thoraxraum durch Hochsteigen des Zwerchfells und Verziehung des Mediastinums verkleinert, die andere Lunge überbläht.

Die kollabierte Lunge zeigt das Bild der akuten Atelektase. Sie ist außerordentlich blutreich und feucht, relativ fest. Von der Schnittfläche läßt sich wenig Flüssigkeit abpressen. Die maximal erweiterten Capillaren hängen in die Alveolarlichtungen hinein, die dadurch komprimiert erscheinen. Alveolen und kleine Bronchien enthalten Ödem, mittlere und große Bronchien oft zähes schleimiges Sekret. In der Pleura findet sich mitunter ein kleiner Erguß.

Die Ursache des akuten Kollapses ist nicht völlig geklärt; verschiedene unterschiedliche Faktoren kommen als auslösende Momente in Betracht. Diese Atelektasen sind seit langem als Folgen von Bauchoperationen und Brusttraumen bekannt, in neuerer Zeit häufiger nach Thoraxoperationen gesehen worden[1]. Sie entwickeln sich im Laufe eines Tages, oft schon in wenigen Stunden und können unter den Zeichen der Atem- und Kreislaufinsuffizienz zum Tode führen oder nach einigen Tagen wieder verschwinden.

Sie treten in ähnlicher Weise nach postdiphtherischer oder aus anderen Ursachen entstandener Zwerchfellähmung auf. COHNHEIM (1882) erwähnt diese Ventilationsstörung bei Trichinose des Zwerchfells. Oft finden sie sich bei Lähmungen des Atemzentrums, etwa nach Traumen oder Tumoren, Gehirnoperation und heute nicht selten als letzte Todesursache bei Atemlähmung nach Poliomyelitis oder bei Schlafmittelvergiftung.

Im Mittelpunkt dieser auslösenden Faktoren steht die primäre Störung der Ventilation entweder als Folge einer Lähmung der Atemmuskulatur oder einer gestörten Zwerchfellfunktion, z. B. nach Bauchoperation, oder als Folge einer Lähmung des Atemzentrums.

Mit der unzureichenden Lungenbelüftung ist stets auch eine ungenügende Expektoration verbunden. Schleimstauungen in den kleinen und mittleren Bronchien, oft auch Sekretion besonders zähflüssigen Schleimes ähnlich wie bei spastischer Bronchitis, lassen die Deutung zu, daß es sich hier im wesentlichen um die Folge einer diffusen Bronchusobstruktion bei erschwerter und unvollständiger Entleerung des Bronchialsekretes handelt. Die Bronchialobstruktion ist intravital durch Bronchoskopie nachgewiesen worden, sie kann durch Bronchialtoilette behoben werden[2].

Ausgedehnte Atelektasen findet man überaus häufig auch dann, wenn die Bronchien mit entzündlichem Exsudat gefüllt sind, das vollständige Verstopfungen oder auch Ventilstenosen in kleinen und mittleren Bronchien hervorruft. Je stärker die Sekretion und je zäher das Sekret, um so häufiger sind die Atelektasen oder bei Ventilstenosen die herdförmigen akuten Überblähungen.

5. Die Streifen- und Plattenatelektasen.

Als Äquivalent oder mildere Form des akuten massiven Lungenkollapses können die streifenförmigen Atelektasen angesehen werden, die kleinere Einheiten als ein Segment umfassen. Im Röntgenbild sind sie gesehen[3] und eingehend bearbeitet worden[4]. Sie bilden bänder- oder plattenförmige Schattenstreifen von 1—5 mm Breite, die vorwiegend in den Unterfeldern der Lunge, oft zwerchfellnahe liegen und mitunter horizontal verlaufen. Daß diese

---

[1] PASTEUR 1910, 1911, A. und P. MOUNIER-KUHN 1955, BIANGALANA und COLOMBO 1952.
[2] JACKSON 1950 u. v. a., Literatur bei LÖFFLER 1956.
[3] HULTÉN 1928, LAURELL 1928, HAUDEK 1931, JACOBAEUS 1932, JACOBAEUS und WESTERMARK 1930, WESTERMARK 1930.
[4] FLEISCHNER 1936, HEUCK 1959, HEINE 1960.

Verschattungen Atelektasen sind, ist in mehreren Fällen von Fleischner (1936) autoptisch erwiesen. Einen dieser Fälle hat Feyrter untersucht und ein atelektatisches Ödem mit geringer Hämorrhagie sowie eine eitrige Bronchitis und Bronchiolitis, aber keinen Verschluß der großen Bronchien gefunden. Diese Atelektasen sind flüchtig, arm an klinischen Symptomen. Sie werden bei Einschränkung der Zwerchfellbewegung, besonders bei Zwerchfellhochstand gefunden und begleiten oft Krankheitsprozesse im Oberbauch. Oberflächliche Atmung, Bronchitis und Bronchiolitis sowie Sekretstauung sind auslösende Faktoren. Thoraxkontusion[1], Kyphoskoliose oder Coronarthrombosen sowie kleine

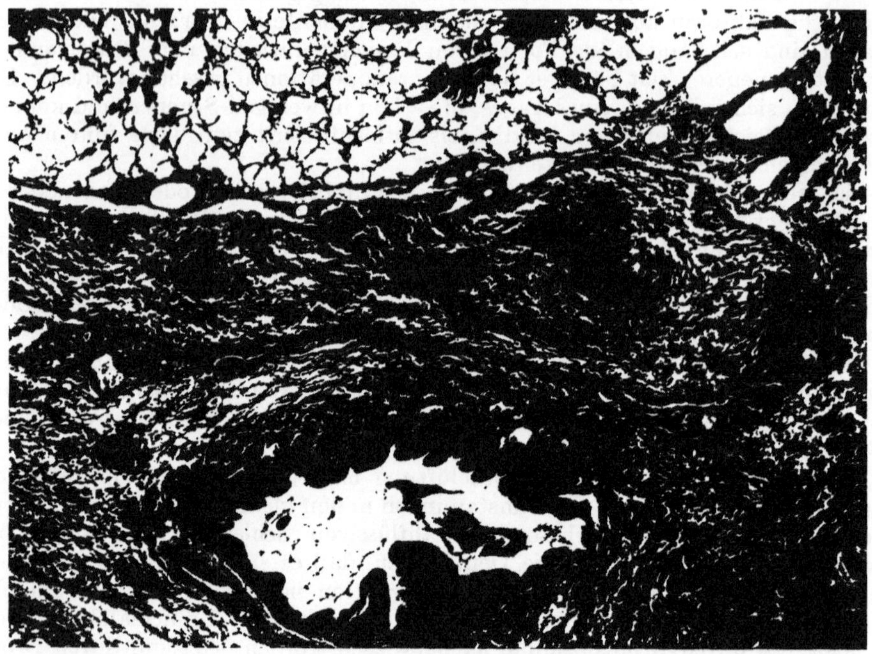

Abb. 44. Streifenatelektase bei chronischer Bronchitis und Bronchiektasen. Überblähung des benachbarten Lungengewebes. E.-Nr. 1238/57.

Pleuraergüsse spielen in der Genese der Atelektase eine Rolle[2]. Sie können Vorläufer von Pneumonien oder Restzustände davon sein (Abb. 44).

Wesentlich für die Pathogenese der Streifenatelektasen ist fast immer die eingeschränkte Ventilation der Unterlappen, die aus vielfachen pulmonalen und extrapulmonalen Ursachen entstanden sein kann. Dabei sammelt sich in den Bronchien Sekret und Exsudat, das durch Obstruktion einen subsegmentalen, selten einen größeren Lungenkollaps auslöst. Die Vorgänge sind ähnlich wie bei massivem Lungenkollaps, nur räumlich weniger ausgedehnt.

Segment- und Streifenatelektasen sind Anlaß zur Auseinandersetzung über die von Reinhardt (1934) aufgestellte und von Kalbfleisch (1941) vertretene These der neuralen metameren Gliederung der Lunge gewesen. Sturm (1948, 1951) hat diese Atelektase als neural ausgelösten, auf einer Kontraktion der glatten Muskulatur der Lunge beruhenden Vorgang angesehen. Eine neural bestimmte segmentale Gliederung der Lunge hat sich jedoch nicht erweisen lassen, und die funktionellen Segmente von Kalbfleisch (1946), Kalbfleisch u.

---

[1] Heuck und Flach 1953.   [2] Fleischner 1936, Heuck 1959, Heine 1960.

HERKLOTZ (1949) werden heute nicht als neural, sondern als bronchial bestimmte Lungeneinheiten aufgefaßt [1].

Dagegen können durch direkte Reizung der Pleura neuroreflektorische Kreislaufstörungen in der Lunge ausgelöst werden [2], die über eine peristatische Hyperämie zu Plasmadiapedese und zu Störungen der Lungenbelüftung führen. Kreislaufstörungen in der Lunge sind auch als Folge von Reizungen an den Organen des Oberbauches im Experiment erzeugt worden [3]. Es ist wahrscheinlich, daß Streifenatelektasen auch auf diesem Wege entstehen können.

Das Reinhardtsche Dellenphänomen läßt sich nach HEUCK (1959) und HEINE (1960) auch an der toten Lunge erzeugen. Dieser Befund wird ebenso wie die durch Knickung oder Stauchung der Lunge intra operationem oder am toten Organ hervorgerufenen Atelektasestreifen als wesentliches Argument für die vorwiegende Bedeutung rein mechanisch wirksamer Faktoren herangezogen.

In der frischen Segment- und Streifenatelektase sind die zu schmalen Spalträumen kollabierten Alveolargänge auf den Hilus ausgerichtet [4]. Die Atelektase ist zwischen Pleura und Hilus ausgespannt, die Pleura in der akuten Phase nur wenig eingezogen. Die Nachbarsegmente rücken dadurch nahe aneinander. Die chronischen Streifenatelektasen schrumpfen dann unter Retraktion in Richtung auf den Hilus, wobei sie die Pleura, ähnlich wie die schrumpfenden Segmentatelektasen, tief einziehen. Der gerichtete Kollaps der Frühphase ist auch noch in der indurierten und geschrumpften Atelektase zu erkennen.

IV. Stenosen und Verschlüsse der kleinen Bronchien und Bronchiolen.

Die überaus häufigen Stenosen und Verschlüsse der kleinen Bronchien und Bronchiolen stehen oft im Mittelpunkt eines krankhaften Lungenprozesses. Mitunter sind sie aber nur Begleiterscheinungen oder bleiben als Residuen einer abgeklungenen Entzündung zurück.

In der Regel sind sie multipel, oft auf so große Gebiete der Endverzweigungen des Bronchialbaumes ausgedehnt, daß man von einer *generalisierten Bronchiolostenose* sprechen kann. Häufiger bleiben sie aber auf einzelne Bronchialgebiete beschränkt oder sind nur an einzelnen Bronchiolen lokalisiert.

Ursachen der Stenosen sind am häufigsten vorübergehende, oft intermittierende Obstruktionen der Lichtung, narbige Deformierung der Bronchialwand oder Obturation und Kompression der Bronchiolen. Dazu tritt als weitere Form die aktive Kontraktion der Bronchialmuskulatur, die nur in diesen muskulären Bronchialabschnitten Stenose und Verschluß der Lichtung herbeiführen kann.

Als Formen der Stenosen kommen im Sinne von JACKSON (1945) die partielle Obstruktion der Lichtung, die Ventilstenose und der totale Verschluß in Betracht.

Die Folgen der Stenose für die Ventilation reichen örtlich von der Atelektase bis zum Emphysem, in ihren allgemeinen Auswirkungen vom funktionell bedeutungslosen Nebenbefund bis zu schwersten Ventilationsstörungen mit dem Ende in der Erstickung. Der poststenotische Lungenabschnitt ist stets hypoventiliert. Dabei ist es unerheblich, ob er gebläht oder kollabiert ist.

a) Anatomische und funktionelle Vorbemerkungen.

Die kleinen Bronchien und Bronchiolen nehmen schon unter normalen Atmungsbedingungen eine Sonderstellung im Bronchialsystem ein. Hier werden

---

[1] ESSER 1951, HUIZINGA 1951, 1952, WEBER 1951 u. a., siehe auch Abschnitt „Myoelastisches System der Lunge", S. 417.
[2] E. REINHARDT, 1934, 1935, LESCHKE 1952, 1953, 1956.
[3] A. BERNARD 1951, STAJANO und SCANDROGLIO 1952, Literatur bei WURM 1954.
[4] WURM 1954.

die größten Strömungswiderstände gemessen (s. S. 468). Nach neueren bronchographischen Untersuchungen[1] sind die Bronchien und der intrathorakale Anteil der Trachea in der Exspirationsphase enger als in der Inspirationsphase. Längen- und Weitedehnung sind an den kleinen Bronchien wesentlich stärker als an den größeren. Die axial in den Lobuli liegenden Lobularbronchien sind im elastischen Fasergerüst der Lunge verspannt und folgen so dem inspiratorischen Dehnungszug, der von der Pleura und ihren hiluswärts einstrahlenden Septen auf das Lungengewebe und auf die Bronchien übertragen wird. In der Exspiration retrahiert sich das elastische Gewebe in Richtung auf den Bronchus- und Gefäßstiel. Die Spannungskräfte, die nach mehreren Richtungen auf die Bronchiolenwand einwirken, werden dabei schwächer, es folgt eine exspiratorische Verkürzung der Bronchien mit Verkleinerung der Lichtung, gleichzeitig aber auch eine Verkleinerung der Alveolargänge und der Alveolen. Solange die Entspannung von der elastischen Retraktionskraft der Lunge abhängt, verlaufen diese Vorgänge an Alveolen und Gangsystem koordiniert. Tritt bei forcierter Ausatmung auch die Exspirationsmuskulatur in Tätigkeit, dann werden die Bronchien ebenso wie das Alveolarsystem unter Druck gesetzt und komprimiert. Diese Kompression ist um so deutlicher, je stärker der intrathorakale Druck ansteigt. Die Störung der Luftströmung in den Bronchiolen bei positiven intrapleuralen Drucken ist aus der Bronchospirographie erschlossen und durch die Bronchographie nachgewiesen worden[2]. Die Änderungen der Lichtungsweite werden dabei als passive, druckabhängige Vorgänge aufgefaßt. Positiver Pleuradruck erhöht den Strömungswiderstand in den kleinen Bronchien. Die auf diesem Wege ausgelöste Bronchiolostenose ist ein Funktionszustand, der an der Leiche nicht mehr erkennbar ist, da mit dem Stillstand der Atembewegung sofort ein Druckausgleich erfolgt.

Neben der passiven Stenosierung durch Kompression sind regulative Änderungen der Lichtungsweite, die auf neuralem Wege oder direkt ausgelöst werden, dort möglich, wo die glatte Muskulatur beherrschendes Wandelement ist. Diese Bronchialprovinz[3] beginnt an den mittleren Bronchien dort, wo sie ihren Knorpel verlieren, und reicht bis in die Bronchioli terminales.

Die in Schraubentouren angeordneten Muskelbündel verlaufen im engen Bronchus steiler als im weiten, ihre Kontraktion verkürzt den Durchmesser der Bronchuslichtung um etwa die Hälfte[4]. Die bei krampfhafter Kontraktion der Muskelwand in Falten gelegte Schleimhaut kann die Lichtung eines Bronchiolus fast verschließen. Unter der Einwirkung von Adrenalin erschlafft die Bronchialmuskulatur[5], während an den Blutgefäßen der Lunge eine Vasoconstriction eintritt. Die nervale Regulation der Bronchialweite verläuft über den Vagus und Sympathicus. Die Reizung des Vagus führt im Tierversuch zum Bronchialmuskelkrampf, Sympathicusreizung in der Regel zur Erweiterung der Bronchien. Die Ergebnisse dieser Versuche sind aber wenig übereinstimmend. Es ist zweifelhaft, ob sie auch für den Menschen gültig sind[6].

b) Arten und Ursachen der Bronchiolostenose.

1. Die Bronchiolokonstriktion.

Im Experiment ist die krampfhafte Konstriktion der Bronchiolen im Schocktod oder beim Asthma bronchiale nachweisbar.

---

[1] Siehe bei Stutz 1949/50.

[2] di Rienzo 1949.

[3] H. H. Weber 1936, 1959.

[4] v. Hayek 1950, 1953.

[5] Einthoven 1892.

[6] Literatur bei Schoedel, dieses Handbuch, V/1, Bucher 1952, Kehler 1953.

α) *Die Schocklunge.*

Im *akuten anaphylaktischen Schock* des Meerschweinchens ist die Lunge maximal gebläht und kollabiert nicht. Die Schocklunge ist groß, hell, blutarm, stark lufthaltig und ganz leicht, alle Lufträume sind maximal gedehnt.

Diese starke Lungenblähung wird allgemein mit einem Ventilmechanismus in den spastisch kontrahierten Bronchiolen erklärt. Bei der maximalen krampfhaften Inspiration wird der Thorax unter Anspannung der gesamten Inspirationsmuskulatur so stark wie möglich ausgeweitet und der erhöhte Bronchialwiderstand überwunden. Eine Exspiration kommt nicht zustande, entweder weil ein Krampf der Atemmuskulatur eine exspiratorische Entspannung, insbesondere eine Erschlaffung des Zwerchfells verhindert oder weil die Ventilstenosen durch den Retraktionsdruck der Lunge nicht überwunden werden (siehe auch unter Asthma bronchiale).

Bei intravenöser Applikation des Antigens ist die spastische Bronchokonstriktion stärker als bei intraperitonealer. Man nimmt an, daß die schockwirksame Substanz bei intravenöser Erfolgsinjektion aus der Intima der Arterien stammt[1]. Bei geringer Dosierung des Antigens, auch bei Applikation durch Inhalation, läuft die anaphylaktische Reaktion protrahiert ab, der Bronchospasmus geht vorüber. Beim Kaninchen ist die Reaktion ähnlich, bei Ratte und Maus sind die Erscheinungen nur gering, dort ist die Lunge nicht Schockorgan.

Die engen Bronchiallichtungen sind beim allergischen Schock mit Sekret gefüllt. In der ödematösen Bronchialschleimhaut finden sich eosinophile Leukocyten[2]. Oft bestehen Hyperämie und Hämorrhagien.

β) *Das experimentelle Asthma bronchiale.*

Ein ähnliches Bild wie im Schock bietet die Lunge bei dem experimentellen, durch Allergene hervorgerufenen *Asthma bronchiale* des Meerschweinchens. Auch hier steht die Bronchokonstriktion im Vordergrund, sie ist aber von einer vermehrten Schleimsekretion in den Bronchien begleitet. Auch hier wird ein Ventilmechanismus als Ursache der Lungenüberblähung angenommen. Der Bronchospasmus ist an der starken Kontraktion der Bronchiolen und kleinen Bronchien auch postmortal daran zu erkennen, daß bei der Bronchographie das Kontrastmittel (Lipiodol) nur schwer und unvollkommen in den Bronchialbaum einfließt. Die in normalen Lungen postmortal leicht zu erzielenden Parenchymfüllungen werden hier nur unter Anwendung von hohem Druck möglich und bleiben unvollkommen. Auch nach Abtragung des Lungenmantels ist keine bessere Bronchialfüllung zu erzielen[3].

Gleichzeitig mit der Bronchokonstriktion tritt auch eine Sperre der Lungengefäße ein. Tusche, die in die Blutbahn eingespritzt wird, fließt nicht in die Lunge hinein, die Lungen bleiben ungefärbt[4].

Das experimentelle Asthma bronchiale läßt sich beim Meerschweinchen auf verschiedene Weise erzeugen.

Bei Inhalation von Histamin[5] entwickelt sich ein reiner Spasmus der Bronchialmuskulatur. Die glatten Muskelfasern der Bronchiolen und kleinen Bronchien sind so stark kontrahiert, daß die Lichtung fast völlig verschlossen ist. Da bei Histamin-Asthma keine vermehrte Schleimsekretion erfolgt, kann man in diesen Versuchen die akute Blähung allein auf die Bronchokonstriktion beziehen. Im Lungenmantel ist diese Erweiterung der Acini besonders stark, im Lungenkern finden sich auch kleine Atelektasen. Dieses Bild ist dem Zustand der Lunge des Menschen beim Tod im Asthmaanfall vergleichbar.

Fast völlige Übereinstimmung im Befund ergibt sich bei der Auslösung des experimentellen Asthmas durch Allergene nach vorausgegangener Allergisierung[6]. Hier entsteht auch ein Schleimhautödem mit vermehrter Schleimsekretion.

Histamin macht beim Meerschweinchen schon in Dosen von 0,1—0,4 mg tödlichen Bronchospasmus, der auch an der isolierten Bronchialmuskulatur auftritt und unabhängig von der Innervation ist. Auch die Arteriolen werden bei Nagetieren durch Histamin stark verengt.

---

[1] J. FORSSMAN 1920.   [2] HANSEN 1957.   [3] WILLIAMSON zit. nach HANSEN 1957.
[4] W. EICKHOFF 1948.   [5] HALPERN 1942.
[6] BUSSON und OGATA 1924, ALEXANDER, BECKE und HOLMES 1926, RATNER, JACKSON und GRUEHL 1927, KALLÓS und PAGEL 1937, COLLDAHL 1943, NOELPP und Mitarbeiter 1950—1954, RATNER 1951, FRIEBEL 1953, 1954.

Aus diesen Versuchen, besonders aus dem Histaminschock, geht einwandfrei hervor, daß beim Meerschweinchen auf die Bronchokonstriktion eine Überblähung der Lunge folgt. Die Strömungsgeschwindigkeit der Luft nimmt gleichzeitig ab und zwar stärker in der Exspiration als in der Inspiration[1].

Für das Asthma des Menschen wird seit Laennec (1826) und Biermer (1865/67) ebenfalls eine bronchospastische Komponente angenommen. Das Vorhandensein der spastischen Bronchialkonstriktion wird aus der Asthmatherapie erschlossen, weil mit Adrenalin und ähnlichen Substanzen, die krampflösend wirken, die Strömungswiderstände im Bronchialbaum innerhalb des Anfalles und auch im Intervall vermindert werden. Die erhöhten Widerstände für die Luftströmung im Bronchialbaum, die in zahlreichen Messungen am Lebenden auch außerhalb des Anfalles festgestellt worden sind, werden als Folge einer spastischen Engstellung der Bronchien angesehen.

Die anatomischen Befunde geben darüber keinen ausreichenden Aufschluß. Am Lebenden ist die Bronchuskonstriktion mit fadendünner Einengung des Bronchuslumens in der Bronchographie festgestellt worden[2]. Eine Hypertrophie der Bronchialmuskulatur, die als Folge der Neigung zu Bronchospasmen postuliert wird und seit Marchand (1916, 1918) mehrfach beschrieben wurde[3], ist kein konstanter Befund[4].

In der Klinik unterscheidet man eine bronchoconstrictorische trockene Form des Asthma von einem hypersekretorischen feuchten Asthma[1]. Bei der hypersekretorischen Form des Asthma sind die kleineren Bronchien hinter den Schleimstenosen deutlich dilatiert, im Bereich der Schleimpfröpfe weitgestellt. Die trockene Form des Asthma soll eine günstigere Prognose haben. Die Bronchokonstriktion spielt beim Tod im Bronchialasthma nach den autoptischen Befunden sehr wahrscheinlich nur eine untergeordnete Rolle, sie tritt jedenfalls hinter der überragenden Bedeutung, die die Schleimobstruktion als Ursache der tödlichen Dyspnoe hat, weit in den Hintergrund (siehe auch spastische Bronchitis).

2. Die akute Obstruktion.

Eine Verstopfung der Bronchiolen kann aus vielen Ursachen heraus entstehen und auf zahlreichen Mechanismen beruhen. Sie kann vorübergehend oder bleibend, vollkommen oder unvollkommen sein.

α) Der akute Schleimverschluß der Bronchiolen.

Akute Verschlüsse der kleinen Bronchien und Bronchiolen beruhen so gut wie ausschließlich auf Verstopfungen der Lichtung durch Schleim oder entzündliches Exsudat. Dieses in seiner Viscosität stark wechselnde Material kann sich in kurzer Zeit in solcher Menge bilden, daß große Strecken des Bronchialbaumes davon ausgefüllt werden. Das angesammelte und nicht ausgehustete Sekret bleibt zunächst dort liegen, wo es gebildet wird. Bei der Bronchitis sind es die mittleren Bronchien, bei der Bronchiolitis vor allem die Bronchiolen, deren engste Stellen durch das Sekret verstopft werden. Schleimpfröpfe legen sich der Bronchialwand an, sind aber auf dieser beweglich und können bei der Atmung und durch den Sekretstrom transportiert werden, der durch die Tätigkeit der Flimmerepithelien unterhalten wird. Ein Hustenstoß kann die Schleimpfröpfe entfernen, eine tiefe Inspiration sie ansaugen oder auch Luft hindurchtreten lassen. Dünnflüssiger Schleim und entzündliches Sekret sind oft mit Luft gemischt, auch im zähen Schleim des Asthmatikers oder bei spastischer Bronchitis kann man Luftblasen

---

[1] Noelpp und Noelpp-Eschenhagen 1956.   [2] di Rienzo 1949, H. H. Weber u. a.
[3] Mönckeberg 1909, Wegelin 1944, Derbes und Mitarbeiter 1951.
[4] Gloor 1954 u. a.

nachweisen, die an der Grenze zur Luft Menisken bilden (Abb. 45). Durch
Mischung von Schleim und Luft in den Bronchien wird der Widerstand
stark erhöht[1]. Der Schleimverschluß ist also keine absolute, unverändert
über längere Zeit andauernde Okklusion der Lichtung, sondern intermittierend
und reversibel. Die Folgen eines Schleimverschlusses sind deshalb sehr wechselnd
und nicht nur von der Menge und Viscosität des Schleimes, sondern auch von der
Atemtiefe abhängig. Eine flache Atmung mit geringer Strömungsintensität wird
die Schleimobstruktion nicht überwinden, eine tiefe und kräftige Ventilation den
Widerstand durchbrechen.

Die wechselnde Viscosität des Bronchialsekrets ist seit langem als mögliche
Ursache einer Bronchialobstruktion in Betracht gezogen worden. Schon LAENNEC

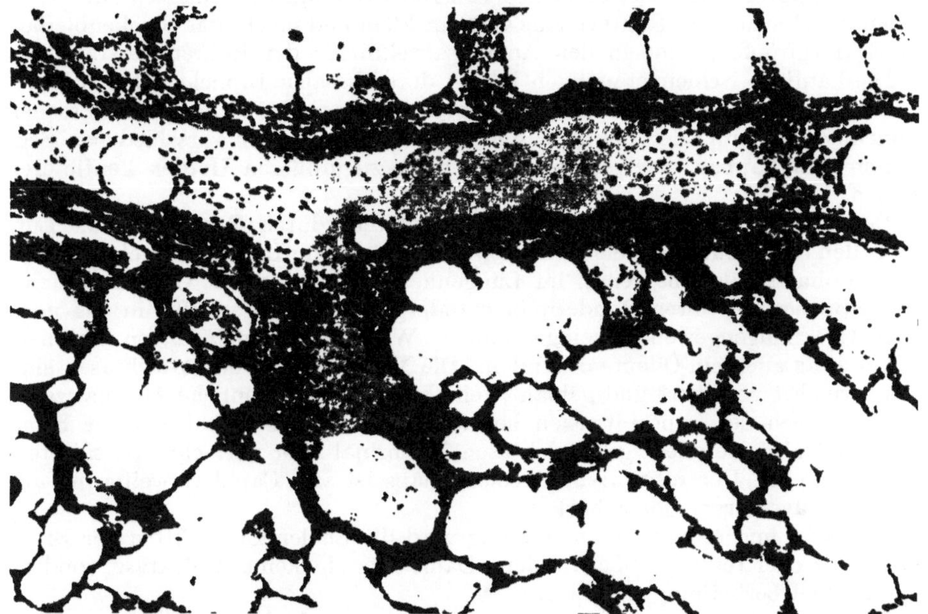

Abb. 45. Schleimobstruktion eines Bronchiolus terminalis bei Asthma bronchiale. Poststenotische Überblähung
der Acini. Ausweitung der Alveolargänge mit Abflachung der Alveolen. Luftbläschen im Schleim.

(1826) hat als Catarrhe sec die Zustände herausgehoben, bei denen das zähe
glasige Sputum als crachet perlée den Hinweis auf die hohe Viscosität des Bronchialsekretes gibt. LIEBERMEISTER (1922) hat die Viscosität des Bronchial-
schleimes durch Einsaugen in enge Röhren bestimmt und besonders hohe Werte
bei asthmoiden Katarrhen gefunden. Zur Fortbewegung des in eine 1—2 mm
weite Capillare eingesogenen Schleimes ist ein Druck von 80 mm Hg (etwa 1 m
H_2O) notwendig. Ähnlich hohe Drucke entstehen in den Bronchialästen nur beim
Hustenstoß[2]. Der Normaldruck in den Alveolen, verstanden als Druckdifferenz
zwischen Alveolarluft und Außenluft, wird in der Ruheatmung bei einem Strömungsvolumen von 0,5 Liter/sec mit 0,5—2 cm H_2O angenommen. Die Schleim-
und Sekretobstruktion der engen Bronchiolen wird durch den normalen Alveolardruck also nicht behoben werden können, besonders wenn der Schleim sehr
viscös ist und sich zusammenhängende Schleimgerinnsel bilden, die bei der Bronchitis plastica große Abschnitte des Bronchialbaumes ausfüllen. Der Druck

---

[1] v. HAYEK 1953, HEINE und NAGEL 1952, 1954, HERTZ und HERTZ 1953.
[2] LIEBERMEISTER 1922.

erhöht sich unter krankhaften Verhältnissen bei Asthma oder Emphysem schon in der Ruheatmung auf das Doppelte bis auf das Vierfache[1].

Die Luftströmung wird bei der Exspiration hiluswärts beschleunigt und erreicht ihren höchsten Wert in der Glottis. Nach Rohrer beträgt die Strömungsgeschwindigkeit beim Hustenstoß im Bronchiolus terminalis 1,2—6 m/sec, in der Trachea 15—35 m/sec und in der Glottis 50,0—120,0 m/sec. Die Hauptbeschleunigung beginnt erst in den Bronchien von 6 mm Weite, dort ist sie nach Rohrer 24,0—62,0 m/sec (s. Abb. 32, S. 469).

Im Gangsystem des Acinus ist die Strömungsgeschwindigkeit mit 0,5 bis 25,0 m/sec auch im Hustenstoß nur gering, ebenso in den Bronchiolen. Die Expulsionskraft, die Geigel (1900) in Blasrohrversuchen mit $17,5 \times 10^6$ erg bei einem exspiratorischen Maximaldruck von 150—160 mm Hg gemessen hat, ist in diesen Abschnitten des Rohrsystems also nur klein und macht das Steckenbleiben der Sekretpfröpfe gerade in den Anfangsabschnitten der Röhren verständlich.

Die häufigen Schleimstauungen in den dorso-basalen Bronchien bei Schwerkranken führen stets zu Atelektasen, die je nach der Größe des verschlossenen Bronchus auf Acini oder Lobuli beschränkt bleiben, aber in verschiedenen Segmenten und Lappen verstreut sein und auch zu größeren Herden konfluieren können.

Der Alveolarkollaps in diesen Herden entsteht durch Resorption der Luft hinter den Stenosen. Die atelektatischen Bezirke sind im Lungenmantel oft scharf durch Lobularsepten begrenzt, im Lungenkern, wo die septale Gliederung fehlt und Läppchen mit ihren Rändern ineinandergreifen, unregelmäßig in das noch lufthaltige Lungengewebe hineingeschoben. Wenn Kreislaufstörungen bestehen, ist fast stets auch ein Ödem vorhanden. Die Nachbarlobuli der Atelektasen sind teils vermehrt ventiliert und gebläht, teils haben sie gewöhnliche Alveolarweite.

Die Folgen der hypostatischen herdförmigen Schleimobstruktion der Bronchien sind also kleinfleckige Atelektasen in normal oder vermehrt ventiliertem Lungengewebe. Der resorptive Alveolarkollaps ist von Capillarerweiterung, oft auch von alveolärem Ödem begleitet.

Bei tiefer und angestrengter Atmung wird die Schleimobstruktion der Bronchien ganz oder teilweise überwunden. Dann entsteht keine Atelektase, sondern eine akute Überblähung der Lunge.

Das klassische Beispiel dafür ist das Asthma bronchiale.

β) Das Asthma bronchiale.

Beim Tod im akuten Asthmaanfall findet sich eine akute Lungenblähung, ein Verschluß der Bronchien mit zähem Schleim, eine eosinophile Bronchitis mit Verschleimung des Bronchialepithels, eine Verbreiterung der Basalmembran sowie ein Zustand vermehrter Sekretion der Schleimdrüsen. Diese seit Marchand (1918), Fraenkel (1909), Mönckeberg (1909) u. a. bekannten Veränderungen sind nach neueren Untersuchungen[2] so typisch für den Asthmatod, daß daraus auch postmortal die Diagnose des Bronchialasthmas gestellt werden darf.

Die zähen elastischen Schleimausgüsse der Bronchien füllen den ganzen Bronchialbaum aus. Sie bilden sich vorwiegend in den kleinen Bronchien von 1 bis 4 mm Durchmesser. An diesen Stellen wird nach den Versuchen mit markierten Antikörpern[3] das Antigen bevorzugt gebunden.

---

[1] Wyss und Schmid 1951, Jeker 1953, Otis, Fenn und Rahn 1950 u. a., Literatur bei Rossier und Mitarbeiter 1956, 1958 sowie bei Noelpp und Noelpp-Eschenhagen 1956.

[2] Riva und Probst 1950, Gloor 1954, Letterer 1957, Gläser 1958, H. Schoen 1958, Giese 1959 (Literatur).

[3] Warren und Dixon 1948.

Die Lungenblähung ist stets hochgradig und diffus. Die Lungenränder überdecken den Herzbeutel. Auch nach der Herausnahme sinken die Lungen nicht
zusammen, die Luft läßt sich auch bei Anwendung von Druck nicht auspressen,
der Luftgehalt der Lungen verringert sich nach längerem Liegen kaum. Das
Lungengewebe kollabiert erst, wenn die Bronchien aufgeschnitten und die Schleimpfröpfe herausgezogen werden.

Unter 94 Asthmatodesfällen fand BULLEN (1952) nur viermal größere, etwas
häufiger kleine Atelektasen. Sie kommen dann vor, wenn pneumonische Komplikationen hinzutreten, gehören also nicht zum reinen Asthmatodesfall.

Die starke Lungenblähung und die Schleimausgüsse der Bronchien sind
kausal voneinander abhängig.

Der asthmatische Anfall beginnt nach dem klinischen Bild mit einer rasch
zunehmenden Dyspnoe[1]. Die Atmung wird keuchend, die Ausatmung ist erschwert und verlängert. Der Thorax wird weit gestellt und schließlich bei nur
kleinen Atemexkursionen in maximaler Inspirationsstellung gehalten. Erst gegen
Ende des Anfalls wird mit dem Husten, der oft schon im Beginn der Dyspnoe
vorhanden ist, ein zähes, klebriges Sputum mit Charcot-Leydenschen Kristallen
und Curschmannschen Spiralen entleert.

Die übermäßige Absonderung des zähen, hochviscösen Schleimes, in dem der
seröse Anteil des Bronchialsekretes stark zurücktritt (Dyskrinie), fällt mit dem
Beginn des Anfalls zusammen. Je mehr Schleim gebildet wird, um so stärker
wird die Dyspnoe. In der angestrengten Inspiration wird die Luft trotz des erhöhten Widerstandes noch angesogen, aber nicht mehr ausgeatmet. Die Schleimpfröpfe wirken wie Ventile, die die Luft in die Alveolen eintreten, aber nicht wieder
zurückströmen lassen. Die Schleimobstruktion der Bronchien wird durch die
elastische Retraktionskraft der Lungen auch unter Mithilfe der Exspirationsmuskulatur nicht überwunden. Die mit der krampfhaften Inspiration einge-
sogene Luft bleibt hinter den Schleimpfröpfen gefangen (Abb. 45).

Die Ventilwirkung der Schleimpfröpfe beruht einmal auf dem Wechsel der
Bronchialweite zwischen Inspiration und Exspiration, die schon unter normalen
Verhältnissen eine deutliche Widerstandserhöhung im Röhrensystem während
der Exspiration bedingt, und zweitens auf der Kompression der kleinen Bronchien
durch die hochgradig geblähten, als Luftkissen wirkenden Acini[2].

Die vermehrte Schleimsekretion im Anfall verstopft nicht alle Bronchien
gleichmäßig. Die kurzen Bronchialäste im Lungenkern sind oft frei von Schleim,
auch im Oberlappen scheint die Schleimobstruktion nicht so gleichmäßig zu sein
wie in den peripheren Teilen des Unterlappens. Nach den anatomischen Befunden
muß angenommen werden, daß ein Teil der Lunge auch im schweren Asthmaanfall noch regelrecht ventiliert wird. In diesem Teil findet wahrscheinlich der
für die Erhaltung des Lebens notwendige Gasaustausch im Anfall statt. Ist der
Anteil der noch durchgängigen Bronchien zu gering, dann folgen Cyanose und
Erstickungstod.

Die große Luftmenge hinter den Stenosen ist für den Gasaustausch nicht
nutzbar. Die maximal geblähten Abschnitte wirken funktionell als Totraum,
in dem kein nennenswerter Luftwechsel vor sich geht.

Die Druck-Volumdiagramme, die aus bronchospirometrischen Messungen
beim Asthmatiker auch während eines Anfalls und beim experimentellen Meer-

---

_[1] Zur Klinik vgl. NOELPP und NOELPP-ESCHENHAGEN 1956 (Literatur), SCHUBERT und FISCHER
1956; kindliches Asthma bei MAI 1951, 1954.
_[2] RIBBERT 1912, 1916.

schweinchenasthma[1] gewonnen worden sind, zeigen einen sehr raschen inspiratorischen Druckanstieg. In der Exspiration fällt der Druck zunächst rasch, dann langsamer ab. Der exspiratorische Schenkel der Kurve zeigt einen Knick, der etwa an der Grenze des ersten Drittels liegt. Statischer und dynamischer Pleuradruck sind erhöht.

Die Abknickung der Kurve im ersten Drittel der Exspirationsphase kann als Folge des Ventilmechanismus aufgefaßt werden, der durch die in der Exspiration einsetzende Bronchuskompression wirksam wird. Sie kann aber auch dadurch entstehen, daß in der Exspiration zunächst die Luft durch die noch freien Bronchien unter raschem Druckabfall abströmt, danach nur noch in geringer Menge aus dem stenotischen Bronchialbezirk entleert wird. Die anatomischen Befunde sprechen für die letzte Interpretation. Entsprechende Messungen an der Leichenlunge liegen noch nicht vor[2].

Im Ende des Anfalls lösen sich die Schleimverschlüsse, der Luftwechsel kommt wieder in Gang.

Der Lösungsvorgang wird durch die Bildung eines dünnflüssigen Sekrets eingeleitet, das von den Bronchialepithelien und von den Schleimdrüsen abgeschieden wird. In dieser Phase schiebt sich zwischen die hochviscösen Schleimpfröpfe und das Bronchialepithel eine dünne Flüssigkeitsschicht, auf der die Schleimpfröpfe durch den Exspirationsdruck herausgleiten. Dieser Wechsel vom trockenen, frustranen Husten zur Expektoration des zähen, klebrigen Sekretes zeigt das Ende des Anfalles, der wenige Minuten oder 1—2 Tage dauern kann. Im Status asthmaticus ist die Lösung verzögert und oft durch medikamentöse Therapie nicht zu fördern, wahrscheinlich, weil die dünnflüssige Phase des Bronchialsekretes nicht in genügender Menge gebildet wird.

Über die Folgen der Bronchialobstruktion und Überblähung für die Lungenelastizität siehe unter bronchostenotischem Emphysem.

γ) Die spastische Bronchitis.

Die akuten und häufiger noch die subakuten und chronisch-rezidivierenden Bronchitiden der muskulären Bronchusabschnitte haben oft einen spastischen Charakter. Die spastische Bronchitis der Kliniker[3] ist in den mittleren und kleinen Bronchien lokalisiert, deren Lichtung durch Kontraktion der Muskelfasern eng gestellt werden kann[4]. Allergische Vorgänge spielen ätiologisch eine bedeutende Rolle, es bestehen also Beziehungen zum Asthma bronchiale. Rossier (1956) unterscheidet eine primär in den Bronchiolen beginnende ascendierende Form von einer primär in den oberen Luftwegen beginnenden descendierenden Bronchitis. Die spastische Komponente einer Bronchitis ist bei der Adrenalin-Medikation zu erkennen, deren spasmolytische Wirkung zu einer wesentlichen Besserung der Ventilation mit erheblicher Steigerung des Atemgrenzwertes führt[5]. Histologisch findet man eine dichte lymphocytär-plasmacelluläre Infiltration der Schleimhaut mit Hyperämie und leichtem Ödem, mitunter auch reichlich

---

[1] Noelpp und Mitarbeiter 1952, 1954, 1956 (Literatur), Gaensler 1950, Gaensler und Mitarbeiter 1952.

[2] Literatur bei Rossier und Mitarbeiter 1956, 1958, Noelpp und Noelpp-Eschenhagen 1956, Wyss 1955 u. a.

[3] Volhard 1921, 1922, Staehelin 1922, 1930, Cocchi 1952, Segal und Dulfano 1953, Löffler 1956, Rossier und Mitarbeiter 1956, Martini und Feller 1956, *Editorial* Lancet 1956, Wenk 1957, Hadorn 1959.

[4] v. Hayek 1952.

[5] Rossier und Méan 1936, 1944, Bühlmann und Wegmann 1951, Wyss und Wilbrandt 1945, Buhr 1958.

eosinophile Leukocyten und in der Lichtung zähes schleimiges Sekret wie bei Asthma.

Die spastische Bronchitis soll auch häufig Silikosen begleiten, wesentlichen Anteil an der Einschränkung der ventilatorischen Funktion haben[1] und bronchographisch erfaßbar sein[2]. Die Frage des Zusammenhanges von spastischer Bronchitis und Staubinhalation wird noch diskutiert[3]. Besserung der Ventilationsleistung und Minderung des Röhrenwiderstandes unter Adrenalin-Medikation werden als Zeichen einer klinisch sonst symptomlosen spastischen Bronchitis angesehen (Bronchitis spastica inappercepta, ROSSIER).

Die spastische Bronchitis endet sehr oft mit einem Emphysem, das als Obstruktionsemphysem selbst bei großer Ausdehnung Herdcharakter behält. Die ungleichmäßige Belüftung der Lungen, die als Verteilungsstörung schon im Beginn des ganzen Prozesses besteht, bleibt bis in die Endphasen führend. Auch in der bereits blasig umgewandelten Lunge bleiben wenig veränderte Lungenbezirke zurück, deren Funktion in der trotz des Emphysems relativ guten globalen Retraktionsleistung der Leichenlunge zum Ausdruck kommt (siehe auch unter Obstruktionsemphysem).

δ) Die Bronchiolitis.

Jede Bronchitis geht in ihrer akuten Phase mit einer Schwellung, Hyperämie und zelligen Infiltration der Schleimhaut einher. Oft ist die Schwellung so stark, daß die Lichtung deutlich eingeengt wird. Die Störungen der Ventilation sind aber nach den klinischen Meßwerten noch gering, solange sich die Infiltration auf die größeren und mittleren Bronchien beschränkt und solange nicht Exsudat die Bronchien verschließt, wie es bei der descendierenden Diphtherie der Fall ist. Dann entstehen stets mehr oder minder ausgedehnte Atelektasen, ähnlich wie bei der einfachen Schleimobstruktion. Erst wenn große Lungenabschnitte von der Ventilation ausgeschlossen sind, folgen Überblähung der restlichen Lungenteile und ventilstenotische Effekte mit lokalem akutem Emphysem.

Anders liegen die Verhältnisse bei der Bronchiolitis. Schleimhautschwellungen in diesem Bereich können die Lichtung bis zum Verschluß einengen, Exsudat und Sekret sie völlig verschließen. Die Bronchiolitis, die ganz überwiegend durch Infektion mit Eitererregern oder Virus, seltener durch Inhalation reizender Gase ausgelöst wird, erstreckt sich immer über große Lungenabschnitte, oft über die ganzen Lungen. Die Bronchiolitis des Kindesalters, die sich an Masern, Keuchhusten und Scharlach anschließt, ist ein Beispiel dafür, ebenso die Bronchiolitis im Greisenalter, die sich oft bei einem Altersemphysem findet. Das, was im klinischen Sprachgebrauch als Emphysembronchitis bezeichnet wird, ist gewöhnlich eine Komplikationsbronchitis[4], die sich sekundär im Verlaufe eines Altersemphysems dann bildet, wenn der schwache Exspirationsstrom das Bronchialsekret nicht mehr herausschleudern kann und Infektionen zu der Sekretstauung hinzutreten.

Die Bronchiolen sind innerhalb der Lobuli im respiratorischen Gewebe verspannt, ihre äußeren Wandschichten gehen ohne Peribronchium in die Septen der Acini und anliegenden Alveolen über. Entzündliche Infiltrate, die sich in der

---

[1] ROSSIER, BUCHER und WIESINGER 1947 u. a., ausführliche Übersicht bei WORTH und SCHILLER 1954.

[2] F. K. FISCHER 1952.

[3] LUCHSINGER und BÜHLMANN 1953, PARRISIUS 1955, HUMPERDINCK 1955, 1956, CARSTENS 1955, 1956, 1957, 1958, GORALEWSKI 1956, GRONEMEYER 1956, WORTH und Mitarbeiter 1956, 1959, VALENTIN 1959, HUSTEN 1956, ZORN 1956, WEICKSEL und BRUGGER 1957, BOEMKE 1959; vgl. auch die Verhandlungen auf der III. Internat. Staublungentagung Münster 1957, Beiträge von HUSTEN, WORTH, SCHILLER, DEENSTRA, GIESE, GILSON, MEY, DÜNNER u. a.

[4] HARTUNG 1958, 1959. GIESE 1959.

Wand ausbreiten (intramurale Bronchiolitis), greifen deshalb leicht auf das interstitielle Lungengewebe über, ebenso auch entzündliche Prozesse, die im lockeren Mesenchym um die Bronchiolen als Peribronchiolitis beginnen. Auch an die Endobronchiolitis, die als katarrhalische Entzündung der Schleimhaut anfängt, schließt sich oft eine zellige Infiltration der übrigen Wandschichten an. Die Wandverdickung ist dabei so beträchtlich, daß die Bronchiolen schon makroskopisch als feine grauweiße Streifen oder im Querschnitt als stecknadelkopfgroße Pünktchen sichtbar werden. Beim Kinde hat ENGEL (1950) Verdickungen der Wand bis zu 1 mm und Einengungen der Lichtung auf 0,2—0,3 mm gemessen.

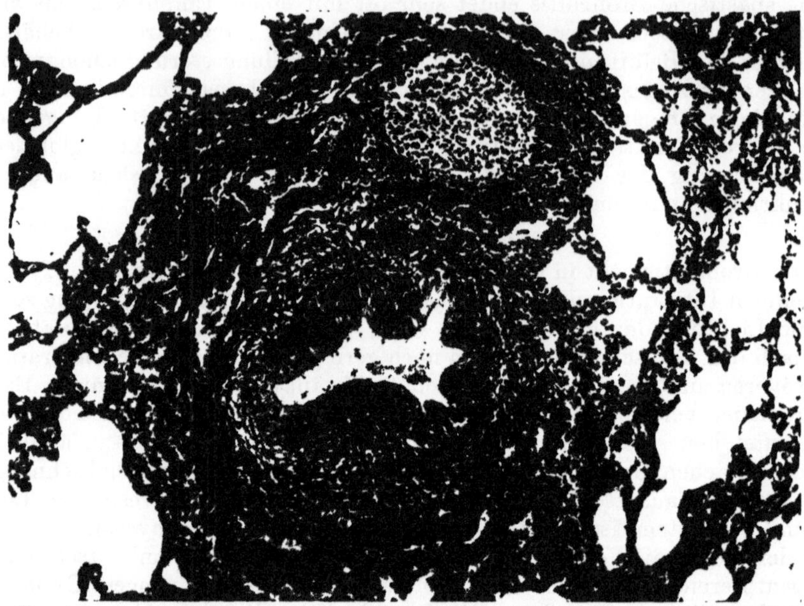

Abb. 46. Chronische Bronchiolitis und Peribronchiolitis nodularis. Lichtung des Bronchiolus lobularis durch Wandinfiltrate um mehr als die Hälfte eingeengt. Bronchiolostenotisches Emphysem. 5jähriges Kind. Kr. 2560/52.

In der subakuten und chronischen Bronchiolitis mit ihrer starken Zellproliferation schwinden die Muskelfasern und auch die elastischen Fasern. Im indifferenten Mesenchym der äußeren Wandschichten und in den anliegenden lymphoiden Zellhaufen bilden sich Lymphfollikel (Bronchiolitis nodularis), die die Bronchiolen komprimieren (Abb. 46). Bei der Bronchiolitis obliterans wächst Granulationsgewebe in die Lichtung, verschließt die Bronchioli terminales und oft auch die Bronchioli respiratorii.

Multiple, oft sehr zahlreiche Bronchiolostenosen und Obliterationen kommen bei Tuberkulose und Silikose vor. Bei der Tuberkulose komprimieren die im Peribronchium sich bildenden Tuberkel die Bronchiolen (Abb. 47), brechen in die Lichtung ein und verschließen die Bronchien auch bei narbiger Rückbildung. In silikotischen Knötchen wird die Wand der eingemauerten Bronchiolen völlig aufgelöst.

3. Chronische Stenosen und Obliteration der kleinen Bronchien und Bronchiolen.

Die chronische Bronchiolitis läuft oft in narbige Stenosierung oder Obliteration der Lichtung aus. Diese Bronchiolostenosen können über große Lungenabschnitte ausgedehnt sein, wie etwa bei der Bronchiolitis obliterans, oder auch nur auf einzelne Äste beschränkt bleiben.

α) *Obliteration und Stenose einzelner Bronchiolen.*

Hinter alten Verschlüssen von Lobularbronchien und Bronchiolen werden fast nie Atelektasen gefunden. Das Hauptbeispiel dafür sind die Restherde bronchogener und hämatogener tuberkulöser Streuungen in den Lungen. Das Granulationsgewebe der produktiven Peri- und Endobronchiolitis tuberculosa durchsetzt herdförmig die Wand der Bronchiolen und hinterläßt bei der Rückbildung, die heute an Resektionspräparaten in allen Stadien verfolgt werden kann, kleine

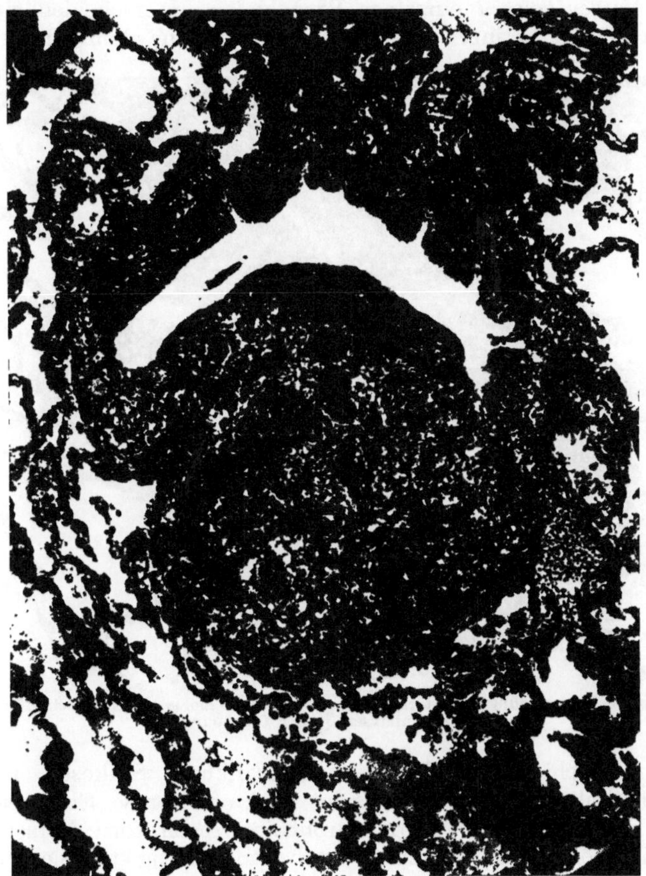

Abb. 47. Sichelförmige Kompression der Lichtung eines Bronchiolus durch einen Tuberkel. E.-Nr. 2127/57.

Narben, in denen kaum noch Reste des Bronchus erkennbar sind. Die Beziehungen zum Bronchiolus müssen in vielen Fällen erst aus der Topographie heraus erschlossen werden. Die Narben liegen zentrolobulär und verschließen je nach ihrer Größe einen wenige Millimeter langen Bronchusabschnitt. Oft obliteriert auch die zugehörige kleine Arterie. Die septalen Begrenzungen der Läppchen des Lungenmantels bleiben erhalten. Die Gänge des Arbor alveolaris werden von der schrumpfenden Narbe gestreckt, die Alveolen abgeflacht. Um die Narbe, die wie eine Spinne im Netz sitzt, bildet sich oft ein Kranz von kleinen Emphysembläschen (s. S. 493, Abb. 22 und 23). Das perinoduläre Emphysem bei der kleinknotigen Silikose entsteht in dieser Weise.

Selten liegt die Dehnungszone am Läppchenrand und bildet dort einen äußeren Kranz geblähter Alveolen, die den Septen unmittelbar anliegen. Loeschcke (1928) hat bereits einen entsprechenden Zustand abgebildet.

Das Ausbleiben der Atelektasen bei diesen Narbenverschlüssen läßt sich nur aus einer kollateralen Belüftung der poststenotischen Abschnitte erklären. Die Konfluenz von Alveolen und Alveolargängen benachbarter Acini ist in diesen Fällen an Schnittreihen nachzuweisen. An Ausgußpräparaten ist sie von Loeschcke (1921, 1928) bei Emphysem dargestellt worden.

Partielle Narbenstenosen einzelner Bronchiolen unterscheiden sich von den totalen Verschlüssen in ihren Folgeerscheinungen nur dem Grade nach. Bei

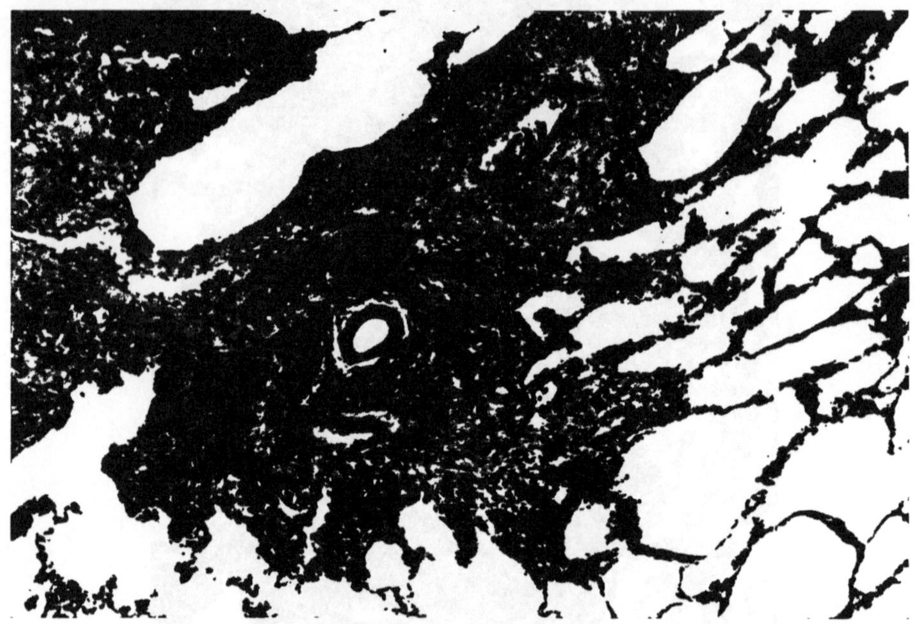

Abb. 48. Fibröse Einscheidung und starre Stenose eines Bronchiolus bei chronischer Bronchiolitis. Narbenemphysem in der Umgebung.

Tuberkulose, Bronchiektasen, Boeckscher Krankheit, Silikosen, interstitiellen Fibrosen und ähnlichen Prozessen findet man oft fibröse Einscheidungen der Bronchiolen, die sich auch auf die Bronchioli respiratorii fortsetzen können (Abb. 48). Die Bronchuslichtungen sind dabei hochgradig stenosiert, oft in kleine Sekundärlichtungen aufgesplittert und drüsenartig umgewandelt (Abb. 49). Der behinderte Luftwechsel ist an der Verkleinerung der zugehörigen Acini erkennbar. Ventileffekte scheinen selten zu sein, kommen aber vor und führen dann zum bronchostenotischen Emphysem, dessen Ausdehnung und Verteilung von dem Grundprozeß abhängig ist.

β) Bronchiolitis obliterans.

Bei der Bronchiolitis obliterans gewinnen diese Stenosen und Verschlüsse erhebliche Ausdehnung. Das Granulationsgewebe, das aus der Wand der entzündeten Bronchien in die Lichtung einwächst, verschließt diese vollständig. Die Verschlüsse sitzen fast stets in den Bronchioli terminales und reichen teilweise auch in die Bronchioli respiratorii hinein. Die Lichtung der Lobularbronchien bleibt meistens offen.

Durch diese Verschlüsse werden Lungenabschnitte von der Größe der Acini und Lobuli von der Luftzufuhr abgeschnitten. Die Erfahrung zeigt, daß hinter solchen absoluten Dauerverschlüssen nur selten Atelektasen liegen. Man findet sie fast nur, wenn das Alveolargerüst gleichzeitig durch eine interstitielle Entzündung sklerosiert oder wenn das Exsudat intraalveolärer Herdpneumonien karnifiziert ist.

Fast regelmäßig kommt es vielmehr zur kollateralen Belüftung von den Nachbaracini über erweiterte Kohnsche Poren. Die Lunge ist nach Abklingen der akuten Erscheinungen makroskopisch annähernd gleichmäßig lufthaltig, ihr Volumen insgesamt eher vermehrt. Aus der aufgeblähten Leichenlunge strömt

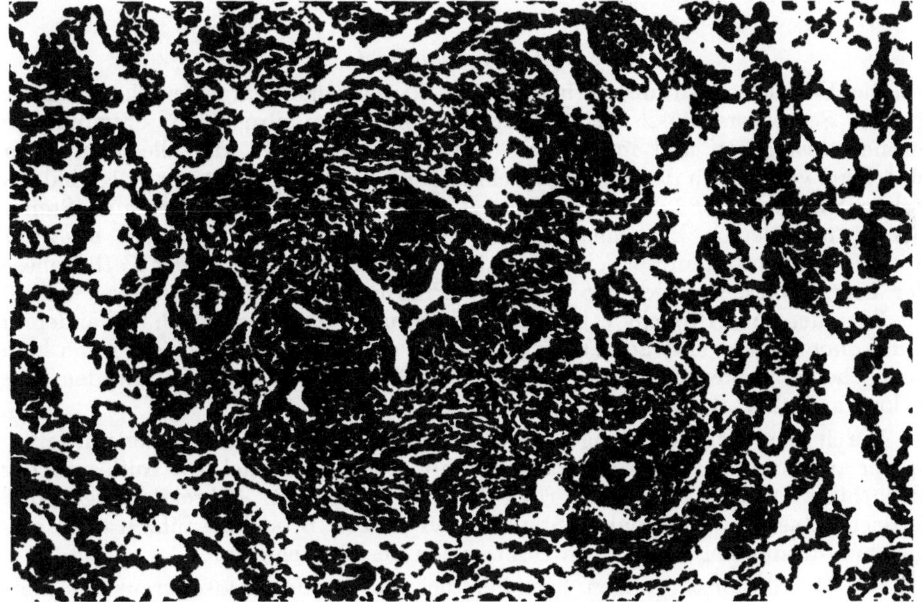

Abb. 49. Drüsenartige Aufsplitterung eines Bronchiolus terminalis bei chronischer Peribronchiolitis. Hypoventilation des umgebenden Gewebes. E.-Nr. 2218/57.

die Luft nach Freigabe des Bronchus aber ungleichmäßig ab, die Luftentleerung ist in den poststenotischen Abschnitten verzögert. Die Alveolen der kollateral belüfteten Acini sind durch die narbige Schrumpfung der obliterierten Bronchioli verzogen, ungleich groß und in der Nähe der Narben mit zusammenhängendem kubischem Epithel ausgekleidet. Ein Gasaustausch mit dem Blut findet an diesen Stellen nicht mehr statt. Die Arteriae terminales, die den obliterierten Bronchiolen anliegen, sind eng gestellt, Intimaproliferationen können ihre Lichtung stenosieren.

Diese sekundäre Pulmonalsklerose kann als Folge der im Interstitium ablaufenden begleitenden Peribronchiolitis oder als ausgleichende Intimaproliferation in funktionell ruhig gestellten Gefäßgebieten angesehen werden (siehe unter Kreislauf in Atelektase).

Als Folge des erhöhten Strömungswiderstandes ist bei ausgedehnter Bronchiolitis obliterans stets ein Cor pulmonale entwickelt.

Oft findet sich in den Endzuständen einer ausgedehnten Bronchiolitis obliterans auch ein Emphysem. Dieses ist teils hinter den Bronchiolostenosen, teils in den Abschnitten mit noch freien Bronchiolen lokalisiert und insoweit als kompensatorisches Emphysem aufzufassen.

Die funktionellen Auswirkungen der Bronchiolitis obliterans, deren Morphologie Behrens u. Fanconi (1958) kürzlich dargestellt haben, sind eine Vermehrung der Residualluft, eine Verminderung der Vitalkapazität und eine verzögerte Retraktion der Lunge, im wesentlichen also Störungen in der Ventilation, zu denen außerdem die Störungen der Lungenzirkulation hinzutreten. Der Atemgrenzwert kann bis auf ein Drittel eingeschränkt sein.

Ein bronchiolostenotisches Emphysem ist bei der Bronchiolitis obliterans vorwiegend kleinblasig. Die kleinen Blasen finden sich diffus verteilt im Lungenkern und im Lungenmantel. Ist die blasige Umwandlung ausgedehnt, dann entsteht eine Wabenlunge, die sich in ähnlicher Weise auch bei der muskulären Lungencirrhose und bei progressiver Lungenfibrose finden kann[1].

γ) Die Bronchiektasie.

Die Ventilationsstörungen bei Bronchiektasie sind komplexer Natur. Hier greifen Sekretverschlüsse der großen und mittleren Bronchien, entzündliche Bronchiolostenosen und interstitielle Fibrosen ineinander, die alle gemeinsam eine Hypoventilation der Lungenabschnitte mit Bronchiektasie zur Folge haben. Schon Reynaud (1835) fand bei der zylindrischen Bronchiektasie eine Stenosierung der kleinen Bronchien. Dieser Befund ist später wiederholt bestätigt worden und kann heute als ein wesentlicher kausaler Faktor in der Pathogenese der Bronchiektasen angesehen werden[2]. Proximal von den Bronchiolostenosen, die Residuen einer Bronchiolitis bei Masern, Keuchhusten, Scharlach und anderem sein können, staut sich Sekret vorwiegend in den basalen Bronchien, wenn kein ausreichend starker exspiratorischer Luftstoß aufgebracht wird, mit dem das Sekret ausgehustet werden kann.

Durch diese Sekretstauungen wird die chronische Entzündung der mittleren, später auch der großen Bronchien unterhalten, die schließlich zur Auflösung der Bronchialwand und zur Erweiterung der Lichtung führt. Sekretstauungen und Bronchiektasen bei hilusnahen Stenosen der großen Bronchien führen auch umgekehrt oft zu einer sekundären Obliteration der Bronchiolen.

Die Ventilationsstörungen betreffen bei der Bronchiektasenkrankheit stets große zusammenhängende Lungenabschnitte und unterscheiden sich dadurch erheblich von den bisher genannten Formen der disseminierten Bronchiolostenosen. Die Möglichkeit der kollateralen Ventilation wird mit zunehmender Zahl der obliterierten Bronchiolen und Sekretverstopfungen mittlerer Bronchien eingeschränkt. Fast nie bildet sich ein bronchostenotisches Emphysem und nur selten eine vollständige Atelektase, bevor die narbige Induration eingetreten ist.

Im Vordergrund steht vielmehr die Hypoventilation mit ihren Folgen für den Gasaustausch und vor allem für die Perfusion der erkrankten Lungenabschnitte. Nach klinischen Untersuchungen[3] fließt das Blut der Pulmonalarterien durch den bronchiektatischen Abschnitt langsamer als durch die gesunden Teile, die Perfusion von der Arteria pulmonalis her ist gedrosselt. Dagegen findet sich stets ein erheblicher Ausbau der Bronchialarterien, die in der Angiographie an Resektionspräparaten der Lunge weite sinusartige Gefäßgeflechte in der Bronchialwand bilden[4]. Ein vermehrter Einstrom von Bronchialarterienblut in die Arteria

---

[1] Meessen 1949, Hamman und Rich 1935, 1944, Haemmerli 1955, Behrens und Fanconi 1958.

[2] Rokitansky 1855, Churchill 1949, Feyrter 1925, Lüchtrath 1950, Galy 1953, Whitwell 1953, Duprez 1951, 1953, Giese 1954, Literatur bei Kartagener 1956.

[3] Bolt 1953, Bolt und Mitarbeiter 1957.   [4] Duprez 1956, Junghanss 1959.

pulmonalis durch die stark vermehrten Anastomosen zwischen Pulmonal- und Bronchialarterien wird angenommen[1]. MEESSEN (1951) spricht von Aortalisation der Lunge[2].

4. Die Kompressionsstenose.

Einengung der Bronchiallichtung als Folge eines von außen auf den Bronchiolus wirkenden Druckes kann organische oder funktionelle Ursachen haben.

Die organisch bedingten Kompressionen beruhen in der Hauptsache auf Schrumpfung peribronchiolärer Schwielen, die aus interstitiellen Herdpneumonien oder aus Granulomatosen (Boecksche Krankheit, Tuberkulose, Syphilis u. a.) entstehen. Ihre Ausdehnung kann bei Staubfibrosen der Lunge besonders groß werden. Unter den Mischstaublungen ist hier besonders die Anthrako-Silikose zu erwähnen, bei der große Staubdepots besonders um die Endabschnitte des Bronchialbaumes abgelagert werden und der Lunge das kleinfleckig schwarze Aussehen geben. Obwohl die Fibrose bei diesen Formen der Anthrakose wegen des geringen Anteils an Quarzstaub nur gering bleibt, kommt es doch zu einer Starre und relativen Kompression der Bronchiolen, deren rhythmische Weiteänderungen bei Inspiration und Exspiration behindert oder aufgehoben werden.

Eine *funktionelle Bronchiolostenose* entsteht, wenn in der Exspiration beträchtliche Druckdifferenzen zwischen Alveolarluft und Bronchuslichtung auftreten. Schon im normalen Exspirationsvorgang beruht die Engstellung der Bronchiolen auf dem Nachlassen des elastischen Lungenzuges und bei der forcierten Ausatmung auf dem positiv werdenden Pleuradruck, der sich auf die Lunge fortpflanzt. Den deutlichsten Ausdruck finden diese dynamischen Bronchiolostenosen in der Differenz zwischen inspiratorischem und exspiratorischem Tiffeneau-Test[3], die normal nur etwa 4% der Vitalkapazität ausmacht. Bei den starren Stenosen ist die Differenz eher vermindert, bei Asthma und Emphysem dagegen wegen des vermehrten Strömungswiderstandes erhöht. Die Differenz beträgt 15% bei leichtem und mittelschwerem Emphysem. Bei einer großen Zahl von Patienten mit schwerem Emphysem fand LICHTERFELD (1960) eine Herabminderung des Exspirationsstoßes um über 35% gegenüber einer fast normalen maximalen Inspirationsgröße.

Bei stärkeren Graden des diffusen Altersemphysems entstehen auf Grund dieser Mechanismen dynamische Ventilstenosen, die auch in ruhiger Exspiration wirksam werden. Die stark gedehnten, zu ungegliederten Luftsäckchen umgebauten Acini retrahieren sich wegen des Elastizitätsverlustes nur in geringem Maße. Die Luft wird durch die Anspannung der Exspirationsmuskulatur mehr oder weniger aus der Lunge ausgepreßt.

Die Bronchiolen, die in den emphysematös umgebauten Acini mit Schwund der septalen Innengliederung auch ihre Verspannungen verloren haben, kollabieren und schließen sich ventilartig mit Einsetzen der Kompression. Die Luft bleibt in den emphysematösen Acini gefangen („air trapping")[4]. Dieser Vorgang wird besonders in den vorderen Lungenrändern wirksam[5] und führt zur blasigen Überformung des ursprünglich gleichmäßigen vesiculären Emphysems[6].

Die funktionelle Ventilstenose ist postmortal an der entspannten Lunge wegen des erfolgten Druckausgleiches nicht zu sehen, im Tiffeneau-Test an der Leichenlunge aber aus dem Verlauf der Exspirationskurve nachweisbar[7].

---

[1] CUDKOWICZ und ARMSTRONG 1953, ARMSTRONG und CUDKOWICZ 1958, LIEBOW und Mitarbeiter 1949, DELARUE 1954, DUPREZ 1956, ADEBAHR 1955, DELARUE und ABELANET 1956, 1959.

[2] SCHOENMACKERS und VIETEN 1952, 1958.   [3] WYSS 1955, LICHTERFELD 1960.

[4] FRY und Mitarbeiter 1954 u. a.   [5] ROHRER 1915, 1925.   [6] HARTUNG 1958.

[7] HARTUNG 1959.

Die Ventilationsleistung mancher Emphysemkranker bessert sich, wenn sie gegen einen Widerstand ausatmen. Dabei steigt der intrabronchiale Druck und verhindert den völligen Ventilschluß des Bronchiolus terminalis.

c) Folgen von Bronchiolostenosen oder Verschlüssen für die Lungenbelüftung.

Jede Änderung der Lichtungsweite einzelner oder zahlreicher Bronchiolen, jede funktionelle Störung der Bronchomotorik behindert die gleichmäßige Belüftung der Lunge und führt zur ventilatorischen Verteilungsstörung (Distributionsstörung), deren Pathophysiologie bereits bei den Stenosen der großen und mittleren Bronchien besprochen wurde (s. S. 485). Die gleichen Vorgänge, die dort an Lappensegmenten und Subsegmenten zur Auswirkung kamen, wiederholen sich hier an den kleinen und kleinsten Lungeneinheiten, nämlich an den Lobuli und Acini.

Die örtlichen Folgen sind abhängig vom Grad und vor allem von der Art der Stenose, die wir hier wie dort in starre Stenose, Ventilstenose und völligen Verschluß unterteilen. Der Zeitfaktor spielt darüber hinaus insofern eine Rolle, als akute Stenosen von kurzer Dauer in ihren Auswirkungen sich unterscheiden von chronischen persistierenden Änderungen der Lichtungsweite. Die Folgen oft rezidivierender akuter Stenosen, z. B. bei Asthma bronchiale und bei spastischer Bronchitis reichen schließlich auch in das Intervall hinein.

Die Spielbreite der konsekutiven Funktionsstörungen wird durch das wechselnde Ineinandergreifen der verschiedenen pathogenetischen Faktoren wesentlich größer als bei Stenosen der oberen und mittleren Luftwege. Je weiter die Stenosen in die Peripherie des Bronchialbaumes rücken, um so bunter und vielfältiger werden ihre Folgeerscheinungen[1].

Von Bronchostenose wird oft auch dann gesprochen, wenn es sich um Folgen einer Bronchiolostenose handelt. Sie können sich äußern als Atelektase mit völliger Luftleere, als Dystelektasen mit vermindertem Luftgehalt und als Emphysem mit vermehrtem Luftgehalt der poststenotischen Abschnitte.

Diese Zustände sind stets herdförmig und stets herdbezogen, also abhängig von Ort und Art der Bronchostenose. Sie können an der Leichenlunge unter den dort gegebenen statischen Bedingungen klar erfaßt und in ihrer Größe bestimmt werden. Ihre funktionelle Bedeutung im Rahmen der örtlichen Ventilation, d. h. des Luftwechsels oder der Belüftung der poststenotischen Abschnitte läßt sich als dynamische Größe nur in groben Zügen abschätzen. Das gilt nicht nur für die Morphologie, sondern auch für die Klinik, mit deren Methoden wohl sehr genaue Bestimmungen der globalen Werte der ganzen Lunge oder großer Lungenteile vorgenommen werden können, die aber für die Funktionsanalyse der hier zur Diskussion stehenden kleinen Abschnitte in der Größenordnung der Lobuli und Acini nicht ausreichen.

Wir dürfen davon ausgehen, daß in diesem Rahmen funktionell zwei in ihrer Folge differente Funktionsstörungen unterschieden werden können. Nämlich 1. die Nichtbelüftung (Nonaeration), deren Ausdruck die vollständige Atelektase ist, und 2. die mangelhafte Belüftung (Hypoventilation), die sowohl zur Dystelektase als auch zum bronchostenotischen Emphysem gehört.

1. Die bronchiolostenotische Atelektase.

Eine bronchiolostenotische Atelektase entsteht fast nur beim akuten vollständigen Verschluß eines Bronchiolus oder eines kleinen Bronchus. Bei erhaltener Zirkulation, die Voraussetzung für die Absorption der Gase aus der Alveolarluft

---

[1] Giese 1960, Hartung 1960.

ist, entwickelt sich in Minuten, längstens bis zu einer Stunde ein vollständiger Kollaps von Acini oder von Lobuli[1]. Das Blut, das durch die Atelektasezone fließt, nimmt nicht am Gasaustausch teil und erscheint als venöse Beimischung im großen Kreislauf.

Da sich bei der Bronchiolitis stets zahlreiche Sekretverschlüsse in den End-ästen des Bronchialbaumes bilden, entstehen auch viele Atelektasen, die vor-wiegend im Lungenmantel und dort besonders in den paravertebralen und dorso-basalen Lungenabschnit-ten liegen. Durch die Summation der vielen kleinen Atelektasen wer-den beträchtliche Lun-genabschnitte von der Ventilation ausgeschlos-sen. Die Reduktion der Atemfläche kann so groß werden, daß schwere Grade von Dyspnoe und Cyanose, ja selbst Erstik-kung eintreten. Bei aus-gedehnten Atelektasen kommt oft eine kompen-satorische Überblähung der Lungenabschnitte hinzu, deren Luftwege noch frei durchgängig sind (Abb. 50).

Die kleinherdigen Atelektasen sind stets reversibel, solange keine Pneumonie hinzutritt. Sie bilden sich nach Lö-sung des Verschlusses sofort zurück, oft genügt eine tiefe Inspiration oder ein Hustenstoß.

Sie verschwinden aber auch, wenn der Verschluß durch Obli-teration des Bronchiolus chronisch wird. Das

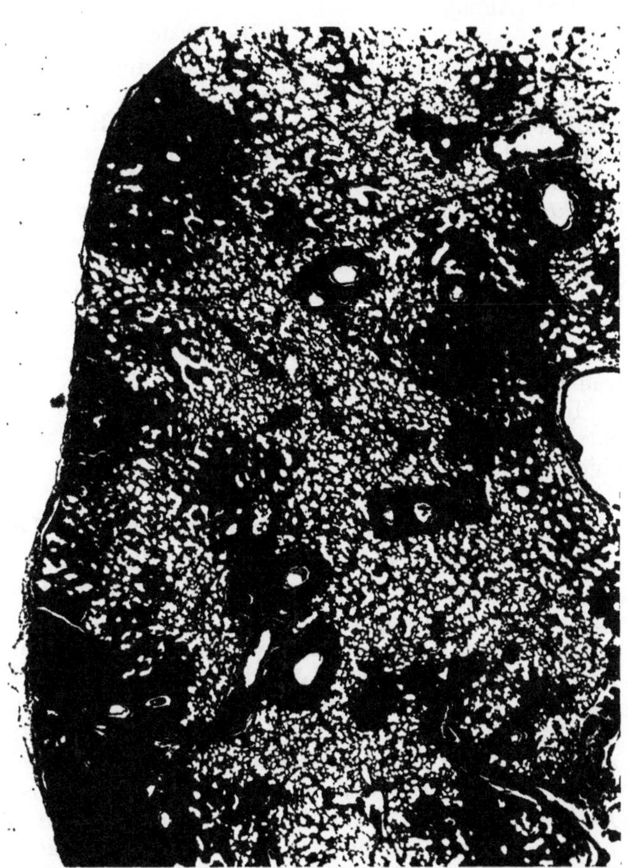

Abb. 50. Ventilatorische Verteilungsstörung. Kleinfleckige Atelektasen und Dystelektasen neben akuter Überblähung bei Bronchiolitis und Keuchhustenpneumonie. 13 Monate altes Kind. S.-Nr. 57/52.

hinter einem alten Bronchiolusverschluß liegende Lungengewebe wird allmählich wieder von Nachbaracini über Kohnsche Poren kollateral belüftet. Die inspira-torische Belüftung ist gegenüber dem benachbarten Lungengewebe mit freien Bronchiolen verzögert, die Entfaltung oft unvollständig. Ebenso hinkt auch die Entlüftung in der Exspirationsphase nach. Diesen Vorgang, der am Lebenden mit Fremdgasmethoden gemessen werden kann, bezeichnen MATTHES u. ULMER (1957) als sukzessive Verteilungsstörung[2]. Bei der Exspiration erscheint zunächst die Luft aus den Lungenabschnitten mit freien Luftwegen, der sich zuletzt die Luft aus den kollateral ventilierten Teilen beimischt. Die verzögerte Auffüllung

---

[1] H. H. LOESCHCKE 1956.   [2] ULMER 1955, 1956, MATTHES, ULMER und WITTEKIND 1959.

und Entleerung poststenotischer Abschnitte läßt sich auch an der Leichenlunge nachweisen.

In den chronisch hypoventilierten, poststenotischen Lungenabschnitten wird stets auch die Perfusion reduziert. Dadurch wird der Anteil der venösen Beimischung geringer als in der akuten Atelektase, es steigt aber der Widerstand im kleinen Kreislauf durch die reflektorische Engstellung der Arteriolen im Bereich der Hypoventilation an. Darum folgt ausgedehnten Bronchiolostenosen so oft das Cor pulmonale.

2. Die Dystelektasen.

Die Dystelektase ist Folge unvollständiger Verschlüsse von Bronchiolen und kleinen Bronchien. Sie bildet sich akut bei eitrig-katarrhalischer Bronchiolitis, ist oft deutlich lobulär angeordnet und in der Regel mit kleinherdigen Atelektasen kombiniert. Ihre chronischen Formen finden sich bei starrer Bronchiolostenose.

Unter Dystelektase versteht Engel (1950) Zustände von Hypoventilation mit konzentrischer Verkleinerung der Acini und Alveolen. Die Stenose läßt inspiratorisch nicht so viel Luft hindurchtreten, wie für die ausreichende Belüftung notwendig ist, während die Exspiration weniger behindert ist. Die Dystelektasen sind, ähnlich wie die bronchiolostenotischen Atelektasen, im Lungenmantel lokalisiert und dort vorwiegend auf die paravertebralen Abschnitte verteilt. Sie bilden sich ganz bevorzugt an solchen Stellen, die schon unter normalen Verhältnissen weniger gut belüftet sind.

In ihren weiteren Folgen sind die auf der Basis chronischer Bronchiolostenosen entstandenen Dystelektasen den Endzuständen alter Obliterationen von Bronchiolen gleichzusetzen.

3. Strömungswiderstände im Bronchialbaum und Lokalisation des Emphysems.

Die bevorzugte Lokalisation des Emphysems in den Lungenrändern und in der Lungenspitze erklärt Rohrer (1915) aus Änderungen des Strömungswiderstandes in den Bronchien.

Die zentral liegenden Läppchen münden fast unmittelbar in einen größeren Bronchus, die peripheren Läppchen hängen an den Endabschnitten des vielfach verzweigten, immer enger werdenden Bronchialbaumes. Der Strömungswiderstand für die Atemluft ist bis zu den peripheren Läppchen doppelt so groß wie zu den zentralen[1]. In den peripheren Läppchen herrscht inspiratorisch der stärkste Unterdruck, exspiratorisch der höchste Überdruck. Die Druckamplitude im Atemcyclus ist hier also höher als in den zentralen Läppchen.

Beim Hustenstoß, bei dem unter hohen Druck gesetzte Luft in der Lunge durch Öffnen der Stimmritze plötzlich ausströmt, entleeren sich wegen des geringeren Strömungswiderstandes zunächst die zentral liegenden Läppchen, während das Volumen der Außenläppchen infolge des darin herrschenden Überdruckes im Laufe des Hustenstoßes noch zunimmt. Die Spitzenaufhellung beim Husten (Kreuzfuchs-Phänomen) wird darauf bezogen.

Bei einer Bronchiolitis ist der Strömungswiderstand zu den äußeren Läppchen um ein Vielfaches höher als zu den zentralen. Daraus ergeben sich große Druckschwankungen, die nach der Ansicht von Rohrer (1915) direkt oder durch Zirkulationsstörungen eine Atrophie der Septen verursachen und so die Entwicklung eines Emphysems fördern.

Alle Zustände, bei denen die Lichtung der Bronchien funktionell durch Bronchokonstriktion (spastische Bronchitis), durch vermehrte Bildung eines hochviscösen Sekrets (Asthma bronchiale) oder durch organische Wandveränderungen

---

[1] Rohrer 1915.

eng gestellt wird, erhöhen die Strömungswiderstände und müssen nach der Vorstellung von ROHRER (1915) zum mindesten als wichtige Teilfaktoren unter den Ursachen des Emphysems angesehen werden.

4. Das bronchiolostenotische Emphysem.

Bei Stenosen kleiner Bronchien und Bronchiolen entwickeln sich oft Ventilmechanismen, die durch Obstruktion der Lichtung, durch organische Wandveränderungen oder durch Kompression entstehen können.

Jedes inspiratorisch wirkende Ventil führt zur Minderbelüftung und schließlich zur Atelektase des poststenotischen Abschnittes.

Bei exspiratorisch wirksamem Ventil füllt sich der poststenotische Abschnitt in der Inspiration mit Luft, die in der Exspiration auf dem Bronchialweg nicht ausströmen kann. Hinter der Stenose kommt es zu einer Luftstauung, in deren Bereich das Fasergerüst der Acini in Dauerspannung gehalten wird. Diese ist in der Inspirationsphase eine Zugspannung, deren übliche Angriffsfläche die Außenwand der Acini und Alveolen ist. In der Exspirationsphase wird sie zu einer Druckspannung, da mit dem Beginn der Exspirationsphase der Dehnungszug nachläßt und nun ein positiver intraalveolärer Druck entsteht, der bei Ruheatmung seinen höchsten Wert im Ende der Exspiration erreicht und bei Anspannung der Exspirationsmuskulatur noch um den positiven Intrapleuraldruck gesteigert werden kann.

α) Die Morphologie des bronchiolostenotischen Emphysems.

Anhaltende Dehnung und Überdehnung mindert die elastischen Eigenschaften des Fasergeflechtes in der Lunge. Der Dehnungsrückstand wird bei Druckentlastung zunehmend größer, die elastische Retraktionskraft nimmt ab. Das Fasersystem paßt sich dem höheren Dehnungsniveau an, das bei inkompletter Ventilwirkung allmählich, bei plötzlich einsetzendem und vollständigem Ventilmechanismus rasch an die obere Grenze der Dehnbarkeit verlagert wird. Das Fasersystem verliert schließlich seine elastischen Eigenschaften.

Die Funktionseinbuße geht einher mit einem Umbau der Acinusstruktur, die sich in wesentlichen Punkten vom senilen Emphysem so deutlich unterscheidet, daß man den bronchostenotischen Ventileffekt aus der veränderten Lungenstruktur mikroskopisch und oft auch schon makroskopisch ablesen kann.

1. Das akute bronchiolostenotische Emphysem. Bei der akuten obstruktiven Bronchostenose, die im Verlaufe eines Asthma bronchiale, einer spastischen Bronchitis, einer schleimig-eitrigen oder einer fibrinösen Bronchiolitis auftritt, werden die Sekretverschlüsse zahlreicher Bronchiolen durch angestrengte und vertiefte Inspiration gesprengt. Die luftgefüllten, überdehnten poststenotischen Lungenbezirke bleiben infolge der exspiratorischen Ventilwirkung auch an der isolierten und kollabierten Leichenlunge in ihrer Form erhalten.

Oft sind nur einzelne Acini, mitunter auch Acinusgruppen und im akuten Asthmaanfall fast die ganze Lunge überbläht. Die Schleim- und Sekretpfröpfe füllen dabei stets die Bronchioli terminales aus, in denen der Ventilmechanismus lokalisiert ist. Die Luftstauung im Acinus erweitert bei der akuten Obstruktion vor allem den Arbor alveolaris, der mit dem Bronchiolus respiratorius I beginnt und in den Alveolargängen endet. Die schwächste Stelle dieses Gangsystems ist der Raum, in dem die rasch aufeinanderfolgenden Teilungen der Bronchioli respiratorii I.—III. Ordnung stattfinden. Hier bilden sich bei positivem intraacinösem Druck blasige Erweiterungen, die LOESCHCKE (1928) als Emphysema bronchiolectaticum bezeichnet hat. Die in die Bronchioli respiratorii hineinreichenden Sekretpfröpfe werden durch den positiven intraacinösen Luftdruck eingedellt (s. Abb. 45, S. 513). Die Alveolarstruktur bleibt erhalten. Das akute Emphysema bronchiolectaticum ist reversibel, wenn der Ventilverschluß schwindet.

Bei ausgedehnten Atelektasen kommt schließlich eine kompensatorische Überblähung der Lungenabschnitte hinzu, deren Luftwege noch frei durchgängig sind.

Eine häufige Komplikation dieser akuten Überdehnungen ist das interstitielle Emphysem. Dieses entsteht, wenn durch Dehnungsrisse der Alveolarwände Luft in das Interstitium eingesogen oder eingepreßt wird. Die einmal in das Interstitium gelangte Luft wird wahrscheinlich in der Phase des positiven Exspirationsdruckes weitergeschoben und kann auf diese Weise in die Pleura, in das Mediastinum und über das Jugulum in die Subcutis gelangen.

Voraussetzung für die Entstehung des interstitiellen Emphysems sind stets ungewöhnlich hohe intraalveoläre Drucke, die vorwiegend bei Ventilstenosen entstehen.

2. Das chronische bronchiolostenotische Emphysem. Voraussetzung für die Entwicklung eines chronischen bronchiolostenotischen Emphysems ist stets ein Ventilmechanismus, der während der Inspiration Luft in den poststenotischen Abschnitt eintreten läßt, aber den exspiratorischen Abstrom behindert oder völlig aufhebt.

Alle Emphyseme, die auf Grund exspirationshemmender Ventilmechanismen entstehen, sind herdförmig und bilden einzelne oder in Gruppen angeordnete, oft kugelige Bläschen. Diese liegen im Beginn ihrer Entwicklung stets im Stamm des Arbor alveolaris, also an der gleichen Stelle, an der sich beim senilen Emphysem das erweiterte Atrium und beim akuten obstruktiven Ventilverschluß das Emphysema bronchiolectaticum bildet. Das Ventil sitzt in der Regel im Bronchiolus terminalis, selten im Bronchiolus lobularis.

Die Bläschen vergrößern sich allmählich durch Dehnung der Wand und durch langsame Ausweitung der Alveolargänge. Reste von Alveolargängen mit den dazugehörigen Alveolen sind oft noch bei erbsen- bis bohnengroßen Emphysemblasen am Rand des Acinus zu finden. Von dieser Größe an setzt sich die Dehnung auch auf die Septen der Acini fort, die bogenförmig ausgebuchtet und durch Erweiterung der Kohnschen Poren gefenstert werden. Durch Verschmelzung benachbarter Acini können schließlich ganze Lobuli zu ständig größer werdenden Blasen umgebildet werden, in denen Reste des Gefäßsystems erhalten bleiben, während das Gangsystem des Arbor alveolaris völlig verschwindet und auch Teile der Bronchioli terminales abgebaut werden (Abb. 51).

Die kleinen Blasen haben eine sehr dünne, durchscheinende Wand. Bei größeren Blasen wird die Wand durch Anteile der Lobularsepten und durch angrenzende Atelektasestreifen dicker, oft milchig-weiß.

Bronchostenotische Blasen sind entsprechend der an den Endabschnitten des Bronchialbaumes ablaufenden Grundkrankheit (Bronchiolitis, Peribronchiolitis) unregelmäßig über die ganze Lunge verstreut, im Lungenmantel aber zahlreicher als im Lungenkern. Im Lungenkern erreichen sie selten mehr als Haselnußgröße. Subpleural können durch allmähliche excessive Dehnung der Pleura apfel- bis faustgroße Blasen entstehen und durch Verdrängung des benachbarten Lungengewebes wie ein intrapulmonaler Pneumothorax wirken[1]. Bronchographische Analysen an der Leichenlunge erlauben die Aussage, daß auch die großen Blasen aus kleinen Lungeneinheiten, in der Regel aus Lobuli hervorgehen[2]. Ebenso

---

[1] West und Mitarbeiter 1951.   [2] Hartung 1958.

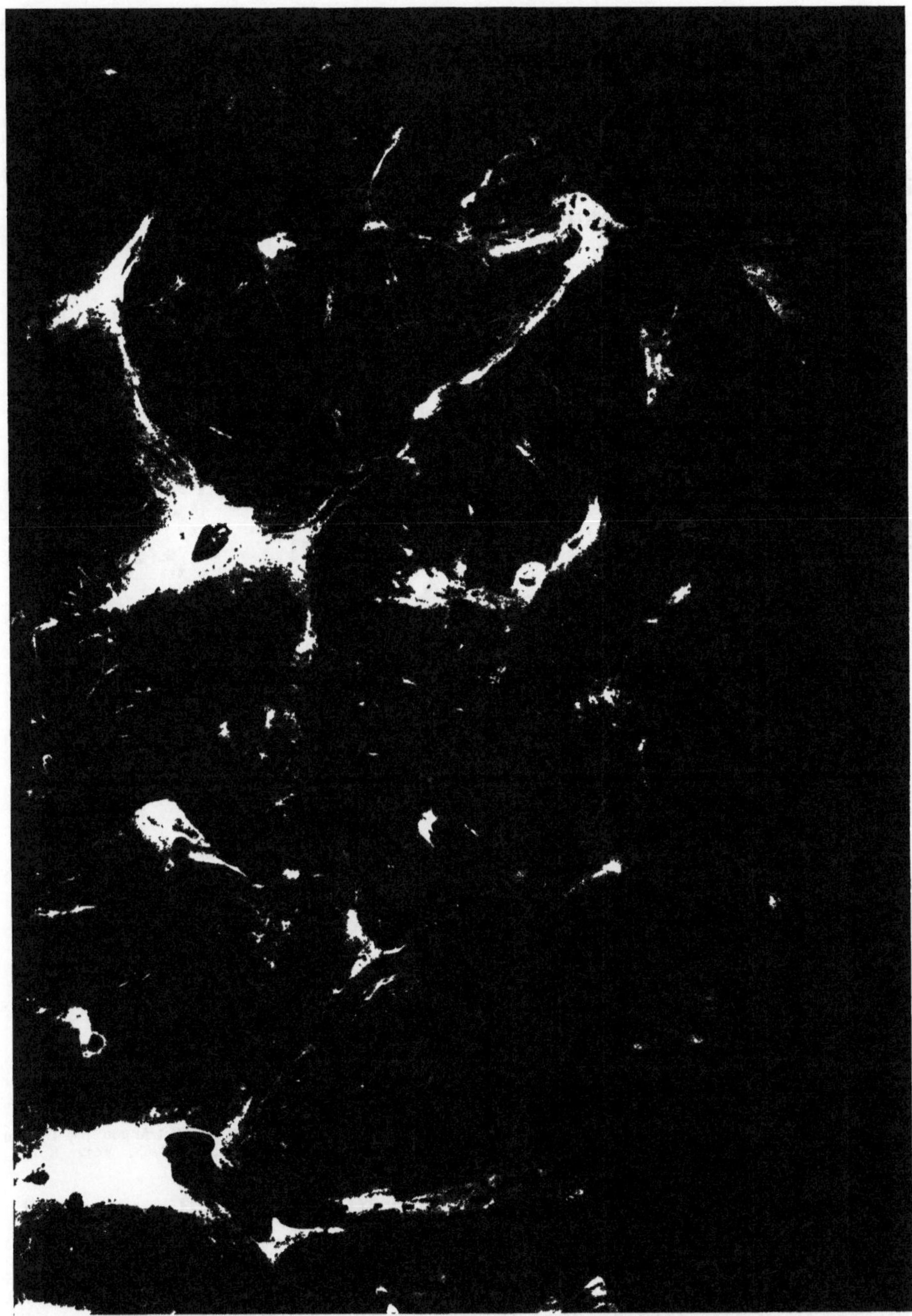

Abb. 51. Lobulär gebundenes bronchiolostenotisches Emphysem. Zentral in den Läppchen Lobulararterien und Bronchiolus lobularis, in den Septen Anschnitte von Venen. S.-Nr. 96/59. Vergr. 3fach.

läßt sich auch bei postmortaler Angiographie nachweisen, daß keine der Blasengröße entsprechende Reduktion von Lungenparenchym erfolgt ist. Man kann die bronchostenotischen großblasigen Umwandlungen der Lunge also nicht als

Lungendystrophie bezeichnen (über die Beziehungen zwischen großblasigem Lungenemphysem und progressiver Lungendystrophie[1]).

β) Die Pathogenese des bronchiolostenotischen Emphysems.

Die ersten eingehenden Untersuchungen zur Frage der Beziehungen zwischen Ventilstenose der Bronchien und Emphysem stammen von Hayashi (1915), der sich bereits auf frühere Hinweise[2] stützt. Ribbert (1916) hat den Ventilmechanismus als entscheidenden Faktor für die Genese aller Emphyseme angesehen.

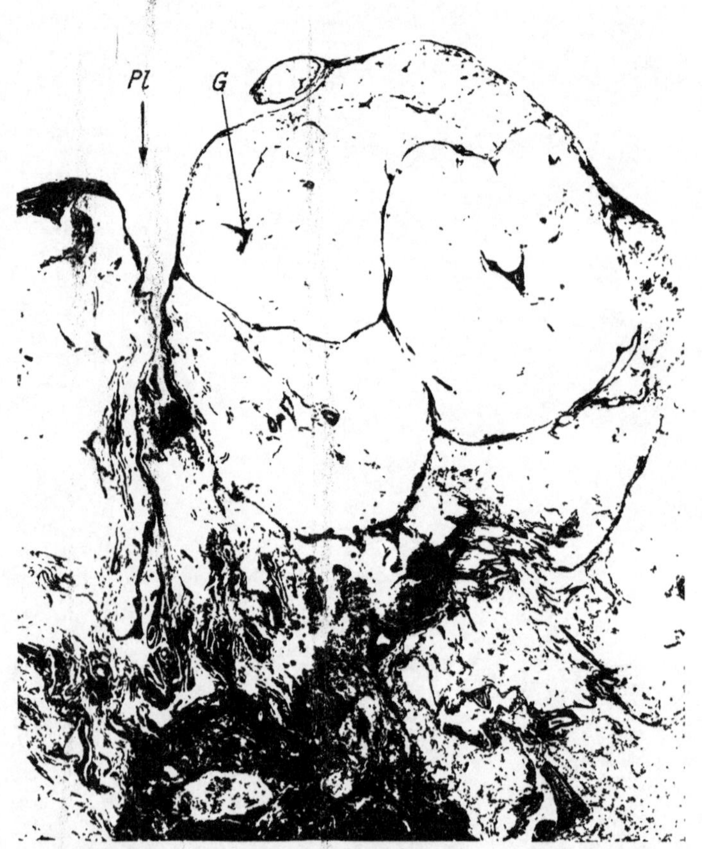

Abb. 52. Blasiges Spitzenemphysem über tuberkulosilikotischer Narbe. Reste von Gefäßsträngen (G) in den überblähten strukturlosen Acini. Einziehung der Pleura (Pl) über der Narbe. S.-Nr. 134/58. Vergr. 3:1.

Dieser Verallgemeinerung hat v. Hansemann (1916) unter Hinweis auf die Untersuchungen von Freund (1906) widersprochen. Auch die späteren Untersuchungen von Loeschcke (1928) zeigen ebenso wie unsere eigenen Befunde, daß eine solche Verallgemeinerung nicht zulässig ist, daß aber die These von Ribbert (1916) für einen beträchtlichen Teil der Emphyseme zutrifft.

1. Bei *kompletter Ventilstenose* füllt sich die poststenotische Blase in der Inspiration und retiniert die Luft. Solange die Blasenwand allseitig geschlossen und

---

[1] Crenshaw 1954, Heilmeyer und Schmid 1956, Trimble 1954, Uehlinger 1957, Heine 1958, Hartung 1958.
[2] Rokitansky 1855, Birch-Hirschfeld 1887, Orth 1905 und Orsós 1907.

noch nicht gefenstert ist, verringert sich die retinierte Luft nur um den Anteil, der von der Blasenwand absorbiert wird.

An der isolierten Lunge sind die Blasen, die Bohnen- bis Kirschgröße erreichen können, daran zu erkennen, daß sie in der kollabierten Lunge bestehen bleiben, sich auch durch Kompression nicht entleeren lassen und bei Anwendung starken Druckes platzen (Abb. 52).

Auch spontane Rupturen solcher Blasen, die sich bevorzugt im Bereich indurierender oder vernarbender Spitzentuberkulosen bilden[1], kommen vor und führen bei subpleuralem Sitz zum Spontanpneumothorax (Abb. 53). KENÉZ, PAPP u. VINCZE (1957) haben entsprechende Befunde an Resektionspräparaten beschrieben.

Über die Druckverhältnisse in diesen allseitig geschlossenen Blasen mit vollständiger Ventilwirkung liegen noch keine Messungen vor. Man darf annehmen, daß der intrabullöse Druck in der Exspiration positiv wird, sobald in den Alveolarräumen und Bronchien der Nachbarschaft die Umkehr vom negativen Inspirationsdruck zum positiven Exspirationsdruck erfolgt[2]. Man muß nach Modellversuchen an Gummiballons[3] sogar damit rechnen, daß nach der Druckumkehr im Bron-

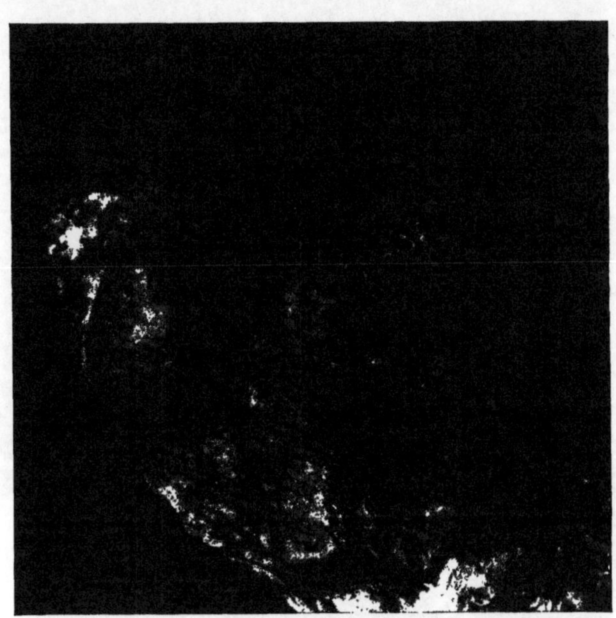

Abb. 53. Isolierte Emphysemblase subpleural am Lappenrand bei Ventilstenose des zugehörigen Bronchiolus. S.-Nr. 58/57.

chialbaum eine Nachdehung der Emphysemblase eintritt, die so stark werden kann, daß die am stenosierten Schenkel hängende Blase platzt. Das wird auch bei Hustenstößen der Fall sein können.

Die allmähliche Vergrößerung der poststenotischen Emphysemblase wird auch damit erklärt, daß der Innendruck einer Blase in umgekehrtem Verhältnis zu ihrem Radius steht (Gesetz von LAPLACE). Je größer der Radius, um so größer wird die Summe der Flächendrucke, die auf ihre Innenwand einwirkt[4]. GOUGH sieht in diesem Druckzuwachs die Ursache sämtlicher blasigen Emphyseme[5]. Auch HEPPLESTON (1953) unterscheidet neben dem zentrolobulären Emphysem ventilstenotische Emphysemblasen.

2. Nur ein kleiner Teil bronchostenotischer Emphysemblasen ist vollständig in sich abgeschlossen (Abb. 54). Die Mehrzahl der Blasen, insbesondere alle großblasigen Emphyseme, haben entweder unvollständig schließende Ventilstenosen oder zusätzliche Verbindungen zur Nachbarschaft (kollaterale Ventilation). Sie sind an der herausgenommenen Lunge daran zu erkennen, daß sich die Luft aus

---

[1] B. FISCHER 1922.　　[2] GONZALES DE VEGA 1951.
[3] ROHRER 1925, EISENREICH 1953, RAU und Mitarbeiter 1957, HEINE 1960 u. a.
[4] GREEN und SHIELD 1950, LENGGENHAGER 1952.
[5] GOUGH 1952, LEOPOLD und GOUGH 1957.

ihnen auspressen läßt oder auch spontan entweicht. Die Entleerung erfolgt aber
stets verzögert gegenüber den Nachbarabschnitten. Die verzögerte Entleerung
läßt sich einfach nachweisen, indem man die isolierte Lunge vom Bronchus her

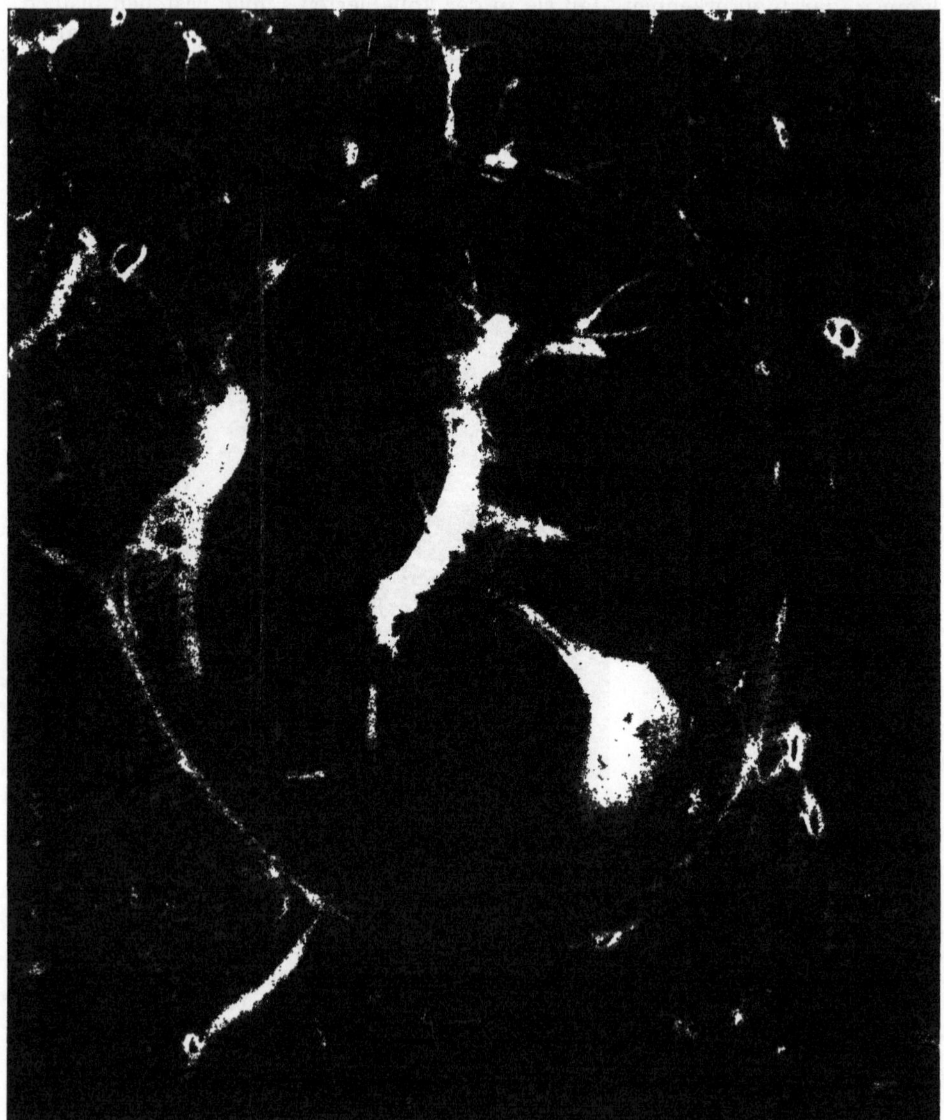

Abb. 54. Isolierte abgeschlossene Emphysemblase eines Acinus mit Rest des Gefäßstieles und Verdrängung des
umgebenden Lungengewebes. Normale Struktur der benachbarten Acini. Enge Ductus alveolares bei post-
mortalem Lungenkollaps. Alveolarstruktur eben erkennbar. S.-Nr. 30/59. Vergr. 7fach (vgl. auch Abb. 3, S. 416).

aufbläst und dann nach Freigabe des Bronchus kollabieren läßt. Die broncho-
stenotischen Blasen bleiben zunächst stehen, verlieren dann aber zunehmend an
Luft. Eine der Ursachen für diesen verzögerten Luftabstrom ist die kollaterale
Ventilation.

HAYASHI (1915) fand bei seinen Untersuchungen des Blasenemphysems
bereits Kommunikationen der Blasen zu belüfteten Nachbargebieten. In seinen

Abbildungen zeigt er kulissenartig hintereinander geschaltete Septen, die er als Klappenbildungen der Zuleitungsbronchien deutet, die man aber in gleicher Weise auch bei Septumfensterung im Rahmen eines senil atrophischen Emphysems finden kann. Die Wand der meisten Emphysemblasen wird teils von Pleura und von Lobularsepten, teils von atelektatischem oder minderbelüftetem Lungengewebe gebildet. Durch Fenster in den Septen und durch die Atelektasezone wird der poststenotische Luftraum hilfsweise, aber nur verzögert und ungenügend entlüftet.

Trotz der Nebenwege bleibt stets eine poststenotische Luftretention, die eine Entspannung der Blasenwand verhindert und Druckdifferenzen zwischen Blase und benachbartem Lungengewebe aufrechterhält. Diese Druckdifferenzen werden um so größer sein, je schlechter die kollaterale Entlüftung ist. Bei frühzeitig eintretender und guter kollateraler Entlüftung kann die Blasenbildung ausbleiben.

Ob für das Wachstum von Emphysemblasen mit kollateraler Entlüftung positive Innendrucke notwendig sind, ist noch umstritten. Intravitale Messungen hierzu liegen am großblasigen Lungenemphysem vor. HAAHTI (1932) fand bei einem Fall intrapleural einen Druck von —12 cm H_2O, in der Blase Drucke zwischen —5 und —3 cm H_2O, die auch nach Absaugen von 750 ml Luft konstant blieben. Ähnlich auch KOROL u. ENSIGN (1934). HEILMEYER u. SCHMID (1956) sowie HAUSSER u. GRIMMINGER (1957) bestimmten Drucke um den Nullwert, die nur um wenige Zentimeter H_2O in der Exspiration überschritten wurden.

Nennenswerte positive Drucke werden in den Blasen bei ruhiger Atmung also nicht entstehen. Sie sind nach dem morphologischen Befund bei negativen Pleuradrucken auch nicht zu erwarten, da die Wände der großen Blasen fast alle elastischen Fasern verloren haben und deshalb auch keine eigene Retraktionskraft mehr entwickeln. Die Blasenwand, die in ihrem größten Umfang aus kollagenem Fasergewebe besteht, wird in der Exspiration nur noch von der elastischen Retraktion des angrenzenden Lungengewebes mitgenommen.

Damit steht auch die Beobachtung in Einklang, daß die vorwiegend subpleural sitzenden Riesenblasen, deren größter Wandanteil von den kollagenen Faserzügen der gedehnten Pleura gebildet wird, keinen nennenswerten Luftwechsel haben[1]. Kollagenes Fasergewebe, das einem ständigen Druck oder Zug ausgesetzt ist, gibt der anhaltenden Dehnung nach. Außerhalb der Lunge sind die Gefäßaneurysmen, Überdehnungen der Haut über Bauchwandbrüchen u. ä. Beispiele dafür.

3. Den gleichen blasenbildenden Effekt haben Ventilstenosen, die durch *Kompression der Bronchiolen* entstehen. Das beste und praktisch wichtigste Beispiel dafür ist das fortgeschrittene Altersemphysem. Die blasige Umwandlung des ursprünglich diffusen Emphysems erfolgt vorwiegend an den Lungenrändern im Bereich langer Endäste des Bronchialbaumes (Abb. 55). Aus klinischen bronchospirometrischen Messungen darf man schließen, daß der Ventileffekt erst im Laufe der Exspiration einsetzt. Wenn die elastische Retraktion des Acinus erschöpft ist, dann wird der an erschlafften Fasersystemen in einem blasigen Hohlraum hängende Bronchiolus nicht mehr unter einem elastischen Spannungszug gehalten. Er kollabiert und wird bei positivem Pleuradruck auch komprimiert (dynamische Bronchiolostenose) (Abb. 56).

Das blasig überformte senile Emphysem unterscheidet sich vom primären bronchostenotischen Emphysem neben dem allgemeinen Elastizitätsverlust der Lunge vor allem auch durch die Lokalisation der Blasen, die stets im Lungenmantel, nie im Lungenkern liegen.

---

[1] HEINE und SCHÜRMEYER 1958.

4. Das vorwiegend kleinblasige Emphysem bei herdförmigen oder diffusen Lungenfibrosen beruht zum Teil auf Narbenzug, zum Teil auf starren Bronchiolo-

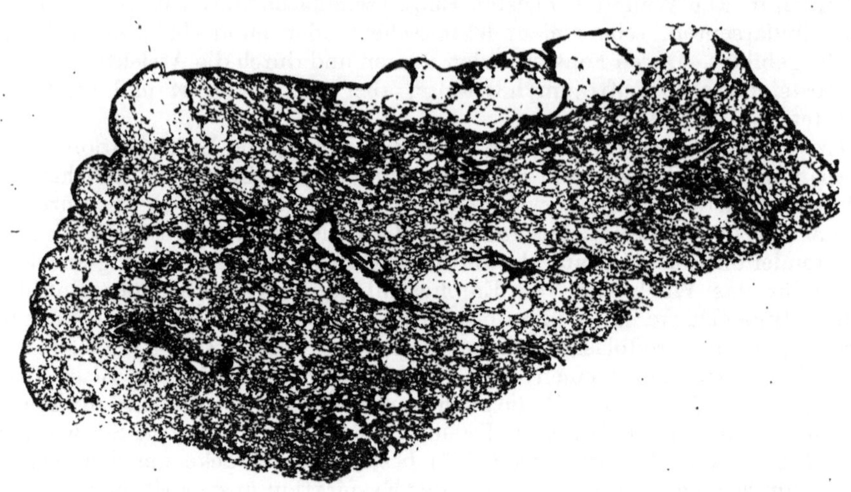

Abb. 55. Blasig überformtes atrophisches Altersemphysem. Blasenbildung vorwiegend in den Lungenrändern bedingt durch dynamische Bronchuskompression während der Exspiration (air trapping). S.-Nr. 451/58.

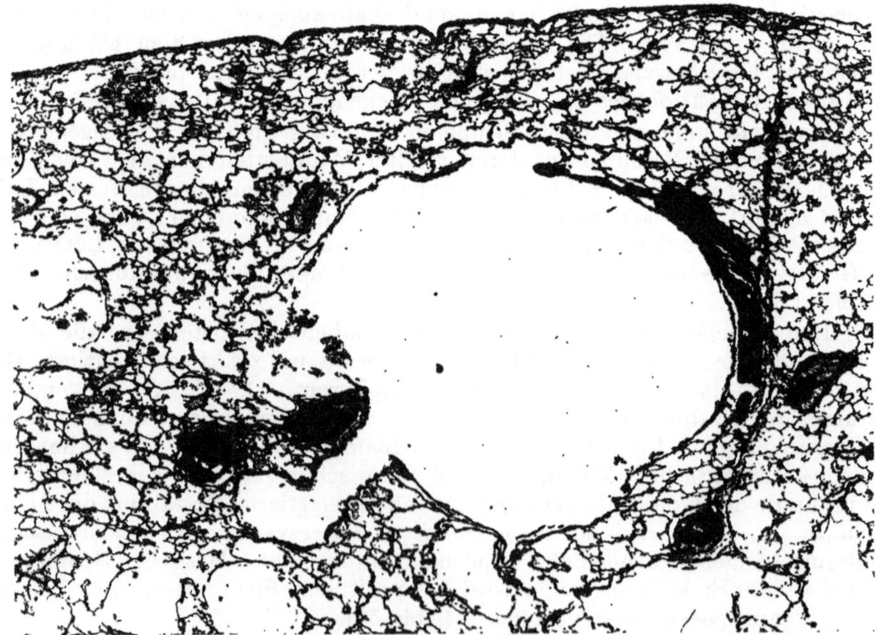

Abb. 56. Emphysemblasen in einem diffusen Emphysem bedingt durch dynamische Bronchiolostenose. S.-Nr. 516/58. Vergr. 7fach.

stenosen. Bei fibröser Peribronchiolitis sind längere Bronchusabschnitte in starre enge Röhren umgewandelt, in deren Bereich der Strömungswiderstand für die inspiratorische und exspiratorische Luftbewegung erheblich vergrößert ist.

Die Frage, warum unter solchen Bedingungen auch ohne Ventileffekte Emphysem entsteht, hat zur Entwicklung mehrerer Theorien geführt.

HECKMANN (1951) hat die Vorstellung, daß blasiges Emphysem nicht im Bereich der Bronchiolostenose, sondern in den gut belüfteten Nachbarabschnitten dadurch entsteht, daß sich Soghöhlen bilden. Diese sollen aus Überdehnung der Lungenabschnitte mit freien Bronchien entstehen. Die anatomischen Befunde sprechen nicht für diese Theorie, da die Emphysemblasen stets hinter den Bronchiolostenosen liegen.

LENGGENHAGER (1952) zeigt an Modellversuchen, daß in einem rhythmisch gefüllten Röhrensystem hinter der Stenose höhere Drucke entstehen als in den weiten Röhrenanteilen. Wenn Wasser im hydrostatischen Widder mit einer engen und einer weiten Röhre durch rhythmisch wiederholte Drucke in Bewegung gesetzt wird, dann entsteht in dem engen Schenkel des Röhrensystems ein höherer Wasserdruck als in dem weiten.

Ein ähnlicher Effekt läßt sich bei rhythmischer Dehnung von Gummifingerlingen zeigen, von denen der eine, an einer verengten Zuleitung hängende sich allmählich immer stärker dehnt, u. U. sogar platzt, während der andere sich rhythmisch dehnt und entdehnt. Entscheidend hierfür sei die größere kinetische Energie der in der nicht stenosierten Leitung bewegten Luftmassen, die wegen geringerer Rohrwiderstände schneller bewegt werden und zu einer vorübergehenden Nachblähung des Ballons hinter der Stenose führen. Ist die Vergrößerung eines Ballons einmal eingetreten, dann wird dieser wegen der größeren Flächendrucksumme bevorzugt weiter aufgebläht. Zu gleichen Ergebnissen ist früher auch schon ROHRER (1925) gekommen.

Aus diesen Versuchen geht hervor, daß bronchostenotisches Emphysem nicht nur durch den in neuerer Zeit von JACKSON (1945) stark in den Vordergrund gerückten Ventilmechanismus, sondern auch aus einer einfachen Verengerung der Lichtung entstehen kann. Weitere Angaben zur Bedeutung der Bronchiolostenose für die Entstehung des blasigen Emphysems bei DUFOURT u. Mitarb. (1952), SPAIN u. KAUFMANN (1954), KOURILSKY u. Mitarb. (1956), BELL (1958), SORS (1958).

γ) Elastizitätsmessungen an Leichenlungen bei bronchostenotischem Emphysem.

Die Auswirkung stärkerer Grade von Narbenemphysem auf die Lungenelastizität wurde bereits bei den fibrotischen Lungen besprochen (S. 436, Tabelle 3). Bei diesen ist die Minimalluftmenge trotz der bestehenden Fibrose nicht selten vergrößert. Der Ablauf der Retraktion ist stark verzögert und unvollständig (positiver Totraumeffekt).

Die Lungen mit bronchostenotischem Emphysem zeigen diese Charakteristika in noch weitaus höherem Maße, erweisen sich im übrigen aber als schlaffe Lungen mit stark herabgesetzten globalen Elastizitätswerten. Gemessen wurden fast ausschließlich bronchostenotische bullöse Emphyseme. Ein besonders hochgradiger Fall von Riesenblasenemphysem ist gesondert dargestellt (Tabelle 7). Der mittlere elastische Widerstand (Elastance) ist auf 1,1 cm H_2O/Liter Dehnung abgesunken. Die mittlere Dehnbarkeit innerhalb des Bereiches der Vitalkapazität (Komplianz) beträgt demnach 0,91 Liter/cm H_2O, liegt also um etwa das Vierfache höher als bei normalen Lungen und noch fast doppelt so hoch wie bei diffusen senilen Emphysemen. Der prozentuale Minimalluftanteil am Kollapsvolumen ist beträchtlich erhöht (57,3%; bei dem Fall von Riesenblasenemphysem in dem untersuchten Oberlappen sogar 75%). Die Volumelastizitätsmoduln liegen noch im Bereich der maximalen Inspirationsstellung unter denen der Exspirationslage bei normalen Lungen (7,1 $\times$ 10^3 dyn/cm², entsprechend etwa 7,2 cm H_2O). Die

Lunge mit Riesenblasenemphysem zeigt innerhalb des Vitalkapazitätsbereiches keinen nennenswerten elastischen Widerstand und erweist sich dadurch als plastisch verformbarer Körper nahezu ohne Eigenelastizität. Die statische Retraktionskraft ist in gleichem Maße herabgesetzt.

Tabelle 7. *Elastizität von Leichenlungen mit bronchostenotischem Emphysem im Vergleich zur Normallunge und zum senilen Emphysem.*

	Normale jugendliche Lungen	Senile Emphyseme	Bronchostenotische Emphyseme	Riesenblasenemphysem
1. Kollapsvolumen ml	1615	2665	2540	8100
2. Minimalluftanteil am Kollapsvolumen %	45,2	52,7	57,3	75,0
3. Mittlerer elastischer Widerstand gegen Dehnung (Elastance) cm HOH/Liter	4,5	2,0	1,1	etwa 0,3
4. Mittlere Dehnbarkeit (Komplianz) Liter/cm HOH	0,22	0,50	0,91	etwa 3,3
5. Volumelastizitätsmoduln $\times 10^3$ dyn/cm²				
Inspirationslage	42,9	13,0	7,1	etwa 3,9
Mittellage	18,0	9,0	5,0	0,0
Exspirationslage	11,9	6,3	3,5	0,0
6. Statische Retraktionskraft (Lungenzug) cm HOH				
Inspirationslage	—12	—5,5	—3,5	—1,0
Exspirationslage	—2	—0,5	—0,4	0,0
7. Tiffeneau-Test, Zweisekundenwert %	46	24	17	9
8. Maximale Atemstromstärke Liter/1. sec	1,1	0,6	0,4	0,2
9. Hysteretischer Dehnungsrückstand (Akkommodationsbreite) %	< 3	10,0	etwa 35	KeineAkkommodation möglich
10. „Totraumeffekt"	Ø	Ø	++	+++
Bemerkungen	—	—	—	Riesenblase etwa 1000 ml

Erläuterung zu dieser Tabelle s. Legende zu Tabelle 2, S. 426.

Alle dynamischen Elastizitätswerte sind stark eingeschränkt, an ihnen erweist sich die Wirkung der nur träge ventilierten Blasenräume. Der Tiffeneau-Test ist erheblich, vielfach extrem erniedrigt (Zweisekundenwert von 17%, bei Riesenblasenemphysem von nur 9%), die Atemstromstärke sehr klein (0,4 bzw. 0,2 Liter/ 1. sec). Die irreversiblen Dehnungsrückstände liegen im Mittel bei 35%, bei dem Riesenblasenemphysem noch höher.

Diese starke Verzögerung des Retraktionsablaufes unter Auftreten hoher, mindestens über 20% der aufgefüllten Luftmenge betragender Restvolumina beruht nicht nur auf der wie bei allen Emphysemen verstärkten elastischen Unvollkommenheit. Ein Teil der Luft wird unter dem Einfluß der exspiratorischen Luftabstrombehinderung festgehalten, vor allem in elastizitätsgeminderten Herden von Narbenemphysem, in kollateral belüfteten Lungenabschnitten oder insbesondere in bronchostenotischen Emphysemblasen. Derartige Gebiete stellen ventilatorischen Totraum dar, der auch mit Fremdgasmischmethoden in der Klinik erfaßt wird. Inwieweit sie durch Störung der Relation zwischen Ventilation und Perfusion auch den funktionellen Totraum vergrößern, ist noch offen.

Ein positiver Totraumeffekt an der Leichenlunge gibt Hinweise dafür, daß sich der ursprüngliche anatomische Totraum auf das krankhaft veränderte Alveolargebiet ausgedehnt hat. Die Größe dieses Totraumanteiles läßt sich aus den Meßergebnissen annähernd abschätzen (Abb. 57; weitere Einzelheiten bei HARTUNG 1959, 1960). Damit wird zugleich eine sehr bedeutende Teilkomponente des funktionellen Totraumes an der Leichenlunge erfaßbar. Es erscheint daher zweckmäßig, trotz der schon bestehenden nomenklatorischen Differenzen an dem Begriff des Totraumeffektes im Sinne des durch anatomische Veränderungen vergrößerten ventilatorischen Totraumes festzuhalten und nicht z. B. nur von einem Blaseneffekt zu sprechen[1], zumal der aus dem Ventilationseffekt über den Gasaustausch definierte funktionelle Totraum der Physiologie und Pathophysiologie in hohem Maße unräumlich ist[2].

V. Die ventilatorische Insuffizienz.

Die in den vorhergehenden Abschnitten dargestellten morphologischen und histomechanischen Untersuchungsbefunde ermöglichen Rückschlüsse auf die intra vitam bestehenden Ventilationsstörungen[3].

In der bewegungsgestörten Lunge (Abschnitt A) ändern sich die statischen Ventilationsvolumina, insbesondere die Größe der Vitalkapazität. Diese ist bei starren oder durch Pleuraschwarte gefesselten Lungen infolge der stark erhöhten elastischen Atemwiderstände inspiratorisch vermindert, bei den schlaffen Lungen und besonders bei den exspirationsgestörten bronchostenotischen Emphysemen durch inspiratorische Verlagerung der Atemmittellage mit Residualluftvermehrung eingeschränkt.

Bedeutsamer noch als diese Verkleinerung des Vitalkapazitätsvolumens ist die Einschränkung der dynamischen Ventilationsgrößen bei allen Störungen im luftleitenden System (Abschnitt B). Sie bestimmen die Atemfrequenz, deren Steigerung in erster Linie zur Erzielung hoher Atemminutenvolumina beiträgt.

Diese durch die morphologisch erkennbaren Strukturänderungen bedingten und mit der histomechanischen Untersuchung erfaßbaren Störungen im mechanischen Verhalten der Lunge während der Ventilationsbewegungen sind die

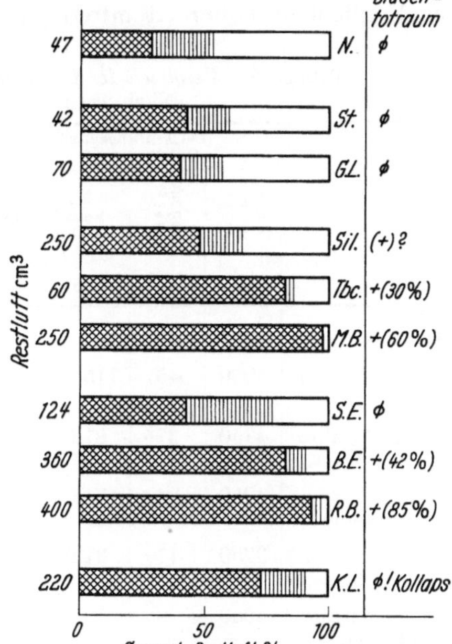

Abb. 57. Darstellung des Totraumanteils an der Restluft bei Volumdehnung mit stufenweise erhöhter Luftfüllung. Schraffiert: 1. Auffüllungsstufe (Einfülldruck etwa 8 cm HOH); gestrichelt: 2. Auffüllungsstufe (Einfülldruck etwa 13 cm HOH); weiß: 3. Auffüllungsstufe (Einfülldruck etwa 20 cm HOH). Die nach der 3., höchsten Auffüllungsstufe gemessene gesamte Restluftmenge ist gleich 100% gesetzt, ihre absolute Größe wird durch die linke Zahlenreihe angezeigt. Ein Einfluß des durch strukturelle Veränderungen im ursprünglichen Alveolarbereich vermehrten anatomischen (ventilatorischen) Totraumes ist erwiesen, wenn bereits nach der 1., niedrigsten Auffüllungsstufe mehr als 70% der gesamten Restluft zurückgehalten werden, während eine rein auf Hysterese beruhende Restluftbildung angenommen werden kann, wenn der Restluftanteil der 1. Auffüllungsstufe weniger als 45% der gesamten Restluftmenge beträgt. Die rechte Zahlenreihe gibt die geschätzte Größe des Totraumanteils an. Alle Werte gelten nur für den jeweils untersuchten Lungenabschnitt (hier Oberlappen). *N* normale Lunge; *St* Stauungslungen; *G.L.* gefesselte Lunge; *Sil.*, *Tbc.*, *M.B.* Narbenlungen mit leichtgradiger Silikose, Miliartuberkulose bzw. M. Boeck; *S.E.* senile, *B.E.* bullöse Emphyseme; *R.B.* Riesenblasenemphysem; *K.L.* postop. Kollaps. (Aus HARTUNG 1959.)

[1] SCHOEDEL 1958, zit. bei HARTUNG 1959.
[2] Siehe S. 472 und bei ROSSIER, BÜHLMANN und WIESINGER 1956, 1958.
[3] GIESE 1960, HARTUNG 1960, UEHLINGER 1960.

Grundlagen der klinisch beobachteten restriktiven und obstruktiven Formen der ventilatorischen Insuffizienz. Die Synthese der statischen und dynamischen Meßwerte von Leichenlungen ermöglicht die Abschätzung der bei den verschiedenen Lungenerkrankungen noch vorhandenen maximalen Ventilationsfähigkeit, die dem klinisch geprüften Atemgrenzwert entspricht (Tabelle 8). Es zeigt sich in Übereinstimmung mit der klinischen Erfahrung, daß bei den starren Lungen auch stärkere Einschränkungen der Vitalkapazität bei ungestörter Dynamik mit der Möglichkeit hoher Atemfrequenzen noch ziemlich weitgehend kompensiert

Tabelle 8. *Vergleich der Leichenlungenwerte mit klinischen Messwerten.*
(Nach Hartung, Ergeb. inn. Med. **15**).

| | Leichenlungenwerte (Hartung 1960) | | | Klinische Meßwerte (Hamm 1958) | | | | |
| | Vitalkapazität[1] | Tiffeneau-Test[2] | Maximale Ventilationsfähigkeit[3] | | Vitalkapazität | Tiffeneau-Test | Atemgrenzwert | | |
	ml	2 sec %	1/min	Verlust %	ml	%	1/min	Verlust %	
Norm, gesamt	4900	41	100	± 0	4810	70,1	100	± 0	Norm, gesamt
Norm, 22 Jahre	5000	46	115	+15,0	5390	74,0	117,4	+17,4	Norm, 16—34 Jahre
Norm, 56 Jahre	4750	37	87,9	—12,1	4205	63,7	81,1	—18,9	Norm, 50—74 Jahre
Senile Emphyseme	4250	24	51,0	—49,0	4070	58,7	74,2	—25,8	leichtes Emphysem[4]
Bronchostenotische Emphyseme	3750	17	31,9	—68,1	3350	46,6	44,2	—55,8	mittelschweres Emphysem[4]
Riesenblasenemphysem	3000	9	13,5	—86,5	2740	29,2	27,4	—72,6	schweres Emphysem[4]
Schwartengefesselte Lunge	1500	42	31,5	—68,5	2350	80,4	55,6	—44,4	Pleuraschwarte, ♀
Zustand nach Pneumektomie	3400	24	40,8	—59,2	2300	84,3	58,9	—41,1	Operationen, ♂
Stauungslunge	3000	36	54,0	—46,0	3560	64,0	72,0	—28,0	„Fibrose", ♂
M. Boeck	3000	19	28,5	—71,5	2160	67,1	47,1	—52,9	„Fibrose", ♀
Vernarbte Miliartbc.	3150	38	59,9	—40,1	3150	61,3	52,9	—47,1	Silikose

[1] Errechnet aus den statischen Werten der Druck-Volumdiagramme unter Berücksichtigung der Dehnbarkeitsgrenze und der Minimalluftvermehrung als Maß des Residualvolumens.
[2] Originalwert des „Tiffeneau-Tests an der Leichenlunge".
[3] Durch den Tiffeneau-Wert gegebener nutzbarer Anteil der vorhandenen Vitalkapazität bei Annahme einer Atemfrequenz von 50/min.
[4] Schweregrade nach Residualvolumen, ähnlich Asthmaemphysem.

werden können, daß aber umgekehrt stärkere Einbußen an dynamischer Ventilationsleistung stets mit bedeutenden Verlusten an Ventilationsfähigkeit einhergehen.

Diese rein quantitativen Aspekte bedürfen einer weiteren Ergänzung. Bei der Besprechung der ventilatorischen Verteilungsstörung (S. 485) und des damit auf das engste verbundenen Totraumproblems (S. 471) wurde bereits auf die vorwiegend qualitativen Störungen eingegangen, die den Nutzeffekt der Ventilation für den Gasaustausch herabsetzen und dadurch eine besondere Bedeutung für die

Lungeninsuffizienz gewinnen. Sie sind das Charakteristikum der obstruktiven bronchostenotischen Emphyseme, bei denen gewöhnlich auch klinisch die schwersten Funktionseinbußen beobachtet werden.

Jede Minderung des Ventilationseffektes durch Totraumvergrößerung hat zwangsläufig eine Steigerung des Minutenvolumens zur Folge, das zur Aufrechterhaltung eines annähernd ausreichenden Gasaustausches geatmet werden muß. Dieser erhöhten Erfordernisventilation stehen die Störungen der Ventilationsmechanik gegenüber, durch die die Ventilationsbewegungen energetisch gesehen unökonomisch werden. Die sog. kritische Grenze der pulmonalen Ventilation, von der an aller zusätzlich geförderte Sauerstoff von der Atemmuskulatur selbst verbraucht wird und die vermehrte Kohlensäureproduktion in der Atemmuskulatur die vollständige Abrauchung der Kohlensäure behindert, kann bis auf das erhöhte Ruheminutenvolumen absinken. Dann ist der Zustand der absoluten ventilatorischen Insuffizienz erreicht. Die Voraussetzungen für derart tiefgreifende Störungen sind sowohl nach den klinischen Erfahrungen, als auch nach den morphologischen und histomechanischen Befunden an Leichenlungen vor allem bei den obstruktiven bronchostenotischen Emphysemen und bei den durch Narbenemphysem komplizierten Lungenfibrosen gegeben. Die diesen in besonderem Maße eigentümlichen Ventilationsstörungen, die zugleich die Stufen auf dem Wege zur absoluten ventilatorischen Insuffizienz darstellen, lassen sich schematisch wie folgt zusammenfassen[1]:

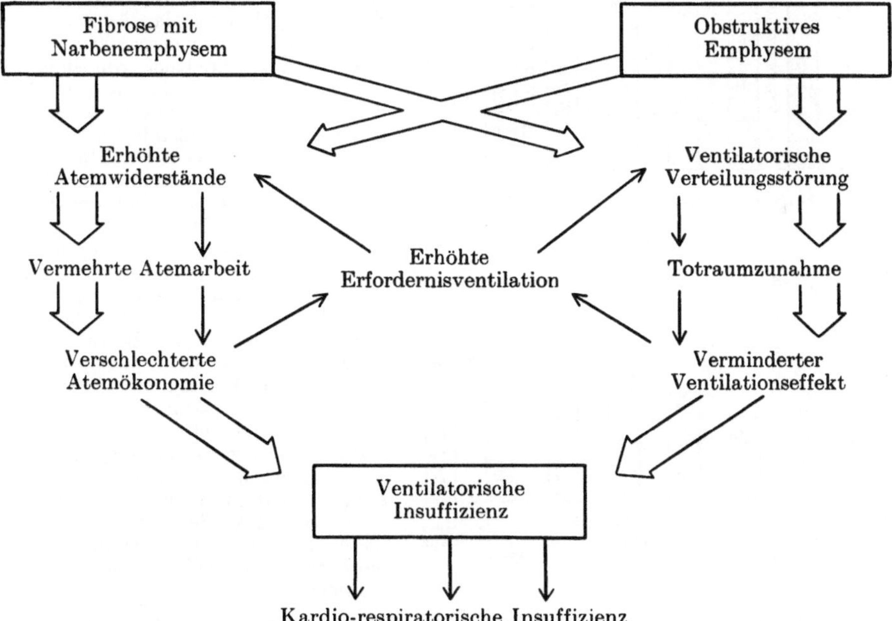

Es sind zugleich die Formen der Lungenerkrankungen, bei denen man anatomisch gewöhnlich ein Cor pulmonale findet. Sie enden fast immer in der kardiorespiratorischen Insuffizienz, deren vielfach eng mit den Ventilationsstörungen verbundene Änderungen der Diffusions- und Perfusionsgrößen in den folgenden Abschnitten behandelt werden.

---

[1] HARTUNG 1960.

C. Störungen der Diffusion.

I. Der alveolocapilläre Gasaustausch.

a) Funktionelle Vorbemerkungen.

Der Gasaustausch zwischen der Alveolarluft und dem Blut in den Lungencapillaren erfolgt nach der vorherrschenden Meinung der Physiologen und Kliniker durch Diffusion[1].

Die ältere Sekretionstheorie von Haldane (1927) und Bohr (1909), nach der die Lungen als Drüsen funktionieren, dabei Gaskonzentrationen entgegen einem Druckgefälle erzeugen und so aktiv am Gasaustausch mitwirken können, hat heute nur wenige Anhänger. Sie wird durch elektronenmikroskopische Befunde an den Mitochondrien unter experimenteller Einwirkung von O_2 und CO_2 erneut zur Diskussion gestellt[2].

Voraussetzung für die Diffusion ist ein Konzentrationsgefälle der auszutauschenden Gase zwischen Blut und Alveolarluft.

In der Ruhe strömen etwa 4 Liter Luft in der Minute durch die Alveolen. Die Alveolarluft hat dabei dauernd einen Sauerstoffdruck von etwa 100 mm Hg und einen Kohlensäuredruck von 40 mm Hg.

Die Lungendurchblutung beträgt in der Ruhe etwa 6 Liter in der Minute. Das in die Lunge einfließende Blut hat einen Sauerstoffdruck von 40 mm Hg und einen Kohlensäuredruck von 45 mm Hg. Im arterialisierten Lungenblut der Lungenvenen sind die Drucke für Sauerstoff 100 mm Hg und für Kohlensäure 40 mm Hg.

Die Differenz der Gasdrucke zwischen Alveolarluft und venösem Lungenblut (alveolo-capillärer Gradient) beträgt in der Ruhe etwa 5 mm Hg für CO_2 und etwa 60 mm Hg für Sauerstoff. Beim Durchfluß des Blutes durch die Capillaren sinkt diese Druckdifferenz ab und am Ende der Capillarstrecke ist ein fast vollständiger Druckausgleich eingetreten. Die Druckdifferenz am Ende der Capillarstrecke wird als endcapillärer Gradient oder Enddruckdifferenz[3] bezeichnet. Ist diese für Sauerstoff größer als 5 mm Hg, dann wird eine Diffusionsstörung angenommen (Abb. 58).

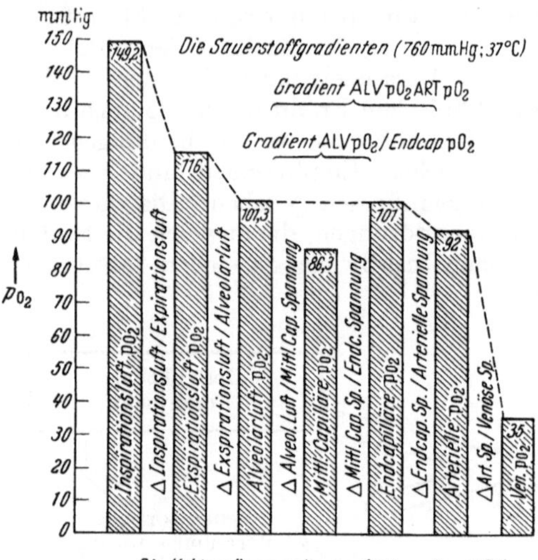

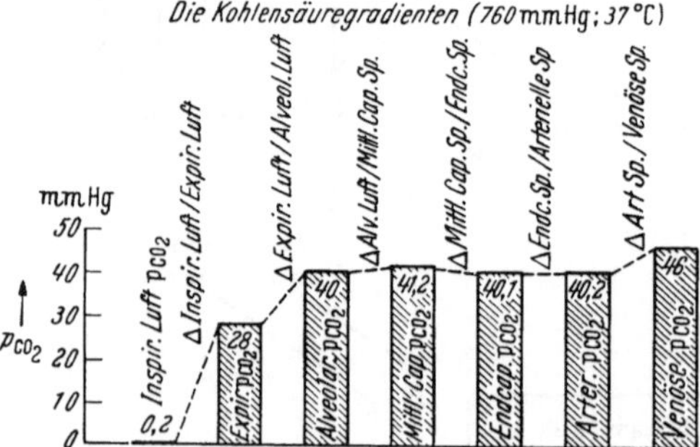

Abb. 58. Differenz der Gasdrucke zwischen Alveolarluft und Lungenblut (alveolocapilläre Gradienten). (Aus Rossier, Bühlmann u. Wiesinger 1958.)

Voraussetzung für einen vollkommenen Druckausgleich zwischen den Gasen der Alveolarluft und dem Blut in den Lungencapillaren ist eine ausreichende Kontaktzeit von etwa 0,1—1 sec sowie eine genügend große Kontaktfläche. Die respiratorische Oberfläche der ganzen Lunge beträgt nach v. Hayek (1953) etwa 30 m² für die Exspiration und höchstens 100 m² für die tiefste Inspiration.

---

[1] Krogh 1909, 1914, 1941, Liljestrand 1925 Literatur, Barcroft 1928, Rossier und Mitarbeiter 1956, Schoedel 1937, 1955, Bartels 1956, 1957, Forster 1957, Matthes 1960.
[2] Schulz 1956, 1958, Meessen und Schulz 1957, Hayek und Mitarbeiter 1958, Meessen 1960.
[3] Bartels 1956, 1957.

Die Gasmenge, die pro Minute und pro mm Hg Druckdifferenz zwischen Alveolarluft und Blut diffundiert, wird als Diffusionskapazität (D), auch Diffusionskonstante oder Diffusionsfaktor bezeichnet. Die Diffusionskapazität für CO_2 (D_{CO_2}) ist 20mal höher als für O_2 (D_{O_2}). Die Diffusionskapazität für O_2 beträgt nach KROGH (1914) 23—43, nach BARTELS (1956, 1957) 13,8—21,5 ml O_2/min/mm Hg.

Die Bindung des Sauerstoffs an das Hämoglobin verläuft in 4 Oxydationsstufen, ein Molekül Hb verbindet sich mit 4 Molekülen Sauerstoff. Das Hämoglobin wirkt als Sauerstoffspeicher[1]. Die O_2-Dissoziationskurve verläuft S-förmig. Oberhalb eines O_2-Druckes von 80 mm Hg Sauerstoff tritt eine Sättigung des Blutes mit O_2 ein, bei geringerem Druck nimmt die Sättigung rasch ab. Je tiefer der alveoläre O_2-Druck absinkt, um so geringer wird die O_2-Druckdifferenz zwischen venösem Blut und Alveolarluft und um so größer der O_2-Gradient am Ende der Capillarstrecke. Bei niederem O_2-Druck in der Alveolarluft reicht also die Kontaktzeit nicht zur völligen Aufsättigung des Blutes mit O_2 aus.

b) Die Morphologie der alveolocapillären Membran.

1. Die Alveolarmembran.

Die Schranke zwischen der Alveolarluft und dem Blut in den Lungencapillaren wird als alveolocapilläre Membran oder kurz als Alveolarmembran bezeichnet. Sie besteht aus dem Alveolarepithel, aus dem Endothel der Capillaren, den zugehörigen Basalmembranen und aus Fasergewebe, das sich in wechselnder Dichte zwischen diesen Hohlräumen ausbreitet.

Die Alveolardeckzellen werden heute auf Grund ihrer submikroskopischen Struktur als Epithelzellen angesehen. Damit hat sich die Auffassung von ASCHOFF (1926), SEEMANN (1929, 1931), HAYEK (1942), BARGMANN (1936) u. a. gegenüber der Deutung von LANG (1926, 1929), MAXIMOW (1926), POLICARD (1926) durchgesetzt, die diese Zellen für Histiocyten gehalten haben.

Die Alveolarepithelien bilden während der Embryonalzeit eine geschlossene Lage kubischer Zellen über den Capillaren der Alveolarwand. Gegen Ende der intrauterinen Entwicklung schieben sie sich in das Niveau der Capillarschicht hinein, legen sich in die Nischen zwischen den Capillaren (Nischenzellen, ASCHOFF 1926) und stecken zuweilen wie Pfröpfe oder Korken so in der Alveolarwand, daß sie mit ihren Fortsätzen in zwei benachbarte Alveolen hineinragen[2]. Mit der Beatmung der Lunge nach der Geburt rücken die Zellen so weit auseinander, daß etwa 95% der Oberfläche des Alveolarraumes von den lang ausgezogenen äußerst dünnen, lichtoptisch nicht mehr erkennbaren 0,05—0,3 μ dicken flügelartigen Fortsätzen der Epithelzellen bedeckt sind. In dem 5—15 μ dicken perinucleären, lichtoptisch sichtbaren Cytoplasma liegt die Masse der Mitochondrien. Die Zellgrenzen schließen fest aneinander. Löst sich eine Zelle ab, dann schieben sich die Fortsätze der Nachbarzellen unter der sich abhebenden Zelle sofort zusammen und decken den Defekt. Die auf Grund lichtoptischer Befunde von HAYEK (1943) vertretene Ansicht, daß die Alveolarepithelien unter dem Einfluß von Adrenalin oder bei Zuständen von Atemnot ihre Fortsätze retrahieren, unter der Einwirkung von Histamin, Atropin und Sauerstoff dagegen ausdehnen, hat sich in elektronenoptischen Untersuchungen nicht bestätigt. Auch im Adrenalinversuch bleibt die lückenlose Auskleidung der Alveolen mit den Epithelfortsätzen erhalten[3], ebenso nach Sauerstoff- und Kohlensäureatmung[4]. Die Alveolarepithelien besitzen eine hohe Plastizität und passen sich den wechselnden Dehnungszuständen der Alveolen an.

Durch die elektronenoptische Untersuchung ist damit auch die alte Streitfrage, ob die gesamte Alveolarwand von Zellen ausgekleidet wird oder ob Capil-

---

[1] BARTELS 1956, 1957, ROSSIER 1956.   [2] MACKLIN 1938, v. HAYEK 1942 u. a.
[3] GIESEKING 1958.   [4] SCHULZ 1956.

larschlingen nackt mit der Alveolarluft in Berührung treten, dahin entschieden, daß die Alveolarwand lückenlos von Epithel bedeckt ist[1].

Zur Alveolarlichtung hin bilden die Epithelien pseudopodienartige, 0,1 bis 0,4 μ lange und 60—120 mμ breite Ausstülpungen, die als Protoplasmafortsätze[2], Cytoplasmafüßchen[3], Microvilli[4] bezeichnet werden. Die bald sehr zahlreich, bald nur gering entwickelten Microvilli tragen zur Vergrößerung der Oberfläche der Alveolarepithelien bei und sind wahrscheinlich für den Stoffaustausch von Bedeutung. Sie können bei Kälteeinwirkung und bei Anoxie schwinden[5].

Die Oberfläche der Alveolarepithelien ist schließlich mit einer dünnen Flüssigkeitsschicht bedeckt, die durch Sekretion der Epithelien entstehen soll[6]. Sie enthält saure Mucopolysaccharide, die mit der PAS-Reaktion nachweisbar sind[7]. Dem Flüssigkeitsfilm, der auf diese Weise die Innenfläche der Alveolen bedeckt, wird eine Bedeutung für die Oberflächenspannung in den Alveolen zugeschrieben[8]. Die Vergrößerung der Alveolen, die Wick 1952 nach Beatmung mit CO_2 an der isolierten Lunge fand, deutet v. Hayek als Folge einer Herabsetzung der Oberflächenspannung zwischen Alveolarwand und Alveolarluft durch die Kohlensäure.

Die Mitochondrien der Alveolarepithelien liegen vorwiegend in der Nähe des Kerns. Sie sind bis zu 2 μ lang, haben eine doppelt konturierte Außenmembran und im Innern ein System von Doppelmembranen, den Cristae mitochondriales. Oft zeigen die Mitochondrien eine Verdichtung und lamelläre Umwandlung der Innenstruktur, die Schulz (1956, 1958) als bandförmige Transformation bezeichnet hat. Diese für die Alveolarepithelien charakteristischen, oft konzentrisch geschichteten osmiophilen Körper, die weder Eisen noch Kalk enthalten, sind mehrfach beschrieben worden[9]. Änderungen in der Sauerstoff- und CO_2-Konzentration der Alveolarluft beeinflussen die Struktur der Mitochondrien. Bei Atmung eines Gasgemisches von Luft und 3% CO_2 kommt es zu einer Verdichtung und bandförmigen Transformation der Mitochondrien, bei O_2-Atmung zu einer Aufhellung, Quellung und Vergrößerung der Mitochondrien mit Verlust der Innenstruktur[10]. Schulz erwägt auf Grund dieser Versuchsergebnisse die Möglichkeit, daß in den Alveolarepithelien durch Veränderungen an den Mitochondrien eine biochemische Regulierung der Lungendurchblutung erfolge.

In der Lunge des Siebenschläfers kommt es im Winterschlaf unter Erhöhung der CO_2-Spannung in der Alveolarluft und Hypoxie ebenfalls zu bandförmiger Transformation der Mitochondrien und in den Lungen von Rattenembryonen zur Bildung von osmiophilen Lamellenkörpern, die aus Mitochondrien abgeleitet werden[11].

Nach v. Hayek u. Mitarb. (1958) entsteht die osmiophile Umwandlung der Mitochondrien bei Erstickung oder auch erst nach dem Tode. In der normalen Lunge soll sie fehlen. Bandförmig transformierte Mitochondrien, die sich in der Erstickung gebildet haben, werden nach Wiederbelebung in etwa 30 min resorbiert[12].

Die Alveolarepithelien liegen einer dünnen Basalmembran auf. Diese stellt sich im elektronenoptischen Bild als ein homogenes, 0,01—0,1 μ dickes Häutchen dar, das scharf gegen die osmiophile basale Grenzschicht der Alveolardeckzellen abgegrenzt ist.

---

[1] Low 1953, Schulz 1956, Gieseking 1956, Bargmann 1956, Dettmer 1956, Schulz 1959 Meessen 1960 u. a.
[2] Policard 1954.   [3] Meessen und Schulz 1957, Schulz 1956.
[4] Karrer 1956, Bargmann und Knoop 1956, v. Hayek und Mitarbeiter 1957.
[5] Lange 1909, v. Hayek und Mitarbeiter 1957.   [6] v. Hayek 1953.
[7] Macklin 1954, Clemens 1956, 1958.   [8] v. Neergaard 1929, v. Hayek 1952.
[9] Schlipköter 1954, Bargmann 1956, Gieseking 1956.
[10] Schulz 1956, Meessen und Schulz 1957.   [11] Schulz 1957.
[12] v. Hayek, Braunsteiner und Pakesch 1958.

2. Die Capillarmembran.

In der Endstrombahn der Lunge unterscheiden wir die Stromcapillaren, in denen ständig Blut fließt, von den Netzcapillaren, die nur fakultativ in den Kreislauf einbezogen sind, zeitweilig abgeschaltet werden können und so als Reservecapillaren dienen (s. unter Perfusionsstörung). Die Netzcapillaren mit einer Lichtungsweite von 6—11 μ liegen in den Alveolarsepten und grenzen so an zwei benachbarte Alveolarräume, mit denen ein Gasaustausch stattfinden kann. Die Stromcapillaren liegen an der Basis der Alveolen und haben auch hier Kontakt mit der Alveolarluft. Ihre Lichtung ist 20—40 μ weit. Die Diffusionsstrecke zwischen Erythrocyten und Alveolarluft ist deshalb innerhalb der Stromcapillaren wesentlich länger als in den Netzcapillaren. Die Kontaktzeit ist wegen der raschen Blutströmung in den Stromcapillaren kürzer als in den Netzcapillaren.

Die Wandstruktur der Netz- und Stromcapillaren zeigt nach lichtoptischen und nach elektronenoptischen Untersuchungen keine Unterschiede. Die Schichtdicke der alveolocapillären Membran ist für Strom- und Netzcapillaren gleich.

Die Capillarwand besteht aus dem Endothel und der Basalmembran. Die Endothelzellen sind nach der Lichtung und an der Basis durch die zarte osmiophile etwa 5 mμ breite Zellmembran begrenzt, die keine Unterbrechungen aufweist. Das Cytoplasma enthält 200 mμ große Mitochondrien und Vacuolen[1]. Im Bereich des Kernes ist die Endothelschicht 3—5 μ, außerhalb des Kernbereiches 0,01—0,2 μ dick. Zum Kernbereich gehören etwa 20% der Capillarwandfläche, der restliche Anteil entfällt auf die dünnen Ausläufer der Endothelzellen. Die Zellgrenzen sind ineinander verzahnt, im Schnitt oft S-förmig. Das Protoplasma ragt an der Berührungsfläche zweier Zellen oft wulstförmig in die Capillarlichtung vor.

Die Endothelzellen liegen einer Basalmembran auf, die im elektronenoptischen Bild[2] als kontrastarmer, homogener, strukturloser „periendothelialer Streifen"[3] den Querschnitt einer Capillare umläuft. Die Basalmembran bildet so eine Hülle um das Endothelrohr. Ein periendothelialer Spaltraum läßt sich in der normalen Lunge an den Netzcapillaren der Alveolarwand nicht darstellen, ist aber von SCHULZ (1956) bei Stauungslungen beschrieben worden.

Die Basalmembranen der Capillaren und der Epithelzellen des Alveolarraumes verschmelzen dort, wo sie sich berühren, zu einer gemeinsamen Membran, deren mittlere Dicke nach eigenen Messungen etwa 0,03—0,1 μ, nach POLICARD (1954) 0,03—0,04 μ, nach KARRER (1956) 0,025 μ und nach SCHULZ (1956) 0,065 μ beträgt. Diese gabelt sich dort, wo Alveolarepithelien und Capillarwand auseinanderrücken, in zwei getrennte Basalmembranen, von denen das Grundhäutchen der Capillaren im allgemeinen dicker ist als das des Alveolarepithels. Der freie Raum zwischen diesen Membranen wird von reticulären und elastischen Fasern sowie von spärlichen interstitiellen Zellen ausgefüllt, deren weit ausgestreckte Ausläufer zwischen den Fasern liegen.

Ob diese Zellen Pericyten, wie SCHULZ (1956) meint (bestritten von v. HAYEK 1953), oder Histiocyten sind, bleibt noch offen. Die reticulären Fasern verbinden benachbarte Blutcapillaren und strahlen in die Basalmembranen ebenso wie in die elastischen Fasern ein.

Die Schichtdicke der gesamten alveolocapillären Membran beträgt nach Messungen im Elektronenmikroskop dort, wo die Capillaren der Alveolarwand dicht anliegen, also in etwa 80% des Alveolarraumes, 0,15—0,5 μ[4]. Nach lichtoptischen Messungen hat man bisher eine Dicke von 1—4 μ angenommen.

---

[1] SCHULZ 1956.
[2] KARRER 1956, POLICARD und COLLET 1956, v. HAYEK und Mitarbeiter 1958, KISCH 1955, 1957.
[3] MEESSEN und SCHULZ 1957.   [4] GIESEKING 1956.

c) Die Permeabilität der alveolocapillären Membran.

Ein wesentlicher Faktor für die Diffusionskapazität zwischen Alveolarluft und capillärer Gefäßstrecke ist die Permeabilität der Austauschfläche. Bisher wurde angenommen, daß der Hauptwiderstand für die Gasdiffusion in der alveolocapillären Membran liegt[1]. Neben dieser sind aber auch das Blutplasma und die Erythrocytenmembran zu berücksichtigen. Aus physiologischen Untersuchungen[2] geht hervor, daß die Diffusion des Sauerstoffs im Plasma, in der Erythrocytenmembran und im Innern der Erythrocyten erheblich verzögert wird. Erythrocytensuspensionen brauchen zur Halbsättigung mit O_2 eine 30mal längere Zeit als Hämoglobinlösungen. Überträgt man die in vitro gewonnenen Meßergebnisse auf die Lunge, dann verhalten sich die Diffusionszeiten Membran:Plasma:Erythrocyt wie 1:10:100[3]. Für einen völligen Druckausgleich zwischen Alveolarluft und Blut in den Lungencapillaren ist nach den Berechnungen von Kreuzer (1953) eine Kontaktzeit von 0,6 sec erforderlich. Kreuzer (1953) legt seinen Berechnungen folgende in Modellversuchen gewonnenen Werte zugrunde:

1. Für die Capillarwand (die der alveolocapillären Membran entspricht) eine 30%ige Serumeiweißlösung von $1\,\mu$ Dicke;
2. für das Plasma eine 7%ige Serumeiweißlösung;
3. für das Gesamtblut eine 4%ige Erythrocytensuspension im Serum;
4. für das Erythrocyteninnere eine 8,5%ige Hb-Lösung;
5. für den Capillar- und Erythrocytenradius $4\,\mu$.

Er kommt damit zu folgenden kürzesten Diffusionszeiten.

1. Zeit für die Capillarwand (= alveolocapilläre Membran)
   von $1\,\mu$ Dicke   0,0017 sec
2. Zeit für $4\,\mu$ Plasma   0,012 sec
3. Zeit für $1\,\mu$ Erythrocyteninneres   0,6137 sec

          0,6274 sec

Da die Kontaktzeit nach Kreuzer (1953) nur 0,1 sec [nach Thews (1956) 0,16 sec] beträgt, ist die Sättigungszeit, die aus der vorstehenden Rechnung hervorgeht, 6mal länger als die Kontaktzeit. Kreuzer (1953) äußert aus diesem Grunde Zweifel daran, ob reine Diffusion für die Sättigung des Blutes ausreicht.

Welche Bedeutung den einzelnen Schichten der alveolocapillären Membran bei der Gasdiffusion zukommt, ist noch ungeklärt. Kreuzer (1953) setzt sie einer 30%igen Eiweißlösung gleich und befindet sich damit in Übereinstimmung mit den Werten, die Krogh (1914) als D_{O_2} für verschiedene Gewebe berechnet hat. Policard (1938, 1955) weist in diesem Zusammenhang auf die osmiophilen, also lipoidhaltigen Grenzmembranen der Epithel- und Endothelzellen hin, die aber nach Kreuzer (1953) für die Diffusion von Gasen und von lipoidlöslichen Stoffen kein Hindernis darstellen.

Die alveolocapilläre Membran bildet nach diesen Meßergebnissen unter Normalverhältnissen eine nur unbedeutende Behinderung des Diffusionsvorganges.

Forster (1957) und ähnlich Matthes (1960) sind dagegen der Meinung, daß diese aus Modellversuchen gewonnenen Werte nicht auf die Verhältnisse in der Lunge angewandt werden können. Sie teilen den gesamten Diffusionswiderstand in einen Membranfaktor und in einen Blutfaktor (sog. intracapillären Diffusionswiderstand), der sich aus der Diffusion im Plasma und aus der chemischen Bindung im Erythrocyten ergibt. Diesen intracapillären Widerstand, der in erheblichem

---

[1] Schoedel 1955.

[2] Pircher 1951, Kreuzer 1953, Roughton und Mitarbeiter 1944/1949, Übersicht bei Matthes 1960.

[3] Bartels 1956, 1957.

Maße auch von dem Erythrocytengehalt (Hämatokrit) des Lungencapillarblutes bestimmt wird, schätzen sie nur auf die Hälfte des gesamten Diffusionswiderstandes. Demnach würden sich unter normalen Bedingungen Membranfaktor und intracapillärer Diffusionswiderstand annähernd die Waage halten.

Die von FORSTER (1957) verwandte Definition des Membranfaktors schließt als wesentlichen Teil auch die Perfusionsgröße der Capillaren ein. Die Differenzen zu der aus den Diffusionsmessungen am Modell einer Eiweißschicht gewonnenen Auffassung von KREUZER (1953) sind dadurch eher verständlich. Daß der Gasaustausch zusätzlicher cellulärer Leistungen etwa im Sinne der Sekretionstheorie bedürfe, erkennt FORSTER (1957) nach den bisher vorliegenden Befunden in Übereinstimmung mit der überwiegenden Mehrzahl der Autoren nicht an.

Man wird also damit zu rechnen haben, daß die alveolocapilläre Membran auch im normalen Zustand zumindest eine zu berücksichtigende Verzögerung des Diffusionsvorganges bewirkt[1]. Ihre erhebliche Bedeutung als Diffusionshindernis unter pathologischen Verhältnissen ist unbestritten. Änderungen der Dicke, der geweblichen Zusammensetzung, des Capillarisierungsgrades oder der Capillarabstände vom alveolären Luftraum werden neben den eigentlichen Perfusionsstörungen stets zu einer Einschränkung der Diffusionskapazität führen.

d) Die Kontaktzeit.

Die Kontaktzeit (t) des Lungenblutes mit der Alveolarluft ist abhängig von der Capillarstrecke (s), die in der Alveolarwand zum Gasaustausch zur Verfügung steht, und von der Strömungsgeschwindigkeit (v) des Blutes in den Capillaren. Daraus ergibt sich die Geschwindigkeitsformel

$$t = s/v.$$

Die Lungencapillaren haben nach der Berechnung von A. MÜLLER (1945) eine Länge von 200—300 μ. Dieser Wert entspricht etwa dem durchschnittlichen Alveolardurchmesser von 250 μ. Für die Lunge der Katze hat VOGEL (1947) kinematographisch eine Capillarlänge von 100—200 μ bestimmt. KREUZER nimmt für seine Berechnungen über die Kontaktzeit eine Capillarlänge von 100—300 μ, im Durchschnitt von 200 μ an.

Der Capillardurchmesser liegt beim Menschen zwischen 6 und 11 μ.

Die Strömungsgeschwindigkeit in den Capillaren beträgt nach den Rechnungen von A. MÜLLER (1945) für die Menschenlunge 0,05 cm/sec.

VOGEL (1947) maß die Strömungsgeschwindigkeit kinematographisch nach Injektion von Tusche in die Katzenlunge. Seine Werte sind 0,1—0,2 cm/sec für die Capillaren und 0,3—0,7 cm/sec für die Arteriolen und Venolen.

Als Kontaktzeit errechnet A. MÜLLER (1945) für den Menschen 0,1—0,3 sec, ROUGHTON (1945) mit der CO-Methode $0,75 \pm 0,25$ sec in der Ruhe und $0,31 \pm 0,1$ sec in der Arbeit.

Das Blutvolumen, das sich in den Lungencapillaren befindet, beträgt in der Ruhe 60 cm³ und bei Arbeit 95 cm³. (Über Capillarzeit s. S. 576.)

e) Die Diffusionskapazität.

Die gesamte Diffusionskapazität ist eine Funktion, die abhängt

1. von der Größe der Kontaktfläche zwischen Blut und Gas, d.h. zwischen Oberfläche durchströmter Alveolarcapillaren und Alveolen,

2. von der Permeabilität der Austauschfläche je Flächeneinheit (Diffusionskonstante),

---

[1] MEESSEN 1960, MATTHES 1960, vgl. auch THEWS, Bad Oeynhauser Gespräche IV, 1961.

3. von den Gasspannungsgradienten zwischen Alveolarluft und Blut und

4. von der Kontaktzeit zwischen Alveolarluft und Capillarblut.

Sie ist also nicht nur abhängig von dem Membranfaktor, sondern wird auch bestimmt von der Ventilation, von der Perfusion und von der Korrelation dieser beiden Größen.

In der Ruhe ist die Diffusionskapazität der Lunge nur zu einem geringen Teil ausgenutzt. Die Reserven sind so groß, daß auch bei körperlicher Arbeit mit einer Steigerung des Sauerstoffverbrauchs auf das 6fache noch eine völlige Aufsättigung des Blutes mit O_2 in der Lunge erfolgt. Diese Leistungssteigerung wird erreicht durch verstärkte Ventilation und durch vermehrte Durchströmung der Lungencapillaren. Damit wird die Austauschfläche vergrößert.

Diffusionsstörungen äußern sich in einer Einschränkung der Diffusionskapazität. Die leichte Diffusionsstörung mindert die Lungenreserven, engt die Anpassungsbreite ein und führt erst in der Arbeit zur Lungeninsuffizienz. Bei schwerer Störung zeigt sich die respiratorische Insuffizienz bereits in der Ruhe.

Die Einschränkung der Diffusionskapazität für O_2 kann bedingt sein

1. durch Reduktion der Austauschfläche zwischen Alveolarluft und Capillarblut. Sie wird damit zu einem Flächenproblem.

2. durch erschwerte Permeabilität der alveolocapillären Membran. Diese entspricht dem Begriff der Pneumonose und wird durch solche Krankheitsprozesse repräsentiert, in denen die Alveolarmembran verdickt und die Distanz zwischen Alveolarluft und Blut vergrößert ist.

Von diesen Diffusionsstörungen im engeren Sinne sind jene Einschränkungen der Diffusionskapazität abzugrenzen, die abhängen

1. von den Änderungen des Gasspannungsgradienten zwischen Alveolarluft und Blut. Diese Störungen sind durch die Bestimmung des Atemvolumens und der Gaskonzentration in der Inspirations- und Exspirationsluft mit klinischen Methoden exakt meßbar. Sie liegen auf der Luftseite und beruhen auf zu geringer Sauerstoffspannung in der Alveolarluft, auf Hypoventilation oder auf ventilatorischen Verteilungsstörungen. Ihre morphologischen Grundlagen werden unter den Ventilationsstörungen besprochen.

2. von der Blutströmung in den Lungencapillaren. Die Strömungsgeschwindigkeit kann so beschleunigt sein, daß die Kontaktzeit des Blutes mit den Gasen der Alveolarluft in der Capillarstrecke für eine volle Aufsättigung mit O_2 nicht ausreicht, oder die Zahl der durchströmten Capillaren kann zu gering sein (funktionelle Reduktion der Kontaktfläche ohne morphologische Veränderungen der alveolocapillären Membran). Diese Störungen des Gasaustausches liegen auf der Blutseite und beruhen auf Änderungen der Zirkulation, die wir unter den Perfusionsstörungen zusammenfassen.

3. von Störungen in der Koordination zwischen alveolärer Belüftung und capillärer Perfusion. Diese Korrelations- oder Verteilungsstörungen teilen sich in eine ventilatorische und in eine zirkulatorische Seite. Sie bilden große, morphogenetisch heterogene Gruppen, die sowohl unter den Ventilationsstörungen als auch unter den Perfusionsstörungen erscheinen.

II. Die Reduktion der Austauschfläche.

a) Die alveolocapilläre Membran als Austauschfläche.

Die Gasmenge, die in der Zeiteinheit durch eine Membran bei gegebenem Konzentrationsgefälle und gegebener Membrandicke diffundiert, ist proportional der Ausdehnung dieser Membran. Die Diffusionskapazität einer Lunge hängt damit in erster Linie von der Größe der Austauschfläche ab.

Die Ausdehnung der Kontaktfläche zwischen Atemgasen und Capillarblut wird sowohl von der Größe des Alveolarraumes als auch von der Weite der Blutcapillaren beeinflußt. Unter Normalverhältnissen bestimmen Inspiration und Exspiration oder Änderungen der Atemmittellage, unter pathologischen Umständen Atelektase und Emphysem die Größe der Austauschfläche von der ventilatorischen Seite her. Die Innenfläche des Alveolarraumes beträgt nach v. Hayek (1953) 30 m² für die Exspiration und höchstens 100 m² für die tiefste Inspiration. Aeby (1880) gibt 40—50 m² für die kollabierte und 103—129 m² für die entfaltete Lunge an. Diese Zahlen werden von Engel (1950) als unrichtig berechnet abgelehnt.

Von dieser Fläche wird nur der Anteil für den Gasaustausch genutzt, in dem die Blutcapillaren unmittelbar an den Alveolarraum angrenzen. Damit wird die Größe der Kontaktfläche abhängig von der Weite des Capillarbettes und auch von der Capillarlänge. Mit der wechselnden Perfusion der Blutcapillaren ändert sich die Größe der Austauschfläche auch von der Blutseite her; sie ist in der Ruhe, in der nur ein Teil der Capillaren geöffnet ist, und bei geringem Durchflußvolumen klein, größer dagegen in der Arbeit, wenn sich auch die Reservecapillaren öffnen.

Unter pathologischen Verhältnissen kommen sowohl gefäßbedingte Vergrößerungen der Kontaktfläche durch Capillarektasie (Stauungslunge) als auch Verkleinerungen durch Reduktion der Capillaren (Emphysem, Lungenfibrose) vor.

Die für die Diffusion zur Verfügung stehende Kontaktfläche wird auch als aktive Lungenoberfläche bezeichnet, die Angaben über ihre Größe schwanken zwischen 20 und 200 m²[1]. Die maximale Aufnahme von Sauerstoff aus der Alveolarluft in das Blut liegt bei 4,5—5,5 l/min. Dieser Wert entspricht der größten Transportkapazität des Blutes für O_2 von etwa 5 l/min. Die Diffusionskapazität wird also durch die Größe der Austauschfläche und durch die Aufnahmefähigkeit des Blutes für O_2 in gleicher Weise begrenzt[2]. Nach Matthes (1960) ist es sogar wahrscheinlich, daß die Grenze der O_2-Aufnahme allein durch die Perfusionsgröße gesetzt wird, während die Diffusionsmöglichkeiten noch weiter gesteigert werden könnten.

b) Die Abhängigkeit der Austauschfläche von Entwicklung, Wachstum und Alterung der Lunge.

1. Entwicklung.

In der fetalen Entwicklung der Lunge beginnen sich während des 6. Embryonalmonats an den Endknospen des Drüsenbaumes die Alveolen zu differenzieren. Gleichzeitig setzt ein starker Wachstumsschub des Mesenchyms und des Capillarnetzes ein. Dadurch wird die Alveolarwand gedehnt. Die Alveolarepithelien, die zunächst eine zusammenhängende Schicht kubischer Zellen bilden, rücken auseinander und lösen sich unter Verfettung teilweise von der Alveolarwand ab. Mit der Streckung der Alveolarwand kommen die Blutcapillaren in eine Schicht mit den Alveolarepithelien zu liegen und treten somit in engste Beziehung zum Alveolarraum, von dem sie nur noch durch die sehr zarten flügelförmigen Fortsätze der Alveolarepithelien geschieden sind. Die schematische Darstellung v. Hayeks (1953) (Abb. 59) illustriert diese Entwicklung, die in der ausgewachsenen Lunge bei Atelektase und Lungenfibrose auch rückläufig in der Weise ablaufen kann, daß der Deckzellenbelag zusammenrückt und die Blutcapillaren unter eine Schicht kubischer Zellen zu liegen kommen. Bei Frühgeburten des

---

[1] Rossier und Bühlmann 1956.
[2] Rossier und Bühlmann 1956, Riley und Mitarbeiter 1951, Shepard und Mitarbeiter 1954.

7. und 8. Monats ist die Entwicklung der Alveolen und ihre Capillarisierung noch nicht abgeschlossen. Die Endsprossen der Bronchioli respiratorii sind nur in geringem Maße alveolär gegliedert und bilden dickwandige, mehr oder minder einheitliche, teilweise noch mit kubischem Epithel ausgekleidete Hohlräume. Die Capillarisierung der Septen ist ebenfalls noch unvollkommen, die aussprossenden Capillaren bilden erst am Ende der fetalen Entwicklung in der Alveolarwand ein einheitliches Netzwerk, das mit dem Auseinanderrücken der Alveolarepithelien unmittelbare Beziehung zum Luftraum erhält. Die hohe Atemfrequenz der Frühgeburten und der Neugeborenen findet ihre Erklärung in der kleinen Kontaktfläche.

In der postfetalen Entwicklung bilden sich in der wachsenden Lunge neue Alveolen und vergrößern damit die Austauschfläche. Der Alveolendurchmesser wächst von 0,05 mm beim Neugeborenen auf 0,2 mm beim 12jährigen Kind.

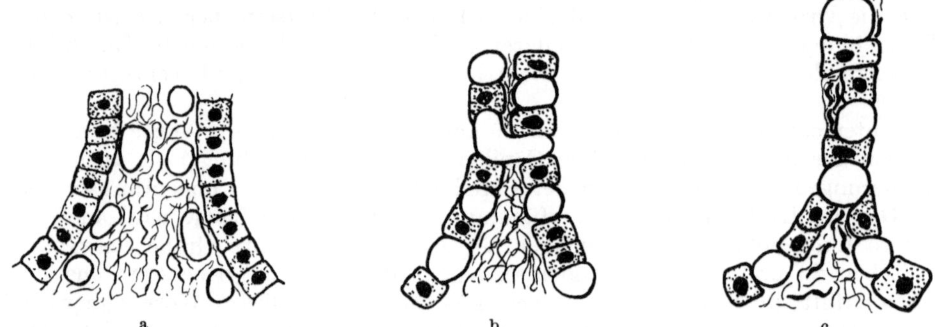

a   b   c

Abb. 59a—c. Schema des Umbaues der embryonalen Wand zweier Alveolen zum Alveolarseptum des Erwachsenen. a Breite Bindegewebsschicht mit Capillaren unter hohem Epithel. b Verminderung des Bindegewebes, Vermehrung der Capillaren (etwa 6.—8. Fetalmonat). c Dichtes Capillarnetz, Epithelzellen auseinandergerückt (postnataler Zustand). (Nach v. Hayek 1953.)

Das Volumen der Lunge nimmt dabei von 100 cm³ auf 1280 cm³ zu, die respirierende Oberfläche des Alveolarraumes von 69,1 cm² auf 235 cm² pro cm³ Volumen und für die ganze Lunge von 1,32 m² auf 30,19 m². Die atmende Oberfläche wird mit dem Wachstum nicht nur absolut größer, sondern es kommt mit der weiteren Differenzierung der Lunge auch zu einer relativen Vergrößerung im Verhältnis zum Körpergewicht um mehr als das Doppelte. Engel (1950) errechnet 4090 cm² respirierende Oberfläche pro kg Körpergewicht beim Neugeborenen und 9400 cm²/kg Körpergewicht beim 12jährigen Kind.

Die Diffusionskapazität der Lunge des Säuglings ist also wegen der relativ kleinen Kontaktfläche etwa um die Hälfte geringer als zur Zeit der Pubertät.

Mit dem relativ stärkeren Wachstum der Lunge und der größeren Austauschfläche sinkt die Atemfrequenz von 40—60 pro min beim Neugeborenen auf etwa 20 Atemzüge pro min in der Pubertät. Gleichzeitig steigt das Atemvolumen eines Atemzuges von 23 cm³ beim Neugeborenen auf 374 cm³ beim 12jährigen Kind. Bezogen auf das Körpergewicht beträgt die Atemgröße beim Säugling etwa 1000—1400 cm³/kg Körpergewicht, beim Erwachsenen nur 300 cm³/kg Körpergewicht, also nur den vierten Teil des Neugeborenen[1].

2. Die Lunge des Erwachsenen.

Mit dem Abschluß der Wachstumsperiode hat die Kontaktfläche ihre größte Ausdehnung erreicht. In der wachsenden Lunge besteht noch ein cranio-caudales

---

[1] Engel 1950.

Gefälle in der Alveolargröße. Die Alveolen der kranialen Lungenabschnitte sind kleiner als die der caudalen. Beim Erwachsenen sind diese Größenunterschiede ausgeglichen, die Alveolen in Ober- und Unterlappen sind gleich groß[1].

Von der mit den zarten Fortsätzen der Alveolarepithelien ausgekleideten Fläche des Alveolarraumes sind etwa 80% als Kontaktfläche zu bezeichnen[2]. Die restlichen 20% der Alveolenoberfläche werden für den Gasaustausch nicht genutzt. Das sind die Zonen, in denen die intercapillären Räume, das interstitielle Fasergerüst und die perinucleären Cytoplasmaanteile von Endothelien und Deckzellen liegen. In der Ruhe ist nur ein Teil der Capillaren durchströmt, die übrigen dienen als Reservecapillaren. Die vollständige Öffnung sämtlicher Capillaren findet man an der Leichenlunge nur bei Lungenstauung, bei zentral ausgelösten Kreislaufstörungen oder im Bereich von Hypostasen. Die Einschränkung der Austauschfläche und die verminderte Gasdiffusion in der Ruhe wird sowohl durch geringere Ventilation als auch durch reduzierte Perfusion erreicht. Beide Vorgänge verlaufen koordiniert.

3. Die Alterslunge.

Die Beobachtung[3] über die Abnahme der Diffusionskapazität der Lunge vom 25. Lebensjahr an gibt zu der Vermutung Anlaß, daß diese Einschränkung mit einer Verminderung der aktiven Lungenoberfläche, also der Kontaktfläche zusammenhängt, nachdem sich für eine Diffusionserschwerung durch Verdickung der alveolocapillären Membran morphologisch kein Äquivalent gefunden hat. Diese Annahme wird von FUEST u. HAAS (1958) durch die vergleichenden Untersuchungen der Capillardichte in der Alveolarwand bestätigt. In gleichem Maße wie sich die Alveolen mit zunehmendem Alter vergrößern, verringert sich relativ die Zahl ihrer Capillaren.

Für die Beziehungen zwischen maximaler Diffusionskapazität, Körpergröße und Alter gibt es die Formel

$$D_{O_2} = (0{,}67 \times \text{Körperlänge/cm}) - 0{,}55 \times (\text{Alter/Jahre} - 40{,}9).$$

Im Alter werden die Alveolarräume gleichsinnig mit dem Verlust an Elastizität der Lunge weiter, ohne daß zugleich auch eine Vermehrung der Capillaren eintritt. Dem vergrößerten Luftraum stehen verhältnismäßig weniger Capillaren gegenüber, das größere Lungenvolumen wirkt funktionell als toter Raum. Ob die im Alter abnehmende Diffusionskapazität Folge dieser Vergrößerung des Alveolarraumes oder Ausdruck einer Verminderung der Lungencapillaren bei Altersemphysem ist, bleibt noch ungeklärt[4]. Nach FORSTER (1957) steht die Unfähigkeit zu genügender Kreislaufsteigerung im Vordergrund.

Auch die ventilatorische Funktion unterliegt einem altersbedingten Wandel, der sich in einer Leistungseinschränkung der Lunge äußert[5].

Die Atemfrequenz erreicht nach den hohen Werten der frühen Kinderjahre ihr Minimum mit 16—18 Atemzügen/min im 3.—5. Lebensjahrzehnt und steigt im Alter wieder gering an. Das Atemzugsvolumen verringert sich von durchschnittlich 530 cm³ in den mittleren Lebensjahren bis auf 430 cm³ im höheren Alter. Die Thoraxexkursionsbreite sinkt von 8—10 cm auf Werte unter 5 cm ab. Die Atmung wird damit oberflächlicher und mehr abdominal. Die maximal atembare Luftmenge (Vitalkapazität), die in den mittleren Lebensjahren etwa 75% der Totalkapazität ausmacht, wird im Alter kleiner; sie sinkt bei Männern auf 75%, bei Frauen auf etwa 52% der früheren Maximalwerte ab. Diese Ein-

---

[1] HAAS 1958. [2] GIESEKING 1960.
[3] KROGH 1914/15, LILIENTHAL und Mitarbeiter 1946, RILEY und Mitarbeiter 1954.
[4] COHN, CAROLL und RILEY 1954. [5] KNOBLOCH und HILSCHER 1958.

buße erfolgt bei nur geringfügiger Änderung der Totalkapazität zugunsten der
Residualluft, deren Anteil an der Totalkapazität von 19,3% (15—25 Jahre) auf
30,8% (55—65 Jahre) zunimmt; auch die Reserveluft wird eingeschränkt. Bei
den dynamischen Werten gibt es eine starke Verminderung des maximalen
Atemminutenvolumens (Atemgrenzwert). Das in der ersten Sekunde nach tiefster
Inspiration maximal ausatembare Luftvolumen (Atemstoßtest nach Tiffeneau)
ist mit den Werten von 85% der Vitalkapazität für Männer bzw. 86% für Frauen
im 3. Lebensjahrzehnt am größten, es sinkt auf 68% (Männer) bzw. 66% (Frauen)
im 7. Lebensjahrzehnt kontinuierlich ab. Trotz dieser signifikanten Einbuße bestehen keine wesentlichen klinischen Symptome, nur die großen funktionellen
Reserven der mechanischen Ventilationsleistung sind eingeschränkt[1]. Nach
eigenen Messungen[2] beträgt der Verlust an ventilatorischer Funktion bei senilem
Emphysem bis 50%.

c) Diffusionsstörungen bei Reduktion der Austauschfläche.

Die Größe der Austauschfläche hängt von dem Dehnungszustand der Lunge
ab. Die innere Oberfläche ist in der kollabierten Lunge kleiner als in der entfalteten. Kollaps und Atelektase verkleinern die Austauschfläche entsprechend der
Abnahme des Lungenvolumens, ebenso Resektion und Pneumektomie entsprechend der Größe des Parenchymverlustes.

Da die Austauschfläche nicht nur von der Alveolenweite, sondern auch von
der Ausdehnung des Capillarbettes bestimmt wird, können schließlich alle indurativen Lungenveränderungen und alle Narben zur Einschränkung der Kontaktfläche führen.

Eine Vergrößerung der Austauschfläche ist nur bis zur maximalen Inspirationslage möglich. Das Volumen pulmonum auctum stellt die obere Grenze der
noch mit einem Nutzeffekt verbundenen Alveolenerweiterung dar. Jede weitere
Dehnung der Alveolarwand, die über eine Abflachung des Alveolarraumes schließlich in einem Alveolarschwund endet, verkleinert wieder die Kontaktfläche durch
Rückbildung und Schwund der Alveolarsepten mit den darin liegenden Capillaren.
Zum großen Lungenvolumen des Emphysems gehört eine kleine Austauschfläche.

1. Parenchymverluste.

Die Austauschfläche der Lunge kann durch zahlreiche Prozesse verkleinert
werden, in deren Verlauf Lungengewebe zerstört oder fibrös umgewandelt wird.
Das funktionierende Parenchym wird dabei um den verlorenen Anteil reduziert.
Die Restlunge übernimmt unter Einschaltung ihrer Reserven den Funktions-
anteil, der auf das verlorene Lungengewebe entfällt. Die ventilatorische Seite
dieses Problems wurde bereits besprochen (s. S. 459 unter zu kleiner Lunge).
Dort ergab sich, daß Vitalkapazität und Atemgrenzwert im Verhältnis zum
Parenchymschwund eingeschränkt sind.

Die Auswirkungen der verkleinerten Austauschfläche sind am besten nach
operativer Entfernung von Lungenteilen zu übersehen.

Bei einseitiger Pneumektomie sinkt die Vitalkapazität etwa um die Hälfte,
der Atemgrenzwert etwa um 30% der Norm. Das Blut wird in der Ruhe noch
ausreichend mit O_2 gesättigt. Bei relativ geringer Belastung entsteht aber
bereits eine O_2-Untersättigung[3]. Diese kann nicht Folge einer ungenügenden
Ventilation sein, da der arterielle CO_2-Druck infolge Hyperventilation absinkt.
Rossier u. Mitarb. (1958) stellen vielmehr eine zu klcine Capillaroberfläche als

---

[1] Knobloch und Hilscher 1958; vgl. auch S. 424—426.   [2] Hartung 1959, 1960.
[3] Maurath und Werber 1951, Maurath 1955, Rossier u. Mitarbeiter 1958.

Hauptursache der O_2-Untersättigung in den Vordergrund. Die Einschränkung der Diffusionskapazität beruht nach SCHERRER (1956) auf einer Verkürzung der Kontaktzeit.

Morphologisch findet man nach Pneumektomie in der Restlunge außer einem Volumen pulmonum auctum einen hohen Blutgehalt und weite Capillaren. Die Auswirkungen der unter Arbeit stets eintretenden Steigerung des Blutdruckes im Pulmonalkreislauf sind in diesen Fällen auch dann gering, wenn sich ein Cor pulmonale entwickelt. Die Arteriolen bleiben weit gestellt und zeigen nur geringe Intimaverdickung. Bei diesem Volumenhochdruck entsteht keine Pulmonalsklerose, die bei Hypoventilation nur selten vermißt wird.

Ebenso wie in der normalen Lunge die maximale Diffusionskapazität bei Arbeit von der Größe der durchbluteten Capillarfläche begrenzt ist, wird auch bei Parenchymverlusten die Leistungsgrenze der Restlunge von der Weite des Gefäßbettes bestimmt. Die ventilatorischen Reserven sind also auch in der Restlunge größer als die zirkulatorischen.

2. Emphysem.

Die Alveolen sind in den Acini zu respiratorischen Einheiten zusammengefaßt, in denen eine annähernd gleichmäßige Durchmischung der Atemgase vorausgesetzt werden kann.

Die Acini, die in der fetalen Lunge zunächst bläschenförmig angelegt sind, werden durch die etwa im 6. Fetalmonat einsetzende Entwicklung der Alveolen und durch Ausdifferenzierung des Arbor alveolaris zu Mikrolungen mit einem reich gegliederten Gangsystem und einer großen inneren Oberfläche.

Nach den Messungen von ENGEL (1950, 1958) beträgt das Volumen eines Acinus 150 mm³, nach seinen Berechnungen an Ausgußpräparaten von MILLER und LOESCHCKE 120 bzw. 187 mm³.

Nach vergleichenden anatomischen Untersuchungen an Tierlungen [1] liegen die Acini bei allen bisher untersuchten Säugetieren in der Größenordnung von 0,1—10 mm³. Der Acinus des Menschen ist also um ein Vielfaches größer. Ebenso sind auch die Alveolen beim Menschen wesentlich größer als beim Tier mit Ausnahme des Elefanten (Tabelle 9).

Tabelle 9. *Größenvergleich respiratorischer Einheiten bei Mensch und Tier.* (Nach ENGEL 1958.)

	Acinus-volumen mm³	Alveolen-durchmesser mm		Acinus-volumen mm³	Alveolen-durchmesser mm
Maus.	0,1	0,005	Katze	1,4	0,17
Hund	0,25	0,1	Ziege.	2,0	0,07
Ratte	0,3	0,05	Ochse	8,0	0,1
Meerschweinchen	0,3	0,06	Elefant	7,0	0,25
Kaninchen . . .	0,5	0,1	Mensch	150,0	0,2

Da die Oberfläche im kleineren Raum relativ größer ist als in einem großen Raum, ist das Verhältnis von Rauminhalt zu innerer Oberfläche in den kleinen Alveolen der Tiere günstiger für den Gasaustausch als in den großen Alveolen des Menschen.

Beim Emphysem verschiebt sich die Relation von Oberfläche zu Rauminhalt in den Acini noch weiter dadurch, daß die Alveolarsepten verstreichen und die Alveolargänge in ungegliederte Röhrchen umgewandelt werden (Abb. 60). Schwinden bei zunehmendem Emphysem schließlich auch die intraacinösen Septen,

---

[1] ENGEL 1958.

dann wird der Acinus zu einer einheitlichen, kaum noch gegliederten Höhle, die der primitiven Sacklunge niederer Tiere, z.B. eines Frosches, entspricht.

Das Ausmaß der Flächenreduktion wird an folgenden Beispielen deutlich:

Wählt man als Modell einen Kubus, der durch 3 Scheidewände in 8 Kammern mit 1 cm Kantenlänge unterteilt ist, so hat jede Kammer eine Oberfläche von 6 cm², der ganze Kubus 8 × 6 cm² = 48 cm². Nimmt man die Scheidewände heraus, dann hat der nunmehr aus

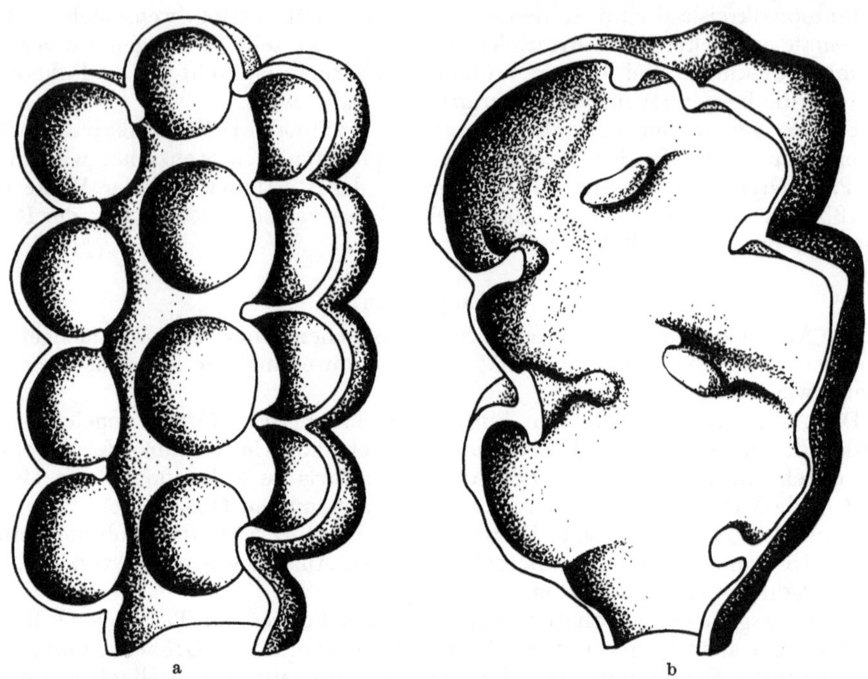

a   b

Abb. 60a u. b. Flächenreduktion in einem Alveolargang bei Emphysem. Schematische Darstellung. a Normaler Alveolargang, um den die Alveolen kabinenartig angeordnet sind. b Stummelförmige Reste der Alveolarsepten nach Umwandlung des Alveolarganges in einen ungegliederten Sack bei Emphysem.

einem Raum bestehende Kubus nur noch eine Oberfläche von 6 × 4 cm² = 24 cm². Die Konfluenz der 8 Kammern bedeutet also eine Reduktion der Oberfläche auf die Hälfte[1].

In dem in Gänge und Alveolen gegliederten Acinus mit seiner im Verhältnis zum Volumen wesentlich größeren inneren Oberfläche kann der Flächenverlust noch stärkere Grade annehmen, wie eine Überschlagsrechnung an einem Acinusmodell zeigt (Tabelle 10).

Tabelle 10. Volumen- und Flächenmaße der normalen Lunge.

Alveole	Durchmesser	0,24 mm
	Volumen	0,0035 mm³
	Fläche	0,09 mm²
	Zahl der Alveolen im Acinus	etwa 21500
	Zahl der Alveolen in der gesamten Lunge	etwa 645 Millionen
Acinus	Durchmesser	6,6 mm
	Volumen	150 mm³
	Fläche	etwa 20 cm²
	Zahl der Acini in der gesamten Lunge	etwa 30000
Gesamte Lunge	Volumen	5000 cm³
	Austauschfläche	etwa 60 m²

Der Acinus mit einem durchschnittlichen Volumen von 150 mm³ hat, vereinfacht als Kugel gedacht, einen Radius von 3,3 mm. Etwa die Hälfte seines Innenraumes entfällt auf das nur teilweise mit Alveolen besetzte Gangsystem, so daß für die Alveolen, die angenähert

---

[1] Uehlinger 1956.

als Halbkugeln angesehen werden können, etwa 75 mm³ Raum im Acinus bleiben. Der mittlere Alveolenradius ist mit 0,12 mm anzusetzen, woraus sich ein Volumen von 0,0035 mm³ und eine Fläche von 0,09 mm² errechnet. Die Gesamtfläche aller Alveolen im Acinus beträgt daher etwa 20 cm², in der gesamten, in Atemmittellage angenommenen Lunge etwa 60 m², wenn man von einer Zahl von 30000 Acini in der Lunge ausgeht.

Verliert nun der Acinus im Zuge des emphysematösen Umbaues bei diffusem senilem Emphysem seine Innengliederung so vollständig, daß er einem leeren Sack gleicht, so beträgt seine Fläche nur noch die einer Kugel mit einem Radius von 3,3 mm, also etwa 1,4 cm², sie ist gegenüber dem in Alveolen gegliederten Acinus um 18,6 cm² = 93% vermindert. Betrifft dieser Acinusumbau die gesamte Lunge in gleichem Maße, so kann die respiratorische Oberfläche der Lunge bis auf 4,2 m², d. h. bis auf 7% ihres normalen Wertes reduziert werden. Eine so starke Flächenreduktion ist auch bei normalen Ventilationswerten nicht mehr mit dem Leben vereinbar. Die Prognose bei Emphysempatienten wird von BATES u. Mitarb. (1956) auf Grund der verbliebenen O_2-Diffusionskapazität gestellt. Durch kombinierte spirometrische und blutgasanalytische Untersuchung ist eine Abgrenzung der ventilatorischen Störungen und der durch Kontaktflächenreduktion bedingten Gasaustauschstörungen möglich[1].

Aus diesen Beispielen geht hervor, daß mit dem emphysematösen Umbau einer Lunge eine erhebliche Verkleinerung der inneren Oberfläche verbunden ist. UEHLINGER (1956) nennt das Emphysem die „Krankheit der Kontaktflächenreduktion", da mit dem Abbau der Alveolarsepten auch ein entsprechender Teil der Capillarfläche durch Schwund der Capillaren in den Septen verlorengeht.

Bei jeder Form des Emphysems ist die Kontaktflächenreduktion morphologisch nachweisbar. Am stärksten ist sie bei dem diffusen atrophischen Emphysem, dessen Hauptvertreter das Altersemphysem ist. Bei schweren Graden dieses Emphysems kann mit einer Flächenreduktion um 50—75% gerechnet werden. Anatomische Messungen liegen noch nicht vor. Bei dem Herdemphysem wird die Fläche weit weniger reduziert, ebenso geht auch beim großblasigen bronchostenotischen Emphysem nur wenig Parenchym verloren (s. unter bronchostenotischem Emphysem). Die schweren Störungen liegen hier vor allem auf der Ventilations- und Perfusionsseite.

Die funktionelle Bedeutung dieses Verlustes an Kontaktfläche scheint geringer zu sein, als man nach dem anatomischen Befund annehmen möchte. Die Erfahrung zeigt, daß ein großer Teil anatomisch deutlicher Emphyseme klinisch unbemerkt bleibt. Unter den Symptomen des diffusen Emphysems steht die Dyspnoe als Zeichen der Ventilationsstörung im Vordergrund. Die Kontaktflächenreduktion schränkt zwar die Reserven ein. Diese sind aber so groß, daß ein Verlust von 50% der 30—120 m² großen Fläche sich noch nicht auf die Sauerstoffsättigung des Blutes auswirkt. Erst bei Reduktion um 75% tritt Insuffizienz bei mäßiger Belastung in Erscheinung. 10% der Kontaktfläche ist der absolute untere Grenzwert[2].

3. Atelektase.

Eine Verkleinerung der Austauschfläche tritt auch dann ein, wenn die Lunge zu wenig belüftet wird.

Die vollständige Atelektase eines größeren Lungenabschnittes kommt im Gasaustausch einem entsprechenden Parenchymverlust gleich. Dieser ventilatorisch tote Raum wird aber noch von Blut durchströmt, das nicht am Gasaustausch teilnimmt und als venöse Beimischung (funktionelles Kurzschlußblut) im linken Herzen erscheint.

In der hypoventilierten Lunge behalten die Alveolen bis zum Kollapszustand ihre Eigenform. Volumen und Austauschfläche verkleinern sich aber nicht in gleichem Maße, sondern die Volumen/Flächenrelation verschiebt sich zugunsten

---

[1] ZUIDEMA und SCHERRER 1955, ROSSIER und Mitarbeiter 1956, 1958, LOTTENBACH 1956, MATTHES und Mitarbeiter 1960.
[2] UEHLINGER 1956.

der Fläche. In der kleinen Alveole der nahezu kollabierten Lunge steht ein sehr kleines Luftvolumen einer relativ großen Austauschfläche gegenüber. Beim Vergleich mit dem Emphysem ergibt sich das Paradoxon, daß bei der großen Emphysemlunge eine absolut zu kleine Austauschfläche einem relativ großen Luftvolumen, bei der kleinen hypoventilierten Lunge ein absolut zu kleines Luftvolumen einer relativ großen Austauschfläche gegenüber steht.

Die Hypoventilation führt neben einer zu geringen O_2-Aufnahme in das Blut auch zu einer verminderten CO_2-Ausscheidung und nachfolgenden Acidose sowie zu Vasoconstriction und damit zum Druckanstieg im kleinen Kreislauf.

Das Hypoventilationssyndrom (Cyanose, Acidose mit Somnolenz, Polyglobulie und pulmonale Hypertonie) wird besonders durch Störungen der Zwerchfellatmung ausgelöst und findet sich oft bei Zwerchfellhochstand. Beispiele dafür sind das Pickwick-Syndrom beim Zwerchfellhochstand durch Adipositas oder die Zwerchfellähmung (s. S. 461 unter diaphragmatogenen Ventilationsstörungen).

III. Permeabilitätsstörungen der alveolocapillären Membran (Pneumonose).

a) Begriffsbestimmung und Abgrenzung.

Die Diffusionsstörungen, die durch verminderte Durchlässigkeit der alveolocapillären Membran für Atemgase bedingt sind, werden als Pneumonosen bezeichnet[1]. Die ersten Versuche einer Abgrenzung der Pneumonose gegen andere Störungen des Gasaustausches stammen von Brauer und seinen Mitarbeitern[2].

Knipping (1935) hat folgende Gruppen aufgestellt, die teils aus allgemeiner klinischer Erfahrung, teils aus Funktionsprüfungen, teils aus anatomischen Befunden abgeleitet sind: 1. Grippepneumonose, 2. Stauungsinduration, 3. krankhafte Ablagerungen und Speicherungen in der Lunge, 4. diabetische Pneumonose und 5. Pneumonose bei Emphysem. Ätiologisch gliedert er in primär pulmonal bedingte Formen und in primär kardial bedingte Lungenveränderungen.

In der Gruppe der Lungenfibrosen erscheinen neben Schäden durch Phosgen und SO_2-Inhalation zahlreiche heterogene, mit Induration des Lungengerüstes einhergehende Prozesse, wie etwa die Silikose, die Boecksche Krankheit, Carcinommetastasen und ähnliche Zustände[3]. Die Fibrosen im engeren Sinne haben fast stets auch erhebliche Störungen der Perfusion durch Capillarreduktion und oft auch örtliche Einschränkungen der Ventilation im Sinne der ventilatorischen Verteilungsstörung zur Folge. Die Abgrenzung des Anteils, der bei diesen Formen der respiratorischen Insuffizienz auf die Diffusion fällt, ist morphologisch kaum möglich.

Beim Versuch einer Gliederung nach morphologischen Gesichtspunkten werden die geweblichen Veränderungen der alveolocapillären Membran im Mittelpunkt stehen. Diese können die Membran in ihrer Gesamtheit oder nur einzelne ihrer Schichten betreffen. Sie können in Quellungen, Einlagerungen flüssiger oder fester Substanzen, in Zellvermehrungen und in Auflagerungen auf die Alveolarwand bestehen. Wir gehen dabei von der Voraussetzung aus, daß jede Verlängerung der Diffusionsstrecke auch gleichzeitig eine Hemmung des Gasaustausches bewirkt, ohne heute schon sagen zu können, von welchem Grade ab mit klinisch in Erscheinung tretenden Funktionsstörungen gerechnet werden kann.

---

[1] Brauer 1932.

[2] Schjerning 1922, Jansen, Knipping und Stromberger 1932, R. Schoen 1930 u. a.

[3] Vgl. Knipping und Bolt dieses Handbuch, Bolt 1960.

Morphologisch können Änderungen in der Struktur und Dicke der Alveolarsepten, deren Folgen eine Verlängerung der Diffusionsstrecke und vielleicht auch eine Vergrößerung des Diffusionswiderstandes durch Änderungen der Medien in der alveolocapillären Membran sind, verhältnismäßig leicht erfaßt werden. Ihre funktionellen Auswirkungen lassen sich einstweilen aber aus methodischen Gründen nur indirekt erschließen.

Die Diffusionserschwerung äußert sich in einer Vergrößerung des endcapillären Spannungsgradienten für O_2 zwischen Blut und Alveolarluft und in einer Minderung des Sauerstoffdruckes im rückfließenden Lungenblut. Der Austausch von Kohlensäure ist wegen ihrer hohen Diffusionsgeschwindigkeit in der Regel unbeeinflußt. Durch Sauerstoffatmung wird die Diffusionskapazität wesentlich verbessert. Bei schweren Membranveränderungen tritt ein vollständiger alveolocapillärer Block ein.

In den meisten Fällen von Pneumonose liegen gleichzeitig Störungen der Blutzirkulation (Perfusion) vor, in deren Folge die Kontaktzeit der Gase mit dem Capillarblut verkürzt ist. Das gilt vor allem für die Lungenfibrose mit starker Reduktion der Blutcapillaren und nachfolgender Hypertonie im kleinen Kreislauf. Die Reduktion der Blutcapillaren muß aber erheblich sein. Erst wenn der capilläre Abschnitt der Lungenstrombahn um zwei Drittel oder mehr eingeschränkt ist, wächst die Strömungsgeschwindigkeit so stark an, daß die verkürzte Kontaktzeit bereits in der Ruhe nicht mehr zur Aufsättigung des Blutes ausreicht.

Bei einer isolierten Membranstörung soll der Druck in der Arteria pulmonalis nicht erhöht sein. Fälle von reinen Diffusionsstörungen ohne gleichzeitige Änderung der Perfusion und ohne ventilatorische Verteilungsstörungen werden in der Klinik nur selten beobachtet[1]. ROSSIER (1956) sagt dazu: Abgesehen von Lungenödem haben wir noch nie eine sichere Diffusionsstörung, die allein oder vorwiegend auf eine eigentliche Membranstörung bei normaler Capillaroberfläche zurückgeführt werden müßte, gesehen[2].

b) Die morphologischen Grundlagen der Pneumonose.

1. Lungenödem.

Das Lungenödem gilt als das Hauptbeispiel der Pneumonose, obwohl auch hier, ähnlich wie bei anderen Ursachen einer Pneumonose, nur selten Störungen der Zirkulation oder Einschränkungen der Ventilation als mitwirkende Faktoren für eine unzureichende Sauerstoffaufnahme in das Blut ausgeschlossen werden können.

Über die morphologischen Veränderungen der alveolocapillären Membran beim Lungenödem sind wir erst aus elektronenoptischen Untersuchungen genauer unterrichtet. Die lichtmikroskopischen Befunde geben keinen ausreichenden Einblick in das Verhalten der einzelnen Schichten beim Durchtritt der Ödemflüssigkeit. Es ist zunächst noch offen, ob alle Formen des Lungenödems, das aus Erhöhung des intracapillären Druckes, aus vermehrter Durchlässigkeit der Capillarwand oder aus Störungen des Lymphabflusses entstehen und durch Einwirkungen zahlreicher heterogener Schädlichkeiten hervorgerufen sein kann, mit gleichartigen Veränderungen der alveolocapillären Membran einhergehen.

MEESSEN und SCHULZ (1957) erzeugten an Ratten akutes Ödem durch intraperitoneale Injektion von Thiosemicarbazid, durch Abschnürung der Vena pulmonalis und durch Einatmung von konzentriertem O_2 oder eines Gasgemisches von Luft mit 3%iger CO_2. GIESEKING (1959) verwandte Adrenalin und Histamin, das intratracheal oder intraperitoneal appli-

---

[1] KNIPPING und BOLT, siehe dieses Handbuch.
[2] ROSSIER, BÜHLMANN und WIESINGER 1956.

ziert wurde. Die gleiche Substanz hatte früher bereits v. Hayek (1943) zum Studium der Ödemgenese in lichtmikroskopischen Untersuchungen verwandt. Kisch (1958) machte gleichartige Versuche am Kaninchen.

Im Beginn des Lungenödems bilden sich im Capillarendothel 0,05—0,1 μ große Vacuolen, in denen das Transsudat als feinflockige Substanz erkennbar ist (Abb. 61). Diese Vacuolen können bis zu 2 μ großen Blasen zusammenfließen, die eine zunächst einfache, später doppeltkonturierte Membran haben. Die Blasen öffnen sich gegen das Interstitium und entleeren ihren Inhalt in das Zwischengewebe. Die Kontinuität der Endothelzellschicht bleibt dabei erhalten, es treten keine Lücken zwischen den Endothelien auf. Die Basalmembran der Endothelien wird vom Transsudat durchflossen, sie stellt ebenso wie die Basalmembran des Alveolarepithels kein Hindernis für den Durchtritt der Flüssigkeit

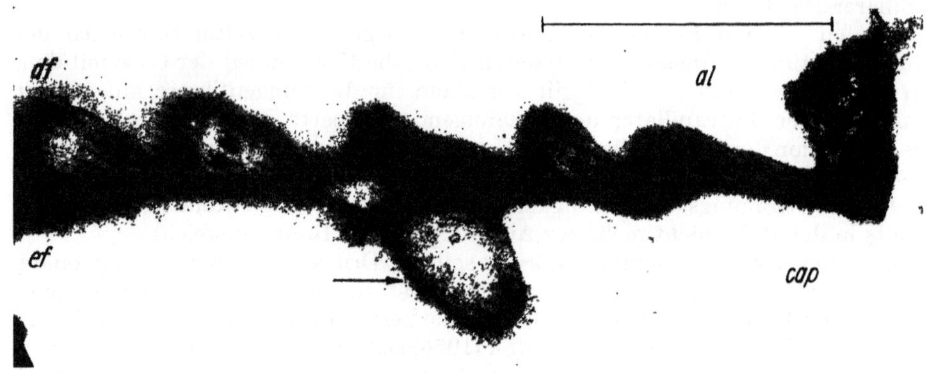

Abb. 61. Experimentelles Lungenödem. Rattenlunge 10 min nach der intratrachealen Injektion von 1 cm³ Adrenalin (1:1000). Vacuolisierung des Endothelcytoplasmas (Pinocytose) (→), beginnende Schwellung des Deckzellfortsatzes. *al* Alveolarraum; *cap* Capillarlichtung; *df* Cytoplasmafortsatz einer Alveolardeckzelle; *ef* flächenhaft ausgebreiteter Cytoplasmafortsatz einer Endothelzelle. Vergr. 38 000 ×.

dar. Bei Versuchen mit Thiosemicarbazid beschreiben Meessen u. Schulz (1957) eine Auflösung der Grenzschicht der Endothel- und Epithelzellen sowie eine Quellung des periendothelialen Streifens. Zu einer interstitiellen Ansammlung größerer Flüssigkeitsmengen kommt es nur dort, wo interstitielles Fasergewebe entwickelt ist, also zwischen den Lungencapillaren und vorzugsweise um die größeren Gefäße. Das reticuläre Fasergeflecht wird von Flüssigkeit durchtränkt, die Elementarfibrillen verquellen und verschmelzen teilweise miteinander. Aus dem Interstitium tritt die Flüssigkeit in die Alveolarepithelien ein, deren Fortsätze bis zu einer Breite von 2,5 μ anschwellen, ohne daß die Zellgrenzen auseinanderweichen[1]. Die Epithelzellen werden dabei nicht von der Basalmembran abgehoben. Bei starker Schwellung der Epithelzellen reißt die äußere Grenzschicht der Epithelzellen ein und gibt der Flüssigkeit den Weg in die Alveole frei (Abb. 62). Der Übertritt der Blutflüssigkeit aus den Capillaren in die Alveolen erfolgt nicht über vorbestehende oder neugebildete intercelluläre Lücken, sondern transcellulär durch Diffusion. In späten Stadien des Ödems entstehen sekundär auch Epitheldefekte.

Im Anfangsstadium des Ödems der Rattenlunge beträgt der mittlere Blut-Luftweg 1,8 μ, im Spätstadium 2,5 μ (gegenüber einer mittleren Norm von 0,15 bis 0,5 μ). Mit dem Einstrom der Flüssigkeit aus dem Interstitium in die Alveolarepithelien bilden sich schlauchartige Einbruchstellen in der basalen Grenzschicht der Alveolarepithelien[2].

---

[1] Gieseking 1959.   [2] Meessen und Schulz 1957.

Die alveolocapilläre Membran ist in ihrer Gesamtheit bei Ödem also erheblich, etwa bis zum 4—5fachen verdickt, die Diffusionsstrecke entsprechend verlängert.

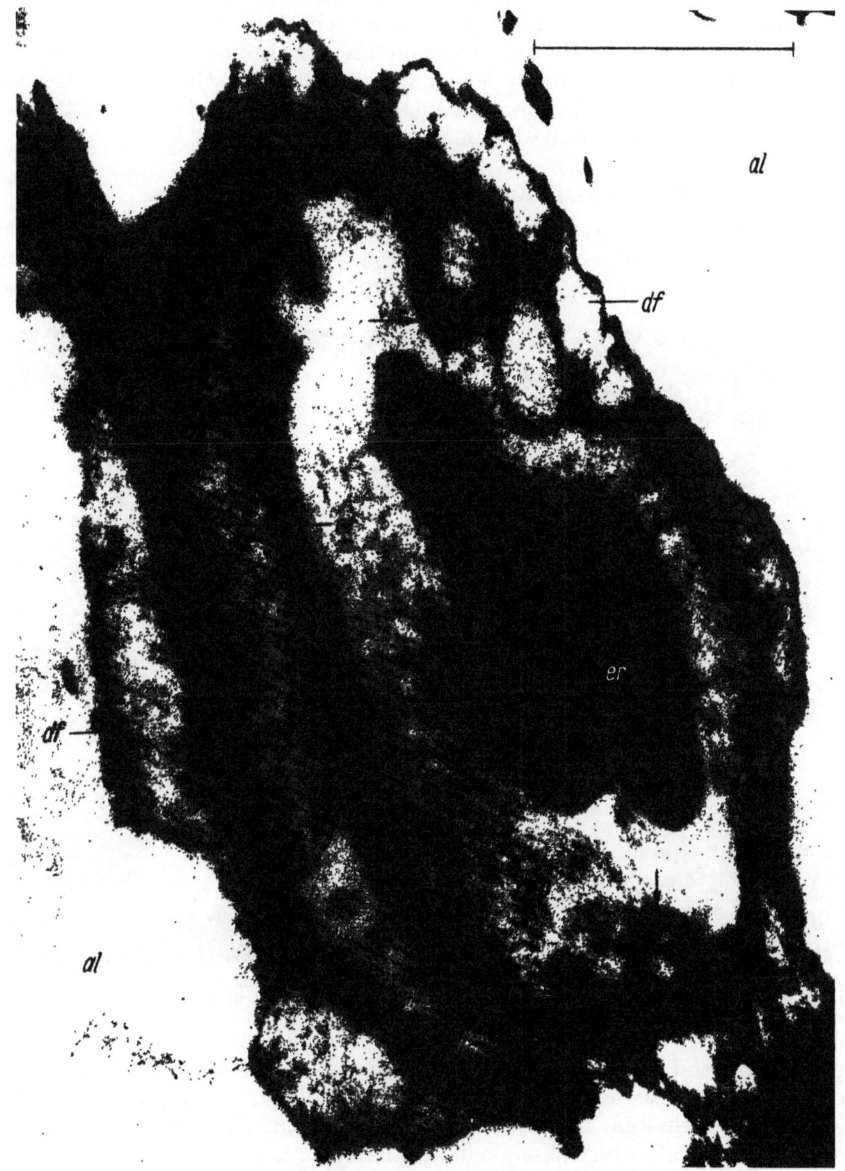

Abb. 62. Experimentelles Lungenödem. Rattenlunge 10 min nach der intratrachealen Injektion von 1 cm³ Adrenalin (1:1000). Vacuolisierung des Endothelcytoplasmas (→), interstitielles Ödem (x), Schwellung und Auflockerung des Cytoplasmas der Alveolardeckzellen. *al* Alveolarraum; *cap* Capillarlichtung; *df* flächenhaft ausgebreiteter, peripherer Cytoplasmafortsatz einer Alveolardeckzelle, durch intraepitheliales Ödem stark geschwollen und aufgelockert; *ef* periphere Cytoplasmazone einer Endothelzelle; *er* Erythrocyt. Vergr. 34000×.

Zu dieser Verlängerung kommt die aus Normalvergleichen zu schließende Erschwerung der Diffusion durch die Ödemflüssigkeit, deren Dichte dem Blutplasma entspricht.

Aus diesen Versuchen geht übereinstimmend hervor, daß die alveolocapilläre Membran von Flüssigkeit durchtränkt wird und aufquillt. Die Diffusionsstrecke wird dadurch verlängert. Der Schluß liegt nahe, daß im Ödem auch dort, wo die Alveolen noch keine vermehrte Flüssigkeit enthalten, eine wesentliche Erschwerung und Verzögerung der Gasdiffusion, insbesondere für O_2 eintritt.

Diese experimentellen Befunde lassen sich auch auf das Ödem beim Menschen übertragen, da in der Dicke der Alveolarwand bei Mensch und Ratte keine nennenswerten Unterschiede bestehen.

2. Diffusionsstörungen durch hyaline Membranen.

In den Lungen von Frühgeburten, seltener von reifen Neugeborenen, bilden sich auf der Wand der Alveolen, der Alveolargänge und der Bronchioli respiratorii oft hyaline Membranen, die in den gewöhnlich nur unvollkommen entfalteten

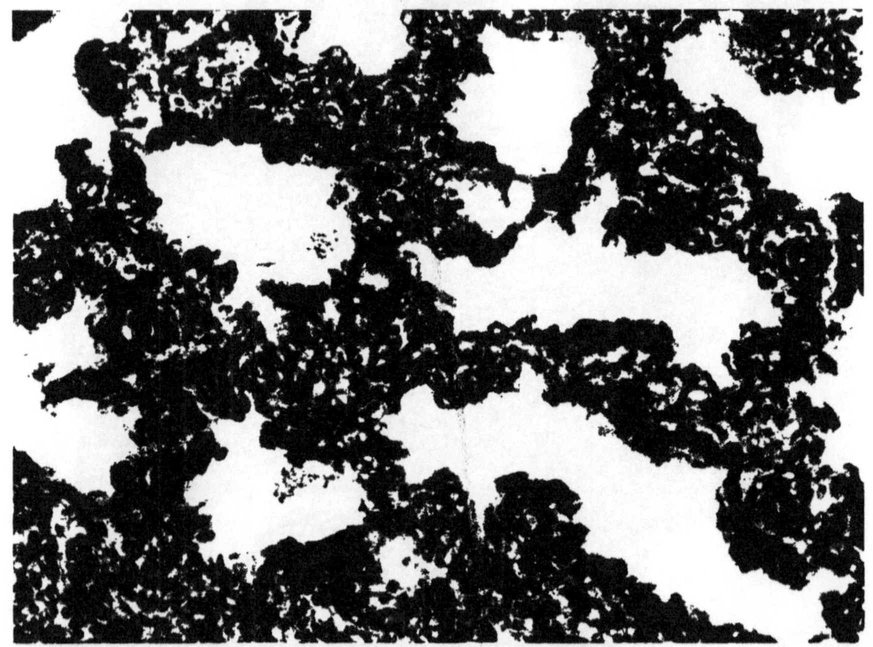

Abb. 63. Hyaline Membranen in der Lunge einer Frühgeburt. Unvollständig entfaltete Alveolen. Zellreiche Septen der noch nicht ausgereiften 41 cm langen Frühgeburt. Gest. 8 Std nach der Geburt. S.-Nr. 197/59. Vergr. 200fach.

Lungen vorwiegend in den beatmeten Lungenabschnitten zu finden sind[1]. Diese homogenen, bis zu 10 und $20\,\mu$ dicken Niederschläge, die Lipoide und Mucopolysaccharide enthalten, liegen der Alveolarwand auf (Abb. 63). Sie entstehen bei vermehrter Capillardurchlässigkeit, als deren Ursache eine allgemeine Ödemneigung Frühgeborener[2], künstliche Sauerstoffbeatmung und Hyperkapnie angeschuldigt werden. Im Tierversuch sind diese hyalinen Membranen bei Sauerstoffvergiftung[3] und durch CO_2-Vergiftung[4] erzeugt worden. Kloos erklärt die Bildung hyaliner Membranen bei O_2-Atmung durch Kohlensäurerückstauung. Unter CO_2-Anreicherung kommt es zu einer Auflockerung und Schwellung der

---

[1] Literaturübersicht bei Kloos 1959.   [2] Veith 1957, Ziegler 1957.
[3] Liebegott 1941, Pichotka 1941, Pichotka und Kühn 1947.
[4] Meessen 1948, Kloos und Wulf 1956.

Gewebsstrukturen mit Verquellung der alveolocapillären Membran, Nekrosen des Alveolarepithels und der Capillarwände.

Die in den Alveolarraum abgeschiedene Ödemflüssigkeit wird in den beatmeten Alveolen eingedickt und legt sich der Alveolarwand an[1].

Neugeborene mit hyalinen Membranen in den Lungen sterben gewöhnlich am 2. Tag nach der Geburt durch Erstickung, deren Ursache neben in der Regel bestehenden Atelektasen die erschwerte Gasdiffusion ist. Die hyalinen Membranen machen einen alveolocapillären Block.

Auch beim Erwachsenen entstehen hyaline Membranen in der Lunge als Folge toxischer Capillarwandschäden und bei chronischem Lungenödem. Bei Urämie, bei diabetischer Acidose, bei Einatmung von Phosgen, Dimethylsulfat, nitrosen Gasen, SO_2 und auch bei infektiös-toxisch bedingten Capillarwandschäden sind hyaline Abscheidungen auf der Alveolarwand und Zellnekrosen beschrieben worden[2]. In der Regel sind bei diesen mehr herdförmigen Membranbildungen andere Alveolarbezirke mit Ödemflüssigkeit gefüllt und dadurch von der Ventilation ausgeschlossen. Todesursache wird hier stets das mehr oder minder ausgedehnte Lungenödem. Die hyalinen Membranen bilden in den noch ventilierten Lungenabschnitten ein zusätzliches Diffusionshindernis.

3. Die Diffusionsstörungen bei Stauungslunge.

Bei allen Zirkulationsstörungen, die mit einer Druckerhöhung im Venensystem einhergehen, erfährt die Lunge Veränderungen, deren Grad von der Schwere und der Dauer der Stauung abhängig ist. Diese Veränderungen spielen sich teils an den Gefäßen und teils am Lungengerüst ab. Das Gefäßsystem wird zunächst im capillären und venösen, später auch im arteriellen Teil erweitert und enthält erheblich mehr Blut als eine normale Lunge. Mit der Angiographie haben SCHOENMACKERS u. VIETEN (1954, 1958) gezeigt, daß die Arterien und Venen bei der Mitralstenose sich nicht gleichmäßig verjüngen, sondern ihr Kaliber an den Teilungsstellen stufenartig verkleinern. Die Arterien sind korkzieherartig geschlängelt, Anastomosen zwischen Bronchial- und Pulmonalarterien werden sichtbar. Das postmortale Angiogramm deckt sich mit den am Lebenden erhobenen Befunden. Die Überlastung des Gefäßsystems äußert sich auch in einer Wandhypertrophie mit Vermehrung der elastisch-muskulösen Anteile. W. W. MEYER und RICHTER (1955, 1956) haben im extrapulmonalen Anteil der Lungenarterie eine Verdoppelung des Gewichtes bei der Mitralstenose feststellen können. Eine sekundäre Sklerose und Atheromatose, ebenso auch herdförmiges Intimaödem der Arterien werden bei schwerer Stauung nie vermißt. Diese Gefäßveränderungen stehen in Korrelation zur Hypertrophie der rechten Herzkammer. Je stärker die Rechtshypertrophie, um so ausgeprägter ist die Gefäßsklerose. Auch für die Venen ist eine Wandsklerose festgestellt worden[3]. Die Veränderungen am Gefäßsystem werden unter den Zirkulationsstörungen genauer besprochen.

Das Lungengerüst wird bei der Stauungslunge durch Faservermehrung diffus verdichtet und versteift. Die chronische Stauungslunge ist groß, derb, infolge des vermehrten Blutgehaltes und der Gerüstsklerose 2—3mal schwerer als eine normale Lunge. Bei der Eröffnung des Thorax retrahiert sie sich nur wenig und kollabiert nach der Herausnahme nicht. Die elastische Dehnbarkeit ist vermindert. Der Luftgehalt ist im ganzen reduziert, der vordere Lungenrand durch

---

[1] v. GAVALLÉR 1956 u. a.
[2] LOESCHCKE 1910, ASCHOFF 1916, W. KOCH 1921, SCHULTZ-BRAUNS 1930, BÜSCHER 1932, PICHOTKA 1941, LIEBEGOTT 1941 u. a.
[3] MEESSEN 1956, VAN BOGAERT 1959.

leichte Blähung abgerundet. Der Endzustand der chronischen Lungenstauung ist die braune Induration.

Vor diesem Hintergrund spielen sich die Vorgänge ab, die wir als Diffusionsstörungen im engeren Sinn bei Lungenstauung bezeichnen wollen. Sie betreffen die Capillarwand, das Alveolarepithel und den Spaltraum zwischen den Basalmembranen des Endothels und des Alveolarepithels. Sie geben die Berechtigung, die Stauungslunge unter Pneumonose abzuhandeln, zumal die Perfusionsstörungen wegen Verlängerung der Kontaktzeit nicht wesentlich zu dem Bilde der Diffusionsstörung beitragen und in vielen Fällen auch nach operativ erreichter hämodynamischer Normalisierung Minderungen der Diffusionskapazität bestehen bleiben.

Die Veränderungen der Capillarwand sind bei chronischer Lungenstauung regelmäßig, wenn auch in verschiedener Stärke gefunden worden. Die Verdickung der Capillarwand steht in Relation zu dem erhöhten Druck in den Capillaren. Bei Stauungslunge und Linksinsuffizienz des Herzens liegt der mittlere pulmonale Capillardruck (p. c. p.), der im Durchschnitt 8,4 mm Hg beim Gesunden beträgt, um 10—20 mm Hg höher[1].

Zu Jeddeloh (1931) hat ebenso wie später andere Autoren[2] auf eine Verdickung der Capillarwand hingewiesen, die Moell (1941) als Ursache der Pneumonose auffaßt. Moell gibt nach Messungen an Paraffin-Schnitten Wanddicken von 2—2,4 μ gegenüber bis 0,4 μ in der normalen Lunge an. Moell fand die Capillarverdickung nicht nur bei Mitralstenose, sondern auch bei anderen Überlastungen des kleinen Kreislaufs.

Durch die elektronenoptischen Untersuchungen sind diese Befunde in ihren Grundzügen bestätigt und erweitert worden. Schulz (1956) konnte an intravital bei Sprengung des stenosierten Klappenringes der Mitralis entnommenen Lungenstückchen feststellen, daß an den Capillarendothelien Verdichtung und Osmiophilie des Cytoplasmas, aber nur geringe Verdickung der Cytoplasmafortsätze von 450 auf 850 Å auftritt. Die Zellverdichtung sieht er als Folge vermehrter Einlagerung von Lipoiden an.

Die Basalmembran der Capillaren schwillt von 0,03—0,1 μ in der normalen Lunge je nach der Schwere der Stauung auf 0,6—1,6 μ an. Die Schwellung der Basalmembran und des Endothels ist damit das Äquivalent der lichtoptisch mit verschiedenen Färbemethoden festgestellten Capillarwandverdickung. Die am Paraffinschnitt gewonnenen Meßergebnisse decken sich etwa mit den elektronenoptischen Befunden. Schulz (1956) gibt für die Mitralstenose durchschnittliche Capillarwanddicken von 2—2,4 μ an. Die Schichtdicke der Basalmembran hängt im übrigen von der Capillarweite ab. In der gedehnten Capillare ist die Basalmembran dünner als in der kollabierten. Mit der Dehnung erfolgt also eine Massenverschiebung der gelartigen Masse aus Eiweiß und Mucopolysacchariden, aus denen sich die Basalmembran aufbaut. Nach Gieseking (1960) nimmt die Schichtdicke der peripheren Endothelzellzonen in chronischen Stauungslungen auf etwa 0,3 μ zu. Die pericapillären Basalmembranen weisen dagegen nur an umschriebenen Stellen Verbreiterungen auf.

Allen akuten Stauungslungen ist weiter die Verlängerung und Erweiterung der Capillaren gemeinsam. Die bei Anstieg des venösen Druckes in Funktion tretenden Regulationsmechanismen der kleinen Venolen und Postcapillaren werden schon frühzeitig durchbrochen. Die Stromcapillaren und das gesamte Maschenwerk der Netzcapillaren werden mit Blut aufgefüllt und gleichzeitig unter erhöhten Druck gesetzt. Dabei wird die Lichtung der Netzcapillaren der Weite

---

[1] Matthes und Mitarbeiter 1959.
[2] Parker und Weiss 1936, O'Neal und Mitarbeiter 1955, Henry 1952, Moschcowitz 1932.

der Stromcapillaren angepaßt. Die in der normalen Lunge 6—12 μ weite und im Querschnitt 1—2 Erythrocyten umfassende Lichtung der Netzcapillaren bekommt einen Durchmesser um 20 μ und mehr und enthält im Querschnitt 3—5, mitunter auch bis zu 10 und 20 Erythrocyten.

Die erweiterten und verlängerten Netzcapillaren wölben sich in die Alveolarlichtung vor[1] und engen die Alveolarlichtung ein. Man kann von einem Prolaps der Capillaren in die Alveolen sprechen. GIAMPALMO u. SCHOENMACKERS (1952), SCHOENMACKERS u. GIAMPALMO (1953) nennen diesen Zustand angiektatische Alveolarkompression (Abb. 64). Dem erweiterten Capillarraum mit der verlang-

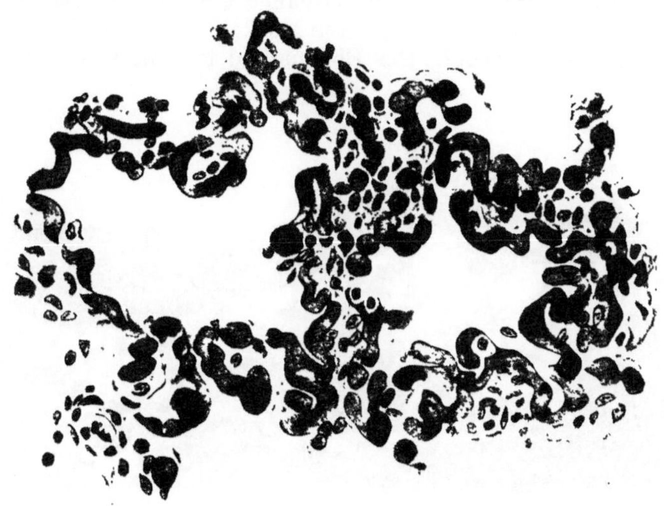

Abb. 64. Angiektatische Alveolarkompression durch Vorspringen der Capillaren in das Alveolarlumen bei Lungenstauung. (Aus CEELEN 1931.)

samten Blutströmung steht der verkleinerte Luftraum gegenüber, zu der Zirkulationsstörung tritt die Einengung des Ventilationsraumes. Die Stauungslunge ist in diesem Zustand durch ein Zuviel an Blut und Zuwenig an Luft charakterisiert.

In den Alveolarsepten kommt es neben der vermehrten serösen Durchtränkung des Spaltraumes zwischen den Capillaren und den Alveolarepithelien, die beiderseits die Alveolarwand bedecken, zu einer deutlichen Vermehrung des reticulären Fasergewebes. In der normalen Lunge sind dort, wo die Capillaren dem Alveolarepithel anliegen, wo also die Basalmembranen der Capillaren und der Epithelschicht miteinander zu einer gemeinsamen Basalmembran verschmelzen, keine Fasern vorhanden. Zwischen den Capillaren liegen dagegen reticuläre und elastische Fasern, die zu einem lockeren Maschenwerk verflochten sind. Der Raum zwischen den Fasern erscheint elektronenoptisch leer, er enthält wahrscheinlich eiweißarme seröse Flüssigkeit[2]. Diese Flüssigkeit ist im Präödem der Stauungslunge vermehrt. Im lichtoptischen Bild gehen diese Zustände von Präödem und von Ödem mit einer Verquellung und Verdickung der Alveolarwand einher, die im ganzen den schon beim Lungenödem beschriebenen Veränderungen gleicht. Diese ödematöse Durchtränkung, die auf einer hydrostatisch bedingten vermehrten Flüssigkeitsdiffusion aus den unter Stauungsdruck stehenden Capillaren beruht,

---

[1] CEELEN 1931, ZU JEDDELOH 1931, MEESSEN 1956.   [2] GIESE und GIESEKING 1957.

tritt intermittierend auf und ist wahrscheinlich eine der Hauptursachen für die
in späten Stadien der Lungenstauung auftretende Zellproliferation.

Bei chronischer Stauung werden Faserstrukturen auch zwischen den Capillaren
und den Fortsätzen der Alveolarepithelien sichtbar. Dadurch rücken die Capillaren im Stadium der Stauungsinduration auseinander und werden gleichzeitig
von der Alveolarwand abgedrängt[1]. Die Capillaren prolabieren nicht mehr in
den Alveolarraum, die Kontaktfläche zwischen Capillaren und Alveolarepithel
wird stark verkleinert. Gleichzeitig ist die Zahl der Netzcapillaren reduziert. Die
Neigung zu den in frühen Stadien der Stauung so häufigen diffusen Blutungen
wird geringer. In der Wand der Alveolargänge und an den Teilungsstellen der
Bronchioli respiratorii sind auch die glatten Muskelfasern vermehrt. Die Alveolar-
knöpfe treten deutlich hervor[2]. Der Endzustand ist eine Gerüstsklerose, die in

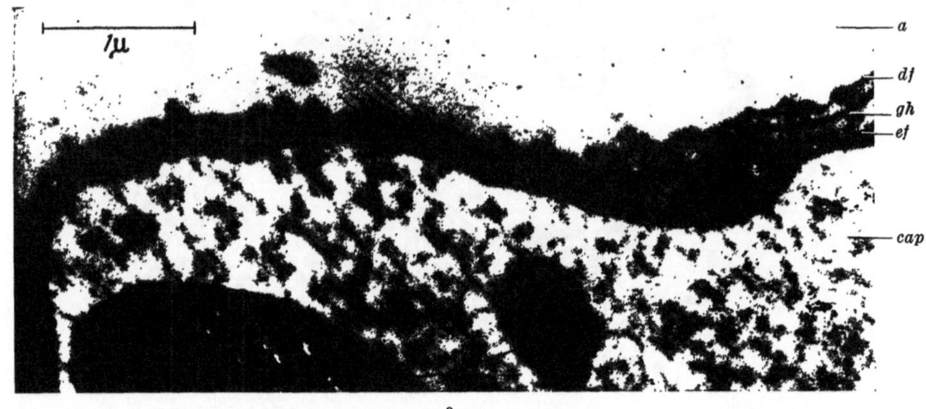

Abb. 65a u. b. a Alveolarmembran in der normalen menschlichen Lunge, Schichtdicke: 0,18—0,55 μ. Vergr.
20 000×. b Teil des Alveolarseptums einer chronischen Stauungslunge. Starke Verbreiterung der Alveolarmembran durch Einlagerung reticulärer und elastischer Fasern zwischen Endothel und Deckzellschicht. Stellenweise Verbreiterung des periendothelialen Grundhäutchens. Schichtdicke der Alveolarmembran: 1,2—2 μ.
Vergr. 20000×. al Alveolarraum, cap Capillarlichtung, dz Teil einer Alveolardeckzelle, df flächenhaft ausgebreiteter Cytoplasmafortsatz einer Alveolardeckzelle, ef flächenhaft ausgebreitete, periphere Cytoplasmazone einer Endothelzelle, gh periendotheliales bzw. subepitheliales Grundhäutchen, rf reticuläre Fasern, el elastische Fasern,
er Erythrocyt, pz Pericyt.

einer mehr herdförmigen Lungenfibrose oder Lungencirrhose endet[3]. Dieses feine
Narbennetz nennen Soulié u. Mitarb. (1954) Pneumonie reticulée hypertrophique
in Anlehnung an ein ähnliches Bild, das Bezançon u. Delarue (1941) bei der
Tuberkulose beschrieben haben.

Die Alveolarepithelien, die mit ihren feinen, lichtoptisch nicht sichtbaren,
aber elektronenmikroskopisch einwandfrei darzustellenden Fortsätzen lückenlos
die Alveolenwand bedecken und feinste pseudopodienartige Ausstülpungen in
die Alveolarlichtung hineinstrecken, sind in der Stauungslunge kaum verändert[4],
aber durch Wandödem teilweise abgehoben. Meessen beschreibt eine Vermehrung
der Protoplasmafortsätze und meint, daß der Gasaustausch mit der so vergrößerten Oberfläche der Alveolarwand verbessert würde. In dem Stadium der fortgeschrittenen Lungenfibrose sind viele Alveolen, deren Wand durch Bindegewebs-
vermehrung starr geworden ist, ganz oder teilweise mit kubischem Epithel ausgekleidet. Dieses bedeutet eine weitere Verdickung der Alveolarwand und eine
zusätzliche Erschwerung des Gasaustausches.

---

[1] Zu Jeddeloh 1931.   [2] Ceelen 1931.   [3] Meessen 1956.
[4] Meessen 1956, Schulz 1956.

MOELL (1941), MEESSEN u. SCHULZ (1957) sehen in der Verdickung der Basalmembran der Capillaren das Haupthindernis für den Gasaustausch und das morphologische Äquivalent einer Pneumonose bei Stauungslunge.

Der Blutluftweg ist, solange die Capillaren in die Alveolen prolabieren, von $0{,}15—0{,}5\,\mu$ in der Norm auf $0{,}6—2{,}45\,\mu$, maximal etwa um das 5—10fache bei

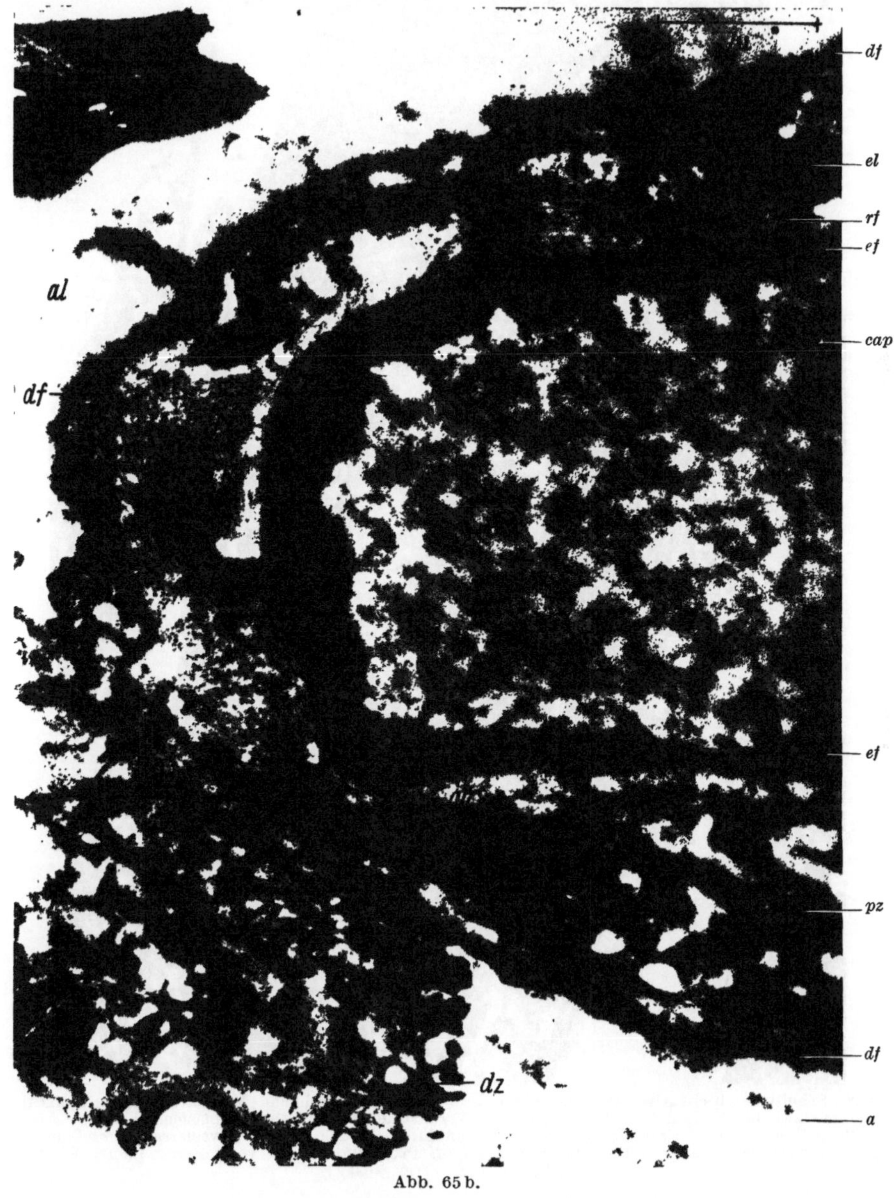

Abb. 65 b.

der Stauungslunge verlängert (Abb. 65). Dazu kommt noch die seröse Durchtränkung und die Faservermehrung im Interstitium bei fortgeschrittenen Graden chronischer Lungenstauung. Bei Umwandlung des Alveolarepithels in eine

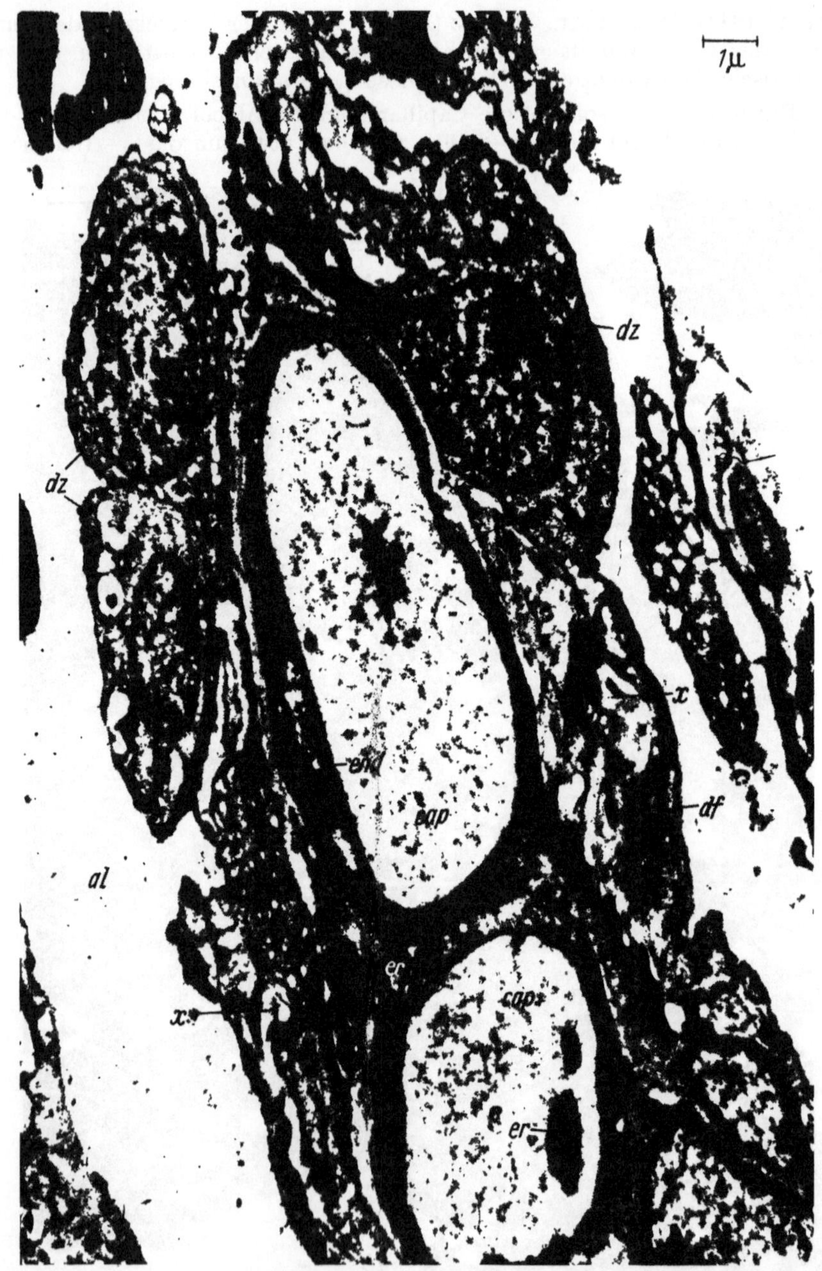

Abb. 66. Schnitt durch ein Alveolarseptum einer chronischen Stauungslunge. Verbreiterung des interstitiellen Spaltraumes zwischen Endothel und Deckzellschicht. Verdichtung des Endothelcytoplasmas. Kubische Alveolardeckzellen. Gesamtdicke der alveolocapillären Membran durchschnittlich 4 μ. *al* Alveolarraum, *cap* Capillarlichtung, *dz* Alveolardeckzellen, *end* Endothelcytoplasma, *df* Deckzellfortsatz, *x* verbreiterter interstitieller Spalt, *er* Erythrocyt. Vergr. 6000×.

Schicht kubischer Zellen wird die alveolocapilläre Membran sogar bis zu 4 und 5 μ dick (Abb. 66).

Ob diese Verlängerung des Blutluftweges den Gasaustausch so erschwert, daß eine Untersättigung des Blutes daraus allein erklärt werden kann, ist zweifelhaft, da nach Modellversuchen an der Norm und Berechnungen[1] der Membranfaktor mit 0,0017 sec nur $^1/_{10}$ des Plasmafaktors (0,012 sec) und weniger als $^1/_{100}$ des Erythrocytenfaktors (0,6137 sec) ausmachen soll.

Setzt man in diese Rechnung die lichtoptisch und elektronenoptisch bei Stauungslunge gemessene Wegstrecke von etwa 2,5 μ ein, dann ergibt sich in der Rechnung von KREUZER (1953) eine Erhöhung des Membranfaktors von 0,0017 sec auf 0,0043 sec. Die gesamte Diffusionszeit von der Alveole in das Erythrocyteninnere verlängert sich damit nur von 0,6274 sec auf 0,6300 sec.

Die Zweifel, die von physiologischer[2] und von klinischer Seite[3] gegenüber der Pneumonose geäußert werden, gründen sich auf diese Rechnung. Wieweit die aus den Modellversuchen gewonnenen Werte auch den Verhältnissen beim Menschen gerecht werden, ist dabei noch offen. Nach den Untersuchungen von FORSTER (1957) am Menschen wird der Membrananteil auf 50% des gesamten Diffusionswiderstandes geschätzt (vgl. S. 544). Damit gewinnt der Membranfaktor eine wesentlich größere Bedeutung als nach der Rechnung von KREUZER (1953) anzunehmen war. Die klinischen Messungen geben nur die Ausgangspositionen, nämlich den Gasgehalt der Alveolarluft und den Grad der Sauerstoffsättigung des rückfließenden Lungenblutes an. Beide sind in der Stauungslunge verändert: die Ventilation durch Einengung und zunehmende Starre des Alveolarraumes, oft noch kompliziert durch intraalveoläres Ödem, die Perfusion durch die außerordentliche Capillarerweiterung und durch das verminderte zirkulierende Blutvolumen.

Dazu kommt eine Erhöhung des O_2-Gradienten, weil der Sauerstoff des Blutes bei Stauungszuständen in der Peripherie stärker ausgeschöpft wird und das in die Lungencapillaren einströmende Blut mehr reduziertes Hämoglobin enthält als in der Norm.

Die Kontaktzeit wird nach der bei Herzklappenfehlern, besonders bei Mitralstenose gemessenen Kreislaufzeit erheblich verlängert sein. Die Angaben über die Kontaktzeit bei Mitralstenose sind aber nicht einheitlich. LANDEN u. BAYER (1952) nehmen an, daß bei Mitralstenose in den Lungencapillaren ein Stauungshochdruck herrscht, der mit einer verlängerten Kontaktzeit verbunden ist. BÜHLMANN u. Mitarb. (1955) sprechen von einem Strömungshochdruck mit einer verkürzten Kontaktzeit.

Die Blutströmungsgeschwindigkeit im kleinen Kreislauf ist bei Mitralfehlern verlangsamt[4], ihre quantitative Abhängigkeit von der Schwere des Klappenfehlers mit der Farbstoffmethode erwiesen[5]. Mit vermindertem Minutenvolumen nimmt die Blutströmungsgeschwindigkeit zu.

Nach dem anatomischen Befund wird nur ein geringer Teil des bei Lungenstauung in den Lungencapillaren und Venen stark vermehrten Blutvolumens in der Zirkulation bewegt. Die Strömungsverlangsamung ist auch mit der selektiven Angiographie sichtbar gemacht worden. Das injizierte Kontrastmittel bleibt unter Sternchenbildungen in Capillarseen stehen[6]. Die Erweiterung der Capillaren hat dazu auch eine Vergrößerung der Austauschfläche zur Folge. Längere Kontaktzeit und größere Austauschfläche werden wahrscheinlich die Verzögerung der Diffusion, die infolge Verdickung der alveolocapillären Membran eintritt, ausgleichen[7].

So bleibt es zweifelhaft, ob bei Stauungslungen vor Eintritt der Induration eine Verzögerung der Gasdiffusion durch Verdickung der alveolocapillären Membran funktionelle Bedeutung im Sinne einer Pneumonose gewinnt. RODE-

---

[1] KREUZER 1953.   [2] SCHOEDEL 1955.   [3] ROSSIER 1956.
[4] BOCK 1951, SWAN und Mitarbeiter 1953, BOLT, KNIPPING und RINK 1955.
[5] BENDER und Mitarbeiter 1957, 1959.   [6] KNIPPING und BOLT, dieses Handbuch.
[7] Lit. bei KNEBEL 1955 und BENDER 1957.

WALD (1957) hat nach Klappensprengung bei Mitralstenose eine Besserung des Gasaustausches gefunden und schließt daraus, daß die Besserung eher auf Änderungen der Kontaktzeit und der Austauschfläche beruht als auf Änderungen der Membrandicke. Andere Beobachtungen haben nach Valvulotomie trotz verbesserter Zirkulation eine deutliche Senkung der Diffusionskapazität mit Vergrößerung der alveoloarteriellen O_2-Druckdifferenz ergeben.

Anders liegen die Verhältnisse, wenn bei fortgeschrittener Stauungsinduration eine allgemeine Gerüstsklerose in zunehmendem Maße Capillaren von der Alveolarwand abdrängt und in der Fibrose zur Verödung bringt. Dann sind infolge der verringerten Austauschfläche durch Reduktion von Netzcapillaren Änderungen

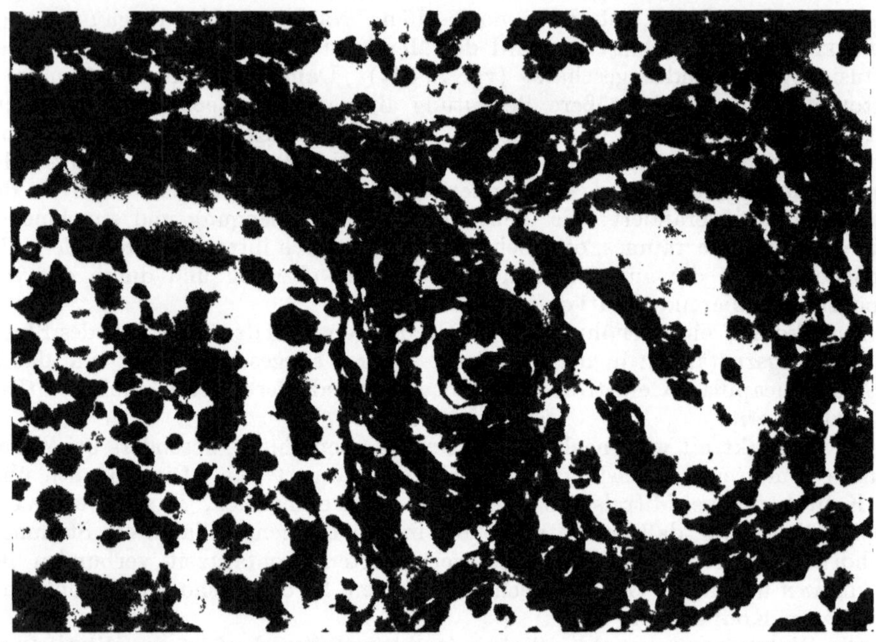

Abb. 67. Chronische Stauungslunge mit Fibrose der Septen und Pulmonalsklerose. Alveolarepithel verdickt und zum Teil von der Alveolarwand abgehoben. Herzfehlerzellen in der Alveolarlichtung. Vergr. 670:1.

der Blutströmung zu erwarten, die in enger Beziehung zu der sekundären Pulmonalsklerose stehen. Diese wird im Endstadium der chronischen Stauungslunge nie vermißt (Abb. 67).

Eine weitere Folge der Lungenstarre ist die Erschwerung der Ventilationsbewegung, die durch erhöhten Gewebswiderstand Dehnbarkeit und elastische Retraktion der Lunge verringert. Alveolarbezirke können durch Fibrose nahezu stillgestellt werden. In solchen Abschnitten bildet das Epithel, das durch das chronische interstitielle Stauungsödem vermehrt abgestoßen wird und vermehrt proliferiert, auf der fibrotischen Alveolarwand dichtliegende kubische Zellreihen. Bei dieser drüsigen Transformation der Alveolen wird der Diffusionsweg so lang, daß ein nennenswerter Gasaustausch mit dem Blut in diesen Alveolengruppen nicht mehr stattfindet.

Bei akuter und chronischer Lungenstauung greifen also verschiedene Vorgänge ineinander:

1. Die Einschränkung der Ventilation durch angiektatische Alveolarkompression und Gerüstsklerose,

2. die ödematöse und sklerotische Verdickung der alveolocapillären Membran,
3. die Änderungen der Blutzirkulation im Capillarbereich.

Diese 3 Faktoren sind beim Gasaustausch so eng miteinander verknüpft, daß eine Abschätzung des Wirkungsgrades der einzelnen Faktoren für sich allein deshalb noch nicht möglich ist[1].

SCHOEN und DERRA (1930) fanden bei Mitralstenose ein arterielles Sauerstoffsättigungsdefizit von etwa 10%. Sie erklärten dieses mit einer erschwerten Sauerstoffdiffusion durch die Alveolarwände. Ob diese Interpretation heute noch aufrechterhalten werden kann, bedarf erneuter Diskussion.

Der Morphologe wird an der Auffassung festhalten, daß in allen Phasen der Stauungslunge vom latenten Präödem bis zur Induration dem Membranfaktor eine überragende Bedeutung unter den Ursachen einer auftretenden Störung des Gasaustausches in der Lunge zukommt.

4. Diffusionsstörungen bei interstitiellen Pneumonien.

Die Frage, ob bei interstitiellen Pneumonien Störungen in der Durchlässigkeit der alveolocapillären Membran eine nennenswerte Rolle beim Gasaustausch zwischen Alveolarluft und Blut spielen, ist ähnlich wie beim Lungenödem von der Morphologie her nur schwer zu beantworten. Die meisten interstitiellen Pneumonien sind herdförmig, oft nicht sehr ausgedehnt. Peribronchiale und perilobuläre interstitielle Pneumonien scheiden aus der Betrachtung aus, weil sie kaum auf die Alveolarsepten übergreifen.

Auch die intralobulären interstitiellen Pneumonien beginnen im lockeren Bindegewebe um den Bronchiolus-Gefäßstiel des Lobulus und Acinus. Selbst die intraacinären Infiltrate liegen vorwiegend in den Wänden des Gangsystems und greifen erst von hier aus auf die Alveolarsepten über. So gibt es z.B. bei den Masern- und Keuchhustenpneumonien stärkere Infiltration nur in den zentroacinären Septen. Regelmäßig sind die Bronchiolen mit Wandinfiltration, vermehrter Sekretion der geschwollenen Epithelien und oft mit erheblicher Stenose der Bronchuslichtung, mitunter sogar mit Schleimobstruktion beteiligt (Abb. 68). Intraalveoläres Exsudat und entzündliche Bronchiolostenose sind bei fast allen interstitiellen Pneumonien als Ursache oft erheblicher Störungen der Ventilation mit im Spiel und lassen sich bei Sauerstoffuntersättigung des Blutes nicht von den reinen Permeabilitätsstörungen abgrenzen. Änderungen der Blutzirkulation in den Capillaren haben bei der akuten interstitiellen Pneumonie nur eine geringe Bedeutung.

Die stärksten Grade interstitieller Infiltration der Alveolarsepten bei freien Bronchiolen finden sich auf der Höhe der interstitiellen plasmacellulären Säuglingspneumonie[2]. Die nach dem Vorschlag von VAN DER MEER u. BRUG (1942) als Pneumocystis Carinii bezeichneten Erreger, die VANĚK und JÍROVEC (1952), JÍROVEC u. VANĚK (1954) als Protozoen, GIESE (1952, 1953) als Pilze ansehen, füllen die Alveolarräume in dichten Kolonien aus. Die Resorption der Stoffwechselprodukte dieser Parasiten ruft die Infiltrate mit Plasmazellen in den Alveolarsepten hervor. Die Plasmazellen füllen das lockere Maschenwerk reticulärer Fasern zwischen den Capillaren aus, drängen die Capillaren auseinander und schieben sich auch zwischen die Alveolarepithelien und Capillaren. Dadurch wird die direkte Kontaktfläche zwischen Alveolen und Capillaren stark eingeengt und die Alveolarwand insgesamt um ein Vielfaches verdickt. Die infiltrierten Lungenabschnitte werden durch die Verdickung der Alveolarwände und durch die Ausfüllung der Alveolarräume mit Parasiten ruhiggestellt, sie nehmen an

---

[1] R. SCHOEN 1930.　　[2] Literatur bei PLIESS 1957.

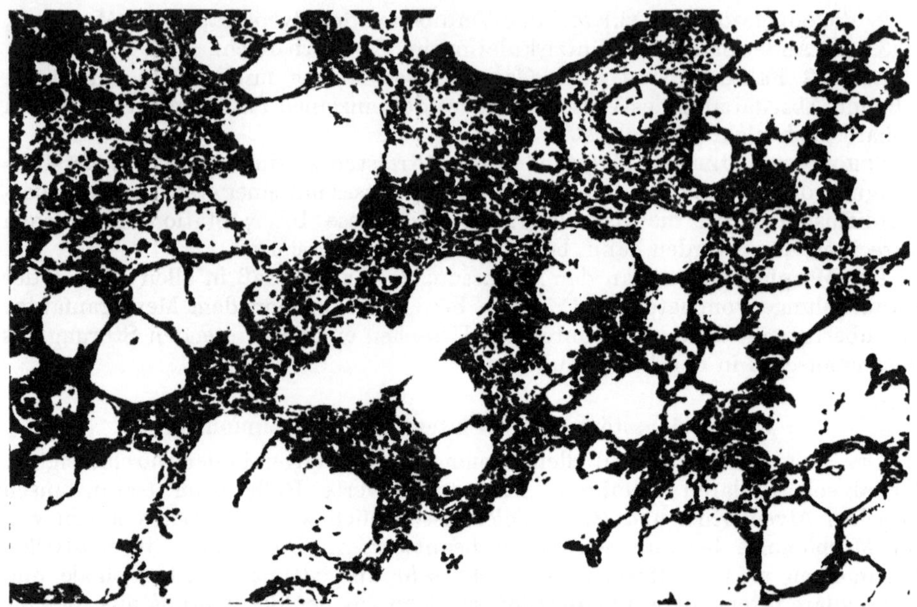

Abb. 68. Interstitielle Masernpneumonie. Zellige Infiltration vorwiegend in den Septen der Bronchioli respiratorii und der Alveolargänge. S.-Nr. 582/58. Vergr. 60fach.

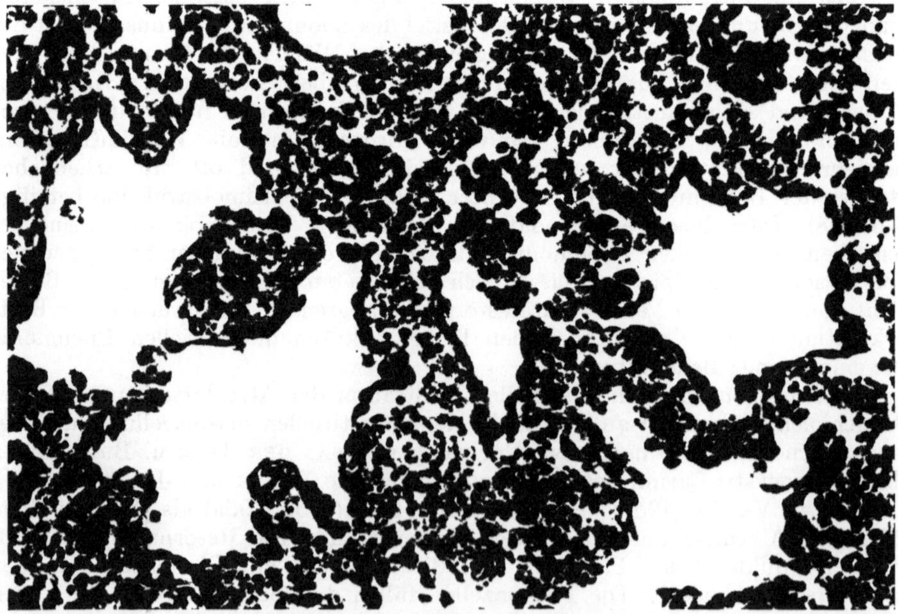

Abb. 69. Verdickung der Alveolarwand bei interstitieller plasmacellulärer Säuglingspneumonie. Kubische Umwandlung des Alveolarepithels. Vergr. 400fach.

der respiratorischen Bewegung der Lunge nicht mehr teil. Die Lunge ist in der Inspirationsstellung fixiert. Die Alveolarepithelien proliferieren und bilden, wie in der fetalen Lunge, Bänder dicht liegender kubischer Zellen (Abb. 69).

So sind also morphologisch alle Voraussetzungen für eine erhebliche Erschwerung und Verzögerung der Gasdiffusion durch die Verdickung der alveolocapillären Membran gegeben. Bedeutung für den Gasaustausch gewinnt die Membranverdickung aber erst, wenn die Parasitenkolonien bei Rückbildung der Pneumonie aus den Alveolen verschwinden und die Ventilation einsetzt. Während die bereits im Beginn der Krankheit eintretende periorale Cyanose und die hohe Atemfrequenz allein durch Einschränkung der Ventilationsfläche erklärt sind, wird bei der Wiederbeatmung der Alveolen eine Diffusionsstörung im Sinne einer Pneumonose so lange anzunehmen sein, als die interstitielle Infiltration der Alveolarsepten andauert. Das Alveolarepithel bildet sich mit der einsetzenden respiratorischen Bewegung der Alveolarwand rasch zu den spärlichen Nischenzellen mit den dünnen cytoplasmatischen Ausläufern zurück.

Die Pneumonose wird im Verlauf der interstitiellen plasmacellulären Pneumonie nur eine zeitlich engbegrenzte, in ihren Folgen schwer abschätzbare Bedeutung haben.

Bei allen anderen Formen der akuten interstitiellen Pneumonien, besonders bei den Viruspneumonien, liegen die Verhältnisse ähnlich. Fast immer stehen dabei Verteilungsstörungen durch Bronchiolostenose oder intraalveoläres Exsudat als Ursache einer O_2-Untersättigung des Blutes so weit im Vordergrund, daß sie den Anteil einer etwa vorhandenen Störung der Membranpermeabilität ganz überdecken.

5. Diffusionsstörungen bei Lungenfibrose.

Unter Lungenfibrosen werden Lungenveränderungen zusammengefaßt, deren bestimmendes Merkmal die Verfestigung des Lungengerüstes ist.

Im Abschnitt über Ventilationsstörungen wurde bereits gezeigt, daß eine fruchtbare Diskussion über die Genese von Atmungsstörungen bei Fibrosen nur dann möglich ist, wenn man diese ätiologisch, pathogenetisch und morphologisch heterogene Gruppe unterteilt.

Dort stand die Einschränkung der ventilatorischen Lungenbewegung, die bis zur völligen Lungenstarre gehen kann, im Mittelpunkt der Betrachtung. Bei diffuser Fibrose laufen Grad und Ausdehnung der Induration parallel mit der Einschränkung der Vitalkapazität, solange die Luftwege frei durchgängig sind. Bei herdförmigen Fibrosen, die sehr häufig Restzustände granulomatöser Prozesse sind, tritt die ventilatorische Verteilungsstörung zu der Lungenstarre, weil Stenosen und Verschlüsse von Bronchiolen und kleinen Bronchien regelmäßige Begleiterscheinungen sind. Bronchostenotisches oder Narbenemphysem bestimmen dabei schließlich die Art der Ventilationsstörung.

Diffusionsstörungen können bei Lungenfibrosen dann angenommen werden, wenn im Laufe des fibrosierenden Prozesses Alveolarwände in der Weise umgebaut werden, daß der Gasaustausch zwischen Alveolarluft und Capillarblut behindert wird. Die vollständige Unterbrechung des Gasaustausches wird als alveolocapillärer Block bezeichnet[1].

Unter den so häufigen herdförmigen und selteneren diffusen Lungenfibrosen haben in diesem Zusammenhang nur solche Prozesse Bedeutung, in denen die Induration im Alveolarbereich erfolgt, denn nur hier kann durch Umgestaltung der alveolocapillären Membran ein Hindernis für den Gasaustausch entstehen. Damit scheiden alle Prozesse aus, bei denen nur interlobuläre und peribronchiale Septen indurieren.

Bei herdförmigen Indurationen, etwa bei großknotiger Silikose, veröden mit den fibrotischen Veränderungen im Lungengerüst gleichzeitig auch die zugehörigen Alveolen. Kleinknotige Silikosen und abheilende Miliartuberkulosen führen durch narbige Schrumpfung der kleinen Einzelherde zu Verziehungen

---

[1] AUSTRIAN, McCLEMENT und Mitarbeiter 1951.

des Lungengerüstes und zu Narbenemphysem, aber nicht zu einer nennenswerten
Fibrosierung der Alveolarsepten außerhalb des Narbenbereiches. Die Lungentuberkulose ist in ihrer exsudativen und produktiven Verlaufsform an das Gangsystem gebunden und stets ein komplexer Vorgang, in dem Alveolarwandver-
dickungen außerhalb der tuberkulösen Herdbildungen nur eine untergeordnete
Rolle spielen. Die Boecksche Krankheit schließlich, die von klinischer Seite so oft
im Zusammenhang mit Diffusionsstörungen genannt wird, ist ebenfalls eine
Granulomatose. Im Bereich der floriden Granulome wird Lungengewebe zerstört, im Narbenstadium, das spontan oder unter Cortisonbehandlung erreicht
wird, beherrscht das kleinblasige Narben- oder Obstruktionsemphysem das Bild.
Die Reihe fibrotischer Lungenprozesse, in denen auf Grund des morphologischen
Befundes keine nennenswerten Diffusionsstörungen aus Verdickung der alveolocapillären Membran angenommen werden können, läßt sich noch erheblich erweitern.

Man versteht unter diesen Umständen die Zurückhaltung vieler Kliniker
gegenüber der Einbeziehung dieser fibrotischen Lungenveränderungen in die
alveolocapillären Membranstörungen (Pneumonosen), die von Baldwin, Cournand u. Richards (1949) vorgeschlagen wurde[1].

Voraussetzung für die Annahme einer Störung des Gasaustausches bei herabgesetzter Diffusionskapazität sind nach Matthes

1. normale oder herabgesetzte arterielle Sauerstoffsättigung in der Ruhe;

2. deutlicher Abfall der arteriellen Sauerstoffsättigung bei körperlicher
Arbeit;

3. in Ruhe und Arbeit normale bzw. infolge kompensatorischer Hyperventilation leicht herabgesetzte arterielle CO_2-Spannung;

4. keine Behinderung der alveolären Ventilation, insbesondere normale bzw.
durch Hyperventilation bestimmte alveoläre Gasspannungen;

5. kein Anhalt für grobe Ungleichmäßigkeit der Zusammensetzung der
Alveolarluft;

6. positiver Effekt von O_2-Atmung.

Nur eine kleine Gruppe aus dem großen Kreis der Lungenfibrosen erfüllt
diese Voraussetzungen, wenn man ausgedehnte Membranverdickung bei freien
Luftwegen ohne ventilatorische Verteilungsstörungen oder Herdemphysem als
Hauptkriterien für die Einordnung ansieht. Dazu gehören die Strahlenfibrosen
der Lungen, die diffuse progressive interstitielle Lungenfibrose und die seltene
Sklerodermie in den Frühstadien.

Die Strahlenfibrose läuft in mehreren Stadien ab[2].

Auf eine sofort an die Bestrahlung anschließende kurzdauernde katarrhalische
Frühreaktion folgen nach einem symptomfreien Intervall von 2—3 Wochen in
der Hauptphase degenerative Gewebsschäden. Capillarwände und Endothelien
quellen auf, ebenso die Alveolarepithelien und die Zellen und Fasern der Alveolarsepten. Aus den erweiterten Blutcapillaren tritt Plasma in die Alveolen und schlägt
sich dort in hyalinen Bändern auf der Alveolarwand nieder. Alveolarepithelien
werden vermehrt abgelöst. An diese 2—3 Monate dauernde exsudative Reaktion
schließen sich die Spätveränderungen an. Diese beginnen mit einer Proliferation
faserbildender Zellen in den Septen, oft in Anlehnung an hyalinisierte und throm-
bosierte Blutcapillaren. Durch die interstitielle Faservermehrung und durch
Organisation hyaliner Membranen werden die Alveolarsepten verdickt. Das neugebildete Fasergewebe hyalinisiert und schrumpft nur wenig. Die Bronchiolen
bleiben durchgängig, es entsteht kein Emphysem.

---

[1] Rossier und Mitarbeiter 1956 (Literatur), Matthes und Mitarbeiter 1960, Matthes 1960.
[2] Engelstad 1934, 1935, Warren 1942, Uehlinger und Schoch 1957.

Im Endstadium ist das strahlengeschädigte Gebiet grau und fest. Luft- und Blutgehalt sind vermindert. In den zugehörigen Blutgefäßen besteht eine Intimafibrose mit Einengung der Lichtung.

Dieses Beispiel zeigt, daß mit der Verdickung der Septen zunächst Alveolarepithel und Capillaren auseinander rücken, und daß mit zunehmender Fibrosierung die zunächst weiten Capillaren eng werden und schließlich schwinden. Die Intimafibrose der zugehörigen Arterien beweist, daß der Blutzustrom zu den Fibrosebezirken erheblich gedrosselt ist. Der alveolocapilläre Block beruht also sowohl auf Membranverdickung als auch auf Capillarreduktion (Abb. 70).

Die progressive interstitielle Fibrose (Typ Hamman-Rich, vgl. S. 438) läuft in der Anfangsphase ähnlich ab wie die Strahlenfibrose in der Hauptphase.

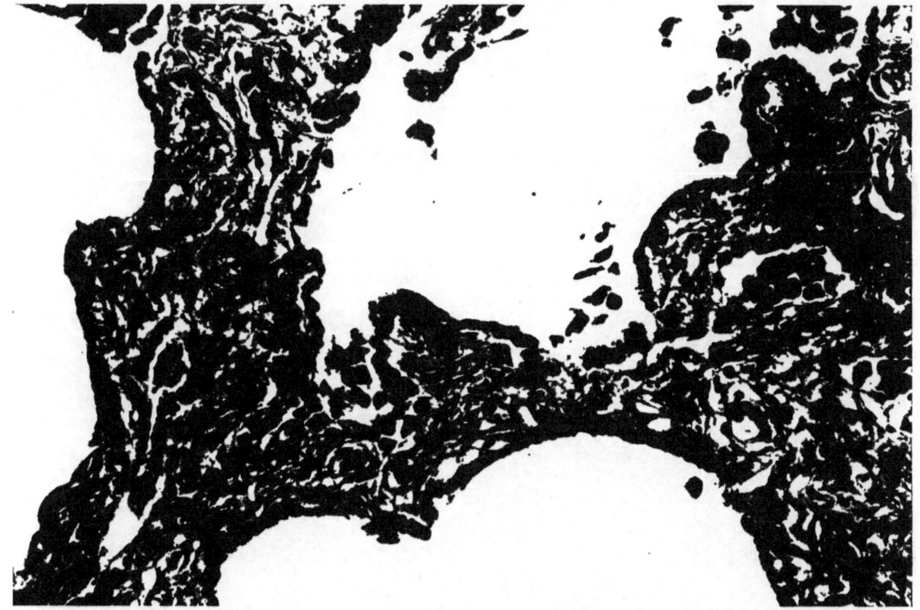

Abb. 70. Lungenfibrose mit alveolocapillärem Block. Starke Verdickung und fibröse Umwandlung der Alveolarsepten. Kubische Umformung des Alveolarepithels. Fast völliger Schwund der Blutcapillaren.

Auf ein exsudatives Vorstadium mit Ödem, Fibrinabscheidung in den Septen und mit hyalinen Membranen auf der Alveolarwand folgt die chronische Entzündung mit lymphocytär-plasmacellulärer Infiltration, Histiocytenproliferation und Neubildung reticulärer, später auch kollagener Fasern.

In den Endstadien treten abweichend von der Strahlenfibrose die narbigen Schrumpfungen mit Bronchiolostenose stark in den Vordergrund. Das komplizierende bronchostenotische und Narbenemphysem überlagert die Diffusionsstörung.

Die Sklerodermie ist in ihrem Ablauf der progressiven interstitiellen Lungenfibrose vergleichbar (Abb. 71). Restzustände von interstitiellen Viruspneumonien, die Lymphangitis reticularis[1] und frühe Stadien der als emphysematöse Wabenlunge endenden Lungencirrhose[2] können ebenfalls dieser Gruppe zugerechnet werden. Die Grenzen sind hier nicht scharf zu ziehen.

---

[1] v. Hansemann 1915.   [2] Rindfleisch 1897, Meessen 1949.

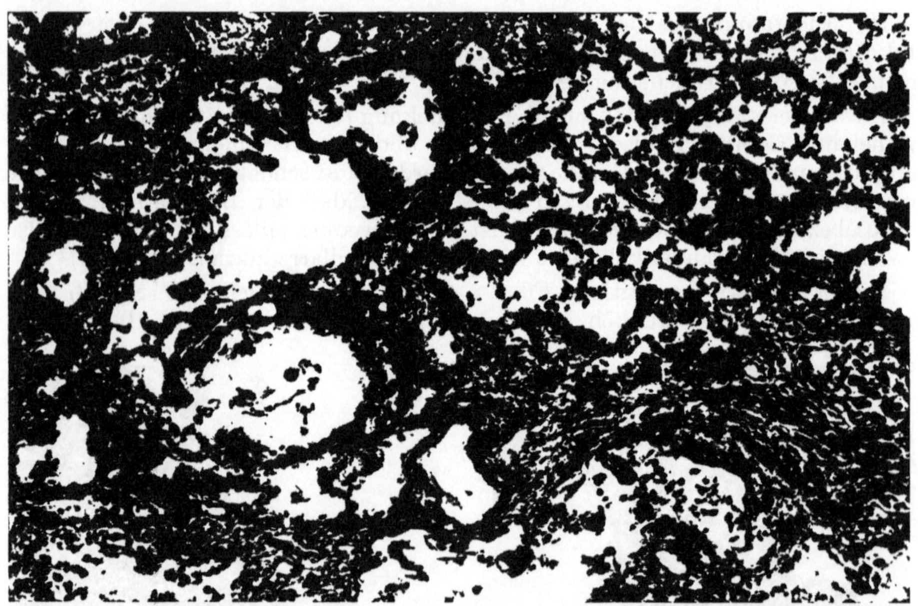

Abb. 71. Interstitielle Lungenfibrose bei Sklerodermie. Zellige Infiltration und unregelmäßige Faservermehrung im Lungengerüst. Beginnendes Emphysem. S.-Nr. 81/56.

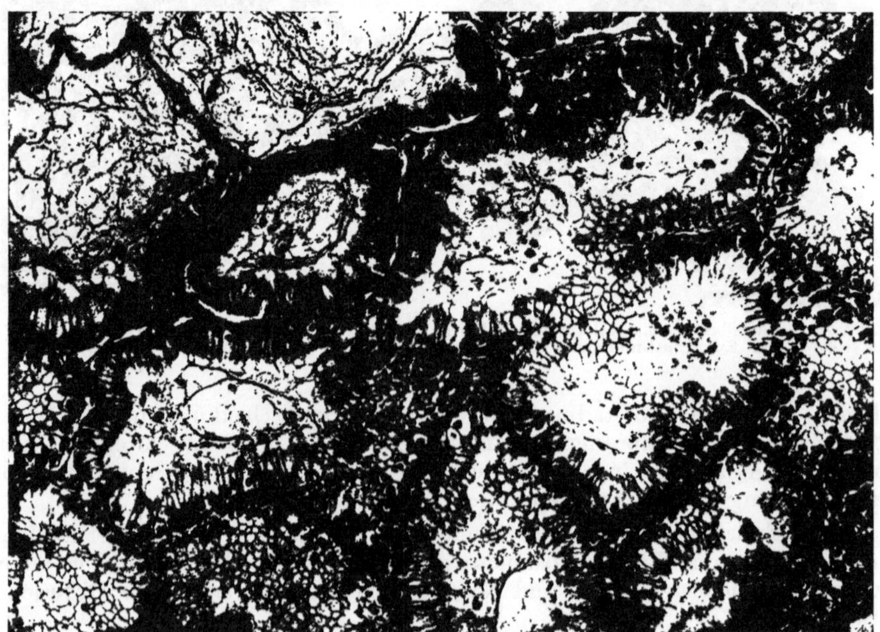

Abb. 72. Lungenadenomatose. Auskleidung der Alveolen mit einreihigem Zylinderepithel in großen Lungenabschnitten. Tod an respiratorischer Insuffizienz. J.-Nr. 1489/53, 38jähriger Mann. Vergr. 158fach.

6. Die Lungenadenomatose.

Diffuse Tumorinfiltrationen werden ebenfalls vielfach den Pneumonosen zugerechnet[1]. Für die Lymphangiosis carcinomatosa ist das nach morphologischen

[1] Knipping und Bolt, dieser Handbuchband.

Befunden nicht berechtigt. Die Krebsausbreitung folgt dabei den Lymphbahnen, die als oberflächliches Lymphgefäßnetz den segmentalen und lobulären Septen folgen oder als tiefes Lymphgefäßnetz Arterien und Bronchien begleiten[1]. Die Alveolarsepten sind dabei nicht infiltriert. Störungen des Gasaustausches können deshalb nicht auf Membranschädigungen zurückgeführt werden.

Dagegen gibt es intraalveolär wachsende Tumorformen, die das Alveolengerüst als Stroma benutzen und die Alveolarlichtungen in mehr oder minder großer Ausdehnung mit einem Krebszellbelag austapezieren. Bei der Lungenadenomatose können auf diese Weise große Lungenabschnitte zwar noch beatmet, aber vom Gasaustausch ausgeschaltet sein (Abb. 72).

Die Jaagziekte (Hetzseuche) der Schafe ist auch eine Lungenadenomatose[2], bei der die Lungeninsuffizienz auf einem alveolocapillären Block beruht.

Alle anderen Formen von Lungentumoren komprimieren die Alveolen oder füllen sie mit Tumorgewebe so dicht aus, daß die Tumorabschnitte nicht mehr belüftet werden. Dazu kommen fast stets Verschlüsse der zugehörigen Bronchien durch das Tumorgewebe und nachfolgende Atelektasen.

So bleibt unter den Geschwülsten nur die Lungenadenomatose, bei der die Voraussetzungen für eine Diffusionsstörung im Sinne der Pneumonose gegeben sind.

D. Störungen der Lungenperfusion.

I. Hämodynamisch bedingte Störungen des Gasaustausches.

Der Gasaustausch zwischen Blut und Alveolarluft geht nur im Capillarbereich vor sich. Das Capillarnetz, eingeschaltet zwischen die zuführende Arteriole und die ableitende Venole, bildet den als Endstrombahn bezeichneten Anteil des pulmonalen Strombogens, der im rechten Ventrikel beginnt und im linken Vorhof endet. Das Verhalten der Endstrombahn der Lunge steht im Mittelpunkt aller Erörterungen über solche Störungen der äußeren Atmung, die auf Änderungen der Blutperfusion beruhen. Die Perfusionsstörungen der Lunge werden deshalb hier nur insoweit besprochen, als sie den Gasaustausch beeinflussen oder vom Atmungsvorgang beeinflußt werden.

Die Ausdehnung des Capillarbettes, der Grad seiner Füllung und die Strömungsgeschwindigkeit in den Capillaren sind entscheidende Faktoren für den Gasaustausch. Zahlreiche krankhafte Prozesse des Lungengewebes, der Pulmonalgefäße oder des Herzens stören Struktur und Strömungsverhältnisse in der Endstrombahn.

Zwei große Gruppen können unterschieden werden:

1. Hämodynamisch bedingte Störungen des Gasaustausches,
2. ventilatorisch bedingte Störungen der Lungenperfusion.

Viele Krankheitsprozesse der Lunge, die mit einer Störung der Ventilation begannen, enden mit einer Insuffizienz des rechten Herzens[3]. Deshalb reicht die Pathologie des kleinen Kreislaufs nicht nur primär, sondern auch sekundär in die Pathologie der äußeren Atmung hinein und ist mit ihr unlöslich verbunden. Ihre Auswirkung ist die kardiorespiratorische Insuffizienz[4].

a) Die Endstrombahn der Lunge.

1. Morphologie.

Die Äste der Arteria pulmonalis folgen dem Verlauf der Bronchien und liegen mit diesen jeweils mitten in dem zugehörigen Versorgungsgebiet. Dieser

---

[1] LAUCHE 1928.   [2] Siehe bei SEDLMEIER 1959.
[3] ROSSIER 1956, R. SCHOEN 1932, HEGGLIN 1956, GROSSE-BROCKHOFF und SCHOEDEL 1957.
[4] UEHLINGER 1956.

gemeinsame Verlauf läßt sich über Segment, Subsegment und Praelobulus bis in den Lobulus verfolgen und endet am Bronchiolus terminalis. Im Lobulus liegen Bronchiolus und kleine Arterien stets axial oder centrolobulär, in der Regel nahe aneinander und durch eine lockere Bindegewebsbrücke verbunden. Am Ende des Bronchiolus terminalis hören diese klaren topographischen Beziehungen zwischen Arterien und Bronchialbaum auf. Der Bronchiolus terminalis geht in den Arbor alveolaris über und führt in das respirierende Lungenparenchym, die begleitende kleine Arterie (Arteria terminalis) teilt sich in 2 Arteriolen, die den Bronchioli respiratorii folgen und sich dann rasch im dichten Capillarnetz verlieren, das die Bronchioli alveolares und die Alveolen umspinnt. Unter Acinus wollen wir den pyramidenförmigen Lungenabschnitt verstehen, der an einem Bronchiolus terminalis hängt und dessen Kantenlänge im Durchschnitt 4—6 mm beträgt (s. auch S. 414). Die Innenfläche des Acinus umfaßt das gesamte Respirationsfeld eines Bronchiolus terminalis. In den Wänden und Septen des in Gänge und Alveolen differenzierten Acinus liegen alle Blutcapillaren, die dem Gasaustausch dienen können.

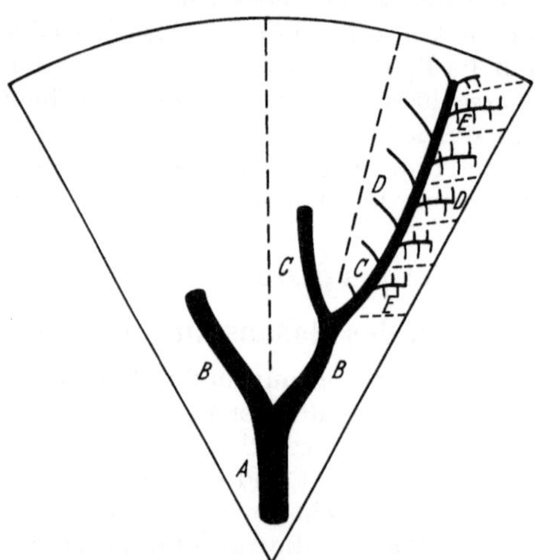

Abb. 73. Angiographische Gliederung des Lungensegmentes. *A* Segmentarterie; *B* Subsegmentarterie; *C* Prälobulararterie; *D* Lobulararterie; *E* Terminalarterie. (Aus Junghanss 1958.)

Aus Arteriogrammen an der Leichenlunge geht hervor, daß die Pulmonalarterien bis zu den Arteriolen untereinander keine Anastomosen besitzen, daß sie also Endarterien sind. Die Aufteilungswinkel der großen Arterien sind bis zu den Prälobulararterien spitz, also hämodynamisch günstig. Von den Prälobulararterien ab werden sie weiter, die Terminalarterien, deren Versorgungsgebiet die Acini sind, haben fast rechtwinklige Abgänge aus den Lobulararterien (Abb. 73). In diesen Abschnitten beginnt wahrscheinlich schon der steile Druckabfall in der Endstrombahn. Die Lichtungen der Prälobulararterien sind 1,2—1,8 mm, der Lobulararterien 0,4—0,8 mm und der Terminalarterien 0,2—0,3 mm weit[1].

Die Endstrombahn der Lunge beginnt mit der Teilung der Arteria terminalis in die Arteriolen. Diese haben sich aus dem Peribronchium gelöst und sind nicht mehr von geschlossenen Lymphbahnen begleitet. Die in der Arteria terminalis noch kräftige Muskelschicht löst sich in den Arteriolen auf, Muskelringe wechseln mit muskelfreien Stellen ab, in denen Elastica externa und interna miteinander verschmelzen[2]. Die Arteriolen verzweigen sich in die Präcapillaren, die in den intraacinösen Septen liegen und in das dichte kommunizierende Capillarnetz der Alveolen übergehen.

Die Alveolocapillaren sammeln sich wieder in den Postcapillaren, die die gleiche Wandstruktur wie die Präkapillaren haben und wie diese zwischen den Alveolargängen liegen. Die Postcapillaren münden in die interacinösen Venolen und diese in die interlobulären Venen. Die kleinen und kleinsten Venen der Lunge besitzen eine elastische Wand. Die elastischen Fasern der Venenwand stehen nicht mit den elastischen Fasern des Lungengerüstes in Verbindung[3]. Nach v. Hayek (1948)

---

[1] Junghanss 1958.   [2] Vandendorpe 1936, Miyata 1939, Merkel 1941, v. Hayek 1953.
[3] Hirsch 1958.

gehen die vorwiegend ringförmig verlaufenden Fasern kontinuierlich in das Faserwerk des umgebenden Lungengewebes über. An der Einmündungsstelle der Postcapillaren in die Venolen sind Muskelringe gefunden worden[1]. In den kleinen Venen können Muskelwülste mit eigener Innervation perlschnurartige Einschnürungen bilden. Die Venen liegen in den Interlobularsepten und begrenzen die Lobuli, deren Länge zwischen 0,8—2,8 cm und deren Breite zwischen 0,6 und 1,5 cm liegen. Das Kaliber der Interlobularvenen entspricht den Lobulararterien. Über die Bronchialvenen und deren anastomotische Verbindungen mit dem Pulmonalsystem siehe FLORANGE (1960), SCHOENMACKERS (1960) und WEIBEL (1959).

Die Gefäße der Endstrombahn sind in das Gefüge des Acinus eingebaut und hängen mit dessen elastisch-reticulärem Fasersystem zusammen[2].

Als durchschnittliche Gefäßweiten lassen sich folgende Zahlen angeben[3]:

Arteria terminalis 150—200 μ, nach Dehnung durch Injektion 200—300 μ;
Arteriole 80—30 μ;
Präcapillare 40—15 μ, gespült bis 70 μ;
Capillare 6—11 μ, gespült 10—12 μ;
Postkapillare etwa 50 μ;
Venole 50—80 μ;
Interlobularvenen 200—300 μ.

MIYATA hat in seinen Messungen Gipfelpunkte der Häufigkeit von Capillarweiten bei 25, 40, 60 und 80 μ gefunden. Die zuführende kleine Arterie hat bis zur Weite von 80 μ eine ununterbrochene Muscularis, unterhalb von 80 μ treten muskelfreie Segmente auf. Präcapillaren und Postcapillaren haben den gleichen Bau und können im histologischen Schnitt höchstens aus ihrer Lage differenziert werden. Sie unterscheiden sich von den sehr viel kleineren Alveolarcapillaren außer der Weite des Kalibers nur noch durch eine leichte Vermehrung der reticulären und elastischen Fasern, die das Gefäß umspinnen.

Zwischen Prä- und Postcapillaren liegen etwa 4—12 Capillaren, in denen der Blutweg etwa 60—250 μ lang ist[4].

2. Funktion.

Das venöse Blut tritt durch die Arteria terminalis in das Zentrum des Acinus ein, durchströmt die Lungencapillaren und fließt arterialisiert zum Acinus- und Lobulusrand, wo es in der Regel von 2 Venen aufgenommen wird.

In welcher Weise der arterielle und venöse Schenkel der Strombahn miteinander in Verbindung stehen, ist noch nicht ausreichend geklärt.

Nach v. HAYEK (1953) gehen aus den weiten Präcapillaren 12—20 kurze Capillaräste direkt ab. Ein bis zwei dieser Äste treten an jede Alveole heran und bilden hier ein enges Netzwerk von 4—12 Capillarmaschen. Die Alveolocapillaren vereinigen sich wieder zu 1—2 Postcapillaren, die in die Venolen einmünden.

Präcapillaren, Capillaren und Postcapillaren haben elektronenoptisch die gleiche Wandbeschaffenheit. Die Bedingungen für die Gasdiffusion sind also in beiden Capillarabschnitten die gleichen, zumal auch die weiten Capillaren an der Basis der Alveolen in die Alveolarwand eingebaut sind und hier Kontakt mit den Gasen der Alveolarluft haben[5].

Aus dieser Darstellung ergibt sich, daß die Lungencapillaren nicht alle dem einfachen klassischen Capillartyp[6] entsprechen, bei dem die Capillaren aus end-

---

[1] v. HAYEK 1943.   [2] MIYATA 1939.
[3] MIYATA 1939, MERKEL 1941, VANDENDORPE 1936, v. HAYEK 1940.
[4] v. HAYEK 1953.   [5] GIESE 1957.   [6] ILLIG 1957.

ständigen Verzweigungen der Arteriolen hervorgehen und ebenso in die endständigen Äste der kleinen Venen münden. Man kann vielmehr nach der Lichtungsweite und nach der Topographie eine Gliederung in 2 Capillarbereiche mit 2 Capillartypen, den *Strom- und den Netzcapillaren*, durchführen[1].

In den terminalen Stromgebieten des großen Kreislaufes ist die Unterscheidung in Strom- und Netzcapillaren eingeführt[2] und erweitert worden[3].

Die Stromcapillaren entspringen aus den Endarteriolen und münden in die Venolen. Man unterscheidet an ihnen

    1. die Metarteriolen mit vereinzelten voll ausgebildeten Muskelzellen,

    2. die proximalen Segmente mit vereinzelten atypischen Muskelzellen und

    3. die muskelfreien distalen Abschnitte.

Die Netzcapillaren bilden Nebenschlüsse der Stromcapillaren. Sie gehen aus Endarteriolen und proximalen Segmenten der Stromcapillaren ab und münden nach netzförmiger Verzweigung untereinander in distale Teile der Stromcapillaren ein. Der Einstrom in Netzcapillaren ist von der Tätigkeit innervierter, muskelhaltiger Abschnitte der Stromcapillaren abhängig.

Die Stromcapillaren haben an ihren Abgangsstellen Schleusenmuskeln, die Netzcapillaren Pförtnerzellen (Tannenberg 1926) oder nach Chambers u. Zweifach (1947) Sphincteren, die nach Illig (1957) aus glatten Muskelzellen bestehen. Chambers u. Zweifach nennen die anastomosenartigen contractilen Verbindungen zwischen kleinen Arterien und Venen auch Gefäßbrücken oder Zentralkanäle. Diese sind für gewöhnlich kontinuierlich, die Netzcapillaren, die Illig auch Sphinctercapillaren nennt, intermittierend durchblutet. Muskelhaltige Anteile der Endstrombahn und Sphincteren sind durch Nervenreizung erregbar, die muskelfreien Capillarabschnitte nicht. Starke Nervenreizung macht Vasodilatation mit Stase, leichte Reizung nach der Rickerschen Stufenregel Fluxion[4]. Arterien, Venen und Capillaren sind reich innerviert, Terminalreticula durch Reiser (1933) und Sunder-Plassmann (1933) auch in der Lunge bis in die Endabschnitte der Gefäßbahn nachgewiesen worden. Auf Adrenalin kontrahieren sich die Sphinctermuskeln bereits bei einer Verdünnung von 1:5—10 Millionen, die Metarteriolen erst bei einer Verdünnung von 1:3—4 Millionen[5]. Die Erregung springt also mit zunehmender Stärke des Reizes herzwärts[6].

In Gefäßgebieten nutritiven Charakters werden in der Regel keine Sphinctercapillaren gefunden. Dort herrscht der klassische dichotomische Verzweigungsmodus vor, d. h. die Capillaren gehen durch Verzweigung aus dem Ende der Arteriolen hervor und bleiben in den Hauptstrom des Blutes zwischen Arterien und Venen eingeschaltet. In Gefäßgebieten ohne nutritive Aufgaben (z. B. Mesenterium der Ratte) kommen arteriovenöse Gefäßbrücken und Sphinctercapillaren in großer Zahl vor[7].

Wieweit diese Untersuchungsergebnisse aus Capillarregionen des großen Kreislaufs auf die Lunge übertragen werden dürfen, ist noch wenig geklärt.

Das engmaschige, reich anastomosierende Capillarnetz der Alveolen mit Lichtungsweiten von 6—11 μ fügt sich ungezwungen in das Netzcapillarsystem ein. Es hat mit diesem gemeinsam den rechtwinkligen Abgang aus noch muskelhaltigen Abschnitten der Endstrombahn, nämlich den Metarteriolen oder Präcapillaren, und es verfügt weiter über Verschlußmechanismen nach Art der Pförtnerzellen. Diese erklären den starken Wechsel in der Perfusion der Alveolocapillaren, der von Wearn u. Mitarb. (1926, 1934), Reinhardt (1934, 1935) an Katzen und Kaninchen durch Thoraxfenster direkt beobachtet worden ist. In der Ruhe ist nur ein kleiner Teil der Netzcapillaren durchstömt. Die Stärke der Perfusion wechselt von Alveole zu Alveole. Man spricht auch von einem Schichtwechsel der Alveolen in der Annahme, daß alternierend bald die eine, bald die andere Alveolengruppe über eine Änderung der Capillardurchblutung für den Gasaustausch herangezogen wird.

In den einzelnen Capillarschlingen einer Alveole wechseln fluxionäre Strömung, Pulsation, Stillstand und reine Plasmaströmung anscheinend regellos in wenigen Minuten ab[8]. Auch rückläufige Blutbewegung kommt vor. Die „Capillarzeit",

---

[1] Giese 1957.   [2] Jacobj 1920, Hill 1921, Krogh 1922, 1929.
[3] Chambers und Zweifach 1940—1947, Shorr 1950, Illig 1957 u. a.
[4] Reinhardt 1935.   [5] Chambers und Zweifach 1944.
[6] Ricker 1924.   [7] Illig 1957.   [8] Wearn und Mitarbeiter 1934.

mit der in klinischen und physiologischen Untersuchungen gerechnet wird, ist nach diesen Beobachtungen bestenfalls ein approximativer Globalwert.

Zu den Stromcapillaren gehören die Endabschnitte der Arteriolen (Metarteriolen), die Präcapillaren und Postcapillaren und die Anfangsabschnitte der Venolen.

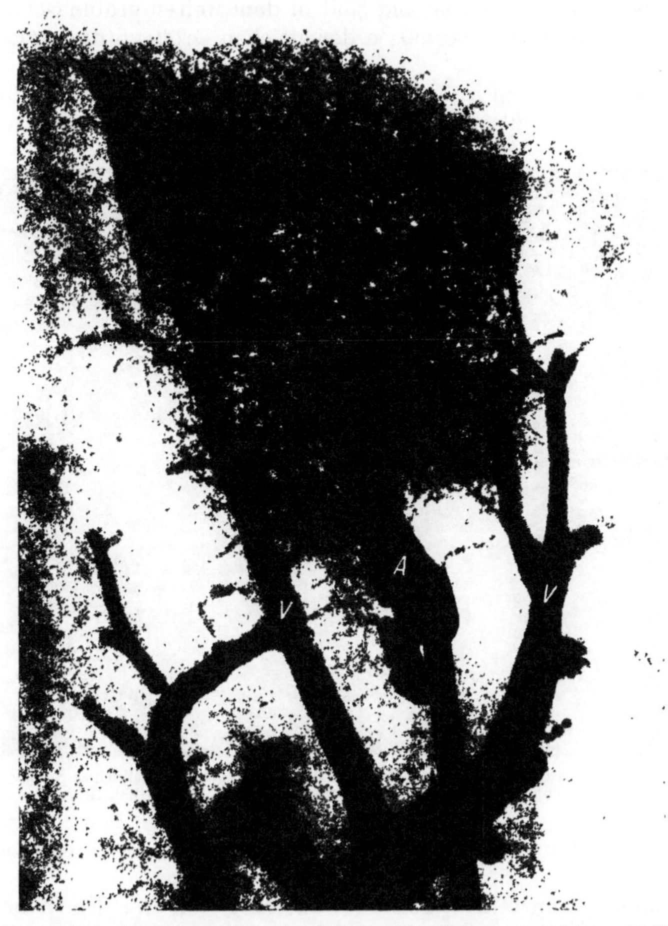

Abb. 74. Isolierte arteriographische Darstellung eines Lobulus. Kanüle in der zentral liegenden Lobulararterie (*A*). Randständig in den Septen die zugehörigen Lungenvenen (*V*). Im Lobulus das Maschenwerk des Stromcapillarnetzes. Netzcapillaren nicht gefüllt. Venöser Rückfluß unter Umgehung des Netzcapillarsystems. Vergr. 3fach

Diese Capillarabschnitte enthalten typische und atypische Muskelzellen, die als Schleusenmuskeln funktionieren und die Perfusion regeln können.

Nach der bisher geltenden Ansicht besteht keine direkte Verbindung zwischen Prä- und Postcapillaren, es wird vielmehr angenommen, daß alles Blut aus den Präcapillaren nur über das System der Netzcapillaren in die Postcapillaren gelangen könne[1].

In eigenen, gemeinsam mit JUNGHANSS[2] durchgeführten angiographischen Untersuchungen an der Leichenlunge konnte gezeigt werden, daß sich bei

---

[1] v. HAYEK 1953.   [2] GIESE 1957, JUNGHANSS 1958.

Verwendung des hochviscösen 40%igen dickflüssigen Jodipinöls als Kontrastmittel im Röntgenbild ein grobmaschiges capilläres Gefäßnetz mit Lichtungsweiten zwischen 20 und 40 μ darstellt. Durch dieses Netz fließt das Kontrastmittel unter Umgehung des Netzcapillarsystems in die Venen ab (Abb. 74). Nimmt man ein dünnflüssiges Kontrastmittel, dann entsteht eine diffuse Füllung des gesamten feinen Capillarnetzes.

An Ausgußpräparaten mit Plastoid sind in dem weiten grobmaschigen Stromcapillarnetz kurze Brückenanastomosen der gleichen Größenordnung nachweisbar (Abb. 75)[1].

Glasperlen, die man dem strömenden Blut beimischt, werden bis zur Größenordnung von 40 μ das Capillarnetz passieren können. Ihr Übergang in die Lungen-

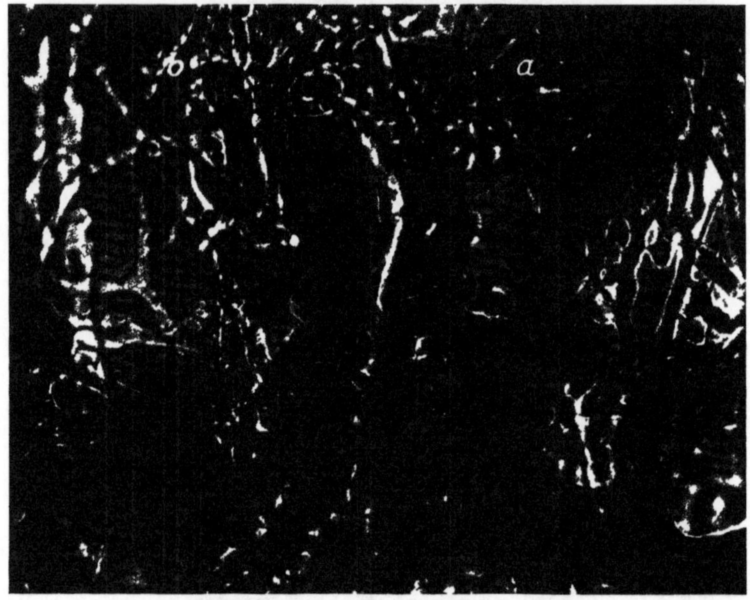

Abb. 75 Plastoidausguß des Lungencapillarnetzes. *a* Grobmaschiges, großkalibriges Stromcapillarnetz. *b* Feinmaschiges, kleinkalibriges Netzcapillarsystem. (Aus Giese 1957.)

venen ist also kein Beweis für die Öffnung präcapillärer arteriovenöser Anastomosen[2].

Diese Befunde vermitteln folgende Vorstellung von der Endstrombahn der Lunge (Abb. 76):

Ein grobmaschiges, 20—40 μ weites Stromcapillarnetz, bestehend aus Metarteriolen, Präcapillaren, Postcapillaren und Anfangsteil der Venolen stellt eine direkte kurze Verbindung zwischen Arterien und Venen im Bereich des Acinus her. Es bewältigt den größten Teil der Ruhezirkulation und hat für die Sauerstoffsättigung ausreichenden Kontakt mit der Alveolarluft. Es ist kontinuierlich durchströmt.

Das engmaschige Netzcapillarsystem mit Lichtungsweiten von 6—11 μ überlagert das Stromcapillarnetz. Es erhält sein Blut im Nebenschluß aus den proximalen Anteilen der Stromcapillaren, verteilt es in der Alveolarwand und gibt es arterialisiert an die distalen Anteile der Stromcapillaren ab. Es nimmt in der Arbeit das vermehrte Herzzeitvolumen auf und dient so als Arbeitskreislauf;

---

[1] Giese 1957, Junghanss 1958.   [2] Vgl. Schoedel 1955, Bostroem und Piiper 1955.

es vermag zeitweilig Blut zu speichern; es wird in der Lungenstauung bei Störungen des Blutdurchflusses bis an die Grenze seiner Kapazität gefüllt; es schwindet im schweren atrophischen diffusen Emphysem bis auf geringe Reste.

Bei schwerem Emphysem atmet die Lunge fast nur mit den Stromcapillaren, ebenso bei Frühgeburten, solange die Alveolen noch nicht ausdifferenziert sind.

Dem Capillarsystem sind die kleinen Arterien vorgeordnet, deren muskuläre Media auf nervale und humorale Reize sowie auf örtlich gebildete Stoffwechselprodukte mit Kontraktion oder Erschlaffung reagiert. Bei Kontraktion entsteht keine Verkürzung der Faser wie bei der quergestreiften Muskulatur, sondern eine Faserquellung[1]. Durch diese wird die Lichtung der Arterien eingeengt, ohne daß sich die äußere Dimension des Gefäßes ändert.

Die alternierende Funktion dieser Gefäßabschnitte, die auch experimentell durch mechanische Pleurareize ausgelöst werden kann[2], erklärt örtliche Unterschiede in der Perfusion kleiner Lungeneinheiten und damit auch die wechselnde O_2-Aufnahme in das Blut.

Allgemeine Vasodilatation und Vasoconstriction wirkt sich in erster Linie auf den Blutdruck im kleinen Kreislauf aus.

Der Hauptwiderstand für die Blutströmung im kleinen Kreislauf kann in den Arteriolen oder in den Capillaren liegen. Wo er lokalisiert ist, hat sich bisher noch nicht genügend klären lassen[3]. Die Unsicherheit hängt mit den methodischen Schwierigkeiten zusammen, die einer Bestimmung des Capillardruckes in der Lunge entgegenstehen. Druckmessungen durch Einführen eines Katheters bis zum Steckenbleiben in einem Pulmonalarterienast geben Werte von 8,4 (4,5—13) mm Hg, die dem etwas niedrigeren linken Vorhofdruck nicht immer entsprechen[4].

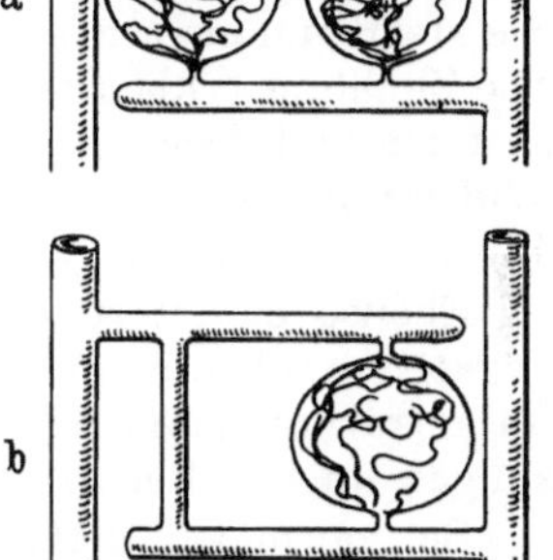

Abb. 76a u. b. Schematische Darstellung der Endstrombahn. a Blutströmung nur über das Netzcapillarsystem möglich. b Blutströmung sowohl über Netzcapillaren als auch über Stromcapillaren möglich. (Aus GIESE 1957.)

Nach MATTHES u. Mitarb. (1960) geben diese Messungen wahrscheinlich nur einen mittleren Gewebsdruck an, der durch die Venenfüllung und durch pulsatorische Schwankungen mitbestimmt ist. Er stellt kein Maß für die Berechnung des Arteriolenwiderstandes dar.

Einen Anhalt für den Ort des Hauptwiderstandes gibt die Messung der Diffusionskapazität, aus der auf die Weite der capillären Strombahn geschlossen werden kann. Da pulmonale Druckerhöhung und Minderung der Diffusionskapazität nicht immer zusammenfallen, kann die Widerstandserhöhung nicht capillär bestimmt sein. Die Verminderung des Capillarwiderstandes bei Belastung erfolgt nicht nur durch Capillardehnung, sondern auch durch Eröffnung neuer Capillargebiete (vgl. Bestimmung des Capillarquerschnittes mittels Messung der Diffusionskapazität[5]).

Verschlossene Capillaren reagieren auf pharmakologische Reize nicht[6]. Pharmaka, die im großen Kreislauf als Vasodilatatoren bekannt sind, haben am Lungenkreislauf beim Gesunden keine Wirkung. Daraus wird der Schluß gezogen, daß die Gefäße des kleinen Kreislaufs unter normalen Verhältnissen

---

[1] HIRSCH 1955.　　[2] REINHARDT 1935.　　[3] PIIPER 1958.
[4] HELLEMS und Mitarbeiter 1949, LAGERLÖF und WERKÖ 1949, FOWLER und Mitarbeiter 1953, CONOLLY und Mitarbeiter 1954, BJÖRK und Mitarbeiter 1954, WIGGERS 1953.
[5] RILEY und Mitarbeiter 1954, BARTELS und Mitarbeiter 1955.　　[6] HALMAGYI 1957.

maximal erweitert sind, denn Vasodilatatoren haben nur auf verengte Gefäße eine Wirkung.

Dagegen wird Vasoconstriction der Arteriolen des kleinen Kreislaufs mit Zunahme des arteriellen Druckes nach Einwirkung von Adrenalin, stärker noch nach Noradrenalin sowohl im Tierversuch als auch beim Menschen beobachtet. Auch der Capillardruck steigt an[1].

Histamin wirkt constrictorisch auf die Pulmonalvenen und -arterien[2].

Die Abnahme des Strömungswiderstandes mit steigenden Gefäßdrucken zeigt sich auch bei Erhöhung des Blutvolumens. Die arteriovenöse Druckdifferenz nimmt mit steigendem Herzzeitvolumen ab[3].

b) Der Blutgehalt der Lunge.

Mit steigendem Durchströmungsdruck nimmt die Blutfüllung der Lunge zu. Sie steigt um etwa 2% an, wenn der arterielle Druck um 1 cm H_2O erhöht wird. Die Zunahme erklärt sich aus der druckabhängigen passiven Dehnung des Gefäßsystems und deckt sich mit der Beobachtung, daß bei zunehmendem Druck der Widerstand geringer wird. Auch bei steigendem venösem Druck erhöht sich die Blutfüllung der Lunge[4].

Ebenso erweitert sich das Gefäßbett der Lunge bei Lungendehnung unter negativem Pleuradruck[5]. Piiper (1957) findet einen besonders starken Anstieg im intrathorakalen negativen Druckbereich von 0—11 cm H_2O (vgl. auch Messungen an der Leichenlunge S. 584).

Bei normalen arteriellen Drucken zwischen 15 und 25 mm Hg (= 20 bis 34 cm H_2O) beträgt der Blutgehalt der Hundelunge 60 ml auf 100 g blutfreies Gewebe bezogen. Auf diese Zahlen gestützt, berechnet Lochner (1957) die Gesamtblutmenge in der menschlichen Lunge auf 600 ml unter Annahme eines Lungengewichtes von 1000 g bei einem 70 kg schweren Menschen. Er kommt dabei auf 12% des gesamten Blutvolumens. Die Blutmenge kann nach Kuno (1918) zwischen 9 und 20% schwanken. Halmagyi (1957) gibt 15% der zirkulierenden Blutmenge als „totale" Blutmenge in der Lunge an, von der sich jeweils nur $^1/_{20}$ als „funktionelle" Blutmenge in den Lungencapillaren befinden sollen[6]. Roughton (1945) berechnet die Blutmenge in den Capillaren ebenfalls auf unter 100 ml.

Die Lungencapillaren enthalten in der Ruhe 60 ml Blut, bei Arbeit 95 ml. Die Kontaktzeit ändert sich dabei gleichzeitig von 0,73 auf 0,34 sec, d.h. die Volumzunahme und die Kontaktzeitverkürzung tragen zur Erhöhung der Lungenfunktion bei Arbeit von der Kreislaufseite her in etwa gleichem Maße bei. Wilson u. Mitarb. (1954) nehmen etwas größere Blutmengen und entsprechend weniger stark verkürzte Kontaktzeiten an. Die vermehrte Füllung des alveolocapillären Gebietes weist ebenfalls auf eine Eröffnung von Reservecapillaren hin.

Von der Gesamtblutmenge soll sich nach Sjöstrand (1951, 1953a, b) ein größerer Teil besonders in den Venolen speichern und als Blutreservoir dienen, von dem aus durch Änderung des Zuflusses zum linken Herzen dessen Schlagvolumen reguliert werden könne. Arterienraum und Venenraum haben etwa gleiche Dimensionen und gleiche physikalische Eigenschaften[7].

Diese Angaben über die Blutmengen konnten in eigenen Untersuchungen mit Backmann (1961) an der Leichenlunge bestätigt und Änderungen des Blutvolumens bei krankhaften Prozessen der Lunge aufgezeigt werden (Tabelle 11).

---

[1] Halmagyi 1957.   [2] Nikulin 1959.   [3] Gauer und Henry 1956.
[4] Lochner 1957.   [5] Ochsner 1952.   [6] Sjöstrand 1951, 1953.   [7] Piiper 1958.

Tabelle 11. *Blutgehalt von Leichenlungen.* (Nach Untersuchungen von BACKMANN.)

	Anzahl, Geschlecht	Mittleres Alter	Frischgewicht	Trockensubstanz vom gesamten Frischgewicht	Blutgehalt auf 100 g blutfreies Frischgewicht	Absoluter Blutgehalt	Blutverteilung zwischen Ober- (bzw. Ober- und Mittel-) und Unterlappen
		Jahre	g	%	ml	ml	
Normale Lungen	2 ♂ 6 ♀	40	648 (470—930)	16,7 (14—19)	68 (48—74)	232	1:1,2
Diffuse Emphyseme	2 ♂ 3 ♀	70	562 (390—730)	14,8 (12—17)	44 (34—58)	162	1:1,5
Stauungslunge	1 ♂	28	1060	12,5	162	633	1:2,3
Verblutung	1 ♂	47	500	18,8	39	139	1:1,5

In den Versuchen wurden zur Erhaltung des Lungenvolumens vor Eröffnung des Thorax die Trachea abgeklemmt und die Gefäße und Bronchien am Hilus unmittelbar nach Eröffnung des Thorax und vor Abtrennung des Herzens verschlossen. Bei 8 normalen Lungen, die nur die gewöhnlichen agonalen Veränderungen aufwiesen, ergab sich bei einem mittleren Frischgewicht von 648 g ein mittlerer Trockensubstanzanteil von 16,7% des Frischgewichtes. Die Werte schwankten zwischen 14 und 19%. Dieser Trockensubstanzanteil entspricht den von RAUEN (1956) angegebenen Normalwerten annähernd.

Als normaler Blutgehalt wurden 68 ml Blut/100 g blutfreies Frischgewicht bei einer Schwankungsbreite zwischen 48 und 74 ml gefunden. Das Verhältnis der Blutmenge im Ober- bzw. bei rechten Lungen im Ober- und Mittellappen gegenüber dem Unterlappen betrug 1:1,2. Diese Werte zeigen zugleich die Spielbreite der agonalen Veränderungen hinsichtlich des wechselnden Gehaltes an Ödemwasser und durch Hypostase beeinflußter Blutverteilung. Eine abnorme Blutverteilung wurde vor allem bei akuter Blähung des Oberlappens und als Folge einer Kompression des Unterlappens durch Herzhypertrophie an der linken Lunge oder durch größere Pleuraergüsse beobachtet. Die Differenzen zwischen linker und rechter Lunge waren unerheblich.

Der relative Blutgehalt von 68 ml auf 100 g blutfreies Lungengewebe ist mit den von LOCHNER (1957) mitgeteilten Werten identisch. Der normale durchschnittliche absolute Blutgehalt der gesamten Lunge beträgt etwa 500 ml, das sind etwa 10% der zirkulierenden Blutmenge. Das von LOCHNER angenommene blutfreie Frischgewicht der Lungen von 1000 g für einen 70 kg schweren Menschen liegt nach den eigenen Messungen und nach den auf ein umfangreiches Material gestützten Wägungen von RÖSSLE u. ROULET (1932) zu hoch. Hieraus ergibt sich die Differenz zu dem von LOCHNER angenommenen absoluten Blutgehalt von 600 ml.

Bei diffusem senilem Emphysem ergab sich ein relativer Blutgehalt von nur 44 ml/100 g blutfreies Frischgewicht, die gesamte Blutmenge war somit um knapp ein Drittel vermindert (Tabelle 11). Dagegen wurde in einer Stauungslunge, die zugleich sehr reichlich Ödemwasser enthielt, eine Vermehrung des Blutgehaltes auf etwa das $2\frac{1}{2}$fache der Norm gemessen. In einem Falle von akuter Verblutung fand sich der Blutgehalt auf nahezu die Hälfte herabgesetzt.

Die Ergebnisse lassen sich dahingehend zusammenfassen, daß die in Leichenlungen gefundene Blutfüllung des Lungengewebes den im Leben gemessenen Werten weitgehend entspricht. Es ist mit einem mittleren Blutgehalt von etwa 500 ml Blut in der gesamten Lunge zu rechnen, das sind etwa 10% der zirkulierenden Blutmenge. Bei Emphysem und bei akuter Verblutung kann der Blutgehalt bis auf die Hälfte herabgesetzt, in Stauungslungen auf über das Doppelte vermehrt sein.

Das kleine Blutvolumen der Emphysemlungen ist Folge der Reduktion des Capillarnetzes, das große Blutvolumen der Stauungslunge Folge der Capillarektasie. Da das Herzminutenvolumen bei Stauungslunge, insbesondere bei Mitralstenosen stark (bis auf 3 Liter) reduziert ist, dienen die erweiterten Capillaren als Speicher für den Blutanteil, den der linke Ventrikel nicht aufnehmen kann. Das Speicherblut in der Stauungslunge ist für den Gasaustausch nutzloser Ballast.

Die in klinischen Messungen festgestellte hohe Strömungsgeschwindigkeit bei Emphysem erklärt sich aus dem geringen Fassungsvermögen des reduzierten Capillarbettes. Die verkleinerte Kontaktfläche und die verkürzte Kontaktzeit wirken in gleicher Weise hemmend auf den Gasaustausch.

c) Die Beziehungen zwischen Lungen- und Körperkreislauf.

Der Lungenkreislauf wird nach neueren Einteilungen in der Kreislaufphysiologie zum Niederdrucksystem (low pressure system) gerechnet[1]. Zu diesem gehören mit dem Lungenkreislauf die gesamten Körpervenen. Es enthält etwa 75—80% der Gesamtblutmenge[2]. Im Niederdruckgebiet werden Gesamtblutvolumen und Gefäßkapazität aufeinander abgestimmt.

Der mittlere Gefäßfüllungsdruck beträgt beim Menschen, kurz nach dem Tode im rechten Vorhof gemessen, 7,6 cm H_2O[3]. Er steigt bei Zunahme des intravasalen Flüssigkeitsvolumens proportional zur vermehrten Menge und bei Erhöhung des Gefäßtonus durch Adrenalingaben bis auf Werte von 16 bis 80 mm Hg an[4].

Die Blutmenge, die sich während des Lebens im Lungenkreislauf zwischen Pulmonal- und Aortenklappen befindet, beträgt etwa 20—25% (zentrales Blutvolumen nach Gauer 1957). Bei Abnahme des Gesamtblutvolumens, etwa nach Aderlaß, sinkt der Mitteldruck des Lungenkreislaufs in gleichem Maße in Lungenarterien, Lungencapillaren und Lungenvenen[5].

Während Adrenalin den Blutdruck über den Gefäßtonus beeinflußt, steigert ihn starke Kälteeinwirkung durch Vermehrung des zentralen Blutvolumens bei Konstriktion der Hautgefäße. Umgekehrt sinkt bei starker Erwärmung der Blutdruck durch Erweiterung der Hautgefäße.

Ähnliche Verschiebungen des Blutvolumens in die intrathorakalen Organe kommen auch bei Übergängen vom Stehen zum Liegen in Betracht. Nach Sjöstrand (1951, 1952, 1953, 1956) kann der Lungenkreislauf auf diese Weise zusätzlich etwa 50 cm³ Blut aufnehmen oder abgeben. Durch Überdruckatmung wird eine etwa gleichgroße Blutmenge aus dem Thorax in die Peripherie verlagert[6]. Nach Versuchen am Hund liegt die vermehrte Blutmenge des Lungenkreislaufs etwa zu gleichen Teilen in Arterien und Venen[7]. Die intrathorakalen Gefäße haben so die Funktion eines Volumenausgleichsgefäßes[8].

Das intrathorakale Blutvolumen hat seinerseits Beziehungen zur Herztätigkeit über die Größe des venösen Blutangebotes und über die Beeinflussung der Herzfrequenz (Bainbridge-Reflex). Nach Lochner u. Schoedel (1950, 1952) besteht eine lineare Korrelation zwischen Blutfüllung des kleinen Kreislaufs und Herzminutenvolumen[9].

---

[1] Gauer und Henry 1956.   [2] Bazett 1949.
[3] Starr 1940, 1949, Starr und Mitarbeiter 1943.   [4] Guyton und Mitarbeiter 1954, Buhr 1954.
[5] Gauer und Henry 1956, Glaser und Mitarbeiter 1954.
[6] Fenn und Mitarbeiter 1947.   [7] Piiper 1958.
[8] Hochrein und Schleicher 1953, Gauer 1957, Gauer und Henry 1956.
[9] Lochner 1957.

d) Blutdruck und Durchflußvolumen im Lungenkreislauf.

1. Physiologische und klinische Meßwerte.

Im Lungenkreislauf steht der arterielle Schenkel als Teilabschnitt des Niederdrucksystems unter einem wesentlich geringeren Druck als im großen Kreislauf (Abb. 77). Nach COURNAND (1950), FOWLER (1953) und ihren Mitarbeitern beträgt der Druck in der Pulmonalarterie beim Menschen:

systolisch 11—29 mm Hg
diastolisch 4—13 mm Hg
Mitteldruck 8—19 mm Hg

Durchschnittswerte sind nach MATTHES u. Mitarb. (1960):

systolisch 22,9 mm Hg
diastolisch 9,1 mm Hg
Mitteldruck 14,4 mm Hg

Im linken Vorhof beträgt der Mitteldruck 5 mm Hg.

Die Lungenarterien zeigen bis weit in die Peripherie elastischen Gefäßtyp mit muskulär variierbarer Elastizität. Die elastischen Fasern werden durch die glatten Muskelfasern gespannt[1]. Der geringe Anteil an kollagenen Fasern und die relativ schwache Muskel-

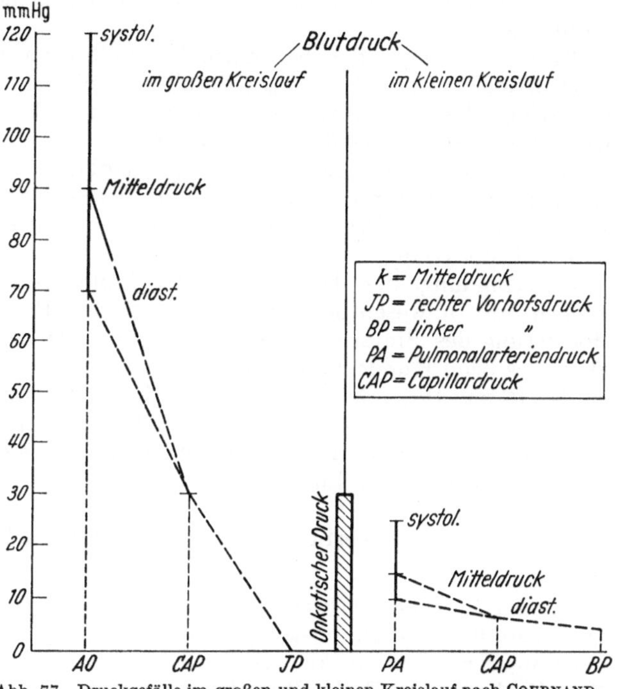

Abb. 77. Druckgefälle im großen und kleinen Kreislauf nach COURNAND. (Aus HALMAGYI 1957.)

schicht erklären die starke Dehnbarkeit auch der kleinen Lungenarterienäste. Aus Strömungsversuchen wird geschlossen, daß das Poiseuillesche Gesetz im kleinen Kreislauf keine volle Gültigkeit hat[2].

Das Speichervolumen des Windkessels beträgt nur 20—30% des Schlagvolumens, im großen Kreislauf dagegen 50%. Der Abstrom am Windkesselende erfolgt daher diskontinuierlich und führt zu einer ausgesprochenen peripheren Volumenpulsation[3]. Die zur Regulation des Druckes befähigten kleinen Arterien unterliegen intermittierender systolischer Dehnung.

Wegen der Elastizitätsverhältnisse und des Niederdruckes ergibt sich eine langsame Pulswellengeschwindigkeit[4].

An der isolierten, von einem Spendertier durchbluteten Hundelunge nimmt der Strömungsdruck mit steigendem Gefäßdruck ab[5]. Diese Widerstandsminderung beruht wahrscheinlich im wesentlichen auf der vermehrten Dehnung der Blutgefäße durch den größeren Druck und ist unabhängig vom Druck in der Pulmonalvene[6].

---

[1] BENNINGHOFF 1935.   [2] WEZLER und SINN 1953.
[3] KNEBEL 1955.   [4] SIEDECK, WENGER und GMACHL 1951.
[5] DALY 1930, WAGNER 1928, WILLIAMS 1954, LOCHNER 1957.   [6] LOCHNER 1957.

Bei vermehrter Strömung, z. B. bei einem verdoppelten Herzminutenvolumen in der Arbeit, bleibt der Mitteldruck in der Arteria pulmonalis unbeeinflußt. Auch bei schwerer Arbeit kommt es zu keiner wesentlichen Druckerhöhung[1].

Die Anpassungsfähigkeit der Lungengefäße ist besser als im großen Kreislauf. Der Lungenkreislauf muß im Gegensatz zu den Stromgebieten des großen Kreislaufes ständig zumindest das Ruheherzminutenvolumen passieren lassen und kann die Durchblutung somit nicht vollständig nach dem Blutbedarf der Lunge regulieren.

In einer Lunge, die bei normaler Belüftung vom Ruheminutenvolumen durchströmt wird, sind nur $1/10$—$1/15$ aller Capillaren von Blut durchflossen[2]. Bei Steigerung des Minutenvolumens werden die Reservecapillaren eröffnet und dadurch die Austauschfläche vergrößert.

Bei organischen Lungenerkrankungen wird die Ausgleichsbreite eingeschränkt. Der Druckanstieg erfolgt deshalb bereits bei geringen Belastungen, wenn in der Ruhe noch normale Druckwerte bestimmt werden. Dies gilt z. B. auch besonders für das Emphysem.

Unterbindung des Hauptastes der Pulmonalarterie oder Pneumektomie ergeben nur unwesentliche Steigerungen des Pulmonalarteriendruckes[3]. Bei Blockierung des Blutzustromes zu einer Lungenhälfte durch die Ballonmethode kommt es beim Hunde zu einem leichten Druckanstieg in der Arteria pulmonalis um 3—10 mm Hg. Dabei bleibt das Herzzeitvolumen praktisch unverändert, d. h., daß die nicht geblockte Lungenhälfte die doppelte Blutmenge aufnehmen kann, ohne daß der Pulmonalarteriendruck nennenswert ansteigt[4]. Der Widerstand in der intakten Lunge muß unter diesen Verhältnissen verringert sein.

2. Perfusionsversuche an der Leichenlunge.

α) Methode.

Die im Tierversuch und am Menschen während des Lebens gewonnenen Ergebnisse über die Durchströmung der Lunge finden eine Ergänzung in Durchströmungsversuchen an der isolierten oder in situ belassenen Leichenlunge. Diese Methode gibt Einblick in den Anteil, den rein mechanisch wirksame Faktoren auf die Lungenperfusion haben. Alle funktionellen regulatorischen Einflüsse, die von der Konzentration der Atemgase in der Alveolarluft und im Blut direkt oder auf dem Nervenwege ausgeübt werden und in die am Lebenden gewonnenen Meßwerte eingehen, bleiben dabei aus dem Spiel.

Die Versuche geben Einblick in den Anteil, den 1. arterieller Druck, 2. Dehnungslage der Lunge und 3. intraalveolärer Druck auf die Durchströmung der Lunge haben.

Der Einfluß dieser physikalischen Größen auf die Gefäßweite wurde bereits von Minkowski (1912), gestützt auf Versuche von D. Gerhardt (1904, 1908, 1910) und Romanoff (1911), hervorgehoben und den unsicheren Ergebnissen aus Durchströmungsversuchen mit pharmakologischer Beeinflussung der Gefäße des kleinen Kreislaufes gegenübergestellt.

In eigenen, mit Hartung und Delfmann (1960) durchgeführten Versuchen wurden Leichenlungen mit einer Testlösung aus Tetrachlorkohlenstoff und Paraffinöl im Verhältnis 6:5 durchströmt. Diese Lösung hatte sich bereits Vivell (1951) bei seinen Durchströmungsversuchen der Coronararterien als zweckmäßig erwiesen.

---

[1] Donald, Bishop und Mitarbeiter 1955, Bühlmann, Schaub und Luchsinger 1955, Hickam und Cargill 1948.
[2] Roughton 1945, v. Euler 1951.
[3] Lichtheim 1876, Cournand 1947.   [4] Leusen und Mitarbeiter 1956, 1957.

Die absoluten Werte, die mit dieser Methode gewonnen werden, weichen erheblich von den während des Lebens gefundenen Größen ab. Derartige Durchströmungsversuche können nur Relativwerte geben, weil sich ein gleichmäßiger, in seiner absoluten Größe dem Verhältnis des Lebenden entsprechender Durchfluß z. T. infolge postmortaler Gerinnselbildung nicht erreichen läßt. In länger andauernden Strömungsversuchen werden die Gefäße, besonders bei Anwendung hoher Einfülldrucke undicht.

Auch an der überlebenden isolierten Hundelunge ist unter normalen Druckbedingungen nur eine Durchströmung von 46% der Durchblutung im Organismus zu erzielen, der mittlere Strömungswiderstand ist dabei auf 220% erhöht[1].

In den eigenen Versuchen an der isolierten menschlichen Leichenlunge war der Durchfluß noch bedeutend niedriger. Er lag unter annähernd normaler Druck- und Dehnungslage (arterieller Druck 22 mm Hg, venöser Druck 0, mittlere

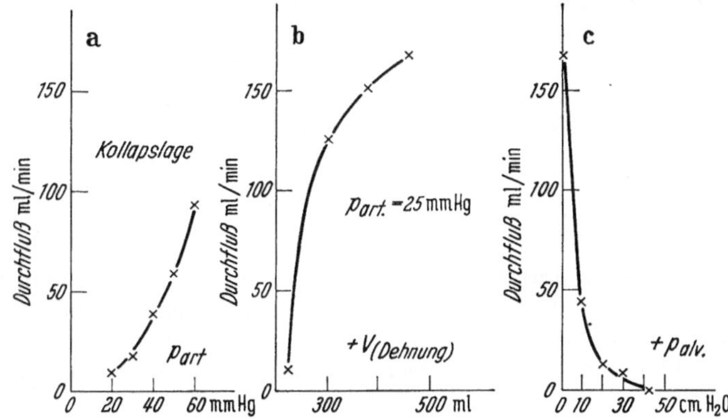

Abb. 78. Beziehungen der Lungenperfusion zu Änderung des arteriellen Druckes (a), des Lungendehnungsgrades (b) und des intraalveolären Druckes (c). Leichenlungenmessungen. (Nach HARTUNG und DELFMANN 1960.)

Dehnungslage entsprechend einem Pleuradruck von —10 cm H₂O) im Mittel bei 13,2% der angenommenen Durchblutungsgröße im Organismus und überschritt auch unter optimalen Bedingungen in keinem Falle eine Durchflußmenge von 25%.

Für die normale Leichenlunge haben sich aber unter verschiedenen Versuchsbedingungen gewonnene Standardwerte ergeben, die regelhafte Beziehungen der Lungenperfusion zu arteriellem Druck, Lungendehnung und intraalveolärem Druck erkennen lassen. Die Abb. 78a—c gibt die typischen Werte von zwei während des gesamten Versuches unter methodisch einwandfreien Bedingungen untersuchten Leichenlungen wieder.

Die an normalen Lungen gewonnenen Werte können mit entsprechenden Messungen an Leichenlungen mit krankhaften Prozessen des Lungengewebes oder der Blutgefäße unmittelbar verglichen werden und geben wertvolle Hinweise auf die mechanisch wirksamen Faktoren bei Störungen der Lungenperfusion.

Eine sinngemäße Übertragung dieser Meßergebnisse an Leichenlungen auf die Verhältnisse am Lebenden ist möglich und — wie an mehreren Beispielen gezeigt werden kann — nützlich für die Klärung der Zusammenhänge zwischen morphologischen Zustandsbildern und gestörter Funktion.

β) Druck und Perfusionsgröße.

Zwischen arteriellem Druck und Durchflußvolumen bestehen an der kollabierten Leichenlunge im physiologischen Druckbereich konstante, im Einzelversuch

[1] PIIPER 1957.

wiederholt reproduzierbare Relationen. Mit der Steigerung des Einfülldruckes von 20 auf 60 mm Hg ergibt sich eine nahezu lineare Zunahme der Durchflußmenge. Bei Drucken zwischen 20 und 40 mm Hg beträgt die Steigerung in den ausgewählten Fällen 680% (s. Abb. 78a). Das Durchflußvolumen wächst in dieser Druckspanne im Durchschnitt auf das Fünf- bis Siebenfache an.

Auch bei weiteren Drucksteigerungen nimmt die Durchflußmenge druckproportional zu. An der Leichenlunge sind zuverlässige Meßwerte nur bis zu Drucken von etwa 60 mm Hg zu gewinnen, da die Blutgefäße bei größeren Drucken undicht werden.

Die Steigerung der Durchflußmenge wird in diesen Versuchen wahrscheinlich im wesentlichen durch Zunahme der Strömungsgeschwindigkeit erreicht, denn man muß annehmen, daß die tonusfreien Gefäße der Leichenlunge, insbesondere die Gefäßstrecke der Arteriolen, schon bei Drucken zwischen 20 und 30 mm Hg bis zur Grenze ihrer regelhaften Kapazität gedehnt sind.

In histologischen Kontrollen durchströmter Lungen ist der gesamte arterielle Schenkel des pulmonalen Strombogens weit gestellt. Am auffälligsten ist diese Weitstellung im Bereich der kleinen Arterien und Arteriolen, die bei Druckbelastung weit stärker gedehnt werden als die proximalen Anteile der Arterien. Im Capillarbereich kommt es auch bei hohen Einfülldrucken nur zu geringen Erweiterungen, solange der venöse Abfluß unbehindert ist. Die Venen können also große Zuflußmengen weiterleiten, ohne daß es zu einer Aufstauung in den Capillaren kommt.

Die kleinen Arterien und Arteriolen sind auch im atonischen, vom Strömungsdruck weitgestellten pulmonalen Strombogen die engste Stelle mit größtem Strömungswiderstand. Diese Abschnitte werden bei hohem Druck und großem Volumen am stärksten belastet. Hier liegt auch die Grenze für das maximal mögliche Durchflußvolumen.

3. Vermehrung des pulmonalen Zirkulationsvolumens.

α) Angeborene Herzfehler.

Eine ständige Vermehrung des Blutvolumens im kleinen Kreislauf belastet die gesamte Lungenstrombahn.

Bei angeborenen Herzfehlern mit Links-Rechts-Shunt, z.B. bei Einmündung der Pulmonalvenen in den rechten Vorhof, bei Vorhofseptumdefekt, bei offenem Ductus Botalli, bei Ventrikelseptumdefekt und bei Truncus arteriosus communis, kann das Blutvolumen im kleinen Kreislauf auf das Doppelte und Dreifache anwachsen. Kurzschlußvolumina von 1,5—6,5 l/min werden noch als gering bezeichnet[1]

Das Verhältnis der Blutströmung zwischen pulmonalem und peripherem Kreislauf beträgt häufig 3 : 1[2].

Der Strömungswiderstand ist bei einem Teil dieser Fehlbildungen nicht erhöht. In einer eigenen Beobachtung von großem Vorhofseptumdefekt und Einmündung einer Lungenvene in den rechten Vorhof hat trotz eines Shunt-Volumens von 6,8 Liter keine pulmonale Hypertonie bestanden. Die kleinen Arterien und Arteriolen waren maximal weit, mit dünner Wand, ohne Intimaproliferation. Auch an den großen Arterien bestand keine Sklerose. Die weite rechte Herzkammer zeigte eine leichte trabeculäre Hypertrophie. Die Lungencapillaren waren geöffnet und leicht erweitert. Es bestand keine Lungenstauung.

In anderen Fällen wird klinisch ein erhöhter oder hoher systolischer Druck gefunden. Dieser ist zu erwarten, wenn das Stromvolumen 10 Liter/min/m² Körperoberfläche übersteigt[3]. Bei mittleren Shuntvolumina steigt der Pulmonalarteriendruck mäßig bis zu etwa 30 mm Hg, bei sehr hohen Shuntvolumina

---

[1] Grosse-Brockhoff 1957.   [2] Halmagyi 1957.   [3] Dexter und Mitarbeiter 1950.

stark an. In diesen Lungen zeigt das pulmonale Gefäßsystem eine vermehrte Blutfüllung. Die Lungen sind dunkelrot und schwer, oft vermindert lufthaltig.

Es besteht also ein reiner Volumenhochdruck. Doch soll auch oft ein Widerstandshochdruck hinzutreten[1].

Aus morphologischen Untersuchungen der Lungenstrombahn geht übereinstimmend hervor, daß die pulmonale Hypertonie mit Gefäßwandveränderungen zusammenfällt, die in den kleinen Arterien beginnen und auf die größeren Arterien fortschreiten. Gleichartige posthypertonische Gefäßveränderungen[2] kommen auch im Gefolge der seltenen genuinen pulmonalen Hypertonie, bei primärer Obliteration von Lungengefäßen und bei Störungen des Blutabflusses aus der Lunge vor.

An den kleinen Arterien kommt es in einem ersten Stadium der Anpassung zur muskulären Mediahypertrophie und Hyperplasie der elastischen Lamellen, an den großen Arterien zu einer diffusen Wandverdickung mit gleichzeitiger Lichtungserweiterung[3].

In den kleinen muskulären Arterien kann auch die fetale Gefäßwandarchitektonik persistieren[4]. Die Gefäße behalten eine dicke muskelkräftige Wand und ein enges Lumen. Durch die Engstellung der kleinen Arterien, die den hämodynamischen Verhältnissen beim Feten entspricht, bleibt der Blutzufluß zu den Lungencapillaren auch nach der Geburt gedrosselt. Mit dem Anstieg des arteriellen Druckes nimmt die Zahl der geöffneten arteriovenösen Anastomosen zu[5].

Im nachfolgenden zweiten Stadium entstehen Wandschäden mit Medianarben und Intimaproliferation, die an den Arteriolen beginnen und in fortgeschrittenen Stadien auf die kleinen Arterien übergreifen. Die Veränderungen an den kleinen Gefäßen verlaufen als Thromboendarteriitis[6] oder als seröse, fibrinöse und nekrotisierende Endarteriitis pulmonalis[7]. ROTTER (1949) ordnet diese Gefäßveränderungen in den Formenkreis der Arteriolosklerose ein, während BREDT einen primären entzündlichen Vorgang annimmt.

Zu dieser Frage, die hier nur kurz gestreift werden kann, sei auf ausführliche Diskussionen darüber hingewiesen[8].

Für den Gasaustausch und die O_2-Sättigung des Blutes sind dagegen die Feststellungen von großer Bedeutung, daß ein kleines Shuntvolumen den Pulmonalkreislauf nur in geringem Maße belastet, ein großes Shuntvolumen zum Volumenhochdruck und zur organischen Stenose im arteriellen Schenkel der Endstrombahn führt.

Dadurch wird ein zunehmender Strömungswiderstand aufgebaut, der das Durchflußvolumen schließlich drosselt und eine Überfüllung der Austauschcapillaren verhindert. Der Druck in den Pulmonalarterien kann dabei auf das Vier- bis Fünffache ansteigen und schließlich bei offenem Ductus Botalli zu einer Shuntumkehr führen[9].

Die Sauerstoffaufnahme in das Blut ist in diesen Fällen in der Ruhe ausreichend. Bei Belastung kann das Volumen nicht mehr im erforderlichen Maße gesteigert werden, es tritt eine kardiale Insuffizienz ein. Herzdekompensation ist nur dann zu erwarten, wenn mehr als 50% des Lungenblutes rezirkulieren[10].

---

[1] BING 1949, 1952, BING und Mitarbeiter 1947, GROSSE-BROCKHOFF 1951, 1957.
[2] KÖNN 1956, 1958.   [3] W. W. MEYER und RICHTER 1955, 1956.
[4] EDWARDS 1950.   [5] LAPP 1950, 1951, GERICKE 1955, KÖHN und RICHTER 1958.
[6] WIESE 1936.   [7] BREDT 1932, 1942, BREDT und STADLER 1940.
[8] HÖRA 1935, STAEMMLER 1937, 1938, 1955, STAEMMLER und SCHMITT 1951, SCHMIDT 1953, KÖNN 1958, KÖHN und RICHTER 1958.
[9] BAYER, GROSSE-BROCKHOFF, LOOGEN und MEESSEN 1957, BAYER, LOOGEN und WOLTER 1954.
[10] BENDER 1959.

β) Aortalisation.

Eine besondere Form der Volumen- und Druckbelastung der Lungengefäße kann mitunter bei der Fallotgruppe vorkommen. Der Blutzufluß in die Pulmonalarterie ist dabei wegen der Pulmonalstenose schon am Einfluß in die Arteria pulmonalis gedrosselt. Dafür kann den Lungen vermehrt Blut durch erweiterte Bronchialarterien und durch zusätzliche Gefäßverbindungen zwischen Aorta und Lunge zugeführt werden. Diesen Vorgang haben GIAMPALMO u. SCHOENMACKERS (1952) als Aortalisation, weitere Verbindungen zwischen Arteria subclavia und Lunge als Spontan-Blalock bezeichnet[1]. Auf diesem Wege wird den Lungencapillaren so viel Blut unter Aortendruck zugeführt, daß eine hochgradige Erweiterung (Pseudoangiomatose) der Capillaren zur Einengung der Alveolen führt (angiektatische Alveolarkompression). Die Vitalkapazität ist dadurch stark eingeschränkt und der Gasaustausch durch gleichzeitige Verdickung der Alveolarmembran gestört.

Das Blut, das den Lungen über die Bronchialarterien zugeleitet wird, kann auf folgenden Wegen in die Strombahn der Pulmonalgefäße gelangen[2]:

1. Über arterioarterielle Anastomosen,
2. über arteriovenöse Anastomosen,
3. über pleurale Anastomosen.

Die arterioarteriellen Anastomosen leiten Aortenblut in die Pulmonalarterien, die es den Capillaren zuführen und so einen Gasaustausch ermöglichen[3].

Das über die arteriovenösen Anastomosen in die Lungenvenen einströmende Blut berührt nicht das Capillargebiet der Lunge und nimmt keinen Sauerstoff auf. Es erscheint als venöse Beimischung im großen Kreislauf.

Bronchialarterien lassen sich im postmortalen Angiogramm von der Arteria pulmonalis aus über Endverzweigungen dieser Äste und pleurale Anastomosen leicht auffüllen. Die Verbindungen liegen im Bereich der Präcapillaren und der Riesencapillaren der Pleura. Bei der Aortalisation strömt das Blut aus den erweiterten Bronchialarterien direkt in das Capillargebiet der Lunge. Vielleicht kommt es auf diesem Weg zu der starken Capillarektasie bei manchen Fällen von Fallotscher Tetralogie und Morbus coeruleus.

γ) Polycythämie.

Bei der Polycythämie ist das gesamte Blutvolumen auf das 3—4fache vermehrt (7,7—23,1 Liter nach HEILMEYER u. BEGEMANN 1951). Der Blutdruck ist trotz dieser starken Volumenvermehrung nicht nennenswert erhöht, teilweise sogar erniedrigt. Die periphere Strombahn ist weit gestellt, die Capillaren sind mit Blut überfüllt, die Strömung ist verlangsamt.

In der Lunge kommt es ebenso wie bei Vorhofseptumdefekten oder Einmündung von Pulmonalvenen in den rechten Vorhof zu einer starken Capillarerweiterung und zur Weitstellung der ganzen Gefäßbahn ohne Rechtshypertrophie.

Im Verlauf der Krankheit entstehen schließlich nach langer Krankheitsdauer und in höherem Lebensalter Blutdrucksteigerungen und Pulmonalsklerose oder proliferierende Thromboendarteriitis obliterans[4]. Diese wird als Folge einer Thromboseneigung bei Polycythämie angesehen.

Die Sauerstoffsättigung des Blutes ist trotz des großen Volumens ebenso wie bei den Shunt-Volumina der Herzfehlbildungen vollständig, solange keine erhebliche Erhöhung des Strömungswiderstandes und damit eine Durchflußerschwerung durch die Lunge hinzutritt.

---

[1] SCHOENMACKERS 1950, MEESSEN 1954, CAIN 1958.
[2] E. MÜLLER 1953, TÖNDURY und WEIBEL 1956, 1958, WEIBEL 1959, FLORANGE 1960.
[3] BLOOMER und Mitarbeiter 1949.   [4] ROTTER und BÜNGELER 1955.

4. Störungen des Blutabflusses (Stauungslunge).

Die häufigsten Ursachen einer Störung des Blutabflusses aus den Lungen sind Mitralklappenfehler, insbesondere die Mitralstenose, oder die Insuffizienz der linken Herzkammer, seltener Vorhofthrombosen, konstriktive Perikarditis oder gelegentlich auch ein Vorhofmyxom[1]. Durch die Rückstauung des Blutes steigt der Druck in Lungenvenen und Capillaren an und löst eine entsprechende Drucksteigerung im arteriellen Schenkel der Strombahn aus. Drucksteigerungen im pulmonalen Venensystem werden also auf die Arterien übertragen. Der Druckgradient zwischen Arterien und Venen bleibt bei leichter Stauung und bei Stauungszuständen von kurzer Dauer unverändert. Bei einem mittleren pulmonalen arteriellen Ruhedruck von 10—18 mm Hg und einem Vorhofdruck von 5 mm Hg beträgt die Druckdifferenz in der Norm 5—13 mm Hg.

Am Beispiel der Lungenstauung bei Mitralstenose hat GROSSE-BROCKHOFF (1954) gezeigt, daß in diesen Fällen das gesamte Druckniveau im Lungenkreislauf um den Betrag der Drucksteigerung in den Lungenvenen bzw. im linken Vorhof angehoben ist[2].

Der mittlere Vorhofdruck liegt bei Mitralstenose selten höher als 35 mm Hg, er kann bis zu 80 mm Hg steigen[3].

Morphologisch findet sich dabei das Bild der schon unter den Diffusionsstörungen S. 559 beschriebenen Stauungslunge mit starker Blutanfüllung des gesamten Capillargebietes. Der Blutgehalt der Lunge ist nach Messungen an der Leiche um das 2—3fache erhöht (s. S. 581).

Die Druckdifferenz in den Pulmonalgefäßen führt zur Öffnung von Anastomosen mit den Bronchialarterien und zur Rückstauung des Blutes in die Gefäße der Bronchialwand, deren Venen teils in die Pulmonalvenen, teils in die Vena azygos einmünden[4].

Auf diesem Wege entsteht die Stauungsbronchitis, die alle stärkeren Grade von Lungenstauung begleitet.

An den großen Lungenvenen treten Intimasklerosen auf, die auch auf die kleinen Lungenvenen übergreifen[5]. Die Venen des Lungenkreislaufes sind, obwohl sie unter erhöhtem Druck stehen, nicht weit gestellt, sondern nach Röntgenuntersuchungen relativ eng[6]. Diese Engstellung ermöglicht die Übertragung und das Wirksamwerden der vom rechten Ventrikel vermehrt geleisteten Druckarbeit auf den linken Vorhof[7].

Auch im Capillarbereich kann der erhöhte Druck auf die Venen übertragen werden, da die Capillaren der Alveolarwand mit der zunehmenden Stauungsfibrose in starre Mäntel aus kollagenem Fasergewebe eingehüllt werden, die dem erhöhten Druck standhalten (Abb. 79, vgl. auch S. 559 u. 566).

Bei lange bestehender Lungenstauung tritt zu dieser Verlagerung des Druckniveaus auch eine Erhöhung des Druckgradienten zwischen Lungenarterien und Venen. Der Druck steigt in den Arterien stärker an als in den Venen, weil sich in den Lungenarterien eine Widerstandszone bildet, in deren Folge der Strömungswiderstand größer wird. TOSETTI (1955) nimmt 3 Widerstandszonen an: Im ersten Stadium kommt es zu Spasmus und Wandhypertrophie der Postcapillaren und Venolen, im zweiten Stadium der Präcapillaren und Arteriolen. Im dritten Stadium treten organische Gefäßveränderungen mit Abnahme der Gefäßelastizität hinzu.

Eine wesentliche Steigerung der arteriovenösen Druckdifferenz fällt zusammen mit organischen Gefäßveränderungen an den Arteriolen und kleinen Arterien.

---

[1] R. SCHOEN 1932, KÖNN 1956.   [2] KLEPZIG und Mitarbeiter 1954.   [3] HALMAGYI 1957.
[4] v. HAYEK 1951.   [5] KÖNN 1956, BRENNER 1935, MEESSEN 1956, 1957, VAN BOGAERT u. a.
[6] MUSSHOFF und Mitarbeiter 1959.   [7] BAYER und Mitarbeiter 1954.

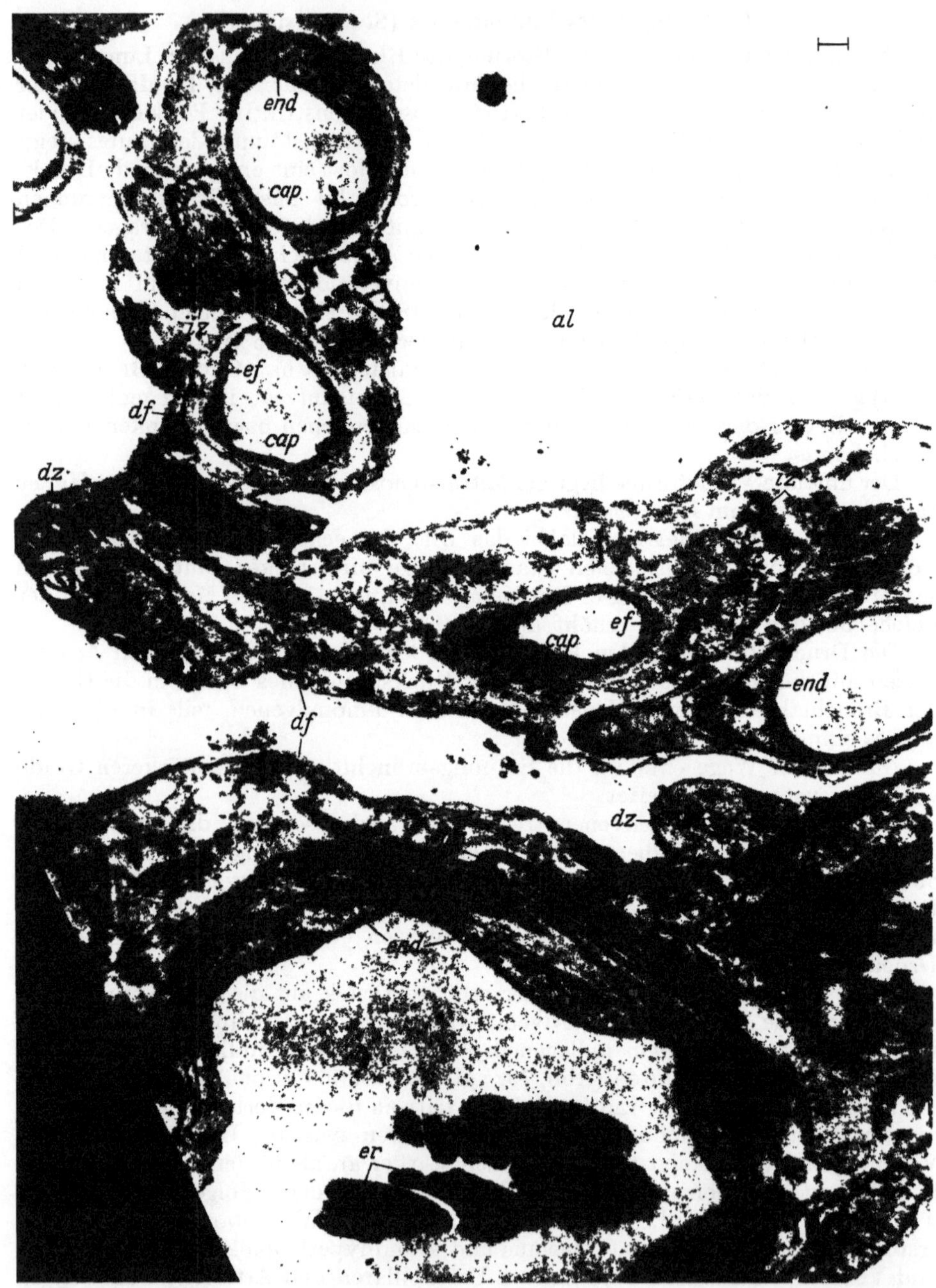

Abb. 79. Alveolarwand bei chronischer Stauung im kleinen Kreislauf. Posthypertonische Umbildung der Endstrombahn. Weit auseinandergedrängte, enggestellte Capillaren mit abgerundetem Querschnitt. Verdickung der endothelialen Wandschicht. Verbreiterung der alveolo-capillären Membran durch ausgedehnte pericapilläre Spalträume, in die reticuläre und besonders reichlich elastische Fasern eingelagert sind. Zahlreiche interstitielle Zellen, die z. T. die Capillaren pericytenähnlich umgreifen (→). Im unteren Bildteil eine Stromcapillare, die von glatten Muskelzellen umgeben ist. Bei (×) interstitielles Ödem. *al* Alveolarraum, *cap* Capillarlichtung, *dz* Alveolardeckzelle, *df* flächenhaft ausgebreitete periphere Cytoplasmazone einer Alveolardeckzelle, *end* Endothelzelle, *ef* flächenhaft ausgebreitete periphere Cytoplasmazone einer Endothelzelle, *iz* interstitielle Zelle, *mz* glatte Muskelzelle, *er* Erythrocyt, *el* elastische Fasern, *rf* reticuläre Fasern. Vergr. 4000×. Patient H. Dr., 29 Jahre. Druckwerte: Pc: 42/33 mm Hg, Art. pulm.: 88/40 mm Hg; re. Ventr.: 92 mm Hg; li. Vorh.: 20 mm Hg.

Nach Thurchetti u. Schirosa (1952) durchlaufen die Gefäßveränderungen ein funktionelles und ein organisches Stadium. Im funktionellen Stadium sind die anatomischen Veränderungen nur gering, die Herzhypertrophie bleibt mäßig. Im organischen Stadium wird die Herzhypertrophie deutlich.

In zahlreichen vergleichenden morphologischen Untersuchungen, die sowohl bei Sektionen[1] als auch an Lungenexcisionen bei Operationen von Herzfehlern durchgeführt wurden[2], ist sichergestellt, daß eine enge Abhängigkeit zwischen den histologischen Veränderungen an den kleinen Lungenarterien und dem Grad der pulmonalen Hypertonie besteht. Die Gefäßveränderungen beginnen mit muskulärer Mediahypertrophie, Verdickung der elastischen Lamellen und fibröser Umwandlung der Adventitia. Dann schließen sich an Muskelschwund und Narbenbildungen der Media, Auflösung der elastischen Lamellen und Intimaproliferation mit starker Einengung der Gefäßlichtung. Die großen Lungenarterien sind stets erweitert und zeigen deutliche Arteriosklerose[3].

Ursache und Bedeutung der Pulmonalsklerose bei venöser Rückstauung in der Lunge sind noch umstritten.

Die kausale Verknüpfung von pulmonaler Venenstauung und Pulmonalsklerose scheint ausreichend bewiesen zu sein, zumal gleichartige Gefäßveränderungen auch ohne rheumatischen Klappenfehler bei Myxom des Herzens[4] und sogar als örtlich beschränkte regionale Pulmonalarteriensklerose bei Tumorkompression pulmonaler Venen gefunden worden sind[5].

Klinische Untersuchungen zeigen, daß der Druck in den Pulmonalarterien nach operativer Sprengung einer Mitralstenose gleichzeitig und proportional zur Senkung des Vorhofdruckes

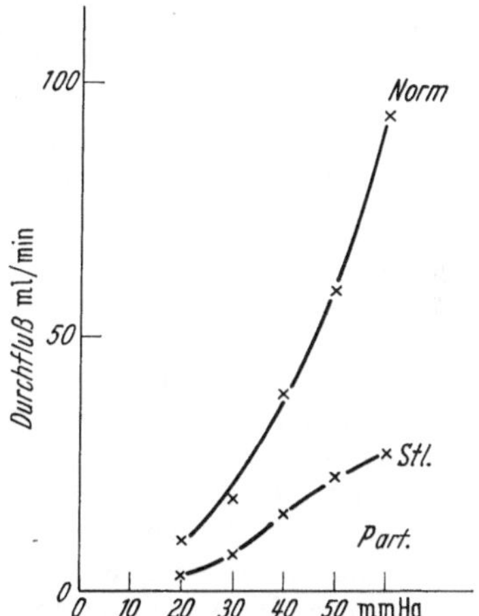

Abb. 80. Verminderte Durchströmbarkeit der Stauungslunge (*StL*) nach Leichenlungenmessungen.

abnimmt, und daß sich auch die Sklerose der kleinen Arterien zurückbildet (Könn 1956, Wade u. Mitarb. 1954 berichten über entgegengesetzte Beobachtungen).

Ungeklärt ist aber, auf welchem Wege die Engstellung kleiner Arterien bei Blutrückstauung ausgelöst wird. Eine reflektorische Arteriolenkonstriktion ist bei Mitralstenose noch nicht nachgewiesen, sie wird von Grosse-Brockhoff (1957) abgelehnt. Ohne diese Annahme wird man aber schwer die Einstellung auf das höhere Druckniveau in den leichten Formen der Mitralstenose erklären können.

Folgen der Stenosen in den kleinen Arterien sind die fortschreitende Erhöhung des Strömungswiderstandes bis zu Werten, die höher liegen als im großen Kreislauf. Dadurch kommt es zu einer starken Reduktion des Kreislaufminutenvolumens, das bis auf die Hälfte der Norm absinken kann. Der Arteriolenwiderstand bremst das Minutenvolumen ab[6].

Durchströmungsversuche an der Leichenlunge zeigen[7] in guter Übereinstimmung mit den vorliegenden klinischen Meßwerten, daß bei chronischen Stauungslungen das Durchflußvolumen der Lunge bis auf weniger als die Hälfte des normalen Volumens reduziert ist (Abb. 80). Sie bestätigen die von Grosse-

---

[1] Henry 1952, Soulié und Mitarbeiter 1954, Heath und Whitaker 1955.
[2] Bayer, Grosse-Brockhoff, Loogen und Meessen 1957, Enticknap 1953.
[3] Literatur bei Könn 1958.   [4] Könn 1956.   [5] Edwards und Burchell 1951.
[6] Lewis und Mitarbeiter 1952, Dexter und Mitarbeiter 1950.
[7] Hartung und Delfmann 1960.

Brockhoff (1957), Bayer u. Mitarb. (1957) mit Nachdruck vertretene Ansicht, daß bei der Mitralstenose in den vorgeschrittenen Stadien organische Gefäßveränderungen der entscheidende Faktor für die Fortentwicklung der pulmonalen Hypertonie sind. Die Gefäßveränderungen setzen nach den Untersuchungen an der Leichenlunge die Grenze für das noch erreichbare Strömungsvolumen, das durch die Kraft des hypertrophierten Herzens in Bewegung gesetzt werden kann. Der Zustand der Capillaren und der erhöhte Capillardruck spielen dabei nur eine untergeordnete Rolle.

Die Verminderung des Kreislaufvolumens setzt die Transportkapazität des Blutes für O_2 herab und ist neben der Pneumonose wesentlicher Faktor für die respiratorische Insuffizienz bei Lungenstauung.

5. Verminderter Blutzufluß.

α) Pulmonalstenose.

Ein zu kleines Blutvolumen erhält die Lunge bei den angeborenen Herzfehlern der Fallot-Gruppe, in deren Mittelpunkt die Pulmonalstenose steht.

In den Lungenarterien wird wegen der herznahen Stenose ein kleines Minutenvolumen unter niedrigem Druck bewegt. Die arteriovenöse Blutdruckdifferenz ist klein, das Blut nimmt in den Capillaren ausreichend Sauerstoff auf. In der Peripherie wird der Sauerstoff des kleinen Blutvolumens stark ausgeschöpft, es entsteht Hypoxie im Gewebe, die eine Hyperventilation veranlaßt. Die Kohlensäurespannung des Blutes wird dadurch erniedrigt. Das zu kleine Minutenvolumen, das wegen der Pulmonalstenose in der Arbeit nicht gesteigert werden kann, ist Ursache der respiratorischen Insuffizienz.

Bei der Fallotschen Tetralogie umgeht ein wechselnd großer Anteil des zirkulierenden Blutes im Rechts-Links-Shunt die Lunge und erscheint ungesättigt als venöse Beimischung im großen Kreislauf[1].

Die Cyanose als Kardinalsymptom dieser Herzfehler beruht auf dem zu kleinen Blutvolumen, das die Lunge durchströmt, und auf der venösen Beimischung durch intrakardialen Rechts-Links-Shunt.

β) Pulmonalsklerose.

Durch zahlreiche Prozesse in der Lunge oder in ihren Gefäßen wird die Strombahn des kleinen Kreislaufs so stark eingeengt, daß der Zustrom zu den Capillaren örtlich oder allgemein abnimmt (Abb. 81).

Bei der diffusen Pulmonalsklerose liegt der Widerstand in den Arteriolen und kleinen Arterien. Die Druckerhöhung vor dem Widerstand wirkt sich nicht auf die Capillarstrecke aus, die Gasdiffusion bleibt ungestört, doch bewirkt nach McIlroy u. Apthorp (1958) die Restriktion des Blutdurchflusses eine Belastungsdyspnoe.

Bei den herdförmigen, mehr oder weniger generalisierten entzündlichen Gefäßerkrankungen der Lunge, wie z.B. der Panarteriitis nodosa und der Endarteriitis obliterans, wird das Strömungsvolumen auf die freien Gefäßabschnitte verlagert. Es entwickelt sich mit großer Regelmäßigkeit eine pulmonale Hypertonie, die aus der Einengung des Strombettes hinreichend erklärt ist. Die Sauerstoffaufnahme ist nicht erschwert, da dem verminderten Strömungsvolumen ein weites unverändertes Capillarbett zu Verfügung steht. Die von dem geringen Blutvolumen durchströmte Fläche kann aber so klein werden, daß Cyanose entsteht. Die Strömung ist bei der hohen arteriovenösen Druckdifferenz beschleunigt.

---

[1] Bing 1949, Grob und Rossi 1949, Abbot 1936, Grosse-Brockhoff 1951, Bayer, Loogen und Wolter 1954.

Die Begrenzung des Durchflußvolumens durch das verengte Gefäßsystem der Lunge ist auch am isolierten Organ festzustellen (Versuchsanordnung s. S. 584) und zur Höhe des Druckes in Beziehung zu setzen.

Bei Lungenfibrosen und Pulmonalsklerosen mit vorbestehender pulmonaler Hypertension läßt sich der erhöhte Strömungswiderstand an der geringen Durchflußmenge und der wesentlich geringeren Wirkung einer Drucksteigerung erkennen. Das ist auch bei einem erhöhten arteriellen Druckniveau, das etwa den anzunehmenden Arbeitsdrucken in diesen Fällen entspricht, deutlich. Die Durchflußmenge ist in Fällen von Lungenfibrose mit Cor pulmonale ähnlich wie bei chronischen Stauungslungen kaum halb so groß wie in den Normalfällen.

Bei Pulmonalarteriensklerose sind die arteriellen Drucke auf ein erhöhtes, anscheinend den vorbestehenden höheren Arbeitsdrucken entsprechendes Niveau verschoben. Die Durchströmung bleibt unter normalen arteriellen Einfülldrucken auch bei optimaler Dehnungslage gering.

Bei Pulmonalsklerose, bei multiplen Embolien und bei diffusen Lungenfibrosen wird die Kontaktzeit zu kurz, wenn die capillare Strombahn und damit die Capillaroberfläche erheblich eingeschränkt ist. In den noch durchgängigen oder durchströmten Capillaren ist der Blutstrom stark beschleunigt. Die Kontaktzeit verhält sich umgekehrt proportional zur Strömungsgeschwindigkeit. In diesen Fällen reicht die Kontaktzeit nicht mehr für eine genügende O_2-Aufnahme aus, das Blut verläßt unvollständig gesättigt die Lunge.

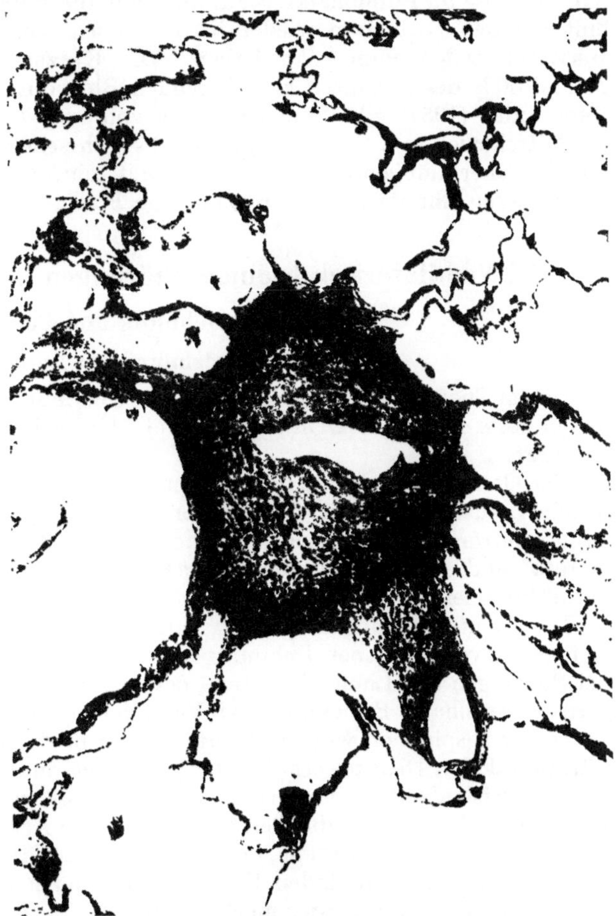

Abb. 81. Anthrako-silikotisches Knötchen mit komprimierter Lobulararterie im Zentrum. Emphysem der Nachbarschaft. S.-Nr. 626/58. Vergr. 20fach.

Der alveoloarterielle O_2-Gradient ist stark vergrößert und beträgt in der Ruhe oft mehr als 30 mm Hg statt 5—7 mm Hg in der Norm[1]. Bei der Arbeit fällt die O_2-Sättigung weiter ab, der alveoloarterielle O_2-Gradient wird größer. Die Kohlensäureabgabe ist in diesen Zuständen wegen der gleichzeitigen Hyper-

---

ROSSIER und Mitarbeiter 1956.

ventilation so stark erhöht, daß alveoläre und arterielle CO_2-Spannung erheblich absinken[1].

Lungenembolien sind eine häufige Ursache für die Entwicklung eines akuten Cor pulmonale[2].

6. Kurzschlußkreislauf (Fehlzirkulation).

Arteriovenöse Fisteln oder Aneurysmen entstehen aus Fehlbildungen der Lungengefäße, oft in Verbindung mit einem Morbus Osler[3]. Sie stellen echte Kurzschlüsse im Pulmonalkreislauf dar, in deren Bereich das zufließende Lungenblut vor den Capillaren wieder in die Venen eingeleitet wird, ohne am Gasaustausch teilgenommen zu haben. Die Kurzschlußmengen liegen zwischen 20 und 60% des gesamten zirkulierenden Blutvolumens der Lungen[4]. Grosse-Brockhoff (1957) gibt Shuntvolumina von 1,9—7,9 Liter/min an. Dabei kann der Mitteldruck in der Arteria pulmonalis wahrscheinlich durch gehäufte Thrombosen kleiner Lungenarterien leicht erhöht sein. Cyanose und Polyglobulie sind bei größeren Shuntvolumina regelmäßige Folge.

II. Ventilatorisch bedingte Störungen der Lungenperfusion.

a) Lungendehnung und Perfusion.

1. Zugdehnung der Lunge.

Die im Thoraxraum ausgespannte Lunge befindet sich unter normalen Verhältnissen stets in einem Dehnungszustand, der sich auch auf die Lungengefäße auswirkt.

Der Gefäßbaum, der anatomisch präparatorisch[5] oder mit Ausgußmethoden[6] in seiner Ausdehnung und Architektonik nur schwer vollkommen darstellbar ist, kann mit röntgenographischen Methoden verhältnismäßig leicht an der Leiche in toto[7] und an der isolierten Lunge[8] oder am Lebenden mit Hilfe des Herzkatheters selektiv[9] sichtbar gemacht werden.

Diese Untersuchungen geben wichtigen Aufschluß über Form und Weite der Gefäße bei verschiedenen Dehnungslagen der Lunge. Sie zeigen weiter, daß auch bei Störungen der Lungenbelüftung oder pathologischen Prozessen des Lungengerüstes regelhafte Beziehungen zu Veränderungen des Gefäßsystems bestehen[10].

In der Inspiration wird der Bluteinstrom in die Lunge mit der Senkung des intrathorakalen Druckes erhöht, die Blutmenge in der Lunge vergrößert und die Lungenkreislaufzeit verlängert[11]. Die Blutcapillaren erweitern sich in der Inspiration[12], ebenso auch die kleinen Arterien und Arteriolen[13]. In der Exspiration kehren sich die Verhältnisse um. Die während der Atembewegung im Brust- und Bauchraum wechselnden Drucke wirken nach Knebel u. Wick (1959) wie ein Druck- und Saugpumpenmechanismus.

Die respiratorisch bedingten Schwankungen des Blutdruckes im kleinen Kreislauf sind nur gering, Rodbard und Mitarbeiter (1956) nennen als obere Grenze 3 mm Hg.

---

[1] Rossier und Mitarbeiter 1956.
[2] Knebel 1956 u. a., Schoenmackers 1958 (Literatur), Ch. Büchner und Könn 1959.
[3] Kucsko 1957.
[4] Maier und Mitarbeiter 1948, Friedlich und Mitarbeiter 1950, Grosse-Brockhoff und Mitarbeiter 1954 u. a.
[5] v. Hayek 1957 (Literatur).   [6] Küttner 1878, Töndury 1956.
[7] Schoenmackers und Vieten 1954.   [8] Miyata 1939, Junghanss 1958.
[9] Bolt, Forssmann und Rink 1957, Semisch und Mitarbeiter 1958.
[10] Schoenmackers und Vieten 1954, Löhr 1956 u. a.   [11] Blumenthal 1954.
[12] Altmann 1954.   [13] Condorelli 1950, Merkel 1949.

Nach direkter Lungenbeobachtung soll in der Inspiration eine Verengung der Capillaren eintreten.[1]

Über die Durchstömungsverhältnisse in der Lunge während der rhythmischen Schwankungen der Dehnungslage in der Inspiration und Exspiration mit den geringen wechselnd negativen und positiven Alveolardrucken wird noch diskutiert. Ebenso ist auch der Mechanismus der Erweiterung des Gefäßbettes und der Ort der Gefäßdrosselung im Kollaps bzw. bei Überdehnung der Lunge noch nicht ausreichend geklärt[2].

Die Meinungsverschiedenheiten erklären sich wenigstens teilweise daraus, daß Lungendehnung durch Zug oder durch Druck in ihrem gegensätzlichen Verhalten nicht genügend beachtet worden sind. In diesem Abschnitt sollen zunächst nur die Strömungsverhältnisse in der unter negativem Pleuradruck stehenden oder in der durch Zug im Unterdruck entfalteten isolierten Lunge besprochen werden.

TENDELOO (1910), VON HAYEK (1953), ALTMANN (1954) u. a. nehmen eine passive Weitstellung durch den an den Gefäßwänden angreifenden elastischen Lungenzug besonders für die kleinen Lungenarterien und Arteriolen an. TENDELOO hat versucht, diese Verhältnisse an in Kautschukblöcken eingeschlossenen elastischen Röhren modellmäßig zu klären. Er kam dabei zu dem Ergebnis, daß die Durchmesservergrößerung durch seitlichen Zug die mit der Längsdehnung verbundene Lichtungseinengung zunächst überwiegt, zumal in den ersten Stadien der Dehnung die Streckung der Gefäße durch Ausgleich der im Kollaps deutlichen Schlängelung erfolgt. CLOETTA (1911 und 1913) hat einen ähnlichen Mechanismus zur Deutung seiner Befunde herangezogen. Man wird aber auch ebenso wie bei den Bronchiolen mit einer öffnenden Wirkung der elastischen und muskulösen Spannungssysteme auf die Terminalarterien im Acinusstiel rechnen müssen[3].

PIIPER (1957) spricht im Zusammenhang mit der Beobachtung, daß die Entfaltung des Lungengewebes offenbar auch mit einer Entfaltung des Gefäßsystems verbunden ist, von einem Formfaktor, den er nicht näher untersucht hat.

Aus eigenen Durchströmungsversuchen[4] an Leichenlungen, die im Unterdruck nach dem Volumenkomplementverfahren stufenweise gedehnt wurden, hat sich gezeigt, daß Änderungen der Dehnungslage einen weit größeren Einfluß auf die Perfusion haben als Steigerungen des arteriellen Einfülldruckes.

In diesen Versuchen wurde der arterielle Druck zwischen 20—30 mm Hg konstant gehalten. Der Dehnungseffekt trat am stärksten beim Übergang von der Kollapslage in einen der Exspirationslage entsprechenden Dehnungszustand auf. Die anfangs geringe Durchflußmenge steigt in dieser Phase sprunghaft auf das 8—12fache des Ausgangszustandes an. Bei weiterer Expansion in den Grenzen der Vitalkapazität erfährt sie bis zu einer der Inspirationslage entsprechenden Dehnung nur noch eine relativ geringe Zunahme bis auf das 10—15-fache des Ausgangswertes (s. Abb. 78, S. 585).

In den ausgewählten Fällen bewirkte die Dehnung vom Kollapszustand bis zur Exspirationslage eine Durchströmungssteigerung von 958%, die weitere Dehnung bis in die Atemmittellage eine erneute Zunahme von 358% des Ausgangswertes. Bei in einzelnen Versuchen weiter getriebener Dehnung wurde eine Umkehr zu niedrigeren Durchflußmengen beobachtet.

Dieser experimentelle Hinweis auf ein Dehnungsoptimum für die Perfusion der Lunge entspricht ähnlichen Beobachtungen im Tierversuch[5], bei denen die größten Durchflußmengen bei einer der Atemmittellage entsprechenden Dehnung gefunden wurden. LOCHNER (1957) fand, daß der Strömungswiderstand in der isolierten Hundelunge bei einem Unterdruck von —7 cm H_2O am geringsten ist.

---

[1] LING 1955, IRWIN und Mitarbeiter 1954, GARCIA RAMOS 1955.
[2] Zusammenfassende Literatur bei ALTMANN 1954.   [3] v. GEHLEN 1940.
[4] HARTUNG und DELFMANN 1960.   [5] CLOETTA 1911, 1913, PIIPER 1957, LOCHNER 1957.

2. Perfusion in Atelektasen.

Die Frage, ob und in welchem Ausmaß Änderungen der Lungenperfusion bei Störungen der Lungenbelüftung auf den Entfaltungszustand der Lunge zurückzuführen sind, läßt sich an den Atelektasen und am Emphysem überprüfen.

Wir unterscheiden eine rote und eine blasse Atelektase (s. S. 497).

In der roten Atelektase ist das luftarme oder luftleere Lungengewebe noch von Blut durchströmt. Der Blutreichtum des feuchten milzähnlichen Lungengewebes beruht auf einer Weitstellung der Lungencapillaren und ist einer akuten Lungenstauung vergleichbar. Die Alveolen sind bei diesen oft unvollständigen und langsam in Tagen entstehenden Atelektasen mit Transsudat gefüllt[1].

Die nachfolgende blasse Atelektase ist grau bis grauschwarz, wenig feucht, oft sogar trocken und zäh. Die Alveolen sind völlig kollabiert, die Alveolarepithelien oft kubisch umgewandelt. Die Netzcapillaren sind fast blutleer.

Das Gefäßbild ist weitgehend abhängig von der Ursache der Atelektase[2].

Bei der Resorptionsatelektase nach Bronchusverschluß werden die Gefäße durch Retraktion des atelektatischen Lungenbezirkes auf den Hilus verkürzt. Sie verlaufen geschlängelt und haben kleine Verzweigungswinkel. Die gewöhnlich rechtwinklig abgehenden Lobular- und Terminalarterien legen sich ihren Stammgefäßen an[3]. Bleibt die Atelektase durch Pleuraverwachsungen gespannt, so rücken die Gefäße zusammen und verlaufen gestreckt. In Kompressionsatelektasen werden die Gefäße gestaucht oder verlagert (s. Abb. 31, S. 466).

In der akuten Atelektase ist der Blutdurchfluß zunächst kaum verringert, es kommt zu einem funktionellen Kurzschluß, d. h. das Blut wird nicht arterialisiert und erscheint als venöse Beimischung im großen Kreislauf[4].

Die kleinen, experimentell durch Pleurareizung erzeugten und durch ein Thoraxfenster beobachteten Atelektasen sind blaurot[5]. Diese Verfärbung ist Ausdruck der noch anhaltenden Blutströmung im Atelektasebereich. Mit der in 10—15 min eintretenden Lösung der Atelektase und Wiederbelüftung der Alveolen verschwindet die blaurote Verfärbung. Bronchokonstriktion kann als wahrscheinliche Ursache dieser Atelektase angesehen werden, Vasodilatation ist ihre unmittelbare Folge.

Nach Unterbindung eines Hauptbronchus beim Hund[6] nimmt die Sauerstoffsättigung sofort um 30% ab. Der Ausfall der einen Lunge wird durch Hyperventilation und vermehrte Perfusion der anderen Lunge kompensiert. Die Durchblutung der freien Lunge steigt sofort um 55% an und liegt in der folgenden Zeit zwischen 50 und 90%. Die Perfusion der Lunge mit unterbundenem Bronchus ist um 20—30% reduziert.

Diese Folgeerscheinungen sind oft schon nach einem Tag, gewöhnlich nach 48 Std, spätestens nach mehreren Tagen verschwunden.

Auch beim Menschen ist nach klinischen Untersuchungen[7] der Blutdurchfluß zunächst kaum vermindert. Es entsteht deshalb eine arterielle Hypoxämie. Im Verlauf einiger Tage erfolgt die Umstellung auf eine Minderdurchblutung der Atelektase.

Bei langsam eintretendem chronischem Bronchusverschluß verlaufen die regulatorischen Kreislaufveränderungen unmerklich.

Die Untersuchungen von Gilroy u. Mitarb. (1951) sprechen dafür, daß die atelektatische Lunge vermehrt von den Bronchialarterien her über arterioarterielle Anastomosen durchblutet wird. In chronischen Atelektasen kommt es zu einer Erweiterung der Bronchialarterien[8]. Dieser vermehrte Zustrom von

---

[1] Spain 1954.   [2] Schoenmackers und Vieten 1958.   [3] Junghanss 1959.
[4] Barcroft 1928, Rossier und Mitarbeiter 1956, Löffler 1956.
[5] Reinhardt 1934, Heuck und Flach 1953, Heuck 1959, Heine 1960.
[6] Andrus 1925.   [7] Gilroy, Wilson und Marchand 1951.
[8] Marchand und Mitarbeiter 1950, Delarue 1954.

Aortenblut, der auch auf dem Wege anderweitiger Kollateralen, z.B. über Pleura-verwachsungen erfolgen kann, erhöht den O_2-Gehalt des Blutes in den Lungen-arterien. In postmortalen Angiogrammen haben sich solche Anastomosen nicht feststellen lassen[1], ebenso nicht in klinischen Angiographien[2].

Die Lungenperfusion kehrt auch in alten Atelektasen in der Regel zur Norm zurück, wenn eine Wiederbelüftung eintritt. Sie bleibt aber irreversibel gestört, wenn die Entfaltung der Lunge durch Fibrose des Lungengerüstes, Pleura-schwarten, Verwachsungen oder andere Ursachen unmöglich wird, oder wenn die Gefäßlichtung durch organische Veränderungen stenosiert ist.

Die Mechanismen, die zur Reduktion der Perfusion in Lungenatelektasen führen, sind noch nicht ausreichend geklärt.

Aus den Durchströmungsversuchen an der Leichenlunge geht eindeutig hervor, daß in einer Lunge, deren Dehnungszustand aus der Atemmittellage heraus stufenweise verringert wird, die Durchflußmenge bei normalen Drucken rasch abnimmt und in der Kollapslage fast versiegt.

Die bei progressiver Lungendehnung aus der Kollapslage erreichte 10—15fache Steigerung des Durchflußvolumens wird bei Absinken der Dehnungslage wieder reduziert.

Damit ist sichergestellt, daß der erhöhte Strömungswiderstand in der Kollaps- und Atelektaselunge zu einem wesentlichen Teil rein mechanisch erklärbar ist und auf dem Wegfall der Zugspannung und der Verkürzung der Lungengefäße beruht. Der verminderte Widerstand kann durch erhöhten Blutdruck teilweise über-wunden werden.

Die Hauptwiderstandszone für die Perfusion scheint im Bereich der Terminal-arterien und Arteriolen zu liegen. Bei Angiographie an Resektionspräparaten oder an Leichenlungen füllt sich die Endstrombahn der Atelektasezone nur unvollständig und erst nach Anwendung eines erhöhten Injektionsdruckes auf. Gefäßabbrüche sind im Bereich der Terminalarterien häufig zu sehen. Das Kaliber der Lobulararterien ist bei einem Injektionsdruck von 25—40 mm Hg von 0,4—0,8 auf 0,6—1,2 mm erweitert, die Lichtung der Terminalarterien beträgt 0,1—0,5 mm. Die Netz- und Stromcapillaren haben mittlere Weiten von 7—8 μ bzw. 15 μ und sind deutlich enger als in der Norm[3].

Am Lebenden wurde mit der selektiven Angiographie ein auffällig verlang-samter Kontrastmitteldurchfluß und ein verspäteter Abfluß in die Pulmonal-venen festgestellt[4]. Diese Ergebnisse stimmen mit den Befunden am post-mortalen Angiogramm überein. Der venöse Rückfluß ist auch dort erschwert und erfolgt verspätet[5].

Wieweit über die mechanisch bedingte Vermehrung des Strömungswider-standes und über die Verzögerung des Durchflusses hinaus regulative Vorgänge auf neuralem Wege durch Reizung der Vasoconstrictoren oder vom Alveolarraum her durch Hypoventilation oder durch Einstrom ungesättigten Arterienblutes in den venösen Schenkel der Endstrombahn einwirken, läßt sich einstweilen noch nicht sagen. Daß solche Einwirkungen stattfinden, ist trotz der bisher noch widerspruchsvollen Versuchsergebnisse sehr wahrscheinlich und in den Atelek-taseversuchen unter dem Pleurafenster direkt zu beobachten[6].

Bei sehr lange bestehenden Atelektasen findet sich an den kleinen und oft auch an den mittleren Arterien eine deutliche Intimaproliferation, die fast bis

---

[1] JUNGHANSS 1959, ARMSTRONG und CUDKOWICZ 1958.
[2] SEMISCH und Mitarbeiter 1958, BOLT und Mitarbeiter 1957, LÖHR und Mitarbeiter 1957.
[3] JUNGHANSS 1959.
[4] BOLT, FORSSMANN und RINK 1957, LÖHR und Mitarbeiter 1957, SEMISCH und Mitarbeiter 1958.
[5] JUNGHANSS 1959. [6] REINHARDT 1934, HEUCK und FLACH 1953.

zur Obliteration gehen kann. Das histologische Bild stimmt teilweise mit den Pulmonalsklerosen aus anderen Ursachen überein, und man darf wohl annehmen, daß die Intimaproliferation aus der Phase der funktionellen Vasoconstriction hervorgeht (Abb. 82).

In vielen, besonders in kleinen Atelektasen wird die Blutzirkulation durch diese Vorgänge so stark gedrosselt, daß abgesehen von der Frühphase der akuten Atelektase keine nennenswerte venöse Beimischung eintritt. In manchen Fällen bildet sich ein erheblicher funktioneller Kurzschluß dadurch heraus, daß die Perfusion des atelektatischen Gebietes anhält. Die venöse Beimischung kann so erheblich werden, daß eine operative Entfernung der Atelektase notwendig wird.

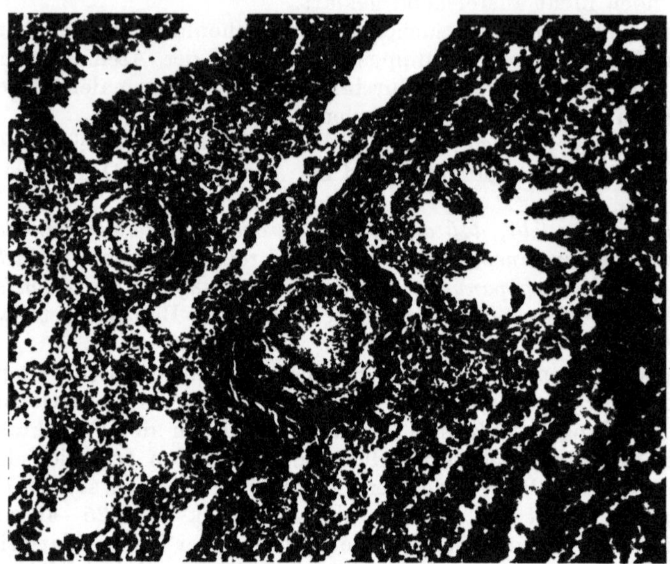

Abb. 82. Hochgradige Intimaproliferation in kleinen Lungenarterien bei chronischer Atelektase unter 24 Jahre liegender Ölplombe. E.-Nr. 6233/56.

Die Atelektase hat in allen Stadien erhebliche Rückwirkungen auf die Lungenperfusion. Die Drosselung der Perfusion in der Atelektase beruht teils auf regulativen Vorgängen, teils auf mechanischer Erschwerung des Durchflusses durch die gestauchten und verkürzten Lungengefäße. Das Hauptgewicht liegt nach den Untersuchungen an der Leichenlunge auf der mechanischen Erschwerung des Blutdurchflusses durch die Atelektasezone.

Bei den Narbenlungen stehen die mechanischen Durchflußstörungen ganz im Vordergrund. Die Entwicklung eines chronischen Cor pulmonale ist dabei ein häufiger Befund[1].

3. Lungenperfusion bei Emphysem.

α) Capillarreduktion.

Im Emphysem erreicht die Lunge die stärkste Entfaltung und damit auch die größte Dehnung des Lungengerüstes und die größte Streckung der Lungengefäße.

Für die Klärung der Beziehungen zwischen Emphysem und Perfusion wird zunächst das genuine konstitutionelle diffuse Emphysem herangezogen, das uns

---

[1] Gerstel 1933, Berblinger 1947, Zorn 1951, Husten 1951, Cicero und Celis 1955, Curti und Mitarbeiter 1955, Gadermann 1957, Esch und Grosse-Brockhoff 1958 (Literatur).

in der reinen Form des Altersemphysems am häufigsten begegnet. Ausgeschlossen werden zunächst die sekundären Emphyseme mit bronchostenotischen Effekten, die unter die Perfusionsstörungen bei positivem intraalveolären Druck fallen und im nächsten Abschnitt besprochen werden.

Das senile diffuse Emphysem ist gekennzeichnet durch Dehnung, Atrophie und Anämie (Morphologie s. S. 427 und S. 551). Im Emphysem kommt es zum Umbau und zu irreversibler Erweiterung der Alveolen tragenden Lufträume. Dabei geht die Alveolarstruktur verloren, die intraacinösen Septen werden

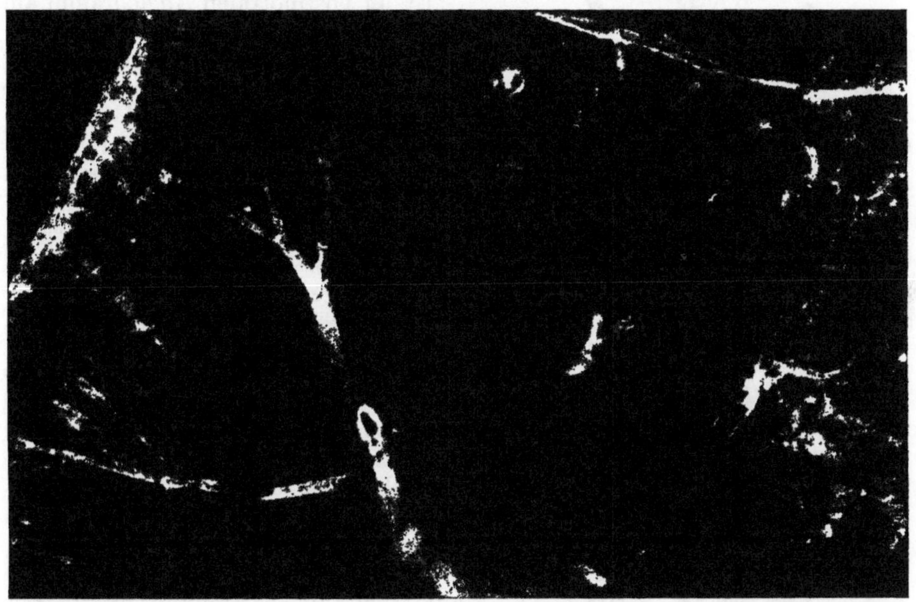

Abb. 83. Hochgradige Atrophie des Lungengewebes bei schwerem senilem Emphysem. Deutliches Hervortreten des Gefäßnetzes bei völligem Schwund der Alveolarstruktur und Ausbau der intraacinösen Septen. Gefäßbild von 2 Acini mit den Aufzweigungen der zentral liegenden Arterie. S.-Nr. 93/59. 78jähriger Mann. Vergr. 10:1.

gefenstert und so weit abgebaut, daß schließlich in den Acini nur noch ein zartes Gitterwerk aus Blutgefäßen übrigbleibt (Abb. 83).

Mit dem Schwund der septalen Gliederung im Acinus ist ein erheblicher Verlust an Austauschfläche verbunden (s. S. 553), in der das dichte Netzwerk der Atemcapillaren liegt[1].

Der Abbau der Alveolarwände geht in der Weise vor sich, daß die Netzcapillaren in der gedehnten Alveolarwand auseinander rücken[2]. Dabei wird die deckende Alveolarzellschicht in eine Porenmembran umgewandelt.

Mit weiterer Dehnung schwinden die 6—11 μ weiten Netzcapillaren, die an die größeren 20—40 μ weiten Stromcapillaren angeschlossen sind. Bei schwerem Emphysem werden auch die Stromcapillaren abgebaut, so daß schließlich nur noch einzelne Gefäße vom Kaliber der Arteriolen und Venolen übrigbleiben. In großen Blasen gehen auch diese Gefäße verloren.

Im Abbau des Gefäßsystems können wir also 3 Stufen unterscheiden:

1. Dehnung und Abbau des Capillarnetzes (Netzcapillaren) der Alveolarwand.
2. Abbau des großmaschigen Stromcapillarnetzes in den intraacinösen Septen.
3. Schwund der gesamten Endstrombahn im großblasigen Emphysem.

---

[1] GIESE 1959. [2] ISAAKSOHN 1871, LOESCHCKE 1928, FUEST und HAAS 1958.

Das hochdifferenzierte Gefäßsystem der Endstrombahn in der Lunge wird im Laufe dieses Umbaues vereinfacht. Mit dem Schwund der Netzcapillaren wird die gesamte terminale Strombahn in ihrer Fläche eingeschränkt und der Blutweg verkürzt. Die am Ende der ersten Abbauphase übrigbleibenden Capillaren sind wesentlich weiter als in der Norm[1]. Sie entsprechen weitgestellten Stromcapillaren (Abb. 84).

Das Gefäßbild beim Emphysem ist im postmortalen Angiogramm am besten darstellbar[2]. Die großen Gefäße erscheinen entsprechend der Lungenvergrößerung verlängert, die Gefäßwinkel und die Gefäßlichtung verkleinert. Das Gefäßbild ist zunächst noch in allen Lungenteilen gleichmäßig, wird aber mit zunehmender Blasenbildung unharmonisch[3]. Bei starkem Capillarschwund wird das angiographische Bild mit einem entlaubten Baum verglichen.

Bei der Angiographie der Endstrombahn[4] bleibt das Lungenfeld infolge des Capillarverlustes hell. Das Kontrastmittel läuft ohne nennenswerten Widerstand in die Arterie ein und tritt sehr rasch in die Venen über, eine dichte capilläre Füllungsphase bleibt aus (Abb. 85). Diese Beobachtung deckt sich mit den Befunden, die bei selektiver Angiographie von Emphysemkranken während des Lebens erhoben werden[5].

Die Bedeutung der Capillarreduktion für die Lungenperfusion und ihre Beziehung zum *Cor pulmonale* wird so unterschiedlich beurteilt, daß aus der Literatur z. Z. kein einheitliches Bild zu gewinnen ist. Der Grund für die differente Beurteilung ist darin zu suchen, daß die verschiedenen Formen des Emphysems in den vorliegenden Statistiken nicht ausreichend differenziert worden sind.

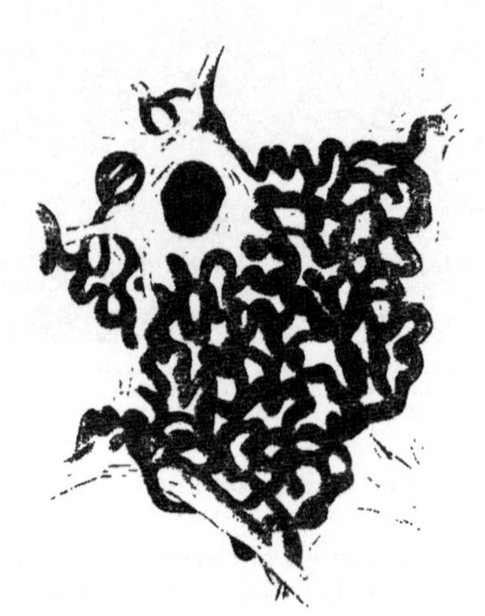

Abb. 84. Oben: Restliches Stromcapillarsystem (*a—c*) nach Schwund der Netzcapillaren beim Emphysem. Unten: Stark gefüllte Netzcapillaren einer normalen Alveolarwand. (Aus Isaaksohn 1871.)

Emphysem allein oder in Kombination mit anderweitigen Lungenerkrankungen ist nach Denolin (1955) die häufigste Ursache eines chronischen Cor pulmonale. Von 619 Obduktionsfällen mit Cor pulmonale war ein Emphysem allein dessen Ursache in 64,3% und als begleitende Komplikation bei anderweitigen Lungenerkrankungen in 87,8% mit beteiligt. Chronisches Emphysem führt nach Matthes, Ulmer und Wittekind (1960) in etwa einem Drittel aller Fälle zum Cor pulmonale, ähnliche Angaben finden sich bei Lin (1956). Giese (1956) gibt in Übereinstimmung

[1] Loeschcke 1921, 1928.   [2] Schoenmackers und Vieten 1958, Bedford 1951.
[3] Schoenmackers und Vieten 1958.   [4] Giese 1957, Junghanss 1959.
[5] Bolt 1955, Bolt und Rink 1951.

mit DELIUS (1955, 1956) 15% an, KERNEN u. Mitarb. (1958) finden es in 36% ihrer Emphysemfälle. Cor pulmonale wird um so häufiger gefunden, je mehr sekundäre Emphyseme mit Bronchostenose und je mehr Narbenemphyseme in die Statistik aufgenommen werden. Nach KIRCH (1955) ist kaum ein Drittel der Fälle von

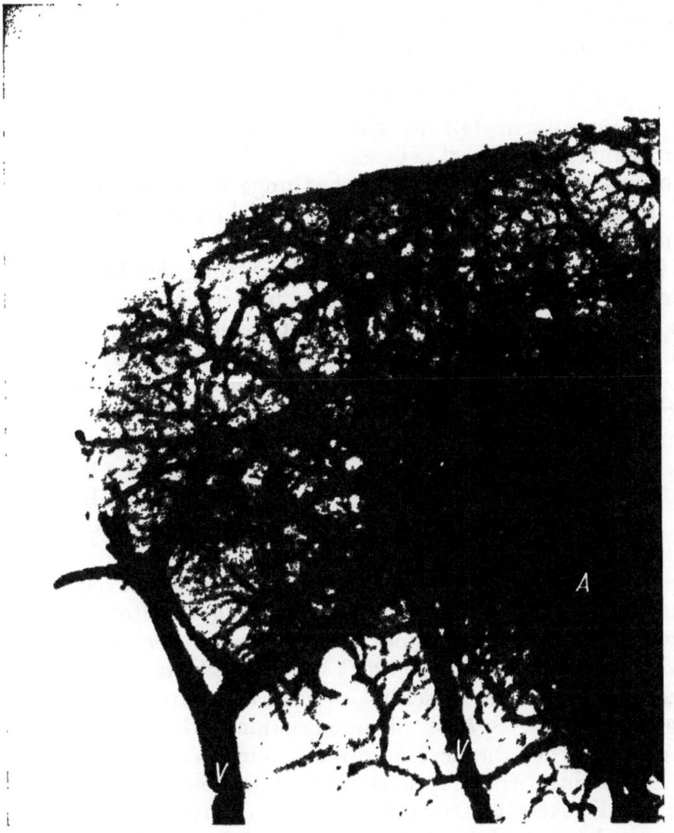

Abb. 85. Arteriogramm eines senilen atrophischen Emphysems (vgl. Abb. 74). Rascher venöser Rückfluß bei ausgedehntem Capillarverlust. *A* Arterie; *V* Vene. S.-Nr. 391/56.

Cor pulmonale Folge von Emphysem. Das ist bei der Häufigkeit schwerer Emphyseme im Obduktionsgut sehr bemerkenswert.

Der Capillarschwund hat eine erhebliche Einengung des Gefäßquerschnittes zur Folge. Daraus erklärt sich die sehr hohe Strömungsgeschwindigkeit mit verkürzter Kontaktzeit[1].

Eine grobe Schätzung des Capillarausfalles bei Emphysematikern ist aus der Diffusionskapazität möglich, da diese von der Größe der Gasaustauschfläche abhängt, die der Lungencapillaroberfläche entspricht.

Beim Gesunden beträgt die Diffusionskapazität für Sauerstoff (D_{O_2}) 20 ml je mm Hg Druckdifferenz. Bei Belastung wird eine beträchtliche Steigerung der Diffusionskapazität beobachtet, die nur durch Eröffnung von Reservecapillaren zustande kommen kann. Das Maximum liegt bei 1200 ml/min O_2-Aufnahme. Oberhalb dieses Sauerstoffverbrauches ist keine weitere Steigerung der Diffusionskapazität möglich[2].

---

[1] BLUMGART und WEISS 1927.   [2] RILEY, SHEPARD und Mitarbeiter 1954.

Donald, Renzetti u. Mitarb. (1952) fanden bei 7 Emphysematikern ohne Cor pulmonale eine Diffusionskapazität von 10,6 ml/mm Hg, bei 8 Emphysematikern mit Cor pulmonale von 6,1 ml/mm Hg. Danach war die Oberfläche der durchströmten Lungencapillaren auf 53% bzw. auf 30% des Normwertes herabgesetzt. Unter der Arbeit steigt die Diffusionskapazität normal auf das 2—3fache an, beim Emphysematiker ist dieser Anstieg nur sehr gering oder fehlt ganz, weil Reservecapillaren kaum zur Verfügung stehen.

β) Strömungswiderstand.

Es wird angenommen, daß der Strömungswiderstand bei Emphysem wegen der Capillarreduktion vermehrt sei.

In Perfusionsversuchen an der Leichenlunge liegen die Durchflußmengen in Fällen von diffusem Emphysem ohne Pulmonalsklerose auch bei niedrigem arteriellem Druck bereits in der Kollapslage relativ hoch. Bei stufenweiser Dehnung der Lunge ist dagegen nur eine geringere Steigerung der Durchflußmenge als in der normalen Lunge zu erreichen. Die Emphysemlunge befindet sich sozusagen in einer Dauerinspirationsstellung und gerät nach Entfernung aus dem Thorax zwar in einen Zustand der Entspannung, aber nicht in einen vollständigen Kollaps. Die Blutgefäße bleiben gestreckt. Diese Versuche zeigen, daß bei unkompliziertem diffusem atrophischem Emphysem der Strömungswiderstand in der Ruhe auch bei beträchtlichem Capillarschwund nicht vermehrt ist.

Die Erklärung dafür könnte im Bau der Endstrombahn liegen.

In dem Abschnitt über die Morphologie der Endstrombahn wurde bereits ausgeführt, daß 2 Auffassungen über die Einschaltung des Capillarsystems in die Lungenstrombahn bestehen:

Nach der einen, vorherrschend vertretenen Ansicht[1] ist das gesamte Capillarsystem endständig zwischen Arterie und Vene eingeschaltet, das Baumuster entspricht etwa der Capillaranordnung im Glomerulus der Niere.

Nach der eigenen Auffassung (1957) sind die engen Capillaren der Alveolarwand (Netzcapillaren) im Nebenschluß an das Stromcapillarnetz der intraacinösen Septen angehängt (vgl. S. 578). Hämodynamisch bedeutet der Schwund des Netzcapillarsystems bei dieser Anordnung keine Vermehrung des Strömungswiderstandes, da das Stromcapillarbett das Ruheminutenvolumen aufnehmen und auch ein in der Arbeit vermehrtes Volumen durch Strömungsbeschleunigung und Capillarerweiterung ohne Widerstandserhöhung fördern kann.

Das Herzminutenvolumen liegt an der Grenze der Norm. Eine generelle Vermehrung, die für das Emphysem angenommen wurde[2], konnte nicht bestätigt werden[3].

Die Höhe des Strömungswiderstandes in der Emphysemlunge kann also nicht allein von der Reduktion der Capillaren abhängen.

Damit stimmt überein, daß bei unkompliziertem atrophischem Emphysem in der Regel kein Cor pulmonale und auch keine Pulmonalsklerose gefunden werden.

Wenn dagegen bei schwerem, insbesondere bei großblasigem Emphysem auch das Stromcapillarnetz abgebaut wird, kann es zu einer so beträchtlichen Verkleinerung des Gefäßquerschnittes kommen, daß auch das Ruheminutenvolumen nur unter Druckerhöhung gefördert wird. Das scheint bei senilem atrophischem Emphysem nur in Ausnahmefällen vorzukommen. Es wird häufiger, wenn bronchostenotische Effekte (Komplikationsbronchitis, trapping s. S. 533) zum genuinen Emphysem hinzutreten.

---

[1] Literatur bei v. Hayek 1953.   [2] McMichael 1950, Harvey und Mitarbeiter 1951.
[3] Matthes, Ulmer und Wittekind 1960.

Ebenso kann auch eine Sklerose der Arterien nicht als Ursache eines Cor pulmonale bei atrophischem Emphysem herangezogen werden, da bei Emphysem mit und ohne Cor pulmonale eine nur unwesentliche Vermehrung organischer Gefäßveränderungen gefunden worden ist[1].

In welcher Beziehung die Bronchialarterien und ihre Anastomosen zu den Pulmonalarterien und zum Cor pulmonale bei Emphysem stehen, ist noch nicht geklärt. Die vermehrten arterioarteriellen Anastomosen, die CUDKOWICZ u. ARMSTRONG (1953) gefunden haben, beziehen sich nach einer neuen Arbeit im wesentlichen auf Fälle mit Bronchiektasen und chronischer Bronchitis[2], Zustände, bei denen Aortalisation in sehr ausgesprochenem Maße vorkommt[3].

b) Der Einfluß des intraalveolären Luftdruckes auf die Lungenperfusion.

1. Experimentelle Untersuchungen.

Im normalen Atemcyclus sind die Druckschwankungen im Alveolarraum bei freien Atemwegen nur gering. In der Inspiration ist der intraalveoläre Druck negativ, in der Exspiration positiv.

Die Druckschwankungen haben in der normalen Ruheatmung eine Amplitude von etwa 5 cm H_2O. Der normale Alveolardruck liegt bei einem Atemstromvolumen von 0,5 l/sec zwischen 0,5 und 2 cm H_2O.[4]

Aus früheren Untersuchungen von GERHARDT (1910) und ROMANOFF (1911) an isolierten und durchströmten Lungen hat sich bereits ergeben, daß die Zunahme des Druckes im Lungenluftraum die Blutströmung erheblich zu erschweren vermag[5].

Bei künstlicher Beatmung am offenen Thorax steigen Druck und Widerstand im Pulmonalkreislauf, das Schlagvolumen der rechten Kammer wird kleiner. Diese Änderungen sind abhängig von positiven intraalveolären Drucken, deren Auswirkungen um so stärker sind, je länger sie andauern[6]. Wenn der positive Druck nur während eines Drittels des Respirationscyclus anhält, fehlt die Blutdruckerhöhung oder bleibt nur ganz gering. Der gleiche Effekt tritt bei Überdruckatmung am geschlossenen System ein. Bei Preßatmung und Husten steigt der Druck im kleinen Kreislauf entsprechend dem intrathorakalen Druck auf ein höheres Niveau. Das Druckgefälle von der Lungenarterie zur Lungenvene bleibt unverändert[7].

In eigenen Perfusionsversuchen[8] an der Leichenlunge hat sich gezeigt, daß schon geringe positive intraalveoläre Drucke die Blutströmung erheblich einschränken, hohe Drucke sie völlig unterbrechen können. Auch hier ergeben sich regelhafte Beziehungen zwischen Durchflußgröße und intraalveolärem Druck.

Steigerungen des alveolären (intrapulmonalen) Druckes können die Durchströmung der Lunge vollständig zum Erliegen bringen. Der positive Alveolardruck erhöht den Strömungswiderstand durch Kompression der Blutgefäße bzw. durch Herabsetzung des transmuralen Druckes wahrscheinlich im Bereich der gesamten Endstrombahn. Er bewirkt eine dem jeweiligen alveolären Druckniveau entsprechende Senkung des transmuralen Druckes. Schon geringe positive Alveolardrucke haben einen pressorischen Effekt auf die Blutströmung.

Bei allen Versuchen an der isolierten Lunge folgen die Weite der Gefäße und damit auch der Strömungswiderstand passiv der Druckdifferenz zwischen Gefäßinnendruck und dem vorwiegend vom Alveolardruck bestimmten Gewebs-

[1] McKEOWN 1952, KERNEN und Mitarbeiter 1958.
[2] ARMSTRONG und CUDKOWICZ 1958.   [3] ADEBAHR 1955 u. a.
[4] NOELPP und NOELPP-ESCHENHAGEN 1956, LOTTENBACH, NOELPP-ESCHENHAGEN und NOELPP 1956.
[5] Siehe auch MINKOWSKI 1912.   [6] ANSCHÜTZ und Mitarbeiter 1955.
[7] HALMAGYI 1957.   [8] HARTUNG und DELFMANN 1960.

druck. Diese Druckdifferenz wird auch als transmuraler Druck bezeichnet (Abb. 86). Jede Steigerung des arteriellen Druckes und bei gleichbleibendem venösem Druck auch der arteriovenösen Druckdifferenz bewirkt demnach nicht nur eine Steigerung der gerichteten treibenden Kräfte für die Blutströmung, sondern über eine Erhöhung des transmuralen Druckes auch eine druckpassive Weiterstellung der Gefäße, unter Umständen auch eine Erschließung zuvor nicht durchströmter Gefäßgebiete. Bei Änderungen der Dehnungslage treten über das elastisch-muskulöse Spannungssystem auf die Gefäße übertragene Formänderungen hinzu. Umgekehrt bewirkt jede Steigerung des Gewebsdruckes durch Erniedrigung des transmuralen Druckes eine Erhöhung der Strömungswiderstände.

Die umgekehrte perfusionsfördernde Wirkung negativer Alveolardrucke hat bereits Romanoff (1911) experimentell nachweisen können. Der negative intraalveoläre Druck fördert z. B. die Entstehung des Ödems bei manchen Formen der Atelektase.

In den eigenen Durchströmungsversuchen sank die Durchflußmenge bei optimaler inspiratorischer Dehnungslage und konstant gehaltenem arteriellem Einfülldruck von etwa 34 cm H_2O ($= 25$ mm Hg) schon bei einer alveolären Drucksteigerung von 10 cm H_2O auf 26%, bei einem alveolären Druck von $+20$ cm H_2O auf 14% der 170 ml/min großen Durchflußmenge bei Versuchsbeginn ab (s.

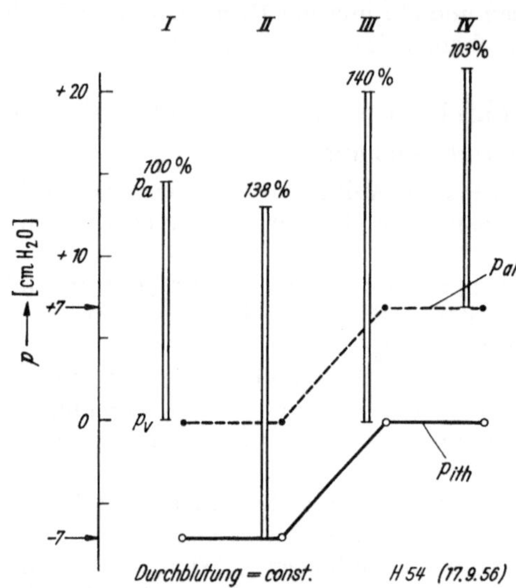

Abb. 86. Zur Bedeutung des transmuralen Druckes für den Widerstand. Der Ordinatenmaßstab gilt für alle Druckwerte. Wegen Konstanz der Durchblutung ist die Länge der Säulen p_a—p_v ein Maß für den Widerstand, dessen Werte auf den Ausgangswert als 100% bezogen sind. (Aus Piiper 1957.)

Abb. 78, S. 585). Die Durchströmung kam bei einem Alveolardruck von $+40$ cm H_2O völlig zum Stillstand. Dieser Druckwert liegt bei den gewählten Versuchsbedingungen nur um wenige cm H_2O unter der Summe des intravasalen Druckes von 34 cm H_2O und des dehnenden Lungenzuges, der einem Intrapleuraldruck von -10 cm H_2O entspricht. Der Verschlußdruck liegt bei dieser Versuchsanordnung bei 5 cm H_2O. Man kann damit rechnen, daß auch die intravitale Strömung bei dieser Druckhöhe unterbrochen wird. Piiper (1957) hat den Verschlußdruck an der isolierten Hundelunge in gleicher Höhe bestimmt.

Die Drosselung wird wieder aufgehoben, sobald das alveoläre Druckniveau um den in der gleichen Größenordnung liegenden arteriellen Öffnungsdruck gesenkt wird. Da die Lungen in Wasser eingeschlossen wurden, waren mit der alveolären Drucksteigerung keine Volumenänderungen verbunden.

Den Einfluß intrabronchialer Druckerhöhung auf die Lungencapillaren hat Schumann (1951) an thorakotomierten Kaninchen bei Überdrucknarkose, im Unterdruck und bei gewöhnlicher Äthernarkose mit Hilfe einer intravitalen Farbstoffinjektion (10% Lithiumcarminlösung) geprüft. Im Unterdruckverfahren und bei Kontrollversuchen sind die Capillaren diffus und stark angefärbt, woraus auf eine gleichmäßige Strömung geschlossen werden kann. Bei Überdruckatmung kommt es nur zu einer geringen und diskontinuierlichen Anfärbung der Capillaren. Die Blutströmung ist also gedrosselt und teilweise unterbrochen.

2. Bronchostenosen und bronchiolostenotisches Emphysem.

Der perfusionsmindernde Einfluß schon relativ geringer positiver Drucke im Alveolarraum hat erhebliche Bedeutung für alle Lungenerkrankungen mit erhöhten Bronchialwiderständen, insbesondere für das bronchostenotische Emphysem, bei dem stark erhöhte Alveolardrucke über längere Perioden in der Exspiration auftreten können. Am Patienten sinkt der Pulmonalarteriendruck ab, wenn die Bronchialwiderstände durch Aleudrin-Inhalationen herabgesetzt werden[1].

Bei Bronchostenosen mit Ventilmechanismen entsteht in der Exspiration ein ansteigender positiver intraalveolärer Druck, der am Ende der Exspiration seinen höchsten Wert erreicht und durch Anspannung der Exspirationsmuskulatur noch gesteigert werden kann.

Das Lungengewebe ist im Bereich einer exspiratorischen Ventilstenose und im bronchostenotischen Emphysem blutarm, blaß, trocken (s. auch unter Bronchiolostenosen S. 527). Die bei akuter bronchostenotischer Überblähung, etwa im Asthmaanfall, maximal gedehnten Alveolarsepten sind fast blutfrei, die Alveolocapillaren leer.

Die experimentellen Untersuchungen lassen die Annahme zu, daß die Störung der Relation zwischen intravasalem Capillardruck und intraalveolärem Druck (d.h. Änderungen des transmuralen Druckes) eine wichtige, vielleicht sogar die Hauptursache für das Versiegen der Perfusion im Bereich des intraalveolären Überdruckes ist.

Im chronischen bronchostenotischen Emphysem entwickeln sich bei Ventilstenosen zahllose kleine Bläschen, deren runde Form Folge des intraalveolären Überdruckes ist. Diese Emphyseme lassen sich morphologisch verhältnismäßig klar von anderen Emphysemformen, insbesondere vom genuinen atrophischen Emphysem abgrenzen[2].

Bei den chronischen bronchostenotischen Emphysemen tritt zu der Überdehnung auch der Abbau der Alveolarsepten und der Verlust an Netzcapillaren. In diesen Fällen bleibt es offen, welcher Anteil der Perfusionsminderung auf druckbedingten Capillarkollaps und wieviel auf den Capillarschwund zu beziehen ist (Abb. 87).

Aus klinischen Untersuchungen[3] geht hervor, daß Emphysem durch Spasmen und Stenosen der Bronchien hervorgerufen und verschlimmert wird. Gelingt therapeutisch eine Lösung der Spasmen, dann bildet sich oft auch die vermehrte Residualluft zurück. Bei spastischer Bronchostenose bestehen stets ventilatorische Verteilungsstörungen. Die Luft wird verzögert in die poststenotischen Bezirke aufgenommen und verzögert wieder abgegeben. In der Ausatmung entleert sich zunächst die Luft aus den stenosefreien Abschnitten, danach aus den poststenotischen Teilen der Lunge. Die Ausatmungsluft zeigt in der ersten Phase der Exspiration die gewöhnliche Gaszusammensetzung, in der zweiten Phase eine CO_2-Anreicherung. MATTHES u. ULMER (1957) nennen diesen Zustand sukzessive Verteilungsstörung, deren Folge fast immer eine Hypoventilation ist. Chronische Hypoventilation führt mit großer Regelmäßigkeit zu pulmonaler Hypertonie und zu Cor pulmonale.

Für diese auch nach morphologischen Befunden häufige Verknüpfung von bronchiolostenotischem Emphysem und pulmonaler Hypertonie mit Cor pulmonale bieten sich folgende Erklärungen an:

1. Erhöhung des intraalveolären Druckes,
2. Hypoventilation,
3. regulative Störungen im Rahmen des v. Eulerschen Prinzips.

[1] BUHR 1953.   [2] GIESE 1959.   [3] MATTHES und ULMER 1957, ROSSIER 1956.

Bei den Klinikern ist heute die Meinung vorherrschend, daß auch in diesen Fällen Hypoventilation Ursache der pulmonalen Hypertonie sei. Welche Bedeutung der erhöhte intraalveoläre Druck hat, ist bisher in diesem Zusammenhang noch nicht diskutiert worden und von morphologischer Seite auch kaum zu entscheiden.

Nach Rimini u. Mitarb. (1957) wird bei einseitiger Überdruckatmung durch Blockierung eines Hauptbronchus ein großer Teil des Blutes zur anderen Lunge

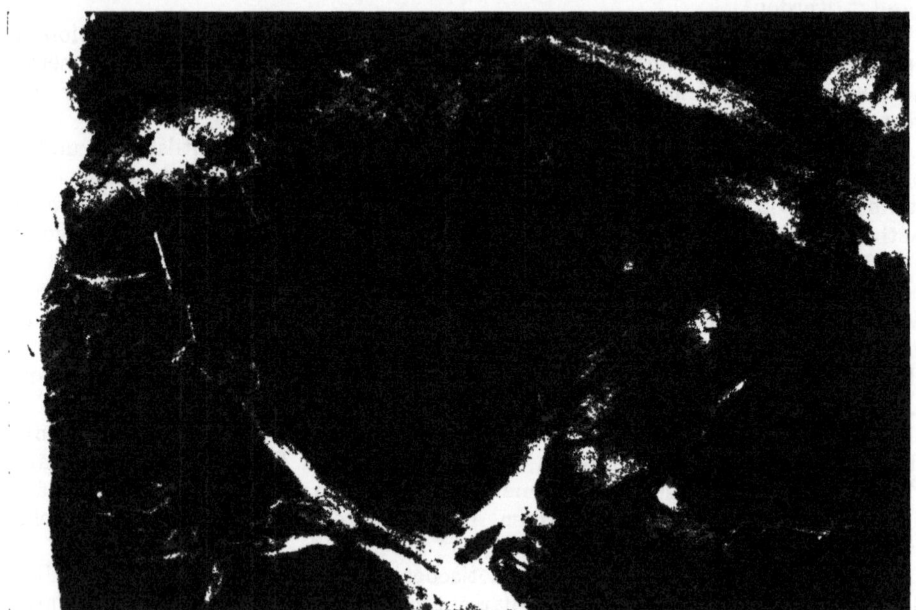

Abb. 87. Bronchostenotisches Emphysem in einem Acinus. Vollständiger Abbau der Alveolarsepten bis auf ein grobes weiträumiges Maschenwerk mit den restlichen Blutgefäßen darin. Völliger Schwund der Netzcapillaren. S.-Nr. 96/59. Vergr. 10fach.

umgeleitet. Die Überdruckatmung hat bereits einen starken Effekt, wenn der intraalveoläre Druck noch nicht den maximalen Pulmonalarteriendruck erreicht oder überschritten hat. Ventilation und Motilität der Überdruckseite sind eingeschränkt.

Damit wird die in Durchströmungsversuchen der isolierten Lunge festgestellte perfusionsmindernde Wirkung des positiven intraalveolären Druckes bestätigt.

Über den Einfluß veränderter Gasspannungen in der Alveolarluft und im Blut kann nur aus physiologischen Experimenten und klinischen Untersuchungen referiert werden.

c) Alveoläre Gasdrucke und Perfusion.

v. Euler u. Liljestrand fanden im Versuch an der Katze, daß der Blutdruck in der Arteria pulmonalis bei Atmung eines Gasgemisches mit erniedrigter O_2-Konzentration ansteigt[1]. Sie bezogen den Druckanstieg auf eine Erhöhung des Widerstandes im kleinen Kreislauf. Diese Befunde, die früher schon von Löhr (1924) erhoben worden sind, wurden an der isolierten Lunge mit kontrollierter Lungendurchblutung[2] und auch am Menschen bestätigt[3].

---

[1] v. Euler und Liljestrand 1946, Liljestrand 1948, v. Euler 1951.

[2] Duke 1950, 1951, Nisell 1950, 1951.

[3] Motley, Cournand und Mitarbeiter 1947, Westcott und Mitarbeiter 1951, Doyle und Mitarbeiter 1952, Siebens und Mitarbeiter 1955 u. a.

Nach NISELL (1952) führt eine Verminderung der alveolären Sauerstoffspannung und ein Ansteigen der Kohlensäurespannung in der Atemluft zu einer Konstriktion der Venolen. Die Venolenconstriction hat eine Steigerung des Capillardruckes zur Folge, die ihrerseits auf reflektorischem Wege eine Konstriktion der Arteriolen und damit eine Erhöhung des Blutdruckes in den Lungenarterien auslöst. Reine Sauerstoffatmung erweitert die Venolen.

Eine verminderte Sauerstoffspannung oder ein erhöhter CO_2-Gehalt im einströmenden Lungenblut erweitert die Arteriolen und läßt die Venolen unbeeinflußt, da im Capillarbereich ein Ausgleich der Gasspannungen zwischen Alveolarluft und Blut eintritt.

In Lungen von Ratten, die mit einem Gasgemisch von 3% CO_2 und Luft beatmet wurden, zeigen die Lungencapillaren eine maximale Dilatation. Das Endothel besteht dann nur noch aus einer 100—150 Å dicken osmiophilen Doppelmembran[1].

Wenn im Tierversuch nur eine Lunge mit einem sauerstoffarmen Gasgemisch beatmet wird, die andere normale Luft erhält, dann kommt es in der hypoxischen Lunge zu einseitiger Durchblutungsminderung, die bis zur Hälfte des Ausgangswertes absinken kann[2].

Auch beim Menschen sind bei einseitiger Hypoxie und kontralateraler Luftoder Sauerstoffatmung ähnliche Befunde erhoben worden[3].

Die Drucksteigerung in der Arteria pulmonalis tritt aber nicht in allen Fällen ein. FISHMAN u. Mitarb. (1952) fanden bei einseitiger Hypoxie keine Druckerhöhung in der Arteria pulmonalis, LEWIS u. GORLIN (1952) bei der Abnahme der O_2-Sättigung im arteriellen Blut auf weniger als 55% eine Vasodilatation.

Bei einseitiger CO_2-Erhöhung in der Atemluft (inspiratorisch etwa 7% CO_2) konnte beim Menschen nur eine sehr geringe, statistisch nicht signifikante Durchblutungsminderung der Lunge gefunden werden[4].

Nach LILJESTRAND (1948) beruht die Abstimmung zwischen der alveolaren Gaskonzentration und dem arteriellen Pulmonaldruck auf einer chemischen Autoregulation des Lungenkreislaufs. Durch Kohlenoxyd und Cyan wird die blutdrucksteigernde Wirkung der Hypoxie aufgehoben[5], bei Narkose abgeschwächt.

Wenn auch die Ergebnisse der experimentellen Untersuchungen und die Befunde am Menschen noch nicht einheitlich sind, darf doch als ausreichend gesichert gelten, daß Hypoxie oder Hyperkapnie auf die Endstrombahn der Lunge vasoconstrictorisch wirken und dadurch eine Hypertonie im kleinen Kreislauf auslösen[6].

An der Tatsache, daß die chronische alveoläre Hypoventilation zu einem chronischen Cor pulmonale führt, besteht kein Zweifel[7]. Die alveoläre Hypoventilation ist durch eine Sauerstoffuntersättigung mit gleichzeitiger Erhöhung der arteriellen CO_2-Spannung charakterisiert.

---

[1] MEESSEN und SCHULZ 1957.
[2] DIRKEN und HEEMSTRA 1948, ATWEL und Mitarbeiter 1951, RAHN und BAHNSON 1953, HEEMSTRA 1954, VENRATH und Mitarbeiter 1955.
[3] WESTCOTT und Mitarbeiter 1951, HERTZ 1956, BÜHLMANN 1956, BÜHLMANN und Mitarbeiter 1956, ULMER und WENKE 1956, 1957.
[4] HERTZ 1957, ebenso RAHN und BAHNSON 1953, STROUD und RAHN 1953, LOCHNER 1957 im Tierversuch.
[5] DUKE und KILLICK 1952.
[6] LOCHNER 1957, ROSSIER 1956, MATTHES und ULMER 1957, HERTZ 1957.
[7] MATTHES, ULMER und WITTEKIND 1960.

Die Beziehungen zwischen Hypoventilation und Perfusion können nach den
angeführten Untersuchungsergebnissen in folgendem Zusammenhang gedacht
werden:

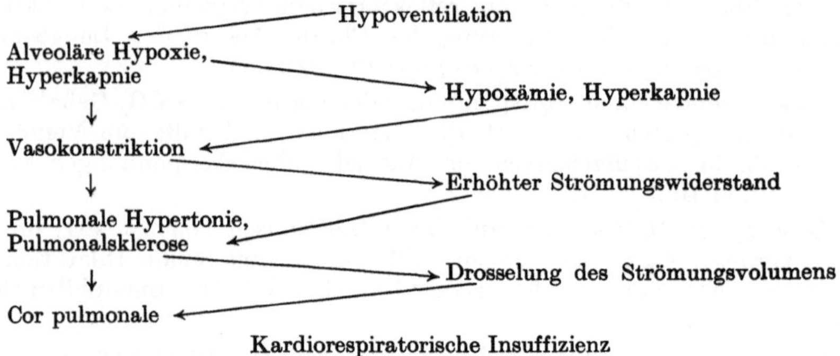

Im Mittelpunkt der durch Hypoxie ausgelösten pulmonalen Hypertonie steht
die Reaktion der Endstrombahn der Lunge. Während unter normalen Bedingungen die kleinen Arterien beim Ansteigen des arteriellen Blutdruckes weit
gestellt werden, der Strömungswiderstand absinkt und das Durchflußvolumen
zunimmt, liegen die Verhältnisse unter pathologischen Bedingungen umgekehrt. Ein durch Hypoxie ausgelöster, über die Norm ansteigender Druck
im kleinen Kreislauf wird hervorgerufen durch eine Engstellung der Arteriolen
und kleinen Arterien. Diesem funktionellen, regulativ bestimmten Stadium folgt
die Pulmonalsklerose mit der organischen Stenose der kleinen Arterien. Der
erhöhte Strömungswiderstand im Lungenkreislauf wird fixiert, das Durchflußvolumen verringert. Im funktionellen Stadium sind Strömungsvolumen und
Blutdruck im Pulmonalkreislauf noch variabel. Im organisch fixierten Stadium
sind allein noch die Größe des Querschnittes und die Kraft des Herzens entscheidend.

Durch den Hypoxie-Reflex wird die Perfusion auf die Ventilation abgestimmt.
Diese Abstimmung kann örtlich auf kleine Lungenabschnitte beschränkt oder
auf die ganze Lunge ausgedehnt sein.

Den örtlichen reflektorischen Einschränkungen der Perfusion liegen fast stets
Bronchiolostenosen oder Schleimverschlüsse, seltener interstitielle Lungenfibrosen mit erschwerter Lungenbewegung zugrunde.

Die kleinste, in dieser Weise reagierende Einheit ist der Acinus, nicht die
einzelne Alveole. Der Acinus ist ein zwar gegliederter, aber doch einheitlicher
Raum, in dem unterschiedliche Gaskonzentrationen wegen des gemeinsamen
weiten Gangsystemes nicht vorstellbar sind.

Das Blut wird durch die örtliche reflektorische Engstellung der Blutgefäße
in die regelrecht belüfteten Lungenanteile abgelenkt. Die Folgen für den Lungenkreislauf sind gering, solange die Ausdehnung der hypoventilierten Lungenabschnitte klein bleibt. Sie gewinnt erst Bedeutung, wenn die Herde sehr zahlreich
und ausgedehnt sind, wie etwa bei der spastischen Bronchiolitis des Kindesalters
und bei der komplizierenden Bronchiolitis des Altersemphysems.

Lokale ventilatorische Verteilungsstörungen können so vorübergehende oder
anhaltende zirkulatorische Verteilungsstörungen auslösen, die bis in die Lungeninsuffizienz hineinreichen. Diese wird um so eher zu erwarten sein, je ausgedehnter die Hypoventilation ist.

Schlußbetrachtung.

Die Leistungen des Thorax-Lungensystems in der äußeren Atmung beruhen auf physikalischen und chemischen Vorgängen, in die neurale und humorale Steuerungen eingreifen. Die Bedeutung der regulativen Steuerung bei Krankheiten im Bereich der Atmungsorgane ist morphologisch so wenig faßbar, daß diese in der vorstehenden, vom morphologischen Standpunkt geführten Diskussion nur gestreift werden konnte. Auf die physiologischen und klinischen Abschnitte dieses Handbuchs muß dazu verwiesen werden.

Um so deutlicher haben sich die physikalischen und chemischen Faktoren in ihrer Bedeutung für den Ablauf des Atmungsvorganges herausgeschält. Man darf am Ende dieser Darstellung sagen, daß die histomechanische Analyse der Lunge eine beachtliche Reihe von Tatbeständen aufgedeckt hat, die als Schlüssel für das Verständnis normaler und gestörter Atmungsfunktion dienen können.

Für den Morphologen haben unter den neuen Forschungsergebnissen die Arbeiten größte Bedeutung, in denen gezeigt werden konnte, daß die histomechanische Analyse der Leichenlunge in ihrer Funktion als Ventilationsorgan Werte gibt, die mit entsprechenden Meßergebnissen der Klinik oder des Tierversuchs volle Übereinstimmung zeigen, und daß auch zahlreiche Störungen in der Perfusion auf mechanische, am toten Organ analysierbare Prinzipien zurückgeführt werden können.

Der Morphologe sieht sich dadurch in den Stand gesetzt, die Funktionsbreite einer Lunge auch am toten Organ abzuschätzen und die Bedeutung von Störungen ihrer Struktur für den Ablauf des Atmungsvorganges zu bestimmen. Morphische und funktionelle Pathologie erscheinen damit in der engen Verbindung, die herzustellen leitendes Prinzip einer Allgemeinen Pathologie ist.

Literatur.

ABBOT, M. E.: Atlas of congenital heart disease. New York: American Heart Assoc. 1936. Congenital heart disease. New York: Nelson 1949. — ADEBAHR, G.: Befunde bei Bronchiektasen nach Untersuchungen an Operationsmaterial. Frankfurt. Z. Path. **66**, 29 (1955). — AEBY, C.: Die Gestalt des Bronchialbaumes und die Homologie der Lungenlappen beim Menschen. Med. Zbl. **16**, 290 (1878). ~ Der Bronchialbaum der Säugetiere und des Menschen, nebst Bemerkungen über den Bronchialbaum der Vögel und Reptilien. Leipzig: Wilhelm Engelmann 1880. — AITKEN, R. S., and E. CLARK-KENNEDY: The concentration of CO_2 in successive portions of an exspired breath. J. Physiol. (Lond.) **64**, 17 (1927). — ALEXANDER, H.: Lungenatelektase. Zbl. Tuberk.-Forsch. **55**, 313 (1942). ~ Atelektasen der Lunge (Tuberkulosebücherei). Stuttgart: Georg Thieme 1951. — ALEXANDER, H. L., W. G. BECKE and J. A. HOLMES: Reactions of sensitized guinea pigs to inhaled antigens. J. Immunol. **11**, 175 (1926). — ALLEN, C. M. VAN: Kollaterale Respiration. 1. Vorhandensein kollateraler Verbindungen zwischen den Lungenläppchen. Z. Anat. Entwickl.-Gesch. **98**, 453 (1932). ~ Kollaterale Respiration. 2. Vorkommen kollateraler Respiration zwischen den Lungenläppchen. Z. Anat. Entwickl.-Gesch. **98**, 466 (1932). — ALLEN, C. M. VAN, and T. S. JUNG: Postoperative atelectasis and collateral respiration. J. thorac. Surg. **1**, 3 (1931). — ALLEN, C. M. VAN, and G. E. LINDSKOG: Collateral respiration in the lung. J. Surg. (New York) **53**, 16 (1931). — ALTMANN, K.: Experimentell-morphologische Untersuchungen über die Beziehungen zwischen der Lungenkapillarweite und dem Lungendehnungsgrad. Z. ges. exp. Med. **122**, 516 (1954). ~ Experimente und Überlegungen zur Frage des Pleuradrucks. Z. ges. exp. Med. **125**, 196 (1955). ANDRUS, W. D. W.: Observations on the cardiorespiratory physiology following the collapse of one lung by bronchial ligation. Arch. Surg. (Chicago) **10**, 506 (1925). — ANGLADE, P. H.: De l'atelectasie pulmonaire. Thése Paris 1935. — ANSCHÜTZ, F., B. DEUBEL, CH. DRUBE u. J. SEUSING: Tierexperimentelle Untersuchungen über die Kreislaufwirkung verschiedener künstlicher Beatmungsmethoden bei nicht eröffnetem Thorax. Z. ges. exp. Med. **125**, 314 (1955). — ANTHONY, A. J.: Funktionsprüfung der Atmung. Leipzig: Johann Ambrosius Barth 1937. — ANTHONY, A. J., u. M. BROGLIE: Grundsätzliches über die Begrenzung der Zwerchfellbewegungen. Klin. Wschr. **1939**, 1126. — ANTHONY, A. J., u. W. LENT: Untersuchungen über die Wirkung erhöhter Atemwiderstände. I. Zur Frage der Wirksamkeit erhöhter Atemwiderstände auf den Gasstoffwechsel. Z. ges. exp. Med. **109**, 624 (1941). — ANTHONY, A. J., W. LENT u. E. M. MÜLLER: Untersuchungen über die Wirkung erhöhter

Atemwiderstände. III. Der Einfluß erhöhter Atemwiderstände auf Herz- und Kreislauf. Z. ges. exp. Med. 109, 650 (1941). — Armstrong, J. B., u. L. Cudkowicz: Die pathologische Anatomie der Bronchialarterien. Ergebn. ges. Tuberk.-Forsch. (Stuttgart) 14, 191 (1958). — Arnstein, A.: Indurative und Zerfallsvorgänge in den mediastinalen Lymphknoten im höheren Alter mit Schädigung benachbarter Organe. Beitr. Klin. Tuberk. 85, 197 (1934). — Aschoff, L.: Über Atherosclerose und andere Sclerosen des Gefäßsystems. Beih. Med. Klin. H. 1 (1908). ~ Elastische Systeme des Tracheobronchialbaumes. Congr. internat. del pathologi, Torino 1912. ~ Über anatomische und histologische Befunde bei Gasvergiftungen. Zit. nach W. Koch 1921. ~ Diskussionsbemerkung zu Lungenemphysem. Tagg. südwestdeutsch. Pathologen, Mannheim 1922. Zbl. allg. Path. path. Anat. 33, 1—20 (1922/23). ~ Über gewisse Gesetzmäßigkeiten der Pleuraverwachsungen. Veröff. Kriegs- u. Konstitutionspath. 3, H. 14 (1923). ~ Bemerkungen zur Physiologie des Lungengewebes. Z. ges. exp. Med. 50, 52 (1926). ~ Über den Lungenacinus. Frankfurt. Z. Path. 48, 449 (1935). — Assmann, H.: Die klinische Röntgendiagnostik der inneren Erkrankungen, 6. Aufl. Berlin: Springer 1950. — Atwell, R. J., J. B. Hickam, W. W. Pryor and E. B. Page: Reduction of blood flow through the hypoxic lung. Amer. J. Physiol. 166, 37 (1951). — Auerbach, O.: Anatomic changes in the lungs following thoracoplasty, study of 134 autopsy cases. J. thorac. Surg. 11, 21 (1941). — Austrian, R., J. H. McClement, A. D. Renzetti jr., K. W. Donald, R. L. Riley and A. Cournand: Clinical and physiologic features of some types of pulmonary diseases with impairment of alveolar capillary diffusion. The syndrom of „alveolar capillary block". Amer. J. Med. 11, 667 (1951).

Baarsma, P. R., and M. N. J. Dirken: Collateral ventilation. J. thorac. Surg. 17, 238 (1948). — Baarsma, P. R., M. N. J. Dirken and E. Huizinga: Collateral ventilation in man. J. thorac. Surg. 17, 252 (1948). — Backmann, G.: Lungenvenen der Wirbeltiere. Lunds Univ. Arsskr., N.F. 33 (1937). Zit. nach Töndury 1956. — Backmann, R.: Blutgehalt und Blutverteilung in den Lungen unter normalen und pathologischen Verhältnissen. Beitr. path. Anat. 124, (1961, im Druck). — Bär, C. G., R. Zeilhofer u. K. Heckel: Über die Beeinflussung des Herzens und der Atmung durch die Trichterbrust. Dtsch. med. Wschr. 1958, 282. — Baldwin, E. F., A. Cournand and D. W. Richards jr.: Pulmonary insufficiency. I. Physiological classification, clinical methods of analysis, standard values in normal subjects. Medicine (Baltimore) 27, 243 (1948). ~ Pulmonary insufficiency. A study of thirty-nine cases of pulmonary fibrosis. Medicine (Baltimore) 28, 1 (1949). ~ Pulmonary insufficiency. III. Study of 122 cases of chronic pulmonary emphysema. Medicine (Baltimore) 28, 201 (1949). — Baltisberger, W.: Über die glatte Muskulatur der menschlichen Lunge. Z. Anat. Entwickl.-Gesch. 61, 249 (1921). — Barcroft, J.: The respiratory function of the blood. Cambridge: Univ. Press 1928. — Bargmann, W.: Zur vergleichenden Histologie der Lungenalveole. Z. Zellforsch. 23, 335 (1935). ~ Die Lungenalveole. In Handbuch der mikroskopischen Anatomie, Bd. V/3. Berlin: Springer 1936. ~ Histologie und mikroskopische Anatomie, 2. Aufl. Stuttgart: Georg Thieme 1956. — Bargmann, W., u. A. Knoop: Vergleichende elektronenmikroskopische Untersuchungen der Lungenkapillaren. Z. Zellforsch. 44, 263 (1956). — Bartels, H.: Neuere Anschauungen über den Vorgang des Gasaustausches in der Lunge. (Referat.) Verh. dtsch. Ges. inn. Med. 62, 25 (1956). ~ Über Möglichkeiten und Grenzen der Beurteilung von Diffusionsbedingungen in der menschlichen Lunge. Bad Oeynhausener Gespräche I, 28 (1956). Berlin-Göttingen-Heidelberg: Springer 1957. — Bartels, H., R. Beer, H. Koepchen, J. Wenner u. J. Witt: Messung der alveolär-arteriellen O_2-Druck-Differenz mit verschiedenen Methoden am Menschen bei Ruhe und Arbeit. Pflügers Arch. ges. Physiol. 261, 133 (1955). — Bartels, J., J. W. Severinghaus, R. E. Forster, W. A. Briscoe and V. V. Bates: The respiratory dead space measured by single breath analysis of oxygen, carbon dioxide, nitrogen or helium. J. clin. Invest. 33, 45 (1954). — Basch, S. v.: Über Lungenschwellung und Lungenstarrheit. Wien. med. Presse 14, 587 (1888). — Bates, D. V., J. M. S. Knott and R. V. Christie: Respiratory function in emphysema in relation to prognosis. Quart. J. Med., N.S. 25, 137 (1956). — Bayer, G.: Regulation der Atmung. In Handbuch der normalen und pathologischen Physiologie, Bd. II. Berlin: Springer 1925. — Bayer, O., F. Grosse-Brockhoff, F. Loogen u. H. Meessen: Vergleichende klinische, pathophysiologische und pathologischanatomische Untersuchungen bei Mitralstenose. Arch. Kreisl.-Forsch. 26, 238 (1957). — Bayer, O., F. Loogen u. H. Wolter: Der Herzkatheterismus bei angeborenen und erworbenen Herzfehlern. Stuttgart: Georg Thieme 1954. — Bayer, O., F. Loogen, H. H. Wolter, R. Rippert, D. Augath u. D. Beier: Zur Pathophysiologie und Klinik der Mitralstenose. Arch. Kreisl.-Forsch. 21, 383 (1954). — Bayliss, L. E., and C. W. Robertson: The viscoelastic properties of the lungs. Quart. J. exp. Physiol. 29, 27 (1939). — Bazett, H. C.: Factors regulating blood pressure. Third Conference. New York: J. Macy jr. Found. 1949. — Bedford, E. D.: Discussion on pulmonary heart disease. Proc. roy. Soc. Med. 44, 597 (1951). Behrens, W.: Anatomischer Beitrag zur Frage der Atelektase. Schweiz. med. Wschr. 1950, 69. — Behrens sen., W., u. A. Fanconi: Bronchiolitis obliterans chronica. Beitr. Klin. Tuberk. 117, 539 (1958). — Beitzke, H.: Respirationsorgane. In Aschoffs Lehrbuch der pathologischen Anatomie, Bd. II. Jena: Gustav Fischer 1909. ~ Zur Mechanik des Gaswechsels beim Lungenemphysem. Tagg. Südwestdtsch. Pathologen, Mannheim 1922. Zbl. allg. Path. path. Anat. **33**, 1—20 (1922/23). ~ Zur Mechanik des Gaswechsels beim Lungenemphysem. Dtsch. Arch. klin. Med. **146**, 91 (1925). ~ Pathologische Anatomie des Tracheo-Bronchialdrüsendurchbruchs. Ergebn. ges. Tuberk.-Forsch. **12**, 17 (1954). — BELL, J. W.: Experimental pulmonary emphysema. Production of emphysematous bullae in the rabbit by infection with tuberculosis. Amer. Rev. Tuberc. **78**, 848 (1958). — BENDER, F.: Die Pulmonalvenentranspositionen und ihre Beziehungen zum Vorhofseptumdefekt. Habil.-Schr. Münster 1959. — BENDER, F., F. HILGENBERG u. G. JUNGEHÜLSING: Fortlaufend registrierte Farbstoffverdünnungskurven bei erworbenen und angeborenen Herzfehlern. Z. Kreisl.-Forsch. **46**, 845 (1957). — BENDER, F., F. HILGENBERG, G. JUNGEHÜLSING, G. MENKHAUS u. E. SCHÜRMEYER: Zur diagnostischen Auswertung von Farbstoffkurven bei angeborenen Herzfehlern mit Links-Rechts-Shunt unter Verwendung von Methylenblau. Z. Kreisl.-Forsch. 1959 (im Druck). — BENNINGHOFF, A.: Über die funktionelle Struktur der Lungengefäße. Z. Kreisl.-Forsch. **27**, 303 (1935). — BERBLINGER, W.: Formen und Ursachen der Herzhypertrophie bei Lungentuberkulose. Bern: Huber 1947. — BERGLUND, G., and P. KARLBERG: Determination of the functional residual capacity in newborn infants; preliminary report. Acta paediat. (Uppsala) **45**, 541 (1956). — BERNARD, A.: Rôle des troubles neuro-vasculaires réflexes dans l'écloison des pneumopathies postopératoires. Acta gastro-ent. belg. **14**, 805 (1951). — BEZANÇON, F., et J. DELARUE: Les scléroses pulmonaires tuberculeuses. Presse méd. **1941**, 1. — BIANCALANA, L.: La sindrome atelectasie del lobo medio. Minerva med. (Torino) **1**, 401 (1952). — BIANCALANA, L., e C. COLOMBO: L'atelectasie polmonare negli interventi di exeresi del polmone. Atti 3. Congr. naz. Chir. torac. **1**, 97 (1952). — BIASI, W. DI: Schwere Silikose. A. Pathologisch-anatomischer Teil. In: KÖNIG u. MAGNUS' Handbuch der gesamten Unfallheilkunde, Bd. II. 1933. ~ Über den Standpunkt des pathologischen Anatomen bei der Begutachtung von Staublungen-Erkrankungen. In: Die Staublungenerkrankungen. Wiss. Forsch.berichte, Naturwiss. Reihe, Bd. 60. Darmstadt: Steinkopff 1950. ~ Probleme der Mischstaubsilikose. Zbl. allg. Path. path. Anat. **100**, 531 (1960). ~ Herdförmige Asbestose — Silikose in Verbindung mit Asbestose. Medizinische **1960**, 1279. — BIERMER, A.: Krankheiten der Bronchien. In: VIRCHOWS Handbuch der speziellen Pathologie und Therapie, Bd. 5, Abt. 1. Erlangen 1865/67. — BING, R. J.: The physiology of congenital heart disease. New York: Nelson 1949. ~ Congenital heart disease. An introduction and classification. Amer. J. Med. **1952**, 77. — BING, R. J., L. D. VANDAM and F. D. GRAY: Physiological studies in congenital heart disease. Bull. Johns Hopk. Hosp. **80**, 107, 121 (1947). — BIRCH-HIRSCHFELD: Pathologische Anatomie, 3. Aufl. 1887. Zit. nach HAYASHI 1915. — BJÖRK, V. O., G. MALMSTRÖM and L. UGGLA: Left atrial and pulmonary „capillary" pressure curves during Valsalva's experiment. Amer. Heart J. **47**, 635 (1954). — BJÖRKMAN, S.: Bronchospirometrie. Acta med. scand., Suppl. **56** (1934). ~ Bronchospirometrie. Eine klinische Methode, die Funktion der menschlichen Lungen getrennt und gleichzeitig zu untersuchen. Stockholm: Aktiebolag Fahlcrantz' Boktryckerie 1934. — BLOOMER, W. E., W. HARRISON, O. F. LIEBOW and A. A. LINDSKOG: Respiratory function and blood flow in the bronchial artery after ligation of the pulmonary artery. Amer. J. Physiol. **157**, 317 (1949). BLUMENTHAL, W.: Die Beeinflussung der Kreislaufzeit durch die Atemlage. Z. Kreisl.-Forsch. **43**, 349 (1954). — BLUMGART, H. L., and S. WEISS: Studies on the velocity of bloodflow. VII. The pulmonary circulation time in normally respiring individuals. VIII. The velocity of bloodflow and its relation to other aspects of the circulation in patients with pulmonary emphysema. J. clin. Invest. **4**, 399 (1927). — BOCK, H. E.: Über die Zirkulationszeit des Blutes in der Lunge. Verh. dtsch. Ges. Kreisl.-Forsch. **17**, 222 (1951). — BÖHMIG, R.: Über die kataplastischen Veränderungen im menschlichen Rippenknorpel. Beitr. path. Anat. **81**, 172 (1928). — BOEMKE, F.: Staublunge und Emphysem aus der Sicht des Pathologen. Herbsttagg Rhein.-Westf. Tbk.vereinigg, Düsseldorf 25. 10. 1958. — BÖNNIGER, M.: Zur Physiologie und Pathologie der Atmung. Z. exp. Path. Ther. **5**, 409 (1909). ~ Zur Aetiologie des Lungenemphysems. Verh. Kongr. inn. Med. **26**, 400 (1909). — BOGAERT, A. VAN: Die Dyspnoe bei den Mitralfehlern. Ärztl. Forsch. **13**, 382 (1959). — BOHN, W.: Über Altersveränderungen am Lungenhilus. Virchows Arch. path. Anat. **318**, 289 (1950). — BOHR, CHR.: Über die Lungenatmung. Skand. Arch. Physiol. **2**, 236 (1891). ~ Die funktionellen Änderungen in der Mittellage und Vitalkapazität der Lungen. Normales und pathologisches Emphysem. Dtsch. Arch. klin. Med. **88**, 385 (1907). ~ Blutgase und respiratorischer Gaswechsel. In: Handbuch der Physiologie des Menschen. Braunschweig: Vieweg & Sohn 1909. ~ Über die Bestimmung der Gasdiffusion durch die Lunge und ihre Größe bei Ruhe und Arbeit. Zbl. Physiol. **23**, 374 (1909). — BOLT, W.: Zum Lungenkreislauf unter Berücksichtigung der Lungenfunktionsprüfung. Beitr. Klin. Tuberk. **110**, 39 (1953). ~ Emphysem (Haemodynamik). Beitr. Klin. Tuberk. **111**, 266 (1954). ~ Pathologische Physiologie des Cor pulmonale. Verh. dtsch. Ges. Kreisl.-Forsch. **21**, 196 (1955). ~ Pathophysiologie der Ventilationsstörungen (Referat). Verh. dtsch. Ges. Path. **44** (1960). — BOLT, W., W. FORSSMANN u. H. RINK: Technik und praktische Bedeutung der Herzkatheterisierung für die funktionelle Diagnostik und die Therapie von Herz- und Lungenerkrankungen. Med. Klin. **1953**, 1614. ~ Selektive Lungenangiographie. Stuttgart: Georg Thieme 1957. — Bolt, W., W. Hollmann, H. Valentin u. H. Venrath: Zur funktionellen Differenzierung kardial oder pulmonal bedingter Lungenveränderungen. Beitr. Klin. Tuberk. 116, 642 (1957). — Bolt, W., u. H. W. Knipping: Zur Klinik des Lungenkreislaufes. Verh. dtsch. Ges. Kreisl.-Forsch. 17, 87 (1951). — Bolt, W., H. W. Knipping u. H. Rink: Funktionsfragen bei der operativen Behandlung der Lungentuberkulose. Thoraxchirurgie 1, 167 (1953/54). ~ Probleme des kleinen Kreislaufs bei Herz- und Lungenkrankheiten. Medizinische 1955, 480. — Bolt, W., u. H. Rink: Selektive Angiographie der Lungengefäße bei Lungentuberkulose. Schweiz. Z. Tuberk. 8, 380 (1951). — Bolt, W., A. Stanischeff u. O. Zorn: Die selektive Angiographie der Lungengefäße. Münch. med. Wschr. 1951, 306. — Borelli, F., e G. Esposito: Sull'alcuni aspetti istoanatomici dell'albero bronchiale doppo exeresi polmonare. (Richerche sperimentali.) Chir. torac. 5, 420 (1952). — Bostroem, B., u. J. Piiper: Über arterio-venöse Anastomosen und Kurzschlußdurchblutung in der Lunge. Pflügers Arch. ges. Physiol. 261, 165 (1955). — Boyden, E. A., and G. J. Scanell: An analysis of variations in the bronchovascular pattern. Amer. J. Anat. 82, 27 (1948). — Braak, J. W. G. ter, u. J. van Niekerk: Der Einfluß des zentripetalen Lungenvagus auf Lage und Bewegung des Zwerchfells. Pflügers Arch. ges. Physiol. 235, 562 (1935). — Brauer, L.: Die respiratorische Insuffizienz. Verh. dtsch. Ges. inn. Med. 44, 120 (1932). — Brauer, L., u. A. Lorey: Die röntgenologische Darstellung der Bronchien mittels Kontrastfüllung. Ergebn. med. Strahlenforsch. 3, 115 (1928). — Braus, H.: Anatomie des Menschen, Bd. 2. Berlin: Springer 1934. — Brecklinghaus, H.: Häufigkeit und Bedeutung von Einbrüchen tuberkulöser Lymphknoten in das Bronchialsystem. Beitr. Klin. Tuberk. 114, 357 (1955). — Bredt, H.: Die primäre Erkrankung der Lungenschlagader in ihren verschiedenen Formen. Virchows Arch. path. Anat. 285, 126 (1932). ~ Entzündung und Sklerose der Lungenschlagader. Virchows Arch. path. Anat. 308, 60 (1942). — Bredt, H., u. L. Stadler: Das Gewebsbild des kleinen Kreislaufes bei entzündlichen Herzfehlern und seine Bedeutung für das klinische Krankheitsbild. Arch. Kreisl.-Forsch. 7, 54 (1940). — Bremer, J. L.: The fate of the remaining lung tissue after lobectomy or pneumonectomy. J. thorac. Surg. 6, 336 (1936/37). — Brenner, O.: Pathology of the vessels of the pulmonary circulation. Arch. intern. Med. 56, 211, 457, 724, 976, 1189 (1935). — Brock, R. C.: The anatomy of the bronchial tree. London: Oxf. Univ. Press 1946. ~ Post-tuberculous bronchostenosis and bronchiectasis of middle lobe. Thorax 5, 5 (1950). — Bronkhorst, W., u. C. Dijkstra: Das neuromuskuläre System der Lunge. Beitr. Klin. Tuberk. 94, 445 (1940). — Brückner, H.: Die Anatomie der Luftröhre beim lebenden Menschen. Z. Anat. 116, 276 (1952). — Brünings, W.: Die direkte Laryngoskopie, Bronchoskopie und Oesophagoskopie. Wiesbaden: J. F. Bergmann 1910. — Bucher, H., u. R. Gloor: Bronchospirometrische Untersuchungen nach abgeschlossener Pneumothoraxbehandlung und nach Dekortikation. Schweiz. Z. Tuberk. 10, 265 (1953). — Bucher, K.: Reflektorische Beeinflußbarkeit der Lungenatmung. Wien: Springer 1952. — Büchner, Ch., u. G. Könn: Temporär chronisches Cor pulmonale im Tierexperiment nach rezidivierender Mikroembolie. Beitr. path. Anat. 121, 170 (1959). — Büchner, F., u. F. Fröhlich: Das System der hellen Zellen. In: Naturforschung und Medizin in Deutschland 1939—1946 (Fiat-Reviews). Allgemeine Pathologie, bearb. von F. Büchner, Bd. 2, S. 177. 1948. — Bühlmann, A.: Experimentelle Untersuchungen über Stenoseatmung. Schweiz. Z. Tuberk. 6, 89 (1949). ~ Formen der Lungeninsuffizienz. Bad Oeynhausener Gespräche I, 112 (1956). Berlin-Göttingen-Heidelberg: Springer 1957. ~ Schweizer Internistenkongreß 1956. Zit. nach Hertz 1957. — Bühlmann, A., C. Maier, M. Hegglin u. R. Kälin: Zur Pathogenese der arteriellen pulmonalen Hypertonie mit besonderer Berücksichtigung des Cor pulmonale beim Emphysem. Cardiologica (Basel) 24, 96 (1954). — Bühlmann, A., C. Maier, M. Hegglin, R. Kälin u. F. Schaub: Beziehungen zwischen Lungenfunktion und Lungenkreislauf. Ein Beitrag zur Genese und Symptomatologie der Hypertonie des kleinen Kreislaufs. Schweiz. med. Wschr. 1953, 1199. — Bühlmann, A., F. Schaub, G. Hossli u. P. Hösli: Haemodynamische Untersuchungen bei allgemeiner und einseitiger Hypoventilation. Helv. med. Acta 23, 545 (1956). — Bühlmann, A., F. Schaub u. P. Luchsinger: Zur Erfolgsbeurteilung der Kommissurotomie bei Mitralstenose. Dtsch. med. Wschr. 1954, 630. ~ Die Hämodynamik des Lungenkreislaufes während Ruhe und körperlicher Arbeit beim Gesunden und bei den verschiedenen Formen der pulmonalen Hypertonie. Schweiz. med. Wschr. 1955, 253. — Bühlmann, A., F. Schaub u. P. H. Rossier: Zur Ätiologie und Therapie des Cor pulmonale. Schweiz. med. Wschr. 1954, 587. — Bühlmann, A., u. T. Wegmann: Bronchialspasmen und Adrenalinversuch. Beitr. Klin. Tuberk. 105, 189 (1951). — Bürger, M.: Altern und Krankheit, 2. Aufl. Leipzig: VEB Thieme 1954. — Büscher: Grün- und Gelbkreuz. Spezielle Pathologie und Therapie der Körperschädigungen durch die chemischen Kampfstoffe. Hamburg 1932. — Buhr, G.: Über den Einfluß der Aleudrin-Aerosol-Inhalation auf die Druckverhältnisse in der Arteria pulmonalis beim Menschen. Z. Kreisl.-Forsch. 42, 669 (1953). ~ Beitrag zur Beeinflußbarkeit des menschlichen Lungenkreislaufs durch vasoaktive Substanzen. Z. Kreisl.-Forsch. 44, 601 (1954). ~ Die Atemwiderstandsmessung in der ärztlichen Begutachtung. Med. Klin. 1958, 2180. — Bullen sen., S. S.: Correlation of clinical and autopsy findings in 176 cases of asthma.

J. Allergy **23**, 193 (1952). — BULLOWA, J. G. M., and C. GOTTLIEB: Roentgenray studies of bronchial movements. Amer. J. med. Sci., Transact. III, Biophysics **2**, 72 (1931). — BURCH-HARDT: Die Luftströmung in der Nase unter pathologischen Verhältnissen. Arch. Laryng. Rhin. (Berl.) **17**, 123 (1905). — BURWELL, C. S., E. D. ROBIN, R. D. WHALEY and A. G. BICKEL-MANN: Extreme obesity associated with alveolar hypoventilation: Pickwickian syndrome. Amer. J. Med. **21**, 811 (1956). — BUSSON, B., u. N. OGATA: Gibt es Beziehungen zwischen den menschlichen Idiosynkrasien und der tierexperimentellen Anaphylaxie? Wien. klin. Wschr. **1924**, 820.

CAIN, H.: Die Lungenstrombahn bei angeborener Pulmonalstenose und Pulmonalatresie. Zbl. allg. Path. path. Anat. **97**, 326 (1958). ~ Haematogene Geschwulstzellenausbreitung in der Lunge, unter besonderer Berücksichtigung sog. regelwidriger Fälle. Z. Krebsforsch. **62**, 323 (1958). — CAMPBELL, E. J. M.: The respiratory muscles and the mechanics of breathing. London: Lloyd-Luke Ltd. 1958. — CARSTENS, M.: Die „Emphysembronchitis" der Bergleute. Eine klinische Studie. Med. wiss. Beitr. Ruhrknappschaft Bochum, H. 6, 17 (1955). — CARSTENS, M., O. BRINKMANN, H. J. LANGE, A. MEISTERERNST u. H. SCHLICHT: Beiträge zur Pathophysiologie der Staublungenkrankheit im Bergbau. I.—IV. Mitteilung. Arch. Gewerbe-path. Gewerbehyg. **16**, 203, 439, 459, 511 (1958). — CEELEN, W.: Die Kreislaufstörungen der Lunge. In: Handbuch der speziellen pathologischen Anatomie und Histologie, Bd. III/3. Berlin: Springer 1931. — CHAMBERS, R., and B. W. ZWEIFACH: Capillary endothelial cement in relation to permeability. J. cell. comp. Physiol. **15**, 255 (1940). ~ Caliber changes of the vessels of the capillary bed. Fed. Proc. **1**, 14(1942).~Topography and function of the mesenteric capillary circulation. Amer. J. Anat. **75**, 173 (1944). ~ Functional activity of blood capillary bed, with special reference to visceral tissue. Ann. N.Y. Acad. Sci. **46**, 683 (1946). ~ Intercellular cement and capillary permeability. Physiol. Rev. **27**, 436 (1947). ~ Blood-borne vasotropic substances in experimental shock. Amer. J. Physiol. **150**, 239 (1947). — CHAPMAN, R. M., B. DILL and A. GRAYBIEL: The decrease in functional capacity of the lungs and heart resulting from deformities of the chest: pulmocardial failure. Medicine (Baltimore) **18**, 167 (1939). — CHIARI, H.: Vikariier-ende Lungenhyperplasie. Verh. dtsch. Ges. Path. **17**, 325 (1914). — CHRISTIE, R. V.: The elastic properties of the emphysematous lung and their clinical significance. J. clin. Invest. **13**, 295 (1934). ~ Chronic hypertrophic emphysema. Its aetiology and the cause of some of its signs and symptoms. Edinb. med. J. **46**, 463 (1939). ~ Emphysema of the lungs. Brit. med. J. **1944**, 143. ~ Dyspnoea in relation to visco-elastic properties of lung. Proc. roy. Soc. Med. **46**, 381 (1953). — CHRISTIE, R. V., and R. MARSHALL: The visco-elastic properties of the lungs in acute pneumonia. Clin. Sci. **13**, 403 (1954). — CHRISTIE, R. V., R. MARSHALL and W. R. STONE: The relationship of dyspnoea to respiratory effort in normal subjects, mitral stenosis and emphysema. Clin. Sci. **13**, 625 (1954). — CHRISTIE, R. V., and J. C. MEAKINS: The intra-pleural pressure in congestive heart failure and its clinical significance. J. clin. Invest. **13**, 323 (1934). — CHURCHILL, E. D.: Pulmonary atelectasis, with special reference to massive collapse of the lung. Arch. Surg. (Chicago) **11**, 489 (1925). ~ The segmental and lobular physiology and pathology of the lung. J. thorac. Surg. **18**, 279 (1949). ~The architectural basis of pulmonary ventilation. Ann. Surg. **137**, 1 (1953). — CHURCHILL, E. D., and R. BEL-SEY: Segmental pneumonectomy in bronchiectasis. The lingula segment of the left upper lobe. Ann. Surg. **109**, 481 (1939). — CICERO, R., and A. CELIS: Ante-mortem and post-mortem angiography of the pulmonary arterial tree in advanced tuberculosis. Amer. Rev. Tuberc. **71**, 810 (1955). — CLEMENS, H. J.: Elektronenoptische Untersuchungen über den Bau der Alveolenwand in der Rattenlunge. Z. Zellforsch. **40**, 1 (1954). ~ Untersuchungen über das maximale Lungenluft-Volumen. Ein Beitrag zum Problem des postnatalen Lungenwachstums. Gegenbaurs morph. Jb. **95**, 447 (1955). ~ Training und Lungenwachstum. Gegenbaurs morph. Jb. **96**, 417 (1956). ~ Vorkommen, Lokalisation und Bedeutung von sauren Muco-polysacchariden in der Lunge. Topochemische Untersuchungen. Acta histochem. (Jena) **2**, 170 (1956). — CLEMENS, H. J., u. R. WILLNOW: Vorkommen, Lokalisation und Bedeutung von sauren Mucopolysacchariden in der Lunge. Ergebn. ges. Tuberk.-Forsch. (Stuttgart) **14**, 651 (1958). — CLÖSGES, J.: Beziehung zwischen Gewicht und Volumen der Lunge. Med. Inaug.-Diss. Düsseldorf 1949. — CLOETTA, M.: Eine neue Methodik zur Untersuchung der Lungenzirkulation. Naunyn-Schmiedeberg's Arch. exp. Path. Pharmak. **63**, 147 (1910). ~ Über die Zirkulation in der Lunge und deren Beeinflussung durch Über- und Unterdruck. Naunyn-Schmiedeberg's Arch. exp. Path. Pharmak. **66**, 409 (1911). ~ Untersuchungen über die Elastizität der Lunge und deren Bedeutung für die Zirkulation. Pflügers Arch. ges. Physiol. **152**, 339 (1913). — COCCHI, U.: Lungenemphysem. In: Lehrbuch der Röntgendiagnostik (SCHINZ-BAENSCH-FRIEDL-UEHLINGER), 5. Aufl., Bd. III/1. Stuttgart: Georg Thieme 1952. — COHN, J. E., D. G. CARROLL and R. L. RILEY: Respiratory acidosis in patients with emphysema. Amer. J. Med. **17**, 447 (1954). — COHNHEIM, J.: Vorlesungen über allgemeine Pathologie, Bd. II: Pathologie der Atmung. Berlin 1882. — COLLDAHL, H.: Gaswechsel und Gewebsatmung beim experimentellen Asthma des Meerschweinchens. Acta physiol. scand. **6**, Suppl. 18 (1943). — COLOMBO, C., E. BEATRICE e L. RULLA: Ricerche istologiche sull'atelectasia pol-monare sperimentale con particolare riguardo alla reversibilità della lesione. Arch. Chir.

Torace 9, 279 (1952). — Condorelli, L.: Physiopathologie de la circulation artérielle pulmo-naire. Schweiz. med. Wschr. 1950, 986. — Conolly, D. C., J. W. Kirklin and E. H. Wood: The relationship between pulmonary artery wedge pressure and left atrial pressure in man. Circulat. Res. 2, 434 (1954). — Cook, C. D., R. B. Cherry, D. O'Brien, P. Karlberg and C. A. Smith: Studies of respiratory physiology in the newborn infant. I. Observations on normal premature and full-term infants. J. clin. Invest. 34, 975 (1955). — Coryllos, P. N.: Postoperative apneumatosis (atelectasis) and postoperative pneumonia. J. Amer. med. Ass. 93, 98 (1929). ~ Alveolar gases exchanges and atelectasis. The mechanism of gas absorption in bronchial obstruction. Arch. Surg. (Chicago) 21, 1214 (1930). ~ Action of the diaphragm in cough. Amer. J. med. Sci. 194, 523 (1937). — Coryllos, P. N., and G. Birnbaum: Obstructive massive atelectasis of the lung. Arch. Surg. (Chicago) 16, 501 (1928). ~ The circulation in the compressed atelectatic and pneumonic lung. Arch. Surg. (Chicago) 19, 1346 (1929). — Cournand, A.: Recent observations on the dynamics of the pulmonary circulation. Bull. N.Y. Acad. Med. 23, 27 (1947). ~ Some aspects of the pulmonary circulation in normal man and in chronic pulmonary diseases. Circulation 2, 641 (1950). — Cournand, A., and F. B. Berry: The effect of pneumonectomy upon cardiopulmonary function in adult patients. Ann. Surg. 116, 532 (1942). — Cournand, A., and D. W. Richards jr.: Pulmonary insuffi-ciency. I. Discussion of physiological classification and presentation of clinical tests. Amer. Rev. Tuberc. 44, 26 (1941). — Crenshaw, L.: Degenerative lung disease. Dis. Chest 25, 427 (1954). — Cudkowicz, L.: Observations on the normal anatomy of the bronchial arteries. Thorax 6, 343 (1951). — Cudkowicz, L., and J. B. Armstrong: The bronchial arteries in pulmonary emphysema. Thorax 8, 46 (1953). — Curti, P.-C., L. Donno et G.-F. Scalfi: Le coeur pulmonaire en phthisiologie. J. méd. Leysin 10, 89 (1955).

Dale, W. A., and H. Rahn: Rate of gas absorption during atelectasis. Amer. J. Physiol. 170, 3 (1952). — Daly, de Burgh, I.: The resistance of the pulmonary vascular bed. J. Physiol. (Lond.) 69, 238 (1930). — Danziger, F.: Untersuchungen über die Luftbewegung in der Nase während des Atmens. Mschr. Ohrenheilk., N.F. 30, 331 (1896). — Dayman, H.: Mechanics of air-flow in health and emphysema. J. clin. Invest. 30, 1175 (1951). — Dean, R. B., and M. B. Visscher: The kinetics of lung ventilation. Amer. J. Physiol. 134, 450 (1941). — Deenstra, H.: Über ungleichmäßige Ventilation und Ventilationsdurchströmungs-verhältnisse bei Patienten mit Silicosis. In: Die Staublungenerkrankungen, Bd. 3, Darm-stadt: Steinkopff 1958. — Delarue, J.: Lesions broncho-pulmonaires et modifications circu-latoires. Atti Soc. lombarda Sci. med. biol. 9, 357 (1954). — Delarue, J., et R. Abelanet: Les bronchiectasies primitives. Étude expérimentale et essai d'interprétation pathogénique. Ann. anat. path., N.S. 1, 257 (1956). — Delarue, J. A., and R. M. Abelanet: Pathogenesis of bronchiectasis. An experimental study. Dis. Chest 35, 394 (1959). — Delius, L.: Klinische Beobachtungen zu den Fragwürdigkeiten des Cor pulmonale. Verh. dtsch. Ges. Kreisl.-Forsch. 21, 337 (1955). ~ Cor pulmonale. In: Klinik der Gegenwart, Bd. I. Berlin u. Wien: Urban & Schwarzenberg 1956. — Delorme, E.: Nouveau traitement des empyèmes chroniques. Gaz. Hôp. (Paris) 67, 94 (1894). — Deming, J., and J. P. Hanner: Respiration in infancy. II. A study of rate, volume and character of respiration in healthy infants during neonatal period. Amer. J. Dis. Child. 51, 823 (1936). — Denolin, H.: Le coeur pulmonaire chronique en médicine interne. Verh. dtsch. Ges. Kreisl.-Forsch. 21, 257 (1955). — Derbes, V. J., N. K. Weaver and A. L. Cotton: Complications of bronchial asthma. Amer. J. med. Sci., N.S. 222, 88 (1951). — Dett-mer, N.: Elektronenmikroskopische Untersuchungen über den Wandbau der Lungenalveole. Beitr. Silikose-Forsch. 45 (1956). — Dexter, L., J. W. Dow, F. W. Haynes, J. I. Whitten-berger, B. Ferris, W. Goodale and H. K. Hellems: Studies of the pulmonary circulation. J. clin. Invest. 29, 602 (1950). — Dina, M. A., e G. Cussini: Il significato delle aderence pleuriche al tavolo anatomico. Pathologica 46, 181 (1954). — Dirken, M. R. S., and H. Heemstra: Alveolar oxygen tension and lung circulation. Quart. J. exp. Physiol. 34, 193 (1948). — Dishoeck, H. A. E. van: Elektrogramm der Nasenflügelmuskeln und Nasenwiderstands-kurve. Acta oto-laryng. (Stockh.) 25, 285 (1937). — Döderlein, W.: Experimentelle Unter-suchungen über die physiologische Bedeutung der Nasennebenhöhlen. Z. Hals-, Nas.- u. Ohrenheilk. 30, 459 (1932). — Donald, K. W., J. M. Bishop, G. Cumming and O. L. Wade: The effect of exercise on the cardiac output and circulatory dynamics of normal subjects. Clin. Sci. 14, 37 (1955). — Donald, K. W., A. Renzetti, R. L. Riley and A. Cournand: Analysis of factors affecting concentrations of oxygen and carbon dioxide in gas and blood of lungs. Results. J. appl. Physiol. 4, 497 (1952). — Donders, F. C.: Beiträge zum Mechanis-mus der Respiration und Zirkulation im gesunden und kranken Zustande. Z. rat. Med., N.F. 3, 287 (1853). ~ Physiologie des Menschen, II. Aufl. 1859. — Doyle, J. T., J. S. Wilson and J. V. Warren: The pulmonary vascular response to short term hypoxia in human subjects. Circulation 5, 263 (1952). — Dreser, H.: Die Bewegung der Atemluft in den Alveolargängen der Lungen. Z. ges. exp. Med. 26, 223 (1922). — Dünner, L.: Pneumokoniosen durch Staub von Getreide und Saaten. In: Die Staublungenerkrankungen, Bd. 3, S. 541. Darmstadt: Steinkopff 1958. — Dufourt, A., J. Brun, J. Viallier, P. Buffard et M. Préault: Emphysème bulleux et emphysème bronchiectasique au cours de l'infection tuberculeuse.

Rev. Tuberc., Sér. V **16**, 635 (1952). — DUKE, H.: Pulmonary vasomotor reactions in isolated perfused cat lungs in response to inhalation of various mixtures of oxygen and nitrogen. J. Physiol. (Lond.) **111**, 17 (1950). ~ Pulmonary vasomotor responses of isolated perfused lungs to anoxia and hypercapnia. Quart. J. exp. Physiol. **36**, 75 (1951). — DUKE, H., and E. M. KILLICK: Pulmonary vasomotor responses of isolated perfused cat lungs to anoxia. J. Physiol. (Lond.) **117**, 303 (1952). — DUKEN, J.: Klinische und experimentelle Studien zur Pathogenese und Diagnostik der Bronchiektasie im Kindesalter. Z. Kinderheilk. **44**, 1 (1927). DUPREZ, A.: Les limites anatomiques de la dilatation des bronches. L'obstruction des petites bronches. J. franç. Méd. Chir. thorac. **5**, 442 (1951). ~ La dilatation des bronches. Acta Tuberc. belg. **44**, 5 (1953). ~ Les modifications des artères bronchiques et pulmonaires au cours de la dilatation des bronches. Rev. belge Path. **25**, 265 (1956).

EBERTH, C. J.: Über Hyperplasie der Muskeln des Lungenparenchyms. Virchows Arch. path. Anat. **72**, 96 (1878). — EBNER, V. v.: Von den Lungen. In: KÖLLIKERS Handbuch der Gewebelehre, 6. Aufl., Bd. 3. Leipzig: Wilhelm Engelmann 1902. — *Editorial*: Die Ätiologie der chronischen Bronchitis (Leitartikel). Brit. med. J. **1956**, 906. Ref. Medizinische **1957**, 473. — EDWARDS, J. E.: Structural changes of the pulmonary vascular bed and their functional significance in congenital heart disease. Proc. Inst. Med. Chicago **18**, 134 (1950). — EDWARDS, J. E., and H. B. BURCHELL: Multilobular pulmonary venous obstruction with pulmonary hypertension. Arch. intern. Med. **87**, 372 (1951). — EGER, W.: Über Bronchiolitis obliterans, hervorgerufen durch eine Cellulosebeize. Mit Bemerkungen zu einer Relationspathologie. Frankfurt. Z. Path. **62**, 551 (1951). — EHRICH, W. E.: Die Entzündung. In: Handbuch der allgemeinen Pathologie, Bd. VII/1. Berlin-Göttingen-Heidelberg: Springer 1956. — EICKHOFF, W.: Die pathologisch-anatomischen Grundlagen der Allergie. Stuttgart: Georg Thieme 1948. — EINTHOVEN, W.: Über die Wirkung der Bronchialmuskeln, nach einer neuen Methode untersucht, und über Asthma nervosum. Arch. f. Physiol. **51**, 367 (1892). — EISENREICH, F. X.: Untersuchungen über die Entstehung von Lungenatelektasen bei Ausschaltung der Lungennerven und unter anderen Bedingungen. Thoraxchirurgie 1, 262 (1953). — ELIASBERG, H., u. W. NEULAND: Die epituberkulöse Infiltration der Lunge bei tuberkulösen Säuglingen und Kindern. Jb. Kinderheilk. **93**, 88 (1920). ~ Zur Klinik der epituberkulösen und gelatinösen Infiltration der kindlichen Lunge. Jb. Kinderheilk. **94**, 102 (1921). — ELLIS, M. P., and A. E. LIVINGTON: A method of directly recording changes in the calibre of the bronchi. J. Physiol. (Lond.) **34**, 223 (1935). — ENGEL, ST.: Lungenmuskulatur. Dtsch. med. Wschr. 1948, 382. ~ Die Lunge des Kindes. Stuttgart: Georg Thieme 1950. ~ ~ The structure of the respiratory tissue in the newly-born. Acta anat. (Basel) **19**, 353 (1953). Zur vergleichenden Anatomie des respiratorischen Gewebes. Ergebn. ges. Tuberk.-Forsch. (Stuttgart) **14**, 1 (1958). — ENGELSTAD, R. B.: Über die Wirkungen der Röntgenstrahlen auf die Lungen. Acta radiol. (Stockh.), Suppl. **19**, 1 (1934). ~ Über die Reaktion der Lungen auf Röntgenbestrahlung. Strahlentherapie **52**, 299 (1935). — ENGHOFF, H.: Zur Frage des schädlichen Raumes bei der Atmung. Eine statistische Studie. Skand. Arch. Physiol. **63**, 15 (1932). ~ Volumen inefficax. Bemerkungen zur Frage des schädlichen Raumes. Uppsala Läk.-Fören. Försh., N.F. **44**, 191 (1938). — ENGSTRÖM, I., P. KARLBERG and S. KRAEPELIN: Respiratory studies in children. I. Lung volumes in healthy children, 6—14 years of age. Acta paediat. (Uppsala) **46**, 277 (1957). — ENTICKNAP, J. B.: Lung biopsy in mitral stenosis. J. clin. Path. **6**, 84 (1953). — EPPINGER, H.: Krankheiten der Lungen (Emphysem der Lungen). Ergebn. allg. Path. path. Anat. 8, 285 (1902). ~ Allgemeine und spezielle Zwerchfellpathologie. Wien 1911. — ESCH, D., u. F. GROSSE-BROCKHOFF: Tuberkulose und Kreislauf. Ergebn. ges. Tuberk.-Forsch. (Stuttgart) **14**, 207 (1958). — ESCHER, F.: Die Tracheal- und Bronchialstenosen. In: Handbuch der inneren Medizin, Bd. IV/2. Berlin-Göttingen-Heidelberg: Springer 1956. — ESSER, CL.: Die Lungensegmente bei den lobären Pneumonien. Dtsch. med. Wschr. 1948, 631. ~ Lungensegmente. Fortschr. Röntgenstr. **71**, 395 (1949). ~ Atypische Pneumonien und Infiltrate. Beitr. Klin. Tuberk. **104**, 182 (1950). ~ Zur Frage des unterschiedlichen Verhaltens bestimmter Lungenabschnitte. Klin. Wschr. **1950**, 81. ~ Topographische Ausdehnung der Bronchien im Röntgenbild mit Berücksichtigung der neuzeitlichen Nomenklatur. Fortschr. Röntgenstr., Erg.-Bd. **66** (1951). ~ Topographische Ausdeutung der Bronchien im Röntgenbild unter besonderer Berücksichtigung des Raumfaktors, 2. Aufl. Stuttgart: Georg Thieme 1957. — EULER, U. S. v.: Physiologie des Lungenkreislaufes. Verh. dtsch. Ges. Kreislauf-Forsch. **17**, 8 (1951). — EULER, U. S. v., and G. LILJESTRAND: Observations on the pulmonary arterial pressure in the cat. Acta physiol. scand. **12**, 301 (1946).

FANO, C. DA: Beitrag zur Frage der kompensatorischen Lungenhypertrophie. Virchows Arch. path. Anat. **207**, 160 (1912). — FARBER, J. E.: Bronchial stenosis and unexpendable lung. Amer. Rev. Tuberc. **43**, 779 (1941). ~ Unexpendable lungs. J. thorac. Surg. **11**, 424 (1942). — FARBER, J. E., and N. S. LINCOLN: The unexpendable lung. I. Statement of the problem. II. Case reports. Amer. Rev. Tuberc. **40**, 704, 710 (1939). — FELIX, W.: Untersuchungen über den Spannungszustand und die Bewegungen des gelähmten Zwerchfells. Z. ges. exp. Med. **33**, 458 (1923). ~ Anatomische, experimentelle und klinische Untersuchungen über den Nervus phrenicus und der Zwerchfellinnervation. Zbl. Chir. **71**, 283 (1927). ~ Topographische Anatomie des Brustkorbes, der Lunge und der Lungenfelle. In: Sauerbruch, Die Chirurgie der Brustorgane, 3. Aufl. Berlin: Springer 1928. ~ Über Relaxatio diaphragmatica. Zbl. Chir. **77**, 1671 (1932). ~ Zur Genese der Relaxatio diaphragmatica. Langenbecks Arch. klin. Chir. **276**, 444 (1953). ~ Über Relaxatio diaphragmatica. Bruns' Beitr. klin. Chir. **186**, 1 (1953). — Fenn, W. O.: Mechanics of respiration. Amer. J. Med. **10**, 77 (1951). — Fenn, W. O., A. B. Otis, H. Rahn, L. E. Chadwick and A. H. Hegnauer: Displacement of blood from the lungs by pressure breathing. Amer. J. Physiol. **151**, 258 (1947). — Feyrter, F.: Über die Masernpneumonie. Virchows Arch. path. Anat. **255**, 753 (1925). ~ Obduktionsbefund, bei Fleischner 1936 mitgeteilt. ~ Über diffuse endokrine Organe. Leipzig: Johann Ambrosius Barth 1938. ~ Zur Pathologie des argyrophilen Helle-Zellen-Organes im Bronchialbaum des Menschen. Virchows Arch. path. Anat. **325**, 723 (1954). — Fischer (-Wasels), B.: Pneumothorax durch Spitzennarbenblasen. Z. klin. Med. **95**, 1 (1922). — Fischer, F. K.: Konstruktiver Lungenbau. In: Lehrbuch der Röntgendiagnostik (Schinz-Baensch-Friedl-Uehlinger), Bd. III, 5. Aufl. Stuttgart: Georg Thieme 1952. ~ Bronchialbaum, Technik der Bronchographie. In: Lehrbuch der Röntgendiagnostik (Schinz-Baensch-Friedl-Uehlinger), 5. Aufl., Bd. III/1. Stuttgart: Georg Thieme 1952. ~ Bronchialerkrankungen. In: Lehrbuch der Röntgendiagnostik (Schinz-Baensch-Friedl-Uehlinger), 5. Aufl., Bd. III/1. Stuttgart: Georg Thieme 1952. — Fischer, P. A.: Zur Morphologie, Häufigkeit und pathogenetischen Bedeutung tuberkulöser lymphadenogener Bronchialwandschädigungen. Beitr. Klin. Tuberk. **113**, 1 (1955). — Fishman, A. P., A. Himmelstein, H. W. Fritts and A. Cournand: Blood flow through each lung in man during unilateral hypoxia. J. clin. Invest. **34**, 637 (1955). — Fishman, A. P., J. H. McClement, A. Himmelstein and A. Cournand: Effects of acute anoxia on the circulation and respiration in patients with chronic pulmonary disease studied during the „steady state". J. clin. Invest. **31**, 770 (1952). — Fleisch, A.: Proprioceptive Atmungsreflexe. Pflügers Arch. ges. Physiol. **219**, 706 (1928). ~ Beeinflussung der proprioceptiven Atmungsreflexe durch Adrenalin und Atropin. Pflügers Arch. ges. Physiol. **224**, 390 (1930). ~ Neuere Ergebnisse über Mechanik und proprioceptive Steuerung der Atmungsbewegung. Ergebn. Physiol. **36**, 249 (1934). — Fleisch, A., u. F. Lehner: Die respiratorische Mittellage. Helv. physiol. pharmacol. Acta **7**, 410 (1949). — Fleischner, F. G.: Atelektase und Lungentuberkulose. Beitr. Klin. Tuberk. **85**, 313 (1934). ~ Atelektase und gerichteter Kollaps der Lunge. Fortschr. Röntgenstr. **53**, 607 (1936). ~ Atelektase und atelektatische Pneumonie bei Ausstoßung oder Durchbruch eines tuberkulösen Drüsenherdes in den Bronchus. Beitr. Klin. Tuberk. **76**, 72 (1936). ~ Bronchial peristalsis. Amer. J. Roentgenol. **62**, 65 (1949). ~ The pathogenesis of chronic substantial (hypertrophic) emphysema. Amer. Rev. Tuberc. **62**, 45 (1950). — Florange, W.: Anatomie und Pathologie der Arteria bronchialis. Ergebn. allg. Path. path. Anat. **39**, 152 (1960). — Föppl, A.: Vorlesungen über technische Mechanik. III. Festigkeitslehre. Leipzig: Teubner 1919. — Folkow, B., and J. R. Pappenheimer: Components of the respiratory dead space and their variation with pressure breathing and with bronchoactive drugs. J. appl. Physiol. **8**, 102 (1955). — Forschbach, J., u. A. Bittorf: Die Beeinflussung der Mittellage der Lunge bei Gesunden. Münch. med. Wschr. **1910**, 1327. — Forssmann, I.: Zit. nach H. Schmidt 1957. — Forster, R. E.: Exchange of gases between alveolar air and pulmonary capillary blood: Pulmonary diffusing capacity. Physiol. Rev. **37**, 391 (1957). — Fowler, N. O., R. N. Westcott and R. C. Scott: Normal pressure in the right heart and pulmonary artery. Amer. Heart J. **46**, 264 (1953.) — Fowler, W. S.: Lung function studies. II. The respiratory dead space. Amer. J. Physiol. **154**, 405 (1948). ~ Respiratory dead space. In: Methods in medical research, Bd. II. Chicago: Year Book Publ. Inc. 1950. — Fraenkel, A.: Ein weiterer Beitrag zur Lehre von der Bronchiolitis obliterans fibrosa acuta. Berl. klin. Wschr. **1909**, 6. ~ Anatomisch-röntgenologische Untersuchungen über die Luftröhre. Fortschr. Röntgenstr. **21**, 267 (1913). — Frank, N. R., D. W. Cugell, E. A. Gaensler and L. B. Ellis: Ventilatory studies in mitral stenosis. A comparison with findings in primary pulmonary diseases. Amer. J. Med. **15**, 60 (1952). — Franke, G.: Experimentelle Untersuchungen über Luftdruck, Luftbewegung und Luftwechsel in der Nase und ihren Nebenhöhlen. Arch. Laryng. Rhin. (Berl.) **1**, 236 (1893). — Fresen, O.: Die gestaltliche Betrachtung des Morbus Boeck. Ergebn. ges. Tuberk.-Forsch. (Stuttgart) **14**, 603 (1958). — Freund, W. A.: Über primäre Thoraxanomalien, speziell über die starre Dilatation des Thorax als Ursache eines Lungenemphysems. Berlin 1906. ~ Über Wechselbeziehungen zwischen Lunge und Thorax beim Emphysem. Bemerkungen zur Arbeit des Herrn H. Loeschcke. Dtsch. med. Wschr. **1911**, 1254. ~ Der heutige Stand der Frage von dem Zusammenhang primärer Thoraxanomalien mit gewissen Lungenkrankheiten. Berl. klin. Wschr. **1912**, 1695. ~ Über das Emphysem. Dtsch. med. Wschr. **1913**, 603. — Friebel, H.: Studien an langdauerndem Asthma des Meerschweinchens. Naunyn-Schmiedeberg's Arch. exp. Path. Pharmakol. **217**, 29 (1953). ~ Über das experimentelle allergische Asthma der Meerschweinchen und seine Beziehungen zum Asthma des Menschen. II. Mitt. Internat. Arch. Allergy **5**, 401 (1954). — Friedlich, A. L., R. J. Bing and S. G. Blount jr.: Physiological study in congenital heart disease; circulatory dynamics in anomalies of venous return to heart including pulmonary arterio-venous fistula. Bull. Johns Hopk. Hosp. 86, 20 (1950). — FRÖHLICH, F.: Die „Helle Zelle" der Bronchialschleimhaut und ihre Beziehungen zumProblem der Chemorezeptoren. Frankfurt. Z. Path. 60, 517 (1949). — FROMME, HENRIETTE: Systematische Untersuchungen über die Gewichtsverhältnisse des Zwerchfells. Virchows Arch. path. Anat. 221, 117 (1916). — FRY, D. L., R. V. EBERT, W. W. STEAD and C. S. BROWN: The mechanics of pulmonary ventilation in normal subjects and in patients with pulmonary emphysema. Amer. J. Med. 16, 80 (1954). — FUEST u. HAAS: Alveolengröße und Kapillarisierungsgrad in menschlichen Lungen verschiedener Altersstufen. Tagg Nord- u. Westdtsch. Path., Kassel, 1958. Zbl. allg. Path. path. Anat. 99, 199 (1959).

GAD, J.: 1879; zit. nach MINKOWSKI u. BITTORF 1912. — GADERMANN, E.: Kardiologische Probleme im Zusammenhang mit Veränderungen im Lungenkreislauf. In: Lungen und kleiner Kreislauf. Bad Oeynhausener Gespräche I, 80 (1956). Berlin-Göttingen-Heidelberg: Springer 1957. — GAENSLER, E. A.: Ventilatory tests in bronchial asthma. J. Allergy 21, 232 (1950). ~ Analysis of the ventilatory defect by timed capacity measurements. Amer. Rev. Tuberc. 64, 256 (1951). ~ Bronchospirometry. I. Review of the literature. J. Lab. clin. Med. 39, 917 (1952). — GAENSLER, E. A., J. V. MALONEY and V. O. BJÖRK: Bronchospirometry. II. Experimental observations and theoretical considerations of resistance breathing. J. Lab. clin. Med. 39, 935 (1952). — GALY, P.: Étude anatomique et pathogénique des bronchiectasies. Ann. Oto-laryng. (Paris) 70, 587 (1953). — GALY, P., et L. PÉROL: Séquelles et complications tardives locales de la primo-infection tuberculeuse. Paris: Doin & Cie. 1952. — GARCIA RAMOS, J.: On the dynamics of the lungs capillary circulation. Amer. Rev. Tuberc. 71, 822 (1955). — GAUBATZ, E.: Über Funktionsprüfungen vor und nach operativer Kollapstherapie. I. Mitt. Beitr. Klin. Tuberk. 88, 730 (1936). ~ Über Funktionsprüfungen vor und nach operativer Kollapstherapie. II. Mitt. Funktionsprüfungen zur Pneumolyse. Beitr. Klin. Tuberk. 91, 201 (1938). — GAUER, O. H.: Die Wechselbeziehungen zwischen Herz- und Venensystem. Verh. dtsch. Ges. Kreisl.-Forsch. 22, 61 (1956). ~ Die Wirkungen von Aderlaß und Transfusion auf die wichtigsten Kreislaufabschnitte. Bibl. haemat., Suppl. ad Acta haemat. (Basel) 6, 61 (1957). — GAUER, O. H., u. J. P. HENRY: Beitrag zur Homöostase des extraarteriellen Kreislaufs. Klin. Wschr. 1956, 356. — GAVALLÉR, B. v.: Die hyalinen Membranen in der Lunge Frühgeborener. Verh. dtsch. Ges. Path. 1956, 191. — GEHLEN, H. v.: Neuere Auffassungen über die Retraktionskraft der Lunge und ihre Grundlagen. Anat. Anz. 87, Erg.-H., 394 (1939). ~ Der Acinus der menschlichen Lunge als elastisch-muskulöses System. Gegenbaurs Morph. Jb. 85, 186 (1940). — GEIGEL, R.: Untersuchungen über die Mechanik der Expectoration. Virchows Arch. path. Anat. 161, 173 (1900). — GERHARDT, D.: Experimentelle Beiträge zur Lehre vom Lungenkreislauf und von der mechanischen Wirkung pleuritischer Ergüsse. Z. klin. Med. 55, 195 (1904). ~ Über den Druck von Pleuraexsudaten. Naunyn-Schmiedeberg's Arch. exp. Path. Pharmak., Suppl. S. 228 (1908) (Festschrift für SCHMIEDEBERG). ~ Über gegenseitige Beeinflussung von Atmungs- und Kreislaufstörungen. Verh. naturforsch. Ges. Basel 21, 313 (1910). — GERICKE, I.: Vergleichende Betrachtungen über die formalen und funktionellen Unterschiede beim Eisenmengerkomplex mit offenem und geschlossenem Ductus arteriosus Botalli. Inaug.-Diss. Berlin-West 1955. — GERLACH, J.: Handbuch der allgemeinen und speziellen Gewebelehre des menschlichen Körpers für Ärzte und Studierende. Mainz: Janitsch 1849. — GERLACH, L.: Über die Beziehungen der Nn. vagi zu den glatten Muskelfasern der Lunge. Pflügers Arch. ges. Physiol. 13, 491 (1876). — GERSTEL, G.: Über die Veränderungen der Lungenblutgefäße bei Staublungenkranken. Veröff. Gewerbe- u. Konstit. path. H. 35, 42 (1933). — GEY, R.: Die Bronchitis deformans. Virchows Arch. path. Anat. 255, 528 (1925). — GHON, A.: Der primäre Lungenherd bei der Tuberkulose des Kindes. Wien: 1912. — GIAMPALMO, A., u. J. SCHOENMACKERS: Die Lunge bei Morbus caeruleus. Beitr. path. Anat. 112, 387 (1952). — GIESE, W.: Die schwielige Induration der Lungenlymphknoten. Beitr. path. Anat. 90, 555 (1933). ~ Die Ätiologie der interstitiellen plasmacellulären Säuglingspneumonie. Mschr. Kinderheilk. 101, 147 (1952). ~ Pathogenese und Ätiologie der interstitiellen plasmazellulären Säuglingspneumonie. Verh. dtsch. Ges. Path. 36, 284 (1953). ~ Bronchiolitis, Bronchiektasen und Pneumonie. Dtsch. med. J. 1954, 279. ~ Wandlungen der Tuberkulose unter dem Einfluß der Chemotherapie. (Referat.) Verh. dtsch. Ges. Path. 39, 74 (1956). ~ Die morphologischen Grundlagen der Ventilationsstörungen bei Emphysem und Bronchitis und ihre Rückwirkungen auf den Kreislauf. (Referat.) Verh. dtsch. Ges. inn. Med. 62, 12 (1956). ~ Pathologische Anatomie und Pathogenese der Pleuritis exsudativa. Wien. med. Wschr. 1957, 999. ~ Über die Endstrombahn der Lunge. In: Lungen und kleiner Kreislauf. Bad Oeynhausener Gespräche I, 45 (1956). Berlin-Göttingen-Heidelberg: Springer 1957. ~ Acinus und Lobulus der Lunge. Zbl. allg. Path. path. Anat. 97, 233 (1957). ~ Der Konstitutionsfaktor beim Emphysem. In: Die Staublungenerkrankungen, Bd. 3. Darmstadt: Steinkopff 1958. ~ Einteilung und Abgrenzung der Emphyseme. Verh. dtsch. Ges. Path. 43, 269 (1959). ~ Alterslunge und Altersemphysem. Medizinische 1959, 2447. ~ Pathomorphologie der Ventilationsstörungen (Referat). Verh. dtsch. Ges. Path. 44 (1960). — Atemorgane. In: Lehrbuch der speziellen Pathologie und Anatomie (KAUFMANN-STAEMMLER). Berlin:

W. de Gruyter & Co. 1960. — Giese, W., u. R. Gieseking: Die submikroskopische Struktur des fibrillären Grundgerüstes der Alveolarwand. Beitr. path. Anat. 117, 17 (1957). — Gieseking, R.: Elektronenoptische Beobachtungen im Alveolarbereich der Lunge. Beitr. path. Anat. 116, 177 (1956). ~ Stoffaufnahme in die Alveolarwand. Beitr. Silikose-Forsch., Sonderbd. 2, 571 (1957). ~ Elektronenoptische Beobachtung der Stoffaufnahme in die Alveolarwand. Verh. dtsch. Ges. Path. 41, 336 (1958). ~ Aufnahme und Ablagerung von Fremdstoffen in der Lunge nach elektronenoptischen Untersuchungen. Ergebn. allg. Path. path. Anat. 38, 92 (1958). ~ Das experimentelle Lungenödem im elektronenoptischen Bild. Verh. dtsch. Ges. Path. 42, 344 (1959). ~ Die chronische Stauungslunge im elektronenoptischen Bild. Beitr. path. Anat. (1960, in Druck). — Gilroy, J. C., V. H. Wilson and P. Marchand: Observations on the haemodynamics of pulmonary and lobar atelectasis. Thorax 6, 137 (1951). — Gilse, P. H. G. van: Die Atmung bei einem Neonatus mit doppelseitiger Choanalatresie. Acta oto-laryng. (Stockh.) 24, 205 (1936). — Gilson, J.: Bronchitis and emphysema in coalworkers pneumoconiosis. In: Die Staublungenerkrankungen, Bd. 3. Darmstadt: Steinkopff 1958. — Gläser, A.: Zur Pathologie der tracheobronchialen Schleimdrüsen. Zugleich ein weiterer Beitrag zur Dyschylie. Beitr. path. Anat. 119, 425 (1958). — Glaser, E. M., D. R. McPherson, K. M. Prior and E. Charles: Clin. Sci. 13, 461 (1954). Zit. nach Halmagyi 1957. — Gloor, F.: Zur Pathologie des Asthma bronchiale. Virchows Arch. path. Anat. 325, 189 (1954). — Gnüchtel, W., B. Löhr u. W. Ulmer: Bronchospirometrische Untersuchungen nach thoraxchirurgischen Eingriffen. I. Der Einfluß der Thorakotomie, Plastik, Segmentresektion und Lobektomie auf die Funktion der einzelnen Lungenflügel. Langenbecks Arch. klin. Chir. 281, 241 (1955). ~ Bronchospirometrische Untersuchungen nach thoraxchirurgischen Eingriffen. II. Vergleich prae- und postoperativer Untersuchungsergebnisse. Langenbecks Arch. klin. Chir. 281, 251 (1955). — Goebel, A.: Die Orthologie und Pathologie der Ausscheidung durch die Lunge. In: Handbuch der allgemeinen Pathologie, Bd. V/2. Berlin-Göttingen-Heidelberg: Springer 1959. — Görgényi-Göttche, O., u. D. Kassay: Atelektasen im Kindesalter. Ergebn. ges. Tuberk.-Forsch. (Stuttgart) 14, 389 (1958). — Gonzáles de Vega, N.: Die irrige Auffassung von der „Insufflations-", Ballon-", Spannungs-" usw. Kaverne. Beitr. Klin. Tuberk. 105, 362 (1951). — Goralewski, G.: Bronchitis-Emphysem-Silikose. Med. Klin. 1956, 2117. — Gordonoff, T.: Gibt es eine Bronchialperistaltik? Z. ges. exp. Med. 97, 1 (1936). ~ Physiologie und Pharmakologie des Expektorationsvorganges. Ergebn. Physiol. 40, 53 (1938). — Gordonoff, T., u. N. Scheinfinkel: Untersuchungen über die angebliche „Bronchialperistaltik". Z. ges. exp. Med. 99, 1 (1936). — Gough, J.: Discussion on the diagnosis of pulmonary emphysema. Proc. roy. Soc. Med. 45, 576 (1952). — Graham, E. A., T. H. Burford and J. H. Mayer: Middle lobe syndrome. Postgrad. Med. 4, 29 (1948). — Grassmann, W.: Bau und Bildung der kollagenen Faser. Beitr. Silikose-Forsch., Sonderbd., Grundfragen zur Silikoseforschung I, S. 137. 1956. — Gray, J. S., and F. S. Grodins: Respiration. Ann. Rev. Physiol. 12, 218 (1951). — Gray, J. S., F. S. Grodins and E. T. Carter: Alveolar and total ventilation and the dead space problem. J. appl. Physiol. 9, 307 (1956). — Green, A. E., and R. T. Shield: Proc. roy. Soc. A 202, 407 (1950). Zit. nach Gough. — Greene, J. A., and R. H. Heeren: Clinical studies of respiration. V. Relation of dyspnea and air hunger to changes of the expiratory volume of the chest. Arch. intern. Med. 57, 100 (1936). — Greene, J. A., and L. W. Swanson: Clinical studies of respiration. VI. Exspiratory inflation during air hunger and dyspnea produced by physical exertion in normal subjects and in patients with heart disease. Arch. intern. Med. 61, 720 (1938). — Grethmann, W.: Zur Pathologie der Miliartuberkulose. Beitr. Klin. Tuberk. 71, 1 (1928). ~ The architecture of the terminal sections of the bronchi of the human lung. Amer. Rev. Tuberc. 31, 261 (1935). — Grob, M., u. E. Rossi: Dis Diagnostik der angeborenen Angiocardiopathien. Helv. med. Acta 4, 189 (1949). — Gronemeyer, W.: Die chronische allergische Bronchitis einschließlich gewerblicher Formen. Verh. dtsch. Ges. inn. Med. 62, 106 (1956). — Grosse-Brockhoff, F.: Einführung in die pathologische Physiologie. Berlin-Göttingen-Heidelberg: Springer 1950. ~ Hämodynamik der Lungenkreislaufstörungen. Verh. dtsch. Ges. Kreisl.-Forsch. 17, 34 (1951). ~ Pathophysiologie des Lungenkreislaufes. In: Lungen und kleiner Kreislauf. Bad Oeynhausener Gespräche I, 64 (1956). Berlin-Göttingen-Heidelberg: Springer 1957. — Grosse-Brockhoff, F., u. G. Iseken: Zur Frage der Häufigkeit der Operationsindikation bei Mitralstenose. Z. Kreisl.-Forsch. 44, 402 (1954). — Grosse-Brockhoff, F., G. Neuhaus u. A. Schaede: Herzbelastung bei arterio-venösen und veno-venösen Anastomosen im großen bzw. im kleinen Kreislauf. Z. Kreisl.-Forsch. 44, 388 (1954). — Grosse-Brockhoff, F., u. W. Schoedel: Der effektive schädliche Raum. Pflügers Arch. ges. Physiol. 238, 501 (1937). ~ Physiologie und Pathophysiologie des Kreislaufes. In: Handbuch der Thoraxchirugie. Berlin-Göttingen-Heidelberg: Springer 1957. — Gruber, G. B.: Zur Kenntnis kranialer Doppelbildung beim Menschen mit Zwerchfellfehlern und mit Herzbeutel-Lunge. Beitr. path. Anat. 110, 346 (1949). ~ Zwerchfellücken, Zwerchfellhernien und Zwerchfelldefekte. Bruns' Beitr. klin. Chir. 186, 129 (1953). — Guyton, A. C., D. Polizo and G. G. Armstrong: Mean circulatory filling pressure measured immediately after cessation of heart pumping. Amer. J. Physiol. 179, 261 (1954).

HAAG, W., u. F. X. EISENREICH: Experimentelle Untersuchungen zur patho-physiologischen Bedeutung der Kollateralventilation. Thoraxchirurgie 4, 52 (1956). — HAAHTI, H. G.: Beobachtungen über einen Fall mit ausgedehnten intrapulmonalen lufthaltigen Hohlräumen. Acta radiol. (Stockh.) 13, 620 (1932). — HAAS, J. H.: Untersuchungen über die Größe der Alveolen in menschlichen Lungen verschiedener Altersstufen. Inaug.-Diss. Köln 1958. — HAASLER, F.: Über kompensatorische Hypertrophie der Lunge. Virchows Arch. path. Anat. 128, 527 (1892). — HADORN, W.: Über die Bestimmung des Exspirationsstoßes (Maximale Ausatmungsstromstärke). Z. klin. Med. 140, 266 (1942). ~ Untersuchungen über das Lungenemphysem. Ein neues Pneumometer zur Messung der maximalen Exspirationsstärke. Helv. med. Acta 10, 81 (1943). ~ Über die Fragwürdigkeit der Diagnose Essentielles Lungenemphysem. Dtsch. med. Wschr. 1959, 213. — HADORN, W., W. BERGER u. F. WYSS: Die quantitative Beurteilung asthmatischer und verwandter Zustände. Int. Arch. Allergy 2, 214 (1951). — HAEFLIGER, E., u. G. MARK: Segment und Lungentuberkulose. Berlin-Göttingen-Heidelberg: Springer 1956. ~ Therapie der Lungentuberkulose. In: Handbuch der inneren Medizin, Bd. IV/3. Berlin-Göttingen-Heidelberg: Springer 1956. — HAEMMERLI, U.: Diffuse progressive interstitielle Lungenfibrose (Hamman-Rich-Syndrom). Schweiz. med. Wschr. 1955, 597. — HALDANE, J. S.: Respiration. New Haven: Yale Univ. Press 1927. — HALDANE, J. S., and J. G. PRIESTLEY: The regulation of the lung-ventilation. J. Physiol. (Lond.) 21, 240 (1905). — HALMAGYI, D. F. J.: Die klinische Physiologie des kleinen Kreislaufs. Jena: VEB Fischer 1957. — HALPERN, B. N.: Les antihistaminiques de synthèse. Essais de chimiothérapie des états allergiques. Arch. int. Pharmacodyn. 68, 339 (1942). — HAMM, J.: Die Bedeutung der Sirographie für die Beurteilung der Lungeninsuffizienz, speziell des Emphysems. Ergebn. inn. Med. Kinderheilk. 10, 299 (1958). — HAMMAN, L., and A. R. RICH: Fulminating diffuse interstitial fibrosis of the lungs. Tr. Amer. clin. climat. Ass. 51, 154 (1935). ~ Acute diffuse interstitial fibrosis of the lungs. Bull. Johns Hopk. Hosp. 74, 177 (1944). — HANSEMANN, D. v.: Über die Poren der normalen Lungenalveolen. S.-B. preuß. Akad. Wiss., phys.-math. Kl. 44 (1895). ~ Untersuchungen über die Entstehung des Lungenemphysems. Berl. klin. Wschr. 1899, 438. ~ Die Lymphangitis reticularis der Lungen als selbständige Erkrankung. Virchows Arch. path. Anat. 220, 311 (1915). ~ Allgemeine aetiologische Betrachtungen mit besonderer Berücksichtigung des Lungenemphysems. Virchows Arch. path. Anat. 221, 94 (1916). — HANSEN, K.: Allergie, 3. Aufl. Stuttgart: Georg Thieme 1957. — HARRIS, W. H., and F. P. CHILLINGWORTH: The experimental production in dogs of emphysema with associated asthmatic syndrom by means of an intratracheal ball valve. J. exp. Med. 30, 75 (1919). — HART, C., u. E. MAYER: Kehlkopf, Luftröhre und Bronchien. In: Handbuch der speziellen pathologischen Anatomie und Histologie (HENKE-LUBARSCH), Bd. III/1. Berlin: Springer 1928. — HARTROFT, S. W.: The microscopic diagnosis of pulmonary emphysema. Amer. J. Path. 21, 889 (1945). — HARTROFT, S. W., and C. C. MACKLIN: Intrabronchial fixation of the human lung for purposes of alveolar measurement. Trans. roy. Soc. Can., Sect. V 37, 75 (1943). — HARTUNG, W.: Über die Bestimmung der Lungenelastizität an der isolierten Leichenlunge. Beitr. path. Anat. 117, 90 (1957). ~ Die Altersveränderungen der Lungenelastizität nach Messungen an isolierten Leichenlungen. Beitr. path. Anat. 118, 368 (1958). ~ Morphologie des bullösen Emphysems, seine Abgrenzung gegen Lungendystrophie. Beitr. Klin. Tuberk. 119, 343 (1958). ~ Elastizitätsmessungen an Leichenlungen als Beitrag zur Pathogenese des Emphysems. Verh. dtsch. Ges. Path. 42, 178 (1959). ~ Über Ausmaß und funktionelle Bedeutung des Elastizitätsverlustes bei verschiedenen Lungenerkrankungen. Beitr. path. Anat. 120, 178 (1959). — Morphologische und histomechanische Analyse der Ventilationsstörungen, unter besonderer Berücksichtigung des Lungenemphysems. Ergebn. inn. Med. Kinderheilk. 15, 273 (1960). ~ Histomechanik der Ventilationsstörungen (Referat). Verh. dtsch. Ges. Path. 44 (1960). — HARTUNG, W. u. L. DELFMANN: Perfusionsversuche an Leichenlungen. Beitr. Klin. Tuberk. 123, 41 (1960). — HARVEY, R. M., and I. M. FERRER: Pulmonary circulation: its relation to altered dynamics. Dis. Chest 25, 247 (1954). — HARVEY, R. M., I. M. FERRER, D. W. RICHARDS jr. and A. COURNAND: Influence of chronic pulmonary disease on the heart and circulation. Amer. J. Med. 10, 719 (1951). — HASLINGER, F.: Die organischen Stenosen der unteren Trachealabschnitte und der Bronchien. Mschr. Ohrenheilk. 63, 357, 560, 617, 782 (1929). — HASLINGER, F., u. K. HITZENBERGER: Das Mediastinalwandern bei künstlicher Bronchusstenose. Wien. klin. Wschr. 1926, 1035. — HAUDEK, M.: Durchwanderungspleuritis bei abdominalen Krankheitsprozessen. Fortschr. Röntgenstr. 45, 1 (1932). — HAUSSER, R., u. A. GRIMMINGER: Über die Luftcystenerkrankung der Lunge. Fortschr. Röntgenstr. 87, 283 (1957). — HAYASHI, J.: Über tödlichen Pneumothorax durch Infarkt und Emphysem. Frankfurt. Z. Path. 16, 1 (1915). — HAYEK, H. v.: Die Läppchen und septa interlobularia der menschlichen Lunge. Z. Anat. 110, 405 (1940). ~ Über periarterielle Lymphräume in der menschlichen Lunge. Anat. Anz. 89, 219 (1940). ~ Bau und Funktion der Alveolarepithelien. Anat. Anz. 93, 149 (1942). ~ Reaktionsfähigkeit der Alveolarepithelien und Lungenödem. Klin. Wschr. 1943, 637. ~ Über die Beziehungen der Alveolarepithelien zu den Kapillaren. Klin. Wschr. 1948, 723. ~ Über Verengung der Bronchi und Bronchioli durch ihre Muskulatur. Wien. klin. Wschr. 1948, 114. ~ Zur Frage der Lungenmuskulatur. Klin. Wschr. 1950, 268. ~ Muskulatur und Lungenparenchym. Z. Anat. 115, 88 (1950). ~ Über die funktionelle Anatomie der Lungengefäße. Verh. dtsch. Ges. Kreisl.-Forsch. 17, 17 (1951). ~ Über reaktive Formveränderungen der Alveolarepithelzellen bei verschiedenem Sauerstoffangebot. Z. Anat. 115, 436 (1951). ~ Die menschliche Lunge und ihre Gefäße, ihr Bau unter besonderer Berücksichtigung der Funktion. Ergebn. Anat. Entwickl.-Gesch. 34, 144 (1952). ~ Zur Anatomie der menschlichen Lunge, der Lungenläppchen und der Alveolenwand unter besonderer Berücksichtigung der Funktion. Wien. klin. Wschr. 1952, 249. ~ Anatomisches zur Frage des Asthma bronchiale. Klin. Wschr. 1952, 625. ~ Über die Veränderlichkeit der Oberflächenspannung in den Alveolen und ihre Bedeutung für die Retraktionskraft der Lunge. Naunyn-Schmiedeberg's Arch. exp. Path. Pharmak. 214, 266 (1952). ~ Die menschliche Lunge. Berlin-Göttingen-Heidelberg: Springer 1953. ~ Die Alveolarepithelien und die pulmonalen Gefäßanastomosen. Ref. Beitr. Silikose-Forsch., Sonderbd., 1955, 229. ~ Anatomische Grundlagen der Lungenfunktion. In: Lungen und kleiner Kreislauf. Bad Oeynhausener Gespräche I, 5 (1956). Berlin-Göttingen-Heidelberg: Springer 1957. — Hayek, H., F. Braunsteiner u. F. Pakesch: Über die Veränderlichkeit der Microvilli der Alveolarepithelien bei Temperaturveränderungen. Wien. Z. inn. Med. 38, 165 (1957). ~ Über das Zugrundegehen und die Neubildung von Mitochondrien in Alveolarepithelzellen. Wien. klin. Wschr. 1958, 951. — Hayward, G. W., and J. M. S. Knott: The effect of excercise on lung distensibility and respiratory work in mitral stenosis. Brit. Heart J. 17, 303 (1955). — Heard, B. E.: Further observations on the pathology of pulmonary emphysema in chronic bronchitis. Thorax 14, 58 (1959). — Heath, D., and W. Whitaker: The pulmonary vessels in patent ductus arteriosus. J. Path. Bact. 70, 285 (1955). ~ The pulmonary vessels in mitral stenosis. J. Path. Bact. 70, 291 (1955). — Heckmann, K.: Der broncho-alveoläre Hypertonus. (Ein Beitrag zur Genese der Höhlenbildungen in den Lungen und des Lungenemphysems.) Münch. med. Wschr. 1951, 910, 962. — Heemstra, H.: Alveolaire zuurstof-spanning en longcirculatie. Groningen: van der Kamp 1948. ~ The development of an increased pulmonary vascular resistance by local hypoxia. Quart. J. exp. Physiol. 39, 83 (1954). — Hegglin, R.: Die Lungenfibrose. In Handbuch der inneren Medizin, 4. Aufl., Bd. IV/2. Berlin: Springer 1956. ~ Die rheumatische Pneumonie. In: Handbuch der inneren Medizin, 4. Aufl., Bd. IV/2. Berlin-Göttingen-Heidelberg: Springer 1956. ~ Die Zirkulationsstörungen der Lunge. (Mit Beiträgen zur pathologischen Anatomie von E. Uehlinger.) In: Handbuch der inneren Medizin, 4. Aufl., Bd. IV/2. Berlin-Göttingen-Heidelberg: Springer 1956. — Heilmeyer, L., u. H. Begemann: Die Polyglobulie und Polycythaemie. In: Blut und Blutkrankheiten. Handbuch der inneren Medizin, 4. Aufl., Bd. II. Berlin-Göttingen-Heidelberg: Springer 1951. — Heilmeyer, L., u. F. Schmid: Die progressive Lungendystrophie. Dtsch. med. Wschr. 1956, 1293, 2118. — Hein, J.: Über den Stand der chirurgischen Behandlung der Lungentuberkulose im In- und Ausland. Beitr. Klin. Tuberk. 104, 37 (1950). — Hein, J., W. Kremer u. W. Schmidt: Die Kollapsbehandlung der Lungentuberkulose. Leipzig: Georg Thieme 1938. — Heine, F.: Das bullöse Lungenemphysem. Beitr. Klin. Tuberk. 119, 298 (1958). ~ Die Pneumothoraxatelektasen. Habil.-Schr. Münster 1960. — Heine, F., W. Benesch u. C. W. Hertz: Untersuchungen zur Methodik der Atemgrenzwertbestimmung. Z. Tuberk. 102, 273 (1953). — Heine, F., u. M. Hell: Über den Einfluß der temporären Phrenicusquetschung auf die Atemfunktion. Beitr. Klin. Tuberk. 109, 266 (1953). ~ Kymographische Studien über den Mechanismus des Waagebalkenphänomens bei gelähmtem Zwerchfell. Beitr. Klin. Tuberk. 116, 376 (1957). — Heine, F., u. O. Nagel: Das EKG nach arterieller Luftembolie. Arch. Kreisl.-Forsch. 17, 378 (1952). — Heine, F., u. E. Schürmeyer: Über spirographische Befunde beim bullösen Lungenemphysem. Beitr. Klin. Tuberk. 119, 337 (1958). — Hellems, H. K., F. W. Haynes and L. Dexter: Pulmonary „capillary" pressure in man. J. appl. Physiol. 2, 24 (1949). — Heller: Klinische und experimentelle Beiträge zur Kenntnis der akuten Lungenatelektase durch obturierenden Fremdkörperverschluß der Bronchien. Z. ges. exp. Med. 2, 453 (1914). — Helliesen, P. J., C. D. Cook, S. Friedlander and S. Agathon: Studies of respiratory physiology in children. I. Mechanics of respiration and lung volumes in 85 normal children 5 to 17 years of age. Pediatrics 22, 80 (1958). — Hellin, D.: Die Folgen von Lungenexstirpation. Eine experimentelle Untersuchung. Naunyn-Schmiedeberg's Arch. exp. Path. Pharmak. 55, 21 (1906). — Hellmann, K.: Untersuchungen zur normalen und pathologischen Physiologie der Nase. Z. Laryng. Rhinol. 15, 1 (1927). — Hellmann, K., u. H. Siegmund: Entzündungen im Bereich der oberen Luft- und Speisewege. In: Pathologie der oberen Luft- und Speisewege (Blumenfeld u. Jaffé). Leipzig: Curt Kabitzsch 1931. — Hempel, J.: Untersuchungen über Veränderungen der Thoraxatmung bei experimentellen Atmungsstörungen. Naunyn-Schmiedeberg's Arch. exp. Path. Pharmak. 169, 254 (1933). — Hempel, K.-J.: Über Knorpelringbildungen der Trachea. Frankfurt. Z. Path. 68, 35 (1957). — Henderson, G., F. P. Chillingworth and J. L. Whitney: The respiratory dead space. Amer. J. Physiol. 38, 1 (1915). — Henderson, Y.: The physiology of atelectasis. J. Amer. med. Ass. 93, 96 (1929). — Henle, J.: Über Tonus, Krampf und Lähmung der Bronchien und über Expektoration. Z. rat. Med. 1, 249 (1844). Zit. nach Gordonoff 1938. — Henrici: Über respiratorische Druckschwankungen in den Nebenhöhlen der Nase. Z. Sinnesphysiol. 41, 283 (1907). — Henry, E. W.: The small pulmonary vessels in mitral stenosis. Brit. Heart J. 14, 406

(1952). — HEPPLESTON, A. G.: The pathological anatomy of simple pneumoconiosis in coal workers. J. Path. Bact. **66**, 235 (1953). — HERBERG, D., G. REICHEL u. W. T. ULMER: Untersuchungen über die Abhängigkeit des absoluten und funktionellen Totraumes von der Ausatemgeschwindigkeit, alveolären Kohlesäurekonzentration, Atemmittellage und vom Lebensalter. Pflügers Arch. ges. Physiol. **270**, 467 (1959/60). — HERTZ, C. W.: Pleuraschwarte und Lungenfunktion. I. Folgezustände nach Pleuritis exsudativa. Beitr. Klin. Tuberk. **112**, 446 (1953). ~ Pleuraschwarte und Lungenfunktion. II. Folgezustände nach Pneumothorax mit röntgenologisch nachweisbarer Pleuraschwarte. Beitr. Klin. Tuberk. **112**, 503 (1954). ~ Die Durchblutungsgröße hypoventilierter Lungenbezirke. Verh. dtsch. Ges. Kreisl.-Forsch. **21**, 447 (1955). ~ Untersuchungen über den Einfluß der alveolaren Gasdrucke auf die intrapulmonale Durchblutungsverteilung beim Menschen. Klin. Wschr. **1956**, 472. ~ Einseitige alveolare CO_2-Erhöhung und Durchblutungsgröße jeder Lungenseite beim Menschen. Klin. Wschr. **1956**, 532. ~ Störungen der Ventilation. In: Lungen- und kleiner Kreislauf. Bad Oeynhausener Gespräche I, 127 (1956). Berlin-Göttingen-Heidelberg: Springer 1957. — HERTZ, C. W., H. DEREN, W. REGEL u. H. WEMMERS: Pleuraschwarte und Lungenfunktion. III. Bronchospirometrische Untersuchungen. Beitr. Klin. Tuberk. **113**, 199 (1955). — HERTZ, C.W., u. G. HERTZ: Luftembolie. Theoretische und experimentelle Untersuchung über das Zustandekommen der Embolisierung von Gefäßen durch Luft. Arch. Kreisl.-Forsch. **19**, 330 (1953). — HERXHEIMER, H.: The influence of costal and abdominal pressure on the action of the diaphragma in normal and emphysematous subjects. Thorax **3**, 122 (1948). — HERZOG, H.: Exspiratorische Stenose der Trachea und der großen Bronchien, hervorgerufen durch eine erschlaffte Pars membranacea. Dtsch. med. Wschr. **1959**, 1766. — HERZOG, H., u. R. NISSEN: Erschlaffung und exspiratorische Invagination des membranösen Teils der intrathorakalen Luftröhre und der Hauptbronchien als Ursache der asphyktischen Anfälle beim Asthma bronchiale und der chronischen asthmoiden Bronchitis des Lungenemphysems. Schweiz. med. Wschr. **1954**, 217. — HERZOG, W., u. F. W. CONRAD: Zur Frage der Lymphknotensilikose mit besonderer Berücksichtigung der Nervenveränderungen durch silikotisch verschwielte Lymphknoten. Arch. Gewerbepath. Gewerbehyg. **14**, 117 (1955). — HESS, W. R.: Die Regulierung der Atmung. Leipzig: Georg Thieme 1931. ~ Die Rolle des Vagus in der Selbststeuerung der Atmung. Pflügers Arch. ges. Physiol. **237**, 24 (1936). — HESS, W. R., u. O. A. M. WYSS: Die Analyse der physikalischen Atmungsregulierung anhand der Aktionsstrombilder des Phrenicus. Pflügers Arch. ges. Physiol. **237**, 761 (1936). — HEUCK, F.: Die Streifenatelektasen der Lunge. Stuttgart: Georg Thieme 1959. — HEUCK, F., u. A. FLACH: Tierexperimentelle und klinische Studien zur Entstehung von plattenförmigen Lungenatelektasen. Z. ges. exp. Med. **122**, 76 (1953). — HICKAM, J. B., and W. H. CARGILL: Effect of exercise on cardiac output and pulmonary arterial pressure in normal persons and in patients with cardio-vasculare disease and pulmonary emphysema. J. clin. Invest. **27**, 10 (1948). — HIERONYMI, G.: Über den altersbedingten Formwandel menschlicher Lungen. Ergebn. allg. Path. path. Anat. (1960, im Druck). HILL, L.: The capillary blood-pressure. J. Physiol. (Lond.) **54**, 24 (1921). — HIRSCH, S.: Über die morphologischen Merkmale der Vasokonstriktion beim Menschen; zugleich ein Beitrag zum Problem der Funktion der glatten Muskelfaser. Acta med. scand. **152**, 381 (1955). ~ Der Wandbau der kleinen Lungengefäße des Menschen unter lebensnahen Präparationsbedingungen. Medizinische **1958**, 680. — HIRSCHMANN, H.: Zur Lehre über den feineren Bau des Lungenparenchyms bei Säugetieren. Virchows Arch. path. Anat. **36**, 335 (1866). — HIS, W.: Zur Bildungsgeschichte der Lungen beim menschlichen Embryo. Arch. Anat. u. Physiol., Anat. Abt. **1887**, 89. — HITZENBERGER, K.: Das Zwerchfell im gesunden und kranken Zustand. Wien: Springer 1927. HOCHREIN, M., u. J. SCHLEICHER: Die Funktion des kardiopulmonalen Systems. Med. Klin. **1953**, 765.— HÖRA, J.: Zur Histologie der klinischen „Primären Pulmonalsklerose". Frankfurt. Z. Path. **47**, 100 (1935). — HÖRSTER, A.: Methoden und bisherige Ergebnisse zur Untersuchung der Frage der Bronchusperistaltik. Inaug.-Diss. Bonn 1941. — HOFBAUER, L.: Störungen der äußeren Atmung. Ergebn. inn. Med. Kinderheilk. **4**, 1 (1909). ~ Zur Pathogenese des Lungenemphysems. Dtsch. med. Wschr. **1912**, 1534. ~ Verbildung des Brustkorbes als Folge von Atemstörungen. Ergebn. allg. Path. path. Anat. **19**, II, 1 (1921). ~ Atmungspathologie und Therapie. Berlin: Springer 1921. ~ Pathologische Physiologie der Atmung. In: Handbuch der normalen und pathologischen Physiologie (BETHE-BERGMANN), Bd. II. Berlin: Springer 1925. — HOFBAUER, L., u. W. KOLMER: Versuch einer klinischen Gruppeneinteilung des Lungenemphysems. Wien. Arch. inn. Med. **15**, 271 (1928). — HOFF, F.: Klinische Physiologie und Pathologie, 2. Aufl. Stuttgart: Georg Thieme 1952. — HOFFMANN, U., u. K. KÜHN: Kollagen. Proc. of the Stockholm Conf. on Electr. Microscopy **1956**, 220. — HUDSON, W. A., and H. A. JARRE: Functional studies of the tracheobronchial tree with the aid of the cinex camera. Brit. J. Radiol. **2**, 523 (1929). — HUIZINGA, E.: Über die Physiologie des Bronchialbaumes. Ned. T. Geneesk. **1937**, 3829. ~ Über die Physiologie des Bronchialbaumes. Pflügers Arch. ges. Physiol. **238**, 767 (1937). ~ La bronchosténose. Bronches 1, 71 (1951). ~ La motilité de la paroi bronchique. Bronches 2, 26 (1952). ~ Bronchography in bronchial cancer and collateral ventilation. J. thorac. Surg. **23**, 445 (1952). — HUIZINGA, E., and E. BEHR: On the division of the lungsegments. Acta radiol. (Stockh.) **21**,

314 (1940). — Huizinga, E., and G. J. Smelt: Bronchography. Assen, Netherlands: Van Gorcum 1949. — Huizinga, E., et C. G. Smit: Collapsus du poumon. Bronches 1, 281 (1951). — Hultén, O.: Beitrag zur Röntgendiagnose der akuten Pankreasaffektionen. Acta radiol. (Stockh.) 9, 222 (1928). — Humperdinck, K.: Chronische Bronchitis, Emphysem. Eine Berufskrankheit der Bergleute? Med. wiss. Beitr. Krankenhaus Bochum 6, 3 (1955). ~ Emphysem-Bronchitis und Berufsarbeit. Med. Klin. 1956, 91. — Hurtado, A., and C. Boller: Studies of total pulmonary capacity and its subdivisions. I. Normal absolute and relative values. J. clin. Invest. 12, 793 (1933). — Hurtado, A., W. W. Fray and W. S. McCann: Studies of total pulmonary capacity and its subdividions. IV. Preliminary observations on cases of pulmonary emphysema and pneumoconiosis. J. clin. Invest. 12, 833 (1933). — Hurtado, A., N. L. Kaltreider, W. W. Fray, W. D. W. Brooks and W. S. McCann: Studies of total pulmonary capacity and its subdivisions. VI. Observations on cases of obstructive pulmonary emphysema. J. clin. Invest. 13, 102 (1934). — Husten, K.: Über den Lungenacinus und den Sitz der acinösen phthisischen Prozesse. Beitr. path. Anat. 68, 496 (1921). ~ Die anatomischen Veränderungen des Herzens bei der Silikose. Beitr. Silikose-Forsch. Ber. Med. Wiss. Tagg 1951, S. 7. ~ Das Emphysem und die chronische Bronchitis des Ruhrbergmanns. Statistische Auswertung von Obduktionsbefunden. Verh. dtsch. Ges. inn. Med. 62, 112 (1956). ~ Das Emphysem und die chronische Bronchitis des Ruhrbergmanns. Statistische Auswertung von Obduktionsbefunden. Knappschaftsarzt H. 8, 11 (1956), Ruhrknappschaft Bochum. ~ Die Abhängigkeit der chronischen Bronchitis und des Lungenemphysems von der Lungenverstaubung und der Silikose. (Referat.) 3. Internat. Staublungentagg, Münster 1957. In: Die Staublungenerkrankungen, Bd. 3, S. 396. Darmstadt: Steinkopff 1958. — Huzly, A.: Posttuberkulöses Syndrom, Mittellappensyndrom, Lappen- und Segmentsyndrom. Tuberk-Arzt 8, 70 (1954). — Huzly, A., u. F. Böhm: Bronchus und Tuberkulose. Stuttgart: Georg Thieme 1955.

Illig, L.: Kapillar-„Kontraktivität", Kapillar-„Sphinkter" und „Zentralkanäle". (A.-V. Bridges.) Klin. Wschr. 1957, 7. — Irwin, J. W., W. S. Burrage, Ch. E. Aimar and R. W. Chestnut jr.: Microscopical observations of the pulmonary arterioles, capillaries, and venules of living guinea pigs and rabbits. Anat. Rec. 119, 391 (1954). — Isaaksohn: Pathologisch-anatomische Veränderungen der Lungengefäße beim Emphysem. Virchows Arch. path. Anat. 53, 466 (1871).

Jaccard, G.: Erkrankungen der Pleura. In: Handbuch der inneren Medizin, 4. Aufl., Bd. IV/4. Berlin-Göttingen-Heidelberg: Springer 1956. — Jackson, Ch.: The bronchial tree; its study by insufflation. Trans. Amer. laryng. Ass. 1918, 319. — Jackson, Ch., and Ch. L. Jackson: Diseases of the nose, throat and ear. Philadelphia 1945. ~ Bronchooesophagology. Philadelphia u. London: W. B. Saunders Company 1950. — Jackson, Ch., and W. E. Lee: Acute massive collapse of the lungs. Ann. Surg. 82, 364 (1925). — Jackson, Ch. L., and J. F. Huber: Correlated applied anatomy of the bronchial tree and lungs with a system of nomenclature. Dis. Chest 9, 319 (1943). — Jacobaeus, H. C.: Der Lungenkollaps bei Lungenkrankheiten. Med. Klin. 1932, 673. ~ Über Lungenkollaps. Verh. dtsch. Ges. inn. Med. 44, 161 (1932). ~ A case of servere bullous emphysema. Acta radiol. (Stockh.) 16, 661 (1935). — Jacobaeus, H. C., and N. Westermark: A further study of massive collapse of the lung. Acta radiol. (Stockh.) 11, 547 (1930). — Jacobj, W.: Beobachtungen am peripheren Gefäßapparat unter lokaler Beeinflussung desselben durch pharmakologische Agentien. Naunyn-Schmiedeberg's Arch. exp. Path. Pharmak. 86, 49 (1920). ~ Pharmakologische Wirkungen am peripheren Gefäßapparat und ihre Beeinflussung auf Grund einer spezifischen Veränderung der Permeabilität der Zellmembran durch Hydroxylionen. Naunyn-Schmiedeberg's Arch. exp. Path. Pharmak. 88, 33 (1920). — Jagič, N., u. G. Spengler: Emphysem und Emphysemherz. Berlin: Springer 1924. — Jansen, K., H. W. Knipping u. K. Stromberger: Klinische Untersuchungen über Atmung und Blutgase. Beitr. Klin. Tuberk. 80, 304 (1932). — Jeddeloh, B. zu: Untersuchungen zur Histologie chronischer Stauungslungen. Beitr. path. Anat. 86, 387 (1931). — Jeker, K.: Die Bestimmung des Strömungswiderstandes im Bronchialsystem des Menschen. Helv. med. Acta 20, 459 (1953). — Jirovec, O.: Über die durch Pneumocystis Carinii verursachte interstitielle Pneumonie der Säuglinge. Mschr. Kinderheilk. 102, 476 (1954). — Jirovec, O., u. J. Vanek: Zur Morphologie der Pneumocystis Carinii und zur Pathogenese der Pneumocystis-Pneumonie. Zbl. allg. Path. path. Anat. 92, 424 (1954). — Jores, L.: Über experimentelles, neurotisches Lungenödem. Dtsch. Arch. klin. Med. 87, 389 (1906). ~ Arterien. In: Handbuch der speziellen pathologischen Anatomie (Henke-Lubarsch), Bd. II. Berlin: Springer 1924. — Junghanss, W.: Die Endstrombahn der Lunge im postmortalen Angiogramm. Virchows Arch. path. Anat. 331, 263 (1958). ~ Das Lungenemphysem im postmortalen Angiogramm. Virchows Arch. path. Anat. 332, 538 (1959). — Jungmann, P.: Beiträge zur Freundschen Lehre vom Zusammenhang primärer Rippenknorpelanomalien mit Lungentuberkulose und Emphysem. Frankfurt. Z. Path. 3, 38 (1909).

Kalbfleisch, H. H.: Die Atelektase, eine Wirkung der Reizung der vegetativ innervierten Teile der Lunge. Allg. path. Schr. (Stuttgart) 2, 5 (1941). ~ An die physiologischen

Segmente der Lunge gebundene pathologische Vorgänge des Organs. Allg. path. Schr. (Stuttgart) 3/4, 5 (1942). ~ Die funktionalen nervalen Segmente bei der chronischen Lungentuberkulose des Menschen. Allg. path. Schr. (Stuttgart) 6, 5 (1947). ~ Über die funktionalen Lungensegmente und andere Zeichen nervaler Einwirkungen bei der chronischen Lungentuberkulose und anderen Lungenkrankheiten, erschlossen aus pathologisch-anatomischen Befunden. Beitr. Klin. Tuberk. 102, 258 (1949). — KALBFLEISCH, H. H., u. G. HERKLOTZ: Experimentelle Untersuchungen über die segmentale Innervation der Lunge. Z. ges. inn. Med. 1, 25 (1946). — KALLÓS, P., u. W. PAGEL: Experimentelle Untersuchungen über Asthma bronchiale. Acta med. scand. 91, 292 (1937). — KAPFERER, J. M.: Der nutzbare Anteil der Vitalkapazität (Tiffeneau-Test). Thoraxchirurgie 1, 547 (1954). — KARRER, H. E.: The ultrastructure of mouse lung. 1. General architecture of capillary and alveolar walls. J. biophys. biochem. Cytol. 2, 241 (1956). ~ The ultrastructure of mouse lung. 2. Some remarks regarding the fine structure of the alveolar basement membrane. J. biophys. biochem. Cytol. 2, 287 (1956). ~ The ultrastructure of mouse lung. 3. Fine structure of the capillary endothelium. Exp. Cell Res. 11, 542 (1956). ~ An electronmicroscopic study of the fine structure of pulmonary capillaries and alveoli of the mouse. Bull. Johns Hopk. Hosp. 98, 65 (1956). — KARTAGENER, M.: Die Bronchitiden. In: Handbuch der inneren Medizin, 4. Aufl., Bd. IV/2. Berlin-Göttingen-Heidelberg: Springer 1956. ~ Die Bronchiektasen. In: Handbuch der inneren Medizin, 4. Aufl., Bd. IV/2. Berlin-Göttingen-Heidelberg: Springer 1956. — KAUFMANN, A.: Zur Frage der glatten Muskulatur der Lunge und ihrer funktionellen Bedeutung. Frankfurt. Z. Path. 63, 122 (1952). — KAUFMANN, E.: Lehrbuch der speziellen pathologischen Anatomie, 9. u. 10. Aufl. Berlin u. Leipzig: W. de Gruyter & Co. 1931. — KAUTZKY, A.: Neuere bronchographische Ergebnisse bei Ektasien der Bronchien. Fortschr. Röntgenstr. 54, 219, 345 (1936). — KAWAMURA, K.: Experimentelle Studien über die Lungenexstirpation. Dtsch. Z. Chir. 131, 189 (1914). — KECK, E.: Sektionsbefunde von 60 Über-90-jährigen. Z. Alternsforsch. 9, 145 (1955). — KEHLER, E.: Neurovegetative Grundprobleme des muskulären und vaskulären Lungensystems. Ärztl. Forsch. 1953, I/197. — KEITH, A.: The mechanism of respiration in man. In: Further advances in physiology. London: E. Arnold 1909. — KENÉZ, J., A. PAPP u. E. VINCZE: Lungentuberkulose und Emphysem. (Eine klinisch-pathologische Studie.) Beitr. Klin. Tuberk. 117, 469 (1957). — KERNEN, J. A., R. M. O'NEAL and D. L. EDWARDS: Pulmonary arteriosclerosis and thromboembolism in chronic pulmonary emphysema. Arch. Path. (Chicago) 65, 471 (1958). — KESSLER, P.: Compensatory phenomena in the residual lung following resection. Acta med. Acad. Sci. hung. 9, 181 (1956). KIENER, M., H. KOBLET u. F. WYSS: Zur Pathologie des stenosierenden Bronchialkollapses mit Lungenemphysem. Schweiz. med. Wschr. 1957, 660. — KILCHES, R.: Zur Frage der Retraktionskräfte der Lunge. Klin. Wschr. 1940, 695. — KIRCH, E.: Die Veränderungen der Herzproportionen bei rechtsseitiger Herzhypertrophie. Zbl. allg. Path. path. Anat. 35, 305 (1924). ~ Entwicklungsablauf der rechtsseitigen tonogenen Herzdilatation bei Mensch und Versuchstier und seine physiologische Erklärung. Virchows Arch. path. Anat. 291, 682 (1933). Dilatation und Hypertrophie des Herzens. Nauheimer Fortbild.lehrg. 14, 47 (1938). ~ Die pathologische Anatomie des Cor pulmonale. Verh. dtsch. Ges. Kreisl.-Forsch. 21, 163 (1955). — KISCH, B.: Electron microscopic investigation of the lungs. (Capillaries and specific cells.) Exp. Med. Surg. 13, 101 (1955). ~ Elektronenmikroskopische Untersuchungen am Lungengewebe. Medizinische 1957, 1564. — KLÄSI, C.: Anatomische Untersuchung über das Entstehen des vesiculären Lungenemphysems. Virchows Arch. path. Anat. 104, 353 (1886). — KLEINSORG, H., u. K. KOCHSIEK: Zur Differenzierung obstruktiver und restriktiver Ventilationsstörungen. Klin. Wschr. 1959, 36. — KLEPZIG, H., H. REINDELL, K. MUSSHOF u. R. WEYLAND: Anpassungsvorgänge des Herzens bei Klappenfehlern. Verh. dtsch. Ges. Kreisl.-Forsch. 20, 111 (1954). — KLINGE, F., u. H. G. FASSBENDER: Pathologische Anatomie der experimentellen Grundlagen. In: Allergie, (HANSEN), 3. Aufl. Stuttgart: Georg Thieme 1957. — KLOOS, K.: Pulmonale hyaline Membranen. (Übersichtsreferat.) Dtsch. med. Wschr. 1959, 78. — KLOOS, K., u. H. WULF: Pulmonale hyaline Membranen bei Neugeborenen. Arch. Kinderheilk. 152, 1 (1956). ~ Pulmonale hyaline Membranen bei Neugeborenen. Naturwissenschaften 1956, 378. — KNEBEL, R.: Haemodynamik des Lungenkreislaufs beim chronischen Cor pulmonale. Verh. dtsch. Ges. Kreisl.-Forsch. 21, 181 (1955). ~ Akutes Cor pulmonale. Dtsch. med. J. 1956, 276. — KNEBEL, R., u. E. WICK: Über das verschiedene Verhalten des transmuralen Venendruckes in der Brusthöhle und im Bauchraum. Ärztl. Forsch. 13, 327 (1959). — KNIPPING, H. W.: Die Pneumonose. Ergebn. inn. Med. Kinderheilk. 48, 249 (1935). — KNIPPING, H. W., W. BOLT, H. VALENTIN u. H. VENRATH: Normale und pathologische Physiologie der Atmung: In: Handbuch der Thoraxchirurgie. Berlin-Göttingen-Heidelberg: Springer 1958. — KNOBLOCH, H., u. W. HILSCHER: Über das Verhalten einiger Funktionen des Respirationstraktus im Alter. Z. Alternsforsch. 11, 351 (1958). — KOCH, W.: Vergiftung durch Gas. In: Handbuch der ärztlichen Erfahrungen im Weltkriege VIII. Leipzig: Johann Ambrosius Barth 1921. ~ Zusammenhangstrennungen, Lageveränderungen und Fremdkörper der Lunge und Bronchien. In: Handbuch der speziellen Pathologie, Bd. III/2. Berlin: Springer

1930. — KÖHN, K., u. M. RICHTER: Die Lungenarterienbahn bei angeborenen Herzfehlern. Stuttgart: Georg Thieme 1958. — KÖLLIKER, A.: Zur Kenntnis des Baues der Lunge. Verh. phys.-med. Ges. Würzb., N.F. 16 (1881). — KÖNN, G.: Über den Einbruch tuberkulös verkäster Lymphknoten in das Bronchialsystem und seine Folgen für die Lungentuberkulose. Beitr. path. Anat. 113, 59 (1953). ~ Die pathologische Morphologie der Lungengefäße beim chronischen Cor pulmonale. Beitr. path. Anat. 116, 273 (1956). ~ Die pathologische Morphologie der Lungengefäßerkrankungen und ihre Beziehungen zur chronischen pulmonalen Hypertonie. Ergebn. ges. Tuberk.-Forsch. (Stuttgart) 14, 101 (1958). ~ Arteriosklerose des Pulmonalsystems. Verh. dtsch. Ges. Path. 41, 77 (1958). — KÖNN, G., u. CH. BÜCHNER: Temporär-chronisches Cor pulmonale nach rezidivierender experimenteller Mikroembolie. Verh. dtsch. Ges. Path. 43, 300 (1959). — KOESTLIN: Arch. physiol. Heilk. 8, 139 (1849). Zit. nach H. MÜLLER 1922. — KOHN, H. N.: Zur Histologie der indurierenden fibrinösen Pneumonie. Münch. med. Wschr. 1893, 42. — KOROL, E., and C. F. ENSIGN: Bullous emphysema (?) or bilateral pneumothorax (?). Radiology 23, 223 (1934). — KOUNTZ, W. B., and H. L. ALEXANDER: Non-obstructive emphysema. J. Amer. med. Ass. 100, 551 (1933). ~ Non-obstructive emphysema. Medicine (Baltimore) 13, 251 (1934). — KOURILSKY, R., S. KOURILSKY, S. LAURENT, J. CHEVREAU, D. BRILLE et C. HATZFELD: Le rôle de l'atteinte bronchiolaire dans l'emphysème pulmonaire chronique. Presse méd. 1956, 324. — KRAMER, R., and A. GLASS: Bronchoscopic localization of lung abscess. Ann. Otol. (St. Louis) 41, 1210 (1932). — KRAUSS, J.: Lungenfunktionsprüfungen. Dtsch. med. Wschr. 1958, 76. — KREUZER, F.: Modellversuche zum Problem der Sauerstoffdiffusion in den Lungen. Helv. physiol. pharmacol. Acta Suppl. 9 (1953). ~ KROGH, A.: The anatomy and physiology of capillaries. New Haven: Yale Univ. Press 1922 u. 1929. ~ Anatomie und Physiologie der Capillaren. Berlin: Springer 1929. ~ The comparative physiology of respiratory mechanisms. Philadelphia: Univ. Penn. Press 1941. — KROGH, A., and M. KROGH: On the rate of diffusion of carbonic oxide into the lungs of man. Skand. Arch. Physiol. 23, 236 (1909). — KROGH, MARIE: The diffusion of gases through the lungs of man. J. Physiol. (Lond.) 49, 271 (1914/15). — KUCSKO, L.: Über Mikround Makroaneurysmen der peripheren Lungenstrombahn. (Vereinig. der path. Anatomen Wiens, wiss. Sitzg vom 30. 10. 1956). Zbl. allg. Path. path. Anat. 96, 302 (1957). — KÜTTNER: Beitrag zur Kenntnis der Kreislaufverhältnisse der Säugetierlunge. Virchows Arch. path. Anat. 73, 476 (1878). — KUHNKE, E.: Elektronenmikroskopische Befunde zur Wirkung der Hyaluronidase auf Kollagenfibrillen. Naturwissenschaften 45, 166 (1958). — KUNO, Y.: J. Physiol. (Lond.) 51, 154 (1918). Zit. nach LOCHNER 1957.

LAENNEC, R. T. H.: Traité de l'auscultation médiate et des maladies du poumon et du coeur, 2e édit. Paris: 1826. — LAGERLÖF, H., and L. WERKÖ: The pulmonary capillary venous pressure pulse in man. Scand. J. clin. Lab. Invest. 1, 147 (1949). — LAGUÉSSE, É., et A. HARDEVILLIER: Présentation d'un acinus pulmonaire. C. R. Congr. Franç. Méd. Lille 1899. — LANDEN, H. C.: Die funktionelle Beurteilung des Lungen- und Herzkranken. Darmstadt: Steinkopff 1955. — LANDEN, H. C., u. O. BAYER: Die Lungenfunktion bei Kranken mit Mitralstenose vor und nach operativer Sprengung der Klappe. Z. Kreisl.-Forsch. 41, 561 (1952). — LANG, F. J.: Über Gewebskulturen der Lunge. Arch. exp. Zellforsch. 2, 93 (1926). ~ Über die Alveolarphagocyten der Lunge. Virchows Arch. path. Anat. 275, 104 (1929). — LANGE: Untersuchungen über das Epithel der Lungenalveole. Frankfurt. Z. Path. 3, 170 (1909). — LAPP, H.: Zur Pathologie der Blutgefäßanastomosen in der Lunge. Verh. dtsch. Ges. Path. 34, 273 (1950). ~ Über die Sperrarterien in der Lunge und die Anastomosen zwischen Arteriae bronchiales und Arteriae pulmonales, über ihre Bedeutung insbesondere für die Entstehung des hämorrhagischen Infarktes. Frankfurt. Z. Path. 62, 537 (1951). ~ Über das Verhalten der Bronchialarterien und ihrer Anastomosen mit der Arteria pulmonalis unter pathologischen Kreislaufbedingungen, insbesondere bei den einzelnen Formen der angeborenen Herzfehler. Verh. dtsch. Ges. Kreisl.-Forsch. 17, 110 (1951). — LAUCHE, A.: Die Entzündungen der Lungen und des Brustfells. In: Handbuch der speziellen pathologischen Anatomie (HENKE-LUBARSCH), Bd. III/1. Berlin: Springer 1928. ~ Das Lungenemphysem. Medizinische 1956, 490. — LAURELL, H.: Über Röntgenuntersuchung bei Typhus abdominalis und bei einigen seiner abdominellen Komplikationen. Acta radiol. (Stockh.) 10, 243 (1929). — LAWTON, R. W., and A. L. KING: Elasticity of the rat lung. Fed. Proc. 8, 92 (1949). — LEHMANN, G.: Die Funktion der menschlichen Nase als Staubfilter. Arbeitsphysiologie 7, 167 (1934). ~ Die Filtrierung der Atemluft und deren Bedeutung für Staubkrankheiten. Berlin: Springer 1938. — LEMOINE, J. M., et J. P. GARAIX: Les dyskinésies a forme hypotonique. Sem. Hôp. Paris 29, 933 (1953). — LENGGENHAGER, K.: Zur Genese des stenotischen Lungenemphysems. Schweiz. med. Wschr. 1952, 542. — LENGYEL, J.: Die elastische Dehnbarkeit der argyrophilen Fasern. Anat. Anz. 74, 330 (1932). — LENT, W.: Untersuchungen über die Wirkung erhöhter Atemwiderstände. II. Die Lungenvolumina und die Lungenventilation. Z. ges. exp. Med. 109, 638 (1941). — LEOPOLD, J. G., and J. GOUGH: The centrilobular form of hypertrophic emphysema and its relation to chronic bronchitis. Thorax 12, 219 (1957). — LEOPOLD, S.: Postoperative massive pulmonary collapse and drow.

ned lung. Amer. J. med. Sci. 167, 421 (1924). — LERNER, L. O.: Gibt es besondere Scheidewände zwischen den Zonen und Segmenten der Lunge? Probl. Tuberk. (russ.) 1951, 49. Ref. Ber. allg. spez. Path. 16, 313 (1953). — LESCHKE, W.: Tierexperimentelle Beiträge zur Frage der segmentalen Innervation der Lungen. Z. ges. inn. Med. 1952, 769; 1953, 249; 1956, 38. — LESTER, C. W., A. COURNAND and R. L. RILEY: Pulmonary function after pneumonectomy in children. J. thorac. Surg. 11, 529 (1941/42). — LETTERER, E.: Die pathologische Anatomie des Asthma bronchiale. Allergie u. Asthma 3, 65 (1957). ~ Allgemeine Pathologie, S. 52. Stuttgart: Georg Thieme 1959. ~ Allgemeine Pathologie. Grundlagen und Probleme. Stuttgart: Georg Thieme 1959. — LEUSEN, J., G. DEMEESTER et K. VUYLSTEEK: Effects de l'occlusion d'une branche de l'artère pulmonaire chez le chien. Acta cardiol. (Brux.) 12, 1 (1957). — LEUSEN, J., u. K. VUYLSTEEK: XX. Internat. Physiol. Kongr. Brüssel 1956. Zit. nach LOCHNER 1957. — LEWIS, B. M., and R. GORLIN: Effects of hypoxia on pulmonary circulation of the dog. Amer. J. Physiol. 170, 574 (1952). — LEWIS, B. M., R. GORLIN, H. E. J. HOUSSAY, F. W. HAYNES and L. DEXTER: Clinical and physiological correlations in patients with mitral stenosis. V. Amer. Heart J. 43, 2 (1952). — LICHTERFELD, A.: Untersuchungen über den inspiratorischen Tiffeneau-Test. Klin. Wschr. 1960, 219. — LICHTHEIM, L.: Die Störungen des Lungenkreislaufes. Berlin 1876. ~ Versuche über Lungenatelektase. Naunyn-Schmiedeberg's Arch. exp. Path. Pharmak. 10, 54 (1879). — LIEBEGOTT, G.: Über Organveränderungen bei langer Einwirkung von Sauerstoff mit erhöhtem Partialdruck im Tierexperiment. Beitr. path. Anat. 105, 413 (1941). — LIEBERMEISTER, G.: Zur normalen und pathologischen Physiologie der Atmungsorgane. I. Über das Verhältnis zwischen Lungendehnung und Lungenvolumen. Zbl. allg. Path. path. Anat. 18, 644 (1907). ~ Zur normalen und pathologischen Physiologie der Atmungsorgane. II. Studien über die Atmungs mechanik bei plötzlich auftretenden Larynxstenosen (nach Beobachtungen an Diphtherie). Dtsch. med. Wschr. 1908, 1669. ~ Zur normalen und pathologischen Physiologie der Atmungsorgane. Frankfurt. Z. Path. 28, 253 (1922). ~ Diskussionsbeitrag zu Emphysem. Tagg Südwestdeutsch. Pathologen, Mannheim 1922. Zbl. allg. Path. path. Anat. 33, 1—20 (1922/23). — LIEBERMEISTER, K.: Über die Lungendurchblutung beim geschlossenen Pneumothorax. Naunyn-Schmiedeberg's Arch. exp. Path. Pharmak. 175, 697 (1934). — LIEBOW, A. A., M. R. HALES, G. E. LINDSKOG, M. R. BLOOMER and W. D. HARRISON: Enlargement of the bronchial arteries and their anastomoses with the pulmonary arteries in bronchiectasis. Amer. J. Path. 25, 211 (1949). — LILIENTHAL, H.: Empyema: Exploration of the thorax with primary mobilization of the lung. Ann. Surg. 62, 309 (1915). — LILIENTHAL, J. L., R. L. RILEY, D. D. PROEMMEL and R. E. FRANKE: An experimental analysis in man of the oxygen pressure gradient from alveolar air to arterial blood during rest and exercise at sea level an at altitude. Amer. J. Physiol. 147, 199 (1946). — LILJESTRAND, G.: Untersuchungen über die Atmungsarbeit. Skand. Arch. Physiol. 35, 199 (1918). ~ Chemismus des Lungengaswechsels. In: Handbuch der normalen und pathologischen Physiologie (BETHE-BERGMANN-EMBDEN-ELLINGER), Bd. II. Berlin: Springer 1925. ~ Regulation of pulmonary arterial blood pressure. Arch. intern. Med. 81, 162 (1948). — LIN, CHI KONG: Cardiac catheterization in acquired lesions of the heart or lungs. Dis. Chest 29, 73 (1956). — LINDSKOG, G., and R. ALLEY: Pharmakological factors influencing collateral ventilation. Meeting Amer. Surg. Assoc. 1948. Zit. nach v. HAYEK 1953. — LING, J. S. L.: Direct microscopic observation of the lung circulation in spontaneously breathing cats. Amer. J. med. Sci. 230, 467 (1955). — LINSER, P.: Über den Bau und die Entwicklung des elastischen Gewebes in der Lunge. Anat. H. 13, 307 (1900). LINZBACH, A. J.: Untersuchungen über die muskuläre Bauchwand und ihren Einfluß auf die Lage der Eingeweide. Virchows Arch. path. Anat. 304, 140 (1939). — LOCHNER, W.: Zur Physiologie des kleinen Kreislaufs. In: Lungen und kleiner Kreislauf. Bad Oeynhausener Gespräche I, 12 (1956). Berlin-Göttingen-Heidelberg: Springer 1957. — LOCHNER, W., u. W. SCHOEDEL: Blutfüllung des kleinen Kreislaufs und Herzminutenvolumen. Pflügers Arch. ges. Physiol. 252, 281 (1950). ~ Die Regulation des Herzzeitvolumens und die Blutfüllung des kleinen Kreislaufs. Pflügers Arch. ges. Physiol. 255, 327 (1952). ~ Die Bedeutung der depressorischen Kreislaufreflexe für die Steuerung des Herzzeitvolumens. Pflügers Arch. ges. Physiol. 255, 333 (1952). — LÖFFLER, W.: Über Atelektase. Bibl. tuberc. (Basel) 4, 13 (1950). ~ Die Lungenatelaktase. In: Handbuch der inneren Medizin, 4. Aufl., Bd. IV/2. Berlin-Göttingen-Heidelberg: Springer 1956. ~ Klinik und Therapie des Emphysems (Referat). Verh. dtsch. Ges. inn. Med. 62, 44 (1956). — LÖFFLER, W., u. F. R. NAGER: Über traumatische Bronchostenose und ihre Behandlung. Schweiz. med. Wschr. 1941, 181. — LÖHR, B.: Der Einfluß gestörter Lungenbelüftung auf den kleinen Kreislauf, Pathophysiologie und Klinik. Münch. med. Wschr. 1956, 838. — LÖHR, H.: Untersuchungen zur Physiologie und Pharmakologie der Lunge. Z. ges. exp. Med. 39, 67 (1924). — LÖHR, H., H. SCHOLTZE u. W. KLINNER: Zur Klärung der angiographischen Symptomatologie bei der Lungentuberkulose. Fortschr. Röntgenstr. 86, 192 (1957). ~ Röntgendiagnostische Probleme der Lunge. Medizinische 1957, 1697. — LÖHR, H., H. SCHOLTZE, W. KLINNER u. R. ZENKER: Zur Indikationsstellung bei der chirurgischen Behandlung der spezifischen und unspezifischen Empyemresthöhle auf Grund der selektiven Lungenangiographie. Langenbecks Arch. klin. Chir. 285, 1 (1957). —

Loeschcke, H.: Beiträge zur Histologie und Pathogenese der Nitritvergiftungen. Beitr. path. Anat. **49**, 457 (1910). ~ Über Wesen und Bedeutung des Zwerchfelltiefstandes beim Emphysematiker. Verh. dtsch. Ges. Path. **16**, 435 (1913). ~ Die Morphologie des normalen und emphysematösen Acinus der Lunge. Beitr. path. Anat. **68**, 213 (1921). ~ Referat über Emphysem, Tagg Südwestdeutsch. Pathologen, Mannheim 1922. Zbl. allg. Path. path. Anat. **33**, 1—20 (1922/23). ~ Methoden zur morphologischen Untersuchung der Lunge. In: Handbuch der biologischen Arbeitsmethoden (Abderhalden), Abt. VIII, Teil 1. Berlin u. Wien: Urban & Schwarzenberg 1924. ~ Störungen des Luftgehaltes der Lunge. In: Handbuch der speziellen pathologischen Anatomie und Histologie (Henke-Lubarsch), Bd. III/1. Berlin: Springer 1928. — Loeschcke, H. H.: Die Absorption von Gas im Organismus als Diffusionsvorgang. Klin. Wschr. **1956**, 801. — Loewy, A.: Über die Bestimmung der Größe des schädlichen Luftraumes im Thorax und der alveolaren Sauerstoffspannung. Pflügers Arch. ges. Physiol. **58**, 416 (1894). — Longacre, J. J., B. N. Carter and L. G. McQuill: An experimental study of some of the physiologic changes following total pneumectomy. J. thorac. Surg. **6**, 237 (1937). — Longacre, J. J., and R. Johansmann: An experimental study of the fate of the remaining lung following total pneumectomy. J. thorac. Surg. **10**, 131 (1940). — Lottenbach, K.: Das Lungenemphysem. In: Handbuch der inneren Medizin, 4. Aufl., Bd. IV/2. Berlin-Göttingen-Heidelberg: Springer 1956. — Lottenbach, K., I. Noelpp-Eschenhagen u. B. Noelpp: Mechanische Aspekte der Lungenfunktion. Theoretischer Beitrag zu den Kapiteln Asthma und Emphysem. In: Handbuch der inneren Medizin, 4. Aufl., Bd. IV/2. Berlin-Göttingen-Heidelberg: Springer 1956. — Low, F. N.: Electron microscopy of the rat lung. Anat. Rec. **113**, 437 (1952). ~ The pulmonary alveolar epithelium of laboratory mammals and man. Anat. Rec. **117**, 241 (1953). ~ The electron microscopy of lung tissue after varied duration of fixation in buffered osmium tetroxide. Anat. Rec. **120**, 827 (1954). — Low, F. N., and M. M. Sampaio: The pulmonary alveolar epithelium as an entodermal derivative. Anat. Rec. **127**, 51 (1957). — Luchsinger, P., u. A. Bühlmann: Die Lungenfunktion bei der Silikose und die Prognose nach Aufhören der Staubarbeit. Z. Unfallmed. Berufskr. **1953**, 282. — Luchsinger, R.: Die Erkrankungen der Nase. In: Handbuch der inneren Medizin, 4. Aufl., Bd. IV/2. Berlin-Göttingen-Heidelberg: Springer 1956. — Lüchtrath, H.: Chronische Bronchitis, Bronchiektasie, bronchiolektatisches Emphysem. Beitr. Klin. Tuberk. **104**, 260 (1950). — Lüchtrath, H., u. H. Friebel: Die Wirkung von Toluylendiisocyanat (Desmodur T) auf die Atemwege. Naunyn-Schmiedeberg's Arch. exp. Path. Pharmak. **227**, 93 (1955). — Luisada, A.: Über Lungendynamik. Ergebn. inn. Med. Kinderheilk. **47**, 92 (1934).

Macklin, C. C.: X-Ray studies on bronchial movements. Amer. J. Anat. **35**, 303 (1925). ~ The musculature of the bronchi and lungs. Physiol. Rev. **9**, 1 (1929). ~ Functional aspects of bronchial muscle and elastic tissue. Arch. Surg. (Chicago) **19**, 1212 (1929). ~ The dynamic bronchial tree. Amer. Rev. Tuberc. **25**, 393 (1932). ~ Bronchial length changes and other movements. Tubercle (Lond.) **14**, 16, 69 (1932). ~ Pulmonic alveolar pores. J. Anat. (Lond.) **69**, 188 (1935). ~ Alveolar pores and their significance in the human lung. Arch. Path. (Chicago) **21**, 201 (1936). ~ Pulmonic alveolar epithelium. J. thorac. Surg. **6**, 82 (1936). ~ The silver lineation of the alveoli. J. thorac. Surg. **7**, 536 (1938). ~ The pulmonary alveolar mucoid film and the pneumonocytes. Lancet **1954 I**, 1099. — MacLeod, J. J. R.: Physiology in modern medicine. London: H. Kimpton 1935. — Märk, W.: Die mechanische Bedeutung der argyrophilen Fasern. Anat. Anz. **94**, 416 (1943). — Magnenat, P.: Étude neurohistologique du poumon. Acta anat. (Basel) **13**, 1/2 (1951). — Mai, H.: Einiges über frühkindliches Asthma. Arch. Kinderheilk. **143**, 65 (1951). ~ Einige Bemerkungen zur Entstehung kindlichen Asthmas. Med. Klin. **1954**, 1097. ~ Asthma und Lungentuberkulose. Ergebn. ges. Tuberk.-Forsch. (Stuttgart) **12**, 175 (1954). — Maier, H., and A. Cournand: Studies of the arterial oxygen saturation in the postoperative period after pulmonary resection. Surgery **13**, 199 (1943). — Maier, H. C., A. Himmelstein, R. L. Riley and J. J. Bunin: Arteriovenous fistula of lung. J. thorac. Surg. **17**, 13 (1948). — Marchand, F.: Ein Beitrag zur Pathologie und pathologischen Anatomie des Bronchialasthma, mit Berücksichtigung der plastischen Bronchitis und der Colica mucosa. Beitr. path. Anat. **61**, 251 (1916). ~ Ein neuer Fall von Asthma bronchiale mit anatomischer Untersuchung. Dtsch. Arch. klin. Med. **127**, 184 (1918). — Marchand, P., J. C. Gilroy and V. H. Wilson: An anatomical study of the bronchial vascular system and its variations in disease. Thorax **5**, 207 (1950). — Marshall, R., W. R. Stone and R. V. Christie: The relationship of dyspnoea to respiratory effort in normal subjects, mitral stenosis and emphysema. Clin. Sci. **13**, 625 (1954). — Martini, P., u. J. Feller: Zum Problem der Bronchitis. Med. Klin. **1956**, 793. — Marx, H.: Die Nasenheilkunde. Jena: Gustav Fischer 1949. — Masshoff, W.: Zur Pathologie des Bronchus bei der Tuberkulose. Med. Mschr. **1955**, 761. ~ Zur Pathomorphologie der Lungentuberkulose. Dtsch. med. Wschr. **1956**, 1873. — Matthes, H.-U.: Die Bedeutung des Atemwiderstandes für die Messung des respiratorischen Stoffwechsels. Arbeitsphysiologie **11**, 117 (1941). — Matthes, K.: Pathophysiologie der Diffusion und Perfusion (Referat). Verh. dtsch. Ges. Path. **44** (1960). —

MATTHES, K., u. W. ULMER: Untersuchungen über die pathophysiologische Bedeutung des Emphysems. I. Verschiedene Emphysemformen. Dtsch. Arch. klin. Med. 204, 275 (1957). ~ Untersuchungen über die pathophysiologische Bedeutung des Emphysems. II. Emphysem und Störungen der Ventilation (Untersuchungen in Ruhe und unter Arbeit). Dtsch. Arch. klin. Med. 204, 284 (1957). ~ Untersuchungen über die pathophysiologische Bedeutung des Emphysems. III. Krankheitsverlauf verschiedener Emphysemformen und deren Beziehung zum chronischen Cor pulmonale. Dtsch. Arch. klin. Med. 204, 298 (1957). — MATTHES, K., W. ULMER u. K. WITTEKIND: Cor pulmonale. In: Handbuch der inneren Medizin, Bd. 9. Berlin-Göttingen-Heidelberg: Springer 1960. — MAURATH, J.: Patho-Physiologie der Atmung in der Lungenchirurgie. Stuttgart: Georg Thieme 1955. — MAURATH, J., u. M. WERBER: Patho-Physiologie der Atmung nach Lob- und Pneumektomie. Dtsch. Z. Chir. 269, 496 (1951). — MAXIMOW, A.: Über undifferenzierte Blutzellen und mesenchymale Keimlager im erwachsenen Organismus. Klin. Wschr. 1926, 2193. — MAXIMOW, A., and W. BLOOM: A textbook of histology. Philadelphia u. London: W. B. Saunders Company 1948. — MAYEDA, S.: Roentgenologic investigations into the peristaltic movements of the human bronchies. Jap. J. med. Sci., III Biophys. 2, 72 (1931). — McILROY, M. B., and G. H. APTHORP: Pulmonary function in pulmonary hypertension. Brit. Heart J. 20, 397 (1958). — McILROY, M. B., and R. V. CHRISTIE: A post-mortem study of the visco-elastic properties of normal lungs. Thorax 7, 291 (1952). ~ A post-mortem study of the visco-elastic properties of the lung in emphysema. Thorax 7, 295 (1952). ~ The work of breathing in emphysema. Clin. Sci. 13, 147 (1954). — McKEOWN, F.: The pathology of pulmonary heart disease. Brit. Heart J. 14, 25 (1952). — McMICHAEL, J.: Heart failure of pulmonary origin. Edinb. med. J. 55, 65 (1948). ~ Pharmacology of the failing human heart. Oxford 1950. — MEAD, J., J. LINDGREN and E. A. GAENSLER: The mechanical properties of lung in emphysema. J. clin. Invest. 34, 1005 (1955). — MEAD, J., and J. L. WHITTENBERGER: Physical properties of human lungs measured during spontaneous respiration. J. appl. Physiol. 5, 779 (1953). — MEER, G., VAN DER, et S. L. BRUG: Infection à pneumocystis chez l'homme et chez les animaux. Ann. Soc. belge Méd. trop. 22, 302 (1942). — MEESSEN, H.: Chronic carbon dioxide poisoning. Arch. Path. (Chicago) 35, 36 (1948). ~ Diskussionsbemerkung zu hyalinen Membranen als CO$_2$-Wirkung. Zbl. allg. Path. path. Anat. 95, 27 (1949). ~ Über Lungencirrhose. Beitr. path. Anat. 110, 1 (1949). ~ Zur pathologischen Anatomie des Lungenkreislaufes. Verh. dtsch. Ges. Kreisl.-Forsch. 17, 25 (1951). ~ Die Lunge bei der Mitralstenose. Dtsch. med. Wschr. 1956, 1445. ~ Zur Pathogenese, Progredienz und Adaptation der angeborenen Herz- und Gefäßfehler. Verh. dtsch. Ges. Kreisl.-Forsch. 23, 188 (1957). ~ Pathomorphologie der Diffusion und Perfusion (Referat). Verh. dtsch. Ges. Path. 44 (1960). — MEESSEN, H., u. H. SCHULZ: Elektronenmikroskopische Untersuchungen des experimentellen Lungenödems. In: Lungen und kleiner Kreislauf. Bad Oeynhausener Gespräche I, 54 (1956). Berlin-Göttingen-Heidelberg: Springer 1957. — MERKEL, H.: Zur Histologie der Lungengefäße. Beitr. path. Anat. 105, 176 (1941). ~ Die Struktur und Funktion des Lungenkreislaufs. Z. Kreisl.-Forsch. 38, 705 (1949). ~ Über die sog. primäre Pulmonalsklerose. Beitr. path. Anat. 109, 437 (1947). — METZ, G. A.: Die Elastizität und die Dehnbarkeit normalen und pathologischen Lungengewebes. Krankh.-forsch. 8, 137 (1930). — METZ, U.: Physikalisch-morphologische Untersuchungen über Festigkeit und Dehnbarkeit der basalen Hirngefäße. Virchows Arch. path. Anat. 317, 385 (1949). — MEY, A. V. M.: Emphysem, Bronchitis und Silikose. In: Die Staublungenerkrankungen, Bd. 3, Darmstadt: Steinkopff 1958. — MEYER, H. E., u. O. H. ROLFS: Ergebnisse bronchographischer Untersuchungen. Beitr. Klin. Tuberk. 92, 1 (1939). — MEYER, W. W., u. H. RICHTER: Gewichtsveränderungen der Arteria pulmonalis mit fortschreitendem Alter und bei Blutdruckerhöhung im kleinen Kreislauf. Verh. dtsch. Ges. Path. 39, 231 (1955), ~ Das Gewicht der Lungenschlagader als Gradmesser der Pulmonalarteriensklerose und als morphologisches Kriterium der pulmonalen Hypertonie. Virchows Arch. path. Anat. 328, 121 (1956). — MEYER, W. W., u. E. SIMON: Die phasenartige Abwandlung der Pulmonalis-Volumendehnbarkeit im Verlauf des Lebens und ihre Bedeutung für das Verständnis einiger krankhafter Arterienveränderungen. Verh. dtsch. Ges. Path. 43, 190 (1959). — MEYLER, L., and E. HUIZINGA: Syndrome of temporary high position of diaphragm; etiologic studies. Ned. T. Geneesk. 1948, 2476. ~ Temporary high position of the diaphragm. J. thorac. Surg. 19, 283 (1950). — MIDDELDORPF, K.: Massiver Lungenkollaps. Dtsch. Z. Chir. 240, 173 (1933). —MILLER, W. S.: Reticulum of the lung. Amer. J. Path. 3, 315 (1927). ~ A further study of emphysematous blebs. Amer. J. Roentgenol. 18, 42 (1927). ~ The lung. Springfield, Ill.: Ch. C. Thomas 1937: 2. Aufl. 1947; 3. Aufl. 1950. — MINK, P. J.: Das Spiel der Nasenflügel. Pflügers Arch. ges. Physiol. 120, 210 (1907). ~ Über die Funktion der Nebenhöhlen der Nase. Arch. Laryng. Rhin. (Berl.) 29, 453 (1915). ~ Die Rolle des kavernösen Gewebes in der Nase. Arch. Laryng. Rhin. (Berl.) 30, 47 (1916). ~ Die respiratorischen Bewegungen des Kehlkopfes. Arch. Laryng. Rhin. (Berl.) 30, 391 (1916). ~ Die respiratorischen Bewegungen des Kehlkopfes, Teil II. Arch. Laryng. Rhin. (Berl.) 31, 125 (1918). ~ Physiologie der oberen Luftwege. Leipzig: Vogel 1920. — MINKOWSKI, O., u. A. BITTORF: Die Pathoogie der Atmung. In: Handbuch der allgemeinen Pathologie (Krehl-Marchand), Bd. II, Abt. I. Leipzig: S. Hirzel 1912. — Miyata, S.: Aufbau und Gestalt der peripheren arteriellen Strombahn des kleinen Kreislaufes. Virchows Arch. path. Anat. 304, 608 (1939). — Mockenhaupt, A., u. J. Mockenhaupt: Lungenfunktion bei Resektionsbehandlung. (Unter besonderer Berücksichtigung von VK u. AGW.) Beitr. Klin. Tuberk. 116, 487 (1957). — Moell, O. H.: Die Veränderungen der Kapillarmembranen der Lunge bei Herzfehlern und ihre Bedeutung für die Pneumonose. Beitr. path. Anat. 105, 366 (1941). — Möllendorff, W. v.: Beiträge zum Verständnis der Lungenkonstruktion. Z. Anat. 111, 224 (1941). — Mönckeberg, I. G.: Zur pathologischen Anatomie des Bronchialasthmas. Verh. dtsch. Ges. Path. 13, 173 (1909). — Moleschott, J.: Ein Beitrag zur Kenntnis der glatten Muskelzellen. Unters. Naturlehre (Gießen) 6 (1860). — Morawitz, P., u. R. Siebeck: Die Dyspnoe durch Stenose der Luftwege. I. Gasanalytische Untersuchungen. Dtsch. Arch. klin. Med. 97, 201 (1909). — Moschcowitz, E.: Der intravasculäre Druck als Ursache der Arteriosclerose. Virchows Arch. path. Anat. 283, 282 (1932). — Motley, H. L., A. Cournand, L. Werkö, A. Himmelstein and D. Dresdale: Influence of short periods of induced anoxia upon pulmonary arterial blood pressure in man. Amer. J. Physiol. 150, 315 (1947). — Mounier-Kuhn, P., et A. Lévy: Le lipoidolage bronchopulmonaire à la sonde sous le contrôle de l'écran radioscopique. Rev. Laryng. (Bordeaux) 52, 427 (1931). — Mounier-Kuhn, P., et A. Mounier-Kuhn: Les bronchopathies postoperatoires et leur traitement. Paris: Masson & Cie. 1955. — Müller, A.: Bemerkungen zum Gasaustausch in den Lungen. Helv. physiol. pharmacol. Acta 3, 203 (1945). — Müller, E.: Zur funktionellen Pathologie der Sperrarterien und der arteriovenösen Kurzschlüsse der Lunge am Beispiel der Geschwulstzellembolie. Frankfurt. Z. Path. 64, 459 (1953). — Müller, H.: Studien über den Pleuradruck. Virchows Arch. path. Anat. 238, 157 (1922). ~ Diskussionsbeitrag zu Emphysem. Tagg. Südwestdeutsch. Pathologen, Mannheim 1922. Zbl. allg. Path. path. Anat. 33, 1—20 (1922/23). — Müller, Leo: Zur Frage der sog. Altersfibrose. Beitr. path. Anat. 82, 57 (1929). — Müller, R. W.: Zur Entstehung der Lungenatelektase. Dtsch. med. Wschr. 1947, 668. — Mülly, K.: Die Erkrankungen und Geschwülste des Mediastinums. In: Handbuch der inneren Medizin, 4. Aufl., Bd. IV/4. Berlin-Göttingen-Heidelberg: Springer 1956. — Mulvihill, D. A., and R. Klopstock: Decortication of the nonexpandable postpneumothorax tuberculous lung. J. thorac. Surg. 17, 723 (1948). — Mundt, E., W. Schoedel u. H. Schwarz: Über die Gleichmäßigkeit der Lungenbelüftung. Pflügers Arch. ges. Physiol. 244, 99 (1940). ~ Über den effektiven schädlichen Raum der Atmung. Pflügers Arch. ges. Physiol. 244, 107 (1940). — Musshoff, K., H. Klepzig, H. Reindell u. R. Weyland: Die Bedeutung des Restblutes für die Formveränderungen des Herzens bei Klappenfehlern. Verh. dtsch. Ges. Kreisl.-Forsch. 20, 114 (1954). — Musshoff, K., H. Krauss, P. Frisch, H. Reindell, H. Klepzig u. G. Engstfeld: Größen- und Formänderungen des Herzens und der Lungengefäße vor und nach Sprengung der Mitralstenose. Dtsch. med. Wschr. 1959, 468.

Neergaard, K. v.: Zur Frage des Druckes im Pleuraspalt. Beitr. Klin. Tuberk. 65, 476 (1927). ~ Neue Auffassungen über einen Grundbegriff der Atemmechanik. Z. ges. exp. Med. 66, 373 (1929). ~ Eine neue Auffassung der Retraktionskraft der Lunge und ihre Bedeutung für den Kollapszustand. Verh. dtsch. Ges. inn. Med. 1929, 249. ~ Über klinische Fragen der Atemmechanik. I. Klinische Messungen pathologisch veränderter Strömungswiderstände in den Atemwegen. Schweiz. med. Wschr. 1930, 429. ~ Über klinische Fragen der Atemmechanik. II. Über das Wesen der Retraktionskraft der Lunge und ihre klinische Messung beim Emphysem. Schweiz. med. Wschr. 1930, 463. — Neergaard, K. v., u. K. Wirz: Über eine Methode zur Messung der Lungenelastizität am lebenden Menschen, insbesondere beim Emphysem. Z. klin. Med. 105, 35 (1927). ~ Messung der Strömungswiderstände in den Atemwegen des Menschen, insbesondere bei Asthma und Emphysem. Z. klin. Med. 105, 51 (1927). ~ Neue Auffassungen über einen Grundbegriff der Atemmechanik. Z. ges. exp. Med. 66, 373 (1929). — Neuhof, H., and R. A. Nabatoff: An angiographic study of the form and function of the remaining lung after pneumectomy. J. thorac. Surg. 17, 799 (1948). — Neumann, R.: „Hiatusinsuffizienz" und sog. „Hiatushernien". Virchows Arch. path. Anat. 289, 270 (1933). Nicod, J.-L.: L'emphysème pulmonaire dans la silicose par sténose mécanique des bronches. Presse méd. 1952, 1682. ~ Silicose, sténose bronchique et emphysème. Schweiz. med. Wschr. 1953, 920. — Niedner, F. F.: Beiträge zur Kenntnis von neurovegetativen Lungenreaktionen. Beobachtungen an der Lunge bei intrathorakalen Operationen. Acta neuroveg. (Wien) 1, 353 (1950). — Nikulin, A.: Veränderungen der Pulmonalarterien nach chronischer Histamininjektion. Beitr. path. Anat. 120, 214 (1959). — Nisell, O.: The action of oxygen and carbondioxide on the bronchioles and vessels of the isolated perfused lungs. Acta physiol. scand. 21, Suppl. 73 (1950). ~ The influence of blood gases on the pulmonary vessels of the cat. Acta physiol. scand. 23, 85 (1951). ~ The influence of carbondioxide on the respiratory movements of isolated perfused lungs. Acta physiol. scand. 23, 352 (1951). ~ Reaction of pulmonary venules of cat; with special reference to effect of pulmonary elastance. Acta physiol. scand. 23, 361 (1951). ~ Some aspects of the pulmonary circulation and ventilation. Int. Arch.

Allergy **3**, 142 (1952). — NISSEN, R.: Die Bronchusunterbindung, ein Beitrag zur experimentellen Lungenpathologie und -chirurgie. Dtsch. Z. Chir. **179**, 160 (1923). ~ Experimentelle Untersuchungen zur Theorie der Entstehung des Lungenemphysems. Dtsch. Z. Chir. **200**, 177 (1927). — NISSEN, R., u. P. COKKALIS: Experimentelle Untersuchungen über mechanische Atemstörungen und einige Folgezustände. Dtsch. Z. Chir. **194**, 50 (1926). — NOELPP, B., u. I. NOELPP-ESCHENHAGEN: Asthma bronchiale. In: Handbuch der inneren Medizin, 4. Aufl., Bd. IV/2. Berlin-Göttingen-Heidelberg: Springer 1956. ~ Das experimentelle Asthma bronchiale des Meerschweinchens. V. Mitt. Int. Arch. Allergy **3**, 302 (1952). — NOELPP, B., I. NOELPP-ESCHENHAGEN u. K. LOTTENBACH: Das Verhalten der elastischen Lungenspannung und des Gewebsdeformationswiderstandes bei der experimentellen asthmatiformen Dyspnoe. Int. Arch. Allergy **5**, 245 (1954). — NOELPP-ESCHENHAGEN, I., B. NOELPP, K. LOTTENBACH u. O. FORSTER: Untersuchungen zur Genese der Dyspnoe. Z. ges. exp. Med. **123**, 258 (1954). — NÜRMBERGER, W.: Tierexperimentelle Studien über die Sportlunge und ihre Rückbildungsfähigkeit. Virchows Arch. path. Anat. **303**, 303 (1939).

OCHSNER jr., A.: Effect of pulmonary blood flow and distension on the capacity of intrapulmonary vessels. Amer. J. Physiol. **168**, 200 (1952). — O'NEAL, R. M., W. A. THOMAS and P. M. HARTROFT: The media of small muscular pulmonary arteries in mitral stenosis. Arch. Path. (Chicago) **60**, 267 (1955). — OPPIKOFER, E.: Paraffin-Wachsausgüsse von Larynx und Trachea bei strumöser Bevölkerung. Arch. Laryng. Rhin. (Berl.) **26**, 399 (1912). ~ Wachsparaffinausgüsse der Luftröhre in situ der Organe hergestellt. Arch. Laryng. Rhin. (Berl.) **27**, 383 (1913). — ORSÓS, F.: Über das elastische Gerüst der normalen und der emphysematösen Lunge. Beitr. path. Anat. **41**, 95 (1907). ~ Die Pigmentverteilung der Pleura pulmonalis und ihre Beziehungen zur Atmungsmechanik und zur generellen mechanischen Disposition der Lungenspitze für die Tuberkulose. Verh. dtsch. Ges. Path. **15**, 136 (1912). ~ Physiologisches und Pathologisches über den Bronchialbaum. Verh. dtsch. Ges. Path. **16**, 419 (1913). ~ Gerüstsysteme der Lunge und deren physiologische und pathologische Bedeutung. Beitr. Klin. Tuberk. **87**, 568 (1936). — ORTH, J.: Beitrag zur Kenntnis des Lungenemphysems. Berl. klin. Wschr. **1905**, 1. — OTIS, A. B., W. O. FENN and H. RAHN: Mechanics of breathing in man. J. appl. Physiol. **2**, 592 (1950). — OTIS, A. B., C. B. MCKERROW, R. A. BARTLETT, J. MEAD, M. B. MCILROY, N. J. SELVERSTONE and E. P. RADFORD: Mechanical factors in distribution of pulmonary ventilation. J. appl. Physiol. **8**, 427 (1956). — OTIS, A. B., and D. F. PROCTOR: Measurement of alveolar pressure in human subjects. Amer. J. Physiol. **152**, 106 (1948).

PAINE, S. R.: The clinical measurement of pulmonary elasticity. J. thorac. Surg. **9**, 550 (1940). — PAKESCH, F., H. v. HAYEK u. H. BRAUNSTEINER: Die Struktur der die Lungenkapillaren bedeckenden Epithelhäutchen. Wien. Z. inn. Med. **38**, 184 (1957). — PARADE, G. W.: Bronchographie. Med. Klin. **1934**, 1483. — PARKER, F., and S. WEISS: The nature and significance of the structural changes in the lungs in mitral stenosis. Amer. J. Path. **12**, 573 (1936). — PAROW, J.: Die mechanische Entstehung und Behandlung des Lungenemphysems. Dtsch. Gesundh.-Wes. **1950**, 1323. ~ Funktionelle Atmungstherapie. Dynamik, Leistungsfähigkeit, Versagen des Atem-Stimmapparates, Bronchialasthma und Lungenemphysem. Stuttgart: Georg Thieme 1953. — PARRISIUS, W.: Ist das Emphysem der Bergleute eine Berufskrankheit? Med. wiss. Beitr. Krankenhaus Bochum H. 6, 5 (1955). — PASTEUR, W.: Respiratory paralysis after diphtheria as a cause of pulmonary complications, with suggestions as treatment. Amer. J. med. Sci. **100**, 242 (1890). ~ Massive collapse of the lung. Lancet **1908 II**, 1351. ~ Active lobar collapse of the lung after abdominal operations. Lancet **1910 I**, 1080. ~ Post-operative lung complications. Lancet **1911 II**, 1329. — PENDL, O.: Über intratracheale Strumen. Mschr. Ohrenheilk. **81**, 16 (1947). — PERLS, M.: Über die Druckverhältnisse im Thorax bei verschiedenen Krankheiten. Dtsch. Arch. klin. Med. **6**, 1 (1869). — PEROMET, R.: La ventilation pulmonaire collatérale. Les dèfaillances. Acta tuberc. belg. **41**, 155 (1950). —PERWITZSCHKY, R.: Die Temperatur- und Feuchtigkeitsverhältnisse der Atemluft in den Luftwegen. Arch. Ohrenheilk. **117**, 1 (1928). — PETERSEN, H.: Über das mechanische Verhalten der elastischen Faser und deren Verwendung in der Konstruktion. Beitr. path. Anat. **76**, 222 (1927). ~ Histologie und mikroskopische Anatomie. München: J. F. Bergmann 1935. — PFANNER, W.: Über Ventilatmung. Med. Klin. **1920**, 1221. — PICHOTKA, J.: Über die histologischen Veränderungen der Lunge nach Atmung von hochkonzentriertem Sauerstoff im Experiment. Beitr. path. Anat. **105**, 381 (1941). — PICHOTKA, J., u. H. A. KÜHN: Experimentelle und morphologische Untersuchungen zur Sauerstoffvergifung. Naunyn-Schmiedeberg's Arch. exp. Path. Pharmak. **204**, 336 (1947). — PIIPER, J.: Verhalten des Strömungswiderstandes und der Blutfüllung am isolierten Lungenlappen des Hundes. Pflügers Arch. ges. Physiol. **264**, 596 (1957). ~ Eine Methode zur Lokalisierung des Strömungswiderstandes. Pflügers Arch. ges. Physiol. **266**, 199 (1958). ~ Über die Lage der Capillaren im Gefäßbett der isolierten Hundelunge. Pflügers Arch. ges. Physiol. **267**, 1 (1958). — PIRCHER, L.: Über die Diffusion des Sauerstoffes. Inaug.-Diss. Fribourg

1951. ~ Physikalische Grundlagen zur Atemmechanik. In: Lungen und kleiner Kreislauf. Bad Oeynhausener Gespräche I, 33 (1956). Berlin-Göttingen-Heidelberg: Springer 1957. — Piso-Borme: Anatomisch-physiologische Studien über die Gegenwart glatter Muskelfasern in den Lungenbläschen der Wirbeltiere. Unters. Naturlehre (Gießen) 6 (1860). — Plenk, H.: Die argyrophilen Fasern (Gitterfasern) und ihre Bildungszellen. Ergebn. Anat. Entwickl.-Gesch., Abt. III 27, 302 (1927). ~ „Aktive Elastizität" der Gitterfasern. Anat. Anz. 69, 25 (1930). — Pliess, G.: Das mikrokulturelle Verhalten von Alveolarzellen und von Pneumocystis Carinii bei der interstitiellen plasmacellulären Säuglingspneumonie. Frankfurt. Z. Path. 68, 153 (1957). ~ Das mikrokulturelle Verhalten von Hefezellen und Bakterien bei der interstitiellen plasmacellulären Säuglingspneumonie. Frankfurt. Z. Path. 68, 185 (1957). ~ Interstitielle plasmacelluläre Säuglingspneumonie als Allgemeinerkrankung. Frankfurt. Z. Path. 68, 565 (1957). — Pohl, R.: Funktionelle Diagnostik am Bronchialsystem. Fortschr. Röntgenstr. 56, 13 (1937). ~ Universelle Erweichungszustände am Tracheobronchialsystem. Fortschr. Röntgenstr. 74, 40 (1951). — Pokorny, C., and C. A. Hellwig: Diffuse interstitial fibrosis of the lungs. Arch. Path. (Chicago) 59, 382 (1955). — Polgar, F.: Studies on respiratory mechanics. Amer. J. Roentgenol. 61, 637 (1949). — Policard, A.: Sur la nature du revétement des alvéoles pulmonaires des mammifères. Bull. Histol. appl. 3, 236 (1926). ~ L'alvéole pulmonaire au microscope électronique. Presse méd. 1954, 1775. ~ Le puomon. Structures et mechanismes à l'état normal et pathologique. Paris: Masson & Cie. 1938; 2. Aufl. 1955. — Policard, A., et A. Collet: Apports de la microscope électronique à la connaissance histophysiologique de la paroi alvéolaire. J. Physiol. (Paris) 48, 687 (1956). — Policard, A., A. Collet, L. Giltaire-Ralyte, Chr. Heuet et C. Desfosset: Recherches au microscope électronique sur le fibres élastiques du poumon. Bull. Micr. appl., Sér. II 4, 139 (1955). — Policard, A., A. Collet, S. Pregernam et C. Benet: Structures alveolaires normales du poumons examinées au microscope électronique. Ann. Rech. méd. 33, 385 (1957). — Policard, A., et P. Galy: Les bronches. Paris: Masson & Cie. 1945. — Ponfick, E.: Ein Fall von angeborener primärer Atrophie der rechten Lunge. Virchows Arch. path. Anat. 50, 633 (1870). — Popovic, L.: Studien aus der Bronchographie. Fortschr. Röntgenstr. 40, 821 (1929). — Putschar, W.: Der funktionelle Skelettumbau und die sog. Belastungsdeformitäten. In: Handbuch der speziellen pathologischen Anatomie, Bd. IX/3. Berlin: Springer 1937.

Rahn, H., and H. T. Bahnson: Effect of unilateral hypoxia on gas exchange and calculated blood flow in each lung. J. appl. Physiol. 6, 105 (1951). — Rahn, H., A. B. Otis, L. E. Chadwick and W. O. Fenn: The pressure volume-diagram of the thorax and lung. Amer. J. Physiol. 146, 161 (1946). — Rahn, J.: Über das Strukturbild der Obstruktionsatelektase in situ. Verh. dtsch. Ges. Path. 43, 271 (1959). — Raither, E.: Studien über Emphysem. Beitr. Klin. Tuberk. 22, 137 (1912). — Ranke, K. E.: Primäraffekt, sekundäre und tertiäre Stadien der Lungentuberkulose auf Grund von histologischen Untersuchungen der Lymphknoten an der Lungenpforte. Dtsch. Arch. klin. Med. 119, 201 (1916). — Ranke, O.: Zur Frage der elastischen Systeme, besonders der Aortenwand. Beitr. path. Anat. 73, 638 (1925). ~ Über die verschiedenen Formen der Kompensation der Arterienwand und ihre Störungen. Beitr. path. Anat. 75, 269 (1926). — Ratner, B.: Experimental asthma. Critical analysis of the literature. Ann. Allergy 9, 677 (1951). — Ratner, B., H. C. Jackson and H. L. Gruehl: Transmission of protein hypersensitiveness from mother to offspring. J. Immunol. 14, 249 (1927). — Rau, G., H. Behn, W. Gebhardt, P. H. Rossier u. A. Bühlmann: Atemmechanische Untersuchungen am Lungenmodell, bei Lungengesunden und bei Patienten mit obstruktivem Emphysem. Schweiz. med. Wschr. 1957, 374. — Rauen, H. M.: Biochemisches Taschenbuch. Berlin-Göttingen-Heidelberg: Springer 1956. — Redenz, E.: Untersuchungen über die elastischen Fasern. I. Untersuchung der isolierten elastischen Fasern des Nackenbandes mit dem Mikromanipulator. Beitr. path. Anat. 76, 226 (1927). ~ Untersuchungen über die elastischen Fasern. II. Dehnung der elastischen Fasern und Platten der Aortenwand mit dem Mikromanipulator. Z. Zellforsch. 4 (1927). — Rein, H.: Einführung in die Physiologie des Menschen, 8. Aufl. Berlin-Heidelberg: Springer 1947. — Reinberg, S. A.: Röntgenstudien über die normale und pathologische Physiologie des Tracheobronchialbaumes. Fortschr. Röntgenstr. 33, 661 (1925). — Reinhardt, E.: Beiträge zur Kenntnis der Lunge als neurovasculares und neuromusculares Organ nach Beobachtungen an der Lunge des lebenden Kaninchens. Virchows Arch. path. Anat. 292, 322 (1934). ~ Lungenkreislauf und Lungenmuskulatur bei Atelektase und Emphysem. Verh. dtsch. Ges. Kreisl.-Forsch. 8, 173 (1935). ~ Die Topik der lobären Pneumonie als Beweis ihrer Entstehung im Z.N.S. Verh. dtsch. Ges. Path. 29, 222 (1936). ~ Die Lunge — ein neurovasculares und ein neuromusculares Organ. Allg. path. Schriftenreihe H. 1, 12 (1941). — Reiser, K. A.: Über die Endausbreitung des vegetativen Nervensystems. Z. Zellforsch. 17, 610 (1933). — Reisseisen: Über den Bau der menschlichen Lunge. Berlin: Rücker 1822. — Reuterwall, O. P.: Über die Elastizität der Gefäßwände und die Methode ihrer näheren Prüfung. Stockholm 1921. ~ Zur Frage der Arterienelastizität. Virchows Arch. path. Anat. 239, 363 (1922). — Reynaud, A. C.: Mémoire sur l'oblitération des bronches. Mém. Acad. Méd. (Paris) 4, 117

(1835). — Ribbert, H.: Die Respirationsorgane. In: Handbuch der allgemeinen Pathologie und pathologischen Anatomie des Kindesalters (v. Brüning u. Schwalbe). Wiesbaden: Bergmann 1912. ∼ Zur Genese des Lungenemphysems. Virchows Arch. path. Anat. 221, 85 (1916). — Ricker, G.: Pathologie als Naturwissenschaft. Berlin: Springer 1924. — Rienhoff, W. F.: Intrathoracic anatomical readjustments following complete ablation of one lung. J. thorac. Surg. 6, 254 (1936/37). — Rienzo, S. di: Radiologic exploration of the bronchus. Springfield 1949. — Riley, R. L.: The work of breathing and its relation to respiratory acidosis. Ann. intern. Med. 41, 172 (1954). — Riley, R. L., and A. Cournand: „Ideal" alveolar air and the analysis of ventilation-perfusion relationships in the lungs. J. appl. Physiol. 1, 825 (1949). ∼ Analysis of factors affecting partial pressures of oxygen and carbon dioxide in gas and blood of lungs. I. Theory. J. appl. Physiol. 4, 77 (1951). — Riley, R. L., A. Cournand and K. W. Donald: Analysis of factors affecting partial pressures of oxygen and carbon dioxide in gas and blood of lungs. II. Methods. J. appl. Physiol. 4, 102 (1951). — Riley, R. L., J. L. Lilienthal, D. D. Proemmel and R. E. Franke: On the determination of the physiologically effective pressures of oxygen and carbon dioxide in alveolar air. Amer. J. Physiol. 147, 191 (1946). — Riley, R. L., R. H. Shepard, J. E. Cohn, D. G. Carroll and B. W. Armstrong: Maximal diffusing capacity of the lung. J. appl. Physiol. 6, 573 (1954). — Rimini, R., J. L. Duomarco, R. Burgos, J. C. Dighiero, J. C. Sapriza and G. H. Surraco: Unilateral positive pressure breathing as a means of partial shift of the pulmonary blood flow. Dis. Chest. 31, 653 (1957). — Rindfleisch, E.: Die Muskulatur der kleinen Bronchien und des Lungenparenchyms. Med. Zbl. 5, 65 (1872). ∼ Lehrbuch der pathologischen Gewebelehre, 6. Aufl. Leipzig: Wilhelm Engelmann 1886. ∼ Über Cirrhosis cystica pulmonum. Zbl. allg. Path. path. Anat. 8, 864 (1897). — Riva, G., u. R. Probst: Der Tod an Asthma bronchiale. Schweiz. med. Wschr. 1950, 1325. — Rodbard, S., I. Kariv and D. F. Heiman: The diagnostic significance of the respiratory fluctuations of the pulmonary arterial pressure in man. Amer. Heart J. 52, 182 (1956). — Rodewald, G.: Untersuchungen über Kurzschlußdurchblutung der Lunge und Diffusionsverhältnisse bei Herz- und Lungenkranken. In: Lungen und kleiner Kreislauf. Bad Oeynhausener Gespräche I, 154 (1956). Berlin-Göttingen-Heidelberg: Springer 1957. — Rössle, R.: Die pathologisch-anatomischen Grundlagen der Epituberkulose. Virchows Arch. path. Anat. 296, 1 (1936). ∼ Die pathologische Anatomie der allergischen Krankheiten des Menschen. In: Allergie (Hansen), 3. Aufl. Stuttgart: Georg Thieme 1957. — Rössle, R., u. F. Roulet: Maß und Zahl in der Pathologie. Berlin u. Wien: Springer 1932. — Rohrer, F.: Der Strömungswiderstand in den menschlichen Atemwegen und der Einfluß der unregelmäßigen Verzweigung des Bronchialsystems auf den Atmungsverlauf in verschiedenen Lungenbezirken. Pflügers Arch. ges. Physiol. 162, 225 (1915). ∼ Die Größe des schädlichen Raumes der Atemwege. Pflügers Arch. ges. Physiol. 164, 295 (1916). ∼ Der Zusammenhang der Atemkräfte und ihre Abhängigkeit vom Dehnungszustand der Atmungsorgane. Pflügers Arch. ges. Physiol. 165, 419 (1916). ∼ Studien über das Wesen und die Entstehung des Lungenemphysems. Münch. med. Wschr. 1916, 1219. ∼ Über die topographische Verteilung der Luftströmungsverhältnisse in der Lunge. Schweiz. med. Wschr. 1921, 741. ∼ Physiologie der Atembewegung. In: Handbuch der normalen und pathologischen Physiologie (Bethe-Bergmann-Embden), Bd. II. Berlin: Springer 1925. — Rokitansky, C.: Handbuch der pathologischen Anatomie, Bd. III. Wien: Braumüller & Seidel 1842. — Romanoff, M.: Experimente über Beziehungen zwischen Atmung und Kreislauf. Naunyn-Schmiedeberg's Arch. exp. Path. Pharmak. 64, 183 (1911). — Rossier, P. H.: Die Pathophysiologie des Emphysems. (Referat). Verh. dtsch. Ges. inn. Med. 62, 34 (1956). ∼ Über Physiopathologie der Atmung. Bibl. tuberc. (Basel) 11, 13 (1956). — Rossier, P. H., H. Bucher u. K. Wiesinger: Studien über die Pathophysiologie der Atmung bei der Silikose. Die Lungenfunktion in Ruhe bei der Silikose. Vjschr. naturforsch. Ges. Zürich 92, 83 (1947). — Rossier, P. H., u. A. Bühlmann: Studien über die Pathophysiologie der Atmung bei der Silikose. Die Lungenfunktion im Arbeitsversuch. Vjschr. naturforsch. Ges. Zürich 95, 51 (1950). ∼ Pathophysiologie der Atmung. In: Handbuch der inneren Medizin, 4. Aufl., Bd. IV/1. Berlin-Göttingen-Heidelberg: Springer 1956. — Rossier, P. H., A. Bühlmann u. P. Luchsinger: Die Pathophysiologie der Atmung bei der Silikose und die Begutachtung der Arbeitsfähigkeit. Dtsch. med. Wschr. 1955, 608. — Rossier, P. H., A. Bühlmann et H. R. Müller: Espace mort et clearance alvéolaire. Schweiz. med. Wschr. 1953, 577, 604. — Rossier, P. H., A. Bühlmann, u. K. Wiesinger: Physiologie und Pathophysiologie der Atmung. Berlin-Göttingen-Heidelberg: Springer 1956; 2. Aufl. 1958. — Rossier, P. H., et H. Méan: L'action de l'adrénaline sur la fonction pulmonaire. Acta Soc. Helv. Sci. Nat. 1936, 356. ∼ Bronchialspasmen und Adrenalinversuch. Praxis 1944, 893. — Rotter, W.: Über die Bedeutung der Ernährungsstörungen insbesondere des O_2-Mangels für die Pathogenese der Gefäßwandveränderungen mit besonderer Berücksichtigung der „Endarteriitis obliterans" und der „Arteriosklerose". Beitr. path. Anat. 110, 46 (1949). — Rotter, W., u. W. Büngeler: Blut und blutbildende Organe. In: Lehrbuch der speziellen pathologischen Anatomie (Kaufmann-Staemmler), 11. u. 12. Aufl., Bd. I/1. Berlin: W. de

Gruyter & Co. 1955. — Rotter, W., H. Wellmer, G. Hinrichs u. W. Müller: Zur Orthologie und Pathologie der Polsterarterien. Beitr. path. Anat. 115, 253 (1955). — Roughton, F. J. W.: The average time spent by the blood in the human lung capillary and its relations to the rates of CO uptake and elimination in man. Amer. J. Physiol. 143, 621 (1945). — Roughton, F. J. W., R. C. Darling and W. S. Root: Factors affecting determination of O_2 capacity, content and pressure in human arterial blood. Amer. J. Physiol. 142, 708 (1944). — Roughton, F. J. W., and J. C. Kendrew: Haemoglobin. London: Butterworthes scientific publications 1949. — Rufer, H. R.: Die Thoraxinnenraummaße und die Zwerchfellgröße bei der Albinoratte in verschiedenen Lebensaltern. Gegenbaurs morph. Jb. 99, 317 (1958). — Russakoff, A.: Über die Gitterfasern der Lunge unter normalen und pathologischen Verhältnissen. Zugleich ein Beitrag zur Kenntnis der feinsten Stützsubstanz einiger Parenchyme. Beitr. path. Anat. 45, 476 (1909).

Sandmann, G.: Über Atemreflexe von der Nasenschleimhaut. Dubois' Arch. 1885, 485. Zit. nach Marx 1949. — Sanen, F. J.: Das Pickwicksche Syndrom (Fettsucht, Hypoventilation, Rechtsinsuffizienz des Herzens, Somnolenz, Hyperkapnie). Med. Klin. 1958, 1360. — Sarnoff, J. S.: Electrophrenical respiration. J. thorac. Surg. 19, 929 (1950). — Sauerbruch, F., u. O. Bruns: Die künstliche Erzeugung von Lungenschrumpfung durch Unterbindung von Ästen der Pulmonalarterie. Mitt. Grenzgeb. Med. Chir. 23, 343 (1911). — Schall, L.: Die Interlobärspalten. Anatomie, Röntgendarstellung und deren klinische Bedeutung. Ergebn. ges. Tuberk.-Forsch. (Stuttgart) 2, 405 (1931). — Schaub, F., A. Bühlmann, R. Kälin u. T. Wegmann: Zur Klinik und Pathogenese des sog. Kyphoskolioseherzens. Schweiz. med. Wschr. 1954, 1147. — Scheideler: Experimentelle Untersuchungen über das Staubbindungsvermögen der menschlichen Nase. Arch. Ohr.-, Nas.- u. Kehlk.-Heilk. 146, 333 (1939). — Scherrer, M.: Die Lungentuberkulose funktionell gesehen. In: Funktion und Klinik der chronisch kranken Lunge. Bibl. tuberc. (Basel) 11, 83 (1956). — Schiller, E.: Tierexperimentelle Beiträge zum Thema Staublunge und Bronchitis. In: Die Staublungenerkrankungen, Bd. 3, S. 435, Darmstadt: Steinkopff 1958. — Schilling, J. N., K. B. Harvey, B. Balke and H. I. Rattunde: Extensive pulmonary resection in dogs: Altitude tolerance, work capacity, and pathologic-physiologic changes. Ann. Surg. 144, 635 (1956). — Schjerning, J.: Über das Problem der Cyanose und den Begriff der Pneumonose. Beitr. Klin. Tuberk. 50, 97 (1922). — Schlipköter, H. W.: Elektronenoptische Untersuchungen ultradünner Lungenschnitte. Dtsch. med. Wschr. 1954, 1658, 1675. — Schmidt, H.: Primäre und sekundäre pulmonale Hypertonie. Dtsch. Arch. klin. Med. 200, 837 (1953). ~ Die essentielle Hypertonie des Lungenkreislaufes und deren Beziehung zur sog. primären Pulmonalsklerose. Arch. Kreisl.-Forsch. 19, 91 (1953). ~ Experimentelle Serologie. In: Allergie (Hansen), 3. Aufl. Stuttgart: Georg Thieme 1957. — Schmidt, M. B.: Rachitis und Osteomalazie. In: Handbuch der speziellen Pathologie, Bd. IX/1. Berlin: Springer 1929. — Schmidt, O. P., u. W. Günthner: Lungenfunktionsprüfungen. (Übersichtsreferat.) Med. Klin. 1959, 753. — Schmorl, G.: Über die Beziehungen anthrakochalikotischer bronchialer Lymphknoten zu Bronchialerkrankungen und über Bronchitis deformans. Münch. med. Wschr. 1925, 757. — Schoedel, W.: Alveolarluft. Ergebn. Physiol. 30, 450 (1937). ~ Neue Gesichtspunkte der Atmungsphysiologie. Beiträge zur Silikose-Forschung, Sonderbd. I, Grundfragen aus der Silikoseforschung. Bochum 1955. ~ Diskussionsbemerkung zum anatomischen und funktionellen Totraum. 1958. Zit. bei Hartung 1959. — Schoen, H.: Pathologische Anatomie des Asthma bronchiale. (Referat.) Tagg Nord- u. Westdtsch. Path., Kassel 1958. Zbl. allg. Path. path. Anat. 99, 198 (1959). — Schoen, R.: Vorgänge im Lungenkreislauf bei Herzkranken. Verh. dtsch. Ges. inn. Med. 41, 422 (1929). ~ Über Störungen des Gasaustausches durch „Pneumonose". Münch. med. Wschr. 1930, 1836. ~ Über die Stauung im Lungenkreislauf. Klin. Wschr. 1930, 1849. ~ Lungendurchblutung und Lungenerkrankungen. Dtsch. med. Wschr. 1932, 574. ~ Tonusprobleme der Atmung. Klin. Wschr. 1936, 1341. — Schoen, R., u. E. Derra: Untersuchungen über die Bedeutung der Cyanose als klinisches Symptom. I. Dtsch. Arch. klin. Med. 168, 52 (1930). ~ Cyanose durch chronische Stauung im Lungenkreislauf, besonders bei Mitralstenose. II. Dtsch. Arch. klin. Med. 168, 176 (1930). — Schoen, R., u. J. Hempel: Über schlaffe und gespannte Apnoe. Weitere Beobachtungen über Änderungen der Tonuslage der Atmungsmuskulatur. Naunyn-Schmiedeberg's Arch. exp. Path. Pharmak. 171, 403 (1933). — Schoenmackers, J.: Die akute Lungenblähung und das interstitielle Emphysem bei intrakraniellen Prozessen. Virchows Arch. path. Anat. 318, 61 (1950). ~ Zur Pathologie der Lungenarterienembolie. (Referat.) Dtsch. med. Wschr. 1958, 115. ~ Über Bronchialvenen und ihre Stellung zwischen großem und kleinem Kreislauf. Arch. Kreisl.-Forsch. 32, 1 (1960). — Schoenmackers, J., u. A. Giampalmo: Über die angiektatische Alveolarkompression bei Morbus caeruleus. Verh. dtsch. Ges. Path. 36, 234 (1953). — Schoenmackers, J., u. H. Vieten: Das Verhalten der Lungengefäße bei verändertem Luftgehalt der Lunge. Untersuchungen am postmortalen Gefäßbild. Fortschr. Röntgenstr. 76, 24 (1952). ~ Das postmortale Angiogramm der Lunge bei Tuberkulose, Silikose und Bronchialcarcinom. Fortschr. Röntgenstr. 76, 51 (1952); 77, 14 (1952). ~ Atlas postmortaler Angiogramme. Stuttgart: Georg Thieme 1954. ~ Vergleichende pathologisch-anatomische und postmortalangiographische Betrachtungen der Lunge. Ergebn. ges. Tuberk.-Forsch. (Stuttgart) 14, 347 (1958). — SCHOSTOK u. STILLER: Referat über die thoraxchirurgische Arbeitstagung in Bad Schachen 1956 mit Beiträgen von MÜLLY, ZUIDEMA, KIRCH, NISSEN, BRUNNER, ADELBERGER, FREY u. a. Thoraxchirurgie 4, 179 (1956/57). — SCHRIEVER, H.: Zur Frage einer Eigenkontraktilität der Lungen. Z. Biol. 95, 566 (1933). — SCHRÖTTER, H. v.: Vorlesungen über die Krankheiten der Luftröhre. Wien 1896. Zit. nach TANNER 1957. — SCHUBERT, R., u. W. FISCHER: Asthma bronchiale und Tod. Medizinische 1956, 1129. — SCHUCHARDT, K.: Hochgradige Atrophie (inveterierte Atelektase) der linken Lunge mit kompensatorischer Hypertrophie der rechten. Virchows Arch. path. Anat. 101, 71 (1885). — SCHÜMMELFEDER, N.: Umfaltungen und Verwachsungen an freien Lungenrändern. Beitr. path. Anat. 116, 422 (1956). — SCHULTZ-BRAUNS, O.: Die tödlichen Vergiftungen durch gasförmige Stickoxyde (Nitrose-Gase) beim Arbeiten mit Salpetersäure. Virchows Arch. path. Anat. 277, 174 (1930). — SCHULTZE, W. H.: Über die Verknöcherung des ersten Rippenknorpels. Langenbecks Arch. klin. Chir. 103, 832 (1914). — SCHULZ, H.: Elektronenoptische Untersuchungen der normalen Lunge und der Lunge bei Mitralstenose. Virchows Arch. path. Anat. 328, 582 (1956). ~ Über den Gestaltwandel der Mitochondrien im Alveolarepithel unter CO_2- und O_2-Atmung. Naturwissenschaften 43, 205 (1956). ~ Elektronenoptische Untersuchungen der Lunge des Siebenschläfers nach Hibernation. Z. Zellforsch. 46, 583 (1957). ~ Die Pathologie der Mitochondrien im Alveolarepithel der Lunge. Beitr. path. Anat. 119, 45 (1958). ~ Die submikroskopische Pathologie der Cytosomen in den Alveolarmakrophagen der Lunge. Beitr. path. Anat. 119, 71 (1958). ~ Die submikroskopische Anatomie und Pathologie der Lunge. Berlin-Göttingen-Heidelberg: Springer 1959. — SCHULZE, F. E.: Die Lungen. In: STRICKERS Handbuch, Lehre von den Geweben. 1871. ~ Beiträge zur Anatomie der Säugetierlungen. S.-B. preuß. Akad. Wiss., phys. math. Kl. 6, 225 (1906). — SCHULZE, W.: Die entzündlichnarbige Bronchostenose und ihre Folgen. Verh. dtsch. Ges. inn. Med. 62, 76 (1956). — SCHUMANN, H. D.: Zur Wirkung intrabronchialer Druckerhöhung auf die Lungencapillaren. Langenbecks Arch. klin. Chir. 268, 554 (1951). — SCHWARTZ, PH.: Automatische endogene lymphadeno-bronchogene Reinfektion in der Initialperiode der Tuberkulose. Folia path. (Istanbul) 1 (1948). ~ Einbrüche tuberkulöser Lymphknoten in das Bronchialsystem und ihre pathogenetische Bedeutung. Beitr. Klin. Tuberk. 103, 192 (1950). ~ Über die bronchogene Ausbreitung der Tuberkulose. Zbl. allg. Path. path. Anat. 90, 245 (1953). ~ Die lymphadenogenen Bronchialschädigungen und ihre Bedeutung für die Entwicklung der Lungenschwindsucht. Beitr. Klin. Tuberk. 110, 106 (1953). ~ Bemerkungen über die Häufigkeit tuberkulöser lymphadenogener Bronchialwandschädigungen im Obduktionsgut mitteleuropäischer Institute für pathologische Anatomie. Tuberk.-Arzt 1953, 221. ~ Die intrathorakale Lymphknotentuberkulose und ihre Beziehungen zu den rückbildungsfähigen Lungenverdichtungen. Tuberk.-Arzt 1953, 368. ~ Lokalisation und Typen lymphadenogener Schädigungen des Tracheobronchialosystems und des Oesophagus. HNO (Berl.) 5, 257 (1956). — SCHWEINITZ, A. v.: Mechanische und chemische Schädigungen der elastischen Fasern. Verh. dtsch. Ges. Path. 43, 69 (1959). ~ SEDLMEIER, H.: Veterinärmedizin. Die primären Lungengeschwülste der Haustiere (Sammelreferat). Münch. med. Wschr. 1959, 2384. — SEEMANN, G.: Über den feineren Bau der Lungenalveole. Beitrag zur Frage des „respiratorischen Epithels". Beitr. path. Anat. 81, 508 (1929). ~ Histobiologie der Lungenalveole. Jena: Gustav Fischer 1931. — SEGAL, M. S., and M. J. DULFANO: Chronic pulmonary emphysema (Modern medical monographs). New York: Grune & Stratton 1953. — SEMISCH, R., J. GESSNER, H.-L. KÖLLING u. H. H. WITTIG: Atlas der selektiven Lungenangiographie. Jena: VEB Fischer 1958. — SHELDON, M. B., and A. B. OTIS: Effect of adrenaline on resistance to gas flow in the respiratory tract and on the vital capacity of normal and asthmatic subjects. J. appl. Physiol. 3, 513 (1951). — SHEPARD, R. H., J. E. COHN, G. COHEN, B. W. ARMSTRONG, D. G. CARROLL, H. DONOSO and R. L. RILEY: The maximal diffusing capacity of the lung in chronic obstructive disease of the airways. Amer. Rev. Tuberc. 71, 249 (1955). — SHORR, E.: Trans. 8. Conf. on liver injury, S. 60. New York: J. Macy jr. Foundation 1950. Zit. nach EHRICH 1956. — SIEBECK, R.: Die Dyspnoe durch Stenose der Luftwege. II. Die Einstellung der Mittellage der Lunge. Dtsch. Arch. klin. Med. 97, 219 (1909). ~ Über die Beeinflussung der Atemmechanik durch krankhafte Zustände des Respirations- und Kreislaufapparates. Dtsch. Arch. klin. Med. 100, 204 (1910). ~ Über den Gasaustausch zwischen der Außenluft und den Alveolen. I. Mitt. Z. Biol. 55, 267 (1910). ~ Über den Gasaustausch zwischen der Außenluft und den Alveolen. II. Mitt. Skand. Arch. Physiol. 25, 81 (1911). ~ Über den Gasaustausch zwischen der Außenluft und den Alveolen. III. Mitt. Dtsch. Arch. klin. Med. 102, 390 (1911). — SIEBENS, A., R. E. SMITH and C. F. STOREY: Effect of hypoxia on pulmonary vessels in man. Amer. J. Physiol. 180, 428 (1955). — SIEDEK, H., R. WENGER u. E. GMACHL: Elektrokymographische Untersuchungen am kleinen Kreislauf. Verh. dtsch. Ges. Kreisl.-Forsch. 17, 170 (1951). — D'SILVA, J. L., D. E. FREELAND and G. KAZANTZIS: The performance of patients with ankylosing spondylitis in the maximum ventilatory capacity test. Thorax 8, 303 (1953). — SIMMONDS, M.: Über Formveränderungen der Luftröhre. Münch. med. Wschr. 1897, 431. ~ Über die Verwendung von Gipsausgüssen zum Nachweis von

Trachealdeformitäten. Verh. dtsch. Ges. Path. 7, 170 (1904). ~ Über Alterssäbelscheiden-trachea. Virchows Arch. path. Anat. 179, 15 (1905). — SIMON, E., u. W. W. MEYER: Das Volumen, die Volumdehnbarkeit und die Druck-Längen-Beziehungen des gesamten aortalen Windkessels in Abhängigkeit von Alter, Hochdruck und Arteriosklerose. Klin. Wschr. 1958, 424. — SJÖSTRAND, F., u. T. SJÖSTRAND: Sinuöse Blutgefäße in der Lunge der Maus. Anat. Anz. 87, 193 (1938). — SJÖSTRAND, T.: Determination of changes in the intrathoracic blood volume in man. Acta physiol. scand. 22, 114 (1951). ~ The regulation of the blood distri-bution in man. Acta physiol. scand. 26, 312 (1952). ~ The significance of pulmonary blood volume in the regulation of the blood circulation under normal and pathologic conditions. Acta med. scand. 145, 155 (1953). ~ Volume and distribution of blood and their significance in regulating the circulation. Physiol. Rev. 33, 202 (1953). ~ Blutverteilung und Regulation des Blutvolumens. Klin. Wschr. 1956, 561. — SKRAMLIK, E. v.: Die Physiologie der Luftwege. In: Handbuch der normalen und pathologischen Physiologie (BETHE-BERGMANN-EMBDEN), Bd. II. Berlin: Springer 1925. ~ Physiologie der Mundhöhle und des Rachens. In: Hand-buch der Hals-, Nasen- und Ohrenheilkunde, Bd. I. Berlin: Springer; München: J. F. Berg-mann 1925. ~ Physiologie des Kehlkopfes. In: Handbuch Hals-, Hasen- und Ohrenheilkunde, Bd. I. Berlin: Springer; München: J. F. Bergmann 1925. — SORS, CH.: Les bronchopneumo-pathies segmentaires. Paris: Foucher 1952. ~ L'emphysème pulmonaire. Étude anatomique et pathogénique. Presse méd. 1958, 1868. — SOULAS, A., et P. MOUNIER-KUHN: Broncho-logie. Paris: Masson & Cie. 1949. — SOULIÉ, P., J. BAILLET, J. CARLOTTI, P. CHICHE, R. PICARD, M. SERVELLE et G. VOCI: Le poumon des mitraux. Essai de confrontation anatomo-physiologique. Arch. Mal. Coeur 46, 393 (1953). — SOULIÉ, P., P. CHICHE, J. BAILETT et R. PICARD: Le poumon des mitraux. La bronchopneumopathie mitrale. Presse méd. 1954, 463. — SPAIN, D. M.: Patterns of pulmonary fibrosis as related to pulmonary function. Ann. intern. Med. 33, 1150 (1950). ~ Acute non-aeration of lung. Pulmonary edema versus atel-ectasis. Dis. Chest 25, 550 (1954). — SPAIN, D. M., and G. KAUFMAN: The basic lesion in chronic pulmonary emphysema. Amer. Rev. Tuberc. 68, 24 (1953). — SPÜHLER, O.: Die Erkrankungen des Zwerchfells. In: Handbuch der inneren Medizin, 4. Aufl., Bd. IV/4. Berlin-Göttingen-Heidelberg: Springer 1956. — STAEHELIN, R.: Pathologie, Pathogenese und Therapie des Lungenemphysems. Ergebn. inn. Med. Kinderheilk. 14, 516 (1915). ~ Über das Lungenemphysem. Klin. Wschr. 1922, 1721. ~ Referat über Emphysem. Tagg Südwest-dtsch. Pathologen, Mannheim 1922. Zbl. allg. Path. path. Anat. 33, 1—20 (1922/23). ~ Die Bronchitis. In: Handbuch der inneren Medizin, Bd. II/2. Berlin: Springer 1930. ~ Das Lungenemphysem. In: Handbuch der inneren Medizin, Bd. II/2. Berlin: Springer 1930. — STAEHELIN, R., u. A. SCHUETZE: Spirographische Untersuchungen an Gesunden, Emphyse-matikern und Asthmatikern. Z. klin. Med. 75, 15 (1912). — STAEMMLER, M.: Die Thromb-endarteriitis obliterans der Lungenarterien. Klin. Wschr. 1937, 1669. ~ Gibt es eine primäre Hypertonie im kleinen Kreislauf? Arch. Kreisl.-Forsch. 3, 125 (1938). ~ Die Kreislauforgane. In: Lehrbuch der speziellen pathologischenAnatomie (KAUFMANN-STAEMMLER), 11./12. Aufl. Berlin: W. de Gruyter & Co. 1955. — STAEMMLER, M., u. K. SCHMITT: Neue Beobachtungen bei sogenannter primärer Pulmonalsklerose. Arch. Kreisl.-Forsch. 17, 264 (1951). — STAJANO, C., et J. J. SCANDROGLIO: L'atelectasie pulmonaire post-traumatique et post-opératoire. Mém. Acad. Chir. 78, 176 (1952). — STANDENATH, F.: Das Bindegewebe. Seine Entwick-lung, sein Bau und seine Bedeutung für Physiologie und Pathologie. Ergebn. allg. Path. path. Anat. 22 (II), 70 (1928). — STARR, I.: Rôle of the „static blood pressure" in abnormal incre-ments of venous pressure, especially in heart failure. II. Clinical and experimental studies. Amer. J. med. Sci., N.S. 199, 40 (1940). ~ Our changing viewpoint about congestive failure. Ann. intern. Med., N.S. 30, 1 (1949). — STARR, I., W. A. JEFFERS and R. H. MEADE jr.: The absence of conspicuous increments of venous pressure after servere damage to the right ventricle of the dog, with a discussion of the relation between clinical congestive failure and heart disease. Amer. Heart J. 26, 291 (1943). — STARR, I., and A. J. RAWSON: Rôle of the „static blood pressure" in abnormal increments of venous pressure, especially in heart failure. I. Theoretical studies on an improved circulation schema whose pumps obey Starling's law of the heart. Amer. J. med. Sci., N.S. 199, 27 (1940). — STEAD, W. W., D. L. FRY and R. V. EBERT: The elastic properties of the lung in normal men and in patients with chronic pulmonary emphysema. J. Lab. clin. Med. 40, 674 (1952). — STEINMANN, E.: Über die Bedeutung der respiratorischen Bifurkationsbewegungen bei Lungenerkrankungen. Schweiz. med. Wschr. 1949, 1126. ~ Die Pathophysiologie des Bronchialbaumes. Fortschr. Hals-Nas.-Ohrenheilk. 3, 40 (1955). — STERNBERG, C.: Über die elastischen Fasern. Virchows Arch. path. Anat. 254, 656 (1925). — STÖHR, PH.: Lehrbuch der Histologie und der mikroskopischen Anatomie. Jena: Gustav Fischer 1903. — STÖSSEL, E. v.: Über muskuläre Cirrhose der Lunge. Beitr. Klin. Tuberk. 90, 432 (1937). — STRAUSS: Über den Einfluß der Dehnung auf die quergestreifte Skelettmuskulatur am Beispiel der Bauchdecken bei Schwangerschaft. Virchows Arch. path. Anat. 266, 4 (1927). — STROUD, R. C., and H. RAHN: Effect of oxygen and carbon dioxide tensions upon the resistance of pulmonary blood vessels. Amer. J.

Physiol. **172**, 211 (1953). — STURM, A.: Die klinische Pathologie der Lunge in Beziehung zum vegetativen Nervensystem. Stuttgart: Georg Thieme 1948. ~ Lunge und vegetatives Nervensystem. Med. Welt **1951**, 969, 1030. ~ Ist die Lunge kontraktil? Schweiz. med. Wschr. **1951**, 859. ~ Die nervalen Faktoren beim Asthma- und Emphysemproblem. Beitr. Klin. Tuberk. **110**, 429 (1954). — STUTZ, E.: Bronchographische Beobachtungen beim Husten. Klin. Wschr. **1948**, 536. ~ Bronchographische Beiträge zur normalen und pathologischen Physiologie der Lungen. Fortschr. Röntgenstr. **72**, 129 (1949); **72**, 309, 447 (1950). ~ Über die Funktion der Lungenmuskulatur. Beitr. Klin. Tuberk. **105**, 221 (1951). — STUTZ, E., u. H. VIETEN: Die Bronchographie. Stuttgart: Georg Thieme 1955. — SUDSUKI, K.: Über Lungenemphysem. Virchows Arch. path. Anat. **157**, 438 (1899). — SUKIENNIKOW, W.: Topographische Anatomie der bronchialen und trachealen Lymphdrüsen. Berl. klin. Wschr. **1903**, 316. — SUNDER-PLASSMANN, P.: Über nervöse Receptorenfelder in der Wand der intrapulmonalen Bronchien des Menschen und ihre klinische Bedeutung, insbesondere ihre Schockwirkung bei Lungenoperationen. Dtsch. Z. Chir. **240**, 249 (1933). ~ Über neurovegetative Receptorenfelder im Kreislaufregulationsmechanismus und durch deren Ausschaltung experimentell erzeugte, morphologisch faßbare Veränderungen im sympathischen Nervensystem. Z. ges. Neurol. Psychiat. **147**, 414 (1933). ~ Der Nervenapparat der menschlichen Lunge und seine klinische Bedeutung. Dtsch. Z. Chir. **250**, 705 (1938). — SWAN, H. J. J., J. ZAPATA-DIAZ and H. WOOD: Dye dilution curves in cyanotic congenital heart disease. Circulation **8**, 70 (1953).

TAKINO, M.: I.—III. Mitt. Acta Sch. med. Univ. Kioto **15**, Fasc. 4 (1933). Zit. nach REINHARDT. — TANNENBERG, J.: Bau und Funktion der Blutkapillaren. Frankfurt. Z. Path. **34**, 1 (1926). — TANNER, E.: Probleme der operierten Lunge. Bibl. tuberc. (Basel) **11**, 102 (1956). ~ Die Tracheobronchialtuberkulose des Erwachsenen. In: Die Tuberkulose und ihre Grenzgebiete in Einzeldarstellungen, Bd. 11. Berlin-Göttingen-Heidelberg: Springer 1957. — TENDELOO, N. PH.: Lungendehnung und Lungenemphysem. Ergebn. inn. Med. Kinderheilk. **6**, 1 (1910). ~ Allgemeine Pathologie, 2. Aufl. Berlin: Springer 1925. ~ Studien über die Entstehung und den Verlauf der Lungenkrankheiten. München: J. F. Bergmann 1931. — TENDELOO, N. PH., J. PH. HENNEMANN u. G. A. METZ: Untersuchungen über Lungenemphysem und Lungenelastizität. I. Elastizität, Dehnbarkeit und Lungenemphysem. II. Elastizität normalen und pathologischen Lungengewebes. Krankheitsforsch. **7**, 163 (1929). — TESCHENDORF, H. J.: Bedeutung und Behandlung der Strahleninduration der Lungen. In: Die Röntgentiefentherapie (H. HOLFELDER). Leipzig: Georg Thieme 1938. — THEWS, G.: Eine Methode zur mathematischen Behandlung der Sauerstoffdiffusion in haemoglobin- und myoglobinhaltigen Lösungen. Naturwissenschaften **1956**, 160. — THIERFELDER, J.: Die Lungenfrisch- und -trockengewichte sowie das anatomische Lungenvolumen bei der Albinoratte in verschiedenen Lebensaltern. Ein Beitrag zur Frage des postnatalen Lungenwachstums. Gegenbaurs Morph. Jb. **99**, 286 (1958). — THIES, O.: Beiträge zur Atemmechanik auf Grund von Leichenversuchen. Virchows Arch. path. Anat. **284**, 772, 796 (1932). — THOMA, R.: Über die Elastizität gesunder und kranker Arterien. Virchows Arch. path. Anat. **116**, 16 (1889). ~ Über die Strömung des Blutes in der Gefäßbahn und die Spannung der Gefäßwand. Beitr. path. Anat. **66**, 377 (1920). — THORÉN, L.: Intratracheal goitre. Acta chir. scand. **95**, 495 (1947). — TIEMANN, F.: Über die Sportlunge. Münch. med. Wschr. **1936**, 1517. — TIFFENEAU, R.: L'examen pulmonaire de l'asthmatique. Déductions, diagnostiques, prognostiques et thérapeutiques. Paris: Masson & Cie. 1957. — TIFFENEAU, R., et P. DRUTEL: Acquisitions nouvelles concernant l'emphysème pulmonaire. Sem. Hôp. Paris **1950**, 396. ~ L'épreuve du cycle respiratoire maximum pour l'étude spirographique de la ventilation pulmonaire. Presse méd. **1952**, 640. — TIFFENEAU, R., et A. PINELLI: Régulation bronchique de la ventilation pulmonaire. J. franç. Méd. Chir. thor. **2—3**, 221 (1948). ~ La capacité pulmonaire utilisable à l'effort, test pour l'exploration de la fonction ventilatoire pulmonaire. Xe Congr. de la Tuberculose. Rev. Tuberc. (Paris) **12**, 555 (1948). — TÖNDURY, G.: Zur Segment-Anatomie der Lungenlappen. Schweiz. Z. Tuberk. **11**, 4, 337 (1954). ~ Anatomische Vorbemerkungen. In: Handbuch der inneren Medizin, Bd. IV/1. Berlin-Göttingen-Heidelberg: Springer 1956. — TÖNDURY, G., u. E. WEIBEL: Über das Vorkommen von Blutgefäßanastomosen in der menschlichen Lunge. Schweiz. med. Wschr. **1956**, 265. ~ Anatomie der Lungengefäße. Ergebn. ges. Tuberk.-Forsch. (Stuttgart) **14**, 59 (1958). — TOEUF, G. DE, et V. CONRAD: Étude expérimentale de la vascularisation du poumon atélectasié. Rev. belge Path. **23**, 31 (1953). — TONNDORF, J.: Der Weg der Atemluft in der menschlichen Nase. Arch. Ohr.-, Nas.- u. Kehlk.-Heilk. **146**, 41 (1939). — TORELLI, G., e A. VALLI: Studio roentgencinematografico della broncografia. Ann. Radiol. diagn. (Bologna) **20**, 205 (1948). — TOSETTI, R.: Les zones de résistance vasculaire pulmonaire au cours du rétrécissement mitral et du coeur pulmonaire chronique des emphysémateux. Arch. Mal. Coeur (Paris) **48**, 346 (1955). — TOUSSAINT-FRANCX, Y., et P. TOUSSAINT: La tuberculose bronchique et la voie d'infection broncho-trachéo-laryngée, exploration comparée sur pièces d'autopsie et sur matériel d'exérèse. Acta tuberc. belg. **46**, 261 (1955). — TRAUBE: 1846. Zit. nach LOEFFLER 1956. — TREN-

Delenburg, P.: Physiologische und pharmakologische Untersuchungen an der isolierten Bronchialmuskulatur. Naunyn-Schmiedeberg's Arch. exp. Path. Pharmak. **69**, 79 (1912). ~ Versuche an der isolierten Bronchialmuskulatur. Zbl. Physiol. **26**, 1 (1913). — Triepel, H.: Einführung in die physikalische Anatomie. Wiesbaden 1902. — Trimble, H. G.: Lungen-Emphysem. Münch. med. Wschr. 1954, 1501. — Turchetti, A., u. G. Schirosa: Essential pulmonary hypertension and its phases of evolution. Cardiologia (Basel) **21**, 129 (1952).

Uehlinger, E.: Die tuberkulöse Spät-Erstinfektion und ihre Frühevolution. Schweiz. med. Wschr. 1942, 701. ~ Die pathologische Anatomie der Bronchustuberkulose. Bibl. tuberc. (Basel) **4**, 31 (1950). ~ Die pathologische Anatomie der tuberkulösen Späterstinfektion. Ergebn. ges. Tuberk.-Forsch. (Stuttgart) **11**, 1 (1953). ~ Die Epidemiologie des Bronchialdurchbruches tuberkulöser Lymphknoten. Beitr. Klin. Tuberk. **110**, 128 (1953). ~ Die Thoraxdeformitäten. In: Handbuch der inneren Medizin, 4. Aufl., Bd. IV/2. Berlin-Göttingen-Heidelberg: Springer 1956. ~ Die pathologische Anatomie und experimentelle Pathologie der Staublungenerkrankungen. In Handbuch der inneren Medizin, 4. Aufl., Bd. IV/3. Berlin-Göttingen-Heidelberg: Springer 1956. ~ Die pathologisch-anatomischen Grundlagen der kardio-respiratorischen Insuffizienz. In: Funktion und Klinik der chronisch kranken Lunge. Bibl. tuberc. (Basel) **11**, 43 (1956). ~ Vanishing lung, progressive Lungendystrophie. In: Röntgendiagnostik (Schinz-Glauner-Uehlinger), Ergebnisse 1952—1956. Stuttgart: Georg Thieme 1957. ~ Pathologische Anatomie und Klinik des Morbus Boeck (Sarkoidose). Regensburg. Jb. ärztl. Fortbild. **6**, 385 (1958). ~ Extrapulmonal bedingte Ventilationsstörungen (Referat). Verh. dtsch. Ges. Path. **44** (1960). — Uehlinger, E., u. G. Schoch: Zur Diagnose und Differentialdiagnose der Lungengerüsterkrankungen: Entzündungen und Dystrophien. In: Röntgendiagnostik (Schinz-Glauner-Uehlinger), Ergebnisse 1952—1956. Stuttgart: Georg Thieme 1957. ~ Das Mittellappensyndrom. In: Röntgendiagnostik (Schinz-Glauner-Uehlinger), Ergebnisse 1952—1956. Stuttgart: Georg Thieme 1957. — Ulmer, W.: Untersuchungen zur Analyse der alveolären Ventilationsstörung bei chronischem Cor pulmonale. Verh. dtsch. Ges. Kreisl.-Forsch. 1955, 360. ~ Untersuchungen über die effektive Ventilationsleistung bei Emphysematikern. Verh. dtsch. Ges. inn. Med. **62**, 68 (1956). ~ Untersuchungen bei Menschen und Hunden über die Wirksamkeit herzsynchroner Mischungsvorgänge in den Atemwegen. Pflügers Arch. ges. Physiol. **268**, 460 (1959). — Ulmer, W., u. G. Lechner: Untersuchungen über die Größe des absoluten Totraumes und dessen Beziehungen zum funktionellen Totraum, zur Ausatemgeschwindigkeit und zum Atemvolumen. Pflügers Arch. ges. Physiol. **268**, 470 (1959). — Ulmer, W., u. M. Stammberger: Untersuchungen über den funktionellen Totraum bei Arbeit und bei willkürlich vertiefter Atmung. Pflügers Arch. ges. Physiol. **268**, 484 (1959). — Ulmer, W., u. A. Wenke: Bronchospirometrische Untersuchungen über Ausmaß und Geschwindigkeit der Durchblutungsregulation des Alveolarraumes in Abhängigkeit von partieller Sauerstoffmangelatmung bei gesunden Versuchspersonen. Internat. Thoraxkongr., Köln 1956. ~ Bronchospirometrische Untersuchungen zur Frage der gasspannungsabhängigen Durchblutungsregulation der Alveolarkapillaren. Arch. Kreisl.-Forsch. **26**, 256 (1957). — Uspenskij, I.: Experimentelle Histamin-Pneumosklerose. Arch. Pat. (Moskau) **14**, 46 (1952). Ref. Ber. allg. spez. Path. **16**, 316 (1953).

Valentin, H., H. Venrath u. J. Kann: Über die Bedeutung von chronischer Bronchitis und Lungenemphysem in der Arbeitsmedizin und die Häufigkeit dieser Krankheitsbilder bei mehr als 1000 Gutachtenpatienten. Arch. Gewerbepath. Gewerbehyg. **17**, 420 (1959). — Vandendorpe, F.: Structure de l'artériole pulmonaire chez l'homme. Ann. anat. path. **13**, 652 (1936). — Vaněk, J.: Interstitielle, nichteitrige Pneumonie. (Diffuse Lungenfibrose und Lungencirrhose.) Zbl. allg. Path. path. Anat. **92**, 405 (1954). — Vaněk, J., u. O. Jírovec: Parasitäre Pneumonie. Interstitielle Plasmazellenpneumonie der Frühgeburten, verursacht durch Pneumocystis Carinii. Zbl. Bakt., I. Abt. Orig. **158**, 120 (1952). — Veith, G.: Über die Albuminocholie bei Frühgeborenen und Säuglingen. Ein Beitrag zum Problem der Unreife. Mschr. Kinderheilk. **105**, 53 (1957). — Venrath, H.: Lungenfunktionsprüfung mit Hilfe von Isotopen. In: Lunge und kleiner Kreislauf. Bad Oeynhausener Gespräche I, 1944 (1956). Berlin-Göttingen-Heidelberg: Springer 1957. — Venrath, H., H. Lechtenbörger, H. Valentin u. H. Bolt: Das Verhalten von Atmung und Kreislauf bei uni- und bilateraler Sauerstoffmangelatmung. Ein Beitrag zur Kompensation akuter Hypoxie durch Kreislaufumstellung. Z. Kreisl.-Forsch. **44**, 544 (1955). — Verzár, F.: Die Regulation des Lungenvolumens. Pflügers Arch. ges. Physiol. **232**, 322 (1933). — Virchow, R.: Gesammelte Abhandlungen zur wissenschaftlichen Medizin. Frankfurt a. M.: Meidinger 1856. ~ Emphysema pulmonum. Berl. klin. Wschr. 1888. — Vivell, O.: Durchströmungsversuche am Coronarsystem bei normalem, hypertrophischem und atrophischem Herzmuskel. Beitr. path. Anat. **111**, 125 (1951). — Vogel, H.: Die Geschwindigkeit des Blutes in den Lungenkapillaren. Helv. physiol. pharmacol. Acta **5**, 105 (1947). — Vogel, J.: Klinische Ergebnisse der Bronchospirometrie unter passiver Beatmung in Narkose und muskulärer Relaxation. Beitr. Klin. Tuberk. **120**, 69 (1959). — Volhard, F.: Über künstliche Atmung durch Ventilation der Trachea und eine einfache Vorrichtung zur rhythmischen künstlichen Atmung. Münch. med. Wschr. **1908**, 209. ~ Diskussionsbemerkung zu Bönniger 1909. Zit. nach Raither 1912. ~ Vortrag über

Lungenemphysem, Verein der Ärzte in Halle a. S. 23. 2. 1921. Ref. Münch. med. Wschr. **1921**, 928. ~ Referat über Emphysem, Tagg. südwestdtsch. Pathologen, Mannheim 1922. Zbl. allg. Path. path. Anat. **33**, 1—20 (1922/23). — WACHOLDER, K.: Die Vitalkapazität als Maß der körperlichen Leistungsfähigkeit. Klin. Wschr. **1928**, 295. — WADE, O. L.: Movements of the thoracic cage and diaphragm in respiration. J. Physiol. (Lond.) **124**, 193 (1954). — WADE, O. L., J. M. BISHOP and K. W. DONALD: The effect of mitral valvotomy on cardiorespiratory function. Clin. Sci. **13**, 511 (1954). — WÄTJEN, J.: Über Lungenhilusveränderungen und ihre Bedeutung bei Staublungen. Arch. Gewerbepath. Gewerbehyg. **12**, 171 (1944). — WAGNER, R.: Über die Beziehungen zwischen Pulmonalisdruck und Minutenvolumen. Z. Biol. **88**, 25 (1929). ~ Über die Widerstände im Lungenkreislauf und über die Mechanismen der zentralnervösen Beeinflussung. Z. Biol. **96**, 410 (1935). ~ Kreislauf und Atmung. Verh. dtsch. Ges. Kreisl-Forsch. **13**, 7 (1940). — WARREN, S.: Effects of radiation on normal tissues. V. Effects on the respiratory system. Arch. Path. (Chicago) **34**, 917 (1942). — WARREN, S., and F. J. DIXON: Antigen tracer studies and histologic observations in anaphylactic shock in the guinea pig. Amer. J. med. Sci. **216**, 136 (1948). — WARREN, S., and O. GATES: Radiation pneumonitis. Experimental and pathological observations. Arch. Path. (Chicago) **30**, 440 (1940). — WAWERLA, W.: Über Veränderungen des elastischen Gewebes in der Lunge bei Fällen von Asthma bronchiale. Virchows Arch. path. Anat. **285**, 12 (1932). — WEARN, J. T., J. S. BARR and W. J. GERMAN: Behavior of the arterioles and capillaries of the lung. Proc. Soc. exp. Biol. (N.Y.) **24**, 114 (1926). — WEARN, J. T., A. C. ERNSTENE, A. W. BROMER, J. S. BARR, W. J. GERMAN and L. J. ZSCHIESCHE: The normal behavior of the pulmonary blood vessels with observation on the intermittence of the flow of blood in the arterioles and capillaries. Amer. J. Physiol. **109**, 236 (1934). — WEBER, E.: Neue Untersuchungen über experimentelles Asthma und die Innervation der Bronchialmuskeln. Arch. Physiol. **63** (1914). — WEBER, H. H.: Die normale Atmung. In: Röntgenkymographische Bewegungslehre innerer Organe (STUMPF-WEBER-WELTZ). Leipzig: Georg Thieme 1936. ~ Bronchographie und Lungenfeinstruktur. Fortschr. Röntgenstr. **75**, 249 (1951). ~ Radiologische Exploration des Hustenaktes. Fortschr. Röntgenstr. **90**, 274, 452 (1959). — WEBER, H. W.: Zur Frage der Segmenteinteilung der Lungen. Verh. dtsch. Ges. Path. **33**, 207 (1949). ~ Über die anatomischen Grundlagen und die Bedeutung der Lungensegmente. Tuberk.-Arzt **4**, 254 (1950). ~ Über Kontraktionsatelektasen. Verh. dtsch. Ges. Path. **34**, 311 (1951). ~ Untersuchungen über die Bedeutung der Lungensegmente. Frankfurt. Z. Path. **62**, 499 (1951). ~ Die Bedeutung der Verzweigungsgebiete der Bronchien I. Ordnung für die Ausbreitung von Krankheitsherden in der Lunge. Frankfurter Z. Path. **62**, 523 (1951). — WEBER, K.-H.: Über die Zwerchfellbeweglichkeit nach thoraxchirurgischen Eingriffen. Beitr. Klin. Tuberk. **118**, 262 (1958). — WEGELIN, C.: Zur pathologischen Anatomie des Asthma bronchiale. Schweiz. med. Wschr. **1944**, 5. — WEIBEL, E.: Die Blutgefäßanastomosen in der menschlichen Lunge. Z. Zellforsch. **50**, 653 (1959). — WEICKSEL, P., u. E. BRUGGER: Die spastische Bronchitis bei Silikose. Verh. dtsch. Ges. inn. Med. **63**, 701 (1957). — WENK, E.: Über das Lungenemphysem. Münch. med. Wschr. **1957**, 1851. — WENZEL, H. G.: Untersuchungen einiger mechanischer Eigenschaften der Haut, insbesondere der Striae cutis distensae. Virchows Arch. path. Anat. **317**, 654 (1950). — WERNLI-HAESSIG, A.: Über die Spätkomplikationen des künstlichen Pneumothorax. Schweiz. Z. Tuberk. **7**, 331 (1950). — WESSELY, E.: Die Luftdruckverhältnisse in den Nebenhöhlen der Nase. Mschr. Ohrenheilk. **55**, 1730 (1921). — WEST, J. R., F. DE BALDWIN, D. W. RICHARDS and A. COURNAND: Physiopathologic aspects of chronic pulmonary emphysema. Amer. J. Med. **10**, 481 (1951). — WESTCOTT, R. N., N. O. FOWLER, R. C. SCOTT, W. D. HAUENSTEIN and J. McGUIRE: Anoxia and human pulmonary vascular resistance. J. clin. Invest. **30**, 957 (1951). — WESTENHÖFER, M.: Über amyzische Atelektase der Lungen. Med. Klin. **1928**, 539. ~ Über den haemorrhagischen Infarkt und die amyzische Atelektase der Lungen. Verh. dtsch. Ges. Path. **28**, 310 (1935). — WESTERMARK, N.: Vergleichende röntgenologische und pathologisch-anatomische Studien von den Bronchien bei Lungentuberkulose unter besonderer Berücksichtigung des Vorkommens von massivem Lungenkollaps. Med. Klin. **1932**, 675. ~ On bronchostenosis, a roentgenological studies. Acta radiol. (Stockh.) **19**, 285, 313 (1938). ~ The motility of the bronchial wall. Bronches **2**, 14 (1952). — WEZLER, K., u. W. SINN: Das Strömungsgesetz des Blutkreislaufs. Aulendorf (Wttbg.):Editio Cantor K.G. 1953. — WHITWELL, F.: A study of the pathology and pathogenesis of bronchiectasis. Thorax **7**, 213 (1952). — WICK, H.: Die Beeinflussung der Tracheobronchial- und Alveolarweite durch lokale Einwirkung des Kohlendioxyds. Arch. int. Pharmacodyn. **88**, 461 (1952). ~ Die Wirkung der Kohlensäure auf die Weite der Lungenalveolen. Über die Änderung der Lungenelastizität durch Kohlensäure. Arch. int. Pharmacodyn. **89**, 1 (1952). — WIESE, F.: Über Thromboendarteriitis obliterans der Lungenarterien, ein Beitrag zur Pathogenese autochthoner Lungenarterien-Thrombose. Frankfurt. Z. Path. **49**, 155 (1936). — WIGGERS, C. J.: Pulmonary wedged catheter pressures. Circulat. Res. **1**, 371 (1953). — WILLIAMS jr., M. H.: Relationships between pulmonary artery pressure and blood flow in the dog lung. Amer. J. Physiol. **179**, 243 (1954). — WILLIAMSON: Zit. nach K. HANSEN 1957. — WILSON, R. H., R. C. EVANS, R. S. JOHNSON and M. E.

Dempsey: An estimation of the effective alveolar respiratory surface and other pulmonary properties in normal persons. Amer. Rev. Tuberc. **30**, 296 (1954). — Winkler, F.: Untersuchungen über die Beziehungen des Abdominaldrucks zur Respiration. Pflügers Arch. ges. Physiol. **98**, 163 (1903). — Wintrich, M. A.: Krankheiten der Respirationsorgane. In: Virchows Handbuch der speziellen Pathologie und Therapie, Bd. V/1. Erlangen: Enke 1854. — Wirz, K.: Das Verhalten des Druckes im Pleuraraum bei der Atmung und die Ursachen seiner Veränderlichkeit. Pflügers Arch. ges. Physiol. **199**, 1 (1923). — Wöhlisch, E., u. R. du Mesnil de Rochemont: Untersuchungen über elastische und thermodynamische Eigenschaften des Bindegewebes (vorläufige Mitteilung). Beitr. path. Anat. **76**, 233 (1927). — Wolpers, C.: Kollagenquerstreifung und Grundsubstanz. Klin. Wschr. **1943**, 624. — Worth, G.: Bronchitis-Emphysem-Silikose (Referat). 3. Internat. Staublungentagg, Münster 1957. In: Die Staublungenerkrankungen, Bd. 3. Darmstadt: Steinkopff 1958. — Worth, G., L. Gasthaus, W. Lühning, K. Muysers, F. Siehoff u. K. Werner: Lungenvolumina und Lungenzeitvolumina bei Kohlenbergarbeitern. Arch. Gewerbepath. Gewerbehyg. **17**, 396 (1969). ~ Kritische Bemerkungen zur Diagnostik des Lungenemphysems bei Kohlenbergarbeitern. Arch. Gewerbepath. Gewerbehyg. **17**, 442 (1959). — Worth, G., u. E. Schiller: Die Pneumokoniosen. Köln: Staufen-Verlag 1954. — Worth, G., H. Valentin, L. Gasthaus, H. Hoffmann u. H. Venrath: Bewirkt die Staubinhalation bei Bergarbeitern eine akute respiratorische Insuffizienz? Arch. Gewerbepath. Gewerbehyg. **14**, 37 (1955). — Worth, G., H. Valentin, L. Gasthaus u. E. Schiller: Hat die Inhalation von Feinstäuben einen unmittelbaren Einfluß auf die Atmung und den Gasstoffwechsel? III. Mitt. Arch. Gewerbepath. Gewerbehyg. **14**, 428 (1956). — Worth, G., H. Valentin, H. Venrath, L. Gasthaus u. H. Hoffmann: Weitere klinische und spirographische Untersuchungen bei Bergleuten vor, während und nach der Untertagearbeit. II. Mitt. Arch. Gewerbepath. Gewerbehyg. **14**, 269 (1956). — Wurm, H.: Tuberkulose und Atelektase. Ergebn. ges. Tuberk.-Forsch. (Stuttgart) **12**, 121 (1954). — Wyss, F.: Asthma bronchiale. Stuttgart: Georg Thieme 1955. — Wyss, F., u. W. Hadorn: Die Pneumometrie. In: Fortschritte der Allergielehre, III. Basel 1952. — Wyss, F., u. J. Regli: Über physiologische und pathologische respiratorische Bronchialkaliberschwankungen. Helv. med. Acta **21**, 479 (1954). — Wyss, F., u. F. Schmid: Beruht die bronchialasthmatische Dyspnoe auf einer Bronchialstenose? Schweiz. med. Wschr. **1951**, 38, 916. — Wyss, F., u. W. Wilbrandt: Die quantitative pneumometrische Beurteilung asthmatischer Zustände und ihre pharmakotherapeutische Beeinflussung. Helv. med. Acta **12**, 819 (1945). — Wyss, H. I.: Bronchiale Perforationsnarben. Beitr. path. Anat. **116**, 625 (1956). — Wyss, O. A. M.: Prinzipielle Betrachtungen über die Funktionsweise der Bronchialmuskulatur. Schweiz. med. Wschr. **1952**, 988.

Zenker, R., G. Heberer u. H. H. Löhr: Die Lungenresektionen (Anatomie, Indikationen, Technik). Berlin-Göttingen-Heidelberg: Springer 1954. — Ziegler, H. K.: Die hyalinen Membranen im Rahmen der Lungenbefunde bei Frühgeborenen. Z. Kinderheilk. **79**, 433 (1957). — Zöllner, N.: Die Diagnostik häufiger Formen der Atmungsinsuffizienz mit einfachen spirometrischen Methoden. Dtsch. med. Wschr. **1958**, 1815, 1852. — Zorn, O.: Herz und Lungenkreislauf bei Silikose. Beitr. Silikose-Forsch. Ber. Med. Wiss. Tagg über Silikose 1951, S. 23. ~ Chronische Bronchitis bei Staubinhalation und ihre Vorbeugung. Verh. dtsch. Ges. inn. Med. **62**, 99 (1956). — Zuidema, P., u. M. Scherrer: Beitrag zur funktionellen Diagnostik des chronisch substantiellen Lungenemphysems. Schweiz. Z. Tuberk. **12**, 215 (1955). — Zuppinger, A.: Die Strahlenveränderungen der Lunge. In: Handbuch der inneren Medizin, 4. Aufl., Bd. IV/2. Berlin-Göttingen-Heidelberg 1956.

Die Orthologie und Pathologie der Kreislauffunktion[*].

Von

Wolf Schoedel-Göttingen

und

Franz Grosse-Brockhoff-Düsseldorf.

Mit 76 Abbildungen.

A. Die Durchblutung der Organe.

I. Grundlagen.

1. Die optimale Einstellung der Durchblutung.

Man kann mit gutem Grund den Kreislauf — wie es in diesem Handbuch geschieht — als einen Hilfsmechanismus des Gewebsstoffwechsels auffassen. Er muß danach so beschaffen sein, daß der Stoffwechselbedarf sämtlicher Organe und sämtlicher Gewebe sichergestellt ist. Die Durchblutung sämtlicher Organe muß ausreichend sein, damit diese Aufgabe erfüllt ist. Man sollte hier gleich einen zweiten teleologischen Satz anführen: Die Kreislaufarbeit sollte so klein wie möglich gehalten werden. Kreislaufarbeit ist in allererster Linie Herzarbeit. Luxusdurchblutung, d. h. Durchblutung der Organe über ihren Stoffwechselbedarf hinaus, würde die Herzarbeit unnötig erhöhen.

Die Durchblutung eines Organs dient zunächst der Deckung seines Stoffwechselbedarfs. Viele Organe erfüllen aber gleichzeitig Aufgaben für andere Organe bzw. den gesamten Organismus. Man kann sie im weitesten Sinne als Regenerationsorgane des Blutes auffassen. Dies gilt für Lunge, Niere, Leber, aber auch für die Haut, indem an dieser Stelle das Blut einen Überschuß von

Tabelle 1. *Abschätzung der Durchblutung und des Sauerstoffverbrauchs der Organe eines 70 kg schweren Menschen.* (Nach M. Schneider, Physiologie des Menschen, 12. Aufl. 1959.)

Organ	Gewicht		Durchblutung			Sauerstoffverbrauch			Art.-ven. Sauerstoffdifferenz
	g	% des Körpergewichts	ml/min	ml/min · 100 g Organgewicht	% des HZV	ml/min	ml/min · 100 g Organgewicht	% des Ges.-O_2-Verbrauchs	ml O_2/100 ml Dbl.
Gehirn	1400	2,0	770	55,0	14,5	45,0	3,2	19,0	5,8
Splanchnicus-Gebiet	2800	4,0	1800	65,0	34,0	84,0	3,0	35,0	4,5
Lunge.	600	0,8	[5250]	[875,0]	[100,0]	12,0	2,0	5,0	[4,5]
Nieren	290	0,4	1100	380,0	21,0	15,0	5,5	6,0	1,5
Herz	320	0,5	200	65,0	4,0	22,5	7,0	9,5	11,0
Innersekretorische Organe	60	0,1	150	250,0	3,0	6,0	10,0	2,5	4,0
Muskulatur	29000	41,0	850	3,0	16,0	43,5	0,15	18,0	5,0
Haut	5000	7,0	125	2,5	2,5	2,5	0,05	1,0	2,0
Skelet.	11000	16,0	160	1,5	3,0	5,5	0,05	2,5	4,0
Übrige Organe . . .	19530	28,2	95		2,0	4,0		1,5	
	70000	100,0	5250		100,0	240,0		100,0	

* Die Bearbeitung dieses Beitrages wurde am 8. 6. 1959 abgeschlossen.

Wärme abgeben kann. Die Organdurchblutung richtet sich in diesen Fällen nicht allein nach den örtlichen Bedürfnissen. Tabelle 1 gibt eine Übersicht über Sauerstoffverbrauch und Durchblutung der wichtigsten Organe. Die angeführten arterio-venösen Sauerstoffdifferenzen lassen erkennen, ob die Durchblutung allein dem Eigenbedarf des Organs dient. Der immer in Tätigkeit befindliche Herzmuskel mit seiner großen arterio-venösen Sauerstoffdifferenz ist ein Beispiel für ein Organ, dessen Durchblutung durch den Eigenstoffwechsel bestimmt ist.

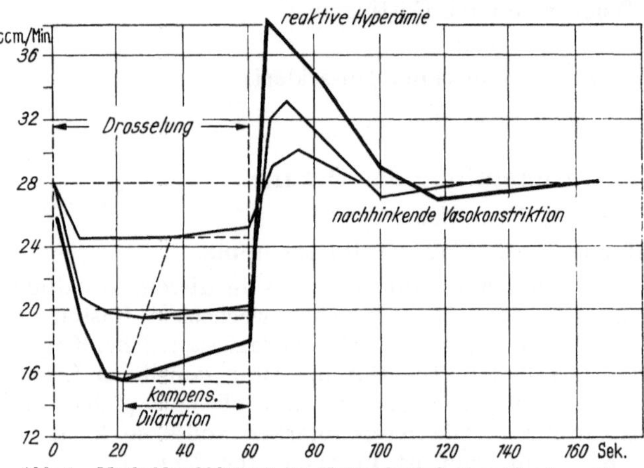

Abb. 1. Muskeldurchblutung im Unterschenkel eines Hundes. Vasomotorische Gegenmaßnahmen bei 3 unterschiedlich starken künstlichen Drosselungen der Blutzufuhr (Rein 1944).

Dagegen haben Haut und Niere eine sehr kleine arterio-venöse Sauerstoffdifferenz. Sie sind Regenerationsorgane und ihre Durchblutung ist nach den Bedürfnissen des ganzen Organismus oder — anders ausgedrückt — nach den Bedürfnissen der Blutregeneration eingestellt.

Werden Organe stärker durchblutet als ihrem Bedarf entspricht, besteht also eine Luxusdurchblutung, so wird dadurch der Kreislauf, insbesondere das Herz, unnötig belastet. Für eine optimale Einstellung der Durchblutung, also eine Vermeidung der Luxusdurchblutung, spricht folgendes Experiment:

Drosselt man mit einer Schraubklemme die Blutzufuhr zum ruhenden Muskel künstlich ab (Abb. 1), so erweitert sich nach kurzer Zeit das Gefäß stromabwärts der Drossel wie man an dem Ansteigen der Durchblutung erkennen kann (kompensatorische Dilatation)[1]. Öffnet man die Drossel wieder, so schießt das Blut in das geöffnete Strombett ein, es folgt die reaktive Hyperämie. Schon sehr geringe Drosselungen lösen diese Gefäßreaktion aus.

Demnach scheint die Durchblutung streng den Erfordernissen angepaßt zu sein. Bei jedem Anstieg des Stoffwechsels muß dann aber die Durchblutung vergrößert werden. Am bekanntesten und wichtigsten ist in diesem Sinne die Arbeitsmehrdurchblutung des Skeletmuskels. Aber nicht in jedem Fall kann die Durchblutung an den momentanen Stoffwechselbedarf angepaßt sein. Insbesondere kann der Strömungswiderstand seinen Minimalwert erreichen, d. h. es können die Gefäße maximal erweitert sein, ohne daß damit der Stoffwechselbedarf schon gedeckt ist. Auch gibt es Fälle, wo starke zentralnervöse Einflüsse die Durchblutung herunterdrücken, so daß der Stoffwechselbedarf momentan nicht gedeckt wird. In diesen Fällen müssen ,,Schulden" eingegangen werden, die in einem späteren Stadium bei länger dauernden Mehrdurchblutungen rückgezahlt werden. Es kommt zunächst zur Anhäufung von Intermediärprodukten, die in einem späteren Stadium bei wieder angepaßter Durchblutung entweder aus dem Organ abtransportiert oder bei nunmehr ausreichend angebotenem Sauerstoff abgebaut werden.

2. Capillarisierung und arterio-venöse Anastomosen.

Damit der Bedarf der Organe mit einer relativ kleinen Durchblutung gedeckt werden kann, muß die Transportfunktion des Blutes möglichst ausgenutzt werden.

---

[1] Rein 1944.

Eine Vorbedingung dafür ist eine gute Capillarisierung. Das Capillarnetz muß dicht genug sein, damit der durch Diffusion erfolgende Stoffaustausch für alle Teile des Gewebes sichergestellt ist. Der Gesamtquerschnitt des Capillarbettes muß hinreichend groß sein, damit die Strömungsgeschwindigkeit des Blutes in den Capillaren niedrig und damit die Kontaktzeit zwischen Blut und Gewebe groß wird. Die Capillarisierung ist ein besonders wichtiger Faktor für die Sauerstoffversorgung des Gewebes. Sie wird an einer anderen Stelle dieses Handbuches ausführlich besprochen [1]. Je höher der Stoffwechsel eines Gewebes, um so dichter ist sein Capillarnetz. Bei Organen, bei denen sich die Intensität des Stoffwechsels mit dem Funktionszustand ändert, ändert sich auch gleichzeitig die Capillarisierung, d. h. die Anzahl der geöffneten Capillaren und ihre Blutfüllung. Dies gilt in besonders starkem Maße für den Skeletmuskel. Eine veränderte Capillarisierung von Organen kann auf den gesamten Kreislauf zurückwirken. Denn je höher die Capillarisierung, um so höher ist auch die Blutfüllung der Organe, es sei denn, daß durch Venomotorik die Blutfüllung der Venen entsprechend herabgesetzt wird. Die Capillarisierung kann damit die Blutverteilung auf die einzelnen Organe und den Rückstrom des Blutes zum Herzen beeinflussen.

Wenn man im allgemeinen annimmt, daß Capillarisierung und Durchblutung dem Organstoffwechsel angepaßt sind, so widersprechen dem anscheinend zahlreiche Befunde über arterio-venöse Kurzschlüsse. Ihrer Struktur nach sind sie nicht dazu geeignet, daß das sie passierende Blut mit dem umgebenden Gewebe in stärkerem Maße in Stoffaustausch tritt. Die Kurzschlußdurchblutung führt dazu, daß dem aus den Capillaren abfließenden Blut ein Teil arteriellen Blutes beigemischt wird, wodurch die Ausnutzung des Blutes verschlechtert wird. Für das Bestehen von arterio-venösen Kurzschlüssen in den verschiedensten Gebieten sprechen einerseits morphologische Befunde, andererseits funktionelle Untersuchungen, die auf arterio-venöse Verbindungen mit sehr großem Querschnitt hinweisen. Der Nachweis solcher Verbindungen gelingt im Tierversuch dadurch, daß man Kugeln verschiedenen Querschnitts in die Arterie injiziert und prüft, ob sie in der Vene wieder zu finden sind [2]. In speziellen Fällen ist es möglich, mit Hilfe von Stoffen, deren Konzentration beim Durchfluß durch die Capillaren einen charakteristischen Endwert erreicht, die Größe der Kurzschlußdurchblutung zu schätzen. So ist es möglich, mit Hilfe der Paraaminohippursäure die Kurzschlußdurchblutung der Niere zu schätzen, da unter den meisten Bedingungen beim Durchfluß durch die Tubuluscapillaren die gesamte Paraaminohippursäure aus dem Blut in die Tubuluszellen übertritt. Die Kurzschlußdurchblutung der Niere beträgt danach weniger als 8% [3]. In ähnlicher Weise kann man die Kurzschlußdurchblutung der Lunge aus den Sauerstoffwerten abschätzen, wenn man die Bedingungen für die Diffusion des Sauerstoffs in der Lunge kennt. Die Kurzschlußdurchblutung der gesunden Lunge scheint danach weniger als 4% zu betragen [4]. Auffallend ist, daß an Niere und Lunge, wo von den Morphologen reichlich arterio-venöse Anastomosen beschrieben werden, der mit funktioneller Methodik ermittelte Anteil der Kurzschlußdurchblutung so niedrig liegt. Es ist nicht auszuschließen, daß die Anastomosen im Zustand, bei dem die Untersuchungen durchgeführt werden, weitgehend geschlossen waren und daß Zustände mit geöffneten arterio-venösen Anastomosen nur noch nicht erfaßt wurden. Ein größeres Ausmaß hat die Durchblutung von arterio-venösen Anastomosen sicherlich in den Fingern

---

[1] OPITZ und LÜBBERS 1956.
[2] BOSTROEM und SCHOEDEL 1953, PIIPER und SCHOEDEL 1954, PRINZMETAL u. a. 1947, 1948, SIMKIN u. a. 1948, PIIPER, SCHNEIDER und SCHOEDEL 1954, SCHOEDEL 1955.
[3] SMITH 1951.   [4] BARTELS u. a. 1955.

und Zehen von Mensch und Tier sowie in den Ohren vom Kaninchen. Abb. 2 zeigt die Verhältnisse in der hinteren Extremität des Hundes, wie sie mit der Kugelmethode gefunden wurden. Die Anastomosen werden unter den meisten Bedingungen durch nervöse Einflüsse verschlossen gehalten. Entnervung führt zu einem starken Anstieg der Anastomosendurchblutung[1]. Einige Autoren schließen aus ihren Befunden auf eine Kurzschlußdurchblutung in der Skeletmuskulatur[2]. Jedoch sind bei den erhobenen Befunden auch andere Deutungen möglich. Anatomische Befunde könnten für eine Zweiteilung des Muskelgefäßsystems in Capillaren und Kurzschlüsse sprechen[3]. Jedoch bedürfen diese Fragen noch weiterer Aufklärung[4].

Über die Funktion der arterio-venösen Anastomosen gibt es zahlreiche Hypothesen, die meist unbefriedigend sind. Es ist naheliegend, daß der Vielfalt der Strukturen[5] eine Vielfalt von Funktionen entspricht, und daß die Verhältnisse auch an den einzelnen Organen verschieden sind. Vielleicht steht die Bedeutung als drüsige Organe[6] und als Teilstrukturen von Receptorensystemen[7] bei den epithelzelligen Anastomosen im Vordergrund. Vielleicht sind andere Kurzschlüsse „Webfehler" im Gefäßsystem oder Folge von Traumen[8]. Ob die dadurch bedingten Fehldurchblutungen unter normalen Verhältnissen größere Ausmaße erreichen, darüber fehlen jegliche Kenntnisse.

Fast alle Vorstellungen über die hämodynamische Bedeutung der arterio-venösen Anastomosen[4] sind unbefriedigend. Man kann sich vorstellen, daß die Kurzschlußdurchblutung eine Art Reservedurchblutung darstellt, die bei Beanspruchung der Organe auf die Capillaren übergeleitet werden kann. Diese Art der Reservedurchblutung wäre dann freilich für den Ruhezustand nichts anderes als eine Luxusdurchblutung und würde zu einer dauernden Belastung des Kreislaufs führen. Auch die Regulierung des arteriellen Druckes über arterio-venöse Anastomosen[9] scheint nicht sehr zweckmäßig. Im Hinblick auf die Kreislaufleistung erfolgt die Einstellung des arteriellen Druckes besser über den Bluteinstrom in das arterielle System als über Änderungen des Abflußwiderstandes. Einleuchtend ist die Funktion der arterio-venösen Anastomosen überall da, wo es auf eine Steigerung des peripheren venösen Druckes wie etwa bei den Schwellkörpern ankommt.

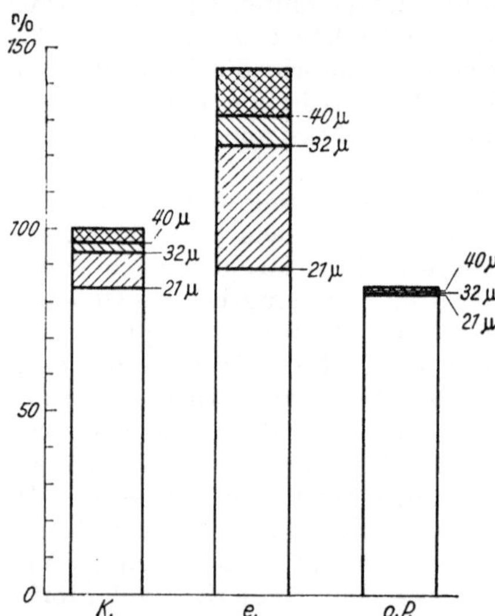

Abb. 2. Durchblutungsanteil der arteriovenösen Anastomosen in der hinteren Extremität des Hundes. Bestimmung mit Wachskugeln von 21, 32 und 40 μ Durchmesser. An der Extremität kann aus dem Durchgang von Kugeln, die größer als 20 μ sind, auf die Durchblutung von arteriovenösen Anastomosen geschlossen werden. In der Abbildung entsprechen also die gesamten schraffierten Flächen der Anastomosendurchblutung. Linke Säule: Kontrollbein, mittlere Säule: entnervtes Bein, rechte Säule: Bein ohne Pfote. Ordinate: Durchblutungsanteile in % der Gesamtdurchblutung des Kontrollbeins. (PIIPER und SCHOEDEL 1954.)

---

[1] PIIPER und SCHOEDEL 1954, FOLKOW 1955.

[2] PAPPENHEIMER 1941, SCHROEDER 1952, BARCROFT und SWAN 1953, WALDER 1955, LAMBERT 1956, MOREIRA u. a. 1956.

[3] ZWEIFACH und METZ 1955a.   [4] CLARA 1956.   [5] CLARA 1956, SPANNER 1952.

[6] STAUBESAND 1950.   [7] ROTTER 1952, ROTTER und WAGNER 1952.

[8] CLARK 1938.   [9] BOSTROEM und SCHNEIDER 1953.

Für die arterio-venösen Anastomosen in den Körperspitzen kann angenommen werden, daß sie für die Temperaturregulation von Bedeutung sind. Sie können dabei sowohl der lokalen Aufwärmung dienen als auch für die Wärmeabgabe des gesamten Organismus von Bedeutung sein[1]. Ihre Durchblutung ist für den Stoffaustausch zwar Kurzschlußdurchblutung, dagegen ist mit ihrer Hilfe ein Wärmeaustausch möglich. Dazu hilft die sehr niedrige Gewebstemperatur an den Körperspitzen. Außerdem wird die Wärme gar nicht allein in der kurzen Strecke der eigentlichen arteriovenösen Anastomose, sondern auch in den zu ihr hin- und von ihr wegführenden Gefäßen, besonders in den Hautvenen ausgetauscht[2]. Durch ihren niedrigen Strömungswiderstand geben die Anastomosen die Möglichkeit, große Blutmengen zum Wärmetransport durch die Körperspitzen hindurchzuschicken, ohne daß die Kreislaufarbeit damit übermäßig groß wird. Die Kurzschlußdurchblutung der Extremitäten ist also gar keine Luxusdurchblutung. Sie dient zwar nicht dem Stoffaustausch, aber dem Wärmeaustausch[3].

3. Durchblutung, Druckgefälle und Strömungswiderstand.

Die Durchblutung der Organe hängt vom arterio-venösen Druckgefälle und dem Strömungswiderstand ab. Änderungen des venösen Druckes sind im allgemeinen zu gering, als daß sie das Druckgefälle und damit die Durchblutung in stärkerem Maße beeinflussen. Dagegen folgt die Durchblutung sehr weitgehend den Änderungen des arteriellen Druckes, soweit nicht Gegenregulationen einsetzen. Da der arterielle Druck die wichtigste geregelte Größe ist, und damit im allgemeinen sehr konstant gehalten wird (S. 678), hängt die Einstellung der Organdurchblutung aber in erster Linie von der Einstellung des Strömungswiderstandes in der Gefäßperipherie ab.

Der periphere Strömungswiderstand ist der Quotient aus Druckgefälle und Durchblutung. Dies gilt für die einzelnen Organe und für den Gesamtkreislauf. In letzterem Falle ist der Gesamtwiderstand der Quotient aus arterio-venösem Druckgefälle und dem Herzzeitvolumen. Der Begriff des peripheren Strömungswiderstandes ist etwas in Mißkredit geraten. Dies beruht besonders darauf, daß Änderungen dieser Größe im allgemeinen auf vasomotorische Vorgänge zurückgeführt wurden, was zwar meistens, aber nicht immer richtig ist.

Verändert man im Experiment planmäßig den Druck und mißt man die zugehörigen Durchblutungswerte, so erhält man die Druck-Durchblutungskurve (p-i-Kurve). Dabei können vasomotorische Vorgänge ausgelöst werden, die dann den Kurvenverlauf beeinflussen. Häufig führt eine Verminderung des Druckes regulatorisch zu einer Senkung des Strömungswiderstandes. Es handelt sich um Gefäßerweiterungen, durch welche trotz des fallenden Druckes die Durchblutung hoch gehalten wird[4]. Untersucht man unter Bedingungen, bei denen regulatorische Vorgänge ausgeschaltet sind, so erhält man häufig Beziehungen zwischen Druck und Durchblutung, wie sie in Abb. 3 wiedergegeben sind. Charakteristisch ist die Versteilung der Kurve mit steigendem Druck. Auch laufen die Kurven nicht durch den Nullpunkt des Koordinatensystems. Die Durchblutung kommt schon zum Stillstand, wenn noch ein bestimmtes Druckgefälle vorhanden ist. Man spricht vom kritischen Schließungsdruck. Er hängt von der Oberflächenspannung zwischen Blut und Gefäßwand, vom Aufbau und Funktionszustand der Gefäßwand und vom Gewebsdruck ab[5].

---

[1] CLARK 1938.   [2] BAZETT 1947.   [3] PIIPER 1956.   [4] FOLKOW 1952.
[5] BURTON 1954, 1951, BURTON und YAMADA 1951, FOLKOW und LÖFVING 1956.

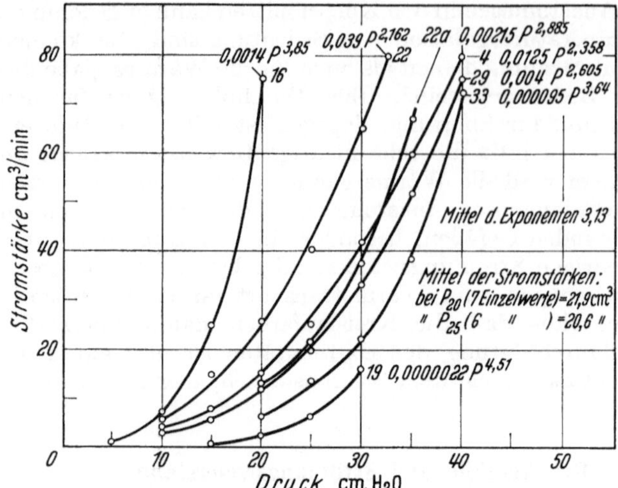

Abb. 3. Druck-Stromstärkekurven, die an Kaninchenlungen gewonnen wurden. Für jede Kurve ist Versuchsnummer und Funktion $(a \cdot p^n)$ angegeben. (Wezler u. Sinn 1953.)

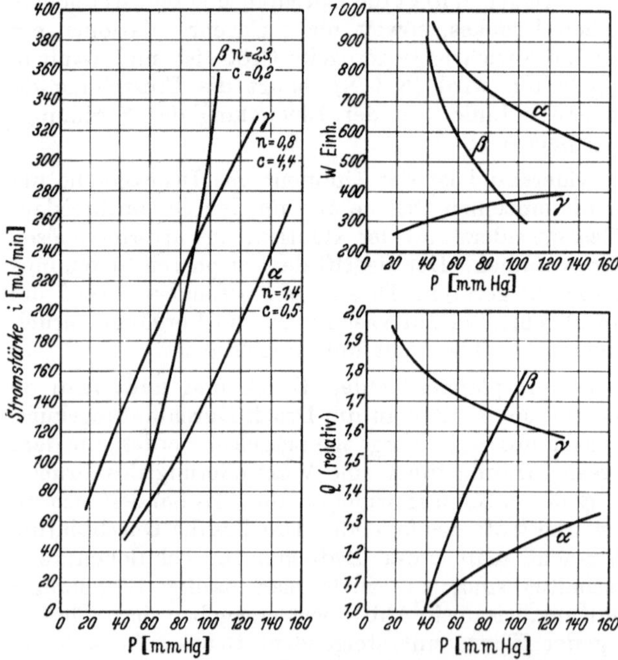

Abb. 4. Beziehungen des Blutdrucks zur Stromstärke, zum relativen Gefäßquerschnitt und zum Strömungswiderstand des arteriellen Kreislaufs. Untersuchungen an der Aorta descendens der Katze. α „unbeeinflußter" Kreislauf; β oligämischer Schock, γ nach Dekapitierung; Druck-Stromstärkekurven; Druck-Widerstandskurven und Druckquerschnittskurven; n Exponent; c Koeffizient der Druck-Stromstärke-Funktion. (Mechelke, Nusser u. Key 1955.)

Die Druckdurchblutungskurve kann meistens (unter Vernachlässigung des kritischen Schließungsdruckes) durch eine Potenzfunktion beschrieben werden:

$$i = a\,p^n$$

(i Stromstärke, p Druck, a und n Konstante)[1].

Bei tierexperimentellen Untersuchungen der Extremitätendurchblutung ist der Exponent um so höher, je geringer der Tonus der Gefäßmuskulatur ist. Frühere Messungen ergaben Werte des Exponenten zwischen 1 und 2. In Ausnahmefällen konnte er bis 5 ansteigen[2]. Unter besseren experimentellen Bedingungen fand man später Exponenten unter 1 (s. S. 646)[3]. Für die Fingerdurchblutung des Menschen fand man Exponenten zwischen 2, 6 und 4[4].

Von besonderer Bedeutung sind die Beziehungen zwischen arteriellem Druck, Herzzeitvolumen (HZV) und Gesamtwiderstand. Bei erhöhtem arteriellem Druck sinkt der Gesamtwiderstand[5]. Anscheinend beruht dies aber weitgehend auf reflektorischen Vorgängen, die von den arteriellen Pressoreceptoren ausgelöst werden. Schaltet man diese Einflüsse aus,

[1] Wezler und Schlüter 1953, Wezler und Sinn 1953.   [2] Green und Mitarbeiter 1944.
[3] Folkow 1949, 1953.   [4] Thauer und Crispens 1955.
[5] Wetterer und Pieper 1955, Mechelke u. a. 1955.

so sind HZV und arterieller Druck angenähert proportional. Der Gesamtwiderstand (Abb. 4) steigt dann mit wachsendem Druck sogar etwas an, was wahrscheinlich auf den steigenden basalen Gefäßtonus bei steigendem intravasalen Druck zurückgeführt werden muß[1] (s. S. 648).

Der Strömungswiderstand hängt sowohl von Eigenschaften des Blutes als auch von solchen des Gefäßsystems ab. Bei heterogenen Flüssigkeiten wie dem Blut ändert sich die Viscosität mit den Strömungsbedingungen. Man kann nur von einer scheinbaren Viscosität sprechen[2]. Die scheinbare Viscosität nimmt mit wachsender Durchblutung ab. Dies bedingt zum Teil die Versteilung der i-p-Kurve mit wachsendem Druck. Im Normalbereich bei Hämatokriten zwischen 30 und 60 ist die scheinbare Viscosität von der Erythrocytenkonzentration nur wenig abhängig[3]. Dies erklärt sich in erster Linie dadurch, daß die Erythrocyten sich hauptsächlich im axialen Strom befinden. Damit wird die Viscosität des Plasmas für die Stromstärke die entscheidende Größe. Ein anderer Umstand ist aber für den Verlauf der i-p-Kurve von noch größerer Bedeutung, die Dehnbarkeit des Gefäßsystems. Hierüber wurden von WEZLER u. Mitarb. eingehende Untersuchungen durchgeführt und theoretische Überlegungen angestellt[4].

Tabelle 2 gibt eine Übersicht über die Faktoren, die den peripheren Strömungswiderstand bestimmen. In den meisten Fällen sind die regulatorischen Einflüsse so stark, daß sie die einfachen physikalischen Gesetzmäßigkeiten überdecken.

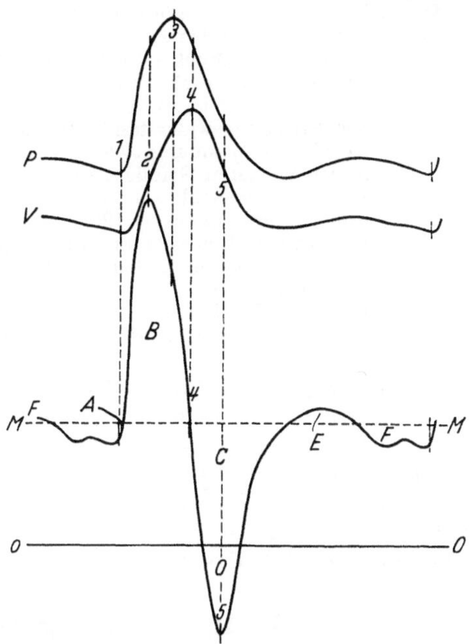

Abb. 5. Schwankungen der Durchblutung in der A. femoralis während einer Herzphase. Obere Kurve P: Druck in der A. femoralis. Mittlere Kurve V: Blutvolumen im arteriellen System peripher der Meßstelle. Unterste Kurve F: Durchblutung. Unterbrochene Linie M—M: mittlere Durchblutung. O—O: Nullinie der Durchblutung. Bei A, C und F verminderte, bei B und E erhöhte Durchblutung gegenüber dem Mittelwert. Die Änderungen der Durchblutungen sind teils auf die Schwankungen des arteriellen Druckes, teils auf die verstärkte oder verminderte Füllung des arteriellen Systems entsprechend der Dehnbarkeit dieser Gefäßabschnitte zurückzuführen. O: Phase des Blutrückstroms. Die eingezeichneten Vertikalen kennzeichnen folgende Zeitpunkte: 1 Beginn der Steigerung von Druck und Durchblutung, 2 maximale Durchblutung bei Druckanstieg und bei Steigerung der arteriellen Blutfüllung, 3 Maximum des Blutdruckes, 4 Maximum der arteriellen Blutfüllung bei stark sinkender Durchblutung, 5 maximaler Blutrückfluß bei starkem Absinken der arteriellen Blutfüllung. (SHIPLEY, GREGG und SCHROEDER 1943.)

Für den Strömungswiderstand und seine Einstellung sind in den meisten Fällen die Arteriolen von entscheidender Bedeutung. Es läßt sich jedoch nicht ausschließen, daß in manchen Organen (Herz, Lunge) die Capillarstrecke den Strömungswiderstand in stärkerem Maße mitbestimmt[5].

In den Extremitäten darf der Strömungswiderstand der großen zuführenden Arterie unter vielen Bedingungen nicht vernachlässigt werden. In anderen

---

[1] LEVY u. a. 1954, MECHELKE u. a. 1955, FOLKOW 1953.
[2] A. MÜLLER 1944, 1948, LAMPORT 1949, FREY-WYSSLING 1952, STACY u. a. 1955.
[3] WHITAKER und WINTON 1933, LEVY und SHARE 1933.
[4] WEZLER und SCHLÜTER 1953, WEZLER und SINN 1953, PHILIPPS u. a. 1955.
[5] ZWEIFACH 1957.

Tabelle 2. *Faktoren, die den peripheren Strömungswiderstand beeinflussen.*

A. *Eigenschaften des Blutes:* Erythrocytenkonzentration und Eiweißkonzentration des Plasmas (A. Müller 1944, 1948, Lamport 1949, Frey-Wyssling 1952).
B. *Eigenschaften des Gefäßsystems:* Anzahl der parallelgeschalteten Röhren, Länge und Weite der einzelnen Gefäßabschnitte.
   I. Physikalische Einflüsse.
      a) Intravasaler Druck (Wezler und Schlüter 1953, Wezler und Sinn 1953).
      b) Extravasaler Druck. Von besonderer Bedeutung für die Durchblutung des Skelet- und Herzmuskels, wobei der Kontraktionszustand der quergestreiften Muskulatur den Strömungswiderstand entscheidend beeinflußt.
      c) Oberflächenspannung zwischen Blut und Gefäßwand. Von besonderer Bedeutung in den kleineren Gefäßen, wo die Oberflächenspannung bei einem kritischen Wert zum Gefäßverschluß führt (Burton 1951, 1954; Burton und Yamada, 1951, Folkow und Löfving 1956).
   II. Regulatorische Einflüsse auf die glatte Muskulatur.
      a) Beeinflussung durch den Gefäßinnendruck (Bayliss 1902, Folkow 1949, 1953, s. auch S. 647).
      b) Einflüsse durch den Gewebsstoffwechsel (s. S. 646).
      c) Nervös-hormonale Einflüsse (s. S. 649).

Gebieten scheinen die Venen (Drosselvenen) für die Einstellung des Strömungswiderstandes von Bedeutung zu sein [1].

Die rhythmischen Schwankungen des arteriellen Druckes mit der Herztätigkeit führen zu rhythmischen Durchblutungsänderungen, besonders in den Arterien. Unter bestimmten Bedingungen kann die Verteilung des Strömungswiderstandes und der Dehnbarkeit der Gefäße entlang dem Gefäßrohr so beschaffen sein, daß das Blut in der Diastole herzwärts zurückfließt (Abb. 5) [2].

II. Die Einstellung der Organdurchblutung.

Die Durchblutungseinstellung erfolgt in einzelnen Kreislaufgebieten nach recht verschiedenen Prinzipien. Für die meisten Organe ist die Anpassung der Durchblutung an den Organstoffwechsel entscheidend. Eine Sonderstellung nimmt die Lunge ein, bei der die Durchblutung dem HZV entspricht. Etwas Ähnliches gilt für die Leber, da das gesamte Blut des Pfortadergebietes durch sie hindurchfließt. Recht wenig ist bekannt über die Einstellung der Durchblutung bei den Regenerationsorganen des Blutes. Die Nierenfunktion scheint die Nierendurchblutung erstaunlich wenig zu beeinflussen [3]. Die Hautdurchblutung unterliegt sehr weitgehend den Einflüssen der Temperaturregulation.

In jedem Falle handelt es sich bei der Durchblutungseinstellung im Sinne der Regeltechnik nicht um eine Regelung, sondern um eine Steuerung. Geregelt wird dagegen die Konzentration bestimmter Stoffe im Gewebe. Ihre Konzentration bestimmt den Grad der Durchblutung und wird auf diese Weise angenähert konstant gehalten.

Die Einstellung der Organdurchblutung wird in den meisten Fällen nicht nur von einem Faktor, sondern von mehreren bestimmt. In erster Annäherung kann man sagen, daß lokale Einflüsse eine durchblutungssteigernde Wirkung auf das Gefäßsystem ausüben, wobei sie die Durchblutung dem erhöhten Stoffbedarf der Peripherie anpassen, während zentrale Einflüsse die Durchblutung hemmen und damit die Belastung des Gesamtkreislaufes klein halten.

1. Lokale Einflüsse.

Die enge Beziehung zwischen Organstoffwechsel und Organdurchblutung spricht für eine lokal-chemische Steuerung [4]. Die Vorstellung ist die, daß die

---

[1] Franklin 1937.   [2] Shipley, Gregg, Schroeder 1943.
[3] Smith 1951.   [4] Rein 1941.

Konzentration von einem oder mehreren chemischen Stoffen im Gewebe „geregelt" wird. Verändert sich bei einem erhöhten Stoffumsatz ihre Konzentration im Gewebe, so löst dies eine Mehrdurchblutung aus, wodurch die alte Konzentration wieder eingestellt wird. Recht viele Stoffwechselprodukte, unter anderem Kohlensäure und Milchsäure, lösen eine Mehrdurchblutung aus, wenn man sie durch Injektionen in die zuführende Arterie mit dem Blute der Peripherie zuführt[1]. Man könnte daraus schließen, daß die Gewebsdurchblutung auch nicht nur durch einen einzigen Stoff gesteuert wird, sondern daß eine ganze Reihe von Stoffwechselprodukten die Einstellung der lokalen Durchblutung bestimmen. In der Sprache des Regeltechnikers würde eine ganze Reihe von Regelkreisen parallel geschaltet sein, die je nach dem Ablauf des Stoffwechsels gemeinsam die Durchblutung hochtreiben oder auch gegensinnige Einwirkungen auf die Durchblutungseinstellung haben können. Der Sauerstoffdruck des Gewebes spielt für die Einstellung der Durchblutung wohl nur eine indirekte Rolle, indem bei Sauerstoffmangel Zwischenprodukte im Gewebe angereichert werden, die dann eine Durchblutungssteigerung hervorrufen. Gegen einen direkten Steuerungseinfluß des peripheren Sauerstoffdruckes sprechen Versuche mit Drosselung der Durchblutung. Die nach Lösung der Drossel auftretende, reaktive Mehrdurchblutung geht mit einer Steigerung der Sauerstoffsättigung im venösen Blut einher. Die reaktive Mehrdurchblutung fällt also im Hinblick auf die Sauerstoffversorgung des Gewebes zu stark aus[2]. Der schwierigere Abtransport der Intermediärprodukte, die während der Drosselung entstanden sind, erfordert die stärkere und längere Hyperämie. Sauerstoffmangel wird dann eine Mehrdurchblutung hervorrufen, wenn der kritische Sauerstoffdruck erreicht wird, d. h., wenn der Sauerstoffdruck im Gewebe so weit abgesunken ist, daß dadurch der oxydative Stoffwechsel herabgesetzt wird. Das tritt im Coronarkreislauf schon bei geringen Senkungen der arteriellen Sättigung ein (s. S. 704). Im Gehirn findet man Durchblutungssteigerungen, wenn der venöse Sauerstoffdruck den Wert von rund 20 mm Hg unterschreitet[3]. Über die Bedeutung des Sauerstoffdruckes für die Lungendurchblutung siehe S. 755.

Um vom Gewebe aus eine Mehrdurchblutung hervorzurufen, ist eine Erweiterung der Arteriolen notwendig. Man nimmt meist an, daß sie über Axonreflexe zustande kommt[4]. Bei der Übertragung könnten cholinergische Mechanismen bedeutungsvoll sein, denn intraarterielle Atropininfusionen verhindern die Entstehung einer reaktiven Hyperämie[5]. Trotz der großen Zahl der Untersuchungen auf diesem Gebiet läßt sich aber nicht ausschließen, daß die gefäßerweiternden Metaboliten direkt auf die Muskulatur der Arteriolenwand und die Capillarsphincter einwirken und so die Steigerung der Durchblutung herbeiführen[6].

Neben der lokal-chemischen Durchblutungssteuerung gibt es noch andere Möglichkeiten, durch die von der Peripherie her die Organdurchblutung beeinflußt wird. Sie zeigen sich besonders bei solchen Organen, bei denen die Durchblutung nicht allein der Deckung des Stoffwechselbedarfs des Organs dient. Die Niere steigert ihren Strömungswiderstand, wenn der arterielle Druck ansteigt und senkt ihn, wenn der arterielle Druck absinkt. Sie hält damit in gewissen Grenzen ihre Durchblutung unabhängig von dem Infusionsdruck[7]. Die Steuerung erfolgt über den intravasalen Druck, wobei der Druck in den Glomerula entscheidend zu sein scheint. Der Mechanismus wird durch KCN und Novocain

---

[1] FLEISCH und SIBUL 1931.   [2] REIN 1944.   [3] OPITZ und SCHNEIDER 1950.
[4] FLEISCH und WEGER 1938.   [5] KEYSSLER und SCHMIER 1951.
[6] FOLKOW 1955 (Literatur!).
[7] HARTMANN u. a. 1936, OCHWADT 1956, SELKURT 1955a.

aufgehoben (Abb. 6). Der Strömungswiderstand wird dabei hauptsächlich in den Vasa afferentia geändert, wie aus dem Verhalten der Inulinclearance hervorgeht. Die Annahme, daß die autonome Widerstandsregulierung der Niere mit Änderungen des intrarenalen Hämatokrits im Zusammenhang steht[1], ist wahrscheinlich nicht berechtigt[2].

Für Durchblutung und Blutgehalt der Lunge scheint eine Steuerung über den Druck keine Bedeutung zu haben. Hier führt jede Erhöhung des intravasalen Druckes zu einer Dehnung des Gefäßsystems, damit zu einer erhöhten Blutfüllung und einem verminderten Strömungswiderstand (s. S. 750). Dagegen soll eine Erhöhung des Druckes im Splanchnicusgebiet zu Venoconstrictionen führen. Bei Erhöhung des Pfortaderdruckes soll deshalb die Blutfüllung dieses Gebietes nur wenig zunehmen[3].

Viel diskutiert ist die Bedeutung des intravasalen Druckes für die Vasomotorik in den Extremitäten. Zahlreiche Untersuchungen, die weitgehend aus den letzten Jahren stammen, wurden teils an Tieren, sehr weitgehend aber an Beinen und Armen des Menschen vorgenommen. Der intravasale Druck ändert sich nicht nur mit dem arteriellen oder venösen Druck.

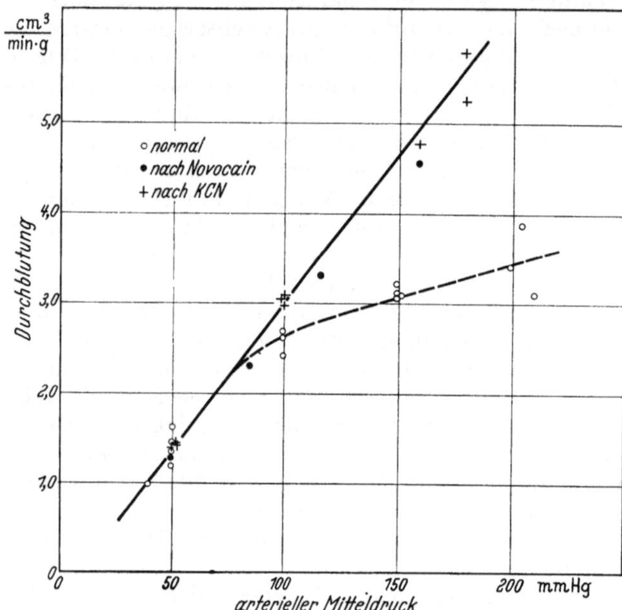

Abb. 6. Beziehung zwischen Druck und Durchblutung an der isolierten Niere. ○ Normalwerte, ● nach intraarterieller Novocain-Infusion (10^{-3} g/cm³), + nach KCN. (Ochwadt 1956.)

Wegen der Hydrostatik ist er auch sehr stark von der Stellung der Extremitäten abhängig, was funktionell von großer Bedeutung ist. Schließlich läßt sich im Experiment die Wandspannung der Gefäße verändern, indem man den um die Extremität befindlichen Außendruck variiert[4]. Findet man bei solchen Untersuchungen Veränderungen des Strömungswiderstandes, so ist zunächst an eine Dehnung oder Entspannung der Gefäße durch den veränderten intravasalen Druck und an Änderungen der scheinbaren Viscosität zu denken (s. S. 645). Es können weiterhin unter den experimentellen Bedingungen die Blutversorgung und die nutritiven Bedingungen der Gewebe verändert und dadurch vasomotorische Vorgänge ausgelöst sein. Eine große Reihe von Untersuchungen erlaubt die Ausschaltung dieser Faktoren. Sie spricht dafür, daß eine Erhöhung des intravasalen Druckes zu einer Steigerung des Strömungswiderstandes führt, oder daß er zum mindesten konstant bleibt[5]. Das widerspricht einer einfachen Abhängigkeit des Strömungswiderstandes von den Dehnbarkeiten der Gefäße.

---

[1] Pappenheimer und Kinter 1956.   [2] Ochwadt 1957.   [3] Selkurt 1955b.
[4] Coles und Greenfield 1956, Coles 1957.
[5] v. Recklinghausen 1906, Folkow 1949, 1953, Coles und Greenfield 1956, Přerovský u. a. 1955.

Abb. 7 stammt von Versuchen, die an den vorderen Extremitäten von Hunden ausgeführt wurden. Die Durchblutung wurde künstlich konstant gehalten und der venöse Druck planmäßig verändert. Unter diesen Versuchsbedingungen sind die Strömungswiderstände den Druckdifferenzen proportional. Außerdem werden die nutritiven Verhältnisse weitgehend konstant gehalten. Wie Abb. 7 zeigt, bleibt bei steigendem venösem Druck der arterio-venöse Widerstand konstant. Der erhöhte intravasale Druck führt also unter diesen Bedingungen nicht zu einer Abnahme, wie das bei einer passiven Dehnung der Gefäße zu erwarten wäre. Letzteres gilt nur für die großen Arterien und großen Venen, in denen bei steigendem intravasalem Druck die Druckdifferenzen vermindert sind. Dagegen nimmt in den kleinen Gefäßen die Druckdifferenz und damit der Widerstand zu, ein Vorgang, der rein druckpassiv nicht zu erklären ist. Die Zunahme des Strömungswiderstandes in den kleinen Gefäßen ist so beachtlich, daß dadurch die Widerstandsabnahme in den großen Gefäßen ausgeglichen wird und der Widerstand über den gesamten Gefäßbereich konstant gehalten wird[1].

Auf welchem Wege intravasale Drucksteigerungen zur Erhöhung des Strömungswiderstandes führen, ist noch unklar. Möglicherweise ist der ganze Mechanismus allein in der glatten Muskelfaser gelegen, die sich auf die erhöhte Spannung hin kontrahiert[2]. Teilweise werden vasomotorische Reflexe angenommen, die von den Venen ausgehen sollen[3]. Die Annahme, es handele sich um zentral-nervöse Einflüsse, wird im allgemeinen abgelehnt, da der Mechanismus beim Menschen nach Sympathektomie noch auslösbar ist[4]. Dem widersprechen aber andere Befunde[5].

2. Zentral-nervöse Einflüsse auf die Einstellung der peripheren Durchblutung.

Den vasomotorischen Nerven kommen zwei Funktionen zu: 1. Sie regulieren die Weite von Arterien und Venen im Dienste des gesamten Kreislaufs. 2. Sie regulieren die Durchblutung derjenigen Organe, bei denen die Durchblutung nicht allein dem lokalen Stoffwechselbedarf dient. Zu 1. Wenn die lokal-chemische Steuerung im allgemeinen die Organdurchblutung zur Deckung des Stoffwechselbedarfs in die Höhe treibt, so hemmt im Gegensatz dazu der nervöse Einfluß die Durchblutung, in erster Linie zur Regelung des arteriellen Druckes. Die vasoconstrictorischen Fasern sind in diesem Sinne die efferenten Bahnen der blutdrucksteuernden Reflexe, die von den Pressoreceptoren im arteriellen System ausgelöst werden. Zu 2. Der typische Fall, in dem durch nervöse

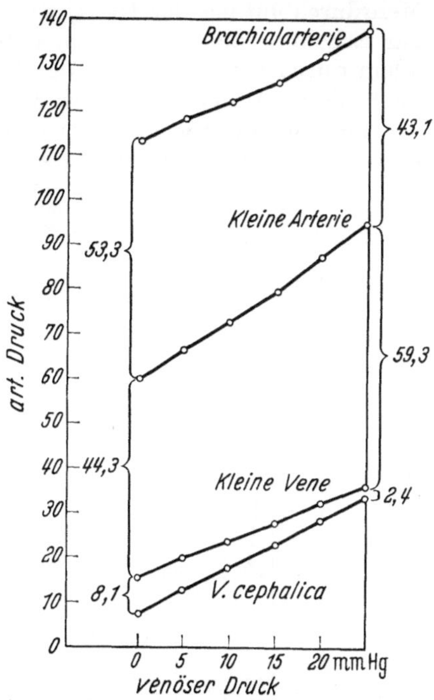

Abb. 7. Wirkung der Steigerung des venösen Druckes auf die Drucke und die Druckgradienten in den großen und kleinen Gefäßen der Katzenextremität bei konstanter Durchblutung. Bei Steigerung des Venendruckes bleibt das Druckgefälle zwischen A. brachialis und V. cephalica praktisch konstant. Während das Druckgefälle in den großen Arterien und Venen abnimmt, steigt es in den kleinen Gefäßen an. Da die Durchblutung konstant gehalten ist, muß auf entsprechende Veränderungen des Strömungswiderstandes geschlossen werden. Die großen Gefäße werden druckpassiv erweitert und damit sinkt ihr Strömungswiderstand. Im Gegensatz dazu nimmt unter Drucksteigerung der Strömungswiderstand in den kleinen Gefäßen zu. (HADDY und GILBERT 1956.)

---

[1] HADDY und GILBERT 1956.   [2] BAYLISS 1902, FOLKOW 1949, 1953, 1955.
[3] GIRLING 1952, GASKELL und BURTON 1953, YAMADA und BURTON 1954, BEACONFIELD und GINSBURY 1955.
[4] BEACONFIELD und GINSBURY 1955, ROSENBERG 1956.
[5] HADDY und GILBERT 1956, PHILLIPS u. a. 1955.

Einflüsse die periphere Durchblutung für die Funktion des Gesamtorganismus eingestellt wird, ist die Steuerung der Hautdurchblutung im Dienste der Temperaturregulation.

Bei den Vasomotoren überwiegen die constrictorischen Fasern[1]. So wird anscheinend die Hautdurchblutung nur durch Vasoconstrictoren gesteuert. Eine Mehrdurchblutung der Haut, wie sie etwa im Dienst der Temperaturregulation zur Erhöhung der Wärmeabgabe an der Körperoberfläche notwendig ist, kommt allein durch ein Nachlassen des Vasoconstrictorentonus zustande[2]. Freilich ist auch dieser Ansicht in letzter Zeit widersprochen worden[3].

Aufhebung des vasoconstrictorischen Dauertonus, etwa durch Sympathektomie, führt zur Durchblutungssteigerung (Abb. 8). Jedoch nimmt nach einiger Zeit die Durchblutung wieder ab. Es stellt sich von neuem ein Gefäßtonus ein[4]. Im Tierexperiment verschwindet die Mehrdurchblutung nach Entnervung bereits nach wenigen Stunden[5]. Die Durchblutung ist dann wieder dem peripheren Stoffwechselbedarf angepaßt, wie sich im Experiment durch Drosselung der arteriellen Blutzufuhr zeigen läßt.

Es besteht kein Zweifel, daß eine nervös bedingte, periphere Mehrdurchblutung nicht nur auf einem Nachlassen des vasoconstrictorischen Tonus, sondern auch auf der Einwirkung von vasodilatatorischen Nervenfasern beruhen kann[6]. Einen letzten Beweis hierfür erbrachten Folkow und Gernandt[7], indem sie die Aktionsströme der Vasodilatatoren im peripheren Nerven aufnahmen. Vasodilatatoren führen zu dem Gefäßsystem der Skeletmuskulatur und wahrscheinlich auch zum Coronargefäßsystem als cholinergische Nerven über den Grenzstrang[8]. Eine Mehrdurchblutung der Skeletmuskulatur kann danach durch zwei verschiedene nervöse Mechanismen ausgelöst sein. Es kann sich um ein Nachlassen des Constrictorentonus

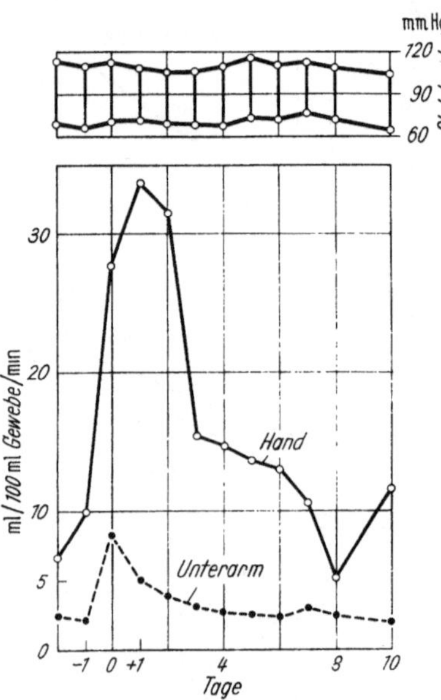

Abb. 8. Wirkung der Sympathektomie auf Muskel- (Unterarm-) und Haut- (Hand-) Durchblutung. Ordinate: Durchblutung in ml/min/100 ml Gewebe. Abszisse: Tage, Operation am Tage — 1. (H. Barcroft, 1952.)

handeln, oder es werden die dilatatorischen Nerven wirksam. Für die Regelung des arteriellen Druckes, wie sie besonders reflektorisch von den Pressoreceptoren aus erfolgt, soll nur die Veränderung des Constrictorentonus von Bedeutung sein. Dagegen steigern die dilatatorischen Nerven die Muskeldurchblutung anscheinend vorsorglich, wenn eine erhöhte Beanspruchung der Muskeln zu erwarten ist[9]. Vasodilatatorische Zentren befinden sich im Hypothalamus[10] und in der Medulla oblongata[11].

Wahrscheinlich spielen nervös-dilatatorische Einflüsse eine Rolle bei der Einstellung der Arbeitsmehrdurchblutung. Elektrische Reizung der motorischen

[1] Folkow 1955. [2] Celander und Folkow 1953, Folkow 1955, Lanier u. a. 1953.
[3] Roddie u. a. 1957. [4] Barcroft 1952.
[5] Mercker und Urbig 1942. [6] Burn 1938, Uvnäs 1954.
[7] Folkow und Gernandt 1952. [8] Folkow und Mitarbeiter 1949.
[9] Lindgren und Uvnäs 1955, Uvnäs 1954, Eliasson u. a. 1952.
[10] Eliasson u. a. 1950. [11] Lindgren und Uvnäs 1953, 1954.

Gebiete in der Großhirnrinde führt zur Durchblutungssteigerung in den zugehörigen Muskeln, auch wenn die Tiere curaresiert sind, die Muskeln also gar nicht in Tätigkeit treten[1]. Es handelt sich wohl um eine Art Mitinnervation gleichzeitig mit der motorischen Innervation. Dieser Mechanismus mag besonders für den Arbeitsbeginn bedeutungsvoll sein. Die Einstellung der Arbeitsmehrdurchblutung wäre damit doppelt gesichert, einerseits im überwiegenden Maße vom Gewebe her über lokal-chemische Einflüsse, andererseits über zentral-nervöse Einflüsse. ASMUSSEN u. Mitarb.[2] nehmen dazu noch eine dritte Art der Auslösung der Arbeitsmehrdurchblutung an. Sie soll auch über Reflexe von der tätigen Extremität aus erfolgen.

3. Zentral-chemische Einflüsse auf die periphere Durchblutung.

Trotz der sehr großen Zahl von Arbeiten auf diesem Gebiet sind wir über die funktionelle Bedeutung zentral-chemischer Einflüsse weitgehend im unklaren. Es sind besonders 2 Gründe, die zu einer kritischen Stellungnahme zwingen. 1. Die Dosierung der Stoffe liegt häufig im Experiment sehr viel höher, als sie normalerweise möglich ist. Das gilt besonders für das Vasopressin, aber auch für die meisten Untersuchungen mit Hormonen des Nebennierenmarks. 2. Die Wirkstoffe greifen teilweise gar nicht primär an den Gefäßen an, sondern sie beeinflussen die Vasomotorik sekundär über Änderungen des Gewebsstoffwechsels. Das gilt mit großer Wahrscheinlichkeit für das Hypoxylienin (auch als Milz-Leber-Mechanismus bezeichnet)[3], aber auch für das Adrenalin[4]. Über die Bedeutung des Serotonins auf den Kreislauf siehe PAGE (1958, Literatur!).

Während das Vasopressin und die Stoffe der Renin-Hypertensingruppe nur constrictorische Wirkungen haben und damit allgemein blutdrucksteigernd wirken, liegen die Verhältnisse bei den Hormonen des Nebennierenmarks komplizierter. Das Adrenalin kann nicht einfach als blutdrucksteigerndes Hormon angesprochen werden. REIN[5] hat das Adrenalin einmal als blutverteilendes Hormon bezeichnet. Zum Teil kommt die Veränderung der Blutverteilung unter Adrenalin dadurch zustande, daß die einzelnen Gefäßgebiete verschieden stark auf constrictorische Einflüsse ansprechen, wobei zwischen nervöser und hormonaler Ansprechbarkeit eine sehr weitgehende Parallelität besteht. So kommt es im Gefäßgebiet der Haut sehr leicht zu starken Konstriktionen, während sie im Coronarkreislauf und im Kreislauf des ZNS nur sehr abgeschwächt auftreten. Das Adrenalin beeinflußt die Durchblutungsverteilung aber andererseits auch dadurch, daß es in manchen Gefäßgebieten und unter bestimmten Bedingungen überhaupt nicht constrictorisch, sondern dilatierend wirkt. Dies gilt besonders für die Coronardurchblutung[6] und teilweise für die Durchblutung der Skeletmuskulatur[7]. In letzterem Fall handelt es sich um direkte lokale Einwirkungen des Adrenalins auf das Gefäßnetz und nicht etwa nur um reflektorische Einflüsse.

Im Skeletmuskel liegt eigentümlicherweise ein Organ vor, dessen Gefäßsystem unter Adrenalin einmal dilatiert, das andere Mal konstringiert. Kleine Dosen wirken häufig dilatierend, große im allgemeinen konstringierend. Daß es sich um zwei grundsätzlich verschiedene Wirkungen handelt, geht aus dem Einfluß anti-adrenergischer Stoffe hervor, die die constrictorische Wirkung aufheben und damit die dilatatorische um so stärker hervortreten lassen[8]. Es ist nicht allein

[1] GREEN und HOFF 1937.　　[2] ASMUSSEN und Mitarbeiter 1943.
[3] REIN 1951b, MEESMANN und SCHMIER 1956a und b.
[4] BÜCHERL und SCHWAB 1952, FOLKOW 1955 (Literatur), HILLE und TESKE 1956, BARCROFT und COBBOLD 1956, LUNDHOLM 1958.
[5] REIN 1937.　　[6] LOCHNER, MERCKER und SCHÜRMEYER 1956.
[7] GOTTSTEIN u. a. 1955, BOCK, HENSEL und RUFF 1955.　　[8] LANNIER u. a. 1953.

die Dosis, die die gegensätzliche Wirkung des Adrenalins am Skeletmuskel erklärt. Auch Stoffwechsellage und Funktion beeinflussen die Adrenalinwirkung. Die constrictorischen Wirkungen sind aufgehoben oder zum mindesten abgeschwächt, wenn der Muskel in Tätigkeit ist. Das kann allein mit einem Überwiegen der durch die lokal-chemischen Reaktionen verstärkten dilatatorischen Einflüsse über die constrictorischen erklärt werden[1]. Andererseits zeigt der ruhende Muskel die Adrenalindilatation nur, wenn er sich in einem guten Zustand befindet[2]. Durch Narkose, schlechte Beatmung und operative Eingriffe wird die dilatatorische Wirkung des Adrenalins am ruhenden Skeletmuskel aufgehoben, und es lassen sich dann nur noch Konstriktionen beobachten. Bestechend ist die Anschauung, daß die dilatatorische Wirkung des Adrenalins ein sekundärer Effekt des durch die hormonalen Einflüsse veränderten Gewebsstoffwechsels ist[3]. Für den Coronarkreislauf scheint diese Erklärung freilich nicht ausreichend[4].

Die Entdeckung des zweiten Hormons des Nebennierenmarks, des Noradrenalins[5], erschwert weiterhin die Beurteilung zentral-chemischer Einflüsse auf die Kreislaufperipherie. Nach histologischen Untersuchungen besitzt das Nebennierenmark zwei getrennte Drüsenanteile, von denen der eine Adrenalin, der andere Noradrenalin produziert[6]. Anscheinend wird die Sekretion beider Drüsen durch unterschiedliche Mechanismen ausgelöst. Reizung von Schmerznervenfasern löst hauptsächlich Adrenalinsekretion aus. Dagegen führt Abklemmung der Carotiden und Asphyxie zu gleichmäßiger Konzentrationssteigerung beider Hormone im Blute. Bei Reizung bestimmter umschriebener Gebiete des Hypothalamus erhält man einmal eine Adrenalin-, das andere Mal eine Noradrenalinsekretion[7]. In grober Annäherung kann man sagen, daß die Bedeutung des Adrenalins auf seiner Stoffwechselwirkung beruht, während das Noradrenalin ähnliche Wirkungen entfaltet wie der Constrictorenanteil des nervösen vasomotorischen Systems. Jeder Versuch, die Bedeutung der Nebennierenmarkhormone zu erfassen, wird noch dadurch erschwert, daß bei verschiedenen Tierarten der Anteil der beiden Hormone im Nebennierenmark sehr stark schwankt[8].

Wieweit die Hormone des Nebennierenmarks „Notstandsfunktionen" haben und den Kreislauf befähigen, mit besonderen Belastungen fertig zu werden, ist heute schwer zu entscheiden. Im allgemeinen sind die direkten Einwirkungen der Hormone auf die Kreislaufperipherie sehr viel weniger bedeutungsvoll als die des Nervensystems[9]. Recht schwierig ist auch die Beurteilung hepato-renaler Stoffe (VEM und VDM), die die Wirkung des Adrenalins auf die Kreislaufperipherie im fördernden und hemmenden Sinne beeinflussen sollen[10].

III. Örtliche Durchblutungsstörungen.

So eindeutig die pathologisch-anatomischen Befunde bei den verschiedenen organischen Gefäßerkrankungen sind, so undurchsichtig werden die Verhältnisse bei den sog. funktionellen Gefäßstörungen. Die vielen ausgearbeiteten Funktionsprüfungen des peripheren Gefäßsystems dienen dazu, funktionelle und organische Störungen voneinander abzugrenzen. Auch ist es mit ihrer Hilfe möglich, den Schweregrad und die therapeutische Beeinflußbarkeit zu prüfen (Messung der Durchblutung mittels Plethysmographie und Calorimetrie, Prüfung der sekun-

---

[1] Mercker und Schoedel 1948.   [2] Gottstein u. a. 1955.
[3] Hille und Teske 1956, Folkow 1955, Lundholm 1958.
[4] Lochner, Mercker und Schürmeyer 1956.
[5] Holtz und Schümann 1948.   [6] Hillarp und Häfkelt 1953.
[7] v. Euler und Folkow 1953, Folkow und v. Euler 1954, Folkow 1955.
[8] v. Euler 1954, Goodall 1951.   [9] Celander 1954.
[10] Zweifach und Metz 1955b (Literatur!).

dären Hyperämie, Kälteteste, Wärmeteste, Veränderungen der Durchblutung durch statische Einflüsse usw.). Die Funktionsprüfungen, so wichtig sie diagnostisch und therapeutisch sind, vermögen aber zum Problem der Entstehung und Pathophysiologie dieser Störungen nur wenig beizutragen. Im Vordergrund der pathologisch-physiologischen Fragestellungen der funktionellen Gefäßstörungen steht die umstrittene Frage nach der Entstehung von *Spasmen*.

Als *Spasmus* bezeichnen wir eine örtlich begrenzte Verengerung im Bereich des Gefäßsystems, die durch Kontraktion der muskulären Gefäßelemente entsteht, und die eine unzureichende Blutversorgung des betreffenden Gewebsabschnittes bedingt. Betroffen können sein: die großen oder größeren Arterien und Venen, die Arteriolen und Venolen sowie die Sphincteren der Capillaren. Diese Gefäßanteile können einzeln für sich oder zusammen am Spasmus beteiligt sein. Spasmen können durch die verschiedensten Reize der Gefäßwand, insbesondere mechanische Reize, Verletzungen, Kälte, nervöse Reize, hormonale Einflüsse ausgelöst werden.

1. Experimentelle Befunde.

Daß mechanische Reize vor allem bei Verletzungen der Gefäßwand Gefäßspasmen herbeiführen, ist aus den Beobachtungen der Gefäßchirurgie hinreichend bekannt. Auch zeigen experimentelle Untersuchungen das Auftreten solcher Gefäßspasmen bei mechanischer Reizung.

So wurden nach nicht zu schwach dosierter mechanischer Reizung von Arterien in der Froschzunge Gefäßkontraktionen beschrieben, die über den gereizten Bezirk hinausgriffen[1]. An den Kaninchenohrgefäßen führen leichte mechanische Reize meist nicht zu einer sichtbaren Reaktion der Arterien. Stärkeren mechanischen Reiz mit Zerrung der Gefäßwände dagegen beantworten die Ohrarterien mit einer Vasoconstriction, die sich bei vorher dilatierten Gefäßen auf einen lokalen Schnürring beschränkt, die sich jedoch bei bestehender Constrictionsbereitschaft auch auf die angrenzenden Arterienabschnitte ausdehnen kann[2].

Recht eindeutig liegen die Verhältnisse bei äußerer Kälteeinwirkung. Hier sind experimentelle Untersuchungen vorhanden, die es ermöglichen, den Mechanismus der Vasoconstriction unter Kälteeinwirkung näher zu analysieren. Schädigungen kleiner Flächen durch Erfrierung mit Kohlensäureschnee erzeugen an den Gefäßen des Kaninchenohres ausgedehnte Spasmen[3]. Man erklärt diese Beobachtung des ausgebreiteten Gefäßspasmus dadurch, daß von einem Schädigungsherd, einem Focus, das zuführende Gefäßsystem auf dem Wege der intramuralen Nerven gegenüber nervösen Reizen so sensibilisiert werden kann, daß es zum Auftreten von Angiospasmen kommt.

Über das Verhalten der Hautvasomotorik beim Menschen unter Kälteeinwirkung liegt eine Reihe von Untersuchungen vor. Ausgangspunkt für die Beurteilung bleibt der klassische Versuch von Lewis[4].

Ein Finger, dessen Hauttemperatur im Eiswasser zunächst auf 0^0 C abgekühlt ist, zeigt nach 4—5 min Eintauchzeit eine spontane Erwärmung bis zu maximal 16^0 C, in der Regel bis zu 10^0 C. Dieses Maximum wird nach etwa 15 min erreicht. Danach fällt die Temperatur zum ursprünglichen Wert wieder ab, und der Cyclus beginnt von neuem.

Es wird angenommen, daß durch die Kälte ein histaminähnlicher Stoff freigesetzt wird, der über einen Axonreflex eine gefäßerweiternde Wirkung entfaltet. Sobald der dilatatorisch wirksame Stoff eine Schwellenkonzentration überschreitet, wird der bestehende kältebedingte vasoconstrictorische Tonus unterbrochen. Ist der Stoff aus der Blutbahn ausgeschwemmt, so kommt es wieder zur Konstriktion. Diese phasenförmig verlaufenden Gefäßreaktionen treten bei Personen mit alten Nervenverletzungen nicht mehr ein. Die Feststellungen von Lewis wurden später vielerorts bestätigt.

---

[1] Krogh 1929.   [2] Meiners 1952.
[3] Tittel 1943/44, Schneider 1952.   [4] Lewis 1928.

Den Sinn dieser Phasen-Reaktion sieht man darin, daß der Körper nicht unter allen Bedingungen die „Schale" zur Erhaltung der „Kern"-Temperatur preisgibt, sondern unter gewissen Umständen der Forderung des Wärmehaushaltes *und* der Verhütung örtlicher Gewebsschädigungen gleichzeitig gerecht zu werden versucht[1].

Untersuchungen über die Blutzirkulation in der Hand bei kalter, normaler und warmer Temperatur ergaben die niedrigsten Durchströmungswerte bei einer Wasserbadtemperatur von 15^0 C (0,9 cm³/100 cm³ Gewebe/min). Bei 5^0 C ist die Durchblutungsgröße wieder wesentlich höher und reicht an die Durchblutungsgröße bei 35^0 C heran (5,9 cm³/100 cm³ Gewebe/min)[2]. Auch andere Untersuchungen ergaben, daß bei mäßiger Kälteapplikation eine starke Vasoconstriction auftritt, während es bei extremen Kältereizen zur Dilatation kommt[3]. Man nimmt an, daß die arterio-venösen Anastomosen an der Phase der Kältedilatation wesentlich beteiligt sind.

Eine besonders wichtige Frage bildet das Vorkommen und das Zustandekommen von *Spasmen* nach *Embolien*. Die diesbezüglichen experimentellen Befunde sind sehr widersprechend. Ebbecke[4] beobachtete bei Fröschen, denen mit Ruß schwarzgefärbte Wachskügelchen in die Blutbahn gespritzt wurden, an den Arterienstellen, an denen sich der Embolus einkeilte, längere Zeit krampfhafte Kontraktionen. Nach experimenteller Luftembolie wurden in den Mesenterialarterien des Kaninchens mikroskopisch Angiospasmen beobachtet[5]. Auf Grund mikroskopischer Lebendbeobachtung der Piagefäße wurden nach experimenteller Embolisierung durch Luft und Tusche sowie nach Embolie durch Blutgerinnsel, durch pulverisierten Bimsstein und pulverisierte Glaswolle und durch Kartoffelstärke Spasmen der Piagefäße beobachtet, die auch die nichtembolisierten Nachbargefäße ergriffen[6]. Demgegenüber zeigen mikroskopische Untersuchungen in neuester Zeit an lebenden Piagefäßen von Kaninchen und Katzen, daß es nach Embolisierung durch Luft, Blutgerinnsel, Knochenmarkfett, flüssiges Paraffin und Kartoffelstärke nicht zu Spasmen der embolisierten oder der benachbarten Gefäße kommt, und daß weiterhin nach Embolisierung durch pulverisierte Glaswolle keine Spasmen auftreten, solange die Glasemboli in den Gefäßen liegen, ohne sie verletzt zu haben[7]. Sobald jedoch ein Glasspieß die Gefäßwand perforiert, sind Angiospasmen zu beobachten. Es muß demnach als problematisch angesehen werden, ob eine Mikroembolie in den Hirngefäßen Spasmen erzeugt. Eine plötzliche Gefäßwandverletzung dagegen ruft mit Sicherheit Angiospasmen hervor. Es erscheint somit nicht berechtigt, aus der klinischen Beobachtung, daß nach einer Embolie manchmal ein größerer Gefäßbereich ausfällt, als dem embolisierten Gefäß entspricht, auf einen ausgebreiteten Spasmus der Nachbargefäße zu schließen. Es kann sich von vornherein um multiple Embolien gehandelt haben, oder es können sich von dem Embolus kleine Teile abreißen und andere Gefäße verstopfen. Schließlich kann sich der festsitzende Embolus durch thrombotische Anlagerung vergrößern und hierdurch weitere Gefäße verlegen. Darüber hinaus dürfte die unterschiedliche anatomische Beschaffenheit des embolisierten Gefäßgebietes eine wesentliche Rolle spielen[7].

Einen breiten Raum nehmen die sog. *Sekundärspasmen* in der Diskussion der organischen Durchblutungsstörungen ein. Bei Gefäßverschluß durch einen Embolus oder durch eine Thrombose, durch Intimawucherungen und durch Mediaverdickungen im Sinne einer Atheromatose oder Endangitis soll es zu solchen Begleitspasmen kommen. Diese sollen nicht nur das erkrankte Gefäß

---

[1] Aschoff 1944.   [2] Spealman 1946.   [3] Aschoff 1944.
[4] Ebbecke 1923.   [5] Chase 1934.
[6] Jacobi und Magnus 1925/26, Villaret und Cadera 1939, Broman 1940.
[7] Schmidt 1955/56.

betreffen, sondern darüber hinaus auch die Nachbargefäße ergreifen und damit der Entstehung eines Kollateralkreislaufs entgegenwirken. Es ist z. B. behauptet worden, daß eine verödete Arterie wie ein vasoconstrictorischer Nerv wirke, der zu einem Spasmus der Kollateralen und damit zu einer verringerten Durchblutung der betroffenen Extremität führt. Aus dieser Vorstellung heraus ist die *Arteriektomie* bei lokalem Verschluß durch Arteriosklerose, Erfrierung, Thrombose usw. durchgeführt worden[1]. Durch die Resektion des verödeten Arterienabschnittes soll die Drosselung der Kollateralen aufgehoben werden.

Man versuchte, diese Auffassung durch Experimente zu stützen, in denen bei Hunden arteriographisch und histologisch beobachtet wurde, daß in einem Hinterbein nach artifizieller Thrombose eines Arteriensegmentes in der Peripherie Veränderungen im Sinne einer Endarteriitis obliterans oder einer Arteriosklerose auftraten, während in dem anderen Bein nach Excision eines, dem thrombosierten Abschnitt entsprechenden Arteriensegmentes solche Veränderungen fehlten[2]. Diese Ergebnisse konnten später von anderen Untersuchern bei ähnlicher Versuchsanordnung nicht bestätigt werden[3]. In neuester Zeit ergaben Untersuchungen an Hunden, Katzen und Kaninchen, denen auf der rechten Seite 3—4 cm der A. iliaca externa thrombosiert und linksseitig ein gleichgroßes Arterienstück reseziert wurde, an Hand von vergleichenden hautthermometrischen, aortographischen und histologischen Untersuchungen, daß kein gefäßverengender Einfluß und keine organische Veränderung der Kollateralen durch den thrombosierten Arterienabschnitt nachzuweisen sind[4]. Wenn trotzdem nach einer Resektion eines thrombosierten Gefäßabschnittes eine Steigerung der Durchblutung beim Patienten eintritt, so ist zu bedenken, daß dieser Eingriff eine partielle Sympathektomie darstellt, die durch Aufhebung eines normalen Vasoconstrictorentonus einen günstigen Einfluß auf die Durchblutung bewirken kann. Die Erfolge sind allerdings vorübergehender Natur; mit der Zeit werden die Gefäße wieder enger (s. S. 650).

2. Klinische Krankheitsbilder[5].

Versucht man die klinischen Krankheitsbilder der örtlichen Durchblutungsstörungen pathophysiologisch zu deuten, so stellt sich die Situation etwa folgendermaßen dar: Gefäßreaktionen, die vom vegetativen Nervensystem ausgehen, sind in der Regel durch ihre kurze Dauer gekennzeichnet. So kommt es bei psychischen Insulten zu kurzdauernden Vasoconstrictionen oder Vasodilatationen der Haut, die generell oder örtlich begrenzt sein können. Welche Reaktion — ob Konstriktion oder Dilatation — eintritt, ist nicht vorauszusagen, sondern vor allem von konstitutionellen Faktoren der betroffenen Person abhängig. Hier sind die örtlich begrenzten Gefäßreaktionen zu nennen, wie sie bei auftretenden psychischen Hemmungen in Form der flüchtigen Gesichtsröte auftreten. Es handelt sich hierbei um Gefäßreaktionen, denen ein eigentlicher Krankheitswert nicht zukommt (über Spasmen der Coronargefäße bei psychischen Insulten s. S. 710).

Die Erkrankungen der peripheren Gefäße manifestieren sich in erster Linie an denjenigen Körperpartien, die der Kälte in besonderem Maße ausgesetzt sind (Finger, Zehen, Nase, Ohren). In der klinischen Literatur ist vielfach die Annahme verbreitet, daß den *arterio-venösen Anastomosen* bei den peripheren Durchblutungsstörungen funktionell eine besondere Rolle zufällt. Die Bedeutung solcher Anastomosen wird vielfach dann angenommen, wenn andere Erklärungsmöglichkeiten für die Störungen der Durchblutung versagen, sie ist aber nicht erwiesen. Man sollte bedenken, wie schwierig der Nachweis der Funktion solcher Anastomosen schon im Tierexperiment ist (s. S. 641).

α) Angiopathien mit Neigung zu erhöhter Verengerungsbereitschaft der Gefäße. Als typische funktionelle Durchblutungsstörung dieser Gruppe gilt die Raynaudsche Krankheit. Geringste äußere Reize, vor allem Kältereize, genügen, um eine

---

[1] Leriche 1937, 1953.
[2] Fontaine und Lucineseo 1936, Fontaine und Schattner 1935.
[3] Strömbeck 1940, Wille-Baumkauff und Büttner 1941.
[4] Herget und Alnov 1953.   [5] Literatur bei Ratschow 1953 und 1959.

Vasoconstriction, vornehmlich an den Fingern bzw. Händen, hervorzurufen. Die Spasmenanfälle können Minuten, Stunden, aber auch Tage dauern. Die Capillaren sind in ihren arteriellen Schenkeln während des Anfalles verengt. In den späteren Stadien erscheinen die venösen Capillaren bzw. Venolen ausgebuchtet. Auch entwickeln sich mit der Zeit anatomische Strukturveränderungen. Da meist das weibliche Geschlecht von dieser Krankheit befallen ist und eine Abhängigkeit der Beschwerden vom menstruellen Cyclus besteht, liegt die Annahme nahe, daß hormonale Faktoren bei der Auslösung mit im Spiele sind. Genaueres ist aber hierüber nicht bekannt. Auch wissen wir bisher nichts Sicheres darüber, an welcher Stelle des Gefäßnervensystems diese besondere Überempfindlichkeit besteht. Es wurden anatomische Veränderungen in den vegetativen Ganglienzellen solcher Kranken beschrieben, die das anatomische Substrat für funktionelle Veränderungen beim Raynaud bilden könnten. Diese Befunde sind aber sehr umstritten. Bei kritischer Sichtung der vorliegenden Befunde hat die Lewissche Annahme immer noch die größte Wahrscheinlichkeit, daß vor allen Dingen die peripheren Gefäße eine abnorme vasoconstrictorische Reaktionsbereitschaft besitzen, und daß diese auch unabhängig vom vegetativen Nervensystem besteht. In diesem Sinne würden auch die Mißerfolge der Sympathektomie beim Morbus Raynaud sprechen. Einige Zeit nach dem operativen Eingriff treten die Beschwerden häufig in der gleichen Stärke wieder auf wie vorher. Als ein besonderes Kennzeichen der Raynaudschen Erkrankung kann das Auftreten einer starken *sekundären* Hyperämie nach Drosselung der Blutzufuhr angesehen werden. Diese sekundäre Hyperämie tritt beim Raynaud oft in stärkerer und ausgeprägterer Form und auch früher auf als normalerweise[1]. Die trophischen Folgen der Gefäßspasmen beim Raynaud sind bei längerer Dauer ein Ödem im Bereich der von den Vasoconstrictionen befallenen Partien, eine Hautatrophie und schließlich eine Sklerodermie.

β) Angiopathien mit Neigung zu abnormen Erweiterungsreaktionen. Hierher gehören die *Akrocyanosen* und die *Erythralgien.* Die Pathophysiologie dieser Störungen ist völlig undurchsichtig. Es muß schon fraglich erscheinen, ob die allgemein übliche Eingruppierung dieser Störungen unter die Gruppe der Angiopathien mit Neigung zu abnormen Erweiterungsreaktionen überhaupt richtig ist. Erweitert sind immer die Venolen. Dagegen sollen die arteriellen Capillarschenkel vielfach konstringiert sein (sog. ,,hypertonisch-atonischer Symptomenkomplex im Capillarbild''[2]. Der mangelnde Venolentonus ist z. T. in konstitutionellen angeborenen Faktoren zu suchen, z. T. besteht auch hier eine fehlerhafte hormonale Steuerung. Das Pubertätsalter ist bevorzugt.

γ) Angitiden und Angiosen. Die im Gefolge der Endangitis obliterans oder der Sklerose der peripheren Gefäße vorkommenden Durchblutungsstörungen sind in erster Linie Folge der anatomischen Strukturveränderungen der Gefäße. Wenn diese Durchblutungsstörungen hier aufgeführt werden, so hat dies zwei Gründe: 1. Es werden ,,neurohormonale'' Zellen in den sympathischen Ganglien beschrieben, die für die Pathogenese dieser Erkrankungen maßgeblich sein sollen[3]. Das Vorkommen solcher Zellen ist aber keineswegs gesichert, ihre Bedeutung, wenn sie überhaupt existieren, erst recht problematisch. 2. Bei diesen Erkrankungen werden in der klinischen Literatur immer wieder Begleitspasmen als maßgeblich für die mangelhafte Durchblutung beschrieben. Die widersprechenden experimentellen Befunde über die Erzeugung solcher Spasmen wurden bereits erörtert. Immerhin gibt es auch klinische Hinweise, die solche Spasmen vermuten lassen. Die oft erhebliche Verbesserung der Durchblutung nach Blockierung oder Durchschneidung der constrictorischen Fasern läßt es zweifelhaft erscheinen, daß diese Erweiterung der Gefäße lediglich durch Auf-

---

[1] Grosse-Brockhoff und Vorlaender 1947.
[2] Ratschow 1953.   [3] Sunder-Plassmann 1943.

hebung eines normalen Vasoconstrictorentonus bedingt ist. Auch ist zu berücksichtigen, daß durch die anatomischen Veränderungen die Gefäßwände so alteriert sind, daß hierdurch die Bedingungen, wie sie für die experimentelle Erzeugung von Spasmen gefordert werden, tatsächlich vorliegen. Man wird demnach die Bedeutung von Begleitspasmen bei den Angitiden der peripheren Gefäße als wahrscheinlich annehmen dürfen, wenn auch ein direkter Beweis hierfür noch aussteht (über Gefäßspasmen bei Endangitis der Gehirngefäße s. S. 660).

Als *Claudicatio intermittens venosa* wird eine Venensperre auf Grund von Venenspasmen bezeichnet, die vor allem nach traumatischen Verletzungen vorkommen. Diese Venenspasmen kommen häufig im Bereich der V. axillaris bei Vorliegen einer Halsrippe vor. Es ist schwierig, die mechanischen Faktoren der Verlegung des Blutrückstromes von Begleitspasmen, die durch die Zerrung der Gefäßwand (Gleiten des Gefäßes über der Halsrippe bei Bewegungen) zu trennen. Jedenfalls spielt der mechanische Faktor eine entscheidende Rolle, da durch Beseitigung der Halsrippe die Störung aufgehoben werden kann. Daß bei entzündlichen Prozessen im Bereich der Venen auch sekundär Spasmen entstehen, ist wohl anzunehmen, doch ist fraglich, ob diese Spasmen für die Durchblutungsstörungen eine wesentliche Rolle spielen.

3. Störungen der Gehirndurchblutung.

Es können nur diejenigen Störungen berücksichtigt werden, die im Zusammenhang mit Erkrankungen der Gefäße des Gehirns stehen (Veränderungen der Gehirndurchblutung bei Hochdruck und Kollaps s. S. 690 und 697). Die Situation ist funktionell pathologisch gegenüber den peripheren Durchblutungsstörungen insofern günstiger, als wir durch die Anwendung der Stickoxydul-Methode nach KETY[1], der O_2-Messung im arteriellen und venösen Blut bei gleichzeitiger Registrierung des arteriellen Druckes, die Möglichkeit haben, auch am kranken Menschen quantitative Einblicke in die Größe der Gehirndurchblutung und des Strömungswiderstandes im Verhältnis zum Energiestoffwechsel des Gehirns zu gewinnen.

Als erstes drängt sich die Frage auf, inwieweit Einschränkungen der Gehirndurchblutung möglich sind, ohne Dauerschäden zu hinterlassen, und wie sich bei solchen Ischämien Durchblutung, Sauerstoffaufnahme und Tätigkeit der Ganglienzellen ändern. Das Zentralnervensystem hat eine besonders geringe Resistenz gegenüber Durchblutungsstörungen (s. Tabelle 3). Speziell ist die Hirnrinde hochgradig empfindlich gegen eine Ischämie.

Wichtig ist die Unterscheidung zwischen *Tätigkeitsumsatz* und *Strukturumsatz* des Gehirns[2]. Unter Strukturumsatz wird der Minimalstoffwechsel verstanden, der zur Aufrechterhaltung der anatomischen Struktur notwendig ist und der eine minimale Durchblutung erfordert. Der Strukturumsatz der Ganglienzellen kann gedeckt werden, wenn die Durchblutung auf $^1/_{12}$ der Norm absinkt. Da die Ausnutzung des Blutes mehr als verdoppelt werden kann, beträgt die O_2-Aufnahme unter diesen Bedingungen immer noch $^1/_5$ der Norm. Wahrscheinlich liegt der Strukturumsatz des Gehirns noch niedriger, er soll etwa 10% des Tätigkeitsumsatzes betragen. Für die Beurteilung der Folgen einer Ischämie hat sich weiterhin der Begriff der „Erholungslatenz"[3] als wichtig erwiesen. Als Kriterium der Erholung nach Ischämie dienen die elektrischen Spontanschwankungen der Rinde und anderer Gebiete. Werden z. B. im Tierexperiment die zuführenden Gefäße abgeklemmt, so verschwinden die Spontanschwankungen nach rund 20 sec fast völlig. Diese Zeit wird als *Überlebenszeit* bezeichnet (auch als *Funktionszeit*). Bei Wiederzufuhr von Blut nach 1 min dauert es rund 20 sec, bis die Spontanschwankungen wieder auftreten. Die so gemessene „Erholungslatenz" nach Ischämie weist eine strenge Korrelation zur *Wiederbelebungszeit* auf. Das ist

---

[1] KETY und SCHMIDT 1948.   [2] OPITZ und SCHNEIDER 1950.   [3] SCHNEIDER 1953.

Tabelle 3. *Resistenz von Warmblütergeweben gegenüber Anoxie oder Ischämie.*
Die Angaben der letzten Spalte beziehen sich auf 100 g frisches Gewebe. (Opitz 1953.)

	Lähmungszeit			Wiederbelebungszeit		Atmung in situ
	Geprüfte Funktion	sec	Methodik	min	Methodik	ml O$_2$/ 100 g/min
Cortex cerebri .	spontan-Pot. EEG	10—30	komplette Ischämie (Kaninchen)	3—5	komplette Ischämie, erste Nekrosen (Katze, Kaninchen)	4—6
Mittelhirn . . .	Corneal-reflex I	25—35	desgl., mechanischer Reiz	5—6	desgl.	etwa 4
	Corneal-reflex II	55—65	desgl., elektrischer Reiz			
Medulla oblongata	Schnapp-atmung	60—120	Dekapitation (Kaninchen)	8—10	desgl.	etwa 3
		60—470	Strangulation (Mensch)			
Rückenmark . .	spinale Reflexe	50—200	Okklusion der Aorta (Katze)	20—25	Okklusion der Aorta (Katze), Nekrosen	etwa 2—3
Herz, Ventrikel .	spontane Kontraktion	400—800	komplette Asphyxie oder Dekapitation (Hund, Kaninchen)	30	Okklusion der Coronargefäße, Nekrosen oder Erholung (Hund)	10
Niere				30 80	erste Nekrosen, 50% Ratten sterben nach Okklusion des Nierenhilus	6—10
Carcinom (Walker)				130	50% Reimplantierbarkeit nach kompletter Ischämie	

die Zeit vom Beginn der Anoxie bis zum Auftreten irreparabler Schäden. Ein geringer Restkreislauf kann für die Erhaltung von Funktion und Struktur von entscheidender Bedeutung sein. Aber besonders ist dem *Zeitfaktor* eine entscheidende Bedeutung zuzumessen. Werden totale Ischämien verschiedener Zeitdauer miteinander verglichen, so steigt mit Zunahme der Ischämiedauer die Erholungslatenz zunächst linear an. Bei einer Dauer von 3 min weist aber die Kurve einen Knick auf (s. Abb. 9). Die Erholungslatenz steigt bei längerer Unterbrechung der Blutzufuhr sehr rasch an. Drosselt man aber die Durchblutung nicht vollständig, so wird die Kurve flacher, der gefährliche Knick wird wesentlich später erreicht. Diese Befunde sind auch von klinischer Bedeutung. Bei *lokalen Ischämien*, die Gebiete betreffen, deren Tätigkeit nicht lebensnotwendig ist, kann erwartet werden, daß auch nach sehr langer Dauer der Lähmung eine Wiederherstellung der Funktion möglich ist, wenn nur in der Zwischenzeit von der Nachbarschaft her der Strukturumsatz gedeckt werden konnte. Damit stehen die klinischen Beobachtungen in guter Übereinstimmung, daß nach cerebralen Insulten unter Umständen noch nach langer Zeit eine gewisse Restitution der Funktionen möglich ist. Für normale Körpertempe-

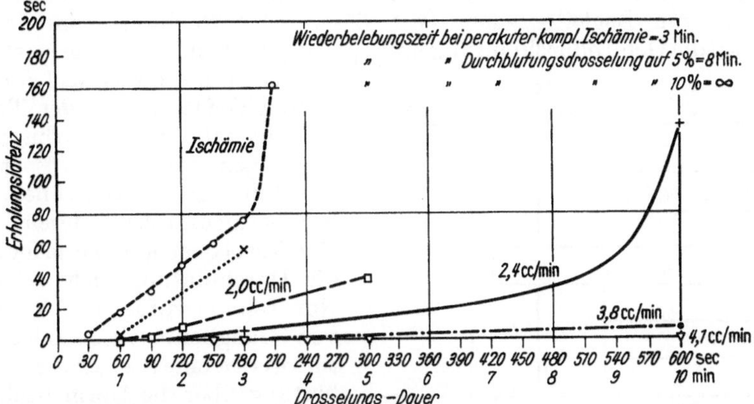

Abb. 9. Abhängigkeit der Erholungslatenz des Cortex von der Dauer der vorangegangenen Ischämie bzw. Oligämie. Versuche am isoliert durchströmten Katzenkopf. Zunächst ist die Abhängigkeit linear, nach einer Zeitdauer, die von der Höhe der Restdurchströmung abhängig ist, findet sich eine starke Versteilung. Damit wächst die Zeit für die volle Erholung rasch an, die „Wiederbelebungszeit" ist bald erreicht. Durch geringe Erhöhung der Restdurchströmung wird der kritische Bereich nach höheren Zeiten verschoben, bei einer solchen von 8—10% der Norm wird die Wiederbelebungszeit unendlich. (M. SCHNEIDER 1953.)

raturen liegt der Strukturumsatz sicher unter $^1/_5$ des normalen Tätigkeitsumsatzes. Bei tieferen Temperaturen wird auch der Strukturumsatz erniedrigt und die Wiederbelebungszeit verlängert. So kann die Wiederbelebungszeit der Ganglienzellen bei totaler Unterbrechung der Blutzufuhr von 3—4 min bei normalen Körpertemperaturen auf etwa das Dreifache steigen, wenn die Körpertemperatur auf etwa 25° C gesenkt wird.

Für Zustände chronischer Ischämie der Gehirngefäße sind vor allem die Krankheitsbilder der *Gefäßsklerose* und der *Endangitis* von Interesse. Bei der Cerebralsklerose wurden deutliche Minderungen der Durchblutung mit Steigerung des Strömungswiderstandes festgestellt, die bei deutlicher Ausprägung auch mit einer Herabsetzung des Sauerstoffverbrauchs einhergehen[1] (s. Abb. 10). Zwischen Abnahme

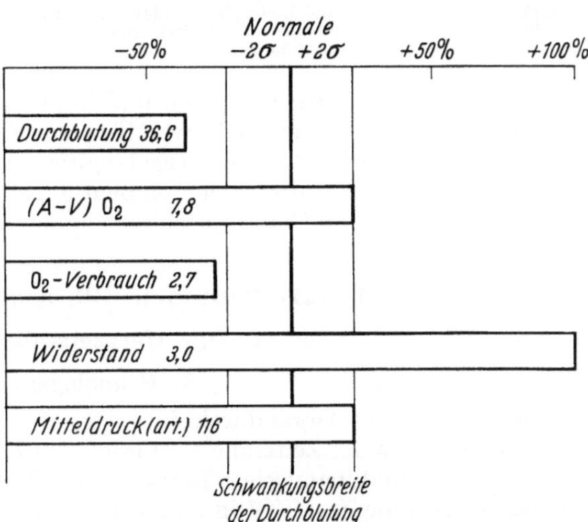

Abb. 10. Hirndurchblutung bei Cerebralsklerose. Mittelwerte von 26 Beobachtungen. Darstellung der Abweichungen vom normalen Mittelwert in %. Die Schwankungsbreite der Durchblutung ($\pm 2\,\sigma$) bei Gesunden ist besonders gekennzeichnet. Die in den Säulen angegebenen Zahlen sind die Mittelwerte (für die Durchblutung in ml/100 g und min, (A—V) O₂ in Vol.-%, für den O₂-Verbrauch in ml/100 g und min, für den Strömungswiderstand in mm Hg/ml/100 g und min und für den arteriellen Mitteldruck in mm Hg.) (BODECHTEL 1953.)

der Durchblutung, Anstieg des Strömungswiderstandes sowie Abnahme der Sauerstoffaufnahme einerseits und den geistigen Funktionen andererseits

[1] BODECHTEL 1953.

scheint eine gewisse Parallelität zu bestehen. Bei der *Endangitis obliterans* der Gehirngefäße liegen die Verhältnisse ähnlich wie bei der Arteriosklerose (s. Abb. 11). Hier erhebt sich wieder die Frage nach dem Vorkommen und der Bedeutung von Begleitspasmen (s. S. 654). Der Nachweis constrictorischer Effekte auf die Gehirndurchblutung unter pathologischen Bedingungen ist dadurch noch mehr erschwert als bei den peripheren Gefäßen, daß der Tonus der Gehirngefäße unter orthischen Bedingungen nicht nervös aufrechterhalten wird. Durchschneidung von Sympathicusfasern, deren Reizung eine Vasoconstriction erbringt, erhöht die Durchblutung nicht oder kaum. Nur selten wurde bei Verwendung von Ganglienblockern oder Sympathicolytica eine Steigerung der Durchblutung über die Norm beobachtet[1]. Beim Vorliegen einer Mangeldurchblutung infolge Gefäßerkrankung ließ sich dagegen durch Pendiomid oder durch Hexamethonium eine Erhöhung der Durchblutung erzielen. Doppelseitige Stellatum-Blockade bewirkt u. U. bei vorher erniedrigter Durchblutung eine Erhöhung der Gesamtdurchblutung bei gleichzeitiger Steigerung der O_2-Aufnahme (s. Tabelle 4).

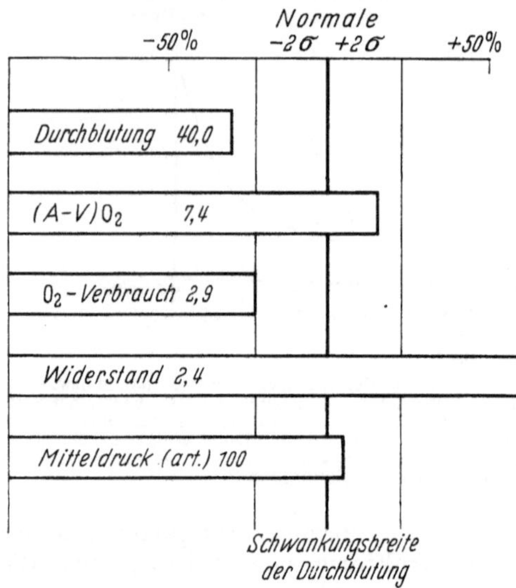

Abb. 11. Hirndurchblutung bei Endangitis obliterans. Mittelwerte aus 9 Beobachtungen. Zeichenerklärung s. Abb. 10. (Bodechtel 1953.)

Auf Grund der experimentellen und klinischen Befunde ist das Vorkommen von Spasmen bei normalen Gehirngefäßen unwahrscheinlich. Begleitspasmen bei organisch veränderten Gefäßen (Endangitis) sind dagegen nicht in Abrede zu stellen, ihre Existenz aber nicht eindeutig bewiesen.

Über Nieren- und Gehirndurchblutung bei Hypertonie siehe S. 689.

B. Herzzeitvolumen, Blutdruck, Blutmenge.

I. Das Herzzeitvolumen.

1. Grundlagen.

Die Summe der Organdurchblutungen ist das HZV, d. h. die Blutmenge, die vom Herzen in der Zeiteinheit gefördert wird. Das HZV ist damit die zentrale Größe jeder hämodynamischen Betrachtung. Man kann Kreislaufvorgänge nicht durchdenken, ohne das HZV in den Mittelpunkt zu stellen. Um so bedenklicher ist es, daß seine Messung in den meisten Fällen nur in Annäherung möglich ist.

In Tabelle 5 sind Herzindices (HZV pro m² Oberfläche) angegeben, die in den letzten Jahren von verschiedenen Autoren mit verschiedenen Methoden am ruhenden Menschen bestimmt wurden. Die in Deutschland viel verwendeten sphygmographischen Methoden haben große Fehlermöglichkeiten. Andererseits treibt häufig die Erregung der Versuchspersonen durch die Herzkatheterisierung das HZV in die Höhe, und so sind die mit der Fick-Methode gewonnenen Werte keine idealen Ruhewerte[2]. Wir müssen uns darüber Rechenschaft geben, daß

---

[1] Schneider 1953.

[2] Asmussen und Nielsen 1955, Christensen 1958, Emmrich u. a. 1958.

Tabelle 4. *Gehirndurchblutung bei Stellatumblockade.*

	Mittlerer arterieller Druck	Durch-blutung	Q_{O_2}	W	Literatur
Normal und Hypertonie	122	57	3,6	2,2	SCHEINBERG
Stellatumblockade, einseitig . .	119	54	3,4	2,3	
Normal und Hypertonie	121	49	3,2	2,5	HARMEL et al.
Stellatumblockade, beidseitig . .	124	48	3,1	2,7	
Cerebrale Gefäßerkrankung . .	111	45,6	2,4	2,6	SHENKIN et al.
Stellektomie, beidseitig	106	55,6	2,9	1,9	

Durchblutung in $cm^3/100$ g und min, $Q_{O_2} = O_2$-Aufnahme in $cm^3/100$ g und min, W = Strömungswiderstand.

die vielen Bemühungen um die Bestimmungen der Normalwerte des HZV am ruhenden Menschen bisher noch zu keinem befriedigenden Ergebnis geführt haben. Teilweise sind die unterschiedlichen Ergebnisse wohl durch Altersunterschiede bedingt. Eine neue amerikanische Untersuchung[1] über das Verhalten des HZV in verschiedenen Altersstufen ist mit sonstigen Ergebnissen schwer zu vergleichen, da die angeführten HZV-Werte auffallend niedrig liegen (s. Tabelle 5 und 6).

Tabelle 5. *HZV und Herzindices an Gesunden bei Ruhe.*

Autoren	Zahl der Unter-suchungen	Methode	HZV l/min		Herzindices l/min/m²	
			Mittel	Extrem-werte	Mittel	Extrem-werte
COURNAND 1950	10	Fick	—	—	3,1	—
DEXTER u. a. 1950	8	Fick	7,4	5,4—9,9	4,2	2,8—5,0
WESTCOTT u. a. 1951	11	Fick	5,4	4,1—8,0	3,1	—
ASMUSSEN und NIELSEN 1952 .	23	Farbstoff	6,9	—	—	—
		Acetylen	6,4	—	—	—
SCHMID und REUBI 1951, 1953 .	9	Wezler-Böger	4,4	3,2—6,4	—	—
		Fick	7,6	5,0—11,0	—	—
MCNEELY u. a. 1954	13	Farbstoff	7,6	2,3—13,2	—	—
BARTELS u. a. 1954	9	Fick	7,5	5,9—9,4	4,6	3,0—5,5
BRANDFONBRENER u. a. 1955 . .	67	Farbstoff	5,1	—	2,9	—

Tabelle 6. *HZV und Alter.*
Mittelwerte für die Dekaden nach BRANDFONBRENER u. Mitarb. (1955).

Dekade	Altersmittelwert der Gruppe	n	Herz-schläge/min	HZV l/min	Herzindex l/min · m²	Schlag-volumen ml
3.	23,6	9	77	6,5	3,7	86
4.	34,1	10	72	6,6	3,5	92
5.	43,3	11	69	5,3	3,0	78
6.	54,8	11	70	4,7	2,8	67
7.	65,4	10	63	4,3	2,6	70
8.	73,3	9	66	4,4	2,5	63
9.	82,0	7	67	3,9	2,4	60
Mittelwerte	52,5	67	69	5,1	2,9	74

Abb. 12 und Tabelle 7 zeigen die Beziehungen zwischen dem HZV und anderen Kreislaufgrößen zum Sauerstoffverbrauch bei körperlicher Arbeit. Neue

---

[1] BRANDFONBRENER u. a. 1955.

mit der Fick-Methode erhobene Befunde zeigen gute Übereinstimmung mit den angeführten Werten[1].

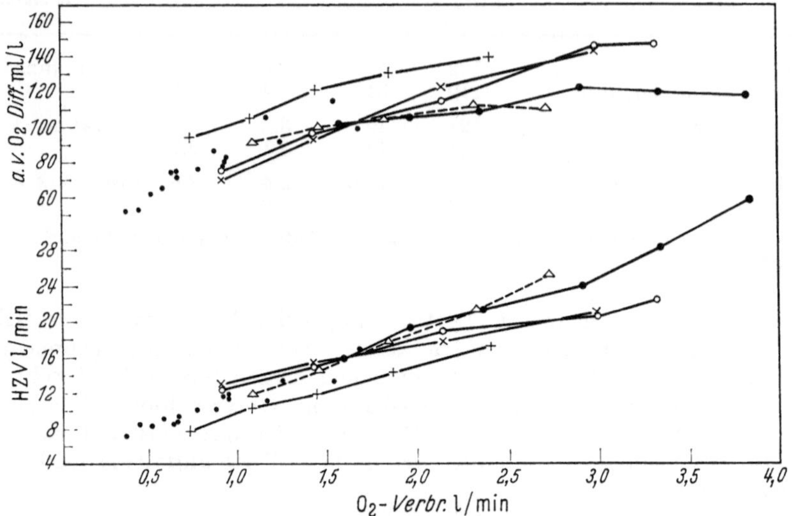

Abb. 12. Herzzeitvolumen und arterio-venöse Sauerstoffdifferenz während Arbeit in Beziehung zur Sauerstoffaufnahme. Die Linien verbinden Mittelwerte von 4 verschiedenen Versuchsreihen, von denen 3 mit der Acetylenmethode, 1 mit der Injektionsmethode ausgeführt wurden. Die kleinen Punkte sind Einzelwerte, die von Riley u. a. und Dexter u. a. mit der direkten Fick-Methode gewonnen wurden. (Asmussen u. Nielsen 1955.)

Tabelle 7. *Kreislauf und O₂-Transport bei Muskeltätigkeit.*
Untersuchungen an 25 gesunden dänischen Studenten. Bestimmung des HZV mit der Injektionsmethode. (Asmussen und Nielsen 1953.)

Mechanische Leistung mkg/min	Anzahl der Bestimmungen	O₂-Verbrauch ml/min	Pulsfrequenz	Schlagvolumen ml	HZV l/min	Art.-ven. O₂-Differenz (mit mittlerem Fehler des Mittelwertes) ml/l
Ruhe	23	267	64	108	6,9	$43 \pm 1,5$
288	7	910	104	118	12,3	$70 \pm 2,7$
540	15	1429	122	126	15,4	$94 \pm 4,9$
900	11	2143	161	117	18,9	$123 \pm 6,1$
1260	18	3007	173	120	20,8	$144 \pm 2,8$

Die Stellung des HZV im Kreislauf sei zunächst durch 4 sehr einfache mathematische Beziehungen gekennzeichnet.

$$1.\ \text{HZV} = \frac{\text{O}_2\text{-Verbrauch}}{\text{arterio-venöse O}_2\text{-Differenz}}.$$

Dieses nach Fick benannte Prinzip[2] ist nicht nur Grundlage für die wichtigsten Bestimmungen des HZV, es kennzeichnet auch gleichzeitig die Beziehungen zwischen HZV und Gewebsstoffwechsel. Ein erhöhter Bedarf der Peripherie kann dadurch gedeckt werden, daß das HZV gesteigert oder dadurch, daß die Transportfunktion des Blutes stärker ausgenützt wird. Letzteres kommt einer Vergrößerung der arterio-venösen Differenz gleich. Beim Fickschen Prinzip steht der Sauerstofftransport stellvertretend für sämtliche Stoffwechselfunktionen. Die Sicherung des Sauerstoffbedarfs der Peripherie ist im allgemeinen und über

---

[1] Donald u. a. 1955.   [2] Fick 1870.

längere Zeiten gesehen die entscheidende Funktion des Blutkreislaufes. Man darf aber dabei nicht übersehen, daß die Einstellung des HZV von anderen Größen mit bestimmt wird, besonders von temperaturregulatorischen Vorgängen.

In Tabelle 8 sind Messungen der arterio-venösen Sauerstoffdifferenz und der venösen Sauerstoffsättigung unter Ruhebedingungen zusammengestellt. (Die Katheterisierung der A. pulmonalis zur Gewinnung von Mischvenenblut dürfte infolge des gesteigerten HZV häufig zu kleinen arterio-venösen Differenzen und zu höheren venösen Sättigungen führen!) Nur ein knappes Drittel des mit dem arteriellen Blut in die Peripherie transportierten Sauerstoffs wird

Tabelle 8. *Gasanalytische Daten aus venösem Mischblut von 9 gesunden jungen Männern.* (BARTELS u. Mitarb. 1955a.)

	Mittelwert	Extremwerte
O_2-Gehalt ml/100 ml	15,1	12,6—16,4
O_2-Sättigung %	76,5	69,4—81,8
CO_2-Gehalt ml/100 ml	51,3	47,1—56,1
Arterio-venöse O_2-Differenz ml/100 ml	4,1	3,3— 5,6

ausgenutzt. Zum Teil beruht das darauf, daß Organe wie Niere und Haut dem Blute nur wenig Sauerstoff entnehmen, da ihre Durchblutung durch andere Funktionen in die Höhe getrieben wird. Andererseits muß aber auch in den Organen, in denen der Sauerstoffbedarf die Durchblutung bestimmt, der Sauerstoffgehalt des venösen Blutes noch relativ hoch sein, damit das Sauerstoffdruckgefälle für jeden Gewebsabschnitt ausreichend ist. Bei erhöhtem Sauerstoffbedarf, besonders bei Muskeltätigkeit, steigt nicht nur das HZV, sondern auch die arteriovenöse Sauerstoffdifferenz an (s. Tabelle 7 und Abb. 12)[1]. Der größte Teil des Blutes fließt in diesem Falle durch die tätige Skeletmuskulatur, die den Sauerstoff sehr weitgehend aus dem Blut herausnimmt[2].

$$2.\ \text{HZV} = \frac{\text{Blutmenge}}{\text{mittlere Kreislaufzeit}}.$$

Die Abhängigkeit des HZV von Blutmenge und mittlerer Kreislaufzeit[3] möchte man, wenn der Zusammenhang nicht so banal wäre, als das eigentliche Kreislaufgesetz bezeichnen. Es besagt nicht mehr und nicht weniger, als daß im Gleichgewichtszustand die Größe der peripheren Durchblutung gleich dem HZV und daß die vom Herzen geförderte Blutmenge gleich dem venösen Rückstrom sein muß. Es bedarf freilich einer genaueren Betrachtung, was unter mittlerer Kreislaufzeit und unter Blutmenge zu verstehen ist (s. S. 670).

$$3.\ \text{HZV} = \frac{\text{Druckgefälle}}{\text{peripherer Strömungswiderstand}}.$$

Diese verkürzte Form der Poiseuilleschen Gleichung, der in der Elektrizitätslehre formal das Ohmsche Gesetz entspricht, gibt die Beziehung zwischen Herzminutenvolumen, Druck und Strömungswiderstand. Sie gilt auch für jede einzelne Komponente des HZV, für die Durchblutung der einzelnen Organe (s. S. 643).

$$4.\ \text{HZV} = \text{Schlagvolumen} \times \text{Schlagfrequenz}.$$

Diese Beziehungen werden im Zusammenhang mit der Herzdynamik besprochen.

---

[1] ASMUSSEN und NIELSEN 1953, DONALD u. a. 1955.
[2] CHRISTENSEN 1937, BARGER u. a. 1956 (Literatur!).
[3] VIERORDT, zit. nach WOLLHEIM 1931, EPPINGER 1931.

2. Die Einstellung des Herzzeitvolumens.

Sowohl das Herz als auch das Gefäßsystem sind an der Einstellung des HZV beteiligt. Primär kommt es auf die Pumpleistung des Herzens an. Aber das Herz kann andererseits nicht mehr fördern, als ihm von der venösen Seite zufließt. Bestimmt nun unter Normal-Bedingungen die Herzleistung oder das venöse Angebot das HZV? Ergebnisse, die am Herz-Lungenpräparat gewonnen wurden, ließen zunächst vermuten, daß das Herz eine Pumpe ist, die angenähert jede Blutmenge fördert, die ihm zufließt, und daß deshalb die Größe des HZV allein vom Gefäßsystem bestimmt wird. Spätere Untersuchungen zeigten jedoch, daß das nervöse und hormonal gesteuerte Herz durchaus unabhängig vom Füllungsdruck die Blutförderung verändern kann. Danach kann im Normalbereich das HZV einmal stärker von seiten des Herzens, ein anderesmal mehr von seiten des Gefäßsystems bestimmt sein. Auf die Bedeutung des Herzens für die Blutförderung muß später ausführlich eingegangen werden (S. 725). Hier sollen zunächst die peripheren Einflüsse besprochen werden.

Die Abhängigkeit des HZV von zirkulierender Blutmenge und mittlerer Kreislaufzeit einerseits, vom Druckgefälle und Strömungswiderstand andererseits zeigen schon sehr einfache Kreislaufmodelle. Das in Abb. 13 skizzierte Modell besteht aus zwei kubischen Gefäßen, von denen das eine die arterielle, das andere die venöse Seite des Gefäßsystems darstellt. Entsprechend der geringen Kapazität der Arterien gegenüber den Venen[1] beträgt die Grundfläche des arteriellen Gefäßes im Modell nur $\frac{1}{3}$ der Grundfläche des venösen Gefäßes. Die beiden Gefäße sind durch eine Röhre verbunden, deren Strömungswiderstand durch einen eingebauten Hahn

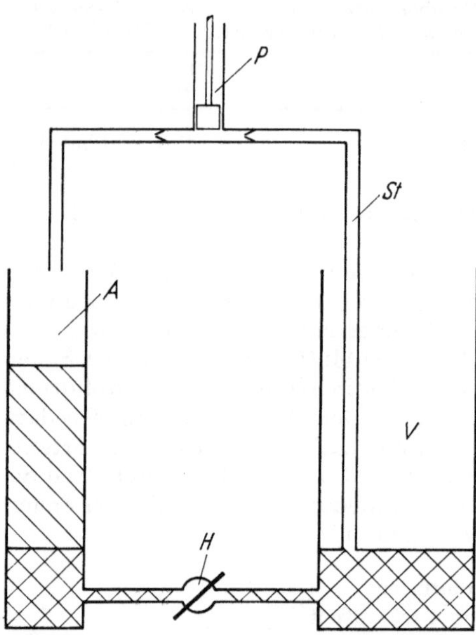

Abb. 13. Einfaches Kreislaufmodell. Die Pumpe P fördert die Flüssigkeit aus dem venösen Gefäß V in das arterielle Gefäß A, sobald das Flüssigkeitsniveau in V das untere Ende des Steigrohres ST erreicht. Die Pumpe P ist ein Modell für ein Herz, das jede Blutmenge fördert, die ihm von der Peripherie angeboten wird. Das arteriovenöse Druckgefälle des Systems ist allein abhängig von der Flüssigkeitsmenge im System. Das Kreislaufzeitvolumen ist durch das arterio-venöse Druckgefälle und den durch den Hahn H variablen Widerstand bestimmt. Gekreuzt schraffiert: ineffektives Blutvolumen; einfach schraffiert: effektives Blutvolumen. Es ist in diesem Modell der arterio-venösen Druckdifferenz proportional.

verändert werden kann. Eine Kolbenpumpe pumpt über ein Steigrohr die Flüssigkeit von der venösen auf die arterielle Seite hinüber. Da ihre Leistung hoch ist und die Strömungswiderstände im Steigrohr und im Stromvolummesser niedrig sind, saugt sie sämtliche Flüssigkeit aus dem venösen Gebiet ab, sobald diese das untere Ende des Steigrohres erreicht. Sie hält damit den Druck im venösen Gefäß, den „Füllungsdruck" konstant und fördert jede Blutmenge, die ihr bei diesem Druck angeboten wird. Auf 2 Vereinfachungen dieses primitiven Modells gegenüber dem menschlichen Kreislauf sei besonders hingewiesen. 1. Die Kapazität des arteriellen und venösen Systems ändert sich in unserem Modell proportional mit dem Druck. (Gibt man dem arteriellen und venösen Gefäß Formen, bei denen sich mit der Höhe der Querschnitt ändert, so können auf diese Weise die Druck-Volum-Beziehungen des Gefäßsystems im Modell berücksichtigt werden[2].) 2. Der Strömungswiderstand ist nicht auf das gesamte Röhrensystem verteilt, sondern liegt praktisch allein in der Bohrung des Hahnes und kann durch Veränderung der Hahnstellung eingestellt werden, ohne daß dadurch die Kapazität des Gefäßsystems beeinflußt wird.

---

[1] Broemser 1939, Green 1950, Landis und Hortenstine 1950, Schleier 1918.
[2] Starr u. a. 1940.

Am Modell hängt das Zeitvolumen allein vom Strömungswiderstand (bei H) und von der arterio-venösen Druckdifferenz ab. Die arterio-venöse Druckdifferenz wird aber durch das effektive Flüssigkeitsvolumen bestimmt, das dem effektiven Blutvolumen im menschlichen Kreislauf entspricht. Die effektive Blutmenge ist derjenige Teil des Blutes, der durch die Herztätigkeit dauernd von der venösen auf die arterielle Seite verschoben wird und damit für die Aufrechterhaltung des arterio-venösen Druckgefälles verantwortlich ist. Das effektive Blutvolumen entspricht der Größe, die BROEMSER[1] als „dauernd verschobenes Volumen" bezeichnet hat. Man kann das effektive Blutvolumen auch definieren als Differenz zwischen der gesamten Blutmenge und dem Volumen des Gefäßsystems bei gegebenem Füllungsdruck des Herzens. Am Modell der Abb. 13 kann man sich den Begriff des effektiven Blutvolumens folgendermaßen klarmachen: Das Modell sei zunächst leer und werde langsam aufgefüllt, bis der Flüssigkeitsspiegel den Einfluß in das Saugrohr erreicht. Die bis dahin aufgefüllte Flüssigkeitsmenge entspricht dem ineffektiven Volumen (in Abb. 13 gekreuzt schraffiert). Solange das ineffektive Volumen noch nicht erreicht ist, fördert die Pumpe keine Flüssigkeit, und das Zeitvolumen ist 0. Erst bei weiterer Auffüllung besteht neben dem ineffektiven ein effektives Volumen (in Abb. 13 einfach schraffiert). Die Pumpe fördert dann Flüssigkeit von

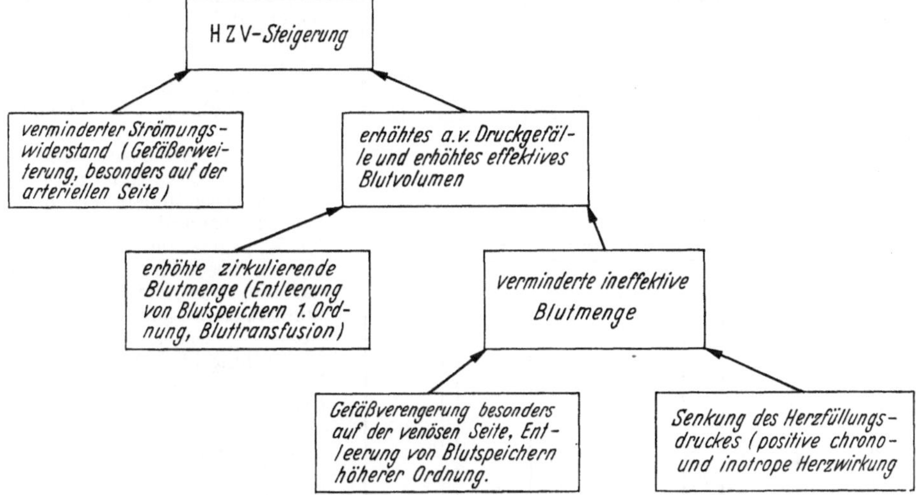

Abb. 14. Möglichkeiten der Steigerung des Herzzeitvolumens.

der venösen zur arteriellen Seite und schafft damit eine arterio-venöse Druckdifferenz. Entsprechend der kleinen Kapazität des arteriellen Systems genügen kleine Steigerungen des effektiven Volumens, um die arterio-venösen Druckdifferenzen stark zu erhöhen. Im Modell ist das geförderte Zeitvolumen dem effektiven Flüssigkeitsvolumen proportional. Für den menschlichen Kreislauf gilt das nicht vollkommen, da die Kapazität der Gefäße mit dem Druck zunimmt. In jedem Falle aber führen kleine Änderungen des effektiven Volumens zu starken Änderungen des arterio-venösen Druckgefälles. Dies erklärt, daß im Verhältnis zur Gesamtblutmenge kleine Blutverschiebungen ausreichen, um starke Rückwirkungen auf die Hämodynamik auszuüben.

Wie im Modell, so läßt sich auch im menschlichen Kreislauf eine Steigerung des HZV auf 2 Grundvorgänge zurückführen, auf eine Erhöhung des arterio-venösen Druckgefälles und auf eine Verminderung des peripheren Strömungswiderstandes (s. Abb. 14). Die arterio-venöse Druckdifferenz wird durch die Steigerung des effektiven Blutvolumens vergrößert, d. h., es wird durch entsprechende Kreislaufumstellungen Sorge getragen, daß dauernd eine größere Blutmenge vom „Niederdruckgebiet" zum „Hochdruckgebiet" verschoben ist. Von funktionell größerer Bedeutung ist die Minderung des peripheren Strömungswiderstandes. Das Blut fließt dann schneller durch die Peripherie, und die Kreislaufzeit wird verkürzt. Dabei steigt die Herzleistung nur proportional dem HZV an. Es ist dies also die ökonomische Form der HZV-Steigerung.

---

[1] BROEMSER 1939.

Zwei Abweichungen des Modells vom menschlichen Kreislauf sind noch besonders zu besprechen: 1. Im Modell wird die Verminderung des Strömungswiderstandes durch Weiterstellung des Hahnes zwischen arteriellem und venösem Gefäß hervorgerufen. Würde nicht das Steigrohr bei erhöhtem Zeitvolumen mehr Flüssigkeit enthalten, so würde sich im Modell der Füllungszustand der beiden Gefäße und damit das arterio-venöse Druckgefälle überhaupt nicht ändern. Wir hätten den idealen Fall, daß von sämtlichen Größen nur HZV und Strömungswiderstand beeinflußt würden, während das arteriovenöse Druckgefälle unverändert bliebe. Das Modell zeigt diese Verhältnisse in guter Annäherung. Die Ursache liegt in der Möglichkeit, den Strömungswiderstand unabhängig vom Fassungsvermögen des Gefäßsystems zu verändern. Beim menschlichen Kreislauf ist das nicht möglich. Die Abnahme des Strömungswiderstandes geht mit einem erhöhten Fassungsvermögen des Röhrensystems einher. Das Modell der Abb. 15 berücksichtigt diese Verhältnisse. Die Kapazität des Gefäßsystems nimmt besonders dadurch zu, daß die Verminderung des Strömungswiderstandes in den Arteriolen den Druck und damit die Blutfüllung im Gebiet der Capillaren und kleinen Venen steigert (Abb. 15). Hinzu kommen kann eine erhöhte Blutfüllung des kleinen Kreislaufs bei gesteigertem HZV[1]. Das effektive Blutvolumen und die arterio-venöse Druckdifferenz würden absinken, wenn nicht entsprechende Regulationen einsetzten. Sie sind dadurch möglich, daß die Arteriolen ein Gebiet hohen Strömungswiderstandes mit geringer Kapazität, die Venen dagegen ein Gebiet großer Kapazität und niedrigen Strömungswiderstandes sind. Eine Erweiterung der Arteriolen senkt den Strömungswiderstand und steigert die Durchblutung. Die dadurch bedingte Kapazitätszunahme kann durch eine Abnahme des Blutfassungsvermögens auf der venösen Seite ausgeglichen werden (Abb. 15b). Da die Venen einen

Abb. 15a u. b. Zur Regulation des effektiven Blutvolumens. Oben: Drucke und Blutverteilung bei enggestellten Arteriolen bzw. wenig geöffnetem Hahn *H*, Schraffierung von rechts nach links. Bei geöffneten Arteriolen bzw. bei geöffnetem Hahn *H* Schraffierung von links nach rechts. Der Anstieg des Druckes im Capillargebiet steigert die Blutmenge im Capillargebiet und vermindert die arterielle Blutmenge und den arteriellen Druck. Unten: Schraffierungen wie im oberen Bild. Ausregulierung der arteriellen Blutfüllung und des arteriellen Druckes durch Verminderung der venösen Blutmenge bei niedrigem Arteriolenwiderstand. *A* arterielles Gebiet; *C* Capillargebiet; *V* venöses Gebiet; *H* Hahn, der den Arteriolen mit veränderlichem Strömungswiderstand entspricht, *W* Strömungswiderstand im venösen Gebiet; *St* Steigrohr; *P* Pumpe.

niedrigen Strömungswiderstand haben, ist an dieser Stelle eine Einengung des Gefäßbettes möglich, ohne daß dadurch der Strömungswiderstand in stärkerem Maße beeinflußt wird.

2. In dem in Abb. 13 skizzierten Kreislaufmodell ist die Pumpe so konstruiert, daß unabhängig von der Kreislaufeinstellung und dem geförderten HZV der venöse Druck in jedem Fall konstant gehalten wird. Das isolierte Herz steigert aber das HZV nur, wenn der Füllungsdruck ansteigt (Straub-Starlingsches Gesetz). Würde diese Gesetzmäßigkeit auch für das

---

Lochner und Schoedel 1952a.

Herz in situ gelten, so müßte man der Pumpe des Modells andere Eigenschaften geben. BROEMSER (1939), STARR (1940) u. a. haben entsprechende Modelle entwickelt. Die Untersuchungen am intakten Tier zeigen aber, daß in sehr vielen Fällen der Füllungsdruck des Herzens durch regulatorische Vorgänge konstant gehalten wird, so daß dem Modell der Abb. 13 eine größere Bedeutung zukommt.

In Abb. 14 ist schon angedeutet, wie das Herz in die Einstellung des HZV eingreift. Wenn durch nervöse oder hormonale Einflüsse die Herzfrequenz und die Herzkraft gesteigert werden, so genügt ein geringerer Füllungsdruck zur Förderung des gleichen HZV. Auf diese Weise wird dauernd eine größere Blutmenge von der venösen auf die arterielle Seite verschoben, das effektive Blutvolumen ist gesteigert (s. S. 734).

II. Blutmenge und Blutverteilung.

1. Größe und Einstellung der Blutmenge.

In Tabelle 9 sind Werte für die Blutmenge des Menschen zusammengestellt. Zweifel an den Methoden zur Bestimmung der Blutmenge sind heute unberechtigt[1]. Die Fehlerbreite ist kleiner als bei anderen Methoden der Kreislaufforschung[2]. Fehler, die dadurch entstehen, daß der Hämatokrit in den einzelnen Kreislaufgebieten verschieden ist, lassen sich vermeiden, wenn man Erythrocyten- und Plasmavolumen gleichzeitig bestimmt.

Man nimmt teilweise an, daß die Einstellung des Blutvolumens einem echten Regelmechanismus unterliegt. Das Blutvolumen wäre damit neben dem arteri-

Tabelle 9. *Mittelwerte von Blutvolumen, Erythrocytenvolumen und Plasmavolumen von 10 gesunden Menschen.*
Erythrocyten- und Plasmavolumen wurden gleichzeitig direkt bestimmt. (GRAY u. FRANK 1953.)

	Mittelwerte	Mittlere Abweichung der Einzelwerte s	Mittlere Abweichung des Mittelwertes s_M
Plasmavolumen (ml)	2795	± 498	157
Erythrocytenvolumen (ml)	2081	± 508	161
Blutvolumen (ml)	4876	± 857	271
Plasmavolumen/kg Körpergewicht (ml/kg) . . .	41,1	$\pm 5,6$	1,7
Erythrocytenvolumen/kg Körpergewicht (ml/kg)	30,3	$\pm 5,6$	1,7
Blutvolumen/kg Körpergewicht (ml/kg)	71,4	$\pm 7,9$	2,5
Venöser Hämatokrit	46,5	$\pm 3,7$	1,0
Hämatokrit im gesunden Organismus	42,3	$\pm 5,5$	1,7

ellen Druck die zweite geregelte Größe im Bereich des Blutkreislaufes. Gegen diese Anschauung gibt es ernste Bedenken. Eine geregelte Größe müßte im Organismus über Receptoren direkt meßbar sein. Das ist aber für das Blutvolumen nicht möglich. Es kann nur bis zu einem gewissen Grade indirekt über die Blutfüllung der intrathorakalen Gefäße und der Herzvorhöfe gemessen werden. Auch die Zusammensetzung des Blutvolumens aus Erythrocytenvolumen und Plasmavolumen mit verschiedenen Einstellmechanismen erschwert die Vorstellung eines echten Regelmechanismus. Schließlich zeigt das Blutvolumen beim Vergleich gesunder Menschen gar nicht unerhebliche Schwankungen, was ebenfalls dagegen spricht, daß das Blutvolumen eine geregelte Größe ist (siehe Tabelle 9 und 10 und Abb. 19).

Der Mechanismus der Einstellung des Blutvolumens ist sicherlich ein sehr komplexer Vorgang. Das beruht schon allein darauf, daß die beiden Teilgrößen

---

[1] GRAY und FRANK 1953.   [2] GREGERSEN 1951, 1953, RAVDIN u. a. 1953.

Erythrocytenvolumen und Plasmavolumen durch verschiedene Mechanismen eingestellt werden. Für die Einstellung des Erythrocytenvolumens ist die Erythropoese wohl die entscheidende Größe, wobei der Sauerstoffdruck im Gewebe von recht großer Bedeutung zu sein scheint[1].

Für die Größe des Plasmavolumens kann für kürzere Zeiten die Verschiebung von Flüssigkeit zwischen extra- und intravasalem Raum eine Rolle spielen[2]. Steigerungen des Capillardruckes führen zur erhöhten Filtration von Flüssigkeit aus dem Gefäßraum in den extravasalen Raum und damit zur Abnahme des Plasmavolumens. Aus diesem Grunde findet man häufig eine Abnahme des

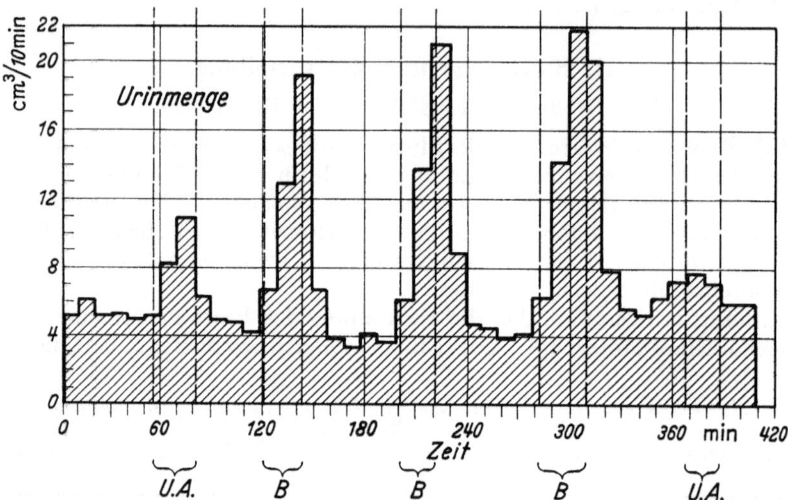

Abb. 16. Urinmenge bei Unterdruckatmung (U.A.) und bei Aufblähen eines Ballons im linken Vorhof (B). (Henry, und Gauer Reeves 1956.)

Plasmavolumens bei körperlicher Arbeit. Jedoch sind diese Änderungen nicht sehr groß. Der rasch ansteigende Druck im Gewebe verhindert eine weitere Filtration. Dabei spielen wahrscheinlich die Fascien der Muskulatur eine wichtige Rolle. Bei ihrer geringen Dehnbarkeit verhindern sie eine Zunahme des Gewebsvolumens, wodurch bei steigendem Capillardruck der Gewebsdruck sehr rasch ansteigt und eine weitere Filtration verhindert. Schließlich führt der Rückstrom der Gewebsflüssigkeit auf dem Lymphweg in das Venensystem zum weiteren Ausgleich zwischen intra- und extravasalem Flüssigkeitsvolumen. Andererseits tritt bei jeder Senkung des Capillardruckes Gewebsflüssigkeit in das Blut über. Nach Blutverlusten kommt diesem Vorgang neben den vasomotorischen Umstellungen eine entscheidende Bedeutung für die Wiederherstellung des effektiven Blutvolumens zu[3].

Für längere Zeiträume ist die Nierentätigkeit der entscheidende Vorgang für die Einstellung des Plasmavolumens. Von großer Bedeutung für die Einstellung des Plasmavolumens scheint die Blutfüllung des intrathorakalen Gefäßsystems zu sein[4]. Vorgänge mit einer gesteigerten Blutfülle des Thorax gehen im allgemeinen mit einer gesteigerten Harnausscheidung, solche mit kleiner Blutfüllung des Thorax mit einer verminderten Harnausscheidung einher. Besonders gut läßt sich dieser Vorgang im Experiment durch Unterdruckatmung auslösen, bei der die Blutfüllung der intrathorakalen Gefäße erhöht ist[5] (Abb. 16). Die

---

[1] Grant und Root 1952.   [2] Landis und Hortenstine 1950.   [3] Chien 1958.
[4] Gauer und Henry 1954.   [5] Gauer u. a. 1954.

reflektorische Steuerung geht anscheinend von Dehnungsreceptoren im linken Vorhof aus[1], wodurch reflektorisch die Sekretion des antidiuretischen Hormons

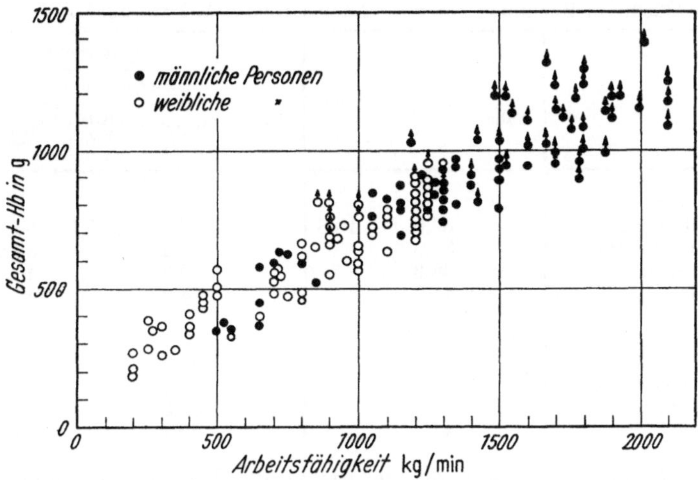

Abb. 17. Beziehung zwischen Hämoglobinmenge und Arbeitsleistung bei einer Pulsfrequenz von 170/min, bei Kindern, Frauen und Männern. Weibliche Versuchspersonen = o; männliche Personen = ●; ♂ und ♂ trainierte Frauen und Männer. (KJELLBERG, RUDHE, SJÖSTRAND 1949.)

gehemmt werden soll. Wahrscheinlich sind auch andere Hormone (Androsteron) an diesen Vorgängen beteiligt[2].

Wenn im allgemeinen die Harnbildung der Blutfüllung der intrathorakalen Gefäße parallel geht, so gibt es eine wichtige Ausnahme: Bei der Herzinsuffizienz ist die Harnmenge auch bei starker Füllung der intrathorakalen Gefäße klein[3]. Über die Ursache hierfür s. S. 746.

Zwischen der Blutmenge im Organismus und der Fähigkeit, körperliche Arbeit zu leisten, besteht eine deutliche Abhängigkeit[4]. Schon nach Blutentnahmen von 500 cm³, wie beim üblichen Blutspenden, zeigt sich eine Abnahme der Leistungsfähigkeit[5]. Abbildung 17 zeigt die Beziehung zwischen Gesamt-Hb-Menge und Arbeitsfähigkeit bei Trainierten und Untrainierten. Im Training nimmt die Gesamt-Hb-Menge zu, bei körperlicher

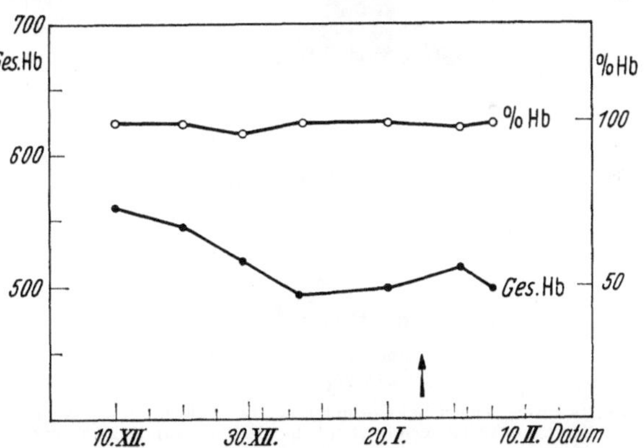

Abb. 18. Verhalten der Gesamthämoglobinmenge und der Hämoglobinkonzentration im Blut bei einer Frau, die wegen einer Beinfraktion 1¹/₂ Monate im Bett liegen mußte. Der Pfeil gibt den Zeitpunkt des 1. Wiederaufstehens an. (SJÖSTRAND 1953.)

Untätigkeit, besonders bei Bettruhe, sinkt sie ab (Abb. 18), eine Tatsache, die bei Veränderungen der Blutmenge von Kranken berücksichtigt werden sollte.

Bei Änderungen der Blutmenge in Abhängigkeit von der Arbeitsbelastung ist der Hämatokrit eine relativ konstante Größe. Es gehen also Änderungen des Erythrocyten- und Plasmavolumens weitgehend parallel. Möglicherweise

---

[1] SIEKER u. a. 1954, HENRY u. a. 1956.
[2] SMITH 1957, SCHWIEGK 1957, SCHMIDT und AVIADO 1958.
[3] ALTSCHULTE 1954.   [4] KJELLBERG u. a. 1949b, SJÖSTRAND 1953.   [5] BALKE u. a. 1954.

Tabelle 10. *Totales Blutvolumen, Erythrocyten- und Plasmavolumen von herzgesunden Patienten und von Herzkranken im kompensierten und dekompensierten Zustand.*
Angaben in ml/kg Körpergewicht. Bei den Patienten mit Herzinsuffizienz ist das Körpergewicht ohne Ödeme in Rechnung gesetzt. (Nach Guyton u. Paul 1955.)

| | Kontrollgruppe | | | Herzkranke | | | | |
| | | | | | dekompensiert | | kompensiert | |
	Fälle	Mittel-wert	mittlere Abwei-chung	Fälle	Mittel-wert	mittlere Abwei-chung	Mittel-wert	mittlere Abwei-chung
Männer	75			46				
Gesamtblutmenge		69,8	± 10,8		90,7	± 18,3	80,4	± 13,3
Erythrocytenvolumen		30,9			40,4		38,8	
Plasmavolumen		38,9			50,3		41,6	
Hämatokrit		44,2			44,6		48,3	
Frauen	32			18				
Gesamtblutmenge		60,6	± 8,9		88,2	± 21,1	70,5	± 13,9
Erythrocytenvolumen		25,1			35,9		31,7	
Plasmavolumen		35,5			52,3		38,8	
Hämatokrit		41,6			40,7		45,0	

beeinflussen die gleichen Vorgänge, die die Größe des Plasmavolumens steuern, über hormonale Vorgänge auch die Erythropoese[1]. Dagegen steigt bei allen Formen der Hypoxie der Hämatokrit an.

Bei den verschiedenartigen Einflüssen auf die Einstellung des Blutvolumens und bei der nicht geringen Streuung der Normalwerte kann es nicht wundernehmen, daß unter patho-

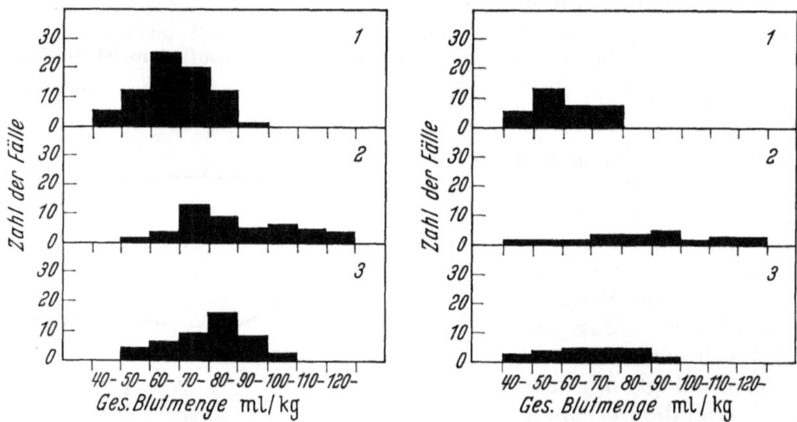

Abb. 19. Blutmengen bei Gesunden (*1*), bei Patienten mit Herzinsuffizienz (*2*) und bei Patienten, bei denen die Herzinsuffizienz erfolgreich behandelt war (*3*), links Männer, rechts Frauen. (Gunton u. Paul 1955.)

logischen Bedingungen auch beim gleichen Krankheitsbild recht verschiedene Blutmengen gefunden werden. Das gilt besonders für die Herzinsuffizienz (Abb. 19, Tabelle 10). Im allgemeinen ist dabei das Blutvolumen gesteigert[2]. Dabei ist der Hämatokrit normal oder leicht gesteigert. Bei Besserung des Krankheitszustandes nimmt das Blutvolumen im allgemeinen ab. Seltener sind Fälle von Herzinsuffizienz mit normalem oder sogar vermindertem Blutvolumen[3].

2. Blutmenge und HZV.

α) *Kreislaufzeit und Blutspeicher.* Das HZV ist der Quotient aus der zirkulierenden Blutmenge und der mittleren Kreislaufzeit. Dabei ist die mittlere

---

[1] Flaks u. a. 1937, Contopoulos u. a. 1953.
[2] Altschute 1954, Kaplan u. a. 1954, Guyton und Paul 1955.   [3] Wollheim 1931.

Kreislaufzeit der Mittelwert der Zeiten, in denen die Partikel der Kreislauf-
flüssigkeit einmal den Kreis durchlaufen. Im ruhenden menschlichen Organismus
kann man im Durchschnitt das HZV mit 6 l/min, die Blutmenge mit 5 Liter
annehmen. Daraus berechnet sich eine mittlere Kreislaufzeit von weniger als
1 min. Soll das HZV gesteigert werden, so kann entweder die zirkulierende Blutmenge gesteigert oder die Strömungsgeschwindigkeit des Blutes erhöht (d. h. die
mittlere Kreislaufzeit verkürzt) werden, oder es kann sich um eine Kombination
beider Vorgänge handeln. Es sind wohl in erster Linie J. BARCROFTs eindrucksvolle Arbeiten über die Speicherfunktion der Milz[1], die zunächst daran denken
ließen, daß eine Steigerung des HZV über eine Vermehrung der zirkulierenden Blutmenge durch Blutentspeicherung zustande kommt. Nun besitzen zwar Hund und
Katze Speichermilzen. Beim Hund können 10—20% der Blutmenge in der Milz
gespeichert sein[2]. Dagegen kommt der menschlichen Milz eine Depotfunktion
nicht zu. Die Erhöhung des HZV bei Muskeltätigkeit geht beim Menschen ohne
Steigerung der zirkulierenden Blutmenge einher. Das Plasmavolumen nimmt im
Beginn der Muskeltätigkeit sogar häufig ab, da als Folge des erhöhten Capillardrucks Flüssigkeit aus dem Gefäßsystem ins Gewebe verschoben wird[3]. Adrenalin-
injektionen steigern über die Entspeicherung der Milz zwar beim Hund, nicht
aber beim Menschen die zirkulierende Blutmenge[4]. Im menschlichen Kreislauf
sind Blutspeicher erster Ordnung, bei denen das Blut in Räumen außerhalb der
eigentlichen Strombahn deponiert ist, ohne Bedeutung. Wenn man beim menschlichen Kreislauf überhaupt von Blutspeichern sprechen will, dann handelt es
sich um solche „zweiter Ordnung": Die Blutbahnen selbst sind stärker mit Blut
gefüllt, als für den Blutbedarf der Organe notwendig ist[5].

Wenn im menschlichen Kreislauf eine Steigerung des HZV nicht mit einer
Vermehrung der zirkulierenden Blutmenge einhergeht, dann kann sie nur durch
Verkürzung der mittleren Kreislaufzeit zustande kommen. Wenn bei Muskeltätigkeit das HZV auf mehr als das Sechsfache des Ruhewertes ansteigt, dann
muß die mittlere Kreislaufzeit unter 10 sec liegen. Die mittlere Kreislaufzeit
ist freilich ein Mittel aus sehr ungleichen Komponenten. Die Coronargefäße sind
vom Blut in weniger als 10 sec passiert und die Kreislaufzeit dieses Blutes beträgt
demnach weniger als 20 sec. Andererseits verteilen sich in die Blutbahn injizierte
Stoffe so langsam im Gesamtblut, daß der Durchfluß durch manche Abschnitte
des großen Kreislaufs schon unter normalen Bedingungen mehr als 8 min dauern
muß. Unter pathologischen Bedingungen können diese Zeiten wahrscheinlich
noch länger sein. Aus solchen Überlegungen heraus sind Versuche verständlich,
die zirkulierende Blutmenge in einen rasch und langsam fließenden Teil auf-
zuteilen, eine „aktive" und eine „passive" Blutmenge. Leider gibt es aber
keine Methode, die beiden Blutbestandteile getrennt zu erfassen. Die Kreislauf-
zeiten der einzelnen Gefäßbezirke gehen so ineinander über, daß eine Abtrennung
der aktiven Blutmenge von der Gesamtblutmenge nicht möglich ist.

Unter Kreislaufzeit versteht man teilweise die Zeit, in der ein Blutbestandteil mit dem
Blutstrom von einer Stelle des Gefäßsystems zu einer anderen gelangt[6]. Man sollte dabei
besser von Durchflußzeiten sprechen. Für derartige Bestimmungen gibt es zahlreiche klinische
Methoden. Für hämodynamische Betrachtungen ist es wichtig zu unterscheiden, ob mit den
jeweils verwendeten Methoden die kürzeste oder die mittlere Durchflußzeit bestimmt wird.

β) Blutspeicherung. Die Begriffe des Blutspeichers und der Blutspeicherung
haben besonders in den dreißiger Jahren eine große Rolle gespielt. Man sah in
der Entspeicherung von Blut die einzige Möglichkeit, das HZV zu erhöhen[7].

---

[1] J. BARCROFT 1926.   [2] GREEN 1950.   [3] CULLUMBINE und KOCH 1949, NYLIN 1947.
[4] NYLIN 1946.   [5] REIN 1933.   [6] TIETZE 1954.
[7] KROGH 1912, PATTERSON, PIPER und STARLING 1914.

Unter gespeichertem Blut ist Blut zu verstehen, das für die Versorgung des Organs nicht benötigt und im Dienste der Kreislaufregulation abgegeben werden kann. Im folgenden seien die Gründe aufgeführt, die uns heute den Begriff Blutspeicherung nur noch mit Vorsicht anwenden lassen.

1. Der Mensch hat keine Blutspeicher erster Ordnung, sondern nur solche höherer Ordnung, bei denen das Blut nicht parallel der Strombahn, sondern in der Strombahn selbst deponiert ist (s. S. 671).

2. Es gibt sicher einige Organe, die bevorzugt im Dienste der Kreislaufregulation Blut aufnehmen oder auch wieder abgeben können, die also im alten Sinne Blutspeicher darstellen. Es ist dies wohl in erster Linie das Splanchnicusgebiet[1]. Eine weitere wichtige Rolle spielt der subpapilläre Plexus der Haut[2]. Letzten Endes kann aber wohl das gesamte Venensystem als Blutspeicher dienen. Durch Änderung der Blutfüllung ihrer Venen können aber unter bestimmten Bedingungen alle Organe zu Blutspeichern werden.

3. Die Mechanismen, die den Blutgehalt der Organe verändern, sind sehr verschieden. Bei Blutspeichern denkt man zunächst an Änderungen der Gefäßkapazität durch vasomotorische Vorgänge oder zumindest durch Einflüsse glatter Muskulatur im Organ (Milz). In anderen Fällen ist aber die Höhe des venösen Druckes für die Blutfüllung des Organs verantwortlich. Das gilt besonders für die Lunge (s. S. 673). Schließlich kann die Blutfüllung durch den hydrostatischen Druck und durch den Druck der umliegenden Organe beeinflußt werden. Letztere beiden Einflüsse sind besonders für die Blutfüllung der Extremitäten von Bedeutung.

4. Es ist häufig nicht zu entscheiden, ob eine erhöhte Blutfüllung eines Organs eine Bereitstellung von Blut für kreislaufregulatorische Zwecke ist, ob also eine Blutspeicherung vorliegt, oder ob die Erhöhung der Blutfüllung ganz anderen Funktionen dient, etwa der speziellen Funktion dieses Organs oder anderen regulatorischen Vorgängen. So kann eine erhöhte Blutfüllung des subpapillären Plexus der Haut eine Blutspeicherung sein. Sie kann aber auch durch die physikalische Temperaturregulation bedingt sein.

5. Nach der „klassischen" Auffassung kann das HZV nur durch Speicherung oder Entspeicherung von Blut verändert werden. Heute müssen wir aber annehmen, daß das nervös und hormonal gesteuerte Herz auch von sich aus unabhängig vom venösen Blutangebot das HZV verändern kann (s. S. 734). Danach kommt bei unserer heutigen Auffassung der Hämodynamik dem Begriff der „Blutspeicherung" nicht mehr die alles beherrschende Bedeutung zu wie vor wenigen Jahrzehnten. Daraus darf freilich nicht geschlossen werden, daß Fragen der Blutverteilung heute unwichtig geworden sind. Versagen der Venomotorik führt auch nach heutiger Anschauung zum Schock[3]. Es gibt aber nebeneinander zwei Mechanismen für die Einstellung des HZV, das venöse Angebot und die gesteuerte Herztätigkeit.

6. Man nimmt häufig an, daß jede erhöhte Durchblutung auch mit einer größeren Blutfüllung einhergeht. Dies muß aber nicht unbedingt der Fall sein. Eine arbeitende Extremität hat in den ersten Minuten trotz gesteigerter Durchblutung keine erhöhte Blutfüllung. Sie kann sogar infolge der Pumpwirkung auf das Venensystem vermindert sein[4]. Auch die Zunahme der Blutfüllung im abführenden Venensystem scheint zunächst gering zu sein. Eine erhöhte Blutfüllung der arbeitenden Extremität stellt sich erst später durch temperaturregulatorische Vorgänge ein[5]. Zum mindesten in einem früheren Stadium körper-

---

[1] Gollwitzer-Meier 1932, Alexander 1954, 1955, 1956.   [2] Wollheim 1933.
[3] Grill 1933, Alexander 1955.   [4] Asmussen 1943, Greenfield und Patterson 1956.
[5] Grill 1933, Christensen und Nielsen 1942.

licher Tätigkeit kann das HZV allein deshalb ansteigen, weil infolge des verminderten peripheren Strömungswiderstandes die Kreislaufzeit verkürzt ist[1]. Jedenfalls erfordert nicht jede Steigerung des HZV die Entleerung von Blutspeichern, es sei denn, man sieht die Venen der arbeitenden Extremitäten in diesem Falle als Blutspeicher an.

Nach all dem ist es meist besser, nicht von Blutspeicherung, sondern einfach vom Blutgehalt eines Organs zu sprechen. Der Blutgehalt der Organe muß im Dienste des Gesamtkreislaufes eingestellt werden, ähnlich wie das für die Durchblutung der Organe gilt. Die Verteilung des Blutes auf die Organe ist ein entscheidender Teilvorgang der Kreislaufregulation, wobei sowohl der Blutbedarf jedes Organs als auch der Zustand des gesamten Kreislaufs berücksichtigt werden muß.

γ) *Die Blutfüllung der Lunge.* Die Lunge ist oft als Blutspeicher angesprochen worden[2]. Die Blutfüllung der Lunge geht nicht allein ihrer Durchblutung, d. h. dem HZV, parallel[3]. Das gilt anscheinend nur bei angespannter Kreislauflage, etwa in Narkose oder bei Laparotomie[4]. Sie ändert sich auch unabhängig vom HZV. Beim Übergang vom Stehen zum Liegen nimmt der Blutgehalt der Beine ab und der der Lunge zu[5]. Auch bei Einwirkung von Kälte ist der kleine Kreislauf stärker mit Blut gefüllt. Letzteres ist eine Folge der verminderten Hautdurchblutung[6]. Bei Muskeltätigkeit ist im allgemeinen die Blutfüllung der Lunge vermindert[7]. Ob vasomotorische Vorgänge an den Füllungsänderungen der Lunge beteiligt sind, ist zweifelhaft. Sehr weitgehend sind sie sicherlich druckpassiv bedingt[8]. Blutfüllungsänderungen der Lunge stehen anscheinend im engen Zusammenhang mit der Funktion des linken Herzens.

Das linke Herz fördert nicht in jedem Fall die gesamte Blutmenge, die ihm angeboten wird. Dabei ist nicht nur an die Auswirkungen des Straub-Starlingschen Gesetzes zu denken, nach dem bei erhöhter Leistung ein erhöhter Füllungsdruck und damit eine erhöhte Blutfüllung im Venensystem der Lunge notwendig ist. Unter Normalbedingungen ist wohl noch wichtiger, daß beim gesteuerten Herzen die geförderte Blutmenge in einem gewissen Grade unabhängig vom Blutangebot sein kann. Wird das Herz vagotonisch gebremst, so steigt der Füllungsdruck und damit auch die Blutfülle der Lunge an. Das angetriebene Herz fördert umgekehrt die gesamte angebotene Blutmenge. Dabei sinken Druck und Blutfüllung in den Lungenvenen. Das Venensystem der Lunge hat dabei für das linke Herz die gleiche Funktion zu erfüllen wie die großen Körpervenen für das rechte Herz. Die Kapazitäten beider Systeme müssen genügend groß sein, damit die Füllungszeiten der Kammern klein bleiben. Ist das Venensystem schlecht gefüllt, so kann nur noch durch die systolische Sogwirkung des Herzens ein hinreichend großes Fördervolumen erhalten werden (s. S. 725)[9].

Man kann im Tierversuch durch Aderlässe und Bluttransfusionen das Blutangebot an das Herz verändern und dabei die Drucke in den Vorhöfen und in der A. pulmonalis verfolgen (Abb. 20)[10]. Dabei ändert sich der zentrale Venendruck mit dem venösen Angebot. Die Druckänderungen in der A. pulmonalis gehen denen des zentralen Venendruckes weitgehend parallel. Das rechte Herz schafft also ziemlich unbeeinflußt vom venösen Angebot eine konstante Druckstufe, die sich auf den zentralen Venendruck aufsetzt. Man kann sagen, daß der kleine Kreislauf funktionell zum ,,Niederdrucksystem" (d. h. zum extraarteriellen System) gehört[11]. Füllungsänderungen im Venensystem des großen Kreislaufs pflanzen sich auf das

---

[1] ASMUSSEN und NIELSEN 1955a.
[2] HOCHREIN und KELLER 1932a und b, HAMILTON 1950, SJÖSTRAND 1953.
[3] LOCHNER und SCHOEDEL 1952a.　　[4] JOHNSON 1951.
[5] HAMILTON und MORGAN 1931, LAGERLÖF u. a. 1951.
[6] GLASER 1949.　　[7] LAMMERANT 1957.　　[8] SARNOFF u. a. 1953.
[9] GAUER 1955.　　[10] HENRY u. a. 1956.　　[11] GAUER und HENRY 1956.

Gefäßsystem der Lunge fort. Dabei können durch die große Dehnbarkeit der Lungengefäße schon bei geringen Druckänderungen, die noch kein Lungenödem bedingen, starke Änderungen der Blutfüllung auftreten.

Am Beispiel der Lunge zeigt sich, daß „Blutspeicherung" nicht durch Vasomotorik bedingt zu sein braucht, sondern daß es sich um Rückstauung von Blut handeln kann. Man kann darüber streiten, ob es glücklich ist, in einem solchen Falle von Blutspeichern zu sprechen.

δ) *Das effektive Blutvolumen.* Man kann versuchen, die gesamte Blutmenge nach ihrer Strömungsgeschwindigkeit in eine zirkulierende und eine deponierte oder auch in eine aktive und passive Blutmenge zu unterteilen. Vom Standpunkt der Hämodynamik ist eine andere Einteilung, die in eine effektive und ineffektive Blutmenge, von größerer Bedeutung. Die ineffektive Blutmenge füllt das Gefäßsystem, ohne daß der Füllungsdruck des Herzens erreicht wird. Das effektive Blutvolumen oder das dauernd (von der venösen auf die arterielle Seite) verschobene Volumen nach Broemser schafft die Druckdifferenz zwischen der arteriellen und der venösen Seite des Gefäßsystems. Die Regelung des arteriellen Druckes (s. S. 678) erfolgt letzten Endes durch die Bereitstellung des nötigen effektiven Blutvolumens.

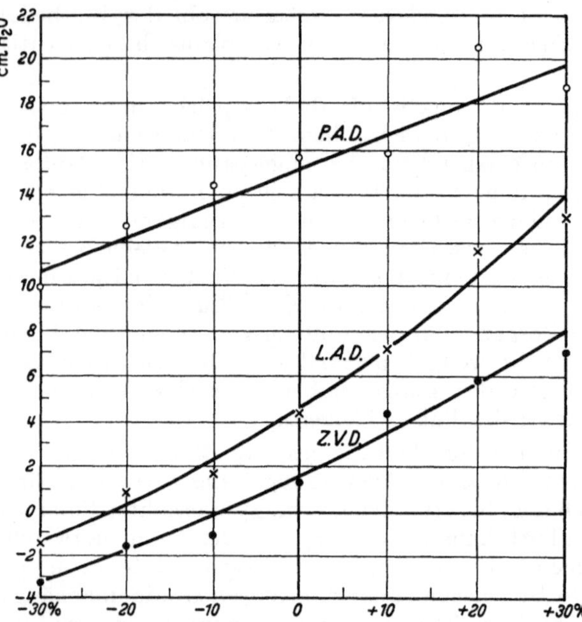

Abb. 20. Zentraler Venendruck (*Z.V.D.*), linker Vorhof- (*L.A.D.*) und Pulmonalarteriendruck (*P.A.D.*) bei Änderungen des Blutvolumens um ± 30% durch Aderlaß und Bluttransfusion (Hund). Mit zunehmendem intrathorakalem Blutvolumen nimmt die arteriovenöse Druckdifferenz ab, da der Strömungswiderstand im erweiterten Lungenstrombett kleiner wird. (Henry, Gauer und Sieker 1956.)

Tabelle 11 gibt das Blutfassungsvermögen der einzelnen Gefäßabschnitte an, wobei der Inhalt der Venen bei 0 mm Hg, der der Arterien bei 100 mm Hg gemessen wurde. Unter diesen Bedingungen fassen die Venen des großen Kreislaufs $^2/_3$, die Arterien noch nicht $^1/_5$ der gesamten Blutmenge. Das kleine Fassungsvermögen und die geringe Dehnbarkeit des arteriellen Systems im Vergleich zum Venensystem muß dazu führen, daß schon geringe Steigerungen der arteriellen Blutmenge eine beachtliche arterio-venöse Druckdifferenz erzeugen können. Abb. 21 gibt die Drucke in den einzelnen Gefäßabschnitten an. Stellt man im Versuch am Hund durch Vagusreizung das Herz still, so gleichen sich arterieller und venöser Druck aus, und es stellt sich im gesamten System ein statischer Druck von etwa 10 mm Hg ein[1]. Auch dieser niedrige statische Druck kennzeichnet das gegenüber dem venösen Teil geringe Fassungsvermögen des arteriellen Systems.

Das effektive Blutvolumen ist also sicherlich gegenüber der gesamten Blutmenge klein. Leider sind nur sehr grobe Schätzungen dieser Größe möglich. Broemser (1939) gibt das dauernd verschobene Volumen mit nur 2% der Gesamtblutmenge an. Es entspricht dies der Blutmenge des arteriellen Windkessels, abzüglich seines Inhaltes beim Druck 0. Die effektive Blutmenge findet sich aber nicht nur in den großen Arterien, sondern auch im Capillargebiet und in den

---

[1] Green 1950, Guyton u. a. 1952.

Tabelle 11. *Dimensionen des Gefäßsystems eines Hundes von 13 kg.* (GREEN 1950.)

Gefäßabschnitt	Durch-messer mm	Anzahl	Gesamt-quer-schnitt cm²	Länge cm	Gesamt-vo-lumen cm³	Gesamtvolumen %
Großer Kreislauf						
Linker Ventrikel (Diastole)	—	—	—	—	25	1,84 ⎫
Aorta	10	1	0,8	40	32	2,34 ⎪
Große Arterien	3	40	3,0	20	60	4,41 ⎪
Arterielle Hauptäste	1	600	5,0	10	50	3,57 ⎪
Sekundäre Äste	0,6	1800	5,0	4	20	1,46 ⎬ 17,79
Tertiäre Äste	0,14	76000	11,7	1,4	16	1,18 ⎪
Endarterien.	0,05	1000000	19,6	0,1	2	0,15 ⎪
Endäste	0,03	13000000	91	0,15	14	1,00 ⎪
Arteriolen	0,02	40000000	125	0,2	25	1,84 ⎭
Capillaren	0,008	1200000000	600	0,1	60	4,41 4,41
Venolen	0,03	80000000	570	0,2	114	8,36 ⎫
Terminaläste	0,075	13000000	570	0,15	85	6,21 ⎪
Terminale Venen	0,13	1000000	132	0,1	13	0,95 ⎪
Tertiäre Venen	0,28	76000	47	1,4	7	0,51 ⎪
Sekundäre Venen	1,5	1800	30	4	120	8,78 ⎬ 66,06
Hauptvenen	2,4	600	27	10	270	19,80 ⎪
Große Venen	6,0	40	11	20	220	16,10 ⎪
Hohlvenen	12,5	1	1,2	40	48	3,51 ⎪
Rechter Vorhof	—	—	—	—	25	1,84 ⎭
Kleiner Kreislauf						
Rechter Ventrikel (Diastole)	—	—	—	—	25	1,84 ⎫ 4,88
Lungenarterien	—	—	—	—	42	3,04 ⎭
Lungencapillaren	—	—	—	—	16	1,17 1,17
Lungenvenen	—	—	—	—	52	3,70 ⎫ 5,54
Linker Vorhof	—	—	—	—	25	1,84 ⎭
Summe					1366	99,85

Venen. Wenn auch die Drucke in diesen Gebieten niedrig sind, so ist andererseits ihr Volumenelastizitätskoeffizient klein, so daß kleine Druckerhöhungen große

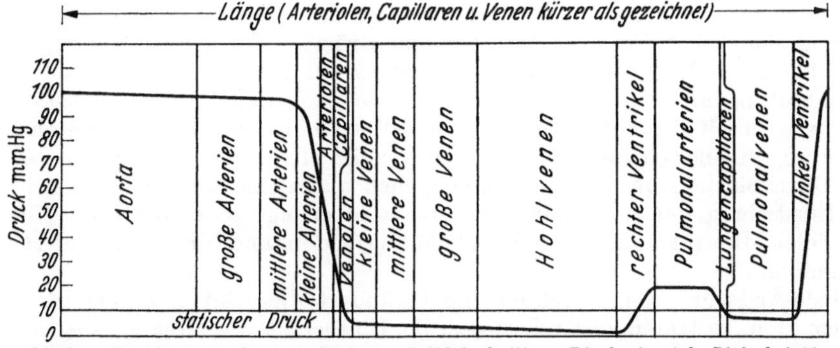

Abb. 21. Mittlerer Blutdruck in den verschiedenen Gefäßabschnitten. Die horizontale Linie bei 10 mm Hg entspricht dem sog. statischen Druck, d. h. dem Druck beim Stillstand des Kreislaufs. (GREEN 1950.)

Änderungen der Blutfüllung hervorbringen. GREEN schätzt das effektive Blutvolumen auf 20% der gesamten Blutmenge nach der Zahl der Pulsschläge, die notwendig sind, um den arteriellen Druck auf 100 mm zu steigern, nachdem vorher durch Vagusreizung das Herz zum Stillstand gebracht und der arterielle Druck auf 20 mm Hg gesenkt wurde. LANDIS und HORTENSTINE (1950) schätzen das effektive Blutvolumen auf ¹/₄ der gesamten Blutmenge. Wenn man Hunden nach Ausschaltung der Pressoreceptoren Blut infundiert, so steigt das HZV 4—5mal stärker an als die zirkulierende Blutmenge[1]. Auch dies deutet auf ein effektives Blutvolumen von 20—25%, wenn man annimmt, daß nach Ausschaltung der Pressoreceptoren kreislaufregulatorische Vorgänge ohne Bedeutung sind, die sonst das Bild komplizieren. Das effektive Blutvolumen ist die Differenz zwischen der gesamten Blutmenge und dem Fassungsvermögen des Gefäßsystems bei Herzfüllungsdruck. Die Einstellung des effektiven Blutvolumens hängt also sowohl von Änderungen des Fassungsvermögens des Gefäßsystems als auch von solchen der Blutmenge ab. Bedarf das Herz zur Blutförderung eines erhöhten Füllungsdruckes, so steigt damit das ineffektive Blutvolumen. Nach grober Schätzung sind $^3/_4$ des Blutes unter normalen Bedingungen ineffektiv. Davon kann ein Achtel bis ein Viertel durch vasomotorische Gefäßverengerungen zur effektiven Blutmenge gemacht werden, etwa nach Blutverlusten oder bei extrem hohem Blutbedarf der Peripherie. Aber auch bei extremer Gefäßverengerung füllt die Hälfte des normalen Blutvolumens den „Totraum" des Gefäßsystems, bleibt also ineffektiv[2]. Bei rascher arterieller Entblutung von Hunden gewinnt man im Mittel nur 60% der gesamten Blutmenge[3].

Das gegenüber der gesamten Blutmenge kleine effektive Blutvolumen erklärt, daß häufig schon kleine Änderungen der Blutmenge durch Bluttransfusion oder Aderlässe das arterio-venöse Druckgefälle und das HZV beeinflussen können. Es muß dies immer dann geschehen, wenn die Änderungen der gesamten Blutmenge nicht durch entsprechende Umstellungen des ineffektiven Blutvolumens aufgefangen werden können. Regulatorische Vorgänge in dieser Richtung scheinen recht häufig träge und unvollkommen abzulaufen. Um so wichtiger ist die Einstellung des gesamten Blutvolumens für das Funktionieren des Kreislaufs. Die Anpassung des Kreislaufs an größere Dauerbelastungen beruht z. T. auf einer Vermehrung des Blutvolumens[4]. Umgekehrt führen beim Menschen Blutentnahmen von 0,5—1 Liter zu einer deutlichen Abnahme der Arbeitsfähigkeit, die auf die schlechtere Regulationsfähigkeit des Kreislaufs zu beziehen ist[5].

3. Durchblutungsverteilung und Blutverteilung.

Die wichtigste Funktion des Kreislaufs ist sicherlich die hinreichende Durchblutung sämtlicher Organe. Da aber aus Gründen der Kreislaufenergetik das HZV klein gehalten werden muß, kommt es auf eine optimale Verteilung der Durchblutung auf sämtliche Organe an. Je nach dem Funktionszustand der Organe wechselt ihr Anteil an der Gesamtdurchblutung. Einer Durchblutungssteigerung in einer Gruppe von Organen wird im allgemeinen eine Einschränkung der Durchblutung in anderen einhergehen (kompensatorische Konstriktion). Die Einstellung der Durchblutungsverteilung erfolgt in erster Linie über die Arteriolen, die sehr weitgehend den Strömungswiderstand für die einzelnen Organe bestimmen.

Jede Änderung der Durchblutung verändert die Blutverteilung im Gefäßsystem, d. h. es treten Veränderungen im Blutgehalt der Organe, aber auch im Blutgehalt der hintereinandergeschalteten Gefäßabschnitte (Arterien, Capillaren Venen) auf. Vasomotorisch weiter gestellte Gefäße fassen mehr, vasomotorisch enger gestellte Gefäße weniger Blut. Ebenso bedeutungsvoll sind aber sekundäre Wirkungen. Veränderte Strömungswiderstände verändern Drucke und Druckgefälle im Blutkreislauf und damit das Blutfassungsvermögen der einzelnen

---

[1] Wang, Einhorn u. a. 1952, Wang und Walcott 1952.
[2] Landis u. a. 1946, Landis und Hortenstine 1950, Rose und Freis 1957.
[3] Wang, Einhorn u. a. 1952, Wang und Walcott 1952.
[4] Sjöstrand 1953.   [5] Balke u. a. 1954.

Gefäßabschnitte. Stärker durchblutete Organe haben zwar nicht in jedem Falle, aber häufig auch einen höheren Blutgehalt (s. S. 672). Das beruht nicht nur auf der aktiven Gefäßerweiterung, sondern besonders auch auf der höheren Blutfülle von Capillaren und Venolen bei Senkung des Strömungswiderstandes in den Arterien und beim Druckanstieg im Bereich der kleineren Gefäße.

Von der gesamten Blutmenge ist unter normalen Bedingungen $^{1}/_{4}$, bei extremer Anspannung des Kreislaufs etwas mehr als die Hälfte verschieblich, d.h. effektiv (s. S. 676). Der übrige Teil des Blutes füllt das Gefäßsystem, ohne daß dabei der Herzfüllungsdruck erreicht wird. Durch folgende Vorgänge wird das effektive Blutvolumen beansprucht:

1. Das arterielle System bedarf zur Aufrechterhaltung des arteriellen Druckes einer bestimmten, zusätzlichen Blutmenge. BROEMSER (1939) schätzte, daß die Auffüllung des Windkessels 2% der Gesamtblutmenge beansprucht. Für das gesamte arterielle System dürfte der Wert wohl höher liegen, aber sicherlich beansprucht das arterielle System das effektive Blutvolumen nur in geringem Maß, auch bei gesteigertem arteriellen Druck.

2. Nach den vorliegenden anatomischen Daten ist das Blutfassungsvermögen der Capillaren recht klein. Es ist noch nicht abzuschätzen, wieweit durch aktive und druckpassive Capillareröffnung oder Capillarerweiterung effektives Blutvolumen beansprucht wird.

3. Durch seine große Kapazität und starke Dehnbarkeit ist das Venensystem das entscheidende Gebiet für alle Blutverschiebungen. Änderungen des peripheren Venendrucks spielen eine wichtige Rolle für die Blutverteilung. Erhöhungen des peripheren Venendrucks können sowohl von der arteriellen als auch von der zentral-venösen Seite her erfolgen. Eine Abnahme des Arteriolen-Widerstandes steigert nicht nur den Capillardruck, sondern auch den in den Venolen. Andererseits führen Steigerungen des zentralen Venendruckes zu Rückstauungen in der Peripherie. Wieweit und an welchen Stellen durch Drosselvenen der venöse Abstrom aus der Peripherie beeinflußt werden kann, und wieweit es dadurch zu Füllungsänderungen im peripheren Venensystem kommt, bedarf noch weiterer Untersuchungen[1].

4. Änderungen des Strömungswiderstandes in der Leber führen zu Erhöhungen des Pfortaderdruckes und damit zu Änderungen der Blutfüllung dieses Gebietes. In früheren Jahren ist die Bedeutung des Splanchnicusgebietes für Blutverschiebungen teilweise überschätzt worden. Man sollte nun aber nicht in den umgekehrten Fehler fallen und diesen Faktor der Blutverteilung völlig vernachlässigen[2]. Besonders scheinen Nachdehnungen der Venen bei länger anhaltenden Drucksteigerungen die Blutfüllung des Pfortadergebietes zu steigern[3].

5. Der kleine Kreislauf ändert seinen Blutgehalt. Sehr weitgehend handelt es sich wohl um passive Änderungen, die durch intrathorakale Druckänderungen und solche des linken Vorhofs in Abhängigkeit von der Herztätigkeit bedingt sind (s. S. 673).

Nicht nur das Gefäßsystem, sondern auch das Herz ist für die Blutverteilung verantwortlich. Die Funktion des linken Herzens bestimmt recht weitgehend die Blutfüllung des kleinen Kreislaufs. Die Funktion des rechten Herzens bestimmt den zentralvenösen Druck und damit die Größe des ineffektiven Blutvolumens. Wird durch nervöse oder hormonale Umstellung der Herztätigkeit der Füllungsdruck vermindert, so steigt damit das effektive Blutvolumen an. Es kommt zu einer veränderten Blutverteilung zwischen der arteriellen Seite und dem „Niederdruckgebiet".

---

[1] FRANKLIN 1937.   [2] ALEXANDER 1955.   [3] ALEXANDER u. a. 1953.

Die für den Organismus und seine Funktionen günstige Blutverteilung erfolgt über nervöse Einflüsse, die sich praktisch auf sämtliche Kreislauforgane, besonders auf das Herz, auf die Arteriolen und auf die Venen auswirken. Die Vorgänge decken sich dabei weitgehend mit denen für die Regulierung des arteriellen Druckes. Das Blut muß so im Kreislauf verteilt sein, daß eine hinreichende effektive Blutmenge vorhanden ist, und damit ist gleichzeitig auch der nötige arterielle Druck eingestellt. Vasomotorische Einflüsse auf das Venensystem sind dabei von besonderer Bedeutung, denn hier sind die Einflüsse auf das Blutfassungsvermögen besonders groß[1]. Aber die anderen Vorgänge sind daneben nicht zu vernachlässigen. Über die Steuerung des Herzens verändert sich die Blutverteilung zwischen arterieller und venöser Seite. Einflüsse auf die Arteriolen verändern zwar in erster Linie die Verteilung der Durchblutung in der Gefäßperipherie. Der veränderte Strömungswiderstand in den Arteriolen beeinflußt aber gleichzeitig auch die Blutfüllung der Capillaren und peripheren kleinen Venen und damit die Blutverteilung in den Organen.

III. Die Regelung des arteriellen Druckes.

Vorbemerkungen. Abb. 22 gibt eine Übersicht über das Verhalten des Druckes in den verschiedenen Kreislaufabschnitten. Der kleine Kreislauf ist gegenüber dem großen durch seinen niedrigen Strömungswiderstand gekennzeichnet. Die Folge davon ist der niedrige Druck in der A. pulmonalis gegenüber dem in der Aorta.

Auf die grundsätzlichen Beziehungen zwischen HZV, Gesamtströmungswiderstand und arterio-venösem Druckgefälle wurde bereits bei der Besprechung der Organdurchblutung eingegangen. Über die Beziehungen zur Herzleistung siehe Abb. 76 (S. 773). Nicht behandelt werden hier die durch die Rhythmik der Herztätigkeit bedingten Blutdruckschwankungen. Sie sind im Zusammenhang mit den physikalischen Bestimmungen des Schlagvolumens häufig und ausführlich diskutiert worden[2].

1. Allgemeines über den Regelkreis.

Noch vor wenigen Jahren verstand man unter Kreislaufregulation alle Einstellungs- und Umstellungsvorgänge im Blutkreislauf. Wenn wir heute unsere Sprache denen der Regeltechniker anpassen, dann ist der Begriff „Kreislaufregulation" anfechtbar. Es handelt sich im Sinne der Regeltechnik durchaus nicht nur um Regelungen, sondern auch um Steuerungen[3]. Es ist zwar fraglich, ob die Sprache der Techniker zur Beschreibung biologischer Vorgänge in jedem Falle geeignet ist. Die Beschreibung biologischer Vorgänge als Abläufe in Regelkreisen ist oft recht unbefriedigend. Bei der vielfachen Verflechtung biologischer Funktionen ist das Herauslösen eines einzelnen Regelkreises in vielen Fällen ein sehr willkürlicher Vorgang. Andererseits scheint es angebracht, bestimmte Begriffe aus der Sprache der Regeltechnik zu übernehmen. So sollte man zwischen Regelung und Steuerung unterscheiden. Unter Regelungen versteht man Vorgänge mit geschlossenem Wirkungsablauf. Die Ausdrücke „Einstellung" oder „Regulation" sollten als übergeordnete Begriffe angewandt werden, wenn noch nicht festgelegt ist, ob es sich um Regelung oder Steuerung handelt[4].

Aufgabe der Regelung ist es, eine Größe konstant zu halten. Deshalb zeichnen sich geregelte Größen durch ihre Konstanz aus. Umgekehrt sind gesteuerte Größen meist recht variabel. Von den Kreislaufgrößen ist der arterielle Blutdruck auffallend konstant. Es ist damit schon wahrscheinlich, daß er eine geregelte Größe ist. Man kann seine Einstellung als ein Schulbeispiel einer

---

[1] Freis und Rose 1957 (Literatur), Gollwitzer-Meier 1932.
[2] Alexander 1953, Kapal u. a. 1950, 1951, Wetterer 1940, 1956, Wetterer und Pieper 1953, Wezler und Böger 1939, Peterson 1952, 1957, Sinn 1956 (Literatur!).
[3] Oppelt 1954.   [4] Wagner 1954, Schoedel 1956.

biologischen Regelung betrachten[1]. Im Gegensatz dazu handelt es sich bei der Einstellung der Organdurchblutung und auch des HZV um Beispiele für Steuerungen. Es besteht in letzterem Falle kein geschlossener Wirkungsablauf. Es ist in erster Linie der Stoffwechsel des Gewebes, der Durchblutung und HZV „steuert".

Die grundsätzlichen Vorgänge für die Regelung des arteriellen Druckes sind seit langem bekannt[2]. Meßstellen des Regelkreises sind die Pressoreceptoren

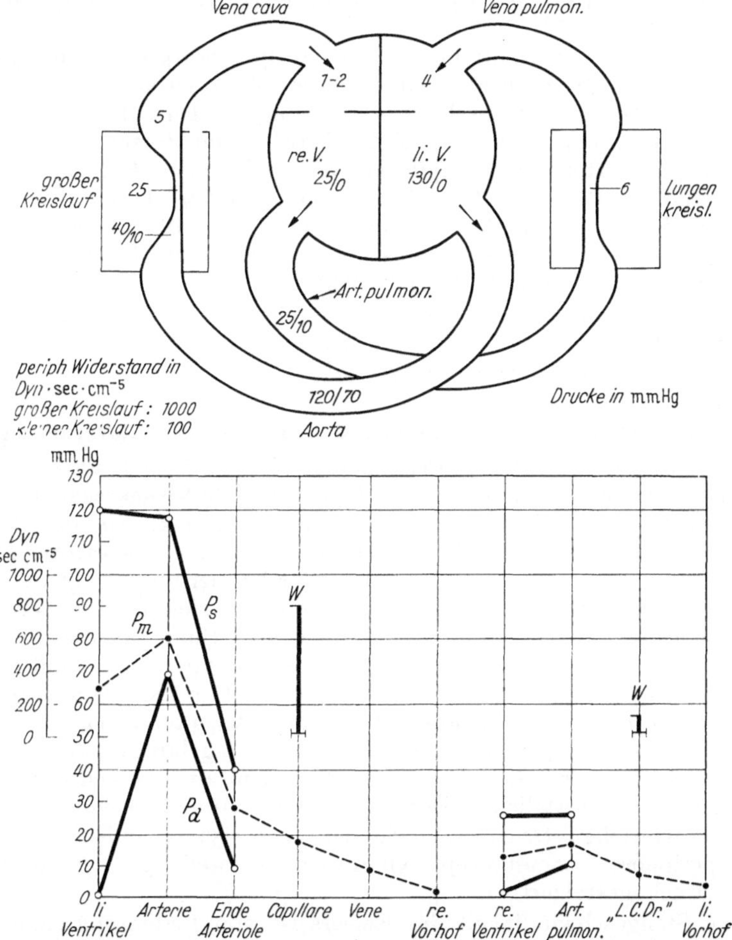

Abb. 22. Schematische Darstellung der Druckverhältnisse im großen und kleinen Kreislauf. P_s systolischer Druck; P_d diastolischer Druck; P_m über die Herzphase gemittelter Druck; W Strömungswiderstand; $L.C.Dr.$ Lungencapillardruck.

am Aortenbogen und am Carotissinus. Sie sind „Eingang" des „Reglers". Dem „Regler" entsprechen bestimmte Bezirke im Zentralnervensystem, besonders Gebiete in der Medulla oblongata. Über die Stellglieder stellt der Regler den Sollwert des arteriellen Druckes ein. Im Unterschied zu den meisten technischen Regelkreisen sind die Stellglieder sehr zahlreich. Fast alle Organe des Blutkreislaufes — Herz und Gefäße — sind Stellglieder für die Regelung des arteriellen Druckes. Sie können den arteriellen Druck beeinflussen, indem sie den Abfluß

[1] WAGNER 1954.   [2] HERING 1927, KOCH 1931, HEYMANS und Mitarbeiter 1933.

aus dem arteriellen System oder den Zufluß zu diesem System verändern. Der erstgenannte Vorgang erfolgt besonders an den Arteriolen, der zweite Vorgang durch Umstellungen im Venensystem und am Herzen. Im allgemeinen werden bei der Regelung vom Regler aus alle Stellglieder gleichzeitig betätigt. Sinkt etwa infolge eines erhöhten Blutbedarfs der Peripherie der arterielle Druck ab, so wird einerseits der periphere Strömungswiderstand durch Konstriktionen im Arteriolengebiet erhöht. Gleichzeitig wird durch venomotorische Vorgänge das Blutangebot an das Herz gesteigert[1] und die Herztätigkeit dem größeren Blutangebot angepaßt.

Damit die Regelung intakt bleibt, müssen die „Störgrößen" kleiner als die „Stellgrößen" sein. So muß etwa ein erhöhter Blutabstrom zur tätigen Skeletmuskulatur (als Störgröße) durch Einschränkung der Durchblutung an anderen Organen und durch einen erhöhten Blutrückstrom zum Herzen und eine erhöhte Blutförderung des Herzens ausgeglichen werden können. Für eine brauchbare Regelung muß der Regler weitere Bedingungen erfüllen. Insbesondere muß die Einstellung mit der nötigen Geschwindigkeit erfolgen. Hierfür sorgen bestimmte Eigenschaften der Pressoreceptoren (s. u.) und der zentralnervösen Schaltung (Regler mit Störgrößenaufschaltung S. 683).

Überschaut man die Eingriffe des ZNS in die Kreislaufeinstellung, so handelt es sich dabei sehr weitgehend um Vorgänge zur Regelung des arteriellen Druckes[2]. Eine Ausnahme ist das Dilatatorensystem[3].

2. Die arteriellen Pressoreceptoren als Meßstellen des Blutdruckreglers.

Von den zahlreichen Receptoren an den Gefäßen[4] sind allein die Pressoreceptoren im arteriellen System Meßstellen der Blutdruckregelung. Nur sie allein messen direkt die Regelgröße, den arteriellen Druck. Von der Gruppe der arteriellen Pressoreceptoren stehen wiederum die am Sinus caroticus und am Aortenbogen ganz im Vordergrund. Nach ihrer Entnervung steigt der arterielle Druck an. Andere arterielle Pressoreceptoren, die sich nach neueren Untersuchungen an der Carotis communis proximal vom Sinus, an der absteigenden Aorta, an den Mesenterialarterien und den Femoralarterien befinden, können also die regelnde Funktion der Pressoreceptoren im Carotissinus und am Aortenbogen nicht übernehmen. Chemoreceptoren und Receptoren im Herzen und an den Venen sind keine eigentlichen Meßstellen des Regelkreises, denn sie messen ja nicht die Regelgröße. Sie können aber trotzdem auf das Zentrum einwirken und die Regelung „verstellen". Der Regler stellt dann einen von der Norm abweichenden arteriellen Druck ein. So wird bei Hypoxyämie im allgemeinen über die peripheren Chemoreceptoren durch „Verstellung" der Regelung der arterielle Druck gesteigert.

Für die Stellgeschwindigkeit des Reglers ist von Bedeutung, daß die Zahl der von den Pressoreceptoren ausgesandten Erregungen nicht nur von der Höhe des arteriellen Druckes, sondern auch von der Geschwindigkeit seiner Veränderung abhängig ist. Ändert man den Druck im Carotissinus sehr plötzlich, so ist die Zahl der ausgesandten Erregungen zunächst sehr hoch, sinkt dann aber auf einen niedrigeren Wert ab, der dauernd gehalten wird (Abb. 23). Jede Änderung des arteriellen Druckes führt damit sehr rasch zu einer relativ starken Reaktion von seiten des Reglers, und dadurch wird die Änderung der Regelgröße rasch aufgefangen. Die Einstellzeit wird kürzer. Die Eigenschaften der Presso-

---

[1] Gollwitzer-Meier 1932, Landis und Hortenstine 1950, Rashkind u. a. 1953, Freis und Rose 1957.
[2] Folkow 1955.   [3] Uvnäs 1954.   [4] Aviado und Schmidt 1955.

receptoren führen zu einer PD-Regelung (Proportional-Differentialregler). Sie läuft nicht nur proportional (P) der Abweichung der Regelgröße von ihrem Soll-

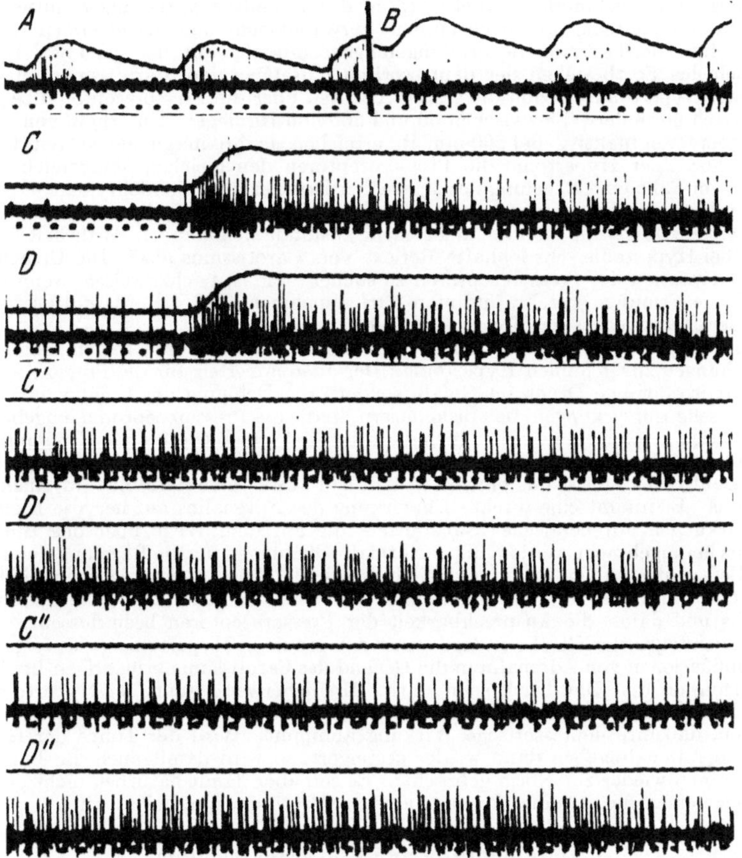

Abb. 23. Aktionsströme der Pressoreceptoren im Carotissinus in Abhängigkeit von der Höhe des Druckes im Carotissinus und der Änderung des Druckes (LANDGREEN u. a. 1953). Die Aktionsströme wurden von einigen wenigen Nervenfasern aufgenommen. Oberste Kurve: Druckablauf, mittlere Kurve: Aktionsströme, untere Kurve: Zeitmarkierung 0,04 sec. *A* Aufnahme bei spontaner Durchblutung, künstlicher Beatmung mit 100% O_2 und einem mittleren arteriellen Druck von 140 mm Hg; *B* Natürliche Durchblutung bei künstlicher Beatmung mit 5,6% Sauerstoff in Stickstoff und einem mittleren arteriellen Druck von 150 mm Hg. Vergleich von *B* mit *A* zeigt, daß es sich um Aktionsströme von Pressoreceptoren und nicht von Chemoreceptoren handelt; *C* Versuche am Sinuspräparat, Steigerung des Druckes im Sinus von 0 auf 120 mm Hg. Im Augenblick des Druckanstiegs ist die Impulsfrequenz besonders hoch und stellt sich später auf eine gleichmäßige Frequenz ein; *C'*, *C''* Fortsetzung von *C*. *D* Aktivierung der Pressoreceptoren durch Acetylcholin; *D'*, *D''* Fortsetzung von *D*. (LANDGREEN, SKOUBY und ZOTTERMAN 1953.)

Wert, sondern ist auch von dem Differentialquotienten der Regelgröße nach der Zeit (D) abhängig[1].

3. Arterielle Pressoreceptoren und Hypertonie.

Es lag zunächst nahe anzunehmen, daß bei der Entstehung der essentiellen Hypertension eine Dysfunktion der arteriellen Pressoreceptoren zum mindesten mitbeteiligt wäre[2]. Der depressorische Einfluß dieser Receptoren könnte vermindert oder aufgehoben sein. Die im Tierexperiment nach Durchtrennung der Aorten- und Sinusnerven auftretende Hypertonie bleibt im allgemeinen nicht lange bestehen[3]. Die Ursache kann in einer unvollkommenen

---

[1] WAGNER 1954. [2] VOLHARD 1942. [3] HEYMANS und BOUCKAERT 1936.

Entnervung der Receptoren oder in einer Regeneration durchschnittener Nervenfasern liegen, oder es könnten die Pressoreceptoren an anderen Abschnitten des arteriellen Systems nach einiger Zeit die Funktion der entnervten Receptoren übernehmen. Das kurzzeitige Fortbestehen des „Entzügelungshochdrucks" (d. h. des Hochdrucks, der nach Entnervung der Pressoreceptoren entsteht) spricht gegen eine Verwandtschaft mit der genuinen Hypertonie.

Gegen eine Gleichsetzung des Entzügelungshochdrucks mit der genuinen Hypertonie spricht auch das Fortbestehen der depressorischen Reflexe vom Carotissinus aus während der genuinen Hypertonie. Schon die ersten Arbeiten über die Pressoreceptoren zeigten, daß ihr Meßbereich normalerweise zwischen 60 und 200 mm Hg liegt[1]. Unterhalb von 60 mm Hg sind die Receptoren inaktiv. Bei 200 mm Hg erreichen sie ihre maximale Aktivität. Würden beim Bestehen einer Hypertonie die Pressoreceptoren den gleichen Meßbereich haben, so wäre in diesem Falle eine Regelung des arteriellen Druckes über sie nicht mehr möglich. Die Pressoreceptoren würden dauernd mit maximaler Frequenz Impulse aussenden, und eine weitere Frequenzsteigerung könnte nicht mehr zustande kommen. In Wahrheit findet man aber auch bei Hypertonie sehr lebhafte Reflexe vom Carotissinus aus[2]. Die Ursache hierfür ist in der Adaptation der Pressoreceptoren zu suchen. Sie ist nachzuweisen, wenn ein Hochdruck mehrere Stunden besteht, und man darf annehmen, daß die Adaptation vollständig ist, wenn der Hochdruck über Monate und Jahre anhält[3].

Untersuchungen über den adäquaten Reiz der Pressoreceptoren zeigen möglicherweise neue Beziehungen zur genuinen Hypertonie. Der adäquate Reiz für die Pressoreceptoren ist nicht der hydrostatische Druck im Gefäß, sondern die Dehnung der Gefäßwand[4]. Werden durch chemische Einwirkungen die Muskelfasern, in die die Pressoreceptoren eingebettet sind, zur Kontraktion gebracht, so werden auch dadurch die Pressoreceptoren in Erregung versetzt. So kommt es zur Senkung des arteriellen Druckes, wenn man Adrenalin oder Noradrenalin von außen auf den Carotissinus einwirken läßt[5]. Palme[6] glaubt freilich an einen anderen Mechanismus. Er nimmt eine direkte Einwirkung des Adrenalins auf nervöse Elemente an. Daß Einwirkungen adrenergischer Substanzen, die auf dem Wege über das Blut an den Carotissinus herangebracht werden, unter Normalbedingungen für die Regelung des arteriellen Druckes Bedeutung haben, kann bezweifelt werden[7]. Aber es ist nicht unmöglich, daß sympathische Einflüsse über das Ganglion cervicale caudale die Wandspannung des Carotissinus und damit die Ansprechbarkeit der Pressoreceptoren beeinflussen[8].

Auf Beziehungen der Gefäßwandspannung zur genuinen Hypertonie weist folgendes hin: Lokale Applikationen von Adrenalin in die Gegend des Carotissinus erniedrigen bei Patienten mit Hypertension den Blutdruck sehr stark. Möglicherweise kann bei Hypertonie in bestimmten Fällen die Erschlaffung der Gefäßwand, in die die Pressoreceptoren eingebaut sind, dazu führen, daß ihre depressorische Wirkung abnimmt. Wird der Tonus der Gefäßwand durch lokale Adrenalingaben dann wieder gesteigert, so wird damit auch die Funktion der Pressoreceptoren wieder zur Norm gebracht[9]. Es soll aber damit natürlich nicht gesagt sein, daß im allgemeinen die genuine Hypertonie vom Carotissinus ausgelöst wird.

4. Durchblutung und Blutdruckregelung.

Die Einstellung des Kreislaufs wird von 2 Vorgängen beherrscht, von der Einstellung der peripheren Durchblutung und von der Regelung des arteriellen Druckes. Die hinreichende Blutversorgung aller Organe ist die Hauptfunktion des Kreislaufs. Der Blutbedarf der Organe ist je nach dem Funktionszustand verschieden. Insbesondere schwankt er mit dem Organstoffwechsel. Die Einstellung der Organdurchblutung auf den Blutbedarf erfolgt über Änderungen des peripheren Strömungswiderstandes. Voraussetzung für die Wirksamkeit dieser Steuerung ist aber ein konstanter, arterieller Druck. Bestände keine Regelung des arteriellen Druckes, so würde die verstärkte Durchblutung der Peripherie zum Absinken des Druckes führen, und damit würde die durchblutungssteigernde Wirkung der peripheren Gefäßerweiterung wieder weitgehend aufgehoben werden.

Sinkt infolge erhöhten Blutbedarfs der Peripherie der periphere Strömungswiderstand ab und droht damit ein Abfall des arteriellen Druckes, so kann die Druckregelung in 2 Richtungen einsetzen. Einmal kann der periphere Strömungs-

---

[1] Hering 1927, Heymans und Mitarbeiter 1933, Koch 1931.
[2] Draper 1950.   [3] Kubicek u. a. 1953.   [4] Hauss u. a. 1949.
[5] Heymans und Mitarbeiter 1950.   [6] Palme 1936, 1944, 1955.
[7] Aviado und Schmidt 1955.   [8] Kezdi 1954.   [9] Kezdi und Hilker 1955.

widerstand in nicht beanspruchten Gefäßgebieten gesteigert werden (kollaterale Vasoconstriction). Diese Regelung wird ausreichen, wenn der Blutbedarf nur in einem sehr kleinen Gefäßgebiet erhöht ist. Zum anderen kann das HZV gesteigert werden, indem das venöse Angebot an das Herz erhöht und das Herz auf die größere Blutförderung eingestellt wird. Diese Regelung wird besonders dann von entscheidender Bedeutung sein, wenn der Blutbedarf sehr vieler Organe gleichzeitig gesteigert ist.

Die Koppelung zwischen der Kreislaufperipherie und dem Kreislaufzentrum ist nach unseren heutigen Vorstellungen eine zum mindesten dreifache.

1. Die „hydrostatische Koppelung" entspricht dem eigentlichen Regelmechanismus für den arteriellen Druck: Ändert sich der arterielle Druck infolge von Widerstandsänderungen in der Peripherie, so werden die peripheren Pressoreceptoren in den Arterien erregt und lösen die Regelung aus.

2. Stoffwechselvorgänge in der Peripherie: Eine erhöhte Kohlensäurebildung im Gewebe steigert den Kohlensäuredruck im Blut, wodurch es zu einer Tonisierung des Kreislaufzentrums kommt. Möglicherweise können auch andere Produkte eines gesteigerten Stoffwechsels den Kreislauf über die Zentrale beeinflussen.

3. Einflüsse von höheren Zentren: Nervöse Vorgänge in der Rinde und im Zwischenhirn stellen vorsorglich das Kreislaufzentrum auf eine zu erwartende Belastung um. Regeltechnisch entspricht dies einer „Regelung mit Störgrößenaufschaltung" (s. S. 680). Gleichzeitig wird über das Dilatatorensystem vorsorglich die periphere Durchblutung in der tätigen Muskulatur erhöht.

Eine vierte Verknüpfung von Peripherie und Kreislaufzentrum ergibt sich wahrscheinlich dadurch, daß bei peripheren Umstellungen Receptoren erregt werden, wobei es dann über afferente Bahnen zu einer Umstellung im Kreislaufzentrum kommt. Zur Sicherstellung des letztgenannten Weges sind aber noch weitere Untersuchungen notwendig.

Nach teleologischen Überlegungen möchte man annehmen, daß die Sicherung des peripheren Blutbedarfs den Vorrang hat vor der Regelung des arteriellen Druckes. Dem scheint aber nicht in allen Fällen so zu sein.

Gibt man Hunden im hämorrhagischen oder traumatischen Schock Dibenamin, so wird der Zustand von den Hunden häufig besser vertragen, obwohl der arterielle Druck dabei weiter absinkt. Es muß also vorher ein Zustand vorhanden gewesen sein, bei dem auf Kosten der Organdurchblutung und zum Nachteil des gesamten Tieres die Regelung des arteriellen Druckes zu stark im Vordergrund stand[1].

Das HZV entspricht der Summe der Organdurchblutungen. Demnach gilt für die Beziehungen zwischen der Einstellung des HZV und der Regelung des arteriellen Druckes das, was oben über die Beziehungen zwischen Organdurchblutung und Blutdruckregelung gesagt wurde. Bei niedrigem, peripherem Gesamtwiderstand und hohem HZV ist entscheidend, daß durch die Mechanismen für die Blutdruckregelung eine ausreichende effektive Blutmenge geschaffen wird (s. S. 674).

IV. Zustände mit verändertem Strömungswiderstand im großen Kreislauf.

Zustände mit verändertem Strömungswiderstand im großen Kreislauf können unter krankhaften Bedingungen aus verschiedenen Gründen auftreten. Einmal beziehen sich diese Veränderungen auf den Gesamtströmungswiderstand, zum anderen auf den Strömungswiderstand einzelner Organe (s. S. 689). Die Frage nach den Veränderungen des Gesamtströmungswiderstandes tritt vor allem bei den *arterio-venösen Fisteln*, bei der *Hypertonie* und der *Hypotonie* auf. Weiterhin

---

[1] REMINGTON u. a. 1950.

ist dieses Problem beim *Schock* und *Kollaps* von großem Interesse. Da beim Schock und Kollaps mit den Veränderungen des Strömungswiderstandes häufig Verminderungen der zirkulierenden Blutmenge und Blutverteilungsstörungen vergesellschaftet sind, sollen diese Störungen gesondert besprochen werden.

1. Arterio-venöse Fisteln im großen Kreislauf.

Typische Beispiele für eine dauernde Erniedrigung des Strömungswiderstandes im großen Kreislauf bilden die arterio-venösen Fisteln, die meist Folge einer Verwundung sind. Seltener treten sie als mykotische Fisteln nach septischen Embolien auf, noch seltener als angeborene Anomalien. Bei den arterio-venösen Fisteln im großen Kreislauf wird infolge der Verkürzung der mittleren Kreislaufzeit dem rechten Herzen dauernd die in der Zeiteinheit durch den Kurzschluß fließende Blutmenge zusätzlich zu seinem annähernd normalen venösen Zufluß angeboten. Da die dem rechten Herzen vermehrt angebotene Blutmenge den

Tabelle 12. *Arterio-venöse Fisteln des großen Kreislaufs.*
(Grosse-Brockhoff, Neuhaus, Schaede 1954.)

Diagnose	Arterieller Druck (RR) mm Hg	Herzindex l/min/m²	Peripherer Strömungs-widerstand mm Hg/l/min und m²
1. Kleine Fistel der A. poplitea	140/80	3,7	28,1
2. Große Fistel zwischen Arcus aortae und V. anonyma	150/60	5,6	18,8
3. Große Fistel zwischen A. renalis und V. cava	180/100	9,7	14,4
4. Große Fistel der A. femoralis	155/85	7,5	16,0
5. Mykotische Fistel der A. femoralis bei schwerer Aorten- und Mitralinsuffizienz nach Endocarditis lenta (dekompensiert)	160/80	2,4	46,5

Lungenkreislauf passiert und zum linken Herzen gelangt, werden beide Herzkammern in gleichem Ausmaß betroffen. Solange das Herz suffizient bleibt, wird von ihm das normale Kreislaufminutenvolumen und das durch den Kurzschluß fließende Zeitvolumen gefördert. Die Erhöhungen des Kreislaufminutenvolumens sind bei großen Fisteln ganz beträchtlich und können bis zum Dreifachen der Norm betragen[1]. Der periphere Widerstand kann bis auf die Hälfte der Norm absinken[2] (s. Tabelle 12). Bei großen Fisteln ist die Blutmenge im allgemeinen erhöht, jedoch ist dies kein regelmäßiger Befund[3]. Obwohl der periphere Strömungswiderstand im großen Kreislauf beträchtlich erniedrigt ist, entwickelt sich infolge der erhöhten Volumenbelastung mit der Zeit nicht nur eine zunehmende exzentrische Dilatation der rechten, sondern auch der linken Herzkammer mit entsprechender Muskelhypertrophie, die schließlich von der

---

[1] Cohen und Mitarbeiter 1948, Friedlich und Mitarbeiter 1950, Grosse-Brockhoff und Mitarbeiter 1954.

[2] Cohen und Mitarbeiter 1948, Friedlich und Mitarbeiter 1950, Grosse-Brockhoff und Mitarbeiter 1954, Gauer und Linder 1948.

[3] Elkin und Mitarbeiter 1947, Sjöstrand 1953.

myogenen Dilatation gefolgt ist. Die arterio-venösen Fisteln sind ein Schulbeispiel dafür, daß der Herzmuskel durch dauernde Volumbelastung ohne andere schädigende Einflüsse mit der Zeit insuffizient wird. Die Dilatation des Herzens entspricht dem Grade der durch den Kurzschluß entstandenen Mehrbelastung. Ebenso ist der Zeitpunkt des Auftretens der Insuffizienzsymptome des Herzens abhängig von der Größe der Fistel, wobei zu berücksichtigen ist, daß mit zunehmendem Alter der Patienten die Insuffizienz früher manifest wird. Bei größeren Fisteln treten die ersten Insuffizienzsymptome beim Erwachsenen etwa 4—5 Jahre nach der Verwundung auf. Sind die ersten Symptome vorhanden, so schreitet die Insuffizienz meist rapide vorwärts. Auf der anderen Seite schwindet die Insuffizienz nach Beseitigung der Fistel innerhalb von Tagen, ja, von Stunden. Auch wird die Herzfigur bereits unmittelbar nach der Beseitigung der Fistel sichtbar kleiner und normalisiert sich innerhalb von einigen Tagen.

Bei plötzlicher Unterbrechung des Kurzschlusses durch Kompression der Arterie oberhalb der Fistel beobachtet man ein Absinken der Herzfrequenz bei gleichzeitiger Verringerung der Blutdruckamplitude (besonders Anstieg des diastolischen Druckes)[1]. Schlagvolumen und Kreislaufminutenvolumen sinken nach Kompression prompt ab. Atropin verhindert das Absinken der Pulsfrequenz nach Kompression, während die Reduktion des Schlag- und Minutenvolumens durch Atropin nicht beeinflußt wird.

2. Hypertonie.

Hypertonie bedeutet zunächst der Wortprägung gemäß lediglich Blutdrucksteigerung. Erhöhungen des Blutdrucks über den Normbereich treten im Gefolge einer Reihe von Erkrankungen auf. In der tabellarischen Übersicht (Tabelle 13)

Tabelle 13. *Faktoren, die zur pathologischen Steigerung des Blutdrucks führen können.*

1. Essentielle Hypertonie	Nebennierenrindencarcinom
2. Renaler Hochdruck:	Thymus-Carcinom mit Cushing-Syndrom
Glomerulonephritis	Placentarstoffe (Eklampsie)
Obstruktion der Nierengefäße	4. Kardiovasculärer Hochdruck:
Pyelonephritis	Aortenisthmusstenose
Harnabflußstörungen	Arterio-venöse Fistel
Cystenniere	Arteriosklerose (?)
Periarteriitis nodosa	5. Neurogener Hochdruck:
PerirenaleNierenparenchymkompression	Chronische Porphyrie
3. Endokriner Hochdruck:	Hirnstammpoliomyelitis
Basophiles Adenom der Hypophyse	Gesteigerter Hirndruck
Nebennierenmarktumor	Sklerose des Sinus caroticus
Nebennierenrindenhyperplasie	Tabes dorsalis
Nebennierenrindenadenom (sog. Conen-Syndrom, Hyperaldosteronismus)	Psychische Erregung

sind die wesentlichen Faktoren aufgeführt, die zu einer Entgleisung der im Normalbereich so gut geregelten Blutdruckgröße führen können. Der Begriff *Hypertonie* wird im klinischen Sprachgebrauch enger gefaßt. Der Kliniker spricht von einer Hypertonie, wenn eine permanente Erhöhung des Mitteldruckes vorliegt. Im wesentlichen handelt es sich um die Formen von Hypertonie, die als „*essentielle*" oder als „*renale*" Hypertonie auftreten. Kurzfristige Steigerungen des Blutdrucks z. B. nach psychischen Emotionen haben noch nichts mit dem

---

[1] WIDGOROWITSCH 1915.

zu tun, was der Kliniker als Hypertonie bezeichnet. Auch Steigerungen des Blutdrucks, wie sie z. B. nach Carotissinus-Blockade auftreten[1], sollten nicht mit Hypertonie im klinischen Sinne verwechselt werden. Wohl gibt es Entzügelungsreaktionen, aber keine Entzügelungshypertonie im klinischen Sinne. (Über die Beziehungen der arteriellen Pressoreceptoren zur Hypertonie s. S. 681.) Erhöhungen des systolischen Druckes allein, wie sie z. B. bei der Sklerose der

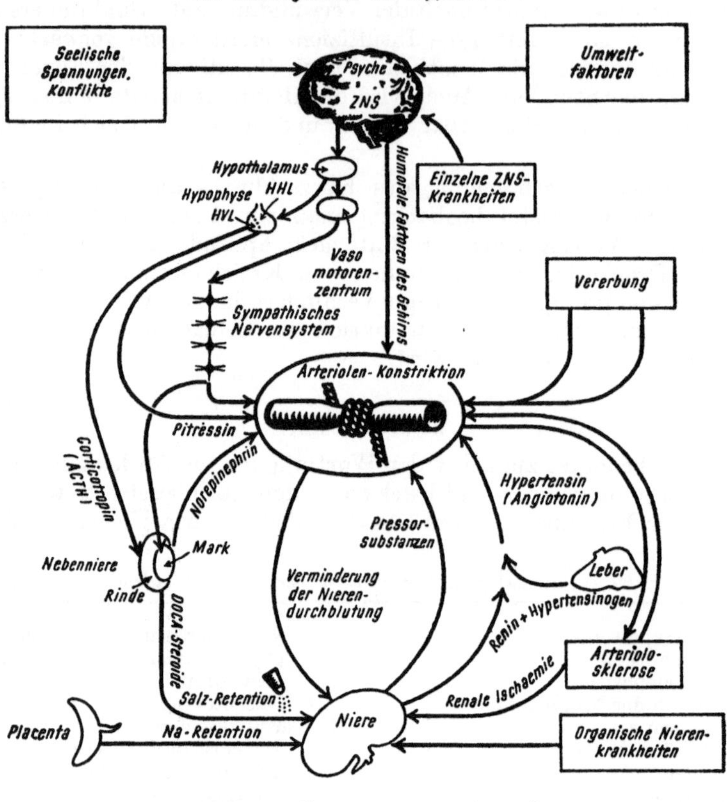

Abb. 24. Zur Pathogenese der Hypertension. (Staub 1954.)

großen Gefäße (Arteriosklerose), bei arterio-venösen Fisteln, bei Aortenklappeninsuffizienz oder Schilddrüsenüberfunktion vorkommen, dürfen nicht in den Krankheitsbegriff Hypertonie eingeordnet werden.

Die nach wie vor unklare *Pathogenese* des Hochdruckes kann nur kurz gestreift werden. Die enge Verflechtung der pathogenen Faktoren (erbliche Belastung, blutdrucksteigernde Substanzen, hormonale Faktoren, äußere Einflüsse) werden durch die Abb. 24 veranschaulicht. Nach den ersten Befunden von Hartwich[2] und später vor allem von Goldblatt[3] konnte durch zahlreiche weitere Experimente bestätigt werden, daß bestimmte Eingriffe an der Niere, die eine Abnahme der Durchblutung zur Folge haben, einen Hochdruck hervorrufen können.

[1] Lampen 1949.   [2] Hartwich 1932.   [3] Goldblatt und Mitarbeiter 1934.

Folgende Maßnahmen sind zur experimentellen Erzeugung einer Hypertonie geeignet:

Drosselung der Nierenarterien, Injektion von Kaolin in die Nierenarterie, Einkapselung der Niere mit verschiedenen Methoden (Cellophanniere, Seidenfadenperinephritis), Unterbindung der Nierenvene, Einengungen im Bereich der Nierenbecken und der ableitenden Harnwege, Sklerose der Niere durch Röntgen-Bestrahlung, durch chemische Einwirkungen, durch Drosselung der Aorta oberhalb der Nieren (unterhalb des Abgangs der Leberarterie) und durch die sog. „endocrine kidney" nach SELYE. Bei all diesen Manipulationen tritt eine Störung der Nierendurchblutung mit Hypoxie und Ausscheidungsstörung der Niere ein. Die Blutdrucksteigerung tritt nach mehr oder weniger langem Intervall auf, sie ist im allgemeinen durch eine Steigerung des peripheren Widerstandes gekennzeichnet. Über das Zustandekommen dieser renalen Hypertonie liegen eine Unmenge von Untersuchungen vor, die auf den Nachweis von Stoffen hinauslaufen, die für die Blutdrucksteigerung verantwortlich sein sollen. Es ist unmöglich, auf die Einzelheiten dieser Stoffe einzugehen, zumal die experimentellen Ergebnisse sehr widersprechend sind. Die größte Bedeutung kommt dem *Renin-Hypertensin-*Mechanismus zu. Die bestechendste und auch in vieler Hinsicht untermauerte Interpretation der experimentellen Befunde scheint die folgende: In der gedrosselten Niere entsteht vermehrt Renin. Renin wandelt encymatisch das im Blut vorhandene Hypertensinogen in Hypertensin I um. Hypertensin I wird durch ein Enzym im Plasma in Hyperntensin II umgewandelt. Hypertensin II besitzt eine ausgeprägte blutdrucksteigernde Wirkung. Normalerweise wird entstandenes Hypertensin durch die Hypertensinase in der Niere abgebaut.

In Analogie zu den Ergebnissen der tierexperimentellen Hochdruckforschung darf man heute auch für die menschliche Pathologie annehmen, daß der Renin-Hypertensin-Mechanismus bei der Auslösung des renal bedingten Hypertonus eine Rolle spielt. Seit Aufdeckung der chemischen Konstitution von Hypertensin I und II[1] ist es unter Einsatz geeigneter Methoden gelungen, im Blut von Tieren mit experimentell erzeugter Hypertonie Renin und Hypertensin in größeren Mengen nachzuweisen als bei Tieren mit normalem Blutdruck[2].

Nicht ausreichend geklärt ist die Frage, ob dieser Mechanismus auch für die Entstehung einer chronischen Hypertonie von Bedeutung ist. Experimentelle Befunde weisen darauf hin, daß Renin-Hypertensin nach einem anfänglichen deutlichen Anstieg beim Drosselungshochdruck bei länger bestehender Hypertonie wieder auf normale Werte zurückgeht[3]. Die Rolle, die bei diesem Paralysierungseffekt dem inzwischen entdeckten „Antirenin"[4] zufällt, ist z. Zt. noch nicht genauer zu umreißen. Neueren Berichten von SKEGGS und KAHN[5] zufolge bestehen auch für eine Wirkung von Hypertensin bei chronischer Hypertonie wichtige Hinweise: Während sich bei Normotonikern durchschnittlich 0,015 E Hypertensin (von 0—0,05 E) pro Liter Blut fanden, wurde bei Patienten mit benigner essentieller Hypertonie ein durchschnittlicher Wert von 0,03 E (d. h. etwa das Doppelte der Kontrollgruppe) festgestellt; bei Patienten mit maligner Hypertension dagegen ein durchschnittlicher Wert von 0,244 E (d. h. fast das 20fache des Wertes der Kontrollgruppe). In wieweit diese Untersuchungsbefunde sich tatsächlich bestätigen werden, muß bei bisher noch fehlenden Nachkontrollen dahingestellt bleiben.

α) *Kreislaufdynamische Veränderungen bei Hypertonie.* Nach kreislaufdynamischen Gesichtspunkten hat man 4 verschiedene Hochdrucktypen unter-

---

[1] SKEGGS und Mitarbeiter 1957.   [2] GROSS 1958.   [3] TAQUINI und Mitarbeiter 1958.
[4] HELMER 1958, WAKERLIN 1958.   [5] SKEGGS und KAHN 1958.

schieden[1]: 1. den Elastizitätshochdruck, 2. den Widerstandshochdruck, 3. den Schlag- oder Minutenvolumenhochdruck, 4. den Kombinationshochdruck.

Die unterschiedliche kreislaufdynamische Charakterisierung der verschiedenen Hochdrucktypen, die als Modellvorstellung durchaus ihre Berechtigung hat, hat auch in der Klinik breitere Anwendung gefunden. Dabei wurden die physikalischen Methoden der Schlag- und Minutenvolumenbestimmung zugrunde gelegt, deren Ergebnisse aber in quantitativer Hinsicht unbefriedigend sind.

Nach den mittels Herzkatheterisierung unter Anwendung des Fickschen Prinzips erhobenen Befunden über die Größe des Kreislaufminutenvolumens muß diese Einteilung des Hochdrucks als recht problematisch angesehen werden. Das Kreislaufminutenvolumen liegt in der überwiegenden Zahl der mittels Herzkatheterisierung untersuchten Fälle im Bereich der normalen Schwankungsbreite[2]. Beim Eintreten von Insuffizienzerscheinungen des Herzens sinkt das Kreislaufminutenvolumen unter die Norm ab.

Der periphere Widerstand ist in der Regel bei der Hypertonie deutlich erhöht[2]. Die Steigerung des peripheren Widerstandes beträgt bis zum Dreifachen der Norm (normaler peripherer Strömungswiderstand etwa 800—1000 dyn sec cm^{-5}). Daß es sich beim Hochdruck in der Regel um einen Widerstandshochdruck handelt, ergibt sich auch daraus, daß nach Sympathektomie das Kreislaufminutenvolumen gleichbleibt, auch wenn der arterielle Mitteldruck erheblich absinkt[3]. Da die Viscosität bei der Hypertonie normal gefunden wurde, muß gefolgert werden, daß die Erhöhung des Strömungswiderstandes durch Engerstellung der arteriellen Strombahn, besonders der Arteriolen, bedingt ist. Da weiterhin in den früheren Stadien der Hypertonie häufig keine anatomischen Veränderungen an den Gefäßen nachweisbar sind, und da durch pharmakologische Maßnahmen (Sedativa, Sympathicolytica, Sympathicusdurchschneidung) der Mitteldruck gesenkt wird, ist anzunehmen, daß diese Engerstellung der Arteriolen zunächst funktioneller Natur ist.

Im Gefolge einer Hypertonie kommt es auch zu Veränderungen der elastischen Eigenschaften des Gefäßsystems. Als Maß für den elastischen Widerstand oder besser gesagt für den Volum-Elastizitäts-Koeffizienten kann die Beziehung Blutdruckamplitude:Schlagvolumen angesehen werden. Eine hohe Blutdruckamplitude, wie sie sich vor allem in den frühen Stadien der essentiellen Hypertonie findet, weist auf eine Erhöhung des Volum-Elastizitäts-Koeffizienten hin. Mit steigendem Volum-Elastizitäts-Koeffizienten steigt die Pulswellengeschwindigkeit an[1].

Zusammenfassend läßt sich sagen, daß bei der Hypertonie die Erhöhung des Strömungswiderstandes ganz im Vordergrund steht, daß aber darüber die Veränderungen der elastischen Eigenschaften der Gefäße nicht übersehen werden dürfen. Das Problem wird dadurch noch kompliziert, daß wir nicht sicher wissen, inwieweit Veränderungen der elastischen Eigenschaften der Gefäße primär vorhanden sein können und inwieweit sie sekundär, d. h. Folge der Druckerhöhung sind. Daß die elastischen Eigenschaften der Gefäße schon im Beginn der Erkrankung verändert sind, erscheint auf Grund der vorliegenden pathologisch-anatomischen Befunde nicht wahrscheinlich. Dagegen ist es sicher, daß ein Hochdruck mit der Zeit zur Mediaverdickung, Hyalinose und Sklerose der Gefäße führt. Im großen und ganzen scheinen graduelle Ausprägung der Hypertonie

---

[1] Wezler und Böger 1939.
[2] Goldring und Chasis 1944, Bolomey und Mitarbeiter 1949, Werkö und Lagerlöf 1949, Varnauskas 1955.
[3] Berglund 1949.

und Schwere der Gefäßveränderungen parallel zu verlaufen. Allerdings gibt es immer wieder Krankheitsfälle, bei denen die Druckerhöhung verhältnismäßig gering, die Gefäßveränderungen dagegen schwerwiegend sind. Bei den anatomischen Veränderungen ist nicht nur die absolute Höhe des Druckes, sondern auch der konstitutionelle Faktor der Gefäßbeschaffenheit mit entscheidend. Letzten Endes kann sich die Arteriosklerose auch unabhängig von einer Blutdruckerhöhung entwickeln. Es wird immer wieder die Frage diskutiert, ob die „Arteriolonekrose“, die wir im klinischen Bild als sog. „maligne Sklerose“ vor uns haben, ein Prozeß sui generis oder einfache Folge der Hypertonie ist. Wenn auch dem „Gefäßfaktor“ bei der Entwicklung der Gefäßveränderungen eine große Rolle zuzuschreiben ist, so spricht doch vieles dafür, daß die Arteriolonekrose letzten Endes eine *Intensitätsvariante* der im Gefolge einer Hypertonie auftretenden anatomischen Gefäßveränderungen ist[1].

β) Nieren- und Gehirnkreislauf bei Hypertonie. Von besonderem Interesse ist das Verhalten der *Nieren-* und der *Hirndurchblutung* beim Hochdruck.

Daß bei „nephrogener“ Hypertonie die Nierendurchblutung vermindert ist, liegt auf der Hand und bedarf keiner besonderen Erörterung. Von größerem Interesse ist die Frage des Verhaltens der Nierendurchblutung bei essentieller Hypertonie. Die Untersuchungen der Nierendurchblutung (Bestimmung des sog. Nierenplasmastroms mit Paraaminohippursäure) und die Bestimmung der Größe des Glomerulumfiltrates (Inulin- oder Kreatinin-Clearance) haben zu folgenden Ergebnissen geführt[2]: Schon in den Frühstadien der essentiellen Hypertonie ist eine Einschränkung der Nierendurchblutung nachweisbar[3]. Die Erniedrigung der Durchblutung ist stärker als die meist erst später festzustellende Abnahme des Glomerulumfiltrates[4]. Bei Eintreten einer Herzmuskelinsuffizienz sinken Durchblutung und Glomerulumfiltrat in stärkerem Grade ab. Die Erniedrigung der Nierendurchblutung bei fehlender Herzinsuffizienz muß auf eine Drosselung der Nierengefäße zurückgeführt werden. Das Kreislaufminutenvolumen ist in diesem Stadium der Hypertonie normal (s. oben). Wahrscheinlich findet die Drosselung in erster Linie im Bereich der Vasa afferentia statt. Allerdings sind die Berechnungen, die zu dieser Schlußfolgerung führen, mit gewissen Unsicherheitsfaktoren behaftet, da einige der hierbei benutzten Größen nicht gemessen werden können. Man darf aber bei der Übereinstimmung der so erhobenen Befunde mit den tierexperimentellen Ergebnissen[5] annehmen, daß diese Aussagen über die Veränderungen der Widerstandsverhältnisse im Nierenkreislauf im großen und ganzen das Richtige treffen.

Es sieht so aus, als ob die Erhaltung einer gewissen Druckkonstanz über der Filtrationsfläche des Glomerulum eine wesentliche Aufgabe des Vas afferens wäre. Es wird vermutet, daß in bestimmten Gefäßabschnitten des Nierenkreislaufs Druckreceptoren vorhanden sind, welche nervös und humoral Weitenänderungen des Vas afferens bewirken. Manches spricht dafür, daß diese Druckreceptoren in den Glomerula gelegen sind (s. Einstellung der Organdurchblutung S. 647). Nach Sympathektomie bleibt die Nierendurchblutung gleich, obwohl der arterielle Mitteldruck abfällt[6]. Es ist anzunehmen, daß auch hierbei druckgesteuerte Änderungen der Widerstandsverhältnisse im Nierenkreislauf im Spiel sind. Das gleiche gilt für die Anwendung blutdrucksenkender Substanzen, wie z. B. der Hydrazin-Phthalacine. Welche Grenzen einer solchen intrarenalen Widerstandsänderung des Nierenkreislaufs bei Steigerung des arteriellen Druckes

---

[1] BÜCHNER 1956, PICKERING 1955.　　[2] Literatur s. SMITH 1951.
[3] GOLDRING und CHASIS 1944.　　[4] VARNAUSKAS 1955.
[5] SELKURT 1955.　　[6] BERGLUND 1949.

gesetzt sind, ist noch nicht klar abzusehen. Nach tierexperimentellen Untersuchungen ist anzunehmen, daß oberhalb 200 mm Hg Durchströmungsdruck (Mitteldruck) die Durchblutung der Niere dem Druck passiv folgt[1]. Oberhalb dieser Grenze reicht also die Eigenregulation nicht mehr aus. Schließlich ist in der menschlichen Pathologie noch zu berücksichtigen, daß sich im Laufe der Zeit Querschnittsänderungen in den Nierenarteriolen ausbilden, die durch die morphologischen Veränderungen der Gefäßwand bedingt sind. Ob durch eine Drosselung der Durchblutung unter die Norm Renin freigesetzt wird, das dann sekundär zu einer weiteren Blutdrucksteigerung führt, ist bisher nicht gesichert. Auch werden die Verhältnisse in diesen Stadien durch das Hinzutreten einer Herzmuskelinsuffizienz sehr unübersichtlich.

Läßt sich in den Frühstadien der Hypertonie eine Durchblutungsminderung der Nieren feststellen, so ist dies *im Gehirn* nicht der Fall. Bei der Hypertonie hält sich die Gehirndurchblutung im Bereich der Norm, solange noch keine stärkeren anatomischen Veränderungen der Gefäße vorliegen. Man darf wohl annehmen, daß die Mechanismen, die zur Widerstandserhöhung im Gesamtkreislauf führen, das Gehirngefäßnetz in etwa gleichem Maße treffen wie die übrigen Gefäßgebiete[2]. Später kristallisieren sich bei der Hypertonie zwei

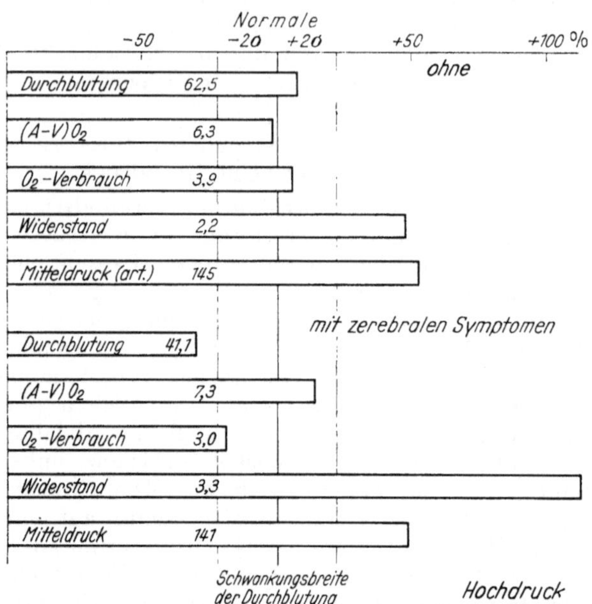

Abb. 25. Die Hirndurchblutung bei Hypertonie. Obere Hälfte: Kranke ohne neurologische Symptome. Untere Hälfte: Kranke mit neurologischen Symptomen. Darstellung der Abweichungen vom normalen Mittelwert in %. Die Schwankungsbreite der Durchblutung bei Gesunden ($\pm 2\ \sigma$) ist besonders gekennzeichnet. Die in Säulen angegebenen Zahlen sind die gefundenen Mittelwerte (Durchblutung in ml/100 g × min) (A—V) O₂ in Vol.-%, O₂-Verbrauch in ml/100 g × min. Widerstand in mm Hg/ml/100 g × min, Mitteldruck (art) in mm Hg. (Bodechtel 1953.)

Gruppen heraus, nämlich 1. Kranke, mit normaler Hirndurchblutung bei erhöhtem Mitteldruck und vermehrtem Strömungswiderstand, 2. Kranke, mit verminderter Hirndurchblutung und stark erhöhtem Strömungswiderstand[3] (s. Abb. 25). Die letzte Gruppe ist die der sog. „Pseudourämie". Zwischen der Schwere der Augenhintergrundsveränderungen und den Veränderungen der cerebralen Durchblutung bestehen keine eindeutigen Korrelationen[4]. Bei denjenigen Kranken, die eine verminderte Hirndurchblutung bei stark erhöhtem Strömungswiderstand und eine Abnahme des Sauerstoffverbrauchs zeigen, handelt es sich um Patienten, bei denen auch anatomische Strukturveränderungen der Gefäße anzunehmen sind. Auffällig ist, daß nach Sympathektomie, auch bei erheblichen Blutdrucksenkungen, nur eine geringe Abnahme der Gehirndurchblutung festgestellt wurde[5]. Hier scheinen Regulationsmechanismen im Spiel zu sein, die wir im einzelnen noch nicht übersehen.

---

[1] Shipley und Study 1951.   [2] Kety 1950.   [3] Bodechtel 1953.
[4] Bodechtel 1953.   [5] Hafkenschiel und Mitarbeiter 1950/51.

3. Hypotonie.

Von einer Hypotonie kann man sprechen, wenn der Ruheblutdruck wesentlich unter dem Altersnormalwert liegt. Zur Kennzeichnung des Krankhaften genügt aber diese Definition nicht. Es gibt viele Menschen mit auffallend niedrigem Blutdruck, die gleichwohl leistungsfähig und keineswegs krank sind; ihr Kreislauf zeigt eine mehr vagotonische Einstellung. Es kommt vielmehr darauf an, ob die Kreislaufregulationen ausreichen, um bei allen Ansprüchen einen genügend hohen Blutdruck und damit eine genügende Durchblutung herstellen zu können. Nur wenn das nicht der Fall ist, können wir von Hypotonie als etwas Krankhaftem sprechen. Eine solche ungenügende Anpassung ist nicht unbedingt an einen niedrigen Ruheblutdruck gebunden, sondern kommt auch bei Menschen mit normalem Ruheblutdruck vor. Ein Hypotoniker im klinischen Sinne ist also unabhängig vom Ruheblutdruck ein Mensch, dessen Regulationen zur Herstellung des notwendigen Blutdrucks nicht ausreichen. Exakte Angaben über die Veränderungen der kreislaufdynamischen Verhältnisse bei Hypotonie, besonders über die Veränderungen des Strömungswiderstandes, liegen bisher nicht vor. Es ist zwar eine große Reihe von Untersuchungen unternommen worden, die mit Hilfe der physikalischen Methoden die kreislaufdynamischen Veränderungen zu erfassen suchte. Doch

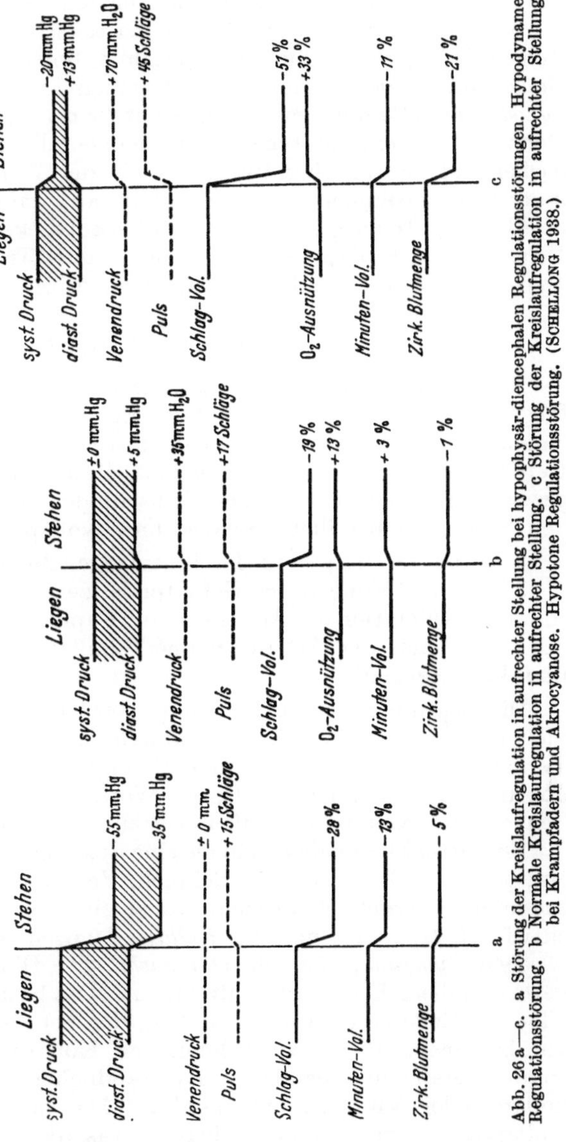

Abb. 26 a—c. a Störung der Kreislaufregulation in aufrechter Stellung bei hypophysär-diencephalen Regulationsstörungen. Hypodyname Regulationsstörung. b Normale Kreislaufregulation in aufrechter Stellung. c Störung der Kreislaufregulation in aufrechter Stellung bei Krampfadern und Akrocyanose. Hypotone Regulationsstörung. (Schellong 1938.)

sind diese Untersuchungen aus den schon genannten Gründen zu einer Aussage über die Größe des Kreislaufminutenvolumens und die Beurteilung des Strömungswiderstandes nicht geeignet. Trotzdem wird die folgende Einteilung in zwei verschiedene Typen wahrscheinlich kreislaufdynamisch das Richtige treffen. [Man unterscheidet die *hypotonen* Regulationsstörungen und die *hypodynamen* Regulationsstörungen[1]. Von der *hypotonen* Regulationsstörung werden vor allem

---

[1] Schellong 1938.

Personen mit äußerlich vielfach schon sichtbaren schlaffen Gefäßen (Varicen, Akrocyanose) betroffen. Es besteht eine konstitutionelle Schwäche der Gefäßwände. Zur Kompensierung der arteriellen Hypotonie besteht eine relative Steigerung des peripheren Strömungswiderstandes (relativ hoher diastolischer Druck, relativ hoher Venendruck). Nach längerem Stehen sinkt bei solchen Personen der systolische Druck, während der diastolische Druck und die Pulsfrequenz ansteigen. Schlagvolumen und Kreislaufminutenvolumen sollen absinken (s. Abb. 26). Doch sind präzise, quantitative Angaben hierüber nicht zu machen. Bei der *hypodynamen* Regulationsstörung steht die nervöse Fehlsteuerung im Vordergrund. Der Vasomotorentonus scheint allgemein herabgesetzt. Beim Stehen sinken systolischer und diastolischer Blutdruck ab, der Venendruck bleibt niedrig, Schlag- und Minutenvolumen sinken ebenfalls ab, während die Pulsfrequenz ansteigt (s. Abb. 26). In ausgesprochenen Fällen entwickelt sich bei diesen Personen unter Belastung ein Kollaps (s. dort). Eine scharfe Trennung der beiden aufgeführten Typen ist in der Klinik nicht möglich, da fließende Übergänge bestehen.

V. Schock und Kollaps.

Bei Schock und Kollaps besteht entweder ein Mangel an Blut oder eine falsche Blutverteilung. Die falsche Verteilung des Blutes kann entweder die hintereinandergeschalteten Gefäßabschnitte (Arterien-Venen) oder parallelgeschaltete Gefäßabschnitte (Splanchnicusgebiet, Haut-Muskelgebiet) betreffen. Wie noch gezeigt wird, sind die einzelnen Kreislaufgebiete in recht verschiedener Weise an den Störungen beteiligt. Schock und Kollaps können herbeigeführt werden:

1. durch Verminderung der Blutmenge (Blutverlust, Verlust an Blutplasma);

2. durch Störungen des Gefäßtonus (zentral bedingte Störungen des Gefäßtonus mit Dilatation der Arteriolen und Capillaren, toxische periphere Lähmungen des Gefäßtonus der Arteriolen und Capillaren, z. B. bei Infektionskrankheiten und Vergiftungen).

Die Begriffe Schock und Kollaps werden in der deutschsprachigen Literatur vielfach synonym verwendet. Dadurch ist manche Verwirrung entstanden. Die Verhältnisse sind jedenfalls in pathophysiologischer Hinsicht klarer, wenn wir uns an Definitionen halten, die den Wortprägungen entsprechen, und nach denen Schock und Kollaps begrifflich getrennt werden müssen. Der *Schock* kann allgemein als eine Schädigung des Kreislaufs auf ein plötzlich eingetretenes Ereignis (z. B. Schreck, Verwundung, Blutverlust, Schmerz, Verbrennung) bezeichnet werden, wobei sich ein komplexes klinisches *Syndrom* entwickelt (s. weiter unten). *Kollaps* dagegen ist identisch mit einem fest umrissenen *Symptom*, nämlich: *Ohnmacht*. Die Ohnmacht kann mit Bewußtseinsverlust einhergehen, muß es aber nicht. Das Symptom Kollaps kann am Anfang oder am Ende eines Schocks stehen, der Schock kann aber auch ohne Kollaps vorübergehen. Wenn wir Schock und Kollaps so definieren und voneinander trennen, erscheinen manche mißverständlichen Bezeichnungen, z. B. Spannungskollaps oder ähnliches, vermeidbar. Die hier gegebene Begriffsprägung des Kollapses stimmt mit dem überein, was die Angelsachsen mit „fainting" bezeichnen. Allerdings ist bei einer solchen Definition eine Reihe von klinischen Zustandsbildern nicht mit erfaßt, die häufig unter der Bezeichnung Kollaps laufen (z. B. verschlechterte Kreislaufverhältnisse bei Infektionskrankheiten, bei Vergiftungen, bei Hormonausfällen). Es dürfte richtiger sein, diese letztgenannten Zustände als allgemeine Kreislaufschäden oder als Insuffizienz des Gefäßsystems (im Gegensatz zur Herzinsuffizienz) zu bezeichnen, den Begriff Kollaps aber bei solchen Zuständen nur dann anzuwenden, wenn das Symptom Ohnmacht auftritt.

1. Der Kreislauf im Schock.

Hämodynamisch ist der Schock gekennzeichnet durch eine *schlechte periphere Durchblutung bei hohem peripherem Widerstand.* Die schlechte periphere Durchblutung ist Folge einer verminderten Blutmenge oder verminderten venösen Rückstroms. Der hohe Strömungswiderstand darf als regulative Maßnahme des Organismus zur Verhinderung eines Kollapses aufgefaßt werden (s. weiter unten). Hierfür wurde auch der Ausdruck „Zentralisation des Kreislaufs" geprägt[1]. Bei den Zuständen der Zentralisation ist freilich im allgemeinen die zentrale Blutmenge in Herz und Lunge stark vermindert, so daß aus diesem Grunde der Ausdruck Zentralisation nicht sehr glücklich ist.

a) Der hämorrhagische Schock.

Während eines Aderlasses bis zu etwa 800 cm³ steigt die Herzfrequenz etwas an, das Kreislaufminutenvolumen sowie der Druck im rechten Vorhof sinken ab. Der arterielle Druck wird dagegen lange Zeit unabhängig vom Absinken des Kreislaufminutenvolumens konstant gehalten[2] (s. Abb. 29). Bei etwa 800 bis 1000 cm³ wird die kritische

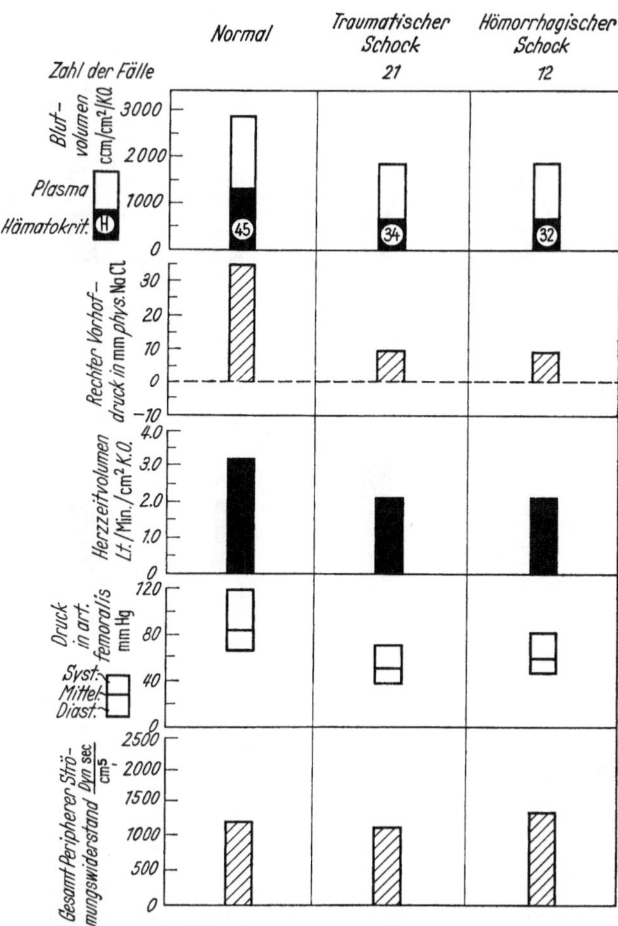

Abb. 27. Vergleich von hämodynamischen Größen beim Gesunden mit solchen im traumatischen und hämorrhagischen Schock. (RICHARDS 1947.)

Grenze erreicht, bei deren Überschreiten es zum Kollaps kommt (s. später). Die Aufrechterhaltung bzw. die Erhöhung des Strömungswiderstandes im Schock ist Folge einer Arteriolenkonstriktion.

b) Der Wundschock.

Der Wundschock ist im wesentlichen mit dem hämorrhagischen Schock vergleichbar. Neben einer Abwanderung von Plasma aus der Wunde ist es die Blutung, die die kreislaufdynamischen Umstellungen bedingt. So sind auch die quantitativen Veränderungen der Blutmenge, des Kreislaufminutenvolumens, des Druckes im rechten Vorhof und des Strömungswiderstandes in etwa

---

[1] DUESBERG und SCHRÖDER 1944. [2] RICHARDS 1947/48.

vergleichbar (s. Abb. 27). Auch beim Wundschock ist es charakteristisch, daß der Strömungswiderstand bis zum Terminalstadium normal oder erhöht bleibt. Die Höhe des systolischen Druckes bietet schon ein gewisses Maß für die Stärke des Blutverlustes[1]. Ist der systolische Druck um 140 mm Hg, so besteht die Wahrscheinlichkeit, daß das zirkulierende Blutvolumen noch über 80% der Norm beträgt. Druckerniedrigungen auf 100 mm Hg bedeuten eine Abnahme der zirkulierenden Blutmenge bis auf 70% der Norm. Ein systolischer Blutdruck unter 85 mm Hg besagt, daß mehr als 25% der zirkulierenden Blutmenge verlorengegangen sind[2]. Wenn auch die Schwere des Schocks im wesentlichen durch die Größe des Blutverlustes bzw. des Flüssigkeitsverlustes aus der Blutbahn bestimmt wird, so darf darüber nicht vergessen werden, daß andere Faktoren wie Angst, Schmerz, Infektionen usw. den Ablauf wesentlich mitbestimmen. Schließlich ist auch die Lokalisation des Traumas maßgebend für die Kreislaufveränderungen. Deswegen ist es nicht verwunderlich, daß die Beziehungen zwischen Blutdruck, Strömungswiderstand, Abnahme des Blutvolumens und Abnahme des Kreislaufminutenvolumens nicht in strenger Korrelation zueinander stehen.

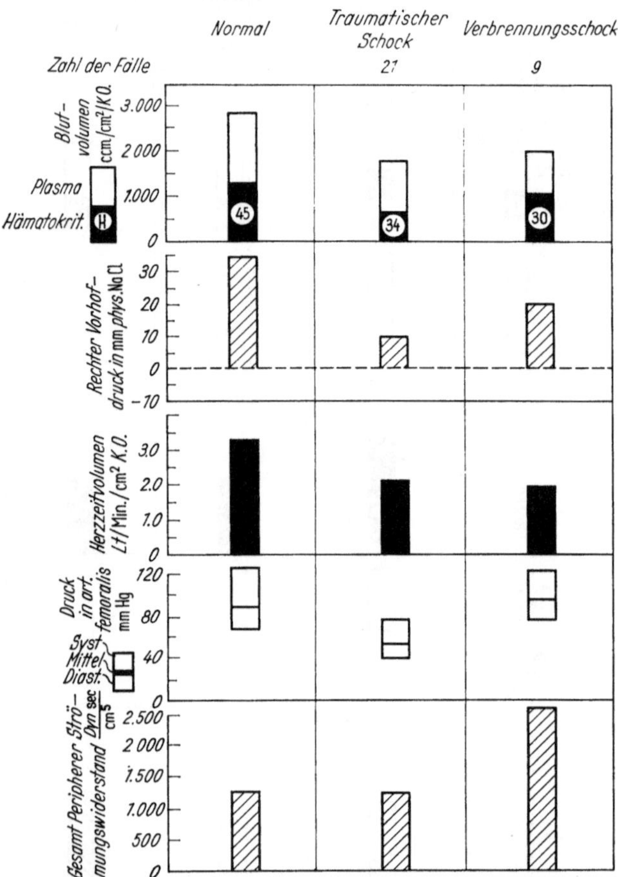

Abb. 28. Vergleich hämodynamischer Größen von Gesunden mit solchen im traumatischen Schock und im Verbrennungsschock. (Richards 1947.)

Bei den Spätkomplikationen ist weiterhin zu beachten, daß durch Erbrechen ein erheblicher weiterer Flüssigkeits- und Salzverlust stattfindet. Schließlich dürfen auch chemische Produkte, die aus den Wunden frei werden und die den Kreislauf schädigen, nicht unberücksichtigt bleiben wie Histamin, Peptide, Adenosintriphosphate. Allerdings besteht über die tatsächliche Auswirkung dieser Stoffe auf den Kreislauf im Schock keine Klarheit[3]. Gegenüber dem Plasma- und Blutverlust sind sie sicher von untergeordneter Bedeutung.

c) Verbrennungsschock.

Beim Verbrennungsschock steht der Verlust von Blutplasma im Vordergrund. Dementsprechend kommt es zu einer relativen Zunahme der corpusculären Blut-

<hr>

[1] Grant und Reeve 1951.   [2] Emerson und Ebert 1945.   [3] Cameron 1954.

elemente (Hämokonzentration). Im übrigen sind die kreislaufdynamischen Veränderungen ganz ähnlich wie beim hämorrhagischen und beim Wundschock[1]. Besonders ausgeprägt ist der Anstieg des Strömungswiderstandes, der bis zum Eintritt des finalen Kollapses hoch bleibt (s. Abb. 28). Komplizierend wirken beim Verbrennungsschock sekundäre Entzündungen, Nierenschädigungen, eine starke Zunahme der Milchsäure im Blut und eine Abnahme des arteriellen und venösen p_H[2]. Eine weitere aggravierende Bedeutung haben histaminartige Stoffe bzw. toxische Produkte aus dem von der Verbrennung betroffenen Wundgebiet[3]. Jedoch ist anzunehmen, daß auch hierbei dem Verlust von Flüssigkeit die überragende Bedeutung zukommt. Wesentlich erscheint noch, daß die Nierendurchblutung weniger als 10% der Norm betragen kann[4], womit die Funktionseinbuße der Niere das Vergiftungsbild der Verbrennung stark beeinflußt (Oligurie bzw. Anurie). Als Zeichen der Tubulusschädigung findet man eine deutliche Verzögerung der Phenolrotausscheidung[5].

2. Der Kreislauf im Kollaps.

Wenn wir den „kardialen" Kollaps nach traumatischen Schädigungen des Herzens und nach Herzinfarkt sowie andere kardiale Synkopen aus unseren Betrachtungen ausschließen, so beruht der Kollaps im wesentlichen auf zwei Ursachen: 1. Auf zu geringem venösem Rückfluß infolge mechanischer Einflüsse. 2. Auf einem plötzlichen Nachlassen des Gefäßtonus infolge des nervösen Versagens der Kreislaufsteuerung.

Zu 1. Ein Schulbeispiel für den Kollaps infolge zu geringen venösen Rückflusses bietet der Valsalvasche Preßversuch. Hierbei wird infolge der intrathorakalen Druckerhöhung der Blutzufluß zum Herzen gestoppt, es kommt zum Kollaps. Ähnlich verhält sich der *orthostatische* Kollaps. Dabei sind häufig Flüssigkeitsverluste mit Verminderung der Blutmenge von Bedeutung. Beim orthostatischen Kollaps besteht oft ein erhöhter Strömungswiderstand im großen Kreislauf. Bei Versuchspersonen, die nach Verabfolgung von Natriumnitrit und aufrechtem Stehen kollabierten, konnte während des Kollapses eine Arteriolenkonstriktion der Haut festgestellt werden[6]. Wie sich die Muskel- und Splanchnicusgefäße verhalten, ist jedoch unbekannt.

Zu 2. Hier liegen Kreislaufuntersuchungen mit Bestimmungen des Kreislaufminutenvolumens nach dem Fickschen Prinzip und Messungen des Drucks im rechten Vorhof vor[7]. Am eindeutigsten sind die Verhältnisse beim Kollaps nach Blutverlust geklärt. In Übereinstimmung damit stehen auch die Untersuchungen über Kreislaufveränderungen bei psychischen Insulten und bei plötzlichem O_2-Mangel, die durch Atmung von sauerstoffarmen Gasgemischen herbeigeführt wurden. Die Kreislaufveränderungen beim Kollaps im Gefolge eines hämorrhagischen Schocks gestalten sich folgendermaßen: Nachdem sich zunächst im Verlauf eines Aderlasses ein Schocksyndrom mit Erhöhung des peripheren Strömungswiderstandes ausgebildet hat, kommt es plötzlich zur Ohnmacht. Im Augenblick der eintretenden Ohnmacht tritt eine Abnahme der Herzfrequenz, des Blutdruckes, des Druckes im rechten Vorhof und des Strömungswiderstandes auf. Das Kreislaufminutenvolumen, das vorher im Stadium des Schocks eine deutliche Erniedrigung erfahren hat, sinkt während des Kollapses nicht weiter ab, sondern steigt im Gegenteil wieder etwas an (s. Abb. 29). Über das Verhalten

---

[1] RICHARDS 1947/48.   [2] CAMERON 1948.   [3] BLALOCK 1931.
[4] SELKURT 1946.   [5] ALLGÖWER und Mitarbeiter 1956.   [6] WEISS und Mitarbeiter 1937.
[7] BARCROFT und Mitarbeiter 1944, WOOD und BURCHELL 1950 (zit. nach BARCROFT und SWAN 1953).

des Herzzeitvolumens bei denjenigen Kollapsformen, die vorher nicht das Stadium des Schocks durchlaufen haben, liegen keine Untersuchungen vor. Bei Versuchen, durch Spinalanaesthesie und aufrechte Körperhaltung Kollapse zu erzeugen, unterschieden sich die Personen, die kollabierten, bezüglich der Größe des Kreislaufminutenvolumens nicht von denen, die nicht kollabierten[1]. Die im Beginn des Kollapses eintretende Bradykardie ist vagal bedingt und kann durch Atropinisierung behoben werden. Dagegen bleibt das Absinken des Blutdrucks durch Atropin unbeeinflußt[2]. Auf Grund dieser Befunde führte Lewis den Ausdruck *vasovagales Syndrom* ein. Die Senkung des Strömungswiderstandes im großen Kreislauf scheint beim Kollaps aus dem hämorrhagischen Schock sowie bei den psychischen und den durch plötzlichen O_2-Mangel bedingten Kollapszuständen obligat. An dem Zustandekommen der Erniedrigung des Strömungswiderstandes sind die verschiedenen Gefäßgebiete nicht gleichmäßig beteiligt. Die Hautgefäße sind auch während der Ohnmacht zum größten Teil konstringiert. Darauf weisen die Gesichtsblässe, plethysmographische Messungen der Hautdurchblutung und Bestimmungen der Hauttemperatur hin. Nur in Ausnahmefällen wurde eine transitorische Dilatation der Hautgefäße im Bereich der Hände festgestellt[3]. Die Vasoconstriction, besonders im Bereich des Gesichtes, tritt auch bei sympathektomierten Patienten während des Kollapses auf[4]. Bei

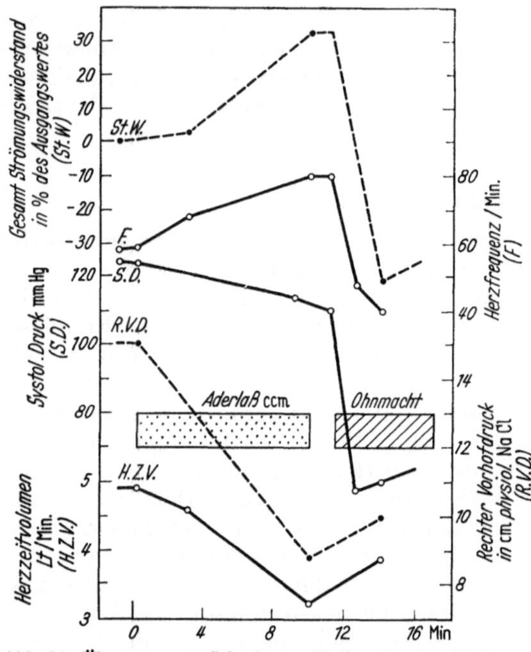

Abb. 29. Übergang vom Schock zum Kollaps im Anschluß an einen Aderlaß. (Barcroft, Edholm, McMichael und Sharpey-Schafer 1944.)

einseitig Sympathektomierten soll sie sogar auf der denervierten Seite stärker ausgeprägt sein. Die Vasoconstriction der Hautgefäße im Bereich des Gesichtes wird mit der vermehrten Ausschüttung von Hypophysenhinterlappenhormon (Vasopressin) in Zusammenhang gebracht (s. weiter unten). Im Gegensatz zur Hautdurchblutung ist die Muskeldurchblutung im Kollaps wesentlich erhöht[5]. Dabei handelt es sich anscheinend nicht nur um das Nachlassen des Konstriktorentonus. Durch Vergleichsuntersuchungen bei normalen und sympathektomierten Patienten während des Kollapses konnte wahrscheinlich gemacht werden, daß die Dilatation der Muskelgefäße durch eine Reizung der zentralen dilatatorischen Regulationsgebiete zustande kommt. Sympathektomierte Patienten zeigen während des Kollapses keine Durchblutungssteigerung, sondern eine Durchblutungsabnahme im Muskel[6]. Die Vasodilatation ist an die Integrität der Benervung der Gefäße gebunden.

---

[1] Pugh und Wyndham 1950.   [2] Lewis 1932.
[3] Edholm 1952.   [4] Barcroft und Edholm 1944.
[5] Barcroft und Mitarbeiter 1944, 1945.   [6] Barcroft und Edholm 1945.

Die Splanchnicusgefäße verhalten sich im Kollaps ähnlich wie die Muskelgefäße. Jedenfalls ist dies für den Kollaps nach hämorrhagischem Schock sichergestellt. Während des Blutverlustes sinkt die Leberdurchblutung bei hohem allgemeinem Strömungswiderstand im Durchschnitt ab (bei Aderlässen von 700 bis 1000 cm³ auf die Hälfte des Normalwertes)[1]. Beim Eintritt des Kollapses kommt es aber nur noch zu einer geringen weiteren Abnahme der Durchblutung, obwohl der Blutdruck stark sinkt. Während des Schockstadiums besteht also eine Vasoconstriction der Splanchnicusgefäße, die beim Eintritt des Kollapses von einer Vasodilatation abgelöst wird. In der *Niere* kommt es ebenfalls während des Kollapses zu einer Vasodilatation[2]. Nicht so eindeutig liegen die Verhältnisse für die *Gehirn*durchblutung[3]. Sicher ist, daß die Gehirndurchblutung während des Kollapses absinkt. Jedoch ist nicht sicher, ob hier ebenfalls eine Vasodilatation stattfindet, oder ob der Strömungswiderstand gleichbleibt bzw. erhöht ist. Über die Größe der *Coronar*durchblutung während des Kollapses liegen keine Messungen vor. Lediglich tierexperimentelle Untersuchungen zeigen, daß beim Kollaps nach hämorrhagischem Schock eine coronare Minderdurchblutung mit den Zeichen einer Herzmuskelinsuffizienz eintreten kann[4]. Wegen der Ähnlichkeit gewisser Symptome — wie z. B. Gesichtsblässe (s. oben), Übelkeit, Erbrechen, Anurie — mit der Pitressinwirkung wird ein vermehrtes Freiwerden von Hypophysenhinterlappenhormonen im Kollaps diskutiert[5]. Im Urin von Patienten, die kollabiert waren, wurde ein wesentlich höherer Gehalt von antidiuretischen Stoffen nachgewiesen[6]. Es bleibt aber fraglich, ob das Hypophysenhinterlappenhormon beim Zustandekommen des Kollaps eine ursächliche Rolle spielt. Es sieht eher so aus, als ob die vermehrte Freisetzung erst sekundär — durch den Kollaps — zustandekommt.

Der Bewußtseinsverlust während des Kollapses ist wahrscheinlich auf eine Hypoxie bzw. Anoxie des Gehirns zurückzuführen. Während des Kollapses sinkt der Sauerstoffgehalt im Venenblut der Gehirngefäße auf Werte ab, die dem sog. kritischen O_2-Druck im Gehirnvenenblut nahekommen[7].

Zu den Kollapsformen, die mit einer plötzlichen Vasodilatation und Erniedrigung des Strömungswiderstandes einhergehen, zählen wahrscheinlich auch die *reflektorischen* Kollapse, wenngleich hierbei Messungen des Kreislaufminutenvolumens fehlen.

Reflektorische Kollapse, wie sie z. B. bei Gewalteinwirkungen besonders auf die Baucheingeweide oder bei Zerrungen am Mesenterium, den Blutgefäßen usw. auftreten, sind typische Beispiele für *vasovagale Synkopen* mit Bradykardie und starkem Absinken des Blutdruckes. Ähnliche vasovagale Reflexvorgänge liegen auch den bei Schmerzreizen auftretenden Kollapsen zugrunde.

Kollapszustände bei Lungenembolien werden teilweise reflektorisch erklärt (Lungenentlastungsreflex)[8]. Die reflektorische Genese solcher Kollapse ist aber noch umstritten. Reflektorische Kollapse können experimentell durch Reizung der Herznerven erzeugt werden. Der Jarisch-Bezold-Reflex hat seinen Ursprung in sensiblen Receptorenfeldern des Herzens[9]. Reizung dieser zentripetal leitenden Fasern führt unter starker Pulsverlangsamung zum Blutdruckabfall. Der häufig auftretende Kollaps im Anschluß an Herzinfarkte soll wenigstens in einem Teil der Fälle mit einer Reizung der afferenten Herznerven in Zusammenhang stehen. Es darf aber nicht übersehen werden, daß der Kollaps bei Herzinfarkt vielfach Ausdruck eines akuten Herzversagens ist.

---

[1] BEARM und Mitarbeiter 1950/51. [2] WARDENER und SWINEY 1951.
[3] LENNOX und Mitarbeiter 1935. [4] SARNOFF und Mitarbeiter 1954.
[5] BARCROFT und SWAN 1953. [6] TAYLOR und NOBLE 1950.
[7] LENNOX und Mitarbeiter 1935. [8] SCHWIEGK 1935. [9] JARISCH 1940.

Pharmakologisch kann der Jarisch-Bezold-Effekt durch *Veratrin* hervorgerufen werden. Durch Vagusausschaltung kann die vasovagale Attacke verhindert werden. Intravenöse Adrenalin-Injektionen führen mitunter zur Reizung der Bezoldschen Receptoren und zu vasovagalen Synkopen[1].

Bei disponierten Patienten (meist Arteriosklerotikern) führen abrupte Kopfbewegungen oder gröbere Manipulationen am Carotissinus zu spontanen oder auch experimentell erzeugbaren, mitunter bedrohlichen synkopalen Zwischenfällen (sog. „*hypersensitives Carotissinussyndrom*"). Man unterscheidet hier drei verschiedene Typen: einen *vagal-kardialen*, einen *depressorischen* und einen *cerebralen* Reflextyp[2]. Beim *vagalen* Typ kommt es durch Druck auf den Carotissinus zu Pulsverlangsamung mit oder ohne Herzblock, zu sekundärer Ischämie des Cerebrums und damit zum Kollaps. Die Ausbildung des Kollapses verläuft in 3 Phasen (s. Abb. 30). In der ersten Phase sind trotz beginnender Bradykardie Gesichtsfarbe, Bewußtsein, Blutdruck und EEG noch unverändert. In der 2. Phase flacht sich die EEG-Kurve ab. Der Patient wird blaß, klagt über Schwindel, der arterielle Druck sinkt ab. Mit zunehmender

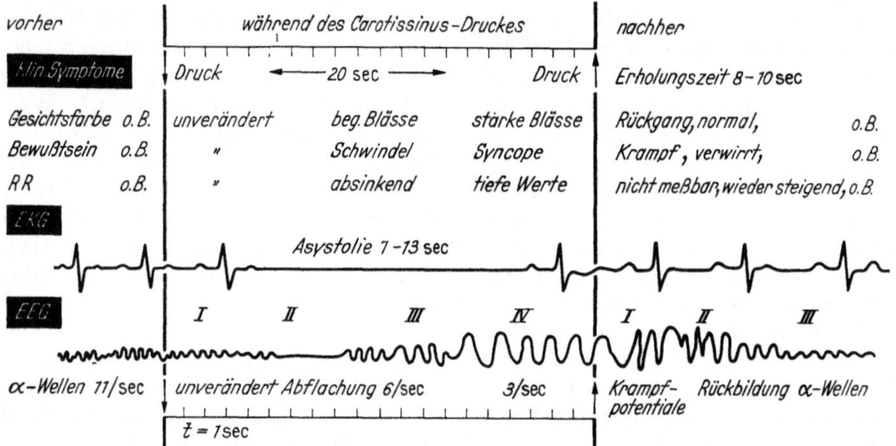

Abb. 30. Klinische Symptomatologie, EKG- und EEG-Veränderungen beim hypersensitiven Carotis-Sinus-Syndrom kardialen Typs. (Franke 1953.)

Herzpause (Asystole von 7—13 sec) zeigen sich in der 3. Phase bei hypoxischen ST- und T-Veränderungen des EKG im EEG hohe Zwischenwellen (besonders hochfrontal). Im Stadium der eigentlichen Synkope treten Totenblässe und kaum meßbarer Blutdruck bei hohen δ-Wellen im EEG auf. Obwohl mit Aufhören des Carotissinusdruckes die Sinusautomatie wieder erwacht, kommt es bei Rückgang der Gesichtsblässe mitunter sogar bei einer gewissen Gesichtsröte zu Krampfpotentialen im EEG. Dabei weist der Patient nach Art eines Adams-Stockeschen Anfalls klonisch-tonische Krämpfe auf. Sodann bildet sich das ganze Bild in etwa 8—10 sec wieder zur Norm zurück. Beim *depressorischen* Typ entwickelt sich auf Carotissinusdruck eine erhebliche Vasodilatation mit Blutdrucksenkung. Es stellt sich eine zentrale Ischämie ein, ohne daß eine erheblichere Pulsverlangsamung vorzuliegen braucht. Beim *cerebralen* Typ kommt es weder zur Pulsverlangsamung noch zur Blutdrucksenkung. Trotzdem entwickelt sich ein kurzdauernder ohnmachtsähnlicher Anfall, der durch Blockierung (Novocain) des Carotissinus beseitigt werden kann.

Der beim „Knockout" auftretende Kollaps wird vielfach als reflektorisch durch Reizung der Carotissinusnerven entstanden erklärt. Es ist jedoch wahrscheinlich, daß dieser Kollaps die Folge eines unmittelbaren Traumas der Ganglienzellen (commotio cerebri) ist. Auch die Bewußtlosigkeit ist hierbei nicht auf eine zentrale Anoxie, sondern eher auf die Commotio zurückzuführen.

Wenn im vorangehenden versucht wurde, die Kreislaufveränderungen im Schock und Kollaps zu analysieren, so bleibt eine solche Darstellung schon deswegen unvollkommen, weil bisher die einzelnen Kreislaufgrößen nur bei bestimmten Schock- und Kollapsformen erfaßt werden konnten. So fehlt vor allem eine zuverlässige Kreislaufanalyse jener Fälle, die durch eine allgemeine Kreislauf-

[1] Konzett und Rothlin 1951.   [2] Weiss und Mitarbeiter 1933, 1936, Franke 1953.

schädigung mit niedrigem Blutdruck und wahrscheinlich auch niedrigem Kreislaufminutenvolumen gekennzeichnet sind, die aber weder als Schock noch als Kollaps bezeichnet werden können. Es handelt sich hierbei vor allem um Zustände starken Flüssigkeitsverlustes (hochgradiges Erbrechen, Durchfälle, ileusartige Krankheitsbilder), komatöse Zustände, Infektionskrankheiten usw. Bei diesen Zustandsbildern ist die Kreislaufschädigung komplexer Natur. Plasmaverlust, Bluteindickung, Veränderungen des Mineralstoffwechsels, Verschiebungen des Blut-p_H, toxische Schädigung der zentralen vasomotorischen Regulationsstellen und der Gefäße kombinieren sich hierbei in unübersichtlicher Weise. Hinzu kommt in vielen Fällen noch eine Schädigung des Herzens, die das Bild weiter kompliziert. Bei diesen Zuständen erschöpft sich unsere Erkenntnis bisher noch im wesentlichen in der klinischen Symptomatologie und der Empirie der therapeutischen Erfahrung.

C. Funktionelle Orthologie und Pathologie des Herzens.

I. Coronardurchblutung.

GREGG[1] behandelt in seiner Monographie eingehend die großen Schwierigkeiten, die bei jeder Untersuchung der Coronardurchblutung auftreten. Es sind das besonders methodische Fragen der Durchblutungsmessung und Schwierigkeiten, die aus dem komplizierten Verlauf des Gefäßsystems abzuleiten sind. Letztere betreffen sowohl die arterielle wie die venöse Seite. Die Größe der Gewebsgebiete, die von den einzelnen Ästen der Coronararterien versorgt werden, schwanken recht stark. Die Verknüpfung dieser Gebiete durch interarterielle Anastomosen kann sehr verschieden sein. Chronische Hypoxie des Herzmuskels führt zu starker Ausbildung von interarteriellen Anastomosen, wodurch die Blutversorgung des gesamten Herzgewebes bei Verschluß eines Hauptastes sichergestellt sein kann[2]. Dagegen reicht bei einem plötzlichen Verschluß eines Hauptastes der Coronardurchblutung die Anastomosierung nicht aus, um den Stoffwechselbedarf der betroffenen Gebiete sicherzustellen[3].

Tabelle 14. *Prozentualer Anteil des Coronarsinus und der einzelnen Herzhöhlen am Gesamtabfluß des venösen Coronarblutes (= 100%).* (LENDRUM, CONDO, KATZ 1945.)

	Coronar-sinus	Rechter Vorhof	Rechter Ventrikel	Linker Vorhof	Linker Ventrikel
Mittelwert	36,4	24,5	30,8	1,4	7,0
$S\,x$	11,8	6,5	5,4	1,7	3,3

Auch die Verhältnisse des venösen Abflusses aus dem Herzen sind kompliziert. Tabelle 14 gibt die verschiedenen Anteile des venösen Abstroms aus dem Coronarsystem in Prozent der Gesamtdurchblutung, wie sie bei Durchströmung isolierter Herzen mit Hundeserum gewonnen wurden[4]. Nach gasanalytischen Untersuchungen wird der Anteil, der in das linke Herz abfließt, auf 16% der Coronardurchblutung geschätzt[5]. Wahrscheinlich ändern sich die Anteile des venösen Abstroms mit der Herzfunktion. Dies kann besonders bei Messungen der Coronardurchblutung mit der Stickoxydulmethode zu falschen Schlüssen führen.

1. Durchblutungswerte.

Tabelle 15 gibt die Werte über die Durchblutung des schlagenden, linken Ventrikels bei angenähert normaler Belastung, wie sie von verschiedenen Autoren

---

[1] GREGG 1950. [2] ECKSTEIN 1955, GIESE und MÜLLER-MOHNSSEN 1958 (Literatur).
[3] MEESMANN und SCHMIER 1955. [4] LENDRUM u. a. 1945.
[5] BARTELS u. a. 1956, ATWELL u. a. 1955.

Tabelle 15. *Werte für die Durchblutung des linken Ventrikels.* (Gregg 1950.)

Autor	Durchblutung des linken Ventrikels ml/min und 100 g	Mittlerer arterieller Druck mm Hg	Bemerkungen
Gregg 1950	74	80	Hund, narkotisiert, Thorax offen, Rotameter an der linken Coronararterie
Gregg 1950	81	80	Hund, narkotisiert, Thorax offen, Stickoxydul-Methode
Eckenhoff u. a. 1948	74	133	Hund, narkotisiert, Stickoxydul-Methode
Goodale u. a. 1948	71	138	Hund, narkotisiert, Stickoxydul-Methode
Harrison u. a. 1936	64	118	Hund, unter Morphin. Ausfluß aus dem Coronarsinus gemessen. Auf Durchblutung des linken Ventrikels umgerechnet
Spencer u. a. 1950	151	119	Hund, ohne Narkose. Stickoxydul-Methode
Bing u. a. 1949	65	92	Mensch, Stickoxydul-Methode

mit sehr verschiedenen Methoden und an recht unterschiedlichen Objekten gewonnen wurden. Die höchsten Werte finden sich bei nicht narkotisierten Hunden. Dies mag z. T. an unvollkommenen Ruhebedingungen liegen. Auch ist bei

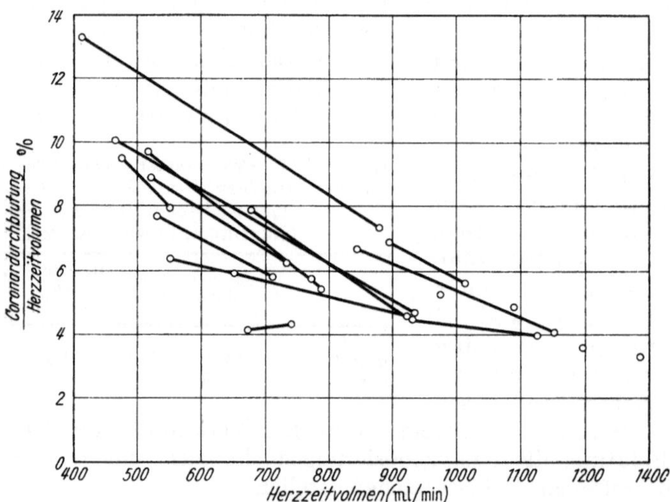

Abb. 31. Beziehung zwischen der Coronardurchblutung und dem Herzzeitvolumen. Mit Strichen verbundene Punkte bezeichnen Beobachtungen im gleichen Versuch. Einzeln stehende Punkte bezeichnen Versuche, in denen nur eine Herzzeitvolumenbestimmung durchgeführt wurde. (Eckenhoff 1947.)

kleineren Tieren der Herzstoffwechsel und die Herzdurchblutung höher als bei großen, was den Vergleich der Werte des Hundes mit solchen des Menschen erschwert. Die gute Übereinstimmung der Ergebnisse, die am nicht narkotisierten ruhenden Menschen und am narkotisierten Hund gewonnen wurden, kann nur als ein Zufall aufgefaßt werden. Zahlen für die Durchblutung des rechten Ventrikels sind für den Menschen nicht zu erhalten. Nach Messungen im Hundeversuch muß man annehmen, daß die Durchblutung des linken und rechten Ventrikels für gleiche Gewichtseinheiten Muskelgewebe angenähert gleich groß ist[1].

Schlecht unterrichtet sind wir über Maximalwerte der Coronardurchblutung. Der Strömungswiderstand des Coronarsystems sinkt im Sauerstoffmangel auf den 4. Teil des Ausgangswertes ab[2]. Nach Adrenalininjektionen wurden beim

---

[1] Gregg 1950.   [2] Allela 1955.

Hund in Narkose Durchblutungen von 300—400 cm^3 pro 100 g und min gefunden[1]. Der Anteil der Coronardurchblutung am HZV schwankt mit dessen Größe. Im allgemeinen beträgt die Coronardurchblutung 4—5% des HZV. Ist das HZV sehr klein, so fließen 9% davon durch die Coronarien (Abb. 31)[2]. Nach Adrenalininjektionen findet man bei gesteigertem HZV eine sehr hohe Coronardurchblutung, etwa 12—13% des HZV[1].

2. Einflüsse auf die Coronardurchblutung.

Abb. 32 gibt eine Übersicht über die mannigfaltigen Einflüsse auf die Coronardurchblutung. Wie bei jedem Organ hängt auch beim Herzen die Durchblutung

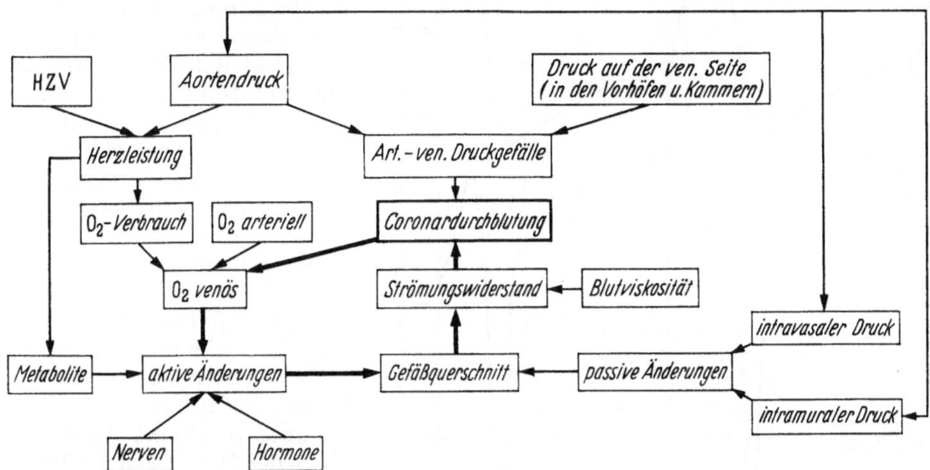

Abb 32. Faktoren, die die Coronardurchblutung bestimmen. Die dick gezeichneten Pfeile kennzeichnen einen Regelkreis, bei dem über die Einstellung der Coronardurchblutung der venöse Sauerstoffdruck des Coronarsystems geregelt wird. (In Anlehnung an KATZ, KATZ und WILLIAMS 1955.)

vom Druckgefälle und vom Strömungswiderstand ab. Der Strömungswiderstand wird nicht allein von der Vasomotorik, sondern auch von einfachen physikalischen Faktoren bestimmt. Die Elastizität des Röhrensystems bedingt bei hohem Innendruck Erweiterung der Gefäße und damit Abnahme des Strömungswiderstandes. Andererseits können die Gefäße durch den Druck im umgebenden Gewebe entspannt oder auch zusammengepreßt werden, und auch dadurch kann der Strömungswiderstand verändert werden. In einer gewissen Parallele zum tätigen Skeletmuskel beeinflußt die Tätigkeit des Herzmuskels den Außendruck auf die Gefäße. Strömungswiderstand und Durchblutung der Coronargefäße ändern sich damit in den einzelnen Phasen der Herztätigkeit.

Ein recht großer Teil der Literatur der Physiologie über die Einstellung der Coronardurchblutung beschäftigt sich mit der Frage, ob die Durchblutung weitgehend durch einfache physikalische Vorgänge — etwa das arterio-venöse Druckgefälle oder den intramuralen Druck in der Herzwand — bestimmt wird, oder ob die Vasomotorik der wichtigere Vorgang ist, und ob auf diese Weise die Durchblutung dem jeweiligen Stoffwechselbedarf des Herzens angepaßt werden kann. Die Frage ist so zu beantworten, daß die vasomotorischen Vorgänge das Bild bestimmen, solange regulatorische Reserven für die Durchblutungseinstellung vorhanden sind. Sind aber diese regulatorischen Möglichkeiten erschöpft, und sind die Gefäße des Herzens bereits auf ihre maximale Weite eingestellt, dann

---

[1] GREGG 1950. [2] ECKENHOFF u. a. 1947.

kann die Durchblutung nur noch durch die Druckverhältnisse bestimmt werden. Kenntnisse über die einfachen physikalischen Einflüsse auf die Coronardurchblutung sind deshalb besonders für pathologische Zustände von großem Interesse.

3. Einfluß der Kontraktion der Herzmuskulatur auf die Coronardurchblutung.

Mißt man die Durchblutung der A. coronaria sinistra mit einer Stromuhr, die eine kurze Einstellzeit hat, so erhält man eine recht komplizierte Kurve (Abb. 33)[1]. Die Durchblutung hat zu Beginn der Diastole ein Maximum und sinkt während der Diastole mit fallendem Aortendruck ab. Während der Systole ist die Durchblutung im Durchschnitt niedriger als während der Diastole. Dies gilt besonders für die Anspannungszeit, in der ein Rückstrom des Blutes beobachtet wird. Der Kurvenablauf wird durch eine ganze Reihe von Faktoren bestimmt. Die Durchblutung ist zunächst abhängig von der Höhe des Aortendrucks. Im besonders starken Maße wird sie aber bestimmt durch die Höhe des Druckes in der Herzwand. Der Einstrom des Blutes in das Coronarsystem verläuft weitgehend dem Gefälle zwischen dem Aortendruck und dem intramuralen Druck parallel. Der in der Systole gesteigerte intramurale Druck vermindert die Coronardurchblutung in diesem Zeitpunkt. Ein weiterer Faktor, der die Durchblutungskurve beeinflußt, ist das Fassungsvermögen des arteriellen Teils des Coronarsystems. Dadurch entsteht ein zweites Maximum der Durchblutung im Beginn der Austreibungszeit. Der rasch ansteigende Druck in der Aorta führt hier zu einem erhöhten Bluteinstrom in das Coronarsystem.

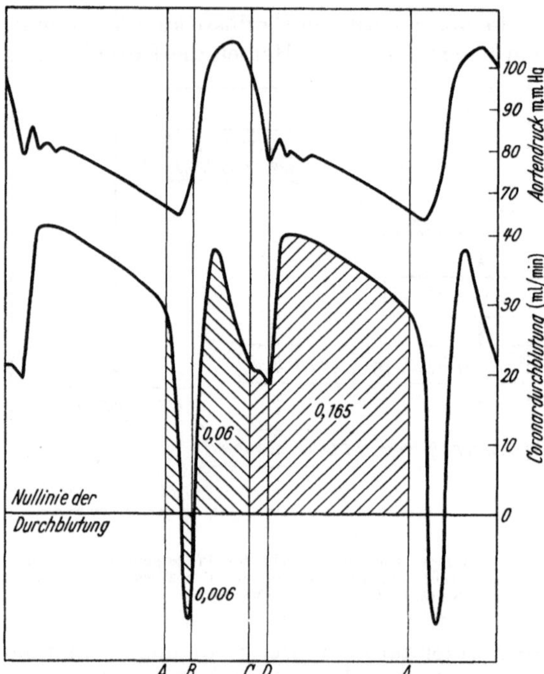

Abb. 33. Durchblutung des Ramus descendens der linken Coronararterie in Abhängigkeit von der Herzphase. Am Ende der Diastole (A) beträgt die Durchblutung 28 ml/min. Am Beginn der isometrischen Kontraktion (A) nimmt die Durchblutung rasch ab, und es tritt ein kurzdauernder Rückstrom auf. Mit dem Beginn der Austreibung (B) setzt die Durchströmung wieder ein und erreicht ein Maximum mit 40 ml/min kurz vor dem Höchstwert des Aortendrucks. Dann nimmt die Durchblutung etwa parallel dem Aortendruck ab, steigt nach dem Schluß der Aortenklappen (D) wieder an und nimmt mit diastolischem Druck bis zum Beginn der nächsten Systole ab. Die Durchflußmenge während jeder Phase kann aus den Flächen errechnet werden. Sie beträgt in der Systole 0,06—0.006 ml = 0,054 ml, in der Diastole 0,165 ml. Da die Herzfrequenz 131/min beträgt, ist die mittlere Durchblutung 29 ml/min. (Green und Gregg 1940.)

Die Höhe des intramuralen Druckes läßt sich abschätzen, wenn man im Experiment das schlagende Herz mit konstantem Druck durchströmt und dabei die Größe des Einstroms mißt[2]. Abb. 34 zeigt den Einstrom bei Infusionsdrucken von 82 und 12 mm Hg in Abhängigkeit von der Herzphase. Bei einem Infusionsdruck von 82 mm Hg kommt der Einstrom während der Systole zum Stillstand. Daraus muß auf einen entsprechenden intramuralen Druck in diesem Zeitpunkt geschlossen werden. Bei 12 mm Hg fließt auch in der Diastole

---

[1] Gregg und Green 1940b.   [2] Gregg und Green 1940a.

kein Blut in das Coronarsystem ein. Diastolisch muß danach in der Herzwand ein Druck von 12 mm Hg herrschen. Nach entsprechenden Versuchen schätzt man den Druck in der Wand des rechten Herzens auf 25 mm Hg systolisch und 15 mm Hg während der Diastole.

Während in der Systole der Einstrom des Blutes in das Coronarsystem gehemmt wird, findet sich in dieser Phase ein gesteigerter Blutabstrom aus dem Sinus coronarius (Abb. 35)[1]. Der steigende, intramurale Druck preßt dann das Venensystem der Coronarien leer und steigert so den Abstrom des Blutes. Man hat die Frage aufgeworfen, ob nicht die rhythmisch tätige Herzmuskulatur die Durchblutung der Coronarien durch eine Art Massage verbessert[2]. Anscheinend ist aber diese Wirkung klein gegenüber der Hemmung des Bluteinstroms durch den erhöhten intramuralen Druck in der Systole[3]. Bringt man im Experiment ein Herz durch Vagusreizung zum Stillstand, so steigt bei konstant gehaltenem Infusionsdruck die Durchblutung der Coronararterien stark an. Der hemmende Effekt der Systolen überwiegt also bei weitem den fördernden Effekt der Massage (Abb. 36). Es ist wenig wahrscheinlich, daß bei diesem Experiment die Steigerung der Durchblutung durch Reizung von vasodilatatorischen Fasern bedingt ist. Der rasche Anstieg der Durchblutung spricht mehr für einen mechanischen Effekt.

Solange das Coronarsystem intakt ist, haben die physikalischen Faktoren für die Herzdurchblutung keine entscheidende Bedeutung, da sie durch vasomotorische Vorgänge am Gefäßsystem ausgeglichen werden können. Wenn aber die vasomotorischen Reserven erschöpft sind, dann gewinnen die physikalischen Einflüsse an Wichtigkeit, und eine Anpassung der

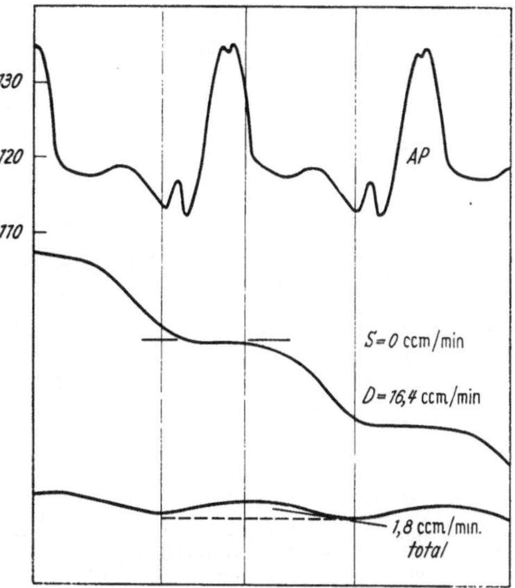

Abb. 34. Zum Strömungswiderstand im Ramus descendens der linken Coronararterie. Obere Kurve (AP): Aortendruck; mittlere Kurve (CF): Stromvolumen der Coronararterie bei konstantem Durchströmungsdruck von 82 mm Hg; untere Kurve: Stromvolumen der Coronararterie bei konstantem Durchströmungsdruck von 12 mm Hg; Zahlenwerte rechts: Durchblutung in der Systolenmitte und in der späten Diastole für die beiden Stromvolumenkurven. Senkrechte Linien markieren die Systole und die Diastole. (Nach GREGG 1950.)

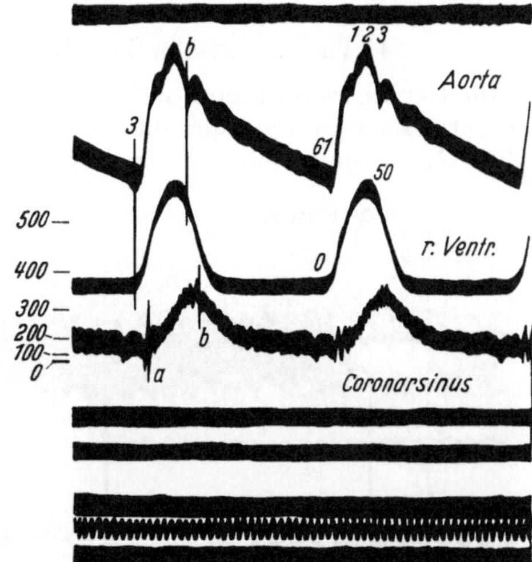

Abb. 35. Blutstrom im Coronarsinus in Abhängigkeit von der Herzphase. Obere Kurve: Aortendruck; mittlere Kurve: Druck im rechten Ventrikel; untere Kurve: Blutstrom im Coronarsinus. Links: Eichung der Durchblutungsmessung in ml/min. (JOHNSON u. WIGGERS 1937.)

Durchblutung an den Herzstoffwechsel ist nicht mehr möglich. Unter diesen Bedingungen muß jede Steigerung der Pulsfrequenz die Versorgung des Herzens

---

[1] JOHNSON und WIGGERS 1937.   [2] OSHER 1953, WIGGERS 1954.
[3] ECKSTEIN u. a. 1950, GREGG 1955.

besonders ungünstig beeinflussen. Bei hoher Pulsfrequenz ist die Systolenzeit groß gegenüber der Diastolenzeit, wodurch der Einstrom in das Coronarsystem gehemmt wird. Dabei fällt die Verschlechterung der Coronardurchblutung mit

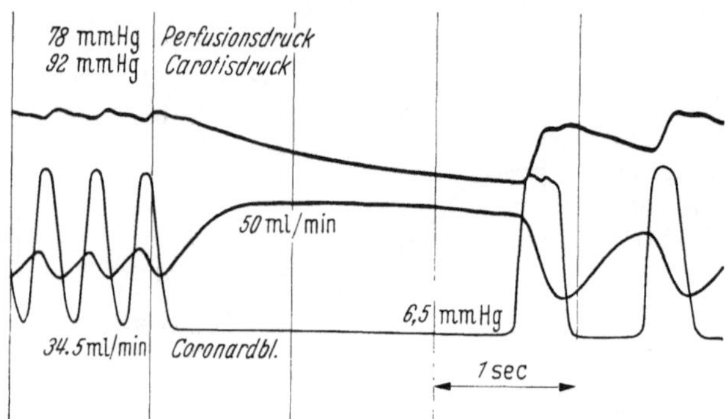

Abb. 36. Wirkung eines kurzdauernden, durch Vagusreizung hervorgerufenen Herzstillstandes auf die Coronardurchblutung bei konstanter Durchströmung des Coronarsystems. Obere Kurve: Druck in der A. carotis; mittlere Kurve: Coronardurchblutung; untere Kurve: Druck im linken Ventrikel. (Shipley und Wilson 1951.)

einem erhöhten Herzstoffwechsel zusammen. Steigt nach Erschöpfen der vasomotorischen Reserven der arterielle Druck an, so wird zwar einerseits durch Erhöhung des arterio-venösen Druckgefälles und durch die Steigerung des intravasalen Druckes die Durchblutung der Coronarien verbessert. Aber die Steigerung des arteriellen Druckes wirkt auf den Kammerdruck und damit auch auf den intramuralen Druck zurück und hemmt auf

diesem Wege den Bluteinfluß in das Coronarsystem. Die Durchblutung steigt deshalb sehr viel weniger an, wie das am stillstehenden Herzen der Fall sein müßte. So ist keine eindeutige Aussage darüber möglich, ob bei Steigerungen des arteriellen Druckes die Versorgung des Herzens durch erhöhte Coronardurchblutung verbessert oder ob sie entsprechend der erhöhten Herzleistung und dem gesteigerten Herzstoffwechsel sogar relativ verschlechtert wird.

4. Vasomotorische Vorgänge im Bereich der Coronarien.

Im Tierexperiment kann man durch Anlegen einer Drossel an einen Hauptast der Coronararterie die Durchblutung des Coronargebietes künstlich herabsetzen (Abb. 37). Schon während der Drosselung findet man einen geringgradigen

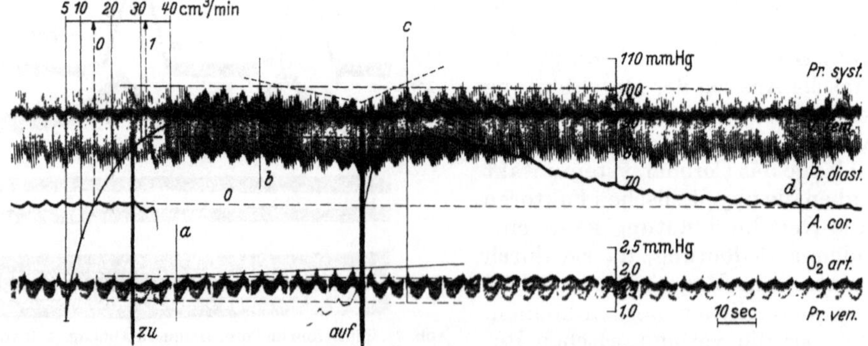

Abb. 37. Drosselung der A. coronaria dextra auf weniger als 4 cm³/min Dauer. Nach 12 sec (bei a) beginnt Anstieg des Druckes im rechten Vorhof, nach 32 sec (bei b) Abnahme des systolischen arteriellen Druckes. Kompensatorische Dilatation setzt sofort ein, kann aber den Durchblutungswert nur wenig verbessern. Entdrosselung ergibt reaktive Hyperämie bis auf 31 cm³/min (bei c), die nach 1 min 50 sec abgeklungen ist und (bei d) in eine längere Durchblutungssenkung übergeht (Rein 1951a).

Wiederanstieg der Durchblutung, der auf einer Verminderung des peripheren Strömungswiderstandes beruht (kompensatorische Dilatation). Entfernt man die Drossel, so schießt die Durchblutung über den Kontrollwert hinaus (reaktive

Mehrdurchblutung)[1]. Das Verhalten bei künstlicher Durchblutungsminderung ist also recht ähnlich wie in anderen Gefäßgebieten, etwa in den Gefäßen der Skeletmuskulatur: Die verminderte Durchblutung führt zu Änderungen von Stoffkonzentrationen im Gewebe, die dann vasomotorische Vorgänge auslösen (s. S. 640). Die Stoffwechsellage im Herzmuskel ist unter physiologischen Bedingungen der entscheidende Faktor für die Einstellung der Coronardurchblutung. Gegensätzliche experimentelle Befunde erklären sich weitgehend daraus, daß unter

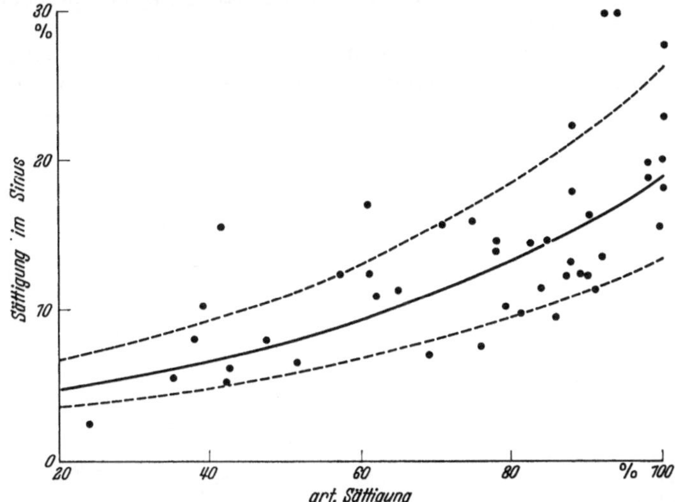

Abb. 38. Beziehung zwischen arterieller O_2-Sättigung und der O_2-Sättigung im Sinus coronarius. Die durchgehende Kurve gibt die Funktion berechnet für eine Kapazität von 25 Vol.-% und für einen mittleren Aortendruck von 100 mm Hg. Die gestrichelten Kurven entsprechen $\pm \bar{s}_{1,234}$. (ALELLA 1954b.)

den Bedingungen des Experimentes im Herzmuskelgewebe ein stärkerer Sauerstoffmangel herrschte und schon von Anfang an das Coronarsystem maximal erweitert war. Dann waren vasomotorische Regulationen nicht mehr möglich, und physikalische Faktoren wie Blutdruck und Gewebsdruck bestimmten allein die Coronardurchblutung. Ist in der Ausgangslage des Experimentes die Sauerstoffversorgung des Herzmuskels aber ausreichend, dann zeigt sich eine weitgehende Parallelität zwischen dem Sauerstoffbedarf des Herzmuskels und der Durchblutung[2]. Der Sauerstoffdruck im Gewebe ist der entscheidende, wenn auch nicht der alleinige chemische Faktor für die Einstellung der Coronardurchblutung. Auch andere Stoffe können an der Durchblutungseinstellung beteiligt sein. Jedoch fehlen uns noch nähere Kenntnisse über diese Mechanismen. Histamin, Acetylcholin, Abbauprodukte der Nucleinsäuren und eine große Reihe weiterer körpereigener Stoffe steigern die Coronardurchblutung, wenn man sie von der arteriellen Seite her dem Coronarsystem zuführt, womit aber noch nicht bewiesen ist, daß sie unter orthischen Bedingungen als Zwischenglieder zwischen dem Gewebsstoffwechsel und der Einstellung der Coronardurchblutung von Bedeutung sind[3].

Hypoxie kann im Gewebe durch verminderten Sauerstoffantransport oder durch erhöhten Sauerstoffverbrauch entstehen. Es wäre wichtig, den Sauerstoffgehalt oder Sauerstoffdruck im Gewebe als steuernden Faktor der Coronardurchblutung zu kennen. Da man ihn nicht direkt messen kann, sind Sauerstoff-

---

[1] REIN 1951.   [2] ALELLA 1958, BRETSCHNEIDER 1958.
[3] WEDD und DRURY 1934, GREENE 1936, MEESMANN und SCHMIER 1956a.

sättigung und Sauerstoffdruck im Coronarvenenblut ein guter Annäherungswert[1]. Freilich ist die Sauerstoffkonzentration im Gewebe als geregelte Größe voraussichtlich auch ein sehr wenig variabler Wert. Damit wird auch die Sauerstoffsättigung des Coronarsinusblutes relativ konstant gehalten, und es bedarf genauer Messungen, um die Beziehungen zwischen dieser Größe und der Coronardurchblutung feststellen zu können. Das zeigt sich deutlich in der Abhängigkeit zwischen arterieller O_2-Sättigung und der O_2-Sättigung des Coronarsinusblutes (Abb. 38). Starken Änderungen der arteriellen Sättigung entsprechen sehr viel geringere Änderungen im Sinusblut[2].

Bei jeder Art verminderten Sauerstoffangebotes von der arteriellen Seite her findet man ein Absinken des Strömungswiderstandes in der Peripherie des Coro-

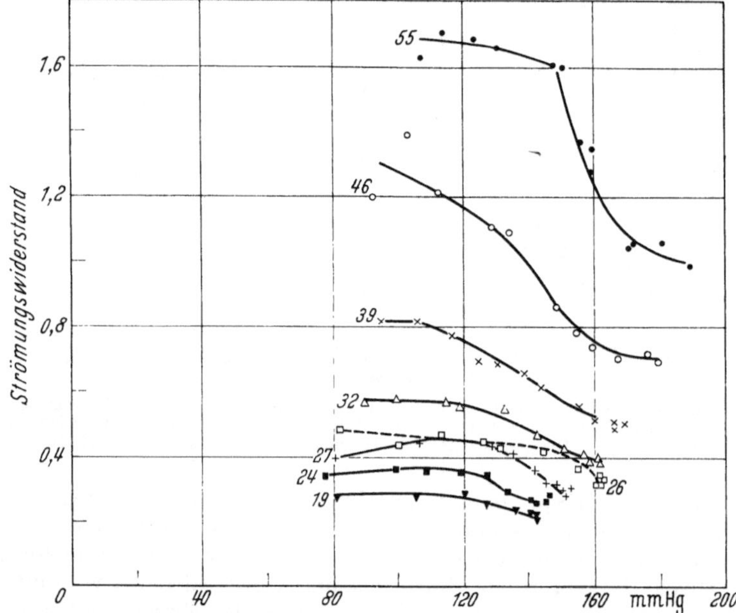

Abb. 39. Abhängigkeit des Strömungswiderstandes im Coronarsystem vom Hämatokrit und vom arteriellen Druck. Die Zahlen an den Kurven geben den Hämatokrit an. Die gestrichelte Linie verbindet Werte, die nach Reinfusion von Erythrocyten gefunden wurden. (Case, Berglund und Sarnoff 1955.)

narsystems. Dies zeigt sich besonders deutlich bei vermindertem Sauerstoffgehalt des arteriellen Blutes. Die Abb. 39 zeigt die Beziehungen zwischen arteriellem Druck und Strömungswiderstand im Coronarsystem bei anämischen Zuständen[3]. Besonders gründlich untersucht sind die Verhältnisse bei arterieller Sauerstoffuntersättigung[4]. Abb. 40 zeigt die Beziehungen zwischen der arteriellen Sättigung und der Leitfähigkeit (dem reziproken Wert des Strömungswiderstandes) im Coronarsystem.

Nicht nur ein vermindertes Sauerstoffangebot von der arteriellen Seite her, sondern auch ein erhöhter Sauerstoffverbrauch des Herzmuskels senkt die Sauerstoffkonzentration im Muskelgewebe. Es ist dies der funktionell entscheidende Faktor für die Anpassung der Herzdurchblutung an die Herzleistung. Gleichgültig ob der Energieumsatz des Herzens mit der Leistung ansteigt, weil der arterielle Druck oder weil das HZV erhöht ist, in jedem Falle steigt auch die

[1] Lochner und Mitarbeiter 1956a.   [2] Alella 1954b.
[2] Case und Mitarbeiter 1955.   [4] Alella 1954, 1955.

Herzdurchblutung an, vorausgesetzt, daß die regulatorischen Reserven noch nicht erschöpft sind. Abb. 41 zeigt die Beziehung zwischen dem Sauerstoffverbrauch des Herzmuskels und seiner Durchblutung[1]. In erster Linie muß die gute Beziehung zwischen diesen beiden Größen auf die steuernden Einflüsse des Gewebsstoffwechsels zurückgeführt werden. Sie zeigen sich besonders in Versuchen, bei denen der Aortendruck planmäßig verändert wurde. Werden in diesen Fällen Versuche mit gleichem Sauerstoffverbrauch des Herzens verglichen, so zeigt sich nur ein recht geringer Einfluß des

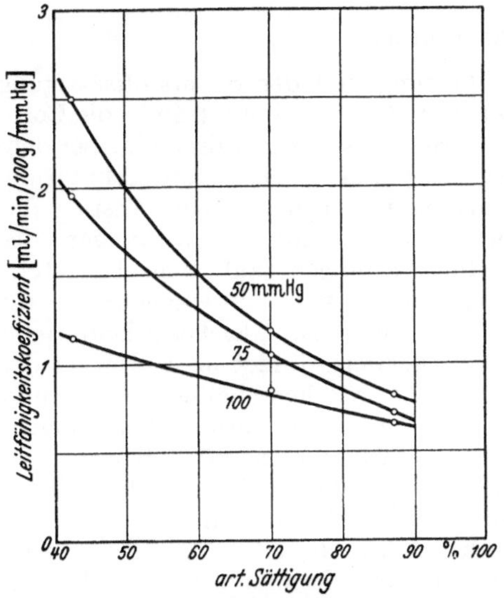

Abb. 40. Die „Leitfähigkeit" der Coronarien (= dem reziproken Werte des Strömungswiderstandes) in Abhängigkeit von der arteriellen O_2-Sättigung bei mittleren Aortendrucken. Mit sinkender arterieller Sättigung steigt die „Leitfähigkeit" an. (ALELLA 1956.)

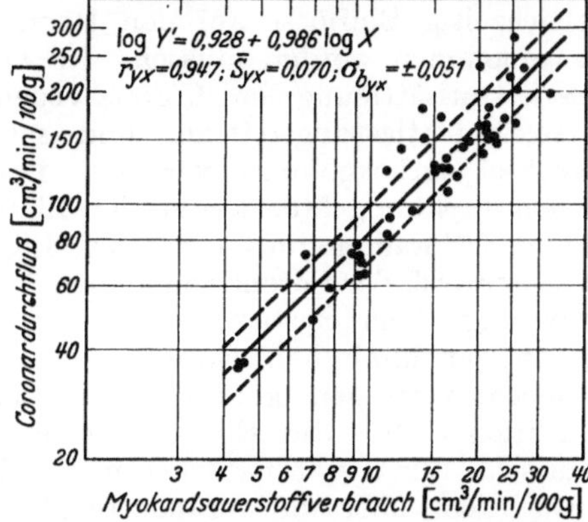

Abb. 41. Logarithmische Beziehung zwischen dem Sauerstoffverbrauch des Herzmuskels und der Coronardurchblutung. Ausgezogene Gerade: Regressionslinie nach der aufgezeichneten Gleichung; gestrichelte Geraden: mittlerer Fehler ($\pm$ S_{yx}). (ALELLA 1955.)

Aortendruckes auf die Coronardurchblutung. Die vom Herzstoffwechsel ausgelösten vasomotorischen Steuerungen gleichen die physikalischen Einflüsse des veränderten Druckgefälles weitgehend aus[2].

5. Hormonale und nervöse Einflüsse auf die Coronardurchblutung.

Für die Einstellung der Coronardurchblutung ist zweifelsohne der Einfluß des Gewebsstoffwechsels im Herzmuskel von entscheidender Bedeutung. Die Coronardurchblutung ist eine Stellgröße in einem Regelkreis, durch die die Konzentration bestimmter Stoffe im Gewebe geregelt wird. Wenn durch nervöse oder hormonale Einflüsse die Durchblutung der Coronarien verändert wird, ohne daß der Herzstoffwechsel im gleichen Sinne beeinflußt wird, so wird das Gleichgewicht zwischen Stoffwechsel und Durchblutung gestört, und Gegenreaktionen werden die äußeren Einwirkungen zum mindesten teilweise wieder aufheben. Zweifelsohne wird aber die Coronardurchblutung auch von außen her über Hormone und Nerven beeinflußt. Möglicherweise spielen solche Vorgänge auch bei der Anpassung der Coronardurchblutung an die veränderte Herzleistung bei Steigerung des HZV oder des arteriellen Druckes eine Rolle. Es ist jedoch nicht leicht, derartige Einflüsse nachzuweisen. Sieht man nach Hormongaben oder Nervenreizungen eine Steigerung der Coronardurchblutung, so braucht das kein direkter vasodilatatorischer Einfluß zu sein. Die äußeren Einflüsse können

---

[1] ECKENHOFF und Mitarbeiter 1947, ALELLA u. a. 1955, FOLTZ und Mitarbeiter 1950.
[2] ALELLA u. a. 1955.

auch primär den Herzstoffwechsel steigern, und die Mehrdurchblutung der Coronarien kann allein darauf zurückzuführen sein. Einen gewissen Anhalt gibt das Verhalten des Coronarvenenblutes. Ein Anstieg seines Sauerstoffdruckes spricht für einen primär dilatierenden Einfluß, während eine Senkung dieser Größe auf eine primäre Steigerung des Herzstoffwechsels hindeutet[1].

6. Chemische Einflüsse.

Nach Untersuchung der Coronardurchblutung und der Sauerstoffsättigung des Coronarvenenblutes muß man annehmen, daß Acetylcholin primär die Coronarien erweitert[2]. Schwieriger liegen die Verhältnisse beim Adrenalin, bei dem gleichzeitig Einflüsse auf den Herzstoffwechsel und die Coronardurchblutung angenommen werden müssen. Im allgemeinen findet man einen Anstieg der Sauerstoffsättigung im Coronarvenenblut. Dies ist auf Auswirkungen des Kreislaufentlastungsreflexes und seine Rückwirkungen auf den Herzstoffwechsel zurückgeführt worden[3]. Doch sprechen neuere Untersuchungen für einen direkten gefäßerweiternden Einfluß des Adrenalins. Gleiches scheint auch für das Noradrenalin zu gelten[4]. Eigentümlicherweise findet man also bei der Vasomotorik der Coronarien keinen Antagonismus zwischen cholinergischem und adrenergischem System, sondern in beiden Fällen Durchblutungssteigerungen. Nach der klinischen Erfahrung, daß Coronarpatienten nervöse Belastungen schlecht vertragen, könnte man erwarten, daß gerade nervös ausgelöste Konstriktionen für die Einstellung der Coronardurchblutung entscheidend sein müssen. Wir wissen natürlich nicht, ob nicht auch in diesen Fällen die Coronarinsuffizienz über die veränderte Herzdynamik und damit über den erhöhten Stoffwechsel der Herzmuskulatur zustande kommt. Das dürfte nicht selten der Fall sein. Es bleibt auffallend, daß im Experiment Coronarkonstriktionen kaum ausgelöst werden können. Eine Ausnahme macht allein das Hypophysin, wobei es vorläufig zweifelhaft bleibt, ob dieser Effekt nicht nur bei sehr hohen Dosierungen im Experiment zustande kommt, und ob für die Einstellung der Coronardurchblutung unter normalen und pathischen Bedingungen dieses Hormon wirklich eine Bedeutung hat.

Über die Pharmakologie der Coronardurchblutung sind neuere Arbeiten vorhanden, auf die ich verweisen möchte[5].

7. Nervöse Einflüsse auf die Coronardurchblutung.

Die Coronargefäße sind reichlich mit Nerven versorgt[6]. Nach den Ergebnissen von Degenerationsexperimenten handelt es sich bei den größeren arteriellen Ästen um vagale und sympathische Fasern, wobei die sympathische Innervation überwiegt. Dagegen werden die kleinen Arterien hauptsächlich vom Vagus aus mit Nerven versorgt. Es ist sehr schwierig, über den Einfluß dieser Nerven auf die Vasomotorik eine Aussage zu machen[7]. Experimentelle Untersuchungen mit Nervenausschaltung und nach Nervenreizung verändern fast regelmäßig auch die Herzdynamik und den Herzstoffwechsel, so daß Durchblutungsänderungen darauf zurückgeführt werden können. Anscheinend verlaufen über den Vagus haupt-

---

[1] Lochner und Mitarbeiter 1956a.
[2] Folkow u. a. 1948, Lochner und Mitarbeiter 1956, Wégria 1951, Heidenreich und Schmidt 1956a.
[3] Gollwitzer-Meier und Kroetz 1939, 1940, Gollwitzer-Meier und Witzleb 1952.
[4] Lochner u. a. 1956b, Feinberg und Katz 1958.
[5] Wégria 1951, Lochner u. a. 1956b, Mercker, Lochner und Bretschneider 1958.
[6] Woollard 1925.   [7] Witzleb 1958.

sächlich cholinergische Fasern mit vasodilatatorischer Wirkung, über den Grenz-strang adrenergische Fasern, die teils eine dilatatorische, teils eine constrictorische Wirkung entfalten [1].

Nach klinischen Erfahrungen möchte man annehmen, daß die Herznerven wichtige reflektorische Einflüsse auf die Herzdurchblutung ausüben, wobei es sowohl zu einer Verbesserung als auch zu einer Verschlechterung der Herzdurch-blutung kommen kann. Die vielen in dieser Richtung angestellten Experimente geben noch keine befriedigende Antwort, denn alle ausgelösten Reflexe beein-flussen gleichzeitig die Herzdynamik und den Herzstoffwechsel [2]. Die Experimente erlauben aber auch nicht den gegensätzlichen Schluß, daß keine primäre reflek-torische Beeinflussung der Herzdurchblutung möglich wäre. Von Interesse sind neue Untersuchungen an Hunden, bei denen zur Beurteilung der Coronardurch-blutung Thermoelektroden eingeheilt waren. Durch elektrische Hautreizung hervorgerufener Schmerz führte zunächst zu einer Verminderung, später zu einer Steigerung der Coronardurchblutung. Bei Zuständen von Furcht war die Coronar-durchblutung vermindert. Es zeigt also hier das Tierexperiment Parallelen zur Auslösung von Angina pectoris durch Emotionen beim Menschen [3].

Von klinischer Seite ist wiederholt behauptet worden, daß Verschluß einzelner Coronaräste reflektorisch zu Vasoconstriction in anderen Abschnitten des Coronar-systems führt. Doch gibt es hierfür keine experimentellen Bestätigungen. Ver-schluß einzelner Coronaräste führt im Gegenteil häufig zu einer verstärkten Durch-blutung der übrigen Äste, was wohl auf interarterielle Anastomosen bezogen werden muß [4].

II. Störungen der Coronardurchblutung.

Die Darstellung der schwerwiegendsten Veränderungen der Coronardurch-blutung infolge Sklerose, Angitis, Thrombose, Infarkt usw. obliegt in erster Linie dem Pathologen. Dabei handelt es sich nicht mehr um eine deskriptive Behandlung des morphologischen Substrates allein, vielmehr stehen die viel-fältigen Fragen der Pathogenese dieser Störungen im Vordergrund pathologisch-anatomischer Forschung. Insofern ist eine morphologische Betrachtung von einer funktionellen nicht zu trennen, wie dies besonders die Arbeiten von BÜCHNER und seiner Schule für die coronaren Durchblutungsstörungen dargetan haben. Im Rahmen dieser Übersicht kann es sich im wesentlichen nur darum handeln, Art und Vorkommen coronarer Durchblutungsstörungen auf funktioneller Basis kurz aufzuzeigen und die Frage zu erörtern, ob sich bei solchen Störungen der Durchblutung Beziehungen zwischen der Größe der Durchblutung und anderen Kreislaufgrößen nachweisen lassen.

Wie aus dem orthisch-funktionellen Teil über die Coronardurchblutung und die Herzenergetik hervorgeht, ist die coronare Durchblutung normalerweise so abge-stimmt, daß die Herzmuskelfasern ausreichend ernährt werden. Während aber bei anderen Organen eine Steigerung der arterio-venösen O_2-Differenz und damit eine stärkere Ausschöpfung des Sauerstoffs bei gleichbleibender Durchblutung möglich ist, ist dies beim Herzen nur in geringem Maße der Fall. Dafür sind die Regulationen im Bereich des Coronarsystems besser ausgeprägt, um die erforderliche Durchblutung des Herzmuskels unter Normalbelastung zu garan-tieren. Störungen im Bereich dieses fein abgestimmten Regulationssystems müssen sich um so folgenschwerer auswirken.

Coronare Durchblutungsstörungen werden auch unter dem Sammelbegriff *Coronarinsuffizienz* zusammengefaßt. Diesen Störungen kommt tatsächlich das

---

[1] KATZ und JOCHIM 1939, HEIDENREICH und SCHMIDT 1956b.   [2] GREGG 1950.
[3] MARSHAK und ARANOVA 1957.   [4] MEESMANN 1958 (Literatur).

Prädikat „*Insuffizienz*" zu, da bereits geringe Abweichungen der Durchblutung von der Norm genügen, um eine akute Ernährungsnot des Herzmuskels zu erzeugen. Freilich sind auch hierbei die Größenordnungen der Durchblutung immer nur in Relation zu der jeweilig geforderten Leistung zu setzen. Man kann dann ganz allgemein von einer Coronarinsuffizienz sprechen, wenn ein Mißverhältnis von Durchblutung und Blutbedarf des Herzmuskels besteht. Es erscheint zweckmäßig, eine „lokalisierte" Coronarinsuffizienz von einer „generellen" Coronarinsuffizienz abzugrenzen.

1. Lokalisierte Coronarinsuffizienz.

Als solche können Zustände von lokal begrenztem O_2-Mangel im Herzen infolge krankhafter Prozesse an den Coronargefäßen oder Fehlsteuerungen der coronaren Durchblutung bezeichnet werden. Wir können schematisch gesehen etwa drei verschiedene Schweregrade unterscheiden[1].

1. Eine infolge einer geringen Minderdurchblutung eintretende Hypoxie des Herzmuskels bewirkt noch keine morphologisch faßbaren bzw. bleibenden Veränderungen des Herzmuskels. Es kommt aber bereits zur Ansammlung von pathologischen Stoffwechselprodukten, die zu einer Reizung der Schmerzreceptoren führen. Werden diese Stoffwechselprodukte durch eine „reaktive" Hyperämie wieder fortgespült, so ist der pectanginöse Anfall beendet, es resultiert keine bleibende Schädigung. Diese Störungen werden vielfach als *Angina pectoris vasomotorica* bezeichnet, womit ihr funktioneller Charakter gekennzeichnet werden soll. Mit dem Ausdruck Angina pectoris vasomotorica wird häufig die Vorstellung von Gefäßspasmen verbunden. Wie weiter unten noch dargelegt werden soll, ist gegenüber der Anwendung des Begriffes Coronarspasmus eine gewisse Zurückhaltung am Platze.

2. Handelt es sich um organisch bedingte Störungen der coronaren Durchblutung in den Endaufzweigungen der Coronargefäße (z. B. Sklerose der distalen Gefäßabschnitte im Gefolge einer Hypertonie), so kommt es zu engumschriebenen bleibenden Durchblutungsstörungen, die Zellnekrosen hinterlassen. Diese treten meist multipel und nacheinander auf, es resultiert als Endergebnis das Bild der Myodegeneratio cordis. Pectanginöse Beschwerden können fehlen, da sich die Prozesse langsam abspielen und die Nekroseherde sehr klein sind.

3. Kommt es zu einem größeren Verschluß eines Coronargefäßes, so entsteht das Bild des akut bedrohlichen Herzinfarktes.

Im Vordergrund der oben genannten Störungen steht pathophysiologisch die Frage nach dem Vorkommen und der Bedeutung von *Coronarspasmen*. Schon beim peripheren Gefäßsystem, bei dem der Nachweis von Spasmen durch direkte Beobachtung möglich ist, erscheint die Bedeutung der Spasmen als Ursache oder als Begleitsymptom einer Durchblutungsstörung umstritten (s. periphere Durchblutungsstörungen). Bei den Coronargefäßen ist die Situation noch schwieriger. Man ist hier allein auf Analogieschlüsse angewiesen. Schon der anatomische Aufbau der Coronargefäße gestaltet die Bedingungen für das Zustandekommen von Spasmen ungünstiger als an den peripheren Gefäßen. Nur die kleinen intramuskulären Aufzweigungen der Coronararterien zeigen den rein muskulären Typ. Im Stamm und in den großen Ästen findet sich dagegen eine sehr stark entwickelte Intima, die stellenweise die Dicke der Media übertrifft, und die in ihrer inneren Schicht Längsmuskelfasern enthält. Eine Elastica externa fehlt. Die Media im Stamm und den großen Gefäßen der Coronararterien nimmt einen kleineren Teil

---

[1] Hauss 1954.

des Querschnittes der Wand ein als die gleichstarker Arterien. Die Zahl ihrer Muskelfasern ist kleiner als die anderer Arterien gleichen Querschnitts. Dies bedeutet, daß die Kranzarterien funktionell betrachtet als muskelschwache Gefäße anzusehen sind. Die Beeinflußbarkeit der Coronardurchblutung durch „aktive" Veränderungen der Weite der Coronararterien ist im physiologischen Bereich und bei funktionellen Durchblutungsstörungen sicher nicht gering (s. Orthologie der Coronardurchblutung). Jedoch fällt die Vorstellung schwer, daß Coronarspasmen allein eine Ischämie bestimmter Herzmuskelabschnitte herbeiführen. Bei den sog. „funktionellen" Durchblutungsstörungen der Herzkranzgefäße sollte über dem „Spasmus" die Bedeutung von Steigerungen der Pulsfrequenz und Absinken des Blutdrucks nicht übersehen werden. Die Bedeutung von Coronarspasmen als Ursache von Durchblutungsstörungen des Herzmuskels ist vor allem von den tierexperimentellen und klinischen Beobachtungen bci stumpfen Herztraumen (Commotio cordis) abgeleitet worden[1]. Abgesehen davon, daß die im Anschluß an ein stumpfes Herztrauma auftretenden Durchblutungsstörungen z. T. direkte Folge einer Prellwirkung auf den Herzmuskel sind, die zu Capillarzerreißungen führen können, dürfen die hierbei auftretenden Durchblutungsstörungen des Herzens nicht ohne weiteres auf Spasmen zurückgeführt werden. Die im Anschluß an solche stumpfen Gewalteinwirkungen auftretenden funktionellen Störungen in Form von Arrhythmien, Blutdruckabfall mit eventuell nachfolgendem Kollaps sind so schwerwiegend, daß hierdurch allein coronare Durchblutungsstörungen stärkeren Grades zustande kommen können. Auch muß betont werden, daß auf Grund der zahlreichen pathologischen Befunde bisher kein eindeutiger Beweis dafür vorliegt, daß ein Coronarspasmus ohne gleichzeitige pathologisch-anatomische Veränderungen der Coronargefäße einen Infarkt mit bleibender Nekrose herbeiführt[2]. Manches spricht dafür, daß ein Begleitspasmus bei vorhandenen anatomischen Veränderungen der Gefäße die Katastrophe auslösen kann. Bewiesen erscheint diese gemeinhin als selbstverständlich geltende These bisher nicht. Die Analogieschlüsse, von denen aus die Notwendigkeit des Bestehens von Coronarspasmen abgeleitet wird, sind nicht ganz überzeugend. Liegen anatomische Veränderungen der Gefäße vor, so können schon geringe Veränderungen der Herztätigkeit wie Blutdruckänderungen, Veränderungen der Pulsfrequenz oder gar Arrhythmien die Infarktkatastrophe herbeiführen, ohne daß ein Spasmus eintreten müßte. Daß beim Zustandekommen des Infarktes funktionelle Störungen eine wesentliche Rolle mitspielen können, liegt auf der Hand. Mit der Annahme eines Spasmus sollte man jedoch vorsichtiger sein, als es üblich ist.

Zu erwähnen ist noch die Bedeutung interarterieller Anastomosen bei eintretender Ischämie des Herzmuskels[3]. Wie die Erfahrungen der Pathologie zeigen, ist die Größe eines Infarktbezirkes häufig kleiner, als es dem regelhaften Versorgungsbereich des von der Blutzufuhr abgeschnittenen Coronararterienastes entspricht. Wie auch aus tierexperimentellen Untersuchungen eindeutig hervorgeht, sind die Herzkranzgefäße keine Endarterien im strengen Sinne. Auf die Bedeutung der arteriellen Anastomosen bei chronischer Hypoxie wurde bereits im funktionellen Teil hingewiesen.

Messungen der Coronardurchblutung bei Patienten mit Coronarinfarkt liegen bisher nur in sehr geringer Zahl vor (besondere Gefährdung der Patienten durch Katheterisierung des Coronarvenensinus!). In einem Falle wurde nach einem Infarkt eine Erniedrigung ($58\ cm^3$ je 100 g Herzmuskel und min) festgestellt[4]. Ob eine solche Erniedrigung der Coronardurchblutung im Anschluß an einen Infarkt die Regel ist, muß dahingestellt bleiben.

---

[1] SCHLOMKA 1934.   [2] BÜCHNER 1956.
[3] ECKSTEIN 1955.   [4] BING und Mitarbeiter 1949.

2. Generelle Coronarinsuffizienz.

Bei dieser Form der Coronarinsuffizienz kommt es zu einer Hypoxie des Herzmuskels, die nicht auf bestimmt abzugrenzende Bezirke eines Coronararteriengebietes beschränkt ist, sondern sich auf größere Gebiete des Herzmuskels oder gleichmäßig auf den gesamten Herzmuskel erstreckt. Dabei kann der Coronarkreislauf und seine Regulation intakt sein. Diese Form der Coronarinsuffizienz ist häufig sekundär und liegt außerhalb des Herzens (z. B. allgemeiner O_2-Mangel, Anämie). Durch die Bezeichnung Coronarinsuffizienz wird hierbei nur das Mißverhältnis zwischen Blutbedarf und Durchblutung zum Ausdruck gebracht. Graduell sind die Erscheinungen des O_2-Mangels bei dieser Form der Coronarinsuffizienz wesentlich geringer als bei der ischämischen Nekrose.

a) Coronarinsuffizienz durch Erniedrigung der arteriellen O_2-Spannung.

Im akuten O_2-Mangel tritt in etwa 7000—8000 m Höhe eine Hypoxie des Herzmuskels auf, die meist auch elektrokardiographisch faßbar ist[1]. Bei Herz- oder Kreislaufgeschädigten werden schon vorhandene elektrokardiographische Zeichen der Hypoxie in Höhen von 4000—5000 m manifest. In der Klinik kommen solche Zustände von Hypoxie des Herzmuskels durch Hypoxämie bei ausgedehnten Pneumonien, Bronchopneumonie, Emphysem, Asthma bronchiale, Lungenödem, offenem Pneumothorax vor. Hierbei wirkt sich eine Kombination einer toxischen Herzmuskelschädigung mit der durch O_2-Mangel bedingten weiteren Schädigung besonders ungünstig aus. Quantitative Angaben über die Größe der Coronardurchblutung bei solchen Zuständen können bisher für den Menschen nicht gemacht werden, da entsprechende Untersuchungen fehlen.

b) Coronarinsuffizienz bei Anämien.

Hierbei liegt eine Reihe von Untersuchungen über die Größe der Coronardurchblutung am Menschen vor[2], die mit den tierexperimentellen Befunden in Einklang stehen. Bei akuten Anämien nach Blutverlust konnten Beziehungen zwischen der Größe der Coronardurchblutung und dem Kreislaufminutenvolumen festgestellt werden. Je größer das Kreislaufminutenvolumen, um so höher die Coronardurchblutung. Auch in anderen Untersuchungen fanden sich bei chronischen hypochromen Anämien Erhöhungen der Coronardurchblutung. Bei Anämien mittleren Grades (Hb 8—9 g-%) wurden Erhöhungen der Coronardurchblutung bis zu 50% festgestellt. Im Mittel ist der Anstieg der Coronardurchblutung jedoch geringer (etwa 20—30%). Trotz der Erhöhung der Coronardurchblutung fand sich bei diesen Anämiegraden bereits eine leichte Senkung des O_2-Verbrauchs des Herzens als Ausdruck einer Hypoxie des Herzmuskels (s. Abb. 42). Bei schwereren Graden von Anämie sind die Zeichen hypoxischer Schädigung des Herzmuskels (Senkung des O_2-Verbrauchs) wahrscheinlich ausgeprägter.

c) Coronarinsuffizienz bei Kollaps (s. unter Kollaps, S. 692).

d) Coronarinsuffizienz bei Überlastung des Herzens. Akute Überlastung.

Tierexperimentelle Untersuchungen haben ergeben, daß bei übermäßigen körperlichen Anstrengungen hypoxische Herzmuskelnekrosen auftreten können[3]. Bei Lungenembolien soll es infolge plötzlicher Drucksteigerung im Lungenkreislauf und Überlastung des rechten Ventrikels zu einer akuten Coronarinsuffizienz

---

[1] Lichti 1934, Opitz und Tillmann 1936.
[2] Bing und Mitarbeiter 1949.   [3] Büchner 1939.

des rechten Herzens kommen. Es ist aber noch nicht zu übersehen, inwieweit beim Zustandekommen der coronaren Durchblutungsstörungen im Gefolge von Lungenembolien Kollapserscheinungen mit Absinken des Kreislaufminutenvolumens und Sauerstoffmangel mit beteiligt oder gar ausschlaggebend sind[1].

e) Chronische Überlastung (s. auch S. 741).

Hierbei liegt mittlerweile eine Reihe von Messungen der Coronardurchblutung beim Menschen vor[2].

Bei der *Hypertonie* wurde die Coronardurchblutung (berechnet auf Gramm Herzgewicht) im Bereich der Norm gefunden. Diese Feststellung steht im Gegen-

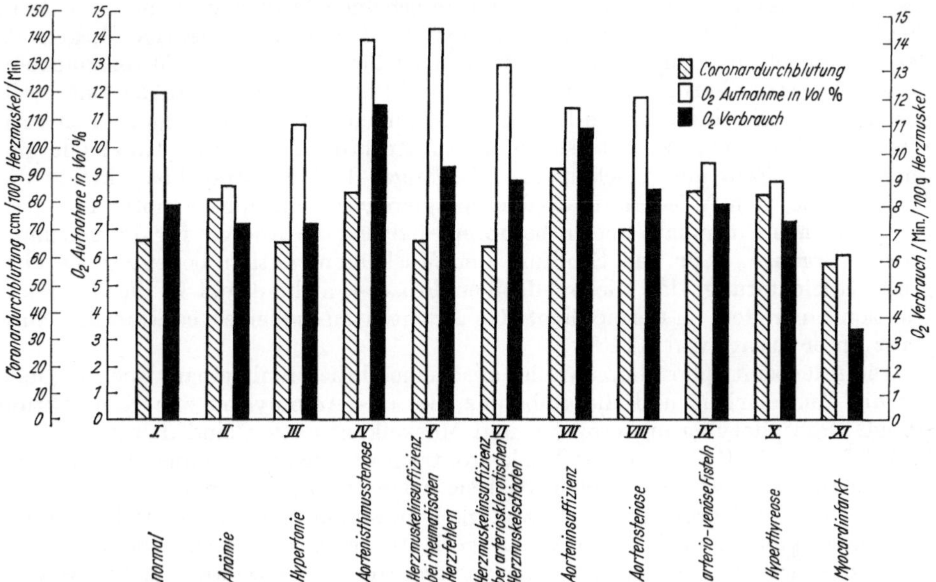

Abb. 42. Coronardurchblutung des linken Ventrikels (pro 100 g und min), O₂-Ausnutzung und O₂-Verbrauch des linken Ventrikels (pro 100 g und min) bei verschiedenen Patientengruppen. (BING u. a. 1949.)

satz zu den Befunden im akuten Tierexperiment, in dem bei plötzlicher Blutdrucksteigerung die Coronardurchblutung zunimmt[3]. Wahrscheinlich begrenzen die anatomischen Verhältnisse beim Hypertoniker die Durchblutung. Im Gegensatz zur Hypertonie der Erwachsenen wurde in mehreren Fällen von *Aortenisthmusstenose* bei Jugendlichen eine erhöhte Coronardurchblutung festgestellt. Man darf folgern, daß bei diesen jungen Patienten das Gefäßsystem noch anpassungsfähiger ist, so daß die auch im Tierexperiment auftretenden Erhöhungen der Coronardurchblutung bei Steigerung des Aortendrucks in solchen Fällen zum Ausdruck kommen.

Bei *Aortenklappeninsuffizienz* wurde in Übereinstimmung mit tierexperimentellen Befunden[4] eine Erhöhung der Coronardurchblutung am Menschen festgestellt. In einem Fall von *Aortenklappenstenose* war die Coronardurchblutung normal. Der Patient klagte aber bei Arbeit über pectanginöse Beschwerden, so daß eine Coronarinsuffizienz bei Belastung sicherlich vorgelegen hat. Bei tierexperimentell erzeugter Aortenklappenstenose wurde eine Erniedrigung der

[1] MEESSEN 1940.   [2] BING und Mitarbeiter 1949.
[3] GREGG und SHIPLEY 1947.   [4] GREEN und GREGG 1940.

Coronardurchblutung gefunden[1]. Bei *arterio-venösen Fisteln* im großen Kreislauf wurde eine eindeutige Erhöhung der Coronardurchblutung festgestellt, ebenso bei *Basedow*.

Über die Beziehungen zwischen coronarer Durchblutung, arterio-venöser O_2-Differenz und O_2-Verbrauch des Herzens bei den genannten Krankheiten gibt die Abb. 42 Auskunft.

III. Die Energetik des Herzens.

In der Feinstruktur und in den physikalisch-chemischen Eigenschaften unterscheidet sich die contractile Substanz des Herzmuskels nicht wesentlich von der des Skeletmuskels[2]. Gewisse Unterschiede scheinen freilich vorhanden zu sein. So soll das Molekulargewicht des Myosins aus dem Herzen niedriger liegen als das des Skeletmuskelmyosins[3]. Auffallend ist der Reichtum an Mitochondrien, die als Träger der Fermente für Oxydation und Phosphorylierung in der Energetik des Herzmuskels eine zentrale Stellung einnehmen[4]. Bei den energetischen Prozessen sind 3 Vorgänge zu unterscheiden: Substratabbau, Auf- und Abbau energiereicher Phosphate und mechanische Vorgänge. Der Substratabbau liefert die Energie, die zum Wiederaufbau der energiereichen Phosphate nötig ist. Die energiereichen Phosphate liefern bei ihrer Spaltung die Energie für die mechanischen Vorgänge. Für das Studium der Muskelkontraktion bedeutete es eine große Erleichterung, daß die oxydativen Prozesse nicht direkt in die der Kontraktion eingreifen. Es ermöglicht das Arbeiten an isolierter contractiler Substanz unter Zusatz von ATP[5].

Die Adenosintriphosphorsäure ist anscheinend die unmittelbare Energiequelle für die Muskelarbeit und die Substanz, die das Actomyosin zur Kontraktion bringt. Phosphorylierungsprozesse und Muskelkontraktion sind damit eng verknüpft[6]. Die ATP-Theorie der Muskelkontraktion wird nicht ohne Widerspruch hingenommen. Wahrscheinlich bedarf sie weiterer Ergänzungen[7].

Die gesamte Energie für die Herztätigkeit entstammt letzten Endes dem Abbau von Substraten. Der Substratabbau verläuft im Herzen nicht anders wie in anderen Geweben[8]. Er erfolgt teils anoxydativ, teils oxydativ. Beim Warmblüterherzen reichen die anoxydativen Prozesse zur Deckung des Energiebedarfs bei weitem nicht aus. Die Sicherung der Sauerstoffzufuhr ist damit Grundbedingung der Herzenergetik.

1. Die energieliefernden Stoffe.

Die Frage, welche Substrate vom Herzmuskel zur Energiegewinnung verwendet werden, ist zunächst an Herzschnitten und am isolierten Herzen untersucht worden. Jetzt sind solche Untersuchungen aber auch am Herzen in situ — sogar am Menschen — möglich, indem man den Coronarsinus katheterisiert und mit der Stickoxydulmethode die Durchblutung des linken Ventrikels bestimmt[9]. Messungen an nicht narkotisierten Patienten ohne Herzinsuffizienz ergaben im Mittel die Zahlen der Tabelle 16[10]. Die angeführten Werte sind Sauerstoffextraktionsquotienten, die nach der Formel

$$\frac{\text{Entnahme von Substanzen} \times O_2\text{-Äquivalent}}{O_2\text{-Verbrauch}}$$

[1] Green und Gregg 1940. [2] Szent Györgyi 1953, Ranney 1955.
[3] Olson 1956. [4] Lehninger 1953. [5] Szent Györgyi 1953.
[6] Szent Györgyi 1953, 1956, Weber und Portzehl 1952.
[7] Fleckenstein 1955, Morales u. a. 1956. [8] Krebs 1954.
[9] Bing und Mitarbeiter 1949. [10] Bing 1955, 1956.

berechnet wurden. Die Bedeutung dieses Ausdruckes ist einfach, wenn man annimmt, daß die vom Herzen aufgenommenen Stoffe sofort und vollständig oxydiert werden. Finden Speicherungs- und Umwandlungsprozesse von Nahrungsstoffen statt, dann wird auch chemische Energie gespeichert. Auch der aufgenommene Sauerstoff ist dann an den Prozessen der Speicherung und Stoffumwandlung beteiligt und dient nicht allein der Energiegewinnung für die mechanischen Leistungen des Herzens. Nach Zufuhr größerer Mengen von Fettsäuren in der Nahrung steigt der Sauerstoffextraktionsquotient der Fettsäuren auf über 100% an. Dies kann nur auf der Grundlage einer Fettsäurespeicherung erklärt werden[1] (s. u.).

Wie Tabelle 16 zeigt, wird nur ein Drittel des oxydativen Stoffwechsels durch Verbrennung von Kohlenhydraten gedeckt[2]. Der übrige Teil besteht aus Nichtkohlenhydraten. Von den verbrauchten Kohlenhydraten fällt etwa die Hälfte auf Glucose, die andere auf Milchsäure. Dies ist eine Bestätigung älterer Befunde am isolierten Herzen, die schon die Fähigkeit des Herzens zeigten, Milchsäure in starkem Maße zur Deckung des Energiebedarfes heranzuziehen. Im einzelnen Fall hängt die Art des verbrauchten Substrats in erster Linie vom Substratangebot, d. h. von den arteriellen Konzentrationen der Stoffe ab[3]. Größe und Art der Herzarbeit und Größe der Coronardurchblutung sind ohne Einfluß auf die Auswahl der vom Herzen verbrannten Stoffe. Die Abhängigkeit der Stoffaufnahme vom arteriellen Angebot gilt besonders für Glucose und Milchsäure[4]. Bei arteriellen Glucosekonzentrationen unter 80 mg-% beträgt die coronare arterio-venöse Konzentrationsdifferenz weniger als 4 mg-%. Steigt die arterielle Glucosekonzentration an, so erhöht sich die Extraktion rasch und erreicht ihren Maximalwert bei Konzentrationen von etwa 110 mg-%. Bei leichteren Graden von Hypoxie und bei schwerer Muskeltätigkeit steigt die Milchsäurekonzentration im Blut, und damit wird auch ein größerer Teil des Energiebedarfs des Herzmuskels durch Lactatabbau gedeckt. Auch Brenztraubensäure wird vom Herzmuskel verbrannt. Wegen der niedrigen arteriellen Konzentration dieses Stoffes spielt die Verbrennung der Brenztraubensäure für die Energiebilanz keine entscheidende Rolle. BING sieht aber in der Brenztraubensäurebilanz des Herzens einen empfindlichen Indicator für Störungen des Myokardstoffwechsels bei Ischämie und Hypoxie. In solchen Fällen wird die Brenztraubensäurekonzentration des Coronarvenenblutes höher als die des arteriellen Blutes. Es wird dann also vom Herzmuskel nicht mehr Brenztraubensäure aus dem Blut aufgenommen und verbrannt, sondern im Gewebe gebildet und an das Blut abgegeben. BING denkt dabei an eine Störung der Cocarboxylaseaktivität. Dieses Co-Ferment wird unter anaeroben Bedingungen durch Dephosphorylierungsprozesse zerstört[5].

Auch bei den Nichtkohlenhydraten besteht eine starke Beziehung zwischen der Substratkonzentration im arteriellen Blut und der Substrataufnahme durch den Herzmuskel. Steigert man den Fettsäuregehalt des Blutes durch fettreiche Ernährung, so findet man für die Fettsäuren Sauerstoff-Extraktionsquotienten

Tabelle 16. *Die relative Beteiligung von Kohlenhydraten und Nichtkohlenhydraten am Gesamtsauerstoffverbrauch des Herzmuskels.* (BING 1956.)

Kohlenhydrate in %		Nichtkohlenhydrate in %	
Glucose	17,90	Fettsäuren	67,0
Brenztraubensäure	0,54	Aminosäuren	5,6
Milchsäure	16,46	Ketonkörper	4,3
Insgesamt	34,90	Insgesamt	76,9

---

[1] BING u. a. 1954.   [2] BING 1955, 1956.   [3] RÜHL 1934.
[4] GOODALE und HACKEL 1953, BING u. a. 1953, ALELLA u. a. 1956.
[5] BING u. a. 1953, EDUARDS u. a. 1954.

im Herzmuskel von über 100%. Die hohe Fettsäureaufnahme ist in diesen Fällen nicht nur durch die Erhöhung des Fettsäurestoffwechsels, sondern auch durch die Fettspeicherung bedingt[1]. Daß der Herzmuskel befähigt ist, Fettsäuren abzubauen, konnte auch an Herzmuskelpräparationen gezeigt werden. Die Herzmitochondrien können Acetat in seine aktive Form umwandeln und damit für eine Oxydation aller Glieder des Citronensäurecyclus sorgen[2]. Die niedrigen R Q, die am isolierten Herzen häufig gefunden wurden, wiesen schon immer auf die große Bedeutung der Fettverbrennung als Energiequelle des Herzens hin. Bing nimmt an, daß schon bei einem leichten Abfall der zirkulierenden Kohlenhydrate der größte Teil der Energieproduktion des Herzens durch Fett aufrechterhalten wird. Schon im nüchternen Zustand der Morgenstunden sollen $^3/_5$ der Energieproduktion aus dem Fettstoffwechsel gedeckt werden.

Im Unterschied zum isolierten Herzen kann das Herz in situ auch große Mengen von Aminosäuren aus dem Coronarblut aufnehmen. Nach Infusion von Aminosäuren fallen bis zu 40% des gesamten kardialen Sauerstoffverbrauchs auf die Verbrennung von Aminosäuren. Auch Ketonkörper werden vom Herzmuskel umgesetzt. Dies ist besonders für den Herzstoffwechsel des diabetischen Patienten bedeutungsvoll[1].

2. Die Sauerstoffversorgung des Herzens.

Der Herzmuskel kann zur Energiegewinnung die verschiedensten Substrate heranziehen. Dadurch ist die Versorgung des Herzens mit Substrat fast in jedem Fall gesichert. Das Warmblüterherz kann aber nur zum ganz geringen Teil seinen Energiebedarf durch anoxydativen Substratabbau decken. Damit wird die Frage der Sauerstoffversorgung entscheidend für die gesamte Herzenergetik. Die häufigste Ursache für ihr Versagen ist die Hypoxie des Herzgewebes.

Tabelle 17 bringt Werte über Sauerstoffverbrauch und Sauerstoffversorgung des menschlichen linken Ventrikels. Es sind Mittelwerte, die an vier kreislaufgesunden Patienten gewonnen wurden[3]. Das venöse Herzblut wurde durch Katheterisierung des Coronarsinus gewonnen. Die Durchblutung des linken Ventrikels wurde mit der Stickoxydulmethode bestimmt. Die Werte stehen in gutem Einklang mit denen anderer Untersuchungen, besonders recht zahlreichen Untersuchungen, die an Hunden vorgenommen wurden[4].

In Tabelle 17 sind zum Vergleich die Werte für die Sauerstoffversorgung des Gehirns angeführt[5]. Das Gehirn ist ja das andere Organ, bei dem die dauernde Sicherung der Sauerstoffversorgung für den Organismus lebensnotwendig ist.

Tabelle 17. *Werte über Sauerstoffversorgung und Sauerstoffverbrauch des menschlichen linken Ventrikels.*

Mittelwerte von 4 Versuchspersonen (Bing u. a. 1949). O_2-Druck des Coronarsinusblutes nomographisch bestimmt (Opitz u. Thews 1952). Im Vergleich dazu Werte für das menschliche Gehirn (Kety u. Schmidt 1948).

	Linker Ventrikel	Gehirn
Coronarsinusblut bzw. Jugularvenenblut		
O_2-Gehalt Vol.-%	5	11
O_2-Sättigung %	28	62
O_2-Druck mm Hg	18	33
Arterio-venöse O_2-Differenz Vol.-%	12	6
Durchblutung von 100 g Gewebe ml/100 g/min	65	54
O_2-Verbrauch von 100 g Gewebe ml/100 g/min	7,8	3,3

---

[1] Bing u. a. 1954.   [2] Ochoa 1944.   [3] Bing u. a. 1949.
[4] Gregg 1950, Mercker, Lochner und Bretschneider 1958.
[5] Kety und Schmidt 1948.

Das Herz kann die Sauerstofftransportfunktion des Blutes sehr viel stärker ausnutzen als das Gehirn. Die arterio-venöse Sauerstoffdifferenz ist doppelt so groß. Sauerstoffsättigung und Sauerstoffdruck liegen im Coronarsinusblut sehr viel niedriger als im Blut der V. jugularis interna.

Wenn andere Organe, etwa Haut oder Niere, den Blutsauerstoff schlecht ausnützen, so erklärt sich das damit, daß bei diesen Organen die Durchblutung gar nicht nach dem Sauerstoffbedarf der Organe eingestellt ist, da in diesen Fällen die Durchblutung anderen Zwecken als der Sauerstoffversorgung dient. Wenn beim Gehirn die Sauerstoffaus-nutzung des Blutes so viel schlechter ist als beim Herzen, so beruht das wohl zum Teil auf dem komplizierten Aufbau des Hirngewebes, wobei der Sauerstoffverbrauch der einzelnen Gewebs- und Zellabschnitte sehr verschieden ist und sehr rasch wechseln kann. Dagegen wird beim Herzmuskel entsprechend der gleichmäßigen Verteilung der Mitochondrien über das gesamte Gewebe der Sauerstoff ziemlich gleichmäßig im gesamten Gewebe des Herzens verbraucht. Der Hauptunterschied zwischen der Sauerstoffversorgung des Gehirns und des Herzens scheint aber darin zu liegen, daß die Sauerstoffversorgung des Herzens in stärkerem Maße durch steuernde Einflüsse dem Sauerstoffbedarf angepaßt werden kann, als das beim Gehirn der Fall ist. Die Capillarisierung des Herzens ist besser als die des Hirngewebes. Bei Eröffnung der Reservecapillaren kommen beim Herzen auf 1 cm³ Gewebe 11000 m Capillaren, in der Hirnrinde aber nur 870 m[1]. Noch

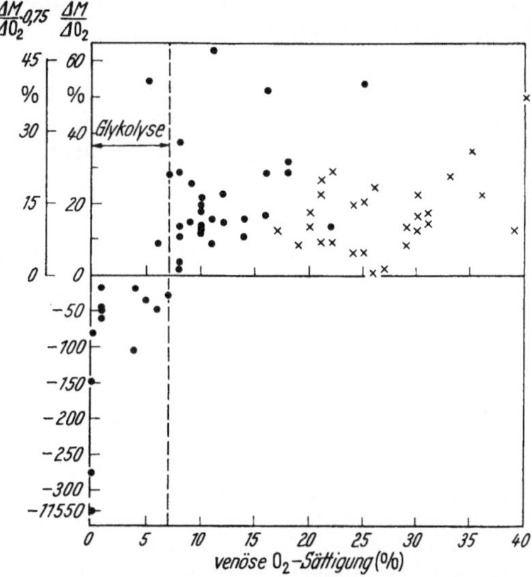

Abb. 43. Beziehung der venösen Sauerstoff-Sättigung des Coronarblutes zu dem Verhältnis „arterio-venöse Milchsäuredifferenz/arterio-venöse Sauerstoffdifferenz $\Delta M/\Delta O2$" im Coronarblut. Bis zu einer Sättigung von 7% besteht keine Abhängigkeit, der Anteil der Milchsäureverbrennung am gesamten aeroben Energiegewinn bleibt unverändert. Unterschreitet die venöse Sauerstoffsättigung jedoch den kritischen Bereich von 7—5%, kehrt sich die arterio-venöse Milchsäuredifferenz als Zeichen einer bilanzmäßigen Glykolyse des Herzmuskels um. Arterielle Hypoxie durch Punkte, Frischluftatmung durch Kreuze gekennzeichnet. Versuche an narkotisierten Hunden. (BRETSCHNEIDER 1958.)

entscheidender ist die gute Einstellbarkeit der Coronardurchblutung, die es ermöglicht, die Sauerstoffzufuhr einem erhöhten Herzstoffwechsel oder einem verminderten Sauerstoffgehalt des arteriellen Blutes anzupassen.

Ist nun die Sauerstoffversorgung des Herzmuskels so eingestellt, daß in jedem Abschnitt der Zelle gerade noch der hinreichende Sauerstoffdruck zur Sicherung der Stoffwechselvorgänge aufrechterhalten wird, oder liegt der Sauerstoffdruck im Gewebe sehr viel höher, als zu diesem Zwecke notwendig wäre? Besteht also im Hinblick auf die Sauerstoffversorgung eine Luxusdurchblutung? Im Gehirn scheint im allgemeinen der Sauerstoffdruck weit über dem kritischen Wert zu liegen[1]. Es ist schwierig, am Herzmuskel die intracellulären O_2-Drucke abzuschätzen, da sowohl die Durchblutung als auch die Sauerstoffaufnahme des Gewebes in unkontrollierbarer Weise mit der rhythmischen Tätigkeit des Herzens sich verändern[2]. Trotzdem muß man auch bei vorsichtiger Abschätzung des Druckgefälles annehmen, daß normalerweise im Innern der Herzmuskelfaser der

---

[1] OPITZ und SCHNEIDER 1950.   [2] OPITZ und THEWS 1952.

Sauerstoffdruck weit über dem kritischen Wert liegt. Wahrscheinlich beträgt das Druckgefälle vom Blute bis ins Gewebsinnere nicht mehr als 5 Torr. Da der Sauerstoffdruck im Coronarvenenblut normalerweise über 20 Torr liegt, ist im Gewebe mit 15 Torr zu rechnen, während der kritische Wert wahrscheinlich unter 5 Torr liegt. Damit erklärt sich auch, daß unter bestimmten Bedingungen der venöse Sauerstoffdruck weiter absinken kann, ohne daß die Funktionsfähigkeit des Herzens dadurch beeinflußt wird. Besonders auffallend ist das bei Muskeltätigkeit. An trainierten Hunden findet man bei Arbeitsleistungen auf dem Laufband regelmäßig einen niedrigeren Sauerstoffdruck als im Ruhezustand[1]. Ein Kennzeichen dafür, ob im Gewebe der kritische Sauerstoffdruck erreicht wird, ist das Verhalten der Lactatbilanz. Senkt man im Tierexperiment den Sauerstoffdruck im Coronarsinusblut, indem man das Versuchstier mit sauerstoffarmen Luftgemischen beatmet, so findet man eine Lactataufnahme des Herzgewebes, solange die venöse Sauerstoffsättigung 5% nicht unterschreitet. Bei niedrigeren Werten wird dagegen vom Herzmuskel Lactat abgegeben[2] (Abb. 43).

3. Energieumsatz, mechanische Leistung, Wirkungsgrad.

Der Energiebedarf des Herzens wird in allererster Linie oxydativ gedeckt. Damit wird der Sauerstoffverbrauch des Herzens ein gutes Maß für den Energieumsatz. Man berechnet im allgemeinen den Energieumsatz nach der folgenden Formel:

$$\text{Energieumsatz (m kg)} = 2{,}057 \times O_2\text{-Verbrauch (ml/min).}$$

Die so berechneten Energieumsätze sind zwar gute Annäherungswerte, andererseits aber nur bedingt richtig. 2,057 ist das Energieäquivalent von 1 cm³ Sauerstoff, wenn als Substrat Kohlenhydrate verbrannt werden. Bei der Berechnung des Energieumsatzes aus dem Sauerstoffverbrauch können Fehler dadurch entstehen, daß andere Substrate verbrannt werden. Von größerer Bedeutung ist es, daß gar nicht in jedem Falle die gesamte oxydativ gewonnene Energie für mechanische Leistung verwandt wird, sondern daß sie teilweise bei der Speicherung oder beim Umbau von Stoffwechselprodukten verbraucht wird.

Zur Berechnung des Wirkungsgrades der Maschine Herz muß man außer dem Energieumsatz auch die mechanische Leistung des Herzens kennen. Für die meisten Fälle berechnet man die Leistung eines Ventrikels in hinreichender Annäherung aus dem HZV und dem arteriellen Druck, gegen den das Blut gefördert werden muß. Unter manchen Bedingungen kann es zweckmäßig sein, bei der Berechnung der mechanischen Leistung außer der Druckvolumleistung auch die Leistung zu berücksichtigen, die für die Beschleunigung des Blutes notwendig ist. Die Berechnung erfolgt dann nach der Formel:

$$L = \dot{Q}P + \frac{m \cdot v^2}{2\,t}$$

(L = Leistung, $\dot{Q}$ = HZV, P = arterieller Druck, m = Masse des ausgeworfenen Blutes v = mittlere Geschwindigkeit in der Austreibungszeit, t = Austreibungszeit). Im allgemeinen ist der zweite Summand der Gleichung klein und kann vernachlässigt werden. Andererseits wird auch bei Berücksichtigung der Beschleunigungsleistung noch nicht die gesamte mechanische Leistung erfaßt. So wird auch durch die viscösen Eigenschaften der Herzwand Energie verbraucht[3].

Die Werte für Energieumsatz und Wirkungsgrad in Tabelle 13 sind für 100 g Ventrikelmuskulatur berechnet. Keine der angeführten 9 Meßreihen ist voll befriedigend. Die an trainierten Hunden ohne Narkose gewonnenen Werte für den Energieumsatz[4] liegen auffallend hoch. Wahrscheinlich war der Ruhezustand der Tiere kein vollkommener. Daraus erklärt sich wohl auch der hohe Wirkungsgrad von 31%. Der Wirkungsgrad des Herzmuskels steigt im allgemeinen an, wenn die Herzleistung vergrößert ist. Außerdem zeigt sich bei Hunden ein Einfluß von Körper- und Herzgewicht auf den Energieumsatz. Größere Tiere haben einen kleineren Umsatz pro 100 g Herzgewicht. Das erschwert den Vergleich mit den am Menschen gewonnenen Zahlen. Bei den am Menschen gewonnenen Werten von Bing u. a.[5] liegen die HZV auffallend niedrig. Wahrscheinlich waren die bei diesen Untersuchungen aus dem rechten Vorhof gewonnenen Blutproben nicht repräsentativ für venöses Mischblut.

---

[1] Lochner und Nasseri 1959.   [2] Hackel und Mitarbeiter 1954, Bretschneider 1958.
[3] Reichel 1953, Literatur bei Rushmer 1956.   [4] Spencer u. a. 1950.   [5] Bing 1949.

Tabelle 18. *Werte für Energieumsatz und Wirkungsgrad des linken Ventrikels.*
Die Werte sind für 100 g Ventrikelmuskulatur angegeben.

	Linker Ventrikel, Hund trainiert, ohne Narkose. (SPENCER u. a. 1950)	Linker Ventrikel, Mensch. (BING u. a. 1949)	Linker Ventrikel, Mensch. (RILEY u. a. 1948)
Mittlerer arterieller Druck mm Hg . .	119	92	84
HZV ml/100 g/min	7700	2820	4000
Mechanische Leistung mkg/100 g/min .	12,5	3,4	4,6
O_2-Verbrauch ml/100 g/min	19,5	7,8	—
Gesamt-Energieumsatz mkg/100 g/min	40,2	16,0	—
Wirkungsgrad %	31	23	—

Es sind aus diesem Grunde in der 3. Spalte der Tabelle 18 die Werte von RILEY u. Mitarb. (1948) angeführt, die mit anderen Berechnungen der mechanischen Leistung des linken Ventrikels gute Übereinstimmung zeigen. Es ist wahrscheinlich, daß von BING u. a. die mechanische Leistung auf Grund ihrer HZV-Werte zu niedrig bestimmt und damit auch ein zu niedriger Wirkungsgrad berechnet wurde.

Mit wachsender Leistung des Herzens wächst im allgemeinen auch sein Sauerstoffverbrauch, jedoch steigt in den meisten Fällen gleichzeitig der Wirkungsgrad an. Erst bei sehr hohen Belastungen wird der Wirkungsgrad wieder geringer. Am deutlichsten zeigt sich dies bei Untersuchungen am Herz-Lungenpräparat (Abb. 44), bei dem die Schlagfrequenz konstant ist. Bedeutende Steigerungen des Wirkungsgrades findet man besonders bei Erhöhung des venösen Zuflusses, dagegen bleibt bei Steigerung des arteriellen Widerstandes der Wirkungsgrad am Herz-Lungenpräparat sehr niedrig[1]. Bei übermäßigen Herzbelastungen wird der Wirkungsgrad wieder kleiner. Das Herz in situ gehorcht im Prinzip den gleichen Gesetzmäßigkeiten. Es findet sich

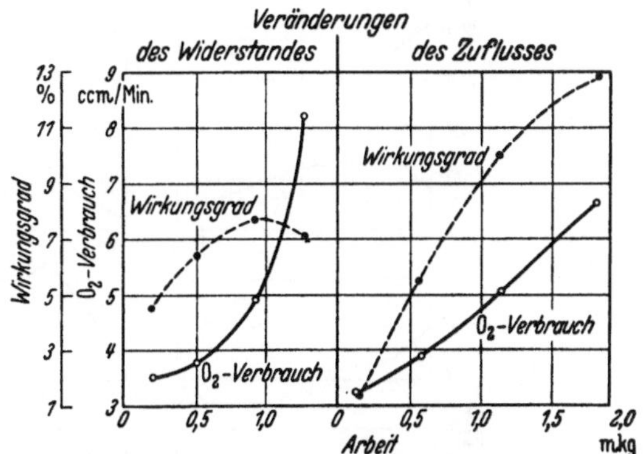

Abb. 44. Veränderungen von Widerstand und Zufluß in ihrem Einfluß auf Sauerstoffverbrauch und Wirkungsgrad des Warmblüterherzens. (GOLLWITZER-MEIER 1939.)

eine starke Erhöhung des Wirkungsgrades bei Steigerung des HZV. Dagegen steigen die Wirkungsgrade weniger an, wenn die Herzleistung durch Steigerung des peripheren Strömungswiderstandes erhöht ist[2] (Abb. 45). Am Menschen erhobene Befunde gehen in die gleiche Richtung. Bei Coronarkatheterisierung von Patienten findet man nach leichter körperlicher Arbeit eine Steigerung der Sauerstoffaufnahme des Herzmuskels, eine erhöhte Coronardurchblutung und im allgemeinen auch eine Zunahme des Wirkungsgrades des Herzmuskels[3].

Daß der Wirkungsgrad des Herzens sich mit der Leistung verändert, ist zum Teil sehr einfach zu erklären. Der Herzmuskel hat wie der Skeletmuskel einen Ruheumsatz. Auch ohne daß er erregt ist, setzt er eine bestimmte Energiemenge um. Dieser Energiebetrag fällt um so stärker ins Gewicht, je niedriger die mechanische Leistung des Herzens ist. Bis vor kurzem nahm man an, daß der Ruhestoffwechsel der Herzmuskulatur sehr hoch läge, und daß er unter normalen Bedingungen bis zur Hälfte des Herzstoffwechsels ausmachen könne[4]. Nach

---

[1] GOLLWITZER-MEIER 1939.   [2] ECKENHOFF u. a. 1947.
[3] LOMBARDO u. a. 1953.   [4] ROHDE 1912, HOFF 1955.

neuen Untersuchungen macht der Ruhestoffwechsel der Herzmuskulatur weniger als 10% des Gesamtumsatzes aus[1] (s. Abb. 46).

Ein weiterer wichtiger Gesichtspunkt für die Betrachtung des Wirkungsgrades ist der der Leerarbeit des Herzmuskels. Ein extremer Fall hierfür ist der des flimmernden Herzens, das je nach dem Grad des Flimmerns einen niedrigeren

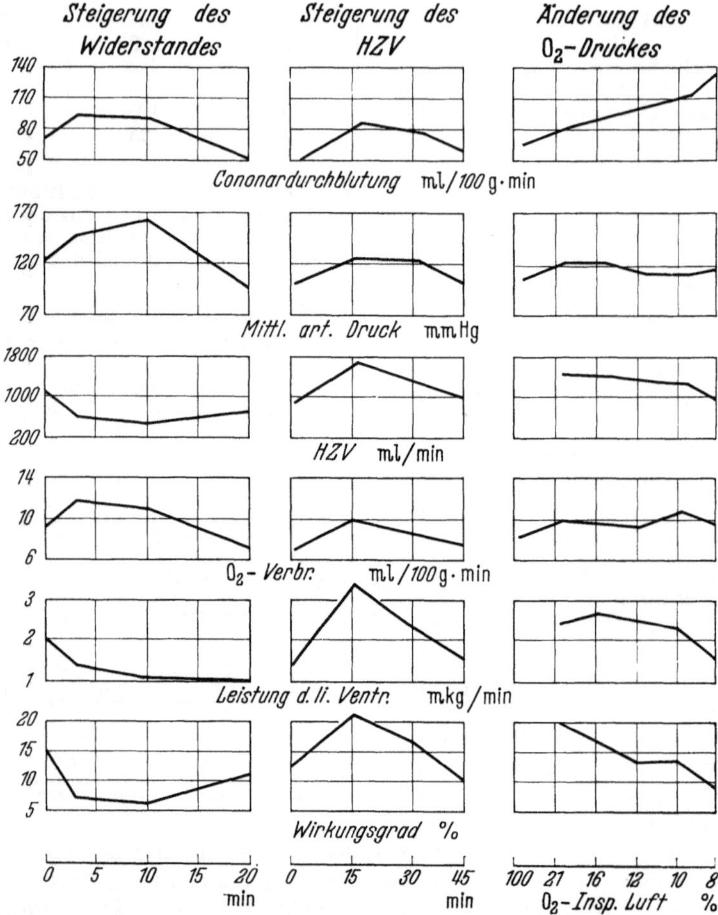

Abb. 45. Wirkungen von Änderungen des peripheren Widerstandes, des Herzzeitvolumens und des arteriellen Sauerstoffdruckes auf Kreislauf und Coronardurchblutung. (Eckenhoff u. a. 1947.)

oder auch einen höheren Energieumsatz hat wie das rhythmisch schlagende Herz, bei dem aber die mechanische Leistung und der Wirkungsgrad 0 sind[2].

Auch beim leer schlagenden Herzen sind Förderleistung und Wirkungsgrad gleich Null. Dabei zeigt sich eine starke Abhängigkeit von Leerleistung und Schlagfrequenz[3] (Abb. 46). Die gesteigerte Leerleistung bei hohen Herzfrequenzen erklärt die niedrigen Wirkungsgrade unter diesen Bedingungen[4]. Am schlagenden

---

[1] Hoffmeister, Kreuzer und Schoeppe 1959, Berglund und Mitarbeiter 1957.

[2] Paul und Mitarbeiter 1954, Jardetzky, Greene und Lorber 1956, Hoffmeister, Kreuzer und Schoeppe 1959.

[3] Hoffmeister und Mitarbeiter 1959.

[4] Alella und Mitarbeiter 1956, Berglund und Mitarbeiter 1958, Maxwell und Mitarbeiter 1958.

Herzen ist bei Förderung des gleichen HZV der Energieumsatz höher, je höher die Herzfrequenz ist. Wenn Adrenalin den Wirkungsgrad verschlechtert, Acetylcholin ihn verbessert, so ist das weitgehend auf die Veränderung der Herzfrequenz zurückzuführen. Wenn am Herz-Lungenpräparat die Wirkungsgrade sehr niedrig sind, so erklärt sich dies in erster Linie aus den hohen Schlagfrequenzen und niedrigen Schlagvolumina. Wie für einen Motor so ist auch für das Herz Voraussetzung für einen guten Wirkungsgrad, daß der richtige Gang eingeschaltet ist. Gangschaltung heißt in diesem Fall Frequenzeinstellung.

Der Energieumsatz der Herzmuskelfaser hängt aber nicht allein von der Zahl der Kontraktionen ab. Für die einzelne Kontraktion ist er im allgemeinen um so höher, je größer seine Ausgangsdehnung ist [1]. Neben der Ausgangslänge ist aber auch der Ablauf der Kontraktion für die Energiefreisetzung von Bedeutung. Für den Sauerstoffverbrauch des Herzens ist es nicht gleichgültig, ob die Arbeit gegen hohen oder niedrigen Druck geleistet wird. „Druckarbeit" erfordert einen höheren Sauerstoffverbrauch als „Volumarbeit" [2] (Abb. 44). Anscheinend ist das Integral der Faserspannung über die Dauer der Systole die entscheidende Größe [3].

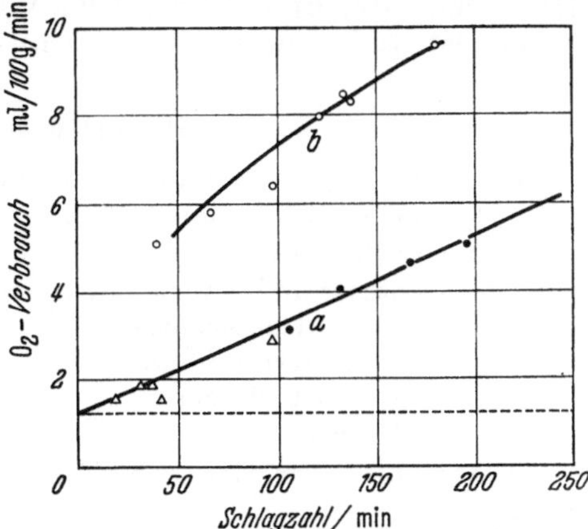

Abb. 46. Abhängigkeit des O₂-Verbrauchs des Herzens von der Schlagfrequenz. - - - Ruheverbrauch (O₂-Verbrauch des stillstehenden Herzens). *a* leer schlagendes Herz, ● eigene Mittelwerte, △ Werte von GREGG (1958). *b* normal schlagendes Herz (Leistung 92 mkg/h) nach Werten von VAN CITTERS et al. (1957), (HOFFMEISTER, KREUZER und SCHOEPPE 1959).

IV. Störungen der Herzenergetik.

Die im funktionellen Teil dargestellten Ergebnisse der experimentellen Erforschung des normalen Herzstoffwechsels rücken auch die Betrachtung der Störungen der Herzenergetik unter krankhaften Bedingungen in ein neues Licht. Durch Katheterisierung des Coronarvenensinus am Menschen gelingt es, die Stoffwechselabläufe, die den Energiestoffwechsel bestreiten, unter krankhaften Bedingungen zu erfassen. Dabei ergeben sich im wesentlichen zwei Hauptprobleme:

1. Kommt es bei verschiedenen Erkrankungen des Herzens zu bestimmten Abweichungen der chemischen Vorgänge im Herzen, die mit der Energie*bildung* verknüpft sind? Ändern sich unter verschiedenen krankhaften Bedingungen die Relationen zwischen den Anteilen der verschiedenen Nährsubstrate wie Eiweiß, Fett und Kohlenhydrate an der Energiebildung? Sind dabei bestimmte Fermententgleisungen nachweisbar?

2. Wie verhält sich der O₂-Verbrauch des geschädigten oder muskelinsuffizienten Herzens? Wie ändert sich der Wirkungsgrad des Herzens unter krankhaften Bedingungen?

Die unter 1. angeführten Fragestellungen betreffen die Störungen der Energie*bildung*, die unter 2. die Störungen der Energie*ausnutzung*.

Wenn auch die diesbezüglichen Forschungsergebnisse noch jüngeren Datums sind, in mancher Beziehung Lücken aufweisen und auch weiterer Bestätigung

---

[1] STARLING und VISSCHER 1926. [2] GOLLWITZER-MEIER 1939, KATZ 1955.
[3] SARNOFF und Mitarbeiter 1958.

bedürfen, so kann auf Grund der bisherigen Untersuchungsergebnisse doch schon manches über die Stoffwechselstörungen des Herzens unter krankhaften Bedingungen ausgesagt werden. Die folgende Einteilung und die Darstellung der Ergebnisse basiert vor allem auf den Arbeiten von Bing u. Mitarb. (auf die zusammenfassende Darstellung von Bing in der Klin. Wschr. 1956, in der auch die Literatur aufgeführt ist, sei besonders hingewiesen).

1. Störungen der Energiebildung.

Diese Störungen werden folgendermaßen unterteilt:

1. Störungen der Energiebildung mit verminderter Herzleistung.
    a) Das Beriberiherz.
    b) Ischämie und Anoxie des Herzmuskels.
        α) Verblutungsschock.
        β) Coronarverschluß.
        γ Kammerflimmern.
        δ) Unterkühlung.
2. Störungen der Energiebildung ohne verminderte Herzleistung. Diabetes mellitus.

1. a) *Beriberiherz.* Bei dieser Ernährungsstörung des Herzens ist die Gewebscocarboxylase durch das Fehlen von Vitamin B_1 (Thiamin, Aneurin) in der Nahrung vermindert. Die Folge ist, daß die Brenztraubensäure nicht zu Acetyl-Coenzym A decarboxyliert werden kann und damit der weitere Abbau der Brenztraubensäure über den Citronensäurecyclus gestört ist.

Wahrscheinlich wird auch der Fettsäureabbau durch Störung des Flavin-Coenzyms betroffen. Die Milchsäureaufnahmefähigkeit des Herzmuskels ist vermindert, möglicherweise durch hemmende Einflüsse des erhöhten Brenztraubensäurespiegels auf die Milchsäure-Dehydrogenase.

1. b) α) *Der Verblutungsschock.* Die deutlichste Veränderung des Myokardstoffwechsels beim Verblutungsschock zeigt sich in einer Verminderung der Brenztraubensäureaufnahme bei gleichzeitig vermehrter Milchsäureaufnahme. Der Brenztraubensäurespiegel des Coronarvenenblutes liegt höher als derjenige des arteriellen Blutes. Trotz einer erhöhten arteriellen Glucosekonzentration sind die Glucoseextraktion und der Glucoseumsatz im Myokard vermindert. Diese Veränderungen bleiben auch nach Retransfusion des entnommenen Blutes bestehen. Offenbar vermag die Blutinfusion die durch die Entblutung hervorgerufenen Stoffwechselstörungen nicht gänzlich zu beseitigen. Für die Entstehung der negativen Brenztraubensäurebilanz wird eine Störung der Cocarboxylase-Aktivität diskutiert. Dieses Co-Ferment (Aneurinpyrophosphat) wird unter anaeroben Bedingungen durch Dephosphorylierungsprozesse zerstört. In gewisser Weise ist die Stoffwechselstörung im hämorrhagischen Schock mit derjenigen bei Beriberi zu vergleichen. Beim hämorrhagischen Schock wird die Cocarboxylase durch die eintretende Hypoxie zerstört, bei Beriberi seine Bildung durch fehlendes Vitamin B_1 verhindert.

1. b) β) *Coronarverschluß.* Hierüber liegen nur tierexperimentelle Ergebnisse vor. Daraus geht hervor, daß die Störung des Brenztraubensäurestoffwechsels beim Coronarverschluß derjenigen im Verblutungsschock ähnlich ist. Offenbar führt aber der experimentelle Coronarverschluß zu noch eingreifenderen Störungen. So finden sich neben den Veränderungen des Brenztraubensäurestoffwechsels erhöhte Glucose- und Milchsäurekonzentrationen im Coronarvenenblut. Durch die ischämische Gewebszerstörung werden strukturgebundene Fermente (Trans-

aminasen, Milchsäuredehydrogenase) frei. Diese lassen sich dann stark vermehrt im Blut nachweisen[1].

1. b) γ) *Kammerflimmern.* Experimentell erzeugtes Kammerflimmern durch Elektroschock an Hunden ergab Folgendes: Die Brenztraubensäure- und Milchsäurekonzentrationen im Coronarvenenblut stiegen auf Werte an, welche über denen des arteriellen Blutes desselben Tieres lagen. Die coronare arterio-venöse Differenz von Glucose und Ketonen verminderte sich. Die Glucose- und Ketonkonzentrationen im Coronarvenenblut lagen bei den meisten Tieren höher als im arteriellen Blut. Auch der Kaliumspiegel war im coronaren Sinusblut erhöht. Es wird angenommen, daß die Coenzyme und ATP nur unter den Bedingungen aktiver Oxydation ihre Funktion erfüllen können. Wird sie bei Kammerflimmern unterbrochen, so werden diese Fermente zerstört, die Störungen werden irreversibel.

1. b) δ) *Auskühlung.* Hierbei finden sich keine meßbaren Veränderungen des qualitativen Herzstoffwechsels. Die Extraktion und Umsetzung von Glucose, Milchsäure und Brenztraubensäure bleibt in ihren Relationen normal. Anscheinend ist der Abfall des Sauerstoffverbrauchs des Herzens geringer als die Erniedrigung des Sauerstoffverbrauchs des gesamten Organismus. Die coronare arterio-venöse Sauerstoffdifferenz soll sich nicht ändern. Die Untersuchungen geben keine Hinweise für das Auftreten einer Hypoxie des Herzmuskels bei Auskühlung.

2. a) *Diabetes mellitus.* Der Zuckerverbrauch des Herzens ist herabgesetzt. Das Herz kann bei Diabetes Glucose wohl verwerten, jedoch in verminderter Menge. Der Milchsäure- und Brenztraubensäureverbrauch ist ebenfalls vermindert. Die Extraktion von Brenztraubensäure im diabetischen Herzen ist erniedrigt. Weiterhin scheint eine ungenügende Verwertbarkeit von Aminosäuren im diabetischen Herzen vorzuliegen. Beim diabetischen Menschen und Hund entnimmt das Herz selbst bei Erhöhung des arteriellen Aminosäurespiegels nur einen relativ kleinen Anteil der Aminosäuren aus dem Coronarblut. Es wird eine Störung der Proteinsynthese vermutet. Schließlich kommt im diabetischen Herzmuskel eine vermehrte Fettspeicherung vor, die auch bei normalen Blutfettkonzentrationen stattfindet. Bei der Vielfältigkeit der gefundenen Störungen ist es nicht möglich zu entscheiden, ob sie auf einen Nenner gebracht werden können, oder ob es sich um eine Reihe nebeneinander bestehender Störungen der enzymatischen Reaktionen der Zelle handelt.

2. Störungen der Energieverwertung.

Abweichungen im Ablauf der energiebildenden Prozesse von der Norm, wie sie oben beschrieben wurden, bedeuten nicht, daß die Energieverwertung ebenfalls gestört ist. So ist z. B. beim Diabetes mellitus trotz ausgeprägter Störungen im Ablauf der energiebildenden Prozesse kein Anhalt gegeben, daß die Energieverwertung, gemessen am Wirkungsgrad, mit dem das Herz arbeitet, gestört ist, solange die coronare Blutversorgung normal bleibt. Wenn beim Beriberiherzen oder bei ischämischen Zuständen des Herzmuskels Störungen der Energiebildung und der Energieverwertung Hand in Hand gehen, so ist zu bedenken, daß es sich hierbei um Sonderfälle handelt, und daß in diesen Sonderfällen wohl nur extreme Grade zu einer Herabsetzung des Wirkungsgrades führen. Auch ist es noch weitgehend unbekannt, warum einige Stoffwechselstörungen bzw. Störungen der Energiebildung von einem verminderten Wirkungsgrad, eventuell sogar von einer Herzmuskelinsuffizienz gefolgt sind, andere hingegen nicht. Das größte

---

[1] La Due, Wroblewski und Karmen 1954, Amelung und Horn 1956.

Kontingent der in der Klinik geläufigen Formen von Herzmuskelschädigungen bzw. Herzmuskelinsuffizienz betrifft die bereits in anderen Kapiteln behandelten Überlastungsschäden, wie sie im Gefolge von arterio-venösen Fisteln, Klappenvitien, Basedow, schweren Anämien usw. auftreten. Es liegen bisher keinerlei Anhaltspunkte dafür vor, daß bei diesen Schädigungen des Herzens Störungen der energieliefernden Prozesse vorhanden sind. Es bestehen keinerlei Unterschiede in der Aufnahme von Glucose, Brenztraubensäure, Milchsäure, Aminosäuren, Fettsäuren oder Ketonkörpern zwischen einem insuffizienten und einem normalen Herzen. Extraktion und Substrataufnahme sind bei der Herzmuskelinsuffizienz normal. Das spontan insuffiziente Herz weist einen normalen ATP-Gehalt auf und ist sogar noch reicher an Kreatin-Phosphorsäure als das nicht insuffiziente Herz. Änderungen der mechanischen Arbeit können ohne Änderungen des energiereichen Phosphatgehaltes auftreten. Die Messungen des Sauerstoffverbrauchs am insuffizienten Herzen ergaben nur leichte Erhöhungen pro Gewichtseinheit, ohne daß aber diese Unterschiede als signifikant anzusprechen sind. Dagegen fand sich in allen Untersuchungen eine deutliche *Herabsetzung des Wirkungsgrades des Herzens im Stadium der muskulären Insuffizienz.* Gegenüber einem durchschnittlichen normalen Wirkungsgrad von 23% wiesen muskelinsuffiziente Herzen eine Erniedrigung des Wirkungsgrades auf 10—17% auf. Im Stadium der Kompensation entsprach der Wirkungsgrad der Norm. Es erscheint noch der Befund bemerkenswert, daß der Sauerstoffverbrauch des hypertrophierten Herzmuskels pro Gewichtseinheit nicht erhöht ist, auch wenn eine deutliche Dilatation der Herzkammern besteht. Dieses Ergebnis steht in einem gewissen Gegensatz zu den tierexperimentellen Untersuchungen von Starling und Visscher (1926) am Herz-Lungenpräparat. Es ist ein Unterschied, ob das Herz plötzlich belastet wird, oder ob sich eine Hypertrophie entwickelt hat. Bei akuter plötzlicher Belastung tritt eine Steigerung des Sauerstoffverbrauchs des Herzens auf, die der Zunahme der diastolischen Kammerfüllung graduell entspricht. Dieser Befund konnte auch am Menschen bestätigt werden. Dauert die Belastung dagegen lange Zeit, und entwickelt sich eine Hypertrophie, so ist der Sauerstoffverbrauch des Herzens zwar insgesamt durch die Gewichtszunahme erhöht, dagegen bleibt der Sauerstoffverbrauch pro Gewichtseinheit normal.

Bing (1956) faßt die experimentellen Ergebnisse der Störungen der Herzenergetik folgendermaßen zusammen: „Es geht aus den Untersuchungen hervor, daß die zu einer Herzinsuffizienz führende Causalfolge entweder mit Stoffwechselstörungen innerhalb des Myocards beginnen kann, die die energiebildenden Vorgänge betreffen oder sie kann in den Strukturen entstehen, die mit der Energiefreisetzung verbunden sind: im kontraktilen Protein. Das letzte Resultat aller pathologischen Abläufe, die zur Herzinsuffizienz führen, ist stets eine Störung der Energiefreisetzung; es ist sehr wohl möglich, daß diese Störungen bedingt sind durch physikalisch-chemische Veränderungen innerhalb der Struktur der kontraktilen Proteine des Myocards."

Inzwischen wird über experimentelle Untersuchungen berichtet, nach denen die physiko-chemischen Eigenschaften des Actomyosins bei chronisch insuffizienten Hundeherzen verändert sind[1]. Das Molekulargewicht von Myosin aus Herzmuskelfasern insuffizienter Herzen wurde erhöht gefunden[2]. Stoffwechselveränderungen der Sarkosome des insuffizienten Herzmuskels sucht man durch Messung des sog. P/O-Quotienten in vitro zu erfassen. Der P/O-Quotient stellt das Verhältnis von der aus der Substratmenge aufgenommenen Menge von anorganischen Phosphationen zu der aufgenommenen Sauerstoffmenge dar und soll normalerweise gleich drei sein. Beim insuffizienten Herzmuskel wurde der P/O-Quotient deutlich erniedrigt gefunden (1,33)[3]. Dieser Befund wird so gedeutet, daß dem insuffizienten Herzen die Fähigkeit verlorengeht, den Sauerstoff in normalem Maße aufzunehmen und andererseits

---

[1] Benson 1955.   [2] Olson 1956.   [3] Lamprecht 1956.

energiereiche Phosphatverbindungen in genügender Menge bereitzustellen. Ferner wurde im hypertrophierten Myokard eine Reduktion der Desoxyribonucleinsäurekonzentration gefunden, ohne daß allerdings eine Abhängigkeit dieser Konzentrationsabnahme vom Ausmaß der Hypertrophie sichergestellt werden konnte[1].

Auch für das Verständnis der Wirkungsweise der Glykoside spielt die Frage eine Rolle, ob sie auf eine physikalisch veränderte, contractile Substanz einwirken, oder ob sie die Energieübertragung vom Phosphatsystem beeinflussen[2]. Wenn der Milz-Lebermechanismus REINs den Wirkungsgrad des Herzens steigert, dann ist ebenfalls an einen Angriff an diesen Stellen zu denken[3].

V. Herzdynamik.

Wenn das Herzzeitvolumen die entscheidende Größe des Blutkreislaufes ist, dann muß man sich die Frage vorlegen, ob diese Größe von seiten des Gefäßsystems oder von seiten des Herzens bestimmt wird. Man kann sich vorstellen, daß die von der Peripherie zugeführte Blutmenge, also der venöse Rückstrom, groß ist, und daß das Herz nur einen Teil dieser Blutmenge auf die arterielle Seite hinüberschafft. Das HZV würde in diesem Fall allein von der Herzfunktion abhängig sein. Die andere Möglichkeit ist die, daß das Herz jede Blutmenge auf die arterielle Seite befördert, die ihm vom Venensystem angeboten wird. In diesem Falle würde das HZV allein von den Funktionen des Gefäßsystems bestimmt. Die Wahrheit liegt in der Mitte. Unter vielen Bedingungen bestimmt das Herz, unter anderen die Kreislaufperipherie die Größe des HZV.

Es ist die Notwendigkeit funktioneller Forschung, daß man einerseits Teile eines Systems isoliert untersucht, andererseits die Funktionen im möglichst unverletzten Organismus zu erfassen sich bemüht. Man muß die Funktionen des isolierten Herzens und die des Herzens in situ kennen. Die Gesetzmäßigkeiten des isolierten Herzens sind gut bekannt. Man hat in letzter Zeit vielfach Zweifel geäußert, ob sie für das Herz in situ Gültigkeit haben. Es ist eine schlechte Formulierung zu sagen, daß die Gesetze des isolierten Herzens in situ außer Kraft gesetzt werden. Sie gelten grundsätzlich weiter, können aber durch zusätzliche Einflüsse überdeckt sein und ihre Bedeutung für den Kreislauf kann damit unter bestimmten Bedingungen gemindert sein.

Über die mechanischen Vorgänge während einer Herzperiode, über die besonders durch Verwendung von Dehnungsmeßstreifen im Tierexperiment Fortschritte erzielt wurden, siehe besonders RUSHMER (1956a). Für manche Betrachtungen der Herzdynamik ist bedeutungsvoll, daß der Ventrikel in der Anpassungszeit seine Form ändert[4], und daß er auf Grund seiner elastischen Eigenschaften nach raschen und starken Entleerungen einen Sog auf die venöse Seite ausüben kann[5].

1. Gesetzmäßigkeiten des isolierten Herzens.

Die contractilen Proteine des Herzens und der Skeletmuskulatur haben weitgehend gleiche chemische und physikalische Eigenschaften[6]. Deshalb gehorchen Skelet- und Herzmuskelfasern sehr weitgehend den gleichen Gesetzmäßigkeiten. Bei beiden Muskelarten zeigt sich besonders eine starke Abhängigkeit der Funktion von der Ausgangsdehnung der Muskelfasern. Je stärker die Faser gedehnt ist, um so stärker ist ihre Arbeitsfähigkeit bei der Kontraktion, um so höher ist die

---

[1] NORY und FRINGS 1960.
[2] HORVÁTH u. a. 1949, SZENT-GYÖRGY 1953, 1956, BING u. a. 1950, ROTHLIN und TAESCHLER 1956, WILBRANDT 1955.
[3] MEESMANN und SCHMIER 1956c.   [4] RUSHMER 1956b.
[5] BRECHER 1958, MEESMANN 1958.   [6] SZENT GYÖRGYI 1953.

dabei freigesetzte Energiemenge, und um so größer ist der Wirkungsgrad der dabei geleisteten Arbeit. Diese Gesetzmäßigkeiten wurden zunächst für den Skeletmuskel festgestellt[1]. Später wurde ihre Gültigkeit am Kaltblüterherzen[2] und am Warmblüterherzen[3] gezeigt. Für das Herz gelten danach folgende Gesetzmäßigkeiten: 1. Je größer das enddiastolische Volumen, umso größer ist die Arbeit pro Herzschlag. Das bedeutet, daß bei zunehmender Füllung des Herzens entweder ein größeres Schlagvolumen gefördert oder gegen einenhöheren arteriellen Druck angearbeitet werden kann. 2. Je größer das enddiastoische Herzvolumen, umso höher ist bei sonst gleichen Bedingungen der Energieumsatz des Herzens. 3. Je größer das enddiastolische Volumen, um so höher ist sein Wirkungsgrad. Viele Nachuntersucher haben diese Gesetzmäßigkeiten bestätigt. Das gilt besonders für Untersuchungen am isolierten Herzen, wobei die verschiedensten Präparate verwendet wurden[4]. Aber auch am Herzen in situ ließen sich entsprechende Befunde erheben, wenn regulatorische Einflüsse auf das Herz ausgeschaltet wurden[5]. Auf die Beziehungen zwischen dem enddiastolischen Volumen zum Sauerstoffverbrauch und zum Wirkungsgrad wurde schon bei der Besprechung der Herzenergetik eingegangen (s. S. 719).

Wenn über die Gültigkeit dieser Gesetzmäßigkeiten am Herzen manchmal Widersprüche auftreten, so beruht das zum Teil auf ungenügender Definition der Begriffe[6]. Unter der mechanischen Arbeit des Herzens kann sehr verschiedenes verstanden werden. Meist wird man sich darauf beschränken müssen, als Index der Herzarbeit das Produkt aus dem Schlagvolumen und dem Druck in der Aorta und A. pulmonalis anzusetzen. Auch ist es zweifelhaft, ob man an Stelle des in vielen Versuchsanordnungen nicht bestimmbaren enddiastolischen Kammervolumens den leichter meßbaren enddiastolischen Kammerdruck einsetzen darf. Das enddiastolische Volumen hängt nicht nur vom Füllungsdruck, sondern auch von der Füllungszeit und von elastischen und plastischen Eigenschaften der Ventrikelwand ab[7].

Es muß betont werden, daß am nichtregulierten Herzen sich zwar sehr exakte Beziehungen zwischen dem enddiastolischen Volumen einerseits und der Herzarbeit, dem Sauerstoffverbrauch und dem Wirkungsgrad andererseits feststellen lassen, daß sich aber diese Beziehungen im Verlauf der Untersuchungen ändern können, und daß sie experimentell beeinflußbar sind. Das versagende Herz zeigt bezogen auf das gleiche endodiastolische Volumen eine geringe Arbeitsfähigkeit, aber ungefähr den gleichen Sauerstoffverbrauch, also einen niedrigeren Wirkungsgrad[6]. Von besonderer Bedeutung sind die Veränderungen der genannten Beziehungen unter Adrenalin. Das zeigt schon Möglichkeiten, wie das Herz in situ reguliert und an die Erfordernisse des Kreislaufs angepaßt werden kann. Unter Adrenalin steigt die isometrische Druckentwicklung[8]. Bei auxotoner Tätigkeit steigt das Schlagvolumen, indem das Herz sich vollkommener kontrahiert und die Restblutmenge kleiner wird. Dabei verbessert sich der Wirkungsgrad[9].

2. Das Herz in situ.

Die am isolierten Herzen gefundenen Gesetzmäßigkeiten zeigten eine Möglichkeit, daß das Herz sich aus sich selbst heraus an veränderte Kreislaufbedingungen

---

[1] Fick 1882, Blix 1895.   [2] Frank 1895.
[3] Straub 1914, Starling 1915. Näheres über die Geschichte der Herzgesetze bei Bauereisen 1957.
[4] Lorber 1953, Ullrich, Rieker und Kramer 1954, Katz 1955.
[5] Sarnoff 1955.   [6] Katz 1955.
[7] Katz 1955, Reichel 1952, 1953, Gehl, Graf und Kramer 1955.
[8] Ullrich, Riecker und Kramer 1954.   [9] Katz 1955, Sarnoff 1955.

anpaßte, übertrieben gesprochen, daß es jede Blutmenge gegen jeden arteriellen Druck förderte. Ein Herz von dieser Anpassungsfähigkeit bedürfte keinerlei Steuerung von außen. In der Tat hat man in den vergangenen Jahrzehnten teilweise geglaubt, daß die nervöse und hormonale Steuerung des Herzens für seine Funktion von untergeordneter Bedeutung wäre. Betrachtet man freilich kritisch die am isolierten Herzen erhobenen Befunde, so merkt man, daß die Anpassungsfähigkeit auf Grund der am isolierten Herzen gefundenen Gesetze doch begrenzt ist. Die erreichten Leistungssteigerungen des isolierten Herzens reichen bei weitem nicht an das heran, was vom Herzen in situ bei Muskeltätigkeit verlangt wird.

RUSHMER[1] gelang es, in die linke Herzkammer von Hunden Dehnungsmeßstreifen einzubauen. Mit ihrer Hilfe konnte er am nichtnarkotisierten Tier fortlaufend die Änderungen des Kammerdurchmessers unter den verschiedenen

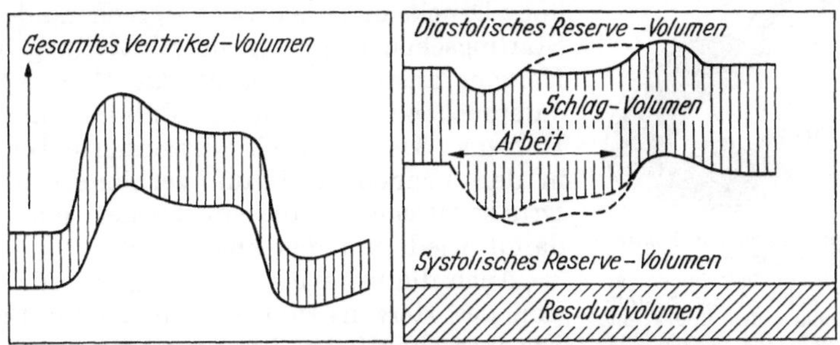

Abb. 47. Verhalten des linken Ventrikels bei Belastung während Muskeltätigkeit. Links: Verhalten, wie es nach den Ergebnissen am isolierten Herzen zu erwarten wäre; rechts: Verhalten, wie es von RUSHMER beim Hund mit geschlossenem Thorax gefunden wurde. (RUSHMER 1955.)

Funktionszuständen verfolgen und daraus auf das Verhalten des Kammervolumens schließen. Im linken Teil der Abb. 47 ist dargestellt, wie sich das Kammervolumen verhalten müßte, wenn es allein den am isolierten Herzen beobachteten Gesetzmäßigkeiten gehorchte. Bei Leistung von körperlicher Arbeit müßten systolisches und diastolisches Volumen stark zunehmen. Im rechten Teil der Abbildung sind die Verhältnisse dargestellt, wie sie von RUSHMER am unnarkotisierten Hund gefunden wurden. Das systolische Volumen ist im Ruhezustand auffallend hoch. Während der Muskeltätigkeit bleibt das diastolische Volumen angenähert gleich, während das systolische Volumen etwas abnimmt. Die Befunde RUSHMERs stehen in gutem Einklang zu dem, was aus zahlreichen röntgenologischen Untersuchungen geschlossen wurde[2]. In Deutschland wiesen besonders DELIUS u. REINDELL auf diese Beziehungen hin[3]. Im Gegensatz zu dem, was nach dem Straub-Starlingschen Gesetz zu erwarten war, ist im allgemeinen bei Muskeltätigkeit das Herzvolumen nicht vergrößert. Auch zeigen Untersuchungen mit Herzkatheterisierung, daß das HZV gesteigert sein kann, ohne daß gleichzeitig der Füllungsdruck des Herzens erhöht ist.

Man darf sich nicht darüber wundern, daß ein Herz, das aus dem Organismus herausgelöst ist, sich anders verhält als ein Herz in situ. Daran ist in erster Linie das Fehlen der nervösen und hormonalen Einflüsse schuld. Es kommt hinzu, daß die Herztätigkeit durch das Vorhandensein des Perikards und durch die Lagerung des Herzens im Thoraxraum beeinflußt wird. Wenn am intakten Kreislauf das

---

[1] RUSHMER 1954, 1955, 1956.
[2] LILJESTRAND u. a. 1938, 1939, SCHWAB 1950 (Literatur), GOLLWITZER-MEIER 1950, SJÖSTRAND 1953, HAMILTON 1955, GREGG u. a. 1955, ASMUSSEN und NIELSEN 1955, KLEPZIG 1955, REINDELL u. a. 1955.
[3] DELIUS und REINDELL 1943, REINDELL und DELIUS 1948.

HZV ansteigt, ohne daß ein erhöhter Füllungsdruck nachweisbar ist, dann beruht das zum Teil auch darauf, daß die Kurve der isometrischen Maxima am Herzen in situ steiler verläuft als am isolierten Herzen. Es bedarf im ersteren Fall nur sehr geringer und kaum nachweisbarer Drucksteigerungen, um die Förderleistung des Herzens zu erhöhen[1].

Beeinflussung der Herztätigkeit durch das Perikard und die Lage im Thorax. Die Bedeutung des Perikards für die Herzfunktion darf nicht unterschätzt werden. Das Perikard schützt das Herz vor einer akuten Überdehnung, bei der nach den am isolierten Herzen gefundenen Gesetzmäßigkeiten Arbeitsfähigkeit und Wirkungsgrad wieder schlechter werden. Außerdem bestimmt es die gesamte Blutfüllung beider Herzhälften. Wenn bei akuter, übermäßiger Belastung des linken Herzens durch hohe Drucke in der Aorta entsprechend den Straub-Starlingschen Gesetzen die Blutfüllung des linken Herzens ansteigt, so sorgt das Perikard für eine entsprechend schlechtere Füllung des rechten Herzens. Der dadurch verminderte Bluteinstrom in den kleinen Kreislauf verhindert übermäßige Druckanstiege in diesem Gebiet und entlastet damit wiederum das linke Herz[2].

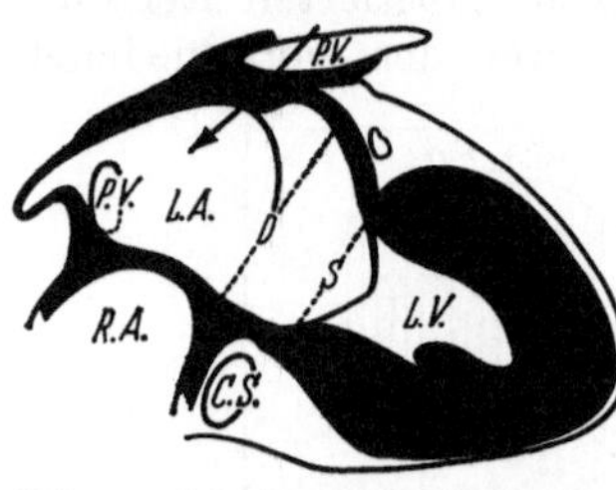

Abb. 48. Schnitt durch das kontrahierte linke Herz des Menschen in situ. Beachte das große Volumen des Vorhofes (*LA*) während der Systole und die Ähnlichkeit des Bildes mit dem der Abb. 49b. Bei Erschlaffung des Ventrikels verlagert sich die Ventrikelebene von der Stellung *S* in die Stellung *D*. Dadurch kann sich der Ventrikel füllen, ohne daß es zu Lateralbewegungen an der Basis des Herzens kommt. Es entsteht ein Bild ähnlich dem der Abb. 49a. *PV* Pulmonalvenen; *LA* linker Vorhof; *LV* linke Kammer; *RA* rechter Vorhof; *CS* Coronarsinus. (Töndury 1951).

Auch die intrathorakale Lage ist für die Funktion des Herzens von entscheidender Bedeutung. Die intrathorakalen Druckverhältnisse bestimmen Größe und Füllung der großen Venen und der Vorhöfe. Auch Stellung und Bewegung der Atrioventrikularebene wird voraussichtlich mitbestimmt (Abb. 48). Das ist besonders für das schnell schlagende, schlecht gefüllte Herz von Bedeutung. Während der Zustrom des Blutes zu dem langsam schlagenden, gut gefüllten Herzen hauptsächlich in der Diastole erfolgt, füllen sich die Kammern des kleinen, schnell schlagenden Herzens hauptsächlich in der Systole durch Verschiebung der Atrioventrikularebene nach der Herzspitze zu, wodurch der Blutstrom in den herznahen Venen in der Systole beschleunigt wird[3] (Abb. 49).

Das gesteuerte Herz. Das Herz in situ steht unter nervösen und hormonalen Einflüssen. Von den chemischen Einflüssen sind die des Adrenalins nach unseren heutigen Kenntnissen die wichtigsten. Der Wirkungsmechanismus des Hypoxyliénins (auch als Milz-Leber-Mechanismus bezeichnet) ist noch nicht zu übersehen[4] (s. auch S. 725). Die nervöse Steuerung des Herzens erfolgt sowohl über adrenergische als auch über cholinergische Fasern, wobei die adrenergischen Fasern im allgemeinen fördernd, die cholinergischen im allgemeinen hemmend auf das Herz einwirken. Die hormonalen und chemischen Einflüsse wirken sowohl auf das Reizleitungssystem, damit auf Erregungsbildung und Erregungsausbreitung, als auch auf die Muskulatur des Herzens und damit auf den Ablauf der Kontraktion. (Über die Wirkung auf die Coronargefäße s. S. 767.)

Herzzeitvolumen, Schlagvolumen, Schlagfrequenz. Der wichtigste Unterschied in der Dynamik des gesteuerten Herzens gegenüber dem ungesteuerten liegt in der Anpassung der Herzfrequenz an die Erfordernisse des Kreislaufs. Nur die Ein-

---

[1] E. A. Müller 1940.   [2] Berglund, Sarnoff und Isaacs 1955.
[3] Böhme 1936, Brecher 1954, Nielson und Kramer 1954, Gauer 1955, 1956.
[4] Rein 1951, Dohrn und Rein 1952, Meesmann und Schmier 1956b.

stellung erhöhter Herzfrequenzen ermöglicht die Förderung großer Herzzeitvolumina, ohne daß die Schlagvolumina übermäßig groß werden müssen. Im
Ruhezustand liegen die Schlagvolumina gesunder ruhender Erwachsener zwischen
60 und 100 cm³ bei Pulsfrequenzen zwischen 50 und 80 Schlägen pro Minute.

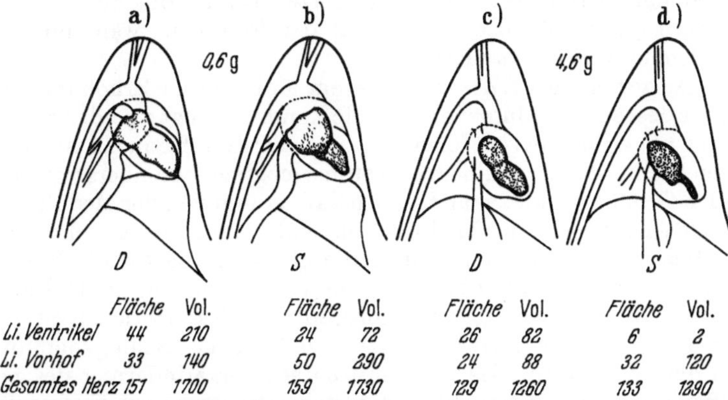

Abb. 49. Röntgenschatten des linken Herzens einer Katze vor und während starker Blutverschiebungen
auf der Zentrifuge. a Präsystole bei einer Beschleunigung von 0,6 g. Das Volumen des linken Ventrikels ist dabei
auf angenähert ³/₅ des totalen Volumens des linken Herzens zu schätzen. b Systole des gleichen Herzschlages.
Der Ventrikel bleibt am Ende der Systole relativ groß. Das Gesamtvolumen des linken Herzens ist gegenüber
der Präsystole praktisch unverändert wegen der starken Vorhoffüllung. c und d Aufnahmen bei Beschleunigung
von 4,6 g. Der Ventrikel entleert sich in der Systole vollkommen. Trotz der starken Blutverschiebung in die
Peripherie bleibt der Schatten des Vorhofes die ganze Zeit sichtbar. (GAUER 1955.)

Die Größe des Schlagvolumens ist dabei von der Körperstellung abhängig. Im
Vergleich zum Liegen wird im Stehen ein kleineres HZV mit höherer Pulsfrequenz
und vermindertem Schlagvolumen gefördert. Bei schweren Arbeiten, die so

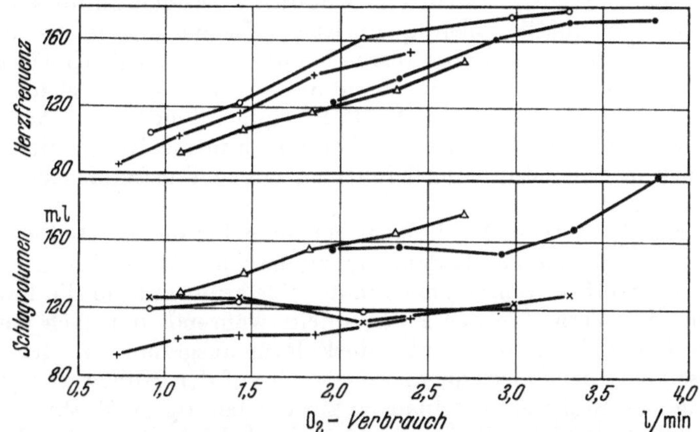

Abb. 50. Pulsfrequenz und Schlagvolumen während körperlicher Arbeit in Beziehung zum Sauerstoffverbrauch.
Die Linien verbinden Werte von 4 verschiedenen Versuchsreihen, von denen 3 mit der Acetylenmethode, 1 mit der
Injektionsmethode (x—x) durchgeführt wurden. (ASMUSSEN u. NIELSEN 1955 a.)

bemessen sind, daß sie über längere Zeit durchgehalten werden können, steigen die
Pulsfrequenzen bis auf 150—180 Schläge an. Bei kurzdauernden erschöpfenden
Arbeiten werden für die Pulsfrequenz auch sehr viel höhere Werte gefunden.
Direkt im Anschluß an Skirennen fand man bei Jugendlichen Werte von 250—270
Schlägen in der Minute[1]. Bei trainierten Männern steigt das Schlagvolumen

---

[1] CHRISTENSEN und HÖBERG 1950.

während schwerer körperlicher Arbeit auf 150—170 ml an und erreicht gelegentlich sogar 200 ml. Untrainierte haben, wenn uns unsere Methoden der HZV-Bestimmung nicht täuschen, auch bei schwerer körperlicher Arbeit nur selten Schlagvolumina über 130 ml. Sie fördern große Herzzeitvolumina durch Steigerung der Herzfrequenz[1] (Abb. 50). Auch trainierte Hunde, die auf dem Laufband laufen, steigern das HZV überwiegend mit der Frequenz, während das Schlagvolumen sich nur wenig verändert[2].

Ob eine Steigerung des HZV in stärkerem Maße durch Erhöhung der Schlagfrequenz oder des Schlagvolumens zustande kommt, hängt von der Steuerung der Herzfrequenz ab. Eine nervöse Beeinflussung der Herzfrequenz ist von den verschiedensten Stellen des Zentralnervensystems möglich, besonders von bestimmten Gebieten der Großhirnrinde, vom Hypothalamus und von der Medulla oblongata. Die steuernden Zentren in der Medulla oblongata stehen unter sehr verschiedenartigen Einflüssen. Weitgehend sind es die gleichen, die für die Steuerung der Vasomotorik von der Medulla oblongata aus von Bedeutung sind. Entscheidend sind die Erregungen, die von den Pressoreceptoren des arteriellen Systems ihren Ausgang nehmen. Hohe Herzfrequenzen und kleine Schlagvolumina finden sich, wenn die Vermehrung des HZV mit so starker Minderung des peripheren Strömungswiderstandes einhergeht, daß gleichzeitig der arterielle Druck absinkt. Wird andererseits das HZV durch ein erhöhtes Blutangebot gesteigert, etwa durch Bluttransfusion oder beim Übergang vom Stehen zum Liegen, so findet man im allgemeinen entsprechend dem erhöhten arteriellen Druck eine niedrige Schlagfrequenz und große Schlagvolumina. Dabei gibt es jedoch einen Wettstreit zwischen den arteriellen Pressoreceptoren und denen in den Herzvorhöfen. Steigerung des Druckes in den Vorhöfen erhöht die Pulsfrequenz (Bainbridge 1915). Ob nach Bluttransfusion die Pulsfrequenz ansteigt oder absinkt, hängt von den gegensätzlichen Auswirkungen der gleichzeitigen Drucksteigerung in den Vorhöfen und im arteriellen System ab[3]. Für die steuernden Einflüsse der arteriellen Pressoreceptoren auf die Pulsfrequenz ist von Bedeutung, daß sie bei erhöhten Druckschwankungen mehr Impulse aussenden als bei einem gleichmäßigen Druck. Erhöhte Druckamplituden beeinflussen auf diese Weise auch bei gleichbleibendem Mitteldruck die Vasomotorik und die Pulsfrequenzsteuerung[4]. Auch die peripheren Chemoreceptoren treiben die Pulsfrequenz in die Höhe. Muskeltätigkeit bei gleichzeitigem Sauerstoffmangel führt zu hohen Pulsfrequenzen und relativ kleinen Schlagvolumina[5].

Impulse aus der tätigen Muskulatur scheinen für die Einstellung der Herzfrequenz eine entscheidende Bedeutung zu haben. Anscheinend erhöht jede Anhäufung von Stoffwechselschlacken in der Skeletmuskulatur die Pulsfrequenz. Abb. 51 zeigt das Verhalten der Pulsfrequenz während und nach einer Arbeit, die fast ausschließlich mit der Wadenmuskulatur ausgeführt wurde. In der Erholungsphase kehrt die Pulsfrequenz sehr rasch auf den Ruhewert zurück, wenn durch Massage die Stoffwechselschlacken aus der betätigten Muskulatur entfernt werden. Andererseits bleibt die Pulsfrequenz hoch, wenn durch Abschnürung der Beine der Abtransport der Stoffwechselschlacken aus der Wadenmuskulatur verhindert wird[6]. Wahrscheinlich wird die Herzfrequenz auch von höheren Abschnitten des Zentralnervensystems beeinflußt. Elektrische Reizung des Hypothalamus führt am wachen Hund im Hinblick auf Frequenz und Kontraktionsablauf zu einer ähnlichen Umstellung der Herztätigkeit, wie sie bei Muskelarbeit beobachtet wird[2].

---

[1] Asmussen und Nielsen 1955.   [2] Rushmer und Smith 1959.
[3] Koepchen, Kramer und Overbeck 1956.   [4] Ead, Green und Neil 1952.
[5] Asmussen und Nielsen 1955b.   [6] E. A. Müller 1955.

Steuerung des Schlagvolumens. Bei der Anpassung der Herztätigkeit an die Erfordernisse des Gesamtkreislaufs steht die Einstellung der Schlagfrequenz ganz im Vordergrund. Daneben gibt es nervöse und hormonale Einflüsse auf die Größe des Schlagvolumens. Sie greifen an der Herzmuskelfaser an. Dabei sind die Beziehungen zu den Grundvorgängen an der contractilen Substanz noch ungeklärt.

Am besten untersucht ist der Einfluß adrenergischer Stoffe. Sie steigern die Herzkraft und die Arbeitsfähigkeit [1]. Diese Erscheinungen sind am ermüdeten Herzen besonders deutlich. Da schon bei erhöhter Schlagfrequenz gewisse Ermüdungserscheinungen der Herzmuskulatur nachweisbar sind, kann an der Bedeutung dieser Stoffe für die Herzfunktion kein Zweifel sein. Bei erhöhter Schlagfrequenz erhält ein adrenergischer Einfluß die Arbeitsfähigkeit des stärker beanspruchten Herzens. Dabei ist besonders an die Freisetzung adrenergischer Stoffe an den Enden der sympathischen Nerven zu denken, weniger an Nebennierenmark-Hormone, die mit dem Blut an die Herzmuskulatur herangebracht werden [2]. Reizung der sympathischen Herznerven führt im Experiment zu einer ähnlichen Umstellung der Herzdynamik, wie sie bei Muskeltätigkeit beobachtet wird [3].

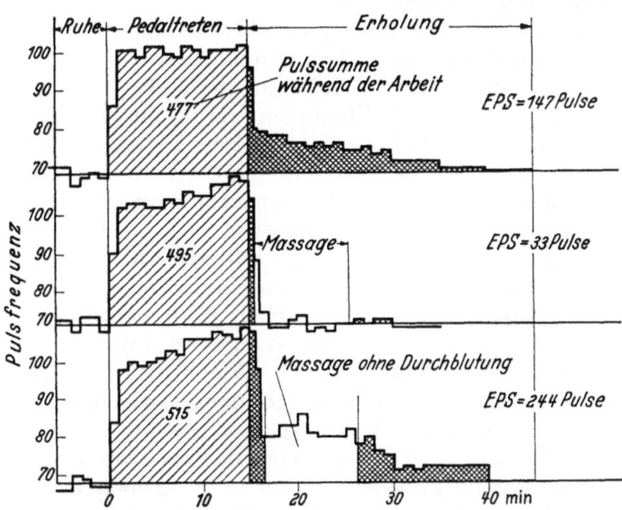

Abb. 51. Einfluß von Massage auf den Pulsabfall nach Muskelarbeit (6,5 g mkg/sec, *EPS* Erholungspulssumme). (E. A. MÜLLER 1955.)

Zweifelhaft sind cholinergische Einflüsse auf die Herzmuskulatur. An der Vorhofmuskulatur sind sie sicherlich vorhanden, dagegen scheinen sie an der Ventrikelmuskulatur des Warmblüters ohne Bedeutung zu sein [4].

Es gibt zwei Möglichkeiten, das Schlagvolumen zu vergrößern: 1. Das Herz kann in der Diastole stärker gefüllt werden (s. S. 732), 2. es kann sich in der Systole vollkommener kontrahieren (s. unten).

Steuernde Einflüsse auf die Herzkontraktion. Wenn man beobachtet, daß am intakten Kreislauf das HZV zunimmt, ohne daß die Herzgröße ansteigt, so beruht das sicherlich weitgehend darauf, daß die Steigerung des HZV im stärkeren Maße über die Frequenzsteigerung als über die Zunahme des Schlagvolumens zustande kommt. Es läßt sich aber nicht ausschließen, daß in diesen Fällen noch andere Faktoren die Herzgröße beeinflussen. Einerseits kann eine höhere Schlagfrequenz dazu führen, daß das Herz in der Diastole nicht völlig erschlafft, und daß aus diesem Grunde das diastolische Volumen verkleinert ist. Andererseits kann das Herz sich in der Systole stärker kontrahieren. Auch das isolierte Herz kontrahiert sich stärker unter dem Einfluß des Adrenalins. Entsprechend kann

---

[1] ULLRICH, RIECKER und KRAMER 1954, SARNOFF 1955.   [2] ANZOLA und RUSHMER 1956.
[3] RUSHMER und WEST 1957.   [4] ULLRICH, RIECKER und KRAMER 1954.

das Herz in situ unter nervösen oder hormonalen Einflüssen sich einmal vollkommener, ein andermal weniger vollkommen zusammenziehen. Es kann auch
auf diese Weise die Größe des Schlagvolumens regulatorisch beeinflußt werden.
Das gebremste Herz enthält eine größere Blutmenge am Ende der Systole und
wirft ein kleineres Schlagvolumen aus. Das angetriebene Herz entleert im Gegensatz dazu sich möglichst vollkommen und steigert so sein Schlagvolumen[1].
Warum unter nervösen Einflüssen sich die Kontraktionsfähigkeit des Herzens
ändert, bedarf weiterer Untersuchungen. Wahrscheinlich sind recht verschiedene
Faktoren daran beteiligt[2].

Würde man das endsystolische Volumen der Herzkammern bei den verschiedenen Funktionszuständen kennen, so wäre damit festgestellt, wieweit die
Straub-Starlingschen Gesetze auch für das Herz in situ ihre Bedeutung haben,
und unter welchen Bedingungen und bis zu welchem Ausmaß steuernde Einflüsse
den Kontraktionsablauf des Herzens beeinflussen[3]. Die Bestimmung des endsystolischen Blutvolumens mit hinreichender Genauigkeit ist aber schwierig.
Mit röntgenologischen Methoden kann man zwar die Größe des gesamten Herzens
bestimmen. Man kann davon ausgehend auch die Blutmenge im ganzen Herzen
abschätzen. Dagegen läßt sich nur sehr angenähert sagen, wieviel von dem Blut
in den Vorhöfen, wieviel in den Kammern gelegen ist. Einen Fortschritt in der
Bestimmung des endsystolischen Kammervolumens brachten Methoden, bei
denen ein Teststoff in die Kammern injiziert und seine Auswaschung aus
der Kammer verfolgt wird[4]. Wie Tabelle 19 zeigt, dürften endsystolisches
Kammervolumen und Schlagvolumen angenähert gleich groß sein. Hohe Werte
des endsystolischen Volumens findet man bei Athleten. Man darf sich nicht
wundern, daß auch bei Hunden das endsystolische Volumen im Vergleich zum
Schlagvolumen groß ist, da sie ja zu großen körperlichen Leistungen befähigt
sind. Das endsystolische Volumen scheint in jedem Falle hinreichend groß zu
sein, um bei Belastungen die Steigerung des Schlagvolumens durch verstärkte
Kontraktion der Kammermuskulatur zu ermöglichen. Athleten, die ihr Schlagvolumen besonders stark erhöhen können, haben im Ruhestand auch ein besonders
großes endsystolisches Blutvolumen der Kammer.

Schlagvolumen und diastolische Füllung. Im allgemeinen wird das Schlagvolumen dadurch vergrößert, daß sich das Herz in der Systole stärker entleert.
Es kann aber auch eine erhöhte diastolische Blutfüllung für die Vergrößerung des
Schlagvolumens von Bedeutung sein. Dies zeigen besonders neue Untersuchungen
an trainierten Hunden, die auf dem Laufband arbeiten[5], bei denen sowohl Abnahmen des endsystolischen Volumens als teilweise auch Zunahmen des enddiastolischen Kammervolumens beobachtet wurden. Wenn beim Menschen im
allgemeinen keine Zunahme des enddiastolischen Volumens gefunden wurde, dann
hängt das wohl damit zusammen, daß die meisten Untersuchungen im Liegen
durchgeführt wurden. Im Liegen sind die Kammern schon im Ruhezustand
maximal gefüllt, so daß beim Einsetzen der Arbeitsleistung keine weitere
Steigerung des enddiastolischen Kammervolumens beobachtet werden kann.

Eine Erhöhung des enddiastolischen Volumens kann durch eine Steigerung
des enddiastolischen Druckes zustande kommen, jedoch ist diese Art der Volumen-
steigerung begrenzt. Das folgt aus dem Verlauf der Ruhedehnungskurve: Höhere
Drucksteigerungen führen nur noch zu geringgradigen Zunahmen des Volumens.
Eine andere Möglichkeit, das enddiastolische Volumen zu verändern, läge darin,

---

[1] Gollwitzer-Meier 1950, Literatur bei Schwab 1950 und bei Schoedel und Kreuzer
1958.
[2] Rushmer 1956.   [3] Kramer 1959.
[4] Bing und Mitarbeiter 1951, Holt 1956, 1957.   [5] Rushmer, Franklin und Ellis 1956.

Tabelle 19. *Größe des endsystolischen Volumens (ESV) und des Verhältnisses von endsystolischem Volumen (ESV) zum Schlagvolumen (SV).*

Methodik	Autor	Objekt	ESV cm³	ESV/SV	Bemerkungen
Schätzung a. d. röntgenolog. bestimmten Herzvolumen	LILJESTRAND u. Mitarb. 1939	Männer, stehend	35	0,4	Nach dem Material der Autoren von GAUER (1955) geschätzt
	KJELLBERG u. Mitarb. 1949 a	Frauen, untrainiert, liegend	30	0,5	Nach dem Material der Autoren von GAUER (1955) geschätzt
		Männer, untrainiert, liegend	51	0,6	
		Männer, trainiert, liegend	83	1,0	
		Männer nach scharfem Training, liegend	101	1,2	
	REINDELL u. Mitarb. 1953	Männer, untrainiert, liegend	88	1,5	Schätzung der Autoren
		Männer, untrainiert, liegend	42	0,5	Nach dem gleichen Material von GAUER (1955) geschätzt
	REINDELL u. Mitarb. 1957	Männer, untrainiert, liegend	—	1,0	Schätzung der Autoren
	REINDELL u. Mitarb. 1953	Athleten, liegend	130	2,2	Schätzung der Autoren
		Athleten, liegend	117	1,4	Nach dem gleichen Material von GAUER (1955) geschätzt
Angiokardiographie	SCHAEDE u. THURN 1957	Patienten ohne Herzbelastung	—	< 1,0	
Auswaschmethode	BING u. Mitarb. 1951	Patienten ohne Herzschädigung, rechter Ventrikel	89	1,7	
Auswaschmethode	HOLT 1956	Hunde in Narkose, linker Ventrikel	38	1,2	Verschiedene Versuchsserien. Daher Absolutwerte des ESV nicht vergleichbar
Auswaschmethode	HOLT 1957 c	Hunde in Narkose, rechter Ventrikel	36	1,6	

daß nervös oder hormonal die Ruhedehnungskurve des Herzens verändert werden könnte. Diese Frage ist viel diskutiert worden. Man spricht von einer Beeinflußbarkeit des Tonus der Herzmuskulatur. Die experimentellen Befunde sprechen eher gegen als für eine regulatorische Beeinflußbarkeit der Ruhedehnungskurve. Dagegen kann bei akuter starker Überlastung die Ruhedehnungskurve nach rechts verschoben werden. Es beruht dies auf plastischen Eigenschaften der Herzmuskulatur[1]. Schließlich führt auch eine chronische Belastung des Herzens zu einer Rechtsverschiebung der Ruhedehnungskurve, die nicht in jedem Fall als pathologisch aufgefaßt werden muß.

Wenn das Sportherz ein großes diastolisches Volumen hat, dann kann es sich dabei um eine Anpassung zur Förderung großer Schlagvolumina handeln[2]. REINDELL und DELIUS sprechen von einer regulatorischen Dilatation. Da man

---

[1] REICHEL 1952, 1953, GEHL, GRAF und KRAMER 1955.
[2] REINDELL und DELIUS 1948, KLEPZIG 1955, KJELLBERG u. a. 1949 a.

im allgemeinen als regulative Vorgänge solche bezeichnet, die rasch ablaufen, chronische dagegen als Anpassung, ist der Name Anpassungsdilatation wohl besser[1]. Es handelt sich beim Sportherzen weniger um eine Dehnung des Herzens als um eine Erweiterung der Herzhöhle durch Umbau der Herzwand.

Für das enddiastolische Volumen und damit für die Größe des Schlagvolumens ist weiterhin entscheidend, ob das Herz in der Diastole wieder vollkommen erschlafft, und ob die Ruhedehnungskurve überhaupt wieder erreicht wird. Bei hohen Schlagfrequenzen braucht dies nicht der Fall zu sein. Nach Untersuchungen am isolierten Herzen müßte man annehmen, daß eine Steigerung der Frequenz auf über 100 Schläge in der Minute deshalb für die Herzleistung ungünstig wäre[2]. Da beim isolierten Herzen bei gesteigerter Schlagfrequenz in der Diastole keine volle Erschlaffung erreicht wird, nimmt das Schlagvolumen bei höheren Frequenzen rasch ab, so daß sich daraus sogar eine Verminderung des HZV ergibt. Beim Herzen in situ müssen die Verhältnisse anders liegen. Bei schwerer körperlicher Arbeit und bei sportlichen Leistungen findet man häufig Herzfrequenzen über 150 bis hinauf zu 200 Schlägen pro Minute. Dabei bleibt der Kreislauf über lange Zeit in gutem Zustand, und es werden auch große HZV gefördert (s. Tabelle 7). Am intakten Kreislauf kann das Herz auch bei großen Frequenzen große Schlagvolumina fördern. Das beruht wohl zum Teil auf dem besseren Zustand der Herzmuskulatur. Ein anderer Faktor ist die bessere diastolische Füllung des Herzens in situ, wobei die Verschiebung der Atrioventrikularebene und der starke Bluteinstrom in die Vorhöfe während der Systole von großer Bedeutung sind (s. S. 728). Schließlich spielen aber für das Herz in situ auch regulatorische Einflüsse eine Rolle, die beim isolierten Herzen fehlen. Bei Einwirkung adrenergischer Stoffe ist die Dauer der Systole stärker verkürzt, als der Frequenzsteigerung entspricht[3]. Auch erschlafft das Herz in der Diastole rascher[4]. Das Adrenalin schafft damit die Möglichkeit, daß auch bei hohen Schlagfrequenzen noch hinreichend große Schlagvolumina gefördert werden können. Über die sympathischen Herznerven kann das Herz im gleichen Sinne beeinflußt werden[5]. Auch elektrische Reize in bestimmten Gebieten des Hypothalamus rufen den gleichen Effekt hervor[6].

Bedeutung der nervösen und hormonalen Herzsteuerung. Die Zusammenhänge zwischen dem Herzen und dem peripheren Kreislauf ergeben sich weitgehend aus den Beziehungen zwischen dem Füllungsdruck des Herzens und seiner Förderleistung. In dem in Abb. 13 gezeigten Modell (s. S. 664) ist die Pumpe so konstruiert, daß sie den Füllungsdruck konstant hält. Das schafft besonders übersichtliche Verhältnisse für Betrachtungen der Kreislaufperipherie. Man kann sich an diesem Modell auch Einflüsse von seiten des Herzens klarmachen, wenn man annimmt, daß durch die nervöse und hormonale Steuerung des Herzens die Höhe des notwendigen Füllungsdruckes im Modell verstellt wird.

Nach der Auffassung der dreißiger Jahre, die heute häufig als „klassisch" bezeichnet wird, beruht das Zusammenwirken von Herz und Kreislaufperipherie auf den Straub-Starlingschen Gesetzen. Die Förderleistung des Herzens ist abhängig von seinem Füllungsdruck. Bei dieser „klassischen" Vorstellung gehen alle Umstellungen des Kreislaufs von der Peripherie aus. Durch Veränderungen der Gefäßkapazität wird dem Herzen eine größere Blutmenge zugeschoben und dadurch der Füllungsdruck und das HZV erhöht. Umgekehrt muß nach der klassischen Anschauung das Herz auch eine größere Blutmenge fördern, wenn das venöse Blutangebot ansteigt. Bluttransfusionen müssen danach den zentralvenösen Druck und das HZV steigern, bis durch regulatorische Vorgänge die Kapazität des Gefäßsystems erhöht und dadurch das Zuviel an Blutangebot wieder beseitigt ist.

---

[1] Dietlen 1951.   [2] Landowne und Katz 1950.   [3] Delius u. a. 1952.
[4] Opdyke 1952, Hild und Herz 1955, Herz 1955, Literatur bei Rushmer 1956.
[5] Anzola und Rushmer 1956.   [6] Rushmer und Smith 1959.

Nach unserer heutigen Anschauung besteht dagegen eine weitgehende Unabhängigkeit zwischen dem venösen Angebot und zentral-venösem Druck einerseits und der Herzleistung andererseits. Diese Unabhängigkeit beruht auf der nervösen und hormonalen Steuerung des Herzens. Das Herz braucht gar nicht die ganze Blutmenge, die ihm von der Peripherie angeboten wird, zu fördern. Es kann durch Vaguseinflüsse abgebremst werden. Es schlägt dann seltener und fördert bei unvollkommener Entleerung ein kleineres Schlagvolumen. Das HZV wird damit unabhängig vom venösen Füllungsdruck. Andererseits kann ein

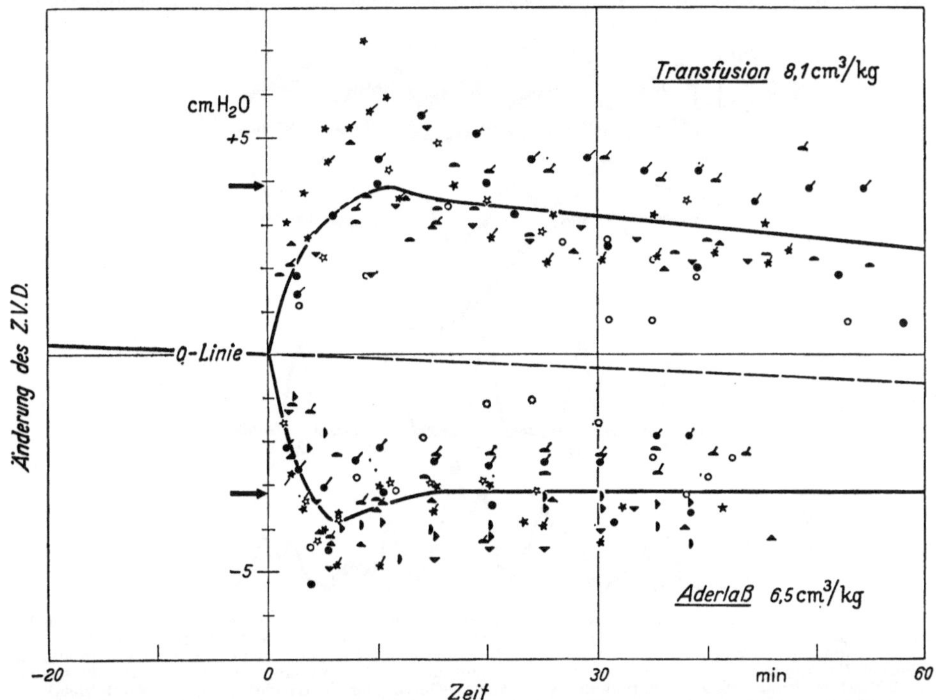

Abb. 52. Das Verhalten des zentralen Venendruckes beim Aderlaß (6,5 ml/kg Körpergewicht) und bei Bluttransfusion (8,1 ml/kg Körpergewicht). Messungen an 12 Versuchspersonen, die auf der Kurve jeweils durch ein besonderes Symbol gekennzeichnet sind. Symbole mit Diagonalstrich beziehen sich auf Wiederholungsexperimente an der gleichen Versuchsperson. Nach einer initialen Phase von 12—15 min während und unmittelbar nach Transfusion oder Aderlaß ändern sich die Drucke für den Rest der Beobachtungszeit nur noch wenig. Die Pfeile zeigen auf die Schnittpunkte der Regressionslinie für die langsame Erholungsphase mit der Nullachse. Sie zeigen die strenge Proportionalität von zentralem Druck und der Änderung des Blutvolumens (3,9/8,1 = 3,2/6,5). Der nahezu horizontale Verlauf der Regressionslinien deutet darauf hin, daß die endgültige Normalisierung des zentralen Venendruckes erst nach Wiederherstellung des normalen Blutvolumens erreicht wird (GAUER, HENRY u. SIEKER 1956).

gesteuertes Herz an einen starken Rückstrom des Blutes aus der Kreislaufperipherie angepaßt werden[1]. Besonders die Frequenzsteigerung führt dazu, daß auch bei gesteigerter Kreislauffunktion das Herz alles Blut fördert, das ihm von der Peripherie angeboten wird, ohne daß unter diesen Bedingungen der venöse Druck ansteigt. Das Herz fördert die größere Blutmenge mit normalem Füllungsdruck. Das Venensystem ist also unter diesen Bedingungen auch nicht stärker mit Blut gefüllt, und das effektive Blutvolumen ist nicht durch stärkere Füllung des Venensystems vermindert.

Die Unterschiede über das Zusammenwirken von Herz- und Kreislaufperipherie nach der klassischen modernen Auffassung führen auch zu neuen Vorstellungen über die Funktionen des Gefäßsystems. Nach der klassischen Vorstellung mußte die Gefäßkapazität eine streng

---

[1] GUYTON 1955.

gesteuerte Größe sein, denn sie bestimmte über den venösen Rückstrom die Größe des HZV. Es wurde angenommen, daß die Blutspeicher oder allgemeiner das Venensystem jede überflüssige Blutmenge aufnehmen konnten, um sie im Falle der erhöhten Kreislauffunktion wieder an das Herz abgeben zu können. Wenn man aber beim Menschen durch Aderlässe oder durch Bluttransfusionen die Blutmenge ändert, so findet man deutliche Änderungen des zentralvenösen Druckes, die über lange Zeit bestehenbleiben[1] (Abb. 52). Das Venensystem schluckt also durchaus nicht sofort das Zuviel an Blut durch Erhöhung seiner Kapazität weg. Zur Normalisierung des zentralen Venendruckes kommt es anscheinend erst durch sehr langsam verlaufende Vorgänge, in erster Linie durch erhöhte Harnproduktion. Der erhöhte Venendruck ist in diesen Fällen Folge der Dämpfung der Herztätigkeit. Das Herz fördert nicht alles Blut, das ihm angeboten wird. Derartige Kreislaufeinstellungen zeigen sich anscheinend

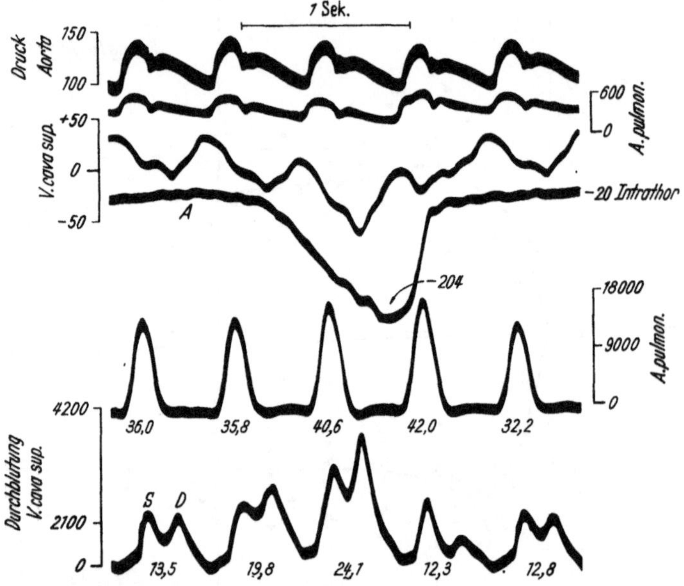

Abb. 53. Wirkung der Spontanatmung auf den venösen Rückfluß und die Durchblutung der A. pulmonalis. Hund von 25 kg. Kurven von oben nach unten: Druck in der Aorta in mm Hg, Druck in der A. pulmonalis, in V. cava sup. und Intrathorakaldruck in mm H_2O, Durchblutung der A. pulm. und der V. cava sup. in ml/min. A Beginn der Inspiration; S Beschleunigung der Durchblutung der V. cava sup. während der Ventrikelsystole; D Beschleunigung der Durchblutung der V. cava sup. während der Ventrikeldiastole. (Brecher 1955.)

nicht nur bei experimenteller Änderung der Blutmenge, sie kommen auch unter regelhaften Bedingungen vor. Sie zeigen sich bei der Umstellung des Blutkreislaufs als Folge des Lagewechsels. Auch bei Blutverlagerungen zwischen den Hautgefäßen und dem übrigen Organismus im Dienste der Temperaturregulation spielen sie eine große Rolle[2]. Es soll damit nicht gesagt werden, daß die Einstellung der Gefäßkapazität für die Kreislaufregulation ohne Bedeutung ist. Es sind aber in jedem Fall zwei Mechanismen möglich, die Veränderung der Förderleistung des Herzens auf Grund seiner nervös-hormonalen Steuerung und die Änderung der Gefäßkapazität. Es bedarf weiterer Untersuchungen, welchem von den beiden Mechanismen in jedem einzelnen Falle die hauptsächliche Bedeutung zuzuschreiben ist.

Nachdem die Straub-Starlingschen Gesetze in den dreißiger Jahren in ihrer Bedeutung für den Kreislauf sicherlich überschätzt worden sind, wird jetzt manchmal die Ansicht geäußert, daß sie für den intakten Kreislauf überhaupt ohne Bedeutung seien. Demgegenüber muß betont werden, daß sie sich immer zeigen, wenn das Spiel der Regulationen aufgehoben ist, oder auch wenn eine gleichmäßige Regulationslage eingehalten wird[3]. Die Straub-Starlingschen Gesetze zeigen sich besonders deutlich in Narkose, wenn die nervös-reflektorischen Steuerungsmechanismen gedämpft sind. Sie treten hervor, wenn die regulatorischen Mechanismen bis an die Grenze des Möglichen beansprucht sind. Sie

---

[1] Gauer, Henry und Sieker 1956.   [2] Glaser 1949.   [3] Hamilton 1955, Sarnoff 1955.

zeigen sich auch bei raschen Änderungen, da die regulatorischen Vorgänge eine
bestimmte Zeit beanspruchen. So läßt Abb. 53[1] erkennen, wie bei der Einatmung
durch die Änderung des intrathorakalen Druckes der Füllungsdruck des Herzens
ansteigt, und wie als Folge der Steigerung des Füllungsdruckes das HZV zunimmt.
Es handelt sich um nichts anderes als um Auswirkungen des Straub-Starlingschen
Gesetzes.

Die Überschätzung der Straub-Starlingschen Gesetze brachte teilweise die
Gefahr mit sich, daß die nervösen Einflüsse auf das Herz für die Steuerung
seiner Funktion unterschätzt wurden. Vergessen wurden sie natürlich nie.
Man hat immer gewußt, daß mit dem Funktionszustand des Kreislaufs sich die
Herzfrequenz ändert, und daß die Frequenz sehr weitgehend nervös gesteuert ist.
Dazu kam in den dreißiger Jahren dieses Jahrhunderts die Beobachtung über das
Fehlen der Herzvergrößerung bei Muskeltätigkeit, das mit den einfachen Herz-
grundgesetzen, wie sie am isolierten Herzen beobachtet werden, nicht zu erklären
war. Heute gibt es viele Befunde, die darauf hinweisen, daß die nervösen Steuerungen des Herzens für die Herzdynamik von entscheidender Bedeutung sind.
Beobachtungen, daß man an trainierten, nichtnarkotisierten Hunden durch
elektrische Reizung im Hypothalamusgebiet eine Umstellung der Herztätigkeit
auf die „Arbeitsdynamik" erreichen kann, und daß bei diesen Tieren auch durch
bedingte Reflexe die Umstellung der Herztätigkeit erreicht wird, sind sicherlich
von großer Wichtigkeit[2]. Eingleisiges Denken ist in der Biologie verboten. Das
gilt auch für die Herzdynamik. Man muß wissen, daß die Gesetzmäßigkeiten, die
in der Struktur der Herzmuskelfaser verankert sind, jederzeit gültig sind. Man
muß sich aber auch bewußt sein, daß das Herz in situ nervösen Einflüssen unterliegt. Besonders durch Veränderung der Herzfrequenz, aber auch durch Einflüsse
auf Kontraktilität der Muskelfasern überdecken diese nervösen Einflüsse nicht
selten die Gesetzmäßigkeiten, die in der Muskelfaser selbst ihren Ursprung haben.

VI. Herzinsuffizienz und Herzmuskelinsuffizienz.

1. Definitionen.

Unklare Definitionen der Herzinsuffizienz sind häufig Ursache von Miß-
verständnissen. So werden z. B. Kreislaufinsuffizienz und Herzinsuffizienz oft
synonym gebraucht. Die Kreislaufinsuffizienz ist aber der übergeordnete Begriff.
Eine Kreislaufinsuffizienz kann vom Herzen ausgehen, sie kann aber ebenso auf
Störungen der peripheren Zirkulation beruhen (z. B. auf einem verminderten
Blutangebot an das Herz beim Schock, beim Kollaps, bei orthostatischen Störungen).

Herzinsuffizienz besagt zunächst nichts anderes als eine Einschränkung der
Leistung des Herzens. Leistungseinschränkung braucht im Ruhezustand nicht
bemerkbar zu sein und kommt häufig erst bei Belastung des Herzens zur Auswirkung. Die Leistungseinschränkung des Herzens kann auf verschiedenen Ursachen beruhen:

a) auf Tachykardien und Arrhythmien, die die Füllungszeiten des Herzens
ungünstig beeinflussen;

b) auf Strombahnhindernissen durch Verwachsungen bei Accretio und Concretio cordis oder auf hämodynamischen Störungen infolge Ventildefekten im
Bereich der Klappen des Herzens;

c) auf einer Herz*muskel*insuffizienz.

Die unter a) und b) aufgeführten Zustände bedingen eine unrationelle Arbeitsweise des Herzens. Diese krankhaften Veränderungen der Herztätigkeit können

---

[1] BRECHER 1955.   [2] RUSHMER und SMITH 1959.

dazu führen, daß das geförderte HZV zu klein wird, so daß der für die periphere Blutversorgung notwendige arterielle Druck nicht aufrecht erhalten wird. Eine solche Leistungseinbuße des Herzens bedeutet aber noch nicht, daß der Herz*muskel* insuffizient ist. Für die klinischen, vor allem therapeutischen Aspekte ist es von sehr großer Bedeutung, die Herz*muskel*insuffizienz von den anderen Formen der Herzinsuffizienz zu trennen. Die Domäne der Digitalistherapie ist die Herzmuskelinsuffizienz, während bei Leistungsminderungen des Herzens, wie sie z. B. durch Arrhythmien oder Strombahnhindernisse oder Ventildefekte zustande kommen, eine therapeutische Wirkung der Digitalis nicht ohne weiteres erwartet werden kann.

Es ist immer wieder versucht worden, für die Herzmuskelinsuffizienz funktionelle Charakteristika ausfindig zu machen, die die Herzmuskelinsuffizienz hämodynamisch von anderen Formen der Herzinsuffizienz abgrenzen lassen. Wurde eine Zeitlang die venöse Rückstauung als das entscheidende Merkmal der Herzmuskelinsuffizienz angesehen (sog. back pressure theorie), so wurde später die Erniedrigung des Kreislaufminutenvolumens als das wichtigste Charakteristikum in den Vordergrund gestellt (sog. forward failure theorie)[1]. Schon aus den obigen Darlegungen geht hervor, daß die Erniedrigung des Kreislaufminutenvolumens allein kein Unterscheidungsmerkmal der Herzmuskelinsuffizienz gegenüber den anderen Formen von Herzinsuffizienz sein kann. Überblickt man weiterhin die Wandlungen der Anschauungen über die Orthologie der Herzdynamik in den letzten 20 Jahren (s. Orthologie der Herzdynamik), so erkennt man, wie schwierig es überhaupt ist, pathophysiologische Kriterien ausfindig zu machen, die nur für die Herzmuskelinsuffizienz Geltung besitzen. Wenn schon im Bereich noch normaler Veränderungen die Auswurfleistung des Herzens unter gleichzeitigen Veränderungen der Füllung und der diastolischen Faserspannung der Kammern bemerkenswerte Schwankungen aufweisen kann, so liegen die Schwierigkeiten einer exakten Abgrenzung der Herzmuskelinsuffizienz vom normalen bzw. von den oben aufgeführten anderen Formen der Herzinsuffizienz erst recht auf der Hand. Die auf den Experimenten von Starling und Straub basierende klassische Lehre, daß ein suffizientes Herz alles Blut, das ihm angeboten wird, wegschafft, daß Erhöhungen der Restblutmenge und Erhöhungen des diastolischen Kammerdrucks generell als Zeichen einer Insuffizienz des Herzmuskels angesehen werden müssen, ist in dieser Form nicht mehr aufrechtzuerhalten. Eine präzise Aussage über die hämodynamischen Kriterien, die die Herzmuskelinsuffizienz von noch normalen Variationen klar abtrennen, kann u. E. nicht gemacht werden. Zur Charakterisierung der hämodynamischen Verhältnisse bei der Herzmuskelinsuffizienz gehen wir besser per exclusionem vor und stellen die Frage, welche hämodynamischen Voraussetzungen bei der Herzmuskelinsuffizienz erfüllt sein müssen. Die Antwort ist recht eindeutig: Eine Herzmuskelinsuffizienz liegt *nur* dann vor, wenn bei körperlicher Beanspruchung oder sogar bei körperlicher Ruhe das Kreislaufminutenvolumen unter dem zu fordernden Sollwert (s. weiter unten) liegt und gleichzeitig der diastolische Druck in der Kammer infolge erhöhter Restblutmenge angestiegen ist. Wenn mit dieser Aussage zunächst nur die Conditio sine qua non für das Vorliegen einer Herzmuskelinsuffizienz erfüllt ist, so fragt es sich weiter, ob regelhafte Schwankungen dieser Größen wenigstens in quantitativer Hinsicht von pathologischen zu unterscheiden sind. Es wurde bereits darauf hingewiesen, daß es im Normalbereich problematisch erscheint, ob man als Maß für die diastolische Füllung bzw. Faserspannung die gemessenen diastolischen Druckwerte

---

Literatur s. Friedberg 1959.

in der Kammer verwerten darf. Bei der manifesten Herzmuskelinsuffizienz ist der enddiastolische Druck in der Kammer (und damit auch der Vorhofdruck) in der Regel deutlich erhöht[1]. Jedoch ist es bisher nicht möglich, eine exakte Grenze festzulegen, wann wir noch von einer regelhaften bzw. regulatorischen Drucksteigerung und wann wir von einer Erhöhung des diastolischen Drucks in der Kammer als Ausdruck einer Leistungsschwäche des Herzmuskels sprechen können. Die Entscheidung ist schon deshalb sehr schwierig, weil bei Hypertrophie der Kammermuskulatur, z. B. infolge Pulmonal- oder Aortenstenose die enddiastolischen Druckwerte beachtlich ansteigen können. So wurden bei Pulmonalstenosen (ohne Ventrikelseptumdefekt) enddiastolische Drucke von mehr als 10 mm Hg gemessen, ohne daß Anzeichen einer Herzmuskelinsuffizienz vorlagen[2]. Bei Widerstandsbelastung der linken Kammer infolge Aortenklappenstenose wurden ohne Vorliegen einer Herzmuskelinsuffizienz analoge Steigerungen des enddiastolischen Drucks in der linken Kammer gefunden[3]. Sowohl bei der Pulmonalstenose wie bei der Aortenstenose wurde eine deutliche Korrelation zwischen dem Grad der Widerstandsbelastung und der Erhöhung des enddiastolischen Drucks in der betroffenen Kammer festgestellt.

Zum Verhalten des Kreislaufminutenvolumens ist folgendes zu bemerken: Das Kreislaufminutenvolumen kann bei der Herzmuskelinsuffizienz unter dem Ruhewert des sog. normalen Herzindex liegen (absolute Erniedrigung des HZV, sog. ,,low output failure"). Bei Zuständen von O_2-Mangel (z. B. Cor pulmonale), bei Stoffwechselsteigerungen (körperlicher Arbeit, Basedow), bei arterio-venösen Fisteln oder bei hochgradigen Anämien kommt es zu starken Erhöhungen des Kreislaufminutenvolumens, die auch im Stadium der Insuffizienz des Herzmuskels noch beachtlich über den als normal geltenden absoluten Zahlen für den Herzindex liegen können (sog. ,,high output failure")[4], und die dennoch für die jeweilige Stoffwechsellage unzureichend sind (relative Erniedrigung des Kreislaufminutenvolumens).

Zusammenfassend ist festzustellen: Eine grundsätzliche Unterscheidung der Herzmuskelinsuffizienz gegenüber dem normalen Schwankungsbereich ist in hämodynamischer Hinsicht nicht möglich. Wohl kann man den Leitsatz aufstellen: Keine Herzmuskelinsuffizienz ohne gleichzeitiges Absinken der geforderten Leistung *und* Anstieg des diastolischen Kammerdrucks. Bei der manifesten Herzmuskelinsuffizienz sind diastolische Kammerdrucke und Vorhofdrucke in der Regel deutlich höher als bei Änderungen der Herzdynamik unter Normalbedingungen. Eine große Schwierigkeit besteht darin, festzustellen, ob die geforderte Leistung erfüllt wird. Einen wichtigen Anhalt gibt der Sauerstoffgehalt des venösen Mischblutes und die arterio-venöse O_2-Differenz.

2. Die Bedeutung der Starling-Straubschen Herzgesetze für die Herzmuskelinsuffizienz.

Während das normale Herz im Bereich normaler Belastungen von den Grundeigenschaften der dem Herzmuskel innewohnenden Anpassungsmöglichkeiten, die Auswurfleistung durch erhöhte diastolische Füllung zu steigern, offenbar nur teilweise Gebrauch macht (s. Herzdynamik), rückt diese in den sog. Starling-Straubschen Herzgesetzen zum Ausdruck kommende Adaptationsmöglichkeit beim geschädigten Herzen mehr und mehr in den Vordergrund. Das muskelschwache Herz, bei dem die nervalhumoralen Anpassungsmöglichkeiten an eine veränderte Leistung bereits erschöpft sind, ist weitgehend darauf angewiesen,

---

[1] COURNAND und Mitarbeiter 1952.　　[2] GROSSE-BROCKHOFF und WOLTER 1958.
[3] FLEMING und GIBSON 1957.　　[4] McMICHAEL 1946, STEAD und Mitarbeiter 1948.

seine Leistung durch Erhöhung der diastolischen Füllung zu steigern. Solange dieser Anpassungsmechanismus ausreicht, um die Peripherie zu versorgen, sprechen wir von Kompensation. Auch diese Unterscheidung hat wichtige praktische Konsequenzen. Bei noch kompensierten Herzen ist Digitalis nutzlos, beim dekompensierten (insuffizienten) Herzmuskel dagegen wirksam.

Die Beziehungen zwischen Steigerung der Auswurfleistung durch Erhöhung der diastolischen Füllung gelten auch im physiologischen Bereich nur innerhalb gewisser Grenzen. Wird im Herz-Lungenpräparat der Venendruck bis zu einem Punkt erhöht, bei dem bereits eine Überdehnung bzw. Überfüllung des Herzens eintritt, so steigt das Schlagvolumen nicht weiter an. Eine weitere Erhöhung des Füllungsdruckes geht dann sogar mit einem eindeutigen Abfall des Schlagvolumens einher[1]. Es darf auf Grund vieler Untersuchungen, in denen der Druckablauf im Herzen und das Kreislaufminutenvolumen mittels Herzkatheterisierung gemessen wurden, als wahrscheinlich angenommen werden, daß beim insuffizienten Herzmuskel das Optimum der diastolischen Füllung eher erreicht ist als beim normalen Herzen[2] (s. Abb. 54). Mit anderen Worten: Das muskelinsuffiziente Herz bedarf zwar einer Erhöhung des Füllungsdruckes um eine geforderte Auswurfleistung zu vollbringen, es schwebt jedoch dabei in der Gefahr, daß das Optimum der Füllung überschritten wird,

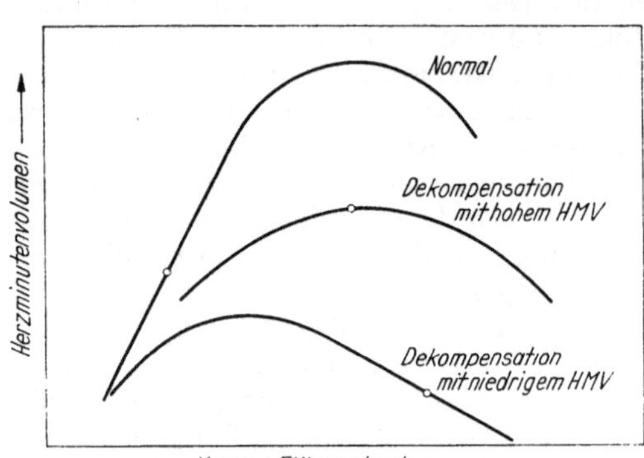

Abb. 54. Hypothetische Kurven über die Beziehungen zwischen dem venösen Füllungsdruck und dem Herzminutenvolumen beim Normalen und bei Dekompensierten mit hohem und niedrigem Minutenvolumen. Die Ausgangslage des Füllungsdruckes ist durch O gekennzeichnet. Das normale Herz kann zugleich mit einem Anstieg des venösen Füllungsdruckes sein Schlagvolumen auf ein hohes Niveau heben. Im Herzversagen der Anämie wird wahrscheinlich das hohe Minutenvolumen wenigstens zum Teil durch den erhöhten Füllungsdruck aufrecht erhalten, doch kann dessen weitere Erhöhung zu einer Abnahme des Minutenvolumens führen. Bei schweren Dekompensationen mit niedrigem Minutenvolumen ist das Herz in den meisten Fällen bereits in einem Zustand, in dem auch kleine Anstiege des Füllungsdruckes zu einem weiteren Abfall des Minutenvolumens führen. (McMichael 1953.)

daß die Kammer überfüllt bzw. überdehnt wird und hierdurch die Leistung weiter absinkt. Erschwerend kommt hinzu, daß durch die infolge der Insuffizienz eingetretene schlechte O_2-Versorgung der kreislaufregulierenden Zentren eine Blutmobilisierung in der Peripherie ausgelöst wird, so daß das venöse Angebot an das Herz übermäßig groß werden kann[3]. Hinzu kommt die Vermehrung der Blutmenge, die in den meisten Fällen von Herzinsuffizienz vorhanden ist[4]. Auch aus diesen Erkenntnissen ergeben sich wiederum wichtige therapeutische Konsequenzen: Im Zustand der Überfüllung des Herzens ist dafür Sorge zu tragen, daß der venöse Füllungsdruck des Herzens herabgesetzt wird. Als therapeutische Maßnahmen kommen besonders in Frage: entsprechende Lagerung des Patienten mit aufgerichtetem Oberkörper bei herabhängenden unteren Extremitäten und ausgiebiger Aderlaß.

3. Verschiedene Formen der Herzmuskelinsuffizienz.

Wir unterscheiden zweckmäßigerweise zwischen einer Überlastungsinsuffizienz und einer Insuffizienz, die durch primäre Schädigung der Muskelfibrillen eintritt.

---

[1] Starling 1915. [2] McMichael und Mitarbeiter 1946.
[3] Wollheim 1931, Freis und Rose 1957, Linhart und Přerosky 1957.
[4] Wollheim 1931, 1950, Brown, Hopper und Wennesland 1957.

a) Überlastungsinsuffizienz.

Bei der Überlastungsinsuffizienz trennen wir *akute* und *chronische* Form voneinander ab.

α) Akute Überlastung. Wird im Herz-Lungenpräparat der Aortenwiderstand durch Einengung des Aortenquerschnitts verändert, so stellen sich die folgenden Veränderungen der Dynamik des Herzens ein, wie sie in der Abb. 55 zum Ausdruck kommen[1]. Unmittelbar nach Erhöhung des Widerstandes steigt der diastolische Kammerdruck als Folge einer Erhöhung der Restblutmenge geringgradig an. Zunächst wird die Erhöhung des Widerstandes durch entsprechende Vergrößerung der diastolischen Füllung bzw. der diastolischen Faserspannung glatt überwunden (Kurve 1—3). Die Kurve 4 dagegen stellt die Veränderung des Druckablaufs bei eintretender Insuffizienz dar. In typischer Weise wird die Druckkurve in der linken Kammer flacher, die Steilheit des Kurvenanstiegs geringer, die Kurve ist im ganzen verbreitert und ihr Gipfel erniedrigt. Durch die erhebliche Vergrößerung des systolischen Blutrückstandes in der Kammer steigen jetzt der diastolische Kammerdruck und der Druck im Vorhof wesentlich an. Erniedrigung des Schlagvolumens und Erhöhung des diastolischen Kammerdruckes und des Vorhofdruckes sind die Kennzeichen der eingetretenen Dekompensation. Wenn diese am Herz-Lungenpräparat gewonnenen Erkenntnisse auch nur mit Vorbehalten auf das im Gesamtkreislauf arbeitende Herz übertragen werden dürfen, so erscheinen die eintretenden hämodynamischen Veränderungen bei akuter Überlastung des Herzens damit im Grundsätzlichen richtig wiedergegeben. Eine akute Überlastungsinsuffizienz durch plötzliche Widerstandserhöhung ist in der Klinik selten. Genannt seien die akute Glomerulonephritis oder andere Blutdruckkrisen im großen bzw. kleinen Kreislauf. Auch wurden akute Insuffizienzen bei übermäßiger Leistung jugendlicher Sportler in seltenen Fällen beobachtet.

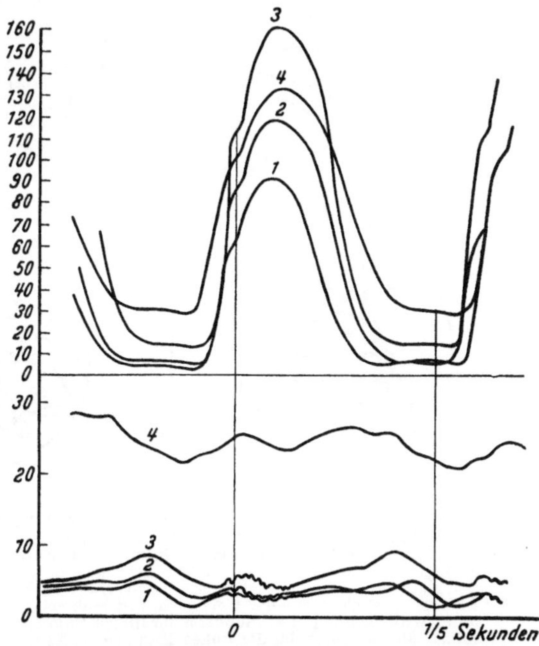

Abb. 55. Druck im linken Ventrikel (oben) und linken Vorhof (unten) bei steigendem Aortenwiderstand. Mit wachsendem Widerstand steigt der Vorhofdruck und der diastolische Ventrikeldruck. Kurve 1—3 bei suffizientem Herzmuskel; Kurve 4 bei insuffizientem Herzmuskel. Die Insuffizienz ist gekennzeichnet durch Verbreiterung der Druckkurve, Steigen des diastolischen und Sinken des systolischen Druckes in der Kammer bei stark erhöhtem Vorhofdruck. (STRAUB 1914.)

β) Chronische Überlastung. Am häufigsten begegnet uns die Herzmuskelinsuffizienz in der Klinik als Folge chronischer Überlastung. Die Belastung tritt entweder in Form einer ausschließlichen oder vorwiegenden *Volumenbelastung* (arterio-venöse Fisteln, Basedow, Anämien, chronischer O_2-Mangel bei Emphysem oder anderen Lungenerkrankungen, Klappeninsuffizienzen) oder in Form vorwiegender oder ausschließlicher *Druckbelastung* auf (z. B. Hypertonie im großen

---

[1] STRAUB 1926.

oder kleinen Kreislauf, Aortenstenose, Pulmonalstenose). Die Überlastung kann sich dabei auf eine Kammer allein beschränken wie z. B. bei der Pulmonalstenose oder dem Cor pulmonale infolge Widerstandserhöhung im kleinen Kreislauf. Häufig sind beide Kammern im gleichen Ausmaß betroffen (z. B. arterio-venöse Fisteln, Basedow). Besteht zunächst eine alleinige Überlastung der linken Herzkammer (z. B. eine Hypertonie im großen Kreislauf, ein Aortenfehler oder eine Mitralinsuffizienz), so kommt es bei eintretender Dekompensation rückwirkend auch zu einer Überlastung der rechten Kammer (s. dazu weiter unten).

Bevor bei einer chronischen Überlastung die Insuffizienz des Herzmuskels eintritt, wird das Stadium der sog. *Adaptation* oder *Kompensation* durchlaufen.

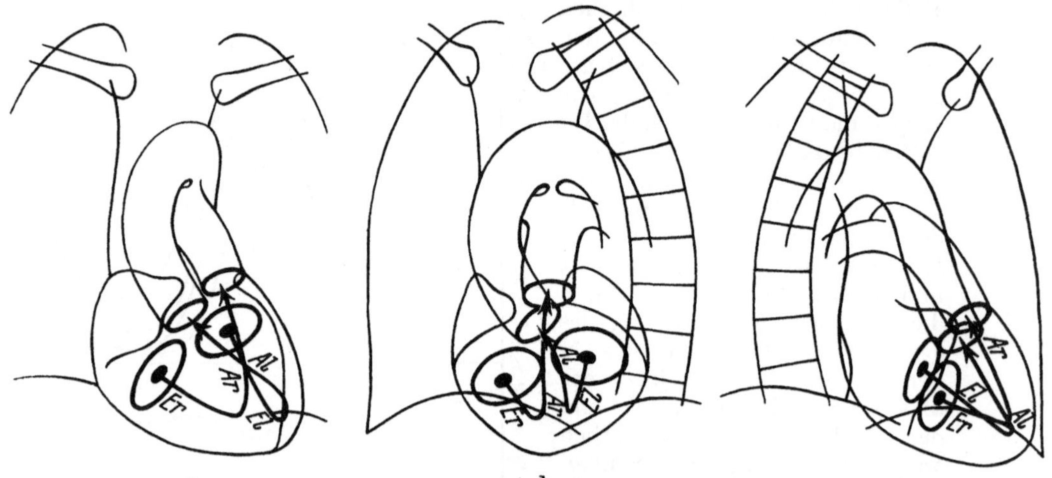

a   b   c

Abb. 56 a—c. Schematische Übersicht der Ein- und Ausflußbahnen des Herzens. Verlaufsrichtung der Ein- und Ausflußbahn beider Kammern. a Im Ventralbild; b in linker vorderer Schrägstellung; c in rechter vorderer Schrägstellung. *Er* Einflußbahn der rechten Kammer; *Ar* Ausflußbahn der rechten Kammer; *El* Einflußbahn der linken Kammer; *Al* Ausflußbahn der linken Kammer. Zu a: Die Einflußbahn der rechten Kammer (*Er*) verläuft nur wenig zur Herzspitze geneigt in fast transversaler Richtung von rechts nach links. Die Ausflußbahn der rechten Kammer (*Ar*) zieht von der Herzspitze fast senkrecht zum Pulmonalisostium und findet auf dem Zwerchfell ein festes Widerlager. Die Einflußbahn der linken Kammer (*El*) verläuft im wesentlichen von hinten oben zur Herzspitze. Die Ausflußbahn der linken Kammer bildet (*Al*) den linken Kammerbogen. Sie erstreckt sich von der Herzspitze nach oben rechts zum Aortenostium. Zu b: Die Einflußbahn der linken Kammer (*El*) erscheint ebenso wie die der rechten (*Er*) stark verkürzt. Zu c: Die Einflußbahn der rechten Kammer (*Er*) erscheint in dieser Projektion wegen ihres annähernd transversalen Verlaufs stark verkürzt. Die Ausflußbahn der rechten Kammer (*Ar*) ist an der linken vorderen Begrenzung des Herzschattens randbildend. Die Einflußbahn der linken Kammer (*El*) bestimmt wegen ihres stark dorsoventralen Verlaufs neben der Größe des dorsal an die Kammer angrenzenden linken Vorhofs die Tiefenausdehnung des Herzschattens. Die Ausflußbahn der linken Kammer (*Al*) erzeugt wegen ihres von links nach vorne nach rechts oben hinten gerichteten Verlaufs bei ihrer Verlängerung in dieser Projektion keine wesentliche Veränderung des Herzschattens, höchstens reicht die Herzspitze tiefer unter das linke Diaphragma herab. Die Querdehnung der Ausflußbahn kann aber zu einer verstärkten Abrundung des linken Herzschattens führen. (Zdansky 1949.)

In dieser Phase entwickelt sich zunächst eine „regulative" Dilatation[1] oder besser Anpassungsdilatation[2] (früher „tonogen" genannt, s. S. 733[3]). Das Herz soll dabei durch die erhöhte diastolische Füllung der gesteigerten Druck- oder Volumenbelastung angepaßt sein. Die Herzfrequenz ist in diesem Zustand häufig, aber nicht regelmäßig gesteigert. Die Anfangsstadien der Anpassungsdilatation entgehen vielfach dem röntgenologischen Nachweis. Mit der Zeit erfährt die Konfiguration des Herzens charakteristische Umwandlungen, je nachdem ob es sich um eine Beanspruchung auf Widerstand oder um eine Volumbelastung handelt (s. Abb. 56). Bei der Widerstandsbelastung wird in erster Linie die Ausflußbahn des Herzens verändert[4]. Die Anpassungsdilatation manifestiert sich hierbei vorwiegend in einer Verlängerung der Ausflußbahn, wodurch die überlastete Kammer

---

[1] Reindell und Delius 1948.　　[2] Dietlen 1951.　　[3] Moritz 1905.　　[4] Kirch 1955.

insgesamt eine Streckung erfährt. Bei stärkeren Graden einer Widerstandserhöhung ist auch eine Dilatation der Einflußbahn, kenntlich an der Zunahme des Querdurchmessers, nachweisbar[1]. Bei der Volumbelastung tritt von Anfang an eine Dilatation der Einflußbahn auf[2]. Hierbei besteht schon im Beginn eine Verbreiterung des Herzens im Querdurchmesser.

Allerdings ist es oft recht schwierig, geringere Dilatationen im Röntgenbild zu erkennen. Wesentlich ist, daß solche regulativen Dilatationen ohne Zeichen einer Insuffizienz des Herzmuskels erhebliche Grade erreichen können. Die Größe der Herzkammer ist also kein Kriterium für die Leistungsfähigkeit des Herzens. Auch große Herzen können durchaus noch leistungsfähig sein. Der Funktionszustand des Herzens läßt sich daher nie auf Grund der Herzgröße beurteilen, sondern nur auf Grund entsprechender Funktionsproben. Der Funktionszustand läßt sich eindeutig bestimmen, wenn man das Kreislaufminutenvolumen und die Druckverhältnisse in den Herzhöhlen kennt. In der Klinik ist man jedoch auf andere Kriterien angewiesen, die indirekt etwas über die Funktionstüchtigkeit des Herzmuskels aussagen (Rückstauungssymptome, Cyanose, Dyspnoe usw.). Die Leistung des Herzens kann unter Ruhebedingungen noch ausreichend sein, während schon bei Belastung durch körperliche Arbeit Insuffizienzsymptome des Herzmuskels in Erscheinung treten. Die Herzmuskelinsuffizienz tritt in der Regel zunächst während körperlicher Belastung auf. Die Insuffizienz des Herzmuskels, die auch bei vollkommener Bettruhe bestehenbleibt, stellt erst das Endstadium dar.

Bei der chronischen Überbelastung erfährt das Herz neben den durch die Anpassungsdilatation bedingten Formveränderungen noch einen weiteren Umbau durch die eintretende Hypertrophie des Muskels. Bei der Entstehung der Hypertrophie des Herzmuskels springt die Bedeutung der Grundeigenschaften des Herzmuskels besonders eindeutig in die Augen. Nicht die in der Zeiteinheit geleistete Arbeit des Herzens ist entscheidend für die Wandstärke seiner Muskulatur. Mehrleistungen des Herzens, die allein durch Erhöhungen der Herzfrequenz zustandekommen, haben keine Hypertrophie zur Folge. Alle jene Mehrleistungen aber bedingen eine Hypertrophie, die mit einer erhöhten diastolischen Anfangsspannung des Ventrikels einhergehen. Ein Herz hypertrophiert, wenn sein Energieumsatz je Kontraktion ansteigt[3].

Die Frage, inwieweit die Hypertrophie die Leistungsfähigkeit des Herzens verbessert, ist immer noch umstritten. Schon beim Sportherzen ist sie nicht eindeutig zu beantworten. Im Tierexperiment konnten keine Beziehungen zwischen dem Grad der Hypertrophie und der Leistungssteigerung gefunden werden[4]. Sicher ist, daß der hypertrophische Herzmuskel in seiner Blutversorgung schlechter gestellt ist als der normale Muskel. Sowohl in tierexperimentellen Untersuchungen[5] als auch in Untersuchungen an Herzen menschlicher Leichen[6] war die Zahl der Capillaren im hypertrophischen Muskel pro Quadratmillimeter Muskel eindeutig herabgesetzt (Abb. 57). In Laufversuchen an Meerschweinchen wurden in neuester Zeit folgende Zahlen ermittelt: Bei hypertrophierten Herzen, deren Gewicht im Durchschnitt 18% über dem normalen Herzgewicht lag, war die Zahl der Capillaren pro mm² um 9%, bei Hypertrophien, deren Durchschnittsgewicht um 26% höher lag als normalerweise, war die Capillarzahl um 18% niedriger als normalerweise. Berechnungen des Verhältnisses der Zahl der Capillaren zur Zahl der Muskelfasern ergaben für hypertrophierte und normale Herzmuskeln annähernd gleiche Werte. Weiterhin zeigten postmortale Durchströmungsversuche des Coronarsystems, daß die absolute Durchblutung infolge Querschnittserweiterung beim hypertrophierten Herzen erhöht sein kann, daß aber die Durchblutung erniedrigt ist, wenn man sie auf die Muskelmasse bezieht[7].

Nur in Ausnahmefällen kommt es zu einer Vermehrung der Faserzahlen und der Capillarzahlen, nämlich dann, wenn das kritische Herzgewicht von 500 g überschritten wird[8]. Es ist

---

[1] Thurn 1956.   [2] Zdlansky 1949.   [3] Weizsäcker 1926.   [4] Hakkila 1955.
[5] Frank 1950, Hakkila 1955.   [6] Roberts und Wearor 1941, Linzbach 1947.
[7] Dock 1956, Vivell 1951.   [8] Linzbach 1950, 1951.

noch umstritten, ob eine Vermehrung der Faser- und Capillarzahlen eintritt, wenn die Überlastung des Herzens bereits im frühen Wachstumsalter einsetzt. Jedoch scheint es nach den
neueren Untersuchungen wahrscheinlich, daß eine Vermehrung der Capillarzahlen auch in
solchen Fällen fehlt[1]. Wahrscheinlich würde der hypertrophierte Muskel von einer solchen
Vermehrung der Capillaren auch keinen Nutzen haben, da für die Diffusionsbedingungen fast
ausschließlich der Querschnitt der Einzelfaser von Bedeutung ist. Der Bindegewebsrahmen,
der die Fasern umgibt, hat bei dem niedrigen Stoffwechsel in diesem Gebiet angenähert den
gleichen Sauerstoffdruck wie das Capillarblut. Damit liegt die Gefahr einer unzureichenden
Sauerstoffversorgung überwiegend in dem verlängerten Diffusionsweg von der Peripherie
der verdickten Faser bis in ihr Zentrum. Es bedarf neuer Berechnungen, um festzustellen,
welche Faserdicken für die Sauerstoffversorgung des Faserinnern kritisch werden[2]. Nach
elektrokardiographischen Befunden soll auch das hypertrophe Sportherz gegen Sauerstoffmangel empfindlicher sein als das normale[3]. Dem ist freilich in letzter Zeit widersprochen
worden[4].

Wenn somit jedenfalls sichergestellt ist, daß der hypertrophierte Herzmuskel bezüglich seiner Ernährungsbedingungen schlechter steht als der normale, so ist trotzdem nicht
in Abrede zu stellen, daß die Herzhypertrophie eine kompensatorische Maßnahme darstellt,

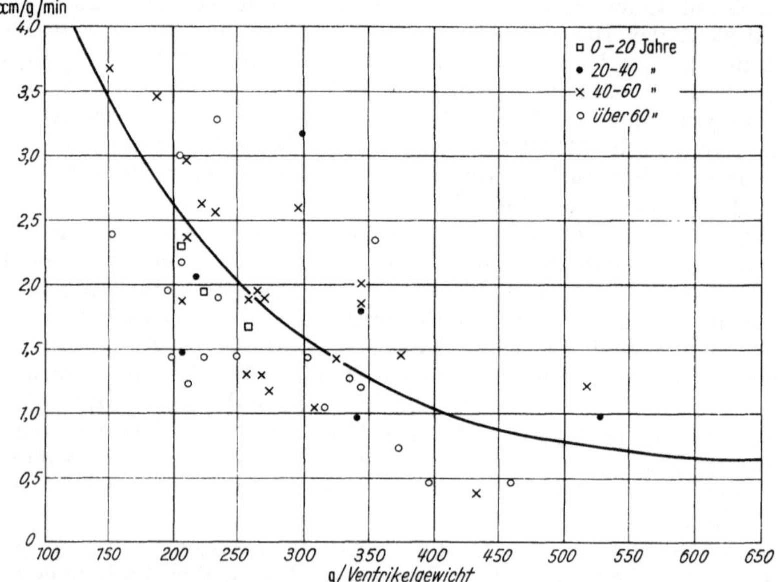

Abb. 57. Die postmortale Durchströmungsfähigkeit des Coronarsystems bei normalen und hypertrophierten
Herzen. Abnahme der Durchströmung pro Gramm Herzgewicht mit zunehmender Herzhypertrophie.
(Vivell 1950.)

die den überlasteten Herzmuskel wenigstens eine Zeitlang in die Lage versetzt, den erhöhten Anforderungen nachzukommen. Vielleicht darf man die Hypertrophie als einen
Kompensationsmechanismus ansehen, der trotz seiner zeitweiligen günstigen Wirkung den
Keim für ein vorzeitiges Versagen der Faser in sich birgt. Die Hypertrophie durch Dicken-
zunahme der einzelnen Fibrillen bedeutet technisch gesprochen eine Materialverschlechterung.
Der Zylinder eines Motors kann zwar eine Zeitlang mit höheren Drucken belastet werden,
wenn der Zylindermantel von minderwertigem Material eine größere Wandstärke besitzt.
Die größere Wandstärke schützt aber nicht vor vorzeitigem Verschleiß.

γ) *Rechts- und Linksinsuffizienzen.* Daß beide Herzkammern in gleichem Ausmaß von einer Überbelastung betroffen werden, trifft nur in den selteneren Fällen
zu (z. B. arterio-venöse Fisteln, Basedow, stärkere Anämien). Meist kommt es
zunächst zu einer muskulären Insuffizienz der linken oder der rechten Kammer.
Hier erhebt sich die Frage, inwieweit beim Eintreten einer Insuffizienz der einen

---

[1] Hakkila 1955.   [2] Opitz und Lübbers 1956, Lübbers 1958.
[3] May 1939, Opitz und Palme 1944.   [4] Klepzig u. a. 1956.

Herzkammer die andere ebenfalls in Mitleidenschaft gezogen wird. Die hämodynamischen Bedingungen sind für die Rechts- und Linksinsuffizienzen in ihrer Rückwirkung auf die überlastungsfreie Kammer verschieden. Eine Insuffizienz der linken Herzkammer wird stets rückwirkend eine vermehrte Arbeit der rechten Herzkammer erfordern. Die mit Beginn der Insuffizienz eintretende Erhöhung des Vorhofdrucks pflanzt sich über die Lungenvenen bis in das arterielle System der Lunge fort. Bei den im Vergleich zum großen Kreislauf niedrigen Druckverhältnissen im kleinen Kreislauf bedeutet eine solche Erhöhung des Drucks in der arteriellen Strombahn der Lunge durch Rückstauung auch quantitativ eine beachtliche Mehrbelastung der rechten Kammer. Demgegenüber wirkt sich eine Insuffizienz der rechten Herzkammer nicht in dieser Weise rückwirkend auf die linke Herzkammer aus. Infolge des steilen Druckgefälles im großen Kreislauf bleiben Druckerhöhungen im venösen Gebiet des großen Kreislaufs praktisch ohne Rückwirkung auf die arterielle Strombahn und den linken Ventrikel. Es gilt somit: Eine Insuffizienz der linken Herzkammer hat stets eine Mehrbelastung der rechten Kammer zur Folge. Eine Rechtsinsuffizienz dagegen bleibt ohne unmittelbare hämodynamische Rückwirkungen auf das linke Herz. Bei der Rechtsinsuffizienz wird das linke Herz schließlich dadurch in Mitleidenschaft gezogen, daß durch die Verminderung des Aortendrucks und womöglich durch eine zusätzliche arterielle Hypoxie die Sauerstoffversorgung des Herzens Schaden leidet.

b) Herzmuskelinsuffizienz durch unmittelbare Schädigung der Muskelfibrillen.

Bei einer Reihe von Erkrankungen kommt es zu einer Herzmuskelinsuffizienz, ohne daß eine Überbelastung vorliegt. Es handelt sich dabei um eine unmittelbare Schädigung der Herzmuskelfibrillen. Ursache für eine solche Schädigung sind besonders Infektionskrankheiten, Zustände von Coronarinsuffizienz, Narkosen, Alkoholschädigungen, Vergiftungen durch Barbiturate oder andere Noxen. In vielen Fällen kann für die Schädigung des Herzmuskels auch ein anatomisch faßbares Substrat gefunden werden (braune Atrophie des Herzens, degenerative Verfettung, Myocarditis rheumatica, Folgen coronarer Durchblutungsstörungen usw.). Die Schädigung der Muskelfibrillen führt zu einer Herabsetzung der Leistungsfähigkeit des Herzens, die je nach dem Grade der Schädigung schon in der Ruhe solche Ausmaße erreichen kann, daß der Herzmuskel den notwendigen Anforderungen nicht mehr nachkommen kann. Unter Absinken des Kreislaufminutenvolumens und Anstieg des diastolischen Kammerdrucks bzw. Vorhofdrucks kommt es zur myogenen Dilatation ohne das kompensatorische Zwischenstadium der Anpassungsdilatation mit nachfolgender Hypertrophie. Es ist viel darüber gestritten worden, ob bei diesen Formen der toxischen Myokardschädigung ein Nachlassen des „Herztonus", d. h. des Spannungszustandes der Muskelfibrillen eine Rolle spielt. Der Pathologe spricht häufig von einem schlaffen Herzen im Gefolge toxischer Schädigung. Der Begriff Herztonus ist aber recht vage und entzieht sich bisher einer exakten Messung. Auch bei diesen Formen der Herzmuskelinsuffizienz ist vor allem das Nachlassen der systolischen Kraftentfaltung des Herzens von entscheidender Bedeutung.

4. Die wesentlichen Folgen der Herzmuskelinsuffizienz.

Die Rückwirkungen der Herzmuskelinsuffizienz sind vielfältig, ihre eingehende Besprechung im Rahmen dieses Überblicks nicht möglich. Abgesehen von der allgemeinen Erschwerung der Versorgung des Gewebes mit Nährstoffen und des Abtransportes von Stoffwechselprodukten stehen im Gefolge einer Herzmuskelinsuffizienz zwei Störungen im Vordergrund: Sauerstoffmangel und Ödem.

a) O_2-Mangel als Folge von Herzmuskelinsuffizienz.

Sinkt das Kreislaufminutenvolumen auf die Hälfte des normalen Wertes ab, so besteht akute Lebensgefahr. Infolge der stärkeren Ausschöpfung des O_2-Gehaltes des Blutes sinkt die O_2-Spannung im Zentralnervensystem so weit ab, daß eine Lähmung der lebenswichtigen Zentren in der Medulla oblongata droht. Erniedrigungen des Kreislaufminutenvolumens auf die Hälfte des Normalwertes werden nur in den Finalstadien der Herzmuskelinsuffizienz beobachtet. Eine Verringerung um ein Drittel ist schon als sehr gefahrvoll anzusehen. Liegt noch eine arterielle Hypoxämie infolge eines gestörten alveolaren Gasaustausches vor, so bedeuten bereits geringe Abnahmen des Kreislaufminutenvolumens unter den normalen Ruhewert eine unmittelbare Gefahr. Bei diesen Formen der Herzmuskelinsuffizienz bleibt das Kreislaufminutenvolumen häufig lange Zeit über der Norm, wie schon oben auseinandergesetzt wurde.

b) Das periphere Ödem.

Die früheren theoretischen Vorstellungen vom kardialen Ödem als Wasserretention infolge Steigerung des venösen Drucks haben sich als unzureichend erwiesen. An dem Zustandekommen des Ödems bei Herzmuskelinsuffizienz ist neben der Erhöhung des venösen Drucks durch Rückstauung eine vermehrte Natrium- bzw. Kochsalzretention wesentlich beteiligt. Die vermehrte Natriumretention kommt auf renalem Wege zustande, einmal durch das Absinken der glomerulären Filtration in der Niere[1], zum anderen durch eine erhöhte Natriumrückresorption in den distalen Tubuli[2]. Worauf die vermehrte Rückresorption von Natrium in den Tubuli beruht, ist noch nicht endgültig geklärt. Mehrere Faktoren sind in Erwägung zu ziehen. Da die Rückresorption von Änderungen des Säure-Basenhaushaltes abhängt[3], ist daran zu denken, daß eine acidotische Stoffwechsellage bei der Herzmuskelinsuffizienz zu vermehrter Rückresorption von Natrium und Wasser führt. Es wurde ferner tierexperimentell festgestellt, daß nach Erniedrigung der venösen O_2-Spannung die Na- und Wasserrückresorption in der Niere ansteigt[4], wobei wahrscheinlich die Ansammlung saurer Stoffwechselprodukte von Bedeutung ist. Schließlich ist eine vermehrte Abgabe von Nebennierenrindenhormonen, insonderheit von *Aldosteron*[5], zu diskutieren, das seinerseits eine vermehrte Natriumrückresorption im Tubulussystem der Niere verursacht. Bei der Herzmuskelinsuffizienz wurden vermehrte Aldosteronausscheidungen im Urin und ein vermehrter Aldosterongehalt in der Ödemflüssigkeit festgestellt[6]. Auf welchem Wege eine vermehrte Aldosteronausscheidung zustande kommt, ist ungeklärt. Offenbar ändert sich die Aldosteronausscheidung in Abhängigkeit von der Blutmenge mit der Na-Zufuhr[7]. Daß es sich um eine vom Hypophysenvorderlappen gesteuerte Nebennierenrindenreaktion handelt, ist unwahrscheinlich. Die Aldosteronausscheidung wird durch ACTH nicht wesentlich erhöht[8]. Ob bei der vermehrten Na- und Wasserrückresorption eine erhöhte Adiuretinproduktion des Hypophysenhinterlappens eine Rolle spielt, ist ungewiß. Unabhängig von diesen z. Zt. noch umstrittenen Fragen nach dem pathogenetischen Mechanismus der Natriumrückresorption in der Niere ergeben sich für die Behandlung des Ödems bei der Herzmuskelinsuffizienz aus den neuen Erkenntnissen schon jetzt wichtige therapeutische Konsequenzen.

---

[1] Merrill 1946, Mokotoff und Mitarbeiter 1948.   [2] Burch und Mitarbeiter 1947.
[3] Pitts und Mitarbeiter 1948.   [4] Briggs und Mitarbeiter 1948.
[5] Luetscher und Mitarbeiter 1954.   [6] Literatur s. Schwiegk 1956.
[7] Axelrad und Mitarbeiter 1954, Gross 1956.
[8] Venning und Mitarbeiter 1954, Simpson und Pait 1955, Liddle und Mitarbeiter 1955.

Ist es z. B. möglich, den Patienten eine weitgehende NaCl-freie Kost zu verabreichen, so kann man ihm ohne größere Gefahr reichlich Flüssigkeitsmengen zuführen. Damit entfällt die für den Patienten oft so schwer erträgliche starke Restriktion der Flüssigkeitszufuhr. Auch erscheint die Verabfolgung von Quecksilberdiuretica in einem neuen Licht. Quecksilberdiuretica können bereits entgegen früheren Anschauungen in den ersten Tagen der Behandlung gegeben werden, da durch sie eine Blockierung der Natriumrückresorption in der Niere erreicht wird und ein wesentlicher Faktor für die Ödementstehung entfällt. Ähnliches gilt für die Verabfolgung von Diamox, Chlorothiazid und Kationen-Austauschern.

5. Energiewechsel des Herzens bei Herzmuskelinsuffizienz.

(s. unter Störungen des Energiestoffwechsels des Herzens).

D. Der Lungenkreislauf.

I. Lungenkreislauf und Gesamtkreislauf.

Die beiden Druckstufen des linken und rechten Herzens teilen den Kreislauf in den großen und kleinen Kreislauf auf. Der Name „kleiner Kreislauf" ist sprachlich ungenau, denn es handelt sich eben nur um einen Abschnitt eines Kreislaufs. Der sog. kleine Kreislauf ist in seiner Bedeutung nur zu verstehen, wenn man sich seine Beziehungen zum Gesamtkreislauf klarmacht. Die Lunge liegt im Hauptschluß des Kreislaufs, und die Lungendurchblutung entspricht dem HZV. Aber nicht nur in der Durchblutung, sondern auch in der Blutfüllung steht die Lunge in Abhängigkeit vom gesamten Kreislauf. Es sind Blutverschiebungen zwischen den beiden Teilkreisläufen möglich. Dabei brauchen Durchblutung und Blutfüllung der Lunge nicht parallel zu gehen. Steigerungen des HZV bei Muskeltätigkeit gehen häufig mit einer Abnahme der Blutfüllung einher (s. S. 673).

Ein Hauptcharakteristikum des kleinen Kreislaufs ist sein niedriger Strömungswiderstand. Dies ist weitgehend durch die kurzen Zu- und Ableitungswege zu den beiden Herzhälften bedingt. Dazu kommt ein im Vergleich zu den meisten Organen des großen Kreislaufs niedriger Strömungswiderstand der Arteriolen. Ihre im großen Kreislauf so wichtige Funktion für die Durchblutungsverteilung auf die einzelnen Parallelleitungen spielt im Lungenkreislauf nur eine untergeordnete Rolle. So kann der Arteriolenwiderstand im Lungenkreislauf niedrig sein.

Die Folge des niedrigen Strömungswiderstandes im Lungenkreislauf ist der niedrige Druck in der A. pulmonalis (s. auch Abb. 22, S. 679). Für manche hämodynamische Betrachtungen ist es günstig, den Gesamtkreislauf nicht in einen großen und kleinen einzuteilen, sondern von einem Hochdruck- und Niederdruckgebiet zu sprechen. Das Hochdruckgebiet entspricht dabei dem arteriellen System des großen Kreislaufs, während das Niederdrucksystem die Venen des großen Kreislaufs und den gesamten kleinen Kreislauf umfaßt[1]. Eine solche Betrachtung sollte freilich nicht dazu führen, daß man die Druckstufe des rechten Herzens zu stark vernachlässigt. Das rechte Herz schafft die Möglichkeit, daß der Druck in den Venen des großen Kreislaufs und damit auch in den Capillaren dieses Systems hinreichend niedrig gehalten wird[2].

Herzzeitvolumen und Lungenkreislauf. Das Lungengefäßsystem liegt im Hauptschluß des Blutkreislaufs. Lungendurchblutung und HZV sind praktisch identisch. Jede Erhöhung des HZV bedeutet im gleichen Maße eine Steigerung

---

[1] GAUER u. a. 1956.   [2] ROSE und Mitarbeiter 1956.

der Lungendurchblutung. Bei Steigerung des HZV steigt im allgemeinen der Druck in der A. pulmonalis im Verhältnis weniger stark an als die Stromstärke. Der Strömungswiderstand des Lungenkreislaufs nimmt also unter diesen Bedingungen ab. Das Gefäßsystem der Lunge paßt sich der größeren Stromstärke an. Nach älteren Messungen an wenigen Versuchspersonen[1] nimmt Cournand[2] an, daß bei Leistung einer mittelschweren, körperlichen Arbeit der Strömungswiderstand im kleinen Kreislauf auf ein Drittel des Ruhewertes heruntergeht, während er im großen Kreislauf nur etwa um die Hälfte absinkt (Tabelle 20).

Tabelle 20. *O_2-Aufnahme und Kreislaufdaten von drei normalen Versuchspersonen in Ruhe und bei leichter (1) bzw. schwerer (2) Arbeit.* (Riley u. a. 1948.)

Nr.	Zustand	Herzfrequenz	O_2-Hb-Sättigung %	O_2-Verbrauch (ml/min/m²)	A-V Differenz (Vol.-%)	Herzzeitvolumen (l/min/m²)	Schlagvolumen (ml)	Blutdruck mm Hg						Widerstand dyn.-sec. cm⁻⁵		Arbeit der Ventrikel	
								A. brachialis			A. pulmonalis			Peripherie	Lunge	links	rechts
								systolisch	diastolisch	mittel	systolisch	diastolisch	mittel			Joule/min	Joule/min
377	Ruhe	47	97	111	4,2	2,62	99	120	59	82	20	10	15	1400	249	51	9
	Arbeit (1)	77	95	436	7,6	5,68	131	144	83	112	24	3	8	900	60	150	10
	Arbeit (2)	105	94	700	9,2	7,53	128	152	100	130	19	9	10	780	57	230	17
378	Ruhe	91	99	147	3,8	3,83	64	122	73	94	19	8	12	1000	135	89	11
	sitzend	100	—	—	—	—	—	—	—	—	18	9	13	—	—	—	—
	Arbeit (1)	127	97	512	8,2	6,17	90	133	88	108	21	5	12	835	93	160	18
	Arbeit (2)	151	96	912	9,9	9,11	111	168	101	131	20	6	8	625	39	292	18
379	Ruhe	73	96	120	3,6	3,35	86	93	63	78	—	—	11	972	144	63	9
	Arbeit (1)*	90	99	269	6,2	4,36	91	97	64	79	—	—	13	752	123	86	14
	sitzend	86	—	—	—	—	—	—	—	—	—	—	13	—	—	—	—
	Arbeit (2)	157	97	824	11,6	7,14	85	140	83	107	—	—	14	634	84	190	25
	Mittel: Ruhe	70	97	126	3,9	3,27	83	112	65	84	20	9	13	1144	176	68	10
	Arbeit (1)	98	97	406	7,3	5,40	104	125	78	100	23	4	11	829	92	132	14
	Arbeit (2)	138	96	812	10,2	7,93	108	153	91	123	19	3	10	680	60	237	20

* Beinarbeit in Rückenlage.

Bei solchen Angaben sollte man nicht vergessen, wie groß die Fehlermöglichkeiten für die Bestimmung des Strömungswiderstandes der Lunge im intakten Organismus sind, und daß auch die Variationsbreite bei gesunden Versuchspersonen sehr groß sein kann. Ein Überblick über die vorliegende Literatur vermittelt heute den Eindruck, daß der Strömungswiderstand bei Veränderung des HZV sich recht verschieden verhalten kann[3]. Anscheinend ist die Körperstellung vor und während der Arbeit für das Verhalten des Strömungswiderstandes in der Lunge von einer gewissen Bedeutung[4]. Der höheren Blutfüllung der Lunge in liegender Stellung entspricht anscheinend ein niedriger Strömungswiderstand. Verschiedenheiten in der Ausgangslage können aber für das Verhalten des Strömungswiderstandes bei Steigerung des HZV wesentlich sein.

An der Einstellung des Lungengefäßsystems auf eine erhöhte Durchblutung ist das Capillargebiet beteiligt. Würde bei Erhöhung des HZV die Capillarisierung der Lunge nicht verändert sein, so würde die Kontaktzeit des Blutes mit der

---

[1] Riley u. a. 1948. [2] Cournand 1954.
[3] Donald u. a. 1955, Slonim u. a. 1954. [4] Dexter u. a. 1951.

Alveolarluft entsprechend der Durchblutungssteigerung abnehmen, und es bestände die Gefahr einer unvollkommenen Arterialisierung des Blutes. Vor mehr als 20 Jahren beobachteten WEARN u. Mitarb.[1] bei der Katze die Lungencapillaren

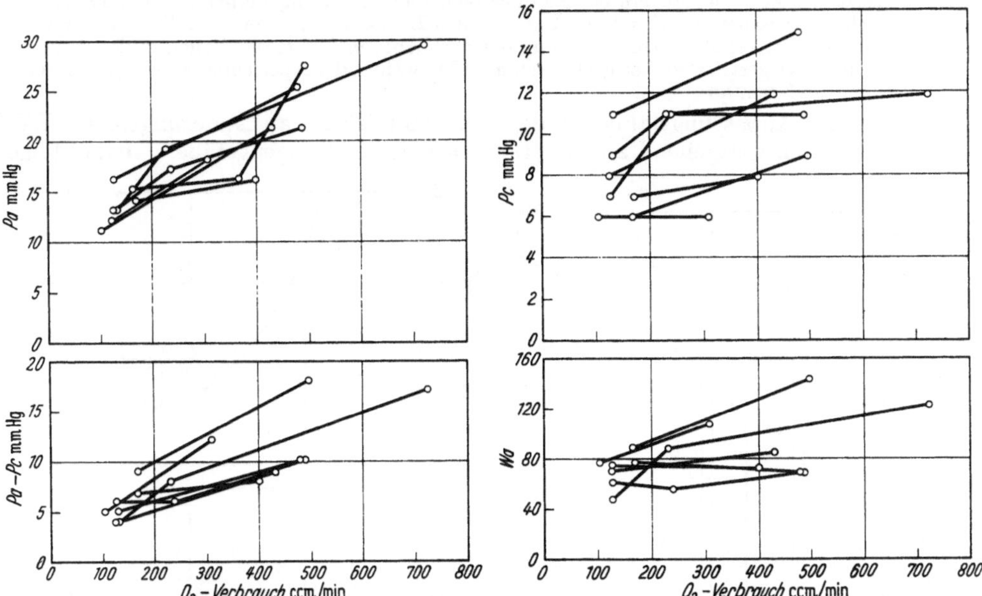

Abb. 58. Wirkung von körperlicher Arbeit auf den mittleren Druck in der A. pulmonalis p_a, den Lungencapillardruck p_c, den Druckgradienten p_a—p_c und den arteriellen Widerstand in der Lunge w_a (DEXTER u. a. 1951).

direkt. Sie stellten fest, daß ihre Zahl stark schwankt und daß im Ruhezustand nur ein kleiner Teil der Gesamtzahl durchblutet ist (Abb. 59). Diese Beobachtungen stehen im guten Einklang mit neuen Untersuchungen über den alveolaren

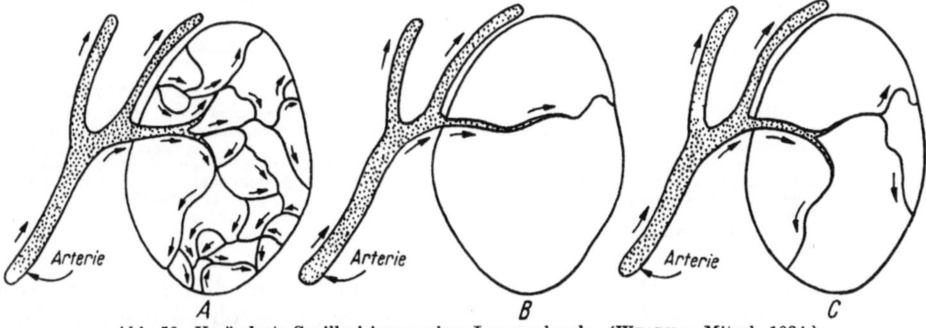

Abb. 59. Veränderte Capillarisierung einer Lungenalveole. (WEARN u. Mitarb. 1934.)

Gasaustausch. Bestimmungen der alveolar-arteriellen Sauerstoffdifferenz bei Muskeltätigkeit weisen darauf hin, daß auch bei gesteigertem HZV die Kontaktzeit von Blut und Alveolarluft genügend lang bleibt, um die Arterialisierung des Blutes zu sichern[2]. Die Diffusionskapazität, d. h. die pro Millimeter Sauerstoffdruck durch die Alveolarwand hindurchtretende Sauerstoffmenge, steigt während Muskeltätigkeit bei jungen Menschen bis auf das Vierfache des Ruhewertes an[3].

---

[1] WEARN und Mitarbeiter 1934.   [2] BARTELS und Mitarbeiter 1955a und b.
[3] RILEY u. a. 1954.

Man kann daraus schließen, daß die Blutfüllung der Lungencapillaren unter diesen Bedingungen um angenähert den gleichen Betrag ansteigt.

Die Anpassungsfähigkeit der Strombahn in der Lunge an eine veränderte Durchblutung zeigt sich auch bei Ausfall einer Lunge oder mehrerer Lungenlappen. Abb. 60 zeigt die Beziehung zwischen der Durchblutung und dem Druck in der A. pulmonalis. Nach Pneumektomie ist trotz erhöhter Durchblutung der verbliebenen Lunge der Druck in der A. pulmonalis nicht gesteigert. Erst bei gesteigertem HZV während körperlicher Arbeit steigt der Druck über die Norm an[1].

Die Anpassungsfähigkeit des Lungenkreislaufs an Änderungen des HZV erklärt sich weitgehend aus der Dehnbarkeit der Lungengefäße[2]. Jede Steigerung

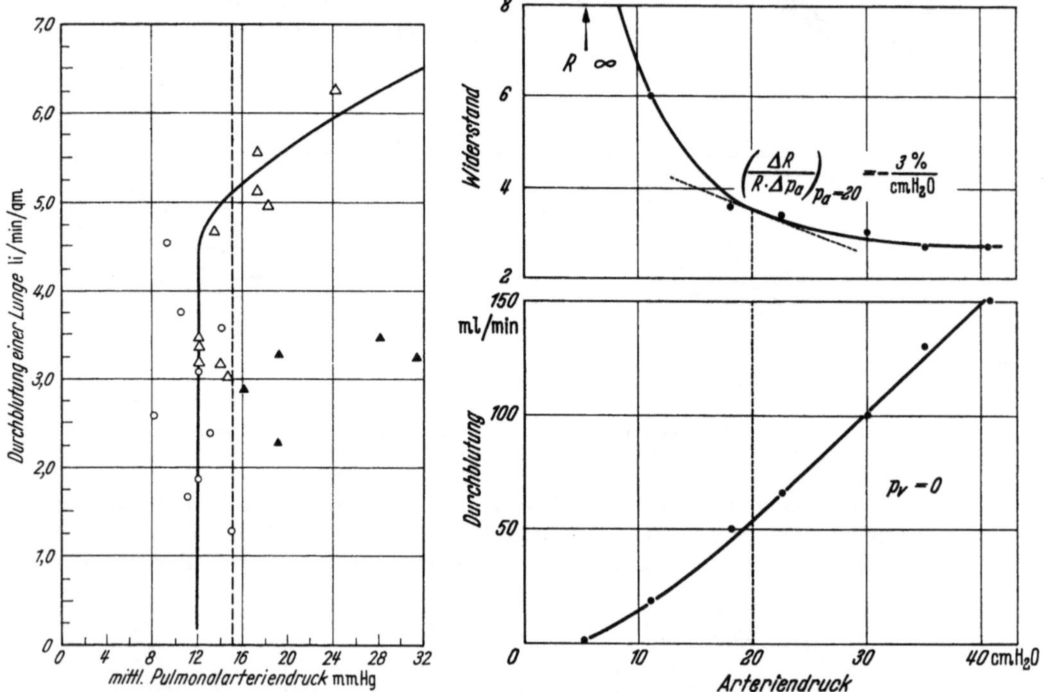

Abb. 60. Beziehung zwischen der Durchblutung einer Lunge und dem Pulmonalarteriendruck. ○ Ärzte mit normaler Lungenfunktion; △ Versuchspersonen mit einer normalen oder fast normalen Lunge nach Pneumektomie; ▲ Versuchspersonen mit chronischem Lungenemphysem oder einer Kreislauferkrankung. (Cournand u. a. 1950.)

Abb. 61. Beziehung zwischen dem Druck in der A. pulmonalis, der Lungendurchblutung und dem Strömungswiderstand in den Lungengefäßen. Untersuchungen an der isolierten Hundelunge. R Strömungswiderstand, p_a Druck in der A. pulmonalis, p_v Druck in der V. pulmonalis. (Piiper 1957.)

des intravasalen Druckes dehnt die Gefäße und vermindert damit den Strömungswiderstand. Das Gefäßsystem der Lunge zeigt diese physikalischen Beziehungen in reiner Form, während sie in anderen Gefäßabschnitten durch vasomotorische Vorgänge weitgehend überdeckt sind. Abnahme des Strömungswiderstandes findet man sowohl bei Steigerung des Druckes in der A. pulmonalis[3] (Abb. 61) als auch beim Druckanstieg in den Lungenvenen[4] (Abb. 62). Sehr deutlich zeigt sich am intakten Organismus die Abhängigkeit von intravasalem Druck und Strömungswiderstand, wenn man die Blutmenge des Versuchstieres durch Blut-

[1] Cournand u. a. 1950, Literatur bei Halmagyi 1957.
[2] Hess 1931, Wagner 1940, Wezler und Sinn 1953.   [3] Williams 1954, Piiper 1957.
[4] Haddy und Mitarbeiter 1953, Piiper 1957, Duke und Carlill 1956.

transfusionen oder Aderlässe ändert[1] (s. Abb. 20, S. 674). Erhöhung der intravasalen Drucke vermindert die Druckdifferenz zwischen A. pulmonalis und linkem Vorhof.

Wir müssen annehmen, daß auch vasomotorische Vorgänge an der Einstellung des Lungengefäßsystems beteiligt sind. Darauf weisen schon anatomische Befunde hin. Die Gefäße zeigen eine glatte Muskulatur, die sich nicht allzu sehr von der des großen Kreislaufs unterscheidet, wenn auch die verstärkte Muskulatur an den Arteriolen beim Menschen und bei vielen Tierarten fehlt. Die Gefäßmuskulatur wird reichlich von Nerven versorgt, so daß man an eine nervöse Steuerung der Gefäßweite denken muß. An der isolierten Lunge lassen sich vasomotorische Vorgänge auch gut nachweisen. Sie weichen nicht allzu sehr von den Verhältnissen im großen Kreislauf ab. Insbesondere führt die Reizung sympathischer Nerven zur Vasoconstriction. Adrenalin und Arterenol verengen im allgemeinen die Gefäße, Acetylcholin erweitert sie[2]. An der Lunge in situ zeigen sich im Prinzip die gleichen vasomotorischen Einflüsse. Jedoch sind solche Untersuchungen recht schwierig und bedürfen strengster Kritik, da man leicht durch gleichzeitige Einflüsse auf Herzdynamik, Hämodynamik und die Lungenmechanik getäuscht werden kann[3]. Von besonderer Bedeutung ist die vasomotorische Wirkung des Sauerstoffmangels (s. S. 755). Auffallend ist die starke vasoconstrictorische Wirkung des Serotonins[4].

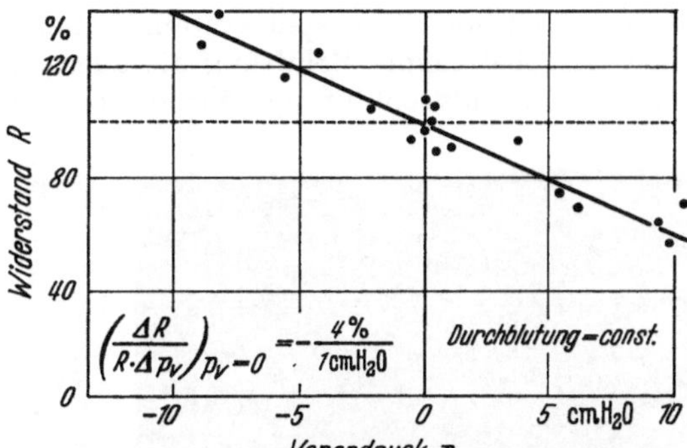

Abb. 62. Beziehungen zwischen dem Druck in der V. pulmonalis und dem Strömungswiderstand in den Lungengefäßen. Untersuchungen an der isolierten Hundelunge. R Strömungswiderstand, p_a Druck in der A. pulmonalis, p_v Druck in der V. pulmonalis. (PIIPER 1957.)

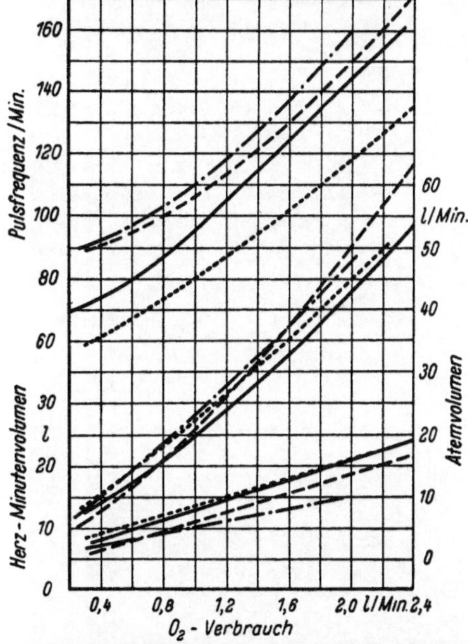

Abb. 63. Die Beziehungen zwischen Atmung und Kreislauf bei vier verschiedenen Versuchspersonen während verschieden starker Muskelarbeit. Als Maß für die Muskelarbeit ist der Sauerstoffverbrauch (Abszisse) angegeben. Die untersten Kurven zeigen das Herzzeitvolumen (dazugehörige Zahlen links), die mittleren das gleichzeitige Verhalten des Atemvolumens. Das oberste Kurvenbündel gibt die Pulsfrequenzen an. (Nach F. A. BAINBRIDGE.)

II. Lungendurchblutung und Lungenbelüftung.

1. Beziehungen zwischen Kreislaufzeitvolumen und Atemzeitvolumen.

Blutkreislauf und Lungenbelüftung sind Teilfunktionen einer Gesamtfunktion, nämlich des Transportes der Atemgase zwischen Außenluft und Gewebe. Wenn der Transport der Atemgase ökonomisch vor sich gehen soll, dann

---

[1] HENRY, GAUER und SIEKER 1956.   [2] DALY 1933, 1958.
[3] BORST, BERGLUND und McGREGOR 1957.   [4] PAGE 1958, ROSE und LAZARO 1958.

müssen die beiden Transportsysteme aufeinander eingestellt sein. Sowohl ein hohes HZV bei kleiner Belüftung als auch eine starke Ventilation der Lunge bei kleiner Lungendurchblutung führen zu einem schlechten Transporterfolg. Die Notwendigkeit einer Koordination von Durchblutung und Belüftung gilt für die ganze Lunge, d. h. für HZV und Atemzeitvolumen. Sie gilt aber auch für jeden einzelnen Lungenabschnitt, für den jeweils Durchblutung und Belüftung aufeinander abgestellt sein müssen (s. S. 754). Die weitgehende Parallelität zwischen HZV und Atemzeitvolumen zeigt sich am deutlichsten bei gesteigertem Sauerstoffverbrauch während körperlicher Arbeit (s. Abb. 63).

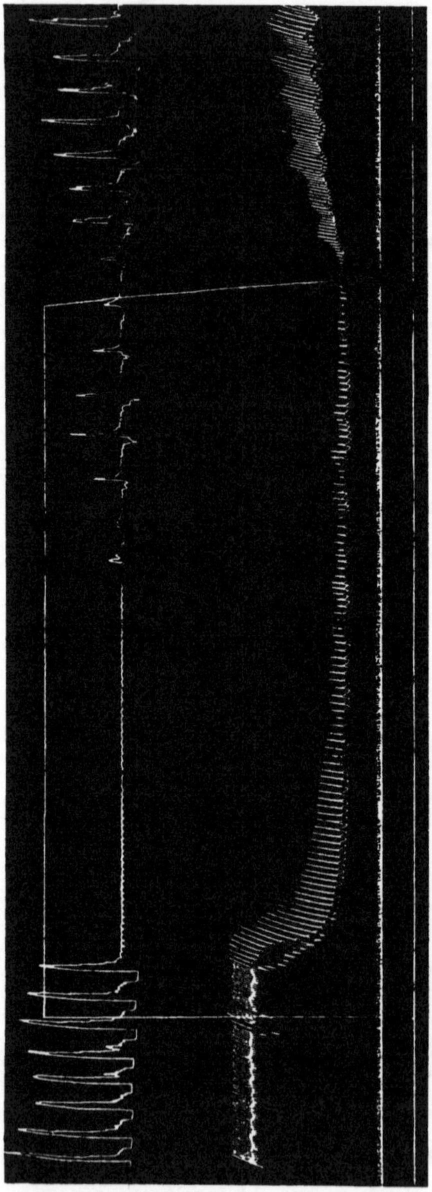

Die Koordination von Kreislauf und Atmung ist in erster Linie dadurch bedingt, daß beide Systeme letztlich durch die gleichen Vorgänge teils chemisch, teils zentral-nervös angetrieben werden (s. u.). Dazu tritt eine gegenseitige Beeinflussung der beiden Funktionen. Eine verstärkte Lungenbelüftung kann unter bestimmten Bedingungen rein mechanisch das HZV steigern (s. S. 757). Wichtiger sind nervös-reflektorische Koppelungen. So führt vertiefte Einatmung zu Vasoconstriction in der Peripherie des großen Kreislaufs[1]. Welche Bedeutung diesem Reflex zukommt, ist freilich schwer zu sagen. Besser untersucht sind reflektorische Einflüsse vom Kreislauf auf die Atmung[2]. Die Pressoreceptoren in der Aorta und im Sinus caroticus sowie die in den Vv. pulmonales beeinflussen nicht nur Kreislaufgrößen, sondern auch die Lungenbelüftung. Im Experiment der Abb. 64 wird der Druck im Sinus caroticus erhöht. Man beobachtet eine Senkung des arteriellen Druckes mit Verlangsamung der Schlagfrequenz des Herzens und gleichzeitig einen Atemstillstand. Sinkt der Druck im isolierten Carotissinus ab, dann kommt es umgekehrt zu einer Steigerung des arteriellen Druckes und einer

Abb. 64. Reflektorische Hemmung der Atmung durch Erhöhung des Druckes im Carotissinus. Versuch am Hund in Narkose. Obere Kurve: Atemtätigkeit; untere Kurve: arterieller Blutdruck des Tieres, in der A. femoralis gemessen. Als nahezu rechtwinklige Figur ist der künstlich gesetzte Druck in einem vom übrigen Kreislauf getrennten Carotissinus, der aber noch in nervöser Verbindung mit dem Zentralnervensystem belassen ist, verzeichnet. Sobald der Sinusinnendruck steigt, fällt der arterielle Druck ab. Gleichzeitig wird die Atemtätigkeit gehemmt. (Koch 1931.)

---

[1] Goetz 1934, Peters 1938, Gilliat 1948.   [2] Aviado und Schmidt 1955.

verstärkten Lungenbelüftung. Man hat geglaubt, daß dieser Reflex für die Umstellung von Kreislauf und Atmung im Beginn der Muskeltätigkeit von entscheidender Bedeutung wäre. Die erhöhte Muskeldurchblutung sollte zum Abfall des arteriellen Druckes führen, und es sollte damit über die arteriellen Pressoreceptoren die Intensivierung von Kreislauf und Atmung ausgelöst werden. Anscheinend setzt aber meistens die zentral-nervöse Regulation so rasch ein, daß es gar nicht zu einem Abfall des arteriellen Druckes im Arbeitsbeginn kommt, so daß dieser Mechanismus im allgemeinen keine Bedeutung für die Umstellung von Kreislauf und Atmung im Beginn der Muskeltätigkeit zu spielen scheint[1].

Entscheidend für das gute Zusammenwirken von Kreislauf und Atmung ist, daß beide Systeme von den gleichen Vorgängen angetrieben werden. Ganz im Vordergrund stehen dabei die Atemgase Kohlensäure und Sauerstoff. Der arterielle Kohlensäuredruck ist das wichtigste Regulans der äußeren Atmung und wirkt gleichzeitig über zentrale Gebiete aktivierend auf den Kreislauf. Er beeinflußt dabei nicht nur den Strömungswiderstand, sondern führt auch zu Gefäßverengerungen auf der venösen Seite des Kreislaufs, wodurch das Blutangebot an das Herz und das HZV gesteigert werden. Die Erhöhung des arteriellen Kohlensäuredruckes steigert also sowohl das Atemzeitvolumen als auch das HZV. In ganz ähnlicher Weise wirkt eine Senkung des arteriellen Sauerstoffdruckes über

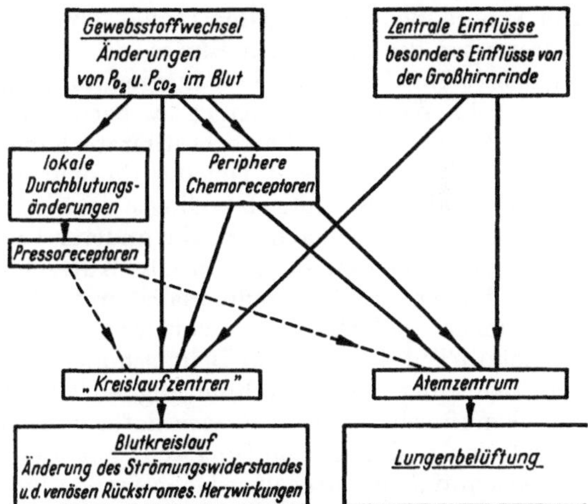

Abb. 65. Koordination von Kreislauf und Atmung durch Einwirkung der gleichen Vorgänge auf das Atemzentrum und die „Kreislaufzentren".

die peripheren Chemoreceptoren im Bereich des Aortenbogens und des Sinus caroticus. Auch hierdurch werden gleichzeitig die äußere Atmung und der Blutkreislauf aktiviert. Bei Muskeltätigkeit werden beide Systeme von den motorischen Gebieten der Großhirnrinde aus angetrieben, indem von da aus sowohl das Atemzentrum als auch die zentral-nervösen Gebiete für die Kreislaufsteuerung Impulse erhalten.

Abb. 65 gibt eine Übersicht über die Umstellung von Kreislauf und Atmung bei Muskeltätigkeit. Sie erfolgt teils von der Zentrale, teils von der Peripherie aus. In letzterem Falle ist es der Gewebsstoffwechsel, der die Intensivierung von Kreislauf und Atmung bewirkt. Der gesteigerte Stoffwechsel führt zur Veränderung der Atemgase im Blut und damit über periphere oder zentrale Chemorezeption zur Umstellung in beiden Systemen. Die Kohlensäure und andere Zwischenprodukte eröffnen lokal in den tätigen Organen die Gefäße und verbessern auf diese Weise ihre Durchblutung. Führt die Verminderung des Strömungswiderstandes in den tätigen Organen zu einer Senkung des arteriellen Druckes (was im allgemeinen freilich nicht der Fall ist), so wirken die arteriellen Pressoreceptoren zusätzlich antreibend auf Atmung und Kreislauf[2].

---

[1] Asmussen und Nielsen 1951.   [2] Rein 1935, 1938.

2. Koordination von Durchblutung und Belüftung in den einzelnen Lungenabschnitten.

Im großen Kreislauf kommt den Arteriolen eine wichtige Funktion zu. Sie sorgen für die richtige Verteilung der Durchblutung auf die einzelnen Organe. Im kleinen Kreislauf führen alle Blutbahnen zum gleichen Organ, und insofern scheint eine Steuerung der Durchblutungsverteilung von geringerer Bedeutung. Das gilt aber nur so lange, als alle Abschnitte der Lunge gleich belüftet sind und damit die gleiche Alveolarluft haben. Im anderen Falle ist eine Anpassung der Durchblutung an die Belüftung der einzelnen Lungenabschnitte notwendig. Passiert eine größere Blutmenge einen schlecht ventilierten Lungenabschnitt, so wird dieses Blut unvollkommen arterialisiert. Es kommt zu dem, was man als „Kurzschlußdurchblutung im weiteren Sinne" bezeichnet[1]. Besser wäre es wohl, in diesem Falle von einer venösen Beimischung (venous admixture) zu sprechen. Die venöse Beimischung der Lunge läßt sich aus den Sauerstoff- und Kohlensäurewerten des arteriellen Blutes, des venösen Blutes und der Alveolarluft berechnen[2]. Im Unterschied zu Lungenkranken, bei denen die venöse Beimischung recht hohe Werte erreichen kann, beträgt sie bei Gesunden nur etwa 2% des HZV. Dabei stammt die so bestimmte Kurzschlußdurchblutung aus recht verschiedenen Quellen. Ein Teil des Coronarblutes fließt über Vv. thebesii in das linke Herz ab. Die dadurch bedingte venöse Beimischung soll etwa ein Drittel des Gesamtbetrages ausmachen[3]. Ein anderer Teil stammt aus dem Bronchialsystem. Ob an der gesunden Lunge direkte Kurzschlüsse des Lungenkreislaufes — also Verbindungen der A. pulmonalis mit der V. pulmonalis unter Umgehung des Lungencapillarbettes — von irgendeiner Bedeutung sind, ist sehr fraglich. Der letzte Teil der venösen Beimischung beruht auf einer schlechten Zuordnung von Belüftung und Durchblutung einzelner Alveolarabschnitte. Auch dieser Anteil muß sehr klein sein, was dafür spricht, daß in allen Lungenabschnitten Ventilation und Durchblutung sehr gut aufeinander abgestimmt sind. Dies ist insofern auffallend, als selbst bei gesunden jungen Menschen die Lungenbelüftung recht ungleichmäßig ist. Bei jungen Männern bedarf es zur Auswaschung des Stickstoffs einer Ventilation, die um 20% größer ist, als wenn die Lungenbelüftung gleichmäßig wäre. Eine nähere Analyse der Clearance-Kurven ergibt, daß ein kleinerer Teil der Lunge (etwa 20%) gegenüber der übrigen Lunge überventiliert wird. Bei älteren Leuten ist die Ungleichmäßigkeit der Lungenbelüftung noch viel ausgesprochener. Die wichtigste Ursache für die ungleichmäßige Lungenbelüftung sind wohl Verschiedenheiten in der Dehnbarkeit des Lungengewebes. Aber auch der zeitliche Ablauf, mit dem das Lungengewebe im Beginn der Inspiration sich dehnt, spielt eine Rolle. Wird doch zunächst die Luft aus dem schädlichen Raum zurückgeatmet[4].

Die Gefahr von Verteilungsstörungen, d. h. fehlender Anpassung von Durchblutung und Belüftung in den einzelnen Lungenabschnitten, wird noch dadurch erhöht, daß sowohl Durchblutungsverteilung als auch Belüftungsverteilung sich mit dem Funktionszustand ändern. Das gilt besonders für veränderte Dehnungszustände der Lunge, die beide Funktionen beeinflussen. Es gilt auch für Lageänderungen, die besonders die Durchblutungsverteilung beeinflussen, in dem die abhängigen Partien aus hydrostatischen Gründen stärker durchblutet sind[5] (s. Tabelle 21).

Wenn beim gesunden Menschen Durchblutung und Belüftung in den einzelnen Lungenabschnitten so gut aufeinander abgestimmt sind, so muß man daran

<hr>

[1] Bartels, Bücherl u. a. 1956.
[2] Bartels und Rodewald 1952, Bartels und Mitarbeiter 1955.
[3] Bartels, Bücherl und Mitarbeiter 1956.   [4] Fowler 1952.   [5] Rahn u. a. 1956.

Tabelle 21. *Belüftung und O_2-Aufnahme der rechten und linken Lungen bei Menschen in Rücken- und rechter Seitenlage, ausgedrückt in Prozent des Gesamtwertes.*

	Rückenlage		Seitenlage		Rückenlage		Seitenlage	
	rechts	links	rechts	links	rechts	links	rechts	links
Belüftung (%)	52	48	54	46	52	48	53	47
$\dot{V}_{O_2}$ (%) . . .	50	50	61	39	49	51	63	37
	Mittel von 10 Studenten				Mittel von 8 Patienten			

denken, daß ein spezieller Regelmechanismus für diese Einstellungen Sorge trägt. Das wäre durch Einflüsse auf die Vasomotorik oder die Bronchomotorik zu erreichen. Man hat in letzter Zeit sich viel mit der Frage beschäftigt, ob dieser Regelmechanismus von den Atemgasen Sauerstoff oder Kohlensäure ausgelöst werden könnte[1].

3. Sauerstoff und Lungendurchblutung.

Die Annahme ist die, daß Sauerstoffmangel in irgendeinem Lungenabschnitt zu einer Vasoconstriction der zugehörigen Gefäße führt, und daß auf diese Weise die Lungendurchblutung der Lungenbelüftung angepaßt wird. Ein schlecht belüfteter Lungenabschnitt bekäme so auch weniger Blut. Diese Hypothese ist bestechend, aber schwer zu beweisen. Die erschreckend große Zahl von Arbeiten auf diesem Gebiet weist schon auf die Schwierigkeiten hin. Am intakten Organismus erfordert eine Bestimmung des Strömungswiderstandes im Lungenkreislauf eine ganze Reihe schwieriger Messungen, die nur in seltenen Fällen gleichzeitig so ausgeführt werden, daß sie brauchbare Resultate liefern (s. S. 751). Aber selbst wenn man Erhöhungen des Strömungswiderstandes im Sauerstoffmangel findet, so braucht die Zunahme des Strömungswiderstandes doch nicht vasomotorisch bedingt zu sein. Insbesondere ändert sich ja der Strömungswiderstand mit dem HZV (S. 750) und mit der Lungenbelüftung (S. 757). Ein unterschiedliches Verhalten der verschiedenen Tierarten scheint eine Aussage weiter zu erschweren. Nach der vorliegenden Literatur scheint es uns wahrscheinlich, daß bei der Katze der Strömungswiderstand im Sauerstoffmangel zunimmt. Das gilt aber anscheinend nicht für den Hund[2], wobei es auch hier gegensätzliche Meinungen gibt[3]. Beim Menschen findet die Mehrzahl der Autoren eine Zunahme des Strömungswiderstandes[4].

Bei den großen Schwierigkeiten, die bei jeder Bestimmung des Strömungswiderstandes in der Lunge auftreten, kommt vergleichenden Messungen eine besondere Bedeutung zu. Insbesondere kann man das Verhalten des Strömungswiderstandes bei Sauerstoffmangel und bei Muskeltätigkeit vergleichen, oder man kann die beiden Lungen vergleichen, wenn sie durch verschiedenartige Beatmung unterschiedliche alveolare O_2-Drucke haben. Abb. 66 zeigt das Verhalten des HZV und des Pulmonalisdruckes bei Muskeltätigkeit oder im Sauerstoffmangel. Bezogen auf die gleiche Steigerung des HZV steigt bei Gesunden der Pulmonalisdruck im Sauerstoffmangel sehr viel stärker an als bei Muskeltätigkeit. Bei Patienten mit nur einer Lunge und reduziertem Gefäßbett steigt dagegen der Druck in der A. pulmonalis in beiden Fällen in gleichem Maße an. Das unterschiedliche Verhalten bei gesunden Personen wird im allgemeinen so gedeutet,

---

[1] v. EULER und LILJESTRAND 1946.   [2] LEUSEN und DEMEESTER 1955 (Literatur).
[3] HÜRLIMANN und WIGGERS 1953.
[4] MOTLEY u. a. 1947, WESTCOTT u. a. 1951, DENOLIN u. a. 1953 (Literatur).

daß der Sauerstoffmangel einen vasoconstrictorischen Effekt hat. Es läßt sich jedoch nicht unbedingt ausschalten, daß umgekehrt die Muskeltätigkeit eine Vasodilatation hervorruft[1].

Durch die Bronchospirometrie wird die Möglichkeit geschaffen, die Verteilung der Durchblutung auf beide Lungen zu bestimmen und zu untersuchen, ob sie sich verändert, wenn eine der beiden Lungen mit sauerstoffarmen Gemischen beatmet wird. Solche Untersuchungen sind gleichzeitig Modellversuche für die Vorstellung, daß über den Sauerstoffdruck der Alveolarluft die Durchblutung einzelner Lungenabschnitte der Lungenbelüftung angepaßt werden kann. Nach

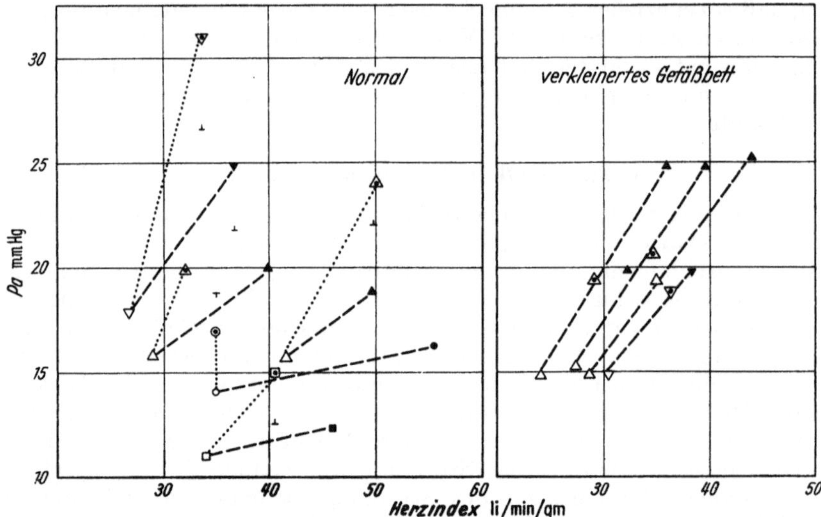

Abb. 66. Beziehungen zwischen dem Druck in der A. pulmonalis und dem Herzzeitvolumen während akuter Hypoxie und während Muskeltätigkeit bei Gesunden (links) und Patienten mit eingeengtem Gefäßbett der Lunge (rechts). Im Sauerstoffmangel ist die Steigerung des Druckes der A. pulmonalis bezogen auf die gleiche Steigerung des Herzzeitvolumens sehr viel größer als bei Muskeltätigkeit.
Ausgangslage: □ ○ △ ▽; Sauerstoffmangel: ⊡ ⊙ △ ▽; Muskeltätigkeit: ■ ● ▲ ▼

den vorliegenden tierexperimentellen Untersuchungen möchte man eine Verschiebung der Durchblutung von der hypoxischen auf die belüftete Lunge annehmen[2]. Leider sind die Befunde am Menschen nicht einheitlich. Jedoch überwiegen die positiven Ergebnisse[3] gegenüber den negativen[4].

Die Befunde über die Einwirkung der Hypoxie auf die Durchblutung und Durchblutungsverteilung sind also recht verwirrend. Insbesondere ist heute nicht zu entscheiden, ob Veränderungen des Strömungswiderstandes vasomotorisch bedingt sind, und ob den Einflüssen des Sauerstoffmangels für die Einstellung des Strömungswiderstandes in der Lunge eine größere Bedeutung zukommt. Bei dieser Situation scheint es auch verfrüht, etwas über den Auslösungsmechanismus zu sagen. Es sei aber darauf hingewiesen, daß an der isolierten Katzen- und Hundelunge Sauerstoffmangel den Strömungswiderstand steigert, was gegen einen reflektorischen Mechanismus spricht[5]. Beim sympathektomierten Menschen soll im Sauerstoffmangel der Druck in der A. pulmonalis ebenso ansteigen wie beim Normalen[6]. Auch das spricht gegen reflektorische Vorgänge. Andererseits

---

[1] Cournand 1954.   [2] Leusen und Demeester 1955 (Literatur).
[3] Hertz 1955, 1956, Ulmer und Wenke 1957.   [4] Fishman u. a. 1955, Cournand 1955.
[5] Nisell 1948, Duke und Killik 1952, Hall 1953.   [6] Cournand 1954.

weisen Untersuchungen am Hund darauf hin, daß die hypoxämische Vasoconstriction reflektorisch von den arteriellen Chemoreceptoren ausgelöst sein kann[1].

Die Befunde über die Wirkung der Kohlensäure auf die Lungengefäße sind ebenfalls widerspruchsvoll. Teilweise wurden constrictorische Effekte und verminderter Blutgehalt der Lungengefäße bei erhöhtem Kohlensäuredruck beobachtet[2].

4. Rückwirkung der Lungenatmung auf den Kreislauf.

Es ist wahrscheinlich, daß bei der Lungenatmung nervös-reflektorische Vorgänge ausgelöst werden, die den Blutkreislauf beeinflussen. Bedeutungsvoller ist aber wohl die rein mechanische Wirkung. Die Lungenatmung muß Druck, Blutstrom, Blutfüllung und Strömungswiderstand in den intrathorakalen Gefäßen und im Herzen beeinflussen. Für eine erste Betrachtung sollen die Wirkungen eines geänderten intrathorakalen Druckes, der über die Atemperiode gemittelt ist, von den Einflüssen atemperiodischer Druckänderungen abgetrennt werden.

Einflüsse eines veränderten intrathorakalen Mitteldruckes. Die Senkung des intrathorakalen Druckes senkt auch den Druck in den intrathorakalen Gefäßen. Das führt zu einem erhöhten Druckgefälle zwischen den Gefäßen innerhalb und außerhalb des Thorax und dadurch zu einem erhöhten Einstrom von Blut in den Thoraxraum. Die Folge ist eine erhöhte Blutfüllung der intrathorakalen Gefäße und des Herzens. Umgekehrt vermindert eine Steigerung des intrathorakalen Druckes das Druckgefälle zwischen den Gefäßen innerhalb und außerhalb des Thorax. Die Folge ist ein verminderter Blutrückstrom und eine verminderte Blutfüllung von Herz und intrathorakalen Gefäßen. Sehr starke Senkungen des intrathorakalen Druckes können zum Kollabieren der extrathorakalen Venen und dadurch zur Hemmung des venösen Rückstroms führen[3].

Änderungen des intrathorakalen Druckes kommen unter verschiedenen Bedingungen vor. Der intrathorakale Druck ist abhängig von der Atemmittellage. Eine erhöhte Atemmittellage, wie sie häufig bei Muskeltätigkeit beobachtet wird, vermindert den intrathorakalen Druck und kann dadurch das Blutangebot an das rechte Herz erhöhen. Inspiratorische Atemwiderstände erniedrigen den intrathorakalen Druck, exspiratorische erhöhen ihn. Bei Atemgeräten wie Gasmasken, Sauerstoffgeräten, Rettungsgeräten und anderen können die zusätzlichen Widerstände der Luftwege den Kreislauf sicherlich recht entscheidend beeinflussen. Eine große Bedeutung kommt dem Verhalten des intrathorakalen Druckes bei jeder Art der künstlichen Beatmung zu[4]. Dabei ist jedoch nicht der absolute Druck entscheidend, sondern das Druckgefälle gegenüber der Umgebung, besonders das Druckgefälle gegenüber dem Abdominalraum, aus dem das Blut zum Herzen zurückströmt. Deshalb üben eine Überdruckatmung von den Luftwegen aus und eine Tankbeatmung mit überwiegendem Unterdruck im Tank die gleichen Wirkungen aus, wenn die Druckgefälle zwischen intra- und extrathorakalem Raum in beiden Fällen gleich sind.

Ob Änderungen des intrathorakalen Druckes überhaupt zur Auswirkung kommen, hängt vom Gesamtzustand des Kreislaufs ab. Nur wenn das Blutangebot an das Herz begrenzender Faktor ist, beeinflußt eine Veränderung des intrathorakalen Druckes den arteriellen Druck und das HZV. So wird man bei einem gesunden, nicht narkotisierten Menschen unter einer bestimmten Form der Überdruckbeatmung keine Kreislaufveränderungen finden, während die gleiche Beatmung bei verschlechtertem Blutrückstrom in Narkose den Kreislauf zum Versagen bringt.

---

[1] Aviado und Mitarbeiter 1954.　　[2] Duke 1949 (Literatur).
[3] Bauereisen und Mitarbeiter 1958.　　[4] Whittenberger 1955.

Im Schema der Abb. 67 sind die verschiedenen Einflüsse des intrathorakalen Druckes zusammengestellt. Von besonderer Bedeutung ist die Beeinflussung des

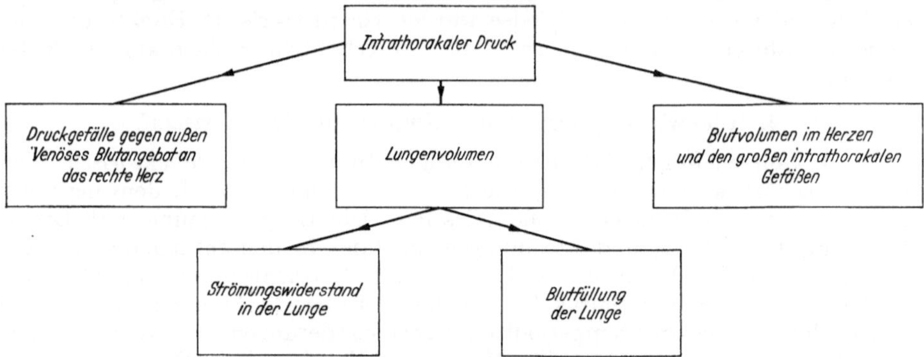

Abb. 67. Schematische Übersicht über die Beziehungen zwischen dem intrathorakalen Druck und der Hämodynamik des Lungenkreislaufs.

venösen Blutangebotes an das rechte Herz. Ein verminderter intrathorakaler Druck läßt vermehrt Blut aus den extrathorakalen Venen des großen Kreislaufs

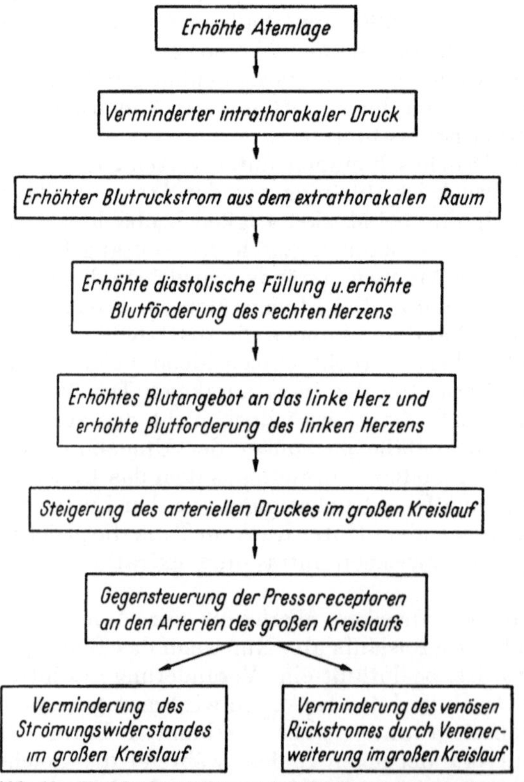

Abb. 68. Kreislaufumstellungen bei Erhöhung der Atemlage.

in die intrathorakalen Venen einströmen (Abb. 68). Das erhöht den Druck im rechten Vorhof und vermehrt die diastolische Füllung des rechten Ventrikels. Ist das rechte Herz leistungsfähig und wird es nicht nervös gebremst, dann wird damit seine Blutförderung gesteigert. Dies erhöht dann auch das Blutangebot und die Blutförderung des linken Herzens. Die dadurch bedingte Drucksteigerung in den Arterien des großen Kreislaufs löst über die dort gelegenen Pressoreceptoren Gegensteuerungen aus: Der periphere Strömungswiderstand des großen Kreislaufs wird gesenkt, über die Venomotorik wird das Blutfassungsvermögen auf der venösen Seite erhöht und damit der venöse Rückstrom zum rechten Herzen wieder herabgesetzt. Aus diesem Grunde findet man stärkere Kreislaufbeeinflussungen durch Veränderungen des intrathorakalen Druckes nur dann, wenn der Kreislauf sich vorher in einem schlechten Zustand befand. Nur unter diesen Bedingungen fehlen die Gegenregulationen, so daß HZV und arterieller Druck ansteigen.

Bei den durch intrathorakale Druckänderungen hervorgerufenen Blutverschiebungen muß folgendes berücksichtigt werden: Nicht die gesamte Blutmenge, die bei Senkung des intrathorakalen Druckes vermehrt dem rechten Herzen zufließt, erreicht das linke Herz. Die Senkung des intrathorakalen Druckes steigert ja die Blutfüllung der intrathorakalen Gefäße und des Herzens. Am isolierten Organ läßt sich zeigen, daß die Blutfüllung der Lunge vom Dehnungszustand abhängig ist (Abb. 69). Auch das gleichzeitig gesteigerte transmurale Druckgefälle (Differenz von Gefäßinnendruck und alveolarem Druck) steigert die Blutfüllung der Lunge[1]. Über die Größe intrathorakaler Blutfüllungsänderungen geben Untersuchungen von FENN u. Mitarb.[2] einen Eindruck. Bei liegenden, gesunden Personen vermindert ein Anstieg des pulmonalen Druckes auf 30 cm Wasser das intrathorakale Blutvolumen um 500 cm³. Das entspricht einer Verminderung des intrathorakalen Blutvolumens auf etwa die Hälfte. Von der verdrängten Blutmenge fanden sich nur etwa 3% in den Extremitäten. Der Hauptteil des Blutes war im Abdomen abgelagert. Änderungen des intrathorakalen Druckes verschieben also teilweise nur das Blut innerhalb des Niederdrucksystems, und zwar zwischen dem Venensystem des großen und dem des kleinen Kreislaufs.

Die größere Kapazität des großen Kreislaufs führt im allgemeinen dazu, daß das erhöhte Blutangebot bei Senkung des intrathorakalen Druckes nicht nur das rechte, sondern auch das linke

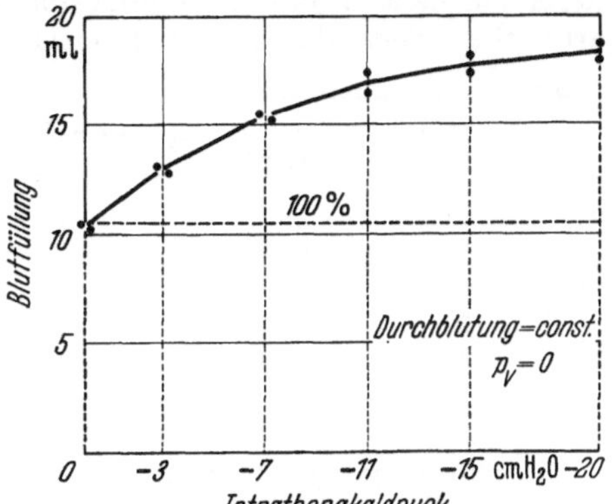

Abb. 69. Beziehungen zwischen dem „intrathorakalen" Druck und der Blutfüllung der Lunge. Untersuchungen an der isolierten Hundelunge. Der „intrathorakale" Druck entspricht dabei dem negativen Druck in der Umgebung der isolierten Lunge. (PIIPER 1957.)

Herz erreicht, und daß auf diese Weise das HZV und der arterielle Druck gesteigert werden können. Es kommt hinzu, daß bei niedrigem intrathorakalem Druck die Arbeitsbedingungen für das Herz günstig sind. Die gute Füllung der Vorhöfe und der angrenzenden Venen verkürzt die Füllungszeit. Auch ist der effektive Druck in den Kammern (die Differenz zwischen dem Kammerdruck und intrathorakalen Druck) erhöht, wodurch nach den Straub-Starlingschen Gesetzen die Leistungsfähigkeit des Herzens verbessert wird.

Wirkungen der vertieften Atmung auf den Kreislauf. Eine vertiefte Atmung schafft größere intrathorakale Druckschwankungen und wirkt damit fördernd auf den Blutkreislauf, vorausgesetzt daß diese Wirkung nicht durch Gegenregulationen aufgehoben wird. In der Inspiration füllt sich wegen des gesteigerten venösen Rückstroms und des erhöhten Blutfassungsvermögens die Lunge mit Blut. In der Exspiration nimmt die Kapazität des kleinen Kreislaufs ab, und damit wird das Blut auf die arterielle Seite des großen Kreislaufs hinübergeschoben. Der Atmungsapparat ist damit nichts anderes als eine Pumpe, wobei die Herzklappen die Ventile sind, die den Blutstrom bloß in einer Richtung passieren lassen. Die äußere Atemmuskulatur leistet dabei Kreislaufarbeit. Ihre Wirkung wird freilich im allgemeinen klein sein, da die Energie zum überwiegenden Teil zur Luftförderung verbraucht wird. Ihre Kreislaufwirksamkeit wird erhöht, wenn der Strömungswiderstand in den Luftwegen gesteigert ist und dadurch die intrathorakalen Druckschwankungen erhöht sind. Der rhythmische Wechsel des intrathorakalen Druckes kann sich aber besonders auch dadurch auswirken, daß er zur

---

[1] OCHSNER 1952, PIIPER 1957.   [2] FENN und Mitarbeiter 1947.

entsprechenden Füllungsänderung der beiden Herzhälften führt. In der Inspiration steigen zunächst Blutangebot und Blutförderung des rechten Herzens. Gegen Ende der Inspiration wirkt sich diese gesteigerte Blutförderung des rechten Herzens auch auf das linke Herz aus. Im Beginn der Exspiration hält die abnehmende Blutkapazität des kleinen Kreislaufs das Blutangebot an das linke Herz zunächst weiterhin hoch, so daß noch in die Exspirationsphase hinein das linke Herz ein erhöhtes Schlagvolumen aufweist. Das mit der Atmung veränderte Blutangebot an das linke Herz ist die hauptsächliche Ursache der respiratorischen Blutdruckschwankungen[1]. Freilich ist dies nicht die einzige Ursache. Es treten nervöse Einflüsse hinzu wie die Koppelung der atmungs- und kreislaufregulierenden Zentren in der Medulla oblongata. Durch die Pressoreceptoren auf der arteriellen Seite des großen Kreislaufs werden die respiratorischen Blutdruckschwankungen gebremst. Gleichzeitig beeinflussen die atemperiodischen Schwankungen des arteriellen Druckes über die Pressoreceptoren die Pulsfrequenz und sind damit teilweise auch für das Auftreten der respiratorischen Arrhythmie, d. h. der rhythmischen Schwankung der Pulsfrequenz mit der Atmung verantwortlich zu machen.

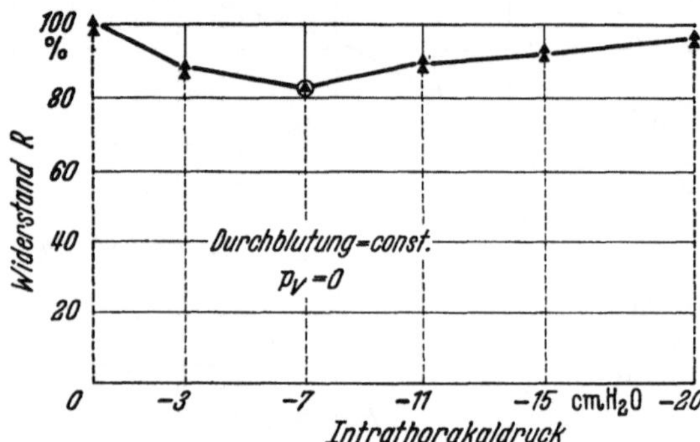

Abb. 70. Beziehung zwischen dem „intrathorakalen" Druck und dem Strömungswiderstand in den Lungengefäßen. Untersuchungen an der isolierten Hundelunge. Der „intrathorakale" Druck entspricht dabei dem negativen Druck in der Umgebung der isolierten Lunge. (Piiper 1957.)

Lungenatmung und Strömungswiderstand im Lungengefäßsystem. Die Lungenatmung verändert mit der Dehnung der Lunge und mit der veränderten Blutfüllung auch den Strömungswiderstand im Lungengefäßsystem. Abb. 70 zeigt die Beziehungen zwischen Lungendehnung und Strömungswiderstand am isolierten Organ[2]. In einem mittleren Dehnungszustand ist der Strömungswiderstand minimal, im Kollaps und bei starker Dehnung dagegen gesteigert. Während die Änderungen der Blutfüllung mit der Lungenatmung für den Kreislauf wahrscheinlich recht häufig von großer Bedeutung sein können, sind die Änderungen des Strömungswiderstandes wohl zu gering, als daß sie den Kreislauf in stärkerem Maße beeinflussen könnten. Wenn jedoch einzelne Lungenabschnitte verschieden stark gedehnt sind, so führt das zu Veränderungen des Strömungswiderstandes in den parallelgeschalteten Gefäßbahnen der Lunge. Das muß für die Durchblutungsverteilung innerhalb des Lungengefäßbettes durchaus von Bedeutung sein. Aus dem Anstieg des Strömungswiderstandes der kollabierten Lunge erklärt sich weitgehend die gute Arterialisierung des Blutes beim Pneumothorax.

III. Das Bronchialgefäßsystem.

Unsere Kenntnisse über die Funktion der Bronchialgefäße sind gering[3]. Die Durchblutung der Bronchialarterien soll 1%[4], nach anderen Angaben 2% des HZV betragen[5]. Bei der Steuerung der Durchblutung scheinen sympathische vasoconstrictorische Nerven von entscheidender Bedeutung zu sein. Auf Pharmaka reagieren die Bronchialgefäße im gleichen Sinne wie andere Gefäßgebiete des

---

[1] Bauereisen 1948.   [2] Piiper 1957 (Literatur).   [3] Daly 1935, Bücherl 1952.
[4] Bruner und Schmidt 1947.   [5] Semming zit. bei Bücherl 1952.

großen Kreislaufs[1]. Es ist nicht ganz exakt, die Bronchialgefäße als Vasa nutritiva der Lunge zu bezeichnen. Neben der mediastinalen Pleura und den Hiluslymphdrüsen versorgen sie nur das Bronchialsystem bis zu den Bronchiolii respiratorii. Das eigentliche Lungenparenchym wird jedoch durch das Pulmonalgefäßsystem oder, soweit die Atemgase in Frage kommen, direkt vom Alveolarraum aus versorgt. Experimente mit akutem Verschluß der Bronchialarterien zeigen, daß beim Hund das Bronchialgefäßsystem für die Versorgung der Hauptbronchi und der Lappenbronchi in der Gegend des Hilus unbedingt notwendig ist, während für die distalen Abschnitte die Blutversorgung des Pulmonalgefäßsystems ausreicht[2]. Möglicherweise spielt an der kranken Lunge die Blutzufuhr über die Bronchialarterien zum Lungenparenchym eine sehr viel wichtigere Rolle[3].

IV. Die Gefäßanastomosen des Lungenkreislaufs.

Es sind zwei Arten von Verbindungen zu unterscheiden: 1. Verbindungen zwischen der A. pulmonalis und der V. pulmonalis. 2. Verbindungen zwischen dem Bronchialgefäßsystem und dem Lungengefäßsystem. In den morphologischen und physiologischen Befunden gibt es so viel Widersprüche, daß es kaum möglich ist, über die Funktion dieser verschiedenen Arten von Anastomosen eine Aussage zu machen. Damit wird es auch schwierig zu beurteilen, ob und wann den Anastomosen bei der Umstellung des Lungenkreislaufs unter pathologischen Bedingungen eine größere Bedeutung zukommt.

Die arterio-venösen Anastomosen. Sie sind nicht nur von den Morphologen beschrieben, sondern es gibt auch eine Reihe von Normalbefunden, die für ihr Vorhandensein sprechen. Insbesondere wurde nachgewiesen, daß größere Glaskugeln das Lungengefäßbett passieren können. Weiterhin wurden sie bei Injektion von Röntgenkontrastmitteln direkt beobachtet. Gegen die Bedeutung der arterio-venösen Anastomosen unter normalen Bedingungen spricht freilich die geringe Beimischung venösen Blutes zum Lungencapillarblut, wie in sehr zahlreichen Untersuchungen festgestellt wurde (s. S. 754). Es ist in letzter Zeit dagegen eingewendet worden, daß unter den emotionalen Einflüssen der Untersuchungsmethoden die Anastomosen sich schließen könnten, daß es andererseits Bedingungen geben könnte, unter denen die Anastomosendurchblutung recht hoch ist. Dabei könnte es von Bedeutung sein, daß die arterio-venösen Anastomosen von den Sperrarterien abgehen und nur bei Eröffnung der Sperrarterien durchgängig sind[4]. Möglicherweise tritt bei akuter Steigerung des Strömungswiderstandes im Capillargebiet eine stärkere Durchblutung der arterio-venösen Anatomosen ein[5]. Möglicherweise kommt den sehr weiten Pleuracapillaren funktionell die Bedeutung von arterio-venösen Anastomosen zu[6].

Verbindungen zwischen dem Bronchialgefäßsystem und dem Lungengefäßsystem. Drei Arten von Verbindungen werden diskutiert. 1. Arterio-arterielle Anastomosen. 2. Veno-venöse Anastomosen. 3. Verbindungen zwischen den beiden Capillargebieten. Dadurch besteht die Möglichkeit, daß aus dem Hochdruckgebiet des großen Kreislaufs arterialisiertes Blut in das Lungengefäßsystem einströmt. Dieser Einstrom erfolgt hauptsächlich über die Capillarsysteme. Bei dem niedrigen Druck im Pulmonalsystem nimmt ein sehr großer Teil des Blutes aus den Bronchialgefäßen seinen Rückweg über die Pulmonalvenen. Nur ein Drittel des Blutes, das die Bronchialarterien passiert, fließt über die Bronchialvenen zurück. Die venöse Beimischung aus dem Bronchialgebiet vergrößert die

---

[1] DALY 1933.   [2] ELLIS und Mitarbeiter 1952.   [3] GIESE 1956.
[4] DALY 1958, CAIN 1958.   [5] NIDEN und AVIADO 1956.
[6] v. HAYEK 1953, LAPP 1951, Literatur bei BÜCHERL 1952.

alveolar-arterielle Sauerstoffdifferenz (s. S. 754). Wenn im allgemeinen beim Gesunden diese Art der venösen Beimischung nur gering ist, so liegt das an dem geringen Anteil der Bronchialdurchblutung am HZV. Die funktionelle Bedeutung der sog. Sperrarterien, die die beiden Gefäßsysteme auf der arteriellen Seite verbinden, und der veno-venösen Anastomosen ist unbekannt. Wahrscheinlich kommt unter pathologischen Bedingungen der Durchblutung dieser Verbindungen eine größere Bedeutung zu. Die Sperrarterien könnten die Möglichkeit schaffen, das unter bestimmten Bedingungen aus dem Hochdruckgebiet des großen Kreislaufs arterialisiertes Blut bestimmten Alveolarabschnitten zugeführt wird[1]. Es könnte aber auch umgekehrt über sie bei hohem Strömungswiderstand der Lungencapillaren Blut aus dem Pulmonalissystem in das Bronchialsystem abfließen, wobei die von den Sperrarterien abgehenden arterio-venösen Anastomosen gleichzeitig eine Abflußmöglichkeit in das Gebiet der V. pulmonalis unter Umgehung des Capillarsystems böten.

V. Die funktionelle Pathologie des Lungenkreislaufs.

Spielt schon normalerweise die humorale und nervöse Regulation des Lungenkreislaufs eine wesentlich geringere Rolle als im großen Kreislauf, so tritt ein *druckpassives* Verhalten des Lungenkreislaufs unter pathologischen Zuständen erst recht in den Vordergrund. Die am meisten interessierenden Größen sind das *Stromvolumen*, der *Blutdruck* und der *Strömungswiderstand*. Man könnte ähnlich wie im großen Kreislauf eine pathophysiologische Einteilung nach diesen Größen vornehmen. Es wäre dann jedoch schwierig, die so wichtigen Zustände der Rückstauung ohne Zwang unterzuordnen. Vor allem aber würde eine solche Einteilung deswegen auf Schwierigkeiten stoßen, weil sich unter pathologischen Verhältnissen anfänglich bestehende niedrige Strömungswiderstände mit der Zeit häufig in hohe Strömungswiderstände umwandeln. Der so wichtige *Zeitfaktor* macht die Situation hämodynamisch für den Lungenkreislauf besonders schwierig, da unter krankhaften Bedingungen vielfach mit der Zeit die Gefäße und das Herz einen anatomischen Umbau erfahren. Es wurde daher eine Einteilung gewählt, die sowohl den strömungsdynamischen Prinzipien wie auch den mit der Zeit eintretenden Abwandlungen der strömungsdynamischen Verhältnisse am ehesten gerecht werden dürfte.

1. Zustände mit gesteigerter Lungendurchblutung.

Die *angeborenen* Herz- und Gefäßanomalien mit „Links-Rechts"-Shunt sind besonders eindrucksvolle Naturbeispiele für Veränderungen der Hämodynamik des Lungenkreislaufs bei gesteigerter Lungendurchblutung. Für die funktionelle Pathologie sind sie aus zweifachen Gründen von besonderem Interesse. Einmal lassen sich bei diesen Anomalien die Beziehungen zwischen Stromvolumen und Widerstand der Strombahn besonders eindeutig aufzeigen, zum anderen sind die Rückwirkungen auf das Herz speziell in Hinsicht auf die Belastung des linken oder des rechten Herzens aufschlußreich[2].

a) Die aorto-pulmonalen Fistelverbindungen.

Diese Anomalien beruhen in der Regel auf einer Persistenz der fetalen Verbindungen zwischen Aorta und A. pulmonalis. Meist bestehen sie in Form des offenen *Ductus arteriosus Botalli*, selten in Form des sog. *aorto-pulmonalen Septumdefektes*. Die Erhöhungen des pulmonalen Stromvolumens können je nach Weite bzw. Länge des Defektes erheblich sein. Mit zunehmendem Lungendurchfluß

---

[1] Giese 1956.   [2] Literatur s. Grosse-Brockhoff 1951, 1957, Loogen 1958.

nimmt der Strömungswiderstand in der Lunge ab (s. Abb. 71). Die Beziehungen zwischen Stromvolumen und Strömungswiderstand gestalten sich hier ganz ähnlich, wie sie auch unter tierexperimentellen Bedingungen festgestellt werden konnten (s. S. 750). Anhaltspunkte für die Wirksamkeit besonderer Regulative sind nicht gegeben. Vielmehr scheinen diese Korrelationen Ausdruck der anatomischen Struktur des Lungengefäßnetzes zu sein. Abb. 72 zeigt die Beziehungen zwischen Größe des Shunts und dem Mitteldruck in der A. pulmonalis bei offenem Ductus arteriosus Botalli. Bei geringerem Kurzschluß (etwa zwischen 1,5—6,5 l/min) sind die Pulmonalisdrucke noch annähernd normal bzw. gering

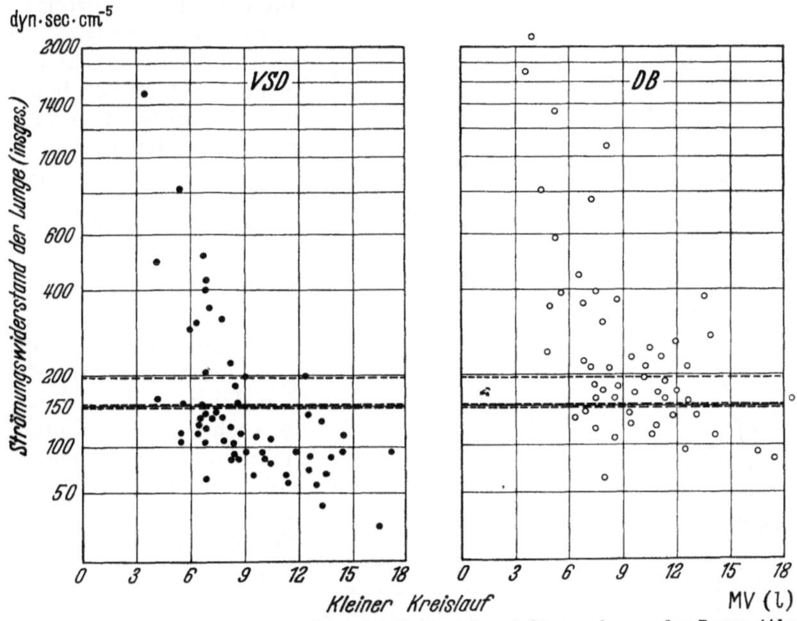

Abb. 71. Beziehung zwischen Strömungswiderstand (Ordinate) und Stromvolumen der Lunge (Abszisse) bei Vorhofseptumdefekt (*VSD*) und offenem Ductus Botalli (*DB*). (GROSSE-BROCKHOFF u. LOOGEN, unveröffentlicht.)

erhöht. In der Mittelgruppe kommt es zu einem mäßigen Anstieg des mittleren Pulmonalarteriendrucks bis zu etwa 30 mm Hg. Bei der obersten Gruppe mit sehr hohen Stromvolumina steigen die Pulmonalisdrucke erheblicher an. Hoher Lungendurchfluß stellt aber nur *einen* möglichen Grund für eine Druckerhöhung im Lungenkreislauf bei offenem Ductus arteriosus Botalli dar. Es entwickelt sich mit der Zeit eine zunehmende Sklerose der kleinen Lungengefäße. Dadurch steigen die Drucke in der A. pulmonalis immer stärker an, die Shunt-Volumina dagegen werden geringer (s. eingeklammerte Punkte der Abb. 72). Es kann der Fall eintreten, daß sich infolge einer massiven Sklerose der Lungengefäße die Stromrichtung im Shunt umkehrt. In diesen Fällen sind dann Druck und Strömungswiderstand im Lungenkreislauf höher als im großen Kreislauf. Die Zeitdauer der Entwicklung eines pulmonalen Hochdruckes bis zum Druckangleich an den Aortendruck kann kurz sein, so daß schon bei Kindern in seltenen Fällen eine Mischungscyanose auftritt.

Die Belastung des Herzens ist beim offenen Ductus Botalli zunächst eine vorwiegende *Volumenbelastung* des *linken* Herzens. Der linke Ventrikel wird vorzeitig insuffizient. Analog den Verhältnissen bei den arterio-venösen Fisteln im großen Kreislauf ist dies wieder ein Beweis mehr dafür, daß eine Herzkammer, in diesem

Falle die linke, insuffizient wird, wenn sie einer dauernden erhöhten Volumenbelastung unterworfen ist. Allerdings sind die Zeiträume bis zum Eintritt der Insuffizienz des Herzmuskels bei den angeborenen Anomalien in der Regel wesentlich länger. Offenbar kann sich der Herzmuskel besser an die Überlastung adaptieren, wenn diese von Geburt an besteht. Die Ursachen einer solchen Adaptation sind noch ungeklärt. Die rechte Herzkammer hat beim offenen Ductus Botalli erst dann Mehrarbeit zu leisten, wenn der Druck in der A. pulmonalis erhöht ist. Je mehr mit der Zeit durch die anatomischen Gefäßveränderungen der Strömungswiderstand der Lungengefäße ansteigt, um so mehr rückt die Mehrarbeit des rechten Ventrikels in den Vordergrund. Schließlich beherrscht in den späten Stadien die Dekompensation der rechten Kammer das klinische Erscheinungsbild.

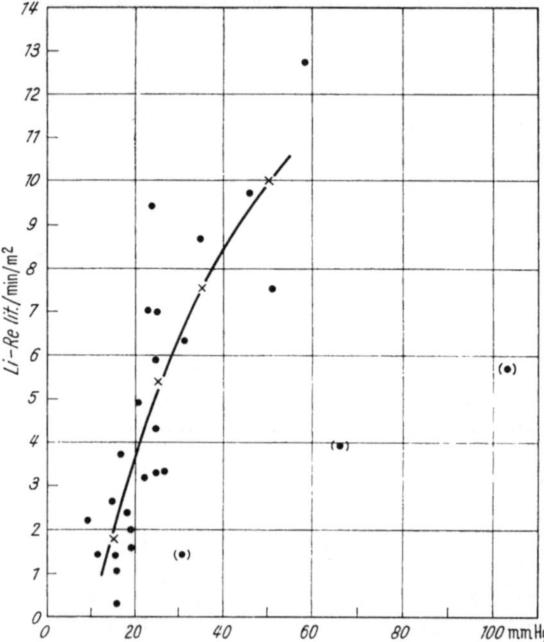

Abb. 72. Beziehungen zwischen der Kurzschlußdurchblutung und dem Mitteldruck in der A. pulmonalis bei offenem Ductus arteriosus Botalli (●). Fälle mit sekundärer Pulmonalsklerose. (Grosse-Brockhoff, Neuhaus u. Schaede 1954.)

b) Vorhofseptumdefekte.

Bei den Vorhofseptumdefekten liegen die strömungsdynamischen Verhältnisse der Lungenstrombahn ähnlich wie beim offenen Ductus arteriosus Botalli. Durch den Links-Rechts-Shunt kommt es auch hier zu erheblichen Zunahmen des pulmonalen Stromvolumens bis auf das Doppelte oder sogar das Dreifache der Norm. Der Mitteldruck in der A. pulmonalis steigt erst deutlich an, wenn das Stromvolumen der Lunge 10 l/min/m² Körperoberfläche übersteigt[1]. Durch die mit der Zeit eintretende Sklerose der kleineren und kleinsten Lungengefäße kommt es zunehmend zu einer Steigerung des Strömungswiderstandes, der in den späten Stadien ebenfalls so beträchtliche Ausmaße erreichen kann, daß es zu einer Umkehr der Stromrichtung im Shunt kommt. Beim Vorhofseptumdefekt besteht im Gegensatz zum offenen Ductus arteriosus Botalli eine *Volumenbelastung* des *rechten* Herzens, die sich in den späteren Stadien mit einer zunehmenden Druckbelastung kombiniert und schließlich zur Rechtsinsuffizienz führt.

c) Ventrikelseptumdefekte.

Bei den kleineren tiefer gelegenen Ventrikelseptumdefekten (Morbus Roger) ist die durch den Links-Rechts-Shunt eintretende Volumenbelastung des rechten Herzens relativ gering. Hierbei gelten für den Lungenkreislauf prinzipiell dieselben Gesetzmäßigkeiten wie beim offenen Ductus Botalli und beim Vorhofseptumdefekt, nur in graduell wesentlich geringerer Ausprägung. Besonderer Erörterung dagegen bedürfen die hochsitzenden Ventrikelseptumdefekte. Man darf wohl heute annehmen, daß es sich auch beim vielumstrittenen Eisenmenger-Syndrom um nichts

---

[1] Dexter und Mitarbeiter 1950.

anderes handelt als um einen hochsitzenden Ventrikelseptumdefekt mit leichter oder stärkerer Rechtsverlagerung der Aorta, bei dem über lange Zeit ein Links-Rechts-Shunt bestanden hat (I. Phase des Krankheitsbildes). Erst wenn infolge fibrotischer bzw. hyaliner oder sklerotischer Veränderungen der Arterien und Arteriolen die Drucke in der Lungenstrombahn den Aortendruck erreichen bzw. überschreiten, entwickelt sich eine *Mischungscyanose* (Rechts-Links-Shunt, II. bzw. III. Phase des Krankheitsbildes). Diese Mischungscyanose kann u. U. schon im frühesten Kindesalter auftreten. Es wurden Krankheitsfälle beschrieben, bei denen bereits im Säuglingsalter Verdickungen der Muscularis der Media und verengte Lumina der kleinen Gefäße festgestellt wurden[1,2]. Ob allerdings die Interpretation[1] dieser Befunde zu Recht besteht, daß nämlich die Lungengefäße beim Eisenmenger infolge einer stärkeren Beanspruchung von Geburt an ihren „fetalen" Charakter bewahren und damit gleichzeitig vor einer zu starken Durchströmung „geschützt" werden, erscheint problematisch.

Die Belastung des Herzens beim Ventrikelseptumdefekt betrifft *beide Kammern*, allerdings in Abhängigkeit vom Lungengefäßwiderstand in verschiedenem Maße. Im Verlauf der Erkrankung wird die Belastung der rechten Kammer durch die Erhöhung des Strömungswiderstandes in der Lungenstrombahn immer größer, so daß in den Endstadien die Dekompensation des rechten Herzens im Vordergrund steht.

d) Falsche Veneneinmündungen.

Einmündungen von Lungenvenen in den rechten Vorhof bzw. in die V. cava.

Hierbei handelt es sich um angeborene veno-venöse Fisteln zwischen den Venen des großen Kreislaufs und des Lungenkreislaufs. Bei den Einmündungen von Lungenvenen in die Hohlvene bzw. den rechten Vorhof besteht auf Grund des Druckgefälles von den Lungenvenen zum rechten Vorhof ein Links-Rechts-Shunt. Es kommt dabei zum Übertritt vollarterialisierten Blutes in das rechte Herz. Auf Grund dieses Links-Rechts-Shunts besteht eine oft hochgradige Steigerung des Lungendurchflusses. Die strömungsdynamischen Verhältnisse sind analog denjenigen beim Vorhofseptumdefekt. Es besteht zunächst eine ausschließliche Volumenbelastung des rechten Herzens, zu der sich erst in den späteren Stadien (anatomische Veränderungen der Lungengefäße) eine Druckbelastung hinzugesellt. Die Volumenbelastung des rechten Herzens kann bis zum Doppelten oder noch mehr betragen.

e) Arterio-venöse Fisteln im Lungenkreislauf.

Diese Anomalien sind im Gegensatz zu denjenigen im großen Kreislauf meist angeboren und nur sehr selten traumatisch entstanden. Sie werden vielfach unter dem Namen „arterio-venöse hypoxiämisierende Lungenangiomatose" beschrieben. Die arterio-venöse Fistel des Lungenkreislaufes hat eine Volumenbelastung beider Ventrikel zur Folge. Es handelt sich hämodynamisch um eine echte Fistel, d. h. es wird Blut unter Umgehung des Capillerkreislaufs auf die andere Kreislaufseite geschleust. Die Kurzschlußmenge ist abhängig von der Zahl der Mißbildungen, der Weite der zu- und abführenden Gefäße und dem bestehenden Druckgradienten. Die Kurzschlußmengen schwanken je nach der Größe der Fistel und ihrem Sitz zwischen etwa 20—60% der gesamten Lungendurchblutung[3] (s. Tabelle 22). Die durch den Kurzschluß der Arterialisierung in den Lungencapillaren entzogene Blutmenge muß zur Aufrecht-

Tabelle 22. *Druck und HZV bei arterio-venöser Lungenfistel.*
(Krankheitsfälle der I. Med. Klinik, Düsseldorf.)

Name und Alter		Druck (mm Hg) in der Pulmonal-arterie	HZV (l/min)	Effektives HZV (l/min)	Shunt (l/min)
W., E.	7 Jahre	50/20	6,4	1,6	4,8
L., I.	21 Jahre	22/8	6,9	5,0	1,9
St., A.	33 Jahre	30/20	6,6	3,4	3,2
Sch., K.	42 Jahre	34/18	17,5	9,6	7,9
K., I.	24 Jahre	15/8	6,7	3,7	3,0
H., H.	35 Jahre	20/8	7,3	3,3	4,0

---

[1] CIVIN und EDWARDS 1950.   [2] MEESSEN 1957.

[3] MAIER und Mitarbeiter 1948, FRIEDLICH und Mitarbeiter 1950, GROSSE-BROCKHOFF und Mitarbeiter 1954, HAUCK und HERTZ 1954, LOOGEN 1955.

erhaltung einer ausreichenden Sauerstoffversorgung der Kreislaufperipherie ausgeglichen werden. Dies kann durch eine verbesserte Utilisation des Sauerstoffs in der Peripherie, eine sekundäre Polycythämie sowie eine entsprechende Vergrößerung des Kreislaufminutenvolumens erreicht werden. Bei größeren Lungenfisteln wird eine Polycythämie nur in Ausnahmefällen vermißt. Die Vergrößerung des Herzminutenvolumens erreicht selten das Ausmaß der Vergrößerungen bei den traumatischen arterio-venösen Fisteln des großen Kreislaufs. Insuffizienzsymptome des Herzmuskels treten daher nicht oder erst viel später in Erscheinung. Durch das gehäufte Auftreten von Verschlüssen kleiner Lungengefäße infolge Thrombosierungen kann der Mitteldruck in der arteriellen Lungenstrombahn trotz der Fistel leicht erhöht sein (s. Tabelle 22). Dadurch ist es wohl zu erklären, daß die graduelle Ausprägung der Mischungscyanose mit der Zeit progredient ist (Erhöhung des Druckgradienten zwischen arterieller und venöser Lungenstrombahn).

2. Rückstauungszustände.

Die hämodynamische Analyse der Rückstauungszustände im Lungenkreislauf setzt einige anatomische Vorbemerkungen voraus. Ausgangspunkt ist dabei die Zweiteilung in den Bronchialkreislauf und in den eigentlichen Lungenkreislauf (s. S. 760). Normalerweise beträgt die Durchblutung der Bronchialgefäße nur 1% der Gesamtlungendurchströmung[1]. Unter pathologischen Umständen kann der Bronchialkreislauf aber eine große Bedeutung für die gesamte Lungendurchströmung erhalten. So sind z. B. bei angeborenen Herzfehlern, die mit einer Atresie der Pulmonalarterien einhergehen, die Bronchialgefäße die einzigen, die für die Oxydation des Blutes in der Lunge zur Verfügung stehen. In solchen Fällen sind die Bronchialgefäße wesentlich großkalibriger, es prägt sich ein sehr starker Kollateralkreislauf zwischen den Bronchialgefäßen und den alveolaren Capillaren aus (sog. Aortalisation des Lungenkreislaufs[2]). Kollateralen zwischen dem Lungenkreislauf und dem Gefäßsystem der Bronchien spielen aber auch unter anderen pathologischen Zuständen eine große Rolle. Während die Venen des Bronchialkreislaufs in den rechten Vorhof einmünden und normalerweise nur ein Teil des Blutes über Kollaterale in den linken Vorkof abfließt, münden die Lungenvenen ausschließlich in den linken Vorhof (s. S. 761). Deshalb müßten sich bei einer Insuffizienz des rechten Herzens die Stauungserscheinungen ausschließlich im Bronchialkreislauf, bei einer Stauung, die vom linken Herzen ausgeht, im Bereich des Alveolarkreislaufs manifestieren. Durch die Kollateralen zwischen Bronchialkreislauf und den Gefäßen der Vasa publica ist aber diese Zweiteilung bei Stauungszuständen teilweise verwischt. Bei der Linksinsuffizienz entwickelt sich sowohl eine Stauung im Gefäßnetz der Alveolen als auch der Bronchien und Bronchiolen, die nur durch die Entwicklung eines ausgeprägten Kollateralkreislaufs zwischen dem Bronchial- und dem Alveolarkreislauf zu erklären ist. Bei Überlastung des rechten Herzens (Cor pulmonale) wird eine Vermehrung der Anastomosen zwischen A. pulmonalis und den Bronchialarterien beschrieben[3].

Die Stauungszustände der Lunge werden zweckmäßigerweise in *akute* und *chronische* Formen eingeteilt.

a) Akute Lungenstauung (Lungenödem).

Die akute Form der Lungenstauung führt zum *Lungenödem*. Man sollte als Lungenödem nur solche Zustände bezeichnen, bei denen es von den alveolaren Capillaren aus zu einem Flüssigkeitsaustritt in die Alveolen kommt. Fälschlicherweise werden häufig auch solche Zustände mit Lungenödem identifiziert, bei denen eine Flüssigkeitsexsudation in die Bronchien und Bronchiolen für den Krankheitsprozeß kennzeichnend ist. In dieser Darstellung kann zur Entstehung

---

[1] Bruner und Schmidt 1947.   [2] Meessen 1951, Schoenmackers und Vieten 1951.
[3] Lapp 1951, Cudkowicz und Armstrong 1953, Giese 1956.

des Lungenödems nur insoweit Stellung genommen werden, als es sich um Auswirkungen hämodynamischer Faktoren handelt. Alle primär hämorrhagischen bzw. entzündlichen oder toxischen Ödemzustände der Lunge infolge unmittelbarer Capillarschädigung schalten hier aus. Die Gefahr eines Lungenödems besteht, wenn der Capillardruck den kolloidosmotischen Druck des Blutes (25 bis 30 mm Hg) erreicht oder überschreitet. Die Gefahr der Entstehung eines Ödems ist in der Lunge wohl deswegen noch besonders groß, weil die Lymphgefäße der Lunge anscheinend unmittelbar vor den Alveolen enden[1]. Die Alveolarwände werden damit bei Erhöhung des Capillardruckes bereits mit Flüssigkeit durchtränkt, bevor es zu einer Drainage dieser Flüssigkeit in die Lymphgefäße kommen kann. Wenn das Auftreten eines Lungenödems im wesentlichen auf eine Gleichgewichtsstörung zwischen Capillardruck und kolloidosmotischem Druck zurückzuführen ist, so sind außerdem noch einige Faktoren zu beachten, die entweder der Entstehung des Ödems Vorschub leisten oder es verhindern können. Sauerstoffmangel an der Capillarmembran stellt einen Faktor dar, der der Entstehung eines Lungenödems Vorschub leistet. Durch Sauerstoffmangel soll die Permeabilität der Lungencapillaren gesteigert und dadurch die Ödementstehung erleichtert werden[2]. Auf der anderen Seite tritt bei Zuständen, bei denen indurative Gewebsveränderungen der Lunge mit Verdickung der Capillarwände zustande gekommen sind, ein Ödem nicht mehr oder nur seltener in Erscheinung. In solchen Fällen kann der Capillardruck den kolloidosmotischen Druck des Blutes deutlich übersteigen (bis zu 40 mm Hg), ohne daß ein Lungenödem eintritt (s. auch S. 768).

Einer besonderen Erörterung bedarf noch die Frage, inwieweit zentralnervöse Faktoren bei der Entstehung eines Lungenödems eine Rolle spielen. Sowohl tierexperimentelle Untersuchungen als auch klinische Beobachtungen lassen darauf schließen, daß durch (extrem starke) Reizung der kreislaufregulierenden, vegetativen Zentralstellen ein Lungenödem auftreten kann[3]. Die Entstehung eines solchen Lungenödems ist teilweise so gedeutet worden, daß durch die zentralnervöse Reizung die Permeabilität der Capillarmembran verändert würde und dadurch ein Lungenödem entstände. Ein Beweis für eine solche „nervale“ Entstehung des Lungenödems wurde aber bisher nicht erbracht. Vielmehr konnte durch Tierexperimente wahrscheinlich gemacht werden, daß durch Reizung der vegetativen Zentralstellen in der Medulla oblongata eine Vasoconstriction im großen Kreislauf auftritt, daß dadurch erhebliche Blutmengen in die Lunge verlagert werden, und daß die hierdurch eintretende Erhöhung des Capillardrucks die Gefahr eines Lungenödems heraufbeschwört[4]. Vasoconstrictionen im großen Kreislauf können nach tierexperimentellen Ergebnissen zu einer Verdoppelung der Blutfülle der Lunge führen. Vasodilatatorische Substanzen oder Spinalanaesthesie führen den umgekehrten Effekt herbei. Dabei sinkt der Capillardruck in der Lunge um so stärker, je höher er vorher war[5]. Je größer die Gefahr des Lungenödems, um so durchgreifender ist die therapeutische Wirksamkeit solcher Maßnahmen. So ist auch die plötzliche und lebensrettende Wirkung eines Aderlasses damit zu erklären, daß die Blutfüllung der Lunge verringert wird. Jedenfalls spielen solche Blutverschiebungen vom großen zum kleinen Kreislauf bei der Ödementstehung eine beachtliche Rolle und verdienen vor allem bei der Therapie entsprechende Berücksichtigung.

b) Chronische Lungenstauung.

Die chronischen Stauungszustände im Lungenkreislauf mit ihren schwerwiegenden hämodynamischen Folgen gehen ebenso wie die akute Stauung vom

<hr>

[1] MILLER 1937.   [2] DRINKER 1950.   [3] CAMERON 1948.
[4] SARNOFF und SARNOFF 1952.   [5] SARNOFF und BERGLUND 1952.

linken Herzen aus. Ihre Ursache ist entweder eine muskuläre Insuffizienz der linken Kammer oder ein Ventildefekt in Form eines Mitralfehlers. Auch sind die Einflußstauungen auf Grund einer Concretio cordis im Bereich des linken Herzens hier einzuordnen. Die Stauungszustände im Lungenkreislauf werden zweckmäßigerweise unterteilt in Stauungszustände ohne Erhöhung des Druckgradienten zwischen arteriellem und venösem Lungengefäßsystem und Stauungszustände mit Erhöhung des Druckgradienten.

α) *Stauungszustände ohne Erhöhung des Druckgradienten.* Druckerhöhungen im Bereich der Lungenvenen führen rückwirkend zu einer Erhöhung des Drucks im arteriellen System. Da die Verhältnisse bei der Mitralstenose recht eindeutig geklärt sind, sollen die hämodynamischen Veränderungen im Gefolge chronischer Stauung an diesem Beispiel erörtert werden. Grundsätzlich gelten diese Feststellungen für alle chronischen Stauungszustände. Ist die Rückstauung jüngeren

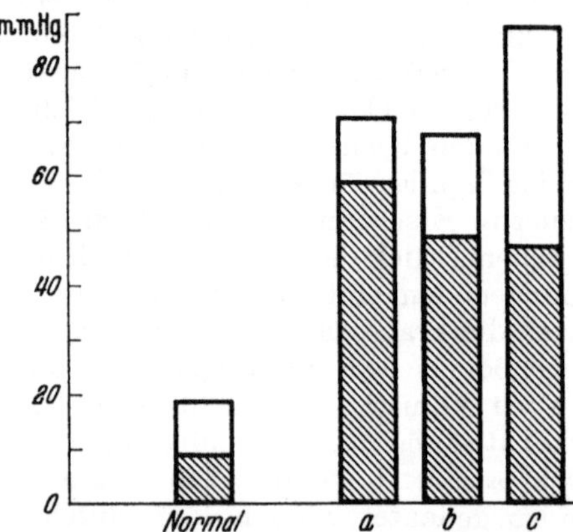

Datums, so bleibt der Druckgradient zwischen arteriellem und venösem Kreislauf praktisch unbeeinflußt. Das gesamte Druckniveau im Lungenkreislauf ist um den Betrag der Drucksteigerung im venösen Gebiet bzw. im linken Vorhof erhöht (s. Abb. 73). Es sind dies jene Krankheitsfälle von Rückstauung, die mit einer großen Blutfülle in der Lunge einhergehen. Es besteht die Gefahr, daß der kolloidosmotische Druck überschritten wird und ein akutes Lungenödem eintritt. Es entwickelt sich ein ausgeprägter Kollateralkreislauf zwischen den alveolaren Capillaren und denen des Bronchialsystems. Die Folgen der Rückstauung manifestieren sich mit der Zeit mehr und mehr im Bronchialkreislauf in Form der Stauungsbronchitis bzw. Stauungsbronchiolitis.

Abb. 73 a—c. Schematische Darstellung verschiedener Formen der Druckerhöhung im Lungenkreislauf bei Mitralstenose an Hand von 3 Beispielen. a: die Druckerhöhung ist ganz ausschließlich durch venöse Rückstauung bedingt; b und c: die Druckerhöhung ist zusätzlich durch eine Widerstandserhöhung im Lungenkreislauf bedingt. Die Höhe der gesamten Säule gibt den Druck in der A. pulmonalis an. Der schraffierte Teil der Säule zeigt den Druck im linken Vorhof, der nichtschraffierte Teil das Druckgefälle im Lungenkreislauf.

β) *Stauungszustände mit Erhöhung des Druckgradienten.* Besteht die Stauung längere Zeit, so ist der Druckgradient zwischen arteriellem und venösem Lungenkreislauf erhöht (s. Abb. 73 und 74). Die Krankheitsfälle mit erhöhtem Druckgradienten haben in der angelsächsischen Literatur den Namen „Protective cases" erhalten. Die Franzosen sprechen von „Barrage artériolaire protégeant". Mit diesen Bezeichnungen will man zum Ausdruck bringen, daß in solchen Fällen durch reflektorische Arteriolenkonstriktion ein Schutzmechanismus in Erscheinung tritt, der die Lunge vor dem Lungenödem bewahren soll. Das Blut könnte dabei über interarterielle Verbindungen aus den Lungenarterien in das Bronchialsystem abgelenkt werden. Gegen eine solche Deutung bestehen jedoch gewisse Bedenken. Abgesehen davon, daß eine reflektorische Arteriolenkonstriktion im Lungenkreislauf bei Mitralstenose bisher nicht erwiesen wurde, müßte ein solcher Mechanismus dazu führen, daß in der Zeiteinheit nur eine kleinere Blutmenge auf dem Wege durch die Lungencapillaren arterialisiert wird. Das linke Herz würde zu wenig Blut fördern, und dadurch würde die Sauerstoffversorgung der Peripherie gefährdet sein. Bei diesen fortgeschrittenen Stauungszuständen mit erhöhtem Druckgradienten ist, wie die Erfahrung zeigt, die Gefahr des akuten

Lungenödems tatsächlich geringer. Der Grund hierfür dürfte aber hauptsächlich in der indurativen Gewebsumwandlung der Lunge mit Verdickung der Capillarwände zu suchen sein. Je stärker die Lungenfibrose, um so seltener das Lungenödem (s. unten). In dieser Phase der Erkrankung nimmt die Blutfüllung der Lunge mehr und mehr ab. Das Blut ist wieder von der Lunge in den großen Kreislauf verlagert. Die Erhöhung des Strömungswiderstandes nimmt mit der Zeit progredient zu. Der Strömungswiderstand in der Lungenstrombahn kann höher werden als im großen Kreislauf (s. Abb. 74). Man sieht dabei, zu welchen Leistungen die rechte Kammer befähigt ist. Insofern erscheint die alte Lehrmeinung von der schwachen rechten und der starken linken Herzkammer korrekturbedürftig. Die Rechtsbelastung steht im Finalstadium der chronischen Stauungslunge ganz im Vordergrund.

Es bleibt die Frage zu erörtern, ob eine enge Korrelation zwischen dem Grad der pulmonalen Hypertension und der Ausprägung der anatomischen Gefäßveränderungen der Lunge besteht. Die Ansichten hierüber sind nicht einheitlich. Während BECKER, BURCHELL u. EDWARDS, GRAHAM u. Mitarb. sowie CURTI u. Mitarb.[1] eine Beziehung zwischen dem Grad der pulmonalen Hypertension und der Ausprägung

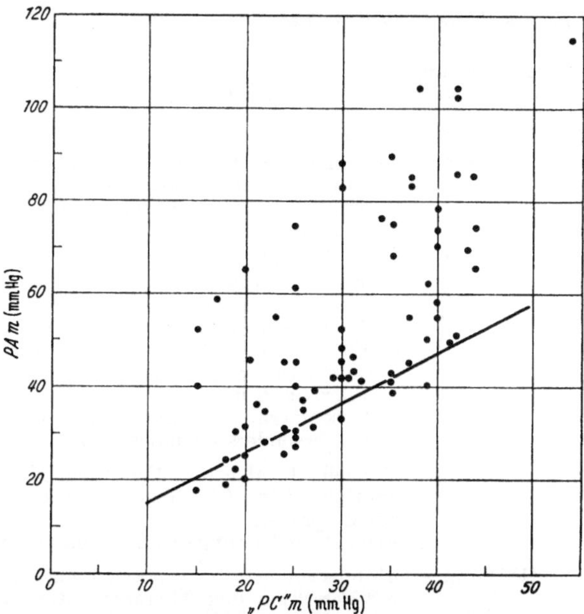

Abb. 74. Das Verhältnis von Mitteldruck in der A. pulmonalis zum Pulmonalcapillardruck (*PC*) bei Mitralstenose. Bei den Patienten ohne Erhöhung des Druckgradienten zwischen arteriellem und venösem System gruppieren sich die Werte um die durchgezeichnete Linie. (GROSSE-BROCKHOFF und LOOGEN 1957.)

der anatomischen Gefäßveränderungen der Lunge vermissen, heben LUKAS u. Mitarb. und DENST u. Mitarb.[2] eine enge Korrelation hervor. Nach den eigenen Erfahrungen sind die Veränderungen der Lungengefäße und des Lungengerüstes um so ausgeprägter, je hochgradiger die pulmonale Hypertonie bzw. die Erhöhung des Strömungswiderstandes ist[3]. Daß solche vergleichenden Untersuchungen nur in grober Annäherung möglich sind und eine große Streubreite aufweisen, liegt auf der Hand. Die Schwierigkeiten bestehen besonders darin, den Grad der Einengung des gesamten Lungenstrombettes aus mikroskopischen Einzelabschnitten abzuschätzen. Das Ergebnis dieser Untersuchungen berechtigt u. E. aber zu der Schlußfolgerung, daß für das Zustandekommen der pulmonalen Hypertonie bei Mitralstenose die funktionelle Engerstellung der Gefäße von geringer Bedeutung ist.

3. Primäre Erhöhungen des Strömungswiderstandes im Lungenkreislauf.

Die Ursachen der primären Widerstandserhöhungen im Lungenkreislauf sind aus der Tabelle 23 ersichtlich.

---

[1] BECKER, BURCHELL und EDWARDS 1951, GRAHAM und Mitarbeiter 1951, CURTI und Mitarbeiter 1953.   [2] LUKAS und Mitarbeiter 1952, DENST und Mitarbeiter 1954.
[3] BAYER, GROSSE-BROCKHOFF, LOOGEN und MEESSEN 1957.

Tabelle 23.

A. Akutes Cor pulmonale

1. Massive Lungenembolie
2. Große Lungenresektion, besonders Pneumektomie, akute Überblähung der verbliebenen Lunge
3. Akute Kompressionsatelektasen größerer Ausdehnung
4. Ventilpneumothorax
5. Lungenödem

B. Subakutes Cor pulmonale

1. Miliartuberkulose
2. Hämatogene Lungenkarzinose
3. Atelektasen größerer Ausdehnung

C. Chronisches Cor pulmonale

I. Gruppe: Verkleinerung der Lungenstrombahn bei normaler alveolarer Belüftung
    1. ohne arterielle Hypoxämie
    2. mit arterieller Hypoxämie infolge Störungen des alveolaren Gasaustausches

Zur Gruppe I gehören hauptsächlich folgende Erkrankungen:
    a) Primäre Pulmonalsklerose
    b) Angitiden verschiedener Genese
    c) Trombosen der Lungengefäße und rezidivierende Embolien
    d) Fibrosen und Granulomatosen (Silikose und andere Staublungen, produktiv-cirrhotische Lungentuberkulose, Boecksches Sarkoid, chronische Fibrosen, Lungencirrhose)
    e) Verkleinerung der Lungenstrombahn nach thoraxchirurgischen Eingriffen, besonders Pneumektomie

II. Gruppe: Mangelhafte alveolare Belüftung mit arterieller Hypoxämie. Emphysem, multiple kleine Obstruktionsatelektasen bei Bronchiolitis, Kyphoskoliose mit Emphysem
Vielfach sind Gruppe I und II miteinander kombiniert

III. Gruppe: Abflußstörungen im venösen Lungenkreislauf. Nach Emphysem, Pleuritis mit Verschwartung, Thoraxoperationen

IV. Gruppe: Funktionelle idiopathische pulmonale Hypertonie?

a) Akute Widerstandserhöhung.

Einen wesentlichen experimentellen Beitrag zu der vielumstrittenen Frage, inwieweit bei akuten Widerstandserhöhungen infolge Embolie reflektorische oder anatomische Faktoren entscheidend sind, liefern die Untersuchungen von Daley, Wade, Maraist und Bing (1951, dort auch weitere Literatur). In Versuchen an Hunden erzielten die Autoren nach Injektion von Lycopodium-Kügelchen in den Hauptast der A. pulmonalis einen beträchtlichen Anstieg des Druckes in der A. pulmonalis. Beidseitige cervicale Vagotomie und ausgedehnte beidseitige thorakale vordere Wurzelresektion beeinflußten den Grad der erzielten pulmonalen Hypertension und des berechneten erhöhten Arteriolenwiderstandes nicht. Injektionen durch einen Katheter, der in der Endarterie lag, riefen einen geringen Anstieg des Pulmonalarteriendruckes hervor. Nach Anlegen einer Ligatur um die den Katheter führende Arterie, die eine Verschleppung der Kügelchen in andere Lungenabschnitte verhinderte, blieb die Blutdrucksteigerung aus. Gleichartige Befunde wurden auch an der isolierten Lunge erzielt. Wiederholte Injektionen von Lycopodium-Kügelchen am Ganztier riefen einen pulmonalen Hochdruck von mehrwöchiger Dauer hervor. Aus diesen Untersuchungen wird geschlossen, daß örtliche Embolien keine generalisierte Vasoconstriction der Lungengefäße bedingen, und daß eine pulmonale Hypertonie im Gefolge von Lungenembolien durch anatomischen Verschluß der Pulmonalarteriolen hervorgerufen wird.

b) Chronische Widerstandserhöhung.

Aus der tabellarischen Zusammenstellung geht schon hervor, daß bei primären chronischen Widerstandserhöhungen entweder der Verlust von Atmungsfläche einschließlich der Gefäße oder selektive anatomische Einengungen der Gefäße durch Hyalinose, endangitische Prozesse und Sklerose die Ursache der Erhöhung des Strömungswiderstandes sind. Häufig kommen Kombinationen dieser beiden ursächlichen Faktoren vor (s. Tabelle 23).

Wenn somit ein großer Teil der primären Erhöhungen des Strömungswiderstandes im Lungenkreislauf, die zum Cor pulmonale führen, durch den pathologisch-anatomischen Gefäßbefund hinreichend erklärt erscheinen, so bleiben zwei Fragen zu beantworten:

1. Gibt es eine „essentielle" Hypertonie im Lungenkreislauf analog derjenigen im großen Kreislauf?

2. Inwieweit sind funktionelle Faktoren an der Steigerung des Strömungswiderstandes in jenen Fällen *mit* beteiligt, bei denen die Gefäße anatomische Einengungen aufweisen?

Zu 1. Für eine essentielle Hypertonie im Lungenkreislauf auf funktioneller Basis tritt eine Reihe von Autoren ein[1]. Diese Autoren ziehen, wenn auch eingeschränkt, Parallelen zur essentiellen Hypertonie im großen Kreislauf. Schon aus den Darlegungen über den anatomischen Bau der Lungengefäße geht hervor, daß solche Analogie-Schlüsse nicht ohne weiteres gezogen werden dürfen. BENNINGHOFF[2] bezeichnet z. B. das arterielle Lungenstromgebiet als Windkessel ohne besondere Eigenmuskelwirkung. Nervöse Regulationen spielen im Vergleich zu den vielfältigen nervösen Steuerungsmechanismen im großen Kreislauf im Lungenkreislauf nur eine untergeordnete Rolle. Unseres Wissens ist bisher kein einschlägiger Krankheitsfall beschrieben worden, bei dem während des Lebens eine pulmonale Hypertonie sichergestellt worden wäre, und bei dem bei systematischer mikroskopischer Untersuchung post mortem keine einengenden Veränderungen an den Lungengefäßen gefunden worden wären. Von pathologisch-anatomischer Seite hat man sich jüngst jedoch auch für die essentielle Hypertonie im Lungenkreislauf als einer neuroregulatorischen Fehlsteuerung eingesetzt[3]. BERBLINGER[4] neigt ebenfalls dazu, bei der Hypertonie im Lungenkreislauf funktionelle Momente in den Vordergrund zu stellen. Die Berechtigung hierzu leitet er aus der häufiger zu beobachtenden Diskrepanz zwischen der Hypertrophie der rechten Herzkammer einerseits und den Lungengefäßveränderungen andererseits ab. Ob aber aus einer solchen Diskrepanz anatomischer Befunde schon auf das Mitspielen nervöser Faktoren bei der Entstehung der pulmonalen Hypertonie geschlossen werden darf, muß dahingestellt bleiben. Eine besondere Rolle spielt bei der Deutung der anatomischen Befunde die beobachtete Mediahypertrophie der kleinen Lungenarterien[5]. Jedoch erscheint das Argument, daß eine solche Mediahypertrophie der Lungengefäße die *Folge* eines Hypertonus sein müßte, nicht überzeugend. Zudem wird auch von pathologisch-anatomischer Seite davor gewarnt, aus einer offenbar schwierig zu beurteilenden Mediahypertrophie der Gefäße weitreichende Schlußfolgerungen zu ziehen[6]. Nach unserem Ermessen kann auf Grund der vorliegenden Befunde die Existenz einer essentiellen Hypertonie im Lungenkreislauf auf funktioneller Basis bisher noch nicht als bewiesen angesehen werden.

---

[1] DELIUS und WITZENHAUSEN 1949, DELIUS 1956, LANGE 1948, DRESDALE und Mitarbeiter 1951, TURCHETTI 1952.

[2] BENNINGHOFF 1930.   [3] STAEMMLER und SCHMITT 1951, SCHMIDT 1953, KIRCH 1955.

[4] BERBLINGER 1947.   [5] SCHMIDT 1953.   [6] BREDT 1932, 1942.

Zu 2. Von manchen Autoren wird eine zusätzliche Erhöhung des Strömungswiderstandes im Lungenkreislauf durch vasomotorische Einflüsse bei schon vorhandener anatomischer Einengung der Gefäße angenommen. Dabei wird in erster Linie der Einfluß eines erniedrigten O_2-Druckes bzw. eines erhöhten CO_2-Druckes in der Alveolarluft diskutiert[1]. Für das Bestehen einer solchen Beziehung zwischen gradueller Ausprägung einer pulmonalen Hypertension und einer Erniedrigung der O_2-Spannung in der Alveolarluft bzw. im arteriellen Blut

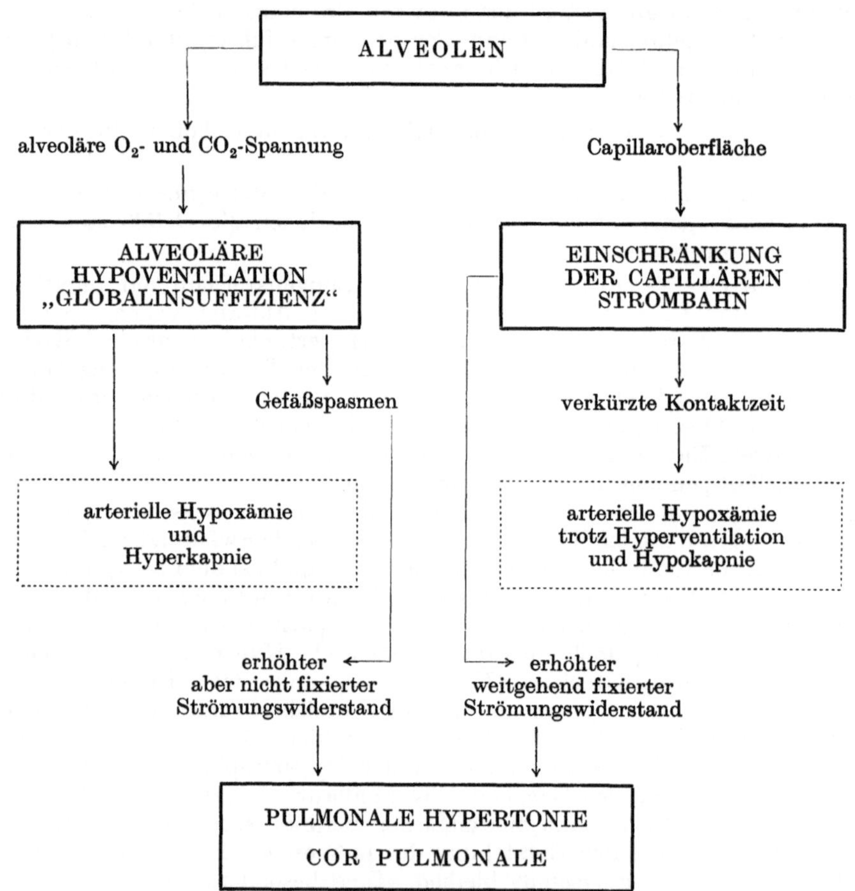

Abb. 75. Schematische Darstellung der hämodynamischen Ätiologie des chronischen Cor pulmonale.

werden folgende Befunde ins Feld geführt: Die Widerstandserhöhung im Lungenkreislauf ist häufig um so ausgeprägter, je hochgradiger die O_2-Untersättigung bzw. die Erniedrigung der O_2-Spannung des arteriellen Blutes ist[2]. Gleiche Beziehungen wurden zwischen Erniedrigung der alveolaren O_2-Spannung, Erhöhung der alveolaren CO_2-Spannung und dem Grad der Drucksteigerung im Lungenkreislauf gefunden[3]. Auf Grund dieser Feststellungen und in Anlehnung an tierexperimentelle Untersuchungen (s. S. 755) stellt man sich den Mechanismus der Erhöhung des Strömungswiderstandes unter krankhaften Bedingungen etwa nach dem Schema der Abb. 75 vor. Gegen die Bedeutung von O_2-Mangel als maßgeb-

[1] Rossier und Bühlmann 1954.   [2] Cournand und Mitarbeiter 1950.
[3] Rossier und Mitarbeiter 1954, Bühlmann und Mitarbeiter 1955.

lichem Faktor für die Erhöhung des Strömungswiderstandes im Lungenkreislauf infolge reflektorischer Engerstellung der Gefäße bestehen bei chronischen Lungenerkrankungen jedoch folgende Bedenken: Die aufgefundenen Beziehungen zwischen der Höhe des Strömungswiderstandes und dem Grad der Erniedrigung der O_2-Spannung in der Alveolarluft bzw. im arteriellen Blut können nebeneinander geordnet sein. Sie besagen noch nicht, daß die Widerstandserhöhung eine Folge der herabgesetzten O_2-Spannung ist. Auch bestehen die Beziehungen zwischen Erhöhung des Strömungswiderstandes und Störungen der O_2- bzw. CO_2-Spannung des arteriellen Blutes längst nicht in allen Fällen[1] (eigene Untersuchungen). Weiterhin erscheint es fraglich, ob die im akuten Tierexperiment

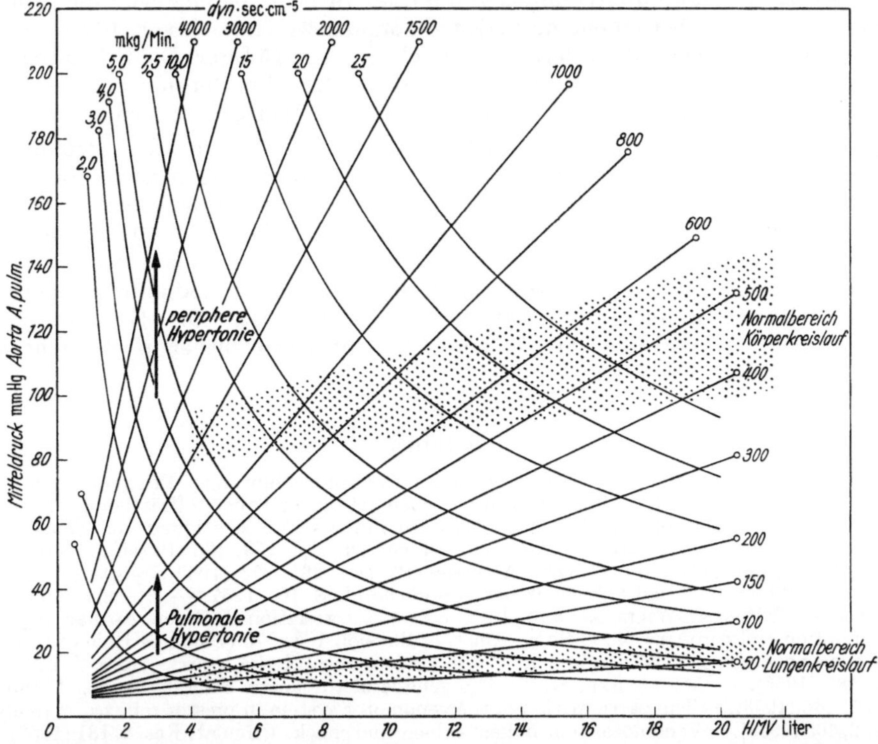

Abb. 76. Beziehungen zwischen Herzminutenvolumen, Herzleistung, Strömungswiderstand und Mitteldruck. Ordinate: Mitteldruck in der A. pulmonalis bzw. Aorta. Abszisse: Herzminutenvolumen. Fächerförmig ausstrahlend: Strömungswiderstände von 50—4000 dyn sec cm⁻⁵. Nach rechts konkav: Herzleistung in mkg/min. Diese Linien verbinden die Punkte, bei denen der rechte bzw. linke Ventrikel bei verschiedenem Widerstand, Herzminutenvolumen und Mitteldruck die gleiche Arbeit leistet. Punktiert: Der Normalbereich für den Körperkreislauf oben und Lungenkreislauf unten. (BÜHLMANN u. Mitarb. 1955.)]

festgestellten Beziehungen zwischen Erniedrigung der alveolaren O_2-Spannung und Erhöhung des Strömungswiderstandes in der Lunge auch für den chronischen Krankheitszustand Gültigkeit haben. Schließlich ist noch zu berücksichtigen, daß der Mechanismus der vasoconstrictorischen Wirkung einer Erniedrigung der alveolaren O_2-Spannung nicht einmal für das akute Experiment klargestellt ist (s. S. 755 und vor allem die letzten kritischen Arbeiten von COURNAND[2]). Aber unabhängig von diesen noch umstrittenen Fragen ist es für die klinischen Belange wichtig, den Faktor O_2-Mangel als wesentliches Krankheitssymptom in Rechnung zu stellen. Gleichgültig, ob die Wirkung von O_2-Mangel eine reflektorische Enger-

---

[1] BOLT 1955.   [2] COURNAND 1956.

stellung der Lungenstrombahn bedingt oder nicht, kann O_2-Mangel den Blutdruck in der Lunge durch Erhöhung des Kreislaufminutenvolumens steigern, wenn die Reservekapazität des Lungenstrombettes bereits stärker beansprucht ist. Die Erhöhung des Kreislaufminutenvolumens stellt eine beachtliche Mehrbelastung des Herzens dar, zumal bei schon vorhandener Widerstandserhöhung im Lungenkreislauf eine Steigerung des Kreislaufminutenvolumens ein weiteres beträchtliches Ansteigen der Pulmonalisdrucke nach sich zieht. Die gegenseitigen Beziehungen zwischen Kreislaufminutenvolumen, Herzarbeit, Strömungswiderstand und Mitteldruck im Lungenkreislauf sind in der Abb. 76 dargestellt[1]. Bei einem Strömungswiderstand von 1000 dyn sec cm^{-5} muß der rechte Ventrikel für ein normales Kreislaufminutenvolumen von 5 Liter in Ruhe bereits etwa die gleiche Arbeit leisten wie bei einem normalen Strömungswiderstand von 100 dyn sec cm^{-5} für das dreimal größere Herzminutenvolumen von 15 Liter. Die Erhöhung des Strömungswiderstandes bei ausgeprägter pulmonaler Hypertension kann enorme Ausmaße erreichen und das Zehnfache des normalen Wertes betragen.

Zusammenfassend kann festgestellt werden: Die Erhöhung des Strömungswiderstandes in der Lungenstrombahn ist in erster Linie abhängig von der Einengung des Strombettes durch anatomische Veränderungen der Gefäße. Sauerstoffmangel kann eine weitere Erhöhung des Blutdrucks bedingen. Jedoch muß es offen bleiben, ob diese Blutdruckerhöhung in der A. pulmonalis Ausdruck einer Vasoconstriction ist, oder ob die durch den O_2-Mangel bedingte Steigerung des Kreislaufminutenvolumens dafür verantwortlich ist. Die Existenz einer „essentiellen" Hypertonie im kleinen Kreislauf kann bisher noch nicht als erwiesen angesehen werden.

Literatur.

Alella, A.: Arterielle O_2-Sättigung und Coronardurchblutung. Pflügers Arch. ges. Physiol. **259**, 422 (1954a). ~ Beziehungen zwischen arterieller Sauerstoffsättigung im Sinus coronarius und Sauerstoffausnutzung im Myocard unter Berücksichtigung von Sauerstoffkapazität und arteriellem Druck. Pflügers Arch. ges. Physiol. **259**, 436 (1954b). ~ Coronardurchblutung und Hypoxie. Pflügers Arch. ges. Physiol. **261**, 373 (1955). ~ Steuerung der Coronardurchblutung. Bad Oeynhausener Gespräche II, S. 10. 1957. — Alella, A., F. L. Williams, C. Bolene-Williams and L. N. Katz: Interrelation between cardiac oxygen consumption and coronary blood flow. Amer. J. Physiol. **183**, 570 (1955). ~ Role of oxygen and exogenous glucose and lactic acid in the performance of the heart. Amer. J. Physiol. **185**, 487 (1956). — Alexander, R. S.: The genesis of the aortic standing wave. Circulat. Res. 1, 145 (1953). ~ The participation of the venomotor system in pressor reflexes. Circulat. Res. 2, 405 (1954). ~ Venomotor tone in hemorrhage and shock. Circulat. Res. 3, 181 (1955). ~ Reflex alterations in venomotor tone produced by venous congestion. Circulat. Res. 4, 49 (1956). — Alexander, R. S., W. S. Edwards and J. L. Ankeney: The distensibility characteristics of the portal vascular bed. Circulat. Res. 1, 271 (1953). — Allgöwer, M., A. Pletscher, J. Siegrist u. A. Walser: Die Behandlung der Verbrennungen. Dtsch. med. Wschr. **1956**, 462. — Altschulte, M. D.: Physiology in diseases of the heart and lungs. Cambridge 1954. — Amelung, D., u. H. D. Horn: Fermentaktivitäts-Bestimmungen im Serum beim Herzinfarkt. Dtsch. med. Wschr. **1956**, 1701. — Anzola, J., and R. F. Rushmer: Cardiac responses to sympathetic stimulation. Circulat. Res. 4, 302 (1956). — Aschoff, J.: Über die Interferenz temperaturregulatorischer und kreislaufregulatorischer Vorgänge in den Extremitäten des Menschen. Pflügers Arch. ges. Physiol. **248**, 197 (1944). — Asmussen, E.: The distribution of the blood between the lower extremities and the rest of the body. Acta physiol. scand. **5**, 31 (1943). — Asmussen, E., E. H. Christensen u. T. Sjöstrand: Über die Abhängigkeit der Lungenvolumen von der Blutverteilung. Skand. Arch. Physiol. **82**, 193 (1939). — Asmussen, E., and M. Nielsen: The arterial blood pressure on transition from rest to work. Acta physiol. scand. **25**, Suppl. 89, 5 (1951). ~ The cardiac output in rest and work determined simultaneously by acetylene and the dye injection methods. Acta physiol. scand. **27**, 217 (1953). ~ Cardiac output during muscular work and its regulation. Physiol. Rev. **35**,

---

[1] Bühlmann und Mitarbeiter 1955.

778 (1955a). ~ The cardiac output in rest and work at low and high oxygen pressures. Acta physiol. scand. **35**, 73 (1955b). — ASMUSSEN, E., M. NIELSEN and G. WIETH-PEDERSEN: On the regulation of circulation during muscular work. Acta physiol. scand. **6**, 353 (1943). — ATWELL, R. J., J. M. RYAN, H. B. HULL and J. F. TOMASHEFSKI: Factors influencing the alveolar-arterial oxygen pressure gradient, role of the left heart. Amer. J. Physiol. **183**, 451 (1955). —AVIADO, D. M., J. S. L. LING, C. W. QUIMBY and C. F. SCHMIDT: Additional role of reflex pulmonary vasoconstriction during anoxia. Fed. Proc. **13**, 4 (1954). — AVIADO, D. M., and C. F. SCHMIDT: Reflexes from stretch receptors in blood vessels, heart and lungs. Physiol. Rev. **35**, 247 (1955). — AXELRAD, B., B. JOHNSON and J. LUETSCHER: Factors regulating the output of sodium-retaining corticoid of human urine. J. clin. Endocr. **14**, 783 (1954).

BAINBRIDGE, F. A.: Diastolic filling. J. Physiol. (Lond.) **49**, 45 (1915). ~ The physiology of muscular excercise. Edit. by ANREP 1923. — BALKE, B., G. T. GRILLER, E. B. KONECCI and U. C. LUFT: Work capacity after blood donation. J. appl. Physiol. **7**, 231 (1954). — BARCROFT, H.: Problems of sympathetic innervation and denervation. Brit. med. Bull. **8**, 363 (1952). — BARCROFT, H., and A. F. COBBOLD: The action of adrenaline on muscle blood flow and blood lactate in man. J. Physiol. (Lond.) **132**, 372 (1956). — BARCROFT, H., and O. G. EDHOLM: On vasodilatation in human skeletal muscle during post-haemorrhagic fainting. J. Physiol. (Lond.) **104**, 161 (1945). — BARCROFT, H., O. G. EDHOLM, J. McMICHAEL and E. P. SHARPEY-SCHAFER: Posthaemorrhagic fainting, study of cardiac output and forearm flow. Lancet **1944 I**, 489. — BARCROFT, H., and H. J. C. SWAN: Sympathetic control of human blood vessels. London 1953. — BARCROFT, J.: Die Stellung der Milz im Kreislaufsystem. Ergebn. Physiol. **25**, 818 (1926). — BARGER, A. C., V. RICHARDS, J. METCALFE and B. GÜNTHER: Regulation of the circulation during exercise. Amer. J. Physiol. **184**, 613 (1956). — BARTELS, H., R. BEER, E. FLEISCHER, H. J. HOFFHEINZ, J. KRALL, G. RODEWALD, J. WENNER u. I. WITT: Bestimmung von Kurzschlußdurchblutung und Diffusionskapazität der Lunge bei Gesunden und Lungenkranken. Pflügers Arch. ges. Physiol. **261**, 99 (1955b). — BARTELS, H., R. BEER, H. P. KOEPCHEN, J. WENNER u. I. WITT: Messungen der alveolar-arteriellen O_2-Druckdifferenz mit verschiedenen Methoden bei Ruhe und Arbeit. Pflügers Arch. ges. Physiol. **261**, 133 (1955a). — BARTELS, H., E. BÜCHERL, M. MOCHIZUKI u. G. NIEMANN: Bestimmung der via venae thebesii in den linken Ventrikel fließenden Blutmenge durch Messung des O_2-Druckes im Blut des linken Vorhofs und einer Arterie beim Menschen. Pflügers Arch. ges. Physiol. **262**, 478 (1956). — BARTELS, H., H. P. KOEPPCHEN, I. LÜHNING, M. MOCHIZUKI u. I. WITT: Die alveolar-arterielle O_2-Druckdifferenz bei Ruhe und Arbeit unter Hypoxie. Pflügers Arch. ges. Physiol. **261**, 535 (1955b). — BARTELS, H., u. G. RODEWALD: Der arterielle Sauerstoffdruck, die alveolar-arterielle Sauerstoffdruckdifferenz und weitere atmungsphysiologische Daten gesunder Männer. Pflügers Arch. ges. Physiol. **256**, 113 (1952). — BAUEREISEN, E.: Atmungseinflüsse auf den arteriellen Blutdruck des Menschen. Arch. Kreisl.-Forsch. **14**, 306 (1948). ~ Die Gesetze der Herzarbeit und ihre Gültigkeit im natürlichen Kreislauf. Klin. Wschr. **1957**, 369. — BAUEREISEN, E., H. BÖHME, H. KRUG, U. PEIPER u. L. SCHLICHER: Der Einfluß der Inspiration auf den Effektivdruck der intrathorakalen Kreislaufabschnitte. Pflügers Arch. ges. Physiol. **266**, 499 (1958). — BAYER, O., F. GROSSE-BROCKHOFF, F. LOOGEN u. H. MEESSEN: Vergleichende klinische, pathophysiologische und pathologisch-anatomische Untersuchungen bei Mitralstenose. Arch. Kreisl.-Forsch. **26**, 238 (1957). — BAYLISS, W. M.: On the local reactions of the arterial wall to changes of internal pressure. J. Physiol. (Lond.) **28**, 220 (1902). — BAZETT, H. C.: Temperaturen in den Blutgefäßen der Extremitäten. Fed. Proc. **6**, 76 (1947). — BEACONFIELD, P., and J. GINSBURY: Effect of changes in limb posture on peripheral blood flow. Circulat. Res. **3**, 478 (1955). — BEARM, A. G., B. H. BILLING, O. G. EDHOLM and S. SHERLOCK: Hepatic blood flow and carbohydrate changes in man during fainting. J. Physiol. (Lond.) **115**, 442 (1951). — BECKER, O. L., H. B. BURCHELL and J. E. EDWARDS: Pathology of the pulmonary vascular tree. II. The occurrence in mitral insufficiency of occlusive pulmonary vascular lesions. Circulation **3**, 230 (1951). — BENNINGHOFF, A.: Blutgefäße und Herz. In Handbuch der mikroskopischen Anatomie des Menschen. Bd. I. 1930. — BENSON, E. S.: Composition and state of protein in heart muscle of normal dogs and dogs with experimental myocardial failure. Circulat. Res. **3**, 221 (1955). — BERBLINGER, W.: Formen und Ursachen der Herzhypertrophie bei Lungentuberkulose. Bern 1947. — BERGLUND, E., H. G. BORST, F. DUFF and G. L. SCHREINER: Effect of heart rate on cardiac work, myocardiol oxygen consumption and corronary blood flow in the dog. Acta physiol. scand. **42**, 185 (1958). — BERGLUND, E., R. G. MONROE u. G. L. SCHREINER: Myocardial oxygen consumption and coronary blood flow during potassium-induced cardiac arrest and during ventricular fibrillation. Acta physiol. scand. **41**, 261 (1957). — BERGLUND, E., S. J. SARNOFF and J. P. ISAACS: Role of the pericardium in regulation of cardiovascular hemodynamics. Circulat. Res. **3**, 133 (1955). — BERGLUND, H.: Sympathicuschirurgie und Hypertension. Verh. dtsch. Ges. Kreisl.-Forsch. **15**, 187 (1949). — BING, R. J.: Myocardial metabolism. Circulation **12**, 635

(1955). ~ Der Myocardstoffwechsel. Klin. Wschr. **34**, 1 (1956). — Bing, R. J., M. M. Hammond, J. C. Handelsman, S. M. Powers, F. C. Spencer, J. E. Eckenhoff, W. T. Goodale, J. H. Hafkenschule and S. S. Kety: Measurement of coronary blood flow, oxygen consumption and efficiency of the left ventricle. Amer. Heart J. **38**, 1 (1949). — Bing, R. J., R. Heimbecker and W. Falholt: An estimation of the residual volume of blood in the right ventricle of normal and diseased human hearts in vivo. Amer. Heart J. **42**, 483 (1951). — Bing, R. J., F. M. Maraist, F. C. Dammann, A. J. Draper, R. Heimbecker, R. Daley, R. Gerard and P. Galazel: Effect of strophantins on coronary blood flow and cardiac oxygen consumption of normal and failing human hearts. Circulation **2**, 513 (1950). — Bing, R. J., A. Siegel, I. Ungar and M. Gilbert: Metabolism of the human heart. Studies on fat, ketone and amino acid metabolism. Amer. J. Med. **16**, 504 (1954). — Bing, R. J., A. Siegel, A. Vitale, F. Balboni, E. Sparks, M. Taeschler, M. Klepper and S. Eckwards: Metabolic studies on the human heart in vivo. Carbohydrate metabolism. Amer. J. Med. **15**, 284 (1953). — Blalock, A.: Experimental shock. The importance of the local loss of fluid in the production of the low blood pressure after burns. Arch. Surg. (Chicago) **22**, 610 (1931). — Blix, M.: Die Länge und Spannung des Muskels. Skand. Arch. Physiol. **5**, 173 (1895). — Bock, K. D., H. Hensel u. J. Ruff: Die Wirkung von Adrenalin und Noradrenalin auf die Muskel- und Hautdurchblutung des Menschen. Pflügers Arch. ges. Physiol. **261**, 322 (1955). — Bodechtel, G.: Zur Klinik der cerebralen Kreislaufstörungen. Mit besonderer Berücksichtigung ihrer kardialen Genese. Verh. dtsch. Ges. Kreisl.-Forsch. **21**, 366 (1953). — Böhme, W.: Über den aktiven Anteil des Herzens an der Förderung des Venenblutes. Ergebn. Physiol. **38**, 251 (1936). — Bolomey, A. A., J. Michie, C. Michie, E. S. Breed, G. E. Schreiner and H. D. Lauson: Simultaneous measurement of effective renal blood flow and cardiac output in resting normal subjects and patients with essential hypertension. J. clin. Invest. **28**, 10 (1949). — Bolt, W.: Pathologische Physiologie des Cor pulmonale. Verh. dtsch. Ges. Kreisl.-Forsch. **21**, 196 (1955). — Borst, H. G., E. Berglund, M. McGregor: The effect of pharmacologic agents on the pulmonary circulation in the dog. J. clin. Invest. **36**, 669 (1957). — Bostroem, B., u. P. W. Schneider: Über die Wirkung depressorischer Reflexe auf die Durchblutung der arteriovenösen Anastomosen der Hundeextremität. Pflügers Arch. ges. Physiol. **257**, 241 (1953). — Bostroem, B., u. W. Schoedel: Über die Durchblutung der arterio-venösen Anastomosen in der hinteren Extremität des Hundes. Pflügers Arch. ges. Physiol. **256**, 371 (1953). — Brandfonbrener, M., M. Landowne and N. W. Shock: Changes in cardiac output with age. Circulation **12**, 557 (1955). — Braunwald, E., H. L. Moscowitz, S. S. Amran, R. P. Lasser, S. O. Sapin, A. Himmelstein, M. M. Ravitch and A. J. Gordon: The hemodynamics of the left side of the heart as studied by simultaneous left atrial, left ventricular, and aortic pressures; particular reference to mitral stenosis. Circulation **12**, 69 (1955). — Brecher, G. A.: Cardiac variations in venous return studied with a new bristle flowmeter. Amer. J. Physiol. **176**, 423 (1954). ~ Critical review of recent work on ventricular diastolic suction. Circulat. Res. **6**, 554 (1958). — Brecher, G. A., and C. A. Hubay: Pulmonary blood flow and venous return during spontaneous respiration. Circulat. Res. **3**, 210 (1955). — Bredt, H.: Die primäre Erkrankung der Lungenschlagader in ihren verschiedenen Formen. (Arteriopathia pulmonalis idiogenica.) Virchows Arch. path. Anat. **284**, 126 (1932). ~ Entzündung und Sklerose der Lungenschlagader. Ein Beitrag zur Kenntnis des Begriffes und der Erscheinungsformen der Endarteriitis und Arteriosklerose. Virchows Arch. path. Anat. **308**, 60 (1942). — Bretschneider, H. J.: Über den Mechanismus der hypoxischen Coronarerweiterung. Bad Oeynhausener Gespräche II, S. 44. 1957. — Bretschneider, H. J., A. Frank, E. Kanzow u. U. Bernard: Über das Verhalten der Milchsäureausnutzung des Koronarblutes zur venösen Sauerstoff-Sättigung. Verh. Dtsch. Ges. Kreislaufforsch. **22**, 300 (1956.) — Briggs, A. P., and D. M. Fowell: Renal and circulatory factors in edema formation of congestive heart failure. J. clin. Invest. **27**, 810 (1948). — Broemser, Ph.: Physiologische Grundlagen der Behandlung der Herzinsuffizienz. Verh. dtsch. Ges. Kreisl.-Forsch. **12**, 289 (1939) — Broman, T.: Über cerebrale Zirkulationsstörungen. Copenhagen 1940. — Brown, E., J. Hooper and R. Wennesland: Blood volume and its regulation. Ann. Rev. Physiol. **19**, 231 (1957). — Bruner, H. D., and C. F. Schmidt: Blood flow in the bronchial artery of the anestethized dog. Amer. J. Physiol. **148**, 648 (1947). — Bücherl, E.: Über die Bronchialgefäße. Klin. Wschr. **30**, 961 (1952). — Bücherl, E., u. M. Schwab: Der Sauerstoffverbrauch des ruhenden Skeletmuskels bei reflektorisch-nervöser Vasokonstriktion. Pflügers Arch. ges. Physiol. **254**, 337 (1952). — Büchner, F.: Die Coronarinsuffizienz. Dresden u. Leipzig 1939. ~ Büchner, F.: Allgemeine Pathologie. München u. Berlin 1956. — Bühlmann, A., C. Maier, M. Hegglin, R. Kälin u. F. Schaub: Beziehungen zwischen Lungenfunktion und Lungenkreislauf. Schweiz. med. Wschr. **1953**, 1199. — Bühlmann, A., F. Schaub u. P. Luchsinger: Die Hämodynamik des Lungenkreislaufs während Ruhe und körperlicher Arbeit beim Gesunden und bei verschiedenen Formen der pulmonalen Hypertonie. Schweiz. med. Wschr. **1955**, 253. — Burch, G., P. Reaser and J. Cronvich: Rates of sodium turnover in normal subjects and in patients with congestive heart failure. J. Lab. clin. Med. **32**, 1169 (1947). — BURN, J. H.: Sympathetic vasodilator fibres. Physiol. Rev. **18**, 137 (1938). — BURTON, A. C.: On the physical equilibrium of small blood vessels. Amer. J. Physiol. **164**, 319 (1951). ~ Relation of structure to function of the tissues of the wall of blood vessels. Physiol. Rev. **34**, 619 (1954). — BURTON, A. C., and S. YAMADA: Relation between blood pressure and flow in the human forearm. J. appl. Physiol. **4**, 329 (1951).

· CAIN, H.: Neben- und Kurzschlüsse im Lungenkreislauf des Menschen. Klin. Wschr. **36**, 321 (1958). — CAMERON, G. R.: Shock. In H. FLOREY, Lectures on general pathology. London 1954. ~ Pulmonary edema. Brit. med. J. **1948**, No 4459, 965. — CASE, R. B., E. BERGLUND and S. J. SARNOFF: Changes in coronary resistance and ventricular function resulting from acutely induced anemia and the effect thereon of coronary stenosis. Amer. J. Med. **18**, 397 (1955). — CELANDER, O.: The range of control exercised by the sympathicoadrenal system. Acta physiol. scand. **32**, Suppl., 116 (1954). — CELANDER, O., u. B. FOLKOW: A comparison of the sympathetic vasomotor fibre control of the vessels within the skin and the muscles. Acta physiol. scand. **29**, 241 (1953). — CHASE, W. H.: Anatomical and experimental observations on air embolism. Surg. Gynec. Obstet. **59**, 569 (1934). — CHIEN, S.: Quantitative evaluation of the circulatory adjustment of splenectomized dogs to hemorrhage. Amer. J. Physiol. **193**, 605 (1958). — CHRISTENSEN, E. H.: Das Herzminutenvolumen. Ergebn. Physiol. **39**, 348 (1937). ~ Die Lebenswandlungen der Kreislauffunktionen in Abhängigkeit von Alter und Geschlecht. Verh. dtsch. Ges. Kreisl.-Forsch. **24**, 60 (1958). — CHRISTENSEN, E. H., u. P. HÖBERG: Physiology of skiing. Arbeitsphysiologie **14**, 292 (1950). — CHRISTENSEN, E. H., u. M. NIELSEN: Investigations of the circulation in the skin at the beginning of muscular work. Acta physiol. scand. **4**, 162 (1942). — CITTERS, R. L. VAN, W. E. RUTH and K. R. REISSMANN: Effect of heart rate on oxygen consumption of isolated dog heart performing no external work. Amer. J. Physiol. **191**, 443 (1957). — CIVIN, W. H., and E. EDWARDS: Pathology of the pulmonary vascular tree. Circulation **2**, 545 (1950). — CLARA, M.: Die arterio-venösen Anastomosen. Wien 1956. — CLARK, G.: Arterio-venous anastomoses. Physiol. Rev. **18**, 229 (1938). — COHEN, S. M., O. G. EDHOLM, S. HOWARTH, J. MCMICHAEL and E. P. SHARPEY-SCHAFER: Cardiac output and peripheral blood flow in arteriovenous aneurysm. Clin. Sci. **7**, 35 (1948). — COLES, D. R.: Heat elimination from the toes during exposure of the foot to subatmospheric pressures. J. Physiol. (Lond.) **135**, 171 (1957). — COLES, D. R., and A. D. M. GREENFIELD: The reactions of the blood vessels of the hand during increases in transmural pressure. J. Physiol. (Lond.) **131**, 277 (1956). — CONTOPOULOS, A. N., D. C. VAN DYKE, M. E. SIMPSON, I. F. GARCIA, R. L. HUFF, B. S. WILLIAMS and H. M. EVANS: Increase in circulating red cell volume after oral administration of pituitary anterior lobe. Blood **8**, 131 (1953). — COURNAND, A.: Some aspects of the pulmonary circulation in normal man and in chronic cardiopulmonary diseases. Circulation **2**, 641 (1950). ~ Shock and circulatory homeostasis. 4th Conference, Josiah Macy foundation 1954. The pulmonary circulation. ~ The mysterious influence of unilateral pulmonary hypoxia upon the circulation in man. Acta cardiol. (Brux.) **10**, 429 (1955). ~ Measurement of total and unilateral pulmonary blood flow during hypoxia in normal man. Europ. Cardiologenkongr. 1956, Stockholm. Abstracts of papers p. 29. — COURNAND, A., M. I. FERRER, R. M. HARVEY and D. W. RICHARDS jr.: Some effects of chronic pulmonary disease upon the heart circulation. Zit. nach COURNAND u. Mitarb. 1950. — COURNAND, A., J. LEQUIME et P. REGNIERS: L'insufficance cardiaque chronique. Études pathophysiologiques. Paris: Masson & Cie. 1952. — COURNAND, A., R. L. RILEY, A. HIMMELSTEIN and R. AUSTRIAN: Pulmonary circulation and alveolar ventilation — perfusion relationsships after pneumoectomy. J. thorac. Surg. **19**, 80 (1950). — CUDKOWICZ, L., and J. B. ARMSTRONG: Bronchial arteries in pulmonary emphysema. Thorax **8**, 46 (1953). — CULLUMBINE, H., and A. C. E. KOCH: The changes in plasma and tissue fluid volume following exercise. Quart. J. exp. Physiol. **35**, 39 (1949). — CURTI, P. C., G. COHEN, B. CASTIEMAN, G. SCANNELL, A. L. FRIEDLICH and G. S. MYERS: Respiratory and circulatory studies of patients with mitral stenosis. Circulation **8**, 893 (1953).

DALEY, R., J. D. WADE, F. MARAIST and R. J. BING: Pulmonary hypertension in dogs induced by injection of lycopodium spores into pulmonary artery, with special reference to the absence of vasomotor reflexes. Amer. J. Physiol. **164**, 380 (1951). — DALY, I. DE B.: Reactions of the pulmonary and bronchial blood vessels. Physiol. Rev. **13**, 149 (1933). ~ The physiology of the bronchial vascular system. Harvey Lect. **31**, 235 (1935). ~ Intrinsic mechanisms of the lung. Quart. J. exp. Physiol. **43**, 2 (1958). — DELIUS, L.: Cor pulmonale. In Klinik der Gegenwart, Bd. I. München u. Berlin 1956. — DELIUS, L., W. BERG und V. WEIBEL: Untersuchungen zur Regulation der Systolendauer. Dtsch. Arch. klin. Med. **199**, 554 (1952). — DELIUS, L., u. H. REINDELL: Die Kreislaufregulation in ihrer Bedeutung für Leistungsfähigkeit und Lebenserwartung. Z. klin. Med. **143**, 29 (1943). — DELIUS, L., u. R. WITZENHAUSEN: Über Entstehungsbedingungen und Folgen der essentiellen und akzidentellen pulmonalen Hypertonie. Z. Kreisl.-Forsch. **38**, 87 (1949). — DENOLIN, H.:

Le coeur pulmonaire chronique en médecine interne. Verh. dtsch. Ges. Kreisl.-Forsch. **21**, 217 (1955). — Denolin, H., A. de Coster et N. Salonikides: Le problème de l'hypertension pulmonaire chronique. Acta clin. belg. **8**, 647 (1953). — Denst, J., A. Edwards, K. T. Neuburger and S. G. Blount: Biopsies of the lung and atrial appendages in mitral stenosis: Correlation of data from cardiac catheterisation with pulmonary vascular lesions. Amer. Heart J. **48**, 506 (1954). — Dexter, L., J. W. Dow, F. W. Haynes, J. L. Whittenberger, B. G. Ferris, W. T. Goodale and H. K. Hellems: Studies of the pulmonary circulation in man at rest. J. clin. Invest. **29**, 602 (1950). — Dexter, L., J. L. Whittenberger, F. W. Haynes, W. T. Goodale, R. Gorlin and C. G. Sawyer: Effect of exercise on circulatory dynamics of normal individuals. J. appl. Physiol. **3**, 439 (1951). — Dietlen, H.: Über das Sportherz. Münch. med. Wschr. **1951**, 2137. — Dock: Allgemeine Pathologie. München u. Berlin 1956. — Doering, P., R. Koch, H. Sanken u. M. Schwab: Die intrarenale Haemodynamik bei essentieller Hypertonie. Klin. Wschr. **1954**, 71. — Dohrn, A., u. H. F. Rein: Über unbekannte Milzfunktionen. Pflügers Arch. ges. Physiol. **255**, 448 (1952). — Donald, K. W., J. M. Bishop, G. Cumming and O. L. Wade: The effect of exercise on the cardiac output and circulatory dynamics of normal subjects. Clin. Sci. **14**, 37 (1955). — Draper, A. J.: The cardioinhibitory carotid sinus syndrome. Ann. intern. Med. **32**, 700 (1950). — Dresdale, D. T., M. Schulz and R. J. Michton: Primary pulmonary hypertension, clinical and hemodynamic study. Amer. J. Med. **11**, 686 (1951). — Drinker, C. K.: Pulmonary edema and inflammation. Cambridge, Mass. 1950. — Duesberg, R., u. W. Schroeder: Pathophysiologie und Klinik der Kollapszustände. Leipzig 1944. — Duke, H. N.: The action of carbon dioxide on isolated perfused dog lungs. Quart. J. exp. Physiol. **35**, 25 (1949). — Duke, H. N., and S. D. Carlill: Pulmonary vasomotor responses to changes of left auricular pressure. J. Physiol. (Lond.) **131**, 12 P (1956). — Duke, H. N., and E. Killik: Pulmonary vasomotor responses of isolated perfused cat lungs to anoxia. J. Physiol. (Lond.) **117**, 303 (1952).

Ead, H. W., J. H. Green and E. Neil: A comparison of the effects of pulsatile and nonpulsatile blood flow through the carotid sinus on the reflexogenic activity of the sinus baroceptors in the cat. J. Physiol. (Lond.) **118**, 509 (1952). — Ebbecke, U.: Gefäßreaktionen. Ergebn. Physiol. **22**, 401 (1923). — Eckenhoff, J. E.: The physiology of the coronary circulation. Anesthesiology **11**, 168 (1950). — Eckenhoff, J. E., J. H. Hafkenschiel, M. H. Harmel, W. T. Goodale, M. Lubin, R. J. Bing and S. S. Kety: Measurement of coronary blood flow by the nitrous oxide method. Amer. J. Physiol. **152**, 356 (1948). — Eckenhoff, J. E., J. H. Hafkenschiel and C. M. Landmesser: The coronary circulation in the dog. Amer. J. Physiol. **148**, 582 (1947). — Eckenhoff, J. E., J. H. Hafkenschiel, C. M. Landmesser and M. Harmel: Cardiac oxygen metabolism and control of the coronary circulation. Amer. J. Physiol. **149**, 634 (1947). — Eckstein, R. W.: Development of interarterial coronary anastomoses by chronic anemia. Circulat. Res. **3**, 306 (1955). — Eckstein, R. W., M. Stroud, C. W. Dowling and W. H. Pritchard: Factors influencing changes in coronary flow following sympathetic nerve stimulation. Amer. J. Physiol. **162**, 266 (1950). — Edholm, O. G.: Physiological changes during fainting. In: Visceral circulation. A. Ciba Foundation Symposium, London, 1952. — Eduards, W. S., A. Siegel and R. J. Bing: Studies on myocardial metabolism. Coronary blood flow, myocardial oxygen consumption and carbohydrate metabolism in experimental hemorrhagic shock. J. clin. Invest. **33**, 1646 (1954). — Eliasson, S., P. Lindgren and B. Uvnäs: Representation in the hypothalamus and the motor cortex in the dog of the sympathetic vasodilator outflow to the skeletal muscles. Acta physiol. scand. **27**, 18 (1952). — Eliasson, S., and G. Ström: On the localisation in the cat of hypothalamic and cortical structures influending cutaneous blood flow. Acta physiol. scand. **20**, Suppl. 70, 113 (1950). — Elkin, D. C., and J. V. Warren: Arteriovenous fistulas. Their effect on the circulation. J. Amer. med. Ass. **134**, 1524 (1947). — Ellis, F. H., J. H. Grindlay and J. E. Edwards: The bronchial arteries. Surgery **31**, 167 (1952). — Emerson, C. P., and R. V. Ebert: Study of shock in battle casualities; measurements of blood volume changes occuring in response to therapie. Ann. Surg. **122**, 745 (1945). — Emmrich, J., H. Steim, H. Klepzig, K. Mushoff, H. Reindell u. B. Baumgarten: Über den Einfluß blutiger Untersuchungsmethoden auf das Herzminutenvolumen. Z. Kreisl.-Forsch. **47**, 326 (1958). — Eppinger, H.: Die gegenseitigen Beziehungen zwischen Minutenvolumen und zirkulierender Blutmenge. In Handbuch der normalen und pathologischen Physiologie. Bd. XVI/2, 1396 (1931). — Euler, U. S. v.: Adrenaline and noradrenaline. Pharmacol. Rev. **6**, 15 (1954). — Euler, U. S. v., u. B. Folkow: Einfluß verschiedener afferenter Nervenreize auf die Zusammensetzung des Nebennierenmarkinkretes bei der Katze. Naunyn-Schmiedeberg's Arch. exp. Path. Pharmak. **219**, 242 (1953). — Euler, U. S. v., u. G. Liljestrand: Observations on the pulmonary arterial blood pressure in the cat. Acta physiol. scand. **12**, 301 (1946).

Feinberg, H., and L. N. Katz: Effect of catecholamines, l-epinephrine and l-norepinephrine on coronary flow and oxygen metabolism of the myocardium. Amer. J. Physiol. **193**, 151 (1958). — Fenn, W. O., A. B. Otis, H. Rahn, L. E. Chadrik and A. H. Hegnauer:

Displacement of blood from the lungs by pressure breathing. Amer. J. Physiol. **151**, 258 (1947). — FERRER, M. I., R. M. HARVEY, R. T. CATCHART, C. A. WEBSTER, D. W. RICHARDS and A. COURNAND: Some effects of digitoxin upon heart and circulation in man, digoxin in chronic cor pulmonale. Circulation **1**, 161 (1950). — FICK, A.: Über die Messung des Blutquantums in den Herzventrikeln. Ber. physik.-med. Ges. Würzburg, 16 (1870). ~ Mechanische Arbeit und Wärmeentwicklung bei der Muskeltätigkeit. Leipzig 1882. — FISHMAN, A. P., A. HIMMELSTEIN, H. W. FRITTS and A. COURNAND: Blood flow through each lung in man during unilateral hypoxie. J. clin. Invest. **34**, 637 (1955). — FLAKS, J., I. HIMMEL et J. ZLOTNIK: Sur l'existence d'une hormone hémopoïétique dans l'hypophyse. Presse méd. **45**, 1261 (1937). — FLECKENSTEIN, A.: Der Kalium-Natrium-Austausch als Energieprinzip in Muskel und Nerv. Berlin 1955. — FLEISCH, A., u. I. SIBUL: Über nutritive Kreislaufregulierung. Pflügers Arch. ges. Physiol. **231**, 787 (1931). — FLEISCH, A., u. P. WEGER: Die nutritive Gewebssensibilität als Grundlage der Arbeitshyperämie. Pflügers Arch. ges. Physiol. **240**, 552 (1938). — FLEMING, P. R., and R. GIBSON: Percutaneous left ventricular puncture in the assessment of aortic stenosis. Thorax **12**, 37 (1957). — FOLKOW, B.: Intravascular pressure as a factor regulating the tone of the small vessels. Acta physiol. scand. **17**, 289 (1949). ~ A study of the factors influencing the tone of denervated blood vessels perfused at various pressures. Acta physiol. scand. **27**, 99 (1953). ~ Nervous control of the blood vessels. Physiol. Rev. **35**, 629 (1955). — FOLKOW, B., and U. S. v. EULER: Selective activation of nor-adrenalin and adrenaline producing cells by hypothalamic stimulation. Circulat. Res. **2**, 191 (1954). — FOLKOW, B., J. FROST, K. HAEGER u. B. UVNÄS: The sympathetic vasomotor innervation of the skin of the dog. Acta physiol. scand. **17**, 195 (1949). — FOLKOW, B., J. FROST and B. UVNÄS: Action of acetylcholine, adrenaline and noradrenaline on the coronary blood flow. Acta physiol. scand. **17**, 201 (1948). — FOLKOW, B., and B. E. GERNANDT: An electrophysiological study of the sympathetic vasodilator fibres of the limb. Amer. J. Physiol. **169**, 622 (1952). — FOLKOW, B., and B. LÖFVING: The distensibility of the systemic resistance blood vessels. Acta physiol. scand. **38**, 37 (1956). — FOLTZ, E. L., R. G. PAGE, W. F. SHELDON, S. K. WONG, W. J. TUDDENHAM and A. J. WEISS: Factors in variation and regulation of coronary blood flow in intact anesthetized dogs. Amer. J. Physiol. **162**, 521 (1950). — FONTAINE, R., E. LUCINESCO, A. SCHATTNER et A. OSWALD: Quelle influence une thrombose limitée exerce-t-elle sur les artères en aval? Presse méd. **1936 II**, 1860. — FONTAINE, R., et R. SCHATTNER: Les bases expérimentales de l'artériectomie. J. Chir. (Paris) **46**, 849 (1935). — FOWLER, W. S.: Intrapulmonary distribution of inspired gas. Physiol. Rev. **32**, 1 (1952). — FRANK, A.: Experimentelle Herzhypertrophie. Z. ges. exp. Med. **115**, 312 (1950). — FRANK, O.: Zur Dynamik des Herzmuskels. Z. Biol. **32**, 370 (1895). — FRANKE, H.: Das Cor pulmonale in der Thoraxchirurgie. Verh. dtsch. Ges. Kreisl.-Forsch. **21**, 300 (1955). — FRANKE, H., u. J. HANN: Die Auswirkungen des hypertensiven Carotis-Sinus-Syndroms kardialen Typs mit längeren Herzpausen auf das Hirnstrombild des Menschen. Verh. dtsch. Ges. Kreisl.-Forsch. **19**, 205 (1953). — FRANKLIN, K. J.: A monograph of veins. Springfield, Ill. 1937. — FREIS, E. D., and J. C. ROSE: The sympathetic nervous system, the vascular volume and the venous return in relation to cardiovascular integration. Amer. J. Med. **22**, 175 (1957). — FREY-WYSSLING, A.: Deformation and flow in biological systems. Amsterdam and New York 1953. — FRIEDBERG, CH. K.: Diseases of the heart. Philadelphia and London 1950. ~ Erkrankungen des Herzens. Deutsch. Übers. von E. GILL. Stuttgart 1959. — FRIEDLICH, A., R. G. BING and S. G. BLOUNT jr.: Physiological studies in congenital heart disease, circulatory dynamics in anomalies of venous return to heart including pulmonary arterio-venous fistula. Bull. Johns Hopk. Hosp. **86**, 20 (1950).

GASKELL, P., and A. C. BURTON: Local postural vasomotor reflexes arising from the limb veins. Circulat. Res. **1**, 27 (1953). — GAUER, O. H.: Volume changes of the left ventricle during blood pooling and exercise in left ventricular performance. Physiol. Rev. **35**, 143 (1955). ~ Wechselbeziehungen zwischen Herz- und Venensystem. Verh. dtsch. Ges. Kreisl.-Forsch. **22**, 61 (1956). — GAUER, O. H., u. J. P. HENRY: Beiträge zur Homöostase des extra-arteriellen Kreislaufs. Klin. Wschr. **34**, 356 (1956). — GAUER, O. H., J. P. HENRY and H. O. SIEKER: Changes in central venous pressure after moderate hemorrhage and transfusion in man. Circulat. Res. **4**, 79 (1956). — GAUER, O. H., J. P. HENRY, H. O. SIEKER and W. E. WENDT: The effect of negative pressure breathing on urine flow. J. clin. Invest. **33**, 287 (1954). — GAUER, O. H., u. F. LINDER: Kreislaufdynamik und vegetativer Tonus der Menschen bei arterio-venösen Fisteln. Klin. Wschr. **26**, 1 (1948). — GEHL, H., K. GRAF u. K. KRAMER: Das Druckvolumdiagramm des Kaltblüterherzens. Die Bedeutung des plastischen Elementes für die Herzmechanik. Pflügers Arch. ges. Physiol. **261**, 270 (1955). — GIESE, W.: Die morphologischen Grundlagen der Ventilationsstörungen beim Emphysem und bei Bronchitis und ihre Rückwirkungen auf den Kreislauf. Verh. dtsch. Ges. inn. Med., 62. Kongr. 12, 1956. — GIESE, W., u. H. MÜLLER-MOHNSSEN: Kollateralkreisläufe im Coronarsystem bei Coronarsklerose. Bad Oeynhausener Gespräche II, S. 159. 1957. — GILLIAT, R. W.: Vasoconstriction in the finger after deep inspiration. J. Physiol. (Lond.) **107**, 76 (1948). —

Girling, F.: Critical closing pressure and venous pressure. Amer. J. Physiol. 171, 204 (1952). — Glaser, E. M.: The effect of cooling and warming on the vital capacity, forerm and hand volume, and skin temperature of man. J. Physiol. (Lond.) 109, 421 (1949). — Goetz, R. H.: Der Fingerplethysmograph als Mittel zur Untersuchung der Regulationsmechanismen in peripheren Gefäßgebieten. Pflügers Arch. ges. Physiol. 235, 271 (1934). — Goldblatt, H., J. Lynch, R. F. Hansel and W. W. Summerville: Studies on experimental hypertension: Production of persistent elevation of systolic pressure by means of renal ischemia. J. exp. Med. 59, 347 (1934). — Goldring, W., and H. Chasis: Hypertension and hypertensive disease. New York: Common Wealth Fund 1944. — Gollwitzer-Meier, K.: Venensystem und Kreislaufregulierung. Ergebn. Physiol. 34, 1145 (1932). ~ Die Energetik des Säugetierherzens. Klin. Wschr. 18, 225 (1939). ~ Pathologische Physiologie der Herzinsuffizienz. Verh. dtsch. Ges. Kreisl.-Forsch. 16, 3 (1950). — Gollwitzer-Meier, K., u. C. Kroetz: Sauerstoffverbrauch und Kranzgefäßdurchblutung des innervierten Säugetierherzens unter Adrenalinwirkung. Pflügers Arch. ges. Physiol. 241, 248 (1939). ~ Kranzgefäßdurchblutung und Stoffwechsel des innervierten Herzens. Klin. Wschr. 19, 580 (1940). — Gollwitzer-Meier, K., u. E. Witzleb: Die Wirkung von l-Noradrenalin auf die Energetik und die Dynamik des Warmblüterherzens. Pflügers Arch. ges. Physiol. 255, 469 (1952). — Goodale, W. T., and D. B. Hackel: Myocardial carbohydrate metabolism in normal dogs with effects of hyperglycemia and starvation. Circulat. Res. 1, 509 (1953). — Goodale, W. T., M. Lubin, J. E. Eckenhoff, J. H. Hafkenschiel and W. G. Bonfield: Coronary sinus cathetrization for studying coronary blood flow and myocardial metabolism. Amer. J. Physiol. 152, 340 (1948). — Goodall, Mc. C.: Studies of adrenaline and noradrenaline in mammalian heart and suprarenals. Acta physiol. scand. 24, Suppl., 85 (1951). — Gottstein, U., H. Hille u. A. Oberdorf: Die Wirkung von Adrenalin und Noradrenalin auf die Durchblutung der Skeletmuskulatur. Pflügers Arch. ges. Physiol. 261, 78 (1955). — Graham, C. K., J. A. Taylor, L. B. Fellis, D. J. Greenberg and S. L. Robbing: Studies in mitral stenosis; correlation of post mortem findings with clinical course of disease in 101 cases. Arch. intern. Med. 88, 532 (1951). — Grant, R. T., and E. B. Reeve: Observations on the general effects of injury in man (with special reference to wound shock). Spec. Rep. Sci. med. Res. Course. (Lond.) No 277, H.M.S.O., London. Zit. nach Cameron. — Grant, W. C., and W. S. Root: Fundamental stimulus for erythropoiesis. Physiol. Rev. 32, 449 (1952). — Gray, S. J., and H. Frank: The simultaneous determination of red cell mass and plasma volume in man with radioactive sodium chromate and chromic chloride. J. clin. Invest. 32, 1000 (1953). — Green, H. D.: Circulatory system: Physical principles. Med. Physics 2, 228 (1950). — Green, H. D., and D. E. Gregg: Changes in the coronary circulation following increased aortic pressure, augmented cardiac output, ischemia and valve lesions. Amer. J. Physiol. 130, 126 (1940). — Green, H. D., and E. C. Hoff: Effects of faradic stimulation of the cerebral cortex on limb and renal volumes in the cat and monkey. Amer. J. Physiol. 118, 641 (1937). — Green, H. D., R. N. Lewis, N. D. Nickerson and A. L. Heller: Blood flow, peripheral resistance and vascular tonus. Amer. J. Physiol. 141, 518 (1944). — Greene, C. W.: Dilation of coronary vessels by certain organic extracts and drugs. J. Pharmacol. exp. Ther. 57, 98 (1936). — Greenfield, A. D. M., and G. C. Patterson: On the capacity and distensibility of the blood vessels of the human forearm. J. Physiol. (Lond.) 131, 290 (1956). — Gregersen, M. J.: Blood volume. Ann. Rev. Physiol. 13, 397 (1951). ~ Effect of circulatory states on determinations of blood volume. Amer. J. Med. 15, 785 (1953). — Gregg, D. E.: Coronary circulation in health and disease. Philadelphia 1950. ~ Some problems of the coronary circulation. Verh. dtsch. Ges. Kreisl.-Forsch. 21, 22 (1955). — Gregg, D. E., and H. D. Green: Effect of viscosity, ischemia, cardiac output and aortic pressure on coronary blood flow measured under a constant perfusion pressure. Amer. J. Physiol. 130, 108 (1940a). ~ Registration and interpretation of normal phasic inflow into a left coronary artery by improved differential manometric method. Amer. J. Physiol. 130, 114 (1940b). — Gregg, D. E., D. C. Sabiston and E. O. Theilen: Performance of the heart: Changes in left ventricular enddiastolic pressure and stroke work during infusion and following exercise. Physiol. Rev. 35, 130 (1955). Gregg, D. E., and R. E. Shipley: Augmentation of left coronary inflow with elevation of left ventricular pressure and observations on the mechanism for increased coronary inflow with increased cardiac load. Amer. J. Physiol. 142, 44 (1947). — Grill, C.: Plethysmographische Untersuchungen über das Arm- und Beinvolumen während und nach der Arbeit, welche die Zirkulationsverhältnisse im Gefäßsystem der Extremitäten beleuchten. Skand. Arch. Physiol. 67, 1 (1933). — Gross, F.: Nebennierenrinde und Wasser-Salz-Stoffwechsel unter besonderer Berücksichtigung von Aldosteron. Klin. Wschr. 1956, 929. — Grosse-Brockhoff, F.: Hämodynamik der Lungenkreislaufstörungen. Verh. dtsch. Ges. Kreisl.-Forsch. 17, 34 (1951). ~ Hämodynamik des Lungenkreislaufs. (Unter besonderer Berücksichtigung pulmonaler Erkrankungen.) Tuberkulosearzt 6, 385 (1952). ~ Klinische Pathologie der erworbenen Herzklappenfehler. Verh. dtsch. Ges. Kreisl.-Forsch. 20, 19 (1954). — Grosse-Brockhoff, F., u. D. Esch: Das Cor pulmonale. Z. Tuberk. 106, 1 (1955). — Grosse-

BROCKHOFF, F., G. NEUHAUS u. A. SCHAEDE: Herzbelastung bei arterio-venösen Fisteln und veno-venösen Anastomosen im großen und kleinen Kreislauf. Z. Kreisl.-Forsch. **43**, 388 (1954). — GROSSE-BROCKHOFF, F., u. O. VORLAENDER: Die reaktive Erwärmung der Haut bei verschiedenen Gefäßkrankheiten. Dtsch. Arch. klin. Med. **194**, 17 (1949). — GROSSE-BROCK-HOFF, F., u. H. H. WOLTER: Der enddiastolische Füllungsdruck bei chronischer Druck- und Volumenbelastung des rechten Ventrikels. Z. Kreisl.-Forsch. **47**, 481 (1958). — GUYTON, A. C.: Determination of cardiac output by equating venous return curves with cardiac response curves. Physiol. Rev. **35**, 123 (1955). — GUYTON, A. C., J. H. SATTERFIELD and J. W. HARRIS: Dynamics of central venous resistance with observations on static blood pressure. Amer. J. Physiol. **169**, 691 (1952). — GUYTON, R. W., and W. PAUL: Blood volume in congestive heart failure. J. clin. Invest. **34**, 879 (1955).

HACKEL, D. B., W. T. GOODALE and J. KLEINERMAN: Effects of hypoxia on the myocardial metabolism of intact dogs. Circulat. Res. **2**, 169 (1954). — HADDY, F. J., and G. S. CAMPBELL: Pulmonary vascular resistance in anesthetized dogs. Amer. J. Physiol. **172**, 747 (1953). — HADDY, F. J., and R. P. GILBERT: The relation of a venous-arteriolar reflex to transmural pressure and resistance in small and large systemic vessels. Circulat. Res. **4**, 25 (1956). — HAFKENSCHIEL, J. H., and C. K. FRIEDLAND: The effect of subtotal adrenalectomy combined with sympathectomy upon the cerebral vascular resistance of patients with severe hypertension. J. clin. Invest. **31**, 635 (1952). — HAKKILA, J.: Studies on the myocardial capillary concentration in cardiac hypertrophy due to training. Ann. med. exp. Fenn. **33**, Suppl., 10 (1955). — HALL, P. W.: Effects of anoxia on postarteriolar pulmonary vascular resistance. Circulat. Res. **1**, 238 (1953). — HALMAGYI, D. F. J.: Die klinische Physiologie des kleinen Kreislaufs. Jena 1957. — HALMER, D. M.: Studies on renin-antibodies. Circulation **17**, 648 (1958). — HAMILTON, W. F.: Circulatory system: Lungs. Med. Physics 2, 207 (1950). ~ Role of Starling concept in regulation of the normal circulation. Physiol. Rev. **35**, 161 (1955). — HAMILTON, W. F., and A. B. MORGAN: Mechanism of the postular reduction in vital capacity, in relation to orthopnea and storage of blood in the lungs. Amer. J. Physiol. **99**, 526 (1931). — HARRISON, T. R., B. F. FRIEDMAN and H. RESNICK: Mechanism of acute experimental heart failure. Arch. intern. Med. **57**, 927 (1936). — HARTMANN, H., S. L. ØRSKOV u. H. F. REIN: Die Gefäßreaktionen der Niere im Verlauf allgemeiner Kreislauf-Regulationsvorgänge. Pflügers Arch. ges. Physiol. **238**, 239 (1936). — HARTWICH, A.: Demonstrationen zum klinischen Referat über Kreislaufwirkungen körpereigener Stoffe. Kongr.-Zbl. ges. Kongr. inn. Med. **44**, 76 (1932). — HAUCK, H. J., u. H.-TH. DANNEEL: Vergleichende Bestimmungen des Herzminutenvolumens zwischen der direkten Fickschen Methode und der physikalischen Methode nach BROEMSER-RANKE. Klin. Wschr. **32**, 687 (1954). — HAUCK, H. J., u. C. W. HERTZ: Das arterio-venöse Lungenaneurysma. Thoraxchirurgie 1, 411 (1954). — HAUSS, W. H.: Angina pectoris. Stuttgart 1954. — HAUSS, W. H., H. KRENZIGER u. H. ASTEROTH: Über die Reizung der Pressoreceptoren im Sinus caroticus beim Hund. Z. Kreisl.-Forsch. **38**, 28 (1949). — HAYEK, H. v.: Die menschliche Lunge. Berlin-Göttingen-Heidelberg 1953. — HEIDENREICH, O., u. L. SCHMIDT: Die Beeinflussung der Coronardurchblutung durch blutdruckwirksame Drogen bei intracoronarer und intravenöser Injektion. Naunyn-Schmiedeberg's Arch. exp. Path. Pharmak. **227**, 250 (1956a). ~ Der Einfluß von Vagusreizung und Carotidenabklemmung auf die Coronardurchblutung. Pflügers Arch. ges. Physiol. **263**, 315 (1956b). — HELMER, O. M.: Studies on renin antibodies. Circulation **17**, 648 (1958). — HENRY, J. P., O. H. GAUER and J. L. REEVES: Evidence of the atrial location of receptors influencing urine flow. Circulat. Res. **4**, 85 (1956). — HENRY, J. P., O. H. GAUER and H. O. SIEKER: The effect of moderate changes in blood volume on left and right atrial pressure. Circulat. Res. **4**, 91 (1956). — HERGET, R., u. P. ALNOV: Experimentelle Untersuchungen über den Einfluß eines thrombosierten Arterienabschnittes auf den Kollateralkreislauf. Bruns' Beitr. klin. Chir. **187**, 212 (1953). — HERING, H. E.: Karotissinusreflexe auf Herz und Gefäße. Dresden 1927. — HERTZ, C. W.: Die Durchblutungsgröße hypoventilierter Lungenbezirke. Verh. dtsch. Ges. Kreisl.-Forsch. **21**, 447 (1955). ~ Untersuchungen über den Einfluß der alveolaren Gasdrucke auf die intrapulmonale Durchblutungsverteilung beim Menschen. Klin. Wschr. **1956**, 472. — HERZ, G.: Die Veränderung der diastolischen Herzfüllung durch Adrenalin. Z. Biol. **108**, 111 (1955). — HESS, W. R.: Die Regulierung der Atmung. Leipzig 1931. — HEYMANS, C., et J. J. BOUCKART: Reflexes vasomoteurs médullaires d'origine barosensible. C. R. Soc. Biol. (Paris) **123**, 986 (1936). — HEYMANS, C., J. J. BOUCKART et P. REGNIERS: Le sinus carotidien et la zone homologue cardio-aortique. Paris 1933. — HEYMANS, C. et G. VAN DEN HEUVEL-HEYMANS: Action of drugs on arterial wall of carotid sinus and blood pressure. Arch. int. Pharmacodyn. **83**, 520 (1950). — HILD, R., u. G. HERZ: Das Druck-Volumen-Diagramm des isolierten Katzenherzens unter dem Einfluß von Adrenalin. Z. Biol. **108**, 42 (1955). — HILLARP, N. A., u. B. HÄFKELT: Evidence of adrenaline and noradrenaline in separate adrenal medullary cells. Acta physiol. scand. **30**, 55 (1953). — HILLE, H., u. H. J. TESKE: Ein Beitrag zum Wirkungsmechanismus von Adrenalin auf die Gefäße der Peripherie. Pflügers Arch. ges. Physiol. **263**, 83 (1956). —

Hochrein, M., u. C. H. J. Keller: Der Einfluß mechanischer Vorgänge auf die mittlere Durchblutung und die Depotfunktion der Lunge. Naunyn-Schmiedeberg's Arch. exp. Path. Pharmak. **164**, 529 (1932a). ~ Über die Beeinflussung der mittleren Durchblutung und der Blutfüllung der Lunge durch pharmakologische Mittel. Naunyn-Schmiedeberg's Arch. exp. Path. Pharmak. **164**, 552 (1932b). — Hoff, H. E.: Nutrition of the heart. In Fultons Textbook of Physiol., 17. Aufl., 699. 1955. — Hoffmeister, H. E., H. Kreuzer u. W. Schoeppe: Der Sauerstoffverbrauch des stillstehenden, des leerschlagenden und des flimmernden Herzens. Pflügers Arch. ges. Physiol. **269**, 194 (1959). — Holt, J. P.: Estimation of the residual volume of the ventricle of the dog's heart by two indicator dilution technics. Circulat. Res. **4**, 187 (1956). ~ Effect of plethora and hemorrhage on left ventricular volume and pressure. Circulat. Res. **5**, 273 (1957). ~ Regulation of the degree of emptying of the left ventricle by the force of ventricular contraction. Circulat. Res. **5**, 281 (1957). — Holt, J. P., and J. Allensworth: Estimation of the residual volume of the right ventricle of the dog's heart. Circulat. Res. **5**, 323 (1957). — Holtz, P., u. H. J. Schümann: Über das Vorkommen von Arterenol in den Nebennieren. Naturwiss. **35**, 191 (1948). — Horváth, I., C. Kirácy and J. Szerb: Action of cardiac glycosides on the polymerisation of actin. Nature (Lond.) **164**, 792 (1949). — Howarth, S., J. McMichael and E. P. Sharpey-Schafer: Circulatory action of theophylline ethylene diamine. Clin. Sci. **6**, 125 (1947). — Hürlimann, A., and C. J. Wiggers: The effects of progressive general anoxia on the pulmonary circulation. Circulat. Res. **1**, 230 (1953).

Jacobi, W., u. G. Magnus: Experimentelle Zirkulationsstörungen an Gehirngefäßen. Langenbecks Arch. klin. Chir. **136**, 211 (1925). ~ Experimentelle Beiträge zur Frage der Hirnembolie. Dtsch. Z. Nervenheilk. **91**, 219 (1926). — Jardetzky, O., E. A. Greene and V. Lorber: Oxygen consumption of the completely isolated dog heart in fibrillation. Circulat. Res. **4**, 144 (1956). — Jarisch, A.: Vom Herzen ausgehende Kreislauf-Reflexe. Arch. Kreisl.-Forsch. **7**, 260 (1940). — Johnson, J. R., and C. J. Wiggers: The alleged validity of coronary sinus outflow as a criterion of coronary reactions. Amer. J. Physiol. **118**, 38 (1937). — Johnson, S. R.: The effect of some anaesthetic agents on the circulation in man. Acta chir. scand. Suppl., 158 (1951).

Kapal, E., F. Martini u. E. Wetterer: Über die Zuverlässigkeit der bisherigen Bestimmungsart der Pulswellengeschwindigkeit. Z. Biol. **104**, 75 (1950). ~ Untersuchungen über die Länge der stehenden Welle im arteriellen System des Menschen. Z. Biol. **104**, 256 (1951). — Kaplan, E., R. C. Pnestow, L. Baker and S. Kruger: Blood volume in congestive heart failure as determined with iodinated human serum albumin. Amer. Heart. J. **47**, 824 (1954). — Kattus, A. A., A. U. Rivin, A. Cohen and G. S. Sofio: Cardiac output and central volume as determined by dye dilution curves. Circulation **11**, 447 (1955). — Katz, A. M., L. N. Katz and F. L. Williams: Regulation of coronary flow. Amer. J. Physiol. **180**, 392 (1955). — Katz, L. N.: Analysis of the several factors regulating the performance of the heart. Physiol. Rev. **35**, 91 (1955). — Katz, L. N., and K. Jochim: Observations on the innervation of the coronary vessels of the dog. Amer. J. Physiol. **126**, 395 (1939). — Kety, S. S.: Circulation and metabolism of the human brain in health and disease. Amer. J. Med. **8**, 205—217 (1950). — Kety, S. S., and C. F. Schmidt: The nitrous oxide method for the quantitative determination of cerebral blood flow in man. J. clin. Invest. **27**, 476 (1948). — Keyssler, H., u. J. Schmier: Reaktionen der peripheren Durchblutung nach Entnervung. Pflügers Arch. ges. Physiol. **253**, 301 (1951). — Kezdi, P.: Control by the superior cervical ganglion of the state of contraction and pulsatile expansion of the carotid sinus arterial wall. Circulat. Res. **2**, 367 (1954). — Kezdi, P., and R. R. J. Hilker: Local application of epinephrine to carotid sinus. Lowering of blood pressure and modification of hyperreactor response in hypertensive patients. Arch. intern. Med. **95**, 720 (1955). — Kirch, E.: Die pathologische Anatomie des Cor pulmonale. Verh. dtsch. Ges. Kreisl.-Forsch. **21**, 163 (1955). — Kjellberg, S. R., U. Rudhe u. T. Sjöstrand: The amount of hemoglobin and the blood volume in relation to the pulse rate and cardiac volume during rest. Acta physiol. scand. **19**, 136 (1949a). ~ Increase of the amount of hemoglobin and blood volume in connection with physical training. Acta physiol. scand. **19**, 146 (1949b). ~ The amount of hemoglobin (blood volume) in relation to the pulse rate and heart volume during work. Acta physiol. scand. **19**, 152 (1949c). — Klepzig, H.: Untersuchungen über die Arbeitsweise des menschlichen Herzens bei vermehrter Belastung. Arch. Kreisl.-Forsch. **23**, 96 (1955). ~ Funktionsdiagnostik des Herzens. Dtsch. med. Wschr. **82**, 1936 (1957). — Klepzig, H., G. Kindermann u. H. Reindell: Zur Frage der Empfindlichkeit des Sportherzens gegen Sauerstoffmangel. Z. Kreisl.-Forsch. **45**, 8 (1956). — Knebel, R.: Hämodynamik des Lungenkreislaufs beim chronischen Cor pulmonale. Verh. dtsch. Ges. Kreisl.-Forsch. **21**, 181 (1955). — Koch, E.: Die reflektorische Steuerung des Kreislaufs. Dresden u. Leipzig 1931. — Könn, G.: Die pathologische Morphologie der Lungengefäße bei chronischem Cor pulmonale. Beitr. path. Anat. **116**, 273 (1956). — Koepchen, H. P., K. Kramer u. W. Overbeck: Herzfrequenz bei Änderung des Blutvolumens. Verh. dtsch. Ges. Kreisl.-Forsch. **22**, 118 (1956). — Konzett, H., u. E. Rothlin: Beobachtungen über vagovasale Synkope-Mechanismen. Z. Kreisl.-Forsch. **40**, 193 (1951). — Kramer, K.: Grundlagen der Herzdynamik. Bad Oeynhausener Gespräche III. 1958. — Krebs, H. A.: Chemical pathways of metabolism, Bd. 1, 109. 1954. — Krogh, A.: On the influence of the venous supply upon the output of the heart. Skand. Arch. Physiol. **27**, 126 (1912). ~ The regulation of the supply of blood to the right heart. Skand. Arch. Physiol. **27**, 227 (1912). ~ Anatomie und Physiologie der Kapillaren. Berlin: 1929. — Kubicek, W. G., F. J. Kottke, D. J. Laker and M. B. Visscher: Adaptation in the pressor-receptor reflex mechanisms in experimental neurogenic hypertension. Amer. J. Physiol. **175**, 380 (1953).

La Due, J. S., F. Wroblewski and A. Karmen: Serum glutamic oxalacetic transaminase activity in human acut transmural myocardial infarction. Science **120**, 497 (1954). Lagerlöf, H., H. Eliasch, L. Werkö and E. Berglund: Orthostatic changes of the pulmonary and peripheral circulation in man. Scand. J. clin. Lab. Invest. **3**, 85 (1951). — Lagerlöf, H., and L. Werkö: Studies on the circulation in man. The auricular pressure pulse. Cardiologia (Basel) **13**, 241 (1949). ~ The pulmonary capillary venous pressure pulse in man. Scand. J. clin. Lab. Invest. **1**, 147 (1949). — Lambert, J.: Réactions vasculaires provoquées dans le muscle strié au repos chez le chien par l'ischémie temporaire expérimentale. Arch. int. Physiol. **64**, 623 (1956). — Lammerant, J.: Le volume sanguin des poumons. Brüssel 1957. — Lampen, H., P. Kezdi u. L. Kaufmann: Entzügelungshochdruck am Menschen. Klin. Wschr. **27**, 272 (1949). — Lamport, H.: Hemodynamics. In Fultons Textbook of Physiol., 16. Aufl., S. 580. Philadelphia and London 1949. — Lamprecht, W.: Zur Wirkung des Strophanthins auf den Herzstoffwechsel. Dtsch. med. Wschr. **81**, 534 (1956). — Landgreen, S., A. P. Skouby u. Y. Zotterman: Sensitization of baroceptors of the carotid sinus by acetylcholine. Acta physiol. scand. **29**, 381 (1953). — Landis, E. M., E. Brown, M. Fauteux and C. Wise: Central venous pressure in relation to cardiac ,,competence", blood volume and exercise. J. clin. Invest. **25**, 237 (1946). — Landis, E. M., and J. C. Hortenstine: Functional significance of venous blood pressure. Physiol. Rev. **30**, 1 (1950). — Landowne, M., and L. N. Katz: Circulatory system: Heart, work and failure. Med. Physics 2, 194 (1950). — Lange, F.: Arterielle Hypertonie der Lungenstrombahn (Cor pulmonale). Dtsch. med. Wschr. **1948**, 204. — Lanier, J. Th., H. D. Green, J. Hardaway, H. D. Johnson and W. B. Donald: Fundamental difference in the reactivity of the blood vessels in skin compared with those in muscle. Circulat. Res. **1**, 40 (1953). — Lapp, H.: Über die Sperrarterien der Lunge und die Anastomosen zwischen A. bronchialis und A. pulmonalis, über die Bedeutung insbesondere für die Entstehung des hämorrhagischen Infarktes. Frankfurt. Z. Path. **62**, 537 (1951). ~ Über das Verhalten der Bronchialarterien und ihrer Anastomosen mit der A. pulmonalis unter pathologischen Kreislaufbedingungen, insbesondere bei den einzelnen Formen der angeborenen Herzfehler. Verh. dtsch. Ges. Kreisl.-Forsch. **17**, 110 (1951). — Lehninger, A. L.: Oxidative phosphorylation. Harvey Lect. **49**, 176 (1953). — Lendrum, B., B. Condo and L. N. Katz: The role of Thebesian drainage in the dynamic of coronary flow. Amer. J. Physiol. **143**, 243 (1945). — Lennox, W. G., F. A. Gibbs and E. L. Gibbs: Relationship of unconsciousness to cerebral blood flow and to anoxemia. Arch. Neurol. Psychiat. (Chicago) **34**, 1001 (1935). — Leriche, R., et R. Fontaine: Conditions nécessaires, résultats et technique de l'artériectomie dans les oblitérations artérielles d'après 80 opérations récentes. Presse méd. **1935 II**, 1953. — Leriche, R., R. Fontaine and S. M. Dupertuis: Arterectomy with follow up studies on 78 operations. Surg. Gynec. Obstet. **64**, 149 (1937). Ref. Zentr.-Org. ges. Chir. **83**, 355 (1937). — Leusen, I., et G. Demeester: Influence de l'hypoxémie sur la circulation pulmonaire chez le chien et chez le chat. Acta cardiol. (Brux.) **10**, 556 (1955). — Levy, M. N., S. H. Brind, F. R. Brandlin and F. A. Phillips: The relationship between pressure and flow in the systemic circulation of the dog. Circulat. Res. **2**, 372 (1954). — Levy, M. N., and L. Share: The influence of erythrocyte concentration upon the pressure flow relationships in the dog's hind limb. Circulat. Res. **1**, 247 (1953). — Lewis, T.: Die Blutgefäße der menschlichen Haut. Berlin 1928. ~ Vasovagal syncope and the carotid sinus mechanism (with comments on Grower's and Nothnagel's syndrome). Brit. med. J. **1932**, 873. — Lichti, J.: Inaug.-Diss. Zürich 1934. Zit. nach Büchner 1956. — Liddle, G., F. Bartter, L. Duncan, J. Barber and C. Delea: Mechanisms regulating aldosterone production in man. J. clin. Invest. **34**, 949 (1955). — Liljestrand, G., E. Lysholm and G. Nylin: The immediate effects of muscular work on the stroke and heart volume in man. Skand. Arch. Physiol. **80**, 265 (1938). — Liljestrand, G., E. Lysholm, G. Nylin and C. G. Zackrisson: Normal heart volume in man. Amer. Heart J. **17**, 406 (1939). — Lindgren, P., and B. Uvnäs: Vasodilator responses in the sceletal muscles of the dog to electrical stimulation in the oblongata medulla. Acta physiol. scand. **29**, 137 (1953). ~ Postulated vasodilator center in the medulla oblongata. Amer. J. Physiol. **176**, 68 (1954). ~ Vasoconstrictor inhibition and vasodilator activation — two functionally separate vasodilator mechanisms in the sceletal muscles. Acta physiol. scand. **33**, 108 (1955). — Linhart, J., and J. Přerovský: Nervous control of venomotor tone in cardiac failure. Rev. Czechoslovak Med. **3**, 3 (1957). — Linzbach, A. J.: Herzhypertrophie und kritisches

Herzgewicht. Klin. Wschr. 1948, 459. ~ Die Muskelfaserkonstante und das Wachstumsgesetz der menschlichen Herzkammern. Virchows Arch. path. Anat. 318, 575 (1950). — Linzbach, A. J., u. M.: Die Herzdilatation. Klin. Wschr. 1951, 621. — Lochner, W., H, Mercker u. E. Schürmeyer: Die Wirkung von Adrenalin, Acetylcholin und Vagusreizung auf die Sauerstoffsättigung des Blutes im Sinus coronarius. Naunyn-Schmiedeberg's Arch. exp. Path. Pharmak. 227, 360 (1956a). ~ Die Wirkung vasoaktiver Pharmaka auf die Sauerstoffsättigung des Coronarsinusblutes. Naunyn-Schmiedeberg's Arch. exp. Path. Pharmak. 227, 373 (1956b). — Lochner, W., u. M. Nasseri: Coronardurchblutung bei Muskeltätigkeit. 1959. — Lochner, W., u. W. Schoedel: Die Regulation des Herzzeitvolumens und die Blutfüllung des kleinen Kreislaufs. Pflügers Arch. ges. Physiol. 255, 327 (1952a). ~ Die Bedeutung der depressorischen Kreislaufreflexe für die Steuerung des Herzzeitvolumens. Pflügers Arch. ges. Physiol. 255, 333 (1952b). — Lombardo, T. A., L. Rose, M. Taeschler, S. Tuluy and R. J. Bing: The effect of exercise on coronary blood flow, myocardial oxygen consumption and cardiac efficiency in man. Circulation 7, 71 (1953). — Loogen, F.: Der pulmonale Hochdruck bei angeborenen Herzfehlern mit hohem pulmonalem Stromvolumen. Arch. Kreisl.-Forsch. 28, 1 (1958). — Loogen, F., u. H. Major: Das arterio-venöse Pulmonalisaneurysma. Münch. med. Wschr. 1955, 21. — Lorber, V.: Energy metabolism of the completely isolated mammalian heart in failure. Circulat. Res. 1, 298 (1953). — Lübbers, D.: Die Gewebsatmung der Herzmuskelfaser. Bad Oeynhausener Gespräche II, S. 32. 1957. — Luetscher, J.: Chromatographic separation of the sodium retaining corticoid from the urine of children with nephrosis, compared with observations on normal children. J. clin. Invest. 33, 276 (1954). — Luetscher, J., B. Johnson, B. Axelrad, J. Cates and G. Sala: Apparent indentity of electrocortin with the sodium retaining corticoid extracted from human urine. J. clin. Endocr. 14, 812 (1954). — Lukas, D. S., J. M. Pearce and F. S. Glann: The relation of anatomic to physiologic changes in the pulmonary vessels in mitral stenosis. J. clin. Invest. 31, 1082 (1952). — Lundholm, L.: The mechanism of the vasodilator effect of adrenaline. Acta physiol. scand. 43, 27 (1958).

Maier, H. C., A. Himmelstein, R. L. Riley and J. J. Bunin: Arterio venous fistula of lung. J. thorac. Surg. 17, 13 (1948). — Marshack, M. E., u. G. N. Aranova: Chronische Versuche über Coronardurchblutung an Hunden. Bull. Eksptl. Biol. i. Med. Suppl. 1, 3 (1957). Zit. nach Simonson, Ann. Rev. Physiol. 20, 143 (1958). — Maxwell, G. M., C. A. Castillo, D. H. White, C. W. Crumpton and G. G. Rowe: Induced tachycardia: its effect upon the coronary hemodynamics, myocardial metabolism and cardiac efficiency of the intact dog. J. clin. Invest. 37, 1413 (1958). —May, S. H.: Elektrocardiographic response to gradually induced oxygen deficiency. Amer. Heart J. 17, 655 (1939). — McMichael, J.: Pharmakologie des Herzversagens. Darmstadt 1953. — McNeely, W. F., and M. A. Gravallese: Cardiac output. J. appl. Physiol. 7, 55 (1954). — Mechelke, K., E. Nusser u. W. Hey: Über die Beziehung zwischen dem Druck und der Stromstärke in der Aorta ascendens bei „unbeeinflußtem" Kreislauf der Katze, im oligämischen Schock und nach Dekapitierung. Pflügers Arch. ges. Physiol. 261, 527 (1955). — Meesmann, W.: Herzdynamik und Coronardurchblutung bei akutem Coronarverschluß. Bad Oeynhausener Gespräche II, S. 120. 1957. ~ Nachweis der diastolischen Sogwirkung der Herzkammer und deren Einfluß auf die intrakardialen Druckabläufe. Z. Kreisl.-Forsch. 47, 534 (1958). — Meesmann, W., u. J. Schmier: Über das Versagen des Herzens bei überkritischer Coronardrosselung. Pflügers Arch. ges. Physiol. 261, 41 (1955). ~ Auswirkungen einer elektrischen Milznervenreizung auf die Coronardurchblutung. Pflügers Arch. ges. Physiol. 263, 293 (1956a). ~ Sauerstoffverbrauch des Herzens im Milz-Leber-Mechanismus. Pflügers Arch. ges. Physiol. 263, 304 (1956b). ~ Herz- und Kreislaufwirkungen körpereigener Stoffe im Vergleich zu den Auswirkungen des „Milz-Leber-Mechanismus. Z. Kreisl.-Forsch. 45, 335 (1956c). — Meessen, H.: Über experimentelle Lungenembolie durch Glasperlen. Arch. Kreisl.-Forsch. 6, 117 (1940). ~ Zur pathologischen Anatomie des Lungenkreislaufs. Verh. dtsch. Ges. Kreisl.-Forsch. 17, 25 (1951). ~ Zur Pathogenese, Progredienz und Adaptation der angeborenen Herz- und Gefäßfehler. Verh. dtsch. Ges. Kreisl.-Forsch. 23, 188 (1957). — Meiners, S.: Über Erregbarkeitssteigerung der Arterien und das Auftreten von Angiospasmen nach lokaler Gewebsschädigung. Pflügers Arch. ges. Physiol. 254, 577 (1952). — Mercker, H., W. Lochner u. H. J. Bretschneider: Die Sauerstoffversorgung des Herzmuskels. Dtsch. med. Wschr. 83, 17 (1958). — Mercker, H., u. W. Schoedel: Die Unterdrückung konstriktorischer Effekte im Gefäßgebiet des tätigen Skeletmuskels. Pflügers Arch. ges. Physiol. 250, 1 (1948). — Mercker, H., u. G. Urbig: Über die Abhängigkeit der reaktiven Hyperämie von der Benervung. Pflügers Arch. ges. Physiol. 245, 756 (1942). — Merrill, A. J.: Edema and decreased renal blood flow in patients with chronic congestive heart failure. Evidence of forward failure as the primary cause of edema. J. clin. Invest. 25, 389 (1946). ~ Mechanisms of salt and water retention in heart failure. Amer. J. Med. 6, 357 (1949). — Miller, W. S.: The lung. Springfield 1937. — Mokotoff, R., and G. Ross: Effect of spinal anesthesia on renal ischemia in congestive heart failure. J. clin. Invest. 27, 335 (1948). — Mokotoff,

R., G. Ross and L. Leiter: Renal plasma flow and sodium reabsorption and excretion in congestive heart failure. J. clin. Invest. **27**, 1 (1948). — Morales, M. F., J. Botts, J. J. Blum and T. L. Hill: Elementary processes in muscle action: an examination of current concepts. Physiol. Rev. **35**, 475 (1956). — Moreira, F., R. F. Mottram and A. Yvonne Werner: The effect of venous pressure on the oxygen content of the venous blood in the deep forearm veins. J. Physiol. **133**, 255 (1956). — Moritz, F.: Über Veränderungen in der Form, Größe und Lage des Herzens beim Übergang aus horizontaler in vertikale Körperstellung. Dtsch. Arch. klin. Med. **82**, 1 (1905). — Motley, H. L., A. Cournand, L. Werkö, A. Himmelstein and D. Dresdale: The influence of short periods of induced acute anoxia upon pulmonary arterial pressures in man. Amer. J. Physiol. **150**, 315 (1947). — Müller, A.: Abhandlung zur Mechanik der Flüssigkeiten mit besonderer Berücksichtigung der Hämodynamik. Strömen heterogener Flüssigkeiten mit Teilchen von gleicher Größenordnung wie der Röhrendurchmesser. Arch. Kreisl.-Forsch. **14**, 80 (1944). ~ Über das Druckgefälle in Blutgefäßen, insbesondere in den Kapillaren. Helv. physiol. Acta **6**, 181 (1948). — Müller, E. A.: Die Beziehungen zwischen Volumen, Leistung, Tonus und Kontraktionsfähigkeit am isolierten Säugetierherzen. Ergebn. Physiol. **43**, 89 (1940). ~ Regulation der Pulsfrequenz in der Erholungsphase nach ermüdender Muskelarbeit. Int. Z. angew. Physiol. **16**, 35 (1955).

Nickerson, J. L., D. C. Elkin and J. V. Warren: The effect of temporary occlusion of arteriovenous fistulas on the heart rate, stroke volume and cardiac output. J. clin. Invest. **30**, 215 (1951). — Niden, A. H., and D. M. Aviado: Effects of pulmonary embolism on the pulmonary circulation with special reference to arteriovenous shunts in the lung. Circulat. Res. **4**, 67 (1956). — Nielson, N. J., u. K. Kramer: Stromvolumpulse der herznahen Venen bei verschiedenen Kreislaufzuständen. Z. Biol. **106**, 389 (1954). — Nisell, O.: Effects of oxygen and carbon dioxide on the circulation of isolated and perfused lungs of the cat. Acta physiol. scand. **16**, 121 (1948). — Nory, H., u. H. D. Frings: Nucleinsäuren im hypertrophischen Herzmuskel. Z. ges. exp. Med. **132**, 538 (1960). — Nory, H., H. D. Frings, A. Walders u. L. Tenderich: Proteinzusammensetzung des Myokards bei experimenteller Herzhypertrophie. Z. ges. exp. Med. **131**, 478 (1959). — Nylin, G.: The effect of adrenalin injected intravenously on the volume of circulating erythrocytes. Acta cardiol. (Brux.) **1**, 225 (1946). ~ The effect of heavy muscular work on the volume of circulating red corpuscles in man. Amer. J. Physiol. **149**, 180 (1947).

Ochoa, S.: Ketoglutaric dehydrogenase of animal tissues. J. biol. Chem. **155**, 87 (1944). — Ochsner, A.: Effects of pulmonary blood flow and distention on the capacity of intrapulmonary vessels. Amer. J. Physiol. **168**, 200 (1952). — Ochwadt, B.: Zur Selbststeuerung des Nierenkreislaufs. Pflügers Arch. ges. Physiol. **262**, 207 (1956). ~ Durchflußzeiten von Plasma und Erythrocyten, intrarenaler Hämatokrit und Widerstandsregulation der isolierten Niere. Pflügers Arch. ges. Physiol. **265**, 112 (1957). — Olson, R. E.: Molecular events in cardiac failure. Amer. J. Med. **20**, 159 (1956). — Opdyke, D. F.: Effect of changes in initial tension, initial volume and epinephrine on ventricular relaxation process. Amer. J. Physiol. **169**, 403 (1952). — Opitz, E.: Der Stoffwechsel des Gehirns und seine Veränderung bei Kreislaufstillstand. Verh. dtsch. Ges. Kreisl.-Forsch. **19**, 26 (1953). — Opitz, E., u. D. Lübbers: Die Physiologie der Zell- und Gewebsatmung. In Handbuch der allgemeinen Pathologie, Bd. IV/2. 1956. — Opitz, E., u. F. Palme: Sauerstoffmangel zur Darstellung der Akklimatisation im Gebirge. Abflachung von T im EKG. Pflügers Arch. ges. Physiol. **248**, 387 (1944). — Opitz, E., u. M. Schneider: Über die Sauerstoffversorgung des Gehirns und den Mechanismus von Mangelwirkungen. Ergebn. Physiol. **46**, 125 (1950). — Opitz, E., u. G. Thews: Einfluß von Frequenz und Faserdicke auf die Sauerstoffversorgung des menschlichen Herzmuskels. Arch. Kreisl.-Forsch. **18**, 137 (1952). — Opitz, E., u. O. Tillmann: Blutkreislauf und Atmung im Unterdruck, Luftfahrtmed. **1**, 69 (1936). — Oppelt, W.: Unser Normblatt. Regelungstechnik H. 2, 26 (1954). — Osher, W. J.: Pressure-flow relationship of the coronary system. Amer. J. Physiol. **172**, 403 (1953).

Page, J. H.: Serotonin. Physiol. Rev. **38**, 277 (1958). — Palme, F.: Einflüsse auf die Funktion der Pressoreceptoren. Z. Kreisl.-Forsch. **28**, 173 (1936). ~ Zur Funktion der branchiogenen Reflexzonen für Chemo- und Pressoreception. Z. ges. exp. Med. **113**, 415 (1944). — Palme, F., u. K. Kalkoff: Die Beurteilung von Zustandsänderungen in der pressorezeptorischen Reflexzone mit Hilfe gleichzeitiger Registrierung von Blutdruck und Aktionspotentialen des undurchschnittenen Sinusnerven. Compt, rend. II. Congr. Intern. d'Angéiol. Fribourg (Schweiz) 1955, S. 60. — Pappenheimer, J. R.: Vasoconstrictor nerves and oxygen consumption in the isolated perfused hindlimb muscles of the dog. J. Physiol. (Lond.) **99**, 182 (1941). — Pappenheimer, J. R., and W. B. Kinter: Hematocrit ratio of blood within mammalian kidney and its significance for renal hemodynamics. Amer. J. Physiol. **185**, 377 (1956). — Patterson, S. W., H. Pieper and E. H. Starling: The regulation of the heard beat. J. Physiol. (Lond.) **48**, 465 (1914). — Paul, H., E. O. Theilen, D. E. Gregg, J. B. Marsh and G. G. Casten: Cardiac metabolism in experimental ventricular fibrillation. Circulat.

Res. 2, 573 (1954). — Peters, G.: Über den Einfluß der Atmung auf das Fingerplethysmogramm. Pflügers Arch. ges. Physiol. 241, 201 (1938). — Peterson, L. H.: Certain physical characteristics of the cardiovascular system and their significance in the problem of calculating stroke volume from the arterial pulse. Fed. Proc. 11, 762 (1952). ~ The dynamics of pulsatile blood flow. Circulat. Res. 2, 127 (1954). ~ Peripheral circulation. Ann. Rev. Physiol. 19, 255 (1957). — Phillips, F. A., S. H. Brind and M. N. Levy: The immediate influence of increased venous pressure upon resistance to flow in the dog's hind leg. Circulat. Res. 3, 357 (1955). — Pickering, G. W.: Hypertonie und Niere. Klin. Wschr. 1955, 370. — Piiper, J.: Hämodynamische Untersuchungen an der isolierten Hundelunge. Pflügers Arch. ges. Physiol. 264, 596 (1957). ~ Durchblutung der arterio-venösen Anastomosen und Wärmeaustausch an der Hundeextremität. Pflügers Arch. ges. Physiol. 268, 242 (1959). — Piiper, J., P. W. Schneider u. W. Schoedel: Kurzschlußdurchblutung. Klin. Wschr. 32, 540 (1954). — Piiper, J., u. W. Schoedel: Untersuchungen über die Durchblutung der arteriovenösen Anastomosen in der hinteren Extremität des Hundes mit Hilfe von Kugeln verschiedener Größe. Pflügers Arch. ges. Physiol. 258, 489 (1954). — Pitts, R. F., and R. S. Alexander: Nature of renal tubular mechanism for acidifying urine. Amer. J. Physiol. 144, 239 (1945). — Pitts, R. F., W. D. Lotspeich, W. A. Schiess and J. L. Ayer: Renal regulation of acid-base balance in man, nature of mechanism for acidifying urine. J. clin. Invest. 27, 48 (1948). — Přerovský, I., J. Linhart, and Z. Feifar: Reflex adjustment of the peripheral circulation in man. Physiol. Bohemoslovenica 4, 389 (1955). — Prinzmetal, M., E. M. Ornitz, B. Simkin and H. C. Bergman: Arterio-venous anastomoses in liver, spleen, and lungs. Amer. J. Physiol. 152, 48 (1948). — Prinzmetal, M., B. Simkin, H. C. Bergman and H. E. Krüger: The collateral circulation of the normal human heart by coronary perfusion with radioactive erythrocytes and glass spheres. Amer. Heart J. 33, 420 (1947). — Pugh, L. G. C., and C. L. Wyndham: Circulatory effects of high spinalanaesthesia in hypertensive and control subjects. Clin. Sci. 9, 189 (1950).

Rahn, H., P. Sadoul, L. E. Farhi and J. Shapiro: Distribution of ventilation and perfusion in the lobes of the dog's lung in the supine and erect position. J. appl. Physiol. 8, 417 (1956). — Ranney, R. E.: Biochemical characteristics of glycerol extracted myocardial fibers. Amer. J. Physiol. 183, 197 (1955). — Rashkind, W. J., D. H. Lewis, J. B. Henderson, D. F. Heiman and R. B. Dietrick: Venous return as affected by cardiac output and total peripheral resistance. Amer. J. Physiol. 175, 415 (1953). — Ratschow, M.: Die peripheren Durchblutungsstörungen. Darmstadt 1953. ~ Angiologie. Stuttgart 1959. — Ravdin, I. S., J. M. Walker and J. E. Rhoads: Blood volume maintenance and regulation. Ann. Rev. Physiol. 15, 165 (1953). — Recklinghausen, H. v.: Unblutige Blutdruckmessung. Naunyn-Schmiedeberg's Arch. exp. Path. Pharmak. 55, 463 (1906). — Reichel, H.: Muskelelastizität. Ergebn. Physiol. 47, 469 (1952). ~ Das plastische und elastische Element des Herzmuskels. Pflügers Arch. ges. Physiol. 257, 202 (1953). — Rein, H. F.: Die Blutreservoire des Menschen. Klin. Wschr. 12, 1 (1933). ~ Die physiologische Verknüpfung von Atmung und Kreislauf. 11. Fortbild.lehrg. Bad Nauheim 1935. ~ Über die physiologischen Aufgaben des Adrenalins als Kreislaufhormon. Verh. dtsch. Ges. Kreisl.-Forsch. 10, 27 (1937). ~ Verknüpfung von Gewebs- und Lungenatmung im besonderen Hinblick auf die Verhältnisse bei der Höhenbeatmung. Luftfahrtmed. 2, 158 (1938). ~ Kreislauf und Stoffwechsel. Verh. dtsch. Ges. Kreisl.-Forsch. 14, 9 (1941). ~ Die bestimmenden Faktoren für die Vasomotorik der Ruhedurchblutung des Skeletmuskels. Pflügers Arch. ges. Physiol. 248, 100 (1944). ~ Über die Drosselungstoleranz und die kritische Drosselungsgrenze der Herz-Coronargefäße. Pflügers Arch. ges. Physiol. 253, 205 (1951). ~ Die Beeinflussung von Coronar- und hypoxiebedingten Myocard-Insuffizienzen durch Milz und Leber. Pflügers Arch. ges. Physiol. 253, 453 (1951). Reindell, H., u. L. Delius: Klinische Beobachtungen über Herzdynamik beim gesunden Menschen. Dtsch. Arch. klin. Med. 193, 639 (1948). — Reindell, H., E. Schildge, H. Klepzig u. H. W. Kirchhoff: Kreislaufregulation. Eine physiologische, pathologische und klinische Studie. Stuttgart 1955. — Reindell, H., R. Weyland, H. Klepzig, E. Schildge u. K. Musshoff: Schweiz. Z. Sportmed. 1, 97 (1953). — Remington, J. W., W. F. Hamilton, H. M. Caddell, G. H. Boyel, M. C. Wheeler and G. W. Pickering: Vasoconstriction as a precipitating factor in traumatic shock in the dog. Amer. J. Physiol. 161, 125 (1950). — Richards jr., D. W.: Effects of hemorrhage on circulation. Ann. N.Y. Acad. Sci. 49, 534 (1947/48). ~ Dynamics of congestive heart failure. Amer. J. Med. 6, 772 (1949). — Riley, R. L., A. Himmelstein, H. L. Motley, H. M. Weiner and A. Cournand: Studies of pulmonary circulation at rest and during exercise in normal individuals and in patients with pulmonary disease. Amer. J. Physiol. 152, 372 (1948). — Riley, R. L., R. H. Shepard, J. E. Cohn, D. G. Carroll and B. W. Armstrong: Maximal diffusing capacity of the lungs. J. appl. Physiol. 6, 573 (1954). — Roberts, J. T., and J. T. Wearor: Quantitative changes in the capillary-muscle relationship in human hearts during normal growth and hypertrophy. Amer. Heart J. 21, 617 (1941). — Roddie, I. C., and J. T. Shepherd: Evidence for critical closure of digital resistance vessels with reduced transmural pressure and passive dilatation with increased venous pressure. J. Physiol. (Lond.) **136**, 498 (1957). — RODDIE, I. C., J. T. SHEPHERD and R. F. WHELAN: The contribution of constrictor and dilator nerves of the skin vasodilatation during body heating. J. Physiol. (Lond.) **136**, 489 (1957). — ROHDE, E.: Über den Einfluß der mechanischen Bedingungen auf den Gaswechsel des Herzens. Naunyn-Schmiedeberg's Arch. exp. Path. Pharmak. **68**, 401 (1912). — ROSE, J. C., and E. D. FREIS: Alterations in systemic vascular volume of the dog in response to hexamethonium and norepinephrine. Amer. J. Physiol. **191**, 283 (1957). — ROSE, J. C., and E. J. LAZARO: Pulmonary vascular responses to serotonin and effects of certain serotonin antagonists. Circulat. Res. **6**, 283 (1958). — ROSE, J. C., E. J. LAZARO and H. P. BROIDA: Dynamics of complete right ventricular failure in dogs maintained with an extracorporeal left ventricle. Circulat. Res. **4**, 173 (1956). — ROSENBERG, E.: Local character of veno-vasomotor reflex. J. Physiol. (Lond.) **185**, 471 (1956). — ROSSIER, A.: Zur Physiopathologie des Emphysems. Verh. dtsch. Ges. inn. Med. 62. Kongr., S. 34, 1956. — ROSSIER, P. H., et A. BÜHLMANN: Cor pulmonale et pathophysiologie alvéolaire. Cardiologia (Basel) **25**, 132 (1954). — ROTHLIN, E., u. M. TAESCHLER: Zur Wirkung der herzwirksamen Glykoside auf den Myocardstoffwechsel. Fortschr. Kardiol. **1**, 189 (1956). — ROTTER, W.: Zur pathologischen Anatomie der arterio-venösen Anastomosen, epitheloiden Gefäßwandzellen und Sperrarterien. Verh. dtsch. Ges. Kreisl.-Forsch. **18**, 278 (1952). — ROTTER, W., u. L. WAGNER: Über die Entwicklung der subungualen Glomera (sog. arterio-venöse Anastomosen) der Zehen. Arch. Kreisl.-Forsch. **18**, 68 (1952). — RÜHL, A.: Über die Bedeutung der Milchsäure für den Herzstoffwechsel. Klin. Wschr. **13**, 1529 (1934). — RUSHMER, R. F.: Continous measurements of left ventricular dimensions in intact unaesthetized dogs. Circulat. Res. **2**, 14 (1954). ~ Applicability of Starling's law of the heart to intact ananaesthetized animals. Physiol. Rev. **35**, 138 (1955). ~ Anatomy and physiology of ventricular function. Physiol. Rev. **36**, 400 (1956a). ~ The initial phase of ventricular systole: Asynchronous myocardial contraction. Amer. J. Physiol. **184**, 188 (1956b). — RUSHMER, R. F., D. L. FRANKLIN and R. M. ELLIS: Left ventricular dimensions recorded by sonocardiometry. Circulat. Res. **4**, 684 (1956). — RUSHMER, R. F., and O. A. SMITH: Cardiac control. Physiol. Rev. **39**, 41 (1959). — RUSHMER, R. F., and T. C. WEST: Role of autonomic hormones on left ventricular performance continuonsly analyzed by electronic computers. Circulat. Res. **5**, 240 (1957).

SANCETTA, S. M., and L. RAKITA: Response of pulmonary artery pressure and total pulmonary resistance of untrained convalescent man to prolonged mild steady state exercise. J. clin. Invest. **36**, 1138 (1957). — SARNOFF, S. J.: Myocardial contractility as described by ventricular function curves. Physiol. Rev. **35**, 107 (1955). — SARNOFF, S. J., and E. BERGLUND: Effect of systemic vasoconstriction and subsequent vasodilatation on flow and pressures in systemic and pulmonary vascular beds. Amer. J. Physiol. **170**, 588 (1952). — SARNOFF, S. J., E. BERGLUND and L. C. SARNOFF: Estimated changes in pulmonary blood volume accompanying systemic vasoconstriction and vasodilation. J. appl. Physiol. **5**, 367 (1953). — SARNOFF, S. J., E. BRAUNWALD, G. H. WELCH, R. B. CASE, W. N. STAINSBY and R. MACRUZ: Hemodynamic determinants of oxygen consumption of the heart with special reference to the tension-time index. Amer. J. Physiol. **192**, 148 (1958). — SARNOFF, S. J., R. B. CASE, P. E. WAITHE and J. P. ISAACS: Insufficient coronary flow and myocardial failure as a complicating factor in late hemorrhagic shock. Amer. J. Physiol. **176**, 439 (1954). — SARNOFF, S. J., and L. C. SARNOFF: Neurohemodynamics of pulmonary edema. Circulation **6**, 51 (1952). SCHAEDE, A., u. P. THURN: Restblut. Fortschr. Röntgenstr. **86**, 696 (1957). — SCHEINBERG, P.: Cerebral blood flow in vascular disease of brain, with observations on effects of stellata ganglion blocks. Amer. J. Med. **8**, 139 (1950). — SCHELLONG, F.: Regulationsprüfung des Kreislaufs. Darmstadt 1938. — SCHLEIER, J.: Der Energieverbrauch in der Blutbahn. Pflügers Arch. ges. Physiol. **173**, 172 (1918). — SCHLOMKA, G.: Commotio cordis und ihre Folgen. Ergebn. inn. Med. Kinderheilk. **47**, 1 (1934). — SCHMID, A., u. F. REUBI: Vergleichende Herzminutenvolumenbestimmung mit der Wezler-Böger-Pulswellenmethode und nach dem direkten Fickschen Prinzip. Cardiologia (Basel) **19**, 42 (1951). — SCHMID, A., F. REUBI u. V. STETTLER: Simultane Herzminutenvolumbestimmung nach Fick und mit der Pulswellenmethode nach Wezler-Böger unter Hydrazinophthalein. Cardiologia (Basel) **23**, 90 (1953). — SCHMIDT, C. F., and D. M. AVIADO: Parallel lines, infinity and cardiovascular reflexes. Circulat. Res. **6**, 229 (1958). — SCHMIDT, H.: Primäre und sekundäre pulmonale Hypertonie. Dtsch. Arch. klin. Med. **200**, 837 (1953). ~ Die essentielle Hypertonie des Lungenkreislaufs. Arch. Kreisl.-Forsch. **19**, 91 (1953). — SCHMIDT, H. W.: Über Embolien in den Arterienkreisen der Pia mater. Z. ges. exp. Med. **125**, 401 (1955). ~ Über Arterienkreise in der Pia mater des Menschen. Dtsch. Z. Nervenheilk. **172**, 526 (1955). ~ Tierexperimentelle Untersuchungen zur Frage der Gefäßspasmen bei Hirnembolie. Dtsch. Z. Nervenheilk. **174**, 499 (1956). — SCHNEIDER, M.: Physiologische Grundlagen der Organdurchblutungsstörungen. Nauheimer Fortbild.lehrg. **18**, 15 (1952). ~ Durchblutung und Sauerstoffversorgung des Gehirns. Verh. dtsch. Ges. Kreisl.-Forsch. **19**, 1 (1953). — SCHOEDEL, W.: Methoden zur Untersuchung von arterio-venösen Anastomosen. 2. Internat. Kongr. Angiologie, Freiburg (Schweiz), 1955. ~ Die Regulation der Atmung. In Handbuch der allgemeinen Pathologie 1956. — Schoedel, W., u. H. Kreuzer: Das Restblut oder endsystolische Volumen der Herzkammern. Dtsch. med. Wschr. 83, 604 (1958). — Schoenmackers, J., u. H. Vieten: Über die Bedeutung der postmortalen Arteriendarstellung für die röntgenologische und pathologisch anatomische Analyse angeborener Herz- und Gefäßfehler. Fortschr. Röntgenstr. 75, 21 (1951). ~ Atlas postmortaler Angiogramme. Stuttgart 1954. — Schroeder, W.: Zur Physiologie der arterio-venösen Anastomosen. Verh. dtsch. Ges. Kreisl.-Forsch. 18, 289 (1952). — Schwab, M.: Die Dynamik des isolierten und des im Organismus schlagenden Herzens. Klin. Wschr. 28, 764 (1950). — Schwiegk, H.: Schock und Kollaps. Klin. Wschr. 1942, 741. ~ Die Auswirkungen von Funktionsstörungen des Herzens auf die Peripherie. Verh. dtsch. Ges. Kreisl.-Forsch. 22, 180 (1956). — Selkurt, E. E.: Der Nierenkreislauf. Klin. Wschr. 1955, 359. ~ Mesenteric blood flow as influenced by elevation of portal venous pressure. Fed. Proc. 14, 136 (1955). — Semming, Å.: Bronchialdurchblutung. Zit. bei Bücherl 1952. — Shipley, R. E., D. E. Gregg and E. F. Schroeder: An experimental study of flow patterns in various peripheral arteries. Amer. J. Physiol. 138, 718 (1943). — Shipley, R. E., and R. S. Study: Changes in renal blood flow, extraction in inulin, glomerular filtration rate, tissue pressure and urine flow with acute alterations of renal artery blood pressure. Amer. J. Physiol. 167, 676 (1951). — Shipley, R. E., and C. Wilson: An improved recording rotameter. Proc. Soc. exp. Biol. (N.Y.) 78, 724 (1951). — Sieker, H. O., O. H. Gauer and J. P. Henry: The effect of continous negative pressure breathing on water and electrolyte excretion by the human kidney. J. Clin. Invest. 33, 572 (1954). — Siemons, K.: Der Kreislauf bei der Endangitis obliterans. Verh. dtsch. Ges. Kreisl.-Forsch. 19, 215 (1953). — Simkin, B., H. C. Bergman, H. Silver and M. Prinzmetal: Renal arteriovenous anastomoses in rabbits, dogs and human subjects. Arch. intern. Med. 81, 115 (1948). — Simpson, S., and J. Pait: Some recent advances in methods of isolation and the physiology and chemistry of electrocortin. Recent Progr. Hormone Res. 11, 183 (1955). — Sinn, W.: Die Elastizität der Arterien und ihre Bedeutung für die Dynamik des arteriellen Systems. Akad. d. Wiss. u. Lit., Mainz, 1956. — Sjöstrand, T.: The regulation of the blood distribution in man. Acta physiol. scand. 26, 312 (1952). ~ Volume and distribution of blood and their significance in regulating the circulation. Physiol. Rev. 33, 202 (1953). — Skeggs, jr., L. T., and J. R. Kahn: Renal pressor system in hypertension: Evidence for circulating hypertensin in chronic renal hypertension. — Mature and activity of purified hypertensin. Circulation 17, 658 (1958). — Skeggs, jr., L. T., J. R. Kahn, K. E. Lentz and N. P. Shumway: The preparation, purification, and amino acid sequence of a polypeptide renin substrate. J. exp. Med. 106, 439 (1957). — Skeggs, jr., L. T., J. R. Kahn and N. P. Shumway: The preparation and function of the hypertensin-converting enzyme. J. exp. Med. 103, 295 (1956). — Slonim, N. B., A. Ravin, O. J. Balchum and S. H. Dressler: The effect of mild exercise in the supine position on the pulmonary arterial pressure of five normal human subjects. J. clin. Invest. 33, 1022 (1954). — Smith, H. W.: The kidney. Structur and function in health and disease. New York 1951. ~ Salt and water volume receptors. Amer. J. Med. 23, 623 (1957). — Spanner, R.: Zur Anatomie der arterio-venösen Anastomosen. Verh. dtsch. Ges. Kreisl.-Forsch. 18, 257 (1952). — Spealman, C. R.: Characteristic of human temperature regulation. Proc. Soc. exp. Biol. (N.Y.) 60, 11 (1946). Spencer, F. C., S. M. Powers, D. L. Merrill and R. J. Bing: Coronary blood flow and cardiac oxygen consumption in unanesthetized dogs. Amer. J. Physiol. 160, 149 (1950). — Stacy, R. W., D. T. Williams, R. E. Worden and R. O. McMorris: Essentials of biological and medical physics. Teil VI: Fluid flow systems in biology. New York-Toronto-London 1955. — Staemmler, M., u. K. Schmitt: Neue Beobachtungen bei sogenannter primärer Pulmonalsklerose (Hypertonie im kleinen Kreislauf). Arch. Kreisl.-Forsch. 17, 264 (1951). — Starling, E. H.: Linacre lecture on the law of the heart. Cambridge 1915. — Starling, E. H., and M. B. Visscher: The regulation of the energy output of the heart. J. Physiol. (Lond.) 62, 243 (1926). — Starr, I., and A. J. Rawson: Theoretical studies on an improved circulation schema whose pumps obey Starling's law of the heart. Amer. J. med. Sci. 199, 27 (1940). — Staub, H.: Pathogenese und Diät der Hypertonie. Dtsch. med. Wschr. 1951, 1. — Staubesand, J.: Über verschiedene Typen arterio-venöser Anastomosen und Glomusorgane im Hahnenkamm. Z. Zellforsch. 35, 265 (1950). — Stead, E. A.: Renal factor in congestive heart failure. Circulation 3, 294 (1951). — Stead, E. A., J. V. Warren and E. S. Brannon: Cardiac output in congestive heart failure. Amer. Heart J. 35, 528 (1948). — Straub, H.: Dynamik des Säugetierherzens. Dtsch. Arch. klin. Med. 115, 531 (1914). ~ Über den kleinen Kreislauf. Der Einfluß des großen Kreislaufs auf den Blutgehalt der Lungen. Dtsch. Arch. klin. Med. 121, 394 (1917). ~ Die Arbeitsweise des Herzens in ihrer Abhängigkeit von Spannung und Länge unter verschiedenen Arbeitsbedingungen. In Bethe-Bergmanns Handbuch der normalen und pathologischen Physiologie, Bd. VII/1, S. 237. 1926. — Strömbeck, J. P.: Effects de la résection artérielle. Acta chir. scand. 83, 510 (1940). — Study, R. S., and R. E. Shipley: Comparison of direct with indirect renal blood flow extraction of inulin and diodrast, before and during acute renal nerve stimulation. Amer. J. Physiol. **163**, 442 (1950). — SUNDER-PLASSMANN, P.: Durchblutungsschäden und ihre Behandlung. Stuttgart 1943. — SZENT-GYÖRGY, A.: Chemical physiology of contraction in body and heart muscle. New York 1953. ∼ General views on the chemistry of muscle contraction. Adv. Cardiol. **1**, 6 (1956).

TAQUINI, A. C., BLAQUIER, P. and A. C. TAQUINI: Studies on the renal humoral mechanism of chronic experimental hypertension. Circulation **17**, 672 (1958). — TAYLOR, N. B. G., and R. L. NOBLE: Appearance of antidiuretic substance in urine of man after various procedures. Proc. Soc. exp. Biol. (N.Y.) **73**, 207 (1950). — THAUER, R., u. W. CRISPENS: Fingertemperatur bei Änderung des hydrostatischen Druckes. Pflügers Arch. ges. Physiol. **261**, 470 (1955). — THURN, P.: Hämodynamik des Herzens im Röntgenbild. Stuttgart: Georg Thieme 1956. — TIETZE, K. H.: Über die Strömungsgeschwindigkeit des Blutes. Leipzig 1954. — TITTEL, S.: Über Reaktionsweise des Gefäßsystems bei lokaler Erfrierung. Z. ges. exp. Med. **113**, 698 (1943/44). — TÖNDURY, G.: Angewandte und topographische Anatomie. Stuttgart 1951. — TURCHETTI, A., u. A. SCHIROSA: Essential pulmonary hypertension and its phases of evolution. Cardiologia (Basel) **21**, 129 (1952).

ULLRICH, K. J., G. RIECKER u. K. KRAMER: Das Druckvolumdiagramm des Warmblüterherzens. Pflügers Arch. ges. Physiol. **259**, 481 (1954). — ULMER, W., u. A. WENKE: Bronchospirometrische Untersuchungen zur Frage der gasspannungsabhängigen Durchblutungsregulation der Alveolarkapillaren. Arch. Kreisl.-Forsch. **26**, 256 (1957). — UVNÄS, B.: Sympathetic vasodilator outflow. Physiol. Rev. **34**, 608 (1954).

VARNAUSKAS, E.: Studies in hypertensive cardiovascular disease. Scand. J. clin. Lab. Invest. **7**, Suppl., 17 (1955). — VENNING, E., A. CARBALLEIRA and J. DYRENFURTH: Excretion of sodium retaining substances. J. clin. Endocr. **14**, 784 (1954). — VILLARET, M., et R. CACHERA: Les embolies cérébrales. Paris 1939. — VIVELL, O.: Durchströmungsversuche am Coronarsystem bei normalem, hypertrophischem und atrophischem Herzmuskel. Beitr. path. Anat. **111**, 125 (1951). — VOLHARD, F.: Nierenerkrankungen und Hochdruck. Leipzig 1942.

WAGNER, R.: Kreislauf und Atmung. Verh. dtsch. Ges. Kreisl.-Forsch. **1940**, 7. ∼ Probleme und Beispiele biologischer Regelung. Stuttgart: Georg Thieme 1954. — WAKERLIN, G. E.: Antibodies to renin as proof of the pathogenesis of cisteined renal hypertension. Circulation **17**, 653 (1958). — WALDER, D. N.: The relationship between blood flow, capillary surface area and sodium clearance in muscle. Clin. Sci. **14**, 303 (1955). — WANG, C. I., S. L. EINHORN, H. J. THOMPSON and W. W. WALCOTT: Bleeding volume of unaesthetized dog. Amer. J. Physiol. **170**, 136 (1952). — WANG, C. I., and W. W. WALCOTT: Effects of anaesthesia on bleeding volume in the dog. Amer. J. Physiol. **170**, 143 (1952). — WARDENER, H. E. DE, and R. R. McSWINEY: Renal haemodynamics in vaso-vagal fainting due to haemorrhage. Clin. Sci. **10**, 209 (1951). — WARREN, J. V., E. S. BRANNON, E. A. STEAD and A. J. MERRIL: Effect of venesection and pooling of blood in extremities on arterial pressure and cardiac output in normal subjects with observations on acute circulatory collapse in 3 instances. J. clin. Invest. **24**, 337 (1945). — WARREN, J. V., D. C. ELKIN and J. L. NICKERSON: The blood volume in patients with arteriovenous fistulas. J. clin. Invest. **30**, 220 (1951). — WARREN, J. V., J. L. NICKERSON and D. C. ELKIN: The cardiac output in patients with arteriovenous fistulas. J. clin. Invest. **30**, 210 (1951). — WEARN, J. T., A. C. ERNSTENE, A. W. BROMER, J. S. BARR, W. J. GERMAN and L. J. ZSCHIESCHE: The normal behavior of the pulmonary blood vessels with observations on the intermittence of the flow of blood in the arterioles and capillaries. Amer. J. Physiol. **109**, 236 (1934). — WEBER, H. H., u. H. PORTZEHL: Kontraktion, ATP-Cyclus und fibrilläre Proteine des Muskels. Ergebn. Physiol. **47**, 369 (1952). — WEDD, A. M., and A. N. DRURY: The action of certain nucleic acid derivations on the coronary flow in the dog. J. Pharmacol. exp. Ther. **50**, 157 (1934). — WEGRIA, R.: Pharmacology of the coronary circulation. Pharmacol Rev. **3**, 197 (1951). — WEISS, S., and J. P. BAKER: Medicine (Baltimore) **12**, 297 (1933). — WEISS, S., R. B. CAPPS, E. B. FERRIS jr. and D. MUNRO: Syncope and convulsions due to a hyperactive carotid sinus reflex. Arch. intern. Med. **58**, 407 (1936). — WEISS, S., R. W. WILKINS and F. W. HAYMER: Nature of circulatory collapse induced by sodium nitrite. J. clin. Invest. **16**, 73, 85 (1937). — WEIZSÄCKER, V. v.: Stoffwechsel und Wärmebildung des Herzens. In BETHE-BERGMANNS Handbuch der normalen und pathologischen Physiologie, Bd. VII/1, S. 689. 1926. — WERKÖ, L., and H. LAGERLÖF: Studies on the circulation in man. Cardiac output and blood pressure in the right auricle, right ventricle and pulmonary artery in patients with hypertensive cardiovascular disease. Acta med. scand. **133**, 427 (1949). — WESTCOTT, R. N., N. O. FOWLER, R. C. SCOTT, V. D. HAUENSTEIN and J. McGUIRE: Anoxia and human pulmonary vascular resistance. J. clin. Invest. **30**, 957 (1951). — WETTERER, E.: Quantitative Beziehungen zwischen Stromstärke und Druck im natürlichen Kreislauf bei zeitlich variabler Elastizität des arteriellen Windkessels. Z. Biol. **100**, 260 (1940). ∼ Die Wirkung der Herztätigkeit auf die Dynamik des Arteriensystems. Verh. dtsch. Ges. Kreisl.-Forsch. **22**, 26 (1956). —

Wetterer, E., u. H. Pieper: Über die Gesamtelastizität des arteriellen Windkessels und ein experimentelles Verfahren zu ihrer Bestimmung am lebenden Tier. Z. Biol. **106**, 23 (1953). ~ Ein indirektes Verfahren zur Bestimmung des diastolischen Abstroms aus dem Arteriensystem und seine Anwendung zum Studium der Druck-Stromstärke. — Beziehung in vivo. Verh. dtsch. Ges. Kreisl.-Forsch. **21**, 430 (1955). — Wezler, K., u. A. Böger: Die Dynamik des arteriellen Systems. Der arterielle Blutdruck und seine Komponenten. Ergebn. Physiol. **41**, 292 (1939). — Wezler, K., u. F. Schlüter: Querdehnbarkeit isolierter kleiner Arterien vom muskulären Typ. Wiesbaden 1953. — Wezler, K., u. W. Sinn: Das Strömungsgesetz des Blutkreislaufs. Aulendorf 1953. — Whitaker, S. R. F., and F. R. Winton: The apparent viscosity of blood flowing in the isolated hindlimb of the dog and its variation with corpuscular concentration. J. Physiol. (Lond.) **78**, 339 (1933). — Whittenberger, J. L.: Artificial respiration. Physiol. Rev. **35**, 611 (1955). — Widgorowitsch, R.: Ein bemerkenswertes Reflexphänomen bei einem Aneurysma der A. femoralis. Dtsch. med. Wschr. **1915**, 711. — Wiggers, C. J.: The interplay of coronary vascular resistance and myocardial compression in regulating coronary flow. Circulat. Res. **2**, 271 (1954). — Wilbrandt, W.: Zum Wirkungsmechanismus der Herzglykoside. Schweiz. med. Wschr. **85**, 315 (1955). — Wille-Baumkauff, H., u. A. Büttner: Untersuchungen zur Ausbildung des Kollateralkreislaufs bei Schlagaderausschneidung und Schlagaderunterbindung. Bruns' Beitr. klin. Chir. **172**, 260 (1941). — Williams, M. H.: Relationships between pulmonary artery pressure and blood flow in the dog lung. Amer. J. Physiol. **179**, 243 (1954). — Witzleb, E.: Nervöse Einflüsse auf die Coronardurchblutung. Bad Oeynhausener Gespräche II, S. 94. 1957. — Wollheim, E.: Die zirkulierende Blutmenge und ihre Bedeutung für Kompensation und Dekompensation des Kreislaufs. Z. klin. Med. **116**, 269 (1931). ~ Die Blutreservoire des Menschen. Klin. Wschr. **12**, 12 (1933). ~ Klinik der Herzinsuffiziens. Verh. dtsch. Ges. Kreisl.-Forsch. **16**, 75 (1950). — Woollard, H. H.: The innervation of the heart. J. Anat. (Lond.) **60**, 345 (1925).

Yamada, S., and A. C. Burton: Effect of reduced tissue pressure on the blood flow of the fingers; the veno-vasomotor reflex. J. appl. Physiol. **6**, 501 (1954).

Zdansky, E.: Röntgendiagnostik des Herzens und der großen Gefäße. Wien 1949. — Zweifach, B. W.: General principles governing the behavior of the microcirculation. Amer. J. Med. **23**, 684 (1957). — Zweifach, B. W., and D. B. Metz: Intrinsic regulation of blood flow in sceletal muscle. Fed. Proc. **14**, 168 (1955a). ~ The relation of blood-borne agents acting on mesenteric vascular bed to general circulatory reactions. J. clin. Invest. **34**, 653 (1955b).

Die allgemeine Pathologie des Blutkreislaufes.

Von

FRANZ BÜCHNER-Freiburg i. Br.

Mit 57 Abbildungen.

Es war eine der wichtigsten Erfindungen des Lebendigen, in die tierischen Organismen ein eigenes System von Gefäßen einzubauen, welche die Aufgabe haben, den Organen eine adäquate Ionen-, Salz- und Nährstofflösung zuzuführen und Stoffwechselprodukte aus den Organen auszuschwemmen. Die vergleichende Anatomie und Physiologie (HESSE 1910, TIGERSTEDT 1921, 1923, VON BRÜCKE 1925, BETHE 1926, VON BUDDENBROCK 1928) sagt uns, daß dieses Gefäßsystem schon bei den Würmern eine Struktur erreichte, die durch den Einbau glatter Muskulatur auf größerer Strecke eine Kontraktion mit einer peristaltischen Welle von hinten nach vorn und einen Rückstrom von vorn nach hinten ermöglichte. Ein zentrales Herz, aus dem das Blut in die Peripherie ausgeworfen und in dem es aus der Peripherie wieder gesammelt wird, finden wir aber erst bei den Crustaceen. Bei ihnen erfolgt auch zum ersten Mal konstant die Koppelung der Atmung an den Kreislauf, indem das gesamte venöse Blut durch ein Kiemensystem getrieben und in diesem arterialisiert wird. Das Crustaceen-Herz ist den Kiemen nachgeschaltet, befördert also nur arterialisiertes Blut. Das Problem der Zentralisierung des Kreislaufmotors wurde dagegen bei den Fischen und damit bei der ersten Stufe der Wirbeltiere so gelöst, daß das Herz, gegliedert in Vorhof, Kammer und Bulbus, den Kiemen vorgeschaltet ist und demgemäß nur venöses Blut in diese hineinpumpt. Im Amphibienherzen wird zum ersten Mal ein zentraler Motor erreicht, der venöses Blut in die Lungen und arterialisiertes Blut in den großen Kreislauf treibt. Bei getrennten Vorhöfen wird diese Arbeit von einer einheitlichen Kammer so geleistet, daß unvollkommene Septen den getrennten Abstrom des venösen Blutes in die Lunge und des arterialisierten Blutes in die Aorta ermöglichen. Das Herz der Vögel und der Säuger vollendet dieses Prinzip durch anatomische Trennung der einen Kammer in einen venösen rechten und einen arteriellen linken Ventrikel.

Durch das System der Gefäße wurden — relativ zur äußeren Oberfläche der Organismen — gewaltige innere Oberflächen und damit Austauschflächen für Nährstoffe, Ionen, Salze, Atemgase und intermediäre Metaboliten geschaffen. Der Erythrocyt machte die in diesem System strömende Flüssigkeit zum Blute. Mit ihm gewannen die Organismen die Fähigkeit, neben dem physikalisch gelösten einen großen Vorrat von chemisch dissoziabel gebundenem Sauerstoff zu transportieren. Das Herz schuf die Möglichkeit, die Flüssigkeit in einem von der Umwelt relativ unabhängigen Kreislaufsystem gerichtet zu bewegen, die Stoffvorräte in diesem System mehrfach umlaufen zu lassen und auszuschöpfen und das Maß des Umlaufes an Leistungsstufen von wechselnder Höhe anzupassen. Die Zentralisation des Atmungsorganes im Kreislauf ermöglichte schließlich eine solche Intensität des aeroben Stoffwechsels, daß ein großer Teil der produzierten Energie zur Eigenerwärmung und damit zur relativen Unabhängigkeit von der Umwelttemperatur verwertet werden konnte.

So wurden durch die zunehmende Differenzierung des Blutkreislaufs große Funktionskreise der Organismen immer umweltunabhängiger, aber zugleich immer kreislaufabhängiger. Das Maß der Lebensäußerungen des tierisch Lebendigen wurde von einer zur anderen Entfaltungsstufe immer mehr von der möglichen Kreislaufleistung gesetzt, das System des Blutkreislaufs wurde neben dem Nervensystem immer mehr der Schrittmacher des gesamten Organismus, wobei das jeweilige Kreislaufsystem eine bestimmte Höhe des Nervensystems ermöglichte, von dessen steuernden und integrierenden Funktionen aber auch intensiv in Dienst genommen wurde.

Ein so zentralisiertes System wie das Blutkreislaufsystem der Säuger und des Menschen ist mit Notwendigkeit besonders störungsfähig. Seine Störung bedeutet zugleich eine besondere Gefahrenquelle für die übrigen Systeme und den gesamten Organismus. Das besagt, daß *der allgemeinen Pathologie des Kreislaufs eine zentrale Stellung in der Pathologie* zukommt.

Das gilt schon von den lokalen Kreislaufstörungen je nach der Wertigkeit des von ihnen befallenen Organes und zwar von der Durchblutungsstörung des ganzen Organs wie von der eines Organsektors. Die Gefährlichkeit und häufige Tödlichkeit von lokalen Kreislaufstörungen des Hirns oder des Herzens ist dafür der eindringlichste Beweis. Noch mehr erwarten wir von den allgemeinen Kreislaufstörungen, von der Insuffizienz des gesamten Kreislaufs, bedrohliche und tödliche Wirkungen. Der Zusammenbruch des Gesamtkreislaufs im Kollaps, in der Herzinsuffizienz und in der Lungenembolie ist daher nicht selten der Schrittmacher des Todes. Bei zahlreichen Krankheiten wird in der letzten entscheidenden Phase das Herz- und Kreislaufsystem in den Mittelpunkt der pathogenetischen Kette gerückt. Die häufige Totenscheindiagnose „Herz- und Kreislaufversagen", oft aus Verlegenheit gestellt, trifft insofern meist das Richtige, als am Ende an diesem System in der Regel die Entscheidung fällt: unter die Tumorkrankheit setzt die Herzschwäche ebenso häufig ihr Siegel wie unter die Erkrankungen der Lungen, der Nieren; die schwere Infektionskrankheit mündet ebenso häufig im Kollaps wie der posttraumatische Zustand.

Unter den *lokalen Kreislaufstörungen* unterschied schon die klassische Pathologie die lokale arterielle Ischämie und die lokale venöse Hyperämie. Die *arterielle Ischämie* kann uns als *absolute Ischämie,* d.h. als völlige Unterbrechung des arteriellen Blutzustromes zu einem Organ oder Organsektor begegnen, am häufigsten als Folge einer *obturierenden arteriellen Thrombose oder Embolie.* Sie verursacht nicht selten die Nekrose des Kernes des zugeordneten ischämisierten Organbezirkes, d.h. einen *Infarkt,* meist einen *anämischen Infarkt.* Die *relative arterielle Ischämie* bedeutet im Unterschied zur absoluten eine krankhafte Einschränkung der arteriellen Blutzufuhr zu einem Organ oder Organteil. Sie hat am häufigsten *Stenosen von Organarterien* zur Voraussetzung. Ihre Folgen sind bei *chronischer relativer arterieller Ischämie* vor allem *Parenchymatrophien* des befallenen Organs, bei *akuter relativer arterieller Ischämie elektive Parenchymnekrosen.* Diese letzteren Folgen arterieller Stenosen haben wir vor allem in den letzten 3 Jahrzehnten beachten gelernt.

Von besonderem Interesse für die Kreislaufpathologie wurde in jüngster Zeit das Phänomen der *temporären arteriellen Ischämie.* In der menschlichen Pathologie kann diese unter 2 Voraussetzungen zustande kommen: 1. *durch thrombotische oder embolische Obturation einer Arterie mit nachfolgender Kompensation der Ischämie durch einen adäquaten Kollateralkreislauf,* 2. durch Thrombose oder Embolie einer Arterie mit *operativer Entfernung des Thrombus oder Embolus,* 3. *durch temporäre spastische Kontraktion einer Arterie.* Die experimentelle Pathologie hat die temporäre arterielle Ischämie vor allem nach temporärer, arterieller Unterbindung untersucht.

Die akute relative arterielle Ischämie und die temporäre absolute Ischämie bieten uns interessante und für die menschliche Pathologie bedeutungsvolle Einblicke in die Abfolge der Stoffwechselstörungen, der Funktionsstörungen und der Strukturstörungen, welche durch die Ischämie gesetzt werden. An diesen Phänomenen wurde vor allem ersichtlich, wie sehr Stoffwechsel- und Strukturstörungen nur zwei Seiten des gleichen krankhaften Ereignisses sind. Das gilt besonders dann, wenn die Störungen der Ultrastruktur der Parenchymzellen mitberücksichtigt werden, wie sie im elektronenmikroskopischen Bild erfaßt werden können.

Als ein wichtiger pathogenetischer Faktor wurde in der neueren Kreislaufpathologie auch die *paradoxe arterielle Durchblutungsinsuffizienz* erkannt. Sie kommt bei akuten und chronischen Überlastungen von Organen vor, deren Blutbedarf so gesteigert wird, daß er von der maximal möglichen arteriellen Durchblutung nicht mehr gedeckt werden kann. Die Organe sind unter solchen Bedingungen relativ zum Normdurchschnitt vermehrt durchblutet, aber nicht adäquat zur Leistung. Unter akuten Bedingungen ist die Wirkung dieses Zustandes mit dem der akuten relativen Ischämie sehr verwandt.

Auf der venösen Seite des Kreislaufs unterscheiden wir unter den lokalen Durchblutungsstörungen die absolute und die relative venöse Hyperämie. Die *absolute venöse Hyperämie* wird als Folge des Verschlusses einer Vene durch Thrombose, Kompression oder Unterbindung beobachtet. Ist ein kollateraler Abstrom des venösen Blutes dabei nicht möglich, so schädigt der Aufstau des venösen Blutes das Parenchym so hochgradig, daß es unter Austritt von Erythrocyten zugrunde geht. So kommt es zum *hämorrhagischen Infarkt durch Venenverschluß*.

Wird der Abstrom venösen Blutes zwar erschwert, aber nicht unterbrochen, so resultiert eine *relative venöse Hyperämie* mit ihren Folgen am Parenchym und an der Permeabilität der Blutcapillaren bis zur serösen Transsudation.

Allgemeine Durchblutungsstörungen begegnen uns einmal als *allgemeine arterielle Oligämie*[1]. Diese kann akut oder subakut dadurch zustande kommen, daß die glatte Muskulatur der peripheren Arterien, besonders der Arteriolen, des großen Kreislaufes insuffizient wird und bei dadurch abfallendem Blutdruck die vis a tergo für die Weiterbeförderung versackender Blutmassen fehlt. Diese allgemeine arterielle Oligämie durch Insuffizienz der arteriellen Peripherie kennzeichnet den *Kollaps*. Die allgemeine arterielle Oligämie kommt aber ebenso bei *akuter Insuffizienz des linken Ventrikels* durch akute Verringerung des Schlag- und Minutenvolumens der linken Kammer zur Beobachtung. Sie tritt schließlich dann ein, wenn durch *embolischen Verschluß größerer Lungenarterien* der Abstrom des Blutes aus der Lunge und damit der Blutzustrom zum linken Ventrikel stark verringert ist.

Allgemeine Durchblutungsstörungen liegen aber auch dann vor, wenn der rechte Ventrikel versagt oder aus anderer Ursache der Einstrom des Blutes aus den großen Venen in das rechte Herz stark eingeschränkt ist. In diesen Fällen begegnet uns die *allgemeine venöse Hyperämie*. Ihre Folgen beschränken sich in der Regel auf die venösen Schenkel der Capillaren und deren Ufer, während die allgemeine arterielle Oligämie sich an der ganzen Capillarstrecke, der arteriellen und der venösen, und ihren Ufern auswirkt.

---

[1] Die klassische Pathologie hat die allgemeine Oligämie mit der allgemeinen Anämie, der Blutarmut, also dem substantiellen Blutmangel gleichgesetzt. Wir wenden den Ausdruck auf Zustände der allgemeinen Einschränkung des *strömenden* Blutes an.

Die absolute arterielle Ischämie.

1. Der arterielle Infarkt.

Die klassische Pathologie hat seit VIRCHOW 1846, 1854 herausgearbeitet, daß der plötzliche Verschluß einer Organarterie durch Thrombose, Embolie oder Unterbindung verschiedene Folgen nach sich ziehen kann. Verfügt das Organ über ausreichende arterielle Anastomosen und ist sein Stoffwechsel weniger anspruchsvoll, so kann die Durchblutung des Versorgungsgebietes der verschlossenen Arterie über die vorhandenen Anastomosen vollwertig aufrechterhalten werden, ohne daß eine Gewebsschädigung eintritt. Das können wir z.B. beim thrombotischen oder embolischen Verschluß einer peripheren Arterie des Fußrückens beobachten oder — bei normalem Lungenkreislauf — beim embolischen Verschluß einer Lungenarterie. Selbst am Hirn mit seinem hohen Blutbedarf ist durch den Circulus arteriosus Willisi die Kollateralversorgung von rechts nach links und vom Versorgungsgebiet der A. carotis interna zu dem der A. vertebrales noch so gesichert, daß beim jüngeren Menschen in der Regel die A. carotis communis oder interna einer Seite unterbunden werden kann, ohne daß dadurch ein morphologisch oder funktionell nachweisbarer Hirnschaden eintritt. Beim Kaninchen ist eine Unterbindung beider Carotiden und A. vertebrales möglich, ohne daß es zum Hirninfarkt oder auch nur zu einer Ganglienzellenschädigung kommt (H. BECKER 1951). Bestehen beim älteren Menschen an den basalen Hirnarterien jedoch arteriosklerotische Stenosen, so können diese genügen, die Anastomosenversorgung nach Unterbindung der A. carotis zur Insuffizienz zu bringen. Aber auch beim jüngeren Menschen ohne Stenosen der Hirnarterien kann schon eine schwere akute Blutung und die dadurch hervorgerufene allgemeine Oligämie, derentwegen z.B. nach Tonsillektomie die A. carotis unterbunden wurde, die Blutversorgung durch den Circulus Willisii so insuffizient machen, daß es zum Hirninfarkt kommt.

An vielen Organen ist der plötzliche embolische oder thrombotische Verschluß einer Organarterie oder einer ihrer Verzweigungen in der Regel von einem keilförmig im Versorgungsgebiet der verschlossenen Arterie entwickelten *anämischen Infarkt* gefolgt. Daß beim Zustandekommen dieser Infarkte der Aufteilung der arteriellen Gefäße und deren Armut an Anastomosen eine große Bedeutung zukommt, beweisen z.B. die embolisch verursachten anämischen Infarkte der Milz nach Thrombosen im linken Herzen: obwohl die Milz als ausschließlich mesenchymales Organ einen weniger intensiven Stoffwechsel hat als die parenchymatösen Organe, wird sie nach Embolie häufig von Infarkten betroffen, da die peripheren Milzarterien nur geringe Anastomosen haben. Erst recht entwickeln sich in der Niere embolische anämische Infarkte, da bei diesem parenchymatösen Organ mit anspruchsvollem Stoffwechsel der Mangel an präcapillären Anastomosen zwischen den Arteriae lobulares eine besondere Infarktbereitschaft bedingt.

Die *Infarktnekrose parenchymatöser Organe* ist eine Totalnekrose von Parenchym und Mesenchym. In der Niere ist sie durch die Koagulationsnekrose der Tubulusepithelien, durch die Nekrose der Glomerula und durch den Untergang des mesenchymalen Gerüstes gekennzeichnet. Beim Herzinfarkt werden die Herzmuskelzellen durch Koagulationsnekrose in kernlose homogene Bänder verwandelt, während gleichzeitig die nekrotischen mesenchymalen Zellen feinkörnig zerfallen. Die Nekrose führt am Herzmuskel zur Ausflutung von Transaminase für die Transaminierung Glutaminat-Oxalazetat ins Blut[1]. Diese Transaminase ist daher vom zweiten Tage an im Blute vermehrt, um nach 3—4 Tagen allmählich

---

[1] LA DUE, WROBLEWSKI und KARMEN 1955.

wieder die Norm zu erreichen[1]. Auch am Hirn ist der Infarkt durch eine Totalnekrose gekennzeichnet, von der die Nervenzellen, ihre Fortsätze, die Gliazellen
und die mesenchymalen Elemente regelmäßig betroffen werden.

Während Niereninfarkte sekundär zur Eintrocknung kommen, wird am Herzinfarkt die trockene Infarktnekrose in der Regel bald durch mehr oder weniger
reichlich eingewanderte Leukocyten aufgelöst. Ist die Leukocyteninvasion
besonders stark, so kann durch Leukocytenfermente eine *Verflüssigung der
Infarktnekrose* eintreten. Die Ruptur des Herzens oder ein Papillarmuskelabriß
mit akuter schwerer Mitralinsuffizienz kann deren Folge sein. Auch bei experimentellem Herzinfarkt am Hund trat dieses Ereignis gelegentlich ein, meist in
der zweiten Woche[2].

Auch am Hirninfarkt nach Embolie oder Thrombose, am häufigsten der
A. cerebri media (VIRCHOW 1847, COHNHEIM 1872, NEUBUERGER 1930, 1944,
SPATZ 1939, MEESSEN und STOCHDORPH 1957) kommt es in der Regel, aber
flüchtig zu einer Leukocyteninvasion in die Infarktnekrose[3]. Gesetzmäßig entwickelt sich dann im Hirninfarkt nach gliös-mesenchymaler Proliferation vom
Infarktrande her zunächst eine partielle Erweichung (Abb. 1) und schließlich
eine totale Verflüssigung der Nekrose, also eine Colliquationsnekrose, deren
Ergebnis nach Wochen oder Monaten eine zunächst mit milchiger, dann mit
liquorartig klarer Flüssigkeit gefüllte vielkammerige Cyste ist[4].

Auch am Tier nehmen Hirninfarkte durch experimentelle Embolie diesen Verlauf. So
fand sich nach Embolie in die A. cerebri media beim Hund nach einem Stadium der weißen
Infarktnekrose, das nach 65 Std erreicht war, schließlich eine Erweichung des Infarktes[5].
Besonders große Erweichungshöhlen konnten auf diese Weise an neugeborenen Hunden nach
Paraffin-Injektion in die rechte A. carotis hervorgerufen werden: schon 6 Tage nach der
Embolie fand sich eine große Erweichungshöhle der rechten Hemisphäre unter Einschluß
des Thalamus und des Hypothalamus mit Erhaltenbleiben eines schmalen Rindenrestes.
Nach 12 Monaten war die befallene Hemisphäre fast ganz in einen blasigen Hohlraum ver-
wandelt, der nur von einer hauchdünnen Membran überzogen war[6].

Der durch Eintrocknung verhärtete Niereninfarkt wird nicht durchorganisiert,
sondern nur am Rande durch Mesenchymsprossung und Entwicklung kollagener
Fibrillen sklerosiert[7]. Am Hirninfarkt wird schon nach wenigen Tagen aus der
Infarktumgebung durch Sprossung von Mesenchym und von Gliazellen die
Infarktorganisation eingeleitet. Dabei werden die freiwerdenden Lipide der Infarktnekrose, besonders auch untergegangener Markscheiden, in den Gliazellen
als Fetttröpfchen gespeichert, so daß schon nach 5—6 Tagen reichlich Fett-
körnchenzellen angesammelt sind, später auch mesenchymale Schaumzellen.
Unter den gliösen Elementen treten die Hortega-Zellen und die Astrocyten in
den Vordergrund[8]. Doch wird der Organisationsvorgang beherrscht von den
Mesenchymwucherungen, die mehr und mehr die Erweichungshöhle durchsetzen
und sich durch Bildung kollagener Fibrillen schließlich zu einem liquorgefüllten
Faserschwamm verfestigen (Abb. 2)[9].

Am Herzmuskel kommt die *Infarktnarbe* auf 2 Wegen zustande: durch
mesenchymale Organisation der Infarktnekrose oder durch Skeletierung des
reticulären Fasergerüstes nach Entparenchymisierung, anschließenden Kollaps
der Reticulinfasern und deren Verfestigung durch Kollagenisierung (Abb. 3)[10].
Beide Narbenformen können sich in der gleichen Infarktnarbe ergänzen. Die

---

[1] FORSTER 1958, HAUSS, GERLACH und SCHÜRMEYER 1958.
[2] MALLORY, WHITE und SALCEDO-SALGAR 1939.
[3] SPIELMEYER 1922, MEESSEN und STOCHDORPH 1957.
[4] SPATZ 1939, MEESSEN und STOCHDORPH 1957.   [5] VILLARET und CATCHERA 1939.
[6] H. BECKER 1949.   [7] RICKER 1924, SCHNAPAUFF 1928.   [8] SPIELMEYER 1922.
[9] SPATZ 1939, MEESSEN und STOCHDORPH 1957.
[10] SARAM 1957, SCHLESINGER und REINER 1955.

Entwicklung der Narbe trat beim Hund bei größeren experimentellen Herz-infarkten innerhalb von 5 Wochen ein, bei kleineren in 2 Wochen[1].

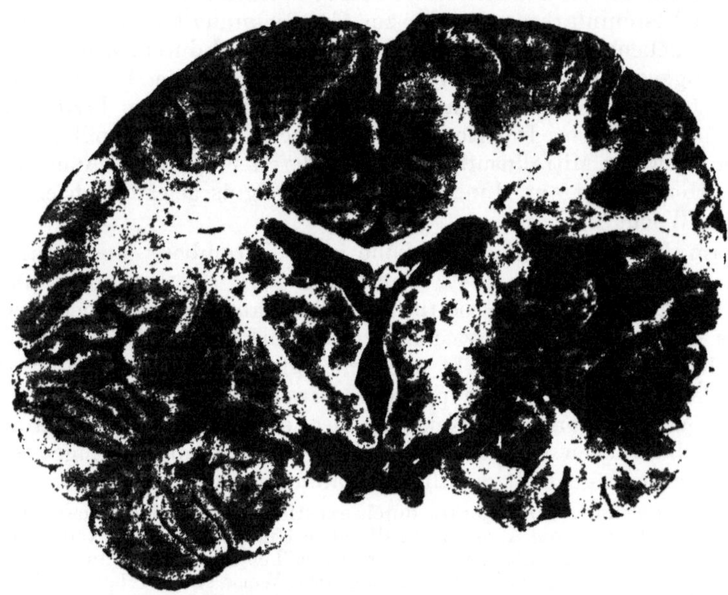

Abb. 1. Hirninfarkt 5 Tage nach Embolie der rechten Arteria cerebri media von der Inselrinde und der Rinde des Schläfenlappens bis in das Putamen in beginnender Erweichung. (Aus H. NOETZEL, Die Pathologie des Nervensystems, Abb. 300 in F. BÜCHNER, Spezielle Pathologie, 3. Aufl. 1960.)

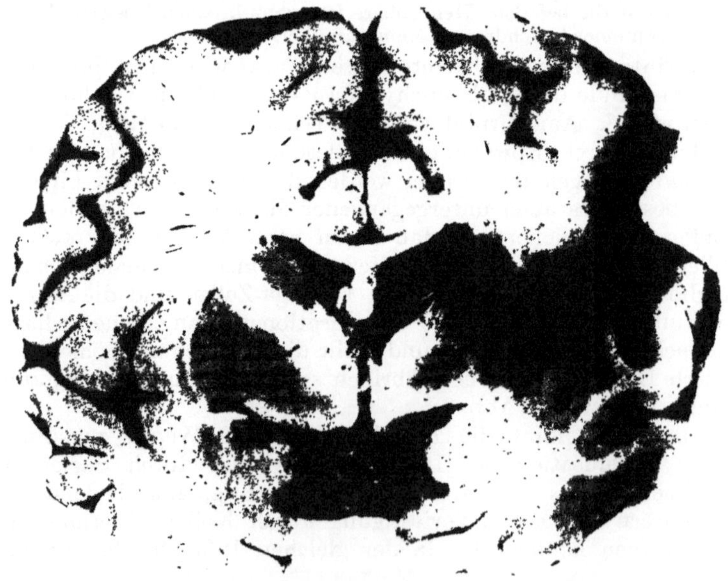

Abb. 2. Narbe eines Hirninfarktes nach arteriosklerotischer Thrombose der A. cerebri media im gleichen Bereich wie in Abb. 1. System von Septen aus lockerem Bindegewebe in der Infarkthöhle. (Aus H. NOETZEL, Die Pathologie des Nervensystems, Abb. 301 in F. BÜCHNER, Spezielle Pathologie, 3. Aufl. 1960.)

Beim Menschen benötigt die Entwicklung der Herzinfarktnarbe je nach der Größe des Infarktes 3—6 Monate[2]. Wird das Organisationsgewebe zu früh belastet, so ist ein mehr oder minder großes *Herzaneurysma* das Ergebnis (Abb. 4).

[1] MALLORY, WHITE und SALCEDO-SALGAR 1929.   [2] BÜCHNER 1955.

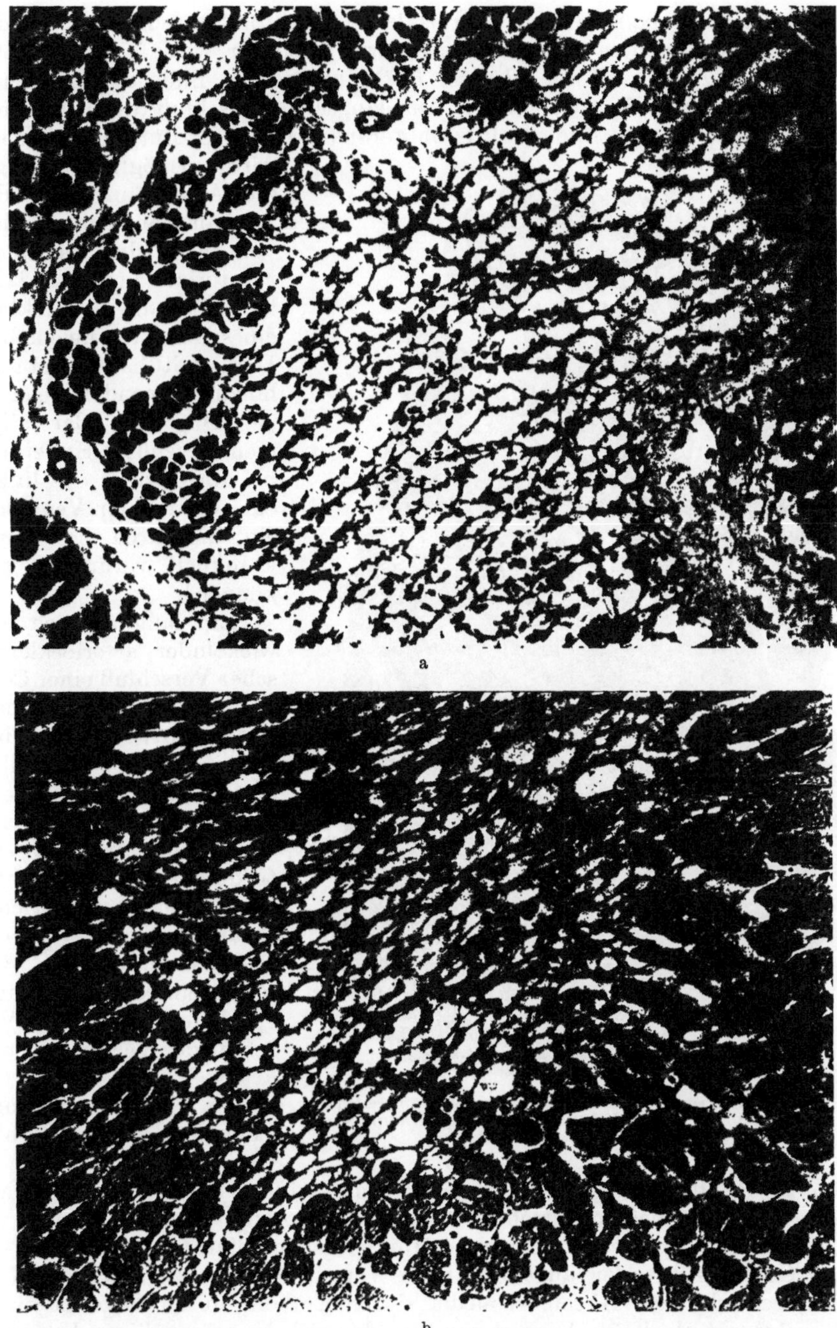

Abb. 3a u. b. a Subakuter Herzinfarkt. Reste der Infarktnekrose (schwarz). Skeletierung des Reticulinfaser-gerüstes im Infarktbereich nach Verflüssigung der Nekrose. b Kollagenisiertes Fasergerüst nach Verflüssigung einer Herzmuskelnekrose in der Nähe eines Herzinfarktes. [Nach M. SARAM, Beitr. path. Anat. 118, 1957 (Abb. 2 und 3)].

Die *große Bedeutung der Plötzlichkeit des Arterienverschlusses* für die Ent-stehung anämischer Infarkte wird durch folgende Beobachtungen besonders ver-anschaulicht:

Die plötzliche embolische oder arteriosklerotisch-thrombotische Verschließung der A. femoralis, poplitea oder tibialis anterior/posterior wird fast regelmäßig von einem *Infarkt der Zehen oder des Fußes* unter dem Bilde des trockenen, seltener des feuchten Brandes gefolgt. Der langsame Verschluß dieser Arterien, wie er besonders bei der Endarteriitis obliterans Winiwarter-Bürger beobachtet wird, ermöglicht dagegen die Ausweitung und den Ausbau von Kollateralen, vor allem über die A. obturatoria. Hier kann daher lange Zeit die Entwicklung eines Infarktes ausbleiben. Dieser tritt häufig erst nach hinzukommender allgemeiner Oligämie oder allgemeiner venöser Hyperämie bei Insuffizienz des linken oder des rechten Ventrikels ein, die durch die Grundkrankheit verursacht sein können[1].

Ein langsam sich entwickelnder arteriosklerotischer Verschluß einer Coronararterie des Herzens kann ohne Entwicklung eines Herzinfarktes zum Ausbau der Anastomosen führen[2]. Dabei kann die Kollateralversorgung über das Ventrikelseptum bei Verschluß des Ramus interventricularis anterior von der rechten Coronararterie aus wirksamer eintreten als in umgekehrter Richtung bei Verschluß der rechten Coronararterie[3].

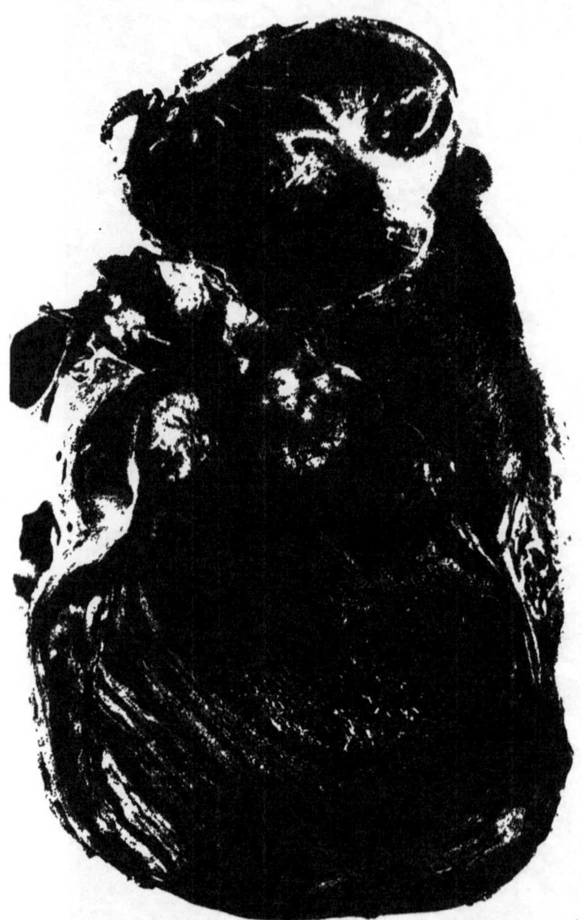

Abb. 4. Großes Aneurysma nach einem die Herzspitze umgreifenden Vorderwandinfarkt des linken Ventrikels mit Aufschichtung eines ausgedehnten Thrombus im Aneurysma.

Im Experiment konnte bei *plötzlichem* Verschluß einer Coronararterie bei 24 von 25 Hunden ein großer, bei einem ein kleiner Herzinfarkt beobachtet werden. Bei allmählichem Verschluß der gleichen Coronararterie im Verlauf von 5 Wochen hatten dagegen nur 4 von 14 Hunden einen Infarkt[4].

Am Gehirn führt der augenblickliche Verschluß einer der basalen Hirnarterien, besonders der A. cerebri media, durch Embolie in der Regel zu einem größeren Infarkt als die im Verlauf von Stunden sich bis zum völligen Verschluß der Arterie entwickelnde arteriosklerotische Thrombose[5].

---

[1] JÄGER 1932.
[2] BLUMGART, SCHLESINGER und DAVIS 1940, BLUMGART, SCHLESINGER und ZOLL 1941.
[3] MÜLLER-MOHNSSEN 1957.   [4] BLUM, SCHAUER und CALEF 1938, ähnlich BURCHELL 1940.
[5] MEESSEN und STOCHDORPH 1957.

Für die *Größe des Herzinfarktes* bei gleichem Sitz des Verschlusses an typischer Stelle, z.B. am oberen Ramus interventricularis der linken Coronararterie, sind außerdem 3 Faktoren von besonderer Bedeutung: 1. Die *Beschaffenheit der übrigen*

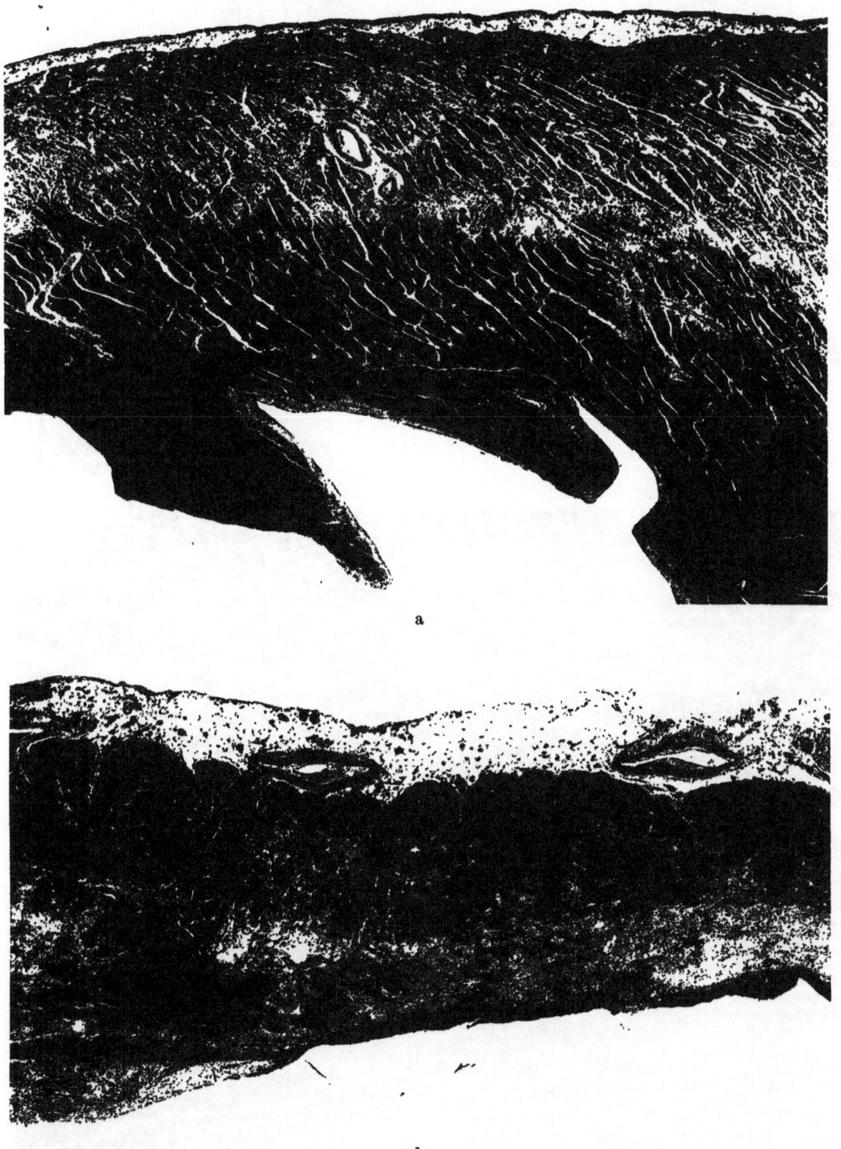

Abb. 5a u. b. a Akuter Vorderwandinfarkt der linken Herzkammer. Obere Bildhälfte (grau): erhaltene äußere epikardnahe Ventrikelwand; untere Bildhälfte (schwarz-grau): Infarktnekrose in der inneren endokardnahen Ventrikelwand. b Vernarbter Vorderwandinfarkt des Herzens. Links von der Bildmitte Infarktnarbe vom Endokard (unten) bis zum Epikard (oben) reichend, sonst Narbe in der inneren Hälfte der Herzwand (grau). (Nach F. BÜCHNER, Spezielle Pathologie, 3. Aufl. 1960, Abb. 26 u. 27.)

Kranzarterien. Sind sie proximal oder in ihrem Verlauf stark stenosiert, so ist die Durchblutung des normalen Versorgungsgebietes der verschlossenen Arterie auf dem Umweg über Anastomosen nur sehr gering: es entwickelt sich

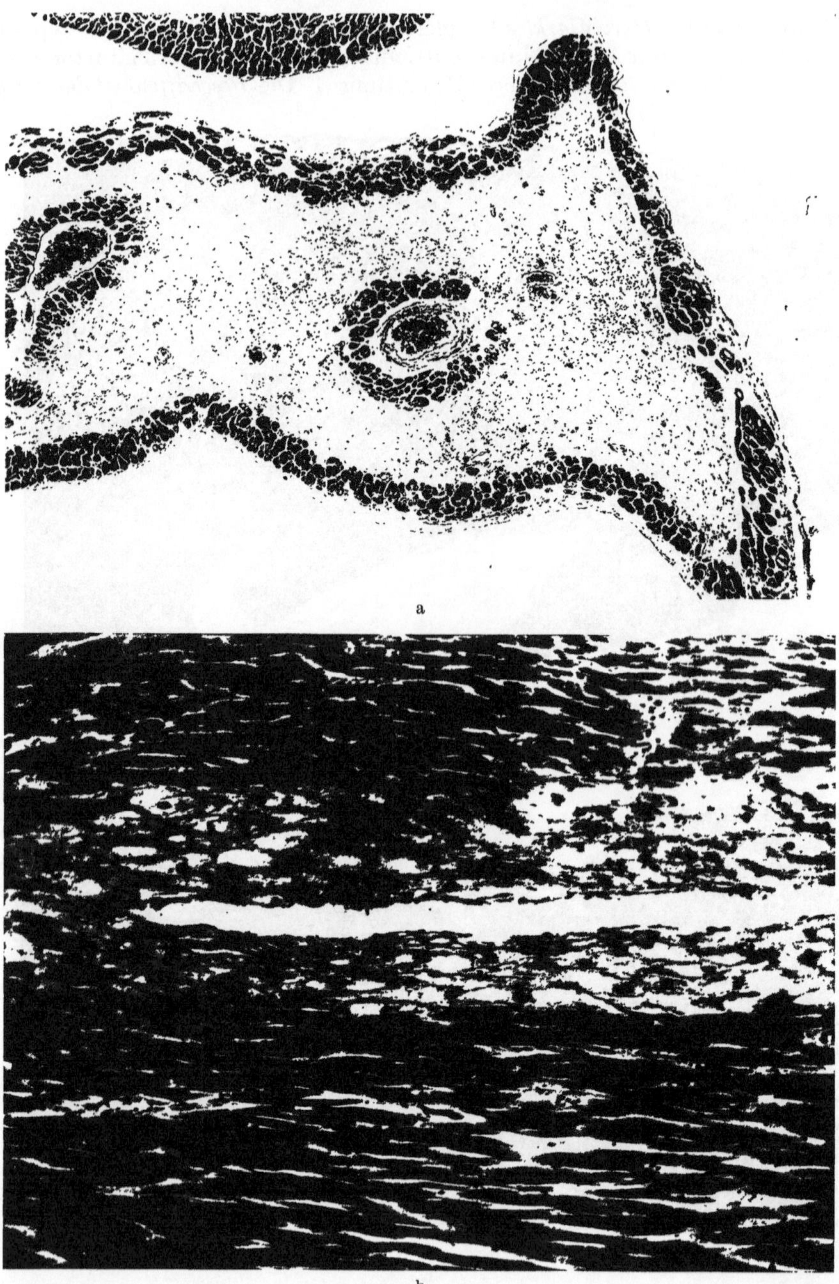

Abb. 6a u. b.   a Erhaltenbleiben einiger Lagen von Herzmuskelzellen (dunkel) subendokardial und perivenös in einer Herzinfarktnarbe (hellgrau).   b Erhaltene, aber stark ödematöse Herzmuskelzellen subendokardial (Mitte) in einer Infarktnekrose (oben und unten).

daher ein großer Infarkt[1]. Sind sie nicht oder nur wenig stenosiert, so ist eine gute Versorgung über Anastomosen mit den Nachbararterien möglich: es resultiert daher in der Regel ein kleinerer Infarkt[1]. 2. Die *durchschnittliche Belastung*

[1] Büchner, A. Weber und Haager 1935, Friedberg 1959.

des Herzens. Arbeitet der Herzmuskel bei Hypertrophie infolge Hypertonie oder Herzklappenfehler an der oberen Grenze seiner Durchblutungsfähigkeit oder hat er diese Grenze schon überschritten, so bewirkt ein hinzutretender Coronarverschluß einen großen Infarkt[1]. Umgekehrt stellen wir fest, daß in der Muskulatur des rechten Ventrikels auch bei Verschluß der ihn ernährenden rechten Kranzarterie durch Thrombose oder Embolie nur selten ein Infarkt eintritt[2]. Der Infarkt liegt in diesen Fällen fast gesetzmäßig im Terminalgebiet der rechten Coronararterie an der Hinterwand des *linken* Ventrikels. Diese Tatsache ist zum wesentlichen darauf zurückzuführen, daß der rechte Ventrikel in der Norm nur etwa $^1/_6$—$^1/_7$ der Druckarbeit des linken Ventrikels zu leisten hat. 3. Die *aktuelle Herzleistung beim thrombotischen oder embolischen Coronarverschluß.* Hütet der Kranke nach Auftreten der ersten Symptome nicht streng das Bett, so resultiert ein großer Infarkt, weil die noch durchgängigen Coronararterien durch ihr eigenes Versorgungsgebiet schon maximal beansprucht sind und für die Anastomosen nichts mehr verfügbar haben. Wird dagegen absolute Bettruhe eingehalten, so kann der Infarkt bei guter Durchgängigkeit der nicht verschlossenen Arterien und mäßiger durchschnittlicher Belastung des Herzmuskels klein bleiben.

Die *Wichtigkeit des jeweiligen Maßes der Kollateralversorgung* wird uns am Herzinfarkt nicht nur in der Flächen-, sondern auch in der Tiefenausdehnung veranschaulicht: bei einem Teil der Infarkte des Herzens beobachten wir nicht selten eine vom Endokard bis zum Epikard reichende Infarktnekrose (Abb. 5b). Bei anderen Infarkten ist dagegen recht häufig nur die innere endokardnahe Hälfte nekrotisch (Abb. 5a), dagegen die epikardnahe erhalten. Dieser Befund ist verständlich, da die Coronararterien vom Epikard her in das Myokard eindringen und in den endokardnahen Schichten ihr Ende finden. Die epikardnahen Myokard-Schichten können daher in günstigen Fällen noch von Anastomosen aus benachbarten Coronararterien mit versorgt werden, nicht dagegen die endokardnahen.

Auch am Hirninfarkt ist der Zustand der übrigen Arterien und damit die Möglichkeit einer Kollateralversorgung von großer Bedeutung. Liegt bei arteriosklerotischer Thrombose der einen A. cerebri media ein arteriosklerotisch stenosiertes extracerebrales Arteriensystem des Gehirns vor, so ist die Kollateralversorgung sehr erschwert und es entwickelt sich in der Regel ein größerer Infarkt. Auch der Zustand des Gesamtkreislaufs, insbesondere das Vorliegen oder das Hinzutreten einer Insuffizienz des linken Ventrikels oder eines peripheren Kollaps bewirkt die Entwicklung eines großen Hirninfarktes[3].

Wie entscheidend für die Entstehung der Infarktnekrose die mangelnde Zufuhr von Sauerstoff und Glucose ist, geht aus 2 charakteristischen Aussparungen in der Nekrose des Herzinfarktes hervor (Abb. 6a und b). Da die Venen im Infarktbereich noch durchströmt werden, können einige Lagen von Herzmuskelzellen rings um die Venenwand durch Diffusion weiter ernährt werden. Sie bleiben daher häufig mitten im Infarkt erhalten, zeigen aber nicht selten feinere Veränderungen ihres Cytoplasmas, insbesondere ein Ödem oder eine Fibrillolyse[4] (Abb. 6a). Ebenso können einige Lagen der innersten Schichten des Myokards vom linken Ventrikel her durch Diffusion versorgt werden, ebenfalls aber die erwähnten Veränderungen des Cytoplasmas erkennen lassen[5] (Abb. 6b).

Die Kollateralversorgung von Organbezirken, die in der Norm von der embolisch oder thrombotisch verschlossenen Arterie ernährt werden, ist besonders bei dem

---

[1] FRIEDBERG 1959.

[2] BÜCHNER, A. WEBER und HAAGER 1935, WARTMANN und HELLERSTEIN 1948 4:160, SAPHIR, PRIEST und Mitarbeiter 1935.

[3] MEESSEN und STOCHDORPH 1957.   [4] BÜCHNER und WEYLAND 1955, SARAM 1957.

[5] LINZBACH 1950, BÜCHNER und WEYLAND 1959.

akuten Herzinfarkt sowie bei dem akuten Infarkt des Gehirns auch dann, wenn
sie aus den anderen nicht verschlossenen Arterien wirksam wurde, zunächst noch
sehr bedroht. Jede akute Mehrbelastung des Herzens, z.B. durch Aufstehen
des Infarktkranken oder schon durch eine mühsame Defäkation, bei der die
normalen Versorgungsbereiche der nicht verschlossenen Herzarterien reichlich Blut benötigen, kann zu einer akuten Insuffizienz der Kollateralversorgung
führen. Die Folge ist dann die Vergrößerung des ursprünglichen Infarktes durch
eine neue Nekroseschale. Klinisch führt dieser *Reinfarkt* erneut zu akuten Infarkt-
zeichen, z.B. zum Wiederanstieg der Transaminase im Blutserum[1] und zu den
typischen Zeichen des Infarktes im Elektrokardiogramm. Auch Hirninfarkte
können durch Mehrbelastung des Organs oder durch hinzutretende Herzinsuffizienz in Schüben wachsen. Die Insuffizienz des linken Ventrikels kann auch beim
Herzinfarkt Ursache einer Infarktvergrößerung sein. So hat der Arzt vieles an
Möglichkeiten in der Hand, durch absolute Ruhighaltung des Kranken und
Stützung seines Kreislaufes Infarkte klein zu halten, während körperliche und
seelische Belastungen besonders den großen Infarkt fördern.

2. Die temporäre absolute arterielle Ischämie.

Von besonderem Interesse für die Frage der Relation von Struktur-, Funktions-
und Stoffwechselstörung nach absoluter Ischämie sind neuere Untersuchungen
über die Wirkung der *temporären Ischämie* an parenchymatösen Organen. Die
Anfälligkeit der verschiedenen Parenchyme gegenüber temporärer absoluter
arterieller Ischämie ist dabei sehr verschieden. Besonders eingehend wurde sie
am *Zentralnervensystem*, vor allem am Gehirn, untersucht. Hier hat Opitz 1952,
1953 einige Grundbegriffe herausgearbeitet, die für die temporäre arterielle
Ischämie aller parenchymatösen Organe von Bedeutung sind: die *Lähmungszeit*,
d.h. die Zeit vom Beginn der Ischämie bis zum Erlöschen der spezifischen Organ-
funktion, die *Erholungszeit*, d.h. die Zeit, innerhalb derer nach Einsetzen der
Lähmung bei wieder normaler Durchblutung das Parenchym sich wieder erholt,
die *Wiederbelebungszeit*[2], d.h. die Dauer der Ischämie, nach der eben noch eine
Wiederbelebung des Parenchyms möglich ist, die *Manifestationszeit*, d.h. die Zeit
vom Eintritt der irreversiblen Schädigung bis zu deren lichtmikroskopischer
Manifestierung. Am *Hirn* sind diese Zeiten ungewöhnlich kurz. So beträgt die
Lähmungszeit, gemessen am Erlöschen der cerebralen Reflexe und der Spontan-
potentiale im EEG, etwa 1 min[3]. Die Wiederbelebungszeit ist nach Experimenten an Katze oder Hund mit temporärer Abklemmung der A. pulmonalis für die
empfindlichsten Nervenzellen des Hirns mit wenig mehr als 3 min zu befristen[4].
Wir selbst sahen nach kurzfristiger Drosselung der Blutzufuhr zum Hirn durch
Halsmanschette von 4 min Dauer bei der Katze schon ein schweres Zellödem und
Nekrosen an Purkinjezellen des Kleinhirns und an Ganglienzellen der Großhirnrinde[5]. Ähnlich schnell wurden Nervenzellnekrosen an der Groß- und Kleinhirnrinde und am Stammhirn des Menschen durch temporär völlige Unterbrechung
des Kreislaufs infolge großer Lungenembolie bei zunächst gelungener Trendelenburgscher Operation in Groß- und Kleinhirnrinde und Hirnstamm beobachtet[6].
Morphologisch stehen am Hirn bei diesen kurzfristigen temporären Ischämien
elektive Parenchymnekrosen ganz im Vordergrund[7], wie sie auch für die akuten
Hypoxydosen an den Parenchymen kennzeichnend sind[8].

---

[1] Forster 1958.   [2] Sugar und Gerard 1938.   [3] Opitz 1952, 1953.
[4] Weinberger, Gibbon und Gibbon 1940, Grenell 1946.   [5] Höfler, vgl. Büchner 1957.
[6] Nystrom 1930, Wustmann und Hallervorden 1935.
[7] Scholz 1949, 1953, 1957.   [8] Büchner 1932, 1939, 1944, 1957.

Am *Herzmuskel* konnte experimentell festgestellt werden, daß eine temporäre Ischämie durch Ligatur einer Coronararterie von 5—20 min Dauer noch keine Nekrose verursacht[1]. Wurde dagegen die 20 min-Grenze überschritten, so entstand eine Infarktnekrose, meist ein massiver Infarkt. Während die Infarktnekrose im Experiment erst nach 28 Std manifest wurde[2], konnte schon in den ersten Stunden fermenthistochemisch eine wesentliche Verringerung des Gehaltes des Herzmuskels an Bernsteinsäure-Dehydrogenase nachgewiesen werden[3].

Noch aufschlußreicher sind die von OPITZ, WG. ROTTER und HILSCHER 1953 inaugurierten Untersuchungen über die temporäre Ischämie der *Niere*.

In diesen Experimenten ergab sich, daß an der Ratte nach temporärer Ischämie der Niere von 10—90 min und wechselnd langer Überlebenszeit nach Lösen der Ligatur (einige Stunden, 1 Tag, 4 Tage) am Hauptstückepithel der Niere fermenthistochemisch in kurzer Zeit eine Verringerung oder ein Schwund der Bernsteinsäure-Dehydrogenase, der alkalischen und der sauren Phosphatase zu beobachten war. Dabei reagierte die Bernsteinsäure-Dehydrogenase am empfindlichsten[4]. Im übrigen erschien das Epithel bei den üblichen lichtmikroskopischen Untersuchungen noch normal. Erst genaue Messungen ergaben eine signifikante Schwellung des Epithels[5]. Als besonders feiner Test für die Einschränkung der Resorptionsleistung dieser Epithelien durch temporäre Ischämie erwies sich in diesen Versuchen die Trypanblauspeicherung, in den neuesten Experimenten[5] auch die Speicherung von Hühnereiweiß: Das normale Hauptstückepithel zeigt nach subcutaner Injektion eine lebhafte Speicherung von Trypanblau oder Hühnereiweiß, mit gesteigerter Ischämiedauer wird diese Speicherung immer geringer. Nach 10 min Ischämie ist die Trypanblauspeicherung nach einem Tag kaum eingeschränkt, nach 20 min Ischämie um 10—15%, nach 40 min Ischämie um 35—40%, nach 60 min Ischämie um 75%. Sie erlischt nach einer Ischämie von 90 min mit einer Überlebenszeit von 1—4 Tagen[6]. Dabei sind allerdings nach 90 min zahlreiche Hauptstückepithelien nekrotisch.

Auch die *Skeletmuskulatur* war Gegenstand gleichsinniger Versuche[7].

An Albinoratten wurde die hintere Extremität für 3—4 Std temporär abgeschnürt; die Tiere wurden 1—28 Tage nach Lösung der Sperre getötet. Sie zeigten herdförmig kleine Muskelfasernekrosen und diffus eine metrisch faßbare Schwellung der Muskelfasern als Ausdruck einer postischämischen energetisch-osmotischen Insuffizienz der Muskelzellen[8]. Histochemisch war auch hier ein Enzymverlust nachweisbar, der für die Bernsteinsäuredehydrogenase und für die alkalische Phosphatase geprüft wurde. Am empfindlichsten reagierte auch hier die Bernsteinsäuredehydrogenase: sie nahm mit einer Latenzzeit von 4 Tagen nach der Ischämie ab und erreichte ein Maximum der Abnahme nach 7—14 Tagen. Der Enzymschwund konnte von einer Atrophie gefolgt sein. Untersuchungen mit der PAS-Reaktion ergaben eine länger dauernde Verminderung der Polysaccharide bis zu völligem Glykogenschwund. Mit chemischer Methodik war schon früher nach 4stündiger temporärer Ischämie ein Schwund von Glykogen, ATP und Phosphokreatin festgestellt worden[9].

Fassen wir die Ergebnisse der dargelegten Untersuchungen über die absolute arterielle Ischämie noch einmal zusammen, so ergeben sich die folgenden Regeln:

1. Wird eine Arterie thrombotisch, embolisch oder durch Ligatur verschlossen, so kann die Versorgung über kollaterale Anastomosen irreversible Veränderungen verhüten. In der Regel kommt es aber bei Unzulänglichkeit von Anastomosen oder bei anspruchsvollerem Organstoffwechsel oder durch das Zusammenwirken beider Faktoren im Versorgungsgebiet der verschlossenen Arterie zu einem mehr oder minder großen Infarkt.

2. Plötzliche Arterienverschlüsse führen eher zum Infarkt als langsame.

3. Die Infarktnekrose betrifft gleichmäßig das Parenchym und das Mesenchym des ischämischen Gebietes.

4. An Herzmuskel und Hirn wird die Größe des Infarktes mitbestimmt von dem Zustand des gesamten Systems der basalen Hirnarterien bzw. der Coronararterien, von der aktuellen Belastung des Gesamtorgans, vom Zustand des gesamten Kreislaufs.

---

[1] BLUMGART, GILLIGAN und SCHLESINGER 1941.
[2] TENNANT, GRAYZEL und Mitarbeiter 1936.   [3] WACHSTEIN und MEISEL 1955.
[4] ZIMMERMANN 1957, SCHLAGETTER und ZIMMERMANN 1957.
[5] ZIMMERMANN, SONNEKALB und WATZ 1960.
[6] ZIMMERMANN 1957, ZIMMERMANN, SONNEKALB und WATZ 1959.
[7] ZIMMERMANN und SCHLEIFER 1959.   [8] Vgl. auch ROTTER 1958, 1959.
[9] HARMAN 1947, HARMAN und GWINN 1949.

5. Eine nur temporäre absolute arterielle Ischämie führt in der Regel nicht zum Infarkt, sondern nach genügend langer Dauer der Ischämie zu disseminierten elektiven Parenchymnekrosen. Dabei besteht eine Empfindlichkeitsskala Hirn, Rückenmark, Herzmuskel, Skeletmuskel, Niere.

6. Die unterschwellige, nicht zur Nekrose führende temporäre arterielle Ischämie manifestiert sich vor allem in der histochemisch nachweisbaren Herabsetzung des Enzymgehaltes, besonders der Bernsteinsäure-Dehydrogenase, an der Niere auch in der Herabsetzung der Speicherungsfunktion der Tubulus-Epithelien.

7. Die akute temporäre arterielle Ischämie führt akut zu einer Verwässerung der zugeordneten Parenchymzellen als Folge einer energetisch-osmotischen Insuffizienz dieser Zellen. Diese Zellveränderung kann die nachfolgende Nekrose einleiten, aber auch in Verbindung mit der Enzymschädigung von einer reversiblen oder irreversiblen Parenchymatrophie gefolgt sein.

Die relative arterielle Ischämie.

Relative Einschränkungen der arteriellen Durchblutung gehören zu den häufigsten Ereignissen in der menschlichen Pathologie. In den meisten Fällen liegen ihnen chronische oder subakute organische Arterienwandveränderungen infolge generalisierter, seltener infolge lokalisierter Arterienerkrankungen zugrunde. Diese Arterienveränderungen werden dann im Sinne einer relativen arteriellen Ischämie wirksam, wenn sie an den Organarterien und ihren Verzweigungen mehr oder minder starke Stenosen setzen. Die Arteriosklerose, die hypertonisch verursachte Arteriolosklerose, die Arteriolonekrose infolge maligner Hypertonie, die Endarteriitis obliterans Winiwarter-Bürger, die Panarteriitis nodosa, die Coronarstenosen bei Mesaortitis syphilitica, die Endarteriitis syphilitica der Hirnarterien, die Wegenersche Arteriitis[1] sind hier zu nennen.

1. Die chronische relative arterielle Ischämie.

Bei den meisten dieser Erkrankungen entwickeln sich die arteriellen Stenosen allmählich. So ist es verständlich, daß sie in einer großen Gruppe ihrer Manifestierungen keine Nekrosen verursachen, sondern *Parenchymatrophien mit mesenchymaler Hyalinisierung und Sklerosierung.*

Im Experiment können wir bei langsam sich steigernder Drosselung einer Nierenarterie diese relative Ischämie an der *Niere* beobachten. So sehen wir z.B. nach Einhüllung der Niere in eine Stoffkapsel eine zunehmende hyalinsklerotische Verdickung der Glomerula und der Bowmanschen Kapseln bis zur totalen Hyalinisierung und Verödung der Malpighischen Körperchen, eine starke Atrophie der Hauptstücke und eine Sklerosierung des Interstitiums[2].

Die gleichen Veränderungen sind uns in der menschlichen Pathologie geläufig als Folge arteriosklerotischer Stenosen an den intrarenalen Arterien. Sie finden sich im Bilde der gebuckelten arteriosklerotischen Schrumpfniere, ebenso aber als Folge arteriolosklerotischer Stenosen der Vasa afferentia bei der granulierten arteriolosklerotischen Schrumpfniere, infolge starker Stenose des Stammes der A. renalis bei der total geschrumpften arteriosklerotischen Schrumpfniere, als Folge hydronephrotischer Ischämisierung der Niere bei der hydronephrotischen und der nephrohydrotischen Schrumpfniere. In unvollständiger Form können wir sie bei Schrumpfniere durch Panarteriitis nodosa der Nieren beobachten[3]. Hier begegnen uns landkartenartig gefleckte, dunkle, flach eingezogene Herde,

---

[1] Wegener 1939, Fahey, Leonhard und Mitarbeiter 1954, Altmann und Schiche 1959.
[2] Iijima 1958.   [3] Staemmler 1955, Suchenwirth 1956.

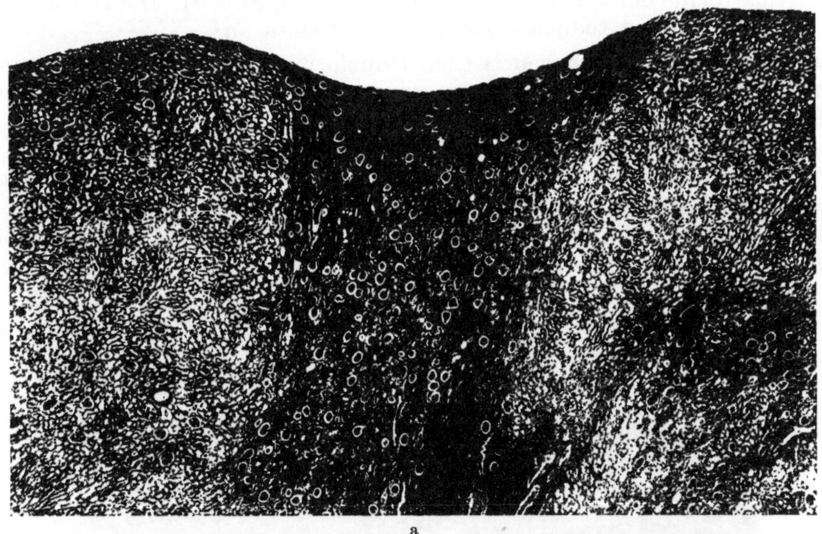

a

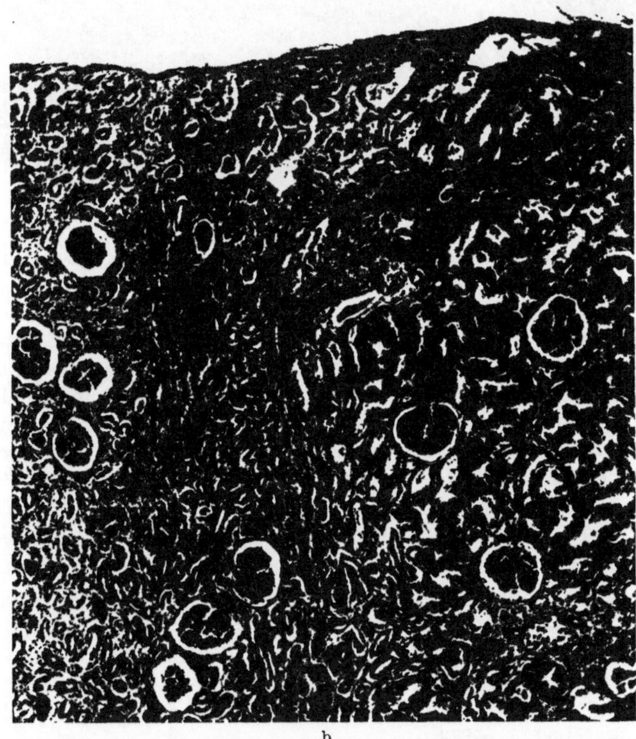

b

Abb. 7a u. b. Unvollkommener Niereninfarkt bei Panarteriitis nodosa. a Schwache Vergrößerung, b Ausschnitt aus a: Links blutgefüllte, etwas atrophische Glomerula, von atrophischen, aber erhaltenen Tubuli umgeben. [Nach R. SUCHENWIRTH, Beitr. path. Anat. 116, 1956, Abb. 5 u. 6.]

die als *„unvollkommene Infarkte"* bezeichnet wurden, mit beginnender hyalin-sklerotischer Umwandlung und Verkleinerung der Glomerula und schon deutlicher

Parenchymatrophie der Hauptstücke (Abb. 7a und b, Abb. 8). Die Herde deuten sich schon bei subakut tödlicher Panarteriitis nodosa an[1].

Nach dem gleichen pathogenetischen Prinzip müssen wir die Veränderungen an den *Inseln des Pankreas* deuten, wie wir sie am häufigsten bei Arteriosklerose oder bei hypertonischer Arteriolosklerose, gelegentlich aber auch bei Panarteriitis nodosa als Folge arterieller Stenosen sehen: Das feine Retikulinfasergerüst der Inseln wird hyalinisiert oder sklerosiert, die Parenchymzellen der Inseln atrophieren oder schwinden.

Diesen kurz skizzierten Bildern sind häufig *schleichend sich entwickelnde Funktionsstörungen* der Nieren bzw. des Inselsystems zugeordnet. An der Niere

Abb. 8. Schrumpfniere mit unvollkommenen Infarkten bei Panarteriitis nodosa, gleicher Fall wie Abb. 7. [Nach R. Suchenwirth, Beitr. path. Anat. 116, 1956, Abb. 4.]

werden bei doppelseitiger Erkrankung je nach der Ausdehnung der Veränderungen die Filtrationsleistung der Glomerula und die Sekretions-Rückresorptionsleistungen der Hauptstücke beeinträchtigt. So kann es bei arteriolosklerotischer, hydronephrotischer und panarteriitischer Schrumpfniere zur schleichenden Urämie kommen, lange vorher aber schon durch Insuffizienz der Wasserrückresorption und damit der Konzentrationsleistung in den Hauptstücken zur Polyurie und zur Isosthenurie. Am Pankreas kann die Veränderung der Inseln bei genügender Ausdehnung eine Insuffizienz der Insulinbildung hervorrufen. Sie kann wesentliche Ursache des arteriosklerotischen und des hypertonischen Diabetes sein.

Dabei können wir bei den arteriosklerotischen und arteriolosklerotischen Stenosen im Pankreas eindrucksvoll die *Bedeutung einer zusätzlichen allgemeinen Oligämie* für den Grad bzw. das Manifestwerden der Inselinsuffizienz beobachten. Seit langem ist es den Internisten bekannt, daß beim akuten Herzinfarkt eine Hyperglykämie mit Glykosurie auftreten kann, unabhängig davon, ob vorher ein Diabetes diagnostiziert wurde[2].

In einer besonderen Untersuchungsreihe wurden 14 Kranke mit Herzinfarkt ohne Diabetes-Anamnese wiederholt einer Glucosebelastung ausgesetzt. Sechs erwiesen sich als manifeste Diabetiker, 4 zeigten abnorme Belastungskurven[3].

---

[1] Suchenwirth 1956.   [2] Levine und Brown 1929.
[3] Goldberger, Alesio und Woll 1945.

Die nächstliegende Deutung dieser Beobachtungen ist unseres Erachtens die, daß bei der Einschränkung des Schlag- und Minutenvolumens und dem Absinken des Blutdruckes infolge des Herzinfarktes die vorher schon bestehenden arteriellen

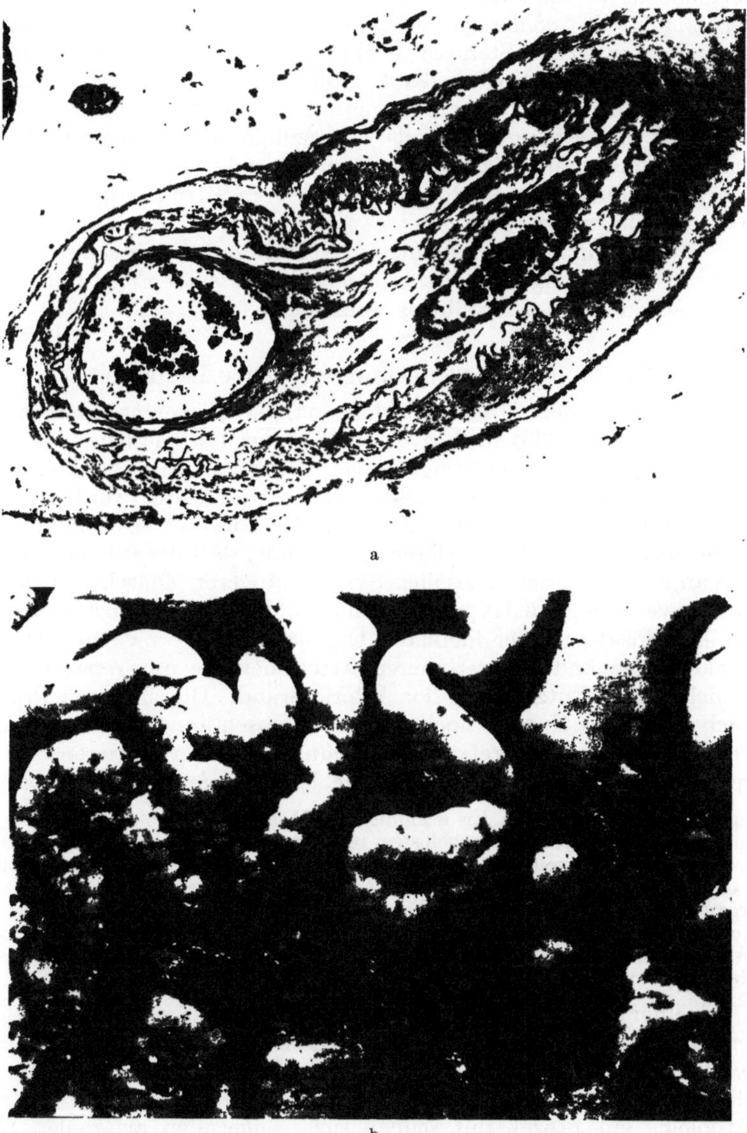

Abb. 9a u. b. a Endarteriitis obliterans einer kleinen Arterie der Leptomeninx an der Konvexität. b Granular-atrophie einiger Hirnwindungen (linke Bildhälfte) infolge Endarteriitis obliterans der vorgeordneten kleinen Arterien der Leptomeninx (nach H. NOETZEL).

Stenosen im Pankreas an den noch funktionstüchtigen Inseln Durchblutungs- und Funktionsinsuffizienzen hervorrufen.

Besonderheiten zeigen die Auswirkungen chronischer relativer arterieller Ischämien am *Hirn*. Hier kann die stenosierende Arteriosklerose der basalen Hirnarterien zu einer *schleichenden Atrophie der Großhirnrinde* führen. Diese ist

durch die Atrophie und den partiellen Schwund der Ganglienzellen der Großhirnrinde ohne Gliafaservermehrung gekennzeichnet. In der Regel entwickelt
sie sich gleichmäßig am ganzen Großhirn, bevorzugt jedoch am Stirnhirn. Sie
ist das morphologische Äquivalent der arteriosklerotischen Altersdemenz.

Bei der *Endarteriitis obliterans* der kleinen Arterien der Hirnkonvexität bewirken die endarteriitischen Stenosen fleckförmige Atrophien der Großhirnrinde
im terminalen Versorgungsbereich der 3 großen Hirnarterien (Abb. 9a und b).
So entstehen grübchenförmige Vertiefungen an der Großhirnrinde mit Ganglien-
zellschwund und Gliawucherung in der Grenzlinie der Versorgungsfelder der
A. cerebri media und anterior bzw. der A. c. media und posterior. Diese Granular-
atrophie ordnet sich in einer sichelförmigen Linie vom Stirnhirn über das Parietal-
hirn zum Occipitalhirn an[1].

Bei der *Panarteriitis nodosa* können die Stenosen meningealer und intracerebraler Arterienaufzweigungen zu *unregelmäßigen kleinherdigen Entmarkungen*,
vor allem im Marklager des Großhirns, führen[2].

2. Die akute stenosenbedingte relative Ischämie.

In einer grundlegenden Studie über die maligne Hypertonie haben SCHÜR-
MANN und MCMAHON (1933) nachgewiesen, daß bei der malignen, schnell sich
steigernden Hypertonie, die bevorzugt jüngere Menschen unter 50 Jahren befällt,
in der Regel Nekrosen parenchymatöser Organe beobachtet werden, besonders
an den Nieren, am Pankreas, an der Leber, am Herzmuskel. Die Befunde fanden
vielfach ihre Bestätigung. Sie erklären sich damit, daß die schnell ansteigende
Hypertonie an dem zarteren arteriellen System jüngerer Menschen nicht wie bei
den langsamer verlaufenden Hypertonien das Bild der Arteriolosklerose und der
peripheren Arteriosklerose der kleineren Organarterien verursacht, sondern das
der Arteriolonekrose und der peripheren Arterionekrose mit reparativer leuko-
zytär-mesenchymaler Entzündung der Arterienwand. Durch diesen Prozeß entwickeln sich in kurzer Zeit so hochgradige Stenosen im peripheren arteriellen
System, daß schwere akute relative Ischämien daraus resultieren. Als deren
Folgen treten im zugeordneten Versorgungsgebiet *multiple Parenchymnekrosen* auf.

Im Zuge der experimentellen Erforschung des Hartwich-Goldblatt-Effektes, d.h. der
Erzeugung einer renin-hypertensinausgelösten renalen Hypertonie durch Drosselung einer
Nierenarterie, meist an der weißen Ratte, kann der Anstieg des Blutdruckes so steil und hoch
sein, daß daraus das Bild einer ausgebreiteten Arteriolonekrose und Arterionekrose der
kleinen Organarterien resultiert, das letztere mit Arterienwandveränderungen wie bei Panarteriitis nodosa des Menschen. Dieser Prozeß führt in kurzer Zeit zu hochgradigen arteriellen
Stenosen und in deren Gefolge zu Nekrosen parenchymatöser Organe z.B. an der Darmwand
oder am Herzmuskel[3].

Auch bei einer schnell fortschreitenden Panarteriitis nodosa des Menschen
können entsprechende stenosebedingte Nekrosen beobachtet werden, z.B. multiple Kleininfarkte an der Niere[4].

Von diesen und wenigen anderen Beispielen abgesehen, ist aber in der menschlichen Pathologie ein Prozeß mit schnell sich steigernden arteriellen Stenosen
selten die Ursache so schwerer akuter Ischämien, daß multiple Nekrosen parenchymatöser Organe die Folge sind. Dagegen können langsam sich entwickelnde
arterielle Stenosen an einigen Organen dann zur *akuten paroxysmalen relativen
arteriellen Ischämie* führen, wenn das von arteriellen Stenosen befallene Organ
starken Belastungsschwankungen ausgesetzt ist. Die Ruhedurchblutung kann an

---

[1] LINDENBERG und SPATZ 1939, NOETZEL und THEODOSSIOU 1957, EICKE 1957, WILDI 1959.
[2] WALTHARD und WALTHARD 1957, MARTIN und NOETZEL 1959.
[3] SUWA 1959.   [4] SUCHENWIRTH 1956.

solchen Organen trotz bestehender Stenosen noch völlig ausreichend sein. *Insuffizient wird die Durchblutung erst, wenn bei akuter Organbelastung aus verschiedener Ursache der Blutbedarf des Organes so ansteigt, daß er infolge der Stenosen nicht mehr gedeckt werden kann.* Die relative arterielle Ischämie tritt also *im Anfall* auf, der bei bestehenden arteriellen Stenosen erst durch die Belastung des Organes ausgelöst wird.

Ein klassisches Beispiel einer solchen paroxysmalen relativen arteriellen Ischämie ist der *Anfall von intermittierendem Hinken durch akute relative Ischämie der Beinarterien.* Der Anfall ist seit langem als typische Manifestierung einer stenosierenden Arteriosklerose, ebenso aber auch einer stenosierenden Endarteriitis obliterans Winiwarter-Bürger der Beinarterien bekannt. Beim Sitzen und Stehen und beim langsamen Gehen im Kurschritt ist bei diesen Kranken die Durchblutung der Beinmuskulatur noch suffizient. Sobald sie schneller gehen oder steigen, kommen sie dagegen infolge akut gesteigerten Blutbedarfes ihrer Beinmuskeln in einen Zustand der Durchblutungsinsuffizienz der unteren Extremitäten. Die akute relative arterielle Ischämie verursacht eine akute Störung des Muskelstoffwechsels und dadurch eine krankhafte Erregung der sensorischen Fasern der Beinmuskulatur. Dadurch wird ein sich steigernder Schmerz ausgelöst, der bei genügender Heftigkeit den Kranken zum Hinken und

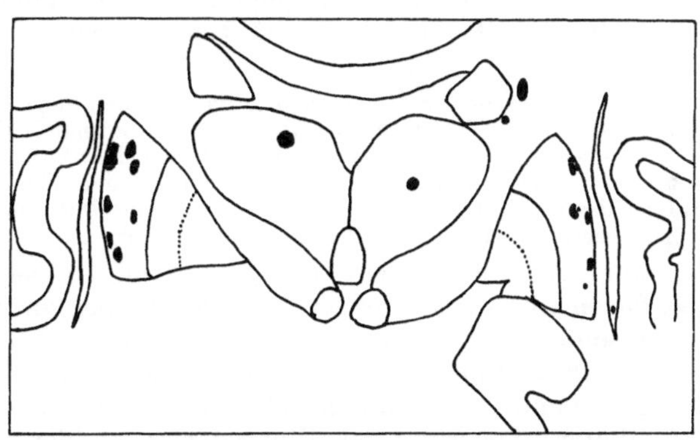

Abb. 10. Skizze einer Frontalstufe des Gehirns bei 74jähriger Frau mit genuiner Hypertonie. Histologisch gesicherte lakunäre Nekrosen infolge arteriosklerotischer Stenosen intracerebraler kleiner Arterien, besonders im Putamen beiderseits. [Nach H. WIRTZ, Beitr. path. Anat. **97**, 1936, Abb. 10.]

schließlich zum Stehenbleiben nötigt. Indem er auf diese Weise die Bewegung einstellt und der Blutbedarf in den Beinmuskeln sich verringert, wird die Durchblutung wieder suffizient, so daß in wenigen Minuten der Schmerz erlischt.

Im Selbstversuch[1] wurde dieser Anfall an der oberen Extremität reproduziert: Drosselten die Untersucher[1] durch den Blutdruckapparat partiell die A. brachialis, so konnten sie durch systematische aktive Bewegung der Unterarmmuskulatur einen schließlich unerträglich heftigen Schmerz auslösen, der nach Einstellen der Bewegung wieder nachließ und verschwand.

Systematische Untersuchungen über die Histologie der Beinmuskeln nach intermittierendem Hinken liegen bisher nicht vor. In Einzelbeobachtungen konnten wir (1939) postnekrotische Narben in der Wadenmuskulatur nachweisen, die wir als Spuren der durchgemachten Anfälle akuter relativer Ischämie deuten.

Anfälle relativer arterieller Ischämien des Gehirns begegnen uns bei der Arteriosklerose der Hirnarterien des Normotonikers und des Hypertonikers. Hier bestehen beim Normotoniker Stenosen an den basalen Hirnarterien des Circulus arteriosus Willisi, beim Hypertoniker zusätzlich, vorherrschend oder ausschließlich Stenosen an den intracerebralen Hirnarterien[2]. Infolge dieser Stenosen kann es vor allem in bestimmten Grisea des Hirns anfallsweise zu akuten Durchblutungsstörungen kommen, besonders im Striatum (Nucleus caudatus und

---

[1] WILLIAM und WEBSTER 1923, LEWIS, PICKERING und ROTHSCHILD 1931.
[2] ANDERS und EICKE 1939, 1940, SCHOLZ und NIETO 1938, SCHIMKAT und KATHKE 1958.

Putamen des Linsenkerns) (Abb. 10), im Thalamus opticus, in grauen Bezirken der Brücke und in Kleinhirnkernen[1]. Die Folge sind ischämische Nekrosen, die in der akuten Phase von perifokalem Ödem begleitet sind und dadurch zu partiellen Blockierungen der Pyramidenbahnen führen. So kommt es zu partiellen Halbseitenlähmungen, z.B. des Gesichts, des Armes, des Beines, d.h. zum *apoplektischen Insult.* Da die Ödeme schnell wieder resorbiert werden, sind die Lähmungen flüchtig und in der Regel nur auf Bruchteile einer Stunde oder auf wenige Minuten beschränkt. Beim Hypertoniker können sich die Nekrosen und damit der apoplektische Insult in der Phase einer vorübergehenden, mitunter therapeutisch herbeigeführten Blutdrucksenkung entwickeln[2]. Durch Anfälle akuter, arteriosklerotisch-arteriolosklerotischer, relativer Ischämie der Großhirnrinde können bei Hypertonikern flüchtige Bewußtlosigkeiten oder leichte Absencen beobachtet werden.

Die Gefährlichkeit einer plötzlich einsetzenden Blutdrucksenkung und Oligämie bei bestehenden Stenosen von Hirnarterien geht aus folgenden Experimenten hervor[3]:

Bei Affen wurde die A. carotis interna der einen Seite bis auf $1/5$ der ursprünglichen Lichtung gedrosselt. Trotzdem wurde noch ein normales Elektrencephalogramm registriert. Wurde aber durch Blutentnahme eine Blutdrucksenkung und eine allgemeine Oligämie gesetzt, so zeigte die zur gedrosselten A. carotis gehörende Hirnhemisphäre typische Veränderungen des EEG. Wurde das vorher entnommene Blut reinfundiert und der Blutdruck wieder normalisiert, so wurde auch das EEG wieder normal.

Auf der anderen Seite begegnen dem Kliniker immer wieder solche Fälle, bei denen eine starke psychische Erregung bei vorbestehender cerebraler Arteriosklerose des Normotonikers oder des Hypertonikers dadurch akut zum apoplektischen Insult führt, daß sie den Stoffwechsel des Gehirns akut auf das Dreifache steigern kann[4]. Die infolge der Stenose ungenügende Blutzufuhr zum Gehirn bei akuter Steigerung des Blutbedarfes ist hier die Ursache der Entwicklung kleiner Parenchymnekrosen in den Stammganglien mit perifokalem Ödem[5].

Ähnliche Anfälle und Nekrosen werden bei der Hypertonie verschiedenen Ursprungs *an der Retina* beobachtet: infolge stenosierender Arteriosklerose und Arteriolosklerose der Retinaarterien kommt es hier morphologisch zu Nekrose und Ödem, klinisch zu partiellen zum Teil reversiblen Gesichtsfeldausfällen[6].

Die akute Coronarinsuffizienz bei Coronarstenosen.

Am eindringlichsten wird uns die pathogenetische Bedeutung des stenosebedingten Anfalles akuter relativer arterieller Ischämie am Herzmuskel im Anfall akuter Coronarinsuffizienz vor Augen geführt. Die Entdeckung dieses Phänomens und seine systematische Durcharbeitung war möglich gemacht, nachdem die Physiologie des Coronarkreislaufs geklärt war. Hier hatten zuerst Hochrein und Keller (1931) und besonders Rein (1931) festgestellt, daß die Coronardurchblutung bei akuter Belastung des Herzmuskels durch körperliche Arbeit akut ansteigt und nach Beendigung der Arbeit in kurzer Frist wieder auf den Normwert sinkt. Dabei nimmt während der akuten Leistungssteigerung des Herzmuskels zunächst die Sauerstoffutilisation im Herzmuskel zu, die Sauerstoffspannung also im venösen Blut des Herzmuskels ab. Diese Senkung der Sauerstoffspannung im venösen Coronarblut löst die Erweiterung und Mehrdurchblutung des Coronarsystems aus. Auch die primäre Senkung der Sauerstoff-

<hr>

[1] Böhne 1927, 1931, Hiller 1935, 1936, Wirtz 1936, Meessen und Stochdorph 1957, Stochdorph und Meessen 1957.
[2] Vgl. Pierach und Heynemann 1959.   [3] Corday, Rothenberg und Putnam 1953.
[4] Max Schneider 1958.   [5] Vgl. Pierach und Heynemann 1959.
[6] de la Fontaine 1927, Aschoff 1934, Liebegott 1957, Marquardt 1957, 1958.

spannung bewirkt eine Zunahme der Coronardurchblutung, die um so steiler ansteigt, je tiefer die Sauerstoffspannung sinkt. *Die Sauerstoffspannung des Coronarblutes ist also der wichtigste regulierende Faktor für den Coronarkreislauf*[1]. Daneben modifiziert der mittlere Aortendruck die Coronardurchblutung: sein Anstieg fördert den Coronarkreislauf, sein Abfall schränkt ihn ein[2].

Nach den Beobachtungen von HOCHREIN und KELLER (1931) sowie von REIN (1931) war zu erwarten, daß bei stenosierender Coronarsklerose oder bei Stenose der Kranzaderabgänge durch Mesaortitis syphilitica akute Mehrbelastungen des Herzmuskels und der dadurch gesteigerte Mehrbedarf von Blut im Herzmuskel Anfälle relativer akuter arterieller Ischämie auslösen und daß diese

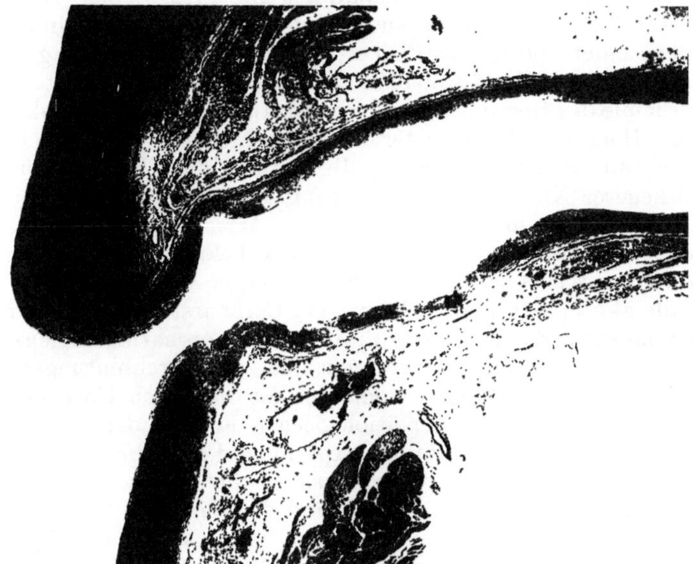

Abb. 11. Starke Stenose des Abganges einer Coronararterie durch Syphilis der Aorta, Coronararterie selbst nicht stenosiert. (Nach F. BÜCHNER, Die Koronarinsuffizienz, 1939, Abb. 10.)

Anfälle bei genügender Intensität und Dauer zu akuten Nekrosen im Herzmuskelparenchym führen müßten. Die systematische histotopographische Stufenuntersuchung des Herzmuskels von Verstorbenen nach Anfällen relativer Ischämie des Myokards infolge stenosierender Coronarsklerose bzw. syphilitischer Stenosen der beiden Coronararterienabgänge (Abb. 11) ergab eine Bestätigung dieser Hypothese: in den inneren Schichten der Muskulatur des linken Ventrikels, besonders in dessen Papillarmuskeln und Trabekeln, fanden sich als *Spuren von Anfällen akuter relativer Ichämie disseminierte elektive Parenchymnekrosen*, als Spuren zurückliegender Anfälle jüngere capillarenreiche Fibroblasten-Narben oder alte capillarenarme Narben aus kollagenen Fibrillen (BÜCHNER 1932). Den Anfall akuter relativer arterieller Ischämie des Herzmuskels infolge von arteriellen Stenosen kennzeichneten wir, in Anlehnung an einen Ausdruck von REIN (1931), als *akute Coronarinsuffizienz* (BÜCHNER 1932), d.h. als einen *Zustand eines akuten Mißverhältnisses von Blutbedarf und Blutangebot im Herzmuskel*[3].

---

[1] ECKENHOFF und Mitarbeiter 1947, REIN 1951, GREGG 1950, ALELLA 1954, 1955, BRETSCHNEIDER 1958, HAUSS 1958.

[2] GOLLWITZER-MEIER und KROETZ 1940, GREGG 1950, HEIDENREICH und SCHMIDT 1956, KIMURA und Mitarbeiter 1957.

[3] Vgl. auch BÜCHNER 1939, 1950, 1957, 1959.

„Die Frage der ‚Insuffizienz' der Coronarregulation wird ohne gleichzeitige Kontrolle der Arbeitsweise und Leistung des Herzens überhaupt nicht zu klären sein. Es eröffnet sich ein weites Arbeitsfeld für die experimentelle Pathologie und Therapie, beispielsweise in *der* Richtung, *Coronarinsuffizienzen* durch Veränderung der Arbeitsweise des Herzens zu beeinflussen" (Rein 1931). „Ist das Gefäß erstarrt und zudem seine Lichtung anatomisch stark eingeengt, so ist die schnelle Anpassung der Coronardurchblutung bei plötzlichem Mehrbedarf unmöglich. Die bekannten häufigsten Grundkrankheiten der Angina pectoris (Coronarsklerose und Syphilis der Aorta) verhindern die schnelle Anpassung der Kranzgefäße an ihre Mehrbelastung bei plötzlicher Mehrarbeit des Herzens. Jede plötzliche Mehrbeanspruchung des Coronarsystems führt daher in solchen Fällen auch ohne Spasmen die Gefahr der *Coronarinsuffizienz* herbei" (Büchner 1932).

In unserem Beitrag über die „Allgemeine Pathologie der cellulären und geweblichen Oxydationen" (dieses Handbuch Bd. IV/2, S. 569, 1957) haben wir uns ausführlich mit der Tatsache auseinandergesetzt, daß Zustände allgemeiner Hypoxämie zu einer Coronarinsuffizienz führen können. Hier dagegen steht für uns zunächst die akute Coronarinsuffizienz als Ausdruck akuter stenosebedingter relativer Ischämie des Herzmuskels im Vordergrund. Daß Anfälle akuter relativer Ischämie des Herzmuskels bei arteriosklerotischen und syphilitischen Coronarstenosen vorkommen und von großer Bedeutung sind, hatte schon eine Reihe älterer und neuerer Kliniker in der Deutung des Angina pectoris-Anfalles angenommen[1]. Ihre Auffassung wurde durch die Arbeiten über das Elektrokardiogramm bei stenosebedingter Angina pectoris bekräftigt[2]. Die histologischen Befunde am Herzmuskel brachten aber zum ersten Mal den exakten Beweis für solche Anfälle akuter relativer Ischämie bei Coronarstenosen und ihre Wirkung auf den Herzmuskel. So rückte das Problem der Coronarinsuffizienz auf längere Zeit in den Mittelpunkt der Erörterungen über die Durchblutungsstörungen des Herzmuskels. In der Pathologie schloß sich an die ersten Untersuchungen eine systematische Durcharbeitung der ätiologischen Formen der Coronarinsuffizienz am menschlichen Herzen[3] und im Tierexperiment[4] an. Unter den in der Pathologie erarbeiteten Gesichtspunkten analysierte die Klinik ihrerseits die Pathogenese sowie die funktionelle Pathologie und die Klinik der Coronarinsuffizienz[5]. In den Vereinigten Staaten haben vor allem Master und sein Arbeitskreis seit 1941 entscheidend in die morphologischen und elektrokardiographischen Untersuchungen eingegriffen[6]. Friedberg 1959 brachte die Ergebnisse der gesamten Forschung in seiner Monographie „Erkrankungen des Herzens" gewichtig zur Darstellung.

Wir haben von unserer ersten Arbeit 1932 an streng zwischen dem Coronarinfarkt als der Folge umschriebener absoluter arterieller Ischämie eines Herzmuskelabschnittes und der das ganze Coronarsystem treffenden relativen arteriellen Ischämie des gesamten Herzmuskels unterschieden, besonders auch in unserer Monographie „Coronarinfarkt und Coronarinsuffizienz" mit A. Weber und Haager (1935) und in unserer Monographie „Die Coronarinsuffizienz" (1939)[6]. Es ist also ein Irrtum, wenn Friedberg (1959) in seiner Monographie

---

[1] Pary 1799, Potain 1880, A. Fraenkel 1891, Huchard 1899, Krehl 1901, Danielopolu 1927, J. Mackenzie 1923, Herrick 1931, Kohn 1931 u. a.

[2] Feil und Siegel 1928, Parkinson und Bedford 1931, Wood, Wolferth und Livezey 1931, Goldhammer und Scherf 1932, Scherf 1932, Rothschild und Kissin 1932, 1933, Dietrich und Schwiegk 1933, Master 1935, Master und Mitarbeiter 1941ff.

[3] Büchner, Weber und Haager 1935, Opitz 1935, Holzmann 1937, Hallermann 1939, Friedberg und Horn 1939, Master und Gubner 1941, Master und Mitarbeiter 1947, 1950, Dack, Master und Mitarbeiter 1949, Horn, Field, Dack und Master 1950, Büchner, Reindell, Klepzig und Weyland 1952 u. a.

[4] Siehe bei Büchner 1932, 1959.

[5] Kroetz 1933, Levy 1936, Weber 1937, Uhlenbruck 1940, Master und Mitarbeiter 1941ff., Holzer und Polzer 1941, Dias 1941, Kienle 1943, 1946, Hochrein 1943, Décourt 1945, Holzmann 1947, Grosse-Brockhoff 1950, Laubry und Soulié 1950, Schaefer 1951, Reindell und Klepzig 1951, Schimert 1951 u. a.

[6] Vgl. Büchner, Allgemeine Pathologie 1950, 1956, 1959, Spezielle Pathologie 1955, 1956, 1960.

„Erkrankungen des Herzens" die Meinung vertritt, wir hätten den Coronarverschluß und den Myokardinfarkt in den Oberbegriff „Coronarinsuffizienz" einbezogen. Seit 1932 vertreten wir vielmehr die 1939 von FRIEDBERG übernommene Auffassung, die Coronarinsuffizienz als pathologisch-physiologisches Phänomen im Sinne einer unzureichenden Coronardurchblutung des Herzmuskels zu definieren und nicht als Krankheitsbild. So stimmen wir auch mit FRIEDBERG (1959) völlig überein, wenn er in seiner Monographie betont: „Von einer Coronarinsuffizienz spricht man, wenn die Coronardurchblutung in quantitativer und qualitativer Hinsicht den Bedarf des Myokards nicht decken kann" (S. 535). „Von einer Coronarinsuffizienz sollte lediglich zur Bezeichnung einer physiologischen Störung gesprochen werden, wenn diese durch eine unzureichende Coronardurchblutung oder eine Sauerstoffarmut des Blutes hervorgerufen wurde" (S. 345).

Die *Nekrosen nach akuter Coronarinsuffizienz* wurden zum Teil als kleine Herzinfarkte bezeichnet. Diese Bezeichnung ist pathologisch-histologisch nicht richtig: Beim Herzinfarkt handelt es sich um eine umschriebene Totalnekrose des Parenchyms und des Mesenchyms im Herzmuskel. Die Nekrosen bei akuter Coronarinsuffizienz sind dagegen *elektive Parenchymnekrosen*, in deren Bereich nur Herzmuskelzellen untergehen, die Mesenchymzellen dagegen den Anfall akuter relativer Ischämie überleben (BÜCHNER 1932 ff.). Das Bild ist verständlich als Ausdruck einer ischämisch bedingten Stoffwechselstörung, bei der der intensive Parenchymstoffwechsel des Herzmuskels fleckweise irreversibel gestört wird, während der weniger intensive Stoffwechsel des Mesenchyms sich nach dem Anfall wieder erholt. Infolgedessen werden die Nekrosebezirke schon in 2—4 Tagen durch Fibroblastenwucherungen ersetzt, in 8—14 Tagen durch Narben aus kollagenen Fibrillen.

Das *Prädilektionsgebiet der Parenchymnekrosen*, die Tatsache also, daß die Nekrosen nach akuter stenosebedingter Coronarinsuffizienz ausgesprochen die Muskulatur des linken Ventrikels und hier die innere Muskelschale, besonders die Papillarmuskeln und Trabekel, bevorzugen (BÜCHNER 1932, MASTER u. Mitarb. 1947) geht zum Teil darauf zurück, daß bei stenosierender Coronarsklerose nicht selten die Äste der linken Kranzader stärker stenosiert sind als die rechte Kranzader. Aber bei gleich starker Stenosierung der rechten und linken Kranzarterien durch Arteriosklerose oder Mesaortitis syphilitica gilt die gleiche Regel. Es müssen also, wie auch aus noch zu erörternden Experimenten hervorgeht, andere Faktoren entscheidender sein. Diese Faktoren sind: 1. Die weit höhere Druckbelastung und der entsprechend höhere Stoffwechsel in der Muskulatur des linken gegenüber denen des rechten Ventrikels. 2. Die Tatsache, daß der hohe systolische Druck im linken Ventrikel die Durchblutung der linken Coronararterie systolisch hemmt, während die rechte Coronararterie bei niedrigem systolischen Druck im rechten Ventrikel systolisch keine wesentliche Verringerung ihrer Durchblutung erfährt (GREGG 1950). 3. Die Tatsache, daß die Verzweigungen der Coronararterien vom Epikard her in die Ventrikel eindringen, von hier aus das Myokard durchsetzen und subendokardial endigen. Für den muskelschwachen rechten Ventrikel ist das in der Regel belanglos, für den muskelstarken linken Ventrikel bedeutet es, daß bei relativer Ischämie die äußeren Wandschichten das arterielle Blut weitgehend abschlucken und die subendokardialen Abschnitte am meisten von der Ischämie betroffen werden.

Die große Bedeutung der funktionellen Belastung eines Organes und seiner Teile für das pathogenetische Wirksamwerden einer akuten relativen Ischämie bis zur Nekrose wird uns also am Phänomen der Coronarinsuffizienz exemplarisch vor Augen geführt. Dabei ist es gleichgültig, auf welche Weise die Mehrbelastung des Herzmuskels, die bei Stenosen im Coronarsystem den Anfall akuter Coronarinsuffizienz bewirkt, zustande kommt. In der Regel ist es eine akute körperliche Arbeit. Dazu müssen wir auch die sekretorische und motorische Mehrarbeit des

Verdauungstraktus während des Verdauungsaktes rechnen, besonders nach größerer und üppiger Mahlzeit[1]. Auch die Wirkung der Kälte ist im gleichen Sinne zu deuten, da die Kälte eine regulatorische Steigerung der Herzarbeit, besonders des Herzminutenvolumens, hervorruft[2]. Schließlich kann die zur akuten Coronarinsuffizienz führende Mehrbelastung des Herzens durch heftige psychische Erregung ausgelöst sein. Raab (1953, 1956) hat die Auffassung entwickelt, daß alle diese verschiedenen Faktoren bei Coronarstenose über den gleichen Mechanismus wirksam werden und eine akute Steigerung der Coronardurchblutung notwendig machen, nämlich über eine akute Ausschüttung von

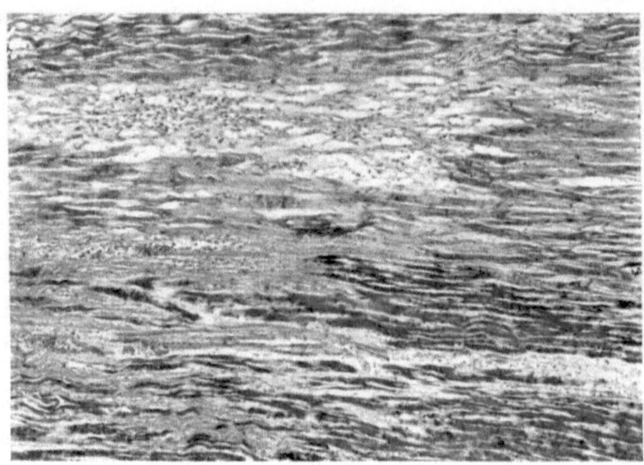

Abb. 12. Papillarmuskel des linken Ventrikels bei Phäochromocytom mit Anfällen von Hypertonie. Blau-grün: Ältere faserreiche Narben, oben lockere junge zellreiche Narbe. Rechts unten orangefarbig: Akute Parenchymnekrose. Rechts oben und am oberen Bildrand: normaler Herzmuskel. Trichromfärbung nach Goldner.

Adrenalin und Noradrenalin aus dem Nebennierenmark und eine dadurch verursachte akute Steigerung der Oxydationen des Herzmuskels (Adrenalin)[3] sowie des Blutdruckes (Noradrenalin). Für diese Auffassung spricht unter anderem die Tatsache, daß beim Phäochromocytom des Nebennierenmarkes Anfälle von akuter Coronarinsuffizienz[4] und Parenchymnekrosen des Herzmuskels[5] (Abb. 12) durch anfallsweise auftretende Ausschüttung von Adrenalin und Noradrenalin hervorgerufen werden. Arteriosklerotische Coronarstenosen sind aber auch hier durch die Grundkrankheit vorgegeben.

Auf der anderen Seite darf nicht übersehen werden, daß bei stärkeren Stenosen im Coronarsystem nicht selten die unter der Wirkung des Vagus erfolgenden nächtlichen Einschränkungen der Durchblutung zur akuten Coronarinsuffizienz führen und mitten in der Nacht den Kranken aus tiefem Schlaf aufwecken. Dementsprechend haben Pierach und Heynemann (1959) den vagalen dem sympathicotonen Typ der Coronarinsuffizienz gegenübergestellt.

Daß bei der stenosebedingten Coronarinsuffizienz aber auch akute Veränderungen im arteriosklerotischen Herd ins Spiel treten können, beweisen 2 Beobachtungen: 1. Eine Eigentümlichkeit arteriosklerotischer Herdbildungen ist es, daß sie recidivierend von einem akuten Ödem mit Quellungsnekrose befallen werden können. An einem coronarsklerotischen Herd kann auf diese Weise aus einer mäßigen, funktionell vielleicht noch bedeutungslosen Enge eine hochgradige, fast verschließende Stenose werden. Wird das Herz in dieser Ödemphase des

---

[1] Vgl. Büchner 1939, Friedberg 1959.   [2] Rein 1931.   [3] Gremels 1933, 1936.
[4] Kalk 1934, Friedberg 1959.   [5] Büchner und Weyland 1959.

arteriosklerotischen Herdes einer starken Belastung ausgesetzt, so kann es akut versagen. Der akute Coronartod ist dann die dramatische Folge. Wir sahen dieses Bild im 2. Weltkrieg nach akutem Coronartod unter über 600 Fällen jüngerer Soldaten (18—39 Jahre) in rund 50% der Fälle als die Todesursache. Die andere Hälfte zeigte zusätzlich eine akute Coronarthrombose[1]. Gleichsinnige Befunde wurden an Soldaten der amerikanischen Wehrmacht erhoben[2]. 2. In seltenen Fällen kann im Bereiche einer arteriosklerotischen Stenose ein Intimariß eintreten, gelegentlich nach Trauma gegen die Herzgegend[3]. Dadurch kann sich in dem Herd ein Hämatom entwickeln, welches plötzlich eine hochgradige Stenosierung hervorzurufen vermag. Bei akuter Belastung des Herzmuskels kann auch hier der akute Coronartod die Folge sein.

Eine Sonderstellung als Ursache von Anfällen akuter Coronarinsuffizienz und eventuell eines akuten Coronartodes nimmt die chronische *Hypertonie* jeder Ätiologie ein. Bei ihr kommt es mit der Zeit sehr häufig als Folge der chronischen Drucküberlastung des arteriellen Systems zu einer stenosierenden Coronarsklerose[4], die besonders in den peripheren Verzweigungen der Coronararterien auftritt (Abb. 13)[5]. Hinzu kommt noch in der Regel eine Arteriolosklerose des Myokards[6]. Dementsprechend sind im Hypertonikerherzen Parenchymnekrosen und deren Narben in der inneren Schale des linken Ventrikels ein häufiger Befund[7].

Anfälle stenosebedingter akuter Coronarinsuffizienz und ihre Folgen am Herzmuskel begegnen uns außer bei der stenosierenden Coronarsklerose und den syphilitischen Stenosen der Coronararterienabgänge auch bei der Panarteriitis nodosa und bei der Endarteriitis obliterans.

Klinisch ist dem Anfall stenosebedingter akuter relativer Ischämie des Myokards, also der akuten Coronarinsuffizienz infolge Stenosen, in der Regel, aber nicht gesetzmäßig, ein Anfall von *Angina pectoris* zugeordnet, also ein Anfall von plötzlichem Schmerz in der Herzgegend mit Engegefühl über der Brust, nicht selten mit akuter Todesangst, wie ihn zuerst HEBERDEN (1772) beschrieben hat. Schon PARY (1799) kannte die Beziehungen dieser Anfälle zur stenosierenden Coronarsklerose und deutete sie als deren Folgen, also als anatomisch fundierte relative Ischämien. Der Anfall zwingt den Kranken, augenblicklich die Belastung des Herzens auf ein Ruhemaß herabzusetzen. Dadurch wird die Coronardurchblutung wieder suffizient, und nach einer durchschnittlichen Dauer von weniger als 3 min[8] erlischt der Schmerz. Mit der Entdeckung der Coronarinsuffizienz trat die *Coronarinsuffizienz-Hypothese des Angina pectoris-Anfalles* in den Vordergrund (BÜCHNER 1932, GOLDENBERG und ROTHBERGER 1933). Sie war schon vorher durch die *Hypoxie-Hypothese des Angina pectoris-Anfalles* von KEEFER und RESNIK 1928 vorbereitet, die ihrerseits durch gleichzeitige Arbeiten wichtige Unterbauungen fand[9].

Hatten schon MACKENZIE 1923 und KOHN 1931 vermutet, daß dem Schmerzanfall und seinen subjektiven Begleitsymptomen eine durch Ischämie des Herzmuskels verursachte akute Stoffwechselstörung des Myokards zugrunde liegt, so gewann diese These dadurch sehr an Wahrscheinlichkeit, daß in den von uns untersuchten Fällen akuter stenosebedingter Coronarinsuffizienz die disseminierten

---

[1] BÜCHNER 1941, E. MÜLLER 1943, 1944, 1949, MEESSEN 1944; vgl. auch BREDT 1949, 1958.
[2] YATER und Mitarbeiter 1947.   [3] PAPACHARALAMPOUS und ZOLLINGER 1953.
[4] FAHR 1923, 1928, 1935, AVERBUCK 1936.
[5] BÄURLE 1950, RAU 1955, SCHIMKAT und KATHKE 1959.   [6] KATHKE 1955.
[7] BÜCHNER, WEBER und HAAGER 1935, HORN, MASTER und Mitarbeiter 1950, BÜCHNER und WEYLAND 1959.
[8] RISEMAN und BROWN 1937.
[9] ROTHSCHILD und KISSIN 1932, BÜCHNER 1932, 1933, DIETRICH und SCHWIEGK 1933, BÜCHNER und von LUCADOU 1934, CHRIST 1934, FRIEDBERG und HORN 1939.

Parenchymnekrosen des Herzmuskels und deren Narben nach Anfällen von Angina pectoris zustande gekommen waren (BÜCHNER 1932). STERNBERG (1924) fand in den von ihm untersuchten Fällen von Angina pectoris regelmäßig eine

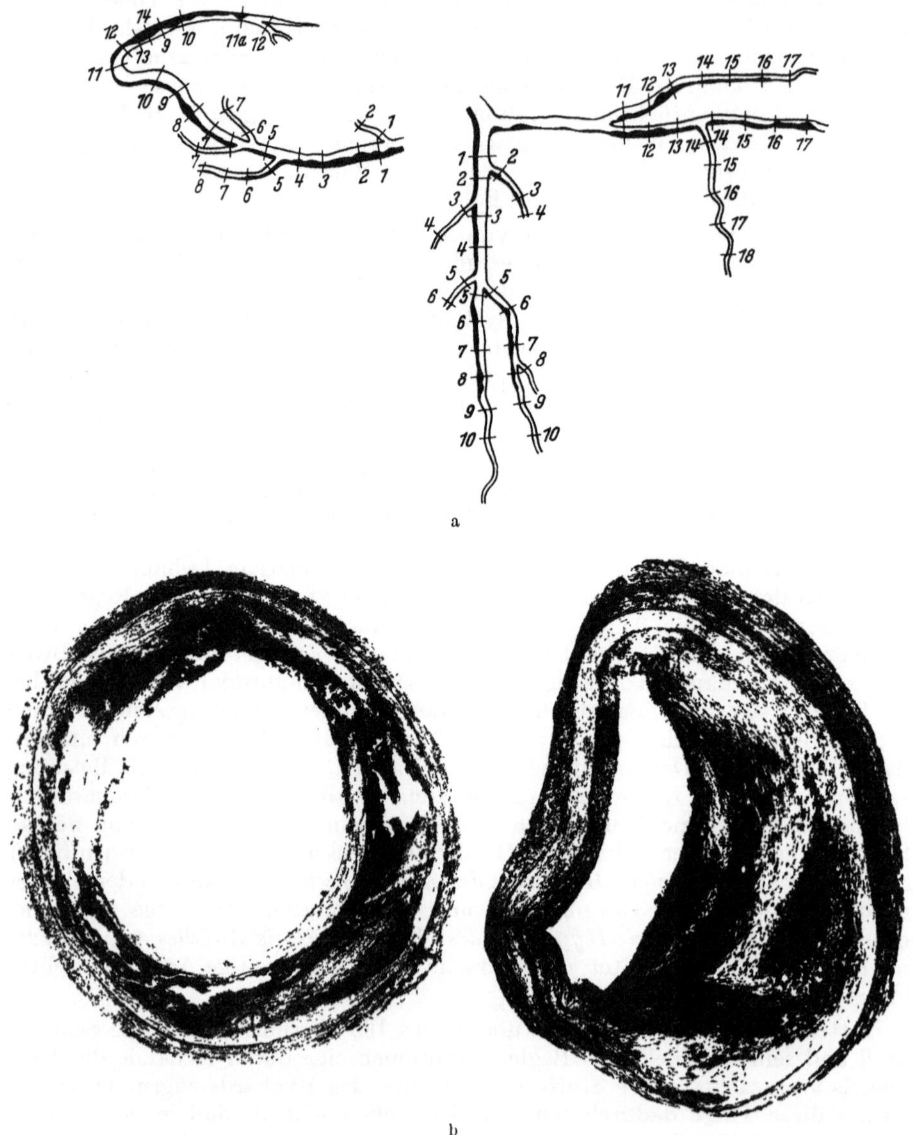

Abb. 13a u. b. a Hypertonische Coronarsklerose bei 48jähriger Frau. Skizze mit Eintragung der histotopographisch gefundenen Stenosen. b Links proximale Coronararterie mäßig stenosiert, rechts distale stark stenosiert. [Nach W. BÄURLE, Beitr. path. Anat. 111, 1950, Abb. 1 u. 6.]

stenosierende Coronarsklerose. BRAUN (1926) untersuchte 127 Fälle von Angina pectoris, alle hatten eine stenosierende Coronarsklerose. KOCH und KONG (1932) sahen das gleiche. Daß langsam eingetretene arteriosklerotische Verschlüsse der Kranzadern ohne Infarkt als Ursachen schwererer Anfälle von Angina pectoris von besonderer Bedeutung sind, haben vor allem die Injektions- und Stufenuntersuchungen des Coronarsystems durch BLUMGART und seine Mitarbeiter seit 1940 bewiesen[1].

Die Bedeutung des *Sauerstoffmangels* im Herzmuskel beim Anfall von Angina pectoris infolge Coronarstenosen und die zugeordneten Befunde des Elektrokardiogramms haben wir ausführlich in unserem Beitrag über die Pathologie der cellulären und geweblichen Oxydationen in diesem Handbuch, Bd. IV/2, dargestellt. Wir dürfen daher hier darauf verweisen[2].

Eine Frage muß aber in diesem Zusammenhang noch erörtert werden. In dem erwähnten Beitrag wurde gezeigt, daß unmittelbar in der akuten Hypoxämie (durch Unterdruck, akute Entblutungsanämie, Kohlenoxydvergiftung) im Elektrokardiogramm beim Menschen und im Experiment charakteristische Veränderungen registriert werden, besonders eine Senkung von ST und T, in der Regel in der Ableitung I und II, und daß diese Abweichungen des Elektrokardiogramms im Verlauf von Minuten oder auch $^1/_2$—1 Std nach Aufhören der Hypoxämie wieder zur Norm zurückkehren. Sie stimmen mit den im spontanen oder provozierten Anfall von Angina pectoris registrierten Kurvenänderungen überein[3]. Im Experiment am Hund waren sie unmittelbar nach mechanischer Einschränkung der Blutzufuhr zur linken Coronaratrerie oder nach Injektion blutdrucksenkender Stoffe (C6, Rauwolfia, Histamin u. a.) zu beobachten, wenn die Coronardurchblutung auf $^1/_3$ der Norm herabgesetzt war[4]. Lichtmikroskopisch treten Parenchym-Nekrosen erst mehrere Stunden nach dem Anfall in Erscheinung. Die Veränderungen des Elektrokardiogramms bei der akuten Coronarinsuffizienz weisen also, wie wir seit 1932 betont haben, nicht vorliegende Nekrosen nach, sondern akute hypoxische Störungen des Herzmuskelstoffwechsels, die in ausgedehnten Abschnitten des Herzmuskels zu einem akuten Energiemangel der Herzmuskelzellen führen[5]. Dieser Energiemangel ist vor allem dadurch hervorgerufen, daß unter der Wirkung akuter Hypoxie des Herzmuskels, wie sie bei akuter Coronarinsuffizienz zwangsläufig gegeben ist, in kurzer Zeit das Kreatinphosphat stark und das Adenosintriphosphat mäßig abnimmt[6], während das anorganische Phosphat ansteigt[7]. Der Energiemangel bewirkt eine Störung der energiefordernden Kaliumaufladung der Herzmuskelzelle entgegen dem Gefälle und der Natriumabgabe in den Intercellularraum entgegen dem Gefälle, also eine Störung des Aufbaues der Ionenmembranen an der Oberfläche der Herzmuskelzelle, dadurch aber Störungen ihres Aktionspotentials[8].

Zwischen dem elektrokardiographischen Befund als dem Zeichen einer ausgedehnten Stoffwechselstörung und dem Befund der lichtmikroskopisch nachweisbaren, mitunter kleinen Gruppen von Parenchymnekrosen klaffte bisher morphologisch eine Lücke. Sie konnte durch jüngste elektronenmikroskopische Untersuchungen geschlossen werden (Abb. 14 und 15)[9]. Schon ein einmaliger Aufstieg des Kaninchens auf 10000—11000 m in der Unterdruckkammer mit sofortigem Ausschleusen des Tieres bewirkt durch akute exogene Hypoxie der Herzmuskelzellen typische Veränderungen[10]: die Mitochondrien schwellen, ihre inneren Lamellen zerfallen und verschwinden. Zwischen den Myokardfibrillen

---

[1] BLUMGART, SCHLESINGER und DAVIS 1940, BLUMGART, SCHLESINGER und ZOLL 1941, FREEDBERG, BLUMGART und Mitarbeiter 1948, BLUMGART, ZOLL und Mitarbeiter 1950, ZOLL, WESSLER und BLUMGART 1951.
[2] BÜCHNER 1957.   [3] Siehe auch FRIEDBERG 1959.   [4] KIMURA und Mitarbeiter 1957.
[5] BÜCHNER und VON LUCADOU 1934, BÜCHNER 1938.
[6] FLECKENSTEIN und Mitarbeiter 1956—1959.
[7] DUSPIVA und NOLTENIUS 1957, 1958, FLECKENSTEIN 1958.
[8] Vgl. FLECKENSTEIN 1942, 1955, 1958.
[9] MÖLBERT 1957, 1958, MÖLBERT und THALE 1958, BÜCHNER, MÖLBERT und THALE 1959, BÜCHNER 1959.   [10] MÖLBERT 1957, 1958.

Abb. 14. Ausschnitt aus einer normalen Herzmuskelzelle eines Kaninchens im elektronenmikroskopischen Bild. In der Mitte dicht zusammengelagerte Mitochondrien mit dicht liegenden inneren Doppellamellen. Rechts und links Teile einer Elementarfibrille mit dunklen Z-Streifen. Vergr. 40000mal. [Nach E. Mölbert, Beitr. path. Anat. 118, 1958, Abb. 1.]

finden sich elektronenoptisch leere, durch Wasseransammlung aufgetriebene Lücken. Diese Veränderungen, die in den inneren Schichten der linken Kammer ihr Maximum haben, nehmen im Verlauf von Stunden zu und gehen dann fleckweise in die Nekrose von Herzmuskelzellen über. Die gleichen Befunde konnten elektronenmikroskopisch am Herzmuskel der Ratte nach Vergiftung mit aerobiose-

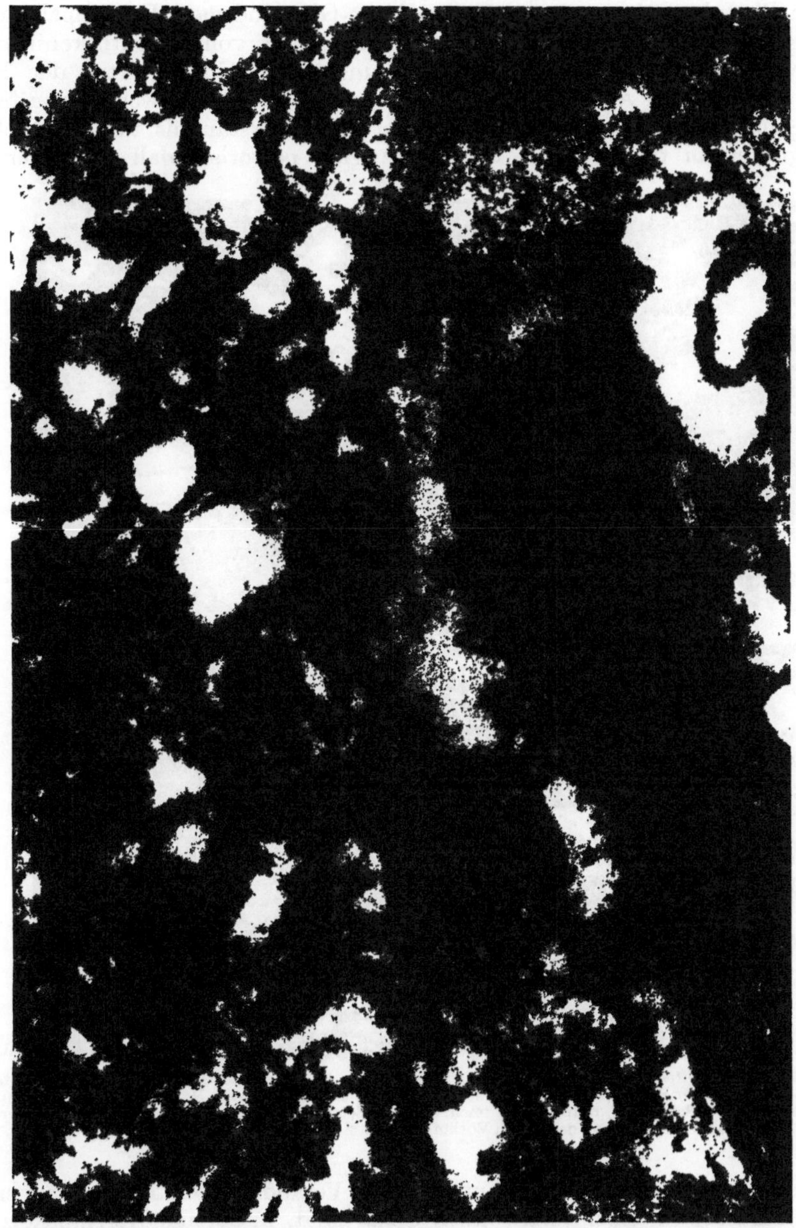

Abb. 15. Ausschnitt einer Herzmuskelzelle nach akuter Hypoxie durch exogenen Sauerstoffmangel. Linke Bildhälfte große Mitochondriengruppe. In den Mitochondrien z. T. nur wenige verkürzte innere Doppellamellen.
Rechts Elementarfibrille. Am rechten Bildrand zwei Mitochondrien mit fast völligem Verlust der inneren Doppellamellen. Zwischen den Mitochondrien der linken Bildhälfte und der Elementarfibrille größere Aussparungen durch
Flüssigkeitsansammlung. Vergr. 45000mal. [Nach E. MÖLBERT, Beitr. path. Anat. 118, 1958, Abb. 4.]

hemmenden Giften beobachtet werden[1], nach Hemmung der Cytochromoxydase
durch Blausäure schon nach 5 min, nach Hemmung der Bernsteinsäuredehydrogenase durch Malonsäure nach 10 min. Ganz Entsprechendes wurde nach

---

[1] MÖLBERT und THALE 1958, BÜCHNER 1959, BÜCHNER, MÖLBERT und THALE 1959.

weißem Phosphor, einem typischen Aerobiose-Gift, und nach Entkoppelung von Atmung und Phosphorylierung durch Überdosierung von Trijodthyronin nachgewiesen[1]. Diese ausgedehnten Veränderungen der Ultrastruktur der Herzmuskelzelle sind der Ausdruck einer akuten energetisch-osmotischen Insuffizienz der Herzmuskelzelle[2]. Sie bahnen ein vertieftes Verständnis für das Elektrokardiogramm in der Hypoxie und im Angina pectoris-Anfall an, indem sie

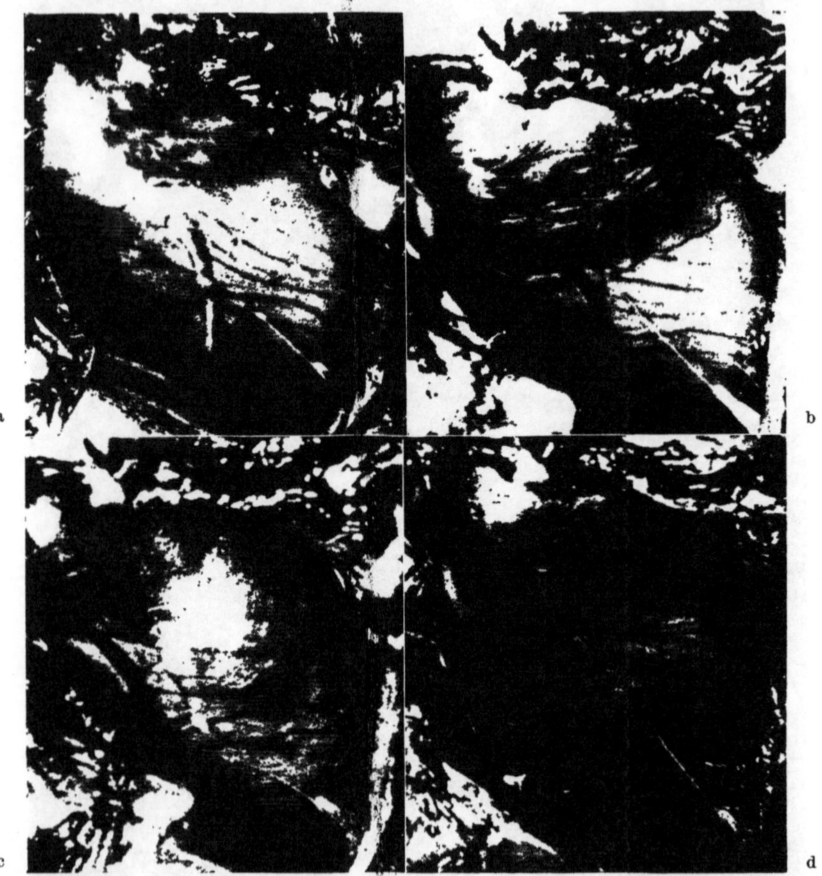

Abb. 16a—d. Freigelegtes Herz des lebenden Kaninchens, oben links bei normaler Atmung, oben rechts nach wenigen Sekunden reiner Stickstoffatmung mit maximaler Erweiterung des linken Vorhofs, unten links 1 min nach Wiederbeatmung mit Sauerstoff, unten rechts nach wenigen Sekunden erneuter Stickstoffatmung mit erneuter starker Erweiterung des linken Vorhofs. (Nach S. IIJIMA 1958, unveröffentlicht.)

zeigen, wie schnell und ausgedehnt schwere Veränderungen der Ultrastruktur des Herzmuskels in einer Phase nachweisbar sind, in der die Herzmuskelzellen lichtmikroskopisch noch unverändert erscheinen[2]. Darüber hinaus machen sie verständlich, warum nicht selten die akute Coronarinsuffizienz in die tödliche Herzinsuffizienz übergeht.

Dies veranschaulicht uns der folgende Versuch[3]: Läßt man ein Kaninchen bei freigelegtem Herzen kurzfristig reinen Stickstoff atmen, so kommt es in Bruchteilen einer Minute zur akuten Insuffizienz des linken Vorhofs mit starker Dilatation und zum deutlichen Hervortreten des linken Herzohrs (Abb. 16b). Die

---

[1] POCHE 1958.   [2] BÜCHNER 1959.   [3] IIJIMA 1958.

Umschaltung auf reine Sauerstoffatmung korrigiert die Insuffizienz des Vorhofs in 1 Minute (Abb. 16c). Bei erneuter reiner Stickstoffatmung kommt es wiederum in Bruchteilen einer Minute zur Vorhof-Insuffizienz (Abb. 16d). Die weitere Beatmung mit reinem Stickstoff ist dann von einer hochgradigen tödlichen Insuffizienz-Dilatation beider Ventrikel gefolgt (Abb. 17). Nach der Anlage des Experimentes bedeutet die akute Stickstoffatmung durch schwere hypoxische Störung des Herzmuskelstoffwechsels eine akute Einschränkung der Energiebildung im Myokard, also eine *akute energetische Insuffizienz des Herzmuskels.*

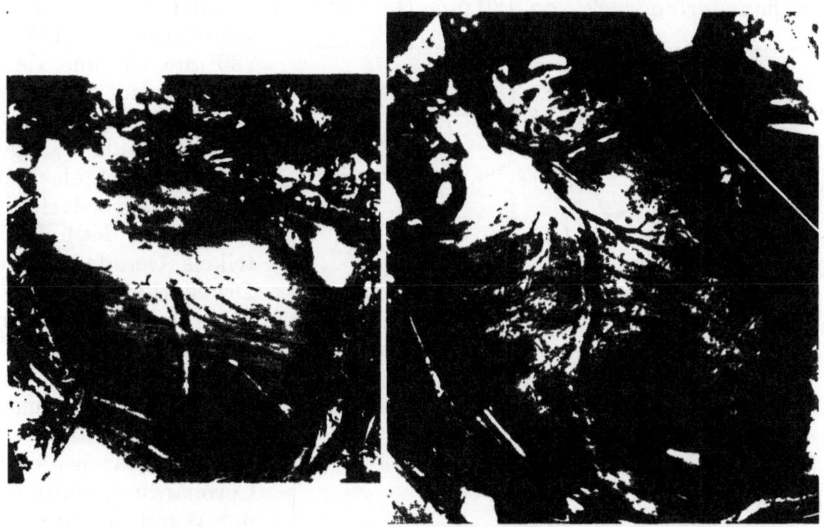

Abb. 17. Herz des lebenden Kaninchens freigelegt. Links bei normaler Beatmung, rechts nach kurzfristiger Stickstoffatmung mit hochgradiger Erweiterung beider Ventrikel (links und rechts gleiche Vergr.). (Nach S. IIJIMA 1958, unveröffentlicht.)

Diese kann nach dem durchgeführten Experiment unmittelbar in eine *akute dynamische Insuffizienz des Herzmuskels* überleiten und zwar zuerst zu einer dynamischen Insuffizienz der Vorhöfe, dann auch der Kammern.

3. Die paradoxe arterielle Ischämie.

Coronarinsuffizienz bei krankhaft erhöhtem Blutbedarf des Herzmuskels.

Die stenosenbedingte akute Coronarinsuffizienz konnten wir als anfallsweise auftretende relative arterielle Ischämie deuten. Bei weiteren Gruppen akuter Coronarinsuffizienz müssen wir dagegen das Prinzip der relativen Ischämie überschreiten und zu einer Vorstellung vordringen, die erst möglich wurde, nachdem die Kreislaufphysiologie erkannt hatte, daß die normale Durchblutung der Organe mit ihrer funktionellen Belastung und damit zugleich mit ihrem Stoffwechsel unmittelbar gekoppelt ist[1]. Mit dieser Erkenntnis zeichnete sich die Möglichkeit ab, daß in einem Organ akut oder chronisch die Funktion und damit der Stoffwechsel krankhaft so überfordert werden, daß die Durchblutung zwar stark gesteigert, aber auch bei morphologisch normalen Arterien trotz maximaler Ausnutzung des zur Verfügung stehenden Strombettes nicht ausreichend ist. Diesen Zustand kennzeichnen wir im folgenden als *paradoxe arterielle Ischämie.* Er ist am besten am Herzmuskel untersucht, und er begegnet uns zunächst bei der *akuten Coronarinsuffizienz infolge krankhafter Veränderungen der Herzklappen.*

---

[1] BARCROFT 1914, W. R. HESS 1923, REIN 1931, 1941.

Bei den Herzklappenfehlern besteht eine krankhafte Mehrbelastung eines oder beider Herzventrikel durch vermehrte Druck- oder Volumenarbeit. An erster Stelle ist hier die schwere *Aortenstenose* zu nennen (FRIEDBERG und HORN 1939). Sie führt dann zu Erscheinungen der Coronarinsuffizienz, wenn das Aortenostium auf mindestens $^1/_4$ der Norm eingeengt ist[1]. Während in der Norm der Gradient zwischen dem systolischen Druck im linken Ventrikel und in der Aorta nur wenige Millimeter beträgt, steigt er bei mäßiger Aortenstenose um 20—50 mm Hg an, bei schwerer um 50—100 mm Hg oder mehr[2]. Es besteht also bei einem normalen systolischen Aortendruck von 120 mm Hg nicht selten im linken Ventrikel ein systolischer Druck von 220 mm Hg und darüber. Das bedeutet eine gewaltige Druckleistung sowie eine entsprechende Steigerung des Stoffwechsels und damit des Blutbedarfes in der Muskulatur des linken Ventrikels. Gerade bei erhöhter Druckarbeit des Herzmuskels steigen die aeroben Stoffwechselprozesse besonders steil an[3]. Hinzu kommt, daß der maximal erhöhte systolische Druck bei der Aortenstenose die Coronardurchblutung in der Wand des linken Ventrikels besonders hemmt (Abb. 18)[4]. Die Coronardurchblutung wird dadurch schon in der Ruhe bis nahe der oberen Grenze der Norm beansprucht. Dabei besteht eine Tendenz zu leichter

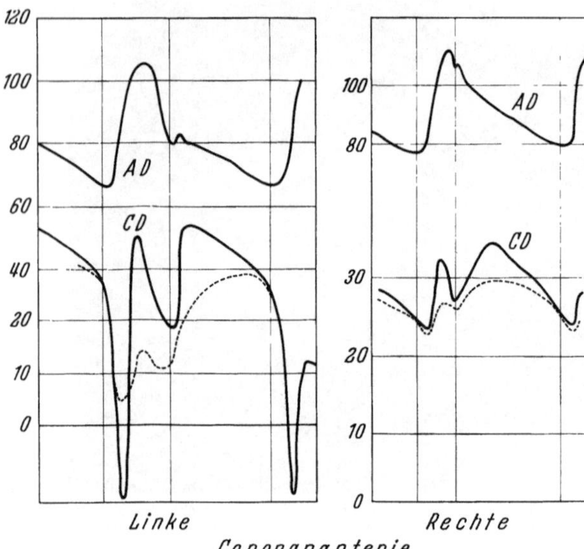

Abb. 18. Coronardurchblutung in der Wand des linken Ventrikels (links) und des rechten Ventrikels (rechts). Deutliche Senkung der Coronardurchblutung in der Wand des linken Ventrikels unter die 0-Linie während der Systole, dagegen kaum in der Wand des rechten Ventrikels. *CD* Coronardurchblutung, *AD* Aortendruck. (Nach GREGG, Coronary Circulation. Philadelphia 1950.)

Hypotonie und deren ungünstiger Wirkung auf die Coronardurchblutung[5]. Mehrbelastungen des Herzens verschiedenen Ursprungs können sich daher bei der Aortenstenose besonders leicht in Anfällen akuter Coronarinsuffizienz manifestieren und den Tod als akuten Coronartod verursachen. Die Neigung zum plötzlichen Tod war seit langem den Ärzten gerade bei diesem Herzfehler geläufig[6]. Auch leiden Kranke mit schwerer Aortenstenose in 10—20% der Fälle an Angina pectoris-Anfällen[7]. So ist es verständlich, daß gerade bei diesem Herzklappenfehler in der Innenschicht der Muskulatur des linken Ventrikels häufig ausgedehnte, meist konfluierende Parenchymnekrosen und deren Narben nachweisbar sind[8] (Abb. 19 und 20). Im Experiment wurde bei starker Aorten-

---

[1] ALLAN 1926, FRIEDBERG 1959.
[2] GOLDBERG, SMITH und Mitarbeiter 1956, NOVACK, COBB und Mitarbeiter 1956, WRIGHT 1956.
[3] GREMELS 1933, GOLLWITZER-MEIER und Mitarbeiter 1936, 1937, KIESE und GARAN 1937, RÜHL 1938.
[4] Vgl. GREGG 1950.   [5] PIERACH und HEYNEMANN 1959.
[6] MARGOLIES und Mitarbeiter 1931, McGINN und WHITE 1934, MARVIN und SULLIVAN 1935, CONTRATTO und LEVINE 1937, BERGERON und Mitarbeiter 1954, vgl. FRIEDBERG 1959.
[7] LIKOFF, BERKOWITZ und Mitarbeiter 1955.
[8] FRIEDBERG und SOHVAL 1939, FRIEDBERG und HORN 1939, BÜCHNER und WEYLAND 1959.

stenose schon in der Ruhe und erst recht bei akuter körperlicher Belastung eine Insuffizienz der Coronardurchblutung registriert[1]. Diese wurde damit erklärt, daß die Erhöhung des Kammerdruckes eine Steigerung des Widerstandes in den peripheren Verzweigungen der Kranzadern verursacht und dadurch die systolische Durchströmung der Coronararterien erschwert[2].

Bei schwerer Aortenstenose ist also zwar die Coronardurchblutung gegenüber der Norm erhöht, aber infolge der ungewöhnlichen Belastung des linken Ventrikels häufig, besonders in Anfällen nicht adäquat, so daß eine Neigung zu Anfällen akuter paradoxer arterieller Ischämie besteht.

Unterschiedlich wird die *Aorteninsuffizienz* in ihrer Bedeutung für entsprechende Anfälle beurteilt. Bei diesem Herzklappenfehler ist die Volumenarbeit des linken Ventrikels gesteigert. Dadurch ist der oxydative Stoffwechsel im Myokard wesentlich erhöht, wenn auch nicht so stark wie bei erhöhter Druckarbeit[3]. Der starke Abfall des diastolischen Blutdruckes und die Herabsetzung des mittleren Aortendruckes kann also in der Zeiteinheit eine Minderdurchblutung verursachen[4]. Tatsache ist, daß bei rheumatischer Aorteninsuffizienz ohne Coronarstenosen in den inneren Schichten der Muskulatur des linken Ventrikels ausgedehnte Parenchymnekrosen und deren Narben nachgewiesen werden können[5]. Bei akut einsetzender Aorteninsuffizienz, wie sie nicht selten bei Endocarditis necroticans ulcerosa lenta infolge akuter Abstoßungen von Klappenfragmenten und akuter Perforation eines Klappenaneurysmas beobachtet wird, sind diese Nekrosen und Narben besonders ausgedehnt und schwer[6] (Abb. 21). Die Häufigkeit der Angina pectoris bei Aorteninsuffizienz ist seit langem bekannt[7] Die experimentellen Beobachtungen widersprechen zum Teil einander. SMITH, MILLER und GRABER (1926) wiesen bei experimenteller Aorteninsuffizienz eine Minderdurchblutung der Coronararterien nach, GREEN (1936) sah dagegen im Experiment in der Diastole eine Minderdurchblutung, in der Systole eine Mehrdurchblutung und insgesamt bei kompensierter Aorteninsuffizienz eine Mehrdurchblutung. Ob diese dem erhöhten Blutbedarf des hypertrophierten linken Ventrikels adäquat ist, mußte er allerdings offenlassen. Am Menschen fanden BING u. Mitarb. (1949) nach Katheterung eine Mehrdurchblutung. FRIEDBERG (1959) übt daher große Zurückhaltung in der Frage der inadäquaten Coronardurchblutung bei Aorteninsuffizienz. Nach unseren morphologischen Befunden müssen wir aber daran festhalten, daß bei der Aorteninsuffizienz Zustände der paradoxen Ischämie im Herzmuskel trotz einer durch erhöhte Volumenarbeit des linken Ventrikels gesteigerten Coronardurchblutung häufig vorkommen.

Über die Hypoxie des Herzmuskels infolge *akuter thrombotischer oder experimenteller Lungenembolie* haben wir uns schon ausführlich in unserem Beitrag zu diesem Handbuch, Bd. IV/2, die Pathologie der cellulären und geweblichen Oxydationen (1957) geäußert. Wir müssen aber auch hier noch einmal darauf eingehen. Folgende Faktoren addieren sich bei der Lungenembolie in ihrer Wirkung auf den Blutbedarf und die Blut- und Sauerstoffversorgung des Herzmuskels: die akute Lungenembolie bedeutet einen schweren organischen Widerstand für die Entleerung des rechten Ventrikels. Dieser Widerstand wird funktionell noch dadurch gesteigert, daß nach Versuchen von EULER und LILJESTRAND (1947) die

---

[1] GREEN 1936, GREEN und GREGG 1940.   [2] FRIEDBERG 1959.
[3] GREMELS 1933, GOLLWITZER-MEIER und Mitarbeiter 1936, 1937, KIESE und GARAN 1937, 1938, RÜHL 1938.
[4] Vgl. GREGG 1950, HEIDENREICH und SCHMIDT 1956.
[5] BÜCHNER 1932, 1939.   [6] BÜCHNER und WEYLAND 1959.
[7] A. FRAENKEL 1891, NOTHNAGEL 1893, J. MACKENZIE 1923, GALLAVARDIN 1925, KEEFER und RESNIK 1928.

mit der akuten Lungenembolie gegebene akute Hypoxie eine akute Vasoconstriction der Pulmonalarterien verursacht. Durch beide Faktoren, die organische und die funktionelle Widerstandserhöhung, wird die Druckarbeit und damit der Blutbedarf des rechten Ventrikels stark gesteigert. Dabei ist aber der Durchstrom des Blutes durch die Lunge verringert, so daß im großen arteriellen Kreislauf eine akute Oligämie und Hypotonie eintreten kann. Die Coronardurchblutung wird dadurch erschwert. Außerdem bewirkt die mangelhafte Durchblutung der Lunge eine allgemeine Hypoxämie. Es besteht also bei akuter Lungenembolie

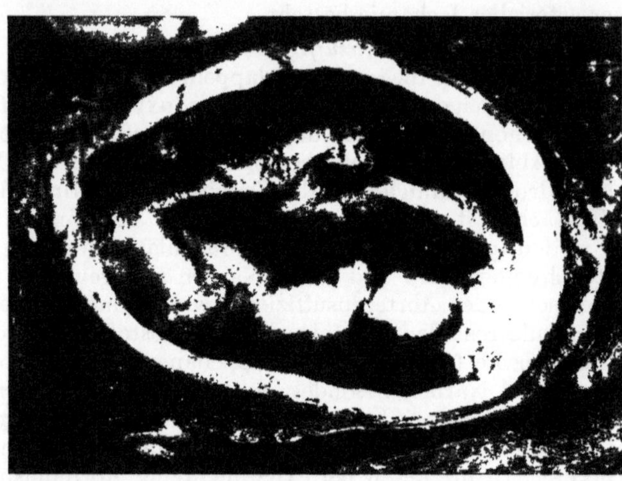

Abb. 19. Schwere Aortenstenose nach Gelenkrheumatismus. Aortenklappe durch Querschnitt der Aorta dicht über dem Klappenansatz freigelegt. (Nach Büchner, F., Spezielle Pathologie, 3. Aufl., Abb. 8, 1960.)

unter anderem in der Wand der rechten Kammer eine paradoxe arterielle Ischämie. Diese führt bevorzugt zu Parenchymnekrosen in der Muskulatur des rechten Ventrikels[1]. Das konnte schon früher[2] und jüngst erneut[3] im Experiment nach rezidivierender Mikroembolie von Fibrinthromben gezeigt werden. Weitere Beobachtungen der menschlichen Pathologie ergaben aber, daß in einer Serie von 12 Fällen mit subakut tödlicher Lungenembolie die Nekrosen bevorzugt in der Muskulatur der Hinterwand des *linken* Ventrikels lagen[4]. In neueren eigenen Untersuchungen konnten wir diesen Befund vereinzelt bestätigen[5]. Wir haben ihn so zu deuten versucht, daß der rechte Ventrikel infolge der Überbelastung durch die akute Lungenembolie aus der rechten Kranzader besonders reichlich Blut abschluckt und das Terminalgebiet der rechten Coronararterie, die Hinterwand des *linken* Ventrikels, in der Blutversorgung besonders beeinträchtigt wird[6].

An 3 Beispielen, der Aortenstenose, der Aorteninsuffizienz und der Lungenembolie, sind wir dem Vorkommen und der Wahrscheinlichkeit von Zuständen der paradoxen arteriellen Ischämie im Herzmuskel begegnet. Es erhebt sich die Frage: Ist der Herzmuskel nicht in jedem Falle von der paradoxen arteriellen Ischämie bedroht, wenn er durch Hypertrophie der linken oder der rechten Kammer oder beider Kammern an Masse zunimmt, also bei jeder Form des *chronischen Cor aortale*, z. B. durch Isthmusstenose der Aorta, durch genuine,

---

[1] Büchner 1938, Weinschenk 1939, Epping 1940.
[2] Balogh 1938, Walder 1939, Meessen 1940, Herbertson 1953.
[3] Könn und Ch. Büchner 1959, Ch. Büchner und Koenn 1959.
[4] Friedberg und Horn 1939, Horn, Dack und Friedberg 1939, s. auch Currens und Barnes 1943, Master und Mitarbeiter 1947, Dack, Master und Mitarbeiter 1949.
[5] Büchner und Weyland 1959.   [6] Büchner 1958.

renale, adrenale, adreno-corticale, hypophysäre Hypertonie, und bei jeder Form
des *chronischen Cor pulmonale*, also z.B. durch Mitralstenose, Myxom des linken

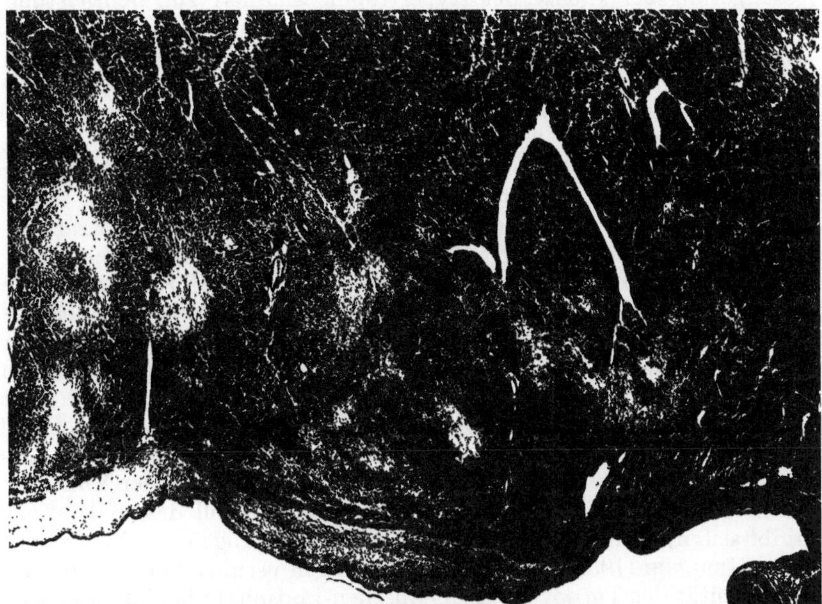

Abb. 20. Stufenschnitt aus der Wand des linken Ventrikels des gleichen Falles von Aortenstenose. Unten verdicktes Endokard, oben epikardnaher Herzmuskel. In der inneren Hälfte der Wand des linken Ventrikels zahlreiche Narben nach ischämischem Untergang von Herzmuskulatur. (Nach BÜCHNER, F., u. R. WEYLAND 1959.)

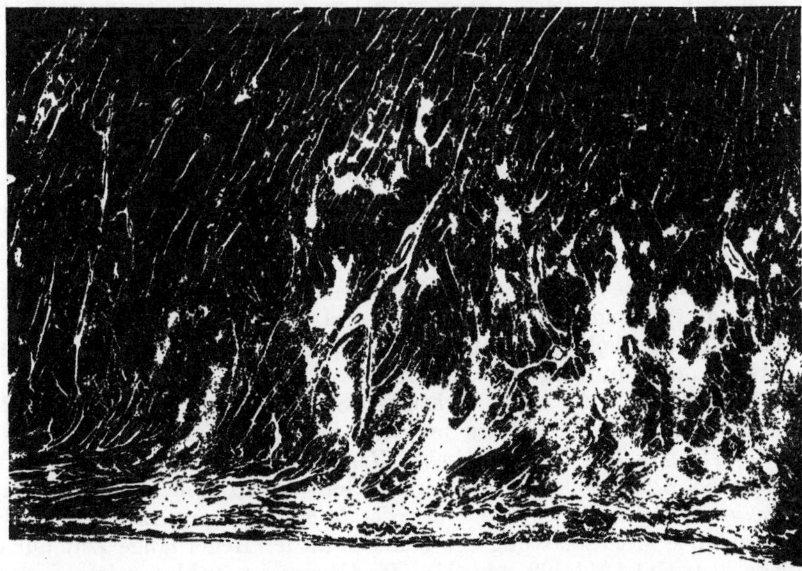

Abb. 21. Stufenschnitt durch die Wand des linken Ventrikels bei schwerer akut einsetzender Aorteninsuffizienz infolge Endocarditis ulcerosa polyposa. Oben epikardnahe Abschnitte, unten Endokard. In der inneren Hälfte der Wand des linken Ventrikels ausgedehnte konfluierende Narbenherde infolge schwerer Ischämie. Keine Coronarverschlüsse und -stenosen. (Nach BÜCHNER, F., u. R. WEYLAND 1959.)

Vorhofs, Panarteriitis oder Endarteriitis der Lungenarterien, rezidivierende
Mikroembolie der Pulmonalarterien. Wir postulieren, daß in all diesen Fällen

chronischer Herzhypertrophie die Durchblutung des Herzmuskels im hypertrophierten Ventrikel gesteigert ist. Aber wir fragen: Bleibt diese Durchblutungssteigerung bei wachsender Hypertrophie adäquat zur Mehrleistung des Herzens oder kommt sie mit der Zeit in die Phase einer paradoxen Ischämie. Wäre dem so, dann müßte die Durchblutungsinsuffizienz zu einer Störung der Energetik des Herzmuskels führen und sich in meßbaren Stoffwechselstörungen des Herzmuskels manifestieren. Das war die Annahme einer Reihe von Klinikern und Pathologen der letzten 3 Jahrzehnte[1].

Vom Standpunkt der Biochemie hat dagegen BING auf Grund seiner Untersuchungen und der seines Arbeitskreises eine Störung der Energetik im hypertrophierten menschlichen Herzmuskel verneint[2]. Er führte bei Kranken mit kompensierter und dekompensierter Herzhypertrophie eine Katheterung des Coronarsinus durch und stellte fest, daß bei ihnen der ATP-Gehalt sowie die Utilisationen von Sauerstoff, Glucose, Pyruvat, Lactat, Fettsäure, Aminosäure und Ketonen die gleichen waren wie bei Herzgesunden. Auch war der respiratorische Quotient normal. Gegenüber diesen Befunden ist zunächst die Frage aufzuwerfen, ob die normale Stoffdifferenz zwischen arteriellem Zustrom und venösem Abstrom im Gesamtorgan einen abnormen Stoffwechsel in Teilen des Myokards ausschließt und ob sich dieser dem Untersucher bei der gewählten Methode entziehen kann. Insbesondere wird durch die von BING angewandte Methode der Turnover der wichtigsten Metaboliten nicht erfaßt. Wie bedeutungsvoll dessen Bestimmung wäre, ergibt sich mit Notwendigkeit aus den Untersuchungen von FLECKENSTEIN, JANKE und GERLACH (1959). Diese Untersuchungen vermitteln erstmalig ein Bild von der Intensität des Turnover der organischen Phosphate bei ihrem konstanten Gehalt am arbeitenden Herzmuskel. Nach diesen Befunden muß mit der Möglichkeit gerechnet werden, daß bei normaler Utilisation der Turnover pro Gewichtseinheit sich im hypertrophierten Herzmuskel an den relativ verringerten Durchstrom anpaßt, indem er sich verlangsamt. Die Herzdynamik müßte dabei herabgesetzt sein, ohne daß der aktuelle Stoffgehalt des Herzmuskels und die Utilisation der Metaboliten krankhaft verändert wäre. BING selbst erörtert diese Möglichkeit nicht. Er sieht vielmehr das Wesen des Insuffizient-Werdens des hypertrophierten Herzmuskels in seiner Unfähigkeit, die im Herzmuskelstoffwechsel freigesetzte Energie zu verwerten. In diesem Sinne deutet er die von ihm gemachte Feststellung, daß das Aktomyosin des krankhaft hypertrophierten Herzmuskels des Menschen sich postmortal schlechter kontrahiert als das des normalen Menschen. Nach experimenteller Herzhypertrophie beim Hunde war die Aktomyosinkonzentration herabgesetzt, ebenso die Reaktion des Aktomyosins auf den Zusatz von ATP[3]. Zur Morphologie der Insuffizienz des hypertrophierten Herzens sagt BING 1959: „The pathologist is unable to find specific changes in heart muscle of patients who died in congestive failure."

Diese Bemerkung trifft etwas richtiges. Sie entbindet uns aber nicht von der intensiven Auseinandersetzung mit den Befunden der *pathologischen Morphologie des Herzmuskels bei chronischer Herzhypertrophie.* Betrachten wir das makroskopische Bild des hypertrophierten Herzens, so stellen wir fest, *daß die Hypertrophie in vielen Fällen auf einen der beiden Herzventrikel beschränkt* ist, da die krankhafte Mehrbelastung des Herzens in der Regel lange Zeit nur einen Herzmuskel betrifft[4] (Abb. 22 und 23). Im Coronarvenenblut, wie es von BING zu seinen Untersuchungen gewonnen wurde, mischt sich also das venöse Blut

---

[1] EPPINGER 1931, HARRISON 1931, 1935, BÜCHNER, WEBER und HAAGER 1935, LINZBACH 1947ff., SCHOENMACKERS 1949 u.a.
[2] BING 1951—1959.   [3] BENSON 1955.
[4] W. MÜLLER 1883, WIDEROE 1911, KIRCH 1921—1955, DÜLL 1941.

aus dem normal belasteten und das aus dem hypertrophierten Ventrikel. So könnten Unterschiede in der Utilisation der Metaboliten durch die Beimischung

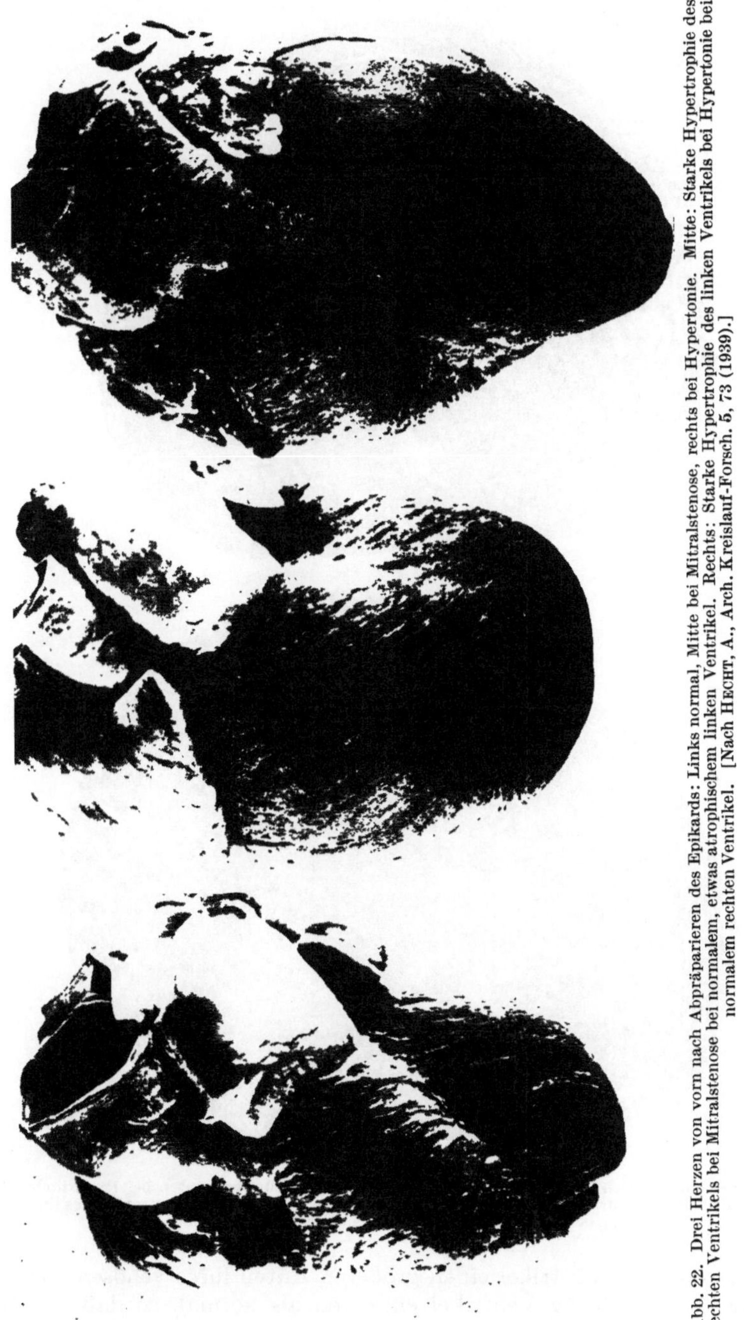

Abb. 22. Drei Herzen von vorn nach Abpräparieren des Epikards: Links normal, Mitte bei Mitralstenose, rechts bei Hypertonie. Mitte: Starke Hypertrophie des rechten Ventrikels bei Mitralstenose bei normalem, etwas atrophischem linken Ventrikel. Rechts: Starke Hypertrophie des linken Ventrikels bei Hypertonie bei normalem rechten Ventrikel. [Nach HECHT, A., Arch. Kreislauf-Forsch. 5, 73 (1939).]

des Venenblutes aus dem normalen Ventrikel verdeckt bleiben. Damit muß besonders bei rechtshypertrophierten Herzen gerechnet werden, bei denen der

Gewichtsanteil des hypertrophierten rechten Ventrikels im Durchschnitt höchstens den des normalen linken erreicht. Hinzu kommt aber die Wahrscheinlichkeit,

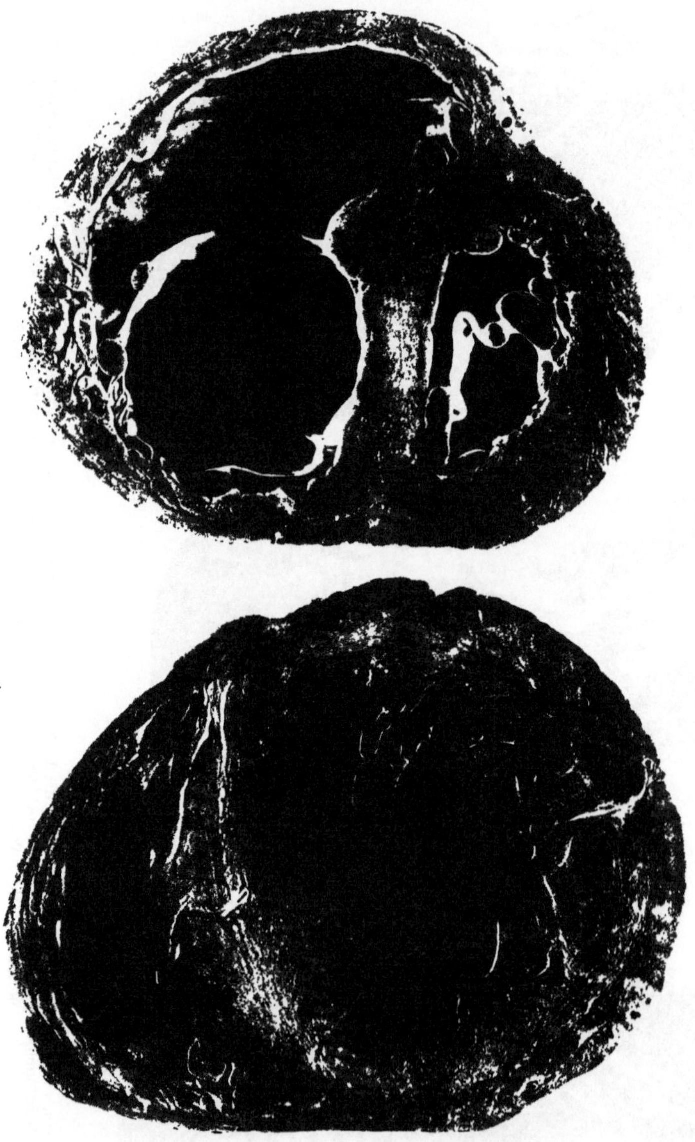

Abb. 23. Querschnitte durch beide Herzkammern: Oben bei Mitralstenose, unten bei Hypertonie. Bei Mitralstenose reine Hypertrophie des rechten Ventrikels, bei Hypertonie fast reine Hypertrophie des linken Ventrikels [Nach Hecht, A., Arch. Kreislauf-Forsch. 5, 73 (1939).]

daß hypertrophierte Ventrikel einen größeren Anteil ihres venösen Blutes durch die Venae Thebesi in die Ventrikel entleeren als normal, so daß das Blut des Sinus coronarius nur zu einem Teil das venöse Blut des hypertrophierten Ventrikels enthält. Angesichts dieser Überlegungen ist es immerhin bemerkenswert, daß im Herzmuskel der Ratte bei experimenteller Hypertrophie durch Drosselungshochdruck eine zunehmende signifikante Verringerung von Kreatinphosphat und weniger von ATP ohne Herzinsuffizienz, insbesondere ohne Lungenödem, gemessen wurde[1]. Anderslautende Ergebnisse scheinen methodenbedingt zu sein[2].

Wichtiger ist aber die Frage nach den Veränderungen der Herzmuskelzellen im hypertrophierten Herzmuskel. Hier hatte schon EPPINGER (1931) die These aufgestellt, daß die Massenzunahme des überlasteten Ventrikels durch echte Hypertrophie der einzelnen Herzmuskelzellen eine zunehmende Verschlechterung der Sauerstoffversorgung der hypertrophierten Zellen herbeiführe. Die gleiche

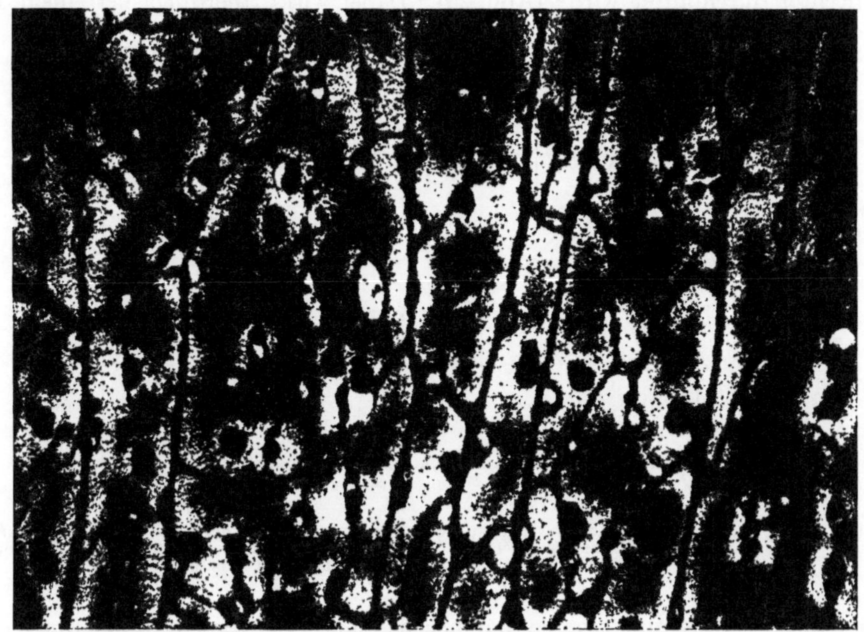

. Abb. 24. Querschnitt durch das Myokard der Ratte mit Silberimprägnation der Capillarwände nach GÖMÖRI. Zahlreiche klaffende Capillaren im Verhältnis 1:1 zu den Querschnitten der Herzmuskelzellen. (Nach SUWA, N., 1959.)

Auffassung suchte HARRISON (1931, 1935) durch Querschnittsmessungen hypertrophischer Fasern zu beweisen. Er war der Meinung, daß von einem bestimmten Grenzwert der Dicke der Herzmuskelzellen an die Sauerstoffversorgung insuffizient würde[3]. Ein weiterer Faktor wurde in der relativ zur Masse kleineren Oberfläche der hypertrophierten Herzmuskelzelle und der dadurch bedingten Erschwerung des Stoffaustausches in die Zelle und aus der Zelle gesehen. Neueste Untersuchungen von LINZBACH (1958) und HORT (1953—1958) haben aber ergeben, daß die Verhältnisse bei der Hypertrophie komplizierter liegen. Zunächst konnten sie feststellen, daß im Erwachsenenherzen auf eine Herzmuskelzelle eine Capillare kommt. [Bei der erwachsenen Ratte wurde fast die gleiche Relation festgestellt[4] (Abb. 24).] Auch bei der physiologischen Hypertrophie durch sportliches Training des Menschen bleibt die Relation 1:1 erhalten, ebenso bei der krankhaften Herzhypertrophie bis zu einem kritischen Herzgewicht von etwa 500 g. Wird dieses überschritten, so kommt es durch Spaltung zu einer echten Hyperplasie, d.h. Vermehrung der Herzmuskelzellen. Mit ihr geht eine

---

[1] DUSPIVA 1959, DUSPIVA und GOHL 1959.   [2] LÜTHY 1959.
[3] Vgl. auch BÜCHNER, WEBER und HAAGER 1935, BÜCHNER 1939, 1949, LINZBACH 1947, NIETH 1949.   [4] SUWA 1959.

Zunahme der Capillaren einher, so daß das Verhältnis 1:1 gewahrt bleibt. Linzbach (1958) ist daher heute der Auffassung, daß der Herzmuskel sich bei Zunahme seiner Masse durch die Folge von Hypertrophie und Hyperplasie der
Herzmuskelzellen und durch die Capillarvermehrung der Gefahr der paradoxen
arteriellen Ischämie zu entziehen sucht[1].

Prüft man freilich die postmortale Durchströmungsfähigkeit des Coronarsystems mit einer Flüssigkeit von der Viscosität des Blutes, so stellt man fest,
daß die Gewichtseinheit des Herzmuskels mit zunehmender Hypertrophie immer
schlechter durchblutet wird[2] (Abb. 25). Dabei wirkt allerdings bei einem Teil

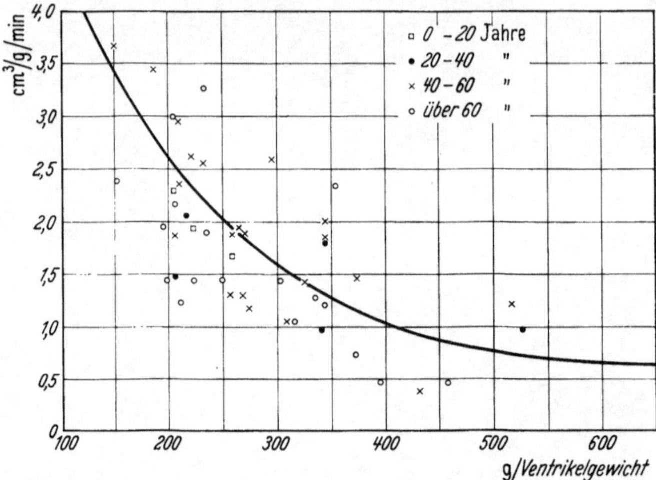

Abb. 25. Die postmortale Durchströmungsfähigkeit des Coronarsystems bei normalen und hypertrophierten
Herzen. Abnahme der Durchströmungsfähigkeit pro Gramm Herzgewicht mit zunehmender Herzhypertrophie.
[Nach Vivell, O., Beitr. path. Anat. 111, 125, 1950, Abb. 2.]

der Fälle von Herzhypertrophie, nämlich bei den Hypertonien, in der Regel eine
hypertonische stenosierende Coronarsklerose zusätzlich als Durchströmungs-
hindernis. Aber bei den Nicht-Hypertonikern mit Hypertrophie ohne Coronarsklerose lagen die Werte ähnlich tief. Die Lösung scheint in Untersuchungen
gefunden zu sein, in denen die lichte Weite der Kranzaderabgänge und ihrer
größeren Äste gemessen wurde[3]. Es stellte sich heraus, daß diese zunächst
parallel mit der Hypertrophie des Herzens zunimmt, dann aber nach Erreichen
eines Maximums sich nicht mehr steigert, während die Herzmuskelmasse sich
weiter vermehrt. In dieser Phase soll es dann zu Durchblutungs- und Stoff-
austauschstörungen im hypertrophierten Herzen kommen[4].

Daß bei höheren Graden der Hypertrophie des Herzmuskels tatsächlich eine
paradoxe arterielle Ischämie im Myokard eintritt, kann zunächst aus systematischen histotopographischen Stufenuntersuchungen des hypertrophierten Herzens
geschlossen werden[5]. Fast in jedem über dem kritischen Gewicht liegenden
Herzen mit krankhafter Hypertrophie kommt es in Schüben zu Parenchymnekrosen von Herzmuskelzellen und zu deren Ersatz durch mesenchymale Faser-
narben, überwiegend in der Muskulatur des hypertrophierten Herzanteils
(Abb. 26). Das gilt von den linkshypertrophierten Herzen ebenso wie von

---

[1] Vgl. auch Wearn 1928, 1939/40.   [2] Dock 1941, Vivell 1950.
[3] Schoenmackers 1949, Vogelberg 1957.   [4] Schoenmackers 1949, Linzbach 1958.
[5] Büchner, Weber und Haager 1935, Linzbach 1947, de Brux 1947, Büchner und
Weyland 1959.

den rechtshypertrophierten. Diese kleinherdigen Zerstörungen von Herzmuskelzellen können nur als die akute Manifestierung einer latenten Bereitschaft zur paradoxen Durchblutungsinsuffizienz oder als Folge von akuten Steigerungen einer manifesten Durchblutungsinsuffizienz verstanden werden. Dafür spricht auch das elektronenmikroskopische Bild bei experimenteller Herzhypertrophie der weißen Ratte durch Drosselungshochdruck: Nach Belastung durch Laufen zeigen hier die Mitochondrien die gleichen schweren Zerstörungen der inneren Lamellen wie sie bei akuter Hypoxie beobachtet wurden[1].

Ebenso sprechen die elektrokardiographischen Befunde und die Ergebnisse der Vektordiagraphie dafür, daß im stark hypertrophierten Herzmuskel mit der Zeit eine paradoxe arterielle Ischämie eintritt. Während vorübergehend die Meinung vertreten wurde, daß bei Hypertrophie allein durch Verlängerung der Wegstrecke für die Erregung oder Verlangsamung der Erregungsausbreitung Senkungen von ST und T bis zum Negativwerden resultieren[2], haben ausführliche neuere Untersuchungen[3], frühere Befunde[4] bestätigt, nach denen diese wie andere Zeichen des Elektrokardiogramms bei Hypertrophie des Herzmuskels eine paradoxe Ischämie anzeigen[5]. Freilich ist bei Auswertung der Kurven sowie des Belastungstestes und des Hypoxämie-Testes, vor allem in der Bewertung der ST-Senkung, besondere Kritik geboten[6]. Von einem stärkeren Ausschlag der Kurve ab ist aber der Test als positiv zu werten[7].

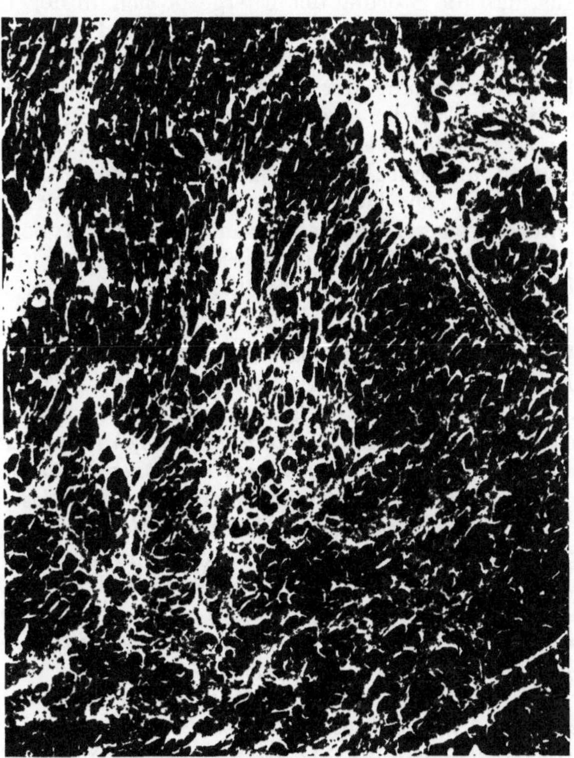

Abb. 26. Ausgedehnte ischämische Narben in der Muskulatur des rechten Ventrikels nach chronischem Cor pulmonale durch rezidivierende Mikroembolie der Pulmonalarterien mit Stenosen im Pulmonalsystem. (Nach BÜCHNER, F., u. R. WEYLAND 1959.)

Die elektrokardiographischen Befunde werden durch die des Vektorkardiogramms wesentlich gestützt: Das Vektorkardiogramm zeigt bei Links- und Rechtshypertrophie häufig einen Schleifenverlauf, der nicht allein durch die Hypertrophie zu erklären und Ausdruck einer Durchblutungsinsuffizienz des hypertrophierten Herzens ist[8]. Auf Grund der morphologischen Befunde müssen wir daher trotz der Beobachtungen von BING und seinen Mitarbeitern an der Auf-

---

[1] MÖLBERT und IIJIMA 1958, 1959.   [2] H. SCHAEFER 1951.
[3] BÜCHNER, KLEPZIG, REINDELL und WEYLAND 1952, 1959.
[4] BÜCHNER, WEBER und HAAGER 1935, HAAS und WEBER 1936, PAPAGEORGIOU und WEBER 1941, REINDELL und BAYER 1943.   [5] Vgl. auch FRIEDBERG 1959.
[6] LEVY und Mitarbeiter 1941, BURCHELL und Mitarbeiter 1948, BIÖRCK 1947.
[7] BÜCHNER, KLEPZIG, REINDELL und WEYLAND 1959, MASTER, ROSENFELD und DONOSO 1959.
[8] BILGER 1958, 1959, BILGER, SANDER, REINDELL und KLEPZIG 1957.

fassung festhalten, daß die Insuffizienz des hypertrophierten Herzmuskels durch eine vorausgehende chronische Coronarinsuffizienz im Sinne einer paradoxen Ischämie und eine dadurch hervorgerufene Insuffizienz der Energetik des Herzmuskels herbeigeführt wird. Dabei dürfte eine Änderung im Kaliumgehalt des hypertrophierten Herzmuskels die Folge, nicht die Ursache einer energetischen Insuffizienz sein, im besonderen die Folge einer Hypoxie[1]. Das schließt nicht aus, daß die Störung der Energetik sich in der Ultrastruktur des Herzmuskels, vor allem am Aktomyosin, auswirkt und dessen Kontraktilität herabsetzt, wie es Bing (1959) feststellte. Elektronenmikroskopisch konnte bei experimenteller Herzhypertrophie der Ratte an den Protofibrillen der Herzmuskelzelle eine später sich wieder ausgleichende Verdickung gemessen werden[2].

Zu paradoxen arteriellen Ischämien kommt es auch im Herzmuskel, im Gehirn und in anderen Parenchymen bei allen *schweren Hypoxämien* verschiedenen Ursprungs. Die Durchblutung ist in diesen Fällen in Anpassung an die Hypoxämie gesteigert, kann aber den durch die Hypoxämie bedingten stark erhöhten Blutbedarf nicht decken. Diese Phänomene sind von uns ausführlich in diesem Handbuch, Bd. IV/2 dargestellt, so daß es genügt, auf diesen Beitrag zu verweisen.

Die wichtigsten Befunde bei relativer arterieller Ischämie seien in den folgenden Leitsätzen noch einmal zusammengefaßt:

1. Stenosebedingte relative Ischämien führen bei chronischer Wirkung an parenchymatösen Organen zu Parenchymatrophien und zu Hyalinisierungen und Sklerosierungen des Mesenchyms, am Hirn zur diffusen Parenchymatrophie ohne Gliose oder zur granulären Parenchymatrophie mit Gliose.

2. Parenchymatrophien können schleichend sich entwickelnde Funktionsstörungen und -ausfälle bewirken. Latente Funktionsschwächen können durch zusätzliche allgemeine Oligämie akut in manifeste funktionelle Insuffizienzen übergehen.

3. Bei mäßigen arteriellen Stenosen kann die arterielle Versorgung des Organs in der Ruhe suffizient sein, durch Belastung infolge erhöhten Blutbedarfes des Organparenchyms dagegen akut insuffizient werden.

4. Solche paroxysmale akute relative arterielle Ischämien sind uns als Folge arterieller Stenosen besonders an der Beinmuskulatur, am Hirn und vor allem am Herzmuskel bekannt, am Herzmuskel unter dem Anfall der akuten Coronarinsuffizienz.

5. Im schweren Anfall akuter Coronarinsuffizienz entwickeln sich lichtmikroskopisch disseminierte kleinherdige elektive Parenchymnekrosen mit einer Manifestationszeit von Stunden.

6. Den lichtmikroskopischen Veränderungen gehen, nach elektronenmikroskopischen Untersuchungen bei exogener Hypoxie oder toxischer Hemmung der Aerobiose, in der akuten Coronarinsuffizienz ausgedehnte Veränderungen der Ultrastruktur der Herzmuskelzelle voraus, die der Ausdruck einer energetisch-osmotischen Insuffizienz der Herzmuskelzellen sind.

7. Die energetisch-osmotische Insuffizienz der Herzmuskelzellen führt in der akuten Coronarinsuffizienz nicht selten unmittelbar in die tödliche dynamische Herzinsuffizienz.

8. Bei chronisch überlasteten Herzen kommt es zur paradoxen arteriellen Ichämie, d.h. zu einer Coronarinsuffizienz trotz krankhaft gesteigerter Coronardurchblutung.

9. Bewiesen ist die paradoxe arterielle Ischämie für die Aortenstenose und für das akute Cor pulmonale, unseres Erachtens auch für die Aorteninsuffizienz. In allen diesen Fällen finden sich als Spuren akuter paradoxer arterieller Ischämie

---

[1] Lagerlöf 1959.　　[2] Mölbert und Jijima 1958.

mehr oder minder ausgedehnte Parenchymnekrosen des Herzmuskels oder deren Narben, besonders nach Aortenstenose, nach akut einsetzender Aorteninsuffizienz infolge Endocarditis ulcerosa polyposa, nach thrombotischer oder experimenteller Lungenembolie.

10. Umstritten ist noch die Frage, ob die krankhafte chronische Hypertrophie des Herzmuskels jeder Ätiologie von einem bestimmten Ausmaß an regelhaft eine paradoxe arterielle Ischämie des Myokards herbeiführt. Den normalen arteriovenösen Differenzen der Metaboliten im ein- und ausströmenden Coronarblut nach BING *stehen die lichtmikroskopisch nachweisbaren ischämischen Veränderungen des Myokards und die elektrokardiographischen Befunde gegenüber.*

Die spastische arterielle Ischämie.

Die Tatsache, daß Arterien sich unter der Wirkung einer lokalen Reizung ihrer glatten Muskulatur vorübergehend krampfhaft kontrahieren und verschließen können, wurde schon in der Mitte des 19. Jahrhunderts durch die Entzündungsexperimente von COHNHEIM (1867, 1873) bekannt. COHNHEIM experimentierte an der Zunge, der Schwimmhaut und an der Nickhaut des lebenden Frosches, zum Teil auch am Ohr des lebenden Kaninchens. In diesen Experimenten wurden an umschriebener Stelle chemische, mechanische oder thermische Reize gesetzt. Dabei kam es zu vorübergehenden Kontraktionen der Arterien, zu Strömungsverlangsamungen oder -steigerungen in den Capillaren, zum Teil zum Stillstand der capillären Durchblutung. Jahrzehnte später haben RICKER und REGENDANZ (1921) die Cohnheimschen Versuche systematisch auf den Warmblüter übertragen und vor allem am freigelegten Pankreas des Kaninchens nachgeprüft.

RICKER hat ebenso wie COHNHEIM in den Arbeiten seines Arbeitskreises die Durchblutungsstörungen ausführlich beschrieben, aber kaum durch Abbildungen belegt. So leiden die älteren Untersuchungen eines so dynamischen Vorganges am Gefäßsystem, wie er bei der Wirkung umschriebener entzündlicher Reize gegeben ist, an dem Mangel an ausreichender Verobjektivierung und Dokumentation der in Rede stehenden Phänomene. Das hat z.B. bei der Analyse der Durchblutungsstörungen bei der allergischen Entzündung dazu geführt, den Angriffspunkt der allergischen Mechanismen zunächst in den Capillaren zu suchen[1], später in den Arterien und Arteriolen[2] und schließlich in jüngster Zeit in den Venen[3].

RICKER und REGENDANZ (1921) haben geglaubt, nach ihren Untersuchungen bei den durch einen örtlichen Reiz ausgelösten Durchblutungsstörungen eine Stufenregel herausarbeiten zu können. Nach dieser Stufenregel soll die Durchblutungsstörung im Wirkungsfeld des Reizes mit einer aktiven Erweiterung und Mehrdurchblutung der Arteriolen beginnen, d.h. mit einer Fluxion. Erst nach Steigerung der Reizwirkung soll dann eine Kontraktion der Arteriolen und dadurch eine Ischämie zustande kommen. Nach weiterer Zunahme der Reizwirkung soll durch Lähmung der glatten Muskelzellen der Arteriolenwand eine Erschlaffung der Arteriolen eintreten und durch sie eine passive Erweiterung und eine erneute Fluxion im Arteriolenbereich. Erst auf dem Höhepunkt der Durchblutungsstörung greife dann der Reiz an der Wand der den Arteriolen vorgeordneten Arterien an. An diesen käme es zu einer Verengerung und schließlich zum Verschluß und dadurch zur spastischen arteriellen Ischämie.

Heute liegt eine Reihe von experimentellen Untersuchungen vor, in denen die Durchblutungsstörungen bei der Entzündung in intravitalen Photogramm-

---

[1] RÖSSLE 1914, FRÖHLICH 1914.   [2] ABELL und SCHENK 1938.
[3] RICH 1951, LECOMTE und HUGUES 1955.

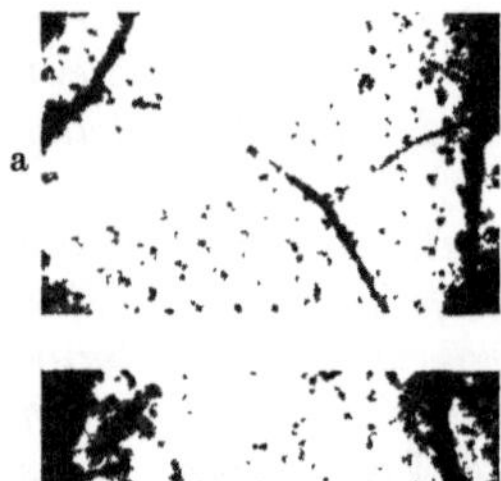

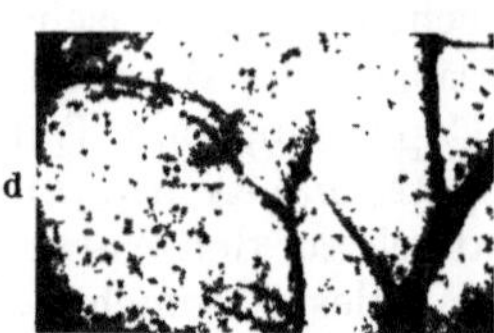

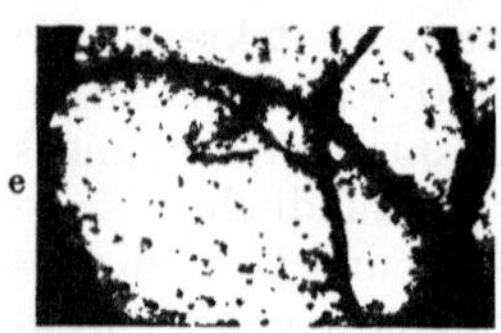

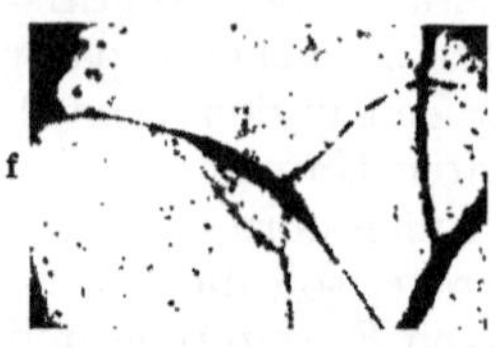

Abb. 27a—f. Intravitales Photogramm der Ohrarterien nach 1 γ Histamin subcutan. a Vor dem Versuche normale Durchblutung, b—d starke Kontraktion der Arterie nach der Injektion mit völliger Durchblutungssperre, e Wiederherstellung der Durchblutung, f Dilatation in dem primär kontrahierten Arterienabschnitt. [Nach IIJIMA, S., Beitr. path. Anat. 119, 433, 1958, Abb. 11.]

serien der Gefäße festgehalten, wurden[1], von TANNENBERG (1927) sowie von MEINERS (1949) auch im Film. Nach den Untersuchungen von HORSTMANN (1955) und IIJIMA (1957) stellen sich die Verhältnisse in vielfacher Übereinstimmung mit den Ergebnissen der anderen Autoren folgendermaßen dar: Am Ohr des lebenden Kaninchens, unserem bevorzugten Untersuchungsobjekt, beobachtet man in der Norm einen periodischen Wechsel der Arterienweite zwischen Erweiterung und Verengerung. Der Wechsel erfolgt in der Regel nach einer Dauer der Erweiterung bzw. Verengerung von 15—20 sec. Diese *physiologische Vasomotion* wird von den verschiedensten Außenfaktoren beeinflußt, z. B. von der Temperatur, der Luftfeuchtigkeit, der Belichtung, von Geräuschen.

Ein *umschriebener Reiz am Kaninchenohr* bewirkt 1. augenblicklich mit dem Einsetzen eines auch nur kurzfristigen mechanischen, thermischen oder chemischen Reizes eine *spastische Kontraktion der Arterie an der Reizstelle* (Abb. 27), 2. eine *Steigerung der Vasomotion* an allen anderen Ohrarterien, *oder* 3. eine *allgemein Arterienerweiterung* am übrigen Ohr. Von einer Stufenfolge: erst Arteriolenveränderungen dann Arterienkontraktion ist nach diesen Experimenten nicht die Rede. Die Dauer des Arterienspasmus ist in der Regel von der Dauer und Intensität des Reizes abhängig. Sie betrug in unseren Versuchen: beim mechanischen Reiz von 5—10 sec in der Regel $1/_2$—1 min, beim Kältereiz von 1 min 2—5 min, nach intracutaner Injektion von 1 γ Histamin 10—20 min. *Die Venen nehmen an der Kontraktion nicht teil* und bleiben während des Versuchs in ihrer Durchblutung fast unverändert.

Histamin breitet sich nach der Injektion entlang der Arterie aus. Dadurch wird seine Wirkung besonders nachhaltig und ausgedehnt. Das geht vor allem aus Experimenten von HAYDON (1958) an der Backentasche des Hamsters hervor.

In diesen Versuchen bewirkte die einmalige Injektion von 0,2 γ Histamin augenblicklich eine Kontraktion der der Histamin-Quaddel benachbarten Arterie, in der Folge eine Ausbreitung der Kontraktion herzwärts und nach distal mit einem Maximum der Ausbreitung nach 20 min, dann eine Wiederfüllung der Arterie nach 34—42 min und eine Wiederherstellung der normalen Durchblutung nach 45 min. In diesen Untersuchungen wurde nach 0,2 γ Histamin kein völliger Verschluß der Arterie mit totaler Entleerung festgestellt, sondern eine hochgradige Verengerung mit segmentärer Steigerung der Ringe und mehrfacher Wiederholung der ringförmigen Kontraktion im gleichen Segment, also keine peristaltische Welle. Während des ganzen Vorganges waren die Venen von unveränderter Weite.

---

[1] LEWIS 1927, 1928, TANNENBERG 1925, 1926, 1927, TANNENBERG und FISCHER-WASELS 1925, 1927, LANG und Mitarbeiter 1930, TITTEL 1944, MEINERS 1949—1952, BELLMAN 1953, ZWEIFACH 1953, ILLIG 1952—1955, STRUCK 1955, HORSTMANN 1955, IIJIMA 1957, HAYDON 1958.

Gleichsinnige Kontraktionen treten primär an den Arteriolen des Reizfeldes auf. Die Kontraktion der Arterie wird in der Regel von einer Dilatation an der

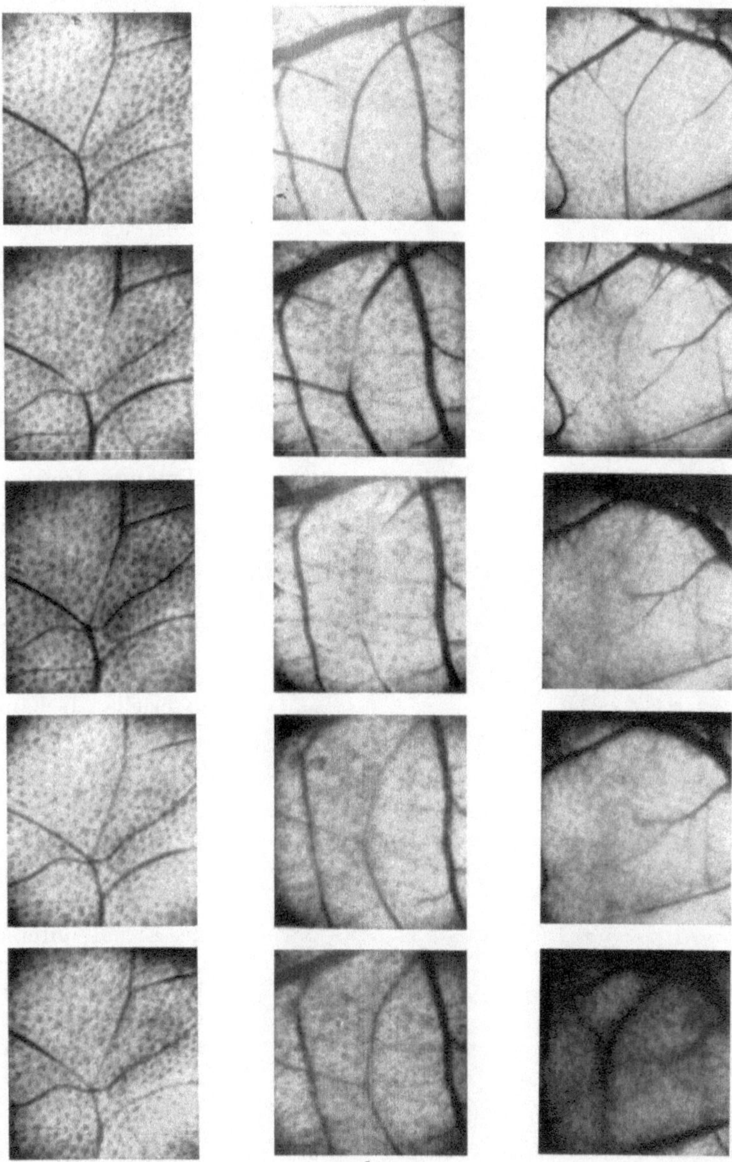

Abb. 28a—c. Intravitale Photogramme von Ohrgefäßen des Kaninchens nach lokaler Injektion von 0,005 cm³ Pferdeserum. a Beim normergischen Tier, b beim sensibilisierten Tier mit Präcipitintiter 1:640, c beim sensibilisierten Tier mit Präcipitintiter 1:2560. a Vorher, nach 5, 10, 30 min; b vorher, nach 2, 10, 20, 40 min; c vorher, nach 2, 30, 60, 150 min. Beim normergischen Tier Durchblutung schon nach 10 min wiederhergestellt, beim sensibilisierten Tier mit niedrigem Präcipitintiter nach 20 min, mit hohem Präcipitintiter nach 60 min noch nicht wiederhergestellt. (Nach IIJIMA, S., Beitr. path. Anat. 118, 67, 1957, Abb. 6.]

Reizstelle und einer Verlagerung des Spasmus nach herzwärts und distal der Reizstelle gefolgt, so daß ein Ringspasmus sichtbar werden kann[1]. Nach kurzer

[1] TITTEL 1944, HORSTMANN 1955, IIJIMA 1957.

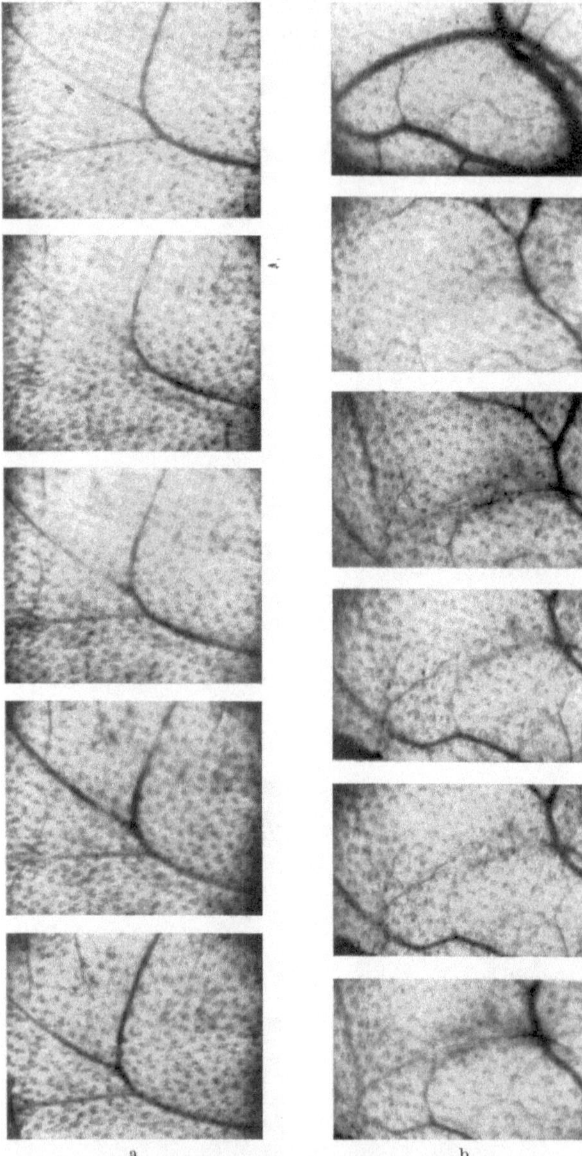

Abb. 29a u. b.   Intravitale Photogramme von Ohrgefäßen des Kaninchens, b nach Sensibilisierung mit Pferdeserum. Wirkung von 1 γ Histamin: a beim normergischen Tier, b beim sensibilisierten Tier in der 3. Woche. a Kontraktion der Arterie an der Reizstelle 5 min nach Injektion, b Kontraktion der Arterie an der Reizstelle bis 90 min nach Injektion. [Nach Iijima, S., Beitr. path. Anat. 118, 241, 1957, Abb. 6.]

Zeit verschwindet auch dieser und die normale Durchblutung wird wieder hergestellt.

Ist die Arterie noch kontrahiert, während die nachgeordneten Arteriolen schon erschlafft sind, so kommt es zunächst zur verlangsamten Durchblutung in den Capillaren. Wird die Arterie spastisch verschlossen, so steht die Durchblutung in den nachgeordneten Arteriolen und Capillaren still. Die gleichsinnige Wirkung verschiedener Reize wird damit erklärt, daß durch sie im Gewebe momentan Histamin freigesetzt wird und dieses die Kontraktion der Arterie an der Reizstelle unabhängig von der Qualität des primären Reizes auslöst.

Eine wesentliche Steigerung erfährt die spastische arterielle Ischämie nach Intensität und Dauer bei der *lokalen Anaphylaxie* (s. Letterer 1956). Experimentell wurde diese schon 1903 von Arthus und Breton nach Sensibilisierung des Tieres gegen artfremdes Eiweiß untersucht. Die dabei auftretenden Durchblutungsstörungen wurden von verschiedenen Autoren analysiert[1], zuletzt in ausgedehnten Experimenten von Iijima 1957, auf die wir uns stützen[2] (Abb. 28). Injiziert man z. B. einem Kaninchen subcutan am Ohr natives Pferdeserum in Mengen von 0,005 cm³, so bewirkt die Erstinjektion in der Regel an der Injektionsstelle eine Arterienkontraktion von 5—10 min. Injiziert man das Pferdeserum wiederholt an anderer Stelle subcutan und nach einer Serie solcher Injektionen

---

[1] Homuth 1930, Nordmann 1931, 1933, Nordmann und Speckmann 1932, Abell und Schenk 1938, Ebert und Wissler 1951.
[2] Vgl. auch Büchner 1959.

schließlich in einer Menge von 0,005 cm³ am Ohr, so bewirken die inzwischen reichlich gebildeten Antikörper in Verbindung mit dem erneut zugeführten Antigen eine hochgradige spastische Kontraktion der benachbarten Arterie. Diese dauert je nach dem Grade der Sensibilisierung, gemessen am Präcipitintiter gegen Pferdeserum, 1—2 Std und ist 30—40 min lang von einer Dilatation der übrigen Ohrarterien begleitet, häufig auch von einer gesteigerten Vasomotion. So ist es verständlich, daß an der Bauchhaut des Kaninchens die lokale Anaphylaxie infolge der langdauernden spastischen arteriellen Durchblutungssperre zur Nekrose des Gewebes führt (Arthussches Phänomen).

Die Steigerung der Arterienkontraktion nach Dauer und Intensität beim anaphylaktischen Tier geht auf eine generalisierte Steigerung der Reaktionsbereitschaft der glatten Muskulatur der Arterien, ja der gesamten glatten Muskulatur[1] durch den Antigen-Antikörperkomplex zurück. Diese wurde besonders am virginellen Uterus des Meerschweinchens ausgetestet[2]. Von hier aus ist es verständlich, daß die Arterien beim anaphylaktischen Tier auch auf die lokale Einwirkung unspezifischer Reize, also mechanischer, thermischer und chemischer Faktoren, mit einer heftigeren und länger dauernden spastischen Ischämie reagieren als beim normergischen Tier (Iijima 1957) (Abb. 29). Sie zeigen also das Phänomen der *Parallergie* (Moro und Keller 1925, Rössle 1933).

Die *spastische arterielle Ischämie* ohne anatomische Arterienveränderungen begegnet uns beim sensibilisierten Organismus noch in einem anderen Phänomen, im Bilde der *allgemeinen Anaphylaxie*, das seit Arthus (1903) sowie Pirquet und Schick (1905) bekannt ist. Wird ein Kaninchen durch eine Serie von subcutanen Injektionen gegen artfremdes Eiweiß sensibilisiert, z.B. gegen Pferdeserum, so entwickelt sich mit zunehmender Steigerung der Antikörperbildung bei dem Tier eine solche Überempfindlichkeit gegen das Antigen, daß dessen intravenöse Injektion in der Regel einen schweren, häufig tödlichen *anaphylaktischen Kollaps* auslöst. Hier kommt das Antigen unmittelbar vom Blutweg aus mit dem Antikörper an der glatten Muskulatur der Lungenarterien zur Wirkung. Die Folge ist eine augenblickliche spastische Kontraktion der Arterien in der gesamten Lungenstrombahn[3]. Dadurch hat der rechte Ventrikel eine extreme Widerstandsarbeit zu leisten, an der er sich in der Regel tödlich erschöpft. In diesen Fällen manifestiert sich die Sperre des Durchstroms der Lunge in wenigen Minuten an den Ohrgefäßen in einer völligen Blutleere der Arterien und schließlich auch der Venen[4] (Abb. 30a). Beim protrahierten anaphylaktischen Versuch kommt neben dem Leerlaufen der Ohrarterien deren spastische Kontraktion besonders deutlich zur Beobachtung (Abb. 30b)[4].

Werden isolierte Organe des Kaninchens mit Pferdeserum durchspült, so wird aus ihnen beim sensibilisierten Tier eine große Menge Histamin freigesetzt, nicht dagegen beim normergischen Tier[5]. Das gleiche ist bei anderen Tierarten festzustellen[3]. Daraus wurde gefolgert, daß der Antigen-Antikörpermechanismus durch Freisetzung von Histamin gefäßwirksam wird[6]. Für diese Hypothese können wir die Tatsache anführen, daß die intravenöse Injektion von Histamin beim Kaninchen ein ähnliches Bild des Spasmus der Pulmonalarterien mit Entleerung der Ohrgefäße verursacht wie die allgemeine Serumanaphylaxie[7].

So können wir diese Erörterungen mit der Feststellung abschließen, daß die spastische arterielle Ischämie bei der normergischen und bei der allergischen

---

[1] Schultz 1910, 1912, Dale 1913, 1920, Ratner 1955, vgl. Letterer 1956.
[2] Schultz 1910, 1912, Dale 1913.   [3] Drinker und Brofenbrenner 1924.
[4] Iijima 1957.   [5] Schachter 1953.
[6] Feldberg und Schachter 1952.   [7] Nikulin 1958.

Entzündung und bei der allgemeinen Anaphylaxie von großer pathogenetischer Bedeutung ist. Gibt es noch spastische arterielle Ischämien anderen Ursprungs?

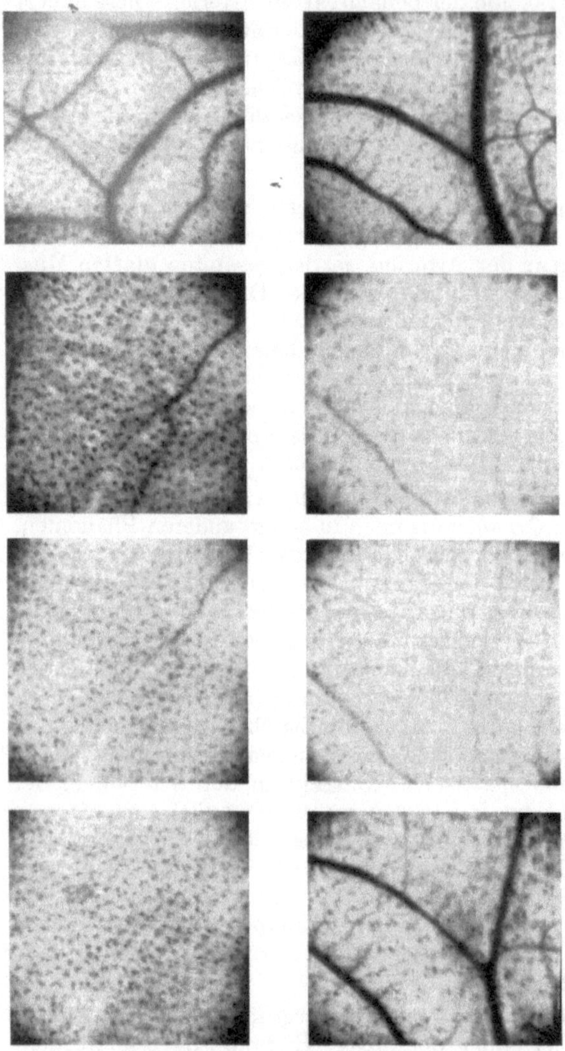

Seit dem vorigen Jahrhundert sind dem Arzte die Kennzeichen der *Raynaudschen Krankheit* bekannt. Es wurde von von Recklinghausen (1883) in einer noch heute gültigen Form folgendermaßen beschrieben:

„Nervöse anämische Individuen, vorzugsweise weiblichen Geschlechts, aber auch kräftige Individuen bekommen besonders des morgens nach dem Aufstehen, offenbar infolge der natürlichen Abkühlung beim Entblößen und Waschen sog. tote Finger in äußerster, oft gelblicher Blässe mit Gefühllosigkeit, zuweilen heftigen Schmerzen. Dieser Zustand kann Stunden dauern. Mit Recht hat Raynaud darauf hingewiesen, daß diese Zustände besonders an den Extremitäten auftreten, daß sie leicht zum symmetrischen Brande führen. Wie die kleineren Arterien bei diesem Zustande sich verengen, konnte Raynaud ophthalmoskopisch an den Netzhautarterien konstatieren."

Hier liegt also ein Krankheitsbild vor, bei dem unter der Wirkung der Kälte vor allem an den Extremitäten eine überschießende spastische arterielle Ischämie eintritt mit der Wirkung, daß infolge des langdauernden arteriellen Spasmus ohne jede anatomische Gefäßveränderung ein *trockener Brand an Händen oder Füßen* auftreten kann. Die spastische Ischämie hat also hier die Wirkung einer absoluten arteriellen Ischämie wie bei arterieller Thrombose oder Embolie.

Grundsätzlich gleichsinnige Veränderungen können wir bei nicht kälte-überempfindlichen

a   b

Abb. 30 a u. b. Verhalten der Ohrgefäße beim sensibilisierten Kaninchen nach intravenöser Erfolgsinjektion von Pferdeserum. a Vor der Injektion, während der Injektion, nach 1,5 min, nach 3 min. Völliger Leerlauf der Ohrarterien im tödlichen anaphylaktischen Schock nach Pferdeserum. b Protrahierter anaphylaktischer Schock nach Pferdeserum. Vorübergehende Entleerung und Kontraktion der Arterien, nicht der Venen, nach 15 min wieder normale Durchblutung. [Nach Iijima, S., Beitr. path. Anat. 118, 67, 1957, Abb. 1 u. 3.]

Menschen bei *Erfrierungen 3. Grades* beobachten. Auch hier kommt es unter der örtlichen Wirkung intensiver Kälte zur spastischen Kontraktion der örtlichen Arterien, die in der Zeit der Wiederaufwärmung überdauert und bei wieder intensiviertem Stoffwechsel nunmehr zum *Kältebrand*, besonders an Fingern und Zehen, Hand und Fuß, führen kann[1].

---

[1] Siegmund 1942, M. Staemmler 1944, H. J. Staemmler 1944, Lang und Mitarbeiter 1944.

Auch bei einer Reihe von *Giften* treten generalisierte, spastische arterielle Ischämien bis zur Entwicklung von Nekrosen auf. Dieses Bild mit dem spastischen Absterben von Fingern und Zehen, den Ohren und der Nasenspitze ist vor allem seit langem vom *Secale* bekannt[1], aber auch beim Nicotin, Adrenalin, Vasopressin, Baryt- und Bleisalz zu beobachten[2].

Noch wichtiger aber ist die Tatsache, daß ein relativ so häufiges Krankheitsbild wie die **Epilepsie** die *Auswirkung spastischer arterieller Ischämien am Gehirn* darstellt und daß durch diese Ischämien *herdförmige Änderungen des Hirnparenchyms* zustande kommen. Das war schon die Auffassung älterer Autoren[3]. Im besonderen aber wurde diese Deutung des Epilepsieschadens des Gehirns ausführlich durch SPIELMEYER (1927, 1928, 1933) sowie durch SCHOLZ (1933, 1949, 1951) begründet. Ischämische Abblassungen der Hirnrinde sind schon früh den Hirnchirurgen am freigelegten Gehirn während des epileptischen Anfalles aufgefallen[4]. Darüber hinaus konnte schon vor Eintreten des Krampfes eine Abblassung der Großhirnrinde beobachtet werden, insbesondere aber auch eine Kontraktion großer arterieller Arterien am freiliegenden Epileptikergehirn nach dem Anfall bis zu einer Dauer von 15—20 min[5].

Im Experiment wurde die spastische Ischämie von Gehirnarterien vor allem nach Cardiazol am Katzenhirn mit der Benzidinmethode zum Nachweis der Erythrocyten erschlossen[6]. Während die Hirnrinde am normalen Katzenhirn bei der Benzidinmethode eine gleichmäßige dichte Füllung der Rindencapillaren mit Erythrocyten erkennen läßt, finden sich nach Cardiazolkrämpfen fleckförmig über die Rinde verteilte Bezirke, in denen die Erythrocyten in den Capillaren völlig fehlen, also zumindest die Capillaren nur von Blutplasma angefüllt waren. Diese Füllungsdefekte überdauerten die Cardiazolkrämpfe beträchtlich. Auch nach Serien von Elektrokrämpfen konnten mit derselben Methode fleckförmige Ischämien des Hirnparenchyms mit einer Dauer bis zu fast $^3/_4$ Std nachgewiesen werden[7].

Daß während des epileptischen Anfalles der Hirnstoffwechsel schwer gestört ist, ergibt sich aus den schweren Veränderungen, insbesondere aus den Krampfströmen, die seit BERGER (1916) vielfach im epileptischen Anfall im EEG nachgewiesen werden konnten. R. JUNG zeigte 1949, daß im Krampfanfall nach den elektrophysiologischen Beobachtungen die Durchschnittsleistung des Hirnparenchyms, insbesondere die cellulären Oxydationen, auf das 50fache ansteigen. Daraus schließt SCHOLZ (1952), daß im epileptischen Anfall und in Krampfzuständen anderer Art in den Ganglienzellen eine *konsumptive Hypoxie als Folge der spastischen Ischämie* besteht.

Der wichtigste Beweis für das Bestehen spastischer Ischämien im Gehirn während des epileptischen Anfalles sind die seit SPIELMEYER (1927) bei der Epilepsie genauer bekannten Parenchymschäden des Gehirns. Insbesondere konnte SPIELMEYER (1928) nachweisen, daß es im epileptischen Krampfanfall im Nissl-Präparat zu charakteristischen *Rindenerbleichungen* kommt, die bei stenosierenden Gefäßprozessen des Gehirns schon früher beschrieben worden waren[8]. Den Erbleichungen liegt im akuten Stadium eine ischämische Nekrose der Ganglienzellen des betroffenen Gebietes zugrunde, bei der die Kerne pyknotisch und in der Rinde vielfach rhombisch deformiert werden. Das Cytoplasma ist im Nissl-Präparat ungefärbt und erweist sich bei der Hämatoxylin-Eosin-Färbung als acidophil, so daß es eosinrot erscheint. Bei der epileptischen Schädigung des Gehirns handelt es sich also um *elektive Parenchymnekrosen*, eine Veränderung, wie sie von SCHOLZ (1949) erstmalig mit aller Klarheit in der Neuropathologie herausgearbeitet und zu der elektiven Parenchymnekrose der Herzmuskelzellen nach akuter Coronar-

---

[1] VON RECKLINGHAUSEN 1883.   [2] MEYER und GOTTLIEB 1936.
[3] PFLEGER 1882, OSLER 1888, SACHS 1892.
[4] Zum Beispiel HORSLEY 1909, KENNEDY 1914, FÖRSTER 1926.
[5] PENFIELD 1933.   [6] DRESZER und SCHOLZ 1939.
[7] ALEXANDER und LOWENBACH 1944, SCHOLZ und JÖTTEN 1951.
[8] P. SCHROEDER 1907, 1916.

insuffizienz in Parallele gesetzt wurde. Scholz gibt diesen Veränderungen 1949 und 1957 die Deutung, daß die spastische Ischämie, die den epileptischen Anfall auslöst und ihm zugeordnet ist, in der Regel nur solange dauert, daß nach der Ischämie die in ihrem Stoffwechsel sehr anspruchsvollen Nervenzellen sich von der Stoffwechselstörung, die sie in der ischämischen Phase durchlaufen, nicht mehr erholen, während die weniger anspruchsvollen Gliazellen und Mesenchymzellen sich in der Regel von der Ischämie erholen und überleben. Gehen auch Gliazellen zugrunde, so ist auch ihre Anfälligkeit und Nekroseneigung abgestuft: zuerst werden neben den Nervenzellen die Oligodendrogliazellen, dann erst die Astrocyten und zuletzt die Mikrogliazellen nekrotisch[1]. Im Experiment konnte gezeigt werden, daß Spasmen der Piaarterien von 5 min Dauer durch direkte elektrische Reizung am Katzenhirn zu elektiven Parenchymnekrosen

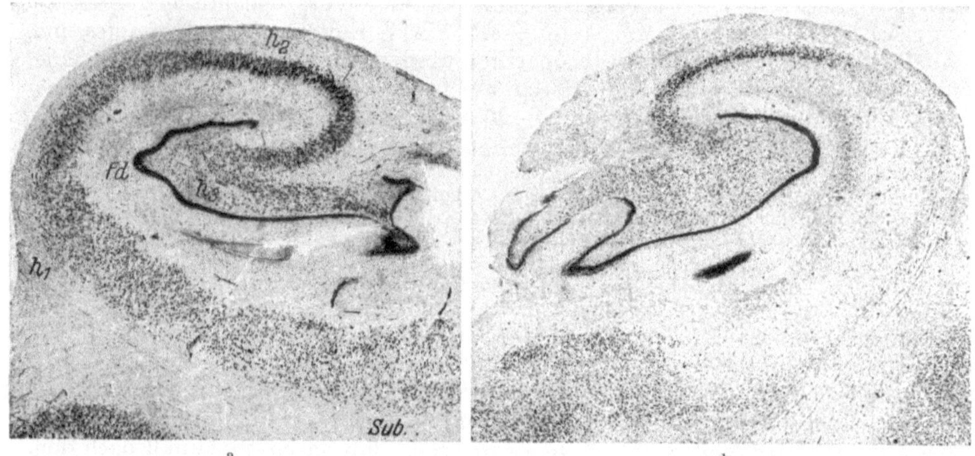

Abb. 31. Links normales Ammonshorn, rechts (spiegelbildlich) Ammonshorn eines Epileptikers. Schwund der Ganglienzellen in den Feldern h 1 und teilweise h 2 nach Anfällen spastischer Ischämie bei Epilepsie. [Aus Scholz, W., Handbuch der speziellen Pathologie, Bd. XIII/1 B, 1957, Abb. 24a u. b.)

führten[2]. Im Anschluß an die Parenchymnekrosen kommt es zu einer Wucherung der Astrocyten und der Mikrogliazellen und dadurch zur Neubildung von Gliafasern. Dabei werden die Ganglienzellen durch Neuronophagie beseitigt. Am Ende resultieren kernarme, faserdichte Narben.

Bei Epileptikern, die viele Anfälle spastischer Ischämie des Gehirns durchgemacht haben, können auf diese Weise in den schweren Anfällen zahlreiche kleine Herde elektiver Parenchymnekrosen entstehen und später in Narbenherde übergehen. Diese Befunde am Epileptikergehirn fanden eine ausführliche Darstellung durch Scholz (1951) an einem großen Beobachtungsgut verstorbener Epileptiker und erneut von Scholz und Hager (1956). Die Veränderungen haben eine *charakteristische Topik*. An erster Stelle ist das Ammonshorn betroffen und zwar in 80% der Fälle[3]. Es zeigt im Narbenzustand das Bild der *Ammonshornsklerose* (Abb. 31), von der besonders der Sommersche Sektor, also das Feld h_1, betroffen ist. *In der Großhirnrinde* finden sich als akutere Veränderungen *Erbleichungen* und *laminäre Ausfälle* (Abb. 32), also schichtförmige, die Nervenzellen bestimmter Rindenschichten elektiv befallende Parenchymnekrosen, wie sie bei der Epilepsie und bei anderen Krampfleiden beschrieben wurden[4]. Durch Narben-

---

[1] Scholz 1957.   [2] Echlin 1940, 1942.   [3] Spielmeyer 1927.
[4] Spielmeyer 1927, 1933, Husler und Spatz 1924, Braunmühl 1928, Scholz 1951.

bildung können sie zu lobären *Ulegyrien*[1] der Großhirnrinde führen[2]. Auch am Kleinhirn kommt es zu ganz entsprechenden Veränderungen, d.h. zur *Atrophie und Sklerose von Kleinhirnläppchen*. Hier werden von der elektiven Parenchymnekrose an erster Stelle die stoffwechselbedürftigsten Purkinje-Zellen, außerdem aber die Ganglienzellen der Körnerschicht betroffen. In besonders schweren Fällen kann durch diesen Prozeß eine *Hemisphärenatrophie* resultieren. Schließlich erkranken bei der Epilepsie noch bevorzugt der *Thalamus opticus* und das *Striatum* im Hirnstamm, das letztere mit einem Narbenbild im Sinne des *Status marmoratus*[3]. Im Kleinhirn wird der *Nucleus dentatus* und in der Medulla oblongata der *Nucleus olivaris inferior* betroffen. Dagegen bleiben auffallenderweise diejenigen Kerne am häufigsten verschont, welche bei allgemeinen Hypoxydosen nicht selten elektiv betroffen werden: der Globus pallidus und das Corpus Luysi[4].

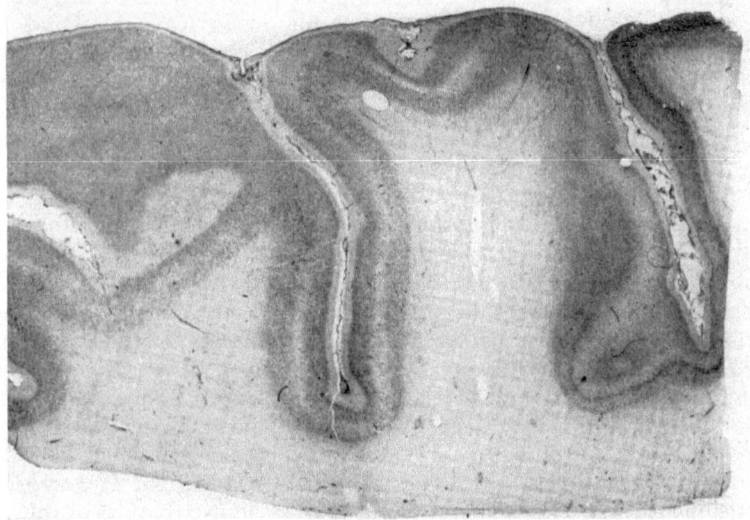

Abb. 32. Großhirnrinde mit laminärer Nekrose der Ganglienzellen im Sinne der laminären Erbleichung (heller Streifen in der sonst dunklen Großhirnrinde durch Nervenzellnekrose) nach 2stündigem epileptischem Anfall. (Aus SCHOLZ, W., u. H. HAGER, Handbuch der speziellen Pathologie, Bd. XIII/4, S. 99, 1956, Abb. 8.)

Ist nach vielen epileptischen Anfällen das Gehirn schwer von solchen Narbenherden, besonders in der Großhirnrinde, betroffen, so kommt es nicht selten zu ausgedehnten Lähmungen, bei Kindern zum Stillstand in der geistigen Entwicklung und schließlich zu Zuständen der Demenz bis zur vollen Idiotie[5]. Zu einem Teil hat die cerebrale Kinderlähmung in diesen epilepsieverursachten Veränderungen ihr anatomisches Substrat[6].

Experimentell konnten elektive Parenchymnekrosen des Hirns nach Krämpfen durch Cardiazol oder Kampfer am Meerschweinchen erzeugt werden[7].

Für das Verständnis der Epilepsie ist es von besonderem Interesse, daß nach akutem Epilepsietod auch am *Herzmuskel* in feinfleckiger Verteilung elektive Parenchymnekrosen beobachtet werden konnten[8]. Ob in diesen Fällen die Herzmuskelnekrosen ihrerseits auf spastische Ischämien von Coronararterienverzweigungen zurückgehen oder durch die extreme Steigerung der Herzarbeit infolge der Krämpfe und eine dadurch zustande kommende paradoxe relative Ischämie

[1] BRESLER 1899.   [2] SCHOB 1930, SCHOLZ 1951.   [3] C. VOGT 1911.
[4] SCHOLZ und HAGER 1956.   [5] SCHOLZ 1951.
[6] HALLERVORDEN 1939, J. E. MEYER 1949.   [7] ROTTER und KRUG 1940.
[8] GRUBER und LANZ 1920, NEUBUERGER 1928, 1933, HADORN und TILLMAN 1935.

hervorgerufen werden, ist bis heute unentschieden. Experimentell konnten durch Cardiazolkrämpfe elektive Parenchymnekrosen des Herzmuskels am Kaninchen hervorgerufen werden[1].

Mit den Beobachtungen bei der Epilepsie sind wir vor die Frage gestellt, ob die spastische arterielle Ischämie nicht eine viel ausgedehntere pathogenetische Bedeutung hat. In den ersten Jahrzehnten unseres Jahrhunderts wurde manches damals ungeklärte Krankheitsbild nach diesem Prinzip gedeutet. Aber für das peptische Geschwür sind inzwischen die Störungen der Sekretion und Motorik des Magens und Zwölffingerdarms pathogenetisch ganz in den Vordergrund getreten, die akute Leberdystrophie konnte für die meisten Fälle als maligne Virus-Hepatitis erkannt werden usw. Lange Zeit wurde ernsthaft die spastisch-ischämische Entstehung eines Teils der *Herzinfarkte* diskutiert. Aber mehr und mehr stellte man die überwältigende Bedeutung der Coronarsklerose mit thrombotischem oder sklerotischem Coronarverschluß für dieses Krankheitsbild fest, nach Friedberg (1959) in über 95% der Fälle. Die wenigen Fälle ausgedehnter infarktartiger Herzmuskelnekrosen bei normalem Coronarsystem erkannte man als Folgen von Kohlenoxydvergiftung, subtotaler großer Lungenembolie oder schwerer Anämie[2]. Auch der *Angina pectoris-Anfall* galt und gilt heute noch zum Teil als Ausdruck nervösausgelöster spastischer arterieller Ischämie des Herzmuskels bei normalem Coronarsystem. Aber auch hier sprechen alle großen autoptisch kontrollierten Untersuchungsreihen gegen diese Auffassung und überwiegend für die stenosebedingte Coronarinsuffizienz als ihre Ursache.

Auch für die Wirkung der Nitrite bei Anfällen von Angina pectoris ist die spastische Theorie des Angina pectoris-Anfalles heute durch andere Vorstellungen abgelöst[3]. Nitrit-Ionen, die sich bei Zufuhr von Natriumnitrit und Amylnitrit, aber auch nach organischen Nitraten wie Glycerintrinitrat (= Nitroglycerin) und Erythrit-tetranitrat, bei alkalischer Reaktion leicht abspalten, vermindern den Tonus der glatten Muskulatur. Ihre wichtigste pharmakologische Wirkung ist eine periphere Gefäßerweiterung, die schon bei therapeutischen Dosen zu einer Blutdrucksenkung von etwa 25 bis 35 mm Hg führt[4]. In Tierversuchen ließ sich zeigen, daß die Coronardurchblutung nach Nitroglycerin oft um das 3—5fache anstieg[5]. Eine direkte Wirkung des Nitrit-Ions auf die glatte Muskulatur der Kranzgefäße spielt dabei sicher eine Rolle, da sich diese sowohl an isolierten Coronararterienstreifen als auch an isolierten Herzen nachweisen läßt. Sie reicht aber zur Erklärung der besonders günstigen Wirkungen von Nitriten bei Angina pectoris-Anfällen nicht aus. Der Coronardurchfluß wird durch Papaverin oder Aminophyllin (= Euphyllin) meist sogar stärker vergrößert als durch Nitroglycerin[6]. Der Vorteil der Nitrite, besonders gegenüber den Xanthinderivaten, liegt darin, daß sie gleichzeitig die Herzarbeit und den Sauerstoffverbrauch des Herzmuskels herabsetzen. Foltz u. Mitarb. fanden, daß die Sauerstoffsättigung im Coronarsinusblut kurz nach der Injektion von Nitroglycerin durchschnittlich um 10% erhöht war[7]. Schließlich sind zur Beurteilung der günstigen Wirkungen von Nitriten auch die Messungen des phasischen Blutflusses durch die Kranzarterien aufschlußreich, die von Boyer und Green (1941) gemacht wurden. Sie fanden, daß der Blutfluß nicht nur in der Diastole, wie das bei Xanthinderivaten der Fall ist, sondern auch in der Systole vermehrt war und zwar so deutlich, daß überhaupt kein Rückfluß auftrat.

---

[1] Meessen 1940.   [2] Kroetz 1936, Friedberg und Horn 1939.
[3] Dargestellt nach freundlicher Beratung durch Herrn Dozenten Dr. Heidenreich-Freiburg i. Br.   [4] Møller 1958.   [5] Wégria, Essex, Herrick und Mann 1940.
[6] Eckenhoff, Hafkenschiel und Mitarbeiter 1947.
[7] Foltz, Rubin, Steiger und Gazes 1950.

Die Vergrößerung des mittleren Coronardurchflusses bei verminderter Herzarbeit, die daraus resultierende erhöhte Sauerstoffsättigung im Sinusblut und die Verbesserung des phasischen Blutstromes gerade in der Systole sind die objektiven pharmakologischen Befunde, die die gute therapeutische Wirkung der Nitrite beim Angina pectoris-Anfall verständlich machen.

Eine ganz andere Frage ist die, wieweit nicht bei stenosierten Arterien an einzelnen Organen, z.B. am Gehirn und am Herzmuskel, die *stenosebedingte Ischämie noch durch eine spastische Ischämie der poststenotischen Arterienverzweigungen gesteigert werden* kann. Im Film hat MEINERS (1949) unter MAX SCHNEIDER gezeigt, daß Sauerstoffmangelatmung durch allgemeine Hypoxämie ischämische Kontraktionen an den Ohrarterien auslösen kann. VON EULER und LILJESTRAND (1947) haben nachgewiesen, daß die Hypoxämie die Pulmonalarterien akut zur Kontraktion bringt und eine akute Hypertonie im rechten Ventrikel und im Stamm der Lungenschlagader verursacht. Diese Beispiele sollten eine systematische Untersuchung auch für das Gehirn und das Coronarsystem veranlassen, wieweit die stenosebedingte Ischämie eine spastisch induzierte Ischämie auslösen und durch sie gesteigert werden kann.

SCHOLZ (1957) vertritt die Auffassung, daß bei allgemeiner Hypoxie die morphologischen Veränderungen am Gehirn entscheidend durch hypoxisch ausgelöste Spasmen kleinerer Hirnarterien mitgestaltet werden, so daß am gleichen Hirn die Folgen der schweren Hypoxydose und die einer zusätzlichen spastischen Ischämie gefunden werden können. In unserem Beitrag über die allgemeine Pathologie der cellulären und geweblichen Oxydationen in diesem Handbuch, Bd. IV/1, ist die Bedeutung dieses Faktors für das Verständnis der Hirnveränderungen bei Hypoxydose gewürdigt, insbesondere auch für das Verständnis der Befunde von ALTMANN und SCHUBOTHE (1942) nach Unterdruck-Hypoxämie bei der Katze. Wir verweisen auf diese Ausführungen.

Für die spastische arterielle Ischämie seien im Rückblick auf das Dargestellte noch einmal folgende Tatsachen hervorgehoben:

1. Lokale mechanische, thermische oder chemische Reizfaktoren rufen augenblicklich an den Arterien des Reizfeldes eine Kontraktion, häufig einen spastischen Verschluß hervor, der je nach der Dauer und Intensität des Reizes verschieden lange fortbesteht. Er ist von einer Dilatation der zunächst kontrahierten Arterienstrecke gefolgt, während sich der Spasmus in der Regel vorübergehend nach proximal und distal verlagert.

2. Bei lokaler Anaphylaxie gegen artfremdes Protein ist nach erneuter Einwirkung des Antigens der arterielle Spasmus intensiver und von wesentlich größerer Dauer, so daß es an der Bauchhaut des Kaninchens im Arthus-Phänomen zur zentralen Nekrose kommt.

3. Bei allgemeiner Anaphylaxie kommt es nach intravenöser Erfolgsinjektion des Antigens zu einer maximalen spastischen Kontraktion der Lungenarterien, die häufig zur akuten Insuffizienz des rechten Herzventrikels führt.

4. Zu Nekrosen führende spastische arterielle Ischämien begegnen uns auch bei der Raynaudschen Krankheit mit trockenem Brand an Händen und Füßen. Ebenso ist der Kältebrand bei der Erfrierung 3. Grades die Folge eines arteriellen Spasmus. Auch eine Reihe von Giften führt über die spastische Ischämie zu Nekrosen an den gipfelnden Teilen.

5. Die Epilepsie geht auf eine spastische arterielle Ischämie der Hirnarterien zurück. Diese verursacht bei genügender Dauer die Entwicklung von Parenchymnekrosen im Grau des Hirns mit charakteristischer Topistik und einer typischen

Empfindlichkeitsskala von der Nervenzelle zur Oligodendroglia-, Makroglia- und Mikrogliazelle.

6. Die allgemeine Hypoxie kann am Hirn durch hypoxisch ausgelöste arterielle Spasmen kompliziert werden, so daß diese das Schädigungsmuster der hypoxischen Veränderungen des Hirnparenchyms mit bestimmen.

Die allgemeine arterielle Oligämie.

So folgenschwer nach unseren bisherigen Darlegungen organbegrenzte akute oder chronische absolute oder relative arterielle Ischämien sein können, so haben sie doch in reinen Fällen einen Vorteil: der Gesamtkreislauf ist bei ihnen intakt, die für die Durchschnittsleistungen des Organismus notwendige Förderarbeit des Herzens, gemessen am Minutenvolumen des Kreislaufs, bleibt in der Regel adäquat und an wechselnde Anforderungen anpassungsfähig.

In der menschlichen und tierexperimentellen Pathologie sind uns aber auch zahlreiche Ereignisse bekannt, bei denen sich der Gesamtkreislauf akut, subakut oder chronisch in einem Zustand der mehr oder weniger bedrohlichen Minderdurchblutung befindet, bei dem vor allem in dem großen arteriellen System das für die Aufrechterhaltung physiologischer Organleistungen notwendige Minutenvolumen nicht mehr kreist, bei denen also eine *allgemeine arterielle Oligämie* besteht. Solche Zustände begegnen uns beim Kollaps, bei der Insuffizienz des linken Ventrikels und beim mangelnden Einstrom von Blut in den linken Ventrikel.

1. Der Kollaps.

Beim *Kollaps* wird die allgemeine arterielle Oligämie nicht durch eine Insuffizienz des Herzmuskels, sondern durch ein *Versagen der Kreislaufperipherie* hervorgerufen. Das wurde auf Grund klinischer Beobachtungen schon 1844 von PFEUFFER klar erkannt. Als Physiologe hat zuerst MAREY (1881) bei der Deutung des Kollaps eine Durchblutungsinsuffizienz des Splanchnicusgebietes in den Vordergrund gerückt und die krankhafte Blutverteilung beim Kollaps mit der bei Pfortaderunterbindung verglichen.

A. Die Pathogenese des Kollaps.

Die *Ursache des Versagens der Kreislaufperipherie* beim Kollaps haben QUINCKE (1869) und NAUNYN (1873) als erste in einer *primären Schädigung des Vasomotorenzentrums der Medulla oblongata* gesehen, ebenso FISCHER (1870) als Chirurg für den postoperativen und den posttraumatischen Kollaps, auch von RECKLINGHAUSEN (1883) als Pathologe. Im Banne dieser Vorstellung blieb die deutsche und später die angelsächsische Kollapsforschung noch bis in den 1. Weltkrieg hinein. So haben ROMBERG (1892) und seine Mitarbeiter[1] ihre experimentelle Beobachtung, daß schwere Kollapszustände durch Bakterientoxine (Pneumokokken, Bac. pyocyaneus, Diphtherietoxin) ausgelöst werden können, hier eingeordnet: Den Angriffsort dieser Gifte haben sie im Vasomotorenzentrum der Medulla oblongata vermutet. CRILE (1899) kam ebenfalls zu dieser Auffassung. Noch HENDERSON hielt sie 1908 für alle Kollapsarten aufrecht.

Neue Vorstellungen bahnten sich erst an, als *die allgemeine arterielle Oligämie beim Kollaps verschiedenen Ursprungs als obligates Kreislaufphänomen* exakt nachgewiesen wurde und in den Mittelpunkt der Kollapsdiskussion rückte, in England zuerst durch ROBERTSON und BOCK (1919), KEITH (1919), ERLANGER, GESELL und GASSER (1919), GASSER, ERLANGER und MEEK (1919), in Deutschland in

---

[1] ROMBERG, PÄSSLER und Mitarbeiter 1899, HEINEKE 1901.

den Arbeitskreisen von EPPINGER (seit 1928[1]) sowie von REIN (seit 1932). Untersucht wurde vor allem der Kollaps infolge Blutung, Trauma, Verbrennung. Dabei wurde festgestellt, daß die Schwere des Kollaps mit der Verminderung der zirkulierenden Blutmenge und mit dem Sinken des Herzminutenvolumens parallel geht[2]. Später ergab sich für den traumatischen Kollaps des Menschen mit der Katheterung oder der Evans-Blau-Methode eine Verminderung der zirkulierenden Blutmenge um 30—40%, d.h. um 1,5—2,0 Liter[3]. Ähnliche Werte wurden bei dem Verbrennungskollaps festgestellt[4].

Im einzelnen stellte man mit der Farbstoff- und der Hämatokrit-Methode bei Menschen mit Blutverlust, Skelettraumen sowie Thorax- und Bauchverwundungen das Eintreten der Kollapssymptome frühestens nach Senkung der zirkulierenden Blutmenge um 15% fest[5]. In einer anderen Untersuchungsreihe wurden bei Schwerverwundeten Senkungen von 2,0—2,5 Liter gemessen[6], in einer dritten Stufe von 14,4—45,9%[7]. Am Hund kam es im experimentellen traumatischen Kollaps zu den charakteristischen klinischen Erscheinungen nach mindestens 30% Einschränkung der zirkulierenden Blutmenge, der Tod trat bei einem Sinken der Blutmenge um 40% und mehr ein[8].

Es lag nahe, von solchen Beobachtungen aus die Hypothese zu entwickeln, daß der *Kollaps in jedem Falle durch Blutverluste nach außen oder durch adäquate innere Verluste von Blutflüssigkeit aus dem Gefäßsystem zustande kommt*[9]. Am eindringlichsten begegnet uns *die Bedeutung dieses hämodynamischen Prinzips für die Kollapsentstehung* bei dem Blutverlust nach außen, dem *Entblutungskollaps*, dem Haemorrhagic shok. Hier fand SCHWIEGK (1942) experimentell am Hund bei einem Blutverlust von etwa 20% noch eine normale zirkulierende Blutmenge. Diese konnte durch Ausschüttung von Blut aus den Blutdepots und durch Einstrom von Flüssigkeit aus den Geweben aufrechterhalten werden. Bei weiterem Blutverlust sank die Blutmenge jedoch unter die Norm, gleichzeitig setzte eine spastische Kontraktion der Arterien in weniger blutbedürftigen Gebieten ein, besonders in den Extremitäten- und Magendarmarterien. Dadurch erfolgte eine Zentralisation des Kreislaufs auf die blutbedürftigsten und lebenswichtigsten Organe, besonders auf Hirn und Herz, so daß diese noch normal durchblutet wurden. Es bestand also eine *kompensierte arterielle Oligämie*. Nahm der Blutverlust weiter zu, so wurde auch in dem eingeschränkten Kreislaufsystem die Blutmenge so stark verringert, daß sich eine *dekompensierte arterielle Oligämie* entwickelte, die den Tod des Tieres herbeiführte. WIGGERS (1950) bezog die Stadien des Entblutungskollaps des Hundes auf den Blutdruck. Bei 30—40% Blutverlust war eine Blutdrucksenkung auf 50 mm Hg erreicht. Bei einem systolischen Blutdruck von 30 mm Hg lagen kritische Blutverluste vor. Demgemäß konnten 3 Stadien des Kollaps unterschieden werden: 1. der latente Kollaps mit einfacher Hypotonie, die sich durch Reinfusion des Blutes beseitigen läßt, 2. der noch reversible Kollaps mit den klinischen Kollapszeichen, bei dem die Reinfusion noch erfolgreich ist, 3. der kritische irreversible Kollaps, bei dem trotz Reinfusion der Tod eintritt.

Auch bei dem *postoperativen Kollaps* handelt es sich in der Regel um den gleichen Mechanismus der Einschränkung der zirkulierenden Blutmenge und zwar durch Blut- und Flüssigkeitsverlust[10].

---

[1] EPPINGER und SCHÜRMEYER 1928, EPPINGER und LEUCHTENBERGER 1932, EPPINGER, KAUNITZ und POPPER 1935.
[2] ROBERTSON und BOCK 1919, KEITH 1919.   [3] COURNAND, RILEY u.a. 1943.
[4] KEELEY, GIBSON und PIJOAN 1939.   [5] EVANS, HOWER, JAMES und ALM 1944.
[6] STEWART 1947.   [7] BEECHER 1949.   [8] GREGERSEN und ROOT 1947.
[9] BLALOCK 1930, 1931 ff., HARRISON 1935, FISHBERG 1940, SCHWIEGK 1942.
[10] FRIEDBERG 1959.

Daß auch beim *posttraumatischen Kollaps* der kreislaufdynamische Faktor eine große Rolle spielt, haben schon ältere Experimente wahrscheinlich gemacht (Blalock 1930, 1931, 1940, 1943).

In diesen Versuchen wurde am Hund ein schweres Trauma an dem einen Hinterbein gesetzt[1]. So kam es zu einer spastischen Kontraktion der Arterien dieses Beines. Dadurch standen die nachgeschalteten Arterien und Capillaren unter der Wirkung einer schweren spastischen Ischämie. Nach Lösung des Spasmus trat in dem durch die Ischämie vorgeschädigten Gewebe eine so starke Insudation von Blutflüssigkeit ein, daß die zirkulierende Blutmenge beträchtlich verringert war. Wurde die Ödembildung im Bein nach Trauma durch Gipsverband unterdrückt, so blieb der Kollaps aus[2].

Ähnlich spielt der kreislaufdynamische Faktor eine große Rolle bei dem *Crush-Syndrom*[3], wie es nach Verschüttung und späterer Entlastung, besonders der unteren Extremitäten, auftritt. Durch die Verschüttung ist die Muskulatur stark ischämisch. Sie wird in großer Ausdehnung nekrotisch und nekrobiotisch. Die Folge ist auch hier eine hochgradige Flüssigkeitsansammlung in den unteren Extremitäten und in der Regel ein Kollaps.

Das Bild wurde von Koslowski (1959) folgendermaßen an der Ratte nachgeahmt: durch eine Klemme wurde am linken Hinterbein eine schwere, später zur Nekrose führende Ischämie gesetzt. Die Klemme wurde nach 6 Std wieder gelöst. Wenige Minuten später kam es durch Wiedereinstrom des Blutes in die vorgeschädigte Muskulatur zu einer rasch zunehmenden Schwellung mit grotesker Auftreibung der Pfoten. Die Schwellung erreichte nach 12 Std ihren Höhepunkt, bestand unverändert etwa 2 Tage und klang dann allmählich wieder ab. Die Ratten zeigten schwere Kollapssymptome.

Ganz ähnlich waren aber auch die Befunde beim *Verbrennungskollaps*[4]. Dabei entsprach der Flüssigkeitsverlust quantitativ der Verminderung der zirkulierenden Blutmenge[5]. Auch beim *Kollaps nach Erfrierung* schafft die spastische Ischämisierung der kältegeschädigten Extremität die Voraussetzungen für ein hochgradiges Ödem nach Lösung der Ischämie und Wiedererwärmung[6], dadurch aber für eine allgemeine Oligämie[7]. Daß hier gerade in der Phase der Wiedererwärmung die energetische Insuffizienz der Muskulatur manifest wird, ist ein Hinweis für deren pathogenetische Bedeutung bei der Ödemgenese[8].

Bei allen diesen Kollapsformen war die *Zentralisation des Kreislaufes* sehr ausgesprochen. So war beim Hund die Durchblutung der A. femoralis um 75% herabgesetzt[9], die Durchblutung der Speicheldrüse um 60%[10].

Lebhaft erörtert wurde die *Frage nach dem Zustandekommen des starken Verlustes von Blutflüssigkeit in das Gewebe* nach Trauma und Verbrennung. Einige Untersucher haben die Meinung vertreten, daß die vorübergehend im Gebiet des Traumas oder der Verbrennung wirksam werdende spastische Ischämie *durch Sauerstoffmangel eine Steigerung der Permeabilität der Capillaren* verursacht[11]. Für diese Auffassung konnte geltend gemacht werden, daß abgekochte und dadurch O_2-freie Ringerlösung bei ihrer Injektion die Durchlässigkeit der Capillaren steigert (Landis 1927, 1928). Eine Spülflüssigkeit von 5 Vol.-% Sauerstoff hatte keine Wirkung bei Durchströmung des Hinterbeins der Ratte, dagegen war die Permeabilität bei 0,88—2,60 Vol.-% deutlich erhöht[12]. In anderen Versuchen

---

[1] Blalock 1931, 1943.   [2] Duncan und Blalock 1942.
[3] Minami 1923, Bywaters 1941, 1945, Bywaters und Mitarbeiter 1941, 1942, 1945, Selberg 1942, Brass 1944, Rothmann 1944, Wg. Rotter 1948, Scriba 1949, Buff 1949, Chiari 1949, Loustalot 1950, Koczewski und Kaiser 1951, Gukelberger 1954.
[4] Blalock 1930, 1931, 1943, Harkins 1941—1945.
[5] Nickerson 1945, Aschworth, Jester und Lloyd 1944.
[6] Siegmund 1942, M. Staemmler 1944, J. Staemmler 1944.
[7] Schwiegk 1942.   [8] Lang und Mitarbeiter 1943.
[9] Baldes, Herrick und Mitarbeiter 1941.   [10] Erlanger, Gesell und Gasser 1919.
[11] Büchner 1940, 1944/1949, Altmann 1946/1949.
[12] Pasquale und Schiller 1951, Hendley und Schiller 1954.

wurden für das venöse Blut 15—25% O_2 statt 65—75% O_2 als wirksam gefunden[1]. Es treten also bei extremen Graden der Hypoxämie bzw. Oligämie Permeabilitätssteigerungen der Capillaren ein, wie das auch schon früher angenommen worden war[2].

Nach elektronenmikroskopischen Untersuchungen der Parenchymzellen der Leber, des Herzmuskels und des Gehirns über die Wirkung des exogenen Sauerstoffmangels und von aerobiosehemmenden Giften auf die Ultrastrukturen der Parenchymzellen[3] dürfte aber ein anderer Faktor von noch größerer Bedeutung für die kollapsverursachende Wirkung der Flüssigkeitsansammlung im Gewebe sein. Nach diesen Untersuchungen führt jede Störung der Aerobiose in den Parenchymzellen in kurzer Frist zu einer Schwellung der Mitochondrien, einer Zerstörung ihrer Cristae sowie zu einer starken diffusen oder vacuoligen Wasseransammlung im Cytoplasma. Das wurde auch schon in lichtmikroskopischen Untersuchungen erkannt[4]. Das Bild ist so zu deuten, daß die Störung der Aerobiose durch Anreicherung von Metaboliten im Cytoplasma eine Hyperosmose auslöst, daß die Bindungsfähigkeit der Makromoleküle für Wasser herabgesetzt ist und daß der Zelle die notwendige Energie fehlt, sich des Wassers zu entledigen. Durch die energetische Insuffizienz versagt außerdem die Aufnahme von Kalium in die Zelle gegen das Gefälle und die Ausscheidung von Natrium aus der Zelle gegen das Gefälle[5]. Die dadurch verursachte Elektrolytverschiebung bewirkt ihrerseits eine Wasserretention im Gewebe. Unter Berücksichtigung dieser Tatsachen ist es naheliegend, mit KOSLOWSKI (1959) die *durch arterielle Ischämie verursachte hypoxische Stoffwechselstörung im Parenchym als wichtigste Ursache des Verlustes an Blutflüssigkeit in das Gewebe* beim Trauma und bei der Verbrennung anzusehen und dieses Prinzip auch auf andere Kollapsformen anzuwenden.

Von anderen Autoren wurde freilich schon seit längerem die Meinung vertreten, daß beim Kollaps und bei den zu beobachtenden Verlusten von Flüssigkeit ins Gewebe *permeabilitätssteigernde Stoffe* regelhaft im Spiele sind und daß der Flüssigkeitsverlust durch die Wirkung dieser Stoffe an den Capillarmembranen zustande kommt. Die Auslösung des Kollaps durch toxische Substanzen war schon in den oben zitierten Experimenten von ROMBERG (1899) und seinen Mitarbeitern[6] nachgewiesen worden: die Injektion von Erregertoxinen, z.B. von Pneumokokken-, Pyocyaneus- und Diphtherietoxin führte zum Kollaps. In der Folge wurde erkannt, daß viele bakterielle Infektionen des Menschen und des Tieres eine Neigung zum Kollaps verursachen. Der Angriffspunkt der Erregertoxine liegt dabei nicht so sehr in den Vasomotorenzentren als vor allem in der Kreislaufperipherie an der glatten Muskulatur der Arteriolen: Durch die Lähmung der Arteriolenmuskulatur verliert das Gefäßsystem den für die Aufrechterhaltung des Blutdrucks und damit der normalen Kreislaufarbeit des Herzens notwendigen Tonus. Der Blutdruckabfall in den Arteriolen verhindert den Durchstrom durch die Capillaren und den venösen Rückstrom zum Herzen. So kommt es zur schnell sich steigernden allgemeinen Oligämie. Ob die den Kollaps verursachenden Erregertoxine allerdings die Capillarpermeabilität erhöhen, ist ungeklärt. Inzwischen traten andere Stoffe in den Vordergrund. Insbesondere hatte DALE mit seinen Mitarbeitern gezeigt[7], daß intravenös zugeführtes *Histamin* den

---

[1] HENRY, GOODMAN und MEEHAN 1947.
[2] ALTMANN 1946, 1949, ALTMANN und BÜCHNER 1948, POPPER 1948.
[3] MÖLBERT und GUERRITORE 1957, MÖLBERT 1957, MÖLBERT 1958, POCHE 1958, BÜCHNER 1959, BÜCHNER, MÖLBERT und THALE 1959, SCHOLZ, BOELLAARD und HAGER 1959.
[4] Vgl. PICHOTKA 1942, ALTMANN 1946/49, BÜCHNER 1957, BECKER und NEUBERT 1959.
[5] FLECKENSTEIN 1942, 1955, DAVIS 1949.   [6] PÄSSLER 1899, HEINEKE 1901.
[7] DALE und RICHARDS 1918, DALE und LAIDLOW 1919, DALE 1929, GADDUM 1936.

Blutdruck senkt und das Bild eines Kollaps mit allgemeiner Oligämie hervorrufen kann. So entwickelte WIGGERS (1923) die Hypothese, daß nach Gewebsverletzun-

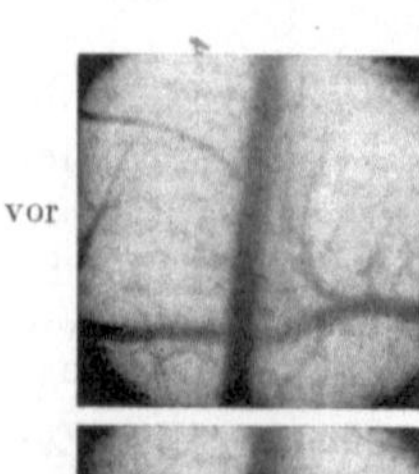

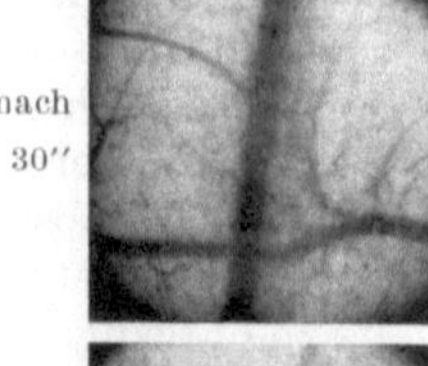

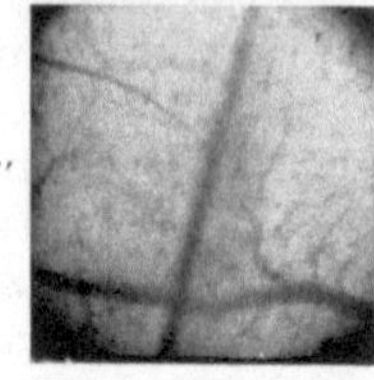

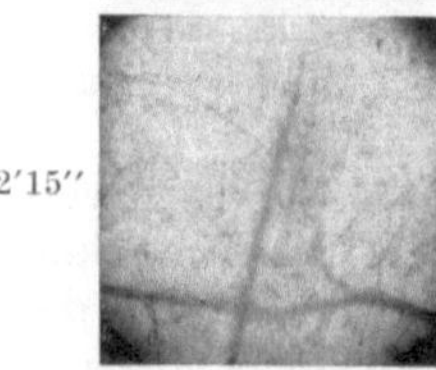

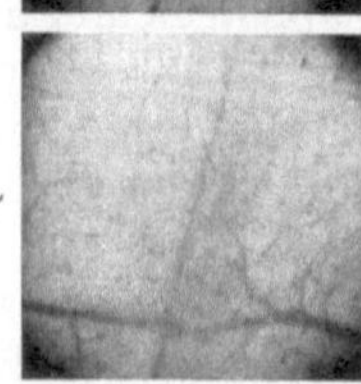

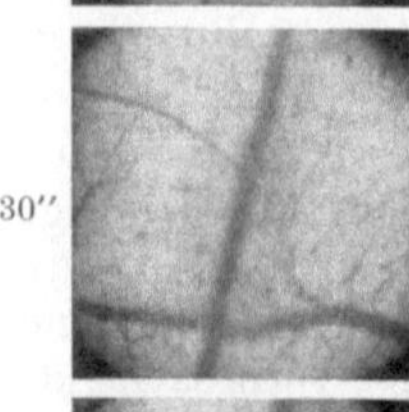

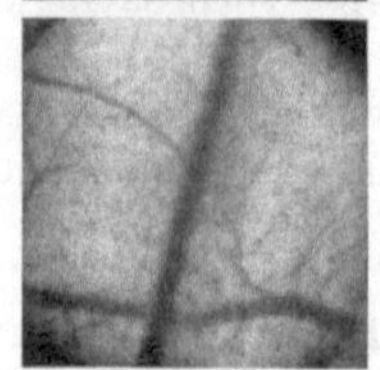

gen, Manipulationen am Darm und Intoxikationen oder nach Blutverlusten durch beschleunigte Proteolyse Histamin und histaminartige Stoffe entstehen und eine Permeabilitätssteigerung an den Capillaren verursachen. Tatsächlich konnte durch die Injektion von Muskel-Autolysat ein entsprechendes Bild hervorgerufen werden (MOON 1934). Mit großen Dosen von Histamin intravenös ließ sich am Hund ein Kollaps mit starker Oligämie reproduzieren[1]. Demgemäß rückten MOON (1934, 1938) sowie EPPINGER u. Mitarb. (1935) die *Histaminhypothese des Kollaps* ganz in den Vordergrund.

Ehe wir dieser Hypothese nachgehen, haben wir zu prüfen, ob nach Injektion von Histamin ein echter Kollaps auftritt. Die Frage ist zum Teil gekoppelt mit der Frage nach dem Wesen des sog. *anaphylaktischen Kollaps*, wie wir ihn oben schon kennengelernt haben. Dabei haben wir betont, daß es am sensibilisierten Kaninchen durch die intravenöse Erfolgsinjektion von Fremdeiweiß, z.B. von Pferdeserum, augenblicklich zu einer krampfhaften Kontraktion der Lungenarterien kommt[2], nach der Hypothese von FELDBERG und SCHACHTER (1952) durch die Freisetzung von Histamin unter der Wirkung des Antigen-Antikörpermechanismus an der Lungenstrombahn. Die Unterbrechung der Lungendurchblutung im anaphylaktischen Kollaps konnten wir mit dem intravitalen Photogramm der Ohrarterien während des Anaphylaxie-Experimentes belegen (Abb. 30)[3]. Nach diesen Experimenten ist das Wesen der Kreislaufstörung im Anaphylaxie-Versuch eine extreme akute Widerstandserhöhung im Lungenkreislauf, ein akutes Cor pulmonale, eine akute Insuffizienz des rechten Ventrikels und in deren Auswirkung eine extreme venöse Hyperämie im Splanchnicusgebiet und in den unteren Extremitäten. Es ist also unexakt, vom anaphylaktischen Kollaps zu sprechen, wenn wir daran festhalten, den Kollaps als primär periphere von der primär kardialen Kreislaufinsuffizienz abzugrenzen. In Wirklichkeit liegt eine extreme akute Rechtsinsuffizienz des Herzens vor.

Injizieren wir beim Kaninchen intravenös Histamin in größerer Dosis, so kommt es wiederum zu einem akuten Spasmus der Pulmonalarterien, zu einer Unterbrechung der Lungendurchblutung und demgemäß zu einer Ischämie in den Ohrarterien (Abb. 33)[4]. Die Drosselung der Pulmonalarterien verursacht auch hier ein akutes Cor pulmonale mit ausgedehnter Entwicklung von Parenchymnekrosen in der Muskulatur des rechten Ventrikels und die zugeordneten

Abb. 33. Intravitale Photogramme der zentralen Ohrarterie vor und nach intravenöser Histamininjektion. Starke Kontraktion der Arterie nach 2 und 3 min. Wiederherstellung der durchschnittlichen Durchblutung nach $4^{1}/_{2}$ min. [Nach A. NIKULIN, Beitr. path. Anat. **120**, 214, 1959, Abb. 1.]

---

[1] EPPINGER und SCHÜRMEYER 1928, EPPINGER und LEUCHTENBERGER 1932, EPPINGER, KAUNITZ und POPPER 1935.   [2] DRINKER und BOFENBRENNER 1924.
[3] IIJIMA 1957.   [4] HERBERTSON 1953, NIKULIN 1959.

Veränderungen des Elektrokardiogramms (Abb. 34)[1]. Auch hier entwickelt sich je nach der Dosis eine akute Rechtsinsuffizienz des Herzens mit venöser Hyperämie der unteren Körperhälfte. Die akute Kreislaufstörung nach intravenöser Zufuhr von Histamin bedeutet also keinen Kollaps, sondern eine akute Rechts-

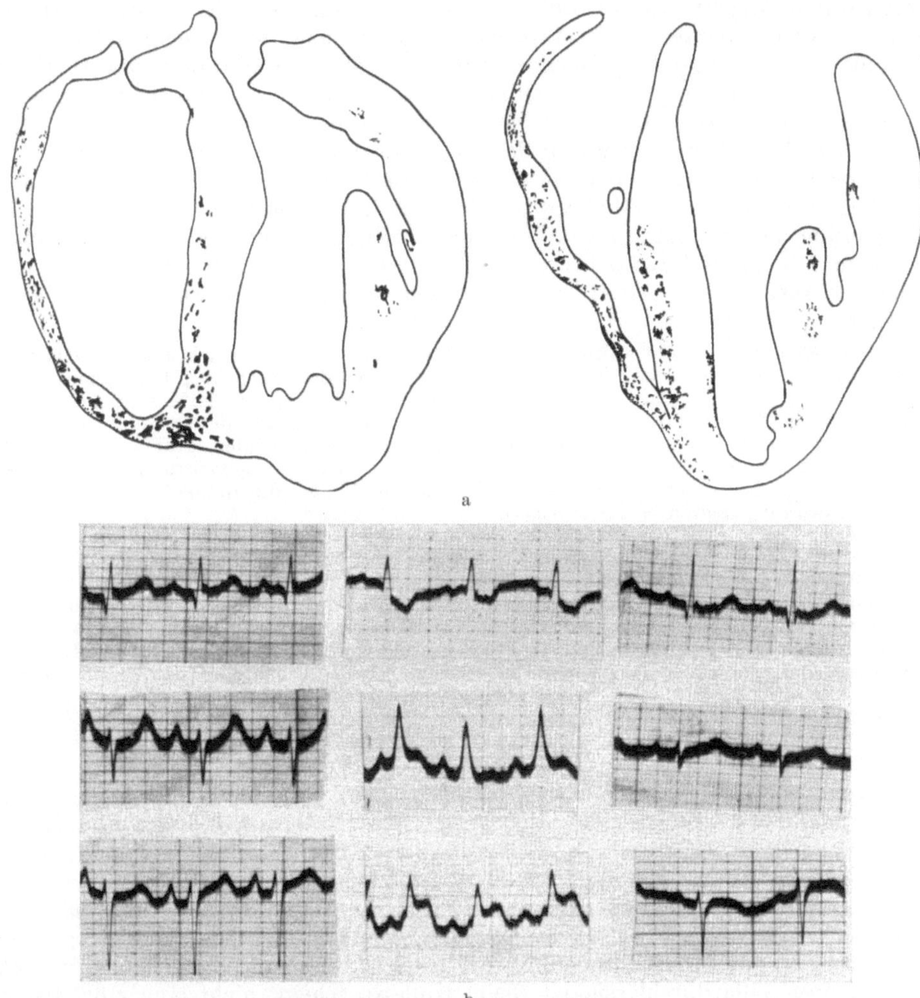

Abb. 34a u. b. a Zahlreiche, in den Stufenskizzen des Herzens durch schwarze Flecken markierte Parenchymnekrosen, bevorzugt in der Muskulatur des *rechten* Ventrikels, nach intravenöser Injektion von Histamin beim Kaninchen. b Elektrokardiogramm des gleichen Tieres: links vor der Injektion, Mitte hoher Abgang von RT in Abb. 3 u. 2 ähnlich der Infarktkurve nach intravenöser Injektion von Histamin beim gleichen Tier, rechts Rückbildung dieser Veränderungen nach dem Versuch. [Nach W. TATERKA, Beitr. path. Anat. 102, 287, 1939, Abb. 34 u. 33.]

insuffizienz des Herzens. Beim Hund ist allerdings die glatte Muskulatur der Lebervenen der Angriffspunkt des Histamins, so daß es zur Lebervenensperre, wiederum mit hochgradiger venöser Hyperämie im Splanchnicusgebiet, kommt, also zu einem kollapsähnlichen Bild, aber nicht zum echten Kollaps.

Daß es unter diesen Bedingungen der hochgradigen venösen Hyperämie nach Histamin zu *akuten Transsudationen* von Blutflüssigkeit aus den extrem gestauten

---

[1] TATERKA 1939, HERBERTSON 1956.

Capillargebieten kommt, also auch im Experiment zu einem hochgradigen Ödem der Magenschleimhaut bei maximaler Stauung in den Schleimhautcapillaren oder zum starken akuten Stauungsödem in der Gallenblasenwand[1], ist verständlich, aber kein Beweis für eine universelle Permeabilitätssteigerung an den Capillaren durch Angriff des Histamins an diesen Strukturen. Es ist die Wirkung starker Steigerung des hydrostatischen Druckes und der zunehmenden Hypoxämie in diesen Capillargebieten[2], außerdem aber die Wirkung der Hypoxie der Parenchyme der gestauten Organe. Dafür sprechen auch Beobachtungen nach temporärer Ischämie der beiden Hinterbeine der Maus. Die mit S 35 radioaktiv markierten Proteine waren danach in der unteren Körperhälfte auf 210% der Norm angereichert, nach Plasmainfusion auf 513%[3].

Daß beim Entblutungskollaps und beim Verbrennungskollaps eine allgemeine Steigerung der Capillarpermeabilität nicht vorliegt, konnte mit radioaktiv markiertem Eiweiß und radioaktiven Farbstoffen nachgewiesen werden: ein vermehrter Austritt dieser Stoffe aus den Capillaren im Kollaps war nicht zu beobachten[4].

Beim Menschen konnte während des Kollaps zunächst eine Vermehrung von Histamin nicht nachgewiesen werden[5]. In neueren Versuchen wurden dann aber kurzdauernde Erhöhungen des Histamingehaltes im Blute in den ersten 24 Std gefunden[6]. Andererseits war kurz vor dem Tode der Histamingehalt erniedrigt[7]. Bei Trennung der Stoffe in der Hochspannungselektrophorese waren nach Verbrennung am Hund in der Haut die Amine vermindert, im Serum Histamin nach 24 Std vermehrt, in der Leber Histamin und Histidin vermehrt; darüber hinaus traten andere H-Substanzen auf, die im biologischen Versuch Histaminwirkung zeigten (J. Rehn 1959).

An der Ratte fand Koslowski 1959 bei 6stündiger temporärer Ischämie eines Hinterbeins nach Lösung der Klemme einen erheblichen Anstieg von H-Substanzen im Blut, der nach 9—12 Std einen Höhepunkt erreichte, nach 24 und fortschreitend nach 48 Std aber von einem Abfall unter den Normwert gefolgt war. Dabei wurden mit der Hochspannungselektrophorese histaminähnliche, aber nicht mit Histamin identische Amine isoliert. Durch den Histamin-Liberator Compound 48/80 dehistaminierte Ratten zeigten bei nachfolgender Kompressionsischämie keine geringere Ödemneigung im geschädigten Bein als nicht vorbehandelte ischämisierte Tiere. Auch konnte durch Antihistaminica das Ödem im ischämisierten Bein nicht wesentlich herabgesetzt werden. Phenazetin-Derivate scheinen den Gehalt des Blutes an histaminartigen Stoffen zu senken, fördern aber eher das Ödem, als daß sie es hemmen.

Koslowski folgert aus seinen verschiedenen Untersuchungsreihen an der Ratte, *daß ein wesentlicher Hinweis für die Mitwirkung von H-Substanzen bei der Entstehung des Extremitäten-Ödems nach 6stündiger, zur Nekrose führender Ischämie nicht gegeben ist und daß die Entstehung des Ödems nur auf dem Hintergrund der durch die Ischämie verursachten energetischen Insuffizienz der Zellen, besonders der des Muskelparenchyms, zu deuten ist.* Vom Erfahrungsgut des Kardiologen her kommt Friedberg (1959) ebenfalls zu der Feststellung: „Die Theorie der allgemeinen Capillardurchlässigkeit (beim Kollaps) scheint nicht länger haltbar zu sein" (S. 358).

Erneut liegt also heute mehr denn je der Akzent der Diskussion über das Kollapsproblem auf der hämodynamischen Hypothese. Als weiterer Beleg für diese Hypothese ist die Gruppe der Erkrankungen mit *enteralem Kollaps* anzuführen. Hier ist vor allem der Kollaps durch starken gastroenteralen Flüssigkeitsverlust bei akuter schwerer Gastroenteritis des Säuglings, bei Paratyphus, bei Cholera mit Erbrechen und Durchfall, bei hohem Ileus zu nennen. Auch der *orthostatische*

---

[1] Eppinger und Leuchtenberger 1932, Eppinger, Kaunitz und Popper 1935.
[2] Büchner 1937, 1944, Altmann und Büchner 1948.
[3] Millican 1954.   [4] Fine, Seligman und Frank 1943.
[5] Barsoum und Gaddum 1936, Dragstedt und Mead 1936.
[6] Birke, Duner, Liljedahl und Mitarbeiter 1957.
[7] Rose und Browne 1940, Lambert und Rosenthal 1943.

Kollaps, zuerst am Aal[1], dann am Kaninchen[2] experimentell hervorgerufen, und auch beim Menschen, besonders bei Leptosomen vorkommend, ist hier einzuordnen, desgleichen der *Kollaps nach Einwirkung besonders starker Fliehkräfte in Richtung Kopf-Beine*[3]. In all diesen Fällen steht die Verminderung der zirkulierenden Blutmenge — durch Wasserverlust, durch Einwirkung der Schwerkraft und durch Wirkung der Fliehkraft — im Mittelpunkt der Pathogenese.

Kehren wir zu den Anfängen unserer Erörterung der Pathogenese des Kollaps zurück, so stellen wir fest, daß bei einer Gruppe von Krankheitsbildern der *Kollaps durch Insuffizienz der Vasomotorenzentren* außer Frage steht. Das gilt vor allem für den Kollaps im hepatischen, diabetischen und im urämischen Koma, für die Spätstadien der unbehandelten Meningitis tuberculosa, für Hirntumoren mit entsprechendem Sitz, für Hirnmassenblutungen und für operative Eingriffe am Gehirn mit Wirkung auf die Hirnbasis. Außerdem ist zu betonen, daß jeder primär oligämische Kollaps durch die oligämische Schädigung der Zentren einen zentral-nervösen Kollaps auslösen und sich durch ihn potenzieren kann. Aus den gleichen Gründen endigt die allgemeine Hypoxämie durch Unterdruck oder sauerstoffarme Gemischatmung in der Regel im zentrogenen Kollaps[4].

Wieweit dabei bestimmte humorale Faktoren zusätzlich ins Spiel treten, wie es Chambers und Zweifach mit ihren Mitarbeitern annehmen, bedarf der weiteren Untersuchung. Zweifach (1952) war der Auffassung, daß der periphere Kreislauf an der proximalen Strombahn bis zu den Arteriolen durch nervöse Regulationen, besonders über den Sympathicus, gesteuert wird, an der terminalen Strombahn, vor allem an den Sphincteren zwischen den Metarteriolen und Capillaren, dagegen durch humorale Faktoren. Beim Kollaps konnten in den Experimenten von Zweifach und seinen Mitarbeitern am freigelegten Mesenterium 2 Phasen unterschieden werden: In der 1. Phase werden die peripheren Arterien und Venen verengert und es erfolgt eine Konstriktion der präcapillaren Arteriolen. Diese Engerstellung der Kreislaufperipherie ermögliche eine Zentralisierung des Kreislaufs. Sie würde durch einen humoral übertragbaren vasoconstrictorischen Faktor, das VEM, ausgelöst. In der 2. Phase des Kollaps bewirke ein vasodepressorischer Faktor, das VDM, eine Erschlaffung der Metarteriolen mit Aufhebung ihrer Reaktionsfähigkeit, dadurch eine Senkung des Blutdruckes und eine starke Verlangsamung der capillären Durchblutung bis zum Strömungsstillstand, besonders in Darm, Leber und Niere. Das VDM soll mit aktiviertem Ferritin identisch sein[5]. Seine biologische Aktivität soll es den Sulfhydrilgruppen verdanken[6]. Das VDM solle durch die Kollapshypoxie in der Niere gebildet werden[7]. Nach wiederholtem Kollaps würde dadurch eine Resistenz eintreten, daß das VDM trotz Hypoxie durch ein inaktivierendes Prinzip in der Leber zerstört wird[8]. In neueren Untersuchungen sind Zweifach und Metz (1956) zu dem Ergebnis gekommen, daß den beiden Substanzen, dem VEM und dem VDM nur eine lokale Bedeutung an der terminalen Strombahn zukommt. Sie haben daher die frühere Hypothese aufgegeben.

B. Die Folgen der allgemeinen arteriellen Oligämie im Kollaps.

Die *klinischen Erscheinungen*, die dem akuten Kollaps zugeordnet sind, haben wir hier und da schon gestreift. Wir müssen sie aber nunmehr kurz zusammengefaßt darstellen.

Wählen wir den traumatischen Kollaps als Beispiel, so stellen wir fest, daß nach schwerer Verwundung oder Verletzung, besonders nach ausgedehnter Zertrümmerung von Muskulatur und Skeletteilen, im Verlauf von Stunden sich ein Zustand entwickelt, bei dem der Kranke uns bei klarem Bewußtsein, mitunter in gehobener Euphorie, mit blasser Haut, beschleunigtem Puls und leicht erhöhtem Blutdruck begegnet. Dieser *initiale Erregungszustand* wurde im deutschen Sprachbereich vielfach als Schock vom Kollaps abgegrenzt, während im angel-

---

[1] Hill zit. nach Meessen 1939.
[2] Eppinger, Kaunitz und Popper 1935, Meessen 1937, 1939 u.a.
[3] Fischer 1938, Gauer 1950.   [4] Noell und M. Schneider 1942, 1948.
[5] Mazur und Shorr 1948.   [6] Mazur, Litt und Shorr 1950.
[7] Shorr, Zweifach und Furchtgott 1945.   [8] Zweifach, Metz, Shorr 1951.

sächsischen Schrifttum Shok in der Regel als Synonym für Kollaps angewandt und das Initialstadium als erstes Stadium des „Shok" gewertet wird. Das Herz ist in dieser Phase noch regulationsfähig, die Vasomotoren des arteriellen Systems sind gut ansprechbar und übererregt.

Mit dem nunmehr folgenden Stadium der *kompensierten Oligämie* beginnt der Kollaps. Die spastisch-regulative Minderdurchblutung der Haut äußert sich in Blässe, Feuchtigkeit und zunehmender Kälte der Haut, besonders Kälte und Kältegefühl an Füßen und Händen und an der Nasenspitze. Hirn und Herz sind trotz des herabgesetzten Minutenvolumens noch normal durchblutet. Dabei ist jedoch der Blutdruck schon gesenkt. Die Niere wird vielfach in die spastische Ischämie einbezogen, wie es auch im intravitalen Angiogramm nach einseitiger Drosselungsischämie eines Hinterbeins bei der Ratte festgestellt werden konnte[1]. Die Nierenischämie führt durch Senkung des Filtrationsdruckes in den Glomerula nicht selten zur Oligurie und Anurie.

Schließt sich das Stadium der *dekompensierten Oligämie* bei weiterer Abnahme der zirkulierenden Blutmenge und des Blutdruckes an, so tritt die Minderdurchblutung des Gehirns klinisch in den Vordergrund: Stimmungsänderungen, Bewußtseinstrübungen, Verwirrtheit bis zur akuten symptomatischen Psychose und Bewußtseinsverlust können sich in mehr oder minder schneller Folge ablösen, mitunter durch epileptische Erregungs- und Krampfanfälle unterbrochen. Lange Zeit bleibt der arterielle Sauerstoffgehalt noch normal, aber die arteriovenöse Sauerstoffdifferenz ist stark vergrößert.

Das *makroskopische Bild bei Tod im schweren Kollaps* (Moon 1934—1937) zeigt folgende Besonderheiten: die oberflächlichen Venen sind kollabiert und leer, die mesenterialen Venen sind stark gefüllt, die Schleimhäute des Magen-Darmtraktus sind cyanotisch-hyperämisch, ödematös und häufig von kleinen Blutungen übersät, ebenso die serösen Häute. Mitunter besteht ein Lungenödem.

Dauert ein Kollaps einige Stunden oder wird er 1—2 Tage überlebt, so kommt ein *für den Kollaps typisches histologisches Bild mit charakteristischer Verteilung der Veränderungen auf die verschiedenen Organe und regelhafter Topik der Veränderungen innerhalb der parenchymatösen Organe zustande.* Am *Herzmuskel*, der systematisch von Meessen 1936—1939, 1945 experimentell im orthostatischen Kollaps und nach anderen Kollapstypen des Kaninchens untersucht wurde, entwickeln sich disseminierte Parenchymnekrosen mit Bevorzugung der inneren Schichten der Muskulatur des linken Ventrikels, die bald durch junges Mesenchym und schließlich durch kollagene Narben ersetzt werden. Daraus geht hervor, daß trotz der Entlastung des Herzens durch verminderte Volumen- und Druckarbeit infolge der Oligämie und Blutdrucksenkung, also trotz stark eingeschränkten Blutbedarfes im Kollaps verschiedener Ätiologie die Coronardurchblutung insuffizient werden kann. Das konnte in den Experimenten von Meessen auch aus den intravitalen Elektrokardiogrammen gefolgert werden: Beim Kollaps verschiedener Ätiologie kam es zur charakteristischen Senkung der ST-Strecke und zur Negativierung der T-Zacke, meist in Ableitung I und II, also zu den gleichen Veränderungen, wie sie uns von der akuten Coronarinsuffizienz des Menschen und im Tierexperiment bekannt sind. Bildete sich der Kollaps, z.B. der orthostatische Kollaps durch Horizontallagerung des Tieres wieder zurück, so wurde das Elektrokardiogramm, meist im Verlauf einer Viertelstunde, wieder normal. Aus beiden Befunden, den histologischen und elektrokardiographischen, wurde auf eine akute energetische Insuffizienz des Herzmuskelparenchyms im Kollaps geschlossen[2]. Die histologischen Veränderungen des Herzmuskels

---

[1] Koslowski 1959.   [2] Meessen 1937, 1939, Büchner 1939.

wurden bald für den Verbrennungskollaps[1] und den Hitzekollaps[2] des Menschen bestätigt.

Später wurde auch von amerikanischen Autoren in einer Serie von Arbeiten das Bestehen einer akuten Coronarinsuffizienz im akuten Kollaps nachgewiesen. Insbesondere bestätigten FRIEDBERG und HORN (1939) die histologischen Befunde von MEESSEN für den akuten Kollaps. Pathologisch-physiologisch fand sich im experimentellen Kollaps nach anfänglicher Verkleinerung des Herzens eine zunehmende Insuffizienz-Dilatation[3]. Die Anpassungsfähigkeit des Herzens an

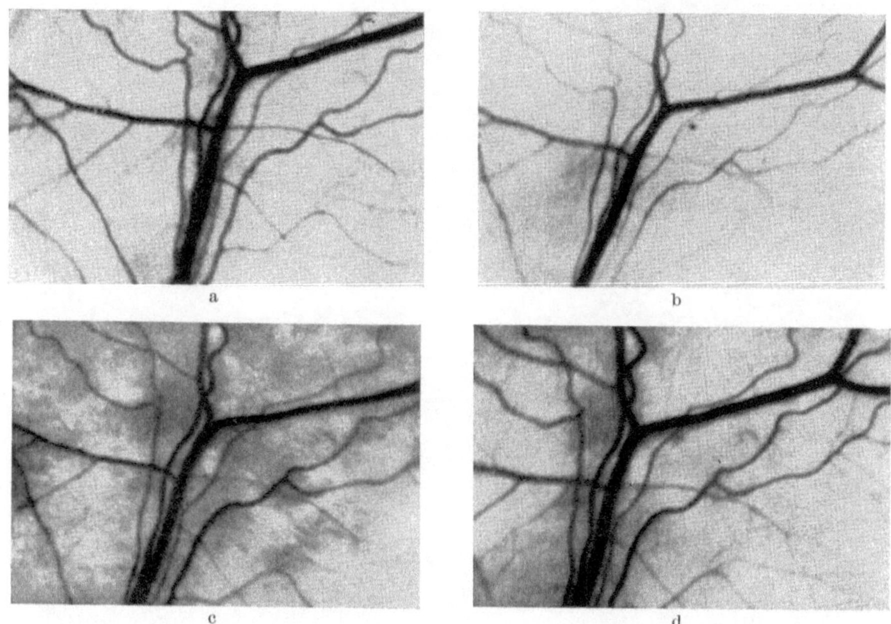

Abb. 35a—d. Intravitale Photogramme des Augenfundus beim Hund a normaler Fundus, b partielle Entleerung kleinerer Arterien im Histaminkollaps, c Zunahme der Gefäßfüllung und reaktive Hyperämie nach Histaminkollaps, d Rückbildung zur Norm (vgl. a). [Nach MEESSEN, H., u. R. SCHMIDT, Arch. f. Kreislauf-Forsch. 10, 255 (1942), Abb. 2.]

gesteigerten venösen Füllungsdruck war herabgesetzt[4]. Beim experimentellen Blutungskollaps zeigte sich die Insuffizienz des Myokards in einer Druckerhöhung in beiden Vorhöfen an[5]. Dabei war die Cocarboxylase verringert[6], die in der Norm hohe Extraktion von Brenztraubensäure war stark herabgesetzt und es bestand ein relativer Sauerstoffmangel[7].

Daß das *Gehirn* im fortgeschrittenen Kollaps von einer starken Oligämie betroffen wird, haben Durchströmungsmessungen ergeben (NOELL und M. SCHNEIDER 1942, KETHY und SCHMIDT 1948, BODECHTEL 1953), ebenso aber auch intravitale Photogramme des Augenhintergrundes bei experimentellem Kollaps bei Hund und Kaninchen (MEESSEN und SCHMIDT 1942). In diesen Photogrammen wurde die reversible Entleerung der Retinaarterien objektiv faßbar (Abb. 35). Histologisch waren in solchen Fällen Nekrosen der Purkinjezellen des Kleinhirns und in der Großhirnrinde nachweisbar[8]. Nach Entblutungskollaps konnten am Gehirn des Kaninchens bevorzugt Ganglienzell-Nekrosen im Ammonshorn sowie in der Rinde von Klein- und Großhirn beobachtet werden[9].

---

[1] ZINCK 1940.   [2] SCHÜRMANN 1938.   [3] KOHLSTAEDT und PAGE 1943, 1944.
[4] WIGGERS 1950.   [5] SARNOFF und Mitarbeiter 1954.   [6] EDWARDS, SIEGEL, BING 1954.
[7] HACKEL und GOODALE 1955.   [8] MEESSEN 1944.   [9] GAVALLÉR 1944.

In der *Leber* führt der Kollaps verschiedener Ätiologie zu Nekrosen oder großtropfigen Verfettungen an den Parenchymzellen der Läppchenzentren, auch im Experiment[1].

Besonders charakteristisch sind die Veränderungen der *Niere* im Kollaps. Sie wurden vor allem bei dem *Crush-Syndrom* beobachtet. Hierbei kommt es an der Niere infolge der regulativen Ischämie und der Kollaps-Oligämie zu

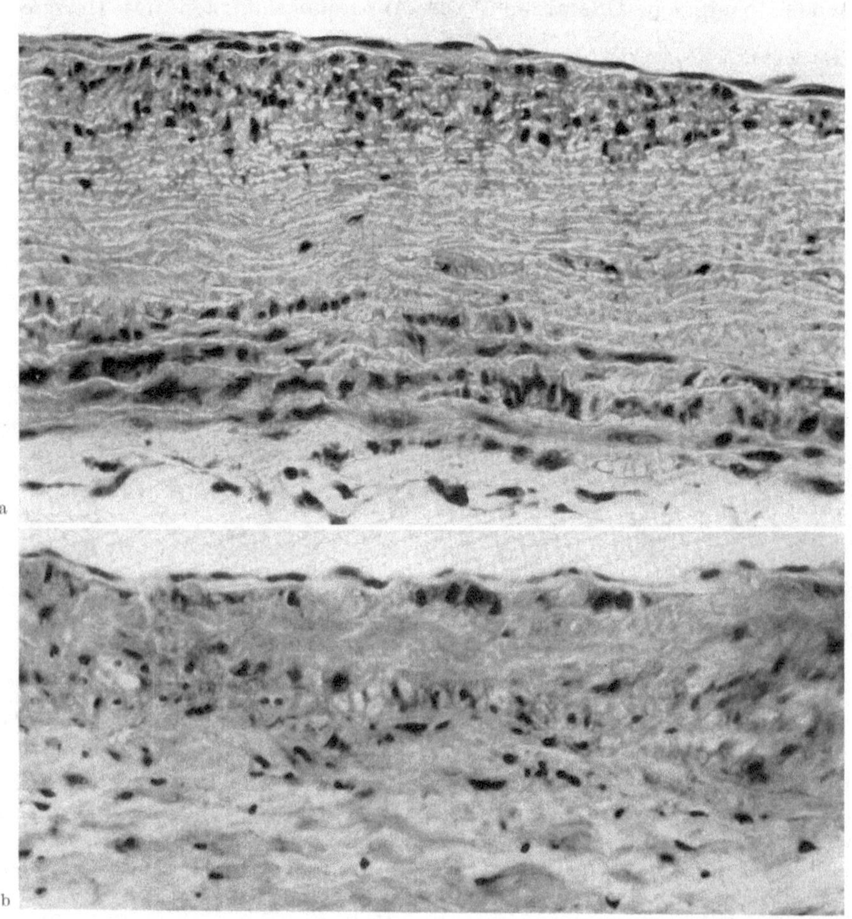

Abb. 36a u. b. a Ausgedehnte bandartige Nekrose der Aorta thoracica mit völligem Kernschwund im Nekrosebereich 24 Std nach 2maligem orthostatischem Kollaps beim Kaninchen. b Bandförmige Nekrose in der Media der Arteria carotis communis mit Schwund der Muskelzellkerne 4 Tage nach 2maligem orthostatischem Kollaps beim Kaninchen. [Nach de Faria, J. L., Beitr. path. Anat. 115, 373, 1955, Abb. 1 u. 4.]

Epithel-Nekrosen in den distalen Hauptstücken, besonders in deren geraden Anteilen[2], also zu einer Veränderung, die von den Angelsachsen als *lower nephron-nephrosis* gekennzeichnet wurde[3]. Das Bild konnte beim Kaninchen durch orthostatischen Kollaps reproduziert werden[4].

Daß auch die *Wandstrukturen des arteriellen Systems* von der Kollaps-Oligämie betroffen werden, haben schon Beobachtungen an den Coronararterien von

[1] Meessen 1937, 1939, Blüthgen 1944, Ellenberg und Osserman 1951.
[2] Bywaters 1944, Lucké 1946, Corcoran und Page 1945, Moon 1953, Rosemann 1960.
[3] Lucke 1946.   [4] Hollmann 1956.

MEESSEN (1939) ergeben: Es fanden sich Wandverquellungen und daran anschließende knötchenförmige Mesenchymzellenwucherungen. In neueren Experimenten konnte festgestellt werden, daß nach orthostatischem Kollaps in der Aorta, zum Teil auch in den Hals- und Femoralarterien des Kaninchens ausgedehnte bandförmige Nekrosen der glatten Muskelzellen unter Erhaltenbleiben der elastischen Elemente entstehen, meist in der mittleren Media (Abb. 36) (DE FARIA 1954, 1955). Ähnliche Nekrosen der glatten Muskulatur konnten auch in der menschlichen Aorta nach tödlichem Kollaps verschiedenen Ursprungs beobachtet werden (Abb. 37)[1].

Nach Entblutungskollaps infolge schwerer Geburt konnte von SHEEHAN 1939 eine Totalnekrose des *Hypophysenvorderlappens* nachgewiesen werden und als

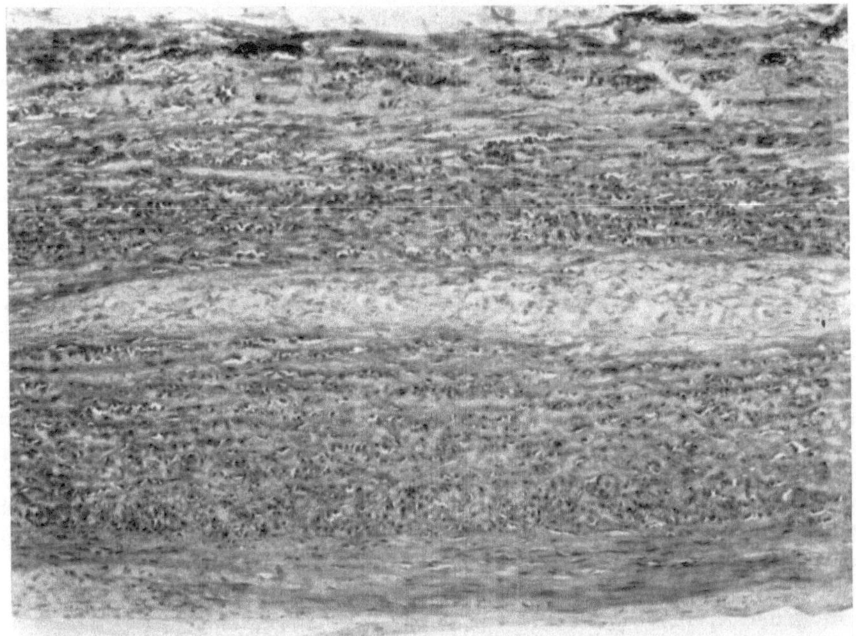

Abb. 37. Bandförmige Nekrose mit Schwund der Muskelfaserkerne in der Mitte der Bauchaorta (helle Zone) nach 24stündigem Kollaps des Menschen. [Nach THIES, W., Beitr. path. Anat. **116**, 431, 1956, Abb. 6.]

deren Folge eine Simondssche Kachexie[2]. Das Bild konnte experimentell am Kaninchen reproduziert werden (DE FARIA 1959).

Insgesamt werden also von der allgemeinen Oligämie im Kollaps verschiedenen Ursprungs bevorzugt die differenzierten Parenchyme des Herzmuskels, des Gehirns, der Leber, der Niere und der glatten Muskulatur des arteriellen Systems, besonders der Aortenmedia, irreversibel getroffen und fleckweise durch elektive Parenchymnekrose vernichtet. Die allgemeine Oligämie ist demnach durch ein ähnliches, zum Teil identisches Schädigungsmuster gekennzeichnet wie die allgemeine Hypoxydose verschiedenen Ursprungs[3]. Nur am Gehirn besteht zum Teil eine andere Topik. Auch sind die Wandveränderungen der Arterien einschließlich der Aorta bevorzugt die Spuren des Kollaps. *Die pathogenetische Verwandtschaft von allgemeiner Oligämie und allgemeiner Hypoxydose wird durch diese Beobachtungen hervorgehoben. Dabei ist freilich zu bedenken, daß von der allgemeinen Oligämie in jedem*

---

[1] ZINCK 1940, THIES 1956, DE FARIA 1957, 1959.
[2] Siehe auch SHEEHAN und MURDOCK 1939.   [3] Vgl. BÜCHNER 1957.

Falle zusätzlich die Substratzufuhr für den aeroben und den anaeroben Stoffwechsel schwer getroffen wird. Das Kennzeichen des Stoffwechsels im akuten Kollaps ist demnach die schwere energetische Insuffizienz aller hochwertigen Parenchyme.

2. Die kardial verursachte allgemeine arterielle Oligämie.

Wenn die allgemeine arterielle Oligämie die entscheidende Durchblutungsstörung beim Kollaps darstellt, so ist es nicht erstaunlich, daß das klinische Erscheinungsbild des Kollaps-Syndroms auch durch eine allgemeine arterielle Oligämie infolge primärer Erkrankung des Herzens hervorgerufen werden kann. Die Übereinstimmung der klinischen Veränderungen sollte uns aber nicht über die grundsätzliche Verschiedenheit in den ätiologischen und pathisch-funktionellen Voraussetzungen hinwegtäuschen. So sollte für die klinische Manifestierung einer kardial bedingten allgemeinen Oligämie auch nicht der Ausdruck „Kollaps" angewendet werden, um dessen klare Abgrenzung von der primären Herzschwäche und um dessen Definition als eines Zustandes der primären Insuffizienz der Peripherie des Kreislaufs jahrzehntelang in der theoretischen und klinischen Forschung gerungen wurde.

Eine kardial verursachte allgemeine Oligämie kann grundsätzlich auf zwei Wegen entstehen: 1. durch eine akute Insuffizienz des linken Ventrikels mit plötzlicher Herabsetzung des Schlag- und Minutenvolumens, d.h. durch eine *akute Insuffizienz der Entleerung des linken Ventrikels,* 2. durch eine *akute Insuffizienz der Füllung des linken Ventrikels* mit dadurch bedingter Herabsetzung des Schlag- und Minutenvolumens[1].

Das klassische Beispiel für die *akute Insuffizienz der Entleerung des linken Ventrikels* beobachtet man beim *akuten Herzinfarkt.* Da der Herzinfarkt fast immer in der Wand des linken Ventrikels entwickelt ist, bedeutet jeder größere Infarkt die Gefahr des akuten Versagens der linken Kammer, zumal in der akuten Phase des Infarktes die Zone der Totalnekrose des Myokards von einer breiten Zone relativer Ischämie umgeben ist, in der zwar das Herzmuskelparenchym zum größeren Teil erhalten bleibt, aber infolge ungenügender Kollateralversorgung nicht vollwertig durchblutet ist. So treten bei einem Teil der Herzinfarkte im akuten Stadium die folgenden Erscheinungen der allgemeinen Oligämie in den Vordergrund[2]: Der Blutdruck sinkt mehr oder minder deutlich, mitunter auf kritische Werte ab, die Haut wird durch Ischämie blaß, kalt und feucht, vor allem an den Händen, Füßen und an der Nase, bis zum Ausbruch von kaltem Schweiß. Als Folge einer Oligämie des Gehirns wird das Bewußtsein getrübt. Selbst Halbseitenlähmungen, bei denen autoptisch Verschlüsse von basalen Hirnarterien ausgeschlossen werden konnten, wurden als Folgen dieser Hirn-Oligämie gedeutet[3]. Als Folge einer Oligämie der Niere kann die Harnausscheidung eingeschränkt sein und in selteneren Fällen völlig sistieren. Bei dieser in allem typischen Kopie des Kollaps-Syndroms besteht höchste Lebensgefahr. Es ist durch das Versagen des Myokards im linken Ventrikel bestimmt und hat nichts mit einem entlastenden Bezold-Jarisch-Reflex zu tun. Da der rechte Ventrikel in der Regel von dem Infarkt und der kollateralen relativen Ischämie nicht mitbetroffen ist, bleibt die Lungendurchblutung erhalten oder sie wird gesteigert. Bei zunehmendem Blutaufstau in der Lunge infolge mangelnder Entleerung der linken Kammer und dann auch des linken Vorhofs addiert sich daher häufig zum Bild der allgemeinen Oligämie das des akuten, kardial bedingten Lungenödems. Dieses fehlt in der Regel bei einer anderen Ursache der kardial verursachten

---

[1] Friedberg 1959.   [2] Hochrein 1937, Friedberg 1959.
[3] Hauss und Kopermann 1950, Rubbar und Angrist 1953.

Oligämie, bei der *diphtherischen Myokardiopathie* mit toxischen Parenchymnekrosen des Herzmuskels. Da diese nicht nur im linken Ventrikel, sondern bevorzugt auch in der Wand des rechten Ventrikels entwickelt sind[1], ist der Bluteinstrom in die Lunge so verringert, daß ein Lungenödem meist ausbleibt. Dagegen beobachten wir dieses neben dem Bilde der allgemeinen Oligämie in der Regel bei akuter Insuffizienz des linken Ventrikels infolge Aorteninsuffizienz und besonders infolge Aortenstenose[2]. Als Abortivformen solcher Oligämien bei Aortenstenose können flüchtige Anfälle von Absenz oder einer Halbseitenlähmung auftreten[3].

Ein schwerster Anfall akuter, kardial bedingter Oligämie begegnet uns auch im *Morgagni-Adams-Stokesschen Syndrom*. Es tritt vor allem auf, wenn bei einem Av-Block vorübergehend der Kammereigenrhythmus versagt. Das kann besonders dann eintreten, wenn ein partieller Av-Block anfallsweise in einen totalen übergeht. Während die Vorhöfe weiterschlagen, sind die Kammern asystolisch. Dadurch sistiert der Auswurf von Blut aus der linken Kammer völlig, es kommt zur totalen Oligämie, insbesondere des Gehirns. Diese bewirkt schlagartig eine Bewußtlosigkeit, das Auftreten epileptiformer Krämpfe und bald auch Cheyne-Stokessches Atmen. Der Kammerstillstand dauert in der Regel höchstens eine Minute, kann aber auch 10 und mehr Minuten erreichen. Bei einem Teil der Fälle versagt schon der Sinusknoten, so daß auch die Vorhöfe asystolisch werden und kein Blut mehr in die Ventrikel einströmt. So steht das Adams-Stokessche Syndrom an der Grenze der Oligämien infolge mangelhaften Blutauswurfes aus dem linken und der *allgemeinen arteriellen Oligämie infolge mangelhaften Blutzustroms in den linken Ventrikel.*

In reiner Form kann uns dieser Zustand beim *Myxom des linken Vorhofs* begegnen. Diese Geschwulst sitzt meist im linken Vorhof gestielt dem Vorhofseptum auf. Je nach ihrer Größe und nach der Lagerung des Patienten kann sie plötzlich ventilartig die Mitralklappe verschließen. Der Einstrom von Blut in den linken Ventrikel sistiert dann und damit der Blutauswurf in das arterielle System. In kurzer Zeit kann sich dabei ein Adams-Stokessches Syndrom einstellen. Das gleiche wird je nach Lagerung gelegentlich bei einem größeren, aus dem Herzvorhof in die Mitralklappe prolabierenden *Thrombus des linken Herzohrs* oder bei einem von diesem abgelösten *Kugelthrombus des linken Vorhofs* beobachtet. In solchen Fällen kann die Blutleere in der arteriellen Peripherie des großen Kreislaufs so hochgradig werden, daß es an gipfelnden Teilen des Organismus zu totalen, wahrscheinlich spastisch gesteigerten Ischämien und in deren Folge zur Nekrose kommt[4]. Auf diese Weise können die Nasenspitze, Teile beider Ohrmuscheln sowie die Endglieder der Finger und der Zehen beiderseits ohne Embolie oder Thrombose in Nekrose übergehen.

Schwerste Füllungsinsuffizienzen des linken Ventrikels begegnen uns ferner bei der *subakuten, subtotalen, thrombotischen Lungenembolie.* Führt die völlige Verlegung des Stammes der rechten und linken Pulmonalarterie infolge totaler Unterbrechung der Lungendurchblutung schlagartig den Tod herbei, so bleibt bei der subtotalen, großen thrombotischen Lungenembolie noch eine Restdurchblutung der Lungen erhalten, jedoch mit unzulänglichem Bluteinstrom in den linken Vorhof und Ventrikel. So kommt es zu einer mehr oder minder schweren, allgemeinen arteriellen Oligämie, zu der sich noch, infolge der gestörten Atmungsfunktion der Lunge, eine Hypoxämie hinzuaddiert. Neben der Senkung des Blutdruckes und der Blässe und Kälte der Haut treten auch hier Zeichen der

---

[1] OHEIM 1938.   [2] McGINN und WHITE 1934, GALLAVARDIN 1937, HAMMARSTEN 1951.
[3] KUMPE und BEAN 1948.   [4] FISHBERG 1940.

schweren Oligämie des Gehirns in den Vordergrund: Verwirrtheitszustände, epileptiforme Anfälle und schließlich tiefe Bewußtlosigkeit.

Die Auswirkungen der kardial verursachten allgemeinen Oligämie an den parenchymatösen Organen sind bisher nicht so systematisch wie bei der Kollaps-Oligämie untersucht. Bekannt ist die Häufigkeit von akuten *läppchenzentralen Nekrosen des Leberparenchyms* infolge akuter Oligämie durch Herzinfarkt[1]. In einer Reihe von Arbeiten wurde die Wirkung der Herzinsuffizienz auf das *Hirn* untersucht. Es wurden Nekrosen der Purkinje-Zellen der Kleinhirnrinde und von Ganglienzellen der Großhirnrinde und des Ammonshorns nachgewiesen[2]. Nach M. Schneider (1958) verkürzt ein kleiner Restkreislauf am Gehirn die Wiederbelebungszeit wesentlich gegenüber einem totalen temporären Kreislaufstillstand.

3. Der temporäre Kreislaufstillstand.

Schon in früheren Beobachtungen wurde die Frage der Wirkung eines temporären Kreislaufstillstandes kasuistisch und systematisch-experimentell untersucht. Dabei erwies sich das Gehirn als das empfindlichste Organ, und die Hirnveränderungen waren der begrenzende Faktor für die Möglichkeit des Überlebens. Wir selbst sahen nach temporärem völligem Stillstand der Hirndurchblutung infolge Adams-Stokesschem Anfall von 7 min Dauer akute Ganglienzellnekrosen in der Großhirnrinde[3]. In einem Einzelfall führte ein Herzstillstand von 10 min bei einem 13jährigen Knaben zu einer Totalnekrose des Großhirns, so daß das Kind als ein Mittelhirnwesen weiterlebt[4]. Nach temporärer völliger Unterbrechung des Kreislaufs infolge Lungenembolie mit technisch geglückter Trendelenburgscher Operation konnte zwar der Kreislauf wiederhergestellt werden. Der über 5 min dauernde Kreislaufstillstand genügte aber, um die Nekrose zahlreicher Ganglienzellen der Groß- und Kleinhirnrinde, des Hirnstammes und der tieferen Zentren zu verursachen und dadurch in wenigen Tagen den Tod herbeizuführen[5].

Im Experiment an der Katze ergab die temporäre Abklemmung des Stammes der Pulmonalarterie von über 3 min Dauer ausgedehnte Nekrosen der Nervenzellen in der Groß- und Kleinhirnrinde, im Nucleus caudatus und im Thalamus opticus. Nach $7^{1}/_{2}$ min war das Weiterleben der Tiere nicht mehr möglich[6]. Ähnlich waren die Befunde am Hund[7].

Das Problem der Folgen des temporären Kreislaufstillstandes an den Parenchymen, besonders am Gehirn, gewann erhöhte Bedeutung durch die moderne Herzchirurgie unter Anwendung eines vorübergehenden Kreislaufstillstandes. Durch die gleichzeitige Unterkühlung wird zwar der Stoffwechsel bedeutend herabgesetzt[8]. So könnte es verständlich sein, daß bei 15° C trotz Kreislaufstillstand von 80' keine neurologischen und keine morphologischen Befunde am Hirn beobachtet wurden[9]. Wir haben jedoch bei 20° C und 30' Kreislaufstillstand irreversible Parenchymveränderungen an Hirn und Herzmuskel gefunden[10].

Auf die Unterschiede im Schädigungsmuster des Gehirns nach schweren allgemeinen Hypoxydosen einerseits und nach schweren allgemeinen Oligämien oder temporärem Kreislaufstillstand haben wir in unserem Beitrag über die Pathologie der cellulären und geweblichen Oxydationen in Bd. IV/2 dieses Handbuches schon hingewiesen[11].

---

[1] Vgl. Büchner 1957.   [2] Bodechtel 1953.
[3] Plambeck 1950.   [4] Monrad-Krohn 1951.
[5] Wustmann und Hallervorden 1935.   [6] Weinberger, Gibbon und Gibbon 1940.
[7] Grenell 1946, Schwiegk 1947.   [8] Brendel 1957, Thauer 1955/56, 1958.
[9] Watanabe 1957, Spohn und Kolb 1959, Wenz, Spohn, Kolb, Heinzel und Kratzert 1959.
[10] Schweikert und Sickinger 1960, Sickinger, Schweikert, Kaniak, Richter, Wiemers und Overbeck 1961.   [11] Büchner 1957.

Bei der allgemeinen arteriellen Oligämie haben wir die folgenden allgemein-pathologisch wichtigen Prinzipien kennengelernt:

1. Eine allgemeine arterielle Oligämie kann der Ausdruck einer akuten, sub-akuten oder länger dauernden allgemeinen Insuffizienz der Peripherie des großen Kreislaufs sein, d.h. eines Kollaps. Die allgemeine arterielle Oligämie kann aber ebenso die Folge einer akuten dynamischen Insuffizienz des linken Ventrikels mit starker Einschränkung des Schlag- und Minutenvolumens sein. Ähnliche Symptome wie beim Kollaps haben hier eine grundsätzlich andere Ursache: die Insuffizienz des Kreislaufmotors. Schließlich kann eine allgemeine arterielle Oligämie die Folge einer mangelhaften Füllung des linken Herzens sein. Diese kann durch subtotale große Lungenembolie durch einen großen Thrombus des linken Vorhofs, durch starke Mitralstenose oder durch starke Verlegung der Mitralklappe infolge eines Myxoms hervorgerufen sein.

2. Beim Kugelthrombus des linken Vorhofs und beim Myxom kann es zu einem temporären Kreislaufstillstand infolge Obturation der Mitralklappe kommen, ebenso im Adams-Stokesschen Anfall durch eine akute Unterbrechung der Erregungsleitung des Herzens. Auch eine große Lungenembolie kann durch zusätzliche spastische Sperre im Pulmonalkreislauf mit sekundärer Lösung des Spasmus einen temporären Kreislaufstillstand bewirken.

3. Beim Kollaps unterscheiden wir ätiologisch den Entblutungskollaps, den posttraumatischen Kollaps, den Verbrennungs-Kollaps, den Kollaps nach Erfrierung, den anaphylaktischen Kollaps, den infektiös-toxischen Kollaps, den zentralnervösen Kollaps.

4. Bei dem Entblutungskollaps steht die Einschränkung der zirkulierenden Blut-menge primär im Vordergrund. Dabei erfolgt vorübergehend eine Kompensation durch Zentralisation des Kreislaufs, d.h. durch Konzentration des Kreislaufs auf den Herzmuskel und das Hirn. Bei weiterem Blutverlust genügt jedoch auch die zentralisierte Blutmenge nicht mehr. Aus der kompensierten wird eine dekompen-sierte Oligämie mit Insuffizienz auch der Durchblutung des Gehirns und des Herz-muskels.

5. Beim posttraumatischen Kollaps und dem Verbrennungskollaps wurde die Wirkung permeabilitätssteigernder Amine bei akutem Gewebszerfall als Kollaps-ursache diskutiert. Die heute vorliegenden blutchemischen Befunde genügen jedoch nicht, diese Hypothese überzeugend zu unterbauen.

6. Auch bei diesen Kollapsformen muß den kreislaufdynamischen Faktoren eine große Bedeutung zugemessen werden: Trauma und Verbrennung lösen spastische Kontraktionen der Arterien in dem Schädigungsfeld aus, so daß die nachgeschalteten Gewebe unter der Wirkung starker Ischämie stehen, besonders ihre Parenchymzellen. In ihnen kommt es daher, vor allem nach Wiedereröffnung des Kreislaufs, zur Einwässerung in den hypoxisch geschädigten Parenchymzellen und durch hypoxische Steigerung der Permeabilität der Capillaren zu großen Flüssigkeitsansammlungen im Interstitium. Die dadurch verursachten starken Flüssigkeitsverluste aus dem strömenden Blut bewirken eine mehr oder weniger intensive allgemeine Oligämie.

7. Bei dem zentralnervösen Kollaps und bei dem infektiös-toxischen Kollaps ist die Erschlaffung der peripheren Arteriolen und Venen die Ursache großer Blut-versackungen in der unteren Körperhälfte und im Splanchnicus-Gebiet mit dem Ergebnis eines zunehmenden relativen Leerlaufs in den zentralen Organen des großen Kreislaufs, insbesondere in Hirn und Herzmuskel.

8. Beim „anaphylaktischen Kollaps" und bei dem sog. Histamin-Kollaps des Kaninchens sind Spasmen der Pulmonalarterien von entscheidender pathogenetischer Bedeutung. Eine dadurch hervorgerufene akute Widerstandserhöhung im Lungen-kreislauf bewirkt eine hochgradige Belastung des rechten Ventrikels. Dadurch kommt es häufig zu dessen Insuffizienz und sekundär zu einem Aufstau venösen Blutes in der unteren Körperhälfte und im Splanchnicus-Gebiet, so daß ein primär peripherer Kollaps vorgetäuscht wird. Infolge der Sperre des Durchstroms durch die Lunge addiert sich eine schwere Oligämie im arteriellen Anteil des großen Kreislaufs hinzu.

9. Die allgemeine arterielle Oligämie verursacht im Kollaps bei genügender Intensität und Dauer des Kollaps und bei genügend langer Überlebenszeit vor allem elektive Parenchymnekrosen an den Nervenzellen des Hirns und an den Herzmuskelzellen mit einem ähnlichen Schädigungsmuster wie bei allgemeiner Hypoxämie. Am Hirn tritt jedoch die Schädigung des Globus pallidus zugunsten der des Putamens zurück. Den irreversiblen Schädigungen der Struktur gehen charakteristische Funktionsstörungen des Hirns und des Herzmuskels voraus, die zum Teil lichtmikroskopisch durch eine akute Einwässerung als Folge akuter Störungen des Parenchymstoffwechsels gekennzeichnet sind. Dabei ist dessen Störung wesentlich intensiver als bei allgemeiner Hypoxämie, da nicht nur die Sauerstoffzufuhr, sondern auch die Substratzufuhr, vor allem für die aerobe und die anaerobe Glucose-Verwertung gestört ist, außerdem aber auch der Abtransport von Intermediärstoffen.

10. Die Leber zeigt die gleichen Veränderungen mit gleicher Topistik wie bei allgemeiner Hypoxämie. In der Niere kann es zur Nekrose der distalen Hauptstückepithelien kommen. Infolge der gleichzeitigen Senkung des Filtrationsdruckes kann die Niere akut versagen bis zur Anurie.

11. In der Wand der Aorta und der größeren Arterien können im Kollaps Zellen der glatten Muskulatur elektiv zugrunde gehen. Ein Durchblutungskollaps nach Geburt kann durch die allgemeine Oligämie zu einer Totalnekrose des Hypophysenvorderlappens führen und eine Simmondsche Kachexie nach sich ziehen.

12. Ein temporärer Kreislaufstillstand kann, vor allem am Hirn und am Herzmuskel, die gleichen Parenchymveränderungen mit gleicher Topistik hervorrufen wie der Kollaps.

13. Bei Unterkühlung wird ein temporärer Kreislaufstillstand zwar länger vertragen als bei normaler Temperatur. Von einer kritischen Zeit ab treten aber auch hier durch schwere Oligämie die gleichen Veränderungen auf, vor allem an den Parenchymzellen des Hirns und des Herzmuskels.

14. Tritt nach Herzoperation im Anschluß an einen temporären Kreislaufstillstand mit Unterkühlung der Tod ein, so ist dieser in den meisten Fällen ein Hirntod.

Die örtlich-regionäre und die allgemeine venöse Hyperämie.

1. Die örtlich-regionäre venöse Hyperämie.

Wird eine Vena femoralis durch einen Thrombus verschlossen, so ist in der Regel distal des Verschlusses der Blutabfluß aus dem betroffenen Bein stark behindert. Infolgedessen kommt es in diesem Gebiet zu einem akuten *Aufstau des venösen Blutes* und durch Steigerung des hydrostatischen Druckes in den Capillaren sowie durch Hypoxie der Capillarwände und durch Hypoxie des Gewebes zu einer Ansammlung von eiweißhaltiger Blutflüssigkeit, d.h. zum *weichen Ödem*, mit ödematöser Auflockerung des Bindegewebes zwischen der Muskulatur sowie in und unter der Haut[1]. Es wird vor allem an den Knöcheln, am Fußrücken, eventuell noch an der Wade sichtbar und tastbar. Beschränkt sich das Ödem auf das Interstitium der Muskulatur, so kann es sich der Beobachtung entziehen. Infolgedessen bleibt die Beinvenenthrombose häufig unerkannt[2]. Wird der verschließende Thrombus sekundär organisiert, so hinterläßt er nach

---

[1] Vgl. Naegeli und Matis 1955.　　[2] Vgl. Staemmler und Wilhelms 1953.

Mesenchymwucherung und partieller Rekanalisation in der Regel eine beträchtliche Narbenstenose in der rekanalisierten Lichtung. Die Venenklappen werden im Zuge des Organisationsvorganges meist insuffizient. So besteht in solchen Fällen fast immer eine dauernde Bereitschaft zur venösen Stauung im befallenen

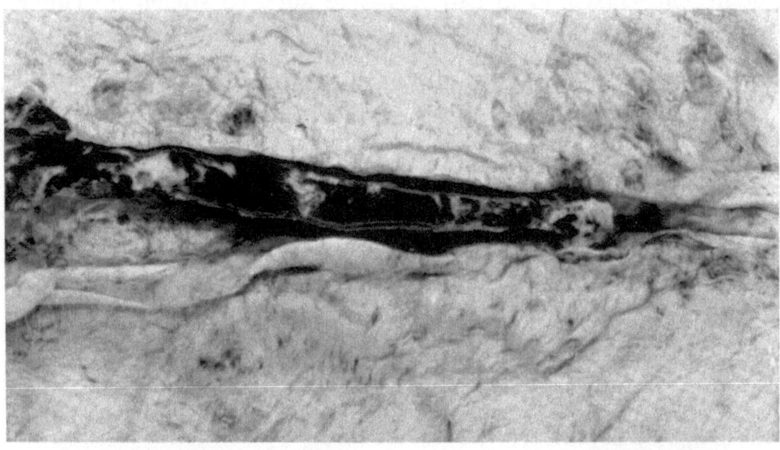

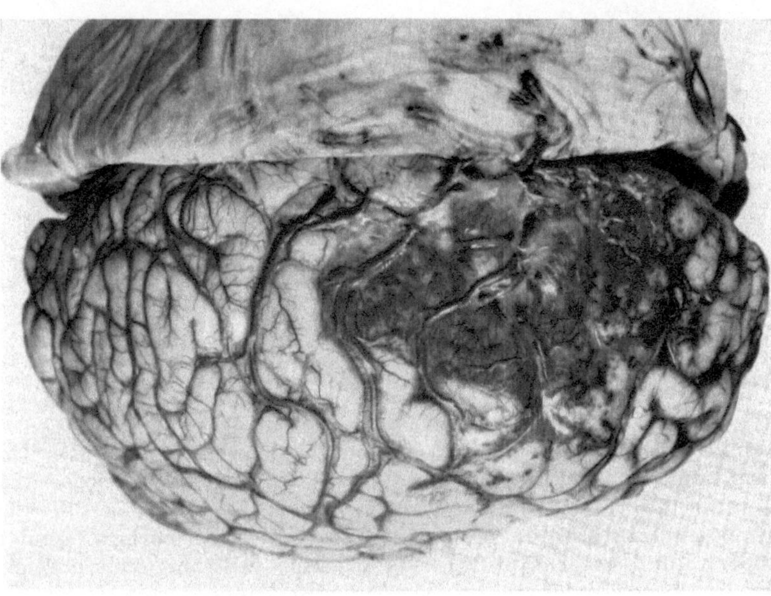

Abb. 38a u. b. a Akute Thrombose im Sinus sagittalis superior der harten Hirnhaut; b Oberfläche eines akuten hämorrhagischen Hirninfarktes infolge der Thrombose des Sinus sagittalis superior der Abb. 38a.

Bein. Diese steigert sich über Tage unter der Wirkung des Gehens und Stehens, sie verringert sich in der Nacht bei motorischer Ruhe der Beine und ihrer Horizontallagerung. Im Tages-Nacht-Rhythmus kann auf diese Weise ein Ödem kommen oder gehen, sich steigern oder verringern. Die große Bedeutung der Schwerkraft und der funktionellen Belastung des Beines ergibt sich vor allem aus dem nicht selten völligen Verschwinden des Ödems bei therapeutischer Hochlagerung und Ruhigstellung der Beine innerhalb weniger Tage. Andererseits führt die schonungslose Belastung der Beine, wie sie nicht selten beruflich erzwungen ist, häufig zum *chronischen harten Ödem mit Ödemsklerose des Mesenchyms.*

Tritt eine Beinvenenthrombose als *fulminante Thrombose der tiefen Beinvenen* mit plötzlichem Verschluß in ganzer Länge auf[1], so stehen im Unterschied zu der lokalen Thrombose der Oberschenkelvenen Kollateralen für den Abfluß des venösen Blutes aus der Tiefe des Beines nicht zur Verfügung. Es kommt also zu einer totalen, nicht zu einer partiellen venösen Stauung im Beingebiet. Die Folge ist daher ein mehr oder minder ausgedehnter *hämorrhagischer Infarkt der Zehen des Fußes und des Unterschenkels* mit ausgedehnten Hämorrhagien in das Gewebe. Wird der Thrombus früh genug operativ entfernt, so kann sich die

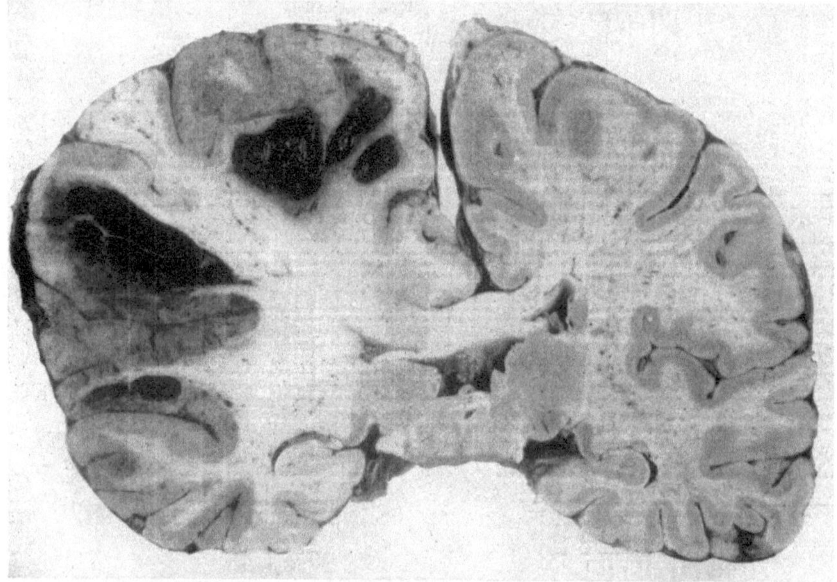

Abb. 39. Akuter hämorrhagischer Infarkt in der rechten Großhirnhemisphäre (seitenverkehrt) mit ausgedehnten Hämorrhagien im Hirnmark und hämorrhagischer Durchsetzung der benachbarten Hirnrinde sowie akutem Ödem im benachbarten Hirnmark. (Abb. 38 und 39 nach Noetzel, H., Die Pathologie des Nervensystems in: Büchner, F. Spezielle Pathologie, 3. Aufl., 1960, Abb. 315—317.)

hämorrhagische Anschoppung noch zurückbilden. Unterbleibt dieser Eingriff, so geht das hämorrhagisch durchsetzte Gewebe zugrunde: Wegen des Abfluß.tops strömt arterialisiertes Blut nicht mehr zu, so daß in kurzer Zeit die Sauerstoff- und Glucosevorräte des stagnierenden venösen Blutes erschöpft sind und sich Intermediärstufen wegen des daniederliegenden Abtransportes anreichern. Die schwere Stoffwechselstörung im hämorrhagisch infarzierten Gebiet führt zur hochgradigen Wasseransammlung und -retention und dadurch zum Bilde des *feuchten Brandes.* Der starke Flüssigkeitsverlust in das Gewebe führt häufig zur *allgemeinen Oligämie* und dadurch zu den Erscheinungen des *akuten Kollaps* (s. S. 844ff.). Dieser ist in einem Viertel der Fälle die Todesursache[2]. Ob zu dem Zustandekommen der Infarktnekrose noch ein reflektorischer Spasmus in der die Vene begleitenden Arteria femoralis, poplitea und tibialis notwendig ist, wie es Leriche 1937 annimmt, ist fraglich. Dagegen spricht die Tatsache, daß wir

---

[1] Grégoire 1938, De Bakey und Ochsner 1948, Naegeli und Matis 1955.
[2] De Bakey und Ochsner 1948.

grundsätzlich das gleiche Bild bei Thrombose des Sinus sagittalis superior am Gehirn beobachten, der nicht von einer Arterie begleitet ist.

Die akute Abflußbehinderung des venösen Blutes durch *Thrombose des Sinus sagittalis superior*[1], wie sie unter anderem bei Polycytämie, bei Dystrophie des Säuglings, bei Eklampsie und bei CO-Vergiftung zu beobachten ist, führt in kurzer Zeit durch Druckerhöhung in den Venen der Konvexität des Großhirns und Hypoxie der Capillarwände und des Parenchyms zu einem Ödem von Rinde und Mark des Großhirns. Dieses kann schon durch Hirndrucksteigerung zu einer akuten Psychose, dann zu Bewußtlosigkeit und innerhalb von 24 Std durch Atem- und Kreislauflähmung zum Tode führen. In der Regel kommt es aber unter Fortschreiten der Thrombose auf die parasagittalen Venen der Meningen

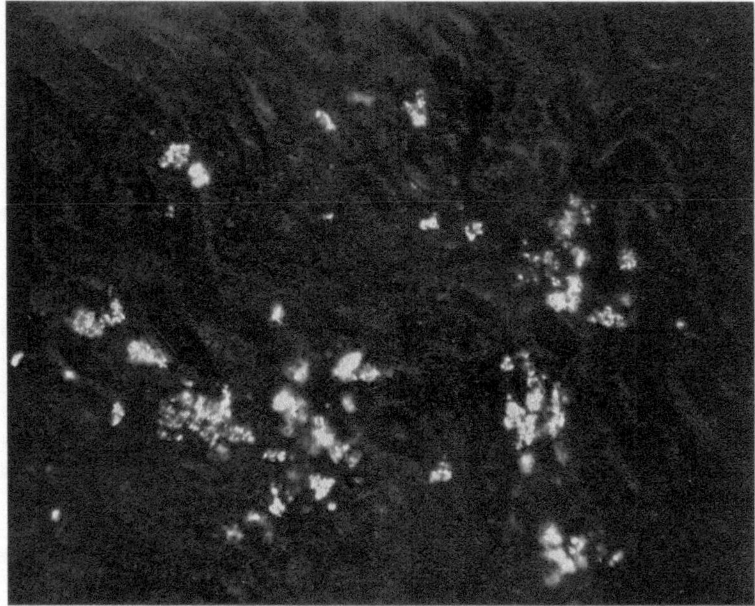

Abb. 40. Polarisationsoptisches Bild der Niere mit reichlicher Ablagerung doppelbrechender Lipoide fleckweise in den Epithelien der Hauptstückepithelien bei klinischer Eiweiß-Lipoid-Nephrose infolge unvollkommener Nierenvenenthrombose.

zu einem *hämorrhagischen Infarkt des benachbarten Großhirns* mit Nekrose des Hirnparenchyms, kompakter Blutung und in der Randzone mit Ringblutungen (Abb. 38 und 39).

Im gleichen Sinne entwickelt sich bei *Thrombose der Nierenvene* ein Ödem und ein *hämorrhagischer Infarkt der Niere,* bei *Thrombose der Nebennierenvenen* deren *hämorrhagische Infarzierung.* Auch die *Mesenterialvenenthrombose* hat den *hämorrhagischen Infarkt,* hier *am Dünndarm,* zur Folge. In seltenen Fällen kann eine unvollständige thrombotische Verschließung einer Nierenvene zu einer hochgradigen Stauungsproteinurie und in deren Folge durch Rückspeicherung zu einer Eiweiß-Lipoidnephrose führen[2] (Abb. 40). Im Experiment konnte dieses Bild neuerdings reproduziert werden[3].

---

[1] NOETZEL 1955, BROBEIL 1955.

[2] HEILMEYER und LIPPROSS 1936, BLAINEY, HARDWICKE und WHITFIELD 1954, DEPARIS, CANIVET, LEVILLAIN und LISSAC 1954, MILLER, HOYT und POLLOCK 1954, KAPLAN, NEWMAN, KAPLAN, BAKER und LEE 1956, MILLIEZ, LAGRUE, DE BAROCHEZ und SAMARCQ 1957, M. STAEMMLER 1958.

[3] HOLLE und DONNER 1957, OMAE, MASSON und CORCORAN 1958.

2. Die allgemeine venöse Hyperämie.

Die Kardinalursache der allgemeinen venösen Hyperämie ist die *akute oder chronische Insuffizienz des rechten Ventrikels und Vorhofes*. Infolge mangelhafter Weiterbeförderung des Blutes aus dem rechten Herzen in die Lunge entwickelt sich dabei langsam oder plötzlich ein akuter Aufstau des Blutes in der oberen und unteren Hohlvene und ihren Quellgebieten.

Von diesem Aufstau werden verschiedene Gefäßgebiete besonders folgenschwer betroffen. So kommt der Aufstau herznah zunächst besonders in der *Leber* zur Wirkung: das venöse Blut wird rings um die Zentralvenen in den Sinusoiden der Läppchenzentren mehr oder minder stark retiniert, Stauungsstraßen können sektorenförmig quer durch die Läppchen die Zentralvenen verbinden. Durch diese Stauung kommt es in den Zentren zur Hypoxie der Leberparenchymzellen. Bedenken wir, daß nach allgemeiner Hypoxämie in kurzer Zeit eine Insuffizienz der Leberzelle für die Galleausscheidung resultiert[1], so verstehen wir, daß bei *akuter Stauungsleber* nicht selten in wenigen Tagen ein Anstieg des indirekt reagierenden Bilirubins im Blutserum, des Urobilinogens im Harn[2] und in einem Teil der Fälle ein *Retentionsikterus*[3] auftritt. (In einem Teil der Fälle ist der auftretende Ikterus allerdings durch Blutzerfall bei hämorrhagischen Lungeninfarkten mit bedingt.) Auch die Fähigkeit zur Glykogensynthese und zur Glucosemobilisierung kann gestört sein, so daß eine *Hypoglykämie* die Folge ist[4]. Die Insuffizienz des Leberparenchymstoffwechsels in den Läppchenzentren führt aber darüber hinaus zu *akuten Stauungsnekrosen der Läppchenzentren*, z.T. auch zu straßenförmigen Nekrosebrücken von Läppchen zu Läppchen. Blut-chemisch manifestieren sich diese akuten Leberparenchymnekrosen in einem *Anstieg der Glutaminat-Pyruvat-Transaminase*[5]. Wird die venöse Stauung chronisch, so tritt keine Regeneration der Läppchenzentren ein, und es kommt durch Kollagenisierung der Reticulinfasern des Mesenchymfaserskelets der Läppchen zur *zentralen Fibrose* oder, nach straßenförmigen Nekrosen, zur *Stauungscirrhose der Leber*.

Bei längerer venöser Stauung treten regelmäßig die Zeichen der *venösen Hyperämie der Niere* in Erscheinung. Diese äußert sich vor allem in einer mäßigen *Albuminurie* mit wenigen Promille Eiweiß im Harn. Sie ist Folge der Hypoxie und der gesteigerten Durchlässigkeit der mit venösem Blut überfüllten Glomerula. Histologisch sieht man das Eiweiß feinkörnig oder homogen in den Bowmanschen Kapseln und in den Tubuli abgelagert. Vieles spricht dafür, daß die venöse Hyperämie außerdem zu einer *gesteigerten Rückresorption von Natrium in der Niere* führt. Das ist vor allem durch Untersuchungen mit Radioisotopen wahrscheinlich gemacht[6]. Bei Herzinsuffizienz infolge experimenteller Klappenfehler am Hund wurde die Steigerung der Rückresorption von Natrium in der Niere exakt nachgewiesen[7].

Es ist naheliegend, außer extrarenalen Faktoren die venös-hyperämische Schädigung des Parenchyms der Niere selbst für die vermehrte Rückresorption des Natriums an den Tubuli verantwortlich zu machen und darin die Manifestierung einer generalisierten Parenchymschädigung mit vermehrtem Austritt von Kalium aus den Zellen und vermehrtem Eintritt von Natrium in die Zellen zu sehen. Daß das Nierenparenchym durch chronische Rechtsinsuffizienz venöshyperämisch-hypoxisch geschädigt wird, geht daraus hervor, daß nicht selten eine fein- bis mitteltropfige basale *Verfettung der Hauptstückepithelien* nach-

---

[1] HANZON 1952.   [2] CHAVEZ, SEPULVEDA und ORTOGA 1943.
[3] KUGEL und LICHTMAN 1943, PARKER und FELDER 1955, FRIEDBERG 1959.
[4] MELLINKOFF und TUMULTY 1952.   [5] FORSTER 1958.
[6] BURCH, REASER und CRONVICH 1947.   [7] BARGER, RUDOLPH und YATES 1954.

gewiesen werden kann, also ein Bild, wie es uns als Folge von Hypoxydosen verschiedenen Ursprungs geläufig ist[1]. Schließlich leidet durch die mangelhafte Durchblutung der Niere die Harnausschwemmung als Ganzes not, so daß der Tages-Nacht-Rhythmus der Harnausscheidung zugunsten einer *Nykturie* gestört ist, sich parallel zur Schwere der Rechtsinsuffizienz eine *Oligurie* entwickelt oder sogar eine mäßige Retention harnpflichtiger Reststickstoffe, also eine *mäßige Azotämie* eintritt.

Von oft nicht genügend berücksichtigter Bedeutung ist die Rückwirkung der Rechtsinsuffizienz auf das *Gehirn*. Schon SCHEINBERG (1950) konnte mit der Stickoxydulmethode von KETY und SCHMIDT (1948) eine Herabsetzung der Hirndurchblutung von 39% in der Phase der Rechtsinsuffizienz nachweisen. BODECHTEL (1953) hat mit der gleichen Methode gezeigt, daß bei kompensiertem chronischem Cor pulmonale wegen chronischen Lungenemphysems die Hirndurchblutung bei bestehender Atmungsinsuffizienz kompensatorisch erhöht war, daß dagegen bei *dekompensiertem chronischem Cor pulmonale* infolge von Emphysem oder Kyphoskoliose eine statistisch signifikante *Herabsetzung der Hirndurchblutung* nachzuweisen war. Bei 21 Fällen von Mitralvitien fand er in der Phase der Kompensation keine nennenswerten Abweichungen der Hirndurchblutung von der Norm; dagegen waren in 11 Fällen mit Herzinsuffizienz die Mittelwerte der Hirndurchblutung stark herabgesetzt[2]. Daß sich bei schweren Rechtsinsuffizienzen diffuse und fleckförmige Ganglienzelluntergänge entwickeln können, hatte BODECHTEL schon 1932 nachgewiesen. Es ist unwahrscheinlich, daß in solchen Fällen eine gleichzeitige Arteriosklerose der Hirnarterien Ursache der Durchblutungsinsuffizienz des Gehirns ist, da Mitralfehler-Kranke selten eine Cerebralsklerose haben (entgegen NOVACK u. Mitarb. 1953).

Andere Erscheinungen der subakuten und chronischen Rechtsinsuffizienz sind so allgemein bekannt, daß es genügt, sie kurz zu erwähnen, besonders die Ansammlung mehr oder minder großer *Transsudate* in den Pleurahöhlen, im Herzbeutel und in der Bauchhöhle sowie *Ödeme*, die sich unter der Wirkung der Schwerkraft vor allem an den Füßen, am Knöchel und am Unterschenkel entwickeln, beim liegenden Kranken aber auch über dem Os sacrum, am Skrotum, an der Haut und Vorhaut des Penis und an der Dorsalfläche der Arme. Bisher wurden diese Veränderungen als Folge des durch die venöse Hyperämie gesteigerten hydrostatischen Druckes und der Stauungs-Hypoxie der Capillarwände angesehen[3]. Neuerdings neigt man jedoch zu der Auffassung, daß der entscheidende Faktor bei der Entstehung dieser Ödeme die infolge der Stauung in der Niere zu beobachtende Steigerung der Natrium-Rückresorption ist. Diese führe zu einer stark gesteigerten Ansammlung von Natrium im Gewebe und dadurch zur Wasserverhaltung. Dem ist jedoch entgegenzuhalten, daß bei der Behinderung des Pfortaderkreislaufes durch Lebercirrhose verschiedenen Ursprungs, durch posthepatitisch-postdystrophische Narbenleber oder durch Pfortaderthrombose im Quellgebiet der Pfortader das gleiche Bild ohne Mitwirkung einer vermehrten Natrium-Rückresorption in der Niere zu beobachten ist. Hier wird uns eindrucksvoll vor Augen geführt, daß das Zusammenwirken von Steigerung des hydrostatischen Druckes, von Hypoxie der Capillarwände in der Darmwand und von hypoxischer Gewebsschädigung ein hochgradiges Ödem und in der Bauchhöhle einen von Punktion zu Punktion schnell sich wieder auffüllenden Ascites bewirkt. Es wäre gezwungen, wollte man der Pfortaderstauung bei Lebercirrhose usw. diese pathogenetischen Potenzen zuerkennen, nicht aber der Pfortaderstauung, wie sie bei Rechtsinsuffizienz zwangsläufig der Leberstauung folgt.

---

[1] Vgl. BÜCHNER 1957.   [2] BODECHTEL 1953.
[3] Zum Beispiel STARLING 1909, ROMBERG 1921.

Ist aber das Starlingsche Prinzip der Transsudat- und Ödementstehung bei der Rechtsinsuffizienz für den Bereich der Pfortader anerkannt, so muß es auch für das große venöse System gültig sein. In dieser Überlegung bestärkt uns die Tatsache, daß wir schwere Beinödeme nach stenosierender Organisation von Thromben der Vena femoralis nur als Folge eines distal des Abstromhindernisses gesteigerten hydrostatischen Druckes, einer venös-hyperämischen Hypoxie der Capillarwände und einer Hypoxie des Gewebes ohne primäre Natriumretention verstehen können.

Die venöse Hyperämie ist durch folgende Eigentümlichkeiten ausgezeichnet:

1. Bei örtlicher venöser Hyperämie, z.B. infolge Venenthrombose, mit erhaltenem kollateralem Abfluß venösen Blutes kommt es infolge Steigerung des hydrostatischen Drucks und infolge Hypoxie an den Capillaren zum Austritt von Blutflüssigkeit, durch Schädigung des Parenchyms zur Einwässerung, durch beide Vorgänge zum akuten Ödem. An der unteren Extremität tritt dieses Ödem in der Regel während der Tagesbelastung auf, um sich nachts wieder zurückzubilden.

2. Bei ungenügendem kollateralem Abfluß kann infolge des thrombotischen Verschlusses einer Vene in dem vorgeschalteten Organ oder in Anteilen des Organes ein hämorrhagischer Infarkt entstehen. Dieser wird am Fuß und Unterschenkel bei fulminanter Thrombose der Schenkelvenen beobachtet, an der Niere bei Thrombose der Nierenvene — bei beiderseitiger Thrombose mit Urämie — an der Nebenniere bei Nebennierenvenenthrombose, am Darm bei Mesenterialvenenthrombose, am Hirn bei Thrombose des Sinus sagittalis superior.

3. Unvollständige Thrombose einer Nierenvene kann zur hochgradigen Stauungsproteinurie und zur Eiweißlipoidnephrose führen.

4. Die allgemeine venöse Hyperämie als Folge akuter oder chronischer Insuffizienz des rechten Herzens bewirkt die Bilder der Stauungsleber mit zentralen Stauungsnekrosen, zum Teil mit Retentionsikterus und Hypoglykämie. Die Folgen können zentrale Fibrose oder Stauungscirrhose der Leber sein.

5. An der Niere verursacht die allgemeine venöse Hyperämie eine Proteinurie und eine gesteigerte Rückresorption von Natrium. Eine mäßige Azotämie kann die Folge sein. Auch das Hirn wird durch die allgemeine venöse Hyperämie stärker geschädigt als dies im allgemeinen bedacht wird. Die Stauungstranssudate und Ödeme ordnen sich in das pathogenetische Gesamtbild ein.

Die Blutungen.

Von Blutungen sprechen wir dann, wenn rotes, also erythrocytenhaltiges Blut die Kreislaufbahn verläßt und nach außen entleert wird. Diese Entleerung kann in das Gewebe, also auch in parenchymatöse Organe, oder in vorgebildete Hohlräume, also in den Magendarmtraktus, in die Luftwege, in die Harnwege, in die Pleura-, Pericard- oder Bauchhöhle oder nach außen erfolgen. Voraussetzungen für Blutungen sind die anatomisch präparierbaren oder nur mikroskopisch nachweisbaren Zerstörungen von Gefäßwänden und Eröffnung von Gefäßlichtungen oder der Durchtritt von Erythrocyten durch unverletzte, in ihrem Strukturgefüge lichtmikroskopisch unveränderte Capillaren. Demgemäß unterscheiden wir mit der klassischen Pathologie die *Blutung per rhexin* und die *Blutung per diapedesin*, die Rhexisblutung und die Diapedesisblutung.

1. Die Rhexisblutungen.

Schwere, nicht selten tödliche Blutungen können sich infolge der Eröffnung arterieller oder venöser Gefäße durch krankhafte Prozesse an den Arterien und Venen oder in ihrer Umgebung entwickeln.

So kann die *Aorta* durch *Mesaortitis syphilitica* in ihrem aufsteigenden Teil oder in ihrem Bogen zu einem Aneurysma ausgeweitet werden. Eines Tages kann es zur Ruptur des Aneurysmas in den Herzbeutel, in die Trachea, in den Oesophagus oder, nach vorhergehender Zerstörung des Sternums, nach außen kommen. Durch *Medionekrosis* schwer geschädigt, kann die Aorta bei Blutdruckerhöhung in den Herzbeutel perforieren. Am Hirn können sich, durch wahrscheinlich angeborene Defekte der Muskulatur der Media oder durch entzündliche, z.B. syphilitische Erkrankungen, *Aneurysmen der basalen Hirnarterien* entwickeln und durch Bersten zu Blutungen in die weichen Hirnhäute oder den Hirnstamm führen[1]. Die *hypertonische Arteriosklerose der intracerebralen Hirnarterien* bewirkt bei plötzlichen zusätzlichen Blutdrucksteigerungen des Hypertonikers große Massenblutungen in den Hirnstamm, die Brücke oder das Kleinhirn[2]. Greift die tuberkulöse Nekrose in der Wand einer Lungenkaverne auf die äußeren Schichten einer noch durchbluteten Arterie über, so kann es an der durch die Nekrose geschwächten Stelle zu einem *tuberkulösen Kavernenaneurysma* kommen. Eine mehr oder minder schwere, mitunter tödliche Blutung kann die Folge sein. Am Grunde *chronischer peptischer Geschwüre* des Magens oder des Zwölffingerdarms kann es an einer in den Geschwürsgrund einbezogenen Arterie zur *peptischen Arrosion* kommen und dadurch zur rezidivierenden, gelegentlich tödlichen Blutung. Bakterienbeladene Emboli können bei der *Thromboendocarditis ulcerosa lenta* Nekrosen und *Aneurysmen* von Arterien verursachen, z.B. der *Arteria lienalis* mit tödlicher Verblutung in die Bauchhöhle. Die *Panarteriitis nodosa* führt nicht selten zu *Aneurysmen der Nierenarterien*, die durch Ruptur schwere Blutungen in das Nierenlager bewirken können. Bei der *geschwürigen Arteriosklerose der Bauchaorta* kommt es nicht selten zum *arteriosklerotischen Aneurysma*, welches durch Perforation im retroperitonealen Gewebe eine tödliche Verblutung verursachen kann.

Aus *varicös erweiterten Venen der weichen Hirnhäute* entwickeln sich mitunter nach Ruptur tödliche Blutungen in die Großhirnrinde und in das anschließende Mark , z.B. bei der Sturge-Weberschen Krankheit. Starke venöse Stauungen im Pfortadersystem, wie sie besonders bei *Lebercirrhose* zustandekommen, führen durch Entwicklung eines Umwegkreislaufs zu *Varixknoten an den unteren Oesophagusvenen*. Aus diesen treten rezidivierende, häufig tödliche Blutungen ein.

Zahlreiche maligne Tumoren haben grundsätzlich die Tendenz in die kleineren Venen, gelegentlich auch in die Arterien, des Geschwulstbereiches einzuwachsen. So kommt es zu rezidivierenden, mitunter tödlichen Blutungen aus dem Magencarcinom, dem Dickdarmcarcinom, dem Bronchialcarcinom, aus den malignen Tumoren der Niere, zur Hämatombildung in Gliomen.

Die dargelegten Beispiele kann jeder Arzt aus der eigenen Erfahrung durch weitere ergänzen.

2. Die Diapedesisblutungen.

Diapedesisblutungen können einmal bei Erkrankungen beobachtet werden, bei denen eine *Veränderung in der Ultrastruktur der Capillarwände* angenommen werden muß. Sie können andererseits eintreten als Folgen von *Störungen des Gerinnungssystems des Blutes*. In beiden Krankheitsgruppen besteht eine Blutungsbereitschaft, eine *hämorrhagische Diathese*. Wenden wir uns zunächst den Störungen der Blutgerinnung als Ursache von hämorrhagischen Diathesen zu, so können wir sie nur von einer kurzen Betrachtung der *Orthologie der Blutgerinnung* her

---

[1] HEYN und NOETZEL 1956.
[2] BÖHNE 1927, 1931, HILLER 1935, 1936, WIRTZ 1936, MEESSEN und STOCHDORPH 1957.

angehen. Wir stützen uns dabei in erster Linie auf die von Biggs und Macfarlane (1957) und von Koller (1958) gegebenen Darstellungen, die ihrerseits von den klassischen Arbeiten von A. Schmidt (1892) und Morawitz (1905) ausgehen. Das Kernstück der Gerinnungslehre dieser Arbeiten erwies sich in der gesamten neueren Forschung als unerschütterlich, insbesondere die Zweistufigkeit des Gerinnungsvorganges im Sinne der Umwandlung von Prothrombin in Thrombin als erster Stufe und der Umwandlung von Fibrinogen in Fibrin als zweiter Stufe. Die moderne Forschung hat im Wesentlichen die Tatsache hinzugefügt, daß die in der Stufe 1 wirksam werdende Thrombokinase einer Serie von Faktoren des Blutplasmas und der Thrombocyten zu ihrer Generation bedarf. Je mehr die Kompliziertheit dieses Systems aufgeklärt werden konnte, um so schwieriger wurde vorübergehend die Verständigung, zumal es sich zeigte, daß der gleiche Faktor mehrfach von verschiedenen Autoren entdeckt und mit verschiedenen Namen belegt wurde. Es bedeutet daher einen entscheidenden Fortschritt, daß eine internationale Nomenklatur-Komission vor kurzem eine Vereinheitlichung der Synonyma durch Numerierung der Faktoren vorgeschlagen hat[1]. So können wir von diesem Vorschlag in unserer Darstellung sogleich Nutzen ziehen.

Im Mechanismus der Blutgerinnung ist das *Fibrinogen* der Faktor I. Es wird als gelöstes Eiweiß unter der Wirkung von *Thrombin* in faseriges *Fibrin* umgewandelt. Diese Umwandlung vollzieht sich so, daß von dem Fibrinogen, einem Linearprotein von etwa 330000 Molekulargewicht, unter der fermentativen Wirkung von *Thrombin* ein *Fibrinopeptid* von 4000—8000 Molekulargewicht abgespalten und zu Fibrinopeptidketten = Fibrin polymerisiert wird[2]. Ein besonderes Ferment dient der Verfestigung des Fibrins[3] unter Gegenwart von Calcium.

Der Faktor II ist das *Prothrombin*, das die spezifische Vorstufe des *Thrombins* darstellt[4]. Es wird durch den Faktor III, die *Thrombokinase*[5] zu Thrombin aktiviert.

Dieser Faktor III tritt in geringer Menge als Gewebsthrombokinase ins Spiel, vor allem aber als Blutthrombokinase[6]. Beide Thrombokinasen enthalten ein Lipoprotein, wahrscheinlich mit Cephalin als Lipoidkomponente[7]. *Gewebsthrombokinase* wird bei jeder Gewebsverletzung, also auch bei jeder Gefäßverletzung, freigesetzt. Ihre Bildung im Gewebe aus dem Gewebefaktor setzt noch *Calcium* als Faktor IV und den Faktor V als einen Beschleunigungsfaktor (Proaccelerin) voraus, ferner den Faktor VII als weiteren Beschleuniger und den Stuart-Prower-Faktor als weiteren Aktivator. Demgegenüber wird die *Blutthrombokinase* aus dem Blutplättchenfaktor durch Verletzung von Thrombocyten, also auch bei jeder Gefäßverletzung, gebildet. Auch hier bedarf es aber der Mitwirkung des Faktor IV (Calcium), V (Beschleunigungsfaktor) und des Stuart-Prower-Faktors. Darüber hinaus treten ins Spiel: Faktor VIII als Anti-Hämophilie-Globulin A, Faktor IX als Anti-Hämophilie-Globulin B und möglicherweise noch andere Faktoren. Die Thrombocyten bewirken außerdem die Retraktion des Fibringerinnsels. Schließlich setzt die Bildung von Prothrombin in der Leber die Mitwirkung von Vitamin K voraus[8]. Wahrscheinlich benötigen aber auch die Vorstufen der Faktoren VII und IX und des Stuart-Prower-Faktors das gleiche Vitamin.

---

[1] Wright 1959.
[2] Lorand 1954, Laki 1954, Sherry, Troll und Glueck 1954, Ferrey 1954.
[3] Lorand 1954, Laki 1954.
[4] Loeliger 1952, Seegers und Alkjaersig 1956, Seegers und Johnson 1956.
[5] Morawitz 1905.   [6] Koller 1954, Biggs und Macfarlane 1957.
[7] Nach Koller 1958.   [8] Dam 1930, 1935.

Bei Verletzungen von Gefäßen steht die Gewebsthrombokinase in wenigen Sekunden, die Blutthrombokinase erst nach einigen Minuten zur Verfügung. Die Gewebsthrombokinase leitet die Gerinnung und damit die Blutstillung ein, die Blutthrombokinase wird aber dann zum entscheidenden Faktor der Blutgerinnung [1].

Dabei werden bei Verletzung von Arterien oder Venen *Agglutinate von Thrombocyten*, also kleinste Thromben, an der Verletzungsstelle gebildet [2], die dann durch Freisetzung des Plättchen-Faktors die Fibringerinnung nach sich ziehen. Dagegen kommt es bei Verletzung von Capillaren unmittelbar zur Bildung eines kleinen abdichtenden Fibrinpfropfes [3].

Nach diesem komplizierten Ineinandergreifen einer ganzen Serie von Faktoren und Mechanismen bei dem Vorgang der Blutgerinnung und damit auch der Blutstillung erwarten wir theoretisch in der *Pathologie der Blutgerinnung* eine ganze Reihe möglicher Störungen mit verwandter Wirkung, nämlich der Neigung zu Blutungen, also zur *hämorrhagischen Diathese*. Bei ihrer Erörterung beziehen wir uns vor allem auf die Monographien von HEILMEYER und BEGEMANN (1951, 1955), HEILMEYER (1960), BIGGS und MACFARLANE (1957), BEGEMANN und HARWERTH (1959).

Die moderne Hämatologie unterscheidet hämorrhagische Diathesen durch Erkrankungen der Blutplättchen, also durch Thrombocytopathien, hämorrhagische Diathesen durch Insuffizienz anderer Gerinnungsfaktoren, also Coagulopathien und hämorrhagische Diathesen durch Capillarwandschäden.

Unter den *Thrombocytopathien* ist am längsten die *Werlhofsche Krankheit* bekannt. Sie ist durch das spontane Auftreten flohstichartiger, fleckförmiger und auch flächenhafter capillärer Hautblutungen und von Blutungen in die Schleimhäute der Nase, der Mundhöhle, des Magendarmkanals, der Harnwege, der Luftwege, bei der Frau auch der Genitalwege mit starken schließlich tödlichen Blutungen aus den Schleimhäuten nach außen gekennzeichnet. Dabei tritt die Krankheit fast in der Hälfte der Fälle vor und in der Pubertät auf. Das Wesen der Erkrankung beruht in dem *Mangel an Thrombocyten*, die von dem Normwert 200000—300000 mm³ unter 50000 mm³ absinken und in akuten Fällen auf 30000—20000 mm³ absinken können. Dabei lassen die Thrombocyten morphologische Veränderungen erkennen, die z.T. durch die Bildung von Riesenplättchen oder von Plättchen mit geringem Granulomer gekennzeichnet sind. Im intravitalen Punktat des Sternalmarks sind die Bildungszellen der Plättchen, die Megacaryocyten, oft vermehrt. Wegen des Plättchenmangels, wahrscheinlich auch wegen der Strukturänderungen der Plättchen, ist die Bildung der Blutthrombokinase gehemmt, aber auch die Bildung des Plättchenfaktors, der die Retraktion des Fibringerinnsels aktiviert. Es ist verständlich, daß die Werlhofsche Krankheit nicht nur als genuine Krankheit, sondern auch als *symptomatische Thrombopenie* auftritt, und zwar bei *Hemmungen der Blutbildung im Knochenmark verschiedener Ätiologie*, z.B. bei der myeloischen und lymphatischen Leukämie, der aplastischen Anämie, den diffusen Myelosen, Retikulosen und Knochenmarkscarcinosen, der Marmorknochenkrankheit Albers-Schönberg. Im Zuge von Infektionen können *Auto-Antikörper gegen Thrombocyten* zur Werlhofschen Krankheit führen, ebenso aber auch *Allergien gegen die verschiedensten Arzneimittel bei wiederholter Anwendung*, z.B. gegen Salvarsan, Sulfonamide, Penicillin, Streptomycin [4].

Das Werlhof-Bild kann aber auch, wiederum durch Insuffizienz der Plättchenfaktoren, durch die *vererbbare Glanzmannsche Thrombasthenie* hervorgerufen

---

[1] KOLLER 1958. [2] APITZ 1942, HUGHUES 1954, 1959. [3] APITZ 1942.
[4] Vgl. PETERS 1949, BEICKERT und NOETZEL 1952, LIEBEGOTT 1955 u.a.

werden. Dabei sind die Plättchen bei normaler Zahl klein, arm an Granulomer oder frei davon, z. T. aber auch riesenhaft bis zu Erythrocytengröße aufgetrieben. Eine ähnliche, dominant vererbbare Thrombopathie ist die von Willebrand und Jürgens 1933 auf den Ålandsinseln und dem finnischen Festland entdeckte Erkrankung[1]. Bei ihr konnten bei regelhaft normaler Thrombocytenzahl jüngst elektronenmikroskopisch viele Mikroplättchen, vereinzelt Riesenplättchen und in den Plättchen schwere Veränderungen am Granulomer, pathologische Trommel-schlegelformen des Granulomer sowie auffallend wenig Mitochondrien nach-gewiesen werden[2].

Coagulopathien mit hämorrhagischer Diathese können angeborene Erkran-kungen sein, in seltenen Fällen durch angeborenen Fibrinmangel, durch wahr-scheinlich angeborenen Mangel an Faktor V, also an dem Beschleunigungsfaktor (Proaccelerin) für die Bildung der Gewebs- und der Blutthrombokinase, durch angeborenen Mangel an Faktor VII als Beschleuniger für die Bildung der Ge-webs- und Blutthrombokinase. Die klassischen Coagulopathien sind die *Hämo-philien* A und B durch Mangel an Faktor VIII bzw. IX, bei denen der Faktor-mangel geschlechtsgebunden recessiv-vererblich auftrtt, so daß nur Männer er-kranken, die Frauen aber als Überträger (Konduktoren) der Anlagen wirken. Hier treten Hautblutungen ganz zurück und schwere tödliche Blutungen nach Trauma (Durchtrennung der Nabelschnur, Zahnextraktion, Gelenk- und Knochen-blutungen) in den Vordergrund.

Außerdem kommen Coagulopathien aber auch durch *Mangel an Faktor II*, *also an Prothrombin*, vor. Er kann *angeboren* vorkommen und sich dann während und in den ersten Tagen nach der Geburt in Blutungen aus der Magen- und Darm-schleimhaut (Melaena neonatorum), in Tentoriumblutungen, Hirnblutungen, Nebennierenblutungen äußern[3]. Zum Teil geht die Krankheit auf eine Schädigung der Leber des Feten bzw. des Neugeborenen zurück, z. T. auch auf einen Mangel an Vitamin K, das erst nach Besiedlung des Neugeborenen-Darmes mit Bakterien gebildet wird, in den ersten Tagen nach der Geburt also fehlen kann. *Bei Er-wachsenen* sehen wir die hämorrhagische Diathese durch Prothrombinmangel vor allem unter zwei Voraussetzungen: 1. durch *mangelnde Resorption von Vitamin K* infolge Acholie und fehlender resorptionsfördernder Gallensäuren im Darm, aber auch bei schweren chronischen Darmkrankheiten, 2. durch *Schädigung des Leber-parenchyms* infolge Leberdystrophie oder Lebercirrhose.

Unabhängig von Störungen der Thrombocyten oder der Gerinnungsfaktoren begegnen uns *hämorrhagische Diathesen* mit capillären Blutungen bei einer Reihe von *Schädigungen der Capillarwand*. So sind die Capillaren beim *Mangel an Vitamin C* ungenügend abgedichtet. Blutungen in das Zahnfleisch, ausgedehnte Blutungen in die Skeletmuskulatur, Periostblutungen und beim Kind Epiphysen-blutungen mit Ablösung des Epiphysenknorpels (Möller-Barlowsche Krankheit) sind die Folgen. Andere hier eingeordnete hämorrhagische Diathesen wie die *Schönlein-Henochsche Purpura rheumatica* und das *Waterhous-Friedrichsensche Syndrom* müssen wir den hämorrhagischen Entzündungen zuweisen, auf deren Darstellung durch Ehrich in diesem Handbuch 1956 verwiesen sei.

Zusammenfassend stellen wir zu den Blutungen folgendes fest:

1. Rhexis-Blutungen können wir bei Ruptur größerer oder kleinerer arterieller Gefäße beobachten, z. B. bei Mesaortitis syphilitica, Medionekrosis der Aorta, Aneurysma einer basalen Hirnarterie, intracerebraler Ruptur einer kleinen Hirn-arterie, peptischem Geschwür, Panarteriitis nodosa von Nierenarterien.

---

[1] Vgl. Jürgens, Lehmann und Mitarbeiter 1957.
[2] Schulz, Jürgens, Hiepler 1958.   [3] Fanconi 1938, Apitz 1943.

2. Aus varicös erweiterten Venen kommt es gelegentlich zu Blutungen an der weichen Hirnhaut oder bei Lebercirrhose am unteren Oesophagus.

3. Diapedesis-Blutungen bei lichtmikroskopisch unveränderter Struktur der Capillarwände sind die Folge von Veränderungen der Ultrastruktur der Capillaren oder von Störungen des Gerinnungssystems des Blutes.

4. Im Anschluß an die moderne Orthologie der Blutgerinnung wurden die hämorrhagischen Diathesen bei Störung der Gerinnungsfaktoren dargestellt.

Die Thrombose.

1. Die Morphologie des Thrombus.

Nach über 150jähriger intensiver Forschung über die Thrombose könnte es überflüssig erscheinen, die Morphologie des Thrombus ausführlicher darzustellen und zu erörtern. Aber die Geschichte der Thrombose-Forschung zeigt, wie mühsam schon allein der Weg zur exakten Beschreibung und Klärung des pathologisch-anatomischen und des pathologisch-histologischen Bildes des Thrombus gewesen ist. Sie zeigt zugleich, wie leicht mit der fortschreitenden Akzentverlagerung von der morphologischen zur biochemischen Betrachtung des Thrombose-Problems bestimmte Grundvorstellungen über die Morphologie des Thrombus verblassen oder sich verfälschen. So ist es unerläßlich, vor allen Erörterungen über die formale und die kausale Pathogenese der Thrombose eine kurze Darstellung des *morphologischen Bildes des Thrombus* zu vermitteln.

Nachdem HUNTER (1793) und CRUVEILHIER (1826) das Vorkommen der intravitalen Blutpfropfbildung entdeckt hatten, gab VIRCHOW (1846, 1854, 1856) zuerst eine genauere Beschreibung dieses Phämonens. Aber so bedeutungsvoll seine Darstellung in der Frage der formalen und der kausalen Pathogenese gewesen ist, in der Beschreibung der Morphologie des Thrombus blieb VIRCHOW in dem Irrtum von HUNTER, CRUVEILHIER und ROKITANSKY befangen, es handle sich bei der Thrombose um eine intravital-intravasale Fibringerinnung und die entscheidende Struktur des Thrombus sei das Fibrin: ,,Die Gerinnung des Blutes innerhalb der Gefäße erfolgt nach denselben Gesetzen wie außerhalb derselben, indem der gelöste Faserstoff seinen Aggregatzustand ändert und fest wird. Dieses Gerinnsel nennen wir Blutpfropf, Thrombus, und demnach schlagen wir für den Vorgang die Bezeichnung Pfropfbildung, Thrombosis vor'' (VIRCHOW 1854). Der Irrtum VIRCHOWs führte zwar dazu, daß HOPPE-SEYLER als Biochemiker am Virchowschen Institut sich mit der Blutgerinnung auseinandersetzte und daß ALEXANDER SCHMIDT unter ihm den bis heute gültigen Kern der Theorie der Blutgerinnung entwickelte[1]. Aber er führte auch zu manchen Umwegen in den Hypothesen über die Thrombusentstehung bis in die jüngste Zeit.

Erst ZAHN (1875) sowie EBERTH und SCHIMMELBUSCH (1888) haben erkannt, daß an der Zusammensetzung der Thromben die *Blutplättchen* wesentlich beteiligt sind. So war 1912 die Zeit gekommen, da ASCHOFF die folgende klassische Beschreibung des makroskopischen und mikroskopischen Bildes des Thrombus geben konnte, das bis heute gültig geblieben ist:

,,Mit FERGE (1909) müssen wir daran erinnern, daß an einem fertig ausgebildeten Thrombus, z.B. der Vena femoralis der proximale, sog. Kopfteil des Thrombus von überwiegend heller Farbe ist, also einen weißen Thrombus repräsentiert, worauf ein gemischtfarbiger Halsteil und ein dunkelroter Schwanzteil folgt. Der weiße Thrombus ist das Bestimmende, der rote nur etwas Akzidentelles. Zunächst muß daran erinnert werden, daß die Zeichnungen an der Oberfläche der Thromben, die Riffelungen, netz- und strichförmigen Zeichnungen gerade an diesem Kopf- und Halsteil zu sehen sind, im roten Schwanzteil schließlich völlig verschwinden. Ein Längsschnitt durch den Kopf- und Halsteil zeigt, daß jene zierlichen

---

[1] Vgl. JORPES 1954.

Oberflächenleisten nichts anderes sind als die Gipfel von Balkensystemen, die in zierlichster Gliederung wie ein Korallenstock das Gerippe des ganzen Thrombus bilden. Alle diese Bälkchen bestehen aus einer feinkörnigen Masse, die nichts anderes darstellt als wolkige Anhäufungen von Blutplättchen. Alle diese Balken sind von einem zierlichen Saume gelapptkerniger Leukocyten umgeben und heben sich von den roten Blutmassen ab, welche die zahllosen Lücken zwischen dem Balkensystem füllen. Das Wichtigste ist, daß in diesem ganzen System das Fibrin so gut wie völlig fehlt. Sobald im Gebiet des weißen, d.h. des primären Thrombus die Gefäßlichtung verschlossen ist, steht die ganze Blutsäule still und unterliegt einer sehr bald einsetzenden Gerinnung. In diesem Schwanzteil des Thrombus können wir keine deutlichen Plättchen-Lamellensysteme mehr erwarten. Dieser rote Thrombus gleicht in seinem mikroskopischen Aufbau im wesentlichen einem postmortalen Gerinnsel. Das Mikroskop läßt erkennen, daß die proximalen festeren Partien reicher an Fibrin sind, während peripherwärts die Zusammensetzung sich immer mehr der des gewöhnlichen Blutes nähert[1]."

Im Sinne dieser Beschreibung unterscheiden wir in der Pathologie seit langem beim Thrombus der Vena femoralis den *Agglutinationsthrombus* als Kopfteil und den *Coagulationsthrombus* als Schwanzteil. *Daß das Agglutinat der Thrombocyten das Essentielle des Thrombus, das Coagulat des Fibrins das Akzidentelle, Sekundäre ist*, zeigt uns das mikroskopische Bild des Thrombus an anderen Standorten: Bei der Thromboendocarditis verrucosa rheumatica stellen die warzigen Auflagerungen am Schließungsrand der Herzklappen in den Frühstadien reine wolkenartige Thrombocyten-Agglutinate dar, denen zwar einige Leukocyten und Erythrocyten, aber kein Fibrin beigemischt sind. (Diese Feststellungen der klassischen Pathologie[2] konnten durch anderslautende Darstellungen[3] nicht widerlegt werden[4].) Ebenso ist aber auch der frische arterielle Thrombus gesetzmäßig aus solchen Thrombocyten-Agglutinaten aufgebaut, z.B. bei akuter Thrombose infolge Coronarsklerose (s. Abb. 42b).

Die *venösen Thromben* haben überwiegend im Quellgebiet der unteren Hohlvene ihren Sitz. Nach großen Statistiken werden hier als Quellthrombosen der Lungenembolien 97—98% aller venösen Thrombosen gefunden[5]. Dabei liegt wiederum das Maximum in den Beinvenen, in denen nach den Statistiken 74, 85 bzw. 89% aller venösen Thrombosen bei Lungenembolie nachgewiesen wurden[6]. Wo die Beckenvenen gesondert aufgeführt waren, waren sie mit 20 bzw. 22% beteiligt[7]. Der Anteil der Thrombose im Plexus prostaticus schwankt in den vorliegenden Sektions-Statistiken zwischen 4,9 und 32%[8]. Für erwachsene Männer halten wir die letztere Zahl für zutreffend. Im höheren Alter ist die Thrombose des Plexus prostaticus bei Verstorbenen nach Krankenlager fast regelmäßig zu finden[9].

Die *Beinvenenthrombose* sitzt am häufigsten in der *Vena tibialis posterior* oder *peronea*, dann in den *Fußvenen* und erst an dritter Stelle in der *Vena femoralis* unterhalb des Poupartschen Bandes[10]. Die Druckempfindlichkeit der Fußsohle[11] oder der Wadenschmerz können daher das erste Thrombosezeichen sein[12]. Im übrigen wird ein großer Teil der Beinvenenthrombosen klinisch nicht erkannt[13]. Jede dieser drei Prädilektionsstellen können im gleichen Fall Sitz von weißen Agglutinationsthromben sein, die nicht selten sekundär durch rote Coagulationsthromben miteinander verbunden werden. So entstehen die *intermittierenden Thromben*[9] und die *Etappenthrombosen*[14]. Thromben von 30—40 cm Länge sind dabei in den Beinvenen keine Seltenheit. Ihre Länge bedeutet zugleich die Voraussetzung für die tödliche Lungenembolie bei ihrer Ablösung und Verschleppung.

[1] Aschoff 1912, S. 8—10, 15, 23 konzentriert.   [2] Ziegler 1888, Aschoff 1912, 1936.
[3] Böhmig und Klein 1953.   [4] Büchner 1955.
[5] Barker und Mitarbeiter 1941, Spohn 1951, Massie 1954.
[6] Spohn 1951, Zeitlhofer und Reifenstuhl 1952, Barker und Mitarbeiter 1941.
[7] Spohn 1951, Massie 1954.
[8] Zeithofer und Reiffenstuhl 1952, Massie 1954.   [9] Aschoff 1911.
[10] Rössle 1935, 1937, Brass 1942, Krieg 1952, Werthemann und Rutishauser 1954.
[11] Denecke 1929, Payr 1930.   [12] Morawitz 1934.
[13] Morawitz 1934, Staemmler und Wilhelms 1953.   [14] Brass 1942.

Demgegenüber stellen die häufigen Thromben im *Plexus prostaticus* beim Mann und im *Plexus vaginalis* bei der Frau die kleinsten unter den venösen Thromben dar. Auch sie werden häufig klinisch nicht erkannt. Das gleiche gilt von den nicht seltenen Thrombosen in den *venösen Sinus der Schädelhöhle*, besonders im Sinus transversus und Sinus sagittalis. Immer wieder begegnen wir in besonderen Fällen der Thrombose der *Vena portae*, der *Vena lienalis* oder der *Mesenterialvenen*.

Die *arteriellen Thrombosen* finden wir am häufigsten in der *Aorta*, vor allem in ihrem abdominalen Anteil, in den *Coronararterien*, und zwar der Häufigkeit nach im Ramus interventricularis der linken Kranzarterie, im Stamm der rechten Kranzarterie und im Ramus interventricularis der linken Kranzarterie, sodann in den *basalen Hirnarterien*, besonders in der Arteria cerebri media und in der Gabel der *Arteria carotis*, ferner in den *Beinarterien* (A. femoralis, poplitea oder tibialis anterior/posterior), in der *Arteria mesenterica cranialis*. Dabei verhielten sich in einer größeren Statistik die Coronar- : Hirnarterien- : Aortenthrombosen wie 23:14:2[1].

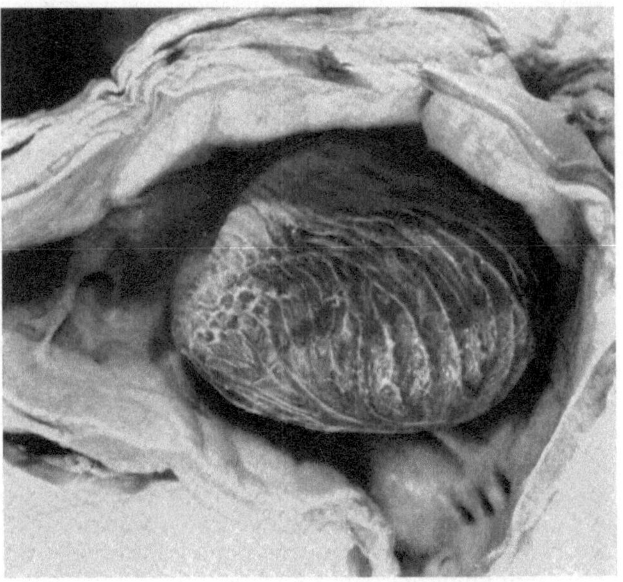

Abb. 41. An der Oberfläche geriffelter Kugelthrombus im linken Vorhof des Herzens bei Mitralstenose. (Nach BÜCHNER, F., Spezielle Pathologie, 3. Aufl., 1960, Abb. 14.)

Thrombosen im Herzen befallen die Herzklappen und zwar ganz überwiegend die des linken Herzens, die Herzvorhöfe, besonders die Vorhofsohren (Abb. 41) und die Herzkammern, vor allem den Spitzenanteil des linken Ventrikels. Hier können flächenhaft Agglutinationsthromben aus Plättchenagglutinaten mit geriffelter, weißgelber Oberfläche in die Herzhöhle hinein entwickelt werden, denen sich sekundär ein die Ventrikellichtung weiter verlegender, rotgrauer Gerinnungsthrombus aus Fibrin und Erythrocyten aufschichtet.

An jedem Thrombus setzen alsbald nach seiner Bildung *sekundäre Veränderungen* ein. Kann das Blutplasma nur unvollkommen in den Agglutinationsthrombus eindringen, so kann ein sekundärer Zerfall der Blutplättchen-Lamellen auftreten und eine eiterähnliche, also *puriforme Erweichung* einsetzen. Dieses Bild wird gelegentlich an Kopfteilen von Beinvenenthromben oder an den parietalen Thromben des Herzens beobachtet. In der Regel aber bewirkt das eindringende Blutplasma eine hyaline Homogenisierung, also eine *Hyalinisierung* der Plättchenlamellen und des dazwischenliegenden Fibrinschwamms. Danach kommt es in den meisten Fällen zur *Organisation des Thrombus*. In das Hyalin sproßt aus der Gefäß- bzw. der Herzwand ein mesenchymales Organisationsgewebe ein. So wird der hyalinisierte Thrombus zuerst von einem Fibroblasten-

---

[1] STAEMMLER und WILHELMS 1953.

schwamm allseitig durchwuchert. Dann entwickeln sich aus Angioblasten junge
Capillaren. Während die Fibroblasten kollagene Fasern bilden, werden die
Capillaren zu sinuösen Bluträumen erweitert, welche die Gefäßlichtung unvollkommen wiederherstellen. Eine Venen- oder Arterienstenose mit mehr oder
minder unvollkommen wiederhergestellter Lichtung ist das Ergebnis dieses Vorganges.

Kleine Thromben, wie sie so häufig im Plexus prostaticus oder vaginalis, zum Teil auch
an den kleinen Venen in der Milz entstehen, können eine andere Umwandlung erfahren.
Auch hier tritt in der Regel eine *Hyalinisierung* des Thrombus ein. Dadurch wird der Thrombus in eine kleine Kugel von der Farbe und der Konsistenz eines Knorpelstückes umgewandelt.
Dann aber erfolgt meist keine Organisation, sondern eine sekundäre Verkalkung des Hyalin.
Sproßt später Mesenchym in diese Kalkkugel ein, so erfolgt dessen *Metaplasie in Knochen-
gewebe,* wie sie uns auch an Herdbildungen anderen Ursprungs nach Verkalkung bekannt ist.

2. Die Ursachen der Thrombose.

Das Bild der mesenchymalen Aufschließung und Organisation des Thrombus
mit seiner lebhaften Sprossung von Fibroblasten und Capillaren, wie wir es eben
kennengelernt haben, hat im Beginn der Thromboseforschung eine große Rolle
in der Erörterung der Ursachen der Thrombose gespielt. Von diesem Bild der
geweblichen Verankerung des Thrombus mit der Venenwand ausgehend, haben
Hunter (1793) und Cruveilhier (1826) die Vorstellung abgeleitet, der Thrombus
sei der Sekundäreffekt und das Produkt einer primären Entzündung der Venenwand, also einer Phlebitis. Hier setzte Virchow (1846, 1854, 1856) mit seiner
Kritik ein. Indem er nachwies, daß die gleichen Mesenchymsprossungen auch
am Embolus der Lunge, ja auch nach experimenteller Lungenembolie nachweisbar sind, folgerte er, daß die Venenwandentzündung bei der Thrombose nicht
der primäre, sondern der sekundäre Vorgang sei, „daß die adhäsive Phlebitis
wesentlich auf der Organisation dieses Thrombus beruhe" (Virchow 1856).

Andere Vorgänger und Zeitgenossen Virchows vertraten die Auffassung, daß
der Thrombose die Wirkung gerinnungsfördernder Substanzen im Blute zugrunde
liege. Sie knüpften damit an Vorstellungen an, die im 17. und 18. Jahrhundert,
ja in einem literarischen Einzelfall noch 1843 für die fälschlich als intravitale
Gerinnungsprodukte angesehenen Herzpolypen entwickelt worden waren[1]. So
stand zur Zeit Virchows neben der Entzündungstheorie die Hypothese von der
primären Dyskrasie als Ursache der Thrombose.

Virchow rückte 1854 diesen Hypothesen gegenüber die *mechanische Theorie
der Thrombose* in den Vordergrund. Für die Bedeutung mechanischer Faktoren
bei der Entstehung eines Thrombus machte Virchow eine Reihe klassischer
Befunde der Pathologie geltend: Die Thromboseneigung bei der Kompression von
Venen durch Geschwülste oder durch den schwangeren Uterus, die Neigung zur
Thrombose in Erweiterungen des Herzens, insbesondere in Herzaneurysmen, in
erweiterten Herzohren und zwischen den Trabekeln erweiterter Herzkammern
sowie in Eweiterungen der Gefäße, vor allem in Varicen. Darüber hinaus führte
er die absolute Verminderung der Herzkraft nach zehrender Krankheit als einen
Faktor an, bei dem die „spontane Phlebitis", d.h. die Spontanthrombose der
Venen als Folge extremer Blutstromverlangsamung so häufig zu beobachten ist.
Ganz auf den Argumenten Virchows fußte von Recklinghausen (1883) in seiner
Allgemeinen Pathologie des Kreislaufs.

Aschoff (1912) gab der mechanischen Theorie eine neue theoretische Unter-
bauung. Indem er im Unterschied zu Virchow die Agglutination der Blutplättchen und nicht die Fibringerinnung als den wesentlichen Vorgang bei der

---

[1] Heynemann 1843.

Thrombusentstehung erkannte[1], suchte er nach Analogien aus der Strömungsphysik. Seine Modellversuche (1911) mit REHBOCK im Flußbaulaboratorium der Technischen Hochschule Karlsruhe hatten das Ergebnis, daß suspendierte Sinkstoffe (Sägespäne) in einem fließenden Gewässer dann zur Ablagerung kamen, wenn durch Errichtung eines Wehrs die Strömungsgeschwindigkeit genügend herabgesetzt wurde. Dabei entstanden netzförmige und streifige Verdichtungen dieser Ablagerungen vor und hinter dem Wehr, die mit den Bildern an der Oberfläche der Thromben große Ähnlichkeit hatten. Aus den Experimenten folgerte ASCHOFF, daß bei Strömungsverlangsamung, nicht bei Stillstand des Blutes, die Thrombocyten als Sinkstoffe zu Thromben ausgefällt werden. Zum Beleg der mechanischen Theorie durch die menschliche Pathologie hat ASCHOFF (1912) weitgehend die Beispiele von VIRCHOW übernommen. Darüber hinaus hat er noch besonders die Bedeutung der Herzinsuffizienz für die venöse Spontanthrombose infolge von Verlangsamungen des Blutstroms hervorgehoben. Auch hat er darauf hingewiesen, daß die Lagerung des Kranken auf einer Seite einseitige Schenkelvenenthrombosen verursacht und die Bevorzugung der linken Seite die häufigere Thrombose der linken Becken- und Schenkelvenen verständlich macht. In einer modernen Statistik war das Verhältnis Links:Rechts: Beiderseits 49:37:14%[2]. Die gleichen Argumente hat ASCHOFF auch 1925, 1934 und 1936 angeführt.

Die Beobachtungen von VIRCHOW, VON RECKLINGHAUSEN und ASCHOFF konnten in der Folge immer wieder bestätigt werden. So genügt es, wenn wir zum Beleg für die Bedeutung mechanischer Faktoren bei der Thromboseentstehung kurz noch einmal auf folgende Beispiele hinweisen: die venöse Thrombose bevorzugt, wie wir sahen, ganz überwiegend das Quellgebiet der Vena cava caudalis gegenüber dem der Cava cranialis. Sie tritt mit besonderer Vorliebe in den Venen der unteren Extremität dann auf, wenn die natürliche Mitwirkung der Beinmuskelbewegungen an der Entleerung der Venen durch Ruhigstellung im Bett stark eingeschränkt oder ausgeschaltet ist, vor allem nach Operationen, Geburten und Traumen. Im Quellgebiet der Vena cava cranialis kommt es besonders dann zur Thrombose, wenn Tumoren eine Vene komprimieren, z. B. eine Struma nodosa die Vena jugularis. In der Schädelhöhle entwickelt sich die venöse Thrombose der Sinus besonders dann, wenn eine Hirnschwellung durch Ödem den Abstrom des Blutes aus den Sinus behindert. Im Ohr des linken Vorhofs entsteht ein Thrombus auffallend häufig dann, wenn der Vorhof infolge einer Mitralstenose insuffizient ist und sich ungenügend entleert. Ganz entsprechend sehen wir die Thrombose an der Spitze des linken Ventrikels bei Insuffizienz der linken Kammer infolge Herzinfarkt oder Myocardiopathia diphtherica.

Seit längerem hat man auch die *arteriellen*, meist auf dem Boden der Arteriosklerose entstehenden *Thrombosen* in die Erörterung der mechanischen Theorie einbezogen. Schon die Tatsache, daß in arteriellen Aneurysmen Thromben häufig der Intima aufgeschichtet werden, z. B. in den syphilitischen Aneurysmen der Aorta ascendens und des Aortenbogens sowie in den arteriosklerotischen Aneurysmen der Bauchaorta, spricht für die Mitwirkung des mechanischen Faktors. Schwieriger aber ist die Frage zu beantworten, welche Bedeutung diesem Faktor für die arterielle Thrombose bei arteriosklerotischer Stenose zukommt. Es liegen jedoch auch hier wichtige Befunde vor. Gefäßkrümmungen und -verzweigungen sind bevorzugte Niederschlagsorte[3]. An der Arteria carotis interna wurden die meisten Thrombosen innerhalb der S-förmigen Krümmung des

---

[1] ZAHN 1875, EBERTH und SCHIMMELBUSCH 1888, ASCHOFF 1912.
[2] OCHSNER und Mitarbeiter 1951.   [3] THOMA 1920.

Syphon gefunden[1]. Zu noch genaueren Vorstellungen haben Modellexperimente an gekrümmten, umschrieben stenosierten Glasröhren und ihren Abgangsstellen geführt[2]. In diesen Versuchen konnte gezeigt und photographisch festgehalten werden, daß hinter Stenosen Unstetigkeiten in der Strömung, insbesondere wandnahe Wirbelbildungen mit abnormen Druck- und Sogwirkungen auf die Wand zustande kommen. Aus den Versuchen wurde gefolgert, daß Strömungsflauten und -schnellen hinter arteriosklerotischen Stenosen durch gegen die Wand gerichtete Strömungen Thrombocyten zu innigem Wandkontakt und zur Agglutination bringen können[3]. Das Aschoffsche Prinzip wird also in diesen Modellversuchen auf die arterielle Thrombose übertragen, ohne daß die Autoren andere Faktoren vernachlässigen.

Diesen anderen Faktoren wollen wir uns im folgenden zuwenden. Schon Virchow (1854) machte die Einschränkung: „Wenn man eine mechanische Theorie aufstellt, so darf man weder die Mischung des Blutes, noch den Zustand der Gefäßwände ausschließen." Aschoff hat schon 1912 neben den mechanischen Faktoren die Veränderung der Gefäßwand und die der Zahl und der Agglutinationsfähigkeit der Blutplättchen besonders betont. 1934 fügte er die Veränderung in der Zusammensetzung der Eiweißkörper des Blutplasmas hinzu.

Daß *Wandveränderungen der Strombahn* eine wichtige Voraussetzung für die Entstehung von Thromben darstellen, hat vor allem Dietrich (1912, 1932, 1934) hervorgehoben. Dietrich beruft sich besonders auf seine Beobachtungen im ersten Weltkrieg, nach denen er die Thrombose besonders bei Infektionen und Wundeiterungen nachweisen konnte. Ferner betont er, daß der akuten Thrombose regelmäßig an der geschädigten Gefäßwand eine homogene Fibrinfällung in schmaler Schicht vorausgehe, auf der erst die Plättchen zum Haften und zur Agglutination kämen. Solche hyaline Fibrinfällungen konnten aber in späteren Nachuntersuchungen bei den verschiedensten Todesursachen des Menschen mit und ohne vorausgehende Infektion, auch bei plötzlichem Unfalltod aus voller Gesundheit, fast in jedem Falle gefunden und als agonales Phänomen gedeutet werden (von Lucadou 1933). Andererseits ließen sich nur zum Teil bei Coronarthrombosen *Fibrinfällungen unter dem Plättchenagglutinat* über dem Gefäßwandendothel nachweisen[4].

Trotz dieser kritischen Einwendungen ist an der Bedeutung der Wandveränderungen der Strombahn für die Thrombose nicht zu zweifeln. Das wird zunächst durch die *Thrombosen innerhalb des Herzens* bewiesen. So haben alle neueren Untersuchungen über die *Thromboendocarditis verrucosa rheumatica* ergeben, daß der Bildung der warzigen Plättchenagglutinate eine Veränderung der Klappe mit Insudation von Blutflüssigkeit und mesenchymaler Wucherung regelmäßig vorausgeht[5]. Erst recht wird bei der *Thromboendocarditis necroticans ulcerosa polyposa* der der Thrombose vorausgehende Klappenschaden in Form bakteriell verursachter Nekrosen und Ulcerationen der Klappe faßbar. Auch bei der Thrombose an der Spitze des linken Ventrikels auf dem Boden des *Herzinfarktes* wäre es falsch, einseitig die infarktbedingte Einschränkung der Herzdynamik zu betonen. Vielmehr ist zu bedenken, daß jeder Herzinfarkt, bei dem zum mindesten die inneren Schichten des Herzmuskels im Infarktbereich nekrotisch sind, zu einer abakteriellen Entzündung des benachbarten Endokards führt. Das Gleiche gilt von der *Myocardiopathia diphtherica* mit ihren ausge-

---

[1] Dörfler 1935, Meyer und Beck 1955.
[2] E. Müller 1955, E. Müller und Otto 1956, Müller-Mohnssen 1957.
[3] Müller-Mohnssen 1957.
[4] Meessen 1944, Apitz 1944.   [5] Klinge 1933, Böhmig und Klein 1953.

dehnten toxischen Nekrosen der Herzmuskelzellen und ihrer Neigung zur Thrombose in der Herzspitze. Und wenn im dilatierten mangelhaft sich entleerenden Ohr des linken Vorhofs bei Mitralstenose Thromben zur Entwicklung kommen, so liegt auch hier ein Endokard vor, das über hypertrophiebedingten Untergängen von Herzmuskelzellen und Sklerosierungen der Vorhofwand sekundär krankhaft verändert ist[1]. Das gleiche gilt von der Thromboseneigung im hypertrophierten rechten Vorhof und in hypertrophierten Ventrikeln.

Noch eindrucksvoller sprechen die Befunde bei *arterieller Thrombose* dafür, daß Wandveränderungen der Strombahn für das Zustandekommen der Thrombose von entscheidender Bedeutung sind. Zwar wurden in jüngster Zeit von WERTHEMANN und RUTISHAUSER (1954) zwei Fälle beschrieben, bei denen eine 27jährige Frau mit frischem Follikelsprung und ein 31jähriger Mann. wahrscheinlich nach Insolation, an einer akuten tödlichen Thrombose der Arteria cerebri media erkrankten, ohne daß nach der histologischen Untersuchung der Thrombose eine Arteriosklerose, eine Arteriitis oder eine andere Wandveränderung der Arterie vorausgegangen war. Von solchen extremen Ausnahmen abgesehen ist aber die arterielle Thrombose der Prototyp der Thrombose auf dem Boden der Wandveränderungen der Strombahn. Das Gros der arteriellen Thrombosen entwickelt sich, besonders an der Aorta, an den Coronararterien, an den basalen Hirnarterien oder der Arteria carotis interna, an den Beinarterien und an der Arteria mesenterica cranialis, auf dem Boden arteriosklerotischer Herde. Dabei kommt dem geschwürigen Aufbruch des arteriosklerotischen Beetes nicht die Bedeutung zu, die ihr früher zugesprochen wurde. Dagegen erwiesen sich bei der Arteriosklerose der Coronararterien des Herzens *akute Ödembildungen und Quellungsnekrosen im arteriosklerotischen Herd* als häufige Voraussetzungen der akuten Coronarthrombose (Abb. 42a und b). Das konnten wir an einer Serie von über 600 Coronartodesfällen jüngerer Soldaten (zwischen 18 und 40 Jahren) im zweiten Weltkrieg nachweisen[2]. In den meisten dieser Fälle war der akute Coronartod im Stadium der akuten Aufquellung und der Quellungsnekrose des coronarsklerotischen Herdes eingetreten, wie sie auch früher schon beschrieben worden waren[3]. Rund in der Hälfte der Fälle, bei über 300 Fällen, war es auf dem Boden der akuten Quellung zur akuten Thrombose gekommen. Die gleichen Befunde wurden an einem großen Beobachtungsgut von akutem Coronartod bei jüngeren Soldaten der amerikanischen Wehrmacht erhoben[4].

Daß solche und andere Wandveränderungen des vorhandenen arteriosklerotischen Herdes akut durch ein schweres Brustwandtrauma und die daraus resultierende allgemeine und örtliche Durchblutungsstörung ausgelöst werden können, beweisen Einzelbeobachtungen (MEESSEN 1940, 1941).

In dem einen Fall führte das Trauma bei einem 30jährigen Soldaten zu multiplen Rippenbrüchen und ohne Herzwandtrauma zu einer akuten Coronarthrombose auf dem Boden eines arteriosklerotischen Herdes, bei der nach 8 Std der Tod eintrat. In dem anderen Falle kam es bei einem 41jährigen Soldaten nach Lungendurchschuß mit Fraktur der 3.—9. Rippe rechts zu multiplen Thrombosen auf bestehenden arteriosklerotischen Herden im Ramus descendens der linken Kranzarterie, in der linken A. carotis communis und in der rechten A. iliaca interna und nach etwa 48 Std zum Tode.

In der Deutung dieser Fälle wurde die Auffassung entwickelt, daß ein Kollaps der verletzten rechten Lunge zur Hypoxämie und dadurch zu akuten Veränderungen an den vorbestehenden arteriosklerotischen Herden geführt habe[5]. Zum Beweis dieser Auffassung wurde darauf hingewiesen, daß auch die akute CO-Hypoxämie bei vorbestehender Coronarsklerose zur akuten Coronarthrombose

---

[1] WIELAND 1956. [2] BÜCHNER 1941. E. MÜLLER 1941, 1944, 1949, 1955, MEESSEN 1944.
[3] LEARY 1934. [4] YATER und Mitarbeiter 1947. [5] MEESSEN 1941.

führen kann[1]. Auch die Neigung zu multiplen arteriosklerotischen Thrombosen bei allgemeiner kardialer Oligämie ist hier einzuordnen[2].

Ein weiterer Beweis für die Bedeutung der Wandschädigung der Arterie als Ursache der akuten Thrombose sind die Befunde bei *akutem Einriß arterio-*

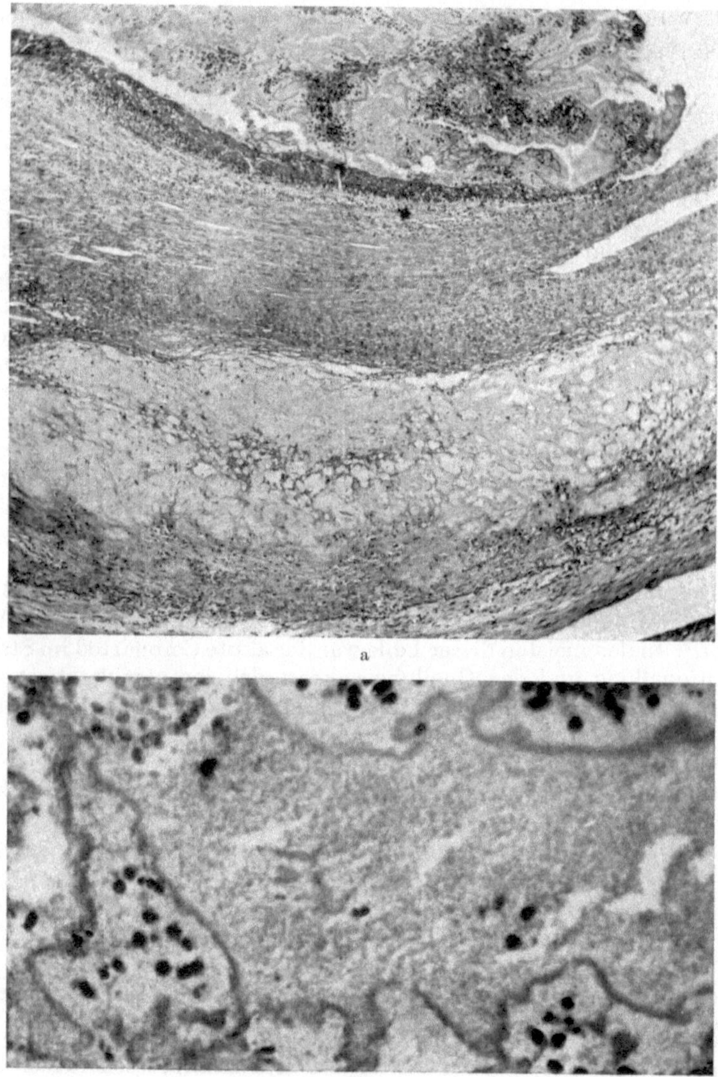

Abb. 42a u. b. a Akute Coronarthrombose (oben) bei ausgedehntem akuten Ödem in der verdickten Intima der Coronararterie (untere Hälfte). b Ausschnitt des frischen Thrombus in starker Vergrößerung. Aufbau aus einem Agglutinat von Thrombocyten.

sklerotischer Herde. Hier konnte gezeigt werden, daß es mitunter bei akuter Anstrengung oder einer akuten Contusion der Herzgegend zum Einriß eines coronarsklerotischen Herdes und zum Hämatom in der Arterienwand kommt,

[1] Morawitz 1934, Kroetz 1936, Hedinger 1923.
[2] Sameni 1961. (noch unveröffentlicht)

und daß sich in der Regel eine akute Thrombose der Coronararterie daran anschließt (PAPACHARALAMPOUS und ZOLLINGER 1953, STAEMMLER 1956). Außerdem kann es aber nach Capillarisierung arteriosklerotischer Herde ohne Intimariß zu intramuralen Hämatomen kommen[1] und durch diese zu akuten Coronarthrombosen[2].

So gewichtig diese Beobachtungen über die Thrombose auf dem Boden arteriosklerotischer Wandveränderungen der Arterien auch sind, so müssen wir uns doch an dieser Stelle mit dem in jüngster Zeit gemachten Versuch auseinandersetzen, den arteriellen Thrombus als das Primäre, den arteriosklerotischen Herd dagegen als das Sekundäre anzusehen, d.h. den arteriosklerotischen Herd als das sekundäre Produkt einer Thrombose oder Embolie auf primär unveränderter Arterienwand zu deuten. Diese Hypothese wurde von DUGUID 1946 für die Arteriosklerose der Coronararterien entwickelt, 1948 auf die Arteriosklerose der Aorta übertragen und 1952 auch auf die Arteriosklerose der Arteria pulmonalis angewandt. Noch jüngst fand sie in MORGAN einen Verfechter auf dem 3. internationalen Kongreß für Kardiologie in Brüssel[3]. Im einzelnen hat DUGUID (1946) an den Kranzadern des Herzens gezeigt, daß ein die Lichtung obturierender Thrombus sich sekundär zu einem sektorförmigen Herd retrahieren kann, daß er als solcher von Intima-Endothel überwuchert wird, dadurch in die Arterienwand gelangt und sekundär in der Tiefe verfetten kann. An dieser Möglichkeit ist nicht zu zweifeln. Sie ist seit langem in der Pathologie der arteriosklerotischen Herdbildungen bekannt[4]. Die Beobachtung berechtigt aber nicht zu der Auffassung, daß die meisten größeren arteriosklerotischen Platten in den Coronararterien die Produkte der Organisation von wandständigen Thromben sind[5]. Diese Auffassung findet ihre Widerlegung besonders in den Beobachtungen des zweiten Weltkrieges, nach denen arteriosklerotische Lipoidherde auffallend häufig schon bei tödlich abgestürzten 20—30jährigen Fliegern zu finden waren[6] und nach denen akute tödliche Coronarthrombosen schon bei 18—30jährigen immer einen arteriosklerotischen Herd einer Coronararterie zur Voraussetzung hatten, meist mit akutem Ödem im arteriosklerotischen Herd (Abb. 43a und b)[7].

Wie leicht auf diesem Gebiet Fehldeutungen möglich sind, hat die Nachprüfung der experimentellen Untersuchungen von DUGUID (1952) zum Problem der Arteriosklerose der Pulmonalarterien ergeben[8]. DUGUID hat nach intravenöser Injektion von Fibringerinnseln am Kaninchen in Einzelschnitten an den Lungenarterien Veränderungen beobachtet, die sehr an arteriosklerotische Herde erinnern. Er vertritt daher die Auffassung, daß pulmonalsklerotische Herde häufig das Sekundärprodukt primärer Thrombosen oder Embolien an der Wand der Pulmonalarterien sind[9]. Die Serienuntersuchung solcher Herde hat aber bei Nachprüfung der Experimente ergeben, daß die arterioskleroseähnlichen Platten in der Serie regelmäßig in gefäßreiche bindegewebige Obturationen der kleinen Pulmonalarterien übergehen, die ihre Herkunft aus der Organisation der Fibrin-Emboli sofort erkennen lassen[8].

Die Neigung zur Thrombose der Aorta thoracica bei Mesaortitis syphilitica, zur Thrombose der basalen Hirnarterien bei syphilitischer oder bei tuberkulöser Arteriitis, zur Thrombose bei Panarteriitis nodosa und bei Endarteriitis obliterans fügt sich zwanglos in die Belege für die Bedeutung des Wandschadens bei der Entstehung der arteriellen Thrombose ein. Ihre Bewährungsprobe aber müßte

---

[1] PATERSON 1936, 1938, 1952, AUFDERMAUR 1952.
[2] ZOLLINGER und PAPACHARALAMPOUS 1953.   [3] MORGAN 1959.
[4] JORES 1924.   [5] DUGUID 1946.   [6] E. MÜLLER 1946/1949.
[7] BÜCHNER 1941, E. MÜLLER 1944, 1949, MEESSEN 1944.
[8] CHR. BÜCHNER und KÖNN 1959, KÖNN und CHR. BÜCHNER 1959.   [9] DUGUID 1952.

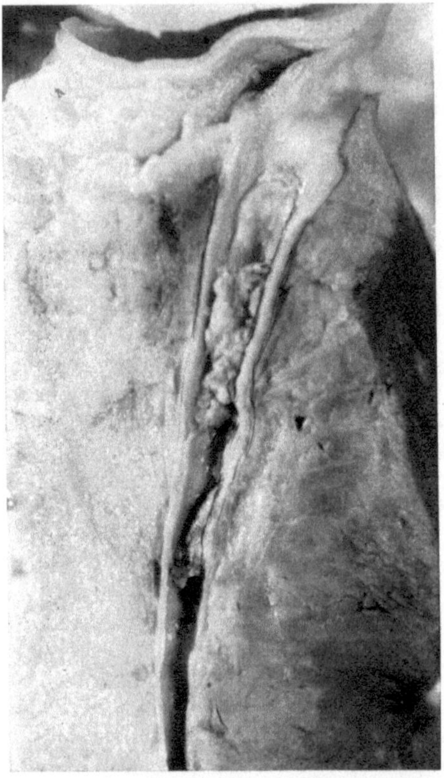

die Gefäßwandhypothese bei der *venösen Thrombose* bestehen. Hier aber liegen die Dinge für den Morphologen am schwierigsten.

Dietrich (1932) hat auf herdförmige Verklumpungen von Endothelkernen in der Intima der Venen aufmerksam gemacht und die Meinung ausgesprochen, daß sie eine Disposition für die venöse Thrombose bewirken. In Nachprüfungen konnte nachgewiesen werden, daß diese Veränderung bei 50—70jährigen einen fast regelmäßigen Befund und offenbar eine Altersveränderung des Endothels der Venen darstellt[1]. Von typischen konstanten, der Thrombose vorausgehenden Veränderungen der Venenwand konnte auch sonst bisher lichtmikroskopisch nichts nachgewiesen werden. Neue Untersuchungen müssen hier einsetzen, insbesondere systematische Untersuchungen des Endothels im Phasenkontrastmikroskop[2] und nach Versilberung[3], aber auch im Elektronenmikroskop. Durch solche Untersuchungen muß abgeklärt werden, ob an den Venen die Schädigung der Kittsubstanz zwischen den Endothelien wirklich die schwache Stelle

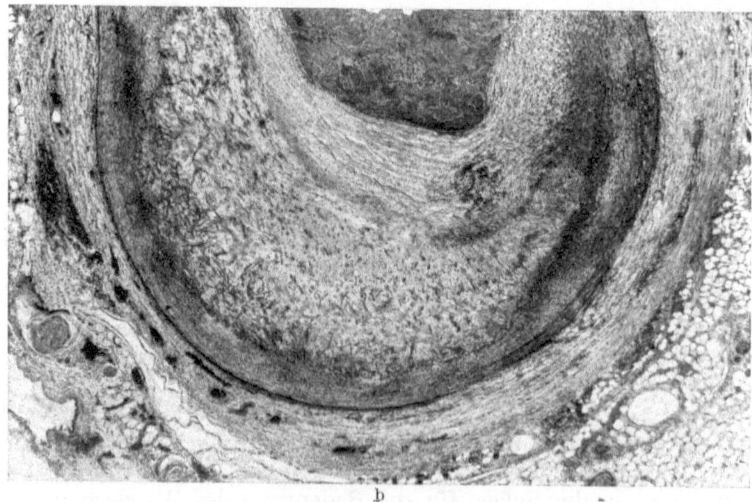

Abb. 43a u. b. a Arteriosklerotischer Thrombus des Ramus interventricularis der linken Kranzarterie in ihrem oberen Verlauf bei 32jährigem Soldaten. b Akute Thrombose auf arteriosklerotischem akut ödematösem Intimaherd bei 25jährigem Soldaten. Plötzlicher Tod am Steuer als LKW-Fahrer. [Nach Büchner, F., Dtsch. Mil. Arzt. 6, 570, 1941, Abb. 3 u. 2.]

bedeutet, an der zuerst Niederschläge von Fibrin und Plättchenagglutinate und damit Thromben entstehen, wie dies jüngst aus morphologischen Untersuchungen

[1] Von Lucadou 1933.   [2] Linzbach 1951.   [3] Impallomeni 1954.

des Venenendothels gefolgert wurde[1]. Daß an den Venen der unteren Extremität unter der Wirkung örtlicher oder allgemeiner Blutstromverlangsamungen bei Bettliegenden und bei Kranken mit Insuffizienz des rechten Herzens feinste Endothelveränderungen eintreten können, ist durchaus wahrscheinlich. Nach den Befunden, die wir heute elektronenmikroskopisch über die Wirkung der Hypoxie auf das Cytoplasma in der Hand haben[2], sind bei der Stauungshyperämie zum mindesten elektronenmikroskopische Veränderungen am Endothel der Venen und damit Störungen der Relation Endothel/Blut zu erwarten. Das gleiche gilt von den Sinus der Schädelhöhle bei Abflußbehinderung durch Hirnödem oder von Venen mit umschriebener Kompression durch eine Geschwulst. Aber die postulierten Befunde liegen bisher nicht vor.

ASCHOFF hat 1912 und später als 3. Faktor für die Entstehung von Thromben die *quantitative und qualitative Veränderung der Blutplättchen* hervorgehoben. Tatsächlich konnte die moderne Hämatologie zeigen, daß Erkrankungen, die durch eine *akute oder chronische Vermehrung der Thrombocyten*, also durch eine *Thrombocytose*, gekennzeichnet sind, eine ausgesprochene Neigung zur Thrombose erkennen lassen. Das gilt vor allem von der *Polycythämie*[3], bei der die starke Wucherung der Erythrocyten mit einer vermehrten Bildung von Megacaryocyten und dadurch mit einer Thrombocytose einhergeht[4]. Das gleiche wird aber auch bei *chronischen Myelosen und Lymphadenosen* als Ursache einer Thromboseneigung beobachtet[5]. Auch nach Milzexstirpation besteht eine Thrombocytose und zugleich eine besondere Thrombosebereitschaft[6]. Und wenn festgestellt werden konnte, daß nach akuten Blutverlusten durch Knochenmarksreizung eine *posthämorrhagische Thrombocytose* und Thromboseneigung hervorgerufen wird[7], so wird auch hier die Bedeutung der Plättchenvermehrung verdeutlicht. Demnach ist bei Fällen wie den dargestellten arteriellen Thrombosen nach Thoraxtrauma und Blutverlust dieser Faktor noch zu den hypoxämisch-oligämisch ausgelösten Quellungen der arteriosklerotischen Intimaherde in Ansatz zu bringen. Auch ist die bei der Sichelzellen-Anämie und bei der Marchia fava-Anämie bekannte Thromboseneigung[8] hier einzuordnen. Ebenso muß auch bei der Thromboseneigung nach CO-Vergiftung[9] die Wirkung der CO-Hypoxie auf das Knochenmark und auf die Plättchenbildung mit in Rechnung gesetzt werden.

Als 4. Faktor wurden in den letzten beiden Jahrzehnten mehr und mehr *Änderungen des Blutplasmas* in den Vordergrund gerückt. Im besonderen vertrat APITZ (1941, 1944) die Auffassung: „Die Thrombose ist ein Blut-, kein Endothelphänomen." Dabei bemühte er sich vor allem darum, die *Bedeutung der Zunahme der Gerinnungsneigung des Blutes für die Thrombose* zu beweisen. Auf Grund von Modellexperimenten entwickelte er die Vorstellung, daß bei der Blutgerinnung das Fibrinogen zunächst in eine gelöste micellare Vorstufe des Fibrins, das *Profibrin*, übergeht, und daß sich das im Blutplasma angereicherte Profibrin an die Blutplättchen anlagert und dadurch deren Agglutination begünstigt. Für die Vermehrung des Profibrins sei in erster Linie die vermehrte Einschwemmung von Gewebsthrombokinase in das Blut und die dadurch verursachte Aktivierung von Prothrombin zu Thrombin verantwortlich. Die Einschwemmung der Gewebsthrombokinase sei besonders bei allen Zuständen mit Einschmelzung und Zertrümmerung von Gewebe gesteigert, im besonderen nach Trauma oder nach

---

[1] IMPALLOMENI 1954.
[2] MÖLBERT und GUERRITORE 1957, MÖLBERT 1958, BÜCHNER, MÖLBERT und THALE 1959, BÜCHNER 1959.
[3] JÜRGENS und BACH 1934.   [4] LÜDEKE 1934.
[5] HITTMAIR 1928, HEILMEYER und BEGEMANN 1951.
[6] ALLEN, BAKER und HINES 1947.   [7] HEILMEYER und BEGEMANN 1951.
[8] BEGEMANN und HARWERTH 1959.   [9] MORAWITZ 1934, KROETZ 1936.

Operation, aber auch bei Tumorzerfall. Die Hypothese von APITZ hat zunächst viele Anhänger gefunden, da sie die Neigung zur Thrombose nach Trauma, Operation und bei Tumorkranken besser als andere Hypothesen verständlich machte. Besonders die Tatsache, daß unter solchen Voraussetzungen nicht die regionale Thrombose im Bereich des Traumas, der Operation oder des Tumors im Vordergrund steht, sondern die *Fernthrombose* mit Bevorzugung der Beinvenen, wurde durch diese Hypothese verständlicher. Die vermehrt im Blute kreisende Gewebsthrombokinase wäre danach der essentielle Faktor bei der Thrombose, die Blutstromverlangsamung, beim Bettlägerigen vor allem im Beingebiet, und die Wandveränderung der Strombahn wären accidentelle Realisationsfaktoren. Als einen besonderen Beleg für seine Auffassung führt APITZ (1941) selbst die Befunde bei der Blutstillung an: Hier kommt es bei Verletzung von Arterien oder Venen an der Stelle der Verletzung zuerst zu einem Agglutinat von Thrombocyten und anschließend zu einem Koagulat von Fibrin (s. S. 869).

Käme der Apitzschen Vorstellung die zentrale Bedeutung zu, die sie in seiner Hypothese einnimmt, so wäre die Thrombose entscheidend an das Phänomen der Blutgerinnung gekoppelt, so wie VIRCHOW es 1854 in der irrigen Ansicht vertreten hat, der Thrombus stelle ein intravital-intravasales Fibringerinnsel dar. Die Geschichte der Thrombose-Forschung stand auf weiten Strecken, so auch in den klassischen Arbeiten von SCHMIDT (1892) sowie von MORAWITZ (1905, 1934) unter dem Einfluß dieser Konzeption. In der jüngsten Thromboseforschung sind hier alle die Bemühungen einzuordnen, welche den Zusammenhang zwischen der Anreicherung von Blutgerinnungsfaktoren und Thrombose zu beweisen suchten. Dabei stellt die Apitzsche These nur *einen* der Gerinnungsfaktoren, die Gewebsthrombokinase, in den Vordergrund. Daneben ist die Anreicherung von Blutthrombokinase durch Zerfall von Thrombocyten und die Aktivierung dieses Plättchenfaktors durch die Plasmafaktoren VIII und IX, möglicherweise auch durch V und VII[1] in Rechnung zu setzen, unter krankhaften Bedingungen also deren Vermehrung.

Mit der Zeit ergaben sich aber gewichtige Einwendungen zum mindesten gegen die allgemeine Bedeutung der Koppelung von Gerinnungsneigung und Thrombose. Das klassische Anticoagulans der modernen Klinik, das *Heparin,* bildet mit einem im Serum vorhandenen Heparinkomplement ein hochwirksames Antithrombin[2]; daneben wirkt es wahrscheinlich in Verbindung mit einem anderen Plasmafaktor als Antithrombokinase. Die Thromboseneigung müßte also durch Heparin absolut unterdrückt werden. Wir haben aber mehrfach nach Heparinbehandlung ausgedehnte Thrombosen beobachtet.

Eine spontane Entkoppelung von Thromboseneigung und Gerinnungsfähigkeit des Blutes begegnet uns häufig bei dem heute in einer größeren Kasuistik bekannten Bilde der *thrombotischen Mikroangiopathie.* Das Krankheitsbild wurde zuerst 1924 von MOSCHKOWICZ als „acute febrile pleiochromic anemia with hyaline thrombosis of the terminal arterioles and capillaries" beschrieben. Die Kasuistik bis 1952 findet sich in der Abhandlung von SYMMERS, die weitere bis 1956 in einer Arbeit von HUNZIKER und OECHSLIN. Inzwischen wurde eine Serie weiterer Fälle bekannt[3]. Das Bild ist vor allem durch zahlreiche *Mikrothromben* in den Arteriolen, den Capillaren und wahrscheinlich auch den Venolen der verschiedensten Organe gekennzeichnet; dabei setzen sich die Thromben sehr wahrscheinlich aus reinen Thrombocyten-Agglutinaten zusammen, die bald hyalinisiert und

---

[1] JÜRGENS 1955.   [2] KOLLER 1958.
[3] SHAPIRO, DOKTOR und CHURG 1957, BÁEZ-VILLASENOR und AMBROSIUS 1957, ANTES 1958, HARRISON, H. N. 1958, WASSERMAN 1958 u. a.

anschließend organisiert werden[1]. Ob der Thrombenbildung eine Hyalinisierung der subintimalen Gefäßwand als präthrombotische Veränderung der Strombahnwand vorausgeht[2], ist noch nicht geklärt, auch nicht durch die neueren Untersuchungen[3]. Die Mikrothromben erinnern an Befunde, wie sie vor längerer Zeit nach Sensibilisierung von Versuchstieren durch Injektion abgetöteter Bakterien beobachtet wurden[4]. Bei den meisten Fällen kommt es zu einer hämorrhagischen Diathese, die auf eine starke Thrombocytenverminderung zurückgeht. Diese Fälle werden als *thrombotische thrombocytopenische Purpura* gekennzeichnet[5]. Die paradoxe Verbindung von hochgradiger Thromboseneigung und Thrombocytopenie wird so gedeutet, daß die Thrombocytenagglutination in den zahllosen Mikrothromben zu einer Herabsetzung der Thrombocyten im strömenden Blut führt. Jedenfalls sind hier Hemmung der Blutgerinnung und extreme Thromboseneigung im gleichen Krankheitsbild vereinigt.

Daß das Profibrin für die Plättchenagglutination kein notwendiger Faktor ist, wurde durch die Tatsache bewiesen, daß bei völligem Mangel an Fibrinogen die Agglutination der Plättchen normal gefunden wurde[6]. Andererseits wurde von JÜRGENS (1952) gezeigt, daß Bakterientoxine und Histamin die Agglutination der Blutplättchen fördern, auch dann, wenn durch Heparin die Blutgerinnung gehemmt wird. Verschiedene Arzneimittel können die Plättchenagglutination begünstigen[7]. Wurden Blutplättchen durch Bienengift oder Histamin agglutiniert, so war elektronenmikroskopisch kein Fibrin oder Profibrin zwischen ihnen nachzuweisen[8].

Nach diesen experimentellen Befunden steht die Frage zur Diskussion, wieweit bei traumatisch oder operativ bedingter Gewebszertrümmerung oder bei tumorbedingtem Gewebszerfall im parenteralen Eiweißabbau entstandene *biogene Amine*, vor allem H-Substanzen und z.B. das *Histamin* selbst, im Blute kreisend zu einer *Steigerung der Agglutinabilität der Blutplättchen* führen und unter Mitwirkung der anderen Faktoren die Neigung zur Thrombose, besonders zur Fernthrombose, fördern (JÜRGENS 1955). In diese Vorstellung würden sich auch Beobachtungen von multiplen arteriellen Thrombosen nach Trauma bei vorbestehender Arteriosklerose, wie wir sie oben wiedergegeben haben (MEESSEN 1941), gut einfügen. Lokalisierte arteriell-arteriosklerotische Thromben, z.B. bei akuter Coronarthrombose, könnten dann möglicherweise durch einen lokalen Einstrom der agglutinationsfördernden Substanzen aus einem ödematösen oder quellungsnekrotischen Intimaherd in das benachbarte Blut zustande kommen, d.h. ohne die universelle Wirkung der Blutfaktoren[7]. Bei Infektionskrankheiten könnte die Neigung zur Thrombose infolge Agglutinationsänderungen der Thrombocyten durch Bakterientoxine oder immunologische Faktoren bewirkt sein, bei allgemeinen Oligaemien durch Hypoxie[9].

In diesem Sinne sprechen die Experimente von JÜRGENS (1955). Er konnte Meerschweinchen durch Rinder-Thrombocyten so sensibilisieren, daß die Tiere nach der Reinjektion von Thrombocyten-Extrakt eine intravitale Plättchenagglutination und zum Teil einen tödlichen Kollaps zeigten. Nach Sensibilisierung von Hunden gegen Thrombocyten von Kaninchen, Meerschweinchen oder Ratten kam es ebenfalls zur intravitalen Plättchenagglutination und darüber hinaus zur Bildung von Plättchenthromben. Auch hier starben die Tiere zum Teil im Kollaps.

Es ist bis heute ungeklärt, welche Rolle *Autoantikörper gegen Thrombocyten* unter pathologischen Bedingungen bei der Steigerung der Agglutinabilität der Thrombocyten und als Ursache einer Thromboseneigung spielen. Die Erforschung

---

[1] SYMMERS 1952.   [2] GORE 1950, ORBISON 1952.
[3] z. B. VON HUNZIKER und OECHSLIN 1957.   [4] DIETRICH 1932.
[5] SINGER, BORNSTEIN und WILE 1947.   [6] PINNIGER und PRUNTY 1946.
[7] JÜRGENS 1955.   [8] JÜRGENS und BRAUNSTEINER 1950.   [9] SAMENI 1961.

der Autohämantikörper könnte hier richtungweisend sein. Nach der zusammenfassenden Darstellung dieses Problembereiches durch Schubothe (1958) sind die von Donath und Landsteiner (1904, 1908) beschriebenen Kältehämolysine echte Autohämantikörper, die als hämolysierende Gegenstoffe gegen die eigenen Erythrocyten gebildet sind. Dagegen können die Kälteagglutinine nicht als Antikörper im engeren Sinne und als Produkte eines Immunisierungsprozesses gedeutet werden, besonders nicht die Steigerung der Bildung von Kälteagglutininen nach manchen Virusinfektionen. Bei der chronischen Kälteagglutininkrankheit wird eine unspezifische, nicht antigenbedingte Entgleisung der Eiweißbildung als Ursache angenommen.

Diese Befunde aus der Pathologie der Agglutination und Auflösung von Erythrocyten legen die Vermutung nahe, daß auch bei den Thrombocyten auf der einen Seite mit der Steigerung der Agglutinabilität und der Auflösung durch Autoantikörperbildung, aber auch durch die verschiedensten unspezifischen, nicht immunologischen Faktoren gerechnet werden muß.

Rückblickend auf die gesamte Erörterung der die Thrombose verursachenden Faktoren stehen wir vor der schon öfter betonten Tatsache, daß Blut, Strombahnwand und Gewebe als eine Einheit gesehen werden müssen (Morawitz 1934) und daß in der Verursachung von Thromben die Störungen der Dynamik des Blutstromes, der Strombahnwand, der Blutplättchen und des Blutplasmas in der Regel unlösbar miteinander verbunden sind. Daß bei allgemeiner Blutstromverlangsamung im venösen System bei Insuffizienz des rechten Ventrikels zwangsläufig elektronenmikroskopische Veränderungen des Endothels der Venen, besonders der Beinvenen, infolge Hypoxie eintreten müssen, haben wir schon betont. Darüber hinaus ist aber auch zu erwarten, daß bei schwerer venöser Stauung hypoxisch ausgelöste Vermehrungen der Thrombocyten und deren hypoxische Schädigung ins Spiel treten. Nach Trauma mit schwerem Blutverlust können wiederum kollapsbedingte Stromverlangsamung, hypoxiebedingte Wandschädigung und hypoxische Änderungen im Plättchensystem gekoppelt sein. Bei schweren Infektionen summieren sich häufig kollapsbedingte Stromverlangsamung mit toxisch bedingter Wandänderung und toxisch verursachter Änderung der Agglutinabilität der Thrombocyten.

Betrachten wir zum Schluß dieses Kapitels das Problem der Thromboseentstehung im Lichte der *Statistik*, so ist zunächst die Tatsache hervorzuheben, daß *nach beiden Weltkriegen* die Aufmerksamkeit der Kliniker und der Pathologen besonders auf die Frage nach der Häufigkeit von Thrombose und Embolie in Deutschland gelenkt wurde. Von Lucadou hat 1931 die auf Sektionsbefunden aufbauenden Statistiken der Pathologen ausgewertet. Er konnte sich dabei auf 73000 Sektionen statistisch verwertbarer Arbeiten stützen[1]. Dabei kam er, wie auch später Bela (1934), zu dem Ergebnis, daß seit 1924 eine statistisch gesicherte Zunahme der Thrombosen und Embolien zu verzeichnen war. Nach dem 2. Weltkrieg wurde die Frage erneut statistisch bearbeitet[2]. Hillemanns erfaßte am Freiburger Pathologischen Institut, unter Ausschluß der unter 20-Jährigen und der Soldaten, 19353 Obduktionen der Jahre 1911—1950 nach statistisch einwandfreien Methoden[3]. Für die tödlichen thrombotischen Embolien stellte er folgende Prozentsätze fest: vor dem 1. Weltkrieg 1912 5%, am Ende des 1. Weltkrieges 1918 1,1%, nach der Inflation (1924) steiler Anstieg bis zu einem Gipfel 1934 von 8,6%, bis zum 2. Weltkrieg 5—6%, in den Hungerjahren nach dem 2. Weltkrieg 2,7%, 1950 6%, 1. Hälfte 1951 6,9%. Es bestanden also statistisch

---

[1] Hoering 1928, Kuhn 1929, Schleussing 1929, Axhausen 1930, Bodon 1931, Wertheimer 1931.
[2] Brass und Sandritter 1949, Hillemanns 1951.   [3] Koller 1943, Hosemann 1949.

gesicherte Häufigkeitsschwankungen der tödlichen Embolien, wie sie auch BRASS und SANDRITTER für Frankfurt 1949 nachgewiesen haben. Die Kurve der Häufigkeit der Fernthrombosen folgte dagegen nach den Untersuchungen von HILLEMANNS (1937—1950) nicht den Wellenbewegungen der Kurve der tödlichen Embolien. Sie war vielmehr vor und nach dem 2. Weltkrieg am Freiburger Obduktionsgut im wesentlichen unverändert die gleiche. Nach den Leichengewichten nahm die Häufigkeit der tödlichen Lungenembolie mit steigendem Körpergewicht erheblich zu; die Dicken neigten doppelt so stark zur tödlichen Lungenembolie wie die Mageren. Eindeutig konnte die Senkung der tödlichen Embolien nach dem 2. Weltkrieg auf die Abmagerung, die steile Wiederzunahme auf die Wiederzunahme der Fettleibigkeit zurückgeführt werden. HILLEMANNS schließt daraus, daß bei Fettleibigkeit zwar die Mobilisationstendenz von Thromben eindeutig erhöht ist, nicht dagegen die Thromboseneigung. Zu ähnlichen Ergebnissen kam RUTISHAUSER (1954) in Basel. Die oft behauptete gesteigerte Neigung der Fettleibigen zur Fernthrombose kann also mit den neuesten statistisch einwandfreien Sektionsstatistiken nicht belegt werden. Dagegen scheinen die Verhältnisse bei der Coronarthrombose anders zu liegen. Hier wurde gezeigt, daß bei Kranken mit akutem Herzinfarkt infolge arteriosklerotischer Thrombose einer Coronararterie die Cholesterinesterwerte des Blutes bei beträchtlicher Streuung der Werte in der Regel über der Norm oder an deren oberer Grenze lagen (GERTTLER und WHITE 1954). Daraus wurde geschlossen, daß bei cholesterinesterreichem Blut, besonders bei Fettleibigkeit, eine Neigung zur Coronarthrombose besteht.

Vielfach erörtert wurde die Frage der Begünstigung von Fernthrombose und Embolie durch meteorologische Einflüsse. Erst in einer neueren Arbeit konnte für Tübingen statistisch einwandfrei gesichert werden, daß Thrombosen mit Vorliebe am Ende einer Hochdruckperiode beim Übergang zu cyclonalem Wetter auftreten, Embolien im besonderen bei stabilen und labilen Aufgleitvorgängen vor Warmfronten und schwachem Warmluftaufgleiten aus Südosten hinter einer nach Osten abgezogenen Kaltfront[1].

Der Forschung seit einem Jahrhundert entnehmen wir für das Phänomen der Thrombose die folgenden Ergebnisse:

1. An jedem Thrombus ist das Agglutinat der Thrombocyten das Essentielle, das Coagulat des Fibrins das nicht in jedem Falle zu beobachtende Accidentelle.

2. Thromben entstehen an Venen, Arterien oder im Herzen mit bestimmten Prädilektionsstellen. In der Regel werden Thromben organisiert, an Organarterien und Venen meist unter Bestehenbleiben einer Stenose.

3. In der Ätiologie der Thromben kommt den von VIRCHOW sowie von ASCHOFF besonders betonten kreislaufdynamischen Faktoren eine zentrale Bedeutung zu.

4. Außerdem setzt die Thrombose in der Regel eine Veränderung der Strombahnwand voraus Diese ist bei den arteriellen Thrombosen mit seltenen Ausnahmen fast regelmäßig makroskopisch oder zumindesten histologisch nachweisbar, ebenso bei den Thrombosen innerhalb des Herzens. Dagegen haben die lichtmikroskopischen Untersuchungen der Venenwand bei venösen Thrombosen bisher keine überzeugenden Befunde ergeben. Von der elektronenmikroskopischen Untersuchung sind Ergebnisse zu erwarten, da die venöse Thrombose in der Regel bei Strömungsverlangsamung und dadurch bewirkter hypoxischer Schädigung der Venenwand auftritt.

5. Die Entstehung arteriosklerotischer Herde durch Organisation primär nicht arteriosklerotisch verursachter arterieller Thrombosen kann in seltenen Fällen angenommen werden: als universelles pathogenetisches Prinzip ist sie auf Grund vieler Beobachtungen unwahrscheinlich.

---

[1] DAUBERT 1955.

6. In der Ätiologie der Thrombosen kann ein dritter Faktor von Bedeutung sein: die quantitative und qualitative Veränderung der Blutplättchen. Alle Zustände, die mit akuter oder chronischer Vermehrung der Thrombocyten einhergehen, bewirken eine Disposition zur Thrombose.

7. Den vorübergehend für die Thromboseätiologie besonders betonten Zunahmen der Gerinnungsneigung des Blutes können wir nach allgemeinen Beobachtungen nicht die entscheidende Bedeutung beimessen. Das immer wieder zu beobachtende Entstehen ausgedehnter Thrombosen unter der Behandlung mit Heparin spricht besonders gegen diese weit verbreitete Hypothese.

8. Dagegen kann durch Amine, Erregertoxine und andere Stoffe die Agglutinabilität der Blutplättchen gesteigert werden.

9. Viele Thrombosen sind nicht als lokalisierte Veränderungen anzusehen, sondern als Ausdruck einer vorübergehenden allgemeinen Thrombosebereitschaft, bei der sich kreislaufdynamische Faktoren mit Strömungsverlangsamung, akute Änderungen der Strombahnwand, Steigerungen der Thrombocytenzahl sowie Steigerungen der Agglutinabilität der Thrombocyten addieren können. So versteht sich auch das nicht seltene multizentrische Auftreten von Thromben.

Die thrombotische Embolie.

Die *wichtigste Folge der Thrombose in den Venen des großen Kreislaufs* ist die *Embolie eines Thrombusfragmentes oder des ganzen Thrombus.* Der für die Embolie vorgezeichnete Weg ist in solchen Fällen die Verschleppung des Thrombus von seiner Ursprungsstelle aus über die Vena cava caudalis oder cranialis und über das rechte Herz in eine Arterie der einen oder anderen Lunge oder in den Stamm und die beiden Hauptäste beider Lungen. Entsprechend der Häufigkeit der venösen Thrombose ist auch die Lungenembolie bei Menschen über 20 Jahren bei den verschiedensten Grundkrankheiten aus natürlicher Ursache oder nach Trauma sehr häufig.

So wurden in einem Sektionsgut von 1932 Obduktionen in 18% der Fälle Lungenembolien gefunden[1], in einem von 176 Fällen in 28%[2], in einem weiteren unter 100 aufeinanderfolgenden Fällen in 39%[3]. Tödliche Lungenembolien (t.E.) fanden wir am Freiburger Institut bei 19353 Gesamtsektionen in einem Zeitraum von 40 Jahren in 754 Fällen, also in 3,9%. Unter 3000 Sektionen Erwachsener ab 20 Jahren der Jahre 1937—1939, 1946—1950 hatten wir in unserem Obduktionsgut 201 = 6,7% tödliche Lungenembolien[4]. Im Baseler Obduktionsgut schwankte die Zahl bei den Erwachsenen über 20 Jahren der Jahre 1910—1952 zwischen 2 und über 5%[5]. Dabei wächst die Gefahr zur tödlichen Embolie signifikant mit dem Alter[6], in Freiburg zwischen 40 und 60 Jahren um das Doppelte[4]. Frauen werden häufiger von der t.E. betroffen als Männer[7]. Bei nachgewiesener venöser Thrombose starben in Freiburg 26,3% Männer, dagegen 35,9% Frauen an tödlicher Lungenembolie[4].

Diese Zahlen, die wir noch aus anderen Statistiken vermehren könnten, mögen einen Eindruck von der Gefährdung durch Lungenembolie, besonders durch die tödliche Lungenembolie verdeutlichen. Bei weitem die häufigsten thrombotischen Emboli der Lungen stammen aus den tiefen Venen des Oberschenkels und nach deren Fortschreiten des Beckens[8]. Ein geringer Prozentsatz kommt aus Thromben des rechten Herzens. Selten ist das Quellgebiet der Vena cava cranialis Sitz der ursächlichen Thrombose.

Die *akut tödliche thrombotische Lungenembolie*[9] tritt am häufigsten dann ein, wenn ein Agglutinations-Thrombus der Oberschenkelvene mit seinem distalen

---

[1] Lubarsch 1918.   [2] Moller 1923.   [3] Schoenmackers 1958.   [4] Hillemanns 1951.
[5] Rutishauser 1954, Werthemann und Rutishauser 1954.
[6] Geissendörfer 1935, Feller 1934, Zinck 1936, Brass und Sandritter 1949, Hillemanns 1951.
[7] Brass und Sandritter 1949, Hillemanns 1951.
[8] Rössle 1937, Neumann 1938.   [9] Virchow 1846, 1856.

Koagulationsthrombus als Ganzes, nicht selten in einer Länge von 30—40 cm, verschleppt und in den Stamm und die beiden Hauptäste der A. pulmonalis eingekeilt wird. Daß in solchen Fällen schlagartig der Kreislauf weitgehend unterbrochen wird, indem dem linken Herzen nur noch wenig Blut zufließt, so daß im großen arteriellen System eine hochgradige Oligämie mit rapidem Blutdruckabfall besteht, bedarf keiner näheren Begründung. Zum Teil ist dieser Blutdruckabfall reflektorisch bedingt[1]. Ob der zuletzt nicht selten noch wahrgenommene Schmerz in der Brust ein Überdehnungsschmerz ist[2], scheint uns zweifelhaft. Näherliegend ist die Deutung, daß ihm die bestehende plötzliche schwere Ischämie des Herzmuskels zugrunde liegt[3]. Zu dieser Wirkung auf den großen arteriellen Kreislauf und die Herzdurchblutung kommt aber noch die Wirkung der extremen Widerstandserhöhung auf den rechten Ventrikel. Er

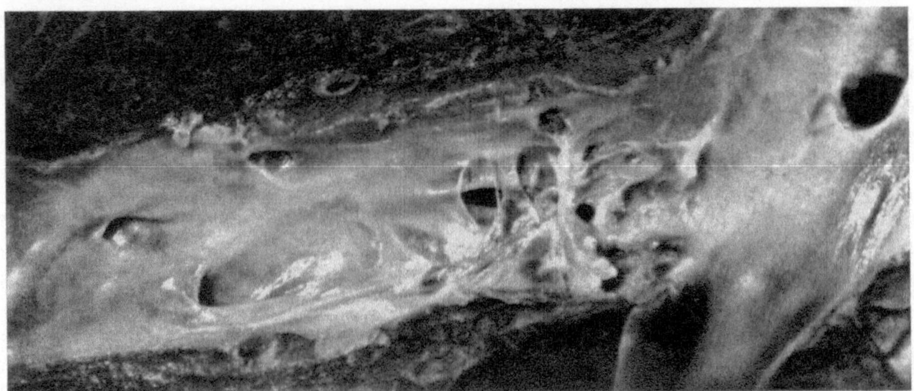

Abb. 44. Strickleiterartiges Narbensystem in einem größeren Ast der Arteria pulmonalis nach Organisation eines Embolus. An anderen Arterien gleicher Befund. Chronisches Cor pulmonale. Herzgewicht: 440 g. [Nach KÖNN, G., Die pathologische Morphologie der Lungengefäßerkrankungen und ihre Beziehungen zur chronischen pulmonalen Hypertonie, Ergebn. ges. Tuberkulose- u. Lungenforsch. 14, 101, 1958, Abb. 10].

zeigt bei der Obduktion das Bild des akuten Cor pulmonale, wie es von KIRCH (1926, 1934) als tonogene Dilatation der Ausflußbahn des rechten Ventrikels beim Menschen und im Experiment beschrieben wurde. Ein 4. Faktor ist die akute Kontraktion der peripheren Pulmonalarterien, wie sie nach den Untersuchungen von U. v. EULER und LILJESTRAND (1947) anzunehmen ist. Diese beiden Autoren sahen beim Hund unter Sauerstoffmangel-Atmung prompt einen Anstieg des Blutdrucks in der Pulmonalarterie als unmittelbaren Effekt der Hypoxie an der glatten Muskulatur der Lungenarterien ohne Mitwirkung eines Reflexes.

Bleiben bei der akut tödlichen Lungenembolie diese verschiedenen Mechanismen der Beobachtung entzogen, so treten sie in ihren Auswirkungen bei *überlebter großer thrombotischer Lungenembolie* und in entsprechenden Experimenten wesentlich deutlicher in Erscheinung. Wir haben darüber ausführlich in Bd. IV/2, S. 604—607 dieses Handbuches nach dem damaligen Stand der Beobachtungen berichtet, so daß wir darauf verweisen können. Hier ist aber folgendes anzufügen:

Häufiger als früher angenommen wurde, bleibt nach großer thrombotischer Lungenembolie noch eine Restdurchblutung erhalten, so daß der Bettliegende damit einen Ruhekreislauf leidlich zu unterhalten vermag. Der Organismus hat dann Zeit, den der Wand der großen Pulmonalarterie anliegenden Embolus mit Mesenchym zu durchwachsen. Das Mesenchym verwandelt sich im Laufe von

---

[1] DALY 1937, SCHWIEGK 1951, DE TACKATS und Mitarbeiter 1939, PARIN 1947.
[2] GROSS 1955.   [3] SCHERF und SCHÖNBRUNNER 1935.

Wochen und Monaten in ein System von weißgrauen kollagenen Narbensträngen, die als Fäden oder Bänder von Wand zu Wand die Lichtung durchziehen, ein System kavernöser Biluträume umschließen und den Durchstrom um so mehr wieder freigeben, je mehr sie schrumpfen (Abb. 44). So besteht in solchen Fällen die Möglichkeit, daß ein vorübergehend hypertrophiertes Cor pulmonale allmählich wieder rückgebildet wird und eine zunächst bestehende Herzerkrankung mit der Zeit wieder verschwindet. Nach unseren Sektionsbeobachtungen werden solche Fälle klinisch häufig während des Lebens nicht erkannt. Sie können aber katamnestisch in diesem Sinne gedeutet werden.

Daß nach der nicht akut tödlichen Lungenembolie in den ersten Tagen und Wochen charakteristische, experimentell reproduzierte Veränderungen des Elektrokardiogramms beobachtet werden können, wurde schon in unserem Handbuchbeitrag über die Hypoxydosen betont (Bd. IV/2). Es handelt sich dabei einmal um die Zeichen des akuten Cor pulmonale: tiefes S_1, tiefes Q_3, RT-Hebung in III mit gegensinniger ST-Strecke in I, negatives T_3, oder nur um die Zeichen der akuten Coronarinsuffizienz mit ST-Senkung und negativem T in einer, zwei oder allen Extremitätenableitungen[1]. Auch haben wir auf die Tatsache hingewiesen, daß infolge Hypoxie der Muskulatur des rechten Ventrikels fleckförmige Parenchymnekrosen von Herzmuskelzellen in der Wand der rechten Kammer nachgewiesen werden konnten (Abb. 50) (beim Menschen: Büchner 1938, Weinschenk 1939, Epping 1940, Büchner und Weyland 1959; experimentell v. Balogh 1938, Walder 1939, Meessen 1940, Herbertson 1953). Amerikanische Untersucher haben in solchen Fällen infarktartige Nekrosen in der Muskulatur des linken Ventrikels, vorwiegend an der Hinterwand, gefunden[2]. Wir konnten im Einzelfall am Menschen diesen Befund bestätigen und fanden nach alter Lungenembolie eine große Infarktnarbe an der linken Hinterwand basal[3]. Wir deuten ihn als Ausdruck dafür, daß bei hochgradiger, akuter Widerstandsarbeit der rechte Ventrikel soviel Blut aus dem Coronarsystem abschluckt, daß der linke Ventrikel ungenügend mit Blut versorgt wird, vor allem im Terminalgebiet der rechten Kranzarterie. Hinzu kommt die Wirkung der mangelhaften Füllung der linken Kammer und der beiden Coronararterien.

Von noch größerer klinischer Bedeutung ist nach den Untersuchungen der letzten Jahre das Bild der *rezidivierenden Lungenembolie*. Da dieses Bild eine der wichtigsten Ursachen der pulmonalen Hypertonie darstellt, werden wir es in dem Kapitel über die pulmonale Hypertonie erörtern.

Embolie von blutfremdem Material.

1. Die Fettembolie.

Die Fettembolie und ihre Folgen sind allgemein so bekannt, daß wir uns in ihrer Darstellung kurz fassen dürfen. Bezüglich der *Fettembolie der Lungen* sei vor allem auf die Darstellung von Ceelen im Handbuch der Speziellen Pathologie III/3 (1931), von Hoffheinz (1933), Kilian (1931), Struppler (1940) verwiesen, für die *Fettembolie des Gehirns* vor allem auf die Berichte von Kilian (1931), Strauss (1933) und besonders von Meessen und Stochdorph (1957). Zum ersten Mal gesehen wurde die capilläre Fettembolie der Lunge von Zenker (1862). Nachdem dann E. Wagner (1862, 1865) mitgeteilt hatte, daß beim Kaninchen nach experimentell herbeigeführtem Femurbruch und Zerstörung des Knochen-

---

[1] Master und Mitarbeiter 1947, Dack, Master und Mitarbeiter 1949.

[2] Friedberg und Horn 1939, Currens und Barnes 1943, Master und Mitarbeiter 1947, Dack, Master und Mitarbeiter 1949, Horn, Master und Mitarbeiter 1950.

[3] Büchner und Weyland 1959.

marks mit einer Sonde in den Lungencapillaren embolisch verschlepptes Knochenmarkfett nachzuweisen ist, hat VON RECKLINGHAUSEN (1863) als erster den Zusammenhang der capillären Fettembolie auf eine Zertrümmerung von Fettmark zurückgeführt. Nach Hufschlagverletzung des Unterschenkels fand er embolisch verschlepptes Fett in der Lunge, im Gehirn und in zahlreichen anderen Organen. Sein Schüler BUSCH hat 1866 diese Beobachtungen durch experimentelle Befunde am Kaninchen nach Zertrümmerung des Femurmarks ergänzt.

Eine Fülle von Untersuchungen hat diese ersten Beobachtungen bestätigt und ergänzt. In der Folge ergab sich, daß eine Fettembolie der Lungen auftreten kann 1. nach traumatischer oder auf andere Weise herbeigeführter krankhafter Zerstörung von fetthaltigem Knochenmark, des Unterhaut-Fettgewebes oder anderer großer Fettlager des Körpers, 2. nach starken Erschütterungen des Knochenmarks und der Fettlager, 3. nach Resorption großer Fettmassen aus den Lymphräumen[1]. Die Erschütterungen von Fettgewebe können schon dann wirksam sein, wenn z.B. bei puerperaler Eklampsie starke Krämpfe zu intensiven Bewegungen der Extremitäten und krampfhaften Kompressionen von Fettgewebe führen[2]. Auch bei Tetanus, bei urämischen Krämpfen, ja sogar bei starker motorischer Unruhe bei Geisteskranken[3] wurden leichte Fettembolien beobachtet[4]. Um so mehr ist es verständlich, daß auch bei Operationen mit Eingriffen am Knochenmark und am Weichteilfettgewebe Fettembolien vorkommen können[5]. Das in die Venen gelangte Fett wird über das rechte Herz in die Lungen verschleppt. Hier fängt es sich in Form wurstförmiger oder gegabelter Gebilde in den Lungencapillaren. Die Fettembolie der Lunge stellt also eine *capilläre Embolie* dar. Am leichtesten ist sie an einem Scherenschnitt von der Lungenschnittfläche im Frischpräparat nachweisbar. Aber auch bei der Sudanfärbung kommt sie deutlich zur Darstellung.

Die Folge der Fettembolie der Lunge ist in kurzer Zeit eine Erschwerung des Gasaustausches innerhalb des Lungengewebes und eine dadurch herbeigeführte Hypoxämie und Hyperkapnie. Darüber hinaus besteht eine Widerstanderhöhung für die Durchblutung der Lunge. Die Folge ist daher eine wesentlich erhöhte Druckarbeit des rechten Ventrikels und ein Cor pulmonale. Auf diese Weise kann es in kurzer Frist zu einer Insuffizienz des rechten Ventrikels und unter dem Einfluß einer allgemeinen venösen Hyperämie zum Tod in der Herzinsuffizienz kommen.

Eine Fettembolie der Lunge wird dann als tödlich angesehen, wenn zwei Drittel aller capillären Gefäßgebiete der Lunge durch die deformierten Fetttropfen verlegt sind[6]. Bleibt der Kranke am Leben, so kann das Fett vorübergehend in den Capillarendothelien der Lunge gespeichert werden[7].

Auf der anderen Seite besteht die Möglichkeit, daß der rechte Ventrikel durch Druckerhöhung den Widerstand im Lungenkreislauf überwindet und das Fett durch die Lungencapillaren hindurch in das Lungenvenenblut treibt. Auf diese Weise kann Fett in das linke Herz und von hier aus in den großen arteriellen Kreislauf gelangen. Ein unmittelbarer Übertritt von Fett aus dem rechten Vorhof in den linken über ein offenes Foramen ovale spielt daneben nur eine untergeordnete Rolle[8].

Die wichtigste Manifestierung der Fettembolie im großen arteriellen System ist die *Fettembolie des Gehirns* (s. MEESSEN und STOCHDORPH 1957). Auch hier handelt es sich um eine *capilläre Fettembolie*, d.h. um die Verlegung von Hirn-

---

[1] LUBARSCH 1905.   [2] VIRCHOW 1886, LUBARSCH 1905.
[3] JOLLY 1881.   [4] CEELEN 1931.   [5] PAYR 1901.
[6] DIETRICH nach CEELEN 1931.   [7] BENEKE 1897.   [8] CEELEN 1931.

capillaren durch wurstförmige und verzweigte in die Capillaren eingekeilte Fetttropfen, wie sie erstmals durch von Recklinghausen (1863) beschrieben wurde.

Neuere systematische Untersuchungen ergaben, daß bei fast 50% der Unfälle mit
Frakturen, die nach 2 Std bis 15 Tagen zum Tode führten, Fett in den Hirncapillaren
nachweisbar war[1]. Im Kriege untersuchte Gehirne nach Flugunfällen zeigten bei 62 von
200 Fällen eine Fettembolie der Lunge und in 15 dieser Lungenfälle eine Fettembolie
des Gehirns[2].

Von der Fettembolie des Gehirns sind die Groß- und Kleinhirnrinde, der
Hirnstamm, das Großhirn- und Kleinhirnmark ziemlich gleichmäßig befallen.
Durch die embolische Verstopfung der Capillaren entwickelt sich in deren Um-
gebung eine kugelförmige Nekrose des Hirngewebes, die in der Hirnrinde als
Erbleichungsherd mit typischem Füllungsdefekt der Capillaren nachweisbar ist.
Diese Befunde wurden in gleicher Weise am Menschen[3] wie auch im Tierversuch[4]
nachgewiesen. Die Ganglienzellen zeigen dabei das Bild der ischämischen Ne-
krose. In den grauen Teilen, insbesondere in Rinde und Thalamus, treten diese
Herde histologisch als Aufhellung und als sog. Mottenfraßherde in Erscheinung[5].
Die oft zahlreichen Markherde sind bei der Fettembolie des Hirns dadurch
gekennzeichnet, daß bei ihnen in unmittelbarer Umgebung der verstopften
Capillare eine kugelförmige Nekrose mit charakteristischer Entmarkung zustande kommt und daß diese Entmarkungsnekrose von einer typischen Ring-
blutung umgeben wird. Dadurch kommt es zu der charakteristischen, schon
makroskopisch die Diagnose ermöglichenden Purpura cerebri, die symmetrisch
im Mark des Großhirns, in den Pyramidenbahnen, im Balken und im Mark des
Kleinhirns nachweisbar ist.

Im klinischen Bild können die Erscheinungen der Fettembolie der Lungen
und die der Fettembolie des Hirns mit apoplektiformen, epileptiformen und
komatösen Symptomen einander ablösen[5].

Fettembolien in anderen Organen des großen Kreislaufs können wir hier
übergehen, da die allgemein-pathologischen Prinzipien, um deren Herausarbeitung
es sich hier gehandelt hat, durch die Befunde an der Lunge und im Hirn genügend
herausgearbeitet sind.

2. Die Luftembolie.

Nach traumatischer oder instrumenteller Eröffnung von Venen, im Uterus
auch nach spontaner Eröffnung venöser Gefäße bei plötzlicher Lösung der Placenta, insbesondere bei Abtreibungen oder Abtreibungsversuchen, kann es zur
Einsaugung von Luft in das venöse Gefäßsystem kommen. Die Folge davon ist
die *Luftembolie*. Sind Venen des großen Kreislaufes eröffnet, so sammelt sich die
Luft im rechten Herzen mehr und mehr an, tamponiert den rechten Vorhof und
Ventrikel aus und führt zu einer Unterbrechung des Kreislaufs und dadurch zum
Tode. Auch nach operativer Eröffnung von Halsvenen kann es zu dieser gefürch-
teten Lufttamponade des rechten Herzens kommen. Die Luft kann aber auch
über den Lungenkreislauf in das linke Herz und aus diesem in das große arterielle
System weiterbefördert werden. Auf der anderen Seite kann bei Eröffnung von
Lungenvenen, z.B. bei Pneumothoraxfüllung oder infolge Lungenzerreissungen
durch Luftstoßwirkung bei Bombennahexplosionen, Luft über die Lungenvenen
und das linke Herz den großen Kreislauf erreichen. In solchen Fällen kommt es
zur embolischen Verschleppung der Luft in das Gehirn. Die Luftbläschen ver-

---

[1] Krauss bei Meessen und Stochdorph 1957.   [2] Krücke 1944, 1948.
[3] Gröndahl 1911, Neubürger 1924, Weimann 1929, 1939, Cammermeyer 1937, Siegmund 1941.
[4] Bodechtel und Müller 1930, Villaret und Catchera 1939, Broman 1939, Harter 1947.
[5] Payr 1898, Gröndahl 1911.

legen dabei vor allem die Capillaren. Diese capilläre Embolie bewirkt, wie die capilläre Fettembolie des Gehirns, im Hirnmark Nekrosen und Ringblutungen (RÖSSLE 1944). Bei plötzlichem Druckfall, besonders bei rapidem Aufstieg in große Höhen oder im Experiment in den Unterdruck, kann sich ebenfalls eine Luftembolie entwickeln, die im Hirn und im Rückenmark präcapilläre und capilläre Gefäße verlegt und wiederum das Bild von Nekrosen mit oder ohne Ringblutungen nach sich zieht (HAYMAKER 1957).

3. Die Fruchtwasserembolie[1].

Zu den seltenen Formen pulmonaler Embolien gehört die Fruchtwasserembolie. Dieses nach einer wenig bekannt gewordenen Mitteilung von J.R. MEYER (1926)[2] zuerst ausführlich von STEINER und LUSHBAUGH (1941) beschriebene, in den meisten Fällen tödliche Krankheitsbild tritt bei Schwangeren unter der Geburt auf. Pathogenetisch entscheidend ist eine plötzliche Verstopfung vieler kleiner Verzweigungen der Lungenarterien durch corpusculäre Fruchtwasserbestandteile. Die in den letzten 15 Jahren bekanntgewordenen mehr als 50 Todesfälle an Fruchtwasserembolie[3] vermitteln ein ziemlich einheitliches Bild über die klinischen Symptome, die pathologisch-anatomischen Veränderungen, die klinischen und anatomischen Bedingungen und die verschiedenen Begleiterscheinungen dieser Embolie.

Die Symptome entsprechen einem sog. Geburtsschock mit plötzlichem Schwindelgefühl, mit Atemnot, leichter Übelkeit und zunehmender Bewußtseinstrübung, nachdem die Schwangerschaft meist komplikationslos abgelaufen und die Geburt normal in Gang gekommen war. Rasch macht sich eine Cyanose bemerkbar; die Gebärende wird tief bewußtlos und nach Absinken des Blutdruckes und Anstieg der Pulsfrequenz tritt der Tod ein. In den meisten Fällen konnte die Diagnose erst nach der Obduktion gestellt werden, da die genannten klinischen Zeichen vieldeutig sind und ein verläßliches, sicheres Symptom für das Vorliegen einer Fruchtwasserembolie nicht bekannt ist.

Eindeutig sind die pathologisch-anatomischen Befunde in den Lungen: Makroskopisch besteht in der Regel ein erhebliches Ödem. In einem Fall[4] wurde eine hämorrhagische Infarzierung beider Lungen beschrieben, in einem anderen[5] eine zentrale Atelektase. Aus den kleinen arteriellen Verzweigungen kann man oft etwa staubkorngroße, gelbliche Partikel auspressen[6], die allerdings zumeist nur wenig auffällig sein dürften. Im Lungenpreßsaft gelingt es dann aber, Fruchtwasserbestandteile, vor allem Hornschüppchen und einzelne Lanugohaare nachzuweisen. Noch klarer ist der Befund bei histologischer Untersuchung: In den feinen Verzweigungen der Lungenarterien finden sich geschichtete, verfettete Hornschüppchen, die zum Teil lamellär aufeinanderliegen und kleine, oft stark ausgeweitete Arterien völlig austamponieren können (Abb. 45a). An anderen Stellen überwiegen Schleimmassen[7], die unter Umständen fädig ausgezogen sind und auf denen gelapptkernige Leukocyten aufgereiht sind (,,Auskämmphänomen" von GROSS und BENZ 1947). Vereinzelt trifft man auch auf Meconiumkörperchen und auf angeschnittene Lanugohaare[8] (Abb. 45b). Diese Befunde sind eindeutig und ermöglichen in jedem Fall eine sichere Diagnose. Vielfach wurden auch zusätzlich frische Agglutinationsthromben in den kleinen Arterienästen gefunden. — Regelhaft ist bei der Obduktion ferner ein dilatiertes, meist schlaffes Herz mit

---

[1] Von Dozent Dr. EKKHARD GRUNDMANN, Pathologisches Institut Freiburg i.Br.
[2] Nach PEREIRA LUZ 1953.
[3] Teilübersichten bei MESTWERDT 1955, LEPAGE und Mitarbeiter 1956, I. MARTIN 1956.
[4] THORNTON 1953.   [5] MATHIESEN 1955.   [6] I. MARTIN 1954, 1956.   [7] SCHUBERT 1956.
[8] LUSHBAUGH und STEINER 1942, I. MARTIN 1954, GRUNDMANN 1957.

viel, meist flüssigem Blut vor allem im rechten Vorhof und in der rechten Kammer. Etwa in der Hälfte der Fälle trat der Tod der Mutter vor Abschluß der Geburt ein, so daß man das abgestorbene Kind im Uterus vorfand.

Die Bedingungen, unter denen die Fruchtwasserembolie erfolgt, sind noch keineswegs vollständig aufgeklärt. Der Weg, den das Fruchtwasser von der Eihöhle in das mütterliche Blut nimmt, war in den Fällen gut zu verfolgen, bei

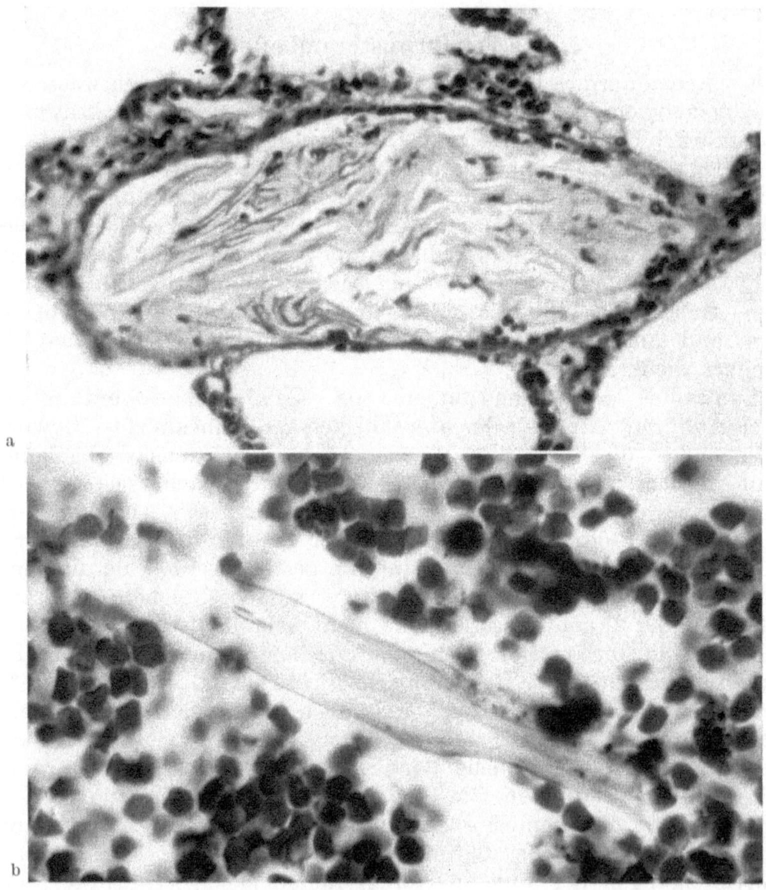

Abb. 45a u. b. a Geschichtete Talgschollen mit einzelnen Leukocyten in einem stark erweiterten kleinen Lungengefäß. b Schräg angeschnittenes Lanugo-Haar in einer Lungenarterie. [Befunde bei Fruchtwasserembolie nach GRUNDMANN, E., Beitr. path. Anat. **117**, 445, 1957, Abb. 2 u. 3.]

denen Defekte in den Eihäuten oder in der Uteruswand festgestellt werden konnten. So haben AHLSTROEM und WIDLUND (1952) eine Fruchtwasserembolie beschrieben, bei der ein 3 cm langer, in Isthmushöhe quer verlaufender Riß in den Eihäuten bestand. Ähnlich fand sich bei der Beobachtung von R. E. MARTIN und FANGER (1954) ein kleiner Eihautriß nahe der Umschlagstelle an der Nabelschnur. Derartige Einrisse sind besonders dann von Bedeutung, wenn die Embolie bei noch stehender Fruchtblase erfolgt ist. Die meisten Todesfälle treten erst nach dem Blasensprung ein, wenn das Fruchtwasser einen direkten Zugang zur Uterusinnenwand finden kann. Das Eindringen in die uterinen Venen ist in den Fällen besonders erleichtert, in denen die placentaren Bluträume, etwa bei vorzeitiger

Placentalösung oder bei Placenta praevia[1], ebenfalls auch nach einer Schnittentbindung[2], eröffnet sind. In anderen Fällen ließen sich Rupturen in der Uteruswand feststellen[3]. Bei der Beobachtung von WATKINS (1948) bestand ein Uterusriß 2—3 cm oberhalb der Cervix von einer Größe von 1—1,5 cm. Die Öffnung führte unmittelbar in das stark geschwollene Ligamentum latum. Die ödematöse Schwellung setzte sich retroperitoneal bis in Nierenhöhe fort und retroperitoneal fanden sich mehr als 50 cm³ Flüssigkeit. STONE u. Mitarb. (1955) fanden bei einem weiteren Todesfall an Fruchtwasserembolie eine unvollständige Uterusruptur von der Größe einer Zangenbranche. Von hier aus gelangte man direkt in die erweiterten Venen des Ligamentum latum und von da in die große untere Hohlvene. Entlang kleiner Cervixrißstellen konnten WYATT und GOLDENBERG (1948) in den uterinen Sinus Fruchtwasserbestandteile erkennen, die von dort aus ebenfalls den Weg in die Lungen genommen hatten.

Diesen Fällen steht aber die Mehrzahl der Beobachtungen gegenüber, in denen keine Defekte in Eihäuten und Uterus gefunden werden konnten. Vielfach mag die Unkenntnis des Krankheitsbildes dazu beigetragen haben, daß kleine Rißstellen unbeachtet blieben. Aber STEINER u. Mitarb., die 1941 eine erste ausführliche Beschreibung von 8 Todesfällen vorgelegt und damals bereits die möglichen Eintrittspforten des Fruchtwassers erörtert hatten, konnten in einem 1949 veröffentlichten weiteren Todesfall selbst nach Injektion mit Farbstofflösungen keine Verletzungen der Eihäute und auch keinen Uterusdefekt nachweisen. Trotzdem fanden sie in den Uterusvenen massenhaft Fruchtwasserbestandteile und in den Lungen das typische Bild einer Fruchtwasserembolie. Auch THORNTON (1953) gelang der Nachweis von Talg und Schleimmassen in der äußerlich intakten Uteruswand[4]. Selbst in Fällen, in denen keine Fruchtwasserembolie eingetreten war, also bei normal entbundenen Frauen, konnten LEARY und HERTIG (1950) Fruchtwasserbestandteile zwischen Amnion und Chorion, in der Decidua am Placentarand und auch in den retroplacentaren Venen nachweisen. Dies gelang nicht nur bei Uterusrupturen[5], sondern auch bei intakter Gebärmutter-Innenwand. Man muß also annehmen, daß unter besonderen, noch nicht vollständig analysierten Bedingungen Fruchtwasser in die Plexus des schwangeren Uterus während des Geburtsaktes eindringen kann.

Dabei kehren in den vielen mitgeteilten Einzelbeobachtungen[6] folgende Befunde immer wieder: 1. Bis auf Ausnahmen[7] begannen die klinischen Symptome erst nach dem Blasensprung, d.h zu einer Zeit in der die trennende Membran zwischen Eihöhlung und Uteruscavum gefallen war. 2. In vielen Fällen wird ausdrücklich hervorgehoben, daß viel Fruchtwasser, manchmal sogar ein Hydramnion vorhanden war. 3. Die Uteruskontraktionen nach dem Blasensprung wurden als besonders stark, ja als tetanoid bezeichnet. Starke Wehen können — besonders bei einem Hydramnion — das Fruchtwasser selbst durch kleine Einrisse in Uterus oder Placenta in die mütterlichen Venengeflechte pressen, vor allem in die oberflächlichen Sinus der Decidua[8], wobei der niedrige Venendruck in den Plexus leicht überschritten werden kann. Man muß berücksichtigen, daß alle diese

---

[1] LUSHBAUGH und STEINER 1942, LOLK und SIKA 1952, SCHUBERT 1956.
[2] Zum Beispiel KOUTZKY und LUKAWSKY 1954.
[3] LUSHBAUGH und STEINER 1942, BOUTON und SAUNDERS 1951.
[4] Siehe auch WYATT und GOLDENBERG 1948.   [5] LANDING 1950.
[6] Zum Beispiel HEMMINGS 1947, JENNINGS und STOFER 1948, SHOTTON und TAYLOR 1949, SCHENKEN und Mitarbeiter 1950, MALLORY und Mitarbeiter 1950, EAMES 1952, CRON und Mitarbeiter 1952, DENNISS und Mitarbeiter 1954, MARTIN 1954, BOWMAN 1955, GRAHAM 1955, WESTBROOK und THOMAS 1956, ATTWOOD 1956, SCHUBERT 1956, GRUNDMANN 1957.
[7] STEINER und Mitarbeiter 1949, AHLSTROEM und WIDLUND 1952.
[8] LEARY und HERTIG 1950.

Faktoren relativ häufig gegeben sind, die Fruchtwasserembolie aber eine seltene Geburtskomplikation darstellt[1]. Wahrscheinlich müssen besondere, heute noch unbekannte Faktoren beteiligt sein, die unter den genannten Bedingungen eine Fruchtwasserembolie der Lungen verursachen.

So wird z. B. von mehreren Autoren die Bedeutung eines besonderen Gerinnungsfaktors im Fruchtwasser diskutiert, der dem Thromboplastin nahestehen soll (Weiner und Reid 1950). Weinert und Reid fanden in vielen kleinen Lungenarterienästen bei Fruchtwasserembolie frische Fibringerinnsel[2], vermuteten dadurch eine relative Fibrinogenverarmung und glaubten auf diese Weise die bei Fruchtwasserembolie mehrfach beobachtete hämorrhagische Diathese erklären zu können. Tatsächlich haben Rendelstein u. Mitarb. (1951) im Fruchtwasser eine hitzestabile und eine hitzelabile Thrombokinase nachweisen können, die dem Heparin antagonistisch wirkte und bei intravenöser Injektion hoher Dosen von Fruchtwasser beim Hund intravasale Fibrinbildung und eine sekundäre Fibrinogenopenie verursachte. Im Gegensatz dazu hat Schneider (1953) — ebenfalls beim Hund — eine gerinnungshemmende Substanz nach Meconiuminjektion nachweisen können, die er später (1955) als Heparin oder zumindest heparinähnliche Substanz identifizierte und die direkt die Hypofibrinogenämie bei Fruchtwasserembolie erklären kann[3]. Lepage u. Mitarb. (1956) sprachen deshalb von einer 2. Periode im Krankheitsbild nach Überstehen des primären Schocks, der Periode schwerster Blutungen wegen der Fibrinogenverarmung. In einer 3. Periode, die allerdings kaum erreicht wurde, stünden anoxische Parenchymschäden der inneren Organe, vor allem der Niere, im Vordergrund.

Im Gegensatz zu den genannten Autoren gelang es anderen Untersuchern[4] nicht, durch Fruchtwasser eine Störung der Blutgerinnung im Tierexperiment zu erzeugen. Da die Tiere Injektionen selbst von viel Fruchtwasser überlebten, hat Hunter (1956) die pathogenetische Bedeutung der Fruchtwasserembolie wie schon vor ihm Mendelson (1948), Dumont (1949) und Tunis (1952) grundsätzlich bezweifelt. Dem stehen aber die über 50 genannten, meist ausführlich beschriebenen Todesfälle und eindeutig positiven Tierexperimente entgegen, in denen Injektionen von ungefiltertem Fruchtwasser bei Kaninchen und bei Hunden[5], bei Kaninchen[6] und bei Ratten[7] zum typischen Schockzustand führten, wonach histologisch die gleichen Lungenveränderungen festgestellt werden konnten wie bei den menschlichen Todesfällen. Schubert (1956) erzeugte beim Hund entsprechende Bilder durch Injektion von mehreren Kubikzentimetern klaren Hühnereiweißes.

Das Experiment von Schubert (1956) verlief noch in anderer Hinsicht bedeutsam: Obwohl beim Hund nie ein offenes Foramen ovale besteht, konnten in den Hirngefäßen Eiweißmassen und kleine, durch diese hervorgerufene Erweichungsherde nachgewiesen werden. Auch in dem von ihm mitgeteilten Obduktionsbefund fanden sich Fruchtwasserbestandteile in den Hirncapillaren, obwohl das Foramen ovale geschlossen war. Diese „gekreuzte Embolie" bei geschlossenem Foramen ovale erklärt sich nach Schubert (1956) dadurch, daß bei Verlegung von Ästen der Pulmonalarterien der Weg über die sog. Sperrarterien zwischen den Pulmonal- und den Bronchialarterien eröffnet wird und auf diese Weise das Blut über arterio-venöse Anastomosen in die Venengeflechte der Bronchialschleimhaut eindringen kann. — Die Fruchtwasserbestandteile im

---

[1] Sheehan 1948, Steiner und Mitarbeiter 1949, May und Winter 1952.
[2] Siehe auch Grundmann 1957.
[3] Eames 1952, Lepage und Mitarbeiter 1955, Bowman 1955, Graham 1955.
[4] Denniss und Mitarbeiter 1954, Hunter und Mitarbeiter 1956.
[5] Steiner und Lushbaugh 1941.   [6] Cron und Mitarbeiter 1952.   [7] Grundmann 1957.

Herzmuskel und in den Nieren konnte I. Martin (1954) bei ihrem Fall eindeutig auf das offene Foramen ovale beziehen.

Als letzte Todesursache wurde von den meisten Autoren[1] ein Fremdkörperschock oder auch eine gegen das Fremdeiweiß gerichtete Überempfindlichkeit angenommen. I. Martin (1954, 1956) erörterte einen cardio-pulmonalen Reflex oder einen durch plötzlichen Druckanstieg im kleinen Kreislauf bedingten reflektorischen Blutdruckabfall im großen. Andererseits konnte Grundmann (1957) bei einem Todesfall an Fruchtwasserembolie frische Herzmuskelnekrosen in der Ausflußbahn der rechten Kammer beobachten, wie sie auch nach thrombotischer Lungenembolie bekannt sind. In den meisten Sektionsfällen wird eine pralle Blutfülle vor allem der rechten Herzkammer erwähnt. Die akute Rechtsbelastung kann noch gesteigert werden durch reflektorische Gefäßspasmen in den Lungenarterien, wie sie nach experimenteller Fruchtwasserembolie Steiner und Lushbaugh nachweisen konnten, oder durch die bereits erörterten Mikrothromben in den feinen pulmonalen Arterienverzweigungen.

In einzelnen Fällen konnte der akute Schock überlebt werden und der Tod trat erst nach Stunden oder Tagen ein[2]. Obwohl die klinische Diagnose immer nur eine Vermutungsdiagnose ist, haben doch mehrere Autoren über nicht tödlich verlaufene Fruchtwasserembolien berichtet. Dabei fand sich im EKG häufig eine Sinustachykardie, verbunden mit den Zeichen eines akuten Cor pulmonale[3], röntgenologisch eine vermehrte Hiluszeichnung und feine Herdschatten in den Lungen, die an eine Miliartuberkulose denken ließen, nach etwa 8 Wochen jedoch völlig verschwunden waren[4]. Bei einer ähnlichen Beobachtung[5] ließ die Intensität der von Anfang an sehr weichen Lungenschatten im Röntgenbild schon nach 5 Tagen deutlich nach[6]. Wie das Tierexperiment gezeigt hat[7], entstehen 3 Tage nach einer Injektion von ungefiltertem Fruchtwasser bei der Ratte in Umgebung der als Fremdkörper wirkenden Fruchtwasserbestandteile riesenzellhaltige Granulome[8], in deren Bereich die Gefäßlichtungen völlig verlegt werden. Bei ausreichendem Befall könnte eine überstandene Fruchtwasserembolie auf diesem Wege ein chronisches Cor pulmonale hervorrufen. Beobachtungen hierüber stehen noch aus.

4. Gewebsembolien.

Seit langem ist es bekannt, daß nach Zertrümmerung z.B. von Leberparenchym oder von Knochenmark kleine Gewebsverbände embolisch in die Lunge verschleppt werden können. Im Rahmen dieses Beitrags ist diese Möglichkeit nur von geringem theoretischem Interesse. Es sei daher nur darauf hingewiesen, daß eine experimentelle Knochenmarksembolie beim Kaninchen nach Tötung durch Nackenschlag relativ häufig vorkommt (Abb. 46) (Chr. Büchner und Könn 1959).

Über die Embolien sind folgende Tatsachen besonders hervorzuheben:

1. Embolien von Fragmenten venöser Thromben oder ganzen venösen Thromben in die Lungenarterien sind auffallend häufig und von großer klinischer Bedeutung.

2. Neben der akut tödlichen großen Lungenembolie ist die Bedeutung der überlebten großen thrombotischen Lungenembolie nicht zu vernachlässigen. Sie kann Ursache einer chronischen pulmonalen Hypertonie sein. Durch Organisation der

---

[1] Zum Beispiel Watkins 1948, Steiner und Mitarbeiter 1949, Sluder und Lock 1952, Stone und Mitarbeiter 1955, Bowman 1955.
[2] Lushbaugh und Steiner 1941, Thornton 1953.   [3] Hager und Davies 1952.
[4] Koutzky und Lukawsky 1954.   [5] Seltzer und Schuman 1947.
[6] Siehe auch Pereira Luz 1953.   [7] Grundmann 1957.
[8] Siehe auch Steiner und Lushbaugh 1941.

Thromben und Rekanalisation der Lungenarterien kann die chronische pulmonale Hypertonie und das zugeordnete Cor pulmonale wieder zurückgebildet werden. Durch rezidivierende Lungenembolie können beide Zustände wiederholt auftreten und Ursache einer schließlich tödlichen chronischen Insuffizienz des rechten Ventrikels werden.

3. Die Fettembolie nach Zertrümmerung von Knochenmark, nach starker Erschütterung des Knochenmarks und der Fettlager oder nach Resorption großer Fettmassen aus den Lymphräumen kann durch Verlegung großer Gebiete der Lungen-

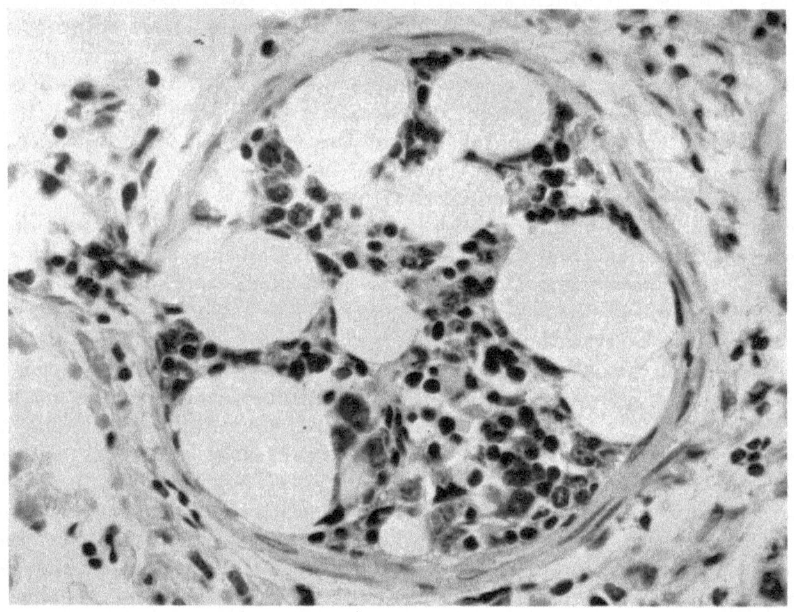

Abb. 46. Knochenmarksembolie mit Fett- und Blutzellen in einer kleinen Lungenarterie beim Kaninchen nach Tötung durch Nackenschlag. (Nach BÜCHNER, CHR., u. G. KÖNN, 1959, noch unveröffentlicht.)

capillaren oder — nach Durchtritt des Fettes durch die Lungenstrombahn — durch capilläre Fettembolie des Hirns lebensbedrohliche und tödliche Erscheinungen hervorrufen.

4. Das gleiche gilt von der Luftembolie, während Gewebsembolien seltener klinisch in Erscheinung treten.

5. In jüngster Zeit wurde die Fruchtwasserembolie in ihrer pathogenetischen Bedeutung erkannt. Durch Eintritt von Fruchtwasser in das Wundbett der Placenta können reichlich Fruchtwasserbestandteile in den kleineren Verzweigungen der Lungenarterien zur Haftung kommen und tödliche Komplikationen herbeiführen, besonders auch durch ihre toxische Wirkung.

Die Hypertonie im großen Kreislauf.

Überblickt man die Erforschung des Problems der krankhaften Blutdruckerhöhung seit der Jahrhundertwende, so kann man zwei allgemein-pathologisch wichtige Feststellungen machen: Zunächst stand die Vorstellung im Vordergrund. daß prähypertonische Veränderungen der Nieren gesetzmäßig die Ursache der Hypertonien seien[1] oder solche der kleinen Arterien vieler Gefäßprovinzen. Dann

---

[1] VOLHARD und FAHR 1914.

aber wurde durch die Arbeiten von JORES (1903, 1924) mehr und mehr erkannt, daß die Gefäß- und Nierenveränderungen bei einem Teil der Hypertonien nicht Ursache, sondern Folge der Blutdruckerhöhung sind. Das Hypertonie-Problem wurde damit zunehmend von der statisch-strukturellen auf die dynamisch-funktionelle Sicht verlagert. Mit diesen Akzentverlagerungen ging zugleich die Erkenntnis einher, daß es keine ätiologisch einheitliche Hypertonie-Krankheit gibt, sondern daß verschiedene Faktoren zu einer akuten und zur chronischen Blutdruckerhöhung führen können. In den Auswirkungen der chronischen Hypertonie münden dann freilich viele ursprünglich getrennte Wege in einen zusammen. Dementsprechend tun wir gut daran, wenn wir unsere Auseinandersetzung mit dem Hypertonieproblem in 2 Abschnitte gliedern: in die Untersuchung der hypertonieverursachenden Faktoren und in die Untersuchung der hypertoniebedingten Veränderungen am arteriellen System. Darüber hinaus wollen wir die Folgen der Hypertonie im einzelnen nicht untersuchen. Wir werden aber feststellen, daß die genauere Kenntnis der Hypertonie-Folgen an den Arterien und Arteriolen des großen Kreislaufs uns den Schlüssel für das Verständnis einer Fülle von relativen Durchblutungsstörungen in die Hand gibt und uns rückblickend noch einmal die große pathogenetische Bedeutung der relativen arteriellen Ischämie in Erinnerung bringt.

1. Ursachen chronischer Blutdruckerhöhung.

Seit langem wurde die Aufmerksamkeit des Arztes auf die Tatsache gelenkt, daß es Hypertoniker-Familien gibt, ja daß bei der genuinen Hypertonie die familiäre Disposition häufig oder gar die Regel ist.

WEITZ stellte schon 1923 bei 82 Kranken mit genuiner Hypertonie fest, daß bei über $^3/_4$ (76,8%) einer oder beide Eltern Hypertoniker waren, während bei 267 normotonischen Kranken kaum $^1/_3$ (30,3%) Hypertoniker-Eltern hatten. O' HARA, WALKER und VICKERS (1924) fanden eine Hypertonie-positive Familiengeschichte bei 68% von 300 Hypertonikern, bei 37,7% von 436 Normotonikern. PLATT (1947) sah bei 78 Hypertonikern in 59% der Fälle Hypertonie bei den Eltern, bei 55 Normotonikern nur in 25,5%. In einer anderen Untersuchungsreihe von Hypertonikern waren unter den Verwandten 1. Grades 109 Hypertoniker, 102 Normotoniker[1].

Eine gewisse Einschränkung erfahren allerdings diese Feststellungen durch die Tatsache, daß bei den Verwandten wegen Hypertonie abgewiesener Gesuchsteller einer Lebensversicherungsgesellschaft und den bei Normotonie aufgenommenen bei je 2188 Gesuchstellern der beiden Gruppen mit gleicher Alters- und Geschlechtsverteilung nur geringe Unterschiede in der Hypertoniehäufigkeit bestanden[2]. Dagegen spricht die Zwillingsforschung wiederum für die erbbedingte Determination der Blutdruckhöhe: bei 112 Homocygoten betrug die Differenz des Blutdruckes der beiden Zwillinge nur 5,1 mm Hg, bei 82 Heterocygoten dagegen 8,2[3], in einer anderen Untersuchungsreihe 6,3 und 11,4[4]. In den Londoner Schulen wurde eine höhere Annäherung der Blutdruckwerte bei den Homocygoten als bei den Heterocygoten gefunden[5]. War einer der Zwillinge Hypertoniker, so betrug für die Homocygoten die Differenz der Blutdruckhöhe 26,4 mm Hg, bei Heterocygoten 36,8[4]. Für die maligne Hypertonie im besonderen wurde bei den Eltern, Geschwistern und Kindern jenseits 30 Jahren wesentlich häufiger eine Hypertonie nachgewiesen als bei einer Kontrollgruppe von Normotonikern[6].

Daß auch *beim Tier* der Blutdruck genetisch grundgelegt ist und in bestimmten Sippen zur krankhaften Erhöhung neigt, zeigen interessante experimentelle Untersuchungen am Kaninchen[7]. Von 553 normalen Tieren hatten 2,7% konstant einen systolischen Blutdruck von 160 mm Hg und darüber. Von dieser Gruppe wurden 8 Paare weitergezüchtet: ihre Nachkommen hatten ebenfalls eine mäßige, wenn auch labile Hypertonie bei beiden Geschlechtern.

Aus allen vorliegenden Untersuchungen ist mit Wahrscheinlichkeit abzuleiten, daß die *Anlage zur genuinen Hypertonie beim Menschen dominant vererblich* ist und daß in den meisten Fällen von genuiner Hypertonie eine genetische Anlage

---

[1] HAMILTON, PICKERING, ROBERTS und SOWRY 1954.   [2] FELDT und WENSTRAND 1943.
[3] VERSCHUER und ZIPPERLEN 1929.   [4] KAHLER und WEBER.   [5] STOCKS 1929.
[6] SOBYE 1948.   [7] ALEXANDER, HINSHAW und DRURY 1954.

mitwirkt. An welchem System sich diese Anlage besonders auswirkt, dürfte uneinheitlich sein. Theoretisch kommt eine gesteigerte Erregbarkeit der glatten Arterienmuskulatur, besonders an den Arteriolen, gegenüber normalen humoralen oder nervösen Impulsen in Frage, ebenso aber auch eine Vermehrung der Impulse des Hormondrüsensystems bzw. einzelner Hormondrüsen, besonders der Hypophyse und der Nebennieren oder seitens der peripheren oder zentralen nervösen Regulation des Blutdrucks.

Daß bei der genuinen Hypertonie die *Hypophyse* und die *Nebennieren* sich in einem Zustand erhöhter Aktivität befinden, geht aus den morphologischen Untersuchungen eindeutig hervor. Seit längerem ist die Tatsache bekannt, daß bei genuiner Hypertonie im Hypophysenvorderlappen der relative Gehalt basophiler Epithelien gegenüber der Norm erhöht ist, also ein *relativer Basophilismus* besteht[1]. Auch konnte, vor allem durch genaue planimetrische Messungen, bei der genuinen Hypertonie eine *Hyperplasie der Nebennierenrinde*[2] und eine *Hyperplasie des Nebennierenmarkes*[3] festgestellt werden. Der Nebennierenrindenhyperplasie ist dabei eine *vermehrte Ausscheidung von Rindenhormonen im Harn* zugeordnet[4]. Mit diesen Befunden ist aber nur ausgesagt, daß sich der Hypophysenvorderlappen sowie Rinde und Mark der Nebennieren *in Anpassung an die Hypertonie* infolge erhöhter Beanspruchung im Zustand der Hyperplasie befinden. Eine etwa genetisch bedingte Übererregbarkeit und erhöhte Strukturentfaltung dieser hormonalen Organe ist damit keineswegs bewiesen. Das ergibt sich vor allem aus der Tatsache, daß auch bei experimentell renaler Hypertonie eine Hyperplasie der Nebennierenrinde eintritt[5].

Daß der genuinen Hypertonie eine erhöhte Erregung der *peripheren oder zentralen Blutdruckregulatoren* zugrunde läge, läßt sich morphologisch bisher nicht wahrscheinlich machen. VOLHARD (1948/49) hat die Hypothese aufgestellt, daß ein Elastizitätsverlust an der Aortenwurzel oder an dem Sinus caroticus beiderseits zu einer Funktionsbeeinträchtigung der depressorischen Nerven führen könne und daß die genuine Hypertonie ein „Entzügelungshochdruck" sei. Für den Sinus caroticus konnte aber gezeigt werden, daß die Erstarrung der Sinuswand und der damit gegebene Verlust an Dehnungsfähigkeit durch Arteriosklerose, die in diesem Gebiet früh, häufig und schwer einzutreten pflegen, in keiner Beziehung zur Hypertonie steht und daß umgekehrt Hypertoniker nicht selten zarte Sinuswandungen beiderseits haben[6]. Auch die Tatsache, daß der experimentelle Entzügelungshochdruck nach Durchtrennung der Depressoren beim Kaninchen nur reversibel auftritt[7] und daß er beim Hund irreversibel nur durch die Durchtrennung der beiderseitigen Carotissinusnerven und der beiden Depressornerven an der Aortenwurzel hervorgerufen werden kann[8], spricht gegen die Bedeutung dieses Mechanismus. An den nervösen Zonen des Zwischenhirns, die nach den Untersuchungen von W. R. HESS (1949) in die Regulierung des Blutdruckes eingreifen, sind ebensowenig primäre, hypertonieverursachende Veränderungen bei genuiner Hypertonie nachzuweisen[9] wie in den blutdruckregulierenden Zonen der Medulla oblongata[10].

Wir können also nur feststellen, daß *hypertonieverursachende morphologische Veränderungen bei der genuinen Hypertonie an keiner der Strukturen* nachgewiesen

---

[1] BERBLINGER 1932, MEESSEN 1935.
[2] LANDAU 1915, VON LUCADOU 1936, LIEBEGOTT 1944, 1952/53, FISHER und HEWER 1947, ROGERS und WILLIAMS 1947, GIAMPALMO 1947, PENDL 1954.
[3] GOLDZIEHER 1931, VON LUCADOU 1936, LIEBEGOTT 1944, 1952/53.
[4] PFEFFER und STAUDINGER jr. 1952.   [5] RATHER 1951.   [6] v. HASSELBACH 1931.
[7] E. KOCH 1931.   [8] HEYMANS und REGNIERS 1933.
[9] WEHRLE 1951.   [10] RUCKERT und DEILMANN 1939.

werden konnten, *die in die Steuerung des Blutdruckes eingreifen*, also *weder an den Arteriolen und kleineren Arterien, noch an Hypophyse und Nebennieren. noch an den Depressornerven und den zentral-nervösen Zonen der Blutdruck- regulation*.

In der psychosomatischen Literatur wird die genuine Hypertonie vielfach als typisches Beispiel einer durch tiefenseelische Störungen verursachten Krankheit gedeutet. ALEXANDER (1951) sieht sie als häufiges Ergebnis des Fortwirkens frühkindlicher Ungeborgenheit im Erwachsenen an. Auf der anderen Seite ist die Häufigkeit der genetischen Disposition zur Hypertonie nicht zu übersehen. Verbinden wir die Erfahrung der Psychotherapeuten mit der der Humangenetiker, so können wir den steilen Anstieg der genuinen Hypertonie in allen Weltstädten und technisierten Ländern während der letzten Jahrzehnte nur so verstehen, daß sich in den Lebensformen und im Daseinsgefüge des Menschen unserer Zeit bei genetischer Anlage die peristatischen Realisatoren für die Manifestierung der Hypertonie wesentlich vermehrt und in ihrer Penetranz gesteigert haben. Nach allen ärtzlichen Erfahrungen sind aber in der modernen Arbeitswelt für den Hypertonie-Gefährdeten offenbar solche freigewählte oder auferlegte psycho- somatische Überforderungen das Entscheidende, die einen Zustand chronischer körperlicher und seelischer Überspannung, Verkrampfung und Ungelöstheit unter- halten, und bei denen die Übersteigerung im Seelischen unmittelbar ihr Korrelat in einer chronischen Übererregtheit der Großhirnrinde und des Zwischenhirns und in einer aus diesen Hirnzentren induzierten Übersteigerung der Kreislauf- arbeit und des Arterien- und Arteriolentonus haben. Hier begegnet uns also die psychosomatische Seinsweise des Menschen unmittelbar in ihrer unauflösbaren und unauslotbaren Einheit[1]. Daher kann auch nur eine grundlegende Änderung der technisch-zivilisatorischen Lebensbedingungen des modernen Menschen, zu- gleich aber seine Heimkehr in die großen Ordnungsgefüge menschlichen Seins mit der Zeit die Hypertonie als Massenerscheinung wieder überwinden.

Daß es *Hypertonien durch primäre diffuse oder tumorhafte Hyperplasien der Nebennierenrinde, des Nebennierenmarkes* und *der basophilen Epithelien des Hypo- physenvorderlappens* gibt, bedarf keiner besonderen Hervorhebung mehr, da sie allgemein im Bilde der Nebennierenrindenhyperplasie und des Nebennieren- rinden-Adenoms bei der *Cushingschen Krankheit* und ihren Abortivformen, im Bilde des *Phäochromocytoms* des Nebennierenmarkes oder an anderen peripheren Ganglien des sympathischen Systems und schließlich im Bilde des *basophilen Adenoms oder der diffusen Wucherung der basophilen Epithelien des Hypophysen- vorderlappens* bekannt sind. Wichtig ist nur, daß mit der Feststellung der diffusen Hyperplasie oder des Adenoms an den genannten Strukturen wahrscheinlich noch nicht das erste Glied in der Ursachenkette der Hypertonie nachgewiesen ist. Es bleibt die Frage, welche Faktoren von Fall zu Fall die Hyperplasie bzw. das Adenom verursacht haben, genetische, embryonal-peristatische, peristatische in der Kindheit, in der Reifezeit oder im Alter, psychosomatische, renale. Daß bei einem Teil der Fälle genetische, embryonal-peristatische oder frühkindlich-peri- statische Einwirkungen entscheidend sind, beweisen die frühkindlichen Fälle von Cushingscher Krankheit und von Phäochromocytom.

Pharmakologisch-experimentell wurde die Hypertonie durch *Nebennierenrinden- hormon* vielfach untersucht.

Zunächst konnte bei Hunden[2], dann bei einseitig nephrektomierten Ratten[3] nach Des- oxycorticosteron (DOCA) eine beträchtliche langdauernde Blutdruckerhöhung hervorgerufen

---

[1] BÜCHNER 1950—1960, ENKE und GERCKEN 1955.
[2] KUHLMAN, RAGAN, FERREBREE, ATCHLEY und LOEB 1939.   [3] SELYE und PENTZ 1943.

werden. Dieser Befund wurde besonders nach Adrenalektomie bestätigt[1]. Andererseits gelang
es bei adrenalektomierten Ratten unter NaCl-armer Kost auch durch *Cortison* Hypertonie zu
erzielen[2], während bei DOCA die NaCl-Armut die Hypertonie verhütete, NaCl-Reichtum sie
förderte[3]. Die Anregung der Regeneration der Nebennierenrinde nach Enucleation eines
Teiles der Nebennieren durch einseitige Nephrektomie und NaCl-Fütterung führte, besonders
bei jungen Ratten, durch Nebennierenhyperplasie zur Hypertonie[4]. Wurde die Nebennierenrinde im Experiment durch Hypophysenvorderlappensubstanz stimuliert und zur Hyperplasie gebracht, so kam es ebenfalls zur Hypertonie.

Es ist verständlich, daß im Zeitalter der therapeutischen Anwendung von
Nebennierenrindenhormonen oder ACTH durch Überdosierungen von ACTH oder
Cortison die Cushingsche Krankheit mit Hypertonie in Einzelfällen zur Ent-
wicklung kam[5].

Von besonderer allgemein-pathologischer Bedeutung sind die Untersuchungen
über die *renale Verursachung von Hypertonie.*

HARTWICH (1930) hatte, angeregt von VOLHARD, nachgewiesen, daß durch
Einengung einer Nierenarterie eine Hypertonie experimentell hervorgerufen werden kann. GOLDBLATT und seine Mitarbeiter (1934) haben diesen Befund bestätigt und systematisch experimentell weiter durchgearbeitet. Im folgenden
sprechen wir daher vom Hartwich-Goldblatt-Phänomen, wenn ein renaler Drosselungshochdruck gemeint ist. In den weiteren Untersuchungen ergab sich, daß
die Blutdruckwirkung der Drosselung der Nierenarterie nicht neural-reflektorisch,
sondern humoral durch Ausschüttung einer Substanz aus der Niere hervorgerufen
wird, die an den Arteriolen verengernd angreift[6] und dadurch einen Widerstandshochdruck bewirkt. Im einzelnen wurde nachgewiesen, daß die Niere bei der
Einengung ihrer Arterie einen Stoff in ihr Venenblut abgibt, der als *Renin* eine
nicht blutdruckwirksame Vorstufe, das *Hypertensinogen,* in das blutdrucksstei-
gernde *Hypertensin* umwandelt. Renin wirkt also bei intravenöser Injektion
als *Hypertensinase* (=Angiotonase), indirekt blutdruckerhöhend, Hypertensin
dagegen als die unmittelbar wirksame Substanz.

Dabei zeigte aus Schweinenieren gewonnenes Renin die folgenden Ergebnisse[7]: *eine*
Renineinheit erhöhte den mittleren Blutdruck beim nichtnarkotisierten Hund um 30 mm.
Bis zu 1,2 E bewirkte Renin eine Blutdrucksteigerung, deren Höhe direkt proportional der
injizierten Reninmenge war. Die langsame und konstante Infusion einer relativ kleinen
Renin-Menge (0,5 E/min) führte zu einer Erhöhung des Blutdruckes für die Dauer des Versuches. Die Dauerinfusion einer relativ großen Reninmenge (2,0 E/min) bewirkte einen
schnellen und starken Anstieg des Blutdruckes. Renin wurde weder bei unbehandelten
Hunden noch nach Injektion größerer Reninmengen im Harn gefunden, es wird also schnell
und zu 100% im Organismus abgebaut.

Über den Ort der Reninbildung innerhalb der Niere konnte festgestellt werden,
daß sich die Hauptmenge des Renins in der Rinde findet und im Mark nur Spuren
nachweisbar sind[8]. Es ließ sich andererseits in einer Fraktion B ein blutdrucksenkender Faktor nachweisen, der ebenfalls in der Rinde wesentlich reichlicher
vorhanden ist als im Mark.

Unter normalen hämodynamischen Bedingungen wird nur wenig Renin aus
der Niere freigesetzt, dagegen unter Senkung des Blutdruckes reichlich[9]. Daraus
wird gefolgert, daß bei Drosselungsischämie eine Hypoxie der Capillarmembranen
der Niere, dadurch aber eine hypoxische Permeabilitätssteigerung der Membranen
und infolge der erhöhten Capillarpermeabilität der Durchtritt großmolekularer
Proteine, also auch von Renin ausgelöst wird.

---

[1] ALLARDYCE, SALTER und RIXON 1951, KNOWLTON und Mitarbeiter 1952, SKELTON 1955.
[2] TOUSSAINT 1951, KNOWLTON, LOEB, STOERK, WHITE und HEFFERNAN 1952.
[3] KNOWLTON und Mitarbeiter 1952, SKELTON 1954.   [4] SKELTON 1956.
[5] SELYE 1950, MASSON, HAZARD, CORCORAN und PAGE 1950.   [6] ABELL und PAGE 1942.
[7] GOLDBLATT, LAMBORM und HAAS 1953.   [8] YOSHIMURA und NEGISHI 1954.
[9] KOHLSTAEDT und PAGE 1957.

Die weitere experimentelle Durcharbeitung des renalen Drosselungshochrucks ergab das folgende:

Wurden bei Hunden beide Nierenarterien eingeengt oder die Bauchaorta oberhalb des Abganges der Nierenarterien, so war die Blutdruckerhöhung besonders hoch und es entwickelte sich eine maligne Hypertonie[1]. Beim Kaninchen trat die Hypertonie noch leichter und schwerer ein, wenn zuerst die eine Niere entfernt und etwa 14 Tage später an der noch vorhandenen Niere die Drosselung herbeigeführt wurde[2]. Wurden bei Ratten oder bei Hunden beide Nieren in Seide eingeschnürt, so daß auf diese Weise eine Ischämie der Nieren eintrat, so kam es ebenfalls zur markanten Hypertonie[3].

Hier ordnen sich Befunde von *Drosselungshochdruck beim Menschen* infolge Stenose *einer* Nierenarterie ein. Insbesondere können arteriosklerotische Stenosen, thrombotische Einengungen die arterielle Durchblutung der Nieren einschränken mit dem Ergebnis, daß eine Hypertonie zur Entwicklung kommt, die dann, wenn die Stenosen nur an der einen Niere entwickelt sind, durch Operation geheilt werden können[4].

Daß die Ischämie der Niere nachwirkt, ergaben die folgenden Versuche:

Wurde bei Ratten die eine Nierenarterie für 3 Std abgeklemmt und anschließend die andere entfernt, so entwickelte sich nach wenigen Tagen eine Hypertonie[5]. Auf der anderen Seite zeigten Tiere, bei denen nach Entfernung der einen und Drosselung der anderen Niere eine Hypertonie entstanden und für einige Zeit (bis zu 2 Monaten) aufrechterhalten war, nach Aufhebung der Drosselung verschiedene Befunde: In einer Untersuchungsreihe wurde bei Kaninchen in kurzer Zeit eine Normalisierung des Blutdruckes beobachtet, in einer anderen, in der die Dauer und Höhe des Blutdrucks größer war, trat ein baldiger Blutdruckabfall nur bei einem Drittel der Tiere ein[6].

Konnte hier noch eine Nachwirkung der Nierenischämie nach Aufhebung der Drosselung für das Weiterbestehen der Hypertonie herangezogen werden, so wird die Auslösung extrarenaler Faktoren durch längerdauernden Drosselungshochdruck mit der Tatsache bewiesen, daß eine durch Drosselung der einen Niere (mit Seide) und Entfernung der anderen verursachte Hypertonie beim Kaninchen oder Hund fast bis zum Tode anhält, wenn die letzte Niere auch noch entfernt wurde[7]. Daraus wird von KOLFF und PAGE (1955) geschlossen, daß im Beginn der renalen Hypertonie das System Renin-Hypertensin entscheidend ist, daß aber bei chronischer renaler Hypertonie die normale Niere die Fähigkeit einbüßt, den Blutdruck auf seinem Normwert zu halten. Ob dieser Effekt auf den Wegfall eines blutdrucksenkenden Faktors der normalen Nierenrinde[8] zurückgeht, ist ungeklärt. Jedenfalls zeigt aber eine Serie von Experimenten, daß die Entfernung beider Nieren auch ohne vorausgehende Drosselung zur Hypertonie führt[9].

Diese konnte besonders dann beobachtet werden, wenn bei Hunden nach doppelseitiger Nephrektomie eine künstliche Niere angelegt oder eine Peritonealspülung durchgeführt wurde, so daß Überlebenszeiten bis zu 19,5 bzw. 21—42 Tagen erzielt wurden[10]. Dabei trat die Hypertonie auch dann ein, wenn mit den Nieren beide Nebennieren entfernt wurden und die Nebennierenrindenhormone nicht substituiert wurden[11]. Durch NaCl-Zufuhr wurde bei solchen Hunden die Hypertonie gefördert[12].

---

[1] GOLDBLATT 1938.
[2] PICKERING und PRINZMETAL 1938, DANIEL, PRICHARD und WARD-McQUAID 1954.
[3] KEMPF und PAGE 1942, SMITH, ZEEK und McGUIRE 1944, SMITH und ZEEK 1947.
[4] MORITZ und OLDT 1937, FREEMAN und HARTLEY 1938, LEITER 1938, OPPENHEIMER, KLEMPERER und MOSKOWITZ 1939, STEWART 1940, RICHARDSON 1943, GYÖRI 1952, GOODMAN 1952, LENG-LÉVY und Mitarbeiter 1952, HILLENBRAND 1956.
[5] KOLETSKY 1950.   [6] DANIEL, PRICHARD und WARD-McQUAID 1954.
[7] PICKERING 1945, DANIEL, PRICHARD und WARD-McQUAID 1954, KOLFF und PAGE 1955.
[8] YOSHIMURA und NEGISHI 1954.
[9] MUIRHEAD, VANATTA und GROLLMAN 1949, MUIRHEAD und Mitarbeiter 1950, MUIRHEAD, TURNER und GROLLMAN 1951.   [10] TURNER und GROLLMAN 1951.
[11] TURNER und GROLLMAN 1951.   [12] MUIRHEAD, JONES und GRAHAM 1953.

Zusammenfassend seien noch einmal folgende ätiologische Faktoren als Ursachen chronischer Blutdruckerhöhung hervorgehoben:

1. Die genuine Hypertonie ist in der Regel eine Erkrankung mit familiärer Disposition und dominantem Erbgang. Beim Tier lassen sich Sippen mit Anlagen zur Blutdruckerhöhung züchten.

2. Bei der genuinen Hypertonie des Menschen finden sich eine Vermehrung der Basophilen des Hypophysenvorderlappens sowie eine Hyperplasie der Nebennierenrinde und des Nebennierenmarkes als Zeichen der Anpassung dieser inkretorischen Strukturen an die gesteigerte Druckarbeit des Herzens. Hypertonieverursachende Veränderungen sind an den inkretorischen Drüsen bei genuiner Hypertonie nicht nachzuweisen.

3. Auch an den peripheren und zentralen nervösen Regulatoren des Blutdruckes ließen sich bisher keine hypertonieverursachenden Strukturveränderungen nachweisen.

4. Bei der genuinen Hypertonie spielen chronische psychosomatische Übersteigerungen und Überforderungen bei vorhandener Hypertonie-Disposition als Realisatoren der Anlage eine große Rolle.

5. Durch Adenome oder Hyperplasie der Basophilen des Hypophysenvorderlappens, durch diffuse oder adenomatöse Hyperplasie der Nebennierenrinde und durch das Phäochromocytom des Nebennierenmarkes oder anderer chromaffiner Gewebe entstehen Krankheiten mit paroxysmaler oder permanenter Hypertonie.

6. Durch ACTH oder Nebennierenrindenhormon lassen sich Blutdruckerhöhungen und chronische Hypertonien hervorrufen.

7. Bei verschiedenen doppelseitigen Nierenkrankheiten entwickeln sich chronische renale Hypertonien. Im Experiment läßt sich eine chronische Hypertonie durch Ischaemie der Nieren, aber auch durch Entfernung beider Nieren unter Dialyse, vor allem mit NaCl-Fütterung herbeiführen. Die Bedeutung des Reninmechanismus wird dadurch sehr eingeschränkt.

8. Beim Menschen kommen operativ heilbare Hypertonien durch einseitige Verengerung einer Nierenarterie vor.

2. Auswirkungen chronischer Hypertonien am arteriellen System.

Seit langem ist den Klinikern wie Pathologen die häufige Koppelung zwischen *Hypertonie und Arteriosklerose* des großen Kreislaufes bekannt. Sie wurde zuerst mit der Annahme gedeutet, daß die Arteriosklerose oder verwandte Arterienerkrankungen die Hypertonie verursachen[1]. Spätere Untersuchungen führten aber zu der Feststellung, daß die Arteriosklerose, wenn sie beim Hypertoniker beobachtet wird, in der Regel eine Folge der Hypertonie darstellt.

Für diese Auffassung konnte zuerst die Tatsache ins Feld geführt werden, daß bei Hypertonikern häufig an den Arteriolen der Niere, des Pankreas, der Leber und anderer parenchymatöser Organe eine *Arteriolosklerose* beobachtet wird, die beim Normotoniker eine große Seltenheit darstellt[2]. Zwar wurde lange Zeit von einzelnen Pathologen ein Zusammenhang zwischen der Arteriolosklerose und Hypertonie verneint[3]. Die Tatsache aber, daß die Arteriolosklerose in Frühfällen der Hypertonie noch vermißt wird[4], daß sie mit der Dauer der Hypertonie an Ausdehnung über die verschiedenen Organe zunimmt, während sich zugleich die einzelnen Herde nach anfänglicher Hyalinose und anschließender Lipoidose

---

[1] Volhard und Fahr 1914, Romberg 1921.
[2] Jores 1903, 1924, Hueck 1920, Aschoff II 1936, Frey 1951.
[3] Besonders Th. Fahr 1925, für den Herzmuskel Odel 1939, Wegelin 1944.
[4] Jores 1903, Hueck 1920, Rühl 1927, 1929.

der Intima bis zur Calcinose weiter verändern, spricht für die Verursachung dieses Prozesses durch Hypertonie. Hinzu kommt, daß die hypertonische Arteriolosklerose auch an früher weniger beachteten Organen bei genuiner wie bei renaler Hypertonie in gleicher Schwere nachweisbar ist, so z.B. im Herzmuskel[1], in der Netzhaut[2] und besonders in der Aderhaut sowie im N. opticus[3]. Beweisend für die Verursachung der Arteriolosklerose durch chronische Hypertonie sind aber die Beobachtungen bei Hypertonie durch Phäochromocytom. Hier konnte die Arteriolosklerose mit Hyalinose und Lipoidose der Intima in einer Serie von Arbeiten an Niere, Pankreas und anderen Organen nachgewiesen werden[4], in einer größeren Anzahl schon bei Kindern und bei Erwachsenen vor dem 30. Lebensjahr. Ebenso wird die Verursachung der Arteriolosklerose durch chronische Hypertonie dadurch bewiesen, daß dieses Bild bei experimentellem Drosselungshochdruck an den Arteriolen vor allem des Magen-Darmkanals und des Pankreas reproduziert werden konnte[5].

Indirekt wurde die Auffassung von der Verursachung der Arteriolosklerose durch Hypertonie auch dadurch bewiesen, daß bei schnell fortschreitender, mit besonders starker Blutdruckerhöhung einhergehender, in der Regel durch Urämie zum Tode führender maligner Hypertonie[6] ein verwandter, aber morphologisch deutlich von der Arteriolosklerose unterschiedener Gefäßprozeß gefunden wird: das Bild der *Arteriolonekrose*. Hier sieht man in der Wand der Arteriolen der Niere und anderer Organe eine körnig-krümelige Nekrose der verdickten Intima, zum Teil verbunden mit Nekrose der glatten Muskelzellen der Media, nicht selten auch mit sekundärer leukocytärer Infiltration der Nekrose oder Ersatz der Nekrose durch Sprossung von Mesenchymzellen aus der benachbarten Intima unter dem Bilde einer Endarteriolitis obliterans. Dieser Befund wurde zuerst von FAHR (1914)[7] als kennzeichnend für die maligne Hypertonie beschrieben und klar von dem der Arteriolosklerose abgegrenzt. In der Folge wurde er von zahlreichen anderen Untersuchern bestätigt. Die meisten Pathologen haben die *Arteriolonekrose* als fortgeschrittenes Stadium der Arteriolosklerose[8] oder als *Intensitätsvariante der Arteriolosklerose* und als die Folge einer besonders schnell und intensiv fortschreitenden Blutdruckerhöhung gedeutet[9]. Gegen diese Auffassung hat FAHR (1925) eingewandt, daß in seinem Beobachtungsgut bei der benignen Hypertonie mit Arteriolosklerose nur 24% der Verstorbenen unter 60 Jahren alt waren, bei der malignen Hypertonie dagegen 92,5%. Eine ähnliche Altersverteilung wurde von späteren Untersuchern festgestellt[10]. Dies spricht jedoch nicht gegen, sondern für die primäre Bedeutung der Blutdruckerhöhung bei der Arteriolonekrose, da bei jüngeren Menschen in der Regel steilere und schnellere Blutdruckanstiege beobachtet werden und die stärker durchsaftete Arteriolenwand leichter der Nekrose anheimfällt. Der Übergang aus der Arteriolosklerose in die Arteriolonekrose wurde durch Vergleich intravitaler Nierenbiopsien mit dem Autopsiebefund neuerdings exakt nachgewiesen[11]. Danach tritt die Arteriolonekrose immer erst in den fortgeschrittenen Stadien der malignen Hypertonie auf.

Experimentell wird die Bedeutung der Hypertonie für die Entstehung der Arteriolonekrose und anderer Wandveränderungen der Arterien im großen

---

[1] ODEL 1940, KATHKE 1955.   [2] DE LA FONTAINE-VERVEY 1927, MARQUARDT 1957.
[3] KOYANAGI 1928, BERGSTRAND 1948, MARQUARDT 1957.
[4] BIEBL und WICHELS 1925, PAUL 1931, VOLHARD 1931, BÜCHNER 1934, GÄRTNER 1936, GEIGER 1939, WEBER 1949, HEIMBUCHER 1950, LIEBEGOTT 1953.
[5] GOLDBLATT 1938.   [6] VOLHARD und FAHR 1914.   [7] VOLHARD und FAHR 1914.
[8] JORES 1903, 1924.   [9] SCHÜRMANN und MACMAHON 1933, PICKERING 1952.
[10] KLEMPERER und OTANI 1931, SCHÜRMANN und MACMAHON 1933, HÜRZELER 1954, ENDES und Mitarbeiter 1955.   [11] ENDES und Mitarbeiter 1955.

Kreislauf durch eine Serie von Arbeiten über den Drosselungshochdruck bewiesen.

Als erster hat GOLDBLATT 1938 an Hunden durch Drosselung beider Nierenarterien oder der Aorta oberhalb beider Arterien die Arteriolonekrose mit Nekrose der Intima und Media und entsprechende Veränderungen an den kleineren Arterien hervorgerufen. Dabei waren die Arteriolen und kleinen Arterien des Magen-Darmtractus, des Pankreas der Gallenblase besonders stark betroffen. Gleiche Veränderungen konnten durch intensiven Drosselungshochdruck an der Ratte nach Stenosierung der Nierenarterien[1] an Ratte und Hund nach Einhüllung der Niere in Seide[2] sowie bei akuter Hypertonie am Hund bzw. am Kaninchen durch beiderseitige Nephrektomie[3] am Kaninchen durch Renininfusion nach Nephrektomie[4] nachgewiesen werden.

In den meisten dieser Experimente traten neben der Arteriolonekrose an den kleineren Arterien Veränderungen mit dem Bilde der *Panarteriitis nodosa* auf[5]. Diese Veränderungen wurden vor allem am Mesenterium, am Hilus der Organe, an den Coronararterien beobachtet. Sie entsprachen dem Bilde der Panarteriitis nodosa des Menschen, während bei der Hypersensibilitäts-Angitis Arterien und Venen befallen waren[6]. Auch die Injektion von Desoxycorticosteron (DOCA) führte zu dem Bild[7]. Die genaue Analyse der Versuchsbedingungen in den verschiedenen Experimenten ergab, daß die Blutdruckerhöhung den ausschlaggebenden Faktor für die Entstehung dieser Veränderungen darstellt und daß die schnell ansteigende Hypertonie besonders ausschlaggebend für sie ist[8], daß sie durch Niereninsuffizienz zusätzlich gefördert wird[9], daß aber die Niereninsuffizienz nicht obligate Voraussetzung ist[10].

Es steht also fest, daß die Hypertonie in der spontanen Pathologie des Menschen die Arteriolosklerose und als ihre Intensitätsvariante die Arteriolonekrose verursachen kann und im Experiment zusätzlich das Bild der Panarteriitis nodosa. Daraus darf gefolgert werden, daß die normale Durchflutung der Gefäßwand durch Blutplasma von der Lichtung nach der Adventitia auf einen optimalen Blutdruck angewiesen ist, und daß bei Druckerhöhung die Durchflutung der Gefäßwand insuffizient wird, so daß Verhaltungen von Plasma zur Hyalinose und sekundären Lipoidose der Intima führen und durch Ernährungsinsuffizienz der Gefäßwand Nekrosen in der Intima und in der glatten Muskulatur der Media entstehen. Dabei mögen zur Dysorie führende Schädigungen des Endothels und krankhafte Insudationen von Blutplasma noch eine zusätzliche Rolle spielen[11]. Welche Bedeutung aber kommt der Hypertonie für die Entstehung der *Arteriosklerose* an der Aorta und den Organarterien zu?

ASCHOFF (1939) hat in seinem letzten Referat über die Arteriosklerose wie in allen seinen vorhergehenden Abhandlungen (1908, 1914, 1930) betont: „Daß

---

[1] WILSON und BYROM 1939, BYROM und DODSON 1948, BALI und GOLDBLATT 1954, KOLETZKY 1955.

[2] SMITH, ZEEK und MCGUIRE 1944, SMITH und ZEEK 1947, ZEEK, SMITH und WEETER 1948, BOHLE, KOHLER und TOMSCHE 1953, LÖRINC und GORACZ 1955.

[3] MUIRHEAD, VANATTA und GROLLMAN 1949, MUIRHEAD, TURNER und GROLLMAN 1951, TURNER und GROLLMAN 1951, DANIEL, PRICHARD und WARD-MCQUAID 1954, KOLFF und PAGE 1955.

[4] PUGH, PICKERING und BLACKET 1952, MASSON, PLAHL, CORCORAN und PAGE 1953.

[5] SMITH, ZEEK und MCGUIRE 1944, SMITH und ZEEK 1947, ZEEK, SMITH und WEETER 1948, TURNER und GROLLMAN 1951, BOHLE, KOHLER und TOMSCHE 1953, BOHLE und TOMSCHE 1953.

[6] ZEEK, SMITH und WEETER 1948.   [7] SELYE und PENTZ 1943, SKELTON 1954, 1955.

[8] SMITH, ZEEK und MCGUIRE 1944, SMITH und ZEEK 1947, BYROM und DODSON 1948, TURNER und GROLLMAN 1951, PUGH, PICKERING und BLACKET 1952, KOLFF und PAGE 1955, LÖRINC und GORACZ 1955.

[9] GOLDBLATT 1938, BALI und GOLDBLATT 1954.

[10] WILSON und BYROM 1939, BYROM und DODSON 1948, KOLETSKY 1955.

[11] HUECK 1920, SCHÜRMANN und MACMAHON 1933.

weder die Altersektasie noch die Arteriosklerose irgend etwas mit dem Blutdruck zu tun hat, haben die Kliniker immer wieder betont. Wir pathologischen Anatomen können diese Beobachtung nur unterstreichen". Sein Korreferent Frey (1939) hat als Kliniker die Behauptung entgegengestellt: „In erster Linie dürfte das Leiden durch eine arterielle Blutdrucksteigerung zur Entstehung gebracht oder in seinem Fortschreiten begünstigt werden." Die Häufigkeit der Verursachung der Arteriosklerose durch Hypertonie hatte Hueck schon 1920 auf Grund pathologisch-anatomischer Untersuchungen betont. Sie wurde durch weitere Arbeiten bewiesen[1].

In der Auseinandersetzung mit der Frage nach der Ursache der hypertonischen Massenblutung wurde dann gezeigt, daß die Hypertonie häufig eine schwere Arteriosklerose der kleineren intracerebralen Arterien bis zu den Präarteriolen und Arteriolen verursacht[2]. Sie kann mit einer Arteriosklerose[3] der basalen Hirnarterien verbunden sein, muß es aber nicht. Sie ist in ihrem Verteilungsschema, in ihrer Gangart[4] für die Hypertonie typisch. Dabei zeigen die kleineren Arterien und Arteriolen alle Übergänge von der subintimalen Hyalinose zur Mesenchymverquellung und zur Medianekrose mit sekundärer Mediafibrose[5]. Hier handelt es sich also um eine Standort-, vielleicht auch um eine Intensitätsvariante des banalen arteriosklerotischen Herdes (Arteriopathia und Arteriolopathia hypertonica[6]).

Ein ähnliches Verteilungsschema zeigt die beim Hypertoniker besonders häufig und früh auftretende hypertonische *Coronarsklerose*. Sie ist nicht nur in den proximalen Abschnitten der Kranzadern, wie in der Regel die Arteriosklerose des Normotonikers, entwickelt, sondern mit besonderer Bevorzugung auch in den extramuralen und intramuralen feineren Verzweigungen des Coronarsystems, also weit in die Peripherie des Coronarsystems ausgedehnt[7].

Eine bis in die Peripherie ausgebreitete Arteriosklerose ließ sich bei der malignen Hypertonie auch an der *Niere* nachweisen, hier wiederum mit typischen Intensitätsvarianten[8].

Fragt man nach dem pathogenetischen Mechanismus, der zu dieser Verursachung der Arteriosklerose und ihrer Varianten führt, so ist es notwendig, vor allem jene diffusen Arterienwandveränderungen hervorzuheben, die vor dem Auftreten der arteriosklerotischen Herd- und Beetbildungen schon bei jeder Hypertonie festzustellen sind: *die Hyperplasie der Media und der Intima* des arteriellen Systems. Schon Thoma (1886—1921), Jores (1898—1924) und Aschoff haben auf dieses der Arteriosklerose in der Regel vorausgehende Phänomen aufmerksam gemacht. Bei der Hypertonie ist es besonders ausgeprägt. Dabei handelt es sich um eine diffuse Vermehrung des elastisch-kollagenen Gewebes in der Intima sowie der elastischen Strukturen und der glatten Muskulatur in der Media. Sekundär kann sich ein Schwund glatter Muskulatur in der Media und ihr Ersatz durch fibröses Gewebe anschließen. Linzbach (1944) hat diesen Anpassungsvorgang der Hyperplasie von Intima und Media in den Mittelpunkt der Pathogenese der hypertonischen Arteriosklerose gerückt, indem er in Anlehnung an Feststellungen von Warburg (1926) folgendes postulierte: Der

---

[1] Rühl 1929, 1938, Wg. Rotter 1944/1949, Albertini 1956, Büchner 1956, Linzbach 1957, Bredt 1957.
[2] Böhne 1927, Rühl 1927, 1929, Neubuerger 1930, Wirtz 1936, Schimkat und Kathke 1958.   [3] Stochdorph und Meessen 1957.   [4] Rühl 1929.
[5] Staemmler 1927, Anders und Eicke 1939, 1940, Spatz 1939, Scholz und Nieto 1938, Stochdorph und Meessen 1957.
[6] Anders und Eicke 1939, 1940.
[7] Hueck 1920, Wg. Rotter 1944/1949, Bäurle 1950, Kathke 1955, Schimkat und Kathke 1959, Rau 1956, Büchner 1956.   [8] Schürmann und MacMahon 1933.

normalen Durchflutung der inneren Aortenwand und der gesamten Arterienwand ist eine für den Stoffwechsel der Gefäßwand optimale Schichtdicke zugeordnet. Von einer bestimmten Grenzschichtdicke an ist der normale Stoffwechsel nicht mehr in allen Wandschichten zu verwirklichen. Durch Überschreitung der Grenzschichtdicke kommt also die Arterienwand zwangsläufig in eine Insuffizienz ihres Stoffwechsels, besonders der oxydativen Prozesse. So kommt es einerseits zu Degenerationen der glatten Muskulatur in der Media[1], andererseits zu Verhaltungen von Plasma in der Intima und dadurch zur Hyalinose, Lipoidose und Calcinose des arteriosklerotischen Herdes. WG. ROTTER (1944/1949) hat daneben vor allem auf die Behinderung der normalen Aorten- und Arterienwanddurchflutung infolge der starken Druckbelastung der Wandstrukturen aufmerksam gemacht. Wieweit daneben noch zusätzliche Störungen im Lipoidstoffwechsel und Vermehrungen der Cholesterinester oder der Lipoproteide die Arteriosklerose des Hypertonikers fördern, steht hier nicht zur Erörterung.

Zusammenfassend kann über die Folgen der Hypertonie am arteriellen System des großen Kreislaufs in der menschlichen Pathologie und im Experiment festgestellt werden:

1. Infolge der Hypertonie jeder Ätiologie kommt es in Anpassung an den abnorm gesteigerten Druck zu einer elastisch-fibrösen Hyperplasie der Intima und zu einer muskulären Hyperplasie der Media der Aorta und der Organarterien bis zu den Arteriolen.

2. Durch Überschreitung der Grenzschichtdicke in der hyperplastischen Aorten- und Arterienwand entwickeln sich herdförmige Defekte in der muskulären Media mit fibrösem Ersatz und arteriosklerotischen Herdbildungen in der Intima.

3. Da die Druckerhöhung sich bis zu den Arteriolen auswirkt, breitet sich die hypertonische Arteriosklerose bis in die periphersten arteriellen intraorganellen Verzweigungen z. B. des Gehirns, des Herzmuskels, der Niere und als Arteriolosklerose bis in die Arteriolen, besonders der Nieren, des Pankreas, des Gehirns aus.

4. Bei schnell sich steigernder intensiver Druckbelastung des arteriellen Systems infolge maligner Hypertonie entwickelt sich in der Regel eine Intensitätsvariante der Arteriolosklerose im Bilde der Arteriolonekrose. Ihr kann statt einer Arteriosklerose eine Arterionekrose der kleinen Organarterien zugeordnet sein.

5. Beim experimentellen Drosselungshochdruck durch Stenosierung der Nierenarterien oder Umwicklung der Nieren mit Seide oder beim Hochdruck durch doppelseitige Nephrektomie oder durch Desoxycorticosteron (DOCA) entwickelt sich je nach Intensität der Blutdruckerhöhung eine Arteriolosklerose oder eine Arteriolonekrose, bevorzugt in den Arteriolen des Magendarmtractus, des Pankreas, der Gallenblase.

6. Darüber hinaus entsteht bei der experimentellen Hypertonie in der Regel eine Panarteriitis nodosa, bevorzugt an den Arterien des Mesenteriums, des Hilus der Organe und des Herzmuskels.

Die pulmonale Hypertonie.

So sehr es heute bewiesen ist, daß die Hypertonie des großen Kreislaufes in der Regel die Folge primär funktioneller Engerstellungen der arteriellen Strombahn, besonders der Arteriolen, ist, so ungeklärt ist bis heute noch die Frage, ob am Pulmonalsystem primär funktionelle Engerstellungen des Gefäßsystems zu einer primär funktionellen pulmonalen Hypertonie führen können, ob es also eine genuine funktionelle Hypertonie des Pulmonalsystems gibt und ob diese häufiger vorkommt.

---

[1] W. W. MEYER 1957.

Nach ihrem Bauplan bieten die Gefäße des Pulmonalsystems durchaus die Voraussetzungen für aktive, funktionell ausgelöste Kaliberschwankungen. Nach BENNINGHOFF 1930, 1935 zeigen die größeren Lungenarterien einen ähnlichen Bau wie die Aorta, sind aber durch reichliche glatte Muskelfasern gekennzeichnet, welche schräg zur Achse des Gefäßrohres in der Media verlaufen. Sie sind Spannungsmuskeln für das elastische Gerüst und stehen im Dienst der Windkesselfunktion der proximalen Anteile der Pulmonalarterien[1]. Auch noch an den kleineren Pulmonalarterienästen bis zu einem Durchmesser von 1 mm herrscht diese Wandstruktur vor. Dagegen zeigen die kleineren Arterien weiter distal in der Media eine typische Ringmuskulatur. In dieser Gefäßstrecke sind also aktive Querschnittsänderungen sehr gut möglich. Auch die Arteriolen sind durch den Einbau glatter Ringmuskulatur gekennzeichnet und zwar in einfacher Schicht bis zu einem Querschnitt von 40 μ, bis zu 20 μ^2. Damit ist also auch im Bereich der Arteriolen der Lungen eine aktive Engerstellung möglich, nicht nur an einzelnen Arteriolen, sondern am ganzen pulmonalen Arteriolensystem.

Hinzu kommt, daß die Lungenvenen zu einem Teil durch eine breite Schicht ringförmig verlaufender glatter Muskulatur Drosselvenen sind[3]. Theoretisch besteht also auch die Möglichkeit einer funktionellen venösen Abflußbehinderung.

Die alten Physiologen waren der Auffassung, daß die Lungendurchblutung infolge der geringen Widerstände und des geringen Druckes druckpassiv erfolgt[4], und daß eine nervöse Steuerung des Pulmonalkreislaufes ohne wesentliche Bedeutung ist[5]. Neuere Untersuchungen rückten aber die Vorstellung einer aktiven Blutverteilungs- und Druckregulierung unabhängig vom Blutvolumen und Druck des großen Kreislaufs in den Vordergrund[6]. Zwar werden vorher kollabierte Capillaren druckpassiv durch stärkere Dehnung der Lunge bei vertiefter Atmung eröffnet, so daß dadurch das Blutvolumen in der pulmonalen Strombahn zunimmt, während der Pulmonaldruck gesenkt wird[7]. Die Möglichkeit aktiver Mitwirkung der Vasomotoren und der Modifikation der druckpassiven Volumen- und Drucksteuerung durch deren wechselnd starke Tonisierung blieb aber zunächst offen[7]. Eindeutig bewiesen wurde die Beeinflußbarkeit der glatten Muskulatur der Pulmonalarterien im Sinne der aktiven Kontraktion oder der aktiven Dilatation durch die Experimente von EULER und LILJESTRAND (1947): Unter Sauerstoffmangelatmung beobachteten sie eine Kontraktion mit Druckanstieg im rechten Ventrikel, unter reiner Sauerstoffatmung eine Dilatation mit Druckabfall im rechten Ventrikel. Nervöse Einflüsse waren dafür nicht entscheidend.

Um die Jahrhundertwende hat die Klinik das Krankheitsbild einer chronischen, primären, schließlich tödlichen pulmonalen Hypertonie entworfen, als AYERZA (1901) das nach ihm benannte Krankheitsbild mit dem Syndrom schwerer Cyanose, Dyspnoe und Polycythämie bei starker anatomisch nicht begründeter Hypertrophie der rechten Herzkammer beschrieb. Inzwischen gelang es nicht nur, dieses Bild immer klarer von der cardial oder pulmonal verursachten anatomisch fundierten pulmonalen Hypertonie abzugrenzen. Es stellte sich durch subtilere histologische Untersuchungen auch heraus, daß viele Fälle anscheinend primär funktioneller pulmonaler Hypertonie in charakteristischen morphologisch und ätiologisch verschiedenartigen organischen Wand- und Lichtungsänderungen des Pulmonalsystems, besonders der kleineren und kleinsten Pulmonalarterien, ihre Ursache haben. Für das Pulmonalsystem wurde damit, im Unterschied zur

---

[1] BENNINGHOFF 1930, 1935, WAGNER 1940, H. SCHMIDT 1953.
[2] MERKEL 1941, VON HAYEK 1953.   [3] BENNINGHOFF 1930, 1935.
[4] TIGERSTEDT 1903.   [5] LICHTHEIM 1876, TIGERSTEDT 1903.
[6] HOCHREIN und KELLER 1932.   [7] R. WAGNER 1940.

Hypertonie des großen Kreislaufs der Akzent mehr und mehr von der funktionellen auf die strukturelle Seite in der Frage der Ätiologie der pulmonalen Hypertonie verlagert. Vom Standpunkt des Pathologen wurden diese Fragen in den letzten Jahren vor allem von Könn (1956, 1957, 1958) durchgearbeitet und dargestellt. Im folgenden stützen wir uns besonders auf seine Abhandlungen.

Die fortschreitende Erforschung dieser Probleme führte aber andererseits auch zu der Erkenntnis, daß die chronische Drucksteigerung im Pulmonalsystem bei genügender Dauer und Intensität ihrerseits eine Reihe von Wandveränderungen der kleineren und kleinsten Arterien verursachen kann, die morphologisch variabler sind als die hypertoniebedingten, in der Regel arteriosklerotischen Veränderungen des großen Kreislaufs. Ja, diese hypertoniebedingten Veränderungen des Pulmonalsystems zeigen zu einem Teil eine auffallende Ähnlichkeit mit den hypertonieverursachenden Veränderungen der kleineren und kleinsten Arterien des Pulmonalsystems. So bedarf es einer besonders sorgfältigen Analyse jedes Einzelfalles und der gesamten Kasuistik, um Ursache und Folge bei der pulmonalen Hypertonie klar voneinander zu trennen. In jedem Falle wird man erwarten dürfen, daß die hypertoniebedingten Gefäßveränderungen an der Steigerung und Fixierung der pulmonalen Hypertonie mitzuwirken vermögen wie z. B. die Arteriosklerose der kleinen Arterien und die Arteriolosklerose bei der Hypertonie im großen Kreislauf[1].

Die organischen Schäden, die eine pulmonale Hypertonie (p. H.) zu verursachen pflegt, können wir in die folgenden Gruppen unterteilen[2]: 1. Kardial verursachte p. H., 2. durch Fehlbildungen der großen Arterien verursachte p. H., 3. durch Veränderungen des Lungengewebes bedingte p. H., 4. durch organische Veränderungen der Pulmonalgefäße bedingte p. H.

Unter den *kardial bedingten pulmonalen Hypertonien* überwiegt der Häufigkeit und Schwere nach die *Mitralstenose*, die in der Phase der Insuffizienz des linken Vorhofs zwangsläufig durch Behinderung des venösen Abflusses aus der Lunge zur p. H. führt. Hier haben schon die alten Kliniker und Pathologen nach der Art des Herzfehlers die p. H. postuliert[3]. Seit der systematischen Herzkatheterung ist die p. H. in solchen Fällen tausendfach exakt gemessen. Drucksteigerungen auf die Höhe des Aortendruckes und darüber sind dabei keine Seltenheit[4]. In anderen Fällen liegt der kardial bedingten p. H. nicht selten eine *chronische Insuffizienz des linken Ventrikels* und Vorhofs infolge großer *Infarktnarbe* in der Muskulatur der linken Herzkammer zugrunde, die ebenfalls eine Abflußbehinderung aus der Lunge verursacht[5]. In seltenen Fällen verursacht ein *Myxom des linken Vorhofs* dadurch eine markante p. H., daß der Tumor die Mitralklappe zum Teil verlegt[6] (Abb. 47b). Als *angeborene Herzfehler* können die Septumdefekte, sowohl ein größerer Defekt des Vorhofseptums als auch ein Defekt des Septum membranaceum, durch einen Links-Rechts-Shunt zur p. H. führen. Beim Defekt des Septum membranaceum erfolgt von der Geburt an eine Aortalisation des Pulmonalsystems, beim Defekt des Vorhofseptums kommt es mit der Zeit zur Druckerhöhung im Pulmonalsystem durch das unphysiologisch große Blutvolumen infolge der Summation des Blutes beider Vorhöfe.

---

[1] Siehe bei Könn 1956—1958.
[2] Vgl. Posselt 1909, Ljungdahl 1915, Steinberg 1929, Brenner 1935, Bredt 1941, Wg. Rotter 1944/1949, Könn 1956, 1957.
[3] Romberg 1891, Torhorst 1904, Posselt 1909, W. Fischer 1909, Parker und Weiss 1936, Heath und Whitaker 1955.
[4] Vgl. Bayer, Loogen und Wolter 1954, Loogen 1958, Klepzig 1955.
[5] Torhorst 1904, Posselt 1909, Ljungdahl 1915, Brenner 1935, Wg. Rotter 1944/1949 Könn 1956.
[6] Schroeder, unveröffentlicht 1952, Könn 1956.

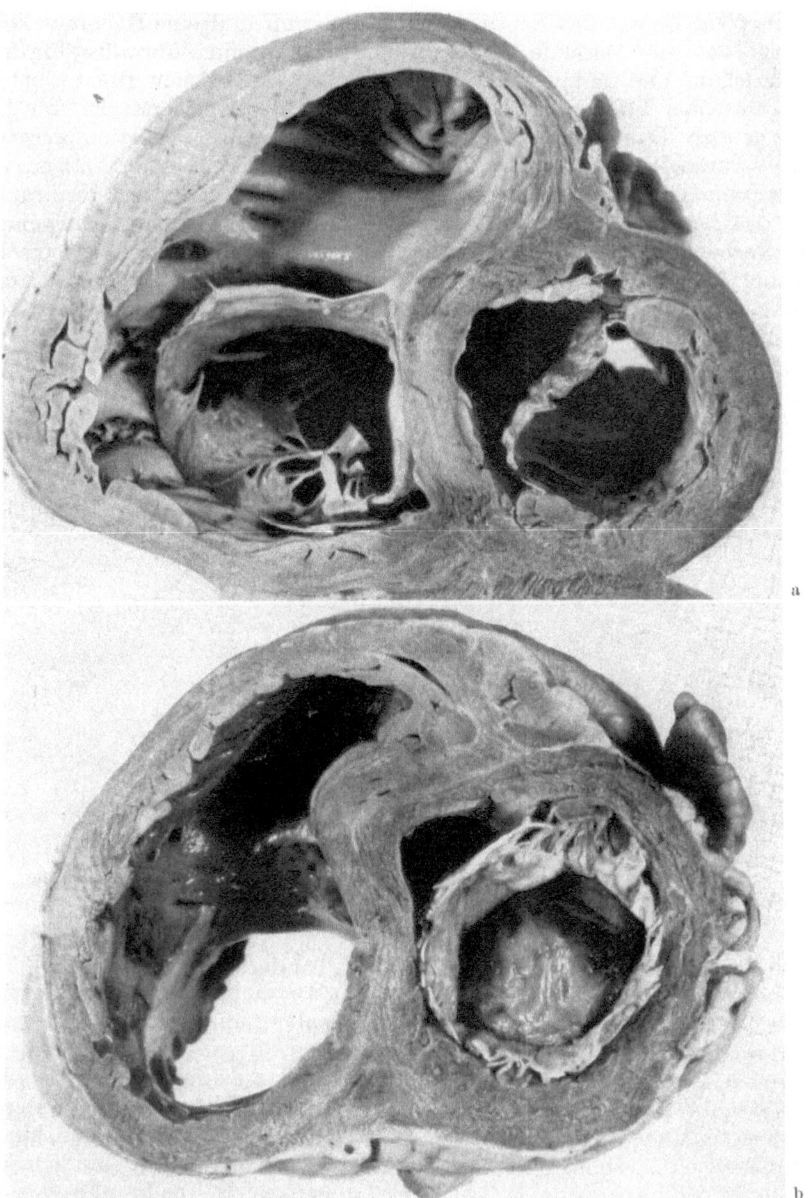

Abb. 47a u. b. a Chronisches Cor pulmonale mit Hypertrophie des rechten Ventrikels (links) infolge Panarteriitis nodosa der Lungenarterien. b Chronisches Cor pulmonale mit starker Hypertrophie des rechten Ventrikels (links) infolge Myxom des linken Vorhofs mit Einengung der Mitralklappe (rechts). (Beobachtungsgut von G. KÖNN.)

In den Erörterungen über die p. H. werden diese beiden angeborenen Septum-defekte neuerdings häufiger herangezogen[1].

Unter den *angeborenen Fehlbildungen der großen arteriellen Gefäße* ist vor allem der Eisenmenger-Komplex als Ursache einer pulmonalen Hypertonie zu nennen.

[1] WELCH und KINNEY 1948, OLD und RUSSEL 1950, EDWARDS 1950, 1957, KIPKIE und JOHNSON 1951, MEESSEN 1954, 1957, BRAUNSTEIN 1954, BERTHRONG und COCHRAN 1955, O'NEAL und THOMAS 1955, COSSEL 1956, DOWNING und WELLER 1956, KÖNN und STORB 1960.

Hier führt ein Defekt des Septum membranaceum und eine Rechtsverlagerung der Aorta, also eine reitende Aorta, in der Regel zu einer Aortalisation des Pulmonalkreislaufs und dadurch zur p.H.[1]. Auch beim offenen Ductus arteriosus Botalli wird das Pulmonalsystem in der Regel durch Überstrom von Aortenblut über den Ductus in die Lungenarterien einer Aortalisation ausgesetzt[2].

Die Verursachung der p.H. durch *chronische Erkrankung des Lungengewebes*, also aus pulmonaler Ursache, ist seit langem bekannt. Hier wird der krankhafte Prozeß des Lungengewebes teils durch Drosselung der kleineren Lungenarterien durch Narbengewebe von außen, teils durch das Übergreifen chronisch entzündlicher Prozesse der Lunge auf die Wand der kleineren Arterien unter Entwicklung einer obliterierenden Endarteriitis wirksam[3] (Abb. 48). Hier ist auch

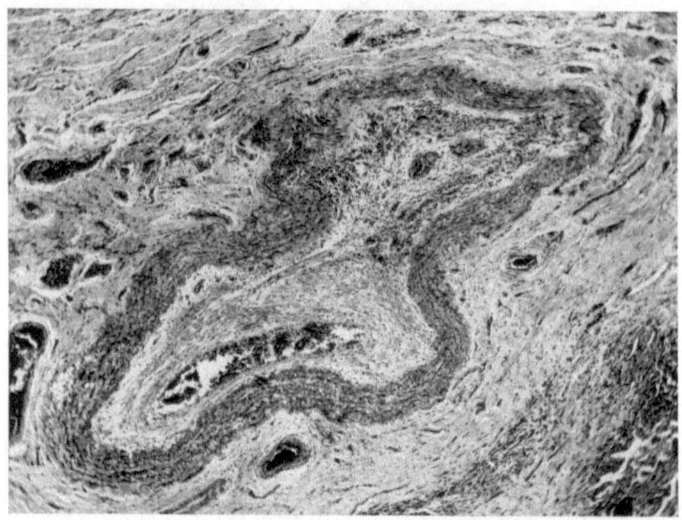

Abb. 48. Endarteriitis obliterans einer mittleren Lungenarterie bei ausgedehnter narbig abgeheilter Lungentuberkulose mit Cor pulmonale. Herzgewicht: 390 g. [Nach Könn, G., Ergebn. ges. Tuberkulose- u. Lungenforsch. **14**, 101, 1958, Abb. 24.]

die p.H. bei chronischer Silikose einzuordnen, bei der es durch die Hyalinisierung der silikotischen Knötchen zunehmend zu einer Drosselung, durch endarteriitische Änderungen zur Stenosierung kleiner und kleinster Lungenarterien kommt[4].

Während die bisher dargestellten kardialen, dysgenetisch-vasculären und pulmonalen Ursachen der p.H. mit bloßem Auge zu erfassen sind, werden die *pulmonal-vasculären Prozesse*, die zu einer p.H. führen können, in der Regel erst durch systematische, mikroskopische, histotopographische Untersuchung des pulmonalen Gefäßsystems nachweisbar. Bei einem Teil der Prozesse jedoch kann schon die Lupenpräparation der kleineren Lungenarterien die krankhaften Gefäßveränderungen sichtbar machen (Koenn 1956).

Zunächst sind hier *entzündliche Wand- und Lichtungsveränderungen der kleineren und kleinsten Lungenarterien* zu nennen. Ayerza (1901) stellte in seinem

---

[1] Stewart und Crawford 1933, Old und Russel 1950, Brown, Heath und Whitaker 1955.

[2] Heath und Whitaker 1955, Brewer 1955, Meessen 1957.

[3] W. Fischer 1909, Ljungdahl 1915, Schultz 1927, Mylius und Schürmann 1930, Giese 1931, Pagel und Henke 1930, Gerstel 1933, Brenner 1935, Parker 1940, Berblinger 1947, Leitner 1949, Nuti und Rellini 1950, Samuelsson 1952, Lavenne und Meersseman 1954, Leinwand, Duryee und Richter 1954, Tosetti 1955.

[4] Giese 1931, Gerstel 1933, Lavenne 1951, Lavenne und Meersseman 1954.

Fall die *Syphilis der Pulmonalarterien* in den Mittelpunkt, obwohl das Protokoll seines Falles histologisch keine Hinweise auf diese Diagnose enthält[1]. Nach einer Reihe von Arbeiten ist aber nicht daran zu zweifeln, daß die syphilitische Arteriitis infolge endarteriitischer Lichtungseinengungen zur p. H. führen kann[2]. Im neueren Schrifttum rücken jedoch andere ätiologische Formen der Arteriitis als Ursache der p. H. in den Vordergrund. Das gilt besonders von der *Panarteriitis nodosa der Lungenarterien* (Abbildung 47a). Während Gru- ber (1926) die Beteiligung der Lungenarterien an diesem Krankheitsbild mit 3,7% angab, stellten spätere Untersucher insgesamt einen Anteil von 25—30% fest[3], bei Kindern allerdings nur 3:30 Fällen mit völliger Autopsie[4]. Es konnten aber auch Einzelfälle[5] und kleinere Beobachtungsreihen[6] mitgeteilt werden, in denen die Panarteriitis nodosa ausschließlich in beiden Lungen entwickelt war und zu einer klassischen p. H. geführt hatte. Dabei waren zum Teil schon lupenmikroskopisch segmentär an den Aufteilungen der kleinen Lungenarterien knötchenförmige Auftreibungen zu erkennen (Könn 1956). Im übrigen zeigen die befallenen kleinen Arterien histologisch segmentär fibrinoide Wandveränderungen und dichte Infiltrate aus neutrophilen

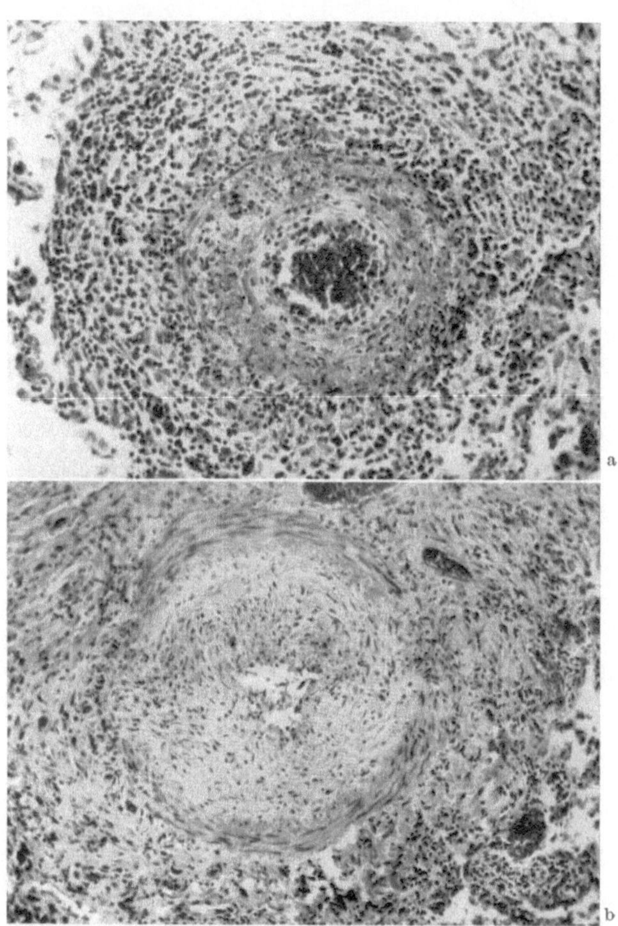

Abb. 49a u. b. Panarteriitis nodosa kleiner Lungenarterien a im floriden, b im Narbenstadium. Chronisches Cor pulmonale. Herzgewicht: 575 g. [Nach Könn, G., Beitr. path. Anat. **116**, 273, 1956, Abb. 2].

und eosinophilen Leukocyten, Lymphocyten und Plasmazellen, aber auch Wandnekrosen oder einen Ersatz der Wand durch Narbengewebe (Abb. 49). Durch Einbeziehung der Intima in die Infiltration oder in die Vernarbung bestanden starke Stenosen der kleinen Arterien. In einem der Fälle hatte sich das Bild im Zuge eines Gelenkrheumatismus von 10jähriger Dauer entwickelt[7], in 3 Fällen

---

[1] Brenner 1935. [2] Arrillaga 1924, Barlaro 1917, Warthin 1919, Escudero 1926.
[3] Harris, Lynch und O'Hare 1939, Andersen 1948, Hicks 1953.
[4] Rothstein und Welt 1933.
[5] Gruber 1926, Sternberg 1925, Bredt 1932, Meessen 1951, Symmers 1952, Staemmler 1954 u. a.
[6] Braunstein 1954, Könn 1955, 1956. [7] Könn 1956.

war es mit einer langdauernden Mitralstenose verbunden[1]. Auf die Mitbeteiligung der arteriovenösen Anastomosen und der Sperrarterien der Lunge an diesem Bilde können wir hier nur kurz verweisen[2].

Auch die *Endarteriitis obliterans* (Winiwarter-Bürger) *der Lungenarterien* kann Ursache einer p. H. sein, wie aus Einzelbeobachtungen hervorgeht[3]. In der Regel ist sie dabei Teilerscheinung einer generalisierten Endarteriitis obliterans. Gelegentlich fand sie sich in der Lunge, während im großen Kreislauf eine Panarteriitis nodosa bestand[4].

Eine seltene, aber interessante vasculäre Ursache der p. H. wurde aus Ägypten als gelegentliche Komplikation der *Bilharziose*, also der Infektion mit dem Schistosomum Bilharzia, mitgeteilt[5]. Die Eier des Schistosomum können, als Emboli in die Lunge verschleppt, an der Wand der Arteriolen eine nekrotisierende Arteriolitis verursachen. Diese kann zu einer obliterierenden Arteriolitis führen, die partiell von einer Rekanalisation gefolgt ist. So kann es bei ausgedehntem Befall der Arteriolen zur klassischen pulmonalen Hypertonie kommen, bei Befall der Lungen durch die Bilharziose in 6,3% der Fälle[6].

Diese Beobachtung leitet uns zu einer der wichtigsten vasculären Ursachen der p. H. über, zur p. H. nach *rezidivierender thrombotischer Streuembolie der Lungen* und Organisation der Emboli (Abb. 50 und 51). Je weiter

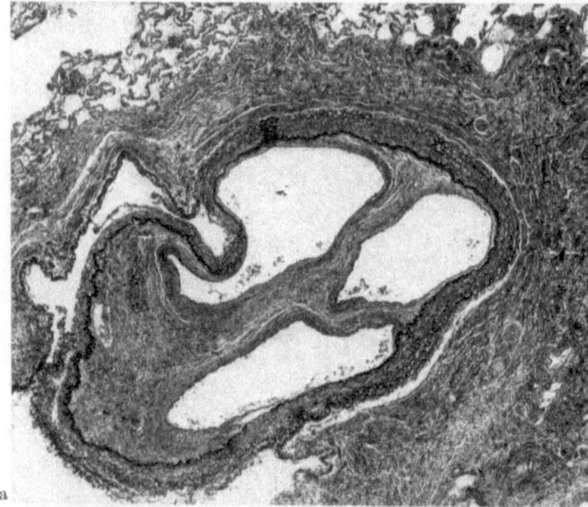

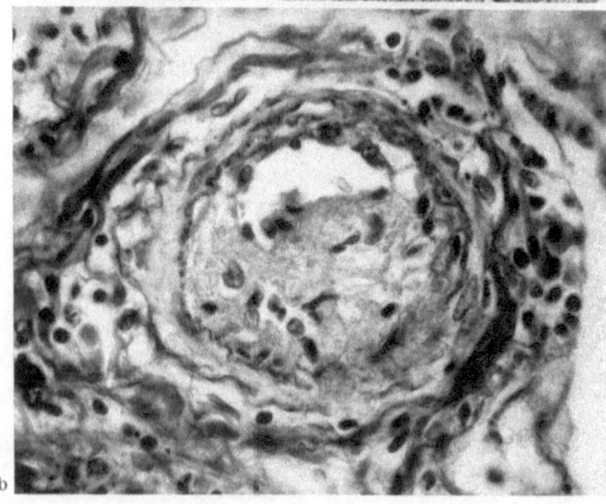

Abb. 50. a Postembolische Narben in einer mittleren Lungenarterie mit cavernösem neugebildetem Gefäßsystem. b Kleinere Lungenarterie, durch Organisation eines Embolus weitgehend obliteriert. Chronisches Cor pulmonale. [Nach Könn, G., Ergebn. ges. Tuberkulose- u. Lungenforsch. 14, 101, 1958, Abb. 12 u. 13.]

peripher die Emboli verschleppt und je zahlreicher sie auf beide Lungen verteilt werden, um so größer ist nach ihrer Organisation und partiellen Rekanalisation ihre permanente stenosierende Wirkung, um so schwerer infolgedessen die p. H. In der Literatur liegt heute eine Serie von Mitteilungen über dieses Krankheitsbild vor[7]. Ob es daneben eine autochthone Thromboendarteriitis obliterans der

[1] Braunstein 1954.   [2] Könn 1955, 1956.
[3] Jäger 1932, Hadorn 1938, Terbrüggen 1951, Könn 1956.
[4] Könn 1956.   [5] Shaw und Ghareeb 1936.   [6] Shaw und Ghareeb 1936.
[7] Eppinger und Wagner 1920, Löwenstein 1922, Ljungdahl 1928, Goedel 1930, Merkel 1947, Spencer 1950, Muirhead, Montgomery und Gordon 1952, Bobeck und Vanek 1953, Barnard 1954, Hiltbold 1954, Lavenne und Meersseman 1954, Lenègre, Gerbaux, Scebat und Lecompte de Floris 1955, Könn 1956, 1958.

Lunge[1] mit dem gleichen Bilde der Organisation und partiellen Rekanalisation thrombotischer Massen gibt, ist bis heute nicht geklärt[2]. Schon die älteren Autoren machen auf die große Schwierigkeit aufmerksam, das Narbenbild der Streuembolie und das der genuinen Thrombose der kleinen Lungenarterien voneinander abzugrenzen[3]. Wir selbst nehmen auf Grund der Untersuchungen von KÖNN (1956, 1957) an, daß die Streuembolie bei weitem die häufigste Ursache dieses Bildes ist; wir können aber nicht ausschließen, daß nach entzündlichen Lungenerkrankungen mit Übergreifen auf die kleinen Arterien das Bild durch genuine Thrombose kopiert werden kann. Ob die Präcipitation von Globulin bei Hyperglobulinämie infolge von Plasmocytose mit anschließender Organisation zu einem ähnlichen Befund führen kann[4], bedarf weiterer Untersuchungen.

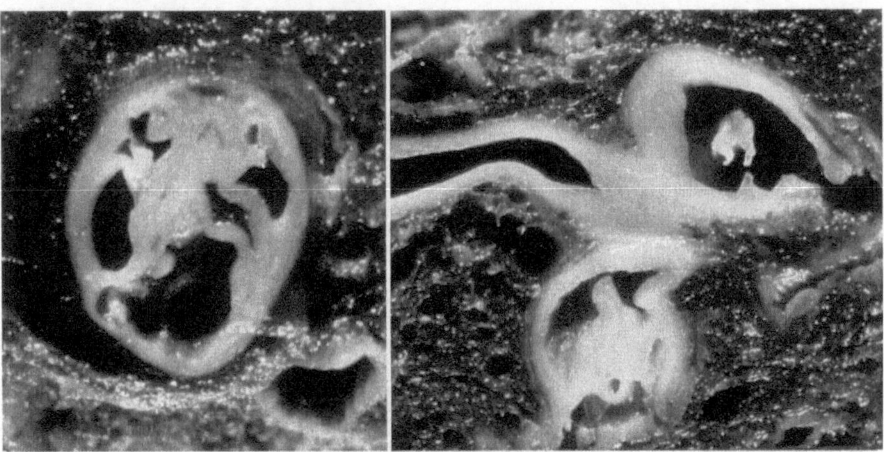

Abb. 51. Mittlere intrapulmonale Arterie bei Lupenpräparation mit grober, unregelmäßiger, narbiger Unterteilung des Gefäßes nach rezidivierender Embolie. Chronisches Cor pulmonale, Herzgewicht: 515 g. [Nach KÖNN, G., Ergebn. ges. Tuberkulose- u. Lungenforsch. 14, 101, 1958, Abb. 16.]

Die experimentelle Forschung hat versucht, durch intravenöse Injektion kleinster Fibringerinnsel aus Kaninchen- oder Menschenblut beim Kaninchen das Bild zu reproduzieren[5]. Zunächst ist das nicht überzeugend gelungen. Dabei war man der Meinung, das Bild der Embolusorganisation sei histologisch mit dem einer Arteriosklerose der Pulmonalarterien identisch[6]. Das führte dann zu der Auffassung, die arteriosklerotischen Herde der Pulmonalarterien seien Sekundärprodukte organisierter Thromben oder Emboli[7]. Neueste Experimente von CHR. BÜCHNER und KÖNN (1959) haben aber eindeutig zu folgenden Ergebnissen geführt: Wurden bei Kaninchen rezidivierende feinste Fibringerinnsel aus Kaninchen- oder Menschenblut in größerer Menge intravenös injiziert, so entwickelte sich nach Organisation der Gerinnsel bei den Tieren zunächst ein chronisches Corpulmonale mit eindeutiger Hypertrophie des rechten Ventrikels und deutlicher Verschiebung der Rechts-Links-Relation zugunsten der rechten

---

[1] WIESE 1936.

[2] HÖRA 1935, HÖNIG 1937, STAEMMLER 1937, MERKEL 1947, TERBRÜGGEN 1951, MUIRHEAD, MONTGOMERY und GORDON 1952, SCHMIDT 1953, LENÈGRE und Mitarbeiter 1955, KÖNN 1956.

[3] MØLLER 1923, BRENNER 1935.   [4] MUIRHEAD, MONTGOMERY und GORDON 1952.

[5] HARRISON 1948, WARTMANN und Mitarbeiter 1951, MUIRHEAD und MONTGOMERY 1951. DUGUID und ANDERSON 1952, HEARD 1952, BARNARD 1954, CHR. BÜCHNER und KÖNN 1959, KÖNN und CHR. BÜCHNER 1959.

[6] DUGUID und ANDERSON 1952.   [7] DUGUID und ANDERSON 1952, MORGAN 1959.

Kammer (Abb. 52a und b). Später als 100 Tage nach der letzten Injektion von
Fibringerinnseln waren aber die neugebildeten Gefäße in den Organisationsnarben

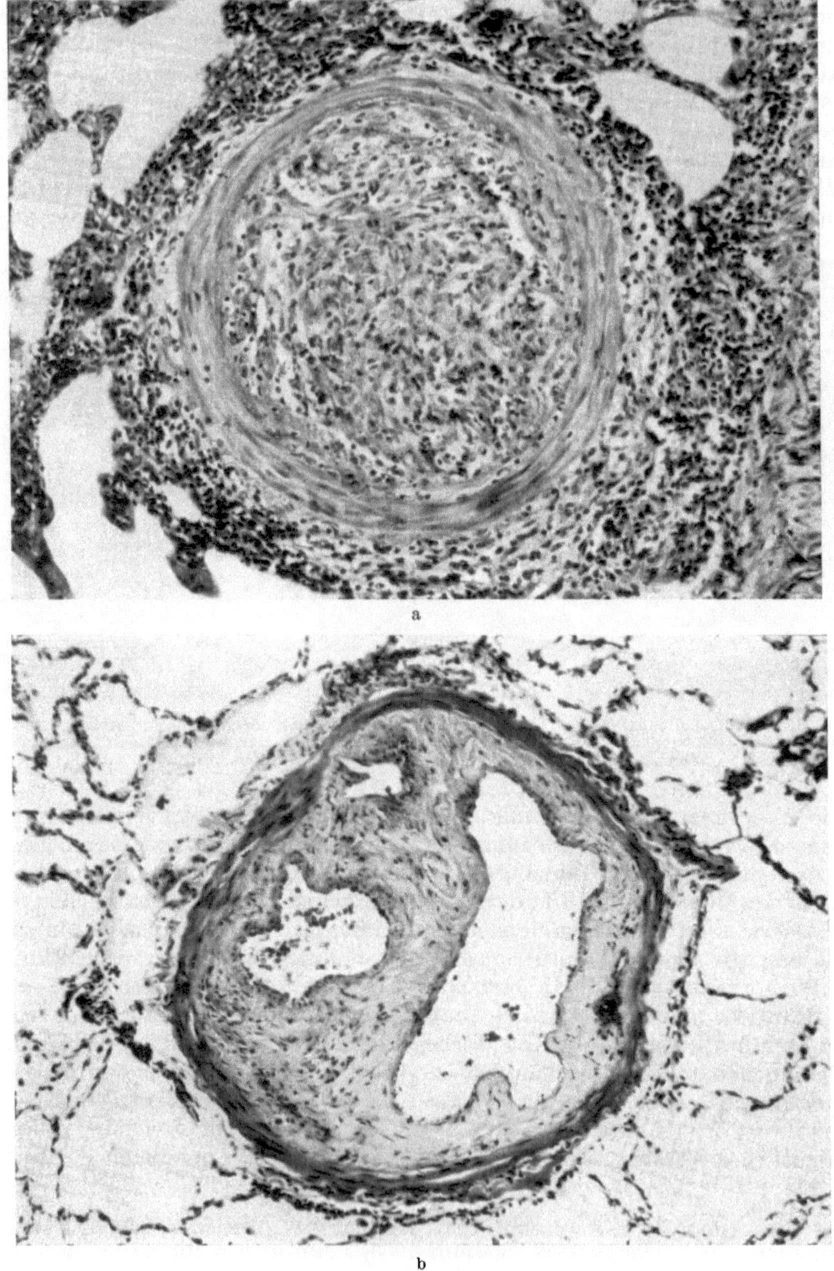

Abb. 52a—c. Experimentelle Fibrinembolie beim Kaninchen. a Durchwachsung des Embolus durch junges
Mesenchym nach 8 Tagen. b Ältere Narbe mit Rekanalisation.

der Gerinnsel so stark ausgeweitet, daß diese kein Hindernis mehr für den Lungenkreislauf bedeuteten (Abb. 52c): das Cor pulmonale, also die Rechtshypertrophie

bildete sich wieder zurück. Als Spuren akuter Überlastungen des rechten Ventrikels nach den Embolien waren in dessen Wand je nach dem Zeitpunkt der Tötung akute Parenchymnekrosen von Herzmuskelzellen oder deren jüngere oder ältere Narben nachzuweisen. Die Herde in den Pulmonalarterien täuschten im Einzelschnitt des Randgebietes arteriosklerotische Polster vor, in der Serie erwiesen sie sich aber als typische Narbenstenosen nach Organisation.

Auf Grund dieser experimentellen Beobachtungen und von Beobachtungen der menschlichen Pathologie vermuten wir, daß es *auch beim Menschen ein*

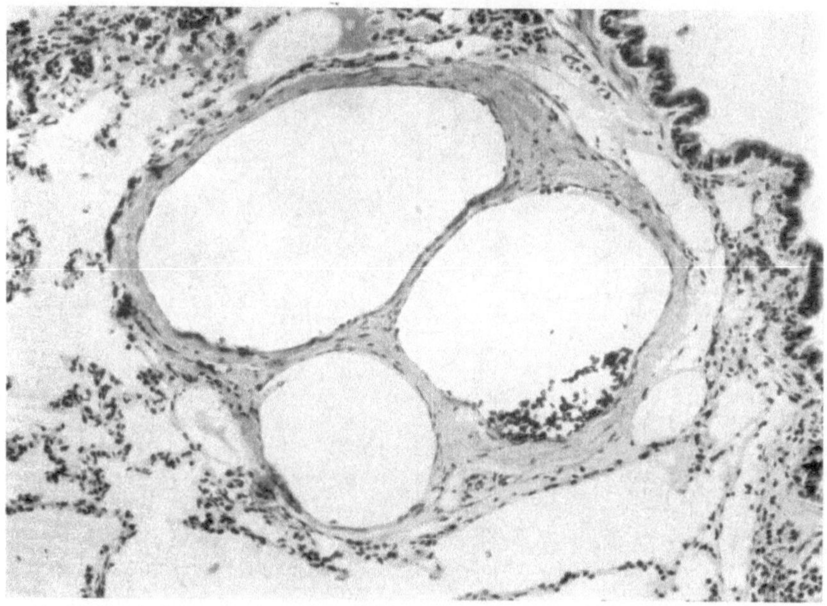

Abb. 52c. Alte Narbe mit Rekanalisation und starker Ausweitung der neugebildeten Gefäße. [Abb. 52a—c nach Büchner, Chr., u. G. Könn, Beitr. path. Anat. **121**, 170, 1959, Abb. 3, 6 u. 8.]

temporär chronisches Cor pulmonale nach rezidivierender Lungenembolie gibt und daß in solchen Fällen im Zuge der Thrombusorganisation eine schwere Herzkrankheit mit pulmonaler Embolie kommen und wieder verschwinden kann.

Darüber hinaus gelang es Berg und Könn soeben, das Bild einer *permanenten pulmonalen Hypertonie mit bleibendem Cor pulmonale* durch experimentelle Streuembolie von nicht organisierbarem Polyvinyl nach intravenöser Injektion am Kaninchen zu erzeugen. In der Muskulatur des rechten Ventrikels fanden sich ausgedehnte Narben nach Parenchymnekrosen.

Die Behinderung der Lungenstrombahn kann in seltenen Fällen auch in den kleinen Lungenvenen liegen. Durch Endophlebitis kommt es hier mitunter zu hochgradigen Stenosen unter Entwicklung von Fremdkörperriesenzellen, selbstverständlich mit dem Ergebnis, daß auch dadurch ein chronisches Cor pulmonale entwickelt wird. Da hier die Druckerhöhung bis in den capillären Anteil der Lunge besteht, kommt es zu rezidivierenden Blutungen in die Alveolen und im Anschluß daran zu hochgradiger Eisenspeicherung in den Alveolarepithelien (Abb. 53) (Ceelen 1931, Könn 1956, 1958).

Das Problem der Ursachen und der Folgen der p. H., besonders der Wandveränderungen an den kleinen Lungenarterien, ist aber dadurch noch besonders kompliziert, daß die p. H. bei genügender Dauer und Intensität an den kleinen

Arterien und an den Arteriolen des Pulmonalsystems charakteristische Wandveränderungen herbeiführt, die zum Teil den Veränderungen sehr ähnlich sind,
die wir soeben als vasculäre Ursachen der p.H. kennengelernt haben (Abb. 54).
Vereinzelt wird zwar die Auffassung vertreten, daß sich die kleineren Arterien

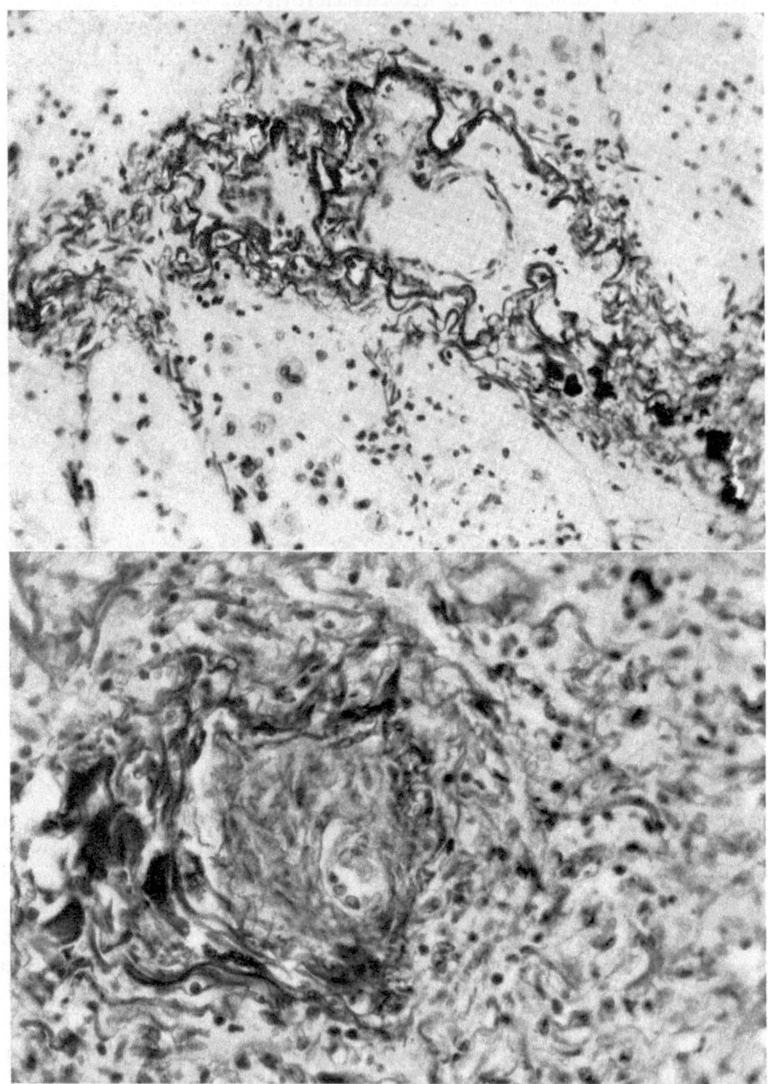

Abb. 53. Endophlebitis obliterans mit beträchtlicher bis stärkster Einengung der kleinen Venen. [Nach Könn, G.,
Ergebn. ges. Tuberkulose- u. Lungenforsch. **14**, 101, 1958, Abb. 22 u. 23.]

bei normalem Pulmonaldruck und bei p.H. in ihren Wandstrukturen nicht
wesentlich unterscheiden[1]. Mehr und mehr wurde aber die Tatsache herausgearbeitet, daß bei langdauernder intensiver p. H. eindeutig sekundäre Wandveränderungen an den kleinen Arterien beobachtet werden können. Zuerst haben
Parker und Weiss (1936) auf solche Befunde bei der Mitralstenose aufmerksam

---

[1] Welch und Kinney 1948.

gemacht. Außerdem führt die chronische p. H. an den größeren und mittleren Pulmonalarterien in der Regel zur typischen Arteriosklerose (Abb. 55—57). Die Befunde wurden in der Folge vielfach bestätigt[1]. KÖNN (1956, 1957, 1958) unterscheidet an diesen hypertoniebedingten Veränderungen das Bild der Anpassungs-

phase mit muskulärer Hypertrophie der Media und Hyperplasie der elastischen Fasern nach Zahl und Dicke und das Bild der Schädigungsphase mit Narben in der Media nach Untergang von Muskulatur und zum Teil stenosierender und obliterierender Intimawucherung. Gegenüber der Auffassung, es handle sich bei diesen Veränderungen um ein Parallelphänomen der zur Mitralstenose führenden Endocarditis oder um eine toxisch verursachte Arteriitis idiopathica unbekannten Ursprungs[2], wurde von verschiedenen Untersuchern darauf aufmerksam gemacht, daß das gleiche Bild auch bei den anderen Gruppen kardial verursachter p. H. und bei p. H. bei angeborenen Fehlern der großen Arterien beobachtet werden kann[3]. Dafür spricht vor allem auch die Tatsache, daß schon bei jüngeren Kindern mit Aortalisation des Pulmonalkreislaufes infolge Septumdefekt, offenem Ductus Botalli oder Eisenmenger-Komplex diese Befunde erhoben werden konnten[4].

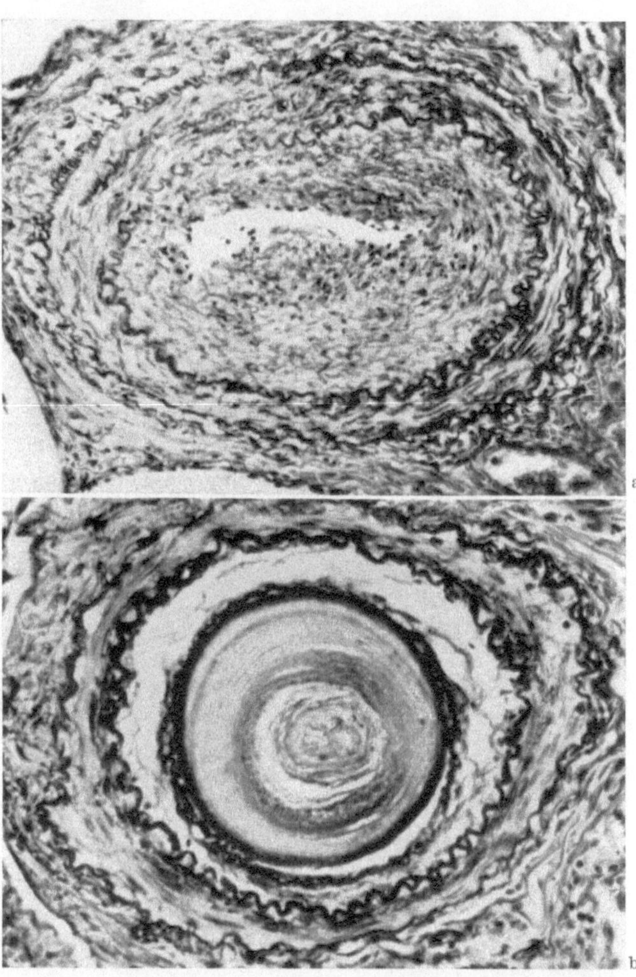

Abb. 54a u. b. Kleine Lungenarterien a mit Lichtungseinengung der Intimaproliferation, b mit hyalinisierter Intima als Folge chronischer pulmonaler Hypertonie. [Nach KÖNN, G., Ergebn. ges. Tuberkulose- u. Lungenforsch. 14, 101, 1958, Abb. 41.]

Es ist verständlich, daß diese Veränderungen sich auch als hypertoniebedingte den hypertonieverursachenden vasculären Prozessen in den primär nicht erkrankten kleineren Arterien hinzugesellen können.

Sehr bemerkenswert ist die Tatsache, daß in einer Reihe von Untersuchungen gezeigt werden konnte, daß sich als Folge einer pulmonalen Hypertonie eine

---

[1] BREDT 1937, 1941, STAEMMLER 1938, WG. ROTTER 1944/1949, KÖNN 1956.
[2] BREDT 1932.　[3] WG. ROTTER 1944/1949, MERKEL 1947, SCHMIDT 1953, KÖNN 1956.
[4] BERTHRONG und COCHRAN 1955, KÖNN 195?, COSSEL 1956, DOWNING und WELLER 1956.

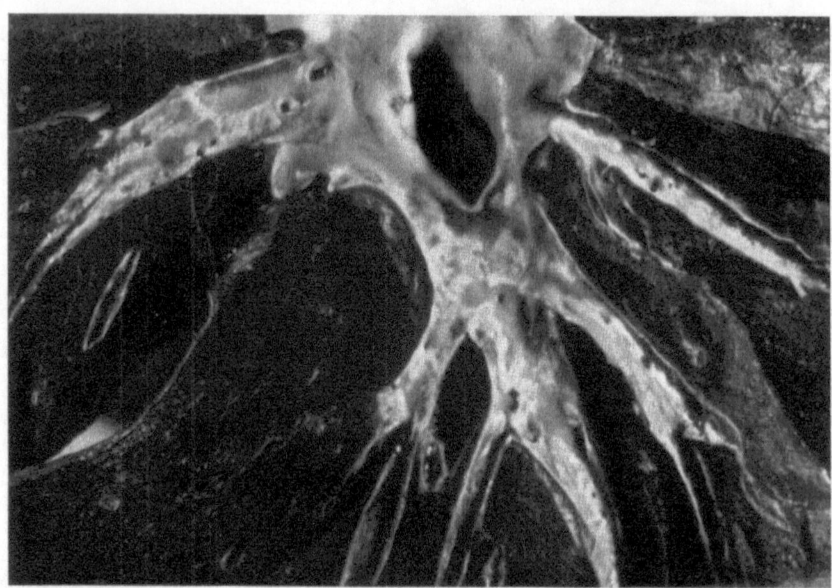

Abb. 55. Starke Arteriosklerose der Pulmonalarterien mit zahlreichen hellen fleckförmigen Lipoidose- und Hyali-
noseherden bei pulmonaler Hypertonie infolge chronischer Insuffizienz des linken Ventrikels bei alter Infarktnarbe.
[Nach Könn, G., Ergebn. ges. Tuberkulose- u. Lungenforsch. 14, 101, 1958, Abb. 30.]

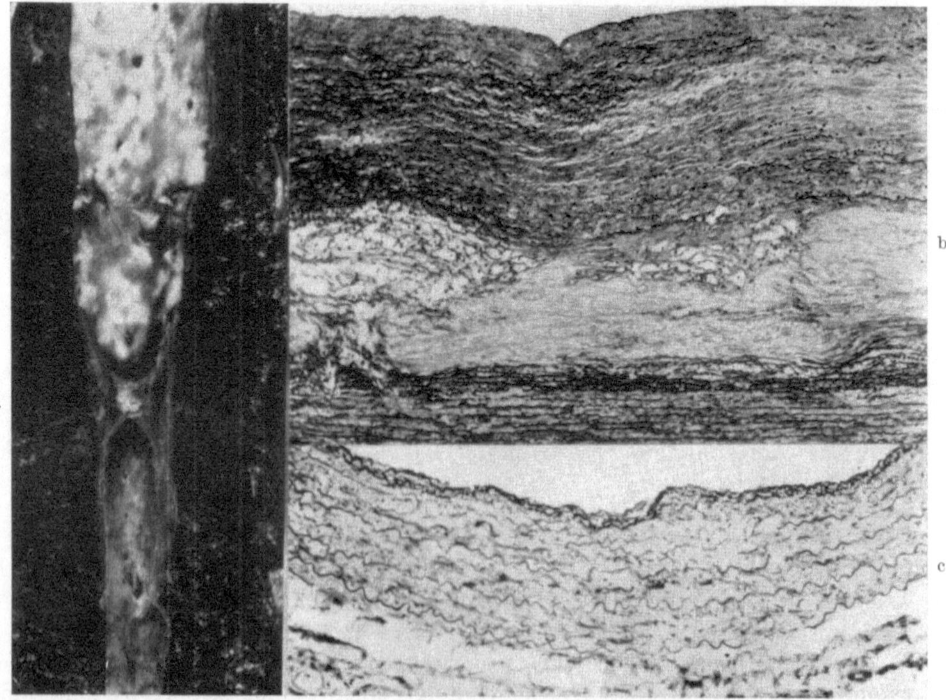

Abb. 56a—c. a Durch Organisationsgewebe (Pfeil!) stark stenosierte kleine Lungenarterie bei multiplen Narbenstenosen der Pulmonalarterien infolge rezidivierender Lungenembolie. Proximal der Stenose schwere Arteriosklerose der Pulmonalarterie. Distal normale Arterie. b Durchschnitt durch den proximalen Arterienabschnitt
mit hochgradiger Wandverdickung und schwerer Arteriosklerose. c Durchschnitt durch den distalen Arterienabschnitt mit normaler dünner Arterienwand. [Chronische pulmonale Hypertonie nach Könn, G., Beitr. path. Anat.
116, 273, 1956, Abb. 25.]

nekrotisierende Arteriitis der kleinen Pulmonalarterien entwickeln kann[1]. Dabei wurde der Befund in diesen Arbeiten vor allem bei Kleinkindern mit angeborenen Shunts beobachtet. Erst durch experimentelle Untersuchungen wird geklärt werden können, ob hier wirklich die p.H. der einzige pathogenetische Faktor ist, oder ob in dem drucküberlasteten Gefäßsystem Erreger einen besonders günstigen Ansiedlungs- oder Angriffspunkt haben, wie uns dies für die Anfälligkeit der drucküberlasteten Herzklappe oder des Ductus Botalli bekannt ist.

Wir stehen jedenfalls am Schluß dieser Erörterungen vor der Frage, ob gelegentlich eine primär-funktionelle p.H. sekundär zu einer nekrotisierenden Arteriitis der kleineren Pulmonalarterien führen kann, so daß das Bild einer

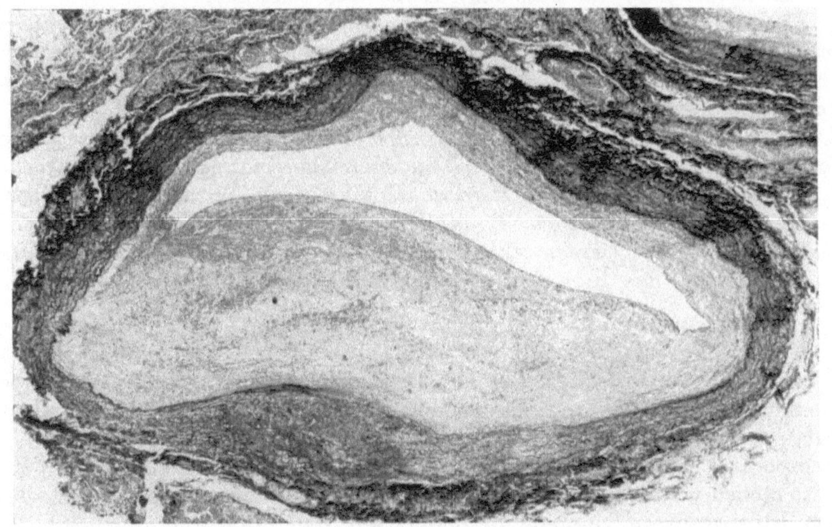

Abb. 57. Großer arteriosklerotischer Herd mit starker Lichtungseinengung infolge chronischer pulmonaler Hypertonie bei Myxom des linken Vorhofes. Herzgewicht: 475 g. [Nach KÖNN, G., Beitr. path. Anat. 116, 273, 1956 Abb. 56.]

primären, die p.H. verursachenden, auf die Lunge beschränkten Panarteriitis nachgeahmt wird. STAEMMLER (1938), W. ROTTER (1944/1949), SCHMIDT (1953), KÖNN (1956) u.a. bejahen diese Möglichkeit unter Hinweis auf einige ihrer Beobachtungen. Auch andere neuere Untersuchungen über hyperplastische, stenosierende Wandveränderungen oder nekrotisierende Arteriitis der kleinen Pulmonalarterien mit p.H. ohne anatomische Ursache der p.H. sprechen dafür[2]. Doch bedarf die Frage weiterer systematischer Untersuchungen beim Menschen und im Experiment.

Über die pulmonale Hypertonie betonen wir zusammenfassend noch einmal das Folgende:

1. Der pulmonalen Hypertonie liegen in der Regel Durchströmungshindernisse am Herzen, im Lungengewebe oder an den Lungengefäßen zugrunde.

2. Jede akute und chronische Insuffizienz des linken Herzens führt zur akuten oder chronischen pulmonalen Hypertonie. Unter den chronischen Insuffizienzen des linken Ventrikels kommt der Mitralstenose und den Zuständen nach Herzinfarkt die entscheidende Rolle zu. Daneben spielt gelegentlich das Vorhofmyxom als Hindernis an der Mitralklappe eine Rolle. Unter den angeborenen Herzfehlern führen vor

---

[1] OLD und RUSSEL 1950, HICKS 1953, KÖNN 1956, DOWNING und WELLER 1956.
[2] BERTHRONG und COCHRAN 1955, DOWNING und WELLER 1956.

allem die angeborenen Septumdefekte durch primäre Steigerung der Lungendurch-
blutung und sekundäre Erhöhung des Widerstandes im pulmonalen System zur
pulmonalen Hypertonie.

3. Chronische Narbenprozesse der Lunge gehen nicht selten mit sekundären
Intimaproliferationen und Lichtungseinengungen an den kleineren Lungengefäßen
einher. Sie wirken als Hindernisse in der Lungenstrombahn und als Ursachen der
pulmonalen Hypertonie.

4. Ohne vorgeschaltete Erkrankung des Lungengewebes können die Lungenarterien
isoliert oder im Zuge einer Erkrankung des gesamten arteriellen Systems an Pan-
arteriitis nodosa, Endarteriitis obliterans oder an Endophlebitis erkranken und durch
die Lichtungseinengung eine pulmonale Hypertonie bewirken.

5. Eine bedeutende Ursache der pulmonalen Hypertonie ist die rezidivierende
thrombotische Lungenembolie, die zahlreiche Stenosen an kleineren Lungenarterien
hinterlassen kann. Sie ist eine der wichtigsten unter den nicht kardial bedingten
Ursachen des chronischen Cor pulmonale.

6. Im Tierversuch konnte das temporäre und das chronische Cor pulmonale
infolge rezidivierender Embolie in den Lungenkreislauf nachgeahmt werden.

7. Die chronische pulmonale Hypertonie führt sekundär zu Veränderungen der
kleineren Lungenarterien durch Wandhyperplasie oder in späteren Stadien durch
Veränderungen im Sinne einer nekrotisierenden Arteriitis. An den größeren Lungen-
arterien bewirkt sie das Bild einer Arteriosklerose.

Rückblick und Ausblick.

Überblicken wir noch einmal die ausführlich dargestellten und erörterten
Phänomene der örtlichen und allgemeinen Durchblutungsstörungen, die absolute,
die relative und die spastische arterielle Ischämie, die allgemeine Oligämie und
den temporären Kreislaufstillstand, die örtliche und die allgemeine venöse Hyperämie, so stellen wir fest, daß diese Zustände in ihren akuten Formen vor allem zu
akuten Stoffwechselstörungen, besonders an den funktionstragenden Parenchymen führen. Die lebenswichtigsten Organe, der Herzmuskel und das Gehirn,
können dieser Störung des aeroben und des anaeroben Stoffwechsels bei genügender Ausdehnung und Intensität erliegen und dadurch den Tod herbeiführen.
In der Phase nach Beginn der akuten Stoffwechselstörung bis zum Tode oder bis
zur Überwindung der Durchblutungsstörung zeigen die betroffenen Organe mehr
oder minder schwere Funktionsstörungen. Wir erkennen also die Funktionsstörungen — am Hirn neurologische und psychotische Symptome, am Herzmuskel
Störungen der Dynamik, an der Leber Störungen in der Galleausscheidung und
des Kohlenhydratstoffwechsels, an der Niere solche der Harnausscheidung — als
unmittelbaren Ausdruck der ischämischen oligämischen oder venös-hyperämischen
Durchblutungsinsuffizienzen.

Dabei beobachten wir nur bei den absoluten Verschlüssen von Organarterien
und Organvenen makroskopisch erfaßbare Totalnekrosen in Teilen des Organs
oder im ganzen Organ. Alle anderen akuten Durchblutungsstörungen manifestieren sich dagegen in der Regel nur in der Dimension des Lichtmikroskops,
und zwar meist als elektive Parenchymnekrosen, d. h. in Nekrosen besonders
stoffwechselbedürftiger und schädigungsgefährdeter Strukturen. Der Nachweis
dieser elektiven Parenchymnekrosen ist deshalb von besonderer Bedeutung, weil
wir in ihnen die *Spuren* der durchlaufenen Stoffwechselstörungen zu erfassen
vermögen. Allerdings betreffen diese morphologisch faßbaren Spuren nur die
Kerngebiete größerer Schädigungsfelder, in denen in der akuten Phase lichtmikroskopisch z. T. reversible Einwässerungen zu beobachten sind.

Wir dürfen erwarten, daß sich die Ausdehnung dieser Felder genauer abgrenzen läßt, wenn wir die noch reversiblen Veränderungen mit den Methoden der Elektronenmikroskopie, des lichtmikroskopischen und des elektronenmikroskopischen Enzymnachweises und der Autoradiographie genauer analysieren. Hier hat sich ein wichtiger Weg zu neuen Forschungen eröffnet, der freilich nicht nur durch die neuen Methoden, sondern vor allem auch durch die bisherige systematische Durcharbeitung der Phänomene mit den klassischen Methoden unter Rückbeziehung auf die Erkenntnisse der modernen Biochemie und Physiologie erschlossen wurde.

Wir konnten feststellen, daß sich auch die Einbeziehung des Thrombose-Problems in stoffwechselpathologische Fragestellungen anbahnt.

Bei den akuten Zuständen der Ischämie, der allgemeinen Oligämie, des temporären Kreislaufstillstandes und der venösen Hyperämie kommt den Störungen des aeroben Stoffwechsels eine entscheidende Bedeutung zu. So sind die Erfahrungen aus der allgemeinen Pathologie der Hypoxydosen, wie sie in Band IV/2 dieses Handbuches dargestellt wurden, zugleich ein wichtiges Modell für das Verständnis der Folgen akuter Kreislaufstörungen. Dementsprechend begegnen wir in den Veränderungen der zellulären Einzelelemente wie in ihrer Topistik, am Einzelorgan und im Gesamtorganismus, verwandten Veränderungen. Auch bei dem Thrombose-Problem stellte sich uns die Frage der Mitwirkung der Hypoxydose als eines wichtigen pathogenetischen Mechanismus.

Die Erörterung über die Hypertonie im großen Kreislauf und über die pulmonale Hypertonie führten uns in der Untersuchung des arteriellen Systems sowie in der des Herzmuskels zu einem Phänomenbereich, in dem die Hypertrophie und Hyperplasie von Strukturen als Anpassung zugleich die Voraussetzung für Schäden dieser Strukturen durch Insuffizienz der Anpassung schaffen. Auf diesem Gebiete begegnen wir also Grundproblemen des pathologischen Wachstums und seiner Grenzen. Auch hier wird erst der systematische Einsatz der modernen Methoden weiterführen.

Dabei wird die weitere Entwicklung einer modernen Pathologie der Faser- und Grundsubstanzen ebenso unerläßlich sein wie in der allgemeinen Pathologie der chronischen Durchblutungsstörungen, bei der wir lichtmikroskopisch vor allem die Sklerose und die hyaline Proteinfällung kennengelernt haben.

So knüpft unser Beitrag Fäden zu vielen anderen Beiträgen dieses Handbuches.

Während des Umbruchs dieses im Frühjahr 1960 abgeschlossenen Beitrages erschienen die Bände „Herz und Kreislauf" des Handbuches der inneren Medizin, 4. Auflage. Ferner konnte ich die Druckfahnen der Monographie von L. ILLIG, „Die terminale Strombahn", Berlin-Göttingen-Heidelberg 1961, einsehen. Herrn ILLIG verdanke ich den Hinweis auf die S. 851 von mir zitierten neuesten Arbeiten von ZWEIFACH und METZ. Andere Änderungen habe ich nicht vorgenommen. Ich verweise aber auf diese wichtigen Werke.

Literatur.

ABELL, R. G., and I. H. PAGE: The reaction of peripheral blood vessels to angiotonin, renin and other pressure agents. J. exp. Med. 75, 305 (1942). — ABELL, R. G., and H. C. SCHENK: Behaviour of blood vessels in anaphylaxis. J. Immunol. 34, 195 (1938). — AHLQVIST, J., and J. BURSTEIN: A case of idiopathic pulmonary hypertension. Acta med. scand. 160, 1—5 (1958). — AHLSTROEM, C. G., u. P. G. WIDLUND: Fruchtwasserembolie. Nord. Med. 47, 361 (1952). — ALBAUM, H. G., and L. J. MILCH: Adenosine triphosphate changes induced by cold, heat and crush injury. Amer. J. Physiol. 178, 293 (1954). — ALBERTINI, A. v.: In Zusammenarbeit mit H. J. BRUNCK u. A. PAPERNITZKI, Die Coronarsklerose in der schweizerischen Bevölkerung. Eine statistische Erhebung an Hand der Sektionsfälle eines

Jahres (1. März 1955 bis 29. Februar 1956). Bull. schweiz. Akad. med. Wiss. **13**, 17 (1956). — Alella, A.: Beziehungen zwischen arterieller Sauerstoffsättigung, Sauerstoffsättigung im Sinus coronarius und Sauerstoffausnutzung im Myokard unter Berücksichtigung von Sauerstoffkapazität und arteriellem Druck. Pflügers Arch. ges. Physiol. **259**, 436 (1954). ∼ Coronardurchblutung und Hypoxie. Pflügers Arch. ges. Physiol. **261**, 373 (1955). ∼ Arterielle Sauerstoffsättigung und Coronardurchblutung. Pflügers Arch. ges. Physiol. **259**, 422 (1954). — Alexander, F.: Psychosomatische Medizin. Berlin 1951. — Alexander, N., L. B. Hinshaw and D. R. Drury: Development of a strain of spontaneously hypertensive rabbits. Proc. Soc. exp. Biol. (N.Y.) **86**, 855 (1954). — Alexander, L., and H. Lowenbach: Experimental studies on electric shock treatment. J. Neuropath. exp. Neurol. **3**, 139 (1944). — Allan, G. F.: A schema of the circulation with experiments to determine the additional load on the apparatus produced by conditions representing valvular lesions. Heart **12**, 181 (1926). — Allardyce, J., J. Salter and R. Rixon: Experimental hypertension. Amer. J. Physiol. **164**, 68 (1951). — Allen, E. V., N. W. Baker and E. A. Hines: Peripheral vascular diseases. Philadelphia and London: 1947. 2. Aufl. 1955. — Allgöwer, M., u. J. Siegrist: Verbrennungen, Berlin-Göttingen-Heidelberg: Springer 1957. — Allison, F., M. R. Smith and W. B. Wood: Studies on the pathogenesis of acute inflammation. I. The inflammatory reaction to thermal injury as observed in the rabbit ear chamber. J. exp. Med. **102**, 655 (1955). — Altmann, H. W.: Über Leberveränderungen bei allgemeinem Sauerstoffmangel, nach Unterdruckexperimenten an Katzen. Frankfurt. Z. Path. **60**, 376 (1946—1949). — Altmann, H. W., u. F. Büchner: Die seröse Entzündung der Organe. Fiat Rev. Allg. Path. **2**, 101 (1948). — Altmann, H. W., u. H. Schiche: Ein Beitrag zur Histologie und zur Einordnung der Wegenerschen Granulomatose. Beitr. path. Anat. **121**, 211 (1959). — Altmann, H. W., u. H. Schubothe: Funktionelle und organische Schädigungen des Zentralnervensystems der Katze im Unterdruckexperiment. Beitr. path. Anat. **107**, 3 (1942). — Anders, H., u. W. J. Eicke: Über Veränderungen an Hirngefäßen bei Hypertonie. Z. ges. Neurol. Psychiat. **167**, 562 (1939). — Anders, H. W., u. W. J. Eicke: Die Hirngefäße beim Hochdruck. Arch. Psychiat. Nervenkr. **112**, 1 (1940). — Andersen, W. A. D.: Textbook of Pathology. St. Louis 1948. — Anderson, I. M., and H. M. R. Coles: Patent ductus arteriosus with pulmonary hypertension a review of 9 cases including one with reversal of blood flow through the ductus. Thorax **10**, 338 (1955). — Antes, E. H.: Thrombotic thrombocytopenic purpura: A review of the literature with report of a case. Ann. intern. Med. **48**, 512 (1958). — Apitz, K.: Über den Bau jüngster Blutplättchenthromben und den Einfluß des Novirudins auf ihre Entstehung. Zbl. allg. Path. path. Anat. **50**, 9 (1931). ∼ Über Profibrin. I. Die Entstehung und Bedeutung des Profibrins im Gerinnungsverlauf. Z. ges. exp. Med. **101**, 552 (1937). ∼ II. Die Bildung von Profibrin bei der Denaturierung des Fibrinogens. Z. ges. exp. Med. **102**, 202 (1938). ∼ Pathologische Physiologie der Blutgerinnung. Kolloid-Z. **85**, 196 (1938). ∼ Die Thrombose als Gerinnung. Klin. Wschr. **1938**, 1785. ∼ Über Profibrin. IV. Die Agglutination von Blutplättchen durch Profibrin. Z. ges. exp. Med. **105**, 89 (1939). ∼ Die intravitale Blutgerinnung. I. Physiologische Grundlagen und Besonderheiten der intravitalen Gerinnung. Ergebn. inn. Med. Kinderheilk. **61**, 54 (1941). ∼ Über Hämophilie beim Weibe. Erbarzt **10**, 219 (1942). ∼ Die Bedeutung der Gerinnung und Thrombose für die Blutstillung. Virchows Arch. path. Anat. **308**, 540 (1942). ∼ Die intravitale Blutgerinnung. III. Dysthrombotische Blutungsübel. Ergebn. inn. Med. Kinderheilk. **63**, 1 (1943). ∼ Über die Ursachen der Arterienthrombose. Virchows Arch. path. Anat. **313**, 28 (1944). ∼ Die intravitale Blutgerinnung. IV. Die Thrombose. Ergebn. inn. Med. Kinderheilk. **64**, 1081 (1945). — Apitz, K., u. A. Thelen: Über Profibrin. III. Bildung und Bestand des Profibrins unter physiologischen Verhältnissen. Z. ges. exp. Med. **103**, 417 (1938). — Arnholdt, F., u. A. Mira-Llinares: Über die Nierenvenenthrombose. Urol. int. (Basel) **5**, 274 (1957). — Arnold, H. A., and A. R. Bainborough: Subacute cor pulmonale following trophoblastic pulmonary emboli. Canad. med. Ass. J. **76**, 478 (1957). — Arnold, O. H.: Neuere Gesichtspunkte zur Genese und Systematik der Krankheiten mit arterieller Hypertonie. Münch. med. Wschr. **1952**, 2358, 2423. — Arnold, O. H., u. K. D. Bock: Zum Begriff der malignen Hypertonie. Z. Kreisl.-Forsch. **43**, 16 (1954). — Arrillaga, F. C.: Thesis No 2536. Buenos Aires 1912. ∼ Sclérose de l'artère pulmonaire secondaire à certains états pulmonaires chroniques. Arch. Mal. Cœur **6**, 518 (1913). ∼ Sclérose de l'artère pulmonaire. Bull. Soc. méd. Hôp. Paris **48**, 292 (1924). — Arthus, M.: Injections répétées de sérum de cheval chez le lapin. C.R. Soc. Biol. (Paris) **55**, 817 (1903). ∼ De l'anaphylaxie à l'immunité. Paris 1921. — Arthus, M., et M. Breton: Lésions cutanées produites par les injections de sérum de cheval chez le lapin anaphylactisé par et pour sérum. C.R. Soc. Biol. (Paris) **55**, 1479 (1903). — Aschoff, L.: Über kapilläre Embolie von riesenkernhaltigen Zellen. Virchows Arch. path. Anat. **134**, 11 (1893). ∼ Über Atherosklerose und andere Sklerosen des Gefäßsystems. Beih. Med. Klin. **1908**, Nr 1. ∼ Thrombose und Sandbankbildungen. Beitr. path. Anat. **52**, 205 (1911). ∼ Thrombose und Embolie. Verh. Naturforscher **83**(I), 344 (1911). ∼ In: Beiträge zur Thrombosefrage. Pathologisch-anatomischer Teil. Leipzig 1912. ∼ Arteriosklerose. Beih. Med. Klin. **1914**,

Nr 1. ~ Über Atherosklerose. Vorträge über Pathologie, 62. Jena 1925. ~ Über Thrombose. Vorträge über Pathologie, 230. Jena 1925. ~ Die Arteriosklerose (Arteriopathia deformans). Ein Ernährungs- und Abnutzungsproblem. Beih. Med. Klin. 26, Nr 1 (1930). ~ Thrombose und Embolie. Verh. dtsch. Ges. Kreisl.-Forsch. 7, 11 (1934). ~ Über die wirklichen und scheinbaren spastischen Gefäßleiden der Retina. Augenärztl. Tagesfragen, Freiburg i. Br. 7, 113 (1934). ~ Kreislaufstörungen (Dyszyklien). In L. ASCHOFF, Pathologische Anatomie, I. 8. Aufl. Jena 1936. ~ Harnapparat. In L. ASCHOFF, Pathologische Anatomie, II. 8. Aufl. Jena 1936. ~ Über Arteriosklerose. Verh. dtsch. Ges. inn. Med. 51, 28 (1939). — ASCHOFF, L., u. S. TAWARA: Die heutige Lehre von den pathologisch-anatomischen Grundlagen der Herzschwäche. Jena 1906. — ASCHWORTH, C. T., A. W. JESTER and LLOYD E. GUY: Local loss of fluid and protein in experimental shock: Relation to decrease of plasma volume and total circulating protein. Amer. J. Physiol. 141, 571 (1944). — ASK-UPMARK, E.: On the „Pulseless Disease" outside of Japan. Acta med. scand. 149, 161 (1954). — ASTRUP, T.: Neuere Aspekte in der Blutgerinnung und der Fibrinolyse und ihren Beziehungen zur Koronarthrombose und Koronarsklerose. Wien. Z. inn. Med. 39, 373 (1958). — ATTWOOD, H. D.: Fatal pulmonary embolism by amniotic fluid. J. clin. Path. 9, 38 (1956). — ATZLER, E., u. G. LEHMANN: Reaktionen der Gefäße auf direkte Reize. In Handbuch der normalen und pathologischen Physiologie, Bd. VII/2, S. 963. 1927. — AUFDERMAUR, M.: Coronarthrombose bei Kranzarterienrissen durch physische und psychische Belastung. Schweiz. med. Wschr. 1952, 1086. — AUSTIN, M. G., and R. F. SCHAEFER: Marfan's syndrome, with unusual blood vessel manifestations. Primary medionecrosis dissection of right innominate, right carotid, and left carotid arteries. Arch. Path. (Chicago) 64, 205 (1957). — AVERBUCK, S. H.: Heart failure in hypertension. Amer. Heart J. 11, 99 (1936). — AXHAUSEN, H.: Zur Frage der Häufung der Thrombosen und Embolien. Virchows Arch. path. Anat. 274, 188 (1930). — AYERZA, L.: Maladie d'Ayerza sclérose secondaire de l'artère pulmonaire (cardiaques noirs). Darin Fall 1 von 1901. Sem. méd. (B. Aires) 23, 386 (1925).

BÄURLE, W.: Die Coronarsklerose bei Hypertonie. Beitr. path. Anat. 111, 108 (1950). — BAEZ, S., B. W. ZWEIFACH, R. PELLON and E. SHORR: A renal factor in vascular response to hemorrhagic and traumatic shock. Amer. J. Physiol. 166, 658 (1951). — BAEZ, S., B. W. ZWEIFACH and E. SHORR: Fed. Proc. 11, 7 (1952). — BAÈZ-VILLASENOR, J., and K. AMBROSIUS: Thrombotic thrombocytopenic purpura: Report of a case with some unusual characteristics. Ann. intern. Med. 46, 378 (1957). — BAKEY, M. E. DE: A critical evaluation of the problem of thromboembolism. Int. Abstr. Surg. 98, 1 (1954). — BAKEY, M. DE, and A. OCHSNER: Phlegmasia cerulea dolens and gangrene associated with thrombophlebitis. Surgery 26, 16 (1948). — BALDES, E. J., J. F. HERRICK, H. E. ESSEX and F. C. MANN: Studies on peripheral blood flow. Amer. Heart J. 21, 743 (1941). — BALI, T., and H. GOLDBLATT: On the pathogenesis of the vascular lesions of malignant hypertension in the rat. Exp. Med. Surg. 12, 460 (1954). — BALOGH, E. v.: Über die röntgenologisch feststellbare anatomische Grundlage des plötzlichen Herztodes bei Luftembolie (mit ergänzenden experimentellen kinematographischen und histologischen Studien). Verh. dtsch. Path. Ges. 31, 371 (1939). — BARATZ, R. A., and R. C. INGRAHAM: Capillary permeability during haemorrhagic shock in the rat. Proc. Soc. exp. Biol. (N. Y.) 89, 642 (1955). — BARCROFT, J.: The respiratory function of the blood. Cambridge 1914. — BARCROFT, J., A. V. BOCK and F. J. W. ROUGHTON: Observations on the circulation and respiration in a case of paroxysmal tachycardia. Heart 9, 7 (1921). — BARENBERG, L. J., N. M. GREENSTEIN, W. LEVY u. S. B. ROSENBLUTH: Nierenvenenthrombose und nephrotisches Syndrom. Amer. J. Dis. Child. 62, 352 (1941). — BARGER, A. C., A. M. RUDOLPH and F. E. YATES: Modern concepts of cardiovascular disease. New York 1954. — BARKER, N. W.: Current status of the problem of thrombosis. Circulation 17, 487 (1958). — BARKER, N. W., K. K. NYGAARD, W. WALTERS and S. T. PRIESTLEY: Statistical study of postoperative venous thrombosis and pulmonary embolism; incidence in various types of operations. Proc. Mayo Clin. 16, 1 (1941). ~ Statistical study of postoperative venous thrombosis and pulmonary embolism; location of thrombosis: relation of thrombosis and embolism. Proc. Mayo Clin. 16, 33 (1941). — BARLARO, D.: Rev. Asoc. méd. argent. 26, 121 (1917). Cit. D. BRACHETTO-BRIAN, Concepto anatomo-pathologico de los cardiacos negros de Ayerza. Rev. Soc. med. int. (B. Aires) 6, 821 (1935). — BARNARD, P. J.: Pulmonary arteriosclerosis and cor pulmonale due to recurrent thromboembolism. Circulation 10, 343 (1954). ~ Thrombo-embolic primary pulmonary sclerosis. Brit. Heart J. 16, 93 (1954). ~ Pulmonary arteriosclerosis due to oxygen, nitrogen, and argon embolism. Experimental study. Arch. Path. (Chicago) 63, 322 (1957). ~ The pathogenesis of experimental thromboembolic pulmonary arteriosclerosis. J. Path. Bact. 73, 17 (1957). ~ Experimental anoxic cardiac enlargement. Lab. Invest. 7, 81 (1958). — BARNES, A. R., and M. B. WHITTEN: Study of the R-T interval in myocardial infarction. Amer. Heart J. 5, 142 (1929). — BAROLDI, G., u. G. SCOMAZZONI: Coronarsklerose und Myokardschäden. Verh. dtsch. Ges. Path. 1958, 138. — BARSOUM, G. S., u. I. H. GADDUM: Nach I. H. GADDUM, Gefäßerweiternde Stoffe der Gewebe. Leipzig 1936. — BAYER, O., F. GROSSE-BROCKHOFF, F. LOOGEN u. H. MEESSEN: Vergleichende klinische, pathophysiologische und pathologisch-anatomische Untersuchungen bei Mitralstenose. Arch. Kreisl.-Forsch. **26**, 238 (1957). — Bayer, O., F. Loogen u. H. H. Wolter: Der Herzkatheterismus bei angeborenen und erworbenen Herzfehlern. Stuttgart 1954. — Beck, C. S.: Symposium on coronary artery disease. Blood supply to ischaemic myocardium distal to the occlusion of a coronary artery. Dis. Chest **31**, 243 (1957). — Becker, H.: Über Hirngefäßausschaltung. I. Extrakranielle Arterienunterbindungen zur Theorie des Sauerstoffmangelschadens am zentral-nervösen Gewebe. Dtsch. Z. Nervenheilk. **161**, 407 (1949). — Becker, V., u. D. Neubert: Über die Entstehung der hydropisch-vakuolären Zellentartung. Beitr. path. Anat. **120**, 319 (1959). — Begemann, H., u. H. G. Harwerth: Praktische Hämatologie. Stuttgart 1959. — Beickert, A.: Zur Entstehung und Bewertung der Arbeitshypertrophie des Herzens, der Nebenniere und Hypophyse. Arch. Kreisl.-Forsch. **21**, 115 (1954). — Beickert, A., u. H. Noetzel: Todesfall bei Penicillinüberempfindlichkeit. Klin. Wschr. **1952**, 37. — Bela, H.: 20 Jahre Thrombosen-Statistik. Virchows Arch. path. Anat. **292**, 629 (1934). — Bell, E. T.: Atherosclerotic gangrene of the lower extremities in diabetic and nondiabetic persons. Amer. J. clin. Path. **28**, 27 (1957). — Bellman, S.: Microangiography. Acta radiol. (Stockh.) Suppl. **102** (1953). — Beneke, R.: Die Fettresorption bei natürlicher und künstlicher Fettembolie und verwandten Zuständen. Beitr. path. Anat. **22**, 343 (1897). — Benninghoff, A.: Blutgefäße. In Handbuch der mikroskopischen Anatomie, Bd. VI, S. 1. 1930. ~ Über die funktionelle Struktur der Lungengefäße. Verh. dtsch. Ges. Kreisl.-Forsch. **1935**, 51. — Benson, E. S.: Composition and state of protein in heart muscle of normal dogs and dogs with experimental myocardial failure. Circulat. Res. **3**, 221 (1955). — Berblinger, W.: Pathologie und pathologische Morphologie der Hypophyse des Menschen. Leipzig 1932. ~ Formen und Ursache der Herzhypertrophie bei Lungentuberkulose. Bern 1947. — Berg, P., u. G. Könn: Noch unveröffentlicht. — Berger, H.: Über das Elektroencephalogramm des Menschen. IX. Arch. Psychiat. Nervenkr. **102**, 538 (1934). — Bergeron, J., W. H. Abelmann, H. Vazquez-Milan and L. B. Ellis: Aortic stenosis — clinical manifestations and course of the disease. Review of on hundred proved cases. Arch. intern. Med. **94**, 911 (1954). — Bergmann, G. v.: Funktionelle Pathologie, 2. Aufl. Berlin 1936. — Bergstrand, H.: Hypertensive vascular changes in the eye. Acta path. microbiol. scand. **25**, 98 (1948). — Berkow, S. G.: Culpability of suprarenals in symptoms and late death from extensive superficial burns. Med. J. Rec. **134**, 386 (1931). — Bernhard-Kreis, E.: Über die Bedeutung des Histamins und seine Wirkung als Ursache des Spättodes nach Verbrennungen. Z. ges. exp. Med. **104**, 756 (1939). — Bernstein, R. E.: Fluid therapy in relation to burn shock and healing. S. Afr. med. J. **26**, 416 (1952). — Berthrong, M., and T. H. Cochran: Pathological findings in 9 children with „primary" pulmonary hypertension. Bull. Johns Hopk. Hosp. **97**, 69 (1955). — Bethe, A.: Vergleichende Physiologie der Blutbewegung. In Handbuch der normalen und pathologischen Physiologie, Bd. VII/1, S. 3. 1926. — Biebl, M., u. P. Wichels: Physiologische und pathologisch-anatomische Betrachtungen im Anschluß an einen Fall von Paragangliom beider Nebennieren. Virchows Arch. path. Anat. **257**, 182 (1925). — Biggs, R., A. S. Douglas, R. G. Macfarlane, J. V. Dacie, W. R. Pitney, C. Merskey and J. R. O'Brien: Christmas disease. A condition previously mistaken for haemophilia. Brit. med. J. **1952** II, 1378. — Biggs, R., and R. G. Macfarlane: Human blood coagulation, 2. Aufl. Oxford: Blackwell 1957. — Bilger, R.: Die Bedeutung der Vektorkardiographie für die Erkennung der Herzhypertrophie. 5. Freiburger Symposion, 70, 1958. — Bilger, R., J. Sander, H. Reindell u. H. Klepzig: Die vektorkardiographischen Befunde bei der krankhaften Belastung des rechten Herzens. Arch. Kreisl.-Forsch. **27**, 117 (1957). — Bing, R. J.: The coronary circulation in health and disease as studied by coronary sinus catheterziation. Bull. N.Y. Acad. Med. **27**, 407 (1951). ~ The role of coronary circulation in shock. Ann. N.Y. Acad. Sci. **55**, 367 (1952). ~ Myocardial metabolism. Circulation **12**, 635 (1955). ~ Disturbances in myocardial metabolism. Advanc. Cardiol. 1, 52 (1956). ~ Der Myokardstoddwechsel. Klin. Wschr. **1956**, 1. ~ Cardiac metabolism in myocardial failure. Advanc. Cardiol. 2, 148 (1959). — Bing, R. J., and M. M. Hammond: Coronary blood flow cardiac oxygen consumption and cardiac efficiency in man. Bull. Johns Hopk. Hosp. **84**, 396 (1949). — Bing, R. J., M. M. Hammond, J. C. Handelsman, S. R. Powers, F. C. Spencer, J. E. Eckenhoff, W. T. Goodale, J. H. Hafkenschiel and S. S. Ketty: The measurement of coronary blood flow oxygen consumption and efficiency of the left ventricle in man. Amer. Heart J. **38**, 1 (1949). — Biörck, G.: Hypoxemia tests in coronary disease. Brit. Heart J. **8**, 17 (1946). ~ Anoxemia and exercise tests in the diagnosis of coronary disease. Amer. Heart J. **32**, 689 (1946). — Birke, G., H. Duner, S. O. Liljedahl, B. Pernow, L.-O. Plantin and L. Troell: Histamine, catechol amines and adrenocortical steroids in burns. Acta chir. scand. **114**, 87 (1957). — Blainey, J. D., J. Hardwicke and A. G. W. Whitfield: The nephrotic syndrome associated with thrombosis of the renal veins. Lancet **1954** II, 1208. — Blalock, A.: Mechanism and treatment of experimental shock. Arch. Surg. (Chicago) **15**, 762 (1927). ~ Experimental shock: A cause of low blood pressure produced by muscle injury. Arch. Surg. (Chicago) **20**, 959 (1930). ~ Experimental shock. Sth. med. J.

(Bgham, Ala.) **23**, 1013 (1930).∼ Trauma to the intestines. (The importance of the local loss of fluid in the production of low blood pressure.) Arch. Surg. (Chicago) **22**, 314, 610 (1931).∼ Principles of surgical care: shock and other problems. St. Louis 1940. ∼ The procurement and use of blood substitutes in the army. Ann. Surg. **115**, 1152 (1942). ∼ The uniform production of experimental shock by crush injury: Possible relationship to clinical crush syndrome. Ann. Surg. **115**, 684 (1942). ∼ Studies on the blood histamine in cases of burns. Ann. Surg. **115**, 390 (1942). ∼ A consideration of the present status of the shock problem. Problems on shock. Surge ry **14**, 487 (1943). — BLALOCK, A., J. W. BEARD and G. S. JOHNSON: Experimental shock. A study of its production and treatment. J. Amer. med. Ass. **97**, 1794 (1931). — BLOCH, E. H.: Microscopic observations of the circulating blood in the bulbar conjunctiva in man in health and disease. Ergebn. Anat. Entwickl.-Gesch. **35**, 1 (1956). — BLÜTHGEN, H.: Beitrag zur Pathologie der Verbrennung. Frankfurt. Z. Path. **58**, 85 (1944). — BLUM, L., G. SCHAUER and B. CALEF: Gradual occlusion of a coronary artery. An experimental study. Amer. Heart J. **16**, 159 (1938). — BLUMGART, H. L., D. R. GILLIGAN and M. J. SCHLESINGER: Experimental studies on the effects of temporary occlusion of coronary arteries. II. The production of myocardial infarction. Amer. Heart J. **22**, 374 (1941). — BLUMGART, H. L., M. J. SCHLESINGER and D. DAVIS: Studies on the relation of the clinical manifestations of angina pectoris, coronary thrombosis and myocardial infarction to the pathologic findings, with particular reference to the significance of collateral circulation. Amer. Heart J. **19**, 1 (1940). — BLUMGART, H. L., M. J. SCHLESINGER and P. M. ZOLL: Multiple fresh coronary occlusions in patients with antecedent shock. Arch. intern. Med. **68**, 181 (1941). — BLUMGART, H. L., P. M. ZOLL, A. S. FREEDBERG and D. R. GILLIGAN: The experimental production of intercoronary arterial anastomosis and their functional significance. Circulation 1, 10 (1950). — BOBEK, K., u. J. VANEK: Chron. Cor pulmonale infolge der Lungenembolisation. Z. ges. inn. Med. **1953**, 596. — BODECHTEL, G.: Gehirnveränderungen bei Herzkrankheiten. Z. ges. Neurol. Psychiat. **140** 657 (1932).∼ Zur Klinik der zerebralen Kreislaufstörungen (mit besonderer Berücksichtigung ihrer kardialen Genese). Verh. dtsch. Ges. Kreisl.-Forsch. **1953**, 109. — BODECHTEL, G., u. G. MÜLLER: Die geweblichen Veränderungen bei der experimentellen Gehirnembolie. Z. ges. Neurol. Psychiat. **124**, 764 (1930). — BODON, G.: Über die Vermehrung der tödlichen Lungenembolien. Langenbecks Arch. klin. Chir. **163**, 329 (1931). — BÖHMIG, R., u. P. KLEIN: Pathologie und Bakteriologie der Endokarditis. Berlin-Göttingen-Heidelberg 1953. — BÖHNE, C.: Beiträge zum Problem der apoplektischen Hirnblutung. Beitr. path. Anat. **78**, 260 (1927). ∼ Die Arten der Schlaganfälle des Gehirns und ihre Entstehung. Beitr. path. Anat. **86**, 566 (1931). ∼ Über die Bedeutung der Hirnerweichung in der Pathogenese der kompakten apoplektischen Hirnblutung. Z. ges. Neurol. Psychiat. **137**, 610 (1931). — BOHLE, A., M. KOHLER u. U. TOMSCHE: Über das Verhalten der epitheloiden Zellen der Vasa afferentia einseitig nephrektomierter Ratten bei renaler Hypertonie durch Einkapselung einer Niere. Beitr. path. Anat. **113**, 414 (1953). — BOHLE, A., u. U. TOMSCHE: Das Verhalten der epitheloiden Zellen der Vasa afferentia der Nierenkörperchen bei experimenteller Hypotonie. Beitr. path. Anat. **113**, 399 (1953). — BOUTON, S. M., and J. R. SAUNDERS: Pulmonary embolism of amniotic fluid. Report of case with reviews of literature. Amer. J. clin. Path. **21**, 566 (1951). — BOWMAN, J. A.: Amniotic fluid embolism. Case report. Amer. J. Obstet. **69**, 905 (1955). — BOYER, N. H., and H. D. GREEN: The effects of nitrites and xanthines on coronary inflow in blood pressure in anesthetizited dogs. Amer. Heart J. **21**, 199 (1941). — BRANDENBURG, W.: Spätfolgen der Luftembolie des Gehirns und ihr pathologisch-anatomisches Bild. Verh. dtsch. Ges. Path. **1958**, 236. — BRASS, K.: Aufbau und Entstehung der Beinvenenthrombose. Frankfurt. Z. Path. **56**, 74 (1942). ∼ Über ein charakteristisches Syndrom bei akuter schwerer Myolyse. Frankfurt. Z. Path. **58**, 387 (1944). — BRASS, K , u. W. SANDRITTER: Statistische Untersuchungen an blanden Fernthrombosen, fulminanten und nicht tödlichen Lungenembolien am Sektionsgut der Jahre 1905—1948. Frankfurt. Z. Path. **61**, 98 (1949). — BRAUN, L.: Über Angina pectoris. Eine historisch-kritische Betrachtung. Wien. klin. Wschr. **1926**, 265, 304. — BRAUNMÜHL, A. v.: Epilepsie. Anatomischer Teil. Z. ges. Neurol. Psychiat. **161**, 292 (1928). — BRAUNSTEIN, H.: Pulmonary periarteritis nodosa. Report of 5 cases, abstracted. Amer. J. Path. **30**, 630 (1954). ∼ Periarteritis nodosa limited to the pulmonary circulation. Amer. J. Path. **31**, 837 (1955). — BRECHT, K., u. S. MEINERS: Über spontane Schwankungen der Gefäßbreite beim Frosch und ihre Beeinflussung durch Cholinderivate und durch Vitamin B_1. Pflügers Arch. ges. Physiol. **245**, 224 (1942). — BREDT, H.: Die primäre Erkrankung der Lungenschlagader in ihren verschiedenen Formen. Virchows Arch. path. Anat. **284**, 126 (1932). ∼ Über Pulmonalsklerose. Verh. dtsch. Ges. Path. **1937**, 398. ∼ Entzündung und Sklerose der Lungenschlagader. Virchows Arch. path. Anat. **308**, 60 (1941). ∼ Über die Sonderstellung der tödlichen jugendlichen Coronarsklerose und der geweblichen Grundlage der akuten Coronarinsuffizienz. Beitr. path. Anat. **110**, 295 (1949). ∼ Die Morphologie der Arteriosklerose. Verh. dtsch. Ges. Path. **42**, 11 (1958). — BRENDEL, W.: Kreislauf und Hypothermie. Verh. dtsch. Ges. Kreisl.-Forsch. **23**, 33 (1957). — BRENNER, O.: Sclerosis of the pulmonary artery with thrombosis.

Lancet **1931** I, 911. ~ Pathology of the vessels of the pulmonary circulation. Arch. intern. Med. **56**, 457, 724, 976, 1189, 1241 (1935). — Bresler: Klinische und pathologisch-anatomische Beiträge zur Mikrogyrie. Arch. Psychiat. Nervenkr. **31**, 566 (1899). — Bretschneider, H. J.: Über den Mechanismus der hypoxischen Coronarerweiterung. Bad Oeynhausener Gespräche II, 44 (1958). — Brewer, D. B.: Fibrous occlusion and anastomosis of the pulmonary vessels in a case of pulmonary hypertension associated with patent ductus arteriosus. J. Path. Bact. **70**, 299 (1955). — Brobeil, A.: Die embolischen und thrombotischen Erkrankungen des Zentralnervensystems. In: Die Thromboembolischen Erkrankungen und ihre Behandlung von Th. Naegeli, P. Matis, R. Gross, H. Runge u. H. Sachs, S. 502. Stuttgart 1955. — Broman, T.: Investigations into the origin of cerebral hemorrhages in experimental animals. Acta psychiat. scand. **14**, 395 (1939). — Bronte-Stewart, B., u. R. H. Heptinstall: The relationship between experimental hypertension and cholesterol-induced atheroma in rabbits. J. Path. Bact. **68**, 407 (1954). — Brown, J. W., D. Heath u. W. Whitaker: Eisenmengers Complex. Brit. Heart J. **17**, 273 (1955). — Brücke, E. Th. v.: Die Bewegung der Körpersäfte. In Handbuch der vergleichenden Physiologie, Bd. I, S. 827. 1925. — Brumfitt, W., u. W. O'Brien: Nierenvenenthrombose und nephrotisches Syndrom. Brit. med. J. **1956** II, 751. — Brunton, T. L.: On the use of nitrite of amyl in angina pectoris. Lancet **1867**, 97. — Brux, J. de: Histo-pathologie du myocarde dans l'insuffisance cardiaque progressive. Ann. anat. path. **17**, 270 (1947). — Bucher, K.: Reflektorische Beeinflußbarkeit der Lungenatmung. Wien 1952. — Buddenbrock, W. v.: Grundriß der vergleichenden Physiologie. Berlin 1928. — Büchner, Chr.: Temporäres chronisches Cor pulmonale nach experimenteller rezidivierender Mikroembolie. Klin. Wschr. **1959**, 621. — Büchner, Chr., u. G. Könn: Temporär-chronisches Cor pulmonale im Tierexperiment nach rezidivierender Mikroembolie. Zugleich ein Beitrag zur Pathogenese der Pulmonalsklerose. Beitr. path. Anat. **121**, 170 (1959). — Büchner, F.: Die Rolle des Herzmuskels bei der Angina pectoris. Beitr. path. Anat. **89**, 644 (1932). ~ Zur Pathogenese der Angina pectoris. Ber. der Med. Ges. Freiburg vom 16. Febr. 1932. Klin. Wschr. **1932**, 1404. ~ Über Angina pectoris. Klin. Wschr. **1932**, 1737. ~ Das morphologische Substrat bei Angina pectoris im Tierexperiment. Beitr. path. Anat. **92**, 311 (1933). ~ Herzmuskelinfarkt und disseminierte Nekrosen des Herzmuskels. Oeynhausener Vortr. **2**, 5 (1933). ~ Herzmuskelschädigungen durch Koronarinsuffizienz. Nauheimer Vortr. **10**, 29 (1934). ~ Spezifische Tumoren des Nebennierenmarks mit Hypertonie. Klin. Wschr. **1934**, 617. ~ Die pathogenetische Bedeutung der Hypoxämie. Klin. Wschr. **1937**, 1409. ~ Die Zeichen der Herzmuskelschädigung durch koronare Insuffizienz im histologischen Bild und im Elektrokardiogramm. Zbl. inn. Med. **58**, 497 (1937). ~ Experimente über Koronarinsuffizienz und ihre morphologische und elektrokardiographische Manifestierung. Verh. dtsch. Ges. inn. Med. **50**, 73 (1938). ~ Die Deutung des Elektrokardiogramms bei den Durchblutungsstörungen des Herzmiskels. Vom Standpunkt des Pathologen. Klin. Wschr. **1938**, 1713, 1745. ~ Die Coronarinsuffizienz. Dresden u. Leipzig 1939. ~ Die pathogenetische Bedeutung allgemeiner und relativer Durchblutungsstörungen. Derm. Wschr. **110**, 54 (1940). ~ Durchblutungsstörungen des Herzmuskels. Dtsch. Mil. arzt, **1941**, 570. ~ Die pathogenetische Bedeutung des allgemeinen Sauerstoffmangels. Verh. dtsch. Path. 1944, S. 20 (1949). (Als Manuskript vervielfältigt 1944.) ~ Über die Ursachen des Versagens des hypertrophierten Herzmuskels. Arch. int. Pharmacodyn. **78**, 115 (1949). ~ Pathologische Anatomie der Herzinsuffizienz. Verh. dtsch. Ges. Kreisl.-Forsch. **16**, 26 (1950). ~ Allgemeine Pathologie. München u. Berlin, 1. Aufl. 1950; 2. Aufl. 1956; 3. Aufl. 1959. ~ Spezielle Pathologie. München u. Berlin, 1. Aufl. 1955; 2. Aufl. 1956; 3. Aufl. 1960. ~ Vom geistigen Standort der modernen Medizin. Freiburg i. Br. 1957. ~ Relative Durchblutungsnot des Herzmuskels. Dtsch. med. Wschr. **1957**, 1037, 1065. ~ Die Pathologie der cellulären und geweblichen Oxydationen. Die Hypoxydosen. In Handbuch der allgemeinen Pathologie, Bd. IV/2, S. 569. 1957. ~ Morphologische Befunde und Elektrokardiogramm bei Durchblutungsstörungen des Herzmuskels. 5. Freiburger Symposion über die Funktionsdiagnose des Herzens, 1957, 4. Berlin-Göttingen-Heidelberg 1958. ~ Die Veränderungen der Ultrastruktur der Herzmuskelzelle bei Störungen der Aerobiose. Eein Beitrag zum Problem der Koronarinsuffizienz. Ärztl. Forsch. **13**, 307 (1959). — Büchner, F., u. W. Lucadou: Elektrokardiographische Veränderungen und disseminierte Nekrosen des Herzmuskels bei experimenteller Coronarinsuffizienz. Beitr. path. Anat. **93**, 169 (1934). — Büchner, F., E. Mölbert u. L. Thale: Das submikroskopische Bild der Herzmuskelzelle nach toxischer Hemmung der Aerobiose. Beitr. path. Anat. **121**, 145 (1959). — Büchner, F., H. Reindell, H. Klepzig u. R. Weyland: Vergleichende elektrokardiographische und morphologische Untersuchungen unter besonderer Berücksichtigung der Brustwandableitungen. Verh. dtsch. Ges. Kreisl.-Forsch. **18**, 141 (1952). — Büchner, F., A. Weber u. B. Haager: Koronarinfarkt und Koronarinsuffizienz. Leipzig 1935. — Büchner, F., u. R. Weyland: Noch unveröffentlicht. 1955. ~ Noch unveröffentlicht 1959. — Bukov, V. A., L. A. Bikov and V. A. Valuk: Concerning a new method of inducing stable hypertension of neurogenic origin in dogs. Arch. Path. (Moskau) **20**, H. 5, 21 (1958). — Burack, W. R., J. P. Pryce and F. John: A reversible nephrotic syndrome associated with congestive heart failure. Circulation **18**, 562 (1958). — BURCH, G., P. REASER and J. CRONVICH: Rates of sodium turnover in normal subjects and in patients with congestive heart failure. J. Lab. clin. Med. **32**, 1169 (1947). — BURCHELL, H. B.: Adjustments in coronary circulation after experimental coronary occlusion. With particular reference to vascularisation of pericardial adhesions. Arch. intern. Med. **65**, 240 (1940). — BURCHELL, H. B., R. D. PRUITT and A. R. BARNES: The stress and the electrocardiogram in the induced hypoxemia test for coronary insufficiency. Amer. Heart J. **36**, 373 (1948). — BURRAGE, W. S., and J. W. IRWIN: Microscopic observations of the pulmonary arterioles, capillaries and venules of living mammals before and during anaphylaxis. J. Allergy **24**, 289 (1953). — BUSCH, F.: Über Fettembolie. Virchows Arch. path. Anat. **35**, 321 (1866). — BUSCH, W., u. K. EISELSBERG: Neue anatomische Untersuchungen über das Cor pulmonale. Cardiologia (Basel) **33**, 137 (1958). — BYROM, F. B., and L. F. DODSON: Causation of acute arterial necrosis in hypertensive disease. J. Path. Bact. **60**, 357 (1948). — BYWATERS, E. G. L.: Effects on kidney of limb compression. Brit. med. J. **1941**, 884. — BYWATERS, E. G. L., G. L. DELORY, O. RIMINGTON and J. SMILES: Methaemoglobin in the urine of air raid causalities with crushing injury. Biochem. J. **54**, 111 (1941). — BYWATERS, E. G. L., and J. H. DIBLE: The renal lesion in traumatic anuria. J. Path. Bact. **54**, 111 (1942).

CALDWELL, R. D., C. W. FITCHETT, E. P. LEHMAN and C. B. MORTON: Observations on portal venous pressure following hepatic artery ligation in experimental animals. Surgery **36**, 1068 (1954). — CAMMERMEYER, J.: Cerebral changes in an acute case of fat embolism. Acta psychiat. scand. **12**, 333 (1937). — CANADA, W. I., F. GOODELE and J. H. CURRENS: Defect of the interatrial septum with thrombosis of the pulmonal artery. Report of 3 cases. New Engl. J. Med. **248**, 309 (1953). — CEELEN, W.: Die Kreislaufstörungen der Lunge. Handbuch der speziellen Pathologie, Bd. III/3, S. 1. 1931. — CHAMBERS, R.: Vasomotion in the hemodynamics of the blood capillary circulation. Ann. N.Y. Acad. Sci. **49**, 549 (1948). — CHAMBERS, R., and B. W. ZWEIFACH: Intercellular cement and capillary permeability. Physiol. Rev. **27**, 436 (1947). — CHAVEZ, I., B. SEPULVEDA and I. A. ORTOGA: The functional value of the liver in heart disease. An experimental study. J. Amer. med. Ass. **121**, 1276 (1943). — CHIARI, H.: Über Veränderungen in der Arteria pulmonalis in Fällen von akuter rheumatischer Endocarditis oder bei Herzfehlern rheumatischen Ursprungs. Klin. Wschr. **1930**, 1862. ~ Über Veränderungen in der Arteria pulmonalis in Fällen von Rheumatismus. Beitr. path. Anat. **88**, 1 (1932). ~ Die pathologische Anatomie der Kriegsverschüttung. Schweiz. med. Wschr. **1949**, 946. — CHOMETTE, G., et R. ABELANET: Infarctus pulmonaire. Étude anatomique et essai d'interprétation physiopathologique. Ann. anat. path., N. s., **3**, 187 (1958). — CHRIST, C.: Experimentelle Kohlenoxydvergiftung, Herzmuskelnekrosen und Elektrokardiogramm. Beitr. path. Anat. **94**, 111 (1934). — CLEMEDSON, C.-J., H. HARTELIUS and G. HOLMBERG: The influence of carbon dioxide inhalation on the cerebral vascular permeability to trypan blue (the bloodbrain barrier). Acta path. microbiol. scand. **42**, 137 (1958). — CODE, C. F.: Histamine in blood. Physiol. Rev. **32**, 47 (1952). — COHNHEIM, J.: Über Entzündung und Eiterung. Virchows Arch. path. Anat. **40**, 1 (1867). ~ Untersuchungen über die embolischen Prozesse. Berlin 1872. ~ Neue Untersuchungen über die Entzündung. Berlin 1873. — *Conference on the Shock Syndrome.* Ann. N.Y. Acad. Sci. **55**, 345 (1952). — CONSTANTINIDES, P., G. SZASZ and F. HARDER: Retardation of atheromatosis and adrenal enlargement by heparin in the rabbit. Arch. Path. (Chicago) **56**, 36 (1953). — CONTRATTO, A. W., and S. A. LEVINE: Aortic stenosis with special reference to angina pectoris and syncope. Ann. intern. Med. **10**, 1636 (1937). — CORCORAN, A. C., and J. H. PAGE: Arch. Surg. (Chicago) **51**, 93 (1945). Nach G. ROSEMANN, Zur Pathogenese der chromoproteinämischen Nephrose. Beitr. path. Anat. **122**, 199 (1960). — CORDAY, E., S. F. ROTHENBERG and T. J. PUTNAM: Cerebral vascular insufficiency; explanation of some types of localized cerebral encephalopathy. Arch. Neurol. Psychiat. (Chicago) **69**, 551 (1953). — COSSEL, L.: Über arteriosklerotische Frühveränderungen im großen und kleinen Kreislauf und Bronchiolitis obliterans bei einem Fall von partiellem Truncus arteriosus communis. Frankfurt. Z. Path. **67**, 247 (1956). — COURNAND, A., R. L. RILEY, S. E. BRADLEY, E. S. BREED, R. P. NOBLE, H. D. LAUSON, M. I. GREGERSEN and D. W. RICHARDS: Studies of the circulation in clinical shock. Surgery **13**, 964 (1943). — CRAIG, J. M., and D. GITLIN: The nature of the hyaline thrombi in thrombotic thrombocytopenic purpura. Amer. J. Path. **33**, 251 (1957). — CRAVER, W. L., and F. GLENN: Massive hemmorhage from peptic ulcer. A cause of myocardial infarction in the aged. Amer. Geriat. Soc. **5**, 969 (1957). — CRILE, G. W.: Surgical shock. Philadelphia 1899. ~ Hemorrhage and transfusion. New York 1909. — CRON, R. S., G. S. KILKENNY, C. WIRTHWEIN and J. R. EVRARD: Amniotic fluid embolism. Amer. J. Obstret. **64**, 1360 (1952). — CROWE, u. W. GREUER: Zur Biologie der Verbrennungsschäden. Zit. nach W. GREUER, Z. ges. exp. Med. **111**, 1 (1943). — CRUCHAUD, S.: Syndrome néphrotique dans un cas de thrombose bilatérale des veines rénales. Helv. med. Acta Ser. A **23**, 495 (1956). — CRUVEILHIER:

Recherches sur le siège immédiat de l'inflammation. Nouv. Bibl. méd. 1826. T. IV. p. 1. Anat. pathol. Liv. IV et XI. (Phlébite). Traité d'anat. path. générale. Paris 1852. T. II. — CURRENS, J. H., and A. R. BARNES: The heart in pulmonary embolism. Arch. intern. Med. 71, 325 (1943).

DACK, S., A. M. MASTER, H. HORN, A. GRISHMAN and L. E. FIELD: Acute coronary insufficiency due to pulmonary embolism. Amer. J. Med. 7, 464 (1949). — DALE, H. H.: Die anaphylaktische Reaktion der glatten Muskulatur des Meerschweinschens. J. Pharmacol. exp. Ther. 4, 167 (1913). ∼ Anaphylaxis. Bull. Johns Hopk. Hosp. 31, 310 (1920). ∼ I. Introduction. Vasomotor hormones. II. Local vasodilator reactions. Histamin. III. Local vasodilator reactions. Histamin. Acethyl-cholin. Conclusion. Lancet 1929, 1179, 1233, 1259. — DALE, H. H., and P. P. LAIDLOW: Histamine shock. J. Physiol. (Lond.) 52, 355 (1919). — DALE, H. H., and A. N. RICHARDS: The vaso-dilator action of histamine and of some other substances. J. Physiol. (Lond.) 52, 110 (1918). — DALY DE BURGH, J.: Quart. J. exp. Physiol. 27, 123 (1937). Zit. nach H. SCHWIEGK, Über Reflexe aus dem kleinen Kreislauf. Verh. dtsch. Ges. Kreisl.-Forsch. 17, 95 (1951). — DAM, H.: Cholesterinstoffwechsel in Hühnereiern und Hühnchen. Biochem. Z. 215, 475 (1929). ∼ Über die Cholesterinsynthese im Tierkörper. Biochem. Z. 220, 158 (1930). ∼ The antihemorrhagic vitamin of the chick. Biochem. J. 29, 1273 (1935). — DAMMANN jr., J. F., J. P. BAKER and W. H. MULLER jr.: Pulmonary vascular changes induced by experimentally produced pulmonary arterial hypertension. Surg. Gynaec. Obstet. 105, 16 (1957). — DAMMIN, G. J., M. L. GOLDMAN, H. A. SCHROEDER and G. PACE: Arterial hypertension in dogs. Lab. Invest. 5, 72 (1956). — DANIEL, P. M., M. M. L. PRICHARD and J. N. WARD-MCQUAID: The renal circulation in experimental hypertension. Brit. J. Surg. 17, 81 (1954). ∼ Total nephrectomy in rabbits with chronic hypertension. Clin. Sci. 13, 247 (1954). ∼ Removal of the clip on the renal artery in rabbits with experimental chronic hypertension. Quart. J. exp. Physiol. 39, 101 (1954). — DANIÉLOPOLU, D.: L'angine de poitrine. Paris 1927. — DAUBERT, K.: Meterorotrope Einflüsse bei der Entstehung der Thromboembolie. In: Die Thrombeoembolischen Erkrankungen und ihre Behandlung von TH. NAEGELI, P. MATIS, R. GROSS, H. RUNGE u. H. SACHS, S. 41. Stuttgart 1955. — DAVIS, H. A.: Shock and allied forms of failure of the circulation. New York 1949. — DÉCOURT, L. V.: Licoes de patologia cardiocirculatoria. Sao Paulo 1945. — DENECKE, K.: Der Plantarschmerz als Frühsymptom einer beginnenden Thrombose der unteren Extremität. Münch. med. Wschr. 1929, 1912. — DENNISS, R. G., W. DOLDIE and C. J. POLSON: Amniotic embolism. A report of two fatalities. J. Obstet. Gynaec. Brit. Emp. 61, 620 (1954). — DEPARIS, M., L. AUQUIER, J. CANIVET, R. LEVILLAIN and J. LISSAC: Thrombose des veines rénales et néphrose lipoïdique. Presse méd. 1954, 1363. — DEROW, H. A., M. J. SCHLESINGER u. H. A. SAVITZ: Nierenvenenthrombose und nephrotisches Syndrom. Arch. inn. Med. 63, 626 (1939). — DEYRUP, I. J.: Circulatory changes following the subcutaneous injection of histamine in dogs. Amer. J. Physiol. 142, 158 (1944). — DIAS, C. B.: A insuficiencia coronaria. Sao Paulo 1941. — DIBLE, J. H.: Organisation and canalisation in arterial thrombosis. J. Path. Bact. 75, 1 (1958). — DIEMER, K.: Retrograde Luftembolie bei Arrosionsaneurysma der Arteria pulmonalis. Virchows Arch. path. Anat. 328, 347 (1956). — DIETRICH, A.: Experimente über Thrombenbildung. Verh. dtsch. path. Ges. 1912, 372. ∼ Thrombose. Ihre Grundlage und ihre Bedeutung. Berlin u. Wien 1932. ∼ Gefäßwand und Thrombose. Verh. dtsch. Ges. Kreisl.-Forsch. 7, 48 (1934). ∼ Reaktive Thrombose im Tierversuch. Virchows Arch. path. Anat. 307, 281 (1941). — DIETRICH, F. M.: Panarteritis der Lunge beim Neugeborenen. Ann. paediat. (Basel) 190, 362 (1958). — DIETRICH, S., u. H. SCHWIEGK: Angina pectoris und Anoxie des Herzmuskels. Z. klin. Med. 125, 195 (1933). ∼ Das Schmerzproblem der Angina pectoris. Klin. Wschr. 1933, 135. — DOBBEN-BROEKEMA, M., and M. N. J. DIRKIN: Influence of the sympathetic nervous system on the circulation in the rabbit's ear. Acta physiol. pharmacol. neerl. 1, 584 (1950). — DOCK, W.: The capacity of the coronary bed in cardiac hypertrophy. J. exp. Med. 74, 177 (1941). — DÖRFLER, J.: Ein Beitrag zur Frage der Lokalisation der Arteriosklerose der Gehirngefäße mit besonderer Berücksichtigung der Arteria carotis interna. Arch. Psychiat. Nervenkr. 103, 180 (1935). — DÖRNER, J., u. H. J. KUSCHKE: Die Beeinflussung der neurogenen Adrenalin- und Arterenoldilatation der Skeletmuskelgefäße durch Novocain, Atropin und Physostigmin, zugleich ein Beitrag zur Frage der Existenz vasodilatatorischer Nerven. Naunyn-Schmiedeberg's Arch. exp. Path. Pharmak. 224, 368 (1955). — DONATH, J.: Beiträge zur Lehre von der paroxysmalen Kältehämoglobinurie. Z. klin. Med. 52, 1 (1904). — DONATH, J., u. K. LANDSTEINER: Über paroxysmale Hämoglobinurie. Münch. med. Wschr. 51, 1590 (1904). ∼ Über paroxysmale Hämoglobinurie. Z. klin. Med. 58, 173 (1905). ∼ Weitere Beobachtungen über paroxysmale Hämoglobinurie. Zbl. Bakt. 45, 204 (1908). — DONTENWILL, W., u. W. ROTTER: Über die Beeinflussung der Reaktion des arteriellen Gefäßsystems bei lokaler Gefrierung durch Antihistaminica. I. Virchows Arch. path. Anat. 322, 428 (1952). — DOUGLAS, W. W.: The role of local sympathetic innervation in pyrogen-induced vasoconstriction occurring in the rabbit ear. J. Physiol.

(Lond.) **126**, 319 (1954). — DOWNING, D. F., and R. W. WELLER: Necrotizing arteritis confined to the pulmonary artery system. J. Dis. Child. **91**, 45 (1956). — DRAGSTEDT, C. A., and F. B. MEAD: Further observations on nature of active substance (anaphylatoxin) in canine anaphylactic shock. J. Immunol. **30**, 319 (1936). — DRESZER, R., u. W. SCHOLZ: Experimentelle Untersuchungen zur Frage der Hirndurchblutungsstörungen beim generalisierten Krampf. Z. ges. Neurol. Psychiat. **164**, 140 (1939). — DRINKER, G. K., u. J. BROFENBRENNER: J. Immunol. **9**, 387 (1924). Zit. nach S. JIJIMA, Die Durchblutungsstörungen am Kaninchenohr bei allgemeiner und lokaler Anaphylaxie. Beitr. path. Anat. **118**, 67 (1957). — DÜLL, M.: Gewichtsbestimmungen der reinen Muskelmasse beider Herzkammern bei normaler und pathologischer Herzbelastung. Beitr. path. Anat. **105**, 337 (1941). — DUESBERG, R., u. W. SCHROEDER: Pathophysiologie und Klinik der Kollapszustände. Leipzig 1944. — DUFF, F., A. D. M. GREENFIELD and R. F. WHELAN: Observations on the mechanism of the vasodilatation following arterial gas embolism. Clin. Sci. **13**, 365 (1954). — DUGUID, J. B.: Thrombosis as a factor in the pathogenesis of coronary atherosclerosis. J. Path. Bact. **60**, 207 (1946). ~ Thrombosis as a factor in the pathogenesis of aortic atherosclerosis. J. Path. Bact. **60**, 57 (1948). ~ Pathogenesis of atherosclerosis. Lancet **1949 II**, 925. ~ The pathogenesis of arterial narrowing (Symposium). Bull. schweiz. Akad. med. Wiss. **13**, 73 (1957). — DUGUID, J. B., and G. S. ANDERSON: The pathogenesis of hyaline arteriolosclerosis. J. Path. Bact. **64**, 519 (1952). — DUMONT, M.: Les embolies pulmonaires amniotiques. Gynéc. et Obstét. **48**, 403 (1949). — DUNCAN, G. W., and A. BLALOCK: The uniform production of experimental shock by crush injury: possible relationship to clinical crush syndrome. Ann. Surg. **115**, 684 (1942). — DUSPIVA, F.: Über den Stoffwechsel adulter und embryonaler Gewebe bei Hypoxie. Klin. Wschr. **1957**, 645. ~ Zur Energetik des Herzmuskels bei experimenteller Hypertrophie. Klin. Wschr. **1959**, 620. — DUSPIVA, F., u. D. GOHL: Der Energiestoffwechsel des hypertrophierten Herzmuskels im Tierexperiment. Beitr. path.Anat. **121**, 124 (1959). ~ Zur Energetik des hypertrophierten Herzmuskels im Tierexperiment. Verh. dtsch. Ges. Path. **1959**, 295. — DUSPIVA, F., u. H. NOLTENIUS: Untersuchungen über den Stoffwechsel bei akuter Hypoxie. Beitr. path. Anat. **118**, 52 (1957).

EAMES, D. H.: Fatal case of obstetric shock due to pulmonary emboli of amniotic fluid. Amer. J. Obstet. **64**, 201 (1952). — EBBECKE, U.: Die lokale vasomotorische Reaktion (L.V.R.) der Haut und der inneren Organe. Pflügers Arch. ges. Physiol. **169**, 1 (1917). — EBERT, R. H., and R. W. WISSLER: In vivo observations of the vasculare reactions to large doses of horse serum using the rabbit ear chamber technique. J. Lab. clin. Med. **38**, 511 (1951). — EBERTH, C. O., u. C. SCHIMMELBUSCH: Die Thrombose. Stuttgart 1888. — ECHLIN, F. A.: Focal cerebral ischemia and reactive gliosis following experimental vascular spasm. Arch. Neurol. Psychiat. (Chicago) **44**, 479 (1940). ~ Vasospasm and focal cerebral ischemia. Arch. Neurol. Psychiat. (Chicago) **47**, 77 (1942). — ECKENHOFF, J. E., and J. H. HAFKENSCHIEL: The effect of nikethamide on coronary blood flow and cardiac oxygen metabolism. J. Pharmacol. exp. Ther. **91**, 362 (1947). — ECKENHOFF, J. E., J. H. HAFKENSCHIEL, C. M. LANDMESSER and M. HARMEL: The coronary circulation in the dog. Amer. J. Physiol. **148**, 582 (1947). ~ Cardiac oxygen metabolism and control of the coronary circulation. Amer. J. Physiol. **149**, 634 (1947). — ECKHARDT, P.: Zur Frage pulmocoronarer Reflexe bei Lungenembolie. Pflügers Arch. **241**, 224 (1938). — EDWARDS, G. A., and C. E. CHALLICE: The fine structure of cardiac muscle cells of newborn and suckling mice. Exp. Cell. Res. **15**, 247 (1958). — EDWARDS, J. E.: Structural changes of the pulmonary vascular bed and their functional significance in congenital heart disease. Proc. Int. Med. Chicago **18**, 134 (1950). ~ The Lewis A. Conner memorial lecture. Functional pathology of the pulmonary vascular tree in congenital cardiac disease. Circulation **15**, 164 (1957). — EDWARDS, J. E., and W. B. CHAMBERLIN: Pathology of the pulmonary vascular tree. III. The structur of the intrapulmonary arteries in cor triloculare biatriatum with subaortic stenosis. Circulation **3**, 524 (1951). — EDWARDS, W. S., A. SIEGEL and R. J. BING: Studies on myocardial metabolism. III. Coronary blood flow, myocardial oxygene consumption and carbohydrate metabolism in experimental haemorrhagic shock. J. clin. Invest. **33**, 1646 (1954). — EHRICH, W. E.: Die Entzündung. In Handbuch der allgemeinen Pathologie, Bd. VII/1, S. 1. 1956. — EICKE, W. J.: Die Endangitis obliterans der Hirngefäße. In Handbuch der speziellen Pathologie, Bd. XIII/1 B, S. 1536. 1957. — EINHAUSER, M.: Behandlung schwerer Verbrennungen mit Nebennierenrindenhormon und Vitamin C im Tierversuch. Klin. Wschr. **1938 I**, 127. ~ Behandlung schwerer Verbrennungen mit Nebennierenrinden und Vit. C im Tierversuch und in der Klinik. Münch. med. Wschr. **1939**, 441. — ELLENBERG, M., and K. E. OSSERMAN: The role of shock in the production of central liver cell necrosis. Amer. J. Med. **11**, 170 (1951). — EMSON, H. E.: Fat embolism studied in 100 patients dying after injury. J. clin. Path. **11**, 28 (1958). — ENDES, P., P. TAKACS-NAGY, P. RUBANYI and P. GÖMÖRI: The pathogenesis of malignant hypertension. Acta morph. Acad. Sci. hung. **5**, 113 (1955). — ENGEL, F. L.: The significance of the metabolic changes during shock. Ann. N.Y. Acad. Sci.

55, 381 (1952). — ENGEL, G. L.: Fainting. Springfield, Ill.: 1950. ~ ENKE, H.,⸀u.⸀G. GERCKEN: Der seelische Befund bei essentiellen Hypertonikern. Psychodiagnostisch-statistische Untersuchungen. Klin. Wschr. **1955**, 551. — EPPING, H.: Untersuchungen über Herzmuskelveränderungen bei chronischer und akuter Überbelastung des rechten Ventrikels. Arch. Kreisl.-Forsch. **6**, 109 (1940). — EPPINGER, H.: Zur Pathologie der Kreislaufcorrelationen. In Handbuch der normalen und pathologischen Physiologie, Bd. **16**/2, S. 1289. 1931. ~ Über Permeabilitätsänderungen im Kapillarbereiche. Verh. dtsch. Ges. Kreisl.-Forsch. **11**, 166 (1938). — EPPINGER, H., H. KAUNITZ u. H. POPPER: Die seröse Entzündung. Eine Permeabilitäts-Pathologie. Wien 1935. — EPPINGER, H., u. R. LEUCHTENBERGER: Zur Pathogenese der Gastritis und des Ulcus ventriculi. Z. ges. exp. Med. **85**, 598 (1932). — EPPINGER, H., u. A. SCHÜRMEYER: Über den Kollaps und analoge Zustände. Klin. Wschr. **1928**, 777. — EPPINGER, H., u. R. WAGNER: Zur Pathologie der Lunge. Wien. Arch. inn. Med. **156**, 83 (1920). — ERLANGER, J., R. GESELL u. H. S. GASSER: Studies in secondary traumatic shock. I. The circulation in shock after abdominal injuries. Amer. J. Physiol. **49**, 90 (1919). — ESCUDERO, P.: Les cardiaques noirs et les maladies de Ayerza. Arch. Mal. Cœur **19**, 439 (1926). — EULER, U. v., and G. LILJESTRAND: Observations on the pulmonary arterial blood pressure in the cat. Acta physiol. scand. **12**, 301 (1947). — EVANS, W., D. S. SHORT and D. E. BEDFORD: Solitary pulmonary hypertension. Brit. Heart J. **29**, 93 (1957).

FAHEY, J. L., E. LEONARD, J. CHURG u. G. GODMAN: Wegeners Granulomatosis. Amer. J. Med. **17**, 168 (1954). — FAHR, G.: Hypertension heart. Amer. J. med. Sci. **175**, 453 (1928). ~ The heart in hypertension. J. Amer. med. Ass. **105**, 1396 (1935). — FAHR, TH.: Kreislaufstörungen in der Niere. In Handbuch der speziellen Pathologie. Niere, Bd. VI/1, S. 121. 1925. ~ Pathologische Anatomie des Morbus Brightii. In Handbuch der speziellen Pathologie. Niere, Bd. VI/1, S. 156. 1925. — FANCONI, G.: Zöliakie. Dtsch. med. Wschr. **1938**, 1565, 1607. — FARIA, LOPES J. DE: Aorten- und Arterienveränderungen nach orthostatischem Kollaps des Kaninchens. Verh. dtsch. Ges. Path. **1954**, 216. ~ Medionekrose der großen und mittelgroßen Arterien nach orthostatischem Kollaps des Kaninchens. Beitr. path. Anat. **115**, 373 (1955). ~ Über die Ätiologie und die formale Pathogenese der Medionekrosis aortae idiopathica. Auf Grund von Aortenveränderungen nach Kollapszuständen. Beitr. path. Anat. **117**, 202 (1957). ~ Medianecrosis aortae after collapse in rabbits. Schweiz. Z. allg. Path. **21**, 103 (1958). ~ Beitrag zur Histopathogenese und Ätiologie der Medionecrosis aortae idiopathica mit Berücksichtigung der Rolle der Aortitis syphilitica. Beitr. path. Anat. **121**, 242 (1959). — FAZEKAS, J. F., J. KLEH and A. E. PARRISH: The influence of shok on cerebral hemodynamics and metabolism. Amer. J. med. Sci. **229**, 41 (1955). — FEIL, H., E. H. CUSHING and J. T. HARDESTY: Accurracy in diagnosis and localisation of myocardial infarction. Amer. Heart J. **15**, 721 (1938). — FEIL, H., u. R. SIEGEL: Electrocardiographic changes during attacks of angina pectoris. Amer. J. med. Sci. **175**, 255 (1928). — FELDBERG, W., and M. SCHACHTER: Histamine release by horse serum from skin of the sensitized dog and non-sensitized cat. J. Physiol. (Lond.) **118**, 124 (1952). — FELDT, R. H., and E. E. W. WENSTRAND: Family history in arterial hypertension. Study of 4376 insurance examinations. Amer. J. med. Sci. **205**, 61 (1943). — FELLER, A.: Thrombose und Embolie. Wien. klin. Wschr. **1934**, 1473. — FERGE, A.: Über den Aufbau und die Entstehung des autochthonen Thrombus. Med.-naturwiss. Arch. **2**, 351 (1909). — FERREY, J. D.: Polymerization of fibrinogen. Physiol. Rev. **34**, 753 (1954). — FINE, J., and A. M. SELIGMAN: Traumatic shock; study of problem of „lost plasma" in hemorrhagic shock by use of radioactive plasma protein. J. clin. Invest. **22**, 285 (1943). — FINE, J., A. M. SELIGMAN and H. A. FRANK: Traumatic shock. An experimental study including evidence against the capillary leakage hypothesis. Ann. Surg. **118**, 238 (1943). — FINNERTY jr., F. A., J. F. FAZEKAS and R. L. GUILLAUDEU: Demonstration of a protective shunting mechanism in collapse. Amer. J. Med. **20**, 947 (1956). — FISCH, U.: Über einen neuen Accelerator der Blutthrombokinasebildung. Thromb. diath. haemorrhag. **2**, 60 (1958). — FISCHER, H., u. P. H. ROSSIER: Starkstromunfälle mit schweren Muskelschädigungen und Myoglobinurie. Helv. med. Acta **14**, 212 (1947). — FISCHER, U.: Luftfahrtmed. **2**, 1 (1938). Zit. nach O. GAUER, The physiological effects of prolonged acceleration. German aviation Medicine. World War II, 1, 554, Washington 1950. — FISCHER, W.: Die Sklerose der Lungenarterien und ihre Entstehung. Dtsch. Arch. klin. Med. **97**, 230 (1909). — FISHBERG, A. M.: Heart faeilure, 2. Aufl. Philadlephia 1940. — FISHER, E. R., and A. C. CORCORAN: Congenital coarctation of the abdominal aorta with resultant renal hypertension. Arch. intern. Med. **89**, 943 (1952). — FISHER, J. A., and T. F. HEWER: The adrenal cortex in essential and renal hypertension. J. Path. Bact. **59**, 605 (1947). — FLECKENSTEIN, A.: Beitrag zum Mechanismus der Muskelkontraktion und zur Entstehung der Aktionströme. Pflügers Arch. ges. Physiol. **246**, 411 (1942). ~ Der Kalium-Natrium-Austausch als Energieprinzip in Muskel und Nerv. Berlin 1955. ~ Die Biochemie der Muskelerregung. Naunyn-Schmiedeberg's Arch. exp. Path. Pharmak. **228**, 46 (1956). — FLECKENSTEIN, A., E. GERLACH u. J. JANKE: Phosphorylierung und aktiver Kationentransport. Schweiz. med. Wschr. **1956**, 1041. — FLECKENSTEIN, A., H. HOCHREIN u. H. KOTOWSKI: Aufhebung der Kaliumlähmung des isolierten Froschherzens durch Adenosintriphosphat. Pflügers Arch. ges. Physiol. **265**, 485 (1958). — FLECKENSTEIN, A., and J. JANKE: The turnover-rates of labile phosphate compounds in skeletal and heart muscle during activity and rest. An investigation with the use of radiophosphorus and paper chromatography. Unit. Nat. Educat. Sci. a. Cult. Org. Internat. Conf. on Radioisotopes in Sci. Res. 1958. — FLECKENSTEIN, A., J. JANKE u. R. E. DAVIES: Der Austausch von radioaktivem Phosphat mit dem α-, β- und γ-Phosphor von ATP und mit Kreatinphosphat bei der Kontraktur des Froschrectus durch Acetylcholin, Nicotin und Succinylbicholin. Naunyn-Schiedeberg's Arch. exp. Path. Pharmak. **228**, 596 (1956). — FLECKENSTEIN, A., J. JANKE u. E. GERLACH: Konzentration und Turnover der energiereichen Phosphate des Herzens nach Studien mit Papierchromatographie und Radiophosphor. Klin. Wschr. **1959**, 451. — FÖRSTER, O.: Die Pathogenese des epileptischen Krampfanfalles. Zbl. ges. Neurol. Psychiat. **44** (1926). — Folkow, B., and B. UVNÄS: Do adrenergic vasodilator nerves exist? Acta physiol. scand. **20**, 329 (1950). — FOLTZ, E. L., A. RUBIN, W. A. STEIGER and P. C. GAZES: The effects of intravenous aminophylline upon the coronary bloodoxygen exchange. Circulation **2**, 215 (1950). — FONTAINE-VERVEY, B. C. DE LA: Über die Arteriolosklerose der Netzhaut und ihre Bedeutung für die Genese der Retinitis albuminurica. Klin. Mbl. Augenheilk. **79**, 148 (1927). — FORSTER, G.: Neuere Enzymreaktionen in der internmedizinischen Diagnostik. Bull. schweiz. Acad. med. Wiss. **14**, 191 (1958). — Fox, CH. L., and H. BAER: Redistribution of potassium, sodium and water in burns and trauma and its relation to the phenomena of shock. Amer. J. Physiol. **151**, 155 (1947). — FRAENKEL, A.: Angina pectoris. Verh. Kongr. inn. Med. **1891**, 228. — FRANCO, A.: Experimental heart failure in rabbits with hypertension. Amer. Heart J. **55**, 239 (1958). — FRANK, H. A.: I. Present-day concepts of shock. New Engl. J. Med. **249**, 445, 486 (1953). — FREEDBERG, A. ST., H. L. BLUMGART, P. M. ZOLL and M. J. SCHLESINGER: The clinical syndrome of cardiac pain intermediate between angina pectoris and acute myocardial infarction. J. Amer. med. Ass. **138**, 107 (1948). — FREEMAN, G., and G. HARTLEY jr.: Hypertension in a patient with a solitary ischemic kidney. J. Amer. med. Ass. **111**, 1159 (1938). — FREEMAN, W. J.: The histologic patterns of ruptured myocardial infarcts. Arch. Path. (Chicago) **65**, 646 (1958). — FREY, W.: Arteriosklerose. Verh. dtsch. Ges. inn. Med. **51**, 51 (1939). — FRIEDBERG, C. K.: Erkrankungen des Herzens. Stuttgart 1959. — FRIEDBERG, C. K., and H. HORN: Acute myocardial infarction not due to coronary artery occlusion. J. Amer. med. Ass. **112**, 1675 (1939). — FRIEDBERG, C. K., and A. R. SOHVAL: Non rheumatic calcific aortic stenosis. Amer. Heart J. **17**, 452 (1939). — FRIES, CH. C., B. LEVOWITZ, S. ADLER, A. W. COOK, K. E. KARLSON and C. DENNIS: Experimental cerebral gas embolism. Ann. Surg. **145**, 461 (1957). — FRÖHLICH, A.: Über lokale gewebliche Anaphylaxie. Z. Immun-Forsch. **20**, 476 (1914). — FUHRMAN, F. A., and J. M. CRISMON: Early changes in distribution of sodium, potassium and water in rabbit muscles following release of tourniquets. Amer. J. Physiol. **166**, 424 (1951). $\sim$ Muscle electrolyts in rats following ischemia produced by tourniquets. Amer. J. Physiol. **167**, 289 (1951).

GADDUM, J. H.: Gefäßerweiternde Stoffe der Gewebe, Eingeleitet von H. H. DALE. Leipzig 1936. — GÄRTNER, W.: Das klinische Bild, insbesondere die Kreislaufstörungen bei Paragangliom der Nebenniere. Z. Kreisl.-Forsch. **28**, 82 (1936). — GALLAVARDIN, L.: Les angines de poitrine. Paris 1925. $\sim$ L'angine de poitrine et ses lésions. D'après une statistique de 44 observations de syndrome angineux avec autopsie. J. Méd. Lyon **1932**, 549. $\sim$ Les syncopes d'effort dans le rétrécissement aortique, leur fréquence et leur valeur diagnostique. Arch. Mal. Cœur **30**, 745 (1937). — GASSER, H. S., J. ERLANGER and W. J. MEEK: Studies in secondary traumatic shock. IV. The blood volume changes and the effect of gum acacia on their development. Amer. J. Physiol. **50**, 31 (1919). — GAUER, O.: The physiological effects of prolonged acceleration. German aviation Medicine. World War II, 1, 554, Washington 1950. — GAVALLÉR, B. V.: Funktionelle und organische Schädigungen des Zentralnervensystems des Kaninchens nach wiederholter Entblutungsanämie. Beitr. path. Anat. **109**, 367 (1944). — GEIGER, H.: Phaeochromocytome als Ursache für paroxysmalen und permanenten Hochdruck. Diss. Freiburg i. Br. 1939. — GEISSENDÖRFER, R.: Thrombose und Embolie. Leipzig 1935. — GERSTEL, G.: Über Veränderungen der Lungenblutgefäße bei Steinstaublungenerkrankungen. Veröff. Gewerbe- u. Konstit. path. **35**, 1 (1933). — GERTTLER, M. M., and P. D. WHITE: Coronary heart disease in young adults. Cambridge, Mass. 1954. — GIBSON, J. H., and E. D. CHURCHILL: The physiology of massive pulmonary embolism. An experimental study of the changes produced by obstruction to the flow of blood through the pulmonary artery and its lobar branches. Ann. Surg. **104**, 811 (1936). — GIESE, W.: Quarzstaub, Schwielenlunge und Lungentuberkulose. Veröff. Gewerbe- u. Konstit.path. **7**, 1 (1931). $\sim$ Die Anastomosen im Koronarkreislauf bei Koronarsklerose. Dtsch. med. Wschr. **1957**, 602, 633. — GOEDEL, A.: Zur Kenntnis der Hypotrophie des rechten Herzens und schwerer Kreislaufstörungen infolge Veränderungen der Lungenschlagaderperipherie. Virchows Arch. path. Anat. **277**, 507 (1930). — GOHRBRANDT, E.: Neueste Ergebnisse in der postoperativen Thromboseentstehung. Med. Klin. **1957**, 990. — GOLDBERG, H., R. SMITH,

J. DICKENS, G. RABER and A. WALDOW: Simultaneous catheteriziation of left and right heart. J. clin. Invest. **35**, 706 (1956). — GOLDBERGER, E., J. ALESIO and F. WOLL: Significance of hyperglycemia in myocardial infarction. N.Y. St. J. Med. **45**, 391 (1945). — GOLDBLATT, H.: Studies on experimental hypertension. VII. Production of the malignant phase of hypertension. J. exp. Med. **67**, 809 (1938). — GOLDBLATT, H., H. LAMBORM and E. HAAS: Physiological properties of renin and hypertensin. Amer. J. Physiol. **175**, 75 (1953). — GOLDBLATT, H., J. LYNCH, R. F. HANZAL and W. W. SUMMERVILLE: Studies on experimental hypertension. I. Production of persistent elevation of systolic blood pressure by means of renal ischemia. J. exp. Med. **59**, 347 (1934). — GOLDENBERG, M., u. C. J. ROTHBERGER: Über Angina pectoris bei Koronarstenose. Z. klin. Med. **123**, 490 (1933). — GOLDHAMMER, M. S., u. D. SCHERF: Elektrokardiographische Untersuchungen bei Kranken mit Angina pectoris. Z. klin. Med. **122**, 134 (1932). — GOLDZIEHER, M. A.: Über die Nebennieren bei Hochdruck und Arteriosklerose. Virchows Arch. path. Anat. **280**, 749 (1931). — GOLLWITZER-MEIER, KL., D. KRAMER u. E. KRÜGER: Der Gaswechsel des suffizienten und insuffizienten Warmblüterherzens. Pflügers Arch. ges. Physiol. **237**, 68 (1936). — GOLLWITZER-MEIER, KL., u. CHR. KROETZ: Kranzgefäßdurchblutung und Gaswechsel des innervierten Herzens. Klin. Wschr. **1940**, 580, 616. — GOLLWITZER-MEIER, KL., u. E. KRÜGER: Zur Verschiedenheit der Herzenergetik und Herzdynamik bei Druck- und Volumenleistung. Pflügers Arch. ges. Physiol. **238**, 269 (1937). — GOODMAN, H. L.: Malignant hypertension with unilateral renal-artery occlusion. New Engl. J. Med. **245**, 8 (1952). — GORE, I.: Disseminated arteriolar and capillary platelet thrombosis. A morphologic study of its histogenesis. Amer. J. Path. **26**, 155 (1950). — GRAHAM, H. K.: Amniotic fluid embolism. Amer. J. Obstet. **70**, 657 (1955). — GRAY, J. D., and S. T. LAUFER: Bernheim's syndrome terminating in nephrosis. Canad. med. Ass. J. **73**, 947 (1955). — GREEN, H. D.: The coronary blood flow in aortic stenosis, in aortic insufficiency and in arteriovenous fistula. Amer. J. Physiol. **115**, 94 (1936). — GREEN, H. D., G. A. BERGERON, J. MAXWELL LITTLE and J. E. HAWKINS: Evidence, from cross transfusion experiments, that no toxic factor is present in ischemic compression shock capable of inducing a shock state in normal dogs. Amer. J. Physiol. **149**, 112 (1947). — GREEN, H. D., and D. E. GREGG: Changes in the coronary circulation following increased aortic pressure augmented cardiac output, ischemia and valve lesions. Amer. J. Physiol. **130**, 126 (1940). — GREEN, H. D., and R. WÉGRIA: Effects of asphyxia, anoxia and myocardial ischemia on coronary blood flow Amer. J. Physiol. **135**, 271 (1942). — GREGERSEN, M. I.: Experimental studies on traumatic and hemorrhagic shock. Ann. N.Y. Acad. Sci. **49**, 542 (1948). — GREGERSEN, M. I., and W. S. ROOT: Experimental traumatic shock produced by muscle contusion with a note on the effects of bullet wounds. A study of the clinical signs of shock in the dog and of the role of blood volume reduction in the development of the shock syndrome. Amer. J. Physiol. **148**, 98 (1947). — GREGG, D. E.: Coronary circulation. Philadelphia 1950. ~ Some problems of the coronary circulation. Verh. dtsch. Ges. Kreisl.-Forsch. **21**, 22 (1955). — GRÉGOIRE, R.: La phlébite bleue. Presse méd. **1938**, 1313. — GREINER, H.: Histologische Befunde bei arterieller Luftembolie. Dtsch. Z. ges. gerichtl. Med. **43**, 415 (1954). — GREMELS, H.: Zur Physiologie und Pharmakologie der Energetik des Säugetierherzens. Naunyn-Schmiedeberg's Arch. exp. Path. Pharmak. **169**, 689 (1933). ~ Über die Steuerung der energetischen Vorgänge am Säugetierherzen. Naunyn-Schmiedeberg's Arch. exp. Path. Pharmak. **182**, 1 (1936). — GRENELL, R. G.: Central nervous system resistance. The effects of temporary arrest of cerebral circulation for periods of two to ten minutes. J. Neuropath. exp. Neurol. **5**, 131 (1946). — GREVEN, K., u. H. FEDERSCHMIDT: Untersuchungen zur Hämodynamik der kleinen und kleinsten Arterien. Pflügers Arch. ges. Physiol. **242**, 617 (1939). — GRIFFIN, G. D. J., H. E. ESSEX and F. C. MANN: Experimental evidence concerning death from small pulmonary emboli. Int. Abstr. Surg. **92**, 313 (1951). — GRÖNDAHL, N. B.: Untersuchungen über Fettembolie. Dtsch. Z. Chir. **11**, 56 (1911). — GROSS, P., and E. J. BENZ: Pulmonary embolism by amniotic fluid. Surg. Gynaec. Obstet. **85**, 315 (1947). — GROSS, R.: Die thromboembolischen Erkrankungen der Lunge. In: Die thromboembolischen Erkrankungen und ihre Behandlung von TH. NAEGELI, P. MATIS, R. GROSS, H. RUNGE u. H. SACHS, S. 299. Stuttgart 1955. — GROSSE-BROCKHOFF, F.: Pathologische Physiologie. Berlin-Göttingen-Heidelberg 1950. ~ Hämodynamik des Lungenkreislaufs. Verh. dtsch. Ges. Kreisl.-Forsch. **17**, 34 (1951). ~ Pathophysiologie des Lungenkreislaufs. Bad Oeynhausener Gespräche I, 64 (1956). — GROSSE-BROCKHOFF, F., u. W. SCHOEDEL: Physiologie und Pathophysiologie des Kreislaufs. In E. DERRAS Handbuch der Thoraxchirurgie, Bd. 1, S. 267—384. 1958. — GRUBER, G. B.: Kasuistik und Kritik der Periarteriitis nodosa. Zbl. Herz- u. Gefäßkr. 18, 145, 165, 185, 205 226, 245, 269 (1926). — GRUBER, G. B., u. H. F. LANZ: Ischämische Herzmuskelnekrose bei einem Epileptiker nach Tod im Anfall. Arch. Psychiat. Nervenkr. **61** (1920). — GRUNDMANN, E.: Zur Fruchtwasserembolie. Beitr. path. Anat. **117**, 445 (1957). — GUKELBERGER, M.: Trauma und Urämie. Schweiz med. Wschr. **1954**, 77. — GYÖRI, E.: Arteriosklerotische Stenosen in Nierenarterien besonders bei Arterienverdoppelungen und ihre Beziehungen zur Hypertonie. Beitr. path. Anat. **112**, 187 (1952).

HAAS, I., u. A. WEBER: Klinische und experimentelle Studien über das Elektrokardiogramm. VI. Über Rechtscoronarinsuffizienz. Z. klin. Med. 131, 132 (1936). ~ Über Rechtscoronarinsuffizienz. Verh. dtsch. Ges. inn. Med. 1936, 343. — HACKEL, D. B., and W. T. GOODALE: Effects of haemorrhagic shock on the heart and circulation of intact dogs. Circulation 11, 628 (1955). — HADORN, W.: Über Endarteriitis obliterans der Organe. Dtsch. Arch. klin. Med. 181, 18 (1938). — HADORN, W., u. A. TILLMAN: Über Beziehungen zwischen Epilepsie und Angina pectoris. Klin. Wschr. 1935, 1308. — HAGER, H. F., and S. D. DAVIES: Nonfatal maternal pulmonary embolism by amniotic fluid. Amer. J. Obstet. 63, 901 (1952). — HAGGART, G. E., and A. M. WALKER: The physiology pulmonary embolism as disclosed by quantitative occlusion of the pulmonary artery. Arch. Surg. (Chicago) 6, 764 (1923). — HAIMOWICI, H.: Stenosing arterial thrombosis. Surgery 36, 1075 (1954). — HALLERMANN, W.: Der plötzliche Herztod bei Kranzgefäßerkrankungen. Stuttgart 1939. — HALLERVORDEN, J.: Kreislaufstörungen in der Ätiologie des angeborenen Schwachsinns. Z. ges. Neurol. Psychiat. 167, 527 (1939). — HALMAGYI, D. F. J.: Die klinische Physiologie des kleinen Kreislaufs. Übers. von STEFAN A. FARAGÓ. Jena 1957. — HAM, A. W.: Coronary and aortic sclerosis, periarteritis nodosa, chronic nephritis and hypertension as sequelae to a single experimentally produced widespread calcium precipitation in the rat. Arch. Path. (Chicago) 29, 731 (1940). — HAMILTON, M., G. W. PICKERING, J. A. F. ROBERTS and G. S. C. SOWRY: The aetiology of essential hypertension. IV. The role of inheritance. Clin. Sci. 13, 273 (1954). — HAMMARSTEN, J. F.: Syncope in aortic stenosis. Arch. intern. Med. 37, 274 (1951). — HANZON, V.: Liver cells secretion under normal and pathologic conditions studied by fluorescence microscopy on living rats. Acta physiol. scand. 28, Suppl. 101 (1952). — HARDERS, H.: Zur Frage der Autoantikörper. Klin. Wschr. 1954, 770. ~ Schlußwort zu der vorstehenden Bemerkung von H. SARRE und K. ROTHER. Klin. Wschr. 1955, 587. — HARKINS, H. N.: Recent advances in the study and management of traumatic shock. Surgery 9, 231, 447, 607 (1941). ~ The treatment of burns. Baltimore 1942. ~ The present status of the problem of termal burns. Physiol. Rev. 25, 531 (1945). ~ The general treatment of the patient with a severe burn. Philadelphia and London 1943. — HARMAN, J. W.: A histological study of sceletal muscle in acute ischemia. Amer. J. Path. 23, 551 (1947). — HARMAN, J. W., and R. P. GWINN: The recovery of the sceletal muscle fibers from acute ischemia as determined by histological and chemical methods. Amer. J. Path. 25, 741 (1949). — HARRIS, A. W., G. W. LYNCH and J. P. O'HARE: Periarteritis nodosa. Arch. intern. Med. 63, 1163 (1939). — HARRISON, C. V.: Experimental pulmonary arteriosclerosis. J. Path. Bact. 60, 289 (1948). ~ Experimental pulmonary hypertension. J. Path. Bact. 63, 195 (1951). ~ Pulmonary hypertension. A symposium. IV. The pathology of the pulmonary vessels in pulmonary hypertension. Brit. J. Radiol. 31, 217 (1958). — HARRISON, FR.: Failure of the circulation. Baltimore 1935. — HARRISON, FR. R., R. ASHMAN and R. M. LARSEN: Congestive heart failure. XII. The relation between the sickness of the cardiac musclefiber and the optimum rate of the heart. Arch. intern. Med. 49, 151 (1931). — HARRISON, H. N.: Thrombotic thrombocytopenic purpura occurring in the puerperium. Associated pancreatic islet-cell necrosis. Arch. intern. Med. 102, 124 (1958). — HART, C.: Über die isolierte Sklerose der Pulmonalarterie. Berl. klin. Wschr. 1916, 304. — HARTER, L.: Über Zirkulationsstörungen des Zentralnervensystems bei experimenteller Fett- und Luftembolie. Virchows Arch. path. Anat. 314, 213 (1947). — HARTFORT, W. ST., and CH. H. BEST: Hypertension of renal origin in rats following less than one week of choline deficiency in early life. Brit. med. J. 1949 I, 4601. — HARTWICH, A.: Der Blutdruck bei experimenteller Urämie und partieller Nierenausschaltung. Z. ges. exp. Med. 69, 462 (1930). — HASSELBACH, H. K. v.: Bestehen Beziehungen zwischen Veränderungen am Sinus caroticus und der Hypertonie? Beitr. path. Anat. 86, 369 (1931). — HASSON, J., J. I. BERKMAN, J. G. PARKER and H. RIFKIN: A clinicopathologic study of chronic renal vein thrombosis in adults. Ann. intern. Med. 47, 493 (1957). — HAUSS, W. H.: Pathophysiologische Probleme bei Coronardurchblutungsstörungen. Bad Oeynhausener Gespräche II, 199 (1958). — HAUSS, W. H., U. GERLACH und E. SCHÜRMEYER: Über die Pathogenese und die klinische Bedeutung der Hyperfermentämie. Dtsch. med. Wschr. 1958, 1310. — HAUSS, W. H., u. H. KOPERMANN: Über das Minutenvolumen beim Myokardinfarkt. Z. Kreisl.-Forsch. 39, 450 (1950). — HAYDON, G.: Noch unveröffentlicht. Siehe F. BÜCHNER, Allgemeine Pathologie, 3. Aufl., S. 334. 1959. — HAYEK, H. v.: Die menschliche Lunge. Berlin-Göttingen-Heidelberg 1953. — HAYMAKER, W.: Decompression sickness. In Handbuch der speziellen Pathologie, Bd. XIII/1 B, S. 1600. 1957. — HEARD, B. E.: An experimental study of thickening of the pulmonary arteries of rabbits produced by the organisation of fibrin. J. Path. Bact. 64, 13 (1952). — HEATH, D., J. W. DUSHANE, E. H. WOOD and J. E. EDWARDS: The aetiology of pulmonary thrombosis in cyanotic congenital heart disease with pulmonary stenosis. Thorax 13, 213 (1958). — HEATH, D., and W. WHITAKER: Hypertensive pulmonary vascular disease. Circulation 14, 323 (1956). ~ The pulmonary vessels in patent ductus arteriosus. J. Path. Bact. 70, 285 (1955). ~ The pulmonary vessels in mitral stenosis. J. Path. Bact. 70, 291 (1955). — HEBERDEN, W.: Some accounts on a disorder of the breast. Med.

Trans. (Lond.) 2 (1772). — HECHT, A.: Zur capillären Gefäßversorgung der subendocardialen Muskelschichten im menschlichen Herzen. Virchows Arch. path. Anat. 331, 26 (1958). — HEGEMANN, G.: Permeabilitätsprobleme bei der Prophylaxe und Therapie des traumatischen Schocks. Langenbecks Arch. klin. Chir. 273, 287 (1953). ~ Allgemeine Operationslehre. Berlin-Göttingen-Heidelberg 1958. — HEIDENREICH, O., u. L. SCHMIDT: Der Einfluß von Vagusreizung und Carotidenabklemmung auf die Coronardurchblutung. Pflügers Arch. ges. Physiol. 263, 315 (1956). — HEILMEYER, L.: Das Blut. In Lehrbuch der speziellen pathologischen Physiologie, 10. Aufl. Stuttgart 1960. — HEILMEYER, L., u. H. BEGEMANN: Blut und Blutkrankheiten. In Handbuch der inneren Medizin, Bd. II., 4. Aufl. 1951. ~ Atlas der klinischen Hämatologie und Cytologie. Berlin-Göttingen-Heidelberg 1955. — HEIMBUCHER, E.: Unveröffentlicht, angeführt bei G. LIEBEGOTT, Die Pathologie der Nebennieren. Verh. dtsch. Ges. Path. 1952, 21. — HEINEKE, H.: Experimentelle Untersuchungen über die Todesursache bei Perforationsperitonitis. Dtsch. Arch. klin. Med. 69, 429 (1901). — HEMMINGS, C. T.: Maternal pulmonary embolism by contents of the amniotic fluid. Amer. J. Obstet. 53, 303 (1947). — HENDLEY, E. D., and A. A. SCHILLER: Change in capillary permeability during hypoxaemic perfusion of rat hindlegs. Amer. J. Physiol. 179, 216 (1954). — HENRY, I., I. GOODMAN and I. MEEHAN: Capillary permeability in relation to acute anoxia and to venous oxygen saturation. J. clin. Invest. 26, 1119 (1947). — HENSCHEN, C.: Die Behandlung der Friedens- und Kriegsverbrennungen. Helv. med. Acta 8, 77 (1941). — HERBERTSON, B. M.: Patchy necrosis of the myocardium of rabbits after anaphylactic shock and after experimental pulmonary embolism. J. Path. Bact. 66, 211 (1953). ~ Patchy myocardial necrosis in rabbits after shock dose of histamine and peptone. J. Path. Bact. 72, 4 (1956). — HERRICK, J. B.: The coronary artery in health and disease. Harvey Lect. Ser. 26, p. 129. Baltimore 1931. — HERRMANN, G., and G. M. DECHERD: The chemical nature of heart failure. Ann. intern. Med. 12, 1233 (1939). — HERRMANN, G., G. DECHERD and T. OLIVER: Creatine changes in heart muscle under various clinical conditions. Amer. Heart J. 12, 689 (1936). — HESS, W. R.: Die Regulierung des peripheren Blutkreislaufs. Ergebn. inn. Med. Kinderheilk. 23, 1 (1923). ~ Die Regulierung des Blutkreislaufes. Leipzig 1930. ~ Das Zwischenhirn. Basel 1949. ~ Der Tierkörper als selbständiger Organismus. In Tierbau und Tierleben von R. HESSE u. FR. DOFLEIN, S. 417ff. Leipzig u. Berlin 1910. — HEYDE u. VOGT: Studien über die Wirkung des aseptischen chirurgischen Gewebszerfalles und Versuche über die Ursachen des Verbrennungstodes. Z. ges. exp. Med. 1, 59 (1913). — HEYMANS, C., and C. HENVEL-HEYMANS: New aspects of blood pressure regulation. Circulation 4, 581 (1951). — HEYMANS, C., et P. REGNIERS: Le sinus carotidien. Paris 1933. — HEYN, K., u. H. NOETZEL: Über verschiedene Formen der Rupturblutungen intracranieller Aneurysmen. Beitr. path. Anat. 116, 61 (1956). — HEYNEMANN, M.: Über die Coagulationen im Herzen. Diss. Würzburg 1843. — HICKS, J. D.: Acute arterial necrosis in the lungs. J. Path. Bact. 65, 333 (1953). — HILL: Zit. nach H. MEESSEN, Experimentelle Untersuchungen zum Collapsproblem. Beitr. path. Anat. 102, 191 (1939). — HILLEMANNS, H. G.: Statistische Untersuchungen über die Häufigkeit der tödlichen Lungenembolien im Freiburger Obduktionsgut der Jahre 1911—1950. Arch. Kreisl.-Forsch. 17, 309 (1951). — HILLENBRAND, H.-J.: Einseitige Nierenerkrankungen und Hochdruck. Z. Urol. 49, 65 (1956). — HILLER, FR.: Zirkulationsstörungen im Gehirn, eine klinische und pathologisch-anatomische Studie. Arch. Psychiat. Nervenkr. 103, 1 (1935). ~ Die Zirkulationsstörungen des Gehirns und Rückenmarks. In Handbuch der Neurologie, Bd. XI, S. 178. 1936. — HILLER, FR.: Die Thrombose der Venen und Sinus des Gehirns. In Handbuch der Neurologie, Bd. XI, S. 178 u. 449. Berlin 1936. — HILTBOLD, P.: Die Sklerose der Pulmonalarterien. Schweiz. med. Wschr. 1954, 161. — HIRSCH, E. F., and R. NAILOR: Atherosclerosis. Arch. Path. (Chicago) 59, 419 (1955). — HITTMAIR, A.: Die Blutplättchen. Folia haemat. 35, 156 (1928). — HOCHREIN, M.: Der Myokardinfarkt. Dresden u. Leipzig 1937. ~ Herzkrankheiten. II. Dresden u. Leipzig 1943. ~ Zur Symptomatologie und Therapie des Cor pulmonale. Med. Klin. 1952, 1551. — HOCHREIN, M., u. J. KELLER: Untersuchungen am Koronarsystem. Naunyn-Schmiedeberg's Arch. exp. Path. Pharmak. 159, 300, 312 (1931). ~ Beiträge zur Blutzirkulation im kleinen Kreislauf. I. Der Einfluß mechanischer Vorgänge auf die mittlere Durchblutung und die Depotfunktion der Lunge. Naunyn-Schmiedeberg's Arch. exp. Path. Pharmak. 164, 529 (1932). ~ II. Über die Beeinflussung der mittleren Durchblutung und der Blutfüllung der Lunge durch pharmakologische Mittel. Naunyn-Schmiedeberg's Arch. exp. Path. Pharmak. 164, 552 (1932). ~ III. Die nervöse Regulation der Durchblutung und Blutfüllung der Lunge. Naunyn-Schmiedeberg's Arch. exp. Path. Pharmak. 166, 229 (1932). — HOCHREIN, M., u. K. SCHNEYER: Der pulmocoronare Reflex. Naunyn-Schmiedeberg's Arch. exp. Path. Pharmak. 187, 265 (1937). — HÖFLER, W.: Siehe F. BÜCHNER, Diskussion zum Referat W. SCHOLZ, Kreislaufschäden des Gehirns und ihre Pathogenese. Verh. dtsch. Ges. Kreisl.-Forsch. 18, 241 (1953). ~ Siehe F. BÜCHNER, Die Pathologie der cellulären und geweblichen Oxydationen. In Handbuch der allgemeinen Pathologie. Bd. IV/2, S. 569. 1957. — HÖNIG, J.: Das Krankheitsbild der Thromboendarteriitis obliterans pulmonalis. Dtsch. Arch. klin. Med. 180, 645 (1937). — Höra, J.: Zur Histologie der klinischen „Primären Pulmonalsklerose". Frankfurt. Z. Path. 47,100 (1935).—Höring, F. O.: Über die Zunahme der tödlichen Lungenembolie und ihre Ursache. Dtsch. Z. Chir. 207 (1928).— Hoffheinz, S.: Die Luft- und Fettembolie. Stuttgart 1933. — Holle, G., R. Burkhardt, S. Arndt u. M. Blödorn: Über manometrische, histochemische, histologische und fasenoptische Befunde bei ischämischer Hypoxydose. (Beitrag zur Morphogenese und zur Frage des örtlichen Gewebstodes.) Virchows Arch. path. Anat. 327, 150 (1955). — Holle, G., u. G. Donner: Das Gefäßsystem der Meerschweinchenniere bei akuter Blutstauung nach Venenligatur. Virchows Arch. path. Anat. 329, 533 (1957). — Hollmann, K. H.: Nierenveränderungen nach orthostatischem Kollaps beim Kaninchen. Frankfurt. Z. Path. 67, 210 (1956). — Holzer, W., u. K. Polzer: Ärztliche Elektrokardiographie. Berlin 1941. — Holzmann, M.: Angina pectoris und Myokardnekrosen im 3. und 4. Dezennium. Helv. med. Acta 4, 791 (1937).~ Klinische Elektrokardiographie. Stuttgart 1947. — Homuth, O.: Zur Kenntnis der Serumwirkung auf die innervierte Blutstrombahn nach Versuchen im lebenden Kaninchen. Z. ges. exp. Med. 73, 251 (1930). — Hope, J.: A Treatise on the diseases of the heart. Philadelphia 1842. — Horn, H., S. Dack and C. K. Friedberg: Cardiac sequelae of embolism of the pulmonary artery. Arch. intern. Med. 64, 296 (1939). — Horn, H., L. E. Field, S. Dack and A. M. Master: Acute coronary insufficiency: pathological and physiological aspects. Amer. Heart J. 40, 63 (1950). — Horn, H., and L. E. Finkelstein: Arteriosclerosis of coronary arteries and mechanism of their occlusion. Amer. Heart J. 19, 655 (1940). — Horsley, V.: The function of the so-called motor area of the brain. Brit. med. J. 1909. — Horstmann, W.: Beobachtungen zur Reaktionsweise des Gefäßsystems am Kaninchenohr bei lokaler Reizung und bei vegetativer Fernreizung. Beitr. path. Anat. 115, 529 (1955). — Hort, W.: Quantitative histologische Untersuchungen am wachsenden Herzen. Virchows Arch. path. Anat. 323, 223 (1953). ~ Morphologische Untersuchungen am Herzen vor, während und nach der postnatalen Kreislaufumschaltung. Virchows Arch. path. Anat. 326, 458 (1955). ~ Quantitative Untersuchungen über die Capillarisierung des Herzmuskels im Erwachsenen- und Greisenalter, bei Hypertrophie und Hyperplasie. Virchows Arch. path. Anat. 327, 560 (1950). ~ Untersuchungen über die Muskelfaserdehnung und das Gefüge des Myokards in der rechten Herzkammerwand des Meerschweinchens. Virchows Arch. path. Anat. 329, 694 (1957). ~ Mikrometrische Untersuchungen an verschieden weiten Meerschweinchenherzen. Verh. dtsch. Ges. Kreisl.-Forsch. 23, 343 (1957). ~ Morphologische Untersuchungen an großen Körpervenen. Verh. dtsch. Ges. Path. 1958, 157. — Hosemann, H.: Die Grundlagen der statistischen Methoden für Mediziner und Biologen. Stuttgart 1949. — Huchard: Traité clinique des maldies du cœur et de l'aorte. Paris 1899. — Hueck, W.: Anatomisches zur Frage nach Wesen und Ursache der Arteriosklerose. Münch. med. Wschr. 1920, 535, 573, 606. — Hürzeler, D.: Untersuchungen über die Pathogenese und den Krankheitsverlauf der malignen Nephrosklerose an Hand von 123 autoptisch veriffizierten Fällen. Helv. med. Acta 21, 576 (1954). — Hugues, J.: Thrombose et hémostase spontanée. I. Internat. Tagg über Thrombose und Embolie. Basel 1954. ~ Metamorphose visqueuse des plaquettes et formation du clou hémostatique. Thromb. diath. haemorrhag. 3, 34 (1959). — Hugues, J., J. Lecomte et Y. Bounameaux: Influence de l'histamine sur l'agglutination des plaquettes et sa signification physiopathologique. Rev. belge Path. 24, 448 (1955). — Huhn, A.: Die Hirnvenen- und Sinusthrombose. Fortschr. Neurol. Psychiat. 25, 440 (1957). — Hunter, J.: Observations on the inflammation of the internal coats of veins. Transact. of Soc. for. the Impr. of med. and chir. Knowledge. Vol. I, p. 18. London 1793. — Hunter, R. M., J. C. Scott, J. P. Schneider and J. A. Krieger: Experimental amniotic fluid infusion. A preliminary report. Amer. J. Obstet. 72, 75 (1956). — Hunter, W. C., V. D. Sneeden, T. D. Robertson and A. G. Suyder: Thrombosis of the deep veins of the leg: Its clinical significance as exemplified in three hundred and fifty-one autopsies. Arch. intern. Med. 68, 1 (1941). — Hunziker, A., u. R. Oechslin: Zur pathologischen Anatomie und Pathogenese der thrombotischen Mikroangiopathie. Beitr. path. Anat. 117, 456 (1957). — Hurt, R. L., and W. J. Hanbury: Intestinal vascular lesions simulating polyparteritis nodosa after resection of coarctation of the aorta. Thorax 12, 258 (1957). — Husler, J., u. H. Spatz: Die Keuchhusteneklampsie. Z. Kinderheilk. 38, 428 (1924).

Iijima, S.: Die Durchblutungsstörungen am Kaninchenohr bei allgemeiner und lokaler Anaphylaxie mit intravitalen Photogrammen. Beitr. path. Anat. 118, 67 (1957). ~ Die Gefäßreaktion des Kaninchenohrs bei Parallergie im intravitalen Photogramm. Beitr. path. Anat. 118, 241 (1957). ~ Die Ohrarterien des Kaninchens bei Masugi-Nephritis und bei experimenteller renaler Hypertonie im intravitalen Photogramm. Beitr. path. Anat. 119, 433 (1958). ~ Unveröffentlicht 1958. — Illig, L.: Diskussionsbemerkung zu: J. Saathoff, Zur Frage des Rickerschen Stufengesetzes. Untersuchungen mit Wärmereiz am Pankreas und Mesenterium des lebenden Kaninchens. Verh. dtsch. path. Ges. 35, 248 (1952). ~ Experimentelle Untersuchungen zum Rickerschen Stufengesetz. Ein Beitrag zur ursächlichen Bedeutung vasomotorischer Reaktionen und Funktionsstörungen für die Genese lokaler

Kreislaufstörungen. Klin. Wschr. **31**, 366 (1953). ~ Demonstration zum Rickerschen Stufengesetz. Verh. dtsch. path. Ges. **37**, 371 (1954). ~ Experimentelle Untersuchungen über die Entstehung der Stase. Ein Beitrag zur Lehre von den örtlichen Kreislaufstörungen. Virchows Arch. path. Anat. **326**, 501 (1955). ~ Die Kapillarmikroskopie der Haut und Schleimhäute. In: Angiologie, S. 367. Stuttgart 1959. ~ Die terminale Strombahn. Capillarbett und Mikrozirkulation. Berlin-Göttingen-Heidelberg 1961. — Impallomeni, G.: Les altérations de l'endothélium dans la thrombose veineuse. I. Internat. Tagg über Thrombose und Embolie, Basel, 1954.

Jacob, H.: Wärme- und Kälteschädigungen des Zentralnervensystems. In Handbuch der speziellen Pathologie, Bd. XIII/3, S. 287. 1955. — Jäger, E.: Zur pathologischen Anatomie der Thrombangitis obliterans bei juveniler Gangrän. Virchows Arch. path. Anat. **284**, 526, 584 (1932). ~ Zur histologischen Ausheilung der Periarteriitis nodosa und deren Beziehung zur juvenilen Atherosklerose. Virchows Arch. path. Anat. **288**, 833 (1933). — Jaques, W. E., and A. L. Hyman: Experimental pulmonary embolism in dogs. A study of the physiologic and anatomic changes following repeated injections of autogenous clots. Arch. Path. (Chicago) **64**, 487 (1957). — Jennings, R. B., J. P. Kaltenbach and G. W. Smetters: Enzymatic changes in acute myocardial ischemic injury. Glutamic oxaloacetic transaminase, lactic dehydrogenase, and succinic dehydrogenase. Arch. Path. (Chicago) **64**, 10 (1957). — Jennings, E. R., and B. E. Stofer: Pulmonary embolism composed of contents of amniotic fluid. Arch. Path. (Chicago) **45**, 616 (1948). — Jiménez Díaz, C., P. de la Barreda, R. Ceballos y R. Ramirez-Guedes: Embolismo primario del circulo menor con sindrome de poliserositis. Rev. clin. esp. **64**, 187 (1957). — Johnson, N. J.: Paradoxical embolism. J. clin. Path. **4**, 316 (1951). — Jolly, F.: Über das Vorkommen von Fettembolie bei aufgeregten Geisteskranken. Arch. Psychiat. Nervenkr. **11**, 201 (1881). — Jores, L.: Über die Neubildung elastischer Fasern in der Intima bei Endarteriitis. Beitr. path. Anat. **24**, 458 (1898). ~ Wesen und Entwicklung der Arteriosklerose. Wiesbaden 1903. ~ Arterien. In Handbuch der speziellen Pathologie, Bd. II, S. 1898. 1924. — Jorpes, J. E.: One hundred years of research on blood coagulation leading to the present day anticoagulant therapy in thrombosis. I. Internat. Tagg über Thrombose und Embolie, Basel, 1954. — Jürgens, R.: Die Blutplättchen und ihre Bedeutung für Blutungsneigung und Thrombusbildung. Verh. dtsch. Ges. inn. Med. **58**, 492 (1952). ~ Koronarthrombose und Gerinnung. Verh. dtsch. Ges. Kreisl.-Forsch. **21**, 77 (1955). ~ Zur Genese der Koronarthrombose. Wien. Z. inn. Med. **39**, 313 (1958). — Jürgens, R., u. K. Bach: Thrombosebereitschaft bei Polycythaemia vera. Dtsch. Arch. klin. Med. **176**, 626 (1934). — Jürgens, R., u. H. Braunsteiner: Zur Pathogenese der Thrombose. Schweiz. med. Wschr. **80**, 1388 (1950). — Jürgens, R., W. Lehmann, O. Wegelius, A. W. Eriksson u. E. Hiepler: Mitteilung über den Mangel an antihämophilem Globulin (Faktor VIII) bei der Aaländischen Thrombopathie (von Willebrand-Jürgens). Thromb. diath. haemorrhag. **1**, 257 (1957). — Jung, R.: Hirnelektrische Untersuchungen über den Elektrokrampf. Die Erregungsabläufe in corticalen und subcorticalen Hirnregionen bei Katze und Hund. Arch. Psychiat. Nervenkr. **183**, 206 (1949).

Kahler, O. H., und R. Weber: Zit. nach M. Hamilton, G. W. Pickering, J. A. F. Roberts and G. S. C. Sowry, The aetiology of essential hypertension. IV. The role of inheritance. Clin. Sci. **13**, 273 (1954). — Kalk, H.: Paroxysmale Hypertension. Blutdruckkrisen und Tumor des Nebennierenmarkes. Klin. Wschr. **1934**, 613. — Kaplan, B. M., J. S. Newman, E. Kaplan, L. A. Baker and J. M. Lee: Bilateral renal vein thrombosis and the nephrotic syndrome. Ann. intern. Med. **45**, 505 (1956). — Karsner, H. T., O. Saphir and T. W. Todd: The state of the cardiac muscle in hypertrophy and atrophy. Amer. J. Path. **1**, 351 (1925). — Kathke, N.: Die Veränderungen der Coronararterienzweige des Myokards bei Hypertonie. Beitr. path. Anat. **115**, 405 (1955). — Katz, L. N., and all.: The Diagnostic value of the electrocardiogramm based on an analysis of 149 autopsy cases. Amer. Heart J. **24**, 627 (1942). — Keefer, C. S., and W. H. Resnik: Angina pectoris. Arch. intern. Med. **44**, 769 (1928). — Keeley, J. L., J. G. Gibson and M. Pijoan: Effect of thermal trauma on blood volume, serum protein, and certain blood electrolytes: experimental study of effect of burns. Surgery **5**, 872 (1939). — Keith, N. M.: Blood-volume changes in wound shock and primary hemorrhage. Spec. Rep. Ser. med. Res. Committee (Lond.) **27**, 36 (1919). — Kellaway, C. H., and W. A. Rawlinson: Studies on tissue injury by heat (1.—3.). Aust. J. exp. Biol. med. Sci. **22**, 63 (1944). — Kempf, G. F., and I. H. Page: Production of experimental hypertension and the indirect determination of systolic blood pressure in rats. J. Lab. clin. Med. **27**, 1192 (1942). — Kennedy, F.: Epilepsy and the convulsive state. Arch. Neurol. Psychiat. (Chicago) **9**, 567 (1914). — Kernen, J. A., R. M. O'Neal and D. L. Edwards: Pulmonary arteriosclerosis and thromboembolism in chronic pulmonary emphysema. Arch. Path. (Chicago) **65**, 471 (1958). — Kese, G.: Die thromboembolische Krankheit während Schwangerschaft und Wochenbett. Die Häufigkeit ihres Vorkommens in Fällen von chronischer Nephritis, Präeklampsie und Eklampsie. Zbl. Gynäk. **80**, 1299 (1958). — Kethy, S. S., and C. F. Schmidt: The effects of altered arterial tensions of carbon dioxide and oxygen on cerebral blood flow and cerebral oxygen consumptions of normal young men. J. clin. Invest. 27, 484 (1948). — KIENLE, F.: Praktische Elektrokardiographie. Leipzig 1943. ~ Das Belastungselektrokardiogramm und das Steh-EKG. Leipzig 1946. — KIESE, M., u. R. S. GARAN: Mechanische Arbeit, Größe und Sauerstoffverbrauch des Warmblüterherzens. Klin. Wschr. 1937, 1219. — KILIAN, H.: Die traumatische Fettembolie. Dtsch. Z. Chir. 231, 97 (1931). — KIMURA, E., T. KANAZAWA, N. SUZUKI, Y. ITO, N. HARIGAI and F. YAMAMOTO: Experimental studies on the coronary insufficiency and the coronary occlusion. II. The relation of the coronary blood flow to the arterial blood pressure, and the effect of the vagus nerves upon it. Tôhoku J. exp. Med. 66, 33 (1957). — KIMURA, E., N. SUZUKI, T. KANAZAWA, Y. ITO, N. HARIGAI, F. YAMAMOTO, S. KUMAGAI, Y. SUZUKI and F. OBARA: Experimental studies on the coronary insufficiency and the coronary occlusion. I. On the relation of the coronary blood flow and the ST-deviation in the electrocardiogram. Tôhoku J. exp. Med. 66, 25 (1957). — KIPKIE, G. F., u. D. S. JOHNSON: Possible pathogenic mechanisms responsible for human periarteritis nodosa. Arch. Path. (Chicago) 51, 387 (1951). — KIRCH, E.: Über gesetzmäßige Verschiebungen der inneren Größenverhältnisse des normalen und pathologisch veränderten menschlichen Herzens. Z. angew. Anat. 7, 235 (1921). ~ Untersuchungen über tonogene Herzdilatation. Verh. dtsch. Ges. Path. 1926, 391. ~ Pathogenese und Folgen der Dilatation und der Hypertrophie des Herzens. Klin. Wschr. 1930, 769, 817. ~ Das Verhalten des Herzens bei Embolien. Verh. dtsch. Ges. Kreisl.-Forsch. 7, 31 (1934). ~ Pathologisch-anatomische Grundlagen der Rechtsinsuffizienz des Herzens. Regensburg. Jb. ärztl. Fortbild. 1952, 471. ~ Pathologische Anatomie des Cor pulmonale. Verh. dtsch. Ges. Kreisl.-Forsch. 21, 163 (1955). — KLEPZIG, H.: Untersuchungen über die Arbeitsweise des menschlichen Herzens bei vermehrter Belastung. Arch. Kreisl.-Forsch. 23, 96 (1955). — KLINGE, F.: Der Rheumatismus. Ergebn. allg. Path. path Anat. 27, 1 (1933). — KNISELY, M. H., and L. WARNER: Methods for the study of the formation of thrombi in vivo. I. Internat. Tagg über Thrombose und Embolie, Basel, 1954. ~ Several steps in the formation of thrombi in vivo. I. Internat. Tagg über Thrombose und Embolie, Basel, 1954. — KNORRE, D.: Vergleichende Untersuchungen über Pulmonalgefäßveränderungen bei Herzklappenfehlern und bei Rechtsherzhypertrophie ohne Herzklappenfehler. Verh. dtsch. Ges. Path. 1958, 126. — KNOWLTON, A. I., E. N. LOEB, H. C. STOERK, J. P. WHITE and J. F. HEFFERNAN: Induction of arterial hypertension in normal and adrenalectomized rats given cortisone acetate. J. exp. Med. 96, 187 (1952). — KOBERNICK, S. D., J. R. MOORE and F. W. WIGLESWORTH: Thrombosis of the renal veins with massive hemorrhagic infarction of the kidneys in childhood. Amer. J. Path. 27, 435 (1951). — KOCH, E.: Die reflektorische Selbststeuerung des Kreislaufs. Dresden u. Leipzig 1931.— KOCH, W., u. L. CHENG KONG: Über die Formen des Koronarverschlusses, die Änderungen im Koronarkreislauf und die Beziehungen zur Angina pectoris. Beitr. path. Anat. 90, 21 (1932).— KOCZEWSKI, B. J., u. K. KAISER: Zur Frage der Nierenschädigung (Crush-Syndrom) nach Kohlenoxydintoxikation. Schweiz. med. Wschr. 1951, 1149. — KÖBERLE, F.: Zur Lehre von der Herzhypertrophie. Münch. med. Wschr. 1957, 247, 296. — KÖHN, K., u. M. RICHTER: Die Lungenarterienbahn bei angeborenen Herzfehlern. (Zwangl. Abh. a. d. Geb. der normalen u. pathol. Anatomie. Hrsg. von W. BARGMANN u. W. DOERR, H. 2.) Stuttgart 1958. ~ Die Veränderungen der Lungenstrombahn bei angeborenen Herzfehlern. Ärztl. Wschr. 1958, 25. — KÖNN, G.: Über eine Erkrankung der Sperrarterien und der arteriovenösen Anastomosen in der Lunge. Beitr. path. Anat. 115, 295 (1955). ~ Wandlungen des morphologischen Bildes der menschlichen Tuberkulose unter der Chemotherapie. Ergebn. ges. Tuberk.-Forsch. 13, 1 (1956). ~ Die pathologische Morphologie der Lungengefäße bei chronischem Cor pulmonale. Beitr. path. Anat. 116, 273 (1956). ~ Arteriosklerose des Pulmonalsystems. Verh. dtsch. Ges. Path. 1957, 77. ~ Die pathologische Morphologie der Lungengefäßerkrankungen und ihre Beziehungen zur chronischen pulmonalen Hypertonie. Ergebn. ges. Tuberk.-Forsch. 14, 100 (1958). ~ Weitere Beiträge zu den Ursachen und Folgen der chronischen pulmonalen Hypertonie. Ber. Med. Ges. Freiburg i. Br. Med. Klin. 1958. ~ Die Pathogenese der chronischen pulmonalen Hypertonie vom Standpunkt des Morphologen. Dtsch. med. Wschr. 1960, 1488, 1495. — KÖNN, G., u. CH. BÜCHNER: Temporär-chronisches Cor pulmonale nach rezidivierender experimenteller Mikroembolie. Verh. dtsch. Ges. Path. 1959, 300. — KÖNN, G., u. R. STORB: Über den Formwandel der kleinen Lungenarterien des Menschen nach der Geburt. Beitr. path. Anat. 123, 212 (1960). — KOHLSTAEDT, K. G., and I. H. PAGE: Hemorrhagic hypotension and its treatment by intraarterial and intravenous infusion of blood. Arch. Surg. (Chicago) 47, 178 (1943). ~ Terminal hemorrhagic shock, circulatory dynamics, recognition and treatment. Surgery 16, 430 (1944). ~ The liberation of renin by perfusion of kidney following reduction of pulse pressure. J. exp. Med. 72, 201 (1957). — KOHN, H.: Zur Angina pectoris. Verh. dtsch. Ges. inn. Med. 1931, 305. — KOLETSKY, S.: Hypertension in rats following complete renal ischemia. Amer. J. Path. 26, 695 (1950). ~ Necrotizing vascular disease in rat. Arch. Path. (Chicago) 59, 312 (1955). ~ Necrotizing vascular disease in rat. II. Role of sodium chloride. Arch. Path. (Chicago) 63, 405 (1957). — KOLETSKY,

S., and D. E. KLEIN: Arterial pressures in tourniquet shock. Proc. Soc. exp. Biol. (N.Y.)
91, 486 (1956). — KOLFF, W. J., and I. H. PAGE: Peristence of experimental renal hypertension after total nephrectomy in dogs. Amer. J. Physiol. 182, 531 (1955). — KOLISKO:
Über Befunde an den Nebennieren bei Verbrennungstod. Vjschr. gerichtl. Med., III. F. 47,
Suppl. 1, 217 (1914). — KOLLER, F.: Arteriosklerose und Thrombogenese (Symposium).
Bull. schweiz. Akad. med. Wiss. 13, 81 (1957). ~ Der heutige Stand der Gerinnungs-
forschung. Thromb. diath. haemorrhag. 2, 407 (1958). — KOLLER, S.: Graphische Tafeln
zur Beurteilung statistischer Zahlen, 2. Aufl. Dresden u. Leipzig 1943. — KOLLER, TH.,
u. W. R. MERZ: Thrombose und Embolie. I. Internat. Tagg über Thrombose und Embolie,
Basel, 1954. — KOLLER, T., H. STAMM, G. A. HAUSER u. M. KLINGLER: Die zerebralen
Venen- und Sinusthrombosen in der Geburtshilfe. Thromb. diath. haemorrhag. 1, 37 (1957). —
KORNFELD, M.: Mikroangiopathia thrombotica. Thrombotische thrombocytopenische
Purpura. Med. Klin. 1958, 1375. — KOSLOWSKI, L.: Autolyse-Krankheiten in der Chirurgie.
Stuttgart 1959. — KOTOWSKI, H., H. ANTONI u. A. FLECKENSTEIN: Elektrophysio-
logische Studien zur Aufhebung der Kaliumlähmung des Froschmyokards durch ATP.
Pflügers Arch. ges. Physiol. 270, 85 (1959). — KOUTZKY, J., u. J. LUKAWSKY: Embolie
durch Amnionflüssigkeit als Ursache von Geburtsschock. Čsl. Gynaek. 19, 334 (1954). —
KOYANAGI, Y.: Über die Pathogenese der Retinitis nephritica. Mbl. Augenheilk. 80, 436
(1928). — KREHL, L.: Beitrag zur Pathologie der Herzklappenfehler. Dtsch. Arch. klin. Med.
46, 454 (1890). ~ Beitrag zur Kenntnis der idiopathischen Herzmuskelerkrankungen. Dtsch.
Arch. klin. Med. 48, 414 (1891). ~ Die Erkrankungen des Herzmuskels und die nervösen
Herzkrankheiten. In NOTHNAGELs Handbuch, Bd. 15, S. 1. 1901. — KRIEG, E.: Die Venen-
entzündung. München u. Berlin 1952. — KRIKENT, R. K.: Zum Problem der Thrombo-
embolien der Nieren. Ter. Arh. 27, H. 3, 74 (1955). — KRÖNKE, E.: Experimentelle
Untersuchungen zum Wirkungsmechanismus der Fettembolie. Langenbecks Arch. klin. Chir.
285, 308 (1957). — KROETZ, CHR.: Herzinsuffizienz und Koronarinsuffizienz. Oynhausener
Vortr. 2, 44 (1933). ~ Angina pectoris und Rauchgasvergiftung. Med. Klin. 1936,
Nr 45. ~ Herzschädigungen nach Kohlenoxydvergiftungen. Dtsch. med. Wschr. 1936,
1365, 1414. — KROGH, A.: The supply of oxygen to the tissues and the regulation of the
capillary circulation. J. Physiol. (Lond.) 52, 457 (1919). ~ Studies on the physiology of the
capillaries. II. The reactions to local stimuli of the blood-vessels in the skin and web of the
frog. J. Physiol. (Lond.) 55, 412 (1921). ~ The anatomy and physiology of capillaries.
II. Aufl. New Haven 1929. — KRÜCKE, W.: Über die Fettembolie des Gehirns nach Flugunfällen. Virchows Arch. path. Anat. 315, 481 (1948). ~ Die Fettembolie des Gehirns.
Verh. dtsch. path. Ges. 1944, 207 (1949). — KUGEL, M. A., and S. S. LICHTMAN: Factors
causing clinical jaundice in heart disease. Arch. intern. Med. 52, 16 (1943). — KUHLMAN, D.,
C. RAGAN, J. W. FERREBREE, D. W. ATCHLEY and R. F. LOEB: Toxic effects of desoxy-
corticosterone esters in dogs. Science 90, 496 (1939). — KUHN, J. K.: Die Bewegung der
Thrombosen und Embolien in den Nachkriegsjahren und ihre Ursachen. Mitt. Grenzgeb.
Med. Chir. 41, 329 (1929). — KUIDA, H., G. J. DAMMIN, F. W. HAYNES, E. RAPAPORT
and L. DEXTER: Primary pulmonary hypertension. Amer. J. Med. 23, 166 (1957). —
KUMPE, C., and W. B. BEAN: Aortic stenosis; study of clinical and pathologic aspects of 107
proved cases. Medicine 27, 139 (1948). — KUPERMAN, I., and G. E. WAKERLIN: Treatment
of experimental renal hypertension in dogs with antirenin. Fed. Proc. 12, 80 (1952).
    LA DUE, J. S., and F. WROBLEWSKI: The significance of the serum glutamic oxalacetic
transaminase activity following acute myocardial infarction. Circulation 11, 871 (1955). —
LAGERLÖF, H. O.: Heart metabolism and myocardial efficiency. Advanc. Cardiol. 2, 165
(1959). — LAKI, K.: Chemistry of prothrombin and some of its reactions. Physiol. Rev. 34,
730 (1954). — LAMBERT, E., and F. R. ROSENTHAL: Study of skin histamine. (With some
results of splanchnic nerve stimulation.) Proc. Soc. exp. Biol. (N.Y.) 52, 302 (1943). —
LAMY, M., J. DE GROUCHY and O. SCHWEISGUTH: Genetic and non-genetic factors in the
etiology of congenital heart disease: a study of 1188 cases. Amer. J. hum. Genet. 9, 17
(1957). — LANCH, M. J. G., ST. S. RAPHAEL and TH. P. DIXON: Fat embolism in chronic
alcoholism. Lancet 1957 II, 123. — LANDAU, M.: Die Nebennierenrinde. Jena 1915. —
LANDING, B. H.: The pathogenesis of amniotic-fluid embolism. II. Uterine factors. New
Engl. J. Med. 243, 590 (1950). — LANDIS, E. M.: The capillary pressure in frog mesentery as
determined by micro-injection methods. Amer. J. Physiol. 75, 548 (1926). ~ Micro-injection
studies of capillary permeability; relation between capillary pressure and rate at which fluid
passes through walls of single capillaries. Amer. J. Physiol. 82, 217 (1927). ~ Micro-injection
studies of capillary permeability; effect of lack of oxygen on permeability of capillary wall to
fluid and to plasma proteins. Amer. J. Physiol. 83, 528 (1928). ~ Capillary pressure and
capillary permeability. Physiol. Rev. 14, 404 (1934). ~ The passage of fluid throught the
capillary wall. Amer. J. med. Sci. 193, 297 (1937). — LANG, K., W. H. A. SCHÖTTLER,
E. SCHÜTTE, H. SCHWIEGK u. U. WESTPHAL: Der Gewebsstoffwechsel bei örtlicher Erfrierung. Klin. Wschr. 1943, 444, 653. — LANGE, F.: Studies on the blood vessels in the

membrane of chick embryo. II. Reactions of the blood vessels in the vascular membrane. J. exp. Med. **52**, 73 (1930). ~ IV. Modification of irritability of the blood vessels. J. exp. Med. **52**, 89 (1930). — LANGE, F., W. EHRICH and A. E. COHN: Studies on the blood vessels in the membranes of the chick embryo I: Absence of nerves in the vascular membrane. J. exp. Med. **52**, 65 (1930). — LARSEN, H. K.: Effect of anoxemia on the human electrocardiogram. Acta med. scand. Suppl. **78** (1938). — LAUBRY, CH., et P. SOULIÉ: Les maladies des coronaires. L'infarctus du myocarde. L'insuffisance coronarienne. 2. Aufl. Paris 1950. — LAVENNE, F.: Le retentissement cardio-vasculaire de la silicose et de l'anthracosilicose. Rev. belge Path. **21**, Suppl. IV, 264 (1951). — LAVENNE, F., et F. MEERSSEMAN: Anatomie pathologique de la circulation pulmonaire. Acta cardiol. (Brux.) **9**, 343 (1954). — LEARY, O. C., and A. T. HERTIG: The pathogenesis of amniotic-fluid embolism. I. Possible placental factors — aberrant squamous cells in placentas. New Engl. J. Med. **243**, 588 (1950). — LEARY, T.: Experimental atherosclerosis in the rabbit compared with human (coronary) atherosclerosis. Arch. Path. (Chicago) **17**, 453 (1934). — LECOMTE, J., u. J. HUGUES: Sur les réactions anaphylactiques des vaisseaux mésentériques du lapin. Int. Arch. Allergy **8**, 72 (1955). — LEDINGHAM, J. M.: Hypertension and disturbances of tissue water, sodium and potassium distribution associated with steroid administration in adrenalectomised rats. Clin. Sci. **13**, 543 (1954). — LEE, K. T., and W. A. THOMAS: Hypertension and coronary arteriosclerosis. Arch. Path. (Chicago) **60**, 616 (1955). — LEINWAND, I., A. W. DURYEE and M. N. RICHTER: Scleroderma (based on a study of over 150 cases). Ann. intern. Med. **41**, 1003 (1954). — LEITER, L.: Unusual hypertensive renal disease. I. Occlusion of renal arteries (Goldblatt-Hypertension). II. Anomalies of urinary tract. J. Amer. med. Ass. **111**, 507 (1938). — LEITNER, ST.: Der Besnier-Boeck-Schaumann, 2. Aufl. Basel 1949. — LENÈGRE, J., et A. GERBAUX: Le cœur pulmonaire chronique par thrombose artérielle pulmonaire. Arch. Mal. Cœur **45**, 289 (1952). — LENÈGRE, J., A. GERBAUX, L. SCEBAT et R. LECOMPTE DE FLORIS: Quatre nouvelles observations de cœur pulmonaire chronique par thrombose artérielle pulmonaire. Arch. Mal. Cœur **48**, 1132 (1955). — LENÈGRE, J., A. MATHIVAT, G. CAROUSO et J. DE BRUX: Pulmonary embolism and infarction in patients with cardiac disease. Their relation to venous thrombosis. Bull. Soc. méd. Hôp. Paris **65**, 219 (1949). — LENGGENHAGER, K.: Entstehung, Erkennung und Vermeidung der postop. Fernthrombose. Stuttgart 1947. — LENG-LÉVY, J., J. VINCENDEAU, J. DAVID-CHAUSSE et R. MALINEAU: Sur un cas clinique d'hypertension artérielle de type Goldblatt. Bull. Soc. méd. Hôp. Paris **68**, 1251 (1952). — LEPAGE, F., L. LEMERRE et A. DUPAY: Ménométrorragies et troubles des fonctions vasculo-sanguines de l'hémostase. Gynéc. et Obstét. **54**, 2 (1955). ~ L'embolie amniotique. Gynéc. et Obstét. **55**, 45 (1956). — LEPAGE, G. A.: Biological energy transformations during shock as shown by tissue analysis. Amer. J. Physiol. **146**, 267 (1946). — LERICHE, FONTAINE u. FRIEDMANN: Zit. nach H. SCHWIEGK, Verh. dtsch. Ges. Kreisl.-Forsch. **17**, 95 (1951). — LERICHE, R.: Quelques considérations de physiologie pathologique sur la thrombose veineuse. I. Internat. Tagg über Thrombose und Embolie, Basel, 1954. — LESSER, M. A.: The treatment of angina pectoris with testosterone-propionate. New Engl. J. Med. **226**, 51 (1942). — LESTER, R., and M. D. DRAGSTEDT: Pathogenesis of gastroduodenal ulcer. Arch. Surg. **44**, 438 (1942). — LETTERER, E.: Über normergische und hyperergische Entzündung. Dtsch. med. Wschr. **78**, 759 (1953). ~ Zur Deutung der Masugi-Nephritis als allergisch-hyperergisches Phänomen. Dtsch. med. Wschr. **1953**, 512. ~ Die allergisch-hyperergische Entzündung. In Handbuch der allgemeinen Pathologie, Bd. VII/1, S. 497. 1956. — LEVINE, S. A., and C. L. BROWN: Coronary thrombosis: its various clinical features. Medicine (Baltimore) **8**, 245 (1929). — LEVY, R. L.: Diseases of the coronary arteries and cardiac pain. New York 1936. — LEVY, R. L., and H. G. BRUENN: Acute fatal coronary insufficiency. J. Amer. med. Ass. **106**, 1080 (1936). — LEVY, R. L., H. G. BRUENN and N. G. RUSSELL jr.: The use of electrocardiographic changes caused by induced anoxemia as a test for coronary insufficiency. Amer. J. med. Sci. **197**, 241 (1939). — LEVY, R. L., and R. L. MOORE: Paravertebral sympathetic block with alcohol for the relief of cardiac pain. J. Amer. med. Ass. **116**, 2563 (1941). — LEVY, R. L., J. E. PATTERSON, T. W. CLARK and H. G. BRUENN: The „anoxemia test" as an index of the coronary reserve: Serial observations on one hundred and thirty-seven patients with their application to the detection and clinical course of coronary insufficiency. J. Amer. med. Ass. **117**, 2113 (1941). — LEVY, R. L., N. E. WILLIAMS, H. G. BRUENN and H. A. CARR: The „anoxemia test" in the diagnosis of coronary insufficiency. Amer. Heart J. **21**, 634 (1941). — LEWIS, B. M., R. GORLIN, H. E. J. HOUSSAY, F. W. HAYNES and L. DEXTER: Clinical and physiological correlations in patients with mitralstenosis. V. Amer. Heart J. **43**, 2 (1952). — LEWIS, R. B., and H. B. GERSTNER: Bloodflow as indicated by temperature changes in rabbit legs before and after exposure to local cold. Amer. J. Physiol. **177**, 501 (1954). — LEWIS, T.: The blood vessels in the human skin and their responses. London 1927. — LEWIS, T., G. W. PICKERING and P. ROTHSCHILD: Observations upon muscular pain in intermittent claudication. Heart **4**, 359 (1931). — LEWIS, TH.: Die Blutgefäße der menschlichen Haut. Berlin 1928. — LIBMAN, E.: Some observations on thrombosis of the coronary arteries. Trans. Ass. Amer. Phycns. **34**, 138 (1939). — Lichtheim, L.: Die Störungen des Lungenkreislaufes. Berlin 1876. — Liebegott, G.: Studien zur Orthologie und Pathologie der Nebennieren. Beitr. path. Anat. **109**, 93 (1944). ~ Die Pathologie der Nebennieren. Verh. dtsch. Ges. Path. **36**, 21 (1953). ~ Zur Pathologie des Penicillinschadens des Zentralnervensystems. Beitr. path. Anat. **115**, 206 (1955). ~ Morphologische Befunde am Auge bei Hypertonie. Ber. 61. Zus.kunft dtsch. Ophthalm. Ges. 1957, S. 197. ~ Die intramurale Coronarsklerose bei Hypertonie. Med. Klin. 1958, 1465. — Likoff, W., D. Berkowitz, C. Denton, H. Goldberg and A. Reale: Transventricular commissurotomy in aortic stenosis. A clinical evaluation. J. Amer. med. Ass. **157**, 1367 (1955). — Lindenberg, R., u. H. Spatz: Über die Thrombarteriitis der Hirngefäße. Virchows Arch. path. Anat. **305**, 531 (1939). — Lindgren, F. T., and J. W. Gofman: The role of lipoproteins in coronary disease. Bull. schweiz. Akad. med. Wiss. **13**, 152 (1957). — Lindner, E.: Der elektronenmikroskopische Nachweis von Eisen im Gewebe. Ergebn. allg. Path. u. path. Anat. **38**, 46 (1958). — Linzbach, A. J.: Vergleich der dystrophischen Vorgänge an Knorpel und Arterien. Virchows Arch. path. Anat. **311**, 432 (1943). ~ Mikrometrische und histologische Analyse hypertropher menschlicher Herzen. Virchows Arch. path. Anat. **314**, 534 (1947). ~ Das ökonomische Prinzip in der Sauerstoffversorgung. Z. ges. inn. Med. **2**, 144 (1947). ~ Herzhypertrophie und kritisches Herzgewicht. Klin. Wschr. **1948**, 459. ~ Die Muskelfaserkonstante und das Wachstumsgesetz der menschlichen Herzkammern. Virchows Arch. path. Anat. **318**, 575 (1950). ~ Untersuchungen über die Grenzschicht zwischen Blut- und Gefäßwand. Verh. dtsch. Ges. Path. **34**, 252 (1951). ~ Quantitative Biologie und Morphologie des Wachstums einschließlich Hypertrophie und Riesenzellen. In Handbuch der allgemeinen Pathologie, Bd. VI/1, S. 180. 1955. ~ Über das Längenwachstum der Herzmuskelfasern und ihrer Kerne in Beziehung zur Herzdilatation. Virchows Arch. path. Anat. **328**, 165 (1956). ~ Die Bedeutung der Gefäßwandfaktoren für die Entstehung der Arteriosklerose. Verh. dtsch. Ges. Path. **41**, 24 (1958). ~ Struktur und Funktion des gesunden und kranken Herzens. In: Die Funktionsdiagnostik des Herzens, S. 94. Berlin-Göttingen-Heidelberg 1958. ~ Die Lebenswandlungen der Struktur des Herzens. Verh. dtsch. Ges. Kreisl.-Forsch. **24**, 3 (1958). — Linzbach, A. J., u. M. Linzbach: Die Herzdilatation. Klin. Wschr. **1951**, 621. — Ljungdahl, M.: Untersuchungen über die Arteriosklerose des kleinen Kreislaufs. Wiesbaden 1915. ~ Gibt es eine chronische Embolisierung der Lungenarterien. Dtsch. Arch. klin. Med. **160**, 1 (1928). — Loeliger, A.: Über den Nachweis eines neuen Gerinnungsfaktors, Faktor VII. Wien. Z. inn. Med. **3**, 169 (1952). — Lörinc, J., and Gy. Goracz: Experimental malignant hypertension. Acta morph. Acad. Sci. hung. **5**, 11 (1955). — Löwenstein, K.: Über Thromboarteriitis pulmonalis. Frankfurt. Z. Path. **27**, 226 (1922). — Lolk, H., u. J. Sika: Fruchtwasserembolie. Ugeskr. Laeg. **1952**, 1799. — Loogen, F.: Der pulmonale Hochdruck bei angeborenen Herzfehlern mit hohem pulmonalem Stromvolumen. Arch. Kreisl.-Forsch. **28**, 1 (1958). — Loomis, D.: Hypertension and necrotizing arteritis in the rat following renal infarction. Arch. Path. (Chicago) **41**, 231 (1946). — Lorand, L.: Interaction of thrombin and fibrinogen. Physiol. Rev. **34**, 742 (1954). — Loustalot, P.: Beitrag zur Frage des Crush-Syndroms. Schweiz. med. Wschr. **1950**, 1045. — Lubarsch, O.: Allgemeine Pathologie. Wiesbaden 1905. ~ Thrombose und Infektion. Berl. klin. Wschr. **1918**, 225. — Lucadou, W. v.: Thrombose und Embolie. Z. Kreisl.-Forsch. **22**, 697 (1931). ~ Endothel und Thrombose. Z. Kreisl.-Forsch. **25**, 785 (1933). ~ Untersuchungen über die Nebenniere, besonders bei chronischer Herzbelastung. Beitr. path. Anat. **96**, 561 (1936). — Lucké, B.: Lower nephron nephrosis (the renal lesions of the crush syndrome, of burns, transfusions and other conditions affecting the lower segments of the nephrons). Milit. Surg. **99**, 371 (1946). — Lüdeke, H.: Thrombophilie und Polycythämie. Virchows Arch. path. Anat. **293**, 218 (1934). — Lüthy, E.: Diskussionsbemerkung. 2. Freiburger Kolloquium über Kreislaufmessungen. 1959. — Lushbaugh, C. C., and P. E. Steiner: Additional observations on maternal pulmonary embolism by amniotic fluid. Amer. J. Obstetr. **43**, 833 (1942).

Mackenzie, J.: Angina pectoris. London 1923. — Malamud: Zit. nach Grosse-Brockhoff, Handbuch der inneren Medizin, Bd. VI/2. 1954. — Mallory, G. K., N. Blackburn, H. J. Sparling and D. A. Nickerson: Maternal pulmonary embolism by amniotic fluid. Report of three cases and discussion of the literature. New Engl. J. Med. **243**, 583 (1950). — Mallory, G. K., P. D. White and J. Salcedo-Salgar: The speed of healing of myocardial infarction. A study of the pathologic anatomy in 72 cases. Amer. Heart J. **18**, 647 (1939). — Mallory, T. B., E. R. Sullivan, Ch. H. Burnett, F. A. Simeoen, S. L. Shapiro and H. K. Beecher: The general pathology of traumatic shock. Surgery **27**, 629 (1950). — Malmström, G.: The cardiological anoxemia test. Acta med. scand. Suppl. **195** (1947). — Mangun, G. N., and V. C. Myers: Purine content of human cardiac and voluntary muscle. J. biol. Chem. **133**, 11 (1940). ~ Normal creatine, phosphorus, and potassium content of human cardiac and voluntary muscle. J. biol. Chem. **135**, 411 (1940). ~ Cardiac muscle. Further studies, investigation of chemical changes in myocardial insufficiency with special reference to adenosintriphosphat. Arch. intern. Med. **78**,

441 (1946). — Mantero, O., G. Baroldi and G. Scomazzoni: The coronary arterial circulation in the hypertrophic heart. Cardiologia (Basel) 32, 48 (1958). — Marey, E. J.: Circulation du sang. Paris 1881. — Margolies, H. M., F. O. Ziellessen and A. R. Barnes: Calcareus aortic valvular disease. Amer. Heart J. 6, 349 (1931). — Marquardt, R.: Die Gefäß- und Netzhautveränderungen des Auges bei Hypertonie. Beitr. path. Anat. 118, 101 (1957). ~ Die arteriosklerotischen Gefäßveränderungen des Auges bei Hypertonie. Verh. dtsch. Ges. Path. 41, 123 (1958). — Marrack, J. R.: The biological significance of complete and incomplete antibodies. I. Congr. Internat. Allergie 1952, p. 249. — Martin, H., u. H. Noetzel: Die Gehirnbeteiligung bei generalisierter Panarteriitis nodosa. Beitr. path. Anat. 121, 347 (1959). — Martin, I.: Zur Kenntnis der Fruchtwasserembolie. Frankfurt. Z. Path. 65, 467 (1954). ~ Die Fruchtwasserembolie als Todesursache während oder nach der Geburt. Geburtsh. u. Frauenheilk. 16, 463 (1956). — Martin, R. E., and H. Fanger: Pulmonary amniotic fluid embolism. Report of a fatal case. Amer. J. Obstet. 67, 1148 (1954). — Marvin, H. M., and A. G. Sullivan: Clinical observations upon syncope and sudden death in relation to aortic stenosis. Amer. Heart J. 10, 705 (1935). — Masshoff, W.: Studien über die Hämolyse. Frankfurt. Z. Path. 61, 1 (1949). — Massie, H.: Beitrag zum Thromboembolieproblem. Dargestellt am Krankengut der Chir. Klin. und am Sektionsgut des Path. Inst. der Univ. Marburg. Inaug.-Diss. Marburg 1954. — Masson, G. M. C., J. B. Hazard, A. C. Corcoran and I. H. Page: Experimental vascular disease due to desoxycorticosterone factors. II. Comparison of pathologic changes. Arch. Path. (Chicago) 49, 641 (1950). — Masson, G. M. C., G. Plahl, A. C. Corcoran and I. H. Page: Accelerated hypertensive vascular disease from saline and renin in nephrectomized dogs. Arch. Path. (Chicago) 55, 85 (1953). — Master, A. M.: The two-step test of myocardial function. Amer. Heart J. 10, 495 (1935). ~ The two-step exercise electrocardiogram: a test for coronary insufficiency. Ann. intern. Med. 32, 842 (1950). — Master, A. M., S. Dack, A. Grishman, L. E. Field and H. Horn: Acute coronary insufficiency: An entity. Shock, hemorrhage and pulmonary embolism as factors in its production. J. Mt Sinai Hosp. 14, 8 (1947). — Master, A. M., S. Dack, H. Horn, B. I. Freedman and L. E. Field: Acute coronary insufficiency due to acute hemorrhage: an analysis of one hundred and three cases. Circulation 1 1302 (1950). — Master, A. M., R. Gubner, S. Dack and H. L. Jaffe: Differentiation of acute coronary insufficiency with myocardial infarctions from coronary occlusion. Arch. intern. Med. 67, 647 (1941). — Master, A. M., and E. T. Oppenheimer: A simple exercise tolerance test for circulatory efficiency with standard tables for normal individuals. Amer. J. med. Sci. 177, 223 (1929). — Master, A. M., I. Rosenfeld and E. Donoso: The Master „2-step" exercise test. Advanc. Cardiol. 2, 243 (1959). — Mathiesen, F. R.: Amniotic emboli. An unusual cause of death. Ugeskr. Laeg. 1955, 320. — May, R., u. J. Thurner: Ein Gefäßsporn in der Vena iliaca communis sinistra als Ursache der überwiegend linksseitigen Beckenvenenthrombosen. Z. Kreisl.-Forsch. 45, 912 (1956). — Mazur, A., J. Litt and E. Shorr: Oxidation and reduction of ferritin sulfhydril groups by liver. J. biol. Chem. 187, 497 (1950). ~ The relation of sulfhydril groups in ferritin to its vasodepressor activity. J. biol. Chem. 187, 485 (1950). ~ Chemical properties of ferritin and their relation to its vasodepressor activity. J. biol. Chem. 187, 473 (1950). — Mazur, A., and E. Shorr: Hepatorenal factors in circulatory homeostasis. IX. The identification of the hepatic vasodepressor substance, VDM, with ferritin. J. biol. Chem. 176, 771 (1948). — McGinn, S., and P. D. White: Clinical observations on aortic stenosis. Amer. J. med. Sci. 188, 1 (1934). — McKeown, F.: The pathology of pulmonary heart disease. Brit. Heart J. 14, 25 (1952). — McLachlin, J., u. J. C. Paterson: Die Ätiologie der Venenthrombose. Klin. Wschr. 36, 645 (1958). — McShan, W. H., R. Potter, A. Goldman, E. G. Shipley and R. K. Meyer: Biological energy transformations during shock as shown by blood chemistry. Amer. J. Physiol. 145, 93 (1945). — Meessen, H.: Zur Pathologie der Hypophyse. Beitr. path. Anat. 95, 39 (1935). ~ Diskussionsbemerkung. Verh. dtsch. Path. Ges. 29, 103 (1937). ~ Über Coronarinsuffizienz nach Histamincollaps und nach orthostatischem Collaps. Beitr. path. Anat. 99, 329 (1937). ~ Koronarinsuffizienz durch Histaminkollaps und durch orthostatischen Kollaps. Verh. dtsch. Ges. Kreisl.-Forsch. 10, 198 (1937). ~ Experimentelle Untersuchungen zum Collapsproblem. Beitr. path. Anat. 102, 191 (1939). ~ Coronarthrombose nach Unfall. Frankfurt. Z. Path. 54, 307 (1940). ~ Über experimentelle Lungenembolie durch Glasperlen. Arch. Kreisl.-Forsch. 6, 117 (1940). ~ Elektrokardiographische und anatomische Untersuchungen an Kaninchen über die Wirkung von Insulinschock und Cardiacolkrampf auf das Herz. Arch. Kreisl.-Forsch. 6, 361 (1940). ~ Arterielle Thrombosen nach Lungenschuß. Beitr. path. Anat. 105, 432 (1941). ~ Über Ursachen und Folgen abnormer Blutverteilung. Ber. naturforsch. Ges. 37, 65 (1941). ~ Über den plötzlichen Herztod bei Frühsklerose und Frühthrombose der Koronararterien bei Männern unter 45 Jahren. Z. Kreisl.-Forsch. 36, 185 (1944). ~ Veränderungen am Zentralnervensystem des Hundes nach Histaminkollaps. Beitr. path. Anat. 109, 352 (1944). ~ Allgemeine Pathologie des Kollapses. Fiat Rev. Allg. Path. 1, 45 (1948). ~ Zur pathologischen

Anatomie des Lungenkreislaufs. Verh. dtsch. Ges. Kreisl.-Forsch. 17, 25 (1951). ~ Pathologische Anatomie des Morbus coeruleus. Langenbecks Arch. klin. Chir. 279, 474 (1954). ~ Die Lunge bei Mitralstenose. Dtsch. med. Wschr. 1956, 1445, 1465. ~ Zur Pathogenese, Progredienz und Adaption der angeborenen Herz- und Gefäßfehler. Verh. dtsch. Ges. Kreisl.-Forsch. 23, 188 (1957). — MEESSEN, H., u. R. SCHMIDT: Über Durchblutungsstörungen der Netzhautgefäße bei experimentellem Kollaps. Arch. Kreisl.-Forsch. 10, 255 (1942). — MEESSEN, H., u. O. STOCHDORPH: Erweichung und Blutung (des Gehirns). In Handbuch der speziellen Pathologie, Bd. XIII/1 B, S. 1384. 1957. ~ Die Embolie durch Luft- und Fetteinschwemmung. In Handbuch der speziellen Pathologie, Bd. XIII/1, S. 1420. 1957. ~ Thromboembolie, die arterielle und venöse Thrombose des Gehirns. In Handbuch der speziellen Pathologie, Bd. XIII/1, S. 1438. 1957. — MEINERS, S.: Über die Erregbarkeitssteigerung der Arterien und das Auftreten von Angiospasmen nach lokaler Gewebsschädigung. Pflügers Arch. ges. Physiol. 254, 557 (1952). — MELLINKOFF, S. M., and P. A. TUMULTY: Hepatic hypoglycemia. Its occurence in congestive heart failure. New Eng. J. Med. 247, 745 (1952). — MENDELSON, C. L.: Pulmonary embolism from amniotic fluid. Amer. J. Obstet. 55, 911 (1948). — MENEELY, G. R., R. G. TUCKER, W. J. DARBY and S. H. AUERBACH: Chronic sodium chloride toxicity in the albino rat. II. Occurence of hypertension and of a syndrome of edema and renal failure. J. exp. Med. 98, 71 (1953). — MERKEL, H.: Über die Bedeutung der sog. paradoxen oder gekreuzten Embolie für die Gerichtliche Medizin (nach einem landgerichtsärztlichen Fortbildungsvortrag). Dtsch. Z. ges. gerichtl. Med. 23, 338 (1934). ~ Zur Histologie der Lungengefäße. Beitr. path. Anat. 105, 176 (1941). ~ Über die sogenannte primäre Pulmonalsklerose. Beitr. path. Anat. 109, 437 (1947). — MESTWERDT, G.: Biologie und Pathologie des Weibes, Bd. X/4, S. 858. München u. Berlin 1955. — MEYER, H. H., u. R. GOTTLIEB: Pharmakologie, 9. Aufl. 1936. — MEYER, J. E.: Zur Ätiologie und Pathogenese des fetalen und frühkindlichen Cerebralschadens. Z. Kinderheilk. 67, 123 (1949). — MEYER, W. W.: Zur Morphologie der hypertonischen Arteriosklerose im kleinen und großen Kreislauf. Zugleich ein Beitrag zur Bedeutung diffuser sklerotischer Arterienveränderungen im Gesamtgeschehen der Arteriosklerose. Bull. schweiz. Akad. med. Wiss. 13, 115 (1957). — MEYER, W. W., u. H. BECK: Das röntgenanatomische und feingewebliche Bild der Arteriosklerose im intrakraniellen Abschnitt der Arteria carotis interna. Virchows Arch. path. Anat. 326, 700 (1954/55). — MEYER, W. W., u. H. RICHTER: Das Gewicht der Lungenschlagader als Gradmesser der Pulmonalarteriensklerose und als morphologisches Kriterium der pulmonalen Hypertonie. Eine quantitativ-anatomische und feingewebliche Untersuchung. Virchows Arch. path. Anat. 328, 121 (1956). — MEYER, W. W., H. RICHTER, P. SCHOLLMEYER u. E. SIMON: Das Fassungsvermögen und die Volumendehnbarkeit des aortalen Windkessels und der Pulmonalis in Abhängigkeit von Alter, Arteriosklerose und Hochdruck. Verh. dtsch. Ges. Kreisl.-Forsch. 23, 346 (1957). — MILLER, G., J. C. HOYT and B. E. POLLOCK: Bilateral renal vein thrombosis and the nephrotic syndrome. Amer. J. Med. 17, 856 (1954). — MILLICAN, R. C.: S^{35}-plasma and erythrocyte distribution in tourniquet-shocked mice. Amer. J. Physiol. 179, 513 (1954). ~ Tourniquet shock in mice. Na^{22} and S^{35}-plasma turn-over in the accumulated fluid in area of injury. Amer. J. Physiol. 179, 520 (1954). — MILLIEZ, P., G. LAGRUE, Y. DE BAROCHEZ and P. SAMARCQ: Les thromboses des veines rénales. I. Aspects cliniques des thromboses des veines rénales. J. Urol. méd. chir. 63, 569 (1957). — MILNE, M. D.: Nierenvenenthrombose und nephrotisches Syndrom. Postgrad. med. J. 30, 640 (1954). — MINAMI, S.: Über Nierenveränderungen nach Verschüttung. Virchows Arch. path. Anat. 245, 247 (1923). — MÖLBERT, E.: Das elektronenmikroskopische Bild der Leberparenchymzelle nach histotoxischer Hypoxydose. Beitr. path. Anat. 118, 203 (1957). ~ Das Leberparenchym bei histotoxischer Oxydationshemmung im elektronenmikroskopischen Bild. Klin. Wschr. 1957, 646. ~ Das elektronenmikroskopische Bild der Leberparenchymzelle nach oxydationshemmenden Cytotoxinen. Verh. dtsch. Ges. Path. 41, 303 (1958). ~ Das elektronenmikroskopische Bild der Herzmuskelzelle nach akuter Hypoxie. Oeynhausener Gespr. 2, 197 (1958). ~ Die Herzmuskelzelle nach akuter Oxydationshemmung im elektronenmikroskopischen Bild. Beitr. path. Anat. 118, 431 (1958). — MÖLBERT, E., u. G. GUERRITORE: Elektronenmikroskopische Untersuchungen am Leberparenchym bei akuter Hypoxie. Beitr. path. Anat. 117, 32 (1957). — MÖLBERT, E., u. S. IIJIMA: Beitrag zur experimentellen Hypertrophie und Insuffizienz des Herzmuskels im elektronenmikroskopischen Bild. Naturwissenschaften 45, 322 (1958). ~ Beitrag zur experimentellen Hypertrophie und Insuffizienz des Herzmuskels im elektronenmikroskopischen Bild. Verh. dtsch. Ges. Path. 42, 349 (1959). — MÖLBERT, E., u. L. THALE: Die Schädigung des Herzmuskels durch Oxydationshemmung im elektronenmikroskopischen Bild. Klin. Wschr. 1958, 337. — MOLLER, K. W.: Pharmakologie. Basel 1958. — MØLLER, P.: Studien über embolische und autochthone Thromben in der Art. pulmonalis. Beitr. path. Anat. 71, 27 (1923). — MONRAD-KROHN, G. H.: Über Anoxia cerebri und Bericht eines ungewöhnlichen Falles. Acta psychiat. scand. 27, 125 (1952). — MONTGOMERY, P., and E. E. MUIRHEAD: A microspectroscopic study of arterioles in benign and malignant hypertension. Amer. J. Path. **33**, 1181 (1954). — MOON, V. H.: Das Schocksyndrom. Dtsch. med. Wschr. **1934**, 1667. ~ Shock. Definition and differentiation. Arch. Path. (Chicago) **22**, 325 (1936). ~ Shock, its mechanism and pathology. Arch. Path. (Chicago) **24**, 642, 794 (1937). ~ Shock and related capillary phenomena. New York 1938. ~ Shock, its dynamics, occurences and management. Philadelphia 1942. ~ The pathology of secondary shock. Amer. J. Path. **24**, 235 (1948). ~ Acute tubular nephrosis, a complication of shock. Ann. intern. Med. **39**, 51 (1953). — MORAWITZ, P.: Die Chemie der Blutstillung. Ergebn. Physiol. 4, 307 (1905). ~ Thrombose. Verh. dtsch. Ges. Kreisl.-Forsch. **1934**, 80. — MORE, R. H., and G. L. DUFF: The renal arterial vasculature in man. Amer. J. Path. **27**, 95 (1951). — MORE, R. M., H. Z. MOVAT and D. M. HAUST: Role of mural fibrin thrombi of the aorta in genesis of arteriosclerotic plaques. Report of two cases. Arch. Path. (Chicago) **63**, 612 (1957). — MORGAN, A. D.: The implications of the thrombogenic theory in coronary disease. Advanc. Cardiol. **2**, 255 (1959). — MORITZ, A. D.: In: Pathology. St. Louis 1948. — MORITZ, A. R., and M. R. OLDT: Arteriolar sclerosis in hypertensive and non hypertensive individuals. J. Path. Bact. **13**, 679 (1937). — MORO, E., u. W. KELLER: Tuberkulöse Hautallergie nach intrakutaner Simultanimpfung von Tuberkulin und Kuhpockenlymphe. Dtsch. med. Wschr. **51**, 1015 (1925). — MOSCHKOWICZ, E.: An acute febrile pleiochromic anemia with hyaline thrombosis of the terminal arteries and capillaries. Arch. intern. Med. **36**, 89 (1925). ~ Vascular sclerosis. New York 1942. — MOYER, T. A.: An assessment of the therapy of burns: A clinical study. Ann. Surg. **137**, 628 (1953). — MÜLLER, E.: Vorweisungen zur Frage der tödlichen Frühsklerose der Herzkranzgefäße. Klin. Wschr. **1941**, 725. ~ Zur Morphogenese der tödlichen Koronarsklerose Jugendlicher. Verh. dtsch. path. Ges. **1944**, 256 (1949). ~ Die tödliche Coronarsklerose bei jüngeren Männern. Beitr. path. Anat. **110**, 103 (1949). ~ Pathologische Anatomie der Koronarthrombose unter besonderer Berücksichtigung der Koronarsklerose und Atheromatose. Verh. dtsch. Ges. Kreisl.-Forsch. **21**, 3 (1955). — MÜLLER, E., u. M. FRIEDLEIN: Meßergebnisse bei coronarsklerotischem Mediaschwund und Intimaumbau und ihre Bedeutung für die vasomotorische Durchblutungsregelung. Frankfurt. Z. Path. **69**, 268 (1958). — MÜLLER, E., u. H. OTTO: Untersuchungen über Art und Bedeutung strömungsmechanischer Vorgänge bei der Coronarthrombose nach Coronarsklerose. Virchows Arch. path. Anat. **328**, 353 (1956). — MÜLLER, W.: Die Massenverhältnisse des menschlichen Herzens. Hamburg 1883. — MÜLLER-MOHNSSEN, H.: Die Topographie der Septumarterien im menschlichen Herzen und ihre Bedeutung für die Entstehung von Kollateralkreisläufen bei Coronarsklerose. Beitr. path. Anat. **118**, 121 (1957). — MUIRHEAD, E. E., A. GROLLMAN and J. VANATTA: Hypertensive cardiovascular disease („Malignant hypertension"): Changes in canine tissues induced by various manipulations of the kidney, with special reference to vascular and myocardial lesions. Arch. Path. (Chicago) **50**, 137 (1950). — MUIRHEAD, E. E., F. JONES and P. GRAHAM: Hypertension in bilaterally nephrectomized dogs in absence of exogenous sodium excess. Arch. Path. (Chicago) **56**, 286 (1953). — MUIRHEAD, E. E., and P. O. MONTGOMERY: Thromboembolic pulmonary arteritis and vascular sclerosis: its experimental production in rabbits by means of intravenously injected human amniotic fluid and autogenous blood clots. Arch. Path. (Chicago) **52**, 505 (1951). — MUIRHEAD, E. E., P. O. MONTGOMERY and C. E. GORDON: Thromboembolic pulmonary vascular sclerosis. Report of a case following pregnancy and of a case associated with cryoglobulinemia. Arch. intern. Med. **89**, 41 (1952). — MUIRHEAD, E. E., L. B. TURNER and A. GROLLMAN: Vascular lesions of dogs maintained for extended periods following bilateral nephrectomy or ureteral ligation. Arch. Path. (Chicago) **51**, 575 (1951). — MUIRHEAD, E. E., J. VANATTA and A. GROLLMAN: Hypertensive cardiovascular disease. Experimental study of tissue changes in bilaterally nephrectomized dogs. Arch. Path. (Chicago) **48**, 234 (1949). — MYERS, J. D., and J. B. HICKAM: An estimation of the hepatic blood flow and splanchnic oxygen consumption in heart failure. J. clin. Invest. **27**, 620 (1948). — MYERS, R.: Experimentelle hämoglobinurische Nephrose beim Meerschweinchen. Inaug.-Diss. Zürich 1950. — MYLIUS, K., u. P. SCHÜRMANN: Universelle, sklerosierende, tuberkulöse, großzellige Hyperplasie, eine besondere Form atypischer Tuberkulose. Beitr. klin. Tuberk. **73**, 166 (1930).

NAEGELI, TH.: Thromboembolische Prozesse im Bereich des Abdomens. In: Die thromboembolischen Erkrankungen und ihre Behandlung, S. 490. Stuttgart 1955. — NAEGELI, TH., u. P. MATIS: Thrombose und Embolie im Bereich der Extremitäten. In: Die thromboembolischen Erkrankungen und ihre Behandlung, S. 253. Stuttgart 1955. ~ Die Thromboembolie als Krankheit. In: Die thromboembolischen Erkrankungen und ihre Behandlung, S. 36. Stuttgart 1955. — NAEGELI, TH., P. MATIS, R. GROSS, H. RUNGE u. H. SACHS: Die thromboembolischen Erkrankungen und ihre Behandlung. Stuttgart 1955. — NAKATA, T.: Das Verhalten der Nebenniere und Milz bei Verbrennung, mit besonderer Berücksichtigung der Todesursache nach Verbrennung und über Korrelation zwischen Nebenniere und Haut. Beitr. path. Anat. **73**, 439 (1925). — NAUNYN, B.: Naunyn-Schmiedeberg's Arch. exp. Path. Pharmak. **1**, 181 (1873). Zit. nach H. EPPINGER, H. KAUNITZ u. H. POPPER, Die seröse

Entzündung. Wien 1935. — Nelson, R. M., and H. E. Noyes: Blood culture studies in normal dogs and in dogs in haemorrhagic shock. Surgery 35, 782 (1954). — Neubürger, K.: Cerebrale Luftembolie. Zbl. ges. Neurol. Psychiat. 38, 480 (1924). ~ Über Herzmuskelveränderungen bei Epileptikern. Verh. dtsch. Path. Ges. 23, 487 (1928). ~ Beiträge zur Histologie, Pathogenese und Einteilung der arteriosklerotischen Hirnerkrankungen. Veröff. Kriegs- u. Konstit.path. 6, H. 26 (1930). ~ Über die Herzmuskelveränderungen bei Epileptikern und ihre Beziehungen zur Angina pectoris. Frankfurt. Z. Path. 46, 14 (1933). ~ Coagulation necrosis in the brain. J. Neuropath. exp. Neurol. 3, 426 (1944). — Neumann, R.: Ursprungszentren und Entwicklungsformen der Beinthrombose. Virchows Arch. path. Anat. 301, 708 (1938). — Nickerson, J. L.: Local fluid loss in trauma. Amer. J. Physiol. 144, 429 (1945). — Nieth, H.: Histologische und cytologische Untersuchungen am menschlichen Herzmuskel nach Hypertrophie und Insuffizienz. Beitr. path. Anat. 110, 618 (1949). — Nikulin, A.: Veränderungen der Pulmonalarterien nach chronischer Histamininjektion. Beitr. path. Anat. 120, 213 (1959). — Noell, W., u. M. Schneider: Über die Durchblutung und Sauerstoffversorgung des Gehirns im akuten Sauerstoffmangel. I. Die Gehirndurchblutung. Pflügers Arch. ges. Physiol. 246, 181 (1942). ~ Quantitative Angaben über Durchblutung und Sauerstoffversorgung des Gehirns. Pflügers Arch. ges. Physiol. 250, 35 (1948). — Noetzel, H.: Die Pathologie des Nervensystems. In F. Büchner, Spezielle Pathologie. Berlin u. München, 1. Aufl. 1955, 3. Aufl. 1960. — Noetzel, H., u. A. Theodossiou: Beitrag zur Morphologie und Pathogenese der generalisierten Endarteriitis obliterans bei 7 Fällen mit Gehirnbeteiligung. Beitr. path. Anat. 117, 109 (1957). — Nordmann, M.: Local reactions in sensitized animals: Arthus phenomenon, „hyperergic inflammation". Physiol. Rev. 11, 41 (1931). ~ Kreislaufstörungen und pathologische Histologie. Ergebn. Kreisl.-Forsch. 4 (1933). — Nordmann, M., u. F. Speckmann: Blutdruck und peripherer Kreislauf bei mit Serum vorbehandelten Kaninchen. Z. ges. exp. Med. 84, 74 (1932). — Nothnagel, G.: Über Gefäßschmerz. Wien. klin. Wschr. 1893, Nr. 46—48. — Novack, P., B. Goluboff, L. Bortin, A. Soffe and H. A. Shenkin: Studies of the cerebral circulation and metabolism in congestive heart failure. Circulation 7, 724 (1953). — Nuti, M., e G. Rellini: Sulle alterazioni istologiche dellarteria polmonare in varie forme di tuberculosi. Ann. Ist. Forlanini 12, 275 (1950). — Nylin, G., and M. Levander: Studies on the circulation with the aid of tagged erythrocyts in a case of orthostatic hypotension (asympathicotonic hypotension). Ann. intern. Med. 28, 723 (1948). — Nystrom, G.: Experiences with the Trendelenburg operation for pulmonary embolism. Ann. Surg. 92, 498 (1930).

Obwegeser, H.: Über die Schönlein-Henochsche Purpura an Hand eines Obduktionsfalles. Beitr. path. Anat. 113, 321 (1953). — Ochsner, A., M. E. de Bakey, P. T. de Camp u. E. de Rocha: Ann. Surg. 134, 405 (1951). Zit. nach R. Gross, Die thromboembolischen Erkrankungen der Lunge. In: Die thromboembolischen Erkrankungen und ihre Behandlung, S. 299. Stuttgart 1955. — Odel, H. M.: Structural changes in the arteriols of the myocardium in diffuse arteriolar disease with hypertension group 4. Coll. Pap. Mayo Clin. 31, 287 (1940). — O'Hara, J. P., W. G. Walker and M. C. Vickers: Heredity and hypertension. J. Amer. med. Ass. 83, 27 (1924). — Oheim, L.: Herzmuskelveränderungen bei Diphtherie, ihre zeitliche Aufeinanderfolge und topographische Verteilung. Beitr. path. Anat. 100, 195 (1938). — Old, J. W., and W. O. Russel: Necrotizing pulmonary arteritis occuring with congenital heart disease (Eisenmengers complex). Amer. J. Path. 26, 799 (1950). — Omae, T., G. M. C. Masson and A. C. Corcoran: Experimental production of nephrotic syndrome following renal vein constriction in rats. Proc. Soc. exp. Biol. (N.Y.) 1958, 821. — O'Neal, R., and W. A. Thomas: The rôle of pulmonary hypertension and thromboembolism in the production of pulmonary arteriosclerosis. Circulation 12, 370 (1955). — Opdyke, D. F., and R. C. Foreman: A study of coronary flow under conditions of hemorrhagic hypotension and shock. Amer. J. Physiol. 148, 726 (1947). — Opitz, E.: Herzmuskelveränderungen durch Störung der Sauerstoffzufuhr. Z. Kreisl.-Forsch. 27, 227 (1935). ~ Energieumsatz des Gehirns in situ unter aeroben und anaeroben Bedingungen. In: Die Chemie und der Stoffwechsel des Nervengewebes, S. 66. Berlin-Göttingen-Heidelberg 1952. ~ Der Stoffwechsel des Gehirns und seine Veränderung bei Kreislaufstillstand. Verh. dtsch. Ges. Kreisl.-Forsch. 19, 26 (1953). — Opitz, E., Wg. Rotter u. W. Hilscher: Über die „Wiederbelebungszeit" der Rattenniere. Verh. dtsch. Ges. Path. 1953, 336 (1954). — Opitz, E., u. M. Schneider: Über die Sauerstoffversorgung des Gehirns und den Mechanismus von Mangelwirkungen. Ergebn. Physiol. 46, 125 (1950). — Oppenheimer, B. S., P. Klemperer and L. Moskowitz: Evidence for the Goldblatt-mechanism of hypertension in human pathology. Trans. Ass. Amer. Phycns 54, 69 (1939). — Orbison, J. L.: Morphology of thrombotic thrombocytopenic purpura with demonstration of aneurisms. Amer. J. Path. 28, 129 (1952). — Ormos, J., G. Lusztig, A. Botos and B. Korpassy: Adrenaline-type arteriosclerosis induced by experimental coarctation of the aorta in rabbits. Acta morph. Acad. Sci. hung. 6, 129 (1956). — Osler, W.: The cerebral palsies of children. Med. News 1888, No 2, 3, 4, 5.

PÄSSLER, H.: Experimentelle Untersuchungen über die allgemeine Therapie der Kreislaufstörung bei akuten Infektionskrankheiten. Arch. klin. Med. **64**, 715 (1899). — PAGE, I. H.: On certain aspects of the nature and treatment of oligemic shock. Amer. Heart J. **38**, 161 (1949). — PAGEL, W., u. F. HENKE: Die Lungentuberkulose. In Handbuch der speziellen pathologischen Anatomie und Histologie, Bd. III/2, S. 307. Berlin 1930. — PAPACHARALAMPOUS, N. X.: Befunde an der Ratte nach langfristigen Versuchen mit intraperitonealen Injektionen von Trypanblau. Beitr. path. Anat. **117**, 85 (1957). — PAPACHARALAMPOUS, N., u. H. U. ZOLLINGER: Morphologie und Pathogenese des subtotalen und totalen Coronarverschlusses. (Intramurales Hämatom, Thrombose, Arteriosklerose, Coronaritis.) Schweiz. med. Wschr. **1953**, 859. — PAPAGEORGIOU, P. D., u. A. WEBER: Klinische und experimentelle Studien über das Elektrokardiogramm. Das sog. Hypertrophie-Elektrokardiogramm. Z. klin. Med. **139**, 259 (1941). — PAPLANUS, S. H., M. J. ZBAR and J. W. HAYS: Cardiac hypertrophy as a manifestation of chronic anemia. Amer. J. Path. **34**, 149 (1958). — PAPPENHEIMER, J. R.: Capillary permeability: deductions concerning the number and dimensions of ultramicroscopic openings in the capillary walls. Ann. N.Y. Acad. Sci. **55**, 465 (1952). — PARDEE, H. E. B.: An electrocardiographic sign of coronary artery obstruction. Arch. intern. Med. **26**, 244 (1920). — PARIN, V. V.: Amer. J. med. Sci. **214**, 167 (1937). Zit. nach H. SCHWIEGK, Über Reflexe aus dem kleinen Kreislauf. Verh. dtsch. Ges. Kreisl.-Forsch. **17**, 95 (1951). — PARK, W. W.: Experimental trophoblastic embolism of the lungs. J. Path. (Chicago) **75**, 257—265 (1958). — PARKER, B. M., and J. R. SMITH: Studies on experimental pulmonary embolism and infarction and the development of collateral circulation in the affected lung lobe. J. Lab. clin. Med. **49**, 850 (1957). — PARKER, F., and S. WEISS: Nature and significance of structural changes in lungs in mitral stenosis. Amer. J. Path. **12**, 573 (1936). — PARKER, J. G., and L. FELDER: Jaundice in cardiac failure without infarction. Ann. intern. Med. **43**, 1031 (1955). — PARKER, R. L.: Pulmonary emphysema. A study of its relations to the heart and pulmonary arterial system. Ann. intern. Med. **14**, 795 (1940). — PARKINSON, J., and D. E. BEDFORD: Electrocardiographic changes during brief attacks of angina pectoris. Lancet **1931 I**, 15. — PARY, C. H.: An inquiry into the symptomes and causes of syncope anginosa commonly called angina pectoris. London 1799. — PASQUALE, E. L. DI, and A. A. SCHILLER: Effect of hypoxemia on edema formation in perfused isolated rat hind limb. Proc. Soc. exp. Biol. (N.Y.) **78**, 567 (1951). — PATERSON, J. C.: Vascularization and hemorrhage of the intima of arteriosclerotic coronary arteries. Arch. Path. (Chicago) **22**, 313 (1936). ~ Capillary rupture with intimal hemorrhage as a causative factor in coronary thrombosis. Arch. Path. (Chicago) **25**, 474 (1938). ~ Factors in the production of coronary artery disease. Circulation **6**, 732 (1952). — PATTERSON, J. E., T. W. CLARK and R. L. LEVY: A comparison of electrocardiographic changes observed during the „anoxemia test" on normal persons and on patients with coronary sclerosis. Amer. Heart J. **23**, 837 (1942). — PAUL, F.: Die krankhafte Funktion der Nebenniere und ihr gestaltlicher Ausdruck. Virchows Arch. path. Anat. **282**, 256 (1931). — PAYR, E.: Über tödliche Fettembolie nach Streckung von Kontrakturen. Münch. med. Wschr. 1898, Nr 28. ~ Über Thromboseembolie. Münch. med. Wschr. **76**, 1574 (1929). ~ Gedanken und Beobachtungen über die Thromboemboliefrage. Anregung zu einer Sammelforschung. Zbl. Chir. **57**, 961 (1930). — PENDL, F.: Myokardstoffwechsel und Herztherapie. Stuttgart 1954. — PENFIELD, W.: The evidence for a cerebral vascular mechanism in epilepsy. Ann. intern. Med. **7**, No 3 (1933). — PEREIRA LUZ, N.: Embolie durch Fruchtwasser und Vernix caseosa. Betrachtungen und Beschreibung eines wahrscheinlichen derartigen Falles. An. Clin. Ginec. Fac. Med. S. Paulo **5**, 78 (1953). — PETERS, G.: Über die Pathologie der Salvarsanschäden des Zentralnervensystems. Beitr. path. Anat. **110**, 371 (1949). — PFEFFER, K. H., u. HJ. STAUDINGER: Über die Ausscheidung von Corticoiden im Urin unter normalen und pathologischen Bedingungen. I. Die Corticoide im Urin bei künstlichem Fieber und anderen Stress-Formen. Klin. Wschr. **1952**, 257. ~ II. Die Corticoide im Urin bei Hypertonikern. Klin. Wschr. **1952**, 306. ~ III. Die Corticoidausscheidung im Urin bei verschiedenem Kochsalzgehalt der Nahrung. Klin. Wschr. **1952**, 307. ~ Corticoidausscheidung im Urin bei einem Fall mit chronischer Nephritis unter Cortisontherapie. Klin. Wschr. **1952**, 304. — PFEIFFER, E. F., u. H. E. BRUCH: Die Autoallergie in der Pathogenese der diffusen Glomerulonephritis. Ergebn. inn. Med., N. F. **4**, 670 (1953). — PFEIFFER, H.: Die Eiweißzerfallsvergiftung. Z. Krankheitsforsch. **1**, 407 (1925). — PFEUFER, K.: Z. ration. Med. **1**, 409 (1844). Zit. nach H. EPPINGER, H. KAUNITZ u. H. POPPER, Die seröse Entzündung. Wien 1935. — PFLEGER, L.: Beobachtungen über Schrumpfung und Sklerose des Ammonshornes bei Epilepsie. Allg. Z. Psychiat. **36** (1880). — PICHOTKA, J.: Tierexperimentelle Untersuchungen zur pathologischen Histologie des akuten Höhentodes. Beitr. path. Anat. **107**, 117 (1942). — PICKERING, G.: The pathogenesis of malignant hypertension. Circulation **6**, 599 (1952). — PICKERING, G. W.: The role of the kidney in acute and chronic hypertension following renal artery constriction in the rabbit. Clin. Sci. **5**, 229 (1945). — PICKERING, G. W., and M. PRINZMETAL: Experimental hypertension of renal origin in the rabbit. Clin. Sci. **3**, 357 (1938). — PIERACH,

A., u. K. HEYNEMANN: Der niedrige Blutdruck und die Hypotonie. Beitr. prakt. Med. 38, 1 (1959). — PINNIGER, J. L., and F. T. G. PRUNTY: Brit. J. exp. Path. 27, 200 (1946). Zit. nach R. JÜRGENS, Zur Pathogenese der Thrombose. In: Thrombose und Embolie. Stuttgart 1954. — PIRANI, C. L., R. JUSTER, H. F. FROEB and C. F. CONSOLAZIO: Use of dextran in hemorrhagic shock. J. appl. Physiol. 8, 193 (1955). — PIRQUET, C., u. B. SCHICK: Zur Theorie der Inkubationszeit. Wien. klin. Wschr. 16, 26, 758 (1903). ~ Die Serumkrankheit. Wien 1905. — PLAMBECK, H.: Veränderungen des menschlichen Gehirns bei chronischem und akutem Sauerstoffmangel. Beitr. path. Anat. 111, 77 (1950). — PLATT, R.: Heredity in hypertension. Quart. J. Med., N. s. 16, 111 (1947). — POCHE, R.: Das submikroskopische Bild der Herzmuskelveränderungen nach Überdosierung von Schilddrüsenhormon. Beitr. path. Anat. 188, 407 (1958). ~ Submikroskopische Beiträge zur Pathologie der Herzmuskelzelle bei Phosphorvergiftung, Hypertrophie, Atrophie und Kaliummangel. Virchows Arch. path. Anat. 331, 165 (1958). — POLLAK, V. E., R. M. KARK, C. L. PIRANI, H. A. SHAFTER and R. C. MUEHRCKE: Renal vein thrombosis and the nephrotic syndrome. Amer. J. Med. 21, 496 (1956). — POPPER, H.: Significance of agonal changes in the human liver. Arch. Path. (Chicago) 46, 132 (1948). — POSSELT, A.: Die Erkrankungen der Lungenschlagader. Ergebn. allg. Path. path. Anat. 13, 298 (1909). — POTAIN: Des différentes formes de l'angine de poitrine. Gaz. Hôp. (Paris) 1880, 96. — PRINZMETAL, M., and H. C. BERGMAN: Heart in experimental shock. J. Mt. Sinai Hosp. 12, 579 (1945). — PUGH, R. C. B., G. W. PICKERING and R. B. BLACKET: The production of vascular lesions and cardiac hypertrophy by infusions of renin and noradrenaline in the rabbit. Clin. Sci. 11, 241 (1952). — PULLMAN, T. N., and W. W. McCLURE: The response of the renal circulation in man to constant-speed infusions of l-Norepinephrine. Circulation 9, 600 (1954).

QUINCKE, H.: Dubois Arch. 1869, 174, 521. Zit. nach H. EPPINGER, H. KAUNITZ u. H. POPPER, Die seröse Entzündung. Wien 1935.

RAAB, W.: Hormonal and neurogenic cardio-vascular disorders. Baltimore 1953. ~ The adrenergic-cholinergic control of cardiac metabolism and function. Advanc. Cardiol. 1, 65 (1956). — RANDALL, H. T.: The shifts of fluid and electrolytes in shock. Ann. N.Y. Acad. Sci. 55, 412 (1952). — RANSTRÖM, S.: Massive fat embolism of the liver. Acta chir. scand. 113, 96 (1957). — RATHER, L. J.: The nature and significance of changes in adrenal cytology, weight, and cortical/medullary ratio in experimental renal hypertension and clinical hypertension. J. exp. Med. 93, 573 (1951). — RATNER, B.: The physiologic pathology of allergic disease. Int. Arch. Allergy 6, 1 (1955). — RAU, H.: Zur Bedeutung der chronischen Blutdruckerhöhung für die Entstehung und Schwere der Arteriosklerose. Klin. Wschr. 1956, 167. — RECKLINGHAUSEN, F. v.: Zur Fettresorption. Virchows Arch. path. Anat. 26, 172 (1863). ~ Handbuch der allgemeinen Pathologie des Kreislaufs und der Ernährung. Stuttgart 1883. — REHN, J.: Untersuchungen zum postoperativen Verhalten der Aminosäuren. Langenbecks Arch. klin. Chir. 290, 466 (1959). ~ Die vermehrte posttraumatische Ausscheidung von biologisch aktiven Peptiden im Urin. Klin. Wschr. 1959, 240. — REHN, J., u. M. J. WHITELAW: Die Verbrennungsbehandlung mit ACTH und Cortison. Langenbecks Arch. klin. Chir. 274, 175 (1953). — REIN, H.: Die Physiologie der Coronardurchblutung. Verh. dtsch. Ges. inn. Med. 1931, 247. ~ Die Physiologie der Herzkranzgefäße. Z. Biol. 92, 101, 115 (1931). ~ Kreislauf und Stoffwechsel. Verh. dtsch. Ges. Kreisl.-Forsch. 14, 9 (1941). ~ Ein Beitrag zur Organisation der Regelungsvorgänge im peripheren Kreislaufapparat. Pflügers Arch. ges. Physiol. 244, 603 (1941). ~ Über die Drosselungstoleranz und die kritische Drosselungsgrenze der Herz-Coronargefäße. Pflügers Arch. ges. Physiol. 253, 205 (1951). — REIN, H., u. M. SCHNEIDER: Die Auswirkung künstlicher Mangeldurchblutung auf den lokalen Stoffwechsel. Pflügers Arch. ges. Physiol. 239, 451 (1938). ~ Die lokale Stoffwechseleinschränkung bei reflektorisch-nervöser Durchblutungsdrosselung. Pflügers Arch. ges. Physiol. 239, 464 (1938). — REINDELL, H., u. O. BAYER: Die elektrokardiographische Überwiegungskurve und ihre Bedeutung für die Frage der Hypertrophie und der Myokardschädigung. Arch. Kreisl.-Forsch. 11, 207 (1943). — REINDELL, H., u. H. KLEPZIG: Die neuzeitlichen Brustwand- und Extremitäten-Ableitungen in der Praxis, 2. Aufl. Stuttgart 1953. — RENDELSTEIN, F. D., H. FRISCHAUF u. E. DEUTSCH: Über die gerinnungsbeschleunigende Wirkung des Fruchtwassers. Acta haemat. (Basel) 6, 18 (1951). — RICH, A. R.: Allergic diseases and diseases accompanied by sensitization. 1. Internat. Allergiekongr., Zürich 1951, 1. Basel u. New York 1952. — RICH, A. R., and J. E. GREGORY: The experimental demonstration that periarteriitis nodosa is a manifestation of hypersensitivity. Bull. Johns Hop. Hosp. 72, 65 (1943). — RICHARDS, D. W.: The effects of hemorrhage on the circulation. Ann. N.Y. Acad. Sci. 49, 534 (1948). — RICHARDSON, G. O.: Atherosclerosis of main renal arteries in essential hypertension. J. Path. Bact. 55, 33 (1943). — RICKER, G.: Pathologie als Naturwissenschaft. Berlin 1922. ~ Pathologie als Naturwissenschaft. Relationspathologie. Berlin 1924. ~ Angriffsort und Wirkungsweise der Reize an der Strombahn. Kritische und antikritische Bemerkungen zu neuesten Abhandlungen über den örtlichen Kreislauf und die Entzündung. Krkh.-Forsch. 1, 457 (1925). — RICKER, G., u. P. REGENDANZ: Beiträge zur Kenntnis der örtlichen Kreislaufstörungen. Nach Untersuchungen am Pankreas und seinem

Bauchfell, an der Conjunctiva und dem Ohrlöffel des Kaninchens. Virchows Arch. path. Anat. **231**, 1 (1921). — RIEHL jr., G.: Experimentelle Untersuchungen über den Verbrennungstod. Naunyn-Schmiedeberg's Arch. exp. Path. Pharmak. **135**, 369 (1928). — RISEMAN, J. E. F., and M. G. BROWN: An analysis of the diagnostic criteria of angina pectoris. A critical study of 100 proved cases. Amer. Heart J. **14**, 331 (1937). — ROBERTSON, H. R., T. S. PERRETT, J. C. COLBECK, J. R. MOORE and D. C. BLAIR: The reaction of ligated peripheral veins to the presence of autogenous clots and thrombi. Surg. Gynec. Obstet. **105**, 727—732 (1957). — ROBERTSON, O. H., and A. V. BOCK: Rept. Special Investig. Comm. on Surgical Shock and Allied Conditions, No 6, London 1919. ~ Blood volume in wounded soldiers. I. Blood volume and related blood changes after hemorrhage. J. exp. Med. **29**, 139 (1919). — RÖSSLE, R.: Über die Merkmale der Entzündung im allergischen Organismus. Verh. dtsch. path. Ges. **17**, 281 (1914). ~ Allergie und Pathergie. Klin. Wschr. **12**, 574 (1933). ~ Über die Häufung von Thrombose und Embolie nach dem Kriege. S.-B. preuß. Akad. Wiss., phys.-math. Kl. **1935**, IV. ~ Über die Bedeutung und die Entstehung der Waden-Venen-Thrombosen. Virchows Arch. path. Anat. **300**, 180 (1937). ~ Über die serösen Entzündungen der Organe. Virchows Arch. path. Anat. **311**, 252 (1944). ~ Über Luftembolie der Capillaren des großen und des kleinen Kreislaufes. Virchows Arch. path. Anat. **313**, 1 (1944). — ROGERS, W. F., and R. H. WILLIAMS: Correlations of biochemical and histological changes in the adrenal cortex. Arch. Path. (Chicago) **44**, 126 (1947). ~ Cholesterol of the human adrenal gland. Its significance in relation to adrenal function and structure. Arch. Path. (Chicago) **46**, 450 (1948). — ROMBERG, E.: Über Sklerose der Lungenarterien. Dtsch. Arch. klin. Med. **48**, 197 (1891). ~ Über die Erkrankungen des Herzmuskels bei Typhus abdominalis, Scharlach und Diphtherie. Dtsch. Arch. klin. Med. **48**, 369 (1891); **49**, 413 (1892). ~ Lehrbuch der Krankheiten des Herzens und der Blutgefäße, 3. Aufl. Stuttgart 1921. — ROMBERG, E., H. PÄSSLER, C. BRUNS u. W. MÜLLER: Untersuchungen über die Allgemeine Pathologie und Therapie der Kreislaufstörung bei akuten Infektionskrankheiten. Dtsch. Arch. klin. Med. **64**, 652 (1899). — ROSE, B., and J. S. L. BROWNE: Alterations in the blood histamine in shock. Proc. Soc. exp. Biol. (N.Y.) **44**, 182 (1940). — ROSEMANN, G.: Zur Pathogenese der chromoproteinämischen Nephrose. Beitr. path. Anat. **122**, 199 (1960). — ROSENBERG, H. S., u. D. G. MCNAMARA: Primary pulmonary hypertension. Pediatrics **20**, 408 (1957). — ROSENTHAL, S. R., F. FINAMORE, F. R. HUNTER, A. S. HUNTER and J. N. ROMAN: On the pathogenesis of death due to burning of the skin. Amer. J. Path. **31**, 568 (1955). — ROTHMANN, A.: Beitrag zur Frage der Myoglobinurie. Verhd. tsch. Ges. Path. **1944**, 156 (1949). — ROTHSCHILD, M. A., and M. KISSIN: Anginal syndrom induced by gradual general anoxaemia. Proc. Soc. exp. Biol. (N.Y.) **29**, 577 (1932). ~ Induced general anoxemia causing S-T deviation in the electrocardiogramm. Amer. Heart J. **8**, 745 (1933). — ROTHSTEIN, J. L., and S. WELT: Periarteritis nodosa in infancy and in childhood; report of two cases with necropsy observations; abstracts of cases in the literature. Amer. J. Dis. Child. **45**, 1277 (1933). — ROTTER, W.: Die Pathologie der physikalischen Umweltfaktoren. Fiat Rev. Gen. Path. **2**, 63 (1948). — ROTTER, WG.: Über die Bedeutung der Ernährungsstörungen, insbesondere des Sauerstoffmangels für die Pathogenese der Gefäßwandveränderungen, mit besonderer Berücksichtigung der „Endarteriitis obliterans" und der „Arteriosklerose". Beitr. path. Anat. **110**, 46 (1949). ~ Über die postischämische Insuffizienz überlebender Zellen und Organe, ihre Erholungszeit und die Wiederbelebungszeit nach Kreislaufunterbrechung. Thoraxchirurgie **6**, 107 (1958). ~ Das morphologische Gewebssubstrat bei gestörter Durchblutung. In: Angiologie. Stuttgart 1959. — ROTTER, W., u. W. BÜNGELER: Blut und blutbildende Organe. In KAUFMANN-STAEMMLER, Lehrbuch der speziellen pathologischen Anatomie, Bd. I/1, S. 642. Berlin 1955. — ROTTER, W., u. P. KRUG: Veränderungen des Gehirns nach Cardiazol- und Campherkrämpfen im Tierversuch. Arch. Psychiat. Nervenkr. **111**, 380 (1940). — ROUS, P., and M. P. GILDING: Is the local vasodilatation after different tissue injuries referable to a single cause? J. exp. Med. **51**, 27 (1930). — RUBBAR, SH., and A. A. ANGRIST: Amer. J. med. Sci. **225**, 20 (1953). — RUBIN, M. I., and M. RAPOPORT: Arteriolosclerosis, hypertension and cerebral atrophy in an infant. J. Pediat. **18**, 643 (1941). — RUCKERT, K. E., u. H. DEILMANN: Histologische Untersuchungen der Medulla oblongata bei Hypertonie. Beitr. path. Anat. **102**, 443 (1939). — RÜHL, A.: Wie weit ist der genuine arterielle Hochdruck anatomisch bedingt? Dtsch. Arch. klin. Med. **156**, 129 (1927). ~ Über die Gangarten der Arteriosklerose. Veröff. Kriegs- u. Konstit. path. H. 21 (1929). ~ Über den Gasstoffwechsel des insuffizienten Herzens. I. Herzinsuffizienz durch Histamin. Naunyn-Schmiedeberg's Arch. exp. Path. Pharmak. **172**, 568 (1933). ~ Wesen und Bedeutung der Gasstoffwechseländerung am insuffizienten Herzen. Naunyn-Schmiedeberg's Arch. exp. Path. Pharmak. **187**, 22 (1937). ~ Warum versagt das Herz des Hypertonikers? Zbl. inn. Med. **1938**, 242. — RUTISHAUSER, G.: Extremitätenthrombose und Lungenembolie bei internen Krankheiten. Gynaecologia (Basel) **138**, 171 (1954).

SAATHOFF, J.: Zur Frage des Rickerschen Stufengesetzes. Untersuchungen mit Wärmereiz am Pankreas und Mesenterium des lebenden Kaninchens. Verh. dtsch. path. Ges. **35**, 245 (1952). — SACHS, B.: Hirnlähmungen der Kinder. Volkmanns Vorträge Nr 46, 47 (1892).—

SAMUELSSON, S.: Primary cor pulmonale. Chronic cor pulmonale resulting from pulmonary hypertension of unknown etiology. Review of literatur. Report of 4 cases. Acta med. scand. **142**, 177 (1952). ~ Chronic cor pulmonale in bronchial asthma, chron. Bronchitis, Bronchiectasis, and pulmonary emphysem. Acta med. scand. **143**, 15 (1952). ~ Chronic cor pulmonale in pulmonary tuberculosis. Acta med. scand. **142**, 315 (1952). — SANBLOM, P.: Nierenvenenthrombose und nephrotisches Syndrom. Acta pediat. (Uppsala) **35**, 160 (1948).— SANDRITTER, W.: Die Morphologie der Thrombolyse an experimentellen Abscheidungs- und Gerinnungsthromben und an menschlichen Thromben. I. Internat. Tagg über Thrombose und Embolie. Basel, 1954. — SANDRITTER, W., F. BECKER u. I. LANGENBERG: Über die Wetterabhängigkeit der Lungenembolie. Klin. Wschr. **35**, 1176 (1957). — SANDRITTER, W., M. HUPPERT u. G. SCHLÜTER: Zur Frage der Fibrinolyse an experimentellen Gerinnungs- und Abscheidungsthromben. Klin. Wschr. **1958**, 651. — SAPHIR, O., L. OHRINGER and H. SILVERSTONE: Coronary arteriosclerotic heart disease in the younger age group: its greater frequency in this group among an increasingly older necropsy population. Amer. J. med. Sci. **231**, 494 (1956). — SAPHIR, O., W. S. PRIEST, W. W. HAMBURGER and L. N. KATZ: Coronary arteriosclerosis, coronary thrombosis and the resulting myocardial changes. An evaluation of their respective clinical pictures including the electrocardiographic records, based on the anatomical findings. Amer. Heart J. **10**, 567, 762 (1935). — SARAM, M.: Über die azelluläre Entstehung von Narben bei Durchblutungsstörungen im Herzmuskel. Beitr. path. Anat. **118**, 275 (1957). — SARNOFF, S. J., R. B. CASE, PH. E. WAITH and J. P. ISAACS: Insufficient coronary flow and myocardial failure as a complicating factor in late haemorrhagic shock. Amer. J. Physiol. **176**, 439 (1954). — SARRE, H., u. K. ROTHER: Bemerkung zur Arbeit H. HARDERS, Zur Frage der Auto-Antikörper. Klin. Wschr. **1955**, 586. — SCHACHTER, M.: Anaphylaxis and histamine release in the rabbit. Brit. J. Pharmacol. **8**, 412 (1952). — SCHAEFER, H.: Das Elektrokardiogramm. Theorie und Klinik. Berlin-Göttingen-Heidelberg 1951. ~ Grundprobleme der vegetativen tonischen Innervation. Acta neuroveg. (Wien) **4**, 201 (1952). — SCHEINBERG, P.: Cerebral blood flow in vascular disease of the brain. With observations on the effects of stellate ganglion block. Amer. J. Med. **8**, 139 (1950). ~ Cerebral circulation in heart faillure. Amer. J. Med. **8**, 148 (1950). — SCHENKEN, J. R., G. P. SLAUGHTER and G. H. DE MAY: Maternal pulmonary embolism of amniotic fluid. Amer. J. clin. Path. **20**, 147 (1950). — SCHERF, D.: Ein Fall von Angina pectoris. Z. klin. Med. **120**, 715 (1932). — SCHERF, D., u. E. SCHÖNBRUNNER: Über Herzbefunde bei Lungenembolien. Z. klin. Med. **128**, 455 (1935). — SCHIMERT, G.: Die Therapie der Coronarinsuffizienz im Lichte einer neueren Betrachtung ihrer Pathogenese. Schweiz. med. Wschr. **1951**, 598. — SCHIMKAT, E., u. N. KATHKE: Vergleichende Untersuchungen über die Coronar- und Cerebralsklerose bei Hypertonie. Beitr. path. Anat. **120**, 26 (1959). — SCHLAGETTER, K., u. H. ZIMMERMANN: Cytologische Untersuchungen an Nierenepithelien. Beitr. path. Anat. **118**, 24 (1957). — SCHLESINGER, M. J., and L. REINER: Focal myocytolysis of the heart. Amer. J. Path. **31**, 443 (1955). — SCHLEUSSING, H.: Thrombose und Embolie vor und nach dem Kriege. Klin. Wschr. **1929**, 2125. — SCHLITTER, J., u. A. A. MÜLLER: Ärztl. Wschr. **10**, 53 (1955). — SCHMIDT, A.: Zur Blutlehre. Leipzig 1892. — SCHMIDT, H.: Über das Wesen der Allergie. Dtsch. med. Wschr. **1950**, 258. ~ Primäre und sekundäre pulmonale Hypertonie. Dtsch. Arch. klin. Med. **200**, 837 (1953). ~ Die essentielle Hypertonie des Lungenkreislaufes und deren Beziehungen zur sog. primären Pulmonalsklerose. Arch. Kreisl.-Forsch. **19**, 91 (1953). — SCHMIDT, J. H.: Fatal bone marrow embolism following thoracotomy. Amer. J. Surg. **95**, 94 (1958). — SCHMITT, K.: Paradoxe Luftembolie mit Auswirkungen auf Herz und Gehirn. Dtsch. Z. Nervenheilk. **177**, 434 (1958). — SCHNAPAUFF, U.: Der Niereninfarkt als Reimplantat. Beitr. path. Anat. **79**, 781 (1928). — SCHNEIDER, C.: Release of anticoagulant during shock of experimental meconium embolism. Amer. J. Obstet. **65**, 245 (1953). ~ Coagulation defects on obstetric shock: Meconium embolism and heparin; fibrin embolism and defibrination. Amer. J. Obstet. **69**, 758 (1955). — SCHNEIDER, M.: Durchblutung und Sauerstoffversorgung des Gehirns. Verh. dtsch. Ges. Kreisl.-Forsch. **19**, 3 (1953). ~ Über die Wiederbelebung nach Kreislaufunterbrechung. Thoraxchirurgie **6**, 95 (1958). — SCHOB, F.: Pathologische Anatomie der Idiotie. In Handbuch der Geisteskrankheiten, Bd. XI, S. 777 (1930). — SCHOENMACKERS, J.: Die Herzkranzschlagadern bei der arterio-kardialen Hypertrophie. Z. Kreisl.-Forsch. **38**, 321 (1949). ~ Zur Anatomie und Pathologie der Coronargefäße. Oeynhausener Gespräche II, 133 (1958). ~ Vergleichende quantitative Untersuchungen über den Faserbestand des Herzens bei Herz- und Herzklappenfehlern sowie Hochdruck. Virchows Arch. path. Anat. **331**, 3 (1958). ~ Zur Pathologie der Lungenarterienembolie. Dtsch. med. Wschr. **1958**, 115. — SCHOENMACKERS, J., u. E. STRATMANN: Koronargefäßsystem und Myocard bei angeborenen Herz- und Gefäßfehlern. Arch. Kreisl.-Forsch. **22**, 153 (1955). — SCHOLZ, W.: Über die Entstehung des Hirnbefundes bei der Epilepsie. Z. Neurol. Psychiat. **145**, 471 (1933). ~ Histologische und topische Veränderungen und Vulnerabilitätsverhältnisse im menschlichen Gehirn bei Sauerstoffmangel, Ödem und plasmatischen Infiltrationen. Arch. Psychiat. Nervenkr. **181**, 621 (1949). ~ Die Krampfschädigungen des Gehirns. Berlin 1951. ~ Kreislaufschäden des Gehirns und ihre Pathogenese. Verh. dtsch.

Ges. Kreisl.-Forsch. 19, 52 (1953). ~ Die nicht zur Erweichung führenden unvollständigen Gewebsnekrosen. Elektive Parenchymnekrose (des Gehirns). In Handbuch der speziellen Pathologie, Bd. XIII/1 B, S. 1284. 1957. — SCHOLZ, W., J. W. BOELLAARD and H. HAGER: Toxicity changes in the central nervous system. Oxygen deficiency and its influence on the central nervous system. Air force office of scientific research 1959. — SCHOLZ, W., u. H. HAGER: Epilepsie. In Handbuch der speziellen Pathologie, Bd. XIII/4, S. 148. 1956. — SCHOLZ, W., u. J. JÖTTEN: Durchblutungsstörungen im Katzengehirn nach kurzen Elektrokrampfserien. Arch. Psychiat. Nervenkr. 186, 264 (1951). — SCHOLZ, W., u. D. NIETO: Studien zur Pathologie der Hirngefäße. I. Fibrose und Hyalinose. Z. ges. Neurol. Psychiat. 162, 675 (1938). — SCHREIBER, S. S., A. BAUMAN, R. S. YALLOW and S. A. BERSON: Blood volume alterations in congestive heart failure. J. clin. Invest. 33, 578 (1954). — SCHREIER, P. C., J. Q. ADAMS, H. B. TURNER and M. J. SMITH: Toxemia of pregnancy as an etiological factor in hypertensive vascular disease. J. Amer. med. Ass. 159, 105 (1955). — SCHROEDER, P.: Hirnveränderungen bei arteriosklerotischer Demenz. Mschr. Psychiat. 22, 451 (1907). ~ Lues cerebrospinalis und ihre Beziehungen zur progressiven Paralyse und Tabes. Dtsch. Z. Nervenheilk. 54, 83 (1916). — SCHRÖDTER, H.: Mitgeteilt in F. BÜCHNER, Spezielle Pathologie, 3. Auf., S. 66. 1960. — SCHUBERT, W.: Fruchtwasserschleimembolie bei klinisch fraglicher Eklampsie. Virchows Arch. path. Anat. 328, 38 (1956). ~ Über einen Emboliemechanismus bei Abtreibung durch Seifenlösung. Virchows Arch. path. Anat. 329, 656 (1957). — SCHUBOTHE, H.: Serologie und klinische Bedeutung der Autohämantikörper. Basel u. New York 1958. — SCHÜRMANN, P.: Der Hitzschlag im Lichte der Kollapsforschung. Veröff. Mil.san.wes. H. 105, 1 (1938). — SCHÜRMANN, P., u. H. E. MacMAHON: Die maligne Nephrosklerose, zugleich ein Beitrag zur Frage der Bedeutung der Blutgewebsschranke. Virchows Arch. path. Anat. 291, 47 (1933). — SCHULTZ, A.: Pathologie der Blutgefäße. Ergebn. allg. Path. path. Anat. 22, Abt. I, 207 (1927). — SCHULTZ, H. W.: The reaction of smooth muscle of guinea-pig sensitised with horse serum. J. Pharmacol. exp. Ther. 1, 549 (1910). ~ Physiological studies in anaphylaxis. IV. Reaction of the cat toward horse serum. J. Pharmacol. exp. Ther. 3, 299 (1912). — SCHULZ, H., R. JÜRGENS u. E. HIEPLER: Die Ultrastruktur der Thrombozyten bei der konstitutionellen Thrombopathie (v. WILLEBRAND-JÜRGENS) mit einem Beitrag zur submikroskopischen Orthologie der Thrombozyten. Thromb. diath. haemorrhag. 2, 300 (1958). — SCHWEIKERT, C. H., u. K. SICKINGER: Pathologisch-histologische Befunde am Hund nach Anwendung eines extracorporalen Kreislaufes in Kombination mit tiefer Hypothermie und temporärem Kreislaufstillstand. Thoraxchirurgie 8, 371 (1960). — SCHWEINBURG, F. B., H. A. FRANK and J. FINE: Bacterial factor in experimental haemorrhagic shock. Evidence for development of a bacterial factor which accounts for irreversibility to transfusion and for the loss of the normal capacity to destroy bacteria. Amer. J. Physiol. 179, 532 (1954). — SCHWIEGK, H.: Shock und Kollaps. Funktionelle Pathologie und Therapie. Klin. Wschr. 1942, 741, 765. ~ Über Reflexe aus dem kleinen Kreislauf. Verh. dtsch. Ges. Kreisl.-Forsch. 17, 95 (1951). — SCOFIELD, G. F., and J. B. BEAIRD jr.: Fatal embolism by amniotic fluid in the lungs. Report of a case. Amer. J. clin. Path. 28, 400 (1957). — SCRIBA, K.: Histologische Organbefunde bei ischaemischer Nekrose der Skeletmuskulatur. Verh. dtsch. Ges. Path. 33, 69 (1950). — SEEGERS, W. H., and N. ALKJAERSIG: The preparation of prothrombin derivatives and a indication of their properties. Arch. biochem. Biophys. 61, 1 (1956). — SEEGERS, W. H., and S. A. JOHNSON: Conversion of prothrombin to autoprothrombin II (platelet cofactor II) and its relation to the blood clotting mechanism. Amer. J. Physiol. 184, 259 (1956). — SELBERG, W.: Tödliche Hämoglubinurie nach Verschüttung. Dtsch. med. Wschr. 1942, 561. — SELTZER, L. M., and W. SCHUMAN: Nonfatal pulmonary embolism by amniotic fluid contents with report of a possible case. Amer. J. Obstet. 54, 1038 (1947). — SELYE, H.: Production of hypertension and hyalinosis by desoxycorticosterone. Brit. med. J. 1950, No 4647. — SELYE, H., and E. I. PENTZ: Pathogenetical correlations between periarteritis nodosa, renal hypertension and rheumatic lesions. Canad. med. Ass. J. 49, 264 (1943). — SHAPIRO, H. D., D. DOKTOR and J. CHURG: Thrombotic thrombocytopenic purpura (Moschcowioz's disease). Report of a case with remission after splenectomy and steroid therapy. Ann. intern. Med. 47, 582 (1957). — SHAPIRO, SH.: Long-term anticoagulant therapy. Med. Clin. N. Amer. 37, 659 (1953). — SHAW, A. F. B., and A. A. GHAREEB: The pathogenesis of pulmonary schistosomiasis in Egypt with special reference to Ayerza's disease. J. Path. Bact. 46, 390 (1936). — SHEEHAN, H. L.: Simmonds disease due to post partum necrosis of anterior pituitary. Quart. J. Med., N. s. 8, 277 (1939). ~ Shock in obstetrics. Lancet 1948 I, 1. — SHEEHAN, H. L., and R. MURDOCK: Postpartum necrosis of the anterior pituitary. Lancet 1939 I, 818. — SHERRY, S., W. TROLL and H. GLUECK: Thrombin as a proteolytic enzyme. Physiol. Rev. 34, 736 (1954). — SHORR, E., B. W. ZWEIFACH and R. F. FURCHTGOTT: On the occurence, sites and modes of origin and destruction, of principles affecting the compensatory vascular mechanisms in experimental shock. Science 102, 489 (1945). — SHORT, D. S.: Survey of pulmonary embolism in general hospital. Brit. med. J. 1952, No 4672, 790. ~ The arterial bed of the lung in pulmonary hypertension. Lancet 1957 II, 12. — SHOTTON, D. M., and C. W. TAYLOR: Pulmonary embolism by amniotic fluid. A report of a fatal case, together with a review of the literature. J. Obstet. Gynaec. Brit. Emp. 56, 46 (1949). — Sickinger, K., C. H. Schweikert, E. G. Kaniak, G. Richter, K. Wiemers u. W. Overbeck: Extracorporaler Kreislauf — tiefe Hypothermie — langdauernder Kreislaufstillstand. Pathologisch-histologische Befunde am Hund. Beitr. path. Anat. 125 (1961). — Siegel, M. L., and H. Feil: Electrocardiographic studies during attacks of angina pectoris and of other paroxysmal pain. J. clin. Inverst. 10, 795 (1931). — Siegmund, H.: Über die Fettembolie nach Verletzungen. Jkurse ärztl. Fortbild. 22, 8 (1941). ~ Zur Pathogenese und Pathologie von örtlichen Kälteschäden. Münch. med. Wschr. 1942, 827. — Sigler, L. H.: Subjective manifestations of acute coronary occlusion or insufficiency. Their relation to area of resulting myocardial injury. Arch. intern. Med. 94, 341 (1954). — Simonart, A.: Au sujet de l'auto-intoxication après brûlure. Bull. Acad. roy. Méd. Belg. 20, 75. — Simonson, E., and A. Keys: The electrocardiographic exercise test: changes in the scala ECG and in the mean spacial QRS and T vectors in two types of exercise; effect of absolute and relative body weight and commend on normal standards. Amer. Heart J. 52, 83 (1956). — Sinapius, D.: Über das Endothel der Venen. Z. Zellforsch. 47, 560 (1958). — Singer, K., F. P. Bornstein and S. A. Wile: Thrombotic thrombocytopenic purpura; hemorrhagic diathesis with generalized platelet thromboses. Blood 2, 542 (1947). — Skelton, F. R.: The influence of 3-methylglucose on the hypertension and cardiovascular-renal changes elicited by desoxycorticosterone acetate in the rat. Endocrinology 55, 288 (1954). ~ Experimental hypertensive vascular disease in the rat. Arch. Path. (Chicago) 60, 190 (1955). ~ Adrenal-regeneration hypertension and factors influencing its development. Arch. intern. Med. 98, 449 (1956). — Sluder, H. M., and F. R. Lock: Sudden maternal death associated with amniotic fluid embolism. Amer. J. Obstet. 64, 118 (1952). — Slyke, D. D. van: Renal tubular failure of shock and nephritis. Ann. intern. Med. 41, 709 (1954). — Smith, C. C., and P. M. Zeek: Studies on periarteritis nodosa. II. The rôle of various factors in the etiology of periarteritis nodosa in experimental animals. Amer. J. Path. 23, 147 (1947). — Smith, C. C., P. M. Zeek and J. McGuire: Periarteritis nodosa in experimental hypertensive rats and dogs. Amer. J. Path. 20b, 721 (1944). — Smith, D. J.: Constriction of isolated arteries and their vasa vasorum produced by low temperature. Amer. J. Physiol. 171, 528 (1952). — Smith, F. M., G. H. Miller and V. C. Graber: The relative importance of the systolic and the diastolic blood pressure in maintaining the coronary circulation. Arch. intern. Med. 38, 109 (1926). — Smith, R. C., H. B. Burchell and J. E. Edwards: Pathology of the pulmonary vascular tree. IV. Structural changes in the pulmonary vessels in chronic left ventricular failure. Circulation 10, 801 (1954). — Sobye, P.: Hereditiy essential hypertension and nephrosclerosis. A genetic clinical study 200 propositi suffering from nephrosclerosis. Diss. Copenhagen 1948. — Soustek, Z.: Hypertensive Arteriolitis im großen Kreislauf. Zbl. allg. Path. path. Anat. 97, 129 (1957). — Spatz, H.: Pathologische Anatomie der Kreislaufstörungen des Gehirns. Z. ges. Neurol. Psychiat. 167, 301 (1939). — Spencer, H.: Primary pulmonary and related vascular changes in the lungs. J. Path. Bact. 62, 75 (1950). — Spielmeyer, W.: Histopathologie des Nervensystems. Berlin 1922. ~ Die Pathogenese des epileptischen Krampfes. Histopathologischer Teil. Z. ges. Neurol. Psychiat. 109, 501 (1927). ~ Über örtliche Vulnerabilität. Z. ges. Neurol. Psychiat. 118, 1 (1928). ~ Funktionelle Kreislaufstörungen und Epilepsie. Z. ges. Neurol. Psychiat. 148, 285 (1933). — Spohn, E., u. E. Kolb: Neue Ergebnisse mit tiefer Hypothermie und lang dauerndem artefiziellem Kreislaufstillstand unter besonderer Berücksichtigung der Toleranz des ZNS. Langenbecks Arch. klin. Chir. 290, 292 (1959). ~ Tiefe Hypothermie unter 20⁰ C. Die Methode von Watanabe, Okamura und Ishikawa. Ihre Leistungsfähigkeit bei Operationen am offenen Herzen im Tierversuch. Langenbecks Arch. klin. Chir. 290, 365 (1959). — Spohn, K.: Die tödlichen Lungenembolien an den Heidelberger Kliniken. Langenbecks Arch. klin. Chir. 269, 518 (1951). — Staemmler, H. J.: Die Entwicklung der Stase in der terminalen Strombahn bei Anwendung von Kältereizen. Virchows Arch. path. Anat. 312, 437 (1944). — Staemmler, M.: Über Veränderungen der kleinen Hirngefäße in apoplektischen und traumatischen Erweichungsherden und ihre Beziehungen zur traumatischen Spätapoplexie. Beitr. path. Anat. 78, 408 (1927). ~ Die Thromboendarteriitis obliterans der Lungenarterien. Klin. Wschr. 1937, 1669. ~ Gibt es eine primäre Hypertonie im kleinen Kreislauf? Arch. Kreisl.-Forsch. 3, 125 (1938). ~ Die Erfrierung. Leipzig 1944. ~ Hypertonie im großen und kleinen Kreislauf. Wien. med. Wschr. 1954, 279. ~ Die Kreislauforgane. In Kaufmann-Staemmler, Lehrbuch der speziellen pathologischen Anatomie, Bd. I/1, S. 1. Berlin 1955. ~ Die Coronarthrombose in der Versicherungsmedizin. Dtsch. Z. ges. gerichtl. Med. 44, 754 (1956). ~ Die Nierenvenenthrombose und ihre Folgen. Dtsch. Arch. klin. Med. 205, 231 (1958). — Staemmler, M., u. P. Wilhelms: Thrombose und Embolie als Todesursachen. Medizinische 1953, 1639. — Starling, E. H.: The fluids of the body. London 1909. — Stead jr., E. A., and R. V. Ebert: Postural hypotension, a disease of the sympathetic nervous system. Arch. intern. Med. 67, 546 (1941). — Steinberg, I., and J. McClenahan: Pulmonary arteriovenous fistula. Amer. J. Med. 19,

549 (1956). — Steinberg, U.: Systematische Untersuchungen über die Arteriosklerose der Lungenschlagadern. Beitr. path. Anat. 82, 307, 443 (1929). — Steiner, P. E., and C. C. Lushbaugh: Maternal pulmonary embolism by amniotic fluid. J. Amer. med. Ass. 117, 1245, 1340 (1941). — Steiner, P. E., C. C. Lushbaugh and H. A. Frank: Fatal obstetric shock from pulmonary emboli of amniotic fluid. Amer. J. Obstet. 58, 802 (1949). — Sternberg, C.: Zur Pathologischen Anatomie der Angina pectoris. Wien. med. Wschr. 74, 2338 (1924). ~ Tödliche Lungenblutung infolge Periarteriitis nodosa. Wien. klin. Wschr. 1925, 729. — Stewart, C. F.: Arteriosclerosis of renal artery orifices with severe hypertension. J. Amer. med. Ass. 114, 2099 (1940). — Stewart, H. L., and B. L. Crawford: Congenital heart disease with pulmonary arteritis. Amer. J. Path. 9, 637 (1933). — Stewart, J. D.: Wound shock. J. Amer. med. Ass. 133, 216 (1947). — Stochdorph, O.: Organgebundene Eigentümlichkeiten der Arteriosklerose der Hirngefäße. Verh. dtsch. Ges. Path. 1958, 145. — Stochdorph, O., u. H. Meessen: Die arteriosklerotische und die hypertonische Gehirnerkrankung. In Handbuch der speziellen Pathologie, Bd. XIII/1, S. 1465. Berlin-Göttingen-Heidelberg 1957. — Stocks, P. (1929): Zit. nach M. Hamilton, G. W. Pickering, J. A. F. Roberts and G. S. C. Sowry, The aetiology of essential hypertension. IV. The role of inheritance. Clin. Sci. 13, 273 (1954). — Stone, S., R. Koucky and H. R. Leland: A fatal case of amniotic fluid embolism. Amer. J. Obstet. 70, 660 (1955). — Strauss, H.: Cerebrale Fettembolie. (Kritisches Sammelreferat.) Zbl. ges. Neurol. Psychiat. 66, 385 (1933). — Streli, R.: Ein Fall zentraler Fettembolie. Klin. Med. 11, 76 (1956). — Struck, G.: Beitrag zur Frage der nervalen Beeinflussung der beginnenden Entzündung. Beitr. path. Anat. 115, 515 (1955). — Struppler, V.: Die Fettembolie. Stuttgart 1940. — Sturm, A.: Die klinische Pathologie der Lunge in Beziehung zum vegetativen Nervensystem. Stuttgart 1948. — Suchenwirth, R.: Über die Eigenständigkeit des Nierenbildes bei Panarteriitis nodosa. Beitr. path. Anat. 116, 613 (1956). — Sugar, O., and R. W. Gerard: Anoxia and brain potentials. J. Neurophysiol. 1, 558 (1938). — Sullivan, B. J., and L. D. Gennaro: Microscopical observations of peripheral circulation at simulated high altitudes. J. Aviat. Med. 24, 131 (1953). — Suwa, N.: Unveröffentlicht 1959. ~ Diskussionsbemerkung zum Vortrag F. Duspiva u. D. Gohl, Zur Energetik des hypertrophierten Herzmuskels im Tierexperiment. Verh. dtsch. Ges. Path. 1959, 300. — Symmers, W. St. C.: Necrotizing pulmonary arteriopathy associated with pulmonary hypertension. J. clin. Path. 5, 36 (1952). ~ Über die thrombotische Mikroangiopathie und ihre Beziehungen zu den sogenannten Kollagenkrankheiten. Verh. dtsch. Ges. Path. 36, 224 (1953).

Takats, G. de, W. C. Beck and G. K. Fenn: Surgery 6 339 (1939). Zit. nach H. Schwiegk, Über Reflexe und dem kleinen Kreislauf. Verh. dtsch. Ges. Kreisl.-Forsch. 17, 95 (195 1). — Tannenberg, J.: Experimentelle Untersuchungen über lokale Kreislaufstörungen. I. Teil. Einleitung. Frankfurt. Z. Path. 31, 173 (1925). ~ IV. Die Leukozytenwanderung und die Diapedese der roten Blutkörperchen. Franfurt. Z. Path. 31, 351 (1925). ~ V. Über Entzündung bei Ausschaltung des Nervensystems durch Lokalanaesthetika. Frankfurt. Z. Path, 31, 385 (1925). ~ Entzündungsversuche im anaphylaktischen Schock. Verh. dtsch. path. Ges. 21, 144 (1926). ~ Bau und Funktion der Blutkapillaren. Frankfurt. Z. Path. 34, 1 (1926). — Tannenberg, J., u. B. Fischer-Wasels: Experimentelle Untersuchungen über lokale Kreislaufstörungen. II. Teil. Das Rickersche Stufengesetz über die Wirkungsweise lokal angewandten Reizes. Frankfurt. Z. Path. 31, 182 (1925). ~ III. Die Stase, zugleich Untersuchungen über die Entstehungsbedingungen eines Kollateralkreislaufes. Frankfurt. Z. Path. 31, 285 (1925). ~ Gefäßnerven und lokale Kreislaufstörung. Frankfurt. Z. Path. 33, 91, 454 (1925). ~ Die lokalen Kreislaufstörungen. In Handbuch der normalen und pathologischen Physiologie, Bd. VII/2, S. 1496. 1927. — Taterka, W.: Vergleichende histotopographische und elektrokardiographische Untersuchungen über linksbetonte und rechtsbetonte Coronarinsuffizienz bei Collaps. Beitr. path. Anat. 102, 287 (1939). — Tennant, R., F. A. Grayzel, F. A. Sutherland and S. W. Stringer: Studies on experimental coronary occlusion. Chemical and anatomical changes in the myocardium after coronary ligation. Amer. Heart J. 12, 168 (1936). — Terbrüggen, A.: Zur pathologischen Anatomie der arteriellen Gefäßerkrankungen. Regensburg. Jb. ärztl. Fortbild. 1951, 90. — Thauer, R.: Ergebnisse experimenteller Kreislaufuntersuchungen bei Hypothermie. Thoraxchirurgie 3, 521 (1955/56). ~ Pathophysiologie der Hypothermie. Thoraxchirurgie 6, 128 (1958). — Thies, W.: Veränderungen der Aortenmedia nach Tod im akuten Kollaps. Beitr. path. Anat. 116, 461 (1956). — Thoma, R.: Untersuchungen über die Histogenese und die Histomechanik des Gefäßsystems. Stuttgart 1893. ~ Über die Strömung des Blutes in der Gefäßbahn und die Spannung der Gefäßwand. Ihre Bedeutung für das normale Wachstum, für die Blutstillung und für die Angiosklerose. Beitr. path. Anat. 66, 92, 259, 377 (1920). ~ Über die Intima der Arterien. Virchows Arch. path. Anat. 230, 1 (1921). — Thompson, R., u. W. Evans: Paradoxical embolism. Quart. J. Med. 23, 135 (1930). — Thornton, L. F.: A fatal case of pulmonary infarction due to embolism of amniotic fluid. Amer. J. Obstet. 66, 871 (1953). — Threlfall, C. J., and H. B. Stoner: Studies on the mechanism of shock.

The effect of limb ischemia on the phosphates of muscle. Brit. exp. Path. **38**, 339 (1957). — Tigerstedt, R.: Skand. Arch. Physiol. **14**, 273 (1903). Zit. nach R. Wagner, Kreislauf und Atmung. Verh. dtsch. Ges. Kreisl.-Forsch. **13**, 7 (1940). ~ Die Physiologie des Kreislaufs. Berlin u. Leipzig 1921—1923. — Tittel, S.: Über die Reaktionsweise des Gefäßsystems bei lokaler Erfrierung. I. Über die Art des Reaktionsablaufes an den einzelnen Abschnitten des Gefäßsystems. Z. ges. exp. Med. **113**, 698 (1943/44). — Tonutti, E.: Zur Analyse der pathophysiologischen Reaktionsmöglichkeiten des Organismus. Diphtherietoxin und Intoxikation nach Verbrennung. Klin. Wschr. **1949**, 569. ~ Toxische Gewebsschäden, Entstehungsmechanismus und Folgerungen. Langenbecks Arch. klin. Chir. **264**, 61 (1950). — Torack, R. M.: The incidence and etiology of pulmonary infarction in the absence of congestive heart failure. Arch. Path. (Chicago) **65**, 574 (1958). — Torhorst, H.: Die histologischen Veränderungen bei der Sklerose der Lungenarterien. Beitr. path. Anat. **36**, 210 (1904). — Tosetti, R.: Les zones de résistance vasculaire pulmonaire an cours du rétrécissement mitral et du cœur pulmonaire chronique des emphysémateux. Arch. Mal. Cœur **48**, 346 (1955). — Tourniaire, A., P. Marion, M. Verrière et G. Tartullier: Cœur pulmonaire aigu intervention-réflexions pathogéniques. Presse méd. **1952**, 1578. — Toussaint, Ch. (1951): Zit. nach Ch. Toussaint, R. Wolter u. P. Sibille, Hypertension et lésions artérielles provoquées chez le rat par l'ingestion de quantités excessives de chlorure de sodium. Rev. belge Path. **23**, 63 (1953). — Toussaint, Ch., R. Wolter et P. Sibille: Hypertension et lésions artérielles provoquées chez le rat par l'ingestion de quantités excessives de chlorure de sodium. Rev. belg. Path. **23**, 63 (1953). — Trueta, J.: The relation of hypertension to the renal circulation. Glasg. med. J. **31**, 217 (1950). — Tunis, B.: Amniotic emboli: Do they really cause sudden death in obstetrics? Amer. J. Obstet. **64**, 72 (1952). — Turner, L. B., and A. Grollman: Role of adrenal in pathogenesis of experimental renal hypertension as determined by a study of the bilaterally adrenalectomized nephrectomized dog. Amer. J. Physiol. **167**, 462 (1951). — Twiss, A., and M. Sokolow: Angina pectoris. Significant electrocardiographic changes following exercises. Amer. Heart J. **23**, 498 (1942).

Uhlenbruck, P.: Die Klinik der Coronarerkrankungen. Berlin 1940.

Verschuer, O. v., u. V. Zipperlen: Die erb- und umweltbedingte Variabilität der Herzform. Z. klin. Med. **112**, 69 (1929). — Villaret, M., et R. Cachera: Les embolies cérébrales. Paris 1939. — Virchow, R.: Über die Verstopfung der Lungenarterie. Frorieps Notizen 1846. Jan. Nr 794. ~ Die Verstopfung der Lungenarterie und ihre Folgen. Traubes Beitr. zur exp. Path. u. Physiol. 1846. H. 2, S. 1. ~ Weitere Untersuchungen über die Verstopfung der Lungenarterie und ihre Folgen. Traubes Beitr. zur exp. Path. u. Physiol. Berl. 1846, H. II. In R. Virchow, Gesammelte Abhandlungen zur wissenschaftlichen Medizin. IV. Thrombose und Embolie. Gefäßentzündung und septische Infection. Frankfurt a. M. 1856. ~ Über die Verstopfung der Lungenarterie. Frorieps Neue Notizen. 1846. Jan. Nr 794. In R. Virchow, Gesammelte Anhandlungen zur wissenschaftlichen Medizin. IV. Thrombose und Embolie. Gefäßentzündung und Septische Infection. Frankfurt a. M. 1856. ~ Über die akute Entzündung der Arterien. Arch. path. Anat. u. Physiol. **1**, 272 (1847). ~ Brandmetastase von der Lunge auf das Gehirn. Arch. path. Anat. u. Physiol. **5**, 275 (1852). ~ Die Pfropfbildungen und Verstopfungen in den Gefäßen. In Handbuch der speziellen Pathologie, Bd. I, S. 156. 1854. ~ Thrombose und Embolie. Gefäßentzündung und septische Infection. IV. In R. Virchow, Gesammelte Abhandlungen zur wissenschaftlichen Medizin. Franfurt a. M. 1856. ~ Form des geronnenen Faserstoffs. Frorieps Neue Notizen aus dem Gebiete der Natur- u. Heilkunde. 1845. Nr 769. In R. Virchow, Gesammelte Abhandlungen zur wissenschaftlichen Medizin. Über den Faserstoff. Frankfurt a. M. 1856. ~ Gesammelte Abhandlungen zur wissenschaftlichen Medizin. Frankfurt a. M. 1856. ~ Über Fettembolie und Eklampsie. Berl. klin. Wschr. **1886**, Nr 30. — Vivell, O.: Durchströmungsversuche am Koronarsystem bei normalem, hypertrophischem und atrophischem Herzmuskel. Beitr. path. Anat. **111**, 125 (1950). — Vogelberg, K.: Die Lichtungsweite der Koronarostien an normalen und hypertrophen Herzen. Z. Kreisl.-Forsch. **46**, 101 (1957). — Volhard, F.: Die doppelseitigen haematogenen Nierenerkrankungen. Die Veränderungen am Herzen und am Gefäßapparat. In Handbuch der inneren Medizin, Bd. VI/1, S. 372. 1931. ~ Über die Pathogenese des roten (essentiellen) arteriellen Hochdrucks und der malignen Sklerose. Schweiz. med. Wschr. **1948**, 1189, 1224. ~ Die Pathogenese des Hochdrucks. Verh. dtsch. Ges. Kreisl.-Forsch. **15**, 40 (1949). — Volhard, F., u. R. Fahr: Die Brightsche Nierenkrankheit. Berlin 1914.

Wachstein, M., and E. Meisel: Succinic dehydrogenase activity in myocardial infarction and in induced myocardial necrosis. Amer. J. Path. **31**, 353 (1955). — Wagner, E.: Arch. Heilk. **3** (1862); **6** (1865). Zit. nach W. Ceelen, Die Kreislaufstörungen der Lunge. In Handbuch der speziellen Pathologie, Bd. III/3, S. 1. 1931. — Wagner, R.: Kreislauf und Atmung. Verh. dtsch. Ges. Kreisl.-Forsch. **13**, 7 (1940). — Wagner, R., D. J. Athanasiou u. E. Bauereisen: Reaktion des arteriellen Blutdruckes beim Menschen auf örtliche Kältereize. Z. Biol. **104**, 214 (1951). — Walder, R.: Elektrokardiographische und histologische

Untersuchungen des Herzens bei experimenteller Luft- und Fettembolie, sowie bei Embolie durch Stärkesuspension. Beitr. path. Anat. 102, 485 (1939). — WALTHARD, B., u. K. M. WALTHARD: Periarteriitis nodosa (des Gehirns). In Handbuch der speziellen Pathologie, Bd. XIII/1 B, S. 1563. 1957. — WARBURG, O.: Über den Stoffwechsel der Tumoren. Berlin 1926. — WARTHIN, A. S.: A case of Ayerza's disease: chronic cyanosis, dyspnoe, and erythemia, associated with syphilis arteriosclerosis of the pulmonary arteries. Trans. Ass. Amer. Phycns 24, 218 (1919). — WARTMANN, W. B., and H. K. HELLERSTEIN: The incidence of heart disease in 2000 consecutive autopsies. Ann. intern. Med. 28, 41 (1948). — WARTMAN, W. B., R. B. JENNINGS and B. HUDSON: Experimental arterial disease: The reaction of the pulmonary arteries to minute emboli of blood clot. Circulation 4, 747 (1951). — WASSERMAN, E.: Thrombohemolytic thrombocytopenic purpura. Case report and review of literature. Amer. J. med. Sci. 24, 648 (1958). — WATANABE, A.: Nippon Kyolu Geka Gakkai Shi. 6, 638 (1957). — WATKINS, E. L.: Sudden maternal death from amniotic fluid embolism. Amer. J. Obstet. 56, 994 (1948). — WEARN, J. T.: The extent of the capillary bed of the heart. J. exp. Med. 47, 273 (1928). ~ Morphological and functional alterations of the coronary circulation. Harvey Lect. 35, 243 (1939/40). ~ Morphological and functional alteration of the coronary circulation. Bull. N.Y. Acad. Med. 17, 754 (1941). — WEBER, A.: Die Elektrokardiographie und andere graphische Methoden in der Kreislaufdiagnostik, 3. Aufl. Berlin 1937. ~ Die klinische Bedeutung der Veränderungen von S-T und T im Extremitätenelektrokardiogramm. Dtsch. med. Wschr. 63, 430 (1937). — WEBER, H. W.: Beitrag zur Kenntnis der Tumoren des chromaffinen Systems und des Sympathicus. Frankfurt. Z. Path. 60, 228 (1949). — WEGELIN, C.: Über Arteriosklerose im Myokard. Schweiz. med. Wschr. 1944, 57. — WEGENER, F.: Über eine eigenartige rhinogene Granulomatose mit besonderer Beteiligung des Arteriensystems und der Nieren. Beitr. path. Anat. 102, 36 (1939). — WÉGRIA, R., H. E. ESSEX, J. F. HERRICK and F. C. MANN: The simultaneous action of certain drugs on the blood pressure and on the flow in the right and left coronary arteries. Amer. Heart J. 20, 557 (1940). — WEHRLE, J.: Histologische Untersuchungen des Zwischenhirns bei genuiner Hypertonie. Beitr. path. Anat. 111, 381 (1951). — WEIMANN, W.: Über Hirnveränderungen bei cerebraler Fettembolie. Dtsch. Z. ges. gerichtl. Med. 13, 95 (1929). ~ Besondere Hirnbefunde bei cerebraler Fettembolie. Dtsch. Z. Nervenheilk. 120, 68 (1939). — WEINBERGER, L., M. GIBBON and J. GIBBON: Temporary arrest of the circulation to the central nervous system. Arch. Neurol. Psychiat. (Chicago) 43, 616, 961 (1940). — WEINER, A. E., and D. E. REID: The pathogenesis of amniotic fluid embolism. III. Coagulant activity of amniotic fluid. New Engl. J. Med. 243, 597 (1950). — WEINSCHENK, K.: Herzmuskelveränderungen bei pathologischer Belastung des rechten Ventrikels. Beitr. path. Anat 102, 477 (1939). — WEIS, FOGH, J.: Aggregation of erythrocytes in small blood vessels. Clinical and experimental studies. Scand. J. clin. Lab. Invest. 9, Suppl. 28, 7 (1957). — WEITZ, W. (1923): Zit. nach M. HAMILTON, G. W. PICKERING, J. A. F. ROBERTS u. G. S. C. SOWRY: The aetiology of essential hypertension. IV. The role of inheritance. Clin. Sci. 13, 273 (1954). — WELCH, K. J., and T. D. KINNEY: The effect of patent ductus arteriosus and interauricular and interventricular septal defects on the development of pulmonary vascular lesions. Amer. J. Path. 24, 729 (1948). — WENZ, W., K. SPOHN, E. KOLB, J. HEINZEL u. R. KRATZERT: Pathologisch-anatomische Befunde nach langdauerndem Kreislaufstop und intracardialen Eingriffen in tiefer Hypothermie unter 20° C am Hund. Langenbecks Arch. klin. Chir. 291, 1 (1959). — WERTHEIMER, C.: Über die Zunahme der Thrombosen und Embolien. Klin. Wschr. 1931, 1387. — WERTHEMANN, A., u. W. RÖSSIGER: Über gewebliche Veränderungen bei wiederholten mehrzeitigen Verbrennungen der Haut der weißen Maus. Z. ges. exp. Med. 73, 631 (1930). — WERTHEMANN, A., u. G. RUTISHAUSER: Zur pathologischen Anatomie der Thrombose. I. Internat. Tagg über Thrombose und Embolie, Basel, 1954. — WESTBROOK, O. C., and J. R. THOMAS: Amniotic fluid embolism complicating late abortion. Amer. J. Obstet. 71, 447 (1956). — WHITLEY, H. J.: The relation between tissue injury and the manifestations of pulmonary fat embolism. J. Path. Bact. 67, 521 (1954). — WHITLEY, H. J., and G. M. WILSON: Wide spread intimal proliferation of arteries with resulting thrombosis. J. Path. 64, 705 (1952). — WIDEROE, S.: Die Massenverhältnisse des Herzens unter pathologischen Zuständen. Christiania 1911. — WIELAND, CH.: Noch unveröffentlicht. 1956. — WIESE, F.: Über Thromboendarteriitis obliterans der Lungenarterien, ein Beitrag zur Pathogenese autochtoner Lungenarterienthrombose. Frankfurt. Z. Path. 49, 155 (1936). — WIGAND, H.: Die nichthämolytischen Bluttransfusionsstörungen. Berlin 1955. — WIGGERS, C. J.: Myocardial depression in shock. A survey of cardiodynamic studies. Amer. Heart J. 33, 633 (1947). ~ The Physiology of Shock. New York 1950. — WIGGERS, C. J., and J. M. WERLE: Amer. J. Physiol. 136, 421 (1942). — WILDI, E.: État granulaire systématisé cardiopathique de l'écorce cérébrale. (Atrophie granulaire.) Étude anatomoclinique. Bull. schweiz. Akad. med. Wiss. 15, 1 (1959). — WILLEBRAND, E., u. R. JÜRGENS: Über eine neue Bluterkrankheit, die konstitutionelle Thrombopathie. Klin. Wschr. 12, 414 (1933a). ~ Über ein neues vererbbares Blutungsübel: Die konstitutionelle

Thrombopathie. Dtsch. Arch. klin. Med. 175, 453 (1933 b). —William, J.A., and W. J.Webster: Sensory phenomena associated with defective blood supply to working muscles. Brit. med. J. 1923, 51. — Williams, G.: Experimental arterial thrombosis. J. Path. Bact. 69, 199 (1955). — Wilson, C., u. F. B. Byrom: Nierenveränderungen bei malignem Hochdruck; ihr experimenteller Nachweis. Zbl. allg. Path. path. Anat. 73, 35 (1939). ~ Nierenveränderungen bei malignem Hochdruck; ihr experimenteller Nachweis. Lancet 236, 136 (1939).— Wilson, C., and G. W. Pickering: Acute arterial lesions in rabbits with experimental renal hypertension. Clin. Sci. 3, 343 (1937/38). — Winter jr., W. J.: Atheromatous emboli; a cause of cerebral infarction. Report of two cases. Arch. Path. (Chicago) 64, 137 (1957). — Wirtz, H.: Die disseminierten Erweichungsherde des Hypertoniker-Gehirns und ihre pathogenetische Bedeutung für die große Hochdruckblutung. Beitr. path. Anat. 97, 219 (1936). — Wissler, R. W., M. L. Eilert, M. A. Schroeder and L. Cohen: Production of lipomatous and atheromatous arterial lesions in the albino rat. Arch. Path. (Chicago) 57, 333 (1954). — Wollheim, E.: Zirkulierende Blutmenge. Kompensation und Dekompensation des Kreislaufes. Verh. dtsch. Ges. inn. Med. 41, 352 (1929). ~ Die zirkulierende Blutmenge und ihre Bedeutung für Kompensation und Dekompensation des Kreislaufes. Z. klin. Med. 116, 269 (1931). — Wood, F. C., C. C. Wolferth and M. M. Livezey: Angina pectoris. Arch. intern. Med. 47, 339 (1931). — Wright, I. S.: The pathogenesis, prevention and medical management of peripheral arterial thrombosis. Amer. J. Med. 23, 704 (1957). ~ Nomenclature of blood clotting factors. Acceptance by the international committee on nomenclature of four factors, their characterization and international number. Thromb. diath. haemorrhag. 3, 435 (1959). — Wustmann, P., u. J. Hallervorden: Beobachtungen bei Trendelenburgschen Embolieoperationen. Dtsch. Z. Chir. 245, 472 (1935). — Wyatt, J. P., and H. Goldenberg: Amniotic fluid embolism. Report of a fatal case. Arch. Path. (Chicago) 45, 366 (1948).

Yater, W. M., A. H. Traum, W. G. Brown, R. P. Fitzgerald, M. A. Geisler and B. B. Wilcox: Coronary artery disease in man 18 to 39 years of age. Amer. Heart J. 36, 334 (1947). — Yoshimura, F., and A. Negishi: Experiments concerning the site of reninformation. Amer. J. Physiol. 178, 251 (1954).

Zahn, W.: Untersuchungen über Thrombose. Bildung der Thromben. Virchows Arch. path. Anat. 62, 81 (1875). — Zeek, P. M., C. C. Smith and J. C. Weeter: Studies on periarteritis nodosa: III. Differentiation between the vascular lesions of periarteritis nodosa and of hypersensitivity. Amer. J. Path. 24, 889 (1948). — Zeitlhofer, I., u. G. Reifenstuhl: Untersuchungen über fulminante tödliche Lungenembolie am Obduktionsmaterial der Jahre 1941—1951. Wien. klin. Wschr. 64, 446 (1952). — Zeman, F., u. A. M. Fishberg: Nierenvenenthrombose und nephrotisches Syndrom. In A. M. Fishberg, Hypertension und Nephritis, 4. Aufl., S. 374. Philadelphia 1944. — Zenker, F.: Beitrag zur normalen und pathologischen Anatomie der Lunge. Dresden 1862. — Ziegler, E.: Über den Bau und die Entstehung der endokarditischen Effloreszenzen. Kongr.-Zbl. ges. inn. Med. 1888. — Zilliacus, H.: The thrombo-embolic disease in preeclampsia. Thromb. diath. haemorrhag. 3, 6 (1959). — Zimmermann, H.: Experimentelle histologische, histochemische und funktionelle Untersuchungen zur Frage der Nierenschädigung nach temporärer Ischämie. Beitr. path. Anat. 117, 65 (1957). — Zimmermann, H., u. D. Schleifer: Morphologie und Histochemie der Skeletmuskulatur nach zeitlicher Durchblutungsdrosselung. Acta histochem. (Jena) 8, 221 (1959). — Zimmermann, H., G. Sonnekalb u. Ch. Watz: Experimentelle Untersuchungen über die Speicherungsfunktion der Rattenniere unter normalen Bedingungen und nach temporärer Ischämie. Beitr. path. Anat. 122, 238 (1960). — Zinck, A. H.: Pathologische Anatomie der Verbrennung. Veröff. Konstit. u. Wehrpath. 46, Jena 1940. — Zinck, K. H.: Läßt sich die Zunahme der fulminanten Embolien durch die Überalterung erklären? Virchows Arch. path. Anat. 296, 289 (1936). ~ Die Verbrennungskrankheit. Hefte Unfallheilk. 47, 10 (1954). — Zoll, P. M., S. Wessler and H. L. Blumgart: Angina pectoris. Amer. J. Med. 11, 331 (1951). — Zollinger, H. U.: Intrarenaler Druck und Niereninsuffizienz; experimentelle Untersuchungen über die akute Hämolyseniere bei der Ratte. Helv. chir. Acta 18, 146 (1951). ~ Anurie bei Chromoproteinurie. Stuttgart 1952. — Zollinger, H. U., u. N. Papacharalampous: Über das appositionelle proximale Wachstum der Coronarthromben. Schweiz. med. Wschr. 1953, 864. — Zuelzer, W. W., R. Kurnetz and R. Fallon: Nierenvenenthrombose und nephrotisches Syndrom. Amer. J. Dis. Child. 81, 27 (1951). — Zweifach, B. W.: Functional deterioration of terminal vascular bed in irreversible hemorrhagic shock. Ann. N.Y. Acad. Sci. 55, 369 (1952). ~ An analysis of the inflammatory reaction through the response of the terminal vascular bed to micro-trauma. Rev. canad. Biol. 12, No 2 (1953). — Zweifach, B. W., R. E. Lee, Ch. Hyman and R. Chambers: Omental circulation in morphinized dogs subjected to graded hemorrhage. Ann. Surg. 120, 232 (1944). — Zweifach, B. W., u. D. B. Metz: Zit. nach I. Illig, Die terminale Strombahn. Berlin-Göttingen-Heidelberg 1961. — Zweifach, B. W., D. B. Metz and E. Shorr: Participation of VEM and VDM mechanisms in drum shock and in development of „resistance" to drum trauma. Amer. J. Physiol. 164, 91 (1951).

Namenverzeichnis.

Die *kursiv* gedruckten Seitenzahlen beziehen sich auf die Literatur.

Abbot, M. E. 592, *609*
Abbott, W. O., u. T. G. Miller 41, *53*
— s. Miller, T. G. 41, *61*
Abderhalden E., u. P. Möller *248*
Abdou, J. A., u. H. Tarver 135, *158*
Abelanet, R. s. Chomette, G. *927*
— s. Delarue, J. 523, *614*
Abelanet, R. M. s. Delarue, J. A. 523, *614*
Abell, R. G., u. I. H. Page 900, *921*
— u. H. P. Schenck 833, 836, *921*
Abelmann, W. H. s. Bergeron, J. 822, *924*
Abels, J. C. s. Rekers, P. E. 50, *63*
Aber, G. M., u. D. S. Rowe 184, *274*
Abernathy, R. S. s. Smith, D. T. 172, *275*
Abrahams, O. L. s. Bothwell, T. H. 206, 208, *251*
Abrams, G. D., u. B. L. Baker 34, *53*
— s. Baker, B. S. 34, *54*
Abrams, J. S. s. Ellison, E. H. 73, *114*
Achard, Ch. *248*
Ackerman, R. F. s. Zilversmit, D. B. *274*
Adamik, E. R. s. Endicott, K. M. 203, *254*
Adams, J. Q. s. Schreier, P. C. *949*
Adams, W. S. s. Figueroa, W. S. 205, *255*
Adebahr, G. 523, 603, *609*
Adison, A. O. s. Boxer, G. E. 185, *251*
Adler, S. s. Fries, Ch. C. *931*
Adlersberg, D. 93, 94, 96, *113*
— E. Grishman u. H. Sobotka 184, *248*
— s. Himes, H. W. 94, *115*
Adolf, W. H. s. Chou, T. 212, *252*
Adrian, E. D. 315, *321*
— u. D. W. Bronk 320, *321*

Aeby, C. 547, *609*
Affeldt, J. E. s. Ferris jr., B. G. *392*
Agathon, S. s. Helliesen, P. J. 456, 486, *620*
Agren, G. 46, *53*
— H. Lagerlöf u. H. Berglund 39, *53*
Aguilar, M. J. s. Crane, J. 107, *114*
Ahlqvist, J., u. J. Burstein *921*
Ahlström, C. G., K. Haeger, D. Jacobsohn u. G. Kahlson 33, *53*
— u. P. G. Widlund 892, 893, *921*
Ahrens, E. H., R. Blomstrand, J. Hinsch, W. Insull, T. T. Tsaltas u. M. L. Peterson 224, *248*
Ahrens, R. s. Portis, S. A. 34, *62*
Aidin, R., B. Corner u. G. Tovey 200, *248*
Aimar, Ch. E. s. Irwin, J. W. 595, *622*
Aitken, R. S., u. E. Clark-Kennedy 473, *609*
Akerd, K. s. Hess, W. R. 305, *322*
Aladjem, F., M. Liebermann u. J. W. Gofman 222, *248*
Alameri, E. H. s. Cohn, E. J. 183, *253*
Albaum, H. G., u. L. J. Milch *921*
Albertini, A. v. 905, *921*
Alberty, R. A. 193, *248*
Albrecht, H., H. Valentin u. H. Venrath *387*
Albright, E. C., F. C. Larson u. W. P. Deiss 214, 215, *248*
— — K. Tomita u. H. A. Lardy *248*
— K. Tomita u. F. C. Larson *249*
— s. Deiss, W. P. 183, 184, *253*
— s. Larson, F. C. 214, 215, 217, *262*
Albright, F., A. F. Forbes, F. C. Bartter, E. C. Reifenstein jr., D. Bryant, L. D. Cox u. E. F. Dempsey *158*

Albrink, M. J., W. W. L. Glenn, J. P. Peters u. E. B. Man 220, *248*
— E. B. Man u. J. P. Peters 220, *249*
— s. Man, E. B. 224, *263*
Alden, G. H. 145, *158*
Alella, A. 700, 705, 706, 707, 774, 811, *922*
— F. L. Williams, C. Bolene-Williams u. L. N. Katz 715, 720, *774*
Alesio, J. s. Goldberger, E. 806, *932*
Alexander, F. 899, *922*
Alexander, H. 501, *609*
Alexander, H. L., W. G. Becke u. J. A. Holmes 511, *609*
— s. Kountz, W. B. *624*
Alexander, J. H., J. B. West, J. A. Wood u. D. W. Richards 312, *321*
Alexander, L., u. H. Lowenbach 839, *922*
Alexander, M. K. s. Priest, W. M. 73, *117*
Alexander, N., L. B. Hinshaw u. D. R. Drury 897, *922*
Alexander, R. S. 672, 677, 678, *774*
— W. S. Edwards u. J. L. Ankeney 677, *774*
— u. M. M. Reydman *387*
— s. Pitts, R. F. *786*
Alhomme, P. s. Facquet, J. *391*
Aliminosa, L. s. Smith, H. W. 185, *270*
Alkjaersig, N. s. Seegers, W. H. 868, *949*
Allan G. F. 822, *922*
Allardyce, J., J. Salter u. R. Rixon 900, *922*
Allen, C. M. van 499, 500, 506, *609*
— u. T. S. Jung *609*
— u. G. E. Lindskog *609*
Allen, E. V., N. W. Baker u. E. A. Hines 881, *922*
Allen, S. W. s. Jandl, J. A. *260*
Allen, T. H., u. P. D. Orahovats 185, *248*
Allensworth, J. s. Holt, J. P. *782*

Gaultier, M., u. P. Maurice 381, *393*
Gavallér, B. v. 559, *617*, 853, *931*
Gay, E. s. Filley, G. F. *392*
Gayet, P., u. M. Guillaumie 40, *58*
Gaza, W. v. 134, 136, 138, *160*
Gazes, P. C. s. Foltz, E. L. 842, *931*
Gebauer, P. W. *393*
Gebhardt, W. s. Rau, G. 487, 531, *630*
Gedigk, P. s. Westphal, U. 184, *273*
Gee, J. B. L. s. Cormack, S. 303, *322*
Geefel, R. van s. Dubois-Manne, R. 81, *114*
Geffen, A. s. Cohen, A. G. *390*
Gegory, R. A. s. Code, C. F. 31, *55*
Gehl, H., K. Graf u. K. Kramer 726, 733, *779*
Gehlen, H. v. 412, 413, 417, 418, 595, *617*
Geigel, R. 514, *617*
Geiger, D. W. s. Sass-Kortsack, A. *268*
Geiger, H. 903, *931*
Geiler, G. s. Seifert, G. 67, 68, *118*
Geisler, M. A. s. Yater, W. M. 815, 877, *954*
Geissendörfer, H. 156, *160*
Geissendörfer, R. 886, *931*
Geist, O. B. s. Sanes, S. 88, *117*
Gellhorn, E., u. W. Budde 6, *58*
Gemmill, C. L., u. D. L. Reeves 301, *322*
Gemzell, C. A. 225, *274*
Gennaro, L. D. s. Sullivan, B. J. *951*
Georg, J. *393*
George, E. P., u. W. Sollich 213, 214, *256*
Gerard, R. s. Bing, R. J. 725, *776*
Gerard, R. W. s. Sugar, O. 802, *951*
Gerbaulet, K., u. W. Fitting 214, *256*
— — u. W. Maurer 213, 214, *256*
— — u. S. Rosenkaimer 214, *256*
— s. Fitting, W. 214, *255*
Gerbaux, A. s. Lenègre, J. 912, 913, *939*
Gercken, G. s. Enke, H. 899, *930*
Gergely, J. s. Ott, H. 223, 232, *265*
Gerhardt, D. 584, 603, *617*
Gericke, I. 587, *617*

Gerlach, E. s. Fleckenstein, A. 817, 826, *930*, *931*
Gerlach, J. 413, *617*
Gerlach, L. 413, *617*
Gerlach, U. s. Hauss, W. H. 795, 811, *933*
German, W. J. s. Wearn, J. T. 576, *637*, 749, *789*
Gernandt, B. E. s. Folkow, B. 650, *779*
Gershon-Cohen, J. s. Shay, H. 32, 33, *63*
Gerstel, G. 491, 598, *617*, 910, *931*
Gerstner, H. B. s. Lewis, R. B. *939*
Gerttler, M. M., u. P. D. White 885, *931*
Gertz, K. H. s. Loeschcke, H. H. 299, 301, 303, 304, 305, *323*
Gesell, R. 302, 320, *322*
— J. Bricker u. C. Magee *322*
— u. E. T. Hansen 320, *322*
— s. Erlanger, J. 844, 846, *930*
Gessner, J. s. Semisch, R. 594, 597, *633*
Geus, A. de 98, *115*
Gey, R. 491, *617*
Geyer, R. P. s. Waddel, W. R. 223, *272*
Ghareeb, A. A. s. Shaw, A. F. B. 912, *949*
Ghon, A. 490, 491, *617*
Giampalmo 898
Giampalmo, A., u. J. Schoenmackers 437, 561, 588, *617*
— s. Schoenmackers, J. 561, *632*
Gibbon, J. s. Landis, E. M. 234, *261*
— s. Weinberger, L. 802, 858, *953*
Gibbon, M. s. Weinberger, L. 802, 858, *953*
Gibbs, E. L. s. Lennox, W. G. 697, *783*
Gibbs, F. A. s. Lennox, W. G. 697, *783*
Gibian, H. 230, *256*
Giblett, E. R., C. G. Hickman u. O. Smithies 207, *256*
— s. Turnbull, A. 204, *275*
Gibson, J. G. s. Gregersen, M. J. 185, *257*
— s. Keeley, J. L. 845, *936*
— s. Vallee, B. L. 181, *272*
Gibson, J. H., u. E. D. Churchill *931*
Gibson, R. s. Fleming, P. R. 739, *779*
Gibson, T., u. P. B. Medawar 138, *160*
Giemsa, G. s. Mayer, M. 185, *264*

Giese 367
Giese, W. 407, 410, 412, 414, 415, 417, 422, 424, 425, 427, 430, 438, 441, 447, 448, 468, 475, 490, 491, 493, 501, 505, 514, 517, 522, 524, 537, 567, 575, 576, 577, 578, 579, 599, 600, 605, *617*, 761, 762, 766, *779*, 910, *931*
— u. R. Gieseking 412, 413, 414, 415, 447, 561, *618*
— u. H. Müller-Mohnssen 699, *779*
Gieseking, R. 541, 542, 543, 549, 555, 556, 560, *618*
— s. Giese, W. 412, 413, 414, 415, 447, 561, *618*
Gieson, D. M. s. Surgenor, D. M. 183, 204, *271*
Gilbert, M. s. Bing, R. J. 222, *250*, 715, 716, *776*
Gilbert, R. P. s. Haddy, F. J. 649, *781*
Gildemeister, H. 184, *256*
Gilder, H., S. F. Redo, D. Barr u. Ch. Gardner Child 231, *256*
Gilding, M. P. s. Rous, P. *947*
Gillespie, J. M. s. Cohn, E. J. *253*
Gilliat, R. W. 752, *779*
Gillich, K. H. 214, 215, *256*
— u. F. W. Aly *256*
— s. Lang, N. *262*
Gilligan, D. R. 185, *256*
— s. Blumgart, H. L. 803, 817, *925*
Gillman, T., u. A. C. Ivy *256*
— s. Endicott, K. M. 203, *254*
Gilman 203
Gilmore, H. R., M. Hamilton, H. Kopelman u. L. Sommer *393*
Gilroy, J. C., V. H. Wilson u. P. Marchand 596, *618*
— s. Marchand, P. 596, *626*
Gilse, P. H. G. van 477, *618*
Gilson, J. 517, *618*
Gilson, J. C., u. P. Hugh-Jones *393*
— s. Lavenne, F. *395*
Giltaire-Ralyte, L. s. Policard, A. 412, 414, 418, 421, *630*
Ginsbury, J. s. Beaconfield, P. 649, *775*
Giovannelli, G. s. Valentin, H. *400*
Girard, F. s. Dejours, P. 311, *322*
Girard, J., P. Louyot, P. Sadoul u. J. P. Grilliat *393*
— s. Simonin, P. *399*
Girling, F. 649, *780*
Gisinger, E. 208, *256*
— s. Braunsteiner, H. 206, *251*

Sachverzeichnis.

65*

66*

Morbus Boeck 436, 443, 523, 538
Morbus Cushing 248
— —, Hypertonie 899, 900, 902
Morbus Osler 367, 383, 594
Morbus Parkinson 212
Morbus Roger 764
Morbus Werlhof 869
Morbus Wilson 210—213, 245
Morgagni-Adams-Stokessches Syndrom 857
Mucoproteide 109
mucosal acceptor 203
mucous cells, *Schleimzellen* 20, 21, 30
Mucoviscidosis 67, 89, 90, 99
— der Erwachsenen 72
—, hoher Elektrolytgehalt 81
—, Leberveränderungen 81 bis 83
—, Schweißtest 82
mucus, *Schleim* 25, 44, 47
Multilumen-Darmsonde 41
— *multilumen intestinal tube* 41
multiple factor theory, Atmungsregulation 303
Mundatmung 476 ff.
muscle, cricopharyngeus 3
—, gastric 5
—, longitudinal, of the distal colon 17
Muscularis mucosae 14, 42
Musculus cricopharyngeus 3
Muskelautolysat 848
Muskelfasern, glatte 412, 413
Muskelfaserschwellung nach temporärer Ischämie 803
Muskeltätigkeit und Atmungsregulation 307
—, Ventilationssteigerung 297
Muzin des Magens 25
Myasthenie, Spirogramm 362
Myelome 149
Myelosen, chronische 881
—, diffuse 869
myenteric plexus 17
— reflex 13, 18, 19
Myocardiopathia diphtherica 857, 875, 876
— —, Thrombose 875
Myocarditis rheumatica 745
Myodegeneratio cordis 710
Myofer, Fremdvehikel 205
myogenic antiperistalsis of colon 17
Myoglobin, Eisen 203
—, Transport 210, 211
Myokard, Arteriolosklerose 815
—, Ischämie, Herzhypertrophie 830
—, kontraktile Proteine 724, 725
—, Totalnekrose 856

Myolyse, toxische 144
Myosin, Herzinsuffizienz 724
Myxom 859
— des linken Vorhofs 825, 857
— — —, pulmonale Hypertonie 908, 919

Nahrungsausnutzung nach totaler Magenresektion 74
Narbenbild der Streuembolie 913
Narbenlunge 423
Narbenstenosen, partielle 520
Narcotica, Atemzentrum 300
Narkosetheorie 236
Nasenatmung, Störung 475
Nasenspitze, Nekrose 857
native proteins 51
Natrium 52, 237
Natriumbicarbonat 37
—, Ausscheidung aus der Zelle 847
—, Rückresorption, gesteigerte 864, 866
Natriumchlorid, *sodium chloride* 52
Natriumdiäthylcarbamat 212
Natriumnitrit, Gefäßerweiterung, periphere 842
Natriumoleat, Thyroxin 216
Natriumretention 746, 866
Natriumrückresorption 170, 746
Nausea 10
N-Ausscheidung im Harn bei Eiweißinfusion 135
Nebenniere, Exstirpation, *adrenalectomy* 34
Nebennierenblutungen 870
Nebennierenhyperplasie, Hypertonie 898, 899, 902
Nebennierenrinde, Pellagra 112
—, Phosphorylierung 97
Nebennierenrindenhormone 176, 224, 225, 746
—, Hypertonie, experimentelle 899, 902
Nebennierenrindeninsuffizienz, Resorptionsstörung 112
Nebennierenmarkhormon, Herzmuskulatur 731
Nebennierenvenenthrombose 863
Nekrosen, extracelluläre Verdauung 144
— parenchymatöser Organe, maligne Hypertonie 808
—, Verdauung toten Materials 143, 144
Nekrosin, Entzündung 155
Nephrektomie, doppelseitige, Hypertonie 901, 902
Nephronen, offene 239
Nephrosen, hämoglobinurische 211

Nephrosen, Hormonjod 215
—, Ödemgenese 198
—, parenterale Eiweißzufuhr 133
Nervensystem, parasympathisches 18, 21, 22, 25
—, sympathisches, *sympathetic nerves* 21, 30, 46
nerves, pelvic visceral, *viscerale Pelvisnerven* 17, 18
Nervi craniosacrales 17
— splanchnici 15, 17, 18, 39
— —, Einfluß auf Magenmotilität, *motility of stomach* 6
nervous control of colonic secretion 47
— and endocrine disturbances, *nervöse und endokrine Störungen* 15
— regulation of gastro-intestinal motility 17
Nervus erigens 47, 48
— opticus, Arteriolosklerose 903
— vagus 17, 23, 30, 39, 45
— —, Durchtrennung, *vagotomy* 9
— —, Reizung, *stimulation* 29, 31, 45
— —, Schluckakt, *deglutition*
Netzcapillaren 576
Netzhaut, Arteriolosklerose 903
Netzhautarterien 838
Neugeborene, Bilirubin 199
neurogenic function, gastrointestinal motility 17
Neuronophagie 840
Neutralisation des Mageninhalts, *neutralization of gastric contents* 32
Nicotin 839
Nicotinsäureamid 112
Niederdruckgebiet, Kreislauf 665, 673, 747
Niere, Arteriosklerose 905, 906
—, Erbrechen, *kidneys, vomiting* 10
—, Hyperämie, venöse 864
—, Infarkte, Eintrocknung 795
—, —, embolische anämische 794
—, Ischämie, relative, experimentelle 804
—, —, spastische 852
—, —, —, Filtrationsdruck in den Glomerula 852
—, —, temporäre 803
—, Kleininfarkt 808
—, Kollaps 854, 860
—, Nekrose der distalen Hauptstückepithelien 860